SECOND EDITION

Volume 1
HEART DISEASE
A Textbook of Cardiovascular Medicine

Edited by

EUGENE BRAUNWALD, M.D.

Hersey Professor of the Theory and Practice of Physic;
Herman Ludwig Blumgart Professor of Medicine, Harvard Medical School;
Chairman, Department of Medicine,
Brigham and Women's and Beth Israel Hospitals, Boston

W. B. SAUNDERS COMPANY

PHILADELPHIA · LONDON · TORONTO · MEXICO CITY · RIO DE JANEIRO · SYDNEY · TOKYO

W. B. Saunders Company: West Washington Square
                           Philadelphia, PA 19105

                           1 St. Anne's Road
                           Eastbourne, East Sussex BN21 3UN, England

                           1 Goldthorne Avenue
                           Toronto, Ontario M8Z 5T9, Canada

                           Apartado 26370 — Cedro 512
                           Mexico 4, D.F., Mexico

                           Rua Coronel Cabrita, 8
                           Sao Cristovao Caixa Postal 21176
                           Rio de Janeiro, Brazil

                           9 Waltham Street
                           Artarmon, N.S.W. 2064, Australia

                           Ichibancho, Central Bldg., 22-1 Ichibancho
                           Chiyoda-Ku, Tokyo 102, Japan

Library of Congress Cataloging in Publication Data
  Main entry under title:

Heart disease.

    Includes bibliographical references and index.
    1. Heart—Diseases. I. Braunwald, Eugene.
[DNLM: 1. Heart diseases—Complications. WG 200
H4364]
RC681.H362   1984   616.1'2   83-2850
ISBN 0-7216-1938-X (single v.)
ISBN 0-7216-1939-8 (v. 1)
ISBN 0-7216-1940-1 (v. 2)
ISBN 0-7216-1941-X (set)

                              ISBN: SINGLE VOLUME   0-7216-1938-X
                              ISBN: VOLUME 1   0-7216-1939-8
                              ISBN: VOLUME 2   0-7216-1940-1
HEART DISEASE   ISBN: SET   0-7216-1941-X

Last digit is the print number: 9   8   7   6   5   4   3   2

Dedicated to the memory of my father,

WILLIAM BRAUNWALD

CONTRIBUTORS

JOSEPH S. ALPERT, M.D.

Professor of Medicine, University of Massachusetts Medical School. Director, Division of Cardiovascular Medicine, University of Massachusetts Medical Center, Worcester, Massachusetts.

Pulmonary Hypertension; Congenital Heart Disease in the Adult; Acute Myocardial Infarction: Pathological, Pathophysiological, and Clinical Manifestations

MURRAY G. BARON, M.D.

Professor of Radiology, Emory University School of Medicine. Associate Chairman of Radiology, Emory University Hospital, Atlanta, Georgia.

Radiological and Angiographic Examination of the Heart

WILLIAM H. BARRY, M.D.

Associate Professor of Medicine, Harvard Medical School. Director, Cardiac Catheterization Laboratory, Brigham and Women's Hospital, Boston, Massachusetts.

Cardiac Catheterization

EUGENE H. BLACKSTONE, M.D.

Cardiovascular Surgical Research Professor, The University of Alabama School of Medicine, University of Alabama, Birmingham, Alabama.

General Principles of Cardiac Surgery

KENNETH M. BOROW, M.D.

Associate Professor of Medicine, Cardiology, University of Chicago. Director, Cardiac Noninvasive Imaging Laboratory, University of Chicago Hospitals and Clinics, Chicago, Illinois.

Congenital Heart Disease in the Adult

EUGENE BRAUNWALD, M.D.

Hersey Professor of the Theory and Practice of Physic, and Herrman Ludwig Blumgart Professor of Medicine, Harvard Medical School. Chairman,

Department of Medicine, Brigham and Women's and Beth Israel Hospitals, Boston, Massachusetts.

The History; The Physical Examination; Contraction of the Normal Heart; Pathophysiology of Heart Failure; Assessment of Cardiac Function; Clinical Manifestations of Heart Failure; The Management of Heart Failure; Pulmonary Edema: Cardiogenic and Noncardiogenic; Pulmonary Hypertension; Congenital Heart Disease in the Adult; Valvular Heart Disease; Coronary Blood Flow and Myocardial Ischemia; Acute Myocardial Infarction: Pathological, Pathophysiological, and Clinical Manifestations; The Management of Acute Myocardial Infarction; Chronic Ischemic Heart Disease; The Cardiomyopathies and Myocarditides; Primary Tumors of the Heart; Pericardial Disease; Traumatic Heart Disease; Cor Pulmonale and Pulmonary Thromboembolism; Hematologic-Oncologic Disorders and Heart Disease; Endocrine and Nutritional Disorders and Heart Disease; Renal Disorders and Heart Disease; General Anesthesia and Noncardiac Surgery in Patients with Heart Disease

MICHAEL S. BROWN, M.D., D.Sc. (Hon.)

Professor, Department of Molecular Genetics, and Director, Center for Genetic Diseases, University of Texas Health Science Center at Dallas. Senior Attending Physician, Parkland Memorial Hospital, Dallas, Texas.

Genetics and Cardiovascular Disease

PETER F. COHN, M.D.

Professor of Medicine and Chief of Cardiology Division, State University of New York Health Sciences Center, Stony Brook, New York.

Chronic Ischemic Heart Disease; Traumatic Heart Disease

WILSON S. COLUCCI, M.D.

Assistant Professor of Medicine, Harvard Medical School. Associate Physician, Brigham and Women's Hospital, Boston, Massachusetts.

Primary Tumors of the Heart

ERNEST CRAIGE, M.D.

Henry A. Foscue Distinguished Professor of Cardiology, University of North Carolina School of Medicine. Director, Cardiac Graphics Laboratory, North Carolina Memorial Hospital, Chapel Hill, North Carolina.

Heart Sounds; Echophonocardiography and Other Noninvasive Techniques to Elucidate Heart Murmurs

ROMAN W. DE SANCTIS, M.D.

Professor of Medicine, Harvard Medical School. Physician and Director of Clinical Cardiology, Massachusetts General Hospital, Boston, Massachusetts.

Diseases of the Aorta

EDWIN G. DUFFIN, Ph.D.

Clinical Research Manager, Pacing Division, Medtronic, Inc., Minneapolis, Minnesota.

Cardiac Pacemakers

HARVEY FEIGENBAUM, M.D.

Distinguished Professor of Medicine, Indiana University School of Medicine. Senior Research Associate, Krannert Institute of Cardiology, Indianapolis, Indiana.

Echocardiography

MANNING FEINLEIB, M.D., Dr. P.H.

Clinical Professor, Georgetown University of Medicine, Washington, D.C. Visiting Lecturer on Epidemiology, Harvard School of Public Health, Boston, Massachusetts. Associate, Johns Hopkins University, Baltimore, Maryland. Director, National Center for Health Statistics, Hyattsville, Maryland.

Risk Factors for Coronary Artery Disease and Their Management

CHARLES FISCH, M.D.

Distinguished Professor of Medicine, Indiana University School of Medicine. Director, Krannert Institute of Cardiology and Division of Cardiology, Indiana University School of Medicine, Indianapolis, Indiana.

Electrocardiography and Vectorcardiography

WILLIAM F. FRIEDMAN, M.D.

J. H. Nicholson Professor of Pediatric Cardiology, University of California, Los Angeles, School of Medicine. Professor and Chairman, Department of Pediatrics, U.C.L.A. Center for Health Sciences, Los Angeles, California.

Congenital Heart Disease in Infancy and Childhood; Acquired Heart Disease in Infancy and Childhood

GOFFREDO G. GENSINI, M.D.

Clinical Professor of Medicine, State University of New York Upstate Medical Center College of Medicine. Director, Monseigneur Toomey Cardiovascular Laboratory and Research Department, Saint Joseph Hospital Health Center, Syracuse, New York.

Coronary Arteriography

JOSEPH L. GOLDSTEIN, M.D., D.Sc. (Hon.)

Paul J. Thomas Professor and Chairman, Department of Molecular Genetics, University of Texas Health Science Center at Dallas. Senior Attending Physician, Parkland Memorial Hospital, Dallas, Texas.

Genetics and Cardiovascular Disease

MICHAEL N. GOTTLIEB, M.D.

Assistant Clinical Professor of Medicine, Harvard Medical School. Associate Physician, Brigham and Women's Hospital, Boston, Massachusetts.

Renal Disorders and Heart Disease

WILLIAM GROSSMAN, M.D.

Professor of Medicine, Harvard Medical School. Chief, Cardiovascular Division, Beth Israel Hospital, Boston, Massachusetts.

Cardiac Catheterization; High–Cardiac Output States; Pulmonary Hypertension

THOMAS P. HACKETT, M.D.

Eben S. Draper Professor of Psychiatry, Harvard Medical School. Chief of Psychiatry, Massachusetts General Hospital, Boston, Massachusetts.

Emotion, Psychiatric Disorders, and the Heart

ROBERT I. HANDIN, M.D.

Associate Professor of Medicine, Harvard Medical School. Director, Hematology Division, Brigham and Women's Hospital, Boston, Massachusetts.

Hematologic-Oncologic Disorders and Heart Disease

B. LEONARD HOLMAN, M.D.

Professor of Radiology, Harvard Medical School. Director, Clinical Nuclear Medicine Services, Brigham and Women's Hospital, Boston, Massachusetts.

Nuclear Cardiology

ROLAND H. INGRAM, Jr., M.D.

Parker B. Francis Professor of Medicine, Harvard Medical School. Director, Respiratory Divisions, Brigham and Women's and Beth Israel Hospitals, Boston, Massachusetts.

Pulmonary Edema: Cardiogenic and Noncardiogenic; Relationship Between Diseases of the Heart and Lungs

NORMAN M. KAPLAN, M.D.

Professor of Internal Medicine, University of Texas Southwestern Medical School. Chief, Hypertension Section, Parkland Memorial Hospital, Dallas, Texas.

Systemic Hypertension: Mechanisms and Diagnosis; Systemic Hypertension: Therapy

JAMES K. KIRKLIN, M.D.

Assistant Professor of Surgery, University of Alabama School of Medicine. Staff Physician, Department of Surgery, University of Alabama Medical Center, Birmingham, Alabama.

General Principles of Cardiac Surgery

JOHN W. KIRKLIN, M.D.

Professor of Surgery, University of Alabama School of Medicine. Director, Division of Cardiothoracic Surgery, Department of Surgery, and Director, Alabama Congenital Heart Disease Diagnosis and Treatment Center, University of Alabama Medical Center, Birmingham, Alabama.

General Principles of Cardiac Surgery

ROBERT I. LEVY, M.D.

Vice President for Health Sciences, Columbia University College of Physicians and Surgeons, New York, New York.

Risk Factors for Coronary Artery Disease and Their Management

BEVERLY H. LORELL, M.D.

Assistant Professor of Medicine, Harvard Medical School. Co-Director, Hemodynamic Research Laboratory, and Attending Cardiologist, Beth Israel Hospital, Boston, Massachusetts.

Pericardial Disease

BERNARD LOWN, M.D.

Professor of Cardiology, Harvard School of Public Health. Senior Physician, Brigham and Women's Hospital, Boston, Massachusetts.

Cardiovascular Collapse and Sudden Cardiac Death

E. REGIS McFADDEN, Jr., M.D.

Associate Professor of Medicine, Harvard Medical School. Director of Research, Shipley Institute of Medicine, Brigham and Women's Hospital, Boston, Massachusetts.

Cor Pulmonale and Pulmonary Thromboembolism; Relationship Between Diseases of the Heart and Lungs

ALBERT OBERMAN, M.D., M.P.H.

Professor and Chairman, Department of Preventive Medicine, The University of Alabama School of Medicine. Active Medical Staff, University of Alabama Hospitals, Birmingham, Alabama.

Rehabilitation of Patients with Coronary Artery Disease

JOSEPH K. PERLOFF, M.D.

Professor of Medicine and Pediatrics, University of California, Los Angeles, School of Medicine. Attending Physician, U.C.L.A. Center for Health Sciences, Los Angeles, California.

Neurological Disorders and Heart Disease; Pregnancy and Cardiovascular Disease

GERALD M. POHOST, M.D.

Associate Professor of Medicine, Harvard Medical School. Director of Nuclear Cardiology, Cardiac Unit, Massachusetts General Hospital, Boston, Massachusetts.

Nuclear Magnetic Resonance Imaging of the Heart

ADAM V. RATNER, B.A.

Special Fellow in Cardiac NMR, Massachusetts General Hospital, Boston, Massachusetts. Fellow, Stanley J. Sarnoff Society of Fellows for Cardiovascular Research, Medical Student, University of Texas Southwestern Medical School, Dallas, Texas.

Nuclear Magnetic Resonance Imaging of the Heart

ROBERT ROBERTS, M.D.

Professor of Medicine, Baylor College of Medicine. Chief of Cardiology, The Methodist Hospital, Houston, Texas.

Hypotension and Syncope

JERROLD F. ROSENBAUM, M.D.

Assistant Professor of Psychiatry, Harvard Medical School. Chief, Clinical Psychopharmacology Unit, Massachusetts General Hospital, Boston, Massachusetts.

Emotion, Psychiatric Disorders, and the Heart

DAVID S. ROSENTHAL, M.D.

Associate Professor of Medicine, Harvard Medical School. Clinical Director, Hematology Division, Brigham and Women's Hospital, Boston, Massachusetts.

Hematologic-Oncologic Disorders and Heart Disease

JOHN ROSS, Jr., M.D.

Professor of Medicine, University of California, San Diego, School of Medicine. Cardiologist, University of California Medical Center, San Diego, California.

Contraction of the Normal Heart

L. THOMAS SHEFFIELD, M.D.

Professor, Department of Medicine, The University of Alabama School of Medicine. Director, ECG Laboratory and Allison Laboratory of Exercise Electrophysiology, University Hospital. Attending Cardiologist, University Hospital and Veterans Administration Hospital, Birmingham, Alabama.

Exercise Stress Testing

EVE E. SLATER, M.D.

Assistant Professor of Medicine, Harvard Medical School. Chief, Hypertension Unit, Massachusetts General Hospital, Boston, Massachusetts.

Diseases of the Aorta

THOMAS W. SMITH, M.D.

Professor of Medicine, Harvard Medical School. Chief, Cardiovascular Division, Brigham and Women's Hospital, Boston, Massachusetts.

The Management of Heart Failure

BURTON E. SOBEL, M.D.

Professor of Medicine and Director of Cardiovascular Division, Washington University School of Medicine. Cardiologist-in-Chief, Barnes Hospital, St. Louis, Missouri.

Cardiac and Noncardiac Forms of Acute Circulatory Failure (Shock); Hypotension and Syncope; Coronary Blood Flow and Myocardial Ischemia; The Management of Acute Myocardial Infarction

EDMUND H. SONNENBLICK, M.D.

Professor of Medicine, The Albert Einstein College of Medicine. Chief, Division of Cardiology, Hospital of the Albert Einstein College of Medicine and The Bronx Municipal Hospital Center, Bronx, New York.

Contraction of the Normal Heart

GENE H. STOLLERMAN, M.D.

Professor of Medicine, Boston University School of Medicine. Attending Physician, University Hospital, Boston, Massachusetts.

Rheumatic and Heritable Connective Tissue Diseases of the Cardiovascular System

LOUIS WEINSTEIN, M.D., Ph.D.

Lecturer in Medicine, Harvard Medical School. Physician and Director of the Clinical Services of the Division of Infectious Disease, Department of Medicine, Brigham and Women's Hospital, Boston, Massachusetts.

Infective Endocarditis

GORDON H. WILLIAMS, M.D.

Professor of Medicine, Harvard Medical School. Chief, Endocrinology-Hypertension Service, Brigham and Women's Hospital, Boston, Massachusetts.

Endocrine and Nutritional Disorders and Heart Disease

ROBERT W. WISSLER, Ph.D., M.D.

Donald N. Pritzker Distinguished Service Professor of Pathology, The Pritzker School of Medicine of the University of Chicago. Physician, University of Chicago Medical Center, Chicago, Illinois.

Principles of the Pathogenesis of Atherosclerosis

MARSHALL A. WOLF, M.D.

Associate Professor of Medicine, Harvard Medical School, Associate Physician-in-Chief, Brigham and Women's Hospital, Boston, Massachusetts.

General Anesthesia and Noncardiac Surgery in Patients with Heart Disease

JOSHUA WYNNE, M.D.

Assistant Professor of Medicine, Harvard Medical School. Director, Noninvasive Cardiac Laboratory, and Associate Physician, Brigham and Women's Hospital, Boston, Massachusetts.

The Cardiomyopathies and Myocarditides

DOUGLAS P. ZIPES, M.D.

Professor of Medicine, Indiana University School of Medicine. Senior Research Associate, Krannert Institute of Cardiology. Attending Physician, University Hospital, Veterans Administration Medical Center, and Wishard Memorial Hospital, Indianapolis, Indiana.

Genesis of Cardiac Arrhythmias: Electrophysiological Considerations; Management of Cardiac Arrhythmias; Specific Arrhythmias: Diagnosis and Treatment; Cardiac Pacemakers

PREFACE TO THE
SECOND EDITION

The rates at which the various branches of medicine progress are by no means uniform. To even the most casual observer, it is evident that cardiology is now moving ahead at an unprecedented velocity. Because of the enormous advances in clinical cardiology and cardiovascular science that have occurred in the four years since publication of the first edition, preparation of the second edition of *Heart Disease* has been a task that has been both more challenging and more intellectually invigorating than I had anticipated. Although the basic format of the book has remained the same, the new edition incorporates extensive changes. Eight entirely new chapters have been added or substituted: Electrocardiography and Vectorcardiography by Charles Fisch; Nuclear Magnetic Resonance Imaging by Adam V. Ratner and Gerald M. Pohost; Genesis of Cardiac Arrhythmias, Management of Cardiac Arrhythmias, Diagnosis and Management of Specific Cardiac Arrhythmias, and The Use of Cardiac Pacemakers, all by Douglas P. Zipes; Rehabilitation of Patients with Coronary Artery Disease by Albert Oberman; Diseases of the Pericardium by Beverly Lorell and Eugene Braunwald; and General Principles of Cardiac Surgery by John W. Kirklin, Eugene H. Blackstone, and James K. Kirklin.

Many new and important areas have been covered, including the use of newly developed imaging techniques—specifically CAT scanning, digital radiography, and nuclear magnetic resonance imaging and much greater emphasis on the applications of two-dimensional echocardiography in cardiovascular diagnosis; the use of intracoronary administration of thrombolytic agents in the treatment of evolving myocardial infarction; the application of Bayesian analysis in the diagnosis of ischemic heart disease by exercise electrocardiography; the use of newer inotropic agents, cardiac transplantation, and mechanical circulatory assistance in the treatment of congestive heart failure; the application of electrophysiological testing in the diagnosis of patients with cardiac arrhythmias; the use of newer antiarrhythmic drugs, electrical stimulation, and surgery in the treatment of previously intractable arrhythmias; current approaches to patients resuscitated from ventricular fibrillation; implications of the results of recent trials relative to the treatment of patients with mild essential hypertension; newer considerations in the selection of artificial heart valves; the role of surgery in the management of infective endocarditis; the basic pharmacology of calcium-channel blocking agents and their use in the treatment of various forms of cardiovascular disease; the role of prostaglandins in thrombosis; and the use of exercise testing in the early postinfarction period for the selection of candidates for coronary artery bypass grafting.

Considerable revisions have been made in both galley and page proofs to accommodate information about the most recent advances in the field; particular emphasis has been placed on insuring a comprehensive and up-to-date bibliography; and several hundred references to publications that appeared in 1983 have been inserted. There are more than 570 new figures and tables.

To the extent that this textbook proves useful to those who wish to broaden their knowledge of cardiovascular medicine and thereby aids in the care of patients afflicted with heart disease, credit must be given to the many talented and dedicated persons involved in its preparation. I offer my deepest appreciation to my fellow contributors for their professional expertise, knowledge, and devoted scholarship, which have so enriched this book. It has been a personal pleasure for me to deal with the W. B. Saunders Company. Mr. John Hanley, President, and Mr. Dereck Jeffers, Medical Editor, have been particularly helpful, as has been their effective production team—Ms. Lorraine Kilmer, Ms. Donna Kennedy, and Mr. Frank Polizzano. Ms. Diane Q. Forti, Special Editor for the first edition, continued to provide outstanding editorial support, while Ms. Patricia Higgins in my office rendered most capable secretarial and editorial services.

Without question, this edition could not have become a reality were it not for the skill and dedication of several very special persons. My responsibilities to the Harvard Medical School and the Brigham and Women's and Beth Israel Hospitals during my leave of absence were shouldered most effectively by my colleagues, Drs. Marshall Wolf, Stephen Robinson, and Steven Come, who provided the Department of Medicine with exemplary leadership. My administrative assistants, Mrs. Mary Jackson at the Brigham and Ms. Judith Walls at the Beth Israel, were enormously helpful in maintaining the orderly flow of activity essential to a busy Department of Medicine. I am deeply indebted to them as well as to Dr. Daniel C. Tosteson, Dean of the Harvard Medical Schoool; Dr. Richard Nesson, President of the Brigham and Women's Hospital; and Dr. Mitchell T. Rabkin, President of the Beth Israel Hospital, for graciously allowing me the freedom to devote myself to this task. My wife, Dr. Nina S. Braunwald, my mother, Mrs. Clare Braunwald, and my children, Karen Gail, Denise Allison, and Adrienne Jill, provided the personal support, encouragement, and understanding so essential for one who adds a task of this dimension to an already crowded professional life.

EUGENE BRAUNWALD

FROM THE PREFACE TO THE FIRST EDITION

Today cardiovascular disease is the greatest scourge afflicting the population of the industrialized nations. As with previous scourges—bubonic plague, yellow fever, and smallpox—cardiovascular disease not only strikes down a significant fraction of the population without warning but causes prolonged suffering and disability in an even larger number. In the United States alone, despite recent encouraging declines, cardiovascular disease is still responsible for almost one million fatalities each year, well over half of all deaths, and almost 5 million persons afflicted with cardiovascular disease are hospitalized each year. The cost of this disease in terms of human suffering is almost incalculable; direct annual costs approximate $18 billion, and indirect annual costs due to morbidity amount to over $10 billion.

Fortunately, research focusing on the causes, diagnosis, treatment, and prevention of heart disease is moving ahead rapidly. In the last 25 years, in particular, we have witnessed an explosive expansion of our understanding of the structure and function of the cardiovascular system —both normal and abnormal—and of our ability to evaluate these parameters in the living patient, sometimes by means of techniques that require penetration of the skin but also, with increasing accuracy, by noninvasive methods. Simultaneously, remarkable progress has been made in preventing and treating cardiovascular disease by medical and surgical means. Indeed, in the United States, the aforementioned steady reduction in mortality from cardiovascular disease during the past decade suggests that the effective application of this increased knowledge is beginning to prolong man's life span—the most valued resource on earth.

An attempt to summarize our present understanding of heart disease in a comprehensive textbook for the serious student of this subject is a formidable undertaking. Following the untimely death of Dr. Charles K. Friedberg, whose masterful text served as a bible to me and to a whole generation of cardiologists during the 1950's and 1960's, the W.B. Saunders Company invited me to accept this responsibility. Younger colleagues, particularly cardiology fellows and medical residents at the Brigham, convinced me of the need for such a book.

Since the early part of this century, clinical cardiology has had a particularly strong foundation in the basic sciences of physiology and pharmacology. More recently, the disciplines of molecular biology, genetics, developmental biology, biophysics, biochemistry, experimental pathology, and bioengineering have also begun to provide critically important information about cardiac function and malfunction. Although it was decided that *Heart Disease: A Textbook of Cardiovascular Medicine* was to be primarily a clinical treatise and not a textbook of fundamental cardiovascular science, an effort has been made to explain, in some detail, the scientific basis of cardiovascular diseases.

Heart Disease is divided into four parts: Part I deals with the examination of the patient in the broadest sense, including clinical findings and the theory and application of modern invasive and noninvasive techniques used to elicit information about the heart and the circulation. Part II is concerned with the pathophysiology, diagnosis, and treatment of the principal abnormalities of circulatory function, including heart failure, shock, arrhythmias, and abnormalities of arterial pressure. Part III consists of descriptions of the principal congenital and acquired diseases affecting the heart, pericardium, aorta, and pulmonary vascular bed in adults and children. Primary disease of other organ systems, such as the nervous, hematopoietic, endocrine, renal, and pulmonary systems, is frequently accompanied by important cardiac complications. Patients with these conditions present particularly challenging problems to both cardiac and noncardiac specialists. Accordingly, Part IV discusses the manner in which diseases of other organ systems affect the circulation and vice versa.

In order to provide a comprehensive, authoritative text in a field that has become as broad and deep as cardiovascular medicine, I chose to enlist contributions from a number of able colleagues. However, it was hoped that my personal involvement in the writing of about half the book would make it possible to eliminate the fragmentation, gaps, inconsistencies, organizational difficulties, and impersonal tone that sometimes plague multiauthored texts. I sought a compromise between a book that is too lengthy (and therefore expensive) as a result excessive repetition and one in which all duplication is eliminated, resulting in fragmented coverage of certain subjects. To help achieve this objective, extensive cross references have been provided within the text.

EUGENE BRAUNWALD

CONTENTS

PART
I

EXAMINATION OF THE PATIENT

1

THE HISTORY

by Eugene Braunwald, M.D.

IMPORTANCE OF THE HISTORY: THE PHYSICIAN'S ROLE

Specialized examinations of the cardiovascular system, presented in Chapters 3 to 11, provide a large portion of the data base required to establish a specific anatomical diagnosis of cardiac disease and to determine the extent of functional impairment of the heart. Although the development of these methods represents one of the triumphs of modern medicine, their appropriate use is *to supplement but not to supplant* a careful clinical examination, which remains the cornerstone of the assessment of the patient with known or suspected cardiovascular disease. There is a temptation in cardiology, as in many other areas of medicine, to carry out expensive, uncomfortable, and occasionally even hazardous procedures to establish a diagnosis when a detailed and thoughtful history and physical examination may be sufficient. Obviously, it is undesirable to subject patients to the unnecessary risks and expenses inherent in many specialized tests when a diagnosis can be made based on an adequate clinical examination or when their management will not be altered significantly as a result of these tests.[1] Intelligent selection of investigative procedures from the broad array now available requires more sophisticated decision-making than was necessary when the choices were limited to the electrocardiogram and chest roentgenogram. The history and physical examination provide the critical information necessary for these decisions.

The Role of the History. The overreliance on laboratory tests has increased as physicians attempt to utilize their time more efficiently by delegating responsibility for taking the history to a physician's assistant or nurse or even by issuing a questionnaire—an approach that I consider to be an undesirable trend insofar as the patient with known or suspected heart disease is concerned. First of all,

it must be appreciated that the history remains the richest source of information concerning the patient's illness, and any practice that might diminish the quality of information provided by the history could ultimately impair the quality of care. Second, the physician's attentive and thoughtful taking of a history establishes a bond with the patient that may be valuable later in securing the patient's compliance in following a complex treatment plan, undergoing hospitalization for an intensive diagnostic work-up or a hazardous operation, and, in some instances, accepting that heart disease is not present at all. It is largely through the direct contact established between the patient and physician during the clinical examination that this confidence can best be established.

Taking a history also permits the physician to evaluate the results of diagnostic tests that have strong subjective components, such as the determination of exercise capacity (see p. 272). Perhaps most importantly, a careful history allows the physician to evaluate the impact of the disease, or the fear of the disease, on the patient's total life and to assess the patient's personality, emotion, and stability; often it provides a glimpse of the patient's responsibilities, fears, aspirations, and threshold for discomfort as well as the likelihood of compliance with one or another therapeutic regimen. Whenever possible, the physician should question not only the patient but also relatives or close friends in order to obtain a clearer understanding of the extent of the patient's disability and a broader perspective concerning the impact of the disease on both the patient and the family. (For example, the patient's spouse is more likely than the patient to provide a history of Cheyne-Stokes [periodic] respiration.)

In interpreting the history obtained from a patient with known or suspected heart disease, it must be appreciated that the combination of the widespread fear of cardiovascular disorders and the deep-seated emotional, symbolic, and sometimes even religious connotations concerning this organ's function may, on the one hand, provoke symptoms that mimic those of organic heart disease in persons with normal cardiovascular systems or, on the other, cause so much fear that serious symptoms are repressed or denied by patients with organic heart disease. Functional complaints referable to the cardiovascular system may also develop in patients with organic heart disease. The unraveling of symptoms and signs due to organic heart disease from those which are unrelated is an important and challenging task, and the history is the most valuable tool in carrying out this task.

Technique. Several approaches can be employed successfully in obtaining a medical history. I believe that the patient should first be given the opportunity to relate his or her experiences and complaints. Although time-consuming and likely to include much seemingly irrelevant information, this technique has the advantage of providing considerable information concerning the patient's intelligence and emotional make-up. After the patient has given an account of the illness, the physician should obtain information concerning the onset and chronology of symptoms; their location, quality, and intensity; the precipitating, aggravating, and relieving factors; and the response to therapy.

Of course, a detailed general medical history including the personal past history, occupational history, nutritional history, and review of systems must be obtained. Concern should focus on a past history of rheumatic fever, chorea, venereal disease or exposure to it, thyroid disease, recent dental extractions or manipulations, earlier examinations that showed abnormalities of the cardiovascular system as reflected in restriction from physical activity at school and in rejection for life insurance, employment, or military service. Personal habits such as exercise, cigarette smoking, alcohol intake, and parenteral use of drugs—illicit and otherwise—should be ascertained, and the exact nature of the patient's work should be assessed. The increasing appreciation of the importance of genetic influences in many forms of heart disease (Chap. 47) underscores the importance of the family history. Details of obtaining the family history in a patient with a possible genetic disorder involving the heart are presented on p. 1611.

A cardinal principle of cardiovascular evaluation is that myocardial or coronary function that may be adequate at rest may be inadequate during exertion; therefore, specific attention should be directed to the influence of activity on the patient's symptoms. Thus, a history of chest pain or discomfort and/or undue shortness of breath that appears only during activity is characteristic of heart disease, whereas the opposite pattern, i.e., the appearance of symptoms at rest and their remission during exertion, is observed only rarely in patients with organic heart disease but is more characteristic of functional disorders. In attempting to assess the severity of functional impairment, the extent of activity and the rate at which it is performed before symptoms develop should be determined and related to a detailed consideration of the therapeutic regimen. For example, the complaint of exertional dyspnea after walking slowly up a flight of stairs in a patient on maximal treatment for heart failure denotes far more severe functional disability than does a similar symptom occur-

ring in an untreated patient who has run up a flight of stairs. It is often useful to ask the patient whether a specific activity that now is difficult, such as climbing two flights of stairs, could be accomplished more easily 3, 6, and 12 months earlier.

As the patient relates the history, important nonverbal clues are often provided. The physician should observe the patient's attitude, reactions, and gestures while being questioned, as well as his or her choice of words or emphasis. Tumulty has likened obtaining a meaningful clinical history to playing a game of chess: "The patient makes a statement and based upon its content, and mode of expression, the physician asks a counter-question. One answer stimulates yet another question until the clinician is convinced that he understands precisely all of the circumstances of the patient's illness."

PRINCIPAL SYMPTOMS OF HEART DISEASE

The principal symptoms of heart disease include dyspnea, chest pain or discomfort, syncope, palpitation, edema, cough, hemoptysis, and excess fatigue. Cyanosis is more often a sign rather than a symptom, but it may be a key feature of the history, particularly of patients with congenital heart disease. Without doubt, history-taking is the most valuable technique available for determining whether or not these symptoms are caused by heart disease. Examples of the manner in which these symptoms may serve as a guide to diagnosis are given in the following pages, and reference is made to other portions of the book that contain more detailed information.

DYSPNEA (see also pp. 492 and 1789)

Dyspnea is defined as an abnormally uncomfortable awareness of breathing; it is one of the principal symptoms of cardiac and pulmonary disease.[2] Since dyspnea can be caused by strenuous exertion in healthy subjects and only moderate exertion in those who are normal but unaccustomed to exercise, it should be regarded as abnormal only when it occurs at rest or at a level of physical activity not expected to cause this symptom. Dyspnea is associated with a wide variety of diseases of the heart and lungs, chest wall, and respiratory muscles as well as with anxiety; the history is the most valuable means of establishing the etiology.

The *sudden* development of dyspnea suggests pulmonary embolism, pneumothorax, acute pulmonary edema, pneumonia, or obstruction of a major airway. In contrast, in most forms of *chronic* heart failure, dyspnea progresses slowly over weeks or months. It should be recognized that such a protracted course may also occur in a variety of other unrelated conditions, including obesity, pregnancy, and bilateral pleural effusions. Inspiratory dyspnea suggests obstruction of the upper airways, whereas dyspnea during expiration characterizes obstruction of the lower airways. Exertional dyspnea suggests the presence of organic diseases, such as left ventricular failure or chronic obstructive lung disease, whereas dyspnea developing at rest may occur in pneumothorax or pulmonary embolism or may be functional. Dyspnea that occurs *only* at rest and is absent on exertion is almost invariably functional. A functional origin is suggested when dyspnea, or simply a heightened awareness of breathing, is accompanied by brief stabbing pain in the region of the cardiac apex or prolonged (more than 2 hours) dull chest pain, and is associated with difficulty in getting enough air into the lungs, claustrophobia, or sighing respirations that are relieved by exertion, by taking a few deep breaths, or by sedation. A history of relief of dyspnea by bronchodilators and corticosteroids suggests asthma as the etiology, whereas relief of dyspnea by rest, digitalis, and diuretics suggests left heart failure.

In patients with *heart failure*, dyspnea is a clinical expression of pulmonary venous and capillary hypertension. It occurs either during exertion or, in resting patients, in the recumbent position and is relieved promptly by sitting upright or standing (orthopnea). The *sudden* occurrence of dyspnea in a patient with a history of rheumatic heart disease suggests the development of atrial fibrillation, rupture of chordae tendineae, or pulmonary embolism.

Paroxysmal nocturnal dyspnea is due to interstitial pulmonary edema secondary to left ventricular failure (p. 493). This condition, beginning usually 2 to 5 hours after the onset of sleep and often associated with sweating and wheezing, is frightening to the patient. Paroxysmal nocturnal dyspnea is relieved by the patient's sitting on the side of the bed or getting out of bed. However, a positional change lasting approximately 20 or more minutes may be required to relieve this symptom, whereas simple orthopnea may be relieved in less than 5 minutes after the patient sits upright. Although paroxysmal nocturnal dyspnea secondary to left ventricular failure is usually accompanied by coughing, a careful history often discloses that the dyspnea *precedes* the cough, not vice versa. In contrast, patients with *chronic pulmonary disease* may also awaken at night, but cough and expectoration often precede the dyspnea. These patients also often have a long history of smoking and a chronic cough with sputum production and wheezing and may be able to breathe more easily while leaning forward. Nocturnal dyspnea in patients with pulmonary disease is usually relieved after the patient rids himself of secretions rather than specifically by sitting up. Details of the value and limitations of the history of dyspnea in differentiating between primary diseases of the heart and lungs[2a] are presented on p. 494 and 1790.

Patients with *pulmonary embolism* usually experience sudden dyspnea that may be associated with apprehension, palpitation, hemoptysis, or pleuritic chest pain. The development or intensification of dyspnea, sometimes associated with a feeling of faintness, may be the only complaint of the patient with pulmonary emboli. Dyspnea accompanying thoracic pain occurs in *acute myocardial infarction*. Occasionally dyspnea is an *"anginal equivalent"* (p. 1337), i.e., a symptom secondary to myocardial ischemia that occurs in place of typical anginal discomfort. This form of dyspnea may be closely associated with a sensation of tightness in the chest, is present on exertion or emotional stress, is relieved by rest but not recumbency, has a duration similar to angina (i.e., 2 to 10 minutes), and is usually responsive to nitroglycerin but not to digitalis. The sudden development of dyspnea in the sitting rather than in the lying position, or in any particular position, suggests the possibility of a *myxoma* (p. 1416) or *ball-valve thrombus* in the left atrium. When dyspnea is relieved by squatting, it is caused most commonly by tetralogy of Fallot or a variant thereof (p. 990).

CHEST PAIN OR DISCOMFORT
(Table 1–1; see also pp. 1335 to 1338)

Although chest pain or discomfort is one of the cardinal manifestations of cardiac disease, it is critical to recognize that it may originate not only in the heart but also in (1) a variety of noncardiac intrathoracic structures, such as the aorta, pulmonary artery, bronchopulmonary tree, pleura, mediastinum, esophagus, and diaphragm; (2) the tissues of the neck or thoracic wall, including the skin, thoracic muscles, cervicodorsal spine, costochondral junctions, breasts,

TABLE 1–1 DIFFERENTIAL DIAGNOSIS OF EPISODIC CHEST PAIN RESEMBLING ANGINA PECTORIS

	DURATION	QUALITY	PROVOCATION	RELIEF	LOCATION	COMMENT
Effort angina	5–15 minutes	Visceral (pressure)	During effort or emotion	Rest, nitroglycerin	Substernal radiates	First episode vivid
Rest angina	5–15 minutes	Visceral (pressure)	Spontaneous (? with exercise)	Nitroglycerin	Substernal radiates	Often nocturnal
Mitral prolapse	Minutes to hours	Superficial (rarely visceral)	Spontaneous (no pattern)	Time	Left anterior	No pattern, variable character
Esophageal reflux	10 minutes to 1 hour	Visceral	Recumbency, lack of food	Food, antacid	Substernal epigastric	Rarely radiates
Esophageal spasm	5–60 minutes	Visceral	Spontaneous, cold liquids, exercise	Nitroglycerin	Substernal radiates	Mimics angina
Peptic ulcer	Hours	Visceral, burning	Lack of food, "acid" foods	Foods, antacids	Epigastric substernal	
Biliary disease	Hours	Visceral (wax and wane)	Spontaneous, food	Time, analgesia	Epigastric ? radiates	Colic
Cervical disc	Variable (gradually subsides)	Superficial	Head and neck movement, palpation	Time, analgesia	Arm, neck	Not relieved by rest
Hyperventilation	2–3 minutes	Visceral	Emotion tachypnea	Stimulus removal	Substernal	Facial paresthesia
Musculoskeletal	Variable	Superficial	Movement palpation	Time, analgesia	Multiple	Tenderness
Pulmonary	30 minutes +	Visceral (pressure)	Often spontaneous	Rest, time, bronchodilator	Substernal	Dyspneic

Reproduced with permission from Christie, L. G., Jr., and Conti, C. R.: Systematic approach to the evaluation of angina-like chest pain. Am. Heart J. *102*:897, 1981.

sensory nerves, or spinal cord; and (3) subdiaphragmatic organs such as the stomach, duodenum, pancreas, and gallbladder.[3-5] Factitious pain or pain of functional origin may also occur in the chest. Although a wide variety of laboratory tests are available to aid in the differential diagnosis of chest pain, the history is without any question the most valuable mode of examination. In obtaining the history of a patient with chest pain, it is helpful to have a mental checklist and to ask the patient to describe the location, radiation, and character of the pain; what causes and relieves the pain; time relationships, including the duration, frequency, and pattern of recurrence of the pain; and associated symptoms. It is also particularly useful to observe the patient's gestures. Clenching the fist in front of the chest while describing the sensation (Levine's sign) is a strong indication of an ischemic origin for the pain.

Quality. It is important to recognize that angina means *choking*, not pain. Thus, the discomfort of angina often is described not as pain at all but rather as an unpleasant sensation; "pressing," "squeezing," "strangling," "constricting," "bursting," and "burning" are some of the adjectives commonly used to describe this sensation. "A band across the chest" and "a weight in the center of the chest" are other frequent descriptions. Often with severe attacks the discomfort may radiate from the chest to the shoulders, extremities, neck, jaws, and teeth. It is characteristic of angina that the intensity of effort required to incite it seems to vary from day to day and throughout the day in the same patient, but often a careful history will uncover explanations for this, such as meals ingested, weather, emotions, and the like. Patients note frequently that activities that may cause angina in the morning or when first undertaken do not do so later in the day. When the threshold for angina is quite variable and defies any pattern, the possibility that myocardial ischemia is caused by coronary spasm should be considered (p. 1336). Thus, a careful history may indicate not only the cause of the pain (i.e., myocardial ischemia) but can even provide a clue to the mechanism of the ischemia (spasm vs. organic obstruction).

When dyspnea is an "anginal equivalent," the patient may describe the midchest as the site of the shortness of breath, whereas true dyspnea is usually not as well localized. Other anginal equivalents are discomfort limited to areas that are ordinarily sites of secondary radiation, such as the ulnar aspect of the left arm and forearm, lower jaw, teeth, neck, or shoulders, and the development of gas and belching, nausea, "indigestion," dizziness, and diaphoresis. Anginal equivalents above the mandible or below the umbilicus are quite uncommon.

The chest discomfort of *pulmonary hypertension* may be identical to that of typical angina; it is caused either by dilatation of the pulmonary arteries or by right ventricular ischemia. The chest discomfort of *unstable angina* and *acute myocardial infarction* (p. 1278) is similar qualitatively to that of angina pectoris in location and character; however, it usually radiates more widely than does angina and is more severe and therefore is generally referred to as pain by the patient. The discomfort generally develops unrelated to unusual effort or emotional stress, often with the patient at rest, or even sleeping. Usually nitroglycerin does not provide complete or lasting relief.

Acute pericarditis (p. 1474) is frequently preceded by a history of a viral upper respiratory infection. The inflammation causes pain that is sharper than is anginal discomfort, is more left-sided than central, and is often referred to the neck or flank. The pain of pericarditis lasts for hours and is little affected by effort but often aggravated by breathing, turning in bed, swallowing, or twisting the body; unlike angina, the pain may lessen when the patient sits up and leans forward.

Aortic dissection (p. 1548) is suggested by persistent pain with radiation to the back and into the lumbar region in an individual with a history of hypertension. An expanding *thoracic aortic aneurysm* may erode the vertebral bodies and cause localized, severe, boring pain that is usually worse at night. An aneurysmally enlarged left atrium in patients with mitral valve disease rarely causes chest pain; instead, patients commonly complain of discomfort in the back or right side of the chest that intensifies on exertion.

Chest-wall pain may be due to *costochondritis* or *myositis* with local costochondral or muscle tenderness, which may be aggravated by moving or coughing. It may also accompany or follow herpes zoster, chest injury, or *Tietze's syndrome* (i.e., discomfort localized in swelling of the costochondral and costosternal joints, which are painful on palpation).

Functional or *psychogenic chest pain* may be one feature of an anxiety state, also called Da Costa's syndrome or neurocirculatory asthenia. It is localized typically to the area of the cardiac apex and consists of a dull, persistent ache that lasts for hours and is often accentuated by or alternates with attacks of sharp, lancinating stabs of inframammary pain of one or two seconds' duration. The condition may occur with emotional strain and fatigue, bears little relation to exertion, and may be accompanied by precordial tenderness. Attacks are usually associated with palpitation, hyperventilation, dyspnea, generalized weakness, and other signs of emotional instability or depression. The pain may not be completely relieved by any medication other than analgesics, but it is partially attenuated by many types of interventions, including rest, exertion, tranquilizers, and placebos. Therefore, in contrast to ischemic pain, functional pain is more likely to show variable responses to interventions on different occasions. Since functional chest pain is often preceded by hyperventilation, which in turn may cause increased muscle tension and be responsible for diffuse chest tightness, some instances of so-called functional chest pain may, in fact, have an organic basis. Chest pain is common in patients with *prolapse of the mitral valve* (p. 1091). The pain varies considerably among patients; it may be similar to that of classic angina pectoris or may resemble the chest pain of neurocirculatory asthenia described above.

Patients who have angina pectoris or have suffered a myocardial infarction often become "heart conscious" and become acutely aware of every kind of chest discomfort. It is particularly challenging to separate organic from functional chest pain in these patients, and the history provides the principal means of determining the extent to which these patients are limited by myocardial ischemia.

Location. Embryonically the heart is a midline viscus; thus, cardiac ischemia produces anginal symptoms that are characteristically felt across both sides of the chest or chiefly substernally. Occasional patients complain of discomfort only to the left or rarely right of the midline. If the pain or discomfort can be localized to the skin or superficial structures, it generally arises from the chest wall. Thus, if the patient can point directly to the site of discomfort, it is usually not angina pectoris, which, like other symptoms arising in deeper structures, tends to be diffuse and eludes precise localization. Pain under or in the region of the left nipple is usually noncardiac in origin and may be functional or due to osteoarthritis, gaseous distention of the stomach, or the splenic flexure syndrome. Although pain due to myocardial ischemia often radiates to the left arm or left shoulder, such radiation also occurs in pericarditis and disorders of the cervical spine. Chest pain that radiates to the neck and jaw occurs in pericarditis as well as in myocardial ischemia. Dissection of the aorta or enlargement of an aortic aneurysm produces pain in the *back* rather than in the front of the chest.

Duration. The duration of the pain is important in determining its etiology. Anginal pain is relatively short, usually lasting from 2 to 10 minutes. However, if the pain is very brief, i.e., a momentary, lancinating, sharp pain, or discomfort that lasts less than 30 seconds, angina can usually be excluded; such a short duration points instead to musculoskeletal pain, pain due to hiatal hernia, or functional pain. Chest pain lasting hours may be seen with acute myocardial infarction, pericarditis, aortic dissection, musculoskeletal disease, herpes zoster, and anxiety.

Precipitating and Aggravating Factors. Angina pectoris occurs characteristically on exertion, particularly when hurrying or walking on an upgrade. Thus, the development of chest discomfort or pain when walking, typically in the cold and against a wind, and after a heavy meal, is characteristic of angina pectoris. An exception is *Prinzmetal's (variant) angina,* which characteristically occurs at rest (p. 1360) and may or may not be affected by exertion; however, it must be remembered that classic (nonvariant) angina, although most often precipitated by effort, not uncommonly may be experienced at rest, as in unstable angina; exertion intensifies the discomfort. Emotional stress also may precipitate angina. Chest pain that occurs after protracted vomiting may be due to the *Mallory-Weiss syndrome,* i.e., a tear in the lower portion of the esophagus. Pain that occurs while bending over is often radicular and may be associated with *osteoarthritis* of the cervical or upper thoracic spine. Chest pain occurring when moving the neck may be due to a *herniated intervertebral disk,* whereas substernal and epigastric discomfort during swallowing may be due to *esophageal spasm. Esophagitis* with or without a hiatal hernia may also be associated with substernal or epigastric burning pain that is brought on by eating or lying down after meals and that may be relieved with antacids; it is often accompanied by acid reflux into the mouth (water brash). Chest pain aggravated by swallowing may also be due to acute pericarditis, whereas pain intensified by coughing may be due to pericarditis, bronchitis, or pleurisy or may be of radicular origin. Pain that occurs when the patient is exhausted is often functional. *Congenital absence of the pericardium* (p. 1517) produces chest pain that is relieved by changing position in bed, is brought on by lying on the left side, and lasts a few seconds. Pain due to the *scalenus anticus*

(thoracic outlet) syndrome may be confused with angina because it is often associated with paresthesias along the ulnar distribution of the arm and forearm. However, in contrast to angina, not only is it typically precipitated by abduction of the arm, lifting a weight, or working with the hands above the shoulders, but it is not brought on by walking.

Relief of Pain. Nitroglycerin and rest characteristically relieve the discomfort of angina in approximately 2 to 5 minutes. If more than 10 minutes transpire before relief, the diagnosis of chronic stable angina becomes questionable and instead suggests unstable angina, acute myocardial infarction, or pain not caused by myocardial ischemia at all. Although nitroglycerin commonly relieves the pain of angina pectoris, the discomfort of esophageal spasm and esophagitis may also be relieved by this drug. Angina pectoris is alleviated by quiet standing or sitting; the recumbent position may not relieve angina. Chest pain secondary to *acute pericarditis* is characteristically relieved by leaning forward, whereas pain that is relieved by food or antacids may be due to *peptic ulcer disease* or esophagitis. Pain that is alleviated by holding the breath in deep expiration is commonly due to *pleurisy.* Some patients with highly nonspecific angina pectoris as well as others with upper gastrointestinal disease or anxiety report relief of symptoms after belching.

Accompanying Symptoms. The physician should always be respectful of the patient who reports the presence of chest pain and profuse sweating. This combination of symptoms frequently signals a serious disorder, often acute myocardial infarction. Severe chest pain accompanied by nausea and vomiting is also often due to myocardial infarction. The latter diagnosis, as well as pneumothorax or pulmonary embolism, is suggested when pain is associated with shortness of breath. Chest pain accompanied by palpitation may be due to the acute myocardial ischemia that results from a tachyarrhythmia-induced increase in myocardial oxygen consumption in the presence of coronary artery disease. Chest pain accompanied by hemoptysis suggests pulmonary embolism with infarction or lung tumor, whereas pain accompanied by fever occurs in pneumonia, pleurisy, and pericarditis. Functional pain is commonly accompanied by frequent sighing, anxiety, or depression.

CYANOSIS (see also p. 949)

Cyanosis is a bluish discoloration of the skin and mucous membranes resulting from an increased amount of reduced hemoglobin or of abnormal hemoglobin pigments in the blood perfusing these areas. There are two principal forms of cyanosis: (1) *central cyanosis,* characterized by decreased arterial oxygen saturation due to right-to-left shunting of blood or impaired pulmonary function, and (2) *peripheral cyanosis,* most commmonly secondary to cutaneous vasoconstriction due to a low cardiac output or exposure to cold air or water; if peripheral cyanosis is localized to an extremity, arterial or venous obstruction should be suspected. A history of cyanosis localized to the hands suggests *Raynaud's phenomenon.* Central cyanosis due to congenital heart disease or pulmonary disease characteristically worsens during exertion, whereas the resting peripheral cyanosis of congestive heart failure may be accentuated only slightly, if at all, during exertion.

Cyanosis usually becomes apparent at a mean capillary concentration of 4 gm/dl reduced hemoglobin (or 0.5 gm/dl methemoglobin). In general, a history of cyanosis in Caucasians is rarely elicited unless arterial saturation is 85 per cent or less; in pigmented races arterial saturation has to drop far lower before cyanosis is perceptible. Cyanosis generally occurs in patients with *congenital heart disease* when the volume of a right-to-left shunt exceeds 25 percent of the left ventricular output. Since it is the *absolute* quantity of reduced hemoglobin in the blood that is responsible for cyanosis, the higher the total hemoglobin content, the greater the tendency toward cyanosis; thus, patients with marked polycythemia become cyanotic at higher levels of arterial oxygen saturation than do patients with normal hematocrit values, and cyanosis may be absent in patients with severe anemia despite marked arterial desaturation.

Although a history of cyanosis beginning in infancy suggests a congenital cardiac malformation with a right-to-left shunt, *hereditary methemoglobinemia* is another, albeit rare, cause of congenital cyanosis; the diagnosis of this condition is supported by a family history of cyanosis in the absence of heart disease.

A history of cyanosis limited to the neonatal period suggests the diagnosis of atrial septal defect with transient right-to-left shunting or, more commonly, pulmonary parenchymal disease or central nervous system depression. Cyanosis beginning at age 1 to 3 months may be reported when spontaneous closure of a patent ductus arteriosus unmasks the reduction of pulmonary blood flow in the presence of right-sided obstructive cardiac anomalies (p. 995). If cyanosis appears at age 6 months or later in childhood, it may be due to the development or progression of obstruction to right ventricular outflow in patients with ventricular septal defect. Development of cyanosis between ages 5 and 15 years suggests an Eisenmenger's reaction with right-to-left shunting as a consequence of a progressive increase in pulmonary vascular resistance (p. 964).

SYNCOPE (see also p. 932)

Syncope, which may be defined as a loss of consciousness, results most commonly from reduced perfusion of the brain. This, in turn, may be due to a reduction of systemic vascular resistance, an elevation of cerebrovascular resistance, hypovolemia, a variety of arrhythmias, and any other condition that causes a sudden reduction of cardiac output and therefore of cerebral blood flow. It should be distinguished from emotional disturbances in which hyperventilation, anxiety, and hysterical fainting are prominent and from seizure disorders, especially petit mal epilepsy.

The history is extremely valuable in the differential diagnosis of syncope (Table 28–1, p. 929). Several daily attacks of loss of consciousness suggest (1) Stokes-Adams attacks, i.e., transient asystole or ventricular fibrillation in the presence of atrioventricular block; (2) other cardiac arrhythmias (Chap. 21); or (3) epilepsy. These diagnoses are suggested when the loss of consciousness is abrupt and occurs over 1 or 2 seconds; a more gradual onset suggests vasodepressor syncope (i.e., the common faint), syncope due to hyperventilation or, much less commonly, hypoglycemia. Cardiac syncope is often of gradual onset without aura,

and is usually *not* associated with convulsive movements, urinary incontinence, and a postictal confusional state. Patients with epilepsy often have a prodromal aura preceding the seizure. Injury from falling is common, as is urinary incontinence and a postictal confusional state, associated with headache and drowsiness. Unconsciousness for a few seconds suggests vasodepressor syncope or syncope secondary to postural hypotension, whereas a longer period suggests aortic stenosis or hyperventilation. *Hysterical fainting* is usually not accompanied by any untoward display of anxiety or change in pulse, blood pressure, or skin color, and there may be a question about whether any true loss of consciousness occurred. It is often associated with paresthesias of the hands or face, hyperventilation, dyspnea, chest pain, and feelings of acute anxiety.

Syncope independent of body position suggests Stokes-Adams attacks, hyperventilation, or epilepsy, whereas syncope of other etiologies usually occurs in the upright position. Syncope occurring upon bending, leaning, or assuming a particular body position should raise the possibility of a left atrial myxoma (p. 1460) or a ball-valve thrombus. Since syncope is an unusual feature of mitral stenosis, when it does occur in a patient thought to have this condition, the possibility of left atrial *myxoma* or *ball-valve thrombus* should be considered. Syncope occurring during or immediately following exertion suggests *aortic stenosis, hypertrophic obstructive cardiomyopathy,* or *primary pulmonary hypertension.* Syncope is rare in patients with angina pectoris unless the latter is secondary to aortic stenosis or hypertrophic obstructive cardiomyopathy. Syncope following insulin administration suggests a hypoglycemic etiology; syncope several hours after eating is characteristic of reactive hypoglycemia. Loss of consciousness following an emotional stress suggests that it is vasodepressor syncope or secondary to hyperventilation.

Patients with *vasodepressor syncope* often have a long history of fainting, commonly associated with emotional or painful stimuli. This, the most usual form of syncope, may be precipitated by the sight or loss of blood or by physical or emotional stress; it can be averted by promptly lying down, and it is characteristically preceded by symptoms of autonomic hyperactivity such as dim vision, giddiness, yawning, sweating, and nausea (p. 934). Syncope secondary to *cerebrovascular disturbance* is often preceded by aphasia, unilateral weakness, or confusion. A history of fainting following sudden movements of the head, shaving the neck, or wearing a tight collar suggests carotid sinus syncope (p. 932). Syncope associated with chest pain may be secondary to massive acute myocardial infarction or infarction associated with arrhythmias; occasionally, following recovery of consciousness, the associated chest pain may be forgotten, and the infarction may be recognized only by means of characteristic changes in serum enzymes and the electrocardiogram.

Consciousness is regained quite promptly in syncope of cardiovascular origin but more slowly with epilepsy. When consciousness is regained after vasodepressor syncope, the patient is usually pale and diaphoretic with a slow heart rate, whereas after a Stokes-Adams attack, the face is often flushed and there may actually be cardiac acceleration. Patients who sustain an injury when falling to the ground during a fainting spell usually have epilepsy or occasionally syncope of cardiac origin, but they rarely have sustained physical damage during reported unconsciousness related to emotional disturbance.

A *family history of syncope* or near syncope can often be elicited in patients with hypertrophic obstructive cardiomyopathy or ventricular tachyarrhythmias associated with Q-T prolongation (pp. 727 and 1626). A family history of epilepsy is positive in approximately 4 per cent of patients with convulsive disorders. Syncope associated with progressive intensification of cyanosis in an infant or child with cyanotic congenital heart disease is likely to be due to cerebral anoxia as a consequence of an increase in the right-to-left shunt, secondary to an increase in the obstruction to right ventricular outflow or a reduction in systemic vascular resistance (p. 950). A history of syncope during childhood suggests the possibility of a cardiovascular anomaly obstructing left ventricular outflow—valvular, supravalvular, or subvalvular aortic stenosis. In patients with hypertrophic obstructive cardiomyopathy, syncope is often post-tussive and occurs in the erect position, when arising suddenly, after standing erect for long periods, and during or immediately after cessation of exertion.

Patients with syncope secondary to *orthostatic hypotension* often have a history of drug therapy for hypertension or of abnormalities of autonomic function, such as impotence, disturbances of sphincter function, peripheral neuropathy, and anhidrosis (p. 930). When syncope is secondary to hypovolemia, there is often a history of melena, anemia, menorrhagia, or treatment with anticoagulants. Syncope associated with *cerebrovascular insufficiency* is frequently associated with a history of unilateral blindness, weakness, paresthesias, or memory defects.

PALPITATION

This common symptom is defined as an unpleasant awareness of the beating of the heart. It may be brought about by a variety of disorders involving changes in cardiac rhythm or rate, including all forms of tachycardia, ectopic beats, compensatory pauses, augmented stroke volume due to valvular regurgitation, hyperkinetic (high–cardiac output) states, and the sudden onset of bradycardia. In the case of premature contractions the patient is more commonly aware of the postextrasystolic beat than of the premature beat itself, and it appears that it is the motion of the heart within the chest that is perceived rather than the increase in cardiac contractility. This explains why palpitation is not a characteristic feature of aortic or pulmonic stenosis or of severe systemic or pulmonary hypertension, conditions characterized by an increased force of cardiac contraction.

When episodes of palpitation last for an instant, they are described as "skipped beats" or a "flopping sensation" in the chest and most commonly are due to extrasystoles. On the other hand, the sensation that the heart has "stopped beating" often correlates with the compensatory pause following a premature contraction. Palpitation characterized by a slow heart rate may be due to atrioventricular block or sinus node disease. When palpitation begins and ends abruptly, it is often due to a paroxysmal tachycardia such as paroxysmal atrial or junctional tachycardia, atrial flutter, or fibrillation, whereas a gradual onset and cessation of the attack suggest sinus tachycardia and/or an anxiety state. A history of chaotic rapid heart action suggests the diagnosis of atrial fibrillation; fleeting and repetitive palpitation suggests multiple ectopic beats. A history of multiple paroxysms of tachycardia, followed by palpitation that occurs only with effort or excitement suggests paroxysmal atrial fibrillation that has become permanent —the palpitation being experienced only when the ventricular rate rises. Some patients have taken their pulse during palpitation or have asked a companion to do so. A rate between 100 and 140 beats/min suggests sinus tachycardia, a rate of approximately 150 beats/min suggests *atrial flutter,* and a rate exceeding 160 beats/min suggests *paroxysmal supraventricular tachycardia.*

A history of palpitation during or after strenuous physical activities is normal, whereas palpitation during mild exertion suggests the presence of heart failure, anemia, or thyrotoxicosis, or that the individual is severely "out of condition." A feeling of forceful heart action accompanied by throbbing in the neck suggests aortic regurgitation. When palpitation can be relieved suddenly by stooping, breathholding, or induced gagging or vomiting, i.e., by vagal maneuvers, the diagnosis of paroxysmal supraventricular tachycardia is suggested. A history of syncope following an episode of palpitation suggests either asystole or severe bradycardia following the termination of a tachyarrhythmia or a Stokes-Adams attack. A history of palpitation associated with anxiety, a lump in the throat, dizziness, and tingling in the hands and face suggests sinus tachycardia accompanying an anxiety state with hyperventilation. Tachycardia associated with angina suggests myocardial ischemia that has been precipitated by increased oxygen demands induced by the rapid heart rate.

As an adjunct to the history, it may be possible to ascertain the rhythm responsible for the palpitation by tapping the finger on the patient's chest in a variety of rhythms and asking the patient to identify the pattern which most closely resembles the abnormal feeling.

In many individuals no obvious cause for palpitation emerges despite careful work-up, including a correlation between episodes of palpitation with a simultaneously recorded ambulatory electrocardiogram (p. 632) or an electrocardiogram recorded by transtelephonic transmission. Anxiety is responsible for the symptom in many such patients, but some of them have known heart disease and may be receiving a vasodilator for the treatment of hypertension or nifedipine for the treatment of myocardial ischemia. In these patients palpitation may be due to postural hypotension resulting in reflex cardiac acceleration.

EDEMA (see also p. 497)

Localization of edema is helpful in elucidating its etiology. Thus a history of edema of the legs that is most pronounced in the evening is characteristic of heart failure or bilateral chronic venous insufficiency. In most patients any visible edema of both lower extremities is preceded by a weight gain of at least 7 to 10 lb. As cardiac edema progresses, it usually ascends to involve the legs, thighs, genitals, and abdominal wall. In patients with heart failure who remain chiefly in bed, the edema localizes particularly in the sacral area. Edema located in both the abdomen and the legs is observed in heart failure and hepatic cirrhosis. Edema may be generalized in the nephrotic syndrome, severe heart failure, and hepatic cirrhosis. A history of edema around the eyes and face is characteristic of the nephrotic syndrome, acute glomerulonephritis, angioneurotic edema, hypoproteinemia, and myxedema. Edema limited to the face, neck, and upper arms may be associated with obstruction of the superior vena cava, most commonly by carcinoma of the lung, lymphoma, or aneurysm of the aortic arch. Edema restricted to one extremity is usually due to venous thrombosis or lymphatic blockage of that extremity.

Accompanying Symptoms. A history of edema associated with dyspnea is most frequently due to heart failure but may also be observed in patients with large bilateral pleural effusions, elevation of the diaphragm due to ascites, angioneurotic edema with laryngeal involvement, and pulmonary embolism. When dyspnea precedes edema, left ventricular dysfunction, mitral stenosis, or chronic lung disease with cor pulmonale is usually responsible. A history of jaundice suggests that edema may be of hepatic origin, whereas edema associated with a history of ulceration and pigmentation of the skin of the legs is most commonly due to chronic venous insufficiency or postphlebitic syndrome. When cardiac edema is *not* associated with orthopnea, it may be due to tricuspid stenosis or regurgitation or constrictive pericarditis; in these conditions edema is not always most prominent in the lower extremities but may be generalized and may even involve the face.

The development of ascites *preceding* edema suggests cirrhosis, whereas a history of ascites *following* edema suggests cardiac or renal disease. *Angioneurotic edema* occurs intermittently, particularly after emotional stress or eating certain foods. *Idiopathic cyclic edema* is associated with menstruation. A history of edema on prolonged standing is observed in patients with chronic venous insufficiency.

COUGH

Cough, one of the most frequent of all cardiorespiratory symptoms, may be defined as an explosive expiration which provides a means of clearing the tracheobronchial tree of secretions and foreign bodies. It can be caused by a variety of infectious, neoplastic, or allergic disorders of the lungs and tracheobronchial tree. Cardiovascular disorders most frequently responsible for cough include those that lead to pulmonary venous hypertension, interstitial and alveolar pulmonary edema, pulmonary infarction, and compression of the tracheobronchial tree by aortic aneurysm. Cough due to pulmonary venous hypertension secondary to left ventricular failure or mitral stenosis tends to be dry, irritating, spasmodic, and nocturnal. When cough accompanies exertional dyspnea, it suggests either chronic obstructive lung disease or heart failure, whereas in a patient with a history of allergy and/or wheezing, cough is often a concomitant of bronchial asthma. A history of cough associated with expectoration for months or years occurs in chronic obstructive lung disease and/or chronic bronchitis.

The character of the sputum may be helpful in the differential diagnosis. Thus, a cough producing frothy, pink-tinged sputum occurs in pulmonary edema; clear, white, mucoid sputum suggests viral infection or longstanding bronchial irritation; thick, yellowish sputum suggests an infectious cause; rusty sputum suggests pneumococcal pneumonia; blood-streaked sputum suggests tuberculosis, bronchiectasis, carcinoma of the lung, and pulmonary infarction.

The combination of cough with *hoarseness* without upper respiratory disease may be due to pressure of a greatly enlarged left atrium on an enlarged pulmonary artery compressing the recurrent laryngeal nerve.

HEMOPTYSIS

The expectoration of blood or of sputum, either streaked or grossly contaminated with blood, may be due to (1) escape of red cells into the alveoli from congested vessels in the lungs (acute pulmonary edema); (2) rupture of dilated endobronchial vessels that form collateral channels between the pulmonary and bronchial venous systems (mitral stenosis); (3) necrosis and hemorrhage into the alveoli (pulmonary infarction); (4) ulceration of the bronchial mucosa or the slough of a caseous lesion (tuberculosis); minor damage to the tracheobronchial mucosa, produced by excessive coughing of any cause can result in mild hemoptysis; (5) vascular invasion (carcinoma of the lung); (6) necrosis of the mucosa with rupture of pulmonary-bronchial venous connections (bronchiectasis).

The history is often decisive in pinpointing the etiology of hemoptysis. Recurrent episodes of minor bleeding are observed in patients with chronic bronchitis, bronchiectasis, tuberculosis, and mitral stenosis. Rarely, these conditions result in the expectoration of large quantities of blood, i.e., more than one-half cup. Massive hemoptysis may also be due to rupture of a pulmonary arteriovenous aneurysm; exsanguinating hemoptysis may occur with rupture of an aortic aneurysm into the bronchopulmonary tree. Hemoptysis associated with a history of expectoration of clear, gray sputum suggests chronic obstructive lung disease and of yellowish-green sputum, pulmonary infection. Hemoptysis associated with shortness of breath suggests mitral stenosis; the hemoptysis is often precipitated by sudden elevations in left atrial pressure during effort or pregnancy and is attributable to rupture of small pulmonary or bronchopulmonary anastomosing veins. Blood-tinged sputum in patients with mitral stenosis may also be due to transient pulmonary edema; in these circumstances it is usually associated with severe dyspnea.

A history of hemoptysis associated with acute pleuritic chest pain suggests pulmonary embolism with infarction. Recurrent hemoptysis in a young, otherwise asymptomatic woman favors the diagnosis of bronchial adenoma. A history of recurrent hemoptysis with chronic marked sputum production suggests the diagnosis of bronchiectasis. Hemoptysis associated with the production of putrid sputum occurs in lung abscess, whereas hemoptysis associated with weight loss and anorexia in a male smoker suggests carcinoma of the lung. When blunt trauma to the chest is followed by hemoptysis, lung contusion is the probable cause. Hemoptysis associated with congenital heart disease and cyanosis suggests Eisenmenger syndrome or Osler-Weber-Rendu disease with pulmonary arteriovenous malformation(s).

A history of drug ingestion may be helpful in elucidating the etiology of hemoptysis; e.g., anticoagulants and immunosuppressive drugs can cause bleeding. A history of ingestion of contraceptive pills may be a risk factor for the development of deep vein thrombosis and subsequent pulmonary embolism and infarction.

OTHER SYMPTOMS

Cardiovascular disorders can cause symptoms emanating from every organ system. Several of these are mentioned here primarily to point out how detailed the history must be of a patient suspected of having cardiovascular disease; fuller discussions are found elsewhere in this text. *Fatigue* is among the most nonspecific of all symptoms in clinical medicine; in patients with an impaired systemic circulation as a consequence of a depressed cardiac output, it may be associated with muscular weakness. In other patients with heart disease, fatigue may be caused by drugs, such as beta-adrenergic blocking agents, by excessive blood pressure reduction in patients treated too vigorously for hypertension or heart failure, and in the latter it may also be caused by excessive diuresis and by diuretic-induced hypokalemia. *Nocturia* is a common early complaint in patients with congestive heart failure. *Anorexia*, abdominal fullness, right upper quadrant discomfort, weight loss, and cachexia are symptoms of advanced heart failure (p. 495). Anorexia, *nausea, vomiting,* and *visual changes* are important signs of digitalis intoxication (p. 525). Nausea and vomiting occur frequently in patients with acute myocardial infarction. *Hoarseness* may be caused by compression of the recurrent laryngeal nerve by an aortic aneurysm, a dilated pulmonary artery, or an enormously enlarged left atrium. A history of *fever* and *chills* is common in patients with infective endocarditis (p. 1149).

The above-mentioned are examples of the wide variety of symptoms not obviously associated with abnormalities of the cardiovascular system that can be of critical importance in differential diagnosis when they are elicited in patients known to have or suspected of having heart disease. They serve to reemphasize that the physician whose responsibility it is to care for patients with heart disease must be first and foremost a broadly based clinician.

THE HISTORY IN SPECIFIC FORMS OF HEART DISEASE

Just as the history is of central importance in determining whether a specific symptom is caused by heart disease, it is equally valuable in elucidating the *etiology* of recognized heart disease. A few examples are given below; considerably greater detail is provided in later chapters that deal with each specific disease entity.

HEART DISEASE IN INFANCY AND CHILDHOOD

The history is particularly helpful in establishing a diagnosis of *congenital heart disease*. In view of the familial incidence of certain congenital malformations (pp. 942 and 1613), a history of congenital heart disease, cyanosis, or heart murmur in the family should be ascertained. Rubella in the first 2 months of pregnancy is associated with a number of congenital cardiac malformations (patent ductus arteriosus, atrial and ventricular septal defect, tetralogy of Fallot, and supravalvular aortic stenosis). A maternal viral illness in the last trimester of pregnancy may be responsible for neonatal myocarditis. Syncope on exertion in a child with congenital heart disease suggests lesions in which the cardiac output is fixed, such as aortic or pulmonic stenosis. Exertional angina in a child suggests severe aortic stenosis, pulmonary stenosis, primary pulmonary hypertension, or anomalous origin of the left coronary artery. A history of syncope or faintness with straining and associated with cyanosis suggests tetralogy of Fallot.

In infants or children with cardiac murmurs, it is important to ascertain as precisely as possible when the murmur was first heard. Murmurs due to either aortic or pulmonic stenosis are usually audible within the first 48 hours of life, whereas those produced by a ventricular septal defect are usually apparent a few days or weeks later. On the other hand, the murmur produced by an atrial septal defect often is not heard until age 2 to 3 months.

Frequent pneumonias early in infancy suggest a large left-to-right shunt, and excessive diaphoresis occurs in left ventricular failure, most commonly due to ventricular septal defect in this age group. A history of squatting is most frequently associated with tetralogy of Fallot or tricuspid atresia (p. 949). Dysphagia suggests the presence of an aortic arch anomaly such as double aortic arch or an anomalous origin of the right subclavian artery passing behind the esophagus. A history of headaches, weakness of the legs, and intermittent claudication is compatible with the diagnosis of coarctation of the aorta (p. 1038). Weakness or lack of coordination in a child with heart disease suggests cardiomyopathy associated with Friedreich's ataxia or muscular dystrophy (p. 1711). Recurrent bleeding from the nose, lips, or mouth associated with dizziness and visual disturbances and a family history of bleeding in a cyanotic child suggest hereditary hemorrhagic telangiectasia (Osler-Weber-Rendu disease) with pulmonary arteriovenous fistula(s). A cerebrovascular accident in a cyanotic patient may be due to cerebral thrombosis or abscess or paradoxical embolization (p. 949).

MYOCARDITIS AND CARDIOMYOPATHY

Rheumatic fever is suggested by a history of sore throat followed by symptoms including rash and chorea (St. Vitus' dance), manifest as a period of twitching or clumsiness for a few months in childhood, as well as by frequent epistaxes and growing pains, i.e., nocturnal pains in the legs (p. 1648). In patients suspected of having myocarditis or cardiomyopathy, a history of Raynaud's phenomenon, dysphagia, or tight skin suggests scleroderma (p. 1663). Pain in the hip or lower back that awakens the patient in the morning and is followed by morning back stiffness suggests rheumatoid spondylitis that is often associated with aortic valve disease (p. 1658). *Carcinoid heart disease* is associated with a history of diarrhea, bronchospasm, and flushing of the upper chest and head (p. 1430). A history of diabetes, particularly if resistant to insulin and associated with bronzing of the skin, suggests *hemochromatosis* that may be associated with heart failure due to cardiac infiltration. *Amyloid heart disease* (p. 1422) is often associated with a history of postural hypotension and peripheral neuropathy. *Hypertrophic cardiomyopathy* (p. 1409), which is generally transmitted as an autosomal dominant trait, is often associated with a family history of this condition and sometimes with a family history of sudden death. The characteristic symptoms are angina, dyspnea, and syncope, which are often intensified paradoxically by digitalis and which occur during or immediately after exercise.

HIGH-OUTPUT HEART FAILURE

Patients with symptoms of heart failure (breathlessness and excess fluid accumulation) with warm extremities often have *high-output heart failure* (Chap. 24). They should be questioned about a history of anemia and of its common causes and accompaniments, such as menorrhagia, melena, peptic ulcer, hemorrhoids, sickle cell disease, and the neurological manifestations of vitamin B_{12} deficiency. Also, in such patients an attempt should be made to elicit a history of thyrotoxicosis (p. 1727) (weight loss, polyphagia, diarrhea, diaphoresis, heat intolerance, nervousness, breathlessness, muscle weakness, and goiter). Patients with beriberi heart disease responsible for high-output heart failure often present with a history characteristic of peripheral neuritis, alcoholism, poor eating habits, diet fads, or upper gastrointestinal surgery.

Patients with chronic *cor pulmonale* (see Chap. 46) frequently have a history of smoking, chronic cough and sputum production, dyspnea, and wheezing relieved by bronchodilators. Alternatively, they may present with a history of pulmonary emboli, phlebitis, and the sudden development of dyspnea at rest with palpitations, pleuritic chest pain, and, in the case of massive infarction, syncope.

PERICARDITIS AND ENDOCARDITIS

In patients in whom *pericarditis* or *cardiac tamponade* is suspected (Chap. 43), an attempt should be made to elicit a history of chest trauma, neoplastic disease of the chest with or without extensive radiation, myxedema, scleroderma, a recent viral infection, tuberculosis, or contact with tuberculous patients. The sequence of development of abdominal swelling, ankle edema, and dyspnea should be determined, since ascites often precedes edema, which in turn may precede exertional dyspnea in patients with chronic constrictive pericarditis. A history of joint symptoms with a face rash suggests the possibility of systemic lupus erythematosus (SLE), an important cause of pericarditis, and it should be recalled that procainamide, hydralazine, and isoniazid can produce an SLE-like syndrome (p. 1660).

The diagnosis of *infective endocarditis* is suggested by a history of fever, severe night sweats, anorexia and weight loss, and embolic phenomena expressed as hematuria, back pain, petechiae, tender finger pads, and a cerebrovascular accident (p. 1149).

Drug-Induced Heart Disease. The increasing appreciation that a wide variety of cardiac abnormalities can be induced by drugs makes a meticulous history of drug intake of great importance.[6] Catecholamines, whether administered exogenously or when secreted by a pheochromocytoma (p. 1734), may produce a myocarditis and arrhythmias. Digitalis glycosides can be responsible for a variety of tachy- and bradyarrhythmias as well as gastrointestinal, visual, and central nervous system disturbances (p. 525). Quinidine may cause Q-T prolongation, ventricular tachycardia of the *torsade de pointes* variety, syncope, and sudden death, presumably due to ventricular fibrillation (p.

TABLE 1–2   A COMPARISON OF THREE METHODS OF ASSESSING CARDIOVASCULAR DISABILITY

CLASS	NEW YORK HEART ASSOCIATION FUNCTIONAL CLASSIFICATION	CANADIAN CARDIOVASCULAR SOCIETY FUNCTIONAL CLASSIFICATION	SPECIFIC ACTIVITY SCALE
I	Patients with cardiac disease but without resulting limitations of physical activity. Ordinary physical activity does not cause undue fatigue, palpitation, dyspnea, or anginal pain.	Ordinary physical activity, such as walking and climbing stairs, does not cause angina. Angina with strenuous or rapid or prolonged exertion at work or recreation.	Patients can perform to completion any activity requiring ≥ 7 metabolic equivalents, e.g., can carry 24 lb up eight steps; carry objects that weigh 80 lb; do outdoor work (shovel snow, spade soil); do recreational activities (skiing, basketball, squash, handball, jog/walk 5 mph).
II	Patients with cardiac disease resulting in slight limitation of physical activity. They are comfortable at rest. Ordinary physical activity results in fatigue, palpitation, dyspnea, or anginal pain.	Slight limitation of ordinary activity. Walking or climbing stairs rapidly, walking uphill, walking or stair climbing after meals, in cold, in wind, or when under emotional stress, or only during the few hours after awakening. Walking more than two blocks on the level and climbing more than one flight of ordinary stairs at a normal pace and in normal conditions.	Patient can perform to completion any activity requiring ≥ 5 metabolic equivalents but cannot and does not perform to completion activities requiring ≥ 7 metabolic equivalents, e.g., have sexual intercourse without stopping, garden, rake, weed, roller skate, dance fox trot, walk at 4 mph on level ground.
III	Patients with cardiac disease resulting in marked limitation of physical activity. They are comfortable at rest. Less than ordinary physical activity causes fatigue, palpitation, dyspnea, or anginal pain.	Marked limitation of ordinary physical activity. Walking one to two block on the level and climbing more than one flight in normal conditions.	Patient can perform to completion any activity requiring ≥ 2 metabolic equivalents but cannot and does not perform to completion any activities requiring ≥ 5 metabolic equivalents, e.g., shower without stopping, strip and make bed, clean windows, walk 2.5 mph, bowl, play golf, dress without stopping.
IV	Patient with cardiac disease resulting in inability to carry on any physical activity without discomfort. Symptoms of cardiac insufficiency or of the anginal syndrome may be present even at rest. If any physical activity is undertaken, discomfort is increased.	Inability to carry on any physical activity without discomfort—anginal syndrome *may be* present at rest.	Patient cannot or does not perform to completion activities requiring ≥ 2 metabolic equivalents. *Cannot* carry out activities listed above (Specific Activity Scale, Class III).

Reproduced by permission of the American Heart Association, Inc., from Goldman L. et al. Comparative reproducibility and validity of systems for assessing cardiovascular functional class: Advantages of a new specific activity scale. Circulation 64: 1227, 1981.

729). Paradoxically the administration of antiarrhythmic drugs is one of the major causes of serious cardiac arrhythmias.[7]

Disopyramide (p. 659), beta-adrenergic blockers (p. 1349), and the calcium channel blocker verapamil (p. 1351) may depress ventricular performance, and in patients with ventricular dysfunction these drugs may intensify heart failure. Alcohol is also a potent myocardial depressant and may be responsible for the development of a cardiomyopathy (p. 1406), arrhythmias, and possibly sudden death. Tricyclic antidepressants may cause orthostatic hypotension and arrhythmias (p. 1838). Lithium, also used in the treatment of psychiatric disorders, can aggravate preexisting cardiac arrhythmias, particularly in patients with heart failure in whom the renal clearance of this ion is impaired.

The anthracycline compounds doxorubicin (Adriamycin) and daunorubicin, which are widely used because of their broad spectrum of activity against various tumors, may cause or intensify left ventricular failure, arrhythmias, myocarditis, and pericarditis (p. 1690). Cyclophosphamide, an antineoplastic alkylating agent, may also cause left ventricular dysfunction. Although not a drug, radiation may cause acute and chronic pericarditis (p. 1509), a pancarditis (p. 1445), and coronary artery disease; further, it may enhance the aforementioned cardiotoxic effects of the anthracyclines.

ASSESSING CARDIOVASCULAR DISABILITY
(Table 1–2)

One of the greatest values of the history is in categorizing the *degree* of cardiovascular disability, so that a given patient's status can be followed over time, the effects of a therapeutic intervention assessed, and patients compared with one another. The Criteria Committee of the New York Heart Association have provided a widely used classification that relates symptoms to "ordinary" activity.[8] The term "ordinary," of course, is subject to varying interpretation, as are terms such as "undue fatigue" that are used in this classification, and this has limited its accuracy and reproducibility. Somewhat more detailed and specific criteria were provided by the Canadian Cardiovascular Society,[9] but this classification and grading is limited to patients with angina pectoris. Recently, Goldman et al.[10]

have developed a new specific activity scale in which classification is based on the estimated metabolic cost of various activities. Although this specific activity scale has not yet been widely used, it appears to be more reproducible and to be a better predictor of exercise tolerance than either the New York Heart Association Classification or the Canadian Cardiovascular Society Criteria.

References

1. Sandler, G.: The importance of the history in the medical clinic and the cost of unnecessary tests. Am. Heart J. *100*:928, 1980.
2. Fishman, A. P.: The first approach to the patient with respiratory signs and symptoms. *In* Fishman, A. P. (ed.): Pulmonary Diseases and Disorders. New York, McGraw-Hill Book Co., 1980, pp. 3–28.
2a. Loke, J.: Distinguishing cardiac versus pulmonary limitation in exercise performance. Chest *83*:441, 1983.
3. Levene, D. L., Billings, R. F., Davies, G. M., Edmeads, J., and Saibil, F. G. (eds.): Chest Pain: An Integrated Diagnostic Approach. Philadelphia, Lea and Febiger, 1977.
4. Levine, H. J.: Difficult problems in the diagnosis of chest pain. Am. Heart J. *100*:108, 1980.
5. Christie, L. G., and Conti, C. R.: Systematic approach to the evaluation of angina-like chest pain. Am. Heart J. *102*:897, 1981.
6. Bristow, M. R. (ed.): Drug-Induced Heart Disease. Amsterdam, Elsevier, 1980, 476 pp.
7. Velebit, V., Podrid, P., Lown, B., Cohen, B. M., and Graboys, T. B.: Aggravation and provocation of ventricular arrhythmias by antiarrhythmic drugs. Circulation *65*:880, 1982.
8. The Criteria Committee of the New York Heart Association: Diseases of the Heart and Blood Vessels; Nomenclature and Criteria for Diagnosis, 6th ed. Boston, Little, Brown and Co., 1964.
9. Campeau, L.: Grading of angina pectoris. Circulation *54*:522, 1975.
10. Goldman, L., Hashimoto, B., Cook, E. F., and Loscalzo, A.: Comparative reproducibility and validity of systems for assessing cardiovascular functional class: Advantages of a new specific activity scale. Circulation *64*:1227, 1981.

GENERAL REFERENCES

Braunwald, E.: Alterations in circulatory and respiratory function. *In* Petersdorf, R. G., et al. (eds.): Harrison's Principles of Internal Medicine, 10th ed. New York, McGraw-Hill Book Co., 1983, pp. 155–181.
Constant, J.: The evolving check list in history-taking. *In* Bedside Cardiology, 2nd ed. Boston, Little, Brown and Co., 1976, pp. 1–22.
Dressler, W.: Clinical Aids in Cardiac Diagnosis. New York, Grune and Stratton, 1970.
Fowler, N. O.: The history in cardiac diagnosis. *In* Fowler, N. O. (ed.): Cardiac Diagnosis and Treatment, 3rd ed. Hagerstown, Md., Harper and Row, 1980, pp. 23–29.
Kraytman, J.: Cardiorespiratory system. *In* The Complete Patient History. New York, McGraw-Hill Book Co., 1979, pp. 11–112.
Oram, S.: Clinical examination. *In* Clinical Heart Disease, 2nd ed. London, William Heinemann, 1981, pp. 45–60.
Parkinson, J.: Cardiac symptoms. Ann. Intern. Med. *35*:499, 1951.
Tumulty, P. A.: Obtaining the history. *In* The Effective Clinician. Philadelphia, W. B. Saunders Co., 1973, pp. 17–28.
White, P. D.: Clues in the Diagnosis and Treatment of Heart Disease. Springfield, Ill., Charles C Thomas, 1955.
Wood, P.: The chief symptoms of heart failure. *In* Diseases of the Heart and Circulation, 3rd ed. Philadelphia, J. B. Lippincott, 1968, pp. 1–25.

2

THE PHYSICAL EXAMINATION

by Eugene Braunwald, M.D.

Two of the most common pitfalls in cardiovascular medicine are the failure by the cardiologist to recognize the effects of systemic illnesses on the cardiovascular system and the failure by the noncardiologist to recognize the cardiac manifestations of systemic illnesses that have major effects on other organ systems. In order to avoid these pitfalls, patients known to have or suspected of having heart disease require not only a detailed examination of the cardiovascular system but a meticulous general physical examination as well. For example, the condition of patients with previously stable rheumatic valvular or coronary artery disease may suddenly deteriorate, not because of the progression of the underlying cardiac condition, but rather because of the development of an unrelated disease—such as a bleeding peptic ulcer or a malignant neoplasm—and a change in the patient's cardiac condition, such as the intensification of angina or dyspnea, may actually signal the presence of the other disorder.

The presence of cardiac disease should prompt a careful search for frequent noncardiac concomitants such as arteriosclerosis of the cerebral vessels and of the arteries of the lower extremities and aorta in patients with ischemic heart disease. Conversely, the very high incidence (approximately 50 per cent) of coronary artery disease in patients with cerebrovascular disorders must be considered in dealing with patients with these disorders. In some patients a cardiovascular abnormality may be responsible for a disorder involving another organ system; for example, retarded physical development and failure to thrive in infants may be secondary to congenital heart disease, and embolic strokes are important complications of rheumatic mitral stenosis and atrial fibrillation, of mitral valve prolapse, and of infective endocarditis.

Examples of disorders which have effects principally on other organs but which often also affect the heart include the following:

1. *Muscular dystrophies* (Chap. 50) causing cardiomyopathies.

2. *Metabolic disorders,* such as hemochromatosis (p. 1425), glycogen storage disease (p. 1051), Gaucher's disease (p. 1425), and Fabry's disease (p. 1425) (myocardial infiltration, heart failure, and conduction defects).

3. *Chromosomal disorders,* such as Turner's syndrome (p. 1614) associated with a variety of congenital cardiac defects, particularly coarctation of the aorta.

4. *Endocrine disorders,* such as acromegaly (p. 1722) associated with accelerated coronary atherosclerosis and myocardial hypertrophy; hyperthyroidism (p. 1727) associated with heart failure and atrial fibrillation, and myxedema (p. 1729) associated with pericardial effusion.

5. *Congenital deafness* (p. 1626) associated with Q-T interval prolongation and serious cardiac arrhythmias.

6. *Raynaud's disease* associated with primary pulmonary hypertension (p. 836), coronary spasm (p. 1360), and sclerodermatous involvement of the heart (p. 1663).

Editor's Note: Examination of the cardiovascular system includes inspection and palpation of the arterial and venous pulses and of the chest as well as auscultation of the heart. The findings elicited on physical examination can be aided enormously by graphic recordings. The details of carrying out the cardiovascular examination and the interpretation of the findings are presented in this chapter and in Chapters 3 and 4. This chapter focuses on the findings elicited by physical examination, while Chapters 3 and 4 deal primarily with the graphic recording of these findings. The three chapters should be considered as a unit, since the subjects covered are similar and the material does not lend itself well to a rigid separation between physical and graphic modes of examination; some degree of overlap in content among these chapters is therefore unavoidable.

7. *Inherited connective tissue disorders,* such as Marfan syndrome (p. 1665), osteogenesis imperfecta (p. 1665), Ehlers-Danlos syndrome (p. 1668), pseudoxanthoma elasticum (p. 1669), associated with aortic dilatation, dissection and regurgitation, mitral valve prolapse, coronary artery disease, and pericarditis; Hurler's syndrome and related disorders of mucopolysaccharide metabolism (p. 1670) associated with arrhythmias, valvular disease, and heart failure.

8. *Collagen vascular diseases:* systemic lupus erythematosus (p. 1660) (valvulitis, myocarditis, and pericarditis), ankylosing spondylitis (p. 1656) (diseases of the aorta and aortic valve), rheumatoid arthritis (p. 1658) (pericarditis and valve disease), vasculitis (p. 1660) (coronary arteritis and myocarditis), polymyositis (p. 1663) (arrhythmias, pericarditis, and myocarditis).

9. *Sarcoidosis* (p. 1426) associated with restrictive cardiomyopathy and arrhythmias.

10. *Chronic hemolytic anemia* (p. 1678) causing cardiac dilatation and myocarditis secondary to transfusional hemosiderosis.

In patients in whom these and related systemic disorders are present or suspected, the physical examination should be conducted so as to allow recognition of the systemic disorder and evaluation of the presence and severity of cardiovascular involvement.

THE GENERAL EXAMINATION

Although one can employ a variety of techniques in carrying out the physical examination, I favor commencing with an assessment of the general appearance of the patient and then employing the regional approach, starting with the head and ending with the lower extremities. It is desirable, whenever possible, to examine the patient on an examining table or bed whose head section may be raised. Examination in a quiet room at a comfortable temperature and in daylight is optimal.

GENERAL APPEARANCE

An assessment of the patient's general appearance is usually begun with a detailed inspection at the time when the history is being obtained.[1,1a] The general build and appearance of the patient, the skin color, and the presence of pallor or cyanosis should be noted, as well as the presence of shortness of breath, orthopnea, periodic (Cheyne-Stokes) respiration (p. 499), and distention of the neck veins. If the patient is in pain, is he or she sitting quietly (typical of angina pectoris); moving about, trying to find a more comfortable position (characteristic of acute myocardial infarction); or most comfortable sitting upright (heart failure) or leaning forward (pericarditis)? Simple inspection will also reveal whether the patient's whole body shakes with each heart beat and whether Corrigan's pulses (bounding arterial pulsations, as occur with the large stroke volume of severe aortic regurgitation, arteriovenous fistula, or complete atrioventricular block) are present in the head, neck, and upper extremities. Marked weight loss, malnutrition, and cachexia, which occur in severe chronic heart failure (p. 499), may also be readily evident on inspection. The cold, sweaty palms and frequent sighing respirations typical of *neurocirculatory asthenia* may be detected, as well as the marked obesity, somnolence, and cyanosis suggestive of the *Pickwickian syndrome* (p. 1596).

The distinctive general appearance of *Marfan syndrome* (p. 1665) is often apparent, i.e., long extremities with an arm span that exceeds the height; a longer lower segment (pubis to foot) than upper segment (head to pubis); arachnodactyly (spider fingers); and a variety of thoracic deformities, including kyphoscoliosis, pectus carinatum, and pectus excavatum. Patients with *muscular dystrophy*—a cause of cardiomyopathy (Chap. 50)—may have difficulty rising from a chair or walking. The diagnosis of *hyperthyroidism,* which frequently causes cardiac disease (p. 1727), can often be suspected from simple inspection (exophthalmos, lid lag, perspiration, a fine tremor). In *Cushing's syndrome,* a cause of secondary hypertension (pp. 885 and 1732), there is trunkal obesity and rounding of the face, with disproportionately thin extremities.

Many congenital somatic abnormalities such as cleft palate or harelip are frequently apparent on simple inspection and are observed in 25 per cent of infants with congenital heart disease; their presence should prompt a search for a cardiac malformation.[2] In the *Ellis–van Creveld syndrome,* dwarfism, polydactyly, and ectodermal dysplasia frequently accompany congenital heart disease. In patients with *coarctation of the aorta,* the lower extremities may be poorly developed, while the upper extremities are normal. Although heart failure may be associated with slight temperature elevation (p. 499), if it exceeds 38°C, it should not be attributed to heart failure alone; it is possible that a complication such as a respiratory or urinary tract infection, endocarditis, or pulmonary embolus is responsible.

HEAD AND FACE

Examination of the face often aids in the recognition of many disorders that can affect the cardiovascular system. *Myxedema* is characterized by a dull, expressionless face; periorbital puffiness; loss of the lateral eyebrows; a large tongue; and dry, sparse hair. An *earlobe crease* occurs more frequently in patients with myocardial infarction than in controls,[3] particularly in patients in whom the myocardial infarction is associated with diabetic retinopathy or hypertension. Furthermore, the presence of an earlobe crease in a relatively young person (i.e., under 45 years) should suggest the possibility of coronary artery disease.

Patients with *rheumatic heart disease* and severe mitral stenosis may exhibit a characteristic facies—a malar flush, cyanotic lips, and slight jaundice due to hepatic congestion.[4] Bobbing of the head coincident with each heart beat (DeMussett's sign) is characteristic of severe aortic regurgitation. Facial edema may be present in patients with *tricuspid valve disease* and *constrictive pericarditis. Infective endocarditis* may result in a "café au lait" complexion. Anemia, cyanosis, and polycythemia may all be suspected from examination of the conjunctivae and oral mucosa. Telangiectasia of the lips and tongue may be associated with pulmonary arteriovenous fistula.

In *Down's syndrome* (mongolism, trisomy 21), which is often associated with congenital heart disease (p. 1613), there is mental deficiency, a prominent medial epicanthus, and a large, often protruding tongue, low-set ears, a poorly formed nasal bridge, and hypoplastic mandible. Adenoma sebaceum of the face may be accompanied by a cardiac *rhabdomyoma* (p. 1461). Approximately 5 per cent of infants with congenital heart disease (most commonly ventricular septal defect) have the so-called cardiofacial syndrome, characterized by unilateral partial lower facial weakness, which may become apparent only when the patient cries.[5] In the so-called *velocardiofacial syndrome*,[6] a cleft of the secondary palate, a long vertical face, and deep overbite with retruded mandible accompany congenital heart disease, most commonly a ventricular septal defect.

Hypertelorism (widely set eyes) is observed in patients with *Noonan's syndrome*,[7] who often have pulmonic stenosis (Figure 47–1, p. 1615); *Turner's syndrome*, often accompanied by coarctation of the aorta (p. 1614); the *multiple lentigines syndrome* (also termed LEOPARD syndrome) (Figure 47–3, p. 1616), often associated with pulmonic stenosis and hypertrophic cardiomyopathy;[8] and *Hurler's syndrome* (arrhythmias and valvular regurgitation) (p. 1670). The facies of one group of patients with a nonfamilial type of *supravalvular aortic stenosis* and mental retardation is quite characteristic (see Figure 29–31, p. 981) and includes hypertelorism; a broad, high forehead; strabismus and epicanthal folds; low-set ears; upturned nose; a long upper lip and wide mouth; and hypoplasia of the mandible, with a pointed chin, small teeth, and dental deformities[9] (p. 982). Patients with *stenosis of the pulmonary artery* and/or its branches often have an unusual facial appearance characterized by a large mouth, a blunt upturned nose, wide-set eyes, internal strabismas, and malformed teeth.[1]

Scleroderma, which can cause several forms of heart disease (p. 1663), can often be recognized in the face, where skin becomes firm, thickened, and leathery in texture and is tightly bound to the underlying subcutaneous tissues. In the late stages of this disease the skin is atrophic, and there is immobility, particularly around the mouth. Patients with *systemic lupus erythematosus* (p. 1660) may present with a butterfly rash on the face. *Acromegaly* (p. 1722) is associated with enlargement of the head, coarse facial features, prognathism, and macroglossia. *Cushing's syndrome*, in which hypertension is often present (p. 1732), is characterized by a moon facies, hirsutism, and acne. *Paget's disease* of bone, which may be associated with a high cardiac output state (p. 817), is characterized by enlargement of the skull. Episodic facial flushing occurs in patients with *carcinoid tumors* (p. 1430) and *pheochromocytoma* (p. 1734). A high, arched palate, prominent ears, and shimmering irides are characteristic of *Marfan syndrome* (p. 1665).

The *muscular dystrophies*, the cardiac manifestations of which are described in Chapter 50, may also affect facial appearance profoundly. Patients with *myotonic dystrophy* (p. 1708) exhibit a dull, expressionless face, with ptosis due to weakness of the levator muscles; the forehead is furrowed, and the temporalis and sternocleidomastoid muscles are atrophied. In the *facioscapulohumeral type* of *muscular dystrophy* (Landouzy-Déjerine) (p. 1708), nearly all the facial muscles are weak, particularly the orbicularis oris, preventing the patients from puckering the mouth and whistling; weakness of the orbicularis oculi, diffuse fattening of the face, and facial asymmetry (particularly around the mouth) are also characteristic.

In patients with *Werner's syndrome*, who are at high risk of developing premature coronary and arterial atherosclerosis, there is premature graying of the hair, frontal baldness, beaking of the nose, cataract formation, and proptosis. Myotonic muscular dystrophy (p. 1708) may also cause premature graying of the hair, frontal thinning or baldness, and early cataracts.

EYES

External ophthalmoplegia and ptosis due to muscular dystrophy of the extraocular muscles occur in the *Kearns-Sayre syndrome*, which may be associated with complete heart block and myocardial failure[10] (p. 1714).

Exophthalmos and stare occur not only in hyperthyroidism, which can cause high-output cardiac failure (p. 1727), but also in advanced congestive heart failure, in which there is severe pulmonary venous hypertension and weight loss (p. 496).[11] The stare is probably due to lid retraction caused by the increased adrenergic tone that accompanies heart failure. Severe tricuspid regurgitation[12] and a carotid artery–cavernous sinus fistula can also cause pulsatile exophthalmos.

Attention should be directed to the *iris* to look for an arcus, a circumferential light ring around the iris. When this ring begins inferiorly, leaving a rim peripherally, and occurs in a young person, it is frequently associated with hypercholesterolemia (Fig. 2–1), xanthelasma (small yellowish deposits of cholesterol on the eyelids), and premature atherosclerosis. (In blacks, an arcus often does not reflect hypercholesterolemia.) Iridodonesis (tremulous iris), in which the iris is not properly supported by the lens because of dislocation or weakness of the suspensory free ligament, occurs in Marfan syndrome. Gray-white spots (Brushfield's spots) in the iris occur in Down's syndrome. Iridocyclitis and enlargement of the lacrimal glands are seen in sarcoidosis, which may be associated with cardiomyopathy (p. 1426).

Blue scleras may be seen in patients with Marfan syndrome (p. 1665), Ehlers-Danlos syndrome (p. 1668), and osteogenesis imperfecta (p. 1668)—disorders that may be associated with aortic dilatation, regurgitation, and dissection and with prolapse of the mitral valve. *Argyll Robertson pupils* (small, irregular, unequal pupils that do not dilate properly on administration of mydriatic drugs and that fail to react to light but constrict on accommodation) are diagnostic of central nervous system syphilis; this may be associated with cardiovascular syphilis, characterized by aneurysm of the ascending aorta, coronary ostial stenosis, and aortic regurgitation (p. 1562). The *cornea* may be clouded in Hurler's syndrome. *Cataracts* are associated with the so-called rubella syndrome, in which a variety of congenital cardiac malformations occur; premature cataracts also occur in Refsum's disease and in myotonic muscular dystrophy, both of which may be associated with cardiomyopathy (p. 1708); *vitreous opacities* are frequent in

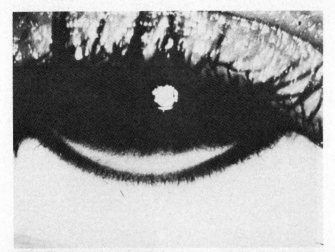

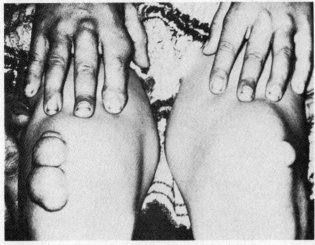

FIGURE 2–1 Arcus juvenilis and xanthelasma of the lids (*top*) and tendinous xanthomas of the knees (*bottom*) in a patient with familial hypercholesteremia. The patient was a 10-year-old girl with a serum cholesterol level of 665 mg per 100 ml. Several other members of the family had a similar syndrome. (From Cogan, D. G.: Ophthalmic Manifestations of Systemic Vascular Disease. Philadelphia, W. B. Saunders Co., 1974, pp. 14 and 15.)

patients with familial amyloidosis, in whom a restrictive cardiomyopathy may be present.

Fundi. Examination of the *fundi* allows classification of arteriolar disease in patients with hypertension (Fig. 2–2*A*) and may be helpful in the recognition of arteriosclerosis. Beading of the retinal artery may be present in patients with hypercholesteremia (Fig. 2–2*B*), and wreathlike arteriovenous anastomoses around the disk are characteristic of Takayasu's disease (p. 1558) (Fig. 2–2*C*). Hemorrhages near the disks with white spots in the center (Roth's spots) occur in infective endocarditis (p. 1151) (Fig. 2–2*D*). Embolic retinal occlusions may occur in patients with rheumatic heart disease, left atrial myxoma, and atherosclerosis of the aorta or arch vessels. Papilledema is present not only in patients with malignant hypertension (Chap. 26) but also in cor pulmonale with severe hypoxia. In coarctation of the aorta, the retinal arteries are particularly tortuous but may not show other changes characteristic of hypertensive retinopathy.[13] In patients with cyanosis and polycythemia, the retinal veins are particularly dilated and edema and retinal papilledema are occasionally present.

SKIN AND MUCOUS MEMBRANES

Central cyanosis (due to intracardiac or intrapulmonary right-to-left shunting) is observed in warm sites, including the conjunctivae and the mucous membranes of the oral cavity, while peripheral cyanosis (due to reduction of peripheral blood flow, such as occurs in heart failure and peripheral vascular disease) is characteristically observed in cool, exposed areas such as the extremities, particularly the nailbeds and nose. Polycythemia can often be suspected from inspection of the conjunctivae, lips, and tongue, which in anemia are pale and in polycythemia are darkly congested.[14] A blotchy cyanotic tinge to the skin associated with episodic flushing, particularly of the face, occurs in patients with *carcinoid tumors,* which may be associated with valvular heart disease (p. 1430).

Bronze pigmentation of the skin and loss of axillary and pubic hair occur in *hemochromatosis* (which may result in cardiomyopathy owing to iron deposits in the heart) (p. 1425). Jaundice may be observed in patients following pulmonary infarction as well as in patients with congestive hepatomegaly or cardiac cirrhosis. *Lentigines,* i.e., small brown macular lesions on the neck and trunk that begin at about age 6 and do not increase in number with sunlight, are observed in patients with pulmonic stenosis and hypertrophic cardiomyopathy[8] (p. 1409).

The skin is ruddy in patients with polycythemia and Cushing's syndrome; sallow and yellowish in both myxedema and in uremia; fine and silky in thyrotoxicosis; coarse and dry in myxedema and acromegaly; thickened and yellow (particularly in the neck and antecubital region) in pseudoxanthoma elasticum; smooth and glossy in longstanding Raynaud's syndrome; and warm and moist in anemia, beriberi, and other high-output states (Chap. 24). Increased sweating, most commonly a cold sweat in the palms, is observed in patients with neurocirculatory asthenia. *Erythema marginatum* (evanescent lesions confined primarily to the trunk) and *subcutaneous nodules* (which occur on the extensor surface of the elbows or over bony prominences such as the spine or skull) may be present in acute rheumatic fever (p. 1648). *Petechiae* occur in infective endocarditis; café-au-lait spots, freckles, and cutaneous neurofibromas occur in patients with pheochromocytoma (p. 1734), while *symmetric vitiligo* of the extremities is seen in patients with hyperthyroidism. Bluish pigmentation of the ear and nose cartilage is characteristic of *ochronosis,* which can produce serious valvular deformities (Chap. 32). Large areas of *psoriasis* or *exfoliative dermatitis* may be responsible for high-output heart failure (p. 820).

Several types of xanthomas, i.e., cholesterol-filled nodules, are found either subcutaneously or over a tendon in patients with hyperlipoproteinemia (Chap. 35). Premature atherosclerosis frequently develops in these individuals. *Tuberoeruptive xanthomas,* present subcutaneously or on the extensor surfaces of the extremities, and *xanthoma striatum palmare,* which produces yellowish, orange, or pink discoloration of the palmar and digital creases, occur most commonly in patients with type III hyperlipoproteinemia (p. 1215). Patients with *xanthoma tendinosum* (Fig. 2–1), i.e., nodular swellings of the tendons, especially of the elbows, extensor surfaces of the hands, and Achilles' tendons, usually have type II hyperlipoproteinemia (p. 1214).

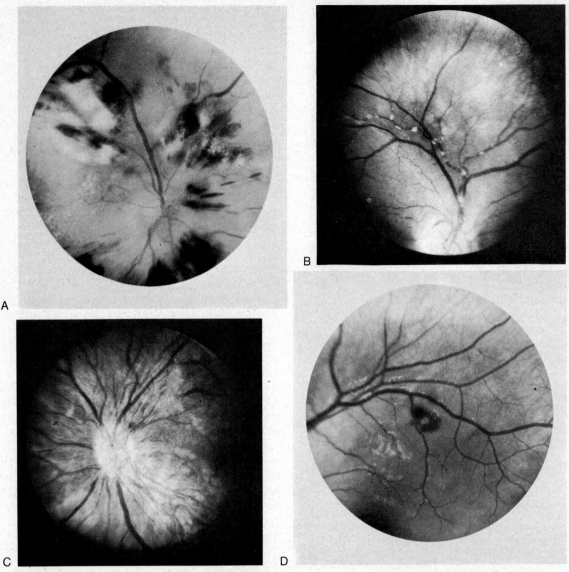

FIGURE 2–2   *A,* Severe hypertensive retinopathy. The patient was a 43-year-old man with the symptoms of malignant hypertension. He subsequently died of massive cerebral hemorrhage. *B,* Beading of the retinal artery in a patient with hypercholesteremia. The patient was a 37-year-old man with a serum cholesterol level of 400 mg per 100 ml. *C,* Proliferative retinopathy of Takayasu-Ohnishi disease. The patient was a 27-year-old Oriental woman with postural amaurosis and hemiplegia. Brachial pulses unobtainable. *D,* Roth spots (hemorrhage with white center) in a patient with subacute bacterial endocarditis. (From Cogan, D. G.: Ophthalmic Manifestations of Systemic Vascular Disease. Philadelphia, W. B. Saunders Co., 1974, p. 52.)

Xanthelasma also occur in this condition but are less specific (Fig. 2–1). *Eruptive xanthomas* are tiny, yellowish nodules, 1 to 2 mm in diameter on an erythematous base, which may present anywhere on the body and are associated with hyperchylomicronemia and are therefore often found in patients with type I and type V hyperlipoproteinemia (p. 1216).

Hereditary telangiectasia are multiple capillary hemangiomas occurring in the skin, nasal mucosa, and upper respiratory and gastrointestinal tracts that resemble the spider nevi seen in patients with liver disease. When present in the lung, they are associated with pulmonary arteriovenous fistulas and cause central cyanosis. Spider nevi on the face occur in patients with *chronic liver disease,* which may be

associated with a high cardiac output state (p. 819). Nicotine staining of the fingers suggests excessive cigarette smoking, an important risk factor for the development of coronary artery disease (p. 1216).

EXTREMITIES

A variety of congenital and acquired cardiac malformations are associated with characteristic changes in the extremities. Among the congenital lesions, short stature, cubitus valgus, and medial deviation of the extended forearm is characteristic of *Turner's syndrome* (p. 1614). Patients with the *Holt-Oram syndrome* (Table 29–2, p. 943), i.e., atrial septal defect with skeletal deformities, often have a thumb with an extra phalanx, a so-called "fingerized thumb," which lies in the same plane as the fingers, making it difficult to appose the thumb and fingers. In addition, they may exhibit deformities of the radius and ulna, causing difficulty in supination and pronation. There is often asymmetry of skeletal involvement, with the left side more severely affected.[15] Polydactyly and hypoplastic fingernails are part of the *Ellis–van Creveld syndrome* (chondroectodermal dysplasia), a disorder frequently associated with atrial or ventricular septal defect (p. 1617). Arachnodactyly is characteristic of the *Marfan syndrome* (p. 1665). Normally, when a fist is made over a clenched thumb, the latter does not extend beyond the ulnar side of the hand, but it usually does so in Marfan's syndrome. When the wrist is encircled by the thumb and little finger of the opposite hand, the little finger will overlap the thumb by at least 1 cm in more than three-fourths of patients with Marfan's syndrome but will rarely do so in individuals without this syndrome.[16] In *osteogenesis imperfecta*, hyperextensibility of the joints is common, but arachnodactyly is not.[17] In patients with *homocystinuria*, the extremities may be elongated and other skeletal abnormalities, such as kyphoscoliosis and pectus carinatum, may be present. Ulnar deviation of the fourth and fifth fingers and flexion at the metacarpophalangeal joints occur in *Jaccoud's arthritis,*[18] a rare concomitant of rheumatic heart disease. In *Down's syndrome*, there is a Simian palm crease, increased space between the fourth and fifth fingers, and a short fifth finger that is curved inward, while in Turner's syndrome the fingers tend to be short.

Raynaud's phenomenon, which sometimes occurs in association with primary pulmonary hypertension (p. 836), scleroderma (p. 1663), and coronary spasm (p. 1360), is characterized by intermittent pallor and/or cyanosis of the extremities precipitated by exposure to cold. With the passage of time, the skin overlying the fingers and under the nails becomes atrophic. Cold, pale or blue hands accompanied by collapse of the forearm veins signifies peripheral vasoconstriction, which may be a normal response to cold, anxiety, or a low cardiac output. In patients with peripheral vascular disease, the ischemic foot typically exhibits paleness on elevation and rubor on dependency.

High cardiac output states (Chap. 24) produce warm, pink hands associated with distention of the forearm veins (signs of vasodilatation). Redness of the palmar eminences may be a sign of severe liver disease, while a fine tremor of the outstretched hands suggests thyrotoxicosis. Peripheral *arteriovenous fistula* or *Paget's disease* of bone may cause local warmth and excessive growth of the affected limb. Systolic flushing of the nailbeds, which can be readily detected by pressing a flashlight against the terminal digits (Quincke's sign), is a sign of aortic regurgitation and of other conditions characterized by a greatly widened pulse pressure. *Differential cyanosis*, in which the hands and fingers (especially on the right side) are pink and the feet and toes are cyanotic, is indicative of patent ductus arteriosus with reversed shunt due to pulmonary hypertension (p. 955); this finding can often be brought out by exercise. On the other hand, *reversed differential cyanosis*, in which cyanosis of the fingers exceeds that of the toes, suggests transposition of the great arteries, pulmonary hypertension,

preductal narrowing of the aorta, and reversed flow through a patent ductus arteriosus.[19]

Clubbing of the fingers and toes[20] (Fig. 2–3). Clubbing of the extremities is characteristic of central cyanosis (cyanotic congenital heart disease or pulmonary disease with hypoxia). It may also appear within a few weeks of the development of infective endocarditis but usually develops after two or three years of central cyanosis. Clubbing is also observed in a variety of suppurative pulmonary lesions and carcinoma of the lung as well as in gastrointestinal disorders, including biliary cirrhosis and regional enteritis; occasionally, it is a harmless familial condition. The earliest forms of clubbing are characterized by increased glossiness and cyanosis of the skin at the root of the nail.[21] Following obliteration of the normal angle between the base of the nail and the skin, the soft tissue of the pulp becomes hypertrophied, the nail root floats freely, and its loose proximal end can be palpated. In the more severe forms of clubbing, bony changes occur, i.e., *hypertrophic pulmonary osteoarthropathy*; these changes involve the terminal digits and in rare instances even the wrists, ankles, elbows, and knees. *Unilateral clubbing* of the fin-

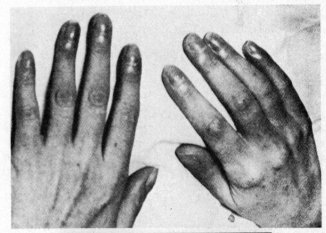

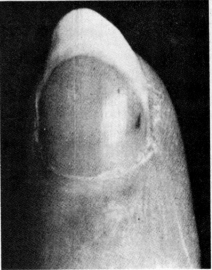

FIGURE 2–3 *Top,* Clubbing of fingers in subacute infective endocarditis. *Bottom,* Splinter hemorrhages due to subacute infective endocarditis. (From Oram, S.: Clinical Heart Disease. London, William Heinemann Medical Books, Ltd., 1971, pp. 289 and 290.)

gers is rare but can occur when an aortic aneurysm interferes with the arterial supply to one arm. Not to be confused with clubbing are the subungual fibromas of the fingers that occur in tuberous sclerosis, a condition often associated with cardiac rhabdomyoma.[22]

Osler's nodes are small, tender, erythematous skin lesions due to infected emboli and occurring most frequently in the pads of the fingers or toes and in the palms of the hands or soles of the feet, whereas *Janeway lesions* are slightly raised, nontender hemorrhagic lesions in the palms of hands and soles of the feet; both these lesions as well as petechiae occur in infective endocarditis (p. 1151). When the latter occur under the nailbeds, they are termed *splinter hemorrhages* (Fig. 2–3).

Edema of the extremities is a common finding in congestive heart failure; however, if it is present in only one leg, it is more likely due to venous obstructive disease than to heart failure. Firm pressure on the pretibial region for 10 to 20 seconds may be necessary for the detection of edema in ambulatory patients. In patients confined to bed, edema appears first in the sacral region. Edema may involve the face in children with heart failure of any etiology and in adults with heart failure associated with marked elevation of systemic venous pressure (e.g., constrictive pericarditis and tricuspid valve disease).

CHEST AND ABDOMEN

Examination of the thorax should begin with observations of the respiratory rate, effort, and regularity. The shape of the chest is important as well; thus, a barrel-shaped chest with low diaphragms suggests emphysema, bronchitis, and possibly cor pulmonale. In chronic obstructive pulmonary disease, accessory muscles are used during inspiration, while expiration is prolonged and often accompanied by wheezing.

Inspection of the chest may reveal a bulging to the right of the upper sternum caused by an aortic aneurysm or a venous collateral pattern caused by obstruction of the superior vena cava, which may also be caused by aortic aneurysm.

Painful enlargement of the *liver* may be due to venous congestion; the tenderness disappears in longstanding heart failure. Hepatic systolic expansile pulsations occur in patients with severe tricuspid regurgitation (Fig. 15–4, p. 497), and presystolic pulsations can be felt in patients with pure tricuspid stenosis and sinus rhythm. Transmitted (as opposed to intrinsic) pulsations of the liver occur in patients with right ventricular enlargement, aneurysmal dilatation of the upper abdominal aorta, and a widened pulse pressure. When firm pressure over the abdomen causes cervical venous distention, i.e, when there is *abdominojugular reflux,* right heart failure is usually present. *Ascites* is also characteristic of heart failure, but is especially characteristic of tricuspid valve disease and chronic constrictive pericarditis.

Splenomegaly may occur in the presence of severe congestive hepatomegaly, most frequently in patients with constrictive pericarditis or tricuspid valve disease. The spleen may be enlarged and painful in infective endocarditis as well as following splenic embolization. Splenic infarction is frequently accompanied by an audible friction rub.

Both *kidneys* may be palpably enlarged in patients with hypertension secondary to polycystic disease. Auscultation of the abdomen should be carried out in all patients with hypertension; a systolic bruit secondary to renal artery stenosis may be audible near the umbilicus or in the flank (p. 880).

Atherosclerotic aneurysms of the abdominal aorta are usually readily detected on palpation (p. 1543), except in markedly obese patients. In patients with *coarctation of the aorta*, no abdominal pulsations are palpable despite the presence of prominent arterial pulses in the neck and upper extremities; arterial pulses in the lower extremities are reduced or absent.

THE JUGULAR VENOUS PULSE

Important information concerning the dynamics of the right side of the heart can be obtained by inspection of the jugular venous pulse.[23,24] Since the venous valves between the superior vena cava and external jugular veins may interfere with pressure estimation in the latter, the *internal* jugular vein is ordinarily employed in the examination. The venous pulse can be analyzed more readily on the right than on the left side of the neck, because the right innominate and jugular veins extend cephalad in an almost straight line along with the superior vena cava, thus favoring transmission of hemodynamic changes from the right atrium, while the left innominate vein may be kinked or compressed by a variety of normal structures, by a dilated aorta, or by an aneurysm.

The patient should be lying comfortably during the examination; clothing should be removed from the neck and upper thorax, and although the head should rest on a pillow, it must not be elevated at a sharp angle from the trunk. The jugular venous pulse may be examined effectively by shining a light tangentially across the neck. Most patients with heart disease are examined most effectively in the 45-degree position, but in patients in whom venous pressure is high, a greater inclination (60 or even 90 degrees) is required to obtain visible pulsations, while in those in whom jugular venous pressure is low, a lesser inclination (30 degrees) is desirable. In order to amplify the pulsations of the jugular veins, it may be helpful to place the patient in the supine position and try to increase venous return by elevating the patient's legs.

The internal jugular vein is located deep within the neck, where it is covered by the sternocleidomastoid muscle and is therefore not usually visible as a discrete structure, except in the presence of severe venous hypertension. However, its pulsations are transmitted to the skin of the neck, where they are usually easily visible. Sometimes considerable difficulty may be experienced in differentiating between the carotid and jugular venous pulses in the neck, particularly when the latter exhibits prominent *v* waves, as occurs in patients with tricuspid regurgitation. However, there are several helpful clues: (1) The arterial pulse is a sharply localized rapid movement that may not be readily visible but that strikes the palpating fingers with considerable force; in contrast, the venous pulse, while more readily visible, often disappears when the palpating finger is placed on the pulsating area. (2) The arterial pulsations do not change when the patient is in the upright position, whereas venous pulsations usually disappear, unless the venous pressure is greatly elevated. (3) Compression of the root of the neck does not affect the arterial pulse but usually abolishes venous pulsations, except in the presence of extreme venous hypertension.

Two principal observations can usually be made from examination of the neck veins: the level of venous pressure and the type of venous wave pattern. In order to estimate jugular venous pressure, the height of the oscillating top of the distended proximal portion of the internal jugular vein, which reflects right atrial pressure, should be determined. The upper limit of normal is 4 cm above the sternal angle, which corresponds to a central venous pressure of approximately 9 cm H_2O, since the right atrium is approximately 5 cm below the sternal angle. When the veins in the neck collapse in a subject in the horizontal position, it is likely that the central venous pressure is subnormal. When obstruction of veins in the lower extremities is responsible for edema, pressure in the neck veins is not elevated and the abdominal-jugular reflux is negative.

The *abdominal-jugular reflux* can be tested by applying firm pressure to the periumbilical region for 30 to 60 seconds with the patient breathing quietly while the jugular veins are observed; increased respiratory excursions or strain should be avoided. In normal subjects jugular venous pressure rises only transiently, while pressure is continued, whereas in right ventricular failure the jugular venous pressure remains elevated.

Pattern of the Venous Pulse.   The events of the cardiac cycle, shown in Figure 12–25, p. 431, provide an explanation for the details of the jugular venous pulse pattern (Figs. 2–4 and 3–34, p. 63). The *a* wave in the venous pulse results from venous distention due to right atrial systole, while the *x* descent is due to atrial relaxation; the *c* wave, which occurs simultaneously with the carotid arterial pulse,[25] is an inconstant wave in the jugular venous pulse and may be due in part to forceful closure of the tricuspid valve; sometimes it is an artifact produced by the adjacent carotid arterial pulse. It is followed by the *x'* descent, caused by the pulling down of the floor of the atrium (descent of the base) by ventricular contraction. (Many investigators refer to this wave as the *x* descent.) The *v* wave results from the rise in right atrial pressure when blood flows into the right atrium during ventricular systole when the tricuspid valve is shut, and the *y* descent, i.e., the downslope of the *v* wave, is related to the decline in right atrial pressure when the tricuspid valve reopens. While all or most of these events can usually be recorded, they are not readily distinguishable on inspection. The descents or downward collapsing movements of the jugular veins are more rapid, produce larger excursions, and are therefore more prominent to the eye than are the ascents (Fig. 2–4). The normal dominant jugular venous descent, the *x'* descent, occurs just prior to the second heart sound, while the *y* descent ends after the second heart sound. With an increase in central venous pressure, the *v* wave becomes higher and the *y* collapse becomes more prominent. The *a* wave can be recognized when it is abnormally prominent; it occurs just before the first heart sound or carotid pulse

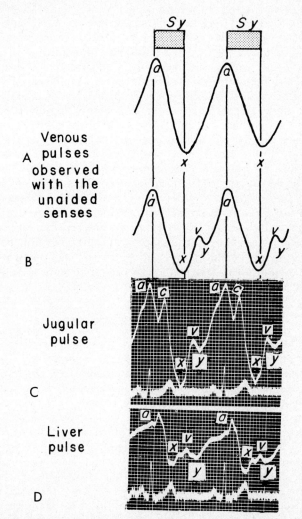

FIGURE 2–4   *A* and *B*, Tracings of the normal venous pulse observed with the unaided eyes. *A*, The outstanding feature is the systolic collapse (*x*), which alternates with a high peak (*a*). *B*, Sometimes in normal subjects a second peak is seen in early diastole (*v*), which is followed by a trough (*y*) that is shallower than the systolic dip (*x*).

C, The graph of the jugular pulse shows, similar to tracing *B*, two peaks (*a* and *v*) and two troughs (*x* and *y*). In addition, a small peak (*c*) interrupts the *x* descent. The *c* wave cannot be perceived with the unaided eye.

D, The most prominent feature of the hepatic pulse, like the jugular pulse, is a systolic dip (*x*). The *a* wave is small. (From Dressler, W.: Clinical Aids in Cardiac Diagnosis. New York, 1970, p. 195, by permission of Grune and Stratton.)

and has a sharp rise and fall. The *v* wave occurs just after the arterial pulse and has a slower, undulating pattern.

Alterations in Disease.   Elevation of jugular venous pressure reflects an increase in right atrial pressure and occurs in heart failure, reduced compliance of the right ventricle, pericardial disease, hypervolemia, and obstruction of the superior vena cava. During inspiration, the jugular venous pressure normally declines but the *amplitude* of the pulsations increases. *Kussmaul's sign* is a paradoxical rise in the height of the jugular venous pressure during inspiration, which occurs frequently in patients with chronic constrictive pericarditis and sometimes in congestive heart failure and tricuspid stenosis. The *x* descent may be prominent in patients with enlarged *a* waves, as well as in patients with right ventricular volume overload (atrial septal defect). Constrictive pericarditis (p. 1488) is characterized by a rapid and deep y descent without a prominent v wave (Fig. 3–38, p. 65); occasionally, the x' descent is prominent in this condition as well. A prominent v wave or cv wave, i.e., fusion of the c and v waves in the absence or attenuation of an x' descent, occurs in tricuspid regurgitation (Fig. 3–37, p. 64, and Fig. 15–5, p. 497); the y descent is gradual in tricuspid stenosis and steep in tricuspid regurgitation. Tall a waves are present in patients with sinus rhythm and tricuspid stenosis or atresia or right ventricular hypertension (Fig. 3–35, p. 63). Cannon (giant) a waves are noted in patients with atrioventricular dissociation when the right atrium contracts against a closed tricuspid valve (see Figure 3–36, p. 64). In atrial fibrillation, the a wave and x descent disappear, and the x' descent becomes more prominent. In right ventricular failure and sinus rhythm, there may be increases in prominence of both the a and v waves.

INDIRECT MEASUREMENT OF BLOOD PRESSURE

Systolic arterial pressure can be estimated without a sphygmomanometer cuff by gradually compressing the brachial artery while palpating the radial artery; the force required to obliterate the radial pulse represents the systolic blood pressure, and with practice, one can often estimate this level within 20 mm Hg. Ordinarily, however, a sphygmomanometer is used to obtain an indirect measurement of blood pressure.[26,27] The cuff should fit snugly around the arm, with its lower edge at least one inch above the antecubital space, and the diaphragm of the stethoscope should be placed close to or under the edge of the sphygmomanometer cuff. The width of the cuff selected should be at least 40 per cent of the circumference of the limb to be used. The standard size, with a 5-inch-wide cuff, is designed for adults with an arm of average size. When this cuff is applied to a large upper arm or a normal adult thigh, arterial pressure will be overestimated;[28] when it is applied to a small arm, the pressure will be underestimated. The cuff width should be approximately 1½ inches in infants and small children, 3 inches in young children (2 to 5 years), and 8 inches in obese adults. The bag should be long enough to extend at least halfway around the limb (10 inches in adults). Mercury manometers are, in general, more accurate and reliable than the aneroid type.

In order to measure arterial pressure in the upper extremity, the patient should be seated or lying comfortably and relaxed, the arm should be slightly flexed and at heart level, and the cuff should be inflated rapidly to approximately 30 mm Hg above the anticipated systolic pressure.[29] These maneuvers, which diminish the volume of blood in the venous bed, decrease the tissue pressure distal to the cuff and thereby increase the flow into the occluded brachial artery. The cuff is then deflated slowly; the pressure at which the brachial pulse can be palpated is close to the systolic pressure. The cuff should be deflated rapidly after the diastolic pressure is noted and a full minute allowed to elapse before pressure is remeasured in the same limb.

To measure pressure in the legs, the patient should lie on his or her abdomen, an 8-inch-wide cuff should be applied with the compression bag over the posterior aspect of the midthigh and should be rolled diagonally around the thigh to keep the edges snug against the skin, and auscultation should be carried out in the popliteal fossa. In order to measure pressure in the lower leg, an arm cuff is placed over the calf, and auscultation is carried out over the posterior tibial artery. Regardless of where the cuff is applied, care must be taken to avoid letting the rubber part of the balloon of the cuff extend beyond its covering and to avoid placing the cuff on so loosely that central ballooning occurs.

Korotkoff sounds. There are five phases of Korotkoff sounds, i.e., sounds produced by the flow of blood as the constricting blood pressure cuff is gradually released. The first appearance of clear, tapping sounds (phase I) represents the systolic pressure. These sounds are replaced by soft murmurs during phase II and by louder murmurs during phase III, as the volume of blood flowing through the constricted artery increases. The sounds suddenly become muffled in phase IV, when constriction of the brachial artery diminishes as arterial diastolic pressure is approached. Korotkoff sounds disappear in phase V, which is usually within 10 mm Hg of phase IV. Diastolic pressure measured directly through an intraarterial needle and external manometer corresponds closely to phase V. In severe aortic regurgitation, however, when the disappearance point is extremely low, sometimes 0 mm Hg, the sound of muffling (phase IV) is much closer to the intraarterial diastolic pressure than is the disappearance point (phase V). When there is a sizable difference between phases IV and V of the Korotkoff sounds (>10 mm Hg), both pressures should be recorded (e.g., 142/54/10 mm Hg). Korotkoff sounds may be difficult to hear and arterial pressure difficult to measure when arterial pressure rises at a slow rate (as in aortic stenosis), when the vessels are markedly constricted (as in hypovolemic shock), and when the stroke volume is reduced (as in severe heart failure). Very soft or inaudible Korotkoff sounds can often be accentuated by dilating the blood vessels of the upper extremities simply by opening and closing the fist repeatedly. In states of shock, the indirect method of measuring blood pressure is unreliable, and arterial pressure should be measured through an intraarterial needle.

The *auscultatory gap* is a silence that sometimes separates the first appearance of the Korotkoff sounds from their second appearance at a lower pressure. This phenomenon tends to occur when there is venous distention or reduced velocity of arterial flow into the arm, as occurs in severe aortic stenosis. If the first muffling of sounds is considered to be the diastolic pressure, it will be overestimated. If the second appearance is taken as the systolic pressure, it will be underestimated. On the other hand, sounds transmitted through the arterial tree from prosthetic aortic valves may be responsible for falsely high readings.

In order to determine arterial pressure in the basal condition, the patient should have rested in a quiet room for 15 minutes. It is desirable to record the arterial pressure in both arms at the time of the initial examination; differences in systolic pressure exceeding 15 mm Hg between the two arms when measurements are made in rapid sequence suggest obstructive lesions involving the aorta or the origin of the innominate and subclavian arteries, or supravalvular aortic stenosis (p. 982). In patients with vertebral-basal artery insufficiency, a difference in pressure between the arms may signify that a subclavian steal is responsible for the cerebrovascular symptoms.[30] In order to determine whether orthostatic hypotension is present, arterial pressure should be determined with the patient in both the supine and the erect positions. However, regardless of the patient's posture, the brachial artery should be at the level of the heart to avoid superimposition of the effects of gravity on the recorded pressure.

Normally, the systolic pressure in the legs is up to 20 mm Hg higher than in the arms, but the diastolic pressure is usually virtually identical. The recording of a higher diastolic pressure in the legs than in the arms suggests that the thigh cuff is too small. When systolic pressure in the popliteal artery exceeds that in the brachial artery by more than 20 mm Hg (Hill's sign), aortic regurgitation is usually present.[31] Blood pressure should be measured in the lower extremities in patients with hypertension to detect coarctation of the aorta or when obstructive disease of the aorta or its immediate branches is suspected.

THE ARTERIAL PULSE

The arterial pulse is determined by a combination of factors, including the left ventricular stroke volume, the ejection velocity, the relative compliance and capacity of the arterial system, and the pressure waves that result from the antegrade flow of blood and reflections of the arterial pressure pulse returning from the peripheral circulation.[32] Bilateral palpation of the carotid, radial, brachial, femoral, popliteal, dorsalis pedis, and posterior tibial pulses should be part of the examination of all cardiac patients. The frequency, regularity, and shape of the pulse wave and the character of the arterial wall should be determined.[33] The carotid pulse (Fig. 2–5A) provides the most accurate representation of the central aortic pulse[33a]. The brachial artery is the vessel ordinarily most suitable for appreciating the rate of rise of the pulse and the contour, volume, and consistency of the peripheral vessels. This artery is located at the medial aspect of the elbow, and it may be helpful to flex the arm in order to palpate it; palpation of the artery should be carried out with the thumb exerting pressure on the artery until its maximal movement is detected (Fig. 2–5B). A normal rate of rise of the arterial pulse suggests that there is no obstruction to left ventricular outflow, whereas a pulse wave of small amplitude with normal configuration suggests a reduced stroke volume.

THE NORMAL PULSE. The pulse in the ascending aorta normally rises rapidly to a rounded dome;[34] this initial rise reflects the peak velocity of blood ejected from the left ventricle. A slight anacrotic notch or pause is frequently recorded, but only occasionally felt, on the ascending limb of the pulse. The descending limb of the central aortic pulse is less steep than is the ascending limb, and it is interrupted by the incisura, a sharp downward deflection related to closure of the aortic valve (Fig. 3–21, p. 54, and Fig. 4–3, p. 70). Immediately thereafter, the pulse wave rises slightly and then declines gradually throughout diastole. As the pulse wave is transmitted to the periphery, its upstroke becomes steeper, the systolic peak becomes higher, the anacrotic shoulder disappears, and the sharp incisura is replaced by a smoother, later dicrotic notch

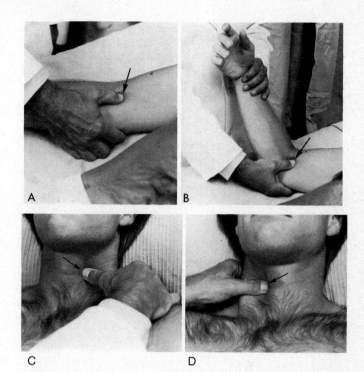

FIGURE 2–5 *A,* Palpation of the right brachial pulse with the thumb while the patient's arm lies at the side with the palm up. *B,* Palpation of the right brachial pulse with the patient's elbow resting in the palm of the examiner's hand. The thumb explores the antecubital fossa (*arrow*), while the patient's forearm is passively raised and lowered to achieve maximum relaxation of muscles around the elbow. *C* and *D,* Palpation of the carotid pulse. The examiner places the right thumb (*arrow*) on the patient's left carotoid artery (*C*). The left thumb (*arrow*) is then applied separately to the right carotid (*D*). (Reproduced with permission from Perloff, J. K. (Ed.): *Physical Examination of the Heart and Circulation,* Philadelphia, W. B. Saunders Co., 1982, pp. 58 and 60.

followed by a dicrotic wave. Normally, the height of this dicrotic wave diminishes with age, hypertension, and arteriosclerosis. In the central arterial pulse (central aorta and innominate and carotid arteries), the rapidly transmitted shock of left ventricular ejection results in a peak in early systole, referred to as the *percussion wave;* a second, smaller peak, the *tidal wave,* presumed to represent a reflected wave from the periphery, can often be recorded but is not normally palpable. However, in older subjects, particularly those with increased peripheral resistance, as well as in patients with arteriosclerosis and diabetes, the tidal wave may be somewhat higher than the percussion wave; i.e., the pulse reaches a peak in late systole. In peripheral arteries, the pulse wave normally has a single sharp peak.

ABNORMAL PULSES. When vascular resistance and arterial stiffness are increased, as in hypertension, there is an increase in pulse wave velocity, and the pulse contour has a more rapid upstroke and greater amplitude. Reduced or unequal carotid arterial pulsations occur in patients with carotid atherosclerosis and with diseases of the aortic arch, including aortic dissection, aneurysm, and Takayasu's disease (Chap. 45). In *supravalvular aortic stenosis* there is a streaming of the jet toward the innominate artery, and the carotid and brachial arterial pulses are stronger on the right than on the left side, and pressures are higher in the right than in the left arm (Fig. 4–6, p. 72, and p. 982). The pulses of the upper extremity may be reduced or unequal in a variety of other conditions, including arterial embolus or thrombosis, anomalous origin or aberrant path of the major vessels, and cervical rib or scalenus anticus syndrome. Asymmetry of right and left popliteal pulses is characteristic of iliofemoral obstruction. Weakness or absence of radial, posterior tibial, or dorsalis pedis pulses on one side suggests arterial insufficiency. In *coarctation of the aorta* the carotid and brachial pulses are bounding, rise rapidly, and have large volumes, while in the lower extremities, the systolic and pulse pressures are reduced, their rate of rise is slow, and there is a late peak. This delay in the femoral arterial pulses can usually be readily detected by simultaneous palpation of the femoral and radial arterial pulses.

In patients with fixed obstruction to left ventricular outflow, the carotid pulse rises slowly (*pulsus tardus*); the upstroke is frequently characterized by a thrill (the *carotid shudder*); and the peak is reduced, occurs late in systole, and is sustained (Figs. 3–22, p. 56; 4–4, p. 70; and 4–7, p. 72). There is a notch on the upstroke of the carotid pulse (anacrotic notch) that is so distinct that two separate waves can be palpated in what is termed an *anacrotic pulse*. *Pulsus parvus* is a pulse of small amplitude, usually because of a reduction of stroke volume. *Pulsus parvus et tardus* refers to a small pulse with a delayed systolic peak, which is characteristic of severe aortic stenosis. This type of pulse is more readily appreciated by palpating the carotid rather than a more peripheral artery. Patients with severe aortic stenosis and heart failure usually exhibit simply a reduced pulse amplitude, i.e., *pulsus parvus*, and the delay in the upstroke is not readily apparent. However, this delay is readily recorded. In elderly patients with inelastic peripheral arteries, the pulse may rise normally despite the presence of aortic stenosis.

The carotid arterial pulse may be prominent or exaggerated in any condition in which pulse pressure is increased, including anxiety or other high cardiac output states (Chap. 24), as well as in bradycardia, and peripheral arteriosclerosis with loss of arterial distensibility. In patients with *mitral regurgitation* or *ventricular septal defect*, the forward stroke volume (from the left ventricle into the aorta) is usually normal, but the fraction ejected during early systole is greater than normal; hence, the arterial pulse is of normal volume (the pulse pressure is normal), but the pulse may rise abnormally rapidly.[35] Exaggerated or bounding arterial pulses may be observed in patients with an elevated stroke volume, with sympathetic hyperactivity, and in patients with a rigid, sclerotic aorta. In *aortic regurgitation*,[31] there is a very brisk rate of rise with an increased pulse pressure (Fig. 3–24, p. 57). The *Corrigan or waterhammer pulse* of aortic regurgitation consists of an abrupt upstroke (percussion wave) followed by rapid collapse later in systole, but no dicrotic notch. Corrigan's pulse reflects a low resistance in the reservoir into which the left ventricle rapidly discharges an abnormally elevated stroke volume, and it can be exaggerated by raising the patient's arm. In *acute* aortic regurgitation, the left ventricle may not be greatly dilated, and premature closure of the mitral valve may occur and limit the volume of aortic reflux;[36] therefore, the aortic diastolic pressure may *not* be very low, the arterial pulse *not* bounding, and the pulse pressure *not* widened despite a serious abnormality of valve

function (p. 1109). "Pistol-shot" sounds heard over the femoral artery when the stethoscope is placed on it (*Traube's sign*), a systolic murmur heard over the femoral artery when it is gradually compressed proximally and a diastolic murmur when the artery is compressed distally (*Duroziez's sign*[31,37]) and Quincke's sign (p. 1110) are also characteristic of severe, chronic aortic regurgitation; of these, Duroziez's sign is the most predictive. Bounding arterial pulses are also present in patients with patent ductus arteriosus or large arteriovenous fistulas; in hyperkinetic states such as thyrotoxicosis, pregnancy, fever, and anemia; in severe bradycardia; and in vessels proximal to a coarctation of the aorta.

In the presence of atrioventricular dissociation, when atrial activity is irregularly transmitted to the ventricles, the strength of the peripheral arterial pulse depends on the time interval between atrial and ventricular contractions. In a patient with rapid heart action, the presence of such variations is suggestive of ventricular tachycardia; with an equally rapid rate, an absence of variation of pulse strength suggests a supraventricular mechanism.

BISFERIENS PULSE. A bisferiens pulse is characterized by two systolic peaks, the percussion and tidal waves, separated by a distinct midsystolic dip; the peaks may be equal or either may be larger. This type of pulse may be detected most readily by palpation of the carotid and less commonly of the radial arteries. It occurs in conditions in which a large stroke volume is ejected rapidly from the left ventricle[38] and is observed most commonly in patients with pure aortic regurgitation (Fig. 3–24, p. 57) and with a combination of aortic regurgitation and stenosis; it may disappear as heart failure supervenes.

A bisferiens pulse is also noted in patients with *hypertrophic obstructive cardiomyopathy*[39] (Figs. 3–23, p. 56, and 4–9, p. 73), but the bifid nature may only be recorded, not palpated; on palpation there may merely be a rapid upstroke. In these patients the initial prominent percussion wave is associated with rapid ejection of blood into the aorta during early systole, followed by a rapid decline as obstruction becomes manifest in midsystole and by a tidal (reflected) wave. The bisferiens pulse of hypertrophic obstructive cardiomyopathy must be distinguished from the anacrotic pulse palpable in some patients with pure aortic stenosis; in both groups of patients with obstruction to left ventricular outflow a double pulse may be palpable. However, in patients with fixed obstruction the pulse rises slowly and the tidal wave is the higher of the two, while in hypertrophic obstructive cardiomyopathy, the pulse rises rapidly and the percussion wave is dominant. In some patients with hypertrophic cardiomyopathy with no or little obstruction to left ventricular outflow, the arterial pulse is normal in the basal state, but obstruction and a bisferiens pulse can be elicited by means of the Valsalva maneuver or inhalation of amyl nitrite. Occasionally, a bisferiens pulse is observed in hyperkinetic circulatory states, and very rarely it occurs in normal individuals.

DICROTIC PULSE. Not to be confused with a bisferiens pulse, in which both peaks occur in systole, is a dicrotic pulse, in which the normally small wave that follows aortic valve closure (i.e., the dicrotic notch) is exaggerated and measures more than 50 per cent of the pulse pressure on direct pressure recordings and in which the dicrotic notch is low (i.e., near the diastolic pressure) (Fig.

3–25, p. 57). It may be present in normal hypotensive subjects with reduced peripheral resistance, as occurs in fever, and it may be elicited or exaggerated by inspiration or the inhalation of amyl nitrite. Rarely, a dicrotic pulse may be noted in healthy adolescents or young adults, but it usually occurs in conditions such as cardiac tamponade, severe heart failure, and hypovolemic shock, in which a low stroke volume is ejected into a soft elastic aorta. A dicrotic pulse is rarely present when systolic pressure exceeds 130 mm Hg.

PULSUS ALTERNANS. Mechanical alternans is a sign of severe depression of myocardial function (p. 1484). Although more readily recognized on sphygmomanometry, when the systolic pressure alternates by more than 20 mm Hg it can be detected by palpation of a peripheral (femoral or radial) pulse or by the recording of an indirect carotid pulse tracing (Fig. 3–26, p. 58). Palpation should be carried out with light pressure and with the patient's breath held in midexpiration to avoid the superimposition of respiratory variation on the amplitude of the pulse. Pulsus alternans is generally accompanied by alternation in the intensity of the Korotkoff sounds and occasionally by alternation in intensity of the heart sounds. Rarely, alternans is so marked that the weak beat is not perceived at all. Aortic regurgitation, systemic hypertension, and reducing venous return by head-tilting or nitroglycerin all exaggerate pulsus alternans and assist in its detection. Pulsus alternans, which is frequently precipitated by a premature ventricular contraction (Fig. 15–7, p. 499), is characterized by a regular rhythm and must be distinguished from pulsus bigeminus (see below), which is usually regularly irregular.

PULSUS BIGEMINUS. A bigeminal rhythm is caused by the occurrence of premature contractions, usually ventricular, occurring after every other beat and results in alternation of the strength of the pulse, which can be confused with pulsus alternans. However, in contrast to the latter, in which the rhythm is regular, in pulsus bigeminus the weak beat always follows the shorter interval. In normal persons or in patients with fixed obstruction to left ventricular outflow, the compensatory pause following a premature beat is followed by a stronger-than-normal pulse. However, in patients with hypertrophic obstructive cardiomyopathy, the postpremature ventricular contraction beat is weaker than normal because of increased obstruction to left ventricular outflow[40] (p. 1418).

PULSUS PARADOXUS. This is a reduction in the strength of the arterial pulse during inspiration or an exaggerated inspiratory fall in systolic pressure (more than 10 mm Hg during quiet breathing). When marked, i.e., an inspiratory reduction of pressure greater than 20 mm Hg, it can be detected simply by careful palpation of the radial or brachial arterial pulse. Milder degrees of a paradoxical pulse can be readily detected on sphygmomanometry: the cuff is inflated to suprasystolic levels and is deflated slowly at a rate of about 2 mm Hg per heart beat; the peak systolic pressure during expiration is noted. The cuff is then deflated even more slowly, and the pressure is again noted when Korotkoff sounds become audible throughout the respiratory cycle. Normally, the difference between the two pressures should not exceed 8 mm Hg during quiet respiration. (Pulsus alternans can also be detected by this maneuver by noting whether peak systolic pressure or the

intensity of the Korotkoff sounds alternates when respiration is held.)

Pulsus paradoxus represents an exaggeration of the normal decline in systolic arterial pressure with inspiration, which results from the reduced left ventricular stroke volume and the transmission of negative intrathoracic pressure to the aorta. It is a frequent finding in patients with cardiac tamponade (p. 1481), occurs less frequently (in about half) in patients with chronic constrictive pericarditis (p. 1489), and is also observed in patients with emphysema and bronchial asthma (who have wide respiratory swings of intrapleural pressure),[41] as well as in hypovolemic shock, pulmonary embolus, pregnancy, and extreme obesity. Aortic regurgitation tends to prevent the development of pulsus paradoxus despite the presence of cardiac tamponade. *Reversed* pulsus paradoxus (an inspiratory rise in arterial pressure) can occur in hypertrophic obstructive cardiomyopathy.[42]

EXAMINATION OF THE HEART

INSPECTION

The cardiac examination proper should commence with inspection of the chest, which can best be accomplished with the examiner standing at the foot of the bed or examining table. Respirations—their frequency, regularity, and depth—as well as the relative effort required during inspiration and expiration, should be noted (p. 496). Simultaneously, one should search for cutaneous abnormalities, such as spider nevi (seen in hepatic cirrhosis and Osler-Weber-Rendu disease). Dilation of veins on the anterior chest wall with caudal flow suggests obstruction of the superior vena cava, while cranial flow occurs in patients with obstruction of the inferior vena cava. Precordial prominence is most striking if cardiac enlargement developed before puberty, but it may also be present, although to a lesser extent, in patients in whom cardiomegaly developed in adult life, after the period of thoracic growth.[43,44]

A heavy muscular thorax, contrasting with less developed lower extremities, suggests coarctation of the aorta, in which visible collateral arteries may be present in the axillae and along the lateral chest wall. The upper portion of the thorax exhibits symmetrical bulging in children with stiff lungs in whom the inspiratory effort is increased. An emphysematous-appearing chest or anterior bulge in the area of the manubrium in a child suggests pulmonary hypertension. A "shield chest" is a broad chest in which the angle between the manubrium and the body of the sternum is greater than normal and is associated with widely separated nipples; it is frequently observed in Turner's and Noonan's syndromes. Careful note should be made of other deformities of the thoracic cage, such as *kyphoscoliosis*, which may be responsible for cor pulmonale (p. 1596); *ankylosing spondylitis*, sometimes associated with aortic regurgitation (p. 1656); and *pectus carinatum* (pigeon chest), which may be associated with Marfan syndrome but does not directly affect cardiovascular function.

Pectus excavatum, a condition in which the sternum is displaced posteriorly, is commonly observed in Marfan syndrome (p. 1665), homocystinuria, Ehlers-Danlos syndrome (p. 1668), Hunter-Hurler syndrome (p. 1670), and a small fraction of patients with mitral valve prolapse (p.

1091). This thoracic deformity rarely compresses the heart or elevates the systemic and pulmonary venous pressures, and the signs of heart disease are more often apparent rather than real. Displacement of the heart into the left thorax, prominence of the pulmonary artery, and a parasternal midsystolic murmur all may falsely suggest the presence of organic heart disease. It may be associated with palpitation, tachycardia, fatigue, mild dyspnea, and some impairment of cardiac function.[45,46] Lack of normal thoracic kyphosis, i.e., the *straight back* syndrome,[1] is often associated with expiratory splitting of the second heart sound, a parasternal midsystolic murmur, and enlargement of the pulmonary artery on x-ray; therefore, it may be confused with atrial septal defect.[47,48]

Cardiovascular pulsations should be looked for on the entire chest but specifically in the regions of the cardiac apex, the left parasternal region, and the third left and second right intercostal spaces. Prominent pulsations in these areas suggest enlargement of the left ventricle, right ventricle, pulmonary artery, and aorta, respectively. A thrusting apex exceeding 2 cm in diameter suggests left ventricular enlargements; systolic retraction of the apex may be visible in constrictive pericarditis. Normally, cardiac pulsations are not visible lateral to the midclavicular line; when present there, they signify cardiac enlargement unless there is thoracic deformity or congenital absence of the pericardium. Shaking of the entire precordium with each heart beat may occur in patients with severe valvular regurgitation, large left-to-right shunts, complete AV block, hypertrophic obstructive cardiomyopathy, and various hyperkinetic states. Aortic aneurysms may produce visible pulsations of one of the sternoclavicular joints of the right anterior thoracic wall.

PALPATION (Table 2–1)

Pulsations of the heart and great vessels that are transmitted to the chest wall are best appreciated when the examiner is positioned on the right side of a supine patient. In order to palpate the movements of the heart and great vessels, the examiner should utilize the fingertips or the area just proximal thereto. Precordial movements should be timed by using the simultaneously palpated carotid pulse or auscultated heart sounds.[49] The examination should be carried out with the trunk elevated to 30 degrees, both with the patient supine and in the partial left lateral decubitus positions; the latter increases the amplitude of the left ventricular impulse. Rotating the patient into the left lateral decubitus position causes the heart to move laterally and increases the palpability of both normal and pathological thrusts of the left ventricle. Indeed, it converts the normal systolic retraction of the apex to an outward expansion. Obese, muscular, and emphysematous persons may have weak or undetectable cardiac pulsations in the absence of cardiac abnormality, while thoracic deformities (e.g., kyphoscoliosis, pectus excavatum) can alter the pulsations transmitted to the chest wall. In the course of cardiac palpation, precordial tenderness may be detected; this important finding (p. 1338) may result from trauma, costochondritis, or Tzietse's syndrome and may be an important indication that chest pain is not due to myocardial ischemia.

THE LEFT VENTRICLE. The *apex beat*, also referred to as the cardiac impulse and the apical thrust, is usually produced by left ventricular contraction and is the lowest and most lateral point on the chest at which the cardiac impulse can be appreciated; normally it is medial

---

TABLE 2–1   CHARACTERISTICS OF PRECORDIAL MOTION IN VARIOUS CARDIAC ABNORMALITIES

AORTIC REGURGITATION	ATRIAL SEPTAL DEFECT	CONGESTIVE CARDIOMYOPATHY	CORONARY ARTERY DISEASE
Apex impulse hyperdynamic in mild to moderate AR Severe AR: LV dilatation results in sustained impulse which is displaced laterally and downward (especially chronic AR) Systolic retraction medial to PMI Palpable *a* wave may be present	Hyperdynamic parasternal impulse PA impulse may be present RV impulse may be sustained if pulmonary hypertension is present and occasionally with large L to R shunt without elevated PA pressure	Sustained and displaced LV impulse, usually felt over 2 interspaces Palpable *a* wave (S_4) and S_3 common Parasternal lift, midsystolic bulge common	Usually normal at rest unless prior MI Palpable S_4 in left decubitus position Ectopic LV bulge thrust if dyssynergy or LV aneurysm. May have transient abnormalities (e.g., bulge, heave) during acute infarction or attack of angina

HYPERTROPHIC CARDIOMYOPATHY	MITRAL REGURGITATION	MITRAL STENOSIS	VALVAR AORTIC STENOSIS
Systolic thrill superior, medial to apex impulse Vigorous LV apical impulse, often sustained Large palpable *a* wave, especially in left decubitus position Occasional mid- or late systolic bulge—"triple ripple"	Apical systolic thrill in severe MR Apex impulse hyperdynamic Severe and/or chronic MR: apex is displaced laterally, sustained with amplitude Can have late parasternal impulse with severe MR without pulmonary hypertension Parasternal (RV) heave if significant pulmonary hypertension S_3 visible and palpable if severe MR S_4 palpable with acute onset MR	Small or impalpable apex impulse but S_1 typically palpable Opening snap palpable medial to apex Apical diastolic thrill in left decubitus position Parasternal lift is common; suggests pulmonary hypertension at rest or with effort	Systolic thrill—aortic area, 2 LICS. Or occasionally at apex Sustained and forceful LV apical impulse Little lateral (leftward) displacement of apex unless LV dilatation has occurred Palpable *a* wave (S_4) is common and indicates severe aortic obstruction

AR = aortic regurgitation; LV = left ventricular; PA = pulmonary artery; RV = right ventricle; MI = myocardial infarction; MR = mitral regurgitation. (Reproduced with permission from Abrams, J.: Examination of the precordium: Primary Cardiol. *8*:156–158, 1982.)

and superior to the intersection of the left midclavicular line and the fifth intercostal space. Although displacement of the apex beat outside the midclavicular line is almost always associated with cardiac enlargement, thoracic deformities—particularly scoliosis, straight back, and pectus excavatum—can result in the lateral displacement of a normal-sized heart. Although the apex beat is also often the point of maximal impulse (PMI), this is not always the case, since the pulsations produced by other structures, e.g., an enlarged right ventricle, a dilated pulmonary artery, or an aneurysm of the aorta, may be more powerful than the apex beat.

The apex cardiogram (p. 58), which traces the movement of the chest wall, often represents the pulsation of the entire left ventricle, not only the movement of the apex itself. Therefore, its contour differs from what is perceived on palpation of the chest or what is recorded by the kinetocardiogram, a device in which the motion of specific points on the chest wall are recorded relative to a fixed point in space,[50] and which therefore presents a more faithful graphic registration of the movements of the palpating finger on the chest wall.

Systolic Motion. During isovolumetric contraction, the heart normally rotates counterclockwise (as one faces the patient), and the lower anterior portion of the left ventricle strikes the anterior chest wall, causing a brief outward motion followed by retraction of the left ventricle and the adjacent chest wall during ejection. The segment of the left ventricle responsible for the apex beat is usually medial to the actual cardiac apex, identified on radiological or angiographic examination. For timing purposes it is useful to correlate pulsations while simultaneously listening to heart sounds; a convenient way to do this is to correlate the observed motion of the stethoscope, placed at the apex, with the auscultatory events.

The peak outward motion of the apex impulse is brief and occurs simultaneously with, or just after, aortic valve opening; then the left ventricular apex moves inward. In asthenic persons, in patients with mild left ventricular enlargement, and in subjects with a normal left ventricle but an augmented stroke volume, as occurs in anxiety and other hyperkinetic states, the cardiac impulse may be overactive; i.e., the outward thrust during systole is exaggerated in amplitude, but it is not sustained during ejection. With moderate or severe left ventricular enlargement, the outward systolic thrust persists throughout ejection, often lasting up to the second heart sound (Figs. 2–6 and 2–7), and this motion may be accompanied by retraction of the left parasternal region. This rocking motion can often be appreciated by placing the index finger of one hand on the apex beat and that of the other hand in the parasternal region and by observing the simultaneous outward motion of the former with retraction of the latter. The left ventricular heave or lift, which is more prominent in left ventricular dilatation than in concentric hypertrophy, is characterized by a sustained outward movement of an area that is larger than the normal apex, i.e., more than 2 cm by 2 cm. An *aneurysm of the left ventricle* also produces a larger-than-normal area of pulsation of the left ventricular apex. Alternatively, it may produce a sustained systolic bulge several centimeters superior to the left ventricular impulse. In patients with *left ventricular dyskinesia*, as occurs in acute myocardial ischemia or following myocardial infarction, there may be two distinct impulses separated from each

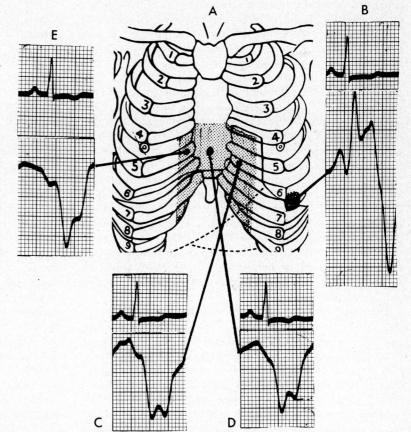

FIGURE 2–6 A large area of systolic retraction is indicated on the chest wall diagram (*A*) by light shading. Graphs taken from three points of this area (*C, D,* and *E*) show a sweeping downward movement during systole as evidence of retraction. The apex beat, felt in the 6th intercostal space, is indicated by an area of heavy shading. A graph of the apical thrust (*B*) shows a sustained upward movement, indicative of a left ventricular overload. The patient was a 40-year-old man with marked rheumatic aortic regurgitation. (From Dressler, W.: Clinical Aids in Cardiac Diagnosis. New York, 1970, p. 83, by permission of Grune and Stratton.)

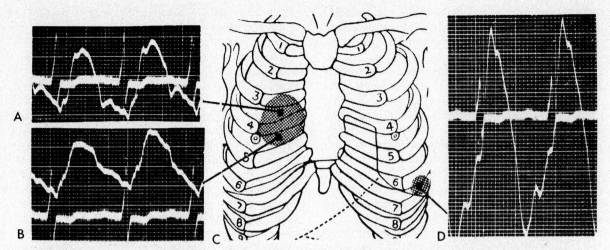

FIGURE 2–7   Diagram of the anterior wall (C) showing two areas of heaving pulsation (indicated by heavy shading). The area on the left side of the chest represents the apical thrust of a hypertrophied ventricle, as is shown on a graph (D). The curve rises 0.05 sec after onset of QRS and forms a broad, high peak during systole. Another area of systolic outward movement is present on the right side of the chest. Two recordings taken from this area (A and B) show curves that differ distinctly from that of the apical thrust. They rise 0.12 sec after QRS and resemble an arterial pulse. The pulsation on the right half of the chest was caused by a dissecting aneurysm of the ascending aorta. (From Dressler, W.: Clinical Aids in Cardiac Diagnosis. New York, 1970, p. 91, by permission of Grune and Stratton.)

other by several centimeters. In *mitral stenosis* there may be a brief prominent apical tap owing to an accentuated first sound, which must be distinguished from the apical thrust of an enlarged left ventricle.

A double systolic outward thrust of the left ventricle is occasionally present in patients with prolapse of the mitral valve (Fig. 3–31, p. 61) and is characteristic of patients with hypertrophic obstructive cardiomyopathy (Fig. 3–30, p. 60) who also often exhibit a typical presystolic cardiac expansion, resulting in three separate outward movements of the chest wall during each cardiac cycle.[39] In *aortic regurgitation* the apex exhibits a prominent outward thrust, but this may be followed by systolic retraction of the anterior chest wall as a consequence of the large stroke volume that evacuates the thorax during systole (Fig. 2–6). *Constrictive pericarditis* (as well as nonconstricting adherent pericarditis) is characterized by systolic retraction of the chest, particularly of the ribs in the left axilla (Broadbent's sign) (Figs. 2–8 and 3–33, p. 62). This inward movement results from interference with the descent of the base of the heart and the compensatory exaggerated motion of the free wall of the left ventricle during ventricular ejection.[51] When left ventricular filling is very rapid during early diastole, as occurs in patients with severe mitral regurgitation, outward movement of the chest wall may be particularly prominent, usually accompanied by a third heart sound (Fig. 3–28, p. 59). A hypokinetic apical impulse is associated with a variety of low cardiac output states, including those secondary to hypovolemia, constrictive pericarditis, and pericardial effusion.

Diastolic Motion. The outward motion of the apex characteristic of rapid left ventricular diastolic filling is accentuated when the inflow of blood into the left ventricle is accelerated, as occurs, for example, in mitral regurgitation or when the left ventricular ejection fraction is reduced. This motion is the mechanical equivalent of and occurs simultaneously with a third heart sound.

When the atrial contribution to ventricular filling is augmented, as occurs in patients with concentric left ventricular hypertrophy, myocardial ischemia, and myocardial fibrosis, a presystolic pulsation (usually accompanying a fourth heart sound) is palpable, resulting in a double outward movement of the left ventricular impulse (Fig. 3–29, p. 60, and 4–4, p. 70). This presystolic expansion is most readily discernible during expiration, when the patient is in the left lateral decubitus position, and it can be confirmed by detecting the motion of the stethoscope placed over the left ventricular impulse or by observing the motion of the tip of a pencil or tongue depressor when the proximal portion is placed near the left ventricular impulse. It can be enhanced by sustained hand grip. Presystolic expansion of the right ventricle occurs in right ventricular hypertrophy and pulmonary hypertension. It may be appreciated by subxiphoid palpation of the right ventricle during inspiration.

The Right Ventricle. A palpable anterior systolic movement (replacing systolic retraction) in the left parasternal region (Fig. 2–9A) usually represents *right ventricular enlargement*, which, in the absence of associated left ventricular enlargement, may be accompanied by reciprocal systolic retraction of the apex. Exaggerated motion of the entire parasternal area usually reflects increased right ventricular recoil due to augmented stroke volume, as occurs in patients with atrial septal defect, while a sustained left parasternal outward thrust reflects right ventricular hypertrophy due to pressure overload, as occurs in pulmonic stenosis. With marked right ventricular enlargement, this chamber occupies the apex and the left ventricle is displaced posteriorly. When both ventricles are enlarged, both the left parasternal and the apical areas may rise with systole, but an area of systolic retraction between them can sometimes be appreciated. In patients with emphysema, an enlarged right ventricle is sometimes detected most readily in the subxiphoid region by palpating the epigastrium and pointing the finger upward (Fig. 2–9B). With marked isolated right ventricular enlargement, the heart may rotate in a clockwise manner, and the right ventricle may form the cardiac apex, producing findings that may

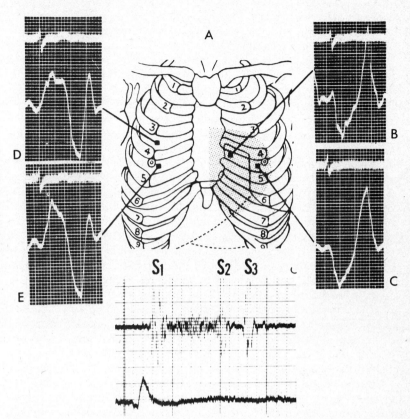

FIGURE 2–8 The chest diagram (*A*) shows an extensive area of systolic retraction on the left side (indicated by light shading). Graphs *B* and *C* were taken from two points of the pulsating area. During systole, both curves move briskly downward and then rise to a sharp peak in early diastole (rebound). Graphs *D* and *E*, taken from two points in the right midclavicular line, show pulsations of opposite direction. The curves move upward during systole and sharply downward during early diastole. The phonocardiogram (*bottom*) shows a holosystolic murmur and a third heart sound "pericardial knock." The tracings are from a 56-year-old woman who suffered from constrictive pericarditis confirmed on postmortem examination. (From Dressler, W.: Clinical Aids in Cardiac Diagnosis. New York, 1970, p. 87, by permission of Grune and Stratton.)

be confused with those of left or biventricular enlargement. When acute myocardial ischemia or myocardial infarction causes dyskinetic movement of the ventricular septum, there may be a transient left parasternal impulse not caused by right ventricular enlargement.

Pulmonary hypertension and/or increased pulmonary blood flow frequently produces a prominent systolic pulsation of the pulmonary artery in the second intercostal space just to the left of the sternum. This pulsation is often associated with a prominent left parasternal impulse,

FIGURE 2–9 *A*, Palpation of the anterior wall of the right ventricle by applying the tips of three fingers in the third, fourth, and fifth interspaces, left sternal edge, during full held exhalation. Patient is supine with the trunk elevated 30 degrees. *B*, Palpation of the inferior wall of the right ventricle in the epigastrium. The flat of the hand is directed upward and toward the left shoulder. The tip of the index finger (arrow) palpates the right ventricle as it descends during full held inspiration. The patient is supine with trunk elevated 30 degrees. *C*, The stethoscope is applied to the cardiac apex while the patient lies in a partial left lateral decubitus position. The examiner's free left hand is used to palpate the carotid artery for timing purposes. *D*, The soft-high frequency early diastolic murmur of either aortic regurgitation or pulmonary hypertensive pulmonary regurgitation is best elicited by applying the stethoscopic diaphragm very firmly to the mid-left sternal edge. The patient leans forward with breath held in full exhalation. (Reproduced with permission from Perloff, J. K. (Ed.): Physical Examination of the Heart and Circulation. Philadelphia, W. B. Saunders Co., 1982.)

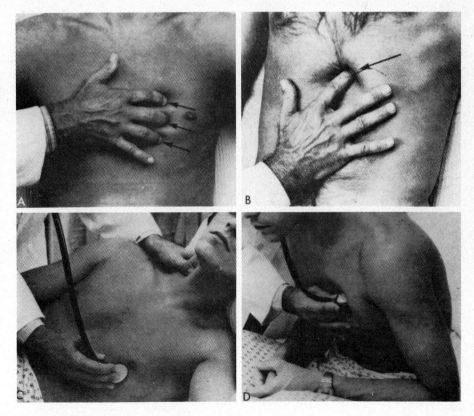

reflecting right ventricular enlargement, and a palpable shock synchronous with the second heart sound, reflecting forceful closure of the pulmonic valve.

Left Atrium. An enlarged left atrium or a large posterior left ventricular aneurysm can make right ventricular pulsations more prominent by displacing the right ventricle anteriorly against the left parasternal area, and in severe mitral regurgitation an expanding left atrium may be responsible for marked left parasternal movement, even in the absence of right ventricular hypertrophy. The left atrial lift, which is transmitted through the right ventricle, commences and terminates after the left ventricular thrust. It can be appreciated by placing the finger of one hand at the left ventricular apex and the finger of the other in the left parasternal region; the movement of the latter finger begins and ends slightly later than that of the former. While this difference in timing may be difficult to appreciate on palpation, particularly when the heart rate is rapid, recordings of chest wall motion in severe chronic mitral regurgitation demonstrate a delayed fall in the left lower precordium compared to the cardiac apex (Fig. 4–16, p. 77). Outward movement of the chest wall that is more marked to the right than to the left of the sternum is usually due to aneurysm of the aorta (Fig. 2–8) or to marked enlargement of the right atrium.

Palpable Sounds. Valve closure, if abnormally forceful, can be appreciated as a tapping sensation. It occurs most prominently in the third left intercostal space in patients with pulmonary hypertension (pulmonic valve closure), in the second right intercostal space in patients with systemic hypertension (aortic valve closure), and at the cardiac apex in patients with mitral stenosis (mitral valve closure). Occasionally, in congenital aortic stenosis, aortic ejection sounds can be palpated at the cardiac apex; ejection sounds originating in a dilated aorta or pulmonary artery can sometimes be felt at the base of the heart.

Thrills. The flat of the hand or the fingertips usually best appreciate thrills, which are palpable manifestations of loud, harsh murmurs with low-frequency components.[52] Since the vibrations must be quite intense before they are felt, far more information can be obtained from the auscultatory than from the palpatory features of heart murmurs. High-pitched murmurs such as those produced by valvular regurgitation, even when loud, are not usually associated with thrills.

PERCUSSION. Palpation is far more helpful than is percussion in determining cardiac size. However, in the absence of an apical beat, as occurs in patients with pericardial effusion, or in some patients with congestive cardiomyopathy, heart failure, and marked displacement of a hypokinetic apical beat, the left border of the heart can be outlined by means of percussion. Also, percussion of dullness in the right lower parasternal area may, in some instances, aid in the detection of a greatly enlarged right atrium. Percussion is of aid in determining visceral situs, i.e., in ascertaining the side on which the heart, stomach, and liver are located. When the heart is in the right chest, but the abdominal viscera are located normally, congenital heart disease is usually present. When both the heart and abdominal viscera are in the opposite side of the chest (situs inversus), congenital heart disease is uncommon.

Cardiac Auscultation

GENERAL PRINCIPLES. Vibrations on the surface of the chest set into motion a column of air that is collected and conducted to the ear by the stethoscope.[53–55] Since high frequencies are damped by a large volume of air between the chest and the ear, the most effective stethoscopes are made of plastic tubing 10 to 12 inches in length with an internal diameter of ⅛ inch; the thicker the tubing, the more room noise is eliminated. The stethoscope should have two chest pieces; a shallow bell and a stiff diaphragm. Since their ability to collect sound is proportional to their diameter, they should be as large as is practical. A small bell and diaphragm are desirable for examining children and thin patients. The ear pieces should be large and comfortable, with their axes parallel to the long axes of the external auditory canals.

High-frequency sounds, such as the first and second heart sounds, and systolic clicks and high-pitched murmurs, such as those of valvular regurgitation, are best appreciated by using the diaphragm, which has a relatively high natural frequency and damps out low frequencies, and by applying firm pressure to the stethoscope. In order to detect low frequencies, the bell of the stethoscope should be applied to the chest with slight pressure, just enough to prevent detection of room noise. When the bell is applied too tightly, the skin under the bell forms a diaphragm, defeating the purpose of the bell by damping out low-frequency sounds. Third and fourth heart sounds and diastolic murmurs originating from the mitral and tricuspid valves are best heard through the bell.

Cardiac auscultation should be carried out in a quiet room with the patient comfortable and the chest exposed.[56,57] Ordinarily the examiner should be on the patient's right side, and the patient should be examined routinely in three positions; supine, sitting, and left lateral decubitus (Figs. 2–9C and D). Occasionally, the effects of squatting, standing, or the prone position (p. 37) and other physiological and pharmacological interventions are studied (pp. 35 and 38). Although the principal areas of cardiac auscultation are the second right interspace ("aortic" area), the second left interspace ("pulmonic" area), the fourth interspace adjacent to the left sternal border ("tricuspid" area), and the cardiac apex ("mitral" area), auscultation should not be limited to these sites, since important findings are sometimes present in other locations, such as the right parasternal region, axilla, neck, and interscapular regions. For example, auscultation just above the sternoclavicular joints is best for detecting a venous hum. Murmurs produced by pulmonary arteriovenous fistula, bronchial collateral vessels, and systemic arterial collaterals in patients with coarctation of the aorta as well as murmurs of pulmonary branch stenosis may be heard over the posterior chest. In some patients with pulmonary emphysema, heart sounds are best heard in the epigastrium. Levine and Harvey have recommended the technique of first listening at the apex, where the first heart sound is normally the loudest sound audible and can usually be readily identified, and then "inching up" the chest along the left sternal border, using the diaphragm and bell alternately.[57] Auscultation should be carried out during normal quiet respiration, during held

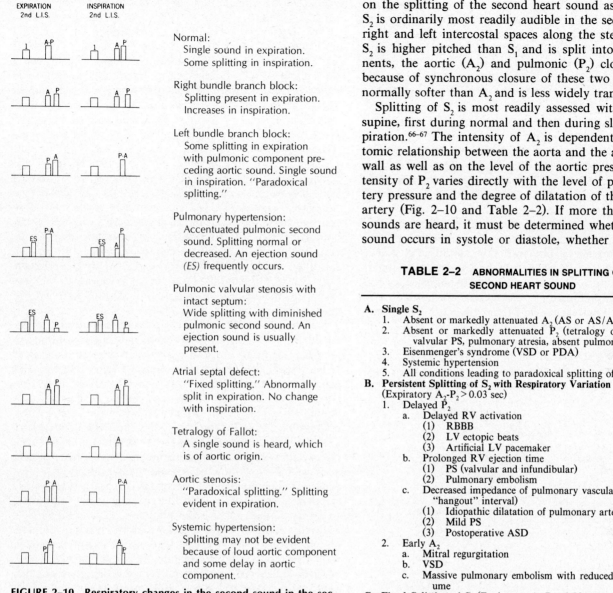

EXPIRATION 2nd L.I.S.	INSPIRATION 2nd L.I.S.	

Normal:
Single sound in expiration.
Some splitting in inspiration.

Right bundle branch block:
Splitting present in expiration.
Increases in inspiration.

Left bundle branch block:
Some splitting in expiration with pulmonic component preceding aortic sound. Single sound in inspiration. "Paradoxical splitting."

Pulmonary hypertension:
Accentuated pulmonic second sound. Splitting normal or decreased. An ejection sound (ES) frequently occurs.

Pulmonic valvular stenosis with intact septum:
Wide splitting with diminished pulmonic second sound. An ejection sound is usually present.

Atrial septal defect:
"Fixed splitting." Abnormally split in expiration. No change with inspiration.

Tetralogy of Fallot:
A single sound is heard, which is of aortic origin.

Aortic stenosis:
"Paradoxical splitting." Splitting evident in expiration.

Systemic hypertension:
Splitting may not be evident because of loud aortic component and some delay in aortic component.

FIGURE 2–10 Respiratory changes in the second sound in the second left intercostal space (2nd L.I.S.) in a variety of conditions. A = aortic second sound; P = pulmonic second sound; ES = early ejection sound. (From Ravin, A., et al.: Auscultation of the Heart. Chicago, Year Book Medical Publishers, 1977, p. 49.)

on the splitting of the second heart sound ascertained.[55–65] S_2 is ordinarily most readily audible in the second or third right and left intercostal spaces along the sternal borders. S_2 is higher pitched than S_1 and is split into two components, the aortic (A_2) and pulmonic (P_2) closure sounds, because of synchronous closure of these two valves.[61] P_2 is normally softer than A_2 and is less widely transmitted.

Splitting of S_2 is most readily assessed with the patient supine, first during normal and then during slow, deep respiration.[66–67] The intensity of A_2 is dependent on the anatomic relationship between the aorta and the anterior chest wall as well as on the level of the aortic pressure. The intensity of P_2 varies directly with the level of pulmonary artery pressure and the degree of dilatation of the pulmonary artery (Fig. 2–10 and Table 2–2). If more than two heart sounds are heard, it must be determined whether the extra sound occurs in systole or diastole, whether it is early or

TABLE 2–2 ABNORMALITIES IN SPLITTING OF THE SECOND HEART SOUND

A. **Single S_2**
 1. Absent or markedly attenuated A_2 (AS or AS/AR)
 2. Absent or markedly attenuated P_2 (tetralogy of Fallot, severe valvular PS, pulmonary atresia, absent pulmonic valve, TA)
 3. Eisenmenger's syndrome (VSD or PDA)
 4. Systemic hypertension
 5. All conditions leading to paradoxical splitting of S_2
B. **Persistent Splitting of S_2 with Respiratory Variation** (Expiratory A_2-$P_2 > 0.03$ sec)
 1. Delayed P_2
 a. Delayed RV activation
 (1) RBBB
 (2) LV ectopic beats
 (3) Artificial LV pacemaker
 b. Prolonged RV ejection time
 (1) PS (valvular and infundibular)
 (2) Pulmonary embolism
 c. Decreased impedance of pulmonary vascular bed (increased "hangout" interval)
 (1) Idiopathic dilatation of pulmonary artery
 (2) Mild PS
 (3) Postoperative ASD
 2. Early A_2
 a. Mitral regurgitation
 b. VSD
 c. Massive pulmonary embolism with reduced LV stroke volume
C. **Fixed Splitting of S_2** (Expiratory A_2-$P_2 > 0.03$ sec; respiratory variation < 0.015 sec)
 1. Inflow into RV constant throughout respiratory cycle (ASD)
 2. Inability of RV to augment stroke volume (severe PS, valvular or infundibular; other causes of RV dysfunction)
D. **Paradoxical Splitting of S_2**
 1. Delayed A_2
 a. Delayed LV activation and contraction (LBBB; RV ectopic beats and artificial pacemaker in RV)
 b. Prolonged LV mechanical systole
 (1) LV outflow obstruction (AS or HOCM)
 (2) Coronary artery disease
 (a) Angina
 (b) Acute myocardial infarction
 (3) Increased LV stroke volume (PDA, AR)
 c. Decreased impedance of systemic vascular bed (increased "hangout" interval)
 (1) Valvular AS; chronic AR; PDA
 2. Early P_2
 a. Early electrical activation and contraction of the RV (Wolff-Parkinson-White syndrome, Type B)

A_2 = aortic valve closure sound; AR = aortic regurgitation; AS = aortic stenosis; ASD = atrial septal defect; HOCM = hypertrophic obstructive cardiomyopathy; LBBB = left bundle branch block; LV = left ventricle; P_2 = pulmonic valve closure sound; PDA = patent ductus arteriosus; PS = pulmonic stenosis; RBBB = right bundle branch block; RV = right ventricle; S_2 = second heart sound; TA = tricuspid atresia; VSD = ventricular septal defect.

normal expiration, and during forced expiration. The effects of variations in respiration and posture on auscultatory findings should be determined.

It is desirable to employ a systematic plan for cardiac auscultation, listening in sequence to the first heart sound (S_1), the second heart sound (S_2), the systolic interval, and then the diastolic interval. An attempt should be made to listen to each component separately.

HEART SOUNDS. S_1 occurs just before the palpable arterial upstroke in the carotid pulse, while S_2 occurs immediately after the peak of the carotid pulse. It is often heard best medial to the apex at the lower sternal border. Splitting of S_1 with a tricuspid component is best heard at the lower left sternal border and it is best detected in inspiration. The intensity, quality, and splitting of each of the sounds should be determined and the effects of respiration late, and whether it is high-pitched (such as a systolic click) or low-pitched (such as a third or fourth heart sound, i.e., S_3 or S_4) (Fig. 2–11). When two heart sounds are heard at the time of S_1, it is often difficult to differentiate between a split S_1, a combination of S_4 and S_1, and a combination of S_1 and an ejection click.[64] The S_4 is usually audible only at the apex and often in the left lateral decubitus position; it is usually low-pitched, associated with palpable presystolic distention of the left ventricle, and attenuated by increased pressure on the bell of the stethoscope. It is rarely heard at the lower left sternal border, where splitting of S_1 is most easily detected. The ejection click is usually louder than the second component of a split S_1 and is often audible at the base of the heart, while splitting of S_1 is rarely heard in this area.

Ejection sounds, which coincide with the full opening of the semilunar valves, are high-pitched and clicking and are heard best with the diaphragm of the stethoscope. Aortic ejection sounds are heard best in the second right interspace and at the apex and are not notably affected by respiration, while pulmonic ejection sounds are heard best in the second left interspace and often diminish in intensity during inspiration. Mid- to late systolic clicks are heard in mitral valve prolapse (p. 1091), are of high frequency, and are also heard best with the diaphragm.

Diastolic Sounds.   Opening snaps (of the mitral or tri-

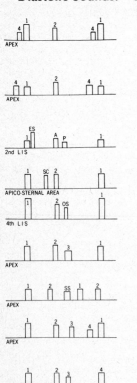

Left-sided fourth heart sound. Louder in expiration. Systemic hypertension, coronary artery disease, myocardiopathy, aortic stenosis.

Left-sided fourth heart sound with prolonged AV conduction. Faint first heart sound.

Pulmonic ejection sound (ES) in mild pulmonary valvular stenosis. Louder in expiration. Delayed pulmonic second heart sound.

Systolic click (SC).

Opening snap (OS) of the mitral valve in mitral stenosis.

Left-sided third heart sound (ventricular filling sound). Left ventricular failure. Mitral regurgitation.

Summation sound (SS) with ventricular failure plus rapid heart rate.

Fourth and third heart sound (quadruple rhythm).

Constrictive pericarditis. Third heart sound occupies a position between an opening snap and the usual third heart sound.

Right-sided fourth heart sound. Louder in inspiration. Pulmonary hypertension, large left-to-right shunt at atrial level.

FIGURE 2–11   Interpretation of extra sounds. 1, 2, 3, and 4 refer to the first, second, third, and fourth sounds. A and P refer to the aortic and pulmonic valve closure sounds, respectively. LIS = left intercostal space; LSB = left sternal border. (From Ravin, A., et al.: Auscultation of the Heart. Chicago, Year Book Medical Publishers, 1977, p. 80.)

cuspid valve) indicate that the valve is mobile. These high-pitched sounds are heard best through the diaphragm.

The diastolic sound during passive filling which occurs during the y descent of the atrial pressure pulse is termed the third heart sound (S_3), while the sound which occurs during ventricular filling caused by atrial contraction is called the fourth heart sound (S_4).[68] When S_3 and S_4 are abnormal, they are referred to as third or fourth heart sound "gallops." S_3 may be normal in children and young adults but when heard in men over the age of 40 years and women over the age of 50 years, they are generally abnormal. Healthy adults may have an S_4, but when heard in the young, this sound is usually abnormal. Since S_3 and S_4 (whether normal or not) are produced by rapid ventricular filling, they are absent in the presence of mitral or tricuspid stenosis. Third and fourth heart sounds are best heard with the bell of the stethoscope, are intensified by the recumbent position and by exercise, such as a few sit-ups, or sustained hand-grip. Inspiration enhances third or fourth heart sounds originating from the right ventricle, but has little detectable effect on such sounds originating from the left ventricle.

S_3 occurs as active ventricular relaxation (reflected in the decline in ventricular pressure) ends and passive filling (reflected in a diastolic rise in ventricular pressure) begins.[67a] It is intensified by rapid early diastolic filling, an elevated atrial pressure, and increased or abnormal diastolic distensibility of the ventricle. Conditions causing ventricular diastolic overload with atrial hypertension are often responsible for an S_3 which is audible in states of increased cardiac output, such as during the third trimester of pregnancy, after exertion, or in anxiety-related tachycardia. It also occurs with impaired left ventricular function of any cause. In the presence of coronary artery disease, an S_3 strongly suggests left ventricular dyskinesia or aneurysm. In patients with aortic regurgitation it usually signifies a reduced ejection fraction and elevated end-systolic volume[69] and in patients with reduced cardiac reserve it correlates well with the response to digitalis.[70]

An S_4 is generally associated with an elevated ventricular end-diastolic pressure and a high ratio of left ventricular wall thickness–to–cavity diameter. As left ventricular distensibility decreases, atrial systole becomes responsible for more than 25 per cent of ventricular filling, and an S_4 may become prominent. Vigorous atrial contraction is necessary to produce an audible S_4, which can be recorded phonocardiographically in about 50 per cent of normal adults, but it is extremely low in intensity and usually not audible. However, a loud, palpable S_4 is almost always abnormal. The common denominators are left ventricular hypertrophy, increased left ventricular end-diastolic pressure, and some restriction to diastolic filling. An S_4 is characteristic of aortic stenosis with a significant left ventricular–aortic pressure gradient, hypertrophic cardiomyopathy, and acute mitral regurgitation. Reduced left ventricular compliance following myocardial infarction often results in an audible S_4. A right ventricular S_4 is common in pulmonary hypertension and pulmonary stenosis.

MURMURS AND OTHER ADVENTITIOUS SOUNDS

Cardiac murmurs should be timed, and their length in the cardiac cycle and their shape, i.e., their intensity (or loudness) as a function of time, should be noted. The *intensity* of a murmur is determined by the quantity and velocity of blood flow across the sound-producing area, by its distance from the stethoscope, and by the transmission qualities of the tissue between the origin of the murmur and the stethoscope.[71] Murmurs are accentuated in thin persons and diminished in patients who are obese, in emphysema, and in the presence of pleural or pericardial fluid.[53] They are accentuated in hyperdynamic states and reduced in hypodynamic states. It is helpful to grade the intensity of murmurs; six grades, as described by Levine, are commonly distinguished.[72] A *Grade 1/6* murmur is the faintest that can be detected, often only after close concentration and adjustment of the stethoscope. A *Grade 2/6* murmur is a faint murmur but can be detected immediately. A *Grade 3/6* murmur is moderately loud, and a *Grade 4/6* murmur is loud. A *Grade 5/6* murmur is a very loud murmur but requires placement of the stethoscope on the chest to be audible. A *Grade 6/6* murmur is so loud that it can be heard even without placing the stethoscope on the chest. The *length* of a murmur depends upon the duration of the events, such as a pressure gradient responsible for it, while the *radiation* of a murmur is determined by its site of origin, its intensity, the direction of the blood flow responsible for the murmur, and the physical characteristics of the chest.[71] The *quality* of murmurs should be described using adjectives such as blowing, harsh, rumbling, musical, and high- or low-pitched. Murmurs with mixed high and medium frequencies sound harsh or rasping, while those with a narrow frequency range, often owing to vibration of an intracardiac structure such as a valve leaflet, are musical or honking in quality.

The interpretation of heart murmurs is based equally on their characteristics (timing, intensity, duration, location, quality, and pitch) and the accompanying auscultatory features, such as the character of the splitting of S_2 as well as the presence of ejection sounds and of S_3 and S_4. The etiology of various murmurs is presented in Table 2–3, and Figures 2–12 and 2–13 illustrate a variety of murmurs and sounds. A discussion of the most important heart murmurs is presented in Chapter 4.

Pericardial friction rubs are the sounds made by two inflamed layers of the pericardium sliding over one another, but they may be present even when there is considerable pericardial effusion. Friction rubs are generally described as scratching, grating, crunching, and creaking; they seem close to the ear and may vary in distribution from a site that is sharply localized to a small area of the precordium to the entire left hemithorax.[73,74] Usually they are most readily audible along the left sternal edge using the diaphragm with firm pressure and are often better heard during deep inspiration and with the patient leaning forward or in the prone position and propped up by the elbows.[75] The sounds are commonly "to and fro" and have either one or two diastolic components. In some patients, however, only a systolic component is audible. Friction rubs may be confused with the to-and-fro murmurs of combined aortic stenosis and regurgitation. Pleural-pericardial friction rubs are caused by the inflamed pleura against the parietal pericardium and are usually heard only during inspiration.

Acute mediastinal emphysema produces loud, bizarre, crunching sounds over the precordium, mainly during sys-

TABLE 2–3 PRINCIPAL CAUSES OF HEART MURMURS

A. Organic Systolic Murmurs
1. Midsystolic (Ejection)
   a. AORTIC
      (1) Obstructive
         (a) Supravalvular—supraaortic stenosis, coarctation of the aorta
         (b) Valvular—AS and sclerosis
         (c) Infravalvular—HOCM
      (2) Increased flow, hyperkinetic states, AR, complete heart block
      (3) Dilatation of ascending aorta, atheroma, aortitis, aneurysm of aorta
   b. PULMONARY
      (1) Obstructive
         (a) Supravalvular—pulmonary arterial stenosis
         (b) Valvular—pulmonic valve stenosis
         (c) Infravalvular—infundibular stenosis
      (2) Increased flow, hyperkinetic states, left-to-right shunt (e.g., ASD, VSD)
      (3) Dilatation of pulmonary artery
2. Pansystolic (Regurgitant)
   a. Atrioventricular valve regurgitation (MR, TR)
   b. Left-to-right shunt to ventricular level

B. Early Diastolic Murmurs
1. Aortic regurgitation (see also Table 32–11, p. 1106)
   a. Valvular: rheumatic deformity; perforation post-endocarditis, post-traumatic, post-valvulotomy
   b. Dilatation of valve ring: aortic dissection, annuloectasia, cystic medial necrosis, hypertension
   c. Widening of commissures: syphilis
   d. Congenital: bicuspid valve, with ventricular septal defect
2. Pulmonic regurgitation (see also p. 1122)
   a. Valvular: post-valvulotomy, endocarditis, rheumatic fever, carcinoid
   b. Dilatation of valve ring: pulmonary hypertension; Marfan's syndrome
   c. Congenital: isolated or associated with tetralogy of Fallot, VSD, pulmonic stenosis

C. Mid-diastolic Murmurs
1. Mitral stenosis
2. Carey-Coomb's murmur (mid-diastolic apical murmur in acute rheumatic fever)
3. Increased flow across nonstenotic mitral valve (e.g., MR, VSD, PDA, high-output states, and complete heart block)
4. Tricuspid stenosis
5. Increased flow across nonstenotic tricuspid valve (e.g., TR, ASD, and anomalous pulmonary venous return)
6. Left and right atrial tumors

D. Continuous Murmurs
1. Patent ductus arteriosus
2. Coronary AV fistula
3. Ruptured aneurysm of sinus of Valsalva
4. Aortic septal defect
5. Cervical venous hum
6. Anomalous left coronary artery
7. Proximal coronary artery stenosis
8. Mammary souffle
9. Pulmonary artery branch stenosis
10. Bronchial collateral circulation
11. Small (restrictive) ASD with MS
12. Intercostal AV fistula

AR = aortic regurgitation; AS = aortic stenosis; ASD = atrial septal defect; AV = arteriovenous; HOCM = hypertrophic obstructive cardiomyopathy; MR = mitral regurgitation; MS = mitral stenosis; PDA = patent ductus arteriosus; TR = tricuspid regurgitation; VSD = ventricular septal defect. (*A* and *C* modified from Oram, S. (ed.): Clinical Heart Disease. London, William Heinemann Medical Books, Ltd., 1981; *D* modified from Fowler, N. O. (ed.): Cardiac Diagnosis and Treatment. Hagerstown, Harper and Row, 1980.)

tole; these are audible most prominently near the apex and sometimes only with the patient in the left lateral recumbent position.[57] *Diaphragmatic flutter* produces regular sounds that are independent of the pulse and are audible over the entire thorax, even in the right axilla, far removed from the heart.[57]

A *cervical venous hum* is a continuous murmur heard best with the stethoscopic bell in the lateral portion of the

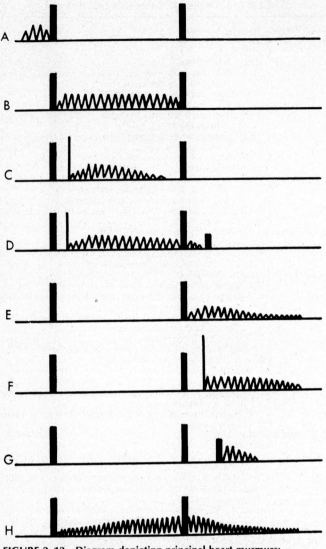

FIGURE 2-12   Diagram depicting principal heart murmurs:

  A, Presystolic murmur of mitral or tricuspid stenosis.

  B, Pansystolic murmur of mitral or tricuspid incompetence or of ventricular septal defect.

  C, Aortic ejection murmur beginning with an ejection click and fading before the second heart sound.

  D, Systolic murmur in pulmonic stenosis spilling through the aortic second sound, pulmonic valve closure being delayed.

  E, Aortic pulmonary diastolic murmur.

  F, Long diastolic murmur of mitral stenosis following the opening snap.

  G, Short mid-diastolic inflow murmur following a third heart sound.

  H, Continuous murmur of patent ductus arteriosus.

  (From Wood, P.: Diseases of the Heart and Circulation. Philadelphia, J. B. Lippincott Co., 1968, p. 75.)

right supraclavicular fossa with the patient sitting or standing and can be confused with the murmur produced by a patent ductus arteriosus.[76] It is due to the rapid downward flow of blood through a jugular vein that becomes artificially stenosed when the patient is in the upright position, and it disappears when the jugular vein is compressed or when the patient assumes the recumbent position. A venous hum can be intensified by tilting the chin upward and can be abolished by pressure over the upper part of the jugular vein. It is common in normal children and in conditions in which the circulation is hyperkinetic such as anemia, thyrotoxicosis, or pregnancy.

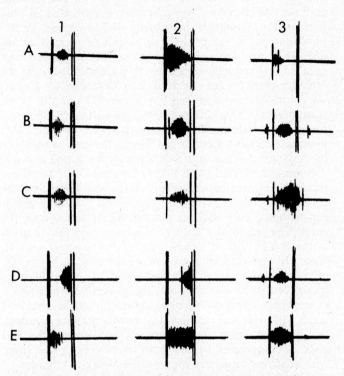

FIGURE 2-13   Sketches of various murmurs and heart sounds.

  A-1, Short, midsystolic murmur, with normal aortic and pulmonic components of S_2—findings consistent with an innocent murmur.

  A-2, Holosystolic murmur that decreases in the latter part of systole—a configuration observed in acute mitral regurgitation.

  A-3, An ejection sound and a short early systolic murmur, plus accentuated, closely split S_2—consistent with pulmonary hypertension, as with Eisenmenger's ventricular septal defect.

  B-1, Early to midsystolic murmur with vibratory component—typical of an innocent murmur.

  B-2, An ejection sound followed by a diamond-shaped murmur and wide splitting of S_2 that may be present with atrial septal defect or mild pulmonic stenosis; an ejection sound is more likely with valvular pulmonic stenosis.

  B-3, Crescendo-decrescendo systolic murmur, not holosystolic; S_3 and S_4 are present—findings consistent with mitral systolic murmur heard in congestive cardiomyopathy or coronary artery disease with papillary muscle dysfunction and cardiac decompensation.

  C-1, Longer, somewhat vibratory crescendo-decrescendo systolic murmur with wide splitting of S_2 sound. If S_2 becomes fused with expiration, atrial septal defect is less likely; if the remainder of the cardiovascular evaluation is normal, this finding is consistent with an innocent murmur.

  C-2, Midsystolic murmur and wide splitting of S_2 that was "fixed"—findings typical of atrial septal defect.

  C-3, Prolonged diamond-shaped systolic murmur masking A_2 with delayed P_2, S_4, and ejection sound—findings typical of valvular pulmonic stenosis of moderate severity.

  D-1, Late apical systolic murmur of prolapsing mitral valve leaflet.

  D-2, Systolic click–late apical systolic murmur of prolapsing mitral leaflet syndrome.

  D-3, S_4 and midsystolic murmur consistent with mitral systolic murmur of cardiomyopathy or ischemic heart disease.

  E-1, Early crescendo-decrescendo systolic murmur ending in midsystole consistent with innocent murmur and small ventricular septal defect.

  E-2 and *E-3*, Holosystolic murmurs consistent with mitral or tricuspid regurgitation and ventricular septal defect. (From Harvey, W. P.: Innocent vs. significant murmurs. Curr. Probl. Cardiol. Vol. 1, No. 8, 1976.)

A *mammary souffle* is a systolic or continuous murmur sometimes heard over the breasts of pregnant or lactating women[77] that can be confused with continuous murmurs produced by pulmonary arteriovenous fistula, patent ductus arteriosus, and other forms of congenital heart disease (Table 2–3D). It is presumably caused by the increased flow of blood through the engorged breast, generally commences just after the first heart sound, is best heard with the patient supine and may disappear in the upright position or with pressure from the stethoscope.

Cardiorespiratory murmurs are systolic (rarely continuous) murmurs heard on inspiration but not when the breath is held or during expiration, and they may result from the movement of air in the bronchial tree during systole and inspiration.[78]

DYNAMIC AUSCULTATION

This is the technique of altering circulatory dynamics by means of a variety of physiological and pharmacological maneuvers and determining their effects on heart sounds and murmurs.[79] As outlined in Figure 2–10 and Tables 2–4 and 2–5, an appreciation of the effects of these interventions can be of great value in the interpretation of a variety of auscultatory findings. The interventions most commonly employed in dynamic auscultation include respiration, postural changes, the Valsalva maneuver, premature ventricular contractions, isometric exercise, and vasoactive agents—amyl nitrite, methoxamine, and phenylephrine.

Respiration

SPLITTING OF S_2. The splitting of S_2 can usually be appreciated best along the left sternal border and is audible when A_2 and P_2 are separated by more than 0.02 sec. During inspiration A_2 ordinarily becomes softer in part because of the increased volume of lung that becomes interposed between the heart and chest wall; P_2 becomes louder because of increased flow into the pulmonary artery. A_2 normally occurs less than 0.02 sec after the pressure in the

left ventricle falls below that in the aorta, while P_2 occurs 0.03 to 0.09 sec after the decline of pressure in the right ventricle below that in the central pulmonary artery; these intervals have been termed the "hang-out" intervals, and their durations are inversely proportional to the impedance to blood flow in the aortic and pulmonic circuits.[80] The lower capacitance and higher resistance of the systemic compared to the pulmonary circulation result in a shorter hang-out interval in the aorta than in the pulmonary artery, and this difference contributes to the normal delay in P_2 compared to A_2 and therefore to the splitting of S_2. As the impedance to pulmonary flow increases with progressive pulmonary hypertension, the hang-out interval in the pulmonary artery shortens (Fig. 2–10D), and there is a reduction in the width of splitting of S_2, so that in severe pulmonary hypertension S_2 may become fused. Several factors play a role in the normal widening of the separation between A_2 and P_2 during inspiration.

During inspiration, venous return to the right side of the heart is augmented, resulting in a higher right ventricular stroke volume and lengthening of the duration of right ventricular ejection. When the respiratory rate is normal, these changes are accompanied by a reduced return of blood to the left side of the heart and a lower left ventricular stroke volume and shorter ejection time. In part, the difference in the effects of respiration on the stroke volumes of the two ventricles is due to the delay in transmission of the augmented right ventricular stroke volume through the pulmonary vascular bed, so that it reaches the left ventricle three or four cardiac cycles later, i.e., during the following expiration.[81] The greater delay in P_2, which accounts for about 75 per cent of the widening of the splitting,[59] results from the increased right ventricular stroke volume and ejection time and an inspiratory decline in pulmonary vascular impedance, with further prolongation of the hang-out interval. The pooling of blood in the lungs during inspiration, with decreased venous return to the left heart, is responsible for shortening of left ventricular systole; earlier occurrence of A_2 accounts for about 25 per cent of the inspiratory augmentation of the width of splitting of S_2.

In normal adults, A_2 and P_2 are separated by 0.04 to

TABLE 2–4 PHYSIOLOGICAL AND PHARMACOLOGICAL MANEUVERS USEFUL IN DIFFERENTIAL DIAGNOSIS OF SIMILAR AUSCULTATORY FINDINGS

AUSCULTATORY PROBLEMS	HELPFUL MANEUVERS*
Systolic murmur of valvular aortic stenosis vs. hypertrophic subaortic stenosis	Sudden squatting, Valsalva maneuver
Systolic murmur of valvular aortic stenosis vs. mid- to late systolic mitral valve dysfunction	Sudden standing, amyl nitrite
Systolic murmur of valvular aortic stenosis vs. mitral regurgitation	Amyl nitrite, phenylephrine, variation in cycle length
Diastolic rumble of mitral stenosis vs. Austin Flint murmur	Amyl nitrite
Diastolic murmur of mitral stenosis vs. tricuspid stenosis	Respiration
Systolic murmur of mitral regurgitation vs. tricuspid regurgitation	Respiration
Supraclavicular bruit vs. aortic stenosis	Extension of shoulder, compression of subclavian artery
Ejection sound in pulmonic stenosis vs. aortic stenosis	Respiration
Small ventricular septal defect vs. pulmonic stenosis	Amyl nitrite, phenylephrine
Large ventricular septal defect with fixed vs. hyperkinetic pulmonary hypertension	Amyl nitrite
Systolic murmur of pulmonic stenosis vs. tetralogy of Fallot	Amyl nitrite
Continuous murmur of patent ductus arteriosus vs. cervical venous hum	Compression of neck veins
Fourth sound plus first sound vs. separation of two components of first heart sound	Respiration, sudden standing, lying with passive leg-raising
Second sound plus opening snap vs. wide separation of second heart sound components	Respiration, phenylephrine, sudden standing

*See Table 2–5 for typical response. (From Criscitiello, M. G.: Physiologic and pharmacologic aids in cardiac auscultation. *In* Fowler, N. O. (ed.): Cardiac Diagnosis and Treatment. Hagerstown, Harper and Row, 1980, p. 89.)

TABLE 2–5   RESPONSE OF MURMURS AND HEART SOUNDS TO PHYSIOLOGICAL AND PHARMACOLOGICAL INTERVENTIONS

CLINICAL DISORDER	INTERVENTION AND RESPONSE
SYSTOLIC MURMURS	
Aortic outflow obstruction	
Valvular aortic stenosis	Louder with passive leg-raising, with sudden squatting, with Valsalva release (after five to six beats), following a pause induced by a premature beat, or after amyl nitrite; fades during Valsalva strain and with isometric handgrip
Hypertrophic obstructive cardiomyopathy	Louder with standing, during Valsalva strain, or with amyl nitrite; fades with sudden squatting, recumbency, or isometric handgrip
Pulmonic stenosis	Midsystolic murmur increases with amyl nitrite except with marked right ventricular hypertrophy; also increases during first few beats after Valsalva release
Mitral regurgitation	
Rheumatic	Murmur louder with sudden squatting, isometric handgrip, or phenylephrine; softens with amyl nitrite
Mitral valve prolapse	Midsystolic click moves toward S_1 and late systolic murmur starts earlier with standing, Valsalva strain, and amyl nitrite; click may occur earlier on inspiration; murmur starts later and click moves toward S_2 during squatting, with recumbency, and often after pause induced by a premature beat
Papillary muscle dysfunction	Late systolic murmur generally softer after a pause induced by a premature beat; response to amyl nitrite variable, depending on acute or chronic nature of this disorder
Tricuspid regurgitation	Murmur increases during inspiration, with passive leg-raising, and with amyl nitrite
Ventricular septal defect	
Small defect with pulmonary hypertension	Fades with amyl nitrite; increases with isometric handgrip or phenylephrine
Large defect with hyperkinetic pulmonary hypertension	Louder with amyl nitrite; fades with phenylephrine
Large defect with severe pulmonary vascular disease	Little change with any of above interventions
Tetralogy of Fallot	Murmur softens with amyl nitrite
Supraclavicular bruit	Altered by compression of subclavian artery; may be eliminated by extension of ipsilateral shoulder
DIASTOLIC MURMURS	
Aortic regurgitation	
Blowing diastolic murmur	Increases with sudden squatting, isometric handgrip, or phenylephrine
Austin Flint murmur	Fades with amyl nitrite
Pulmonary regurgitation	
Congenital	Early or mid-diastolic rumble increases on inspiration and with amyl nitrite
Pulmonary hypertension	High-frequency blowing murmur not altered by above interventions
Mitral stenosis	Mid-diastolic and presystolic murmurs louder with exercise, left lateral position, coughing, isometric handgrip, or amyl nitrite; phenylephrine widens A_2-OS interval; inspiration produces sequence of A_2-P_2-OS
Tricuspid stenosis	Mid-diastolic and presystolic murmurs increase during inspiration, with passive leg-raising, and with amyl nitrite
CONTINUOUS MURMURS	
Patent ductus arteriosus	Diastolic phase amplified with isometric handgrip or phenylephrine; diastolic phase fades with amyl nitrite
Cervical venous hum	Obliterated by direct compression of jugular veins or by Valsalva strain
ADDED HEART SOUNDS	
Gallop rhythm	
Ventricular gallop (S_3) and atrial gallop (S_4)	Accentuated by lying flat with passive leg-raising; decreased by standing or during Valsalva; right-sided gallop sounds usually increase during inspiration; left-sided during expiration.
Summation gallop	Separates into ventricular gallop (S_3) and atrial gallop (S_4) sounds when heart rate slowed by carotid sinus massage
Ejection sounds	Ejection sound in pulmonary stenosis fades and occurs closer to the first sound during inspiration

From Criscitiello, M. G.: Physiologic and pharmacologic aids in cardiac auscultation. *In* Fowler, N. O. (ed.): Cardiac Diagnosis and Treatment. Hagerstown, Harper and Row, 1980, p. 88).

0.05 sec during inspiration, with a single S_2 heard during expiration (split ≤ 0.02 sec). Occasionally there may be residual audible splitting in expiration (0.03 to 0.04 sec) in the supine position, but in normal adults auditory expiratory splitting disappears in the sitting or standing position. Expiratory splitting heard in both the supine and upright positions is uncommon in normal subjects of any age. Expiratory splitting of ≥ 0.03 sec, with an increase of ≤ 0.015 sec in the width of splitting, is considered to be "fixed" splitting.

There are four types of abnormal splitting of S_2: (1) Absent splitting (single S_2), (2) splitting that is persistent during expiration, (3) fixed splitting, and (4) paradoxical splitting. The major causes of each are presented in Table 2–2, and further discussion of this subject can be found on pp. 45–47.

S_3, S_4, AND EJECTION SOUNDS. When third and fourth sounds originate from the left ventricle, they are characteristically augmented during expiration and diminished during inspiration, whereas they exhibit the opposite response when they originate from the right side of the heart. Like other left-sided events, the opening snap of the mitral valve may become softer during inspiration and louder during expiration owing to respiratory alterations in venous return, whereas the opening snap of the tricuspid valve behaves in the opposite fashion. Inspiration also diminishes the intensity of valvular pulmonic ejection sounds, since the elevation of right ventricular diastolic pressure causes partial presystolic opening of the pulmonic valve and therefore less upward motion of the valve during systole. On the other hand, respiration does not affect the intensity of nonvalvular pulmonic ejection sounds or of aortic ejection sounds.

MURMURS. Respiration exerts more pronounced and consistent alterations on murmurs originating from the right than the left side of the heart. During inspiration, the diastolic murmurs of tricuspid stenosis and pulmonic regurgitation, the systolic murmurs of tricuspid regurgitation[82] and of mild or moderate pulmonic stenosis, and the pre-systolic murmur of Ebstein's anomaly are all accentuated. During expiration, the increased venous return to the left side of the heart may result in mild accentuation of the diastolic murmur of mitral stenosis and the systolic murmurs of mitral regurgitation, ventricular septal defect, and valvular aortic stenosis. The inspiratory reduction in left ventricular size in patients with mitral valve prolapse increases the redundancy of the mitral valve and therefore the degree of valvular prolapse; consequently, the midsystolic click and the systolic murmurs occur earlier during systole and frequently become accentuated[83] (p. 1092). The effects of inspiration on auscultatory findings may be accentuated by the use of the Müller maneuver, i.e., forced inspiration against a closed glottis. Deep, maintained expiration tends to accentuate soft, early diastolic murmurs of aortic or pulmonic regurgitation.

Postural Changes

Assumption of the lying from the standing or sitting position results in an increase in venous return, which augments first right ventricular and, several cardiac cycles later, left ventricular stroke volume. The principal auscultatory changes include widening of the splitting of S_2 in all phases of respiration and augmentations of right-sided S_3 and S_4 and, several cardiac cycles later, left-sided S_3 and S_4.[84] The systolic murmurs of valvular pulmonic and aortic stenosis, the systolic murmurs of mitral and tricuspid regurgitation and ventricular septal defect, and most functional systolic murmurs are augmented. On the other hand, since left ventricular end-diastolic volume rises, the systolic murmur of hypertrophic obstructive cardiomyopathy is diminished, and the midsystolic click and systolic murmur associated with mitral valve prolapse are delayed and sometimes attenuated.[79,83]

Sudden standing or sitting up from a lying position has the opposite effect; in patients in whom there is relatively wide splitting of S_2 during expiration—a finding that may be confused with fixed splitting—the width of the splitting is reduced, so that a normal pattern emerges during the respiratory cycle. No change in splitting occurs in patients with true fixed splitting.

SQUATTING. A change from standing to squatting increases venous return and systemic resistance simultaneously. Stroke volume and arterial pressure rise, and the latter may induce a transient reflex bradycardia. The auscultatory features include augmentation of S_3 and S_4 (from both ventricles) and as a consequence of an increased in stroke volume, the systolic murmurs of aortic and pulmonic stenosis and the diastolic murmurs of mitral and tricuspid stenosis become louder.[79] The elevation of arterial pressure increases blood flow through the right ventricular outflow tract of patients with the tetralogy of Fallot and increases the volume of mitral regurgitation and of the left-to-right shunt through a ventricular septal defect, thereby increasing the intensity of the systolic murmur in these conditions. Also, the diastolic murmur of aortic regurgitation is augmented consequent to an increase in aortic reflux. The combination of elevated arterial pressure and increased venous return increases left ventricular size,

which reduces the obstruction to outflow and therefore the intensity of the systolic murmur of hypertrophic obstructive cardiomyopathy;[85] the midsystolic click of mitral valve prolapse and the systolic murmur are delayed.

Assumption of the left lateral recumbent position accentuates the intensity of S_1, S_3, and S_4 originating from the left side of the heart; the opening snap and the murmurs associated with mitral stenosis and regurgitation; the midsystolic click and late systolic murmur of mitral valve prolapse; and the Austin Flint murmur associated with aortic regurgitation. Sitting up and leaning forward make the diastolic murmurs of aortic and pulmonic regurgitation more readily audible.

THE VALSALVA MANEUVER. During phase I, the initial phase of the Valsalva maneuver, intrathoracic pressure rises, producing a transient increase in left ventricular output. During phase II, the straining phase, systemic venous return declines; filling of the right and then of the left side of the heart are reduced; and the stroke volume and mean arterial and pulse pressures fall and heart rate increases. As a consequence, S_3 and S_4 become attenuated and the A_2–P_2 interval narrows.[59] As stroke volume and arterial pressure fall, the systolic murmurs of aortic and pulmonic stenosis and of mitral and tricuspid regurgitation, and the diastolic murmurs of aortic and pulmonic regurgitation and of tricuspid and mitral stenosis all diminish. However, as left ventricular volume is reduced, the systolic murmur of hypertrophic obstructive cardiomyopathy becomes louder,[86] and the systolic click and murmur of mitral valve prolapse commence earlier. During phase III, the release of the Valsalva maneuver, the aortic and pulmonic components of S_2 normally become more widely separated.[59,87] During the first few beats of phase IV, the overshoot following release of the Valsalva murmurs and filling sounds (S_3 and S_4) originating from the right side of the heart return to normal and may be transiently accentuated. Filling sounds and murmurs originating from the left side of the heart also return to pre-Valsalva levels after six to eight beats and then may be transiently augmented.

An abnormal "square-wave" response to the Valsalva maneuver (see Figure 15–9, p. 501) occurs in patients with atrial septal defect, mitral stenosis, and heart failure of any etiology. With such a response, the above-described changes in hemodynamics and therefore in the auscultatory findings do *not* occur.

POSTPREMATURE VENTRICULAR CONTRACTIONS. When a premature contraction is followed by a significant pause, both an increase in ventricular filling and an augmentation of cardiac contractility occur. Consequently, during the postpremature beat, the systolic murmurs of aortic and pulmonic stenosis and of hypertrophic obstructive cardiomyopathy are augmented,[40] while the systolic murmurs of rheumatic mitral regurgitation and of ventricular septal defect are not altered significantly. The systolic murmur of tricuspid regurgitation and the diastolic murmur of aortic regurgitation become louder consequent to increased right ventricular filling and an elevated arterial pressure, respectively. The increase in left ventricular size delays the systolic click and the systolic murmur of mitral valve prolapse. Similar auscultatory changes follow prolonged diastolic pauses in atrial fibrillation and sinus arrhythmia.

ISOMETRIC EXERCISE. This can be carried out

simply and reproducibly using a calibrated handgrip device, but isometric exercise should be avoided in patients with ventricular arrhythmias and myocardial ischemia. Handgrip should be sustained for 20 to 30 seconds, but a Valsalva maneuver during the handgrip must be avoided. Isometric exercise results in significant increases in systemic vascular resistance, arterial pressure, heart rate, cardiac output, left ventricular filling pressure, and heart size. As a consequence, (1) S_3 and S_4 originating from the left side of the heart become accentuated, (2) the systolic murmur of aortic stenosis is diminished as a result of a reduction of the pressure gradient across the aortic valve, (3) the diastolic murmur of aortic regurgitation and the systolic murmurs of rheumatic mitral regurgitation and ventricular septal defect increase, (4) the diastolic murmur of mitral stenosis becomes louder consequent to the increase in cardiac output, and (5) the systolic murmur of hypertrophic obstructive cardiomyopathy and the systolic click and murmur secondary to mitral valve prolapse are delayed because of the increased left ventricular volume.

Pharmacological Agents

Inhalation of *amyl nitrite* for 10 to 15 seconds produces marked vasodilatation, resulting first in a reduction of systemic arterial pressure, then in a reflex tachycardia, followed in turn by an increase in stroke volume and in venous return.[88-91] S_1 is augmented and A_2 is diminished. The opening snaps of the mitral and tricuspid valves become louder, and as arterial pressure falls, the A_2-opening snap interval shortens. An S_3 originating in either ventricle is augmented, owing to greater rapidity of ventricular filling, but since mitral regurgitation is reduced, the S_3 associated with this lesion is diminished. The systolic murmurs of valvular aortic stenosis, pulmonic stenosis, hypertrophic obstructive cardiomyopathy, and functional systolic murmurs are all accentuated because of the increase in left ventricular contractility and stroke volume. The reduction of arterial pressure increases the right-to-left shunt and decreases the blood flow from the right ventricle to the pulmonary artery and diminishes the systolic ejection murmur in patients with tetralogy of Fallot.[92] The increase in cardiac output augments the diastolic murmurs of mitral and tricuspid stenosis and of pulmonary regurgitation and the systolic murmur of tricuspid regurgitation. However, as a result of the fall in systemic arterial pressure, the systolic murmurs of mitral regurgitation and ventricular septal defect, the diastolic murmurs of aortic regurgitation, and the Austin Flint murmur as well as the continuous murmurs of patent ductus arteriosus and of systemic arteriovenous fistula are all diminished.[93] The reduction of cardiac size results in an earlier appearance of the midsystolic click and systolic murmur of mitral valve prolapse; the intensity of the systolic murmur exhibits a variable response.

Methoxamine and *phenylephrine* increase systemic arterial pressure. In general, methoxamine, 3 to 5 mg intravenously, elevates arterial pressure by 20 to 40 mm Hg for 10 to 20 minutes, but phenylephrine is preferred because of its shorter duration of action; 0.5 mg of phenylephrine administered intravenously elevates systolic pressure by approximately 30 mm Hg for only 3 to 5 minutes.[89] Both drugs cause a reflex bradycardia and decreased contractility and cardiac output. The intensity of S_1 is usually re-

duced, A_2 becomes softer, and the A_2-mitral opening snap interval becomes prolonged. The responses of S_3 and S_4 are variable. As a result of the increased arterial pressure, the diastolic murmur of aortic regurgitation; the systolic murmurs of mitral regurgitation, ventricular septal defect, and tetralogy of Fallot; and the continuous murmur of patent ductus arteriosus and systemic arteriovenous fistula all become louder.[93,94] On the other hand, as a consequence of the increase in left ventricular size, the systolic murmur of hypertrophic obstructive cardiomyopathy becomes softer, and the click and murmur of mitral valve prolapse syndrome are delayed. The reduction in stroke volume diminishes the systolic murmur of valvular aortic stenosis.[79]

References

1. Perloff, J. K.: Physical examination of the heart and circulation. Philadelphia, W. B. Saunders Co., 1982.
1a. Silverman, M. E.: Causes of valve disease: Visual clues. J. Cardiovasc. Med. *8*: 340, 1983.
2. Greenwood, R. D., Rosenthal, A., Parisi, L., Flyer, D. C., and Nadas, A. S.: Extracardiac abnormalities in infants with congenital heart disease. Pediatrics *55*:485, 1975.
3. Shoenfeld, Y., Mor, R., Weinberger, A., Avidor, I., and Pinkhas, J.: Diagonal ear lobe crease and coronary risk factors. J. Am. Geriatr. Soc. *28*:184, 1980.
4. Wood, P.: Diseases of the Heart and Circulation. 3rd ed. Philadelphia, J. B. Lippincott, 1968, p. 625.
5. Cayler, G. G., Blumenfeld, C. M., and Anderson, R. L.: Further studies of patients with the cardiofacial syndrome. Chest *60*:161, 1971.
6. Young, D., Shprintzen, R. J., and Goldberg, R. B.: Cardiac malformations in the velocardiofacial syndrome. Am. J. Cardiol. *46*:643, 1980.
7. Noonan, J. A.: Hypertelorism with Turner phenotype. Am. J. Dis. Child. *116*: 373, 1968.
8. St. John Sutton, M. G., Tajik, A. J., Giuliani, E. R., Gordon, H., and Su, W. P. D.: Hypertrophic obstructive cardiomyopathy and lentiginosis: A little known neural ectodermal syndrome. Am. J. Cardiol. *47*:214, 1981.
9. Beuren, A. J., Schultze, C., Eberle, P., Harmjanz, D., and Aptiz, J.: The syndrome of supravalvular aortic stenosis, peripheral pulmonary stenosis, mental retardation and similar facial appearance. Am. J. Cardiol. *13*:471, 1964.
10. Clark, D. S., Myerburg, R. J., Morales, A. R., Befeler, B., Hernandez, F. A., and Gelband, H.: Heart block in Kearns-Sayre syndrome. Chest *68*:727, 1975.
11. Cogan, D. G.: Ophthalmic Manifestations of Systemic Vascular Disease. Philadelphia, W. B. Saunders Co., 1974.
12. Earnest, D. L., and Hurst, J. W.: Exophthalmos, stare, increase in intra-ocular pressure and systolic propulsion of the eyeballs due to congestive heart failure. Am. J. Cardiol. *26*:351, 1970.
13. Walker, G. L., and Stanfield, T. F.: Retinal changes associated with coarctation of the aorta. Trans. Am. Ophthalmol. Soc. *50*:407, 1952.
14. Fishman, A. P.: Cyanosis. *In* Fishman, A. P. (ed.): Pulmonary Diseases and Disorders. New York, McGraw-Hill Book Co., 1980, pp. 78 and 79.
15. Smith, A. T., Sack, G. H., Jr., and Taylor, G. J.: Holt-Oram syndrome. J. Pediatr. *95*:538, 1979.
16. Walker, B. A., and Murdoch, J. L.: The wrist sign. Arch. Intern. Med. *126*:276, 1970.
17. Criscitiello, M. G., Ronan, J. A., Besterman, E. M., and Schoenwetter, W.: Cardiovascular abnormalities in osteogenesis imperfecta. Circulation *31*:255, 1965.
18. Zvaifler, N. J.: Chronic postrheumatic fever (Jaccoud's) arthritis. N. Engl. J. Med. *267*:10, 1962.
19. Buckley, M. J., Mason, D. T., Ross, J., Jr., and Braunwald, E.: Reversed differential cyanosis with equal desaturation of the upper limbs. Syndrome of complete transposition of the great vessels with complete interruption of the aortic arch. Am. J. Cardiol. *15*:111, 1965.
20. Finger clubbing. Lancet *1*:1285, 1975.
21. Lanken, P. N., and Fishman, A. P.: Clubbing and hypertrophic osteoarthropathy. *In* Fishman, A. P. (ed.): Pulmonary Diseases and Disorders. New York, McGraw-Hill Book Co., 1980, pp. 84–91.
22. Pomerleau, O. F., and Schwarz, H. J.: Tuberous sclerosis with unusual findings: A case report. J. Maine Med. Assoc. *60*:137, 1969.
23. Constant, J.: Arterial and venous pulsations in cardiovascular diagnosis. J. Cardiovasc. Med. *5*:973, 1980.
24. Swartz, M. H.: Jugular venous pressure pulse: Its value in cardiac diagnosis. Primary Cardiol. *8*:197, 1982.
25. Rich, L. L., and Tavel, M. E.: The origin of the jugular C wave. N. Engl. J. Med. *284*:1309, 1971.
26. Bordley, J., III, Connor, C. A. R., Hamilton, W. F., Kerr, W. J., and Wiggers, C. J.: Recommendations for human blood pressure determinations by sphygmomanometers. Circulation *4*:503, 1951.
27. London, S. B., and London, R. E.: Critique of indirect diastolic end point. Arch. Intern. Med. *119*:39, 1967.
28. Maxwell, M. H., Schroth, P. C., Waks, A. U., Karam, M., and Dornfeld, L.

P.: Error in blood-pressure measurement due to incorrect cuff size in obese patients. Lancet 2:33, 1982.

29. Kirkendall, W. M., Burton, A. C., Epstein, F. H., and Freis, E. D.: Recommendations for human blood pressure determination by sphygmomanometers. Circulation 36:980, 1967.

30. Sproul, G.: Basilar artery insufficiency secondary to obstruction of left subclavian artery. Circulation 28:259, 1963.

31. Sapira, J. D.: Quincke, de Musset, Duroziez, and Hill: Some aortic regurgitations. South. Med. J. 74:459, 1981.

32. Abrams, J.: The arterial pulse. Primary Cardiol., 8:138, 1982.

33. Schlant, R. C., and Feiner, J. M.: The arterial pulse—clinical manifestations. Curr. Probl. Cardiol. Vol. 1, No. 5, 1976, 50 pp.

33a. Perloff, J. K.: The physiologic mechanisms of cardiac and vascular physical signs. J. Am. Coll. Cardiol. 1:184, 1983.

34. Marshall, H. W., Helmholz, H. F., Jr., and Wood, E. H.: Physiological consequences of congenital heart disease. In Hamilton, W. F., and Dow, P. (eds.): Handbook of Physiology. Section 2, Circulation. Vol. I. Washington, D.C., American Physiological Society, 1962, pp. 417–487.

35. Elkins, R. C., Morrow, A. G., Vasko, J. S., and Braunwald, E.: The effects of mitral regurgitation on the pattern of instantaneous aortic blood flow. Clinical and experimental observations. Circulation 36:45, 1967.

36. Kelly, E. R., Morrow, A. G., and Braunwald, E.: Catheterization of the left side of the heart: A key to the solution of some perplexing problems in cardiovascular diagnosis and management. N. Engl. J. Med. 262:162, 1960.

37. Rowe, G. G., Afonso, S., Castillo, C. A., and McKenna, D. H.: The mechanism of the production of Duroziez's murmur. N. Engl. J. Med. 272:1207, 1965.

38. Fleming, P. R.: The mechanism of the pulsus bisferiens. Br. Heart J. 19:519, 1957.

39. Braunwald, E., Lambrew, C. T., Rockoff, S. D., Ross, J., Jr., and Morrow, A. G.: Idiopathic hypertrophic subaortic stenosis. I. A description of the disease based upon an analysis of 64 patients. Circulation 30 (Suppl. 4):3, 1964.

40. Brockenbrough, E. C., Braunwald, E., and Morrow, A. G.: A hemodynamic technic for the detection of hypertrophic subaortic stenosis. Circulation 23:189, 1961.

41. Rebuck, A. S., and Pengelly, L. D.: Development of pulsus paradoxus in the presence of airways obstruction. N. Engl. J. Med. 288:66, 1973.

42. Massumi, R. A., Mason, D. T., Zakauddin, V., Zelis, R., Otero, J., and Amsterdam, E. A.: Reversed pulsus paradoxus. N. Engl. J. Med. 289:1272, 1973.

43. Davies, H.: Chest deformities in congenital heart disease. Br. J. Dis. Chest 53:151, 1959.

44. Perloff, J. K.: Diagnostic inferences drawn from observation and palpation of the precordium with special reference to congenital heart disease. Adv. Cardiopulm. Dis. 4:13, 1969.

45. Reusch, C. S.: Hemodynamic studies in pectus excavatum. Circulation 24:1143, 1961.

46. Beiser, G. D., Epstein, S. E., Stampfer, M., Goldstein, R. E., Noland, S. P., and Levitsky, S.: Impairment of cardiac function in patients with pectus excavatum. N. Engl. J. Med. 287:267, 1972.

47. deLeon, A. C., Perloff, J. K., Twigg, H. L., and Majd, M.: The straight back syndrome. Clinical cardiovascular manifestations. Circulation 32:193, 1965.

48. Siegel, J. S., and Schechter, E.: The straight back syndrome. Am. J. Med. 42:309, 1967.

49. Abrams, J.: Examination of the precordium. Primary Cardiol. 8:156, 1982.

50. Bancroft, W. H., Jr., Eddleman, E. E., Jr., and Larkin, L. N.: Methods and physical characteristics of the kineto-cardiographic and apex cardiographic systems for recording low-frequency precordial motion. Am. Heart J. 73:756, 1967.

51. Dressler, W.: Clinical Aids in Cardiac Diagnosis. New York, Grune and Stratton, 1970, 246 pp.

52. Counihan, T. B., Rappaport, M. B., and Sprague, H. B.: Physiologic and physical factors that govern the clinical appreciation of cardiac thrills. Circulation 4:716, 1951.

53. Rappaport, M. B., and Sprague, H. B.: Physiologic and physical laws that govern auscultation, and their clinical application: The acoustic stethoscope and the electrical amplifying stethoscope and stethograph. Am. Heart J. 21:257, 1941.

54. Faber, J. J., and Burton, A. C.: Spread of heart sounds over chest wall. Circ. Res. 11:96, 1962.

55. Stein, P. D.: A Physical and Physiological Basis for the Interpretation of Cardiac Auscultation. Mt. Kisco, N.Y., Futura Publishing Co., 1981, 288 pp.

56. Leatham, A.: Auscultation of the Heart and Phonocardiography. Edinburgh, Churchill Livingstone, 1975, p. 181.

57. Levine, S. A., and Harvey, W. P.: Clinical Auscultation of the Heart. 2nd ed. Philadelphia, W. B. Saunders Co., 1959, 657 pp.

58. Luisada, A. A., and Portaluppi, F.: The Heart Sounds. New York, Praeger Publishers, 1982, 246 pp.

59. Aygen, M. M., and Braunwald, E.: The splitting of the second heart sound in normal subjects and in patients with congenital heart disease. Circulation 25:328, 1962.

60. Beck, W., Schrire, V., and Vogelpoel, L.: Splitting of the second heart sound in constrictive pericarditis, with observations on the mechanism of pulsus paradoxus. Am. Heart J. 64:765, 1962.

61. Leatham, A.: The second heart sound: Key to auscultation of the heart. Acta Cardiol. 19:395, 1964.

62. Yurchak, P. M., and Gorlin, R.: Paradoxical splitting of the second heart sound in coronary heart disease. N. Engl. J. Med. 269:741, 1963.

63. Leatham, A.: Auscultation of the heart since Laennec. Thorax 36:95, 1981.

64. Abrams, J.: The first heart sound. Primary Cardiol. 8:15, 1982.

65. O'Toole, J. D., Reddy, S. P., Curtiss, E. I., Griff, F. W., and Shaver, J. A.: The contribution of tricuspid valve close to the first heart sound: An intracardiac micromanometer study. Circulation 53:752, 1976.

66. Shaver, J. A., and O'Toole, J. D.: The second heart sound: Newer concepts. Part I: Normal and wide physiological splitting. Mod. Concepts Cardiovasc. Dis. 46:7, 1977.

67. Shaver, J. A., and O'Toole, J. D.: The second heart sound: Newer concepts. Part II: Paradoxical splitting and narrow physiological splitting. Mod. Concepts Cardiovasc. Dis. 46:13, 1977.

67a. Oxawa, Y., Smith, D., and Craige, E.: Origin of the third heart sound. II. Studies in hyman subjects. Circulation. 67:399, 1983.

68. Abrams, J.: The third and fourth heart sounds. Primary Cardiol. 8:47, 1982.

69. Abdulla, A. M., Frank, M. J., Erdin, R. A., Jr., and Canedo, M. I.: Clinical significance and hemodynamic correlates of the third heart sound gallop in aortic regurgitation: A guide to optimal timing of cardiac catheterization. Circulation 64:463, 1981.

70. Lee, D. C-S., Johnson, R. A., Bingham, J. B., Leahy, M., Dinsmore, R. E., Goroll, A. H., Newell, J. B., Strauss, H. W., and Haber, E.: Heart failure in outpatients: A randomized trial of digoxin versus placebo. N. Engl. J. Med. 306:699, 1982.

71. Rushmer, R. F., and Morgan, C.: Meaning of murmurs. Am. J. Cardiol. 21:722, 1968.

72. Freeman, A. R., and Levine, S. A.: The clinical significance of the systolic murmur. A study of 1000 consecutive "noncardiac" cases. Ann. Intern. Med. 6:1371, 1933.

73. Holldack, K., Heller, A., and Groth, W.: The pericardial friction rub in the phonocardiogram. Am. J. Cardiol. 4:351, 1959.

74. Harvey, W. P.: Auscultatory findings in diseases of the pericardium. Am. J. Cardiol. 7:15, 1961.

75. Dressler, W.: Effect of respiration on the pericardial friction rub. Am. J. Cardiol. 7:130, 1961.

76. Fowler, N. O., and Gause, R.: The cervical venous hum. Am. Heart J. 67:135, 1964.

77. Tabatznik, B., Randall, T. W., and Hersch, C.: The mammary souffle of pregnancy and lactation. Circulation 22:1069, 1960.

78. Harvey, W. P.: Innocent versus significant murmurs. Curr. Probl. Cardiol. Vol. 1., No. 8, 1976, 51 pp.

79. Delman, A. J., and Stein, E.: Dynamic Cardiac Auscultation and Phonocardiography: A Graphic Guide. Philadelphia, W. B. Saunders Co., 1979, pp. 559–792.

80. Shaver, J. A., O'Toole, J. D., Curtiss, E. I., Thompson, M. E., Reddy, P. S., and Leon, D. F.: Second heart sound. In Physiologic Principles of Heart Sounds and Murmurs. New York, American Heart Association, Monograph No. 46, 1975, pp. 58–67.

81. Goldblatt, A., Harrison, D. C., Glick, G., and Braunwald, E.: Studies on cardiac dimensions in intact, unanesthetized man. II. Effects of respiration. Circ. Res. 13:455, 1963.

82. Rios, J. C., Massumi, R. A., Breesmen, W. T., and Sarin, R. K.: Auscultatory features of acute tricuspid regurgitation. Am. J. Cardiol. 23:4, 1969.

83. Fontana, M. E., Wooley, C. F., Leighton, R. F., and Lewis, R. P.: Postural changes in left ventricular and mitral valvular dynamics in the systolic click-late systolic murmur syndrome. Circulation 51:165, 1975.

84. Rodin, P., and Tabatznik, B.: The effect of posture on added heart sounds. Br. Heart J. 25:69, 1963.

85. Nellen, M., Gotsman, M. S., Vogelpoel, L., Beck, W., and Schrire, V.: Effect of prompt squatting on the systolic murmur in idiopathic hypertrophic obstructive cardiomyopathy. Br. Med. J. 3:140, 1967.

86. Braunwald, E., Oldham, H. N., Jr., Ross, J., Jr., Linhart, J. W., Mason, D. T., and Fort, L., III: The circulatory response of patients with idiopathic hypertrophic subaortic stenosis to nitroglycerin and to the Valsalva maneuver. Circulation 29:422, 1964.

87. van der Hauwaert, L. G.: The effect of the Valsalva maneuver on the splitting of the second sound. Acta Cardiol. 19:518, 1964.

88. Barlow, J., and Shillingford, J.: The use of amyl nitrite in differentiating mitral and aortic systolic murmurs. Br. Heart J. 20:162, 1958.

89. Beck, W., Schrire, V., Vogelpoel, L., Nellen, M., and Swanepoel, A.: Hemodynamic effects of amyl nitrite and phenylephrine on the normal human circulation and their relation to changes in cardiac murmurs. Am. J. Cardiol. 8:341, 1961.

90. Schrire, V., Vogelpoel, L., Beck, W., Nellen, M., and Swanepoel, A.: The effects of amyl nitrite and phenylephrine on the intracardiac murmurs of small ventricular septal defects. Am. Heart J. 62:225, 1961.

91. Vogelpoel, L., Schrire, V., Nellen, M., and Swanepoel, A.: The use of amyl nitrite in the differentiation of Fallot's tetralogy and pulmonary stenosis with intact ventricular septum. Am. Heart J. 57:803, 1959.

92. Vogelpoel, L., Schrire, V., Nellen, M., and Swanepoel, A.: The use of phenylephrine in the differentiation of Fallot's tetralogy from pulmonary stenosis with intact ventricular septum. Am. Heart J. 59:489, 1960.

93. Criscitiello, M.: Physiologic and pharmacologic aids in cardiac auscultation. In Fowler, N. O. (ed.): Cardiac Diagnosis and Treatment. 3rd ed. Hagerstown, Harper and Row, 1980, pp. 77–90.

94. Crevasse, L.: The use of a vasopressor agent as a diagnostic aid in auscultation. Am. Heart J. 58:821, 1959.

3

HEART SOUNDS:

PHONOCARDIOGRAPHY; CAROTID, APEX, AND JUGULAR VENOUS PULSE TRACINGS; AND SYSTOLIC TIME INTERVALS

by Ernest Craige, M.D.

Phonocardiography, or the graphic representation of heart sounds and murmurs, has been practiced since the turn of the century.[1] As commonly used, the term phonocardiography also embraces pulse tracings—carotid, apex, and jugular venous—so that a relatively complete graphic reproduction of auscultatory, visible, and palpable signs of cardiac origin can be provided.[2–6] With the addition of echocardiography to the armamentarium of noninvasive techniques it has become possible to display the echo signal in conjunction with the older graphic methods of multichannel records, the result being an enormously increased diagnostic potential. The combined method is called *echophonocardiography.*[7,8]

In this chapter we will describe the technique of recording phonocardiograms with carotid, apex, and jugular venous pulsations and will discuss the utility of the combined method—echophonocardiography—in the identification and interpretation of heart sounds. In Chapter 4 the role of echophonocardiography in studies of heart murmurs will be considered. The techniques, usefulness, and limitations of echocardiography are presented in Chapter 5.

CARDIAC VIBRATIONS AND THEIR REGISTRATION BY GRAPHIC METHODS

Contraction and relaxation of the heart produces vibrations over the precordium which are perceived by auscultation and palpation, as discussed in Chapter 2. The spectrum of vibrations reaching the chest wall is dominated by the very low frequencies perceived at the bedside as palpable phenomena.[2] A recording that would represent the cardiac vibrations exactly as received and without filtration would not be useful, since the enormous size of the low-frequency vibrations would preclude an adequate representation of the less intense higher frequencies, appreciated acoustically as heart sounds and murmurs. Therefore the recording apparatus, like the human ear itself, must be provided with a system of filters, so that the resulting graphic record may more nearly approximate the sound spectrum perceived by the ear.[9,10]

The principal energy of the palpable movements of the heart emanates from very low-frequency vibrations, i.e., at the lower end of the 0 to 30 cps range.[11] The lower threshold of audibility, although variable, is approximately at 30 cps and extends up to several thousand cycles per second. However, most vibrations of cardiac origin that appear to be of diagnostic importance are in the spectrum of 30 to 1000 cps.[12] Thus, the phonocardiograph should be able to filter out the very low-frequency vibrations which can be represented as a displacement tracing or apexcardiogram. The remaining higher frequency vibrations can then be suitably amplified, so that the resulting graphic records may simulate the phenomena appreciated by auscultation. By a selective filtration system, the lower frequencies in the audible range may be permitted to dominate the tracing, such as might be useful in recording third and fourth heart sounds and low-frequency rumbling murmurs. Alternatively, suppression of low frequencies and amplification of high-frequency vibrations results in optimal presentation of the first and second heart sounds, ejection sounds, opening snaps, and murmurs such as those of mitral and aortic regurgitation.[2]

PHONOCARDIOGRAPHIC TECHNIQUE

Facilities and Equipment. One of the main reasons for disappointment with phonocardiograms is the inadequacy of tracings due to faulty technique or poor recording conditions. The room must be quiet or sound-conditioned, with a sound-absorbent ceiling and wall covering, drapes over the windows, and a carpet, and mechanical noises, such as humming and rattling of air conditioners or fans, must be eliminated in order to obtain tracings free of background noise. To avoid a confusion of wires, transducers should be hung from racks appropriately located on the wall near the patient's head.

The bed should be comfortable, allow elevation of the patient's head, and be high enough so that the examiner can conveniently auscultate and apply the necessary transducers. Usually the patient is supine, with the head elevated for comfort or as required for optimal visualization or registration of venous or carotid pulsations. During recording of the carotid pulse, a pillow should be placed beneath the patient's shoulders in order to hyperextend the neck and thereby thrust the carotid artery forward, supported firmly by the transverse processes of the cervical spine. It may be necessary for the patient to assume the left lateral decubitus position to enhance auscultatory and palpable phenomena at the cardiac apex.

Paper speed is usually set at 100 mm/sec, which is optimal for measurement of systolic time intervals[13] as well as for observation of the relationship of heart sounds and valvular and ventricular events. However, slower paper speeds may be preferable for displaying the effects of respiration or other physiological or pharmacological maneuvers or in scanning the heart by means of the accompanying echocardiogram.

Although a variety of microphones for heart-sound registration is available, we prefer the air-coupled type, attached to the lightly lubricated chest wall by means of a rubber suction bulb.* Any excess hair that might interfere with the firm, air-tight attachment of the microphone should be removed. Smaller transducers are essential for infants and small children and are also useful where prominent ribs preclude adequate contact with the microphone rim.

Transducers for pulse tracings—carotid, apex, or venous—are commonly of the piezoelectric crystal type. A funnel or tambour is applied to the pulsation under study, and changes in air pressure are conducted via a rubber tube to the crystal device for conversion to electrical signals. The transducer-recording system must have an adequate time constant of 3.0 sec or more. With some of the older equipment, too short a time constant resulted in distortion of the curves and subtle temporal displacement of important landmarks in the carotid and apex tracings.[11,14,15] The principles of physics pertinent to this subject are beyond the scope of this chapter; however, a simple test of one's apparatus for the adequacy of the duration of the time constant consists merely of observing the effect on the oscilloscope of sustained pressure applied to the funnel or tambour of the transducer. If after a rapid rise of the signal on the oscilloscope, there is an immediate (0.3 sec or so) fall to the baseline, despite continued pressure on the sensing head of the transducer, then obviously the apparatus will yield a systematic distortion of the pulsatile phenomena being recorded. This distortion is equivalent to a partial differentiation of the signal.[16] A plateau will appear as an inverted V, and a shallow trough may become a deep crevasse. Besides these morphological alterations, the timing of landmarks (which constitutes one of the principal uses of pulsatile records) may be disturbed, resulting in erroneous interpretations. A time constant of 3.0 sec or more is adequate for recording carotid, apex, and venous pulsations. An infinite time constant may be theoretically superior but is usually

impractical, owing to the wide swings of the baseline associated with respiration that make interpretation difficult.

Respiration can be monitored by means of a nasal thermistor probe. This produces a satisfactory curve that can be superimposed on the other parameters of a multichannel tracing. Alternatively, a strain-gauge device that reponds to chest expansion may be employed, but this has the disadvantage that the expansile belt may interfere with placement of the transducers on the chest wall. The technique and equipment required for echocardiography are described in Chapter 5.

A number of satisfactory recorders are available, and the choice depends on such factors as obtaining satisfactory phonocardiograms and echocardiograms, price, availability of service, and size and portability of the equipment. The recorder should be capable of multichannel registration at a variety of paper speeds. Some recorders provide immediate processing, although this may sacrifice the vivid contrast of black and white tracings. The latter usually require a separate photographic developer.

Recording Technique. In view of the many possible combinations of transducers and chest-wall locations, the registration of graphic tracings must be preceded by a bedside assessment of the problem. Ideally, the clinician should be present in the noninvasive

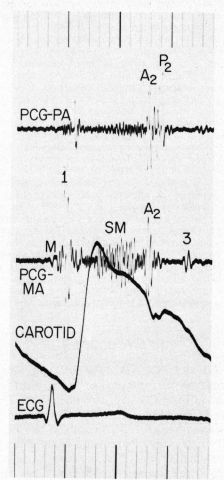

FIGURE 3–1 Phonocardiogram in mild mitral regurgitation. Two phonocardiograms are taken simultaneously, one at the second left intercostal space (PCG-PA) and one at the cardiac apex (PCG-MA). This demonstrates the wide transmission of the aortic component of the second heart sound (A_2) while the pulmonic component (P_2) is confined to the upper left sternal edge. A late systolic murmur (SM) and third sound (3) are best seen at the apex. Also, the initial low-frequency component (M) of the first sound (1) is seen at the same location. In the illustrations in this chapter, the following symbols will be used to indicate location of the microphones on the chest wall: AA = second right intercostal space; PA = second left intercostal space; LSE = lower left sternal edge (third or fourth left intercostal space); MA = cardiac apex. (Time lines = 0.04 sec.)

---

*Leatham microphone, Irex Company, Ramsey, New Jersey.

laboratory to supervise application of the microphones to the most informative locations on the chest wall. If this is not possible, the areas best suited for registration can be designated with a mark, or at least the problem should be indicated clearly, so that laboratory personnel can make the most appropriate choices. It must be emphasized that informative tracings cannot be provided by a technician applying transducers to the chest wall in a routine, unsupervised manner. Phonocardiograms thus recorded are more often misleading than helpful in cardiac diagnosis. In general, it is preferable to record from two microphones simultaneously in order to clarify the transmission of certain sounds such as P_2 and to separate such sounds from others occurring in close temporal proximity, such as opening snaps, third sounds, and the like (Fig. 3–1).[17]

The most commonly used sites for application of the microphones are those generally employed in auscultation: the second right interspace, often called the "aortic area"; the second left interspace, or the "pulmonary area"; the lower left sternal edge and xiphoid region, or the "tricuspid area"; and the cardiac apex, or the "mitral area." The designation of these anatomical locations on the thoracic wall as "valve areas" is an oversimplification that may be misleading, since there is no exclusive transmission of acoustical events from any particular valve to a certain area on the chest wall. Thus the designations "AA," "MA," and other similar symbols for second right interspace, cardiac apex, and so on are used in the illustrations in Chapters 3 and 4 simply for economy of space.

Occasionally, there may be a competition for chest-wall space between microphones and ultrasound transducers, especially in children. In such instances, some judgment regarding priorities for positions will have to be exercised. Following the application of the microphones, it is imperative to listen through an amplifying stethoscope plugged into the recorder in order to determine whether the auscultatory phenomena in question can be heard and adequately visualized on the oscilloscope. This precaution also helps to eliminate artifacts due to hair or poor contact with the chest wall and to identify artifacts due to bowel sounds or percussion noises from hyperdynamic chest-wall movement. All these extraneous sounds are more easily identified by means of auscultation than by means of a graphic record, in which their rhythmic recurrence with the heartbeat may simulate some important intracardiac manifestation. Most phonocardiographic recordings are equipped with a system of filters that can be used to suppress the low-frequency vibrations of cardiac origin which would otherwise dominate the tracing. The resultant spectrum of vibrations simulates more closely the sounds perceptible to the human ear. A choice of filters can be made in order to accentuate low-frequency diastolic sounds and rumbles or, alternatively, the higher frequency valvular sounds (i.e., S_1, S_2, opening snaps) or murmurs (e.g., that of aortic regurgitation). However, even the best equipment commercially available will fail to record adequately faint, high-pitched murmurs.

HEART SOUNDS

FIRST HEART SOUND.   The first heart sound (S_1) is best recorded at the cardiac apex and is identified by its relationship to the ECG and carotid upstroke (Fig. 3–1). It consists phonocardiographically of an initial inaudible low-frequency vibration, "M," occurring at the onset of ventricular systole, then two intense high-frequency bursts of vibrations at the time of atrioventricular valve closure, followed by a few variable low-intensity vibrations (Fig. 3–2).[18,19]

The genesis of heart sounds, particularly the origin of S_1, has been a controversial issue since the early part of the nineteenth century. Arguments have centered on the question of whether or not the atrioventricular valves make a significant contribution to sound genesis. The classic theory relates the principal high-frequency vibrations of S_1 to mitral and tricuspid closure, respectively.[20–22] An alternative hypothesis attributes the high-frequency elements of S_1 to the movement and acceleration of blood in early systole, the first element being related to left ventricular dP/dt

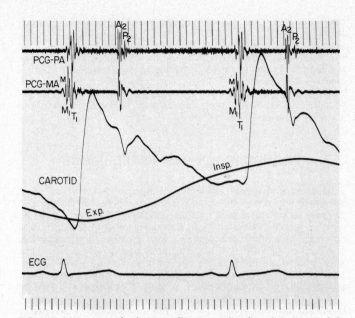

FIGURE 3–2 Normal phonocardiogram. The first heart sound is best seen at the cardiac apex (PCG-MA) and consists of a low-frequency component (M), followed by two high-frequency bursts of vibrations (M_1, T_1), and finally a few low-intensity, low-frequency vibrations in early systole. Normal widening of the A_2- P_2 interval with inspiration is demonstrated.

and the second to ejection of blood into the root of the aorta.[23,24] In the past this problem was studied by means of hemodynamic investigations with catheterization of the relevant heart chambers combined with phonocardiography. The delay occasioned by the transmission of pressure pulses through fluid-filled catheters makes routine catheterization unsuitable for such observations. High-fidelity tracings obtained via catheter-tipped micromanometers demonstrate the pressure crossover points between left atrium and ventricle, signaling the moment of *onset* of valve closure that inevitably must precede final closure by an appreciable interval.[25–28]

The technique of echophonocardiography is particularly applicable to studies of this problem,[29,30] since valvular and acoustical events are transmitted from their source to graphic registration with essentially no time delay, thereby facilitating the accumulation of data necessary for resolution of the problems associated with the origin of heart sounds (Fig. 3–3). Variation in intensity of the major elements of S_1 has been studied in cases of complete heart block[31,32] and ventricular premature beats.[33] The relative contribution of the velocity of mitral valve closure as opposed to the force of left ventricular contraction in the determination of the intensity of S_1 has been investigated in a rapidly fluctuating situation such as atrial fibrillation, and velocity of mitral valve closure was found to have the dominant role. These studies are consistent with the classic theory that presumes that atrioventricular closure and the ensuing tension of valvular structures are associated with the initiation of vibrations appreciated acoustically as S_1.[8,29,30,32] The observation of Traill and Fortuin of a loud "presystolic first heart sound" in diastole simultaneous with premature closure of the mitral valve in severe aortic regurgitation provides additional evidence favoring the valvular origin of S_1.[34]

Normal Splitting of S₁. The two major components of S₁ are separated by a narrow interval of 0.02 to 0.03 sec in most normal subjects.[22] This degree of separation is difficult to perceive by means of auscultation, and phonocardiography may record the two elements of S₁ blurring into a continuum of vibrations. Normal splitting is recorded most satisfactorily in the pediatric age group. The mitral component, M_1, is the louder and is best recorded at the cardiac apex. The tricuspid component, T_1, that immediately follows is best recorded at the left lower sternal border.

Abnormal Splitting of S₁. Abnormal splitting of S₁ may result from either electrophysiological or hemodynamic changes that alter the timing of atrioventricular valve closure.

Electrical Factors. These include abnormalities associated with bundle branch block,[35,36] ectopic ventricular beats, ventricular tachycardia, idioventricular rhythm, preexcitation, and ventricular pacing.[37] Wide splitting with preservation of the normal sequence (M_1 to T_1) may be recorded in right bundle branch block, ectopic beats or idioventricular rhythms originating in the left ventricle, pacing from the left ventricle, or preexcitation patterns that result in left ventricular contraction before right. Reversed splitting may occur with the opposite of the above situations, i.e., ectopic rhythms and paced beats originating in the right ventricle. It does not follow, however, that reversed splitting necessarily occurs in left bundle branch block (LBBB), since the *onset* of the left ventricular pressure rise often starts on time despite the *delay* in the completion of depolarization of the left side, which causes the characteristic electrocardiographic pattern.[38] Burggraf has shown that in LBBB there may be a normal sequence (M_1 followed by T_1) or a simultaneous M_1T_1 or a reversal of the two elements.[39] Typically, the low amplitude of S₁ in LBBB makes identification of individual components more difficult.

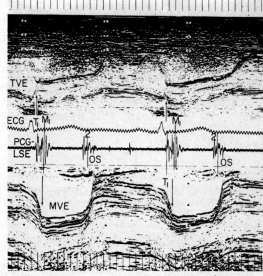

FIGURE 3-4 Reversed splitting of S₁ in mitral stenosis. A dual echophonocardiogram shows a widely split S₁ with T_1 identified by its coincidence with tricuspid valve closure (↑) preceding M_1, which occurs at the time of mitral valve closure (↓). An opening snap (OS) follows S₂ and is identified by its occurrence at the time of full opening of the mitral valve in early diastole.

Hemodynamic Factors. Hemodynamic abnormalities that result in alteration in the timing of M_1 and T_1 include mitral stenosis and left atrial myxoma. In mitral stenosis, pressure in the left ventricle must rise to higher than normal levels before pressure in the left atrium is exceeded and the mitral valve starts to close.[40] In severe cases the delay in the timing of mitral valve closure, and therefore of M_1, may result in reversed splitting of S₁ (Fig. 3-4). Similarly, in left atrial myxoma, M_1 is delayed as the result of a hemodynamic situation simulating that of mitral stenosis. With extrusion of the tumor from ventricle to atrium, a loud, late S₁ is audible and usually palpable.

Mixed Electrical and Hemodynamic Factors. In Ebstein's anomaly (pp. 996 and 1040) the combination of right bundle branch block (RBBB) and an unusually large, deformed tricuspid valve results in a greatly delayed T_1.[41] Closure of the large anterior tricuspid leaflet in association with a loud, high-frequency sound as long as 0.14 sec after closure of the mitral valve provides a characteristic echophonocardiographic picture (Fig. 3-5).[41,42] The diagnostic specificity of these findings obviates cardiac catheterization in most instances.

Intensity of S₁. Several factors are of importance in determining the intensity of the major components of S₁, and these include the ability of the atrioventricular valves to close, their mobility, the velocity of their closing movement, and the strength of ventricular systole. "Closure" of the atrioventricular valves as perceived echocardiographically occurs at the "*c*-point," where the leaflets are seen to approximate each other in early systole. Echocardiography cannot distinguish between *apposition* of the leaflets and the *tension* on the bellies of the leaflets which immediately follows. Presumably it is the latter event that is associated with vibrations perceived as sound.

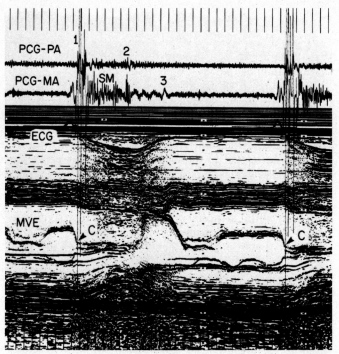

FIGURE 3-3 An echophonocardiogram showing the relationship between mitral valve closure and a very loud first heart sound (1). PCG at the cardiac apex (MA) shows a holosystolic murmur of mild mitral regurgitation. The C points indicate apposition of the leaflets of the mitral valve on the mitral valve echogram (MVE).

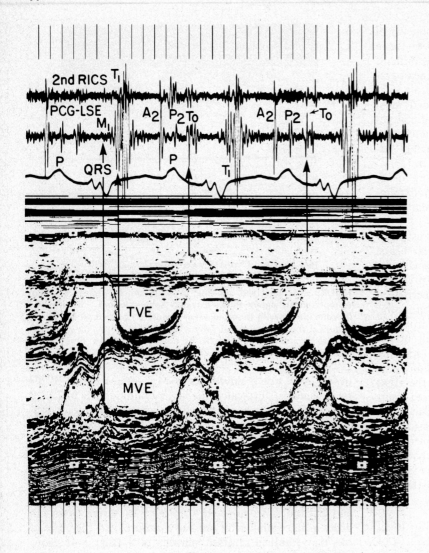

FIGURE 3–5   Ebstein's anomaly. Echophonocardiogram of the tricuspid valve (TVE) and mitral valve (MVE) showing delayed closure of the large tricuspid valve 0.12 sec from onset of the QRS complex. Closure of the tricuspid valve is associated with a very loud T_1 or "sail sound," which dwarfs the mitral component of S_1 (M_1). Additional sounds include tricuspid opening (T_0) synchronous with the E-point of the tricuspid echo.

Ability of the AV Valves to Close. In mitral regurgitation, in which closure of the valve is ineffectual, S_1 may be soft. This is best illustrated in rheumatic valvular disease, in which shortening and thickening of the chordae tendineae preclude normal closure. In prolapse of the mitral valve, however, the valve may seat normally in early systole, an event associated with a loud S_1 (Fig. 3–1), although prolapse of the valve and regurgitation may occur later in systole.[43]

Mobility of the Valve. A calcified valve that is completely immobilized is associated with a soft or absent S_1.

Velocity of Closure. This is the most important factor in determining the intensity of S_1. Clinical observations pertinent to this subject have indicated that the velocity of closure of the mitral valve varies on a beat-to-beat basis. Such opportunities for study are afforded by cases of complete heart block[31,32] and atrial fibrillation.[8] A high velocity of closure has been found to correlate with a loud S_1 and a slow velocity of closure with a soft S_1. When the valve is completely closed at the onset of ventricular systole, as with a long P-R interval[32] or with severe, acute aortic regurgitation,[44] S_1 may be silent or, occasionally, audible in diastole,[34] depending on the velocity of the closing movement. These observations support the clinical teaching of Wolferth and Margolies, who many years ago proposed

that the intensity of S_1 depends on mitral (atrioventricular) valve position at the onset of systole.[45]

The loudness of T_1 in atrial septal defect may be explained by the same hypothesis, since the valve is held open by the augmented flow from right atrium to right ventricle, until final closure occurs with right ventricular systole.[46,47] The loud M_1 characteristic of mitral stenosis may also be related to the fact that the valve is held open by the transvalvular pressure gradient until a very sharp, high-velocity closing movement of the valve apparatus is effected by ventricular systole (Fig. 3–4). If a loud M_1 is present in mitral stenosis, one may assume that some portion of the valve is capable of moving (bulging) in the direction of the atrium even though the mouth of the valve may be largely immobilized by fibrosis and even calcification.

Strength of Ventricular Systole. Although obviously closure of the AV valves is dependent on ventricular systole, the contribution of the *force of ventricular contraction* to the intensity of S_1 is less than that of the *velocity of valve closure*.[8,48] Thus, in atrial fibrillation, the long diastoles which, according to the Starling principle, should lead to the most forceful contractions are not necessarily followed by the loudest first heart sounds.[8] In fact a sound may at times be observed when the mitral valve closes precocious-

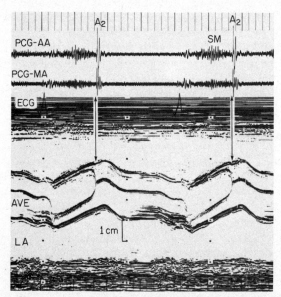

FIGURE 3–6 Echophonocardiogram illustrating the relationship between closure of the aortic valve and onset of the high-frequency vibrations of A₂. An ejection systolic murmur (SM) is noted in the phonocardiogram from the second right intercostal space. AVE = aortic valve echo; LA = left atrium.

ly in diastole when no ventricular contraction at all has taken place.[34,49] In left bundle branch block a variety of factors may contribute to the characteristic softness of S_1, including extracardiac abnormalities such as emphysema in older subjects, impaired ventricular contraction due to myocardial disease, and partial closure of the valve prior to ventricular systole owing to a long P-R interval plus a further delay between onset of the QRS complex and initiation of ventricular systole in some cases of LBBB.[36,39]

SECOND HEART SOUND. The classic explanation of the origin of the two components of the second heart sound relates these events to closure of the aortic and pulmonic valves, respectively, thus warranting the designations "A_2" and "P_2."[20,22,50] The coincidence of the onset of A_2 and aortic valve closure is clearly demonstrable in combined echophonocardiographic recordings (Fig. 3–6). In vitro studies of Stein and associates utilizing high-speed cinematographic techniques have confirmed and delineated in precise detail the role of valvular vibrations in the origin and intensity of A_2.[51,52] Careful investigations by Hirschfeld et al. utilizing high-fidelity aortic root pressure tracings in conjunction with echo- and phonocardiograms demonstrate the simultaneous occurrence of aortic valve closure, the onset of A_2, and the incisura in the pressure record.[53] These observations reinforce the traditional concept of the role of the aortic valve in the genesis of A_2.[54]

The pulmonic component of the second heart sound (P_2) is generally attributed to closure and tensing of the pulmonic valve.[20,22,50] This relationship is more difficult to demonstrate by echophonocardiography than the analogous events on the left side of the heart, because one can rarely visualize more than one cusp of the pulmonic valve and therefore the exact moment of closure cannot be accurately pinpointed. In Figure 3–7, however, from a patient with chronic rheumatic heart disease, the closing point of the valve cusps can be seen and is synchronous with P_2.

By auscultation or phonocardiography the two elements of the second heart sound are best appreciated in the pulmonary area or second left intercostal space where normal splitting is demonstrated on inspiration. The aortic component of S_2 can be identified by its occurrence just before the incisura of the carotid pulse tracing and by its wide transmission to the cardiac apex. P_2, on the other hand, is usually recorded only at the upper left sternal edge, unless it is of abnormal intensity.

Therefore the method recommended above, of utilizing two sound transducers simultaneously, is ideally suited for recording the timing, relative intensity, transmission, and behavior in conjunction with respiration of the two elements of S_2.[22] Quiet deep breathing with the mouth open is the best method of producing the desired physiological alterations, since it will be relatively free from obscuring artifacts.

Normal Splitting of S₂. In newborn infants S_2 is initially single.[55] However, during the first day of life, with falling resistance in the pulmonary circuit, the inspiratory separation of A_2 and P_2 becomes perceptible phonocardiographically. Normally, thereafter, fusion of the elements of S_2 occurs with expiration, and separation varying from 0.02 to 0.06 sec occurs with inspiration.[56]

In older subjects in whom auscultation and phonocardiographic observations may be obscured by emphysema,

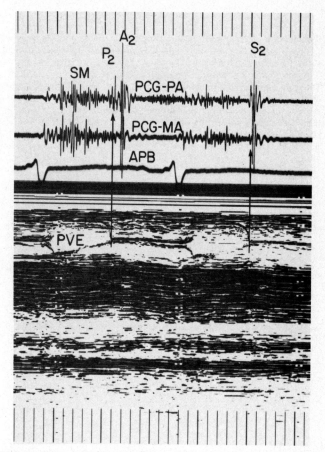

FIGURE 3–7 Echophonocardiogram from a patient with severe chronic rheumatic heart disease. There is reversed splitting of S_2 such that P_2 precedes A_2 in the first beat. In the second beat, which is premature (APB), the two elements of S_2 fuse. A simultaneous echo of the pulmonary valve (PVE) shows that P_2 occurs coincident with closure of the two visible cusps.

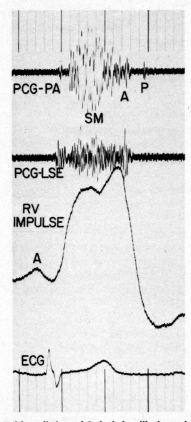

FIGURE 3–8 Wide splitting of S₂ in infundibular pulmonic stenosis. There is an associated ventricular septal defect with left-to-right shunting. The separation of A₂- P₂ is 0.08 sec, a figure consistent with the systemic pressures encountered in the right ventricle (RV).[57] There is an ejection murmur in the second left intercostal space (PA) from the RV outflow obstruction, whereas at the lower sternal edge (LSE), the murmur has a holosystolic configuration, suggesting that it is largely the result of the ventricular septal defect. The RV impulse recorded at LSE shows a prominent *a* wave (A) and a sustained systolic thrust consistent with right ventricular hypertrophy.

only one element of S₂ may by audible, giving the erroneous impression that splitting is no longer present.

Wide Splitting of S₂ with Respiratory Variation. As with splitting of S₁, wide splitting of S₂ may occur for either electrical or hemodynamic reasons.

Electrical Factors. Those factors contributing to prolongation of the interval between A₂ and P₂ include right bundle branch block, pacing of the left ventricle, preexcitation, and ventricular premature beats originating on the left side of the heart. Under these circumstances graphic records demonstrate a further prolongation of the A₂-P₂ interval with inspiration, even though this is usually difficult to perceive by means of auscultation.

Hemodynamic Factors. Those factors that increase the splitting of S₂ include the following.

OBSTRUCTION TO RIGHT VENTRICULAR OUTFLOW. Valvular pulmonic stenosis results in prolongation of right ventricular systole, with delay and diminution of P₂. The magnitude of the separation of A₂-P₂ can be used to estimate the severity of the stenosis, being greater with higher right ventricular pressures (Fig. 3–8).[57] With infundibular stenosis, a similar separation of the components of S₂ is seen.

SHORTENING OF LEFT VENTRICULAR EJECTION TIME. In severe mitral regurgitation, the left ventricular ejection time is abnormally short and A₂ is early, resulting in a prolongation of the interval between A₂ and P₂. Respiratory variation is preserved.

Broad Fixed Splitting of S₂. In atrial septal defect there is, in most instances, broad and fixed splitting of S₂ (Fig. 3–9).[58] Fixed separation of A₂-P₂ is defined as a gap that varies no more than 0.01 sec with inspiration and expiration. The mechanism for the broad and fixed characteristics of the second heart sound has been studied in Murgo's laboratory by means of carefully monitored beat-to-beat simultaneous measurements of flow, pressure, and systolic time intervals in the right and left heart.[59] These

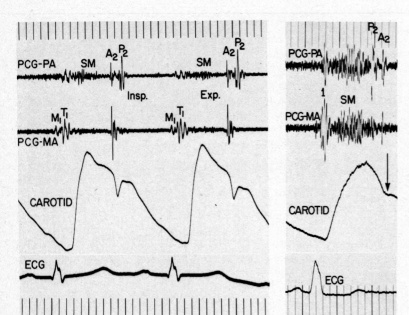

FIGURE 3–9 *Left,* Atrial septal defect showing a midsystolic murmur (SM) and "fixed" splitting of S₂ in the second left intercostal space (PCG-PA). The separation of A₂ and P₂ is 0.06 sec in inspiration and expiration. The first heart sound shows a relatively loud tricuspid component (T₁). *Right,* Aortic stenosis, with reversed splitting of S₂. There is a prominent midsystolic murmur. A₂ is identified by its occurrence immediately prior to the incisura (arrow) on the carotid pulse tracing. P₂ is seen to fall still earlier by 0.04 sec. The carotid upstroke is slow and is shattered by coarse vibrations.

investigators have shown that during expiration the right heart ejection dynamics in patients with atrial septal defect are normal and the wide expiratory split is explained by an abnormally shortened left ventricular ejection time. During inspiration, P_2 is delayed in patients with atrial septal defect and in normal subjects. However, unlike in normal subjects, A_2 does not move to an earlier position during inspiration in patients with atrial septal defect. A_2 thus retains a relatively constant interval with P_2. These findings are consistent with the 1960 phonocardiographic studies Shafter.[60]

Paradoxical Splitting of S_2. Reversal in the normal sequences of A_2-P_2 can occur from either electrical or hemodynamic causes.

Electrical Factors. Electrical disturbances that alter the normal sequence of depolarization of the ventricles include left bundle branch block (Fig. 3–10) and ectopic beats, paced beats, or idioventricular rhythm originating on the right side of the heart. Preexcitation may also result in a precedence of right ventricular systole and reversal of S_2.

Hemodynamic Factors. Mechanical factors that are associated with prolongation of left ventricular ejection time include outflow obstruction of the left ventricle, as in aortic stenosis (Fig. 3–9), or hypertrophic obstructive cardiomyopathy (HOCM). Paradoxical splitting of S_2 is found only in the most severe cases. In patent ductus arteriosus, the increased stroke volume of the left ventricle may also lengthen left ventricular ejection time, resulting in a reversal of A_2-P_2. However, the accentuation of the murmur at

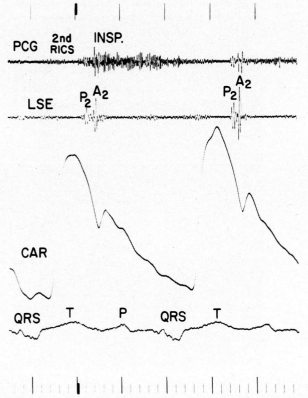

FIGURE 3–10 Reversed splitting of S_2 in left bundle branch block. PCG at left sternal edge (LSE) shows P_2 before A_2, the latter being identified by its occurrence immediately before the incisura in the carotid pulse tracing. With inspiration the gap between P_2 and A_2 narrows, illustrating the physical sign that would permit the detection of reversed splitting by auscultation.

the time of S_2, which is characteristic of this defect, obscures the details of S_2 both on auscultation and on the phonocardiogram.

Single S_2. The second sound may seem to be single on auscultation or on the phonocardiogram because (1) it is indeed single, (2) one of its two elements is inaudible, or (3) both components occur simultaneously. The most common cause for an *apparently* single S_2 is inability to hear or record the fainter of the two elements of the sound (usually P_2) due to emphysema, obesity, or other technical problems. A truly single S_2, however, is seen in tetralogy of Fallot or pulmonary atresia, in which A_2 is loud and is usually easily recorded, whereas pulmonary closure is so soft that it escapes detection. Fusion of the two elements of S_2 resulting in a very loud single S_2 occurs with ventricular septal defect with pulmonary hypertension.

Intensity of S_2. Recording the two elements of S_2 is best accomplished with the microphone at the upper left sternal border. Although P_2 is best appreciated in this location and is poorly transmitted elsewhere, it ordinarily does not exceed A_2 in intensity in normal subjects, even at the upper left sternal edge. When it is shown by graphic records to exceed A_2 in amplitude or to be unusually widely transmitted, such as to the cardiac apex, one must suspect pulmonary hypertension or atrial septal defect.[61] An exaggerated P_2 is, however, only a crude indicator of pulmonary hypertension. In atrial septal defect, P_2 may be accentuated and widely transmitted even when the pulmonary arterial pressure is normal.

A diminished P_2 is found in pulmonic stenosis, either valvular or infundibular, since this obstructing lesion results in low pressure in the pulmonary artery and therefore a diminished force effecting closure of the valve (Fig. 3–8).

Accentuation of A_2, like other phonocardiographic observations of heart-sound intensity, is usually a subjective assessment owing to variations in thickness of the chest wall and other technical factors that make quantitation virtually impossible. Nevertheless, an increase in A_2 can frequently be noted in systemic hypertension, coarctation of the aorta, and corrected transposition of the great arteries.

Reduction in intensity of A_2 occurs in aortic stenosis in adults, in whom the valve is often immobilized by calcification. In children with congenitally deformed but still mobile valve cusps, the intensity of A_2 is usually normal. A soft A_2 may be found in aortic regurgitation. Sabbah et al. attribute this to (1) the lower diastolic pressure in the aorta that results in a diminished rate of change in the driving pressure, i.e., the diastolic pressure gradient between the aorta and the left ventricle that effects valve closure; and (2) a diminished ability of the abnormal valve to become tense and vibrate after closure.[62]

EJECTION SOUNDS. Ejection sounds of aortic origin are of high frequency and occur early in systole, usually 0.12 to 0.14 sec after the Q wave of the electrocardiogram. These sounds are most prominent in association with a deformed aortic valve, as in congenital aortic stenosis, bicuspid configuration (Fig. 3–11),[63–65] or rheumatic heart disease. A mobile valve is necessary for sound production, since with heavy calcification and immobilization of the valve the ejection sound disappears. Aortic ejection sounds from deformed valves are widely

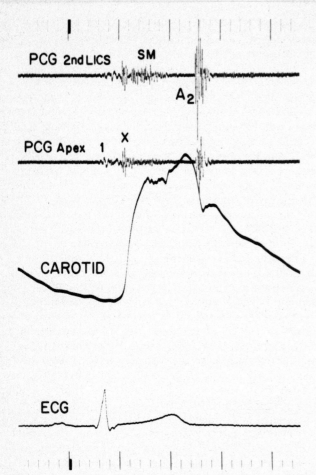

FIGURE 3–11 Aortic ejection sound of valvular origin in a 22-year-old man. The ejection sound (X) is widely transmitted over the precordium and is well seen at cardiac apex. An early to midsystolic murmur is recorded at the base of the heart (PCG 2nd LICS). The carotid tracing is deformed with a delayed peak. These findings are best explained by a bicuspid aortic valve with mild stenosis.

transmitted over the precordium and are well recorded at the cardiac apex. They also occur in association with systemic hypertension and other conditions in which the aortic root may be dilated. Such ejection sounds have a similar timing but are usually less prominent than those due to valvular disease. Under these conditions the sound is not as widely transmitted as with a deformed valve and may be confined to the upper right sternal border (Fig. 3–12). The intensity of aortic ejection sounds does not vary with respiration.

The clinical conditions in which pulmonic ejection sounds occur are similar to those in which aortic ejection sounds are found—valve abnormalities, such as congenital pulmonic stenosis; pulmonary hypertension;[66-68] and idiopathic dilatation of the pulmonary artery. These sounds are usually confined to the upper left sternal border. Their timing is earlier than that of aortic ejection sounds, usually occurring 0.09 to 0.11 sec after the Q wave. The pulmonic ejection sound associated with valve stenosis fluctuates with respiration, being loudest during expiration, and this fluctuation is attributed to the position of the valve at the onset of right ventricular systole.[68] With inspiration, blood is drawn into the right ventricle, augmenting the effect of atrial systole and resulting in partial opening of the pul-

monic valve prior to ventricular systole. The consequently diminished additional movement of the valve imparted by ventricular systole is associated with a muted ejection sound. With expiration, on the other hand, the valve opens swiftly from a fully closed position, and at the sudden termination of its opening movement, a maximal ejection sound ensues. The decrease in intensity of the ejection sound in pulmonic valve stenosis with inspiration contrasts with the behavior of T_1, which increases with inspiration. Careful attention to this detail may be helpful in indentifying auscultatory events in early systole. The ejection sound of pulmonic valve stenosis occurs slightly earlier with severe obstruction. The ejection sound of pulmonary hypertension, however, is delayed slightly when the level of pressure in the pulmonary artery is high (Fig. 3–13).[69,70]

Although some details of the controversies concerning the origin of the first and second sounds may seem merely "academic," the principles involved are of considerable clinical importance, especially in recognition of ejection sounds, which begin at the exact time of *maximal opening* of the semilunar valves (Fig. 3–13). Ejection sounds are called "valvular" when found in association with abnormal valves and "vascular" when valves are normal, but the physiology is otherwise disturbed. In either case it can be

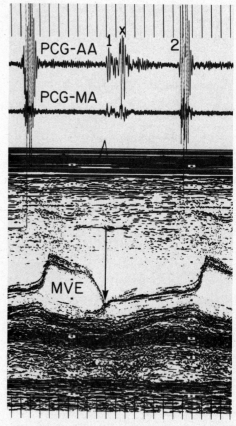

FIGURE 3–12 Aortic ejection sound of "vascular" origin in a patient with syphilitic aortitis and dilated aorta. An ejection sound (X) is seen to follow the first sound and mitral valve closure in the mitral valve echo (MVE = arrow) by 0.06 sec. It is coincident with full opening of the aortic valve (not illustrated) and is not widely transmitted, being clearly recorded only in the second right intercostal space (AA). The second sound is very prominent in the phonocardiogram and had a ringing "tambour" quality on auscultation.

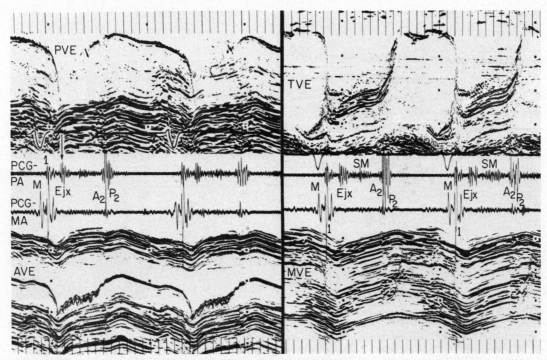

FIGURE 3–13 Ejection sound associated with pulmonary hypertension. The patient had mitral stenosis, and a Hancock porcine aortic valve had been inserted in the mitral position. Dual echophonocardiograms identify the various sounds occurring in early systole.

Left, Dual echophonocardiogram of pulmonic valve (PVE) and of patient's own aortic valve (AVE). The pulmonic valve achieves a fully open position coincident with the ejection sound (Ejx), which is much delayed at 0.17 sec from the onset of QRS, consistent with the pulmonary hypertension.[70] The aortic valve (AVE) opens earlier and thus cannot be responsible for the Ejx. The low-frequency vibration M occurs before S_1 (1) and is attributed to ventricular muscular contraction.[19]

Right, Dual echophonocardiogram of same patient showing the tricuspid valve (TVE) and prosthetic valve (MVE) closing simultaneously coincident with S_1. The echocardiographic representation of the valves has been magnified to facilitate examination of details of their movements. The QRS complex in the left-hand panel has been retouched to permit its identification within a mass of echoes.

shown by echophonocardiography that the high-frequency ejection sound starts at the moment of full opening of the aortic or pulmonic valve.[71] Although it is generally accepted that the "valvular" ejection sound is caused by halting of the "doming" valve, the origin of the "vascular" sounds is not clear, and their presence is by no means invariable in systemic or pulmonary hypertension. It may be that the vascular ejection sounds do in fact originate from the semilunar valve cusps that have undergone geometric changes as a result of being seated in a dilated great vessel. Under these circumstances, the cusps of a normal semilunar valve could not lie against the wall of the great vessel during ejection but rather would be suspended in a triangular pattern tangential to the ring. Thus, being drawn taut in early systole, they might be expected to vibrate and produce an ejection sound analogous to that of the bicuspid valve, the geometry of which similarly prevents complete opening.

OPENING SNAPS. Mitral opening snaps can best be recorded approximately midway between the pulmonary and mitral areas, i.e., over the midprecordium.[72] High-frequency settings of the recording apparatus are preferred for these sounds. Tricuspid opening snaps can occasionally be recorded at the lower left sternal edge in the presence of tricuspid stenosis, atrial septal defect, or Ebstein's anomaly (Fig. 3–5).[46] Echophonocardiographic studies

show that opening snaps from either side of the heart occur at exactly the time of maximal opening of the respective atrioventricular valve in early diastole (Fig. 3–14).[73] Recognition of these relationships allows identification of sounds in this phase of the cardiac cycle with considerably more precision than has been possible with phonocardiography alone. The genesis of mitral and tricuspid opening snaps, once a fully open position of the valve is achieved, is of importance in the establishment of general principles of the genesis of sound, since it parallels the situation described above in connection with ejection sounds and their relationship to full opening of the semilunar valves. Opening snaps are characteristic of a stenotic though still pliable valve, but they are also seen in circumstances in which there is swift opening of a nonstenotic valve, such as occurs in severe mitral regurgitation or atrial septal defect.[74]

An acoustically similar sound is the tumor "plop" of a left atrial myxoma. This occurs when the tumor has moved in early diastole and comes to a sudden halt at the full extent of its excursion into the ventricle. The anatomical correlates of this sound can easily be demonstrated by echophonocardiography (Fig. 3–15).[8]

CLICK MURMUR SYNDROME (see also Chap. 31). The midsystolic click, which is one of the principal diagnostic features of prolapse of the mitral valve, has been

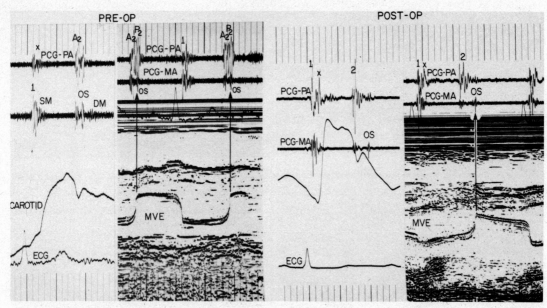

FIGURE 3–14   Mitral stenosis. The two left panels (pre-op) illustrate an opening snap (OS) occurring 0.04 sec after A_2, its identity confirmed by coincidence with full opening of the mitral valve (arrow). P_2 is visible only in the phonocardiogram at PA, occupying the space between A_2 and OS. An ejection sound (x) is seen in the tracing from the second left interspace (PA), reflecting pulmonary hypertension. Following successful valvulotomy (post-op), the OS moves out to 0.10 sec from A_2. The differences in carotid pulse wave contour in the two tracings are accounted for by technical imperfections in the pre-op record, since there was no evidence of aortic valve disease.

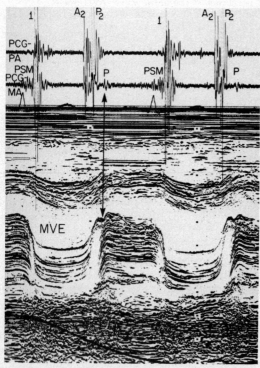

FIGURE 3–15   Left atrial myxoma. A young woman with a large myxoma resulting in symptoms of pulmonary congestion. S_1 is accentuated and delayed and is preceded by a brief "presystolic" crescendo murmur (PSM) occurring as the tumor mass (dense echoes in MVE) is thrust by ventricular contraction into the orifice of the mitral valve, thereby obstructing inflow from the atrium. P_2 is accentuated because of pulmonary hypertension and is widely transmitted to the cardiac apex (MA). It is followed by a tumor "plop" (P), which occurs 0.10 sec from A_2 and is coincident with completion of the ventricular excursion of the tumor mass (arrow).

shown to coincide with the time of maximal valve prolapse (Fig. 3–31).[75] This observation is consistent with the thesis advanced above that high-frequency sounds of cardiac origin occur when a valve has moved in response to hemodynamic forces and is suddenly checked in its course.

THIRD AND FOURTH HEART SOUNDS.   In contrast to S_1, S_2, ejection sounds, and opening snaps, which are predominantly of high frequency, third (S_3) and fourth (S_4), or atrial, sounds are of low frequency. The left-sided S_3 occurs in association with rapid filling of the ventricle, as in normal youthful subjects, mitral regurgitation (Fig. 3–1), or thyrotoxicosis.[76] In other pathological conditions, such as left ventricular failure, the term "gallop" is applied to the analogous sound,[77] but once again its pathogenesis is related to ventricular filling in early diastole. In pericardial constriction, ventricular filling is also confined to early diastole and terminates with a sharp S_3 or pericardial "knock" (Fig. 3–16).[78] In all these situations, the phonocardiogram records a low-frequency vibration (S_3) simultaneously with the peak of the rapid filling wave of the apex cardiogram. The echocardiographic correlation, however, is less helpful than with the high-frequency sounds discussed above. The third sound may be associated with a change in the E–F slope of mitral valve closure, but this probably reflects a change in the pattern of ventricular filling rather than being indicative of a direct causative relationship. The onset of the third heart sound has been reported to bear a close relationship to halting of the rapid posterior motion of the left ventricular wall in early diastole,[79] although this relationship has been questioned by other investigators.[80] Recent studies by Ozawa et al.[80a] attribute the sound to a sudden inherent limitation in the long axis filling movement of the left ventricle, a view consistent with traditional concepts dating from Potain in the nineteenth century.

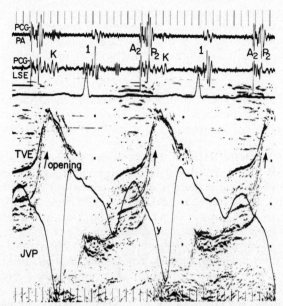

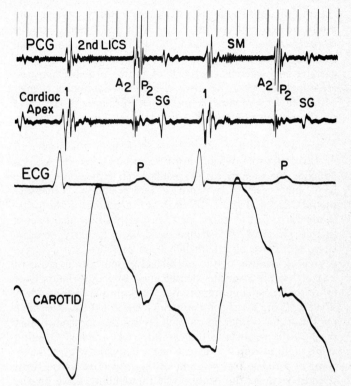

FIGURE 3–16 Pericardial knock. The relationship of the third sound or knock (K) associated with constrictive pericarditis to the jugular venous pulse (JVP) and movements of the tricuspid valve TVE is shown. The valve opens completely (arrows) before the knock. The latter, however, is closely related temporally to the nadir of the y descent of the JVP. P_2 is accentuated and widely transmitted, consistent with the pulmonary hypertension that was found at cardiac catheterization.

Fourth sounds, or atrial sounds, occur under circumstances of altered compliance of the ventricle, either left or right.[81] Thus, in coronary heart disease, HOCM, aortic stenosis, and systemic hypertension, a left-sided S_4 is a common feature (Fig. 3–17). A right-sided S_4 may be found under analogous circumstances, as in pulmonary hypertension or pulmonic valve stenosis.[82]

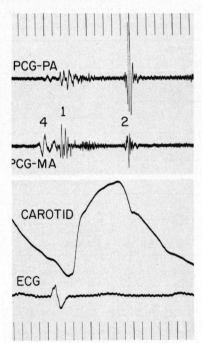

FIGURE 3–17 Fourth heart sound (4) in association with systemic hypertension and left ventricular hypertrophy. The low frequency of S_4 is apparent, compared with S_1 and S_2.

FIGURE 3–18 Summation sound, often called summation gallop, (SG) in a young woman with second-degree AV block characterized by Wenckebach periods. Atrial systole occurs in early diastole owing to the long P-R interval, and the augmented left ventricular filling results in a summation sound.

Identification of S_4 in a graphic tracing is best accomplished by noting its coincidence with the peak of the a wave in the accompanying apexcardiogram.[83] The echophonocardiogram is also less useful here than in identification of the high-frequency sounds discussed previously. The left-sided S_4 occurs during the phase of atrial reopening of the mitral valve and is temporally related to the a point of the mitral valve motion. The combination of a long P-R interval and a rapid heart rate may result in telescoping of diastolic events in such a way that third and fourth sounds may merge to form a loud summation sound (Fig. 3–18).[84]

ECHOPHONOCARDIOGRAPHY FOR THE IDENTIFICATION OF HEART SOUNDS. The finding on auscultation of two discrete sounds in quick succession at the onset of systole presents a common auscultatory problem. This combination could be due to normal splitting of S_1, with both mitral (M_1) and tricuspid (T_1) elements being well heard, as in normal youthful subjects (Figs. 3–2, 3–4, and 3–5), atrial septal defect, or right bundle branch block. Alternatively, a somewhat similar combination of sounds could be produced by S_4-S_1 or by S_1 and an ejection sound, as with a bicuspid aortic valve or valvular pulmonic stenosis (Figs. 3–11 to 3–14, and 3–17). A sequence of S_1 and an early systolic click of mitral origin can also present in this fashion. Although the associated findings, on physical examination, x-ray, and electrocardiogram may clarify this problem, one may wish to resort to echophonocardiography for a more certain solution. M_1 and T_1 can be identified by their coincidence with full closure of the mitral and tricuspid valves, respectively. Aortic and pulmonic ejection sounds occur with full opening of the respective semilunar valve. Fourth sounds, or atrial sounds, occur at the peak of the *a* wave of the apexcardiogram, whereas the click of mitral prolapse may be identified as occurring after the above-mentioned events. Mitral clicks sometimes coincide with prolapse of the valve on the echocardiogram, but this relationship is not invariable.

A similar problem often exists at the end of systole and in early diastole when various combinations of A_2, P_2, opening snaps, and third sounds from either side of the heart may lead to a confused interpretation of bedside physical signs (Figs. 3–14 to 3–16). Opening of the prosthetic valve in the mitral or tricuspid position also occurs in this phase of the cardiac cycle. A very early opening snap, indicative of a high left atrial pressure and a severe degree of stenosis of the mitral valve, may occur close to P_2, so that the accurate identification of these sounds is of more than academic importance. A_2 is most precisely identified as being synchronous with closure of the aortic valve on the echocardiogram as well as by its occurrence just prior to the incisura in the carotid artery tracing. Opening snaps and prosthetic valve sounds coincide with achievement of a fully open position of the respective valve; third sounds occur at the peak of the rapid filling wave on the apexcardiogram. P_2, then, is often identified by exclusion because of the difficulty in delineating closure of the pulmonic valve echocardiographically.

CONCEPTS OF THE GENESIS OF HEART SOUNDS. From the observations summarized in the preceding pages, we offer the following hypotheses to explain the origin of heart sounds that may be divided into high- and low-frequency categories. Of the high-frequency sounds, the first and second heart sounds are causally related to completed closure of the atrioventricular and similunar valves, respectively. High-frequency sounds occur at the time of complete opening of these valves and are recognized as ejection sounds or opening snaps. A high-frequency sound occurs at the time of completion of prolapse of the mitral valve in the mitral valve prolapse syndrome. The majority and possibly all of these sounds are valvular in origin. In contrast, low-frequency sounds are probably related to alterations in patterns of ventricular filling, which may in turn cause alterations in motion of the atrioventricular valves. Thus, the high-frequency sounds may be regarded as "valvular" and the low-frequency sounds as "ventricular."

FRICTION RUBS. The principal elements of a pericardial friction rub occur during those phases of the cardiac cycle in which there is maximal movement of the heart in the pericardial sac. These are atrial systole, ventricular systole, and passive ventricular filling in early diastole. This timing of auscultatory events can be portrayed graphically if desired. Unfortunately, however, phonocardiography does not reproduce the unique auscultatory quality of a rub, and therefore it usually adds nothing to a bedside assessment made by a competent examiner.

PROSTHETIC VALVE SOUNDS. Surgical implantation of prosthetic valves and pacemakers has resulted in a whole array of new auscultatory phenomena. The sounds produced by prostheses vary, depending on their location, their manner of opening and closing, and their constituents—plastic, steel, or biological tissues.[84a] In general, the metal balls used in Starr-Edwards valves produce the loudest, most distinctive sounds on both opening and closing.[85] Tilting disk valves (e.g., Björk-Shiley or Lillihei-Kaster) produce loud, crisp sounds on closing but little or no sound on opening.[86] Porcine heterograft valves produce a sound similar to that of a normal valve on closing, but they may open silently.[87] The timing of prosthetic valve movements may occasionally provide information regarding malfunction, since the movements of prostheses are in response to rapidly fluctuating pressures in adjacent heart chambers. For example, the expected time of opening of most of the currently used prostheses in the mitral posi-

Prosthesis type	Mitral Prosthesis	Acoustic Characteristics	Aortic Prosthesis	Acoustic Characteristics
Ball Valves	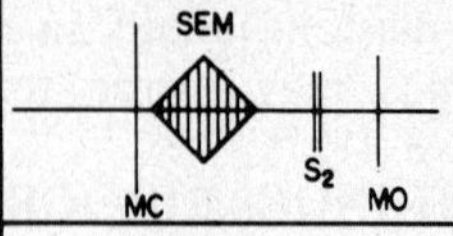 SEM	1) A_2–MO interval 0.07–0.11 sec. 2) MO > MC 3) II–III/VI Systolic ejection murmur (SEM) 4) No diastolic murmur	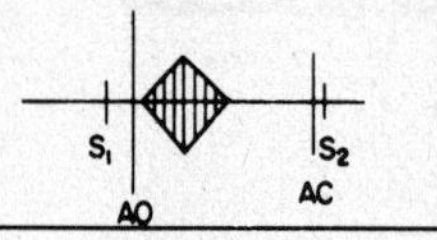 SEM	1) S_1–AO interval 0.07 sec. 2) AO > AC 3) II/VI harsh SEM 4) No diastolic murmur
Disc Valves	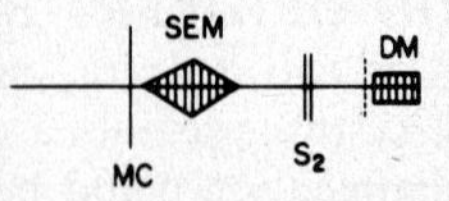 SEM DM	1) A_2–MO interval 0.05–0.09 sec. 2) MO is rarely heard 3) II/VI SEM is usually heard 4) I–II/VI diastolic rumble is usually heard	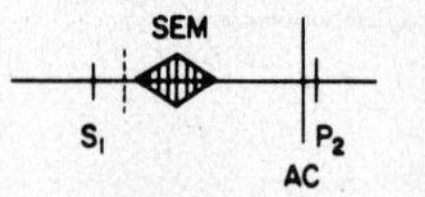 SEM	1) S_1–AO interval 0.04 sec. 2) AO is uncommonly heard, AC is usually heard 3) II/VI SEM is usually heard 4) Occasional diastolic murmur
Porcine Valves	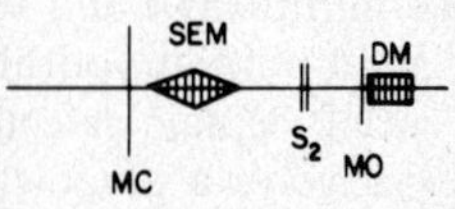 SEM DM	1) A_2–MO interval 0.1 sec. 2) MO is audible 50% 3) I–II/VI apical SEM 50% 4) Diastolic rumble $\frac{1}{2}$–$\frac{2}{3}$	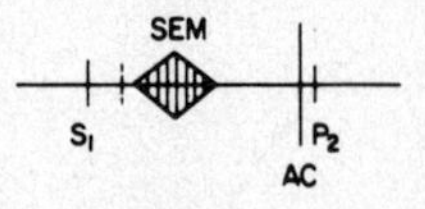 SEM	1) S_1–AO interval 0.03–0.08 sec. 2) AO is uncommonly heard, AC is usually heard 3) II/VI SEM in most 4) No diastolic murmur
Bileaflet Valve (St. Jude)			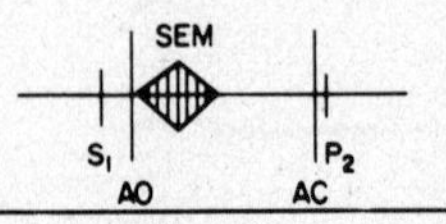 SEM	1) AO and AC commonly heard 2) A soft SEM is common

FIGURE 3–19 Summary of the acoustic characteristics of each valve prosthesis according to type and location. SEM = systolic ejection murmur; DM = diastolic murmur; S_1 = first heart sound; S_2 = second heart sound; P_2 = pulmonic second sound; A_2 = aortic second sound; AO = aortic valve opening sound; AC = aortic valve closure sound; MO = mitral valve opening sound; MC = mitral valve closure sound. (Reproduced with permission from Smith, N. D., Raizada, V., and Abrams, J.: Auscultation of the normally functioning prosthetic valve. Ann. Intern. Med. *95*:594, 1981.)

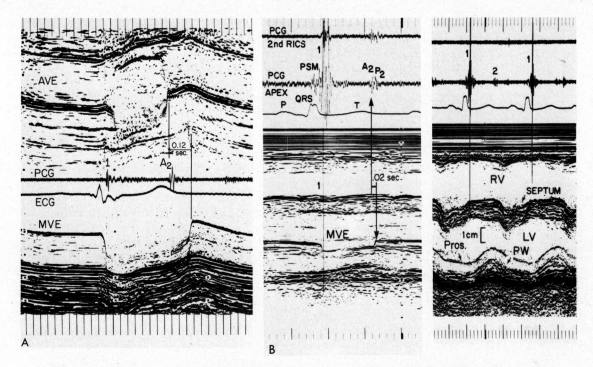

FIGURE 3–20 *A,* Echophonocardiogram from a patient with a normally functioning Lillihei-Kaster prosthesis in the mitral position. The dual echo shows the aortic valve above (AVE) and mitral prosthesis below (MVE). A_2 is coincident with aortic valve closure and is followed after 0.12 sec by full opening of the prosthesis.

B, Left, A Starr-Edwards prosthesis in the mitral position, malfunctioning due to thrombosis causing obstruction. The valve closes with a loud sound (1) preceded by a presystolic crescendo murmur (PSM) resembling that of mitral stenosis. The prosthesis opens only 0.02 sec after A_2, indicating an extremely short isovolumetric relaxation time, which in turn suggests a high left atrial pressure.

Right, In the same patient the echo shows a dilated right ventricle (RV) with paradoxical septal movement consistent with the clinically evident tricuspid regurgitation. The left ventricle (LV) is relatively small, a point discounting paravalvular leak and favoring obstruction at the valve level as an explanation for the suspected left atrial hypertension.

tion is approximately 0.08 sec following the aortic component of S_2 (Figs. 3–19 and 3–20A).[85-87] This period reflects the isovolumetric relaxation time of the left ventricle, and a major factor determining its length is left atrial pressure. Obstruction of the prosthesis by a thrombus or a paravalvular leak will produce elevation of left atrial pressure, and isovolumetric relaxation time will be abbreviated.[88] Once one has established that there may be malfunction of the prosthesis, differential diagnosis of mitral obstruction due to thrombosis from mitral regurgitation resulting from paravalvular leak requires a further step—examination of the left ventricular chamber by echocardiography. Obstruction of the valve simulates mitral stenosis, and one would expect to find no increase in ventricular size from control records and no evidence of hyperdynamic ventricular wall movements (Fig. 3–20B). With paravalvular leak, however, the stroke volume of the left ventricle will be augmented, resulting in exaggerated movements of the posterior wall of the left ventricle and normalization of the septal movements, which are ordinarily hypokinetic or even paradoxical following open-heart prosthetic valve surgery (Chap. 5).[89,90]

For an analysis of prosthetic valve function by the method described above, a combination of echo-and phonocardiography is necessary, since A_2 is detected on the sound record, and the opening of many of the valves in current use is silent and must be documented by a simultaneous echocardiogram.[88]

PACEMAKER SOUNDS. A sharp, high-frequency sound of very brief duration is occasionally audible overlying a transvenous pacemaker placed in the right ventricle. This sound, which may be accompanied by a slight twitch of skeletal muscle in the underlying area of the chest wall, is coincident with the pacemaker spike and is believed to arise from the stimulation of intercostal muscle.[91]

CAROTID PULSE TRACINGS

The carotid pulse is recorded by placement of the transducer firmly over the arterial pulsation, previously identified by palpation. As noted above, its prominence can be enhanced by hyperextension of the neck.

NORMAL CAROTID PULSE. The normal carotid pulse tracing (Figs. 3–1 and 3–2) has a rapid, smooth upstroke, beginning approximately 0.12 to 0.15 sec from the onset of the QRS complex in adults; it reaches a peak within 0.12 sec. Following the period of rapid ejection of blood from the left ventricle, the pulse wave declines to the dicrotic notch, or incisura, which is caused by aortic valve closure. Owing to the transmission time of the pulse wave from the aortic root to the site of application of the transducer over the carotid artery, there is a variable delay from the aortic closure sound, A_2, to the incisura of approximately 0.02 to 0.03 sec (Figs. 3–1 and 3–2). During diastole, the carotid pulse wave usually falls gently until the next systolic pulse. The shape of carotid pulse curves varies widely among different normal individuals and even in the same subject, depending on the mode of application of the transducer. Therefore experience with the range of normality in this, as well as in other laboratory tests, is necessary in order to appreciate truly abnormal curves and also to avoid erroneous diagnoses associated with normal variants.

APPLICATIONS OF CAROTID PULSE TRACINGS

Timing of Acoustic Events. The incisural notch occurs approximately 0.02 to 0.03 sec after aortic valve closure and A_2. Therefore the carotid pulse tracing is a reliable marker for this important auscultatory and phonocardiographic event (Figs. 3–1 and 3–2) and is a most valuable basic ingredient in the phonocardiographic examination.

Systolic Time Intervals

Systolic time intervals (STI) have been used sporadically for a century as a measure of left ventricular performance.[92–95] It is only in recent years however, that validation of the significance of STI has been obtained through comparative studies with various invasive indices of ventricular function (Chap. 14). This has led to widespread acceptance of STI as a simple, inexpensive, and nontraumatic method of estimating left ventricular performance and following the patient's progress over time. Many investigators have contributed to our rapidly increasing knowledge of the significance and utility of STI in clinical medicine. In particular, Weissler, Lewis, and associates have been responsible for popularization of this noninvasive method, and the reader is referred to their extensive publications for further details on the subject.[13,96–105,107,110]

The three basic STI are the preejection period (PEP), the left ventricular ejection time (LVET), and the total electromechanical interval (QS_2) (Fig. 3–21). In order to avoid misleading errors, the technique of recording must be carried out with meticulous attention to detail. STI are obtained from simultaneous fast-speed (100 mm/sec) recordings of the electrocardiogram, the phonocardiogram, and the carotid pulsation.[13] The ECG lead that most clearly displays the onset of left ventricular depolarization is

chosen. The phonocardiogram must provide a clear view of the initial high-frequency vibrations of the aortic component of the second heart sound (A_2). The carotid pulsation is generally recorded with a funnel-shaped pick-up attached by polyethylene tubing to a transducer with an adequate time constant, as discussed earlier in this chapter under Technique in Phonocardiography. For clear and accurate measurement of STI, one should employ tracings with the following characteristics: (1) a clear initial depolarization force departing acutely from a flat baseline on the electrocardiogram, to mark the beginning of QRS; (2) a sharp inscription of the initial high-frequency vibrations of A_2; and (3) a clearly discernible rapid upstroke and pointed single incisural notch on the carotid arterial pulse tracing. Amplification of the carotid signal should be adequate to provide a pulse wave of at least 5 cm in height.[98]

The QS_2 is measured from the onset of the QRS to the earliest high-frequency vibrations of A_2. LVET is measured from the beginning upstroke to the trough of the incisural notch of the carotid pulse tracing (Fig. 3–21). The PEP is that interval from the beginning of ventricular depolarization to the beginning of ventricular ejection. PEP is derived by subtracting LVET from QS_2, this step being necessary in order to eliminate the delay in transmission of the arterial pulse from the aortic root to the position on the carotid artery of the transducer. The PEP is made up of the electromechanical interval plus the isovolumetric contraction time. The electromechanical interval is relatively constant in most individuals, except where there is left ventricular conduction delay, as in left bundle branch block. Therefore, variations in isovolumetric contraction time constitute the principal information of physiological significance in measurements of the PEP.

In applying STI measurements, correction must be made for differences in heart rate. When heart rate is derived from the R-R interval, a simple linear equation best describes the relationship of STI to rate. The regression equations of Weissler have been generally adopted (Table 3–1) for this purpose.

In applying STI clinically, derivations from normal regressions can be indicated by expressing each of the systolic time intervals as an "index" value, as shown in Table 3–1. By calculating the index value, one obtains an estimate

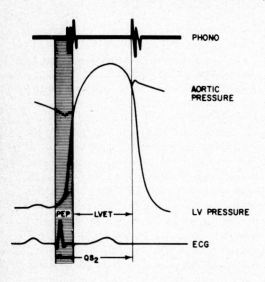

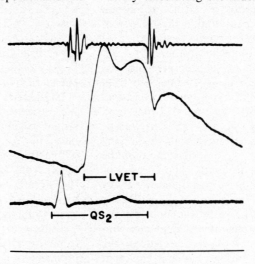

$$PEP = QS_2 - LVET$$

Figure 3–21 On the left is a diagram of the left ventricular events which constitute the STI. On the right is a recording of a phonocardiogram, external carotid pulse, and electrocardiogram at 100 mm/sec paper speed. The subintervals of the STI are indicated on both. (From Lewis, R. P., et al.: A critical review of the systolic time intervals. Circulation 56:146, 1977. By permission of the American Heart Association, Inc.)

TABLE 3–1   CALCULATION OF STI INDEX VALUES FROM RESTING REGRESSION EQUATIONS

Sex	Equation	Normal Index (msec)	SD
M	$QS_2I = 2.1\ hr + QS_2$	546	14
F	$QS_2I = 2.0\ hr + QS_2$	549	14
M	$LVETI = 1.7\ hr + LVET$	413	10
F	$LVETI = 1.6\ hr + LVET$	418	11
M	$PEPI = 0.4\ hr + PEP$	131	10
F	$PEPI = 0.4\ hr + PEP$	133	10

Key: I=index; SD=standard deviation; M=male; F=female; hr=heart rate.
From Weissler, A.M., et al.: Bedside technics for the evaluation of ventricular function in man. Am. J. Cardiol. *23*:577, 1969.

of the deviation from normal that cannot be explained by the heart rate. Thus, for example, a QS_2 index (QS_2I) of 506 msec in a man is easily recognized as being 40 msec shorter than the expected normal value of 546 msec.

At rates below 110 beats/min, the PEP and LVET shorten proportionately as heart rate increases. Therefore, a simple and increasingly popular method of expressing variations in STI in the normal range of heart rates is by the ratio of PEP/LVET. This ratio may identify left ventricular dysfunction when either the PEPI or the LVETI or both are still within the limits of normal. Since in many types of left ventricular dysfunction PEP lengthens and LVET shortens, higher ratios for PEP/LVET are abnormal. The PEP/LVET ratio is normally approximately 0.34 to 1,[98] with the upper limit being 0.42 to 1.[100]

Factors Influencing the STI. Factors known to influence the PEP and LVET are listed in Table 3–2. With left ventricular failure, regardless of cause, PEPI lengthens and LVETI shortens. Prolongation of PEPI is principally due to a reduced rate of left ventricular pressure rise during isovolumetric systole (LV dP/dt).[13] PEPI can also be prolonged by delayed electrical activation, as in LBBB. Under these circumstances, obviously a prolongation of PEPI cannot be used as an indicator of diminished left ventricular performance, since the problem may be simply due to electrical delay. An estimate of the delay can be obtained from the apexcardiogram.[96]

TABLE 3–2   FACTORS INFLUENCING SYSTOLIC TIME INTERVALS

	Increase (↑)	Decrease (↓)
PEP	LV muscle failure Left bundle branch block ↓Preload Negative inotropic agents	Aortic valve disease ↓LV isovolumic pressure Positive inotropic agents
LVET	Aortic valve disease ↓Afterload	LV muscle failure ↓Preload Positive inotropic agents Negative inotropic agents
QS₂	Left bundle branch block Aortic valve disease	Positive inotropic agents

From Lewis, R.P., et al.: A critical review of the systolic time intervals. Circulation *56*:146, 1977, by permission of the American Heart Association, Inc.

The shortening of LVETI that occurs with heart failure is a complex result of alterations in the rate and extent of fiber shortening of the left ventricle as well as delay in the onset of ejection due to prolongation of PEPI. Of these several factors, probably the most influential is a diminished extent of fiber shortening.[99] Thus, a shortened LVETI or abnormally elevated PEP/LVET ratio may be found in the presence of a diminished stroke volume. It is of interest to note that the absolute size of the stroke volume does not determine LVET, but rather the size of the stroke volume relative to the end-diastolic volume.[99] Studies relating the PEP/LVET ratio to left ventricular ejection fraction determined by quantitative angiography have shown a close correlation.[101] The relationship has been obtained in patients having valvular and nonvalvular heart disease with a wide variation in functional impairment.

The duration of systole (QS_2I) is remarkably constant for any individual patient. Many types of heart disease result in directionally opposite changes in PEPI and LVETI. QS_2I may therefore be relatively unaffected.[102] However, with inotropic stimulation, such as with digitalis or catecholamines, QS_2I is shortened.[103]

Clinical Applications of Systolic Time Intervals

EVALUATION OF LEFT VENTRICULAR PERFORMANCE IN CHRONIC MYOCARDIAL DISEASE.   In a wide variety of heart diseases involving the left ventricle, including myocarditis, cardiomyopathy, coronary artery disease, hypertensive heart disease, and mitral valve disease, a deterioration in left ventricular performance may be manifest in an elevated PEP/LVET ratio. As mentioned above, this ratio correlates best with the angiographic ejection fraction.[100,101,104] Frequently, when overt manifestations of heart failure have been eliminated with diuretics, the persisting severe left ventricular dysfunction continues to be reflected in an abnormal PEP/LVET ratio.[105] On the other hand, a fundamental change such as a subsidence of myocarditis or relief of a reversible cardiomyopathy can be monitored by means of a gradually falling PEP/LVET ratio in serial observations. The STI have been used to estimate prognosis in patients following healed myocardial infarction, with an abnormal PEP/LVET ratio being found to indicate a significantly worse prognosis over a 5-year period.[100] These results are consistent with the generally agreed upon observation that left ventricular function is a major prognostic factor in coronary artery disease.

AORTIC VALVE DISEASE.   In aortic valve disease, either stenosis or regurgitation, there is a shortening of PEPI and a lengthening of LVETI such that the PEP/LVET ratio tends to fall.[98] The PEPI is short in aortic stenosis owing to the rapid dP/dt and low aortic diastolic pressure. Significant outflow tract obstruction lengthens LVETI. This observation has led to the use of STI as an additional noninvasive parameter for estimating severity of aortic stenosis.[106] Where left ventricular dysfunction has complicated the course of aortic stenosis, opposing trends are found, with PEPI lengthening and LVETI shortening. The net result is that PEP/LVET cannot be reliably used to assess left ventricular function in aortic stenosis.

In aortic regurgitation there is also a shortening of PEPI because of the low diastolic pressure and a lengthening of

LVETI.[98] Although a tendency can be found for PEP/LVET to fall with severe aortic regurgitation, the quantitative value of such a measurement has not been established.

Use of STI in Clinical Pharmacology. One of the most promising areas for the use of STI in the future is in clinical pharmacology. Extensive studies have been performed demonstrating the effects of digitalis glycosides on STI.[107–109] These show that QS_2I responds by shortening in the presence of inotropic stimulation. Propranolol, on the other hand, has been shown to lengthen QS_2I when excessive adrenergic tone is present, and it has been suggested that the STI may become a useful measure for determining the adequacy of beta blockade of angina pectoris.[110] Similarly, the STI can be used to measure the cardiotoxic effect of antineoplastic agents[111,112] and of antiarrhythmic agents and the cardiostimulatory effects of dobutamine and of various vasodilators.

In summary, studies in the past 20 years have established that externally derived systolic time intervals accurately reflect their invasively determined counterparts. The STI have been shown to correlate well with widely accepted measures of left ventricular function, such as the ejection fraction, in a great variety of clinical disorders. The effects of an increasing array of pharmacological agents on the STI are being carefully evaluated, and results are being made available for clinical use. Therefore, STI have become a valuable adjunct to the clinical evaluation of patients and in following their course over prolonged periods, since the measurements are harmless and inexpen-

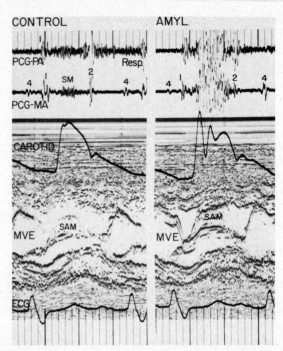

FIGURE 3–23 Hypertrophic obstructive cardiomyopathy (HOCM). *Left,* The control echophonocardiogram shows a fourth sound (4) at MA. The PCG-PA is obscured by a respiratory artifact (Resp). A midsystolic ejection murmur coincides with systolic anterior movement of the MVE (SAM). The carotid pulse contour is within normal limits. *Right,* Following inhalation of amyl nitrate (AMYL) the murmur becomes louder and the carotid pulse becomes deformed with a spike-and-dome pattern characteristic of HOCM. These changes are coincident with a more prominent SAM, which appears to be in contact with the interventricular septum.

sive. The method, like any laboratory test, can be abused if performed indiscriminately or with less than impeccable techniques and instrumentation. Only temporal data are obtained by STI. Therefore, the method is not useful in differential diagnosis, since heart diseases of a variety of etiologies have similarly disturbed measurements. Valvular disease such as aortic stenosis or regurgitation affects the STI profoundly and often in a direction opposite to the effects of myocardial disease. The same is true of certain drugs and catecholamines. Therefore, these deceptively simple measurements actually require a very sophisticated overall appreciation of the entire clinical and pharmacological situation if they are to be used effectively and in the patient's best interest.

CAROTID PULSE CONTOUR PATTERNS

Variability in morphological and temporal details of the carotid pulse may result from technical aspects of the recording, including the choice and application of transducers.[13] In spite of these problems, however, a considerable amount of qualitative information can be derived from alterations in carotid pulse wave tracings in various disease states. A slowly rising carotid pulse deformed by a shudder—the graphic representation of a thrill—is characteristic of valvular or subvalvular diaphragmatic aortic stenosis (Fig. 3–22). Unfortunately, efforts to quantitate the severity of aortic stenosis by the contour of the carotid pulse, the rapidity of its upstroke, or the achievement of its peak[106] have been disappointing.[113] In elderly patients with arterio-

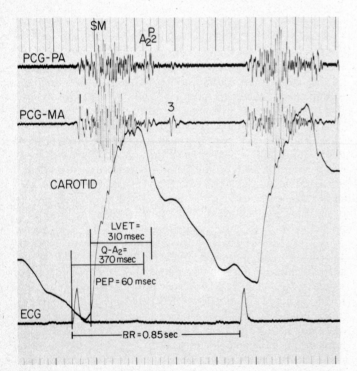

FIGURE 3–22 Valvular aortic stenosis in an 11-year-old boy with moderately severe obstruction (gradient=50 to 60 mm Hg across the aortic valve). A loud midsystolic murmur is seen in all valve areas. The carotid upstroke is delayed and shattered by coarse vibrations. A_2 is well preserved. A third sound (3) is present, probably a normal finding in this youthful subject. The STI indicate a short PEP and prolonged LVET.[13]

sclerotic and therefore inelastic peripheral vasculature, the upstroke of the carotid pulse may be relatively swift despite severe obstruction. Conversely, in some cases of severe aortic regurgitation without any systolic gradient across the valve, the physical and graphic signs during systole may nevertheless simulate those of aortic stenosis.

A spike-and-dome pattern characterizes the carotid pulse wave of HOCM (Fig. 3–23). A bisferiens pulse is characteristic of aortic regurgitation or mixed aortic stenosis and regurgitation (Fig. 3–24). A large dicrotic wave is sometimes seen in cardiomyopathy and other low-output conditions such as postoperatively in valve replacement for aortic or mitral regurgitation (Fig. 3–25).[114,115] Further examples of the use of carotid pulse tracings in combination with other noninvasive techniques, including echocardiograms, are illustrated in Chapter 4.

Abnormalities of Pulse Frequency, Regularity, and Amplitude

Inequality of Pulses. By using two pulse-sensitive transducers simultaneously, one can document inequality of the carotid pulses in arteriosclerotic occlusive disease, dissecting aneurysm, or supravalvular aortic stenosis. Diminished amplitude and delay in the femoral arterial pulse in coarctation of the aorta can be demonstrated by the simultaneous recording of the femoral and the brachial or carotid pulses.

Changes in Amplitude with Normal Rhythm. The reduction in amplitude of the pulse on inspiration character-

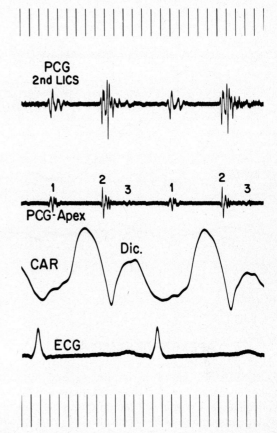

FIGURE 3–25 Dicrotic wave (Dic.) in the pulse tracing of a man with cardiomyopathy.

istic of *paradoxical pulse* is readily documented by carotid pulse recording performed in conjunction with a pneumogram. The patient should be instructed to breathe slowly and more deeply than usual during the registration of this phenomenon.

Pulsus alternans can also be confirmed by arterial pulse tracings and is often accentuated during the first few beats following a premature ventricular beat (Fig. 3–26). Since the peripheral pulses are more sensitive for the detection of pulsus alternans than is the carotid pulse, one may find it useful to apply the pulse transducer over the femoral artery. The graphic record demonstrates not only the alternating height of the pulse waves but also a beat-to-beat alteration in the rate of rise of the pulse wave as well as in systolic time intervals. The stronger beats display a shorter PEP and longer LVET and therefore a lower PEP/LVET ratio than do the weaker beats, reflecting the higher level of the contractile state in the former.[116]

Ectopic Rhythms. With ventricular tachycardia, variations in the amplitude of the pulse from beat to beat reflect the rapidly changing sequence of atrial and ventricular systole and the results of more effective ventricular contraction when fortuitously there is a properly timed atrial systole. The totally irregular rhythm and beat-to-beat changes in the amplitude of the pulse characteristic of atrial fibrillation can be documented by carotid pulse tracings. Similarly, the ineffective systoles occasioned by premature beats are easily demonstrable.

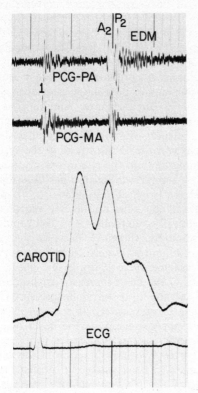

FIGURE 3–24 Pulsus bisferiens in aortic regurgitation. The carotid pulse is bifid, and there is a large excursion reflecting the wide pulse pressure. The phonocardiogram establishes that both humps of the carotid pulse are systolic in time (i.e., prior to A₂), thus separating the bisferiens pulse from a large dicrotic wave (Fig. 3–27), with which it may be confused at the bedside. There is no incisura, owing to aortic incompetence. EDM = early diastolic murmur.

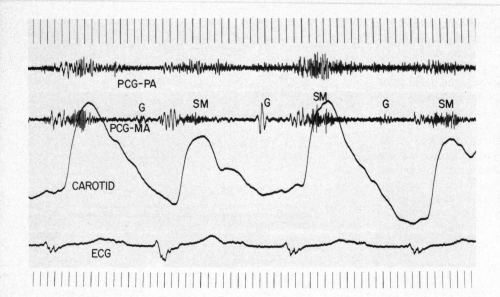

FIGURE 3–26 Pulsus alternans in a man with aortic stenosis and left ventricular failure. The first and third beats are of greater amplitude than are the second and fourth beats. The stronger beats are also marked by a louder murmur (SM) and less abnormality of STI. The diastolic sound (G) is louder after the second (weak) beat. It is a summation sound caused by merging of S_3 and S_4, resulting from the combined effect of a rapid heart rate and a prolonged P-R interval.

APEXCARDIOGRAPHY[117]

TECHNIQUE. The apex impulse is best appreciated on palpation as well as for recording purposes by having the patient lie in a partial left lateral decubitus position. A triangular supporting pillow beneath the back promotes comfort and relaxation. The optimal registration of the apexcardiogram may require that the patient hold his breath in partial exhalation. The transducer funnel or tambour may be held by hand over the left ventricular apex. Alternatively, a strap can be used to hold the transducer in place, but this technique makes it more difficult to keep the device in proper position. The transducer used in apexcardiography senses the *relative* position of the diaphragm of the transducer with respect to its rim. (With a funnel device, the skin serves as a diaphragm.) Thus, ordinarily the rim of the sensing head of the transducer rests on the ribs, and its diaphragm moves with the soft tissues in the intercostal space. Reproducibility in recording the apexcardiogram is adversely affected by differences in the patient's position, the pressure with which the transducer is applied, and, most of all, failure to place the transducer precisely over the point of maximum impulse. Other methods of recording precordial motion include kinetocardiography[118] and cardiokymography.[119] These methods avoid the problem of relative movement of the chest wall with respect to the rim of the transducer mentioned above and record, instead, absolute movement. Kinetocardiography accomplishes this by attaching the transducer to a fixed point in space, a technique that is useful but too cumbersome for routine use. Cardiokymography employs a capacitance transducer that is held slightly separated from the chest wall.[119] The apparatus is light and easily applied and has recently been found to be of value in detecting wall-motion abnormalities after exercise in patients with ischemic heart disease.[120] Although each of these techniques is useful, space does not permit a discussion of the normal patterns and variations observed in disease states. The following paragraphs therefore will deal with apexcar-

diography, which is the most widely used method of recording precordial movement.

NORMAL APEXCARDIOGRAM. The apexcardiogram is a graphic representation of precordial movement. As the name implies, it is usually recorded over the left ventricular apex.[117] However, the same technique and equipment can be used to record movements at the left sternal edge, reflecting right ventricular hypertrophy or pulsations of a dilated pulmonary artery.[82,121] The heave resulting from an anteriorly situated ventricular aneurysm can also be appreciated.

The physiological correlations of the major landmarks of the apexcardiogram have been carefully worked out by Willems et al.[122,123] by means of simultaneous registration of the left ventricular apexcardiogram and high-fidelity left ventricular pressures in dogs. These studies showed a very precise synchronism in the upstroke of the systolic wave of the apexcardiogram and the rise in left ventricular pressure (Fig. 3–27). A similar relationship has been reported in humans.[124] The early diastolic nadir or "0"-point in the apexcardiogram and that in the left ventricular pressure are also practically simultaneous.[122] The rapid upstroke of the apexcardiogram therefore initiates the isovolumetric phase of systole and is largely completed during this portion of the cardiac cycle. During this phase the external circumference of the heart increases as the ventricle changes its shape and the intraventricular pressure rises. The upstroke terminates in normal subjects with the "E"-point, which occurs approximately at the onset of ejection. The E-point, however, is often obliterated in disease states that result in hypertrophy or dysfunction of the ventricle. During the remainder of systole in normal subjects, the apexcardiogram describes a declining plateau as the volume of the heart diminishes. A more abrupt decline begins to occur just before the second heart sound. A nadir or 0-point is reached in early diastole at approximately the time of opening of the mitral valve. This is followed by a rapid filling wave and a slow filling wave, reflecting analogous events in the left ventricular pressure curve. In late diastole, the *a* wave is recorded, reflecting movement of a small amount of blood into the left ventricle as a result of atrial systole. In normal subjects the *a* wave is of modest height, usually less than 15 per cent in amplitude with respect to the total height of the apexcardiogram.

In a combined tracing, with phonocardiograms and carotid pulse tracing, the systolic upstroke of the apexcardiogram can be used to divide the preejection period into its two major components—the electromechanical interval and the isovolumetric contraction time (Fig. 3–27). Such a division would be useful in LBBB, in which the electromechanical interval might constitute a disproportionate part of the PEP. The 0-point in early diastole should not be used as a marker for mitral valve opening, since its relation to this event is only an approximation, and a more accurate reflection of valve movement is provided by the echocardiogram (Figs. 3–4 and 3–14). The diastolic waves of the apexcardiogram, i.e., the rapid filling wave and the *a* wave, are the low-frequency counterparts of the third and fourth, or atrial, sounds, respectively. Therefore the apexcardiogram can be used to identify diastolic auscultatory events (Figs. 3–28 and 3–30).

APEXCARDIOGRAPHY IN DISEASE. The systolic portion of the apexcardiogram has only a limited number of patterns of diagnostic utility. These can be broadly clas-

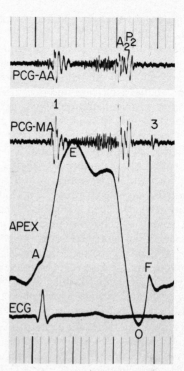

FIGURE 3–28 Hyperdynamic apexcardiogram in mitral regurgitation. The configuration of the tracing in systole is qualitatively similar to a normal curve, although the amplitude was clearly exaggerated by palpation. The rapid filling wave (F) is higher than normal and terminates in a sharp point coincident with its audible counterpart, the third heart sound (3).

sified as (1) *normal* (described above), (2) *hyperdynamic*, and (3) *sustained.*[125]

Hyperdynamic movement is perceived at the bedside as a thrust of exaggerated height but one which falls away immediately from the palpating fingers. It is found in conditions characterized by an increased stroke volume such as in normal subjects after exercise, in thyrotoxicosis, or in mitral regurgitation (Fig. 3–28).[125,126] The graphic tracing shows a systolic wave of normal shape but of increased amplitude (although this is difficult to measure) and a prominent rapid filling wave.

The *sustained* impulse is the graphic equivalent of a heave or thrust, as may be found in left ventricular hypertrophy, such as that associated with hypertension or aortic stenosis (Fig. 3–29). The systolic portion of a sustained apical impulse is characterized by a plateau or a dome-shaped or rising curve, in contrast to the gentle systolic decline seen in the normal or hyperdynamic tracing. An accompanying finding is a prominent *a* wave. A somewhat similar heave is found in cardiomyopathy or chronic ischemic heart disease. A variant of the sustained impulse occurs in HOCM, in which the systolic portion may be bifid in configuration preceded by a large *a* wave, thus giving a triple-humped appearance (Fig. 3–30).

In the mitral prolapse or click murmur syndrome, a collapse or deep notch in the apex impulse may occasionally be noted coinciding with the click as recorded on an accompanying phonocardiogram (Fig. 3–31).[127] Left atrial myxoma may cause a very deep notch on the systolic upstroke of the apexcardiogram. This notch occurs at the time of extrusion of the tumor from ventricle to atrium

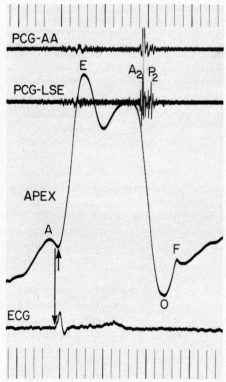

FIGURE 3–27 Normal apexcardiogram. A low-amplitude *a* wave (A) in presystole follows the P wave of the ECG, which is not visible in this lead. The onset of the QRS (downward arrow) is followed after a brief electromechanical interval (0.02 sec) by the onset of the swift upward movement of the apex tracing (upward arrow), culminating in the E point at approximately the time of beginning ejection into the aorta. A generally declining curve during systole ends with an abrupt downward fall at the time of A_2. The nadir (0) is reached at approximately the time of mitral valve opening. The rapid filling wave (F) occurs during early diastolic filling of the left ventricle.

and is accompanied by audible vibrations that prolong the intense first heart sound.[128]

Exaggeration of the height of the rapid filling wave and assumption of a sharper configuration of its peak are characteristic of mitral regurgitation or left-to-right shunts such as patent ductus arteriosus and ventricular septal defect, which result in augmentation of ventricular filling in early diastole (Fig. 3–28). Unfortunately, owing to the wide range of normal findings, as well as the difficulty in quantitating apexcardiogram, there is no clear cut-off point between the pathological conditions listed above and the prominent rapid filling wave seen in a healthy young subject who might be expected to have a normal third heart sound. Similarly, a heightened *a* wave is found in a variety of conditions having in common diminished compliance of the left ventricle.[81,129] These include left ventricular hypertrophy, as in systemic hypertension, aortic stenosis, and HOCM; or myocardial disease, as in ischemic heart disease and cardiomyopathy (Figs. 3–29 and 3–30). The height of the *a* wave is generally estimated from the ratio of "*a*" to the total amplitude of the apexcardiogram "H", as in Figure 3–30. In normal individuals a small *a* wave (<15 per cent of the total amplitude) is found.[129] In many conditions in which the *a* wave is prominent, however, such as in aortic stenosis, the systolic portion of the apexcardiogram is proportionately exaggerated, so that the ratio may remain normal. Absence of an *a* wave is to be expected in conditions that limit inflow into the left ventricle, such as mitral stenosis and constrictive pericarditis. In the important, although unusual, circumstance of acute severe aortic regurgitation in which left ventricular pressure exceeds left atrial pressure in the latter part of diastole, with resulting pre-

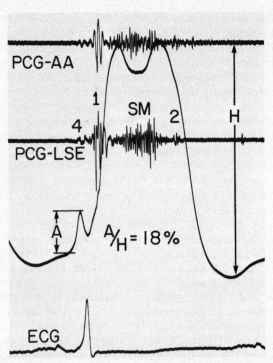

FIGURE 3–30 Apexcardiogram in HOCM. The *a* wave (A) is exaggerated in height, being 18 per cent of the entire amplitude of the apexcardiogram (H), and has an unusually rapid upstroke that culminates in a sharp peak, coinciding with the fourth heart sound (4). The systolic phase of the apexcardiogram has a bifid appearance with a prominent late systolic hump. The saddle-shaped decline in midsystole coincides in time with the systolic murmur and carotid pulse deformity, which, in turn, are related to the obstruction occasioned by the systolic anterior motion of the mitral valve, as illustrated in Figure 3–23.

mature closure of the mitral valve in diastole, the *a* wave is also absent.[130,131]

PULSATILE MOVEMENTS IN OTHER PRECORDIAL LOCATIONS. Following preliminary examination by palpation, useful patterns of precordial movement may be obtained by placement of the transducer over locations other than the apex.

Normal Right Ventricular Movement. In children, a gentle thrust can be appreciated in the third and fourth interspaces at the left sternal edge.[14] Tracings obtained at this location are qualitatively similar to the normal apexcardiogram, although of low amplitude. By this noninvasive method, an electromechanical interval of 0.03 sec from onset of the QRS of the electrocardiogram to the beginning of right ventricular systole in normal children has been established.[14] In older normal subjects it is usually impossible to feel or record a right ventricular impulse.

Right Ventricular Hypertrophy. In right ventricular hypertrophy a heave at the left sternal edge can be perceived by palpation.[82,132] This can usually be recorded with the patient supine and the sensing head of the transducer firmly applied to the interspace where the systolic impulse has been detected. Occasionally in emphysematous patients, the optimal site may be just beneath the xiphoid.

Pulmonary Hypertension. When severe pulmonary hypertension has been present sufficiently long to produce right ventricular hypertrophy, the right apexcardiogram demonstrates a sustained movement in systole.[82] This sys-

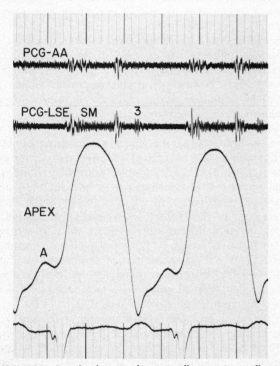

FIGURE 3–29 Sustained type of apexcardiogram in cardiomyopathy. The systolic portion of the tracing is dome-shaped, the graphic representation of a heave. It is preceded by a prominent *a* wave (A). The PCG shows a holosystolic murmur (SM) and a third sound (3).

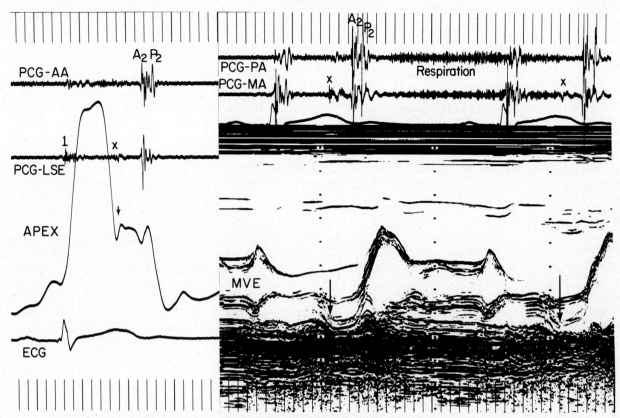

FIGURE 3-31 Mitral valve prolapse. The apexcardiogram (APEX) on the left shows a notch (arrow) in midsystole at the time of the click (X), followed by a plateau. In the echophonocardiogram on the right, X coincides with the downward movement or prolapse of the valve (arrow).

tolic thrust is usually preceded by a large *a* wave in presystole, reflecting altered compliance of the hypertrophied ventricle. Other manifestations of pulmonary hypertension may include forceful pulsations of the dilated pulmonary artery[29,121] and increased amplitude of P_2, signs which may be palpated and recorded at the upper left sternal edge. The arterial origin of the pulsatile tracing in this location can be determined by the delayed timing of its upstroke with reference to a simultaneously obtained electrocardiographic Q wave. This affords an opportunity to record right ventricular ejection time by a noninvasive method. The heave of the right ventricle itself is perceived lower along the left sternal edge and follows the Q wave more closely after a usual electromechanical interval of only ± 0.03 sec.[14]

Pulmonic Stenosis (see also pp. 986 and 1037). In children with valvular pulmonic stenosis, precordial movement over the right ventricle may provide a valuable ancillary means of estimating the severity of the obstruction. When right ventricular systolic pressure exceeds approximately 60 mm Hg, one can usually record a convex or sustained systolic movement at the left sternal edge.[132] Usually the systolic expansion is preceded by an *a* wave of increased size, reflecting altered compliance of the hypertrophied ventricle. The accompanying phonocardiogram from the pulmonary area demonstrates a wide separation of A_2 and P_2, as mentioned above.[57]

Tetralogy of Fallot (see also pp. 990 and 1034). Although the degree of infundibular stenosis in this condition may be extreme and right ventricular pressures are equal to those on the left, the precordial movement in cyanotic children with tetralogy of Fallot is remarkably quiet.[117] There is usually a brief shock or vibration that can be palpated and recorded at the time of S_1 and S_2. The systolic phase is marked by a plateau or even a concave pattern in the graphic record. There is no atrial sound and no exaggeration of the *a* waves in the right apexcardiogram or the jugular venous pulse tracing. These differences in the pulsatile records in cyanotic forms of tetralogy of Fallot and pure valvular pulmonic stenosis probably result from the escape route afforded by the right-to-left shunt through the septal defect, which may serve to decompress the right ventricle.

Tricuspid Regurgitation (see also pp. 1, 17). Tricuspid regurgitation usually appears as a complication of left-sided disease such as mitral stenosis with pulmonary hypertension. Under these circumstances a right ventricular heave may be appreciated on palpation and in graphic records, as described above (see Fig. 3-37).[133] In pure tricuspid regurgitation in which the valve has been destroyed by infective endocarditis or injured by trauma but in which pulmonary hypertension is absent, a different precordial pulsatile pattern is encountered. The grossly evident precordial "heave" proves to be *diastolic* in time, whereas systole is marked by a retraction or inward movement (Fig. 3-32).[117,133,134] These events mirror the massive filling and emptying of the right ventricle and graphically appear as a mirror image of the pulsatile movements of the great veins and the liver.

Constrictive Pericarditis (see also Chap. 43). Although in some longstanding cases of constrictive pericarditis the precordium may be immobile, a little appreciated

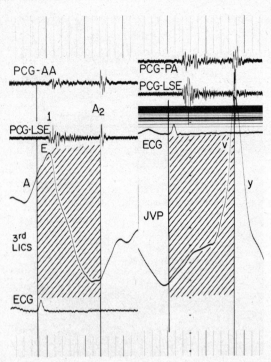

FIGURE 3–32 Precordial movement in pure tricuspid regurgitation in a young woman with infective endocarditis on the tricuspid valve due to heroin addiction. The right ventricular impulse tracing (left) taken at the left sternal edge shows a brief outward (upward) move during the isovolumetric phase of systole (E), merging with the preceding *a* wave. This is followed by a deep inward (downward) movement during the remainder of systole, reflecting reduction of right ventricular volume. Systole is shaded to facilitate comparison with JVP (right), which shows a reciprocal relationship to the precordial pattern, with a large late systolic *v* wave due to tricuspid regurgitation.

but frequently encountered sign is an inward systolic movement, as in pure tricuspid regurgitation (Fig. 3–33).[134] The outward heave is in early diastole and corresponds in time to the pericardial knock. Palpation alone may be misleading, with inadvertent inversion of the phases of the cardiac cycle, unless one is careful to use the heart sounds or the carotid pulse as a temporal landmark. An explanation for the unusual pattern of precordial movement in constrictive pericarditis has been provided by El-Sharif and El-Said, who propose that the pulsatile record is a reflection of filling and emptying of the heart, its usual outward thrust during the isovolumetric phase of systole being inhibited by the constriction.[135]

Left Ventricular Aneurysm (see Chap. 38). A large anterior myocardial infarction may lead to formation of an aneurysm with a palpable systolic heave in an ectopic location, usually over the midprecordium. Graphic records over such a bulge made with the patient supine usually reveal a bifid impulse made up of a large *a* wave followed by a sustained plateau during ventricular systole.[136] This finding in association with a QS pattern in precordial electrocardiographic leads and persistent ST elevation is strongly suggestive of aneurysm. Regarding the physiological derangement, additional information obtained by noninvasive means is provided by systolic time intervals. Prolongation of PEP and shortening of LVET accurately predict a seriously disturbed state of left ventricular function.[100]

Mitral Regurgitation (see also Chap. 31). In severe mitral regurgitation, either acute or chronic, there may be a striking lift of the whole precordium in systole. This is attributed to expansion of the posteriorly located left atrium, causing the heart to push forward against the thoracic cage. This movement peaks late in systole coincident with the *v* wave in the left atrial pressure pulse and thus differs morphologically from the more localized heave of right ventricular hypertrophy, which reaches its maximal height earlier in systole.[137]

SUMMARY. In summary, although the time of onset of the swift upstroke and the diastolic nadir of the left ventricular pressure pulse as well as certain diastolic details are accurately depicted in the apexcardiogram, the morphology of the tracings is extremely complex and as yet incompletely understood. Many factors such as ballistic recoil of the heart, filling and emptying, rotation, and the manner of coupling to the chest wall as well as technical factors with regard to equipment and application of transducers affect the curves. However, it is encouraging that a more rational explanation of the apexcardiogram is emerging from the carefully controlled studies in which the various features of the apex tracings are related to hemodynamic data[82,122,123,138] and that other methods of analysis, such as cardiokymography, are proving to be of diagnostic utility in ischemic heart disease.[120] Thus, it is possible that graphic studies of precordial motion may cease to be regarded as a minor empirical adjunct to noninvasive assessment and may assume a more important role in cardiac diagnosis.

JUGULAR VENOUS PULSE (JVP)

TECHNIQUE. The jugular venous pulse is recorded by pressing the funnel of the pulse transducer in the fossa above the clavicle between the attachments of the sternocleidomastoid muscle. Care must be taken to direct the transducer to exclude, if possible, the underlying arterial pulsation. The venous pulse obtained in this manner closely resembles the pressure curve of the right atrium.

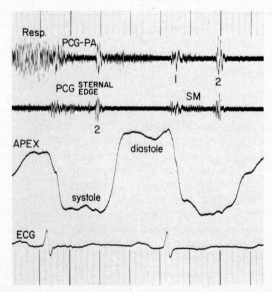

FIGURE 3–33 Precordial movement in constrictive pericarditis. The precordium moves inward (downward on graphic record) during systole and outward during diastole, probably resulting from volume changes in the right ventricle.[135]

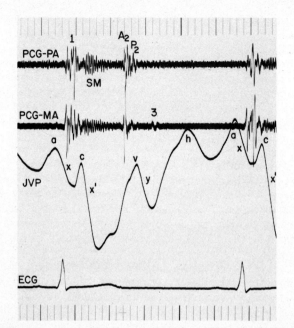

FIGURE 3–34 Normal jugular venous pulse (JVP) tracing in a young person with a functional systolic murmur (SM). The major features of the JVP are as follows: *a* wave, resulting from right atrial systole; *x* descent, atrial relaxation; *c* wave, tricuspid closure resulting from right ventricular contraction; *x′* descent, descent of the base plus continuing effect of atrial relaxation, associated with antegrade flow from the great veins; *v* wave, passive accumulation of blood in the right atrium while tricuspid valve is closed; *y* descent, filling of the right ventricle following opening of the tricuspid valve; *h* wave, a stasis wave in the venous system, apparent only at slower heart rates.

le and emptying of the atrium, the *v* wave collapses, providing in graphic tracings the *y* descent—a prominent negative wave. In normal subjects the *y* descent is not of the magnitude of the *x′* descent described above. In subjects with slow heart rates there may be another positive wave (*h*) later in diastole, resulting from passive distention of the venous system (Fig. 3–34).[139]

ABNORMALITIES OF THE JVP. In all efforts to use the JVP in cardiac diagnosis, the enormous variability of the pulse contour and relative height and depth of its constituents must be realized. This is true among different subjects as well as in the same patient on successive occasions or with minor alterations in technique. Therefore only rather gross alterations in pulse morphology as described below can be utilized safely if one is to avoid overreading the tracings. Nevertheless, examination of the venous pulse either at the bedside or in graphic records has a long history of utility in assessing arrhythmias and in anticipating physiological derangements involving the right side of the heart. In circumstances in which there is some impediment to right atrial systole, as with tricuspid stenosis or right ventricular hypertrophy resulting from pulmonic valvular stenosis or pulmonary hypertension, the *a* wave may increase in amplitude (Fig. 3–35). Persistent or intermittent *exaggeration of the a wave* may also reflect contraction of the atrium against a closed tricuspid valve due to electrocardiographic abnormalities that distort the usual sequence of atrioventricular (AV) contraction. These include AV nodal and ventricular tachycardia, premature ventricular beats, and atrioventricular dissociation (Fig. 3–

NORMAL JVP. The normal JVP consists of three peaks (*a, c,* and *v*) and three descents (*x, x′,* and *y*) (Fig. 3–34).[139,140] The *a* wave is the result of right atrial systole. It follows the P wave of the electrocardiogram and is slightly delayed from its counterpart in the right atrial pressure pulse by transmission to the jugular venous system. Relaxation of the atrium results in an insignificant downward movement, the *x* descent. In patients with a normal P-R interval, the *x* descent is quickly interrupted by a second peak of minor dimension, the *c* wave. This occurs as a result of tricuspid valve closure and therefore accompanies T_1, or the tricuspid component of the first heart sound. The *c* wave is often confused in JVP recordings because of interference from the underlying carotid arterial pulse. Its identity as a separate and distinct wave can be clarified in circumstances in which the carotid pulse is delayed, as in left bundle branch block.[141]

Following the *c* wave, there is in normal subjects a prominent *x′* descent, a downward movement which usually dominates the venous pulse record. The *x′* descent occurs during ventricular systole and is attributed to the "descent of the base"—a movement of the atrial floor in the direction of the ventricle due to contraction of the latter chamber. A mass of blood is thus drawn in an antegrade direction from the venous system to the right atrium, with resulting collapse of the JVP.[142] There follows, during the latter portion of ventricular systole, a positive wave *v*, which results from passive accumulation of blood in the right atrium while the triscuspid valve remains closed. With opening of the tricuspid valve in early diasto-

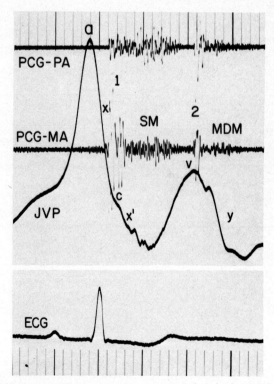

FIGURE 3–35 Jugular venous pressure (JVP) in mitral stenosis with pulmonary hypertension. The JVP is dominated by a very large *a* wave resulting from diminished compliance of the right ventricle associated with pulmonary hypertension. The peaked *a* wave represents a brief period of retrograde flow from right atrium to great veins.[141]

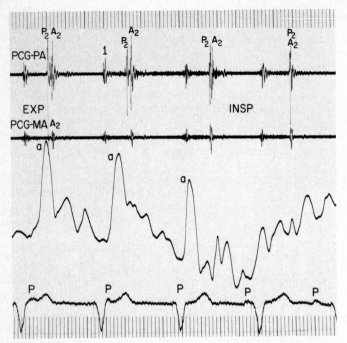

FIGURE 3-36 Jugular venous pressure (JVP) showing "cannon" *a* waves in a patient with a transvenous pacemaker in the right ventricle. In the first three cycles, atrial systole coincides with ventricular systole, so that the right atrium is contracting against a closed tricuspid valve. There is reversed splitting of S₂, with P₂ preceding A₂ in expiration (EXP), but narrowing of separation occurs with inspiration (INSP).

36). An intermittent accentuation of the *a* wave in ventricular tachycardia indicates that atria and ventricles are out of phase, and it may therefore be of some help in certain clinical circumstances in distinguishing ventricular tachycardia from atrial tachycardia with bundle branch block. A prominent *a* wave may be found in association with *left*

ventricular hypertrophy, presumably reflecting encroachment by the hypertrophied interventricular septum on the right ventricle—the Bernheim effect.

In tricuspid regurgitation, the *v* wave is unusually prominent, the *x'* descent becomes shallower, and with increasing hemodynamic deterioration the *c* and *v* waves merge to form a prominent ascending plateau (Fig. 3–37). Under these circumstances the *v* wave no longer reflects merely the normal passive accumulation of blood in the right atrium and venous system while the tricuspid valve is closed in systole; rather, it is due to a massive retrograde wave through an incompetent valve into the great veins. Unfortunately, the time-honored custom of using the letter *v* for both the normal systolic peak and the abnormal regurgitant wave when the valve is incompetent has interfered with understanding the genesis of these waves of the JVP in health and disease.

The *x* descent that results from atrial relaxation is seldom of any prominence and can reach significant proportions only when atrial and ventricular systoles are separated, as with a long P-R interval or in complete heart block.

The *x'* descent is normally one of the most prominent features of the JVP. It becomes shallow or is eliminated in tricuspid regurgitation. It may be deep in some cases of constrictive pericarditis.[143]

The *y* descent is less steep in tricuspid stenosis. Unfortunately, this assessment must be subjective, since the waves of the JVP cannot be quantitated and the relative swiftness of their movements is dependent on apparatus, technique, and paper speed. In constrictive pericarditis, however, a rapid, deep *y* descent interrupting an otherwise high plateau of the venous pulse provides a pattern familiar to hemodynamicists, since it simulates the "square-root sign" recorded in diastolic pressure tracings from all the heart chambers (Fig. 3–38).

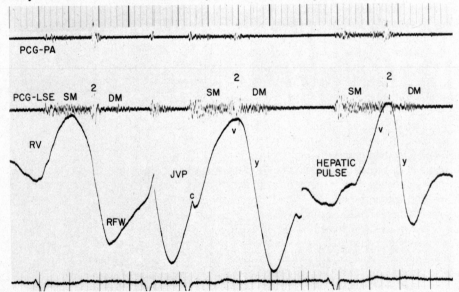

FIGURE 3-37 Tricuspid regurgitation secondary to mitral stenosis and pulmonary hypertension. *Left,* RV impulse showing a sustained heave, palpable at the left sternal edge. The PCG shows systolic and diastolic murmurs of tricuspid regurgitation at the left sternal edge (LSE). This right ventricular heave is a consequence of right ventricular hypertrophy secondary to pulmonary hypertension and is in contrast to the inward systolic movement seen in tricuspid regurgitation due to intrinsic abnormality of the tricuspid valve, with normal RV pressures as seen in Figure 3–32. *Center,* JVP shows an enormous *v* wave due to tricuspid regurgitation and retrograde flow. *Right,* Hepatic pulse is similar to JVP, although its ascent is slightly delayed.

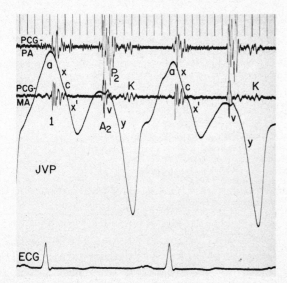

FIGURE 3–38 Jugular venous pressure (JVP) in constrictive pericarditis. In this severe and longstanding case, the x' descent has become very shallow and the y descent is the principal feature, indicating that antegrade flow from the venous system to the right heart is now limited to early diastole.[142] A pericardial knock (K) is seen at approximately the nadir of the y descent.

SUMMARY

Phonocardiograms and pulse-wave tracings of carotid, apex, and venous origin have a number of uses which may be summarized as follows:

1. *As an objective record of physical signs.* Although descriptions and diagrams in patients' charts are helpful in evaluating changes occurring over time, a more accurate and detailed collection of data can be provided by graphic records of sounds, murmurs, and pulsatile phenomena. These are often valuable in studying the progression of disease or the effects of pharmacological and surgical interventions.
2. *To determine temporal relationships:*
   a. Systolic time intervals as ordinarily measured require a combination of phonocardiogram, carotid pulse tracing, and electrocardiogram.
   b. Other temporal relationships such as A_2-OS time can be only roughly estimated by auscultation but can be accurately determined by phonocardiography.
3. *In the identification of heart sounds.* Difficulties may be encountered in determining the identity of sounds clustered around the beginning or end of systole. Such problems can be clarified by phonocardiography in combination with other graphic methods. In particular, the major elements of S_1, ejection sounds, opening snaps, and low-frequency sounds (S_3, S_4) can be accurately identified by combined multichannel tracings.
4. *In affording clues to specific diagnoses from distinctive heart-sound or pulse-wave patterns.* Although many phonocardiographic and pulse-wave patterns lack specificity, they may be quite useful in confirming suspected diagnoses such as aortic stenosis, HOCM, constrictive pericarditis, and so on, as outlined above.
5. *In teaching bedside diagnostic skills.* The utility of graphic methods, either "live" on an oscilloscope or in permanent form on paper, is well established as a powerful tool in facilitating the acquisition and enhancement of skills in physical diagnosis at all levels of training.

Phonocardiography is *not* useful as a means of determining the presence or absence of barely detectable murmurs. Very soft murmurs often merge with background vibrations in the tracing and therefore cannot be identified with any more certainty than by auscultation.

Acknowledgments

The author is indebted to his colleague Dr. Peter Mills and many others who collaborated in the collection from our own laboratory of data used in this chapter. Dr. Mills is the coauthor of a paper on this subject[8] that has been freely quoted in this and the following chapter. Dr. Richard P. Lewis has been very helpful with the section on systolic time intervals. I am also very grateful for the technical assistance of Ms. Sally Moos and Ms. Carla Wolfe of the Cardiac Graphics Laboratory at North Carolina Memorial Hospital, Chapel Hill, North Carolina, who are responsible for the records used as illustrations in Chapters 3 and 4.

References

1. Einthoven, W., and Geluk, M. A. J.: Die Registrierung der Herztöne. Pflüger's Arch. Physiol. *57*:617, 1894.
2. McKusick, V. A.: Cardiovascular Sound in Health and Disease. Baltimore, Williams and Wilkins, 1958.
3. Fishleder, B. L.: Exploración cardiovascular y fono mecanocardiografía clínica. México, La Prensa Médica Mexicana, 1966.
4. Tavel, M. E.: Clinical phonocardiography and external pulse recording, 3rd ed. Chicago, Year Book Publishers, 1978.
5. Esper, R. J., and Madoery, R. J.: Progresos en auscultación y fono mecanocardiografía. Buenos Aires, López Libreros, 1974.
6. Leatham, A.: Auscultation of the Heart and Phonocardiography. London, Churchill Livingstone, 1975.
7. Craige, E.: On the genesis of heart sounds: Contributions made by echocardiographic studies. Circulation *53*:207, 1976.
8. Mills, P., and Craige, E.: Echophonocardiography. Prog. Cardiovasc. Dis. *20*: 337, 1978.
9. Zalter, R., Hodara, H., and Luisada, A. A.: Phonocardiography. I. General principles and problems of standardization. Am. J. Cardiol. *4*:3, 1959.
10. Lewis, D. H.: Phonocardiography. *In* Hamilton, W. F., and Dow, P. (eds.): Handbook of Physiology. Section 2, Circulation. Vol. I. Washington, D. C., American Physiological Society, 1962, p. 685.
11. Kesteloot, H., Willems, J., and Van Vollenhoven, E.: On the physical principles and methodology of mechanocardiography. Acta Cardiol. *24*:147, 1969.
12. Butterworth, J. S., Chassin, M. R., McGrath, R., and Reppert, E. H.: Cardiac Auscultation. New York, Grune and Stratton. 1960.
13. Lewis, R. P., Rittgers, S. E., Forester, W. F., and Boudoulas, H.: A critical review of the systolic time intervals. Circulation *56*:146, 1977.
14. Craige, E., and Schmidt, R. E.: Precordial movements over the right ventricle in normal children. Circulation *32*:232, 1965.
15. Mashimo, K., Tanabe, T., Kinoshita, S., Sakamoto, S., and Tsushima, N.: An instrumental aspect of apexcardiography: Decay characteristic of transducers and its clinical implication. Jap. Heart J. *7*:536, 1966.
16. Leech, G.: The apexcardiogram: Recording technique and relation to cardiac function. Application notes for cardiovascular instrumentation. Vol. 1, No. 4. Irex Medical Systems, Upper Saddle River, New Jersey, 1973.
17. Leatham, A.: Phonocardiography. Br. Med. Bull. *8*:333, 1952.
18. Rappaport, M. B., and Sprague, H. B.: The graphic registration of the normal heart sound. Am. Heart J. *23*:591, 1942.
19. Armstrong, T. G., and Gotsman, M. S.: Initial low frequency vibrations of the first heart sound. Br. Heart J. *35*:691, 1973.
20. Rouanet, J.: Analyse des bruits du coeur. Thesis No. 252, Paris, 1832. (Reprinted in reference 2 above.)
21. Dock, W.: Mode of production of the first heart sound, Arch. Intern. Med. *51*: 737, 1933.
22. Leatham, A.: Splitting of the first and heart sounds. Lancet *2*:607, 1954.
23. Luisada, A. A., MacCanon, D. M., Kumar, S., and Feigen, L. P.: Changing views on the mechanism of the first and second heart sounds. Am. Heart J. *88*: 503, 1974.
24. Di Bartolo, G., Nunez-Dey, D., Muiesan, G., MacCanon, D. M., and Luisada, A. A.: Hemodynamic correlates of the first heart sound. Am. J. Physiol. *201*: 888, 1961.

25. Laniado, S., Yellin, E. L., Miller, H., and Frater, R. W. M.: Temporal relation of the first heart sound to closure of the mitral valve. Circulation 47:1006, 1973.

26. Lakier, J. B., Fritz, V. U., Pocock, W. A., and Barlow, J. B.: The mitral components of the first heart sound. Br. Heart J. 34:160, 1972.

27. Lakier, J. B., Bloom, K. R., Pocock, W. A., and Barlow, J. B.: Tricuspid component of first heart sound. Br. Heart J. 35:1275, 1973.

28. O'Toole, J. D., Reddy, P. S., Curtiss, E. L., Griff, F. W., and Shaver, J. A.: The contribution of tricuspid valve closure to the first heart sound. An intracardiac micromanometer study. Circulation 53:752, 1976.

29. Waider, W., and Craige, E.: The first heart sound and ejection sounds: Echophonocardiographic correlation with valvular events. Am. J. Cardiol. 35:346, 1975.

30. Craige, E.: Echocardiography in studies of the genesis of heart sounds and murmurs (Chapter 2). In Yu, P., and Goodwin, J. (eds.): Progress in Cardiology. Vol. 4. Philadelphia, Lea and Febiger, 1975.

31. Shah, P. M., Kramer, D. H., and Gramiak, R.: Influence of the timing of atrial systole in mitral valve closure and on the first heart sound in man. Am. J. Cardiol. 26:231, 1970.

32. Burggraf, G. W., and Craige, E.: The first heart sound in complete heart block. Circulation 50:17, 1974.

33. Kostis, J. B.: Mechanisms of heart sounds. Am. Heart J. 89:546, 1975.

34. Traill, T. A., and Fortuin, N. J.: Presystolic mitral closure sound in aortic regurgitation with left ventricular hypertrophy and first degree heart block. Br. Heart J. 48:78, 1982.

35. Brooks, N., Leech, G., and Leatham, A.: Complete right bundle branch block: Echophonocardiographic study of first heart sound and right ventricular contraction tones. Br. Heart J. 41:637, 1979.

36. Hultgren, H. N., Craige, E., and Bilisoly, J.: The late first heart sound in left bundle branch block. Circulation 64 (Suppl. 4):27, 1981.

37. Haber, E., and Leatham, A.: Splitting of heart sounds from ventricular asynchrony in bundle-branch block, ventricular ectopic beats, and artificial pacing. Br. Heart J. 27:691, 1965.

38. Braunwald, E., and Morrow, A. G.: Origin of heart sounds as elucidated by analysis of the sequence of cardiodynamic events. Circulation 18:971, 1958.

39. Burggraf, G. W.: The first heart sound in left bundle branch block: An echophonocardiographic study. Circulation 63:429, 1981.

40. Wooley, C. F.: Intracardiac phonocardiography; intracardiac sound and pressure in man. Circulation 57:1039, 1978.

41. Crews, T. L., Pridie, R. B., Benham, R., and Leatham, A.: Auscultatory and phonocardiographic findings in Ebstein's anomaly. Correlation of first heart sound with ultrasonic records of tricuspid valve movement. Br. Heart J. 34:681, 1972.

42. Tajik, A. J., Gau, G. T., Giuliani, E. R., Ritter, D. G., and Schattenberg, T. T.: Echocardiogram in Ebstein's anomaly with Wolff-Parkinson-White preexcitation syndrome, type B. Circulation 47:813, 1973.

43. Dashkoff, N., Fortuin, N. J., and Hutchins, G. M.: Clinical features of severe mitral regurgitation due to floppy mitral valve. Circulation 50 (Suppl. 3):60, 1974.

44. Mann, T., McLaurin, L., Grossman, W., and Craige, E.: Acute aortic regurgitation due to infective endocarditis, N. Engl. J. Med. 293:108, 1975.

45. Wolferth, C. C., and Margolies, A.: Certain effects of auricular systole and prematurity of beat on the intensity of the first heart sound. Trans. Am. Assoc. Physicians 45:44, 1930.

46. Leatham, A., and Gray, I.: Auscultatory and phonocardiographic signs of atrial septal defect. Br. Heart J. 18:193, 1956.

47. Lopez, J. F., Linn, H., and Shaffer, A. B.: The apical first heart sound as an aid in the diagnosis of atrial septal defect. Circulation 26:1296, 1962.

48. Stept, M. E., Heid, C. E., Shaver, J. A., Leon, D. F., and Leonard, J. J.: Effect of altering P-R interval on the amplitude of the first heart sound in the anesthetized dog. Circ. Res. 25:255, 1969.

49. Mills, P. G., Chamusco, R. F., Moos, S., and Craige, E.: Echophonocardiographic studies of the contribution of the atrioventricular valves to the first heart sound. Circulation 54:944, 1976.

50. Lewis, J. K., and Dock, W.: The origin of the heart sounds and their variations in myocardial disease. J.A.M.A. 110:271, 1938.

51. Sabbah, H. N., and Stein, P. D.: Investigation of the theory and mechanism of the origin of the second heart sound. Circ. Res. 39:874, 1976.

52. Stein, P. D: A Physical and Physiological Basis for the Interpretation of Cardiac Auscultation: Evaluations Based Primarily on the Second Heart Sound and Ejection Murmurs. Mount Kisco, N.Y., Futura Publishing Co., 1981.

53. Hirschfeld, S., Liebman, J., Borkat, G., and Bormuth, C.: Intracardiac pressure-sound correlates of echocardiographic aortic valve closure. Circulation 55:602, 1977.

54. Potain, P. C.: Note sur les dédoublements normaux des bruits du coeur. Bull. Mém. Soc. Méd. Hôp. (Paris) 3:138, 1866.

55. Craige, E., and Harned, H. S.: Phonocardiographic and electrocardiographic studies in normal newborn infants. Am. Heart J. 65:180, 1963.

56. Harris, A., and Sutton, G. C.: Second heart sound in normal subjects. Br. Heart J. 30:739, 1968.

57. Leatham, A., and Weitzman, D.: Auscultatory and phonocardiographic signs of pulmonary stenosis. Br. Heart J. 19:303, 1957.

58. Leatham, A., and Gray, I.: Auscultatory and phonocardiographic signs of atrial septal defect. Br. Heart J. 18:193, 1956.

59. Damore, S., Murgo, J. P., Bloom, K. R., and Rubal, B. J.: Second heart sound dynamics in atrial septal defect. Circulation 64(Suppl. 4):28, 1981.

60. Shafter, H. A.: Splitting of the second heart sound. Am. J. Cardiol. 6:1013, 1960.

61. Perloff, J. K.: Auscultatory and phonocardiographic manifestations of pulmonary hypertension. Prog. Cardiovasc. Dis. 9:303, 1967.

62. Sabbah, H. N., Khaja, F., Anbe, D. T., and Stein, P. D.: The aortic closure sound in pure aortic insufficiency. Circulation 56:859, 1977.

63. Ross, R. S., and Criley, J. M.: Cineangiocardiographic studies of the origin of cardiovascular physical signs. Circulation 30:255, 1964.

64. Hancock, E. W.: The ejection sound in aortic stenosis. Am. J. Med. 40:569, 1966.

65. Leech, G., Mills, P., and Leatham, A.: The diagnosis of a non-stenotic biscuspid aortic valve. Br. Heart J. 40:941, 1978.

66. Leatham, A., and Vogelpoel, L.: Early systolic sound in dilatation of the pulmonary artery. Br. Heart J. 16:21, 1954.

67. Minhas, K., and Gasul, B. M.: Systolic clicks: Clinical phonocardiographic and hemodynamic evaluation. Am. Heart J. 57:49, 1959.

68. Hultgren, H. N., Reeve, R., Cohn, K., and McLeod, R.: The ejection click of valvular pulmonic stenosis. Circulation 40:631, 1969.

69. Mills, P., Amara, I., McLaurin, L. P., and Craige, E.: Noninvasive assessment of pulmonary hypertension from right ventricular isovolumic contraction time. Am. J. Cardiol. 46:272, 1980.

70. Curtiss, E. I., Reddy, P. S., O'Toole, J. D., and Shaver, J. A.: Alterations of right ventricular systolic time intervals by chronic pressure and volume overloading. Circulation 53:997, 1976.

71. Mills, P. G., Brodie, B., McLaurin, L. P., Schall, S., and Craige, E.: Echocardiographic and hemodynamic relationships of ejection sounds. Circulation 56:430, 1977.

72. Margolies, A., and Wolferth, C. C.: The opening snap in mitral stenosis. Am. Heart J. 7:443, 1932.

73. Craige, E.: Editorial. On the genesis of heart sounds: Contribution made by echocardiographic studies. Circulation 53:207, 1976.

74. Millward, D. K., McLaurin, L. P., and Craige, E.: Echocardiographic studies to explain opening snaps in presence of nonstenotic mitral valves. Am. J. Cardiol. 31:64, 1973.

75. Criley, J. M., Lewis, K. B., Humphries, J. O., and Ross, R. S.: Prolapse of the mitral valve: Clinical and cine-angiocardiographic findings. Br. Heart J. 28:488, 1966.

76. Nixon, P. G. F.: The genesis of the third heart sound. Am. Heart J. 65:712, 1963.

77. Harvey, W. P., and Stapleton, J.: Clinical aspects of gallop rhythm with particular reference to diastolic gallops. Circulation 18:1017, 1958.

78. Tyberg, T. I., Goodyer, A. V. N., and Langou, R. A.: Genesis of pericardial knock in constrictive pericarditis. Am. J. Cardiol. 46:570, 1980.

79. Sakamoto, T., Ichiyasu, H., Hayashi, T., Kawarakani, H., Amano, K., and Hada, Y.: Genesis of the third heart sound. Jap. Heart J. 17:150, 1976.

80. Prewitt, T., Gibson, D., Brown, D., and Sutton, G.: The "rapid filling wave" of the apex cardiogram: its relation to echocardiographic and cineangiographic measurements of ventricular filling. Br. Heart J. 37:1256, 1975.

80a. Ozawa, Y., Smith, D., and Craige. E.: Localization of the origin of the third heart sound. Circulation 66 (Suppl. 2):210, 1982.

81. Gibson, T. C., Madry, R., Grossman, W., McLaurin, L. P., and Craige, E.: The A wave of the apexcardiogram and left ventricular diastolic stiffness. Circulation 49:441, 1974.

82. Kesteloot, H., and Willems, J.: Relationship between the right apexcardiogram and the right ventricular dynamics. Acta Cardiol. 22:64, 1967.

83. Craige, E.: The fourth heart sound. In Leon, D. F., and Shaver, J. A. (eds.): Physiologic Principles of Heart Sounds and Murmurs. New York, American Heart Association Monograph, No. 46, 1975, p. 74.

84. Shah, P. M., and Jackson, D.: Third heart sound and summation gallop. In Leon, D. F., and Shaver, J. A. (eds.): Physiologic Principles of Heart Sounds and Murmurs. New York, American Heart Association Monograph No. 46, 1975, p. 79.

84a. Smith, N. D., Raizada, V., and Abraus, J.: Auscultation of the normally functioning prosthetic valve. Ann. Intern. Med. 95:594, 1981.

85. Hultgren, H. N., and Hubis, H.: A phonocardiographic study of patients with the Starr-Edwards mitral valve prosthesis. Am. Heart J. 69:306, 1965.

86. Gibson, T. C., Starek, P. J. K., Moos, S., and Craige, E.: Echocardiographic and phonocardiographic characteristics of the Lillehei-Kaster mitral valve prosthesis. Circulation 49:434, 1974.

87. Smith, N. D., Raizada, V., and Abrams, J.: Auscultation of the normally functioning prosthetic valve. Ann. Intern. Med. 95:594, 1981.

88. Brodie, B. R., Grossman, W., McLaurin, L. P., Starek, P. J. K., and Craige, E.: Diagnosis of prosthetic mitral valve malfunction with combined echophonocardiography. Circulation 53:93, 1976.

89. Miller, H. C., Gibson, D. G., and Stephens, J. D.: Role of echocardiography and phonocardiography in diagnosis of mitral paraprosthetic regurgitation with Starr-Edwards protheses. Br. Heart J. 35:1217, 1973.

90. Burggraf, G. W., and Craige, E.: Echocardiographic studies of left ventricular wall motion and dimensions after valvular heart surgery. Am. J. Cardiol. 35:473, 1975.

91. Harris, A.: Pacemaker "heart sound." Br. Heart J. 29:608, 1967.

92. Garrod, A. H.: On some points connected with the circulation of the blood, arrived at from a study of the sphygmograph-trace. Proc. R. Soc. Lond. 23:140, 1874-1875.

93. Bowen, W. P.: Changes in heart rate, blood pressure and duration of systole resulting from bicycling. Am. J. Physiol. 11:59, 1904.

94. Wiggers, C. J.: Studies on the consecutive phases of the cardiac cycle. II. The laws governing the relative durations of ventricular systole and diastole. Am. J. Physiol. *56*:439, 1921.

95. Lombard, W. P., and Cope, O. M.: The duration of the systole of the left ventricle of man. Am. J. Physiol. *77*:263, 1926.

96. Lewis, R. P., Leighton, R. F., Forester, W. F., and Weissler, A. M.: Systolic time intervals. *In* Weissler, A. M. (ed.): Noninvasive Cardiology. New York, Grune and Stratton, 1974, p. 301.

97. Weissler, A. M.: Current concepts in cardiology. Systolic time intervals. N. Engl. J. Med. *296*:321, 1977.

98. Lewis, R. P., Diagnostic value of systolic time intervals in man. *In* Fowler, N.O. (ed.): Diagnostic Methods in Cardiology. Philadelphia, F.A. Davis Co., 1975, pp. 245–264.

99. Lewis, R. P.: The use of systolic time intervals for evaluation of left ventricular function. *In* Noble, O., and Fowler, N. O (ed.): Noninvasive Diagnostic Methods in Cardiology. Philadelphia, F. A. Davis, 1983.

100. Weissler, A. M., O'Neill, W. W., Sohn, Y. H., Stack, R. S., Chew, P. C., and Reed, A. H.: Prognostic significance of systolic time intervals after recovery from myocardial infarction. Am. J. Cardiol. *48*:995, 1981.

101. Garrard, C. L., Jr., Weissler, S. M., and Dodge, H. T.: The relationship of alterations in systolic time intervals to ejection fraction in patients with cardiac disease. Circulation *42*:455, 1970.

102. Weissler, A. M., Harris, W. S., and Schoenfeld, C. D.: Systolic time intervals in heart failure in man. Circulation *37*:149, 1968.

103. Lewis, R. P., Boudoulas, H., Forester, W. F., and Weissler, A. M.: Shortening of electromechanical systole as a manifestation of excessive adrenergic stimulation in acute myocardial infarction. Circulation *46*:856, 1972.

104. Lewis, R. P., Boudoulas, H., Welch, T. G., and Forester, W. F.: Usefulness of systolic time intervals in coronary artery disease. Am. J. Cardiol. *37*:787, 1976.

105. Unverferth, D. V., Lewis, R. P., Leier, C. V., Magorien, R. D., and Fulkerson, P. K.: The use of echocardiography and systolic time intervals in monitoring therapy of congestive heart failure. J. C. U. *8*:479, 1980.

106. Bonner, J. A., Sacks, H. N., and Tavel, M. E.: Assessing the severity of aortic stenosis by phonocardiography and external carotid pulse recordings. Circulation *48*:247, 1973.

107. Weissler, A. M., Snyder, J. R., Schoenfeld, C. D., and Cohen, S.: Assay of digitalis glycosides in man. Am. J. Cardiol. *17*:768, 1966.

108. Carliner, N. H., Gilbert, C. A., Pruitt, A. W., and Goldbert, L. I.: Effect of maintenance digoxin therapy on systolic time intervals and serum digoxin concentrations. Circulation *50*:94, 1974.

109. Forester, W. F., Lewis, R. P., Weissler, A. M., and Wilke, T. A.: The onset and magnitude of the contractile response to commonly used digitalis glycosides in normal subjects. Circulation *49*:517, 1974.

110. Boudoulas, H., Beaver, B. M., Kates, R. E., and Lewis, R. P.: Pharmacodynamics of inotropic and chronotropic responses to oral propranolol. Studies in normal subjects and in patients with angina. Chest *73*:146, 1978.

111. Bristow, M. R., Mason, J. W., Billingham, M. E., and Daniels, J. R.: Doxorubicin cardiomyopathy: Evaluation by phonocardiography, endomyocardial biopsy and cardiac catheterization. Ann. Intern. Med. *88*:168, 1978.

112. Al-Israil, S. A. D., and Whittaker, J. A.: Systolic time interval as index of schedule-dependent doxorubicin cardiotoxicity in patients with acute myelogenous leukemia. Br. Med. J. *1*:1392, 1979.

113. Ichiyasu, H., and Craige, E.: Assessment of the severity of aortic stenosis from the carotid pulse tracing. Jap. Heart J. *21*:465, 1980.

114. Orchard, R. C., and Craige, E.: Dicrotic pulse after open heart surgery. Circulation *62*:1107, 1980.

115. Ewy, G. A., Rios, J. C., and Marcus, F. I.: The dicrotic arterial pulse. Circulation *39*:655, 1969.

116. Hada, Y., Wolfe, C., and Craige, E.: Pulsus alternans determined by biventricular simultaneous systolic time intervals. Circulation *65*:617, 1982.

117. Craige, E.: Apexcardiography. *In* Weissler, A. M. (ed.): Noninvasive Cardiology. New York, Grune and Stratton, 1974, p. 1.

118. Eddleman, E. E.: Ultra low frequency precordial movements—kinetocardiograms. Am. J. Cardiol. *4*:649, 1959.

119. Vas, R., Diamond, G. A., Wyatt, H. L., Protasio, L., da Luz, P. L., Swan, H. J. C., and Forrester, J. S.: Noninvasive analysis of regional myocardial wall motion: Cardiokymography. Am. J. Physiol. *233*:700, 1977.

120. Silverberg, R. A., Diamond, G. A., Vas, R., Tzivoni, D., Swan, H. J. C., and Forrester, J. S.: Noninvasive diagnosis of coronary artery disease: The cardiokymographic stress test. Circulation *61*:579, 1980.

121. Sakamoto, T., Matsuhisa, M., Inoue, K., Hayashi, T., and Ito, U.: Clinical and hemodynamic observation of indirect pulmonary artery pulse tracing. Cardiovasc. Sound Bull. *3*:127, 1973.

122. Willems, J. L., Kesteloot, H., and De Geest, H.: Influence of acute hemodynamic changes on the apexcardiogram in dogs. Am. J. Cardiol. *29*:504, 1972.

123. Willems, J. L., De Geest, H., and Kesteloot, H.: On the value of apexcardiography for timing intracardiac events. Am. J. Cardiol. *28*:59, 1971.

124. Bush, C. A., Lewis, R. P., Leighton, R. F., Fontana, M. E., and Weissler, A. M.: Verification of systolic time intervals and true isovolumic contraction time from the apexcardiogram by mitromanometer catheterization of the left ventricle and aorta. Circulation *41* (Suppl. 3):121, 1970.

125. Sutton, G. C., Prewitt, T. A., and Craige, E.: Relationship between quantitated precordial movement and left ventricular function. Circulation *41*:179, 1970.

126. Sutton, G. C., Craige, E., and Grizzle, J. E.: Quantitation of precordial movement. II. Mitral regurgitation. Circulation *35*:483, 1967.

127. Lucardie, S. M., and Durrer, D.: The late systolic murmur. Arch. Kreislaufforsch. *53*:174, 1967.

128. Algary, W. P., and Craige, E.: Left atrial myxoma. Diagnosis with the help of the phonocardiogram and apexcardiogram. Arch. Intern. Med. *129*:470, 1972.

129. Voigt, G. C., and Friesinger, G. C.: The use of apexcardiography in the assessment of left ventricular diastolic pressure. Circulation *41*:1015, 1970.

130. DiMattéo, J., LaFont, H., Hui Bon Hoa, F., et al.: La courbe méchanique ventriculaire dans l'insuffisance aortique. Arch. Mal. Coeur *60*:1320, 1967.

131. Fortuin, N. J., and Craige, E.: On the mechanism of the Austin Flint murmur. Circulation *45*:558, 1972.

132. Schmidt, R. E., and Craige, E.: Precordial movements over the right ventricle in children with pulmonary stenosis. Circulation *32*:241, 1965.

133. Armstrong, T. G., and Gotsman, M. S.: The left parasternal lift in tricuspid incompetence. Am. Heart J. *88*:183, 1974.

134. Mounsey, J. P. D.: Inspection and palpation of the cardiac impulse. Prog. Cardiovasc. Dis. *10*:187, 1967.

135. El-Sherif, A., and El-Said, G.: Jugular, hepatic, and praecordial pulsations in constrictive pericarditis. Br. Heart J. *33*:305, 1971.

136. Craige, E., and Fortuin, N. J.: Noninvasive measurement of ventricular function in chronic ischemic heart disease. *In* Likoff, W., Segal, B. L., Insull, W., and Moyer, J. H. (eds.): Atherosclerosis and Coronary Heart Disease. New York, Grune and Stratton, 1972, p. 221.

137. Basta, L. L., Wolfson, P., Eckbert, D. L., and Abboud, F. M.: The value of left parasternal impulse recordings in the assessment of mitral regurgitation. Circulation *48*:1055, 1973.

138. Manolas, J., Wirz, P., and Rutihauser, W.: Relationship between duration of systolic upstroke of apexcardiogram and internal indexes of myocardial function in man. Am. Heart J. *91*:726, 1976.

139. Constant, J.: The x′ descent in jugular contour nomenclature and recognition. Am. Heart J. *88*:372, 1974.

140. Benchimol, A., and Tippit, H. C.: The clinical value of the jugular and hepatic pulses. Prog. Cardiovasc. Dis. *10*:159, 1967.

141. Rich, L. L., and Tavel, M. E.: The origin of the jugular C wave. N. Engl. J. Med. *284*:1309, 1971.

142. Sivaciyan, V., and Ranganathan, N.: Transcutaneous Doppler jugular venous flow velocity recording: Clinical and hemodynamic correlates. Circulation *57*:930, 1978.

143. Kesteloot, H., and Denef, B.: Value of reference tracings in the diagnosis and assessment of constrictive epi- and pericarditis. Br. Heart J. *32*:675, 1970.

•

4

ECHOPHONOCARDIOG-RAPHY AND OTHER NONINVASIVE TECHNIQUES TO ELUCIDATE HEART MURMURS

by Ernest Craige, M.D.

Most cardiac murmurs are believed to arise from disturbances of blood flow manifest as turbulence. Turbulence is defined as an irregular condition of motion in which velocity and pressure show a random variation in relation to time and space coordinates.[1] Fluctuating velocities and pressures due to turbulence presumably produce local vibrations at the wall of the vessel or heart chamber which then are transmitted to the chest wall and perceived as murmurs.[2] Maximum turbulence is found in the recipient vessel or chamber, such as, for example, in the root of the great vessels in aortic or pulmonic stenosis, in the left atrium in mitral regurgitation, and in the cavity of the left ventricle in aortic regurgitation.[3] Noninvasive cardiac diagnostic methods—specifically echophonocardiography—can be used to illustrate the common types of heart murmurs encountered in clinical· practice.

SYSTOLIC MURMURS[4,5]

CLASSIFICATION OF SYSTOLIC MURMURS. The convenient classification of systolic murmurs into two main categories—*ejection* and *regurgitant*—as popularized by Leatham, has improved our understanding of pathogenetic mechanisms as well as facilitated communication among observers.[4] In general, "ejection murmurs" are midsystolic in timing and are the result of ejection of blood into the root of one of the great vessels. A classic example of an ejection murmur is that associated with stenosis of one of the semilunar valves (Fig. 4–1). The term "regurgitant murmur" has been used to describe a holosystolic murmur that may be found when the pressure relationships between the donor chamber (ventricle) and the recipient chamber (atrium, or lower pressure ventricle) fa-

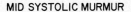

MID SYSTOLIC MURMUR

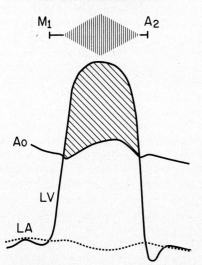

FIGURE 4–1 Midsystolic murmur in aortic stenosis, with pressure records from left ventricle (LV), left atrium (LA), and aorta (A$_o$). In early systole, LV pressure rises swiftly and opens the aortic valve, whereupon ejection into the root of the aorta can begin; only then does the midsystolic or ejection murmur start, peaking at the time of maximum gradient across the valve (shaded area). At the end of systole, the falling pressure in the LV results in diminishing flow across the aortic valve, and the murmur fades away before A$_2$.

vor retrograde flow *throughout* systole (Fig. 4–2). With improved understanding of variations in the hemodynamic patterns of mitral valve disease, it has become apparent that the physical signs associated with mitral regurgitation may also vary greatly. For instance, in acute mitral regurgitation, the murmur may be prominent in early and midsystole but may terminate before the second heart sound. In mitral valve prolapse, on the other hand, the murmur may be confined to late systole. These alterations from the classic pattern are readily explicable on the basis of known information concerning the anatomical and physiological derangements in these conditions. Thus, ef-

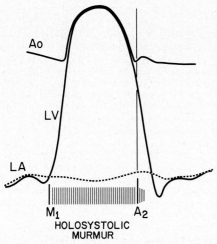

FIGURE 4–2 Holosystolic murmur. In mitral regurgitation LV pressure rises and immediately exceeds LA pressure. Thus the regurgitant murmur begins with M$_1$, continues throughout systole, and may continue even slightly beyond A$_2$, because the falling pressure in the LV still exceeds that of the LA, thus favoring continuing regurgitation.

forts to describe these abbreviated murmurs within the framework of the "ejection" and "regurgitant" terminology has led to a confusing misuse of terms, such as "ejection-type" murmur to describe a murmur that results from regurgitation but is less than holosystolic in duration.

Therefore, in this chapter, simple descriptive terms, such as "early systolic," "late systolic," "holosystolic," and "midsystolic," will be used to indicate the position of systolic murmurs in the cardiac cycle. Murmurs that begin with the first heart sound and proceed to the second sound on their side of origin are called holosystolic. A murmur that begins with the first heart sound and finishes in either mid- or late systole but well before the second heart sound on its side of origin is designated an early systolic murmur. Conversely, with a late systolic murmur, early systole is silent, the murmur generally beginning in mid- to late systole and proceeding to the second heart sound on its side of origin. If the murmur begins at an interval after the first heart sound and ends before the second, and both early and late systole are murmur-free, the murmur is designated "midsystolic."

MIDSYSTOLIC MURMURS

Physiological Murmurs. The commonest murmur is soft, midsystolic in time, and not associated with any cardiac abnormality. Such functional or innocent murmurs are usually best heard and recorded at the left sternal edge in either the second or the third left intercostal space. Most commonly they consist phonocardiographically of random noise, i.e., vibrations of various frequencies.[6] The intensity of physiological murmurs can be magnified by physical activity, excitement, pregnancy, anemia, thyrotoxicosis, fever, and so on, presumably owing to increases in the volume and velocity of ejection. In thin subjects or individuals with a depressed sternum, proximity of the stethoscope or microphone to the source of the murmur may result in even greater intensity. The source of physiological midsystolic murmurs is thought to be the right ventricular outflow tract and root of the pulmonary artery, because their area of maximal intensity is at the left sternal edge overlying these anatomical structures. The innocent murmurs, maximal lower over the midprecordium, are often more musical or even grunting in quality and appear on the phonocardiogram in crescendo-decrescendo silhouette, with vibrations of a constant frequency rather than random noise (Fig. 4–3). Appreciation of the innocent nature of the murmurs described above is facilitated by the absence of other evidence of heart disease by means of physical examination, electrocardiogram, and chest x-ray. From a phonocardiographic point of view, the midsystolic timing of the murmur is important in differentiating it from the holosystolic murmur of an interventricular septal defect. The basal systolic murmur of an atrial septal defect, however, represents an exaggerated flow murmur in midsystole resulting from augmentation of right ventricular stroke volume. It therefore resembles an innocent murmur. Attention to the details of the second heart sound, however, should clarify this problem, since the wide, fixed splitting of S$_2$, which is characteristic of atrial septal defect (see Figure 3–9A, p. 46), would not be found with an innocent or physiological murmur. Other causes of midsystolic murmurs resulting from ejection across deformed or

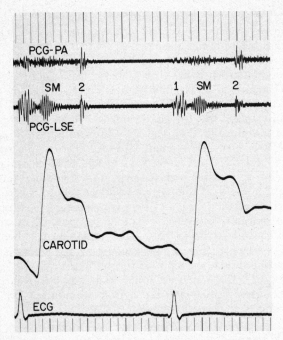

FIGURE 4–3   Functional murmur in a healthy 20-year-old man. The midsystolic timing of the murmur and vibratory appearance are characteristic of many innocent murmurs. The phonocardiogram is otherwise normal, as is the carotid pulse tracing. PCG-PA =phonocardiogram in second left intercostal space; PCG-LSE =phonocardiogram at left sternal edge.

obstructing outflow tracts and semilunar valves are described in the following paragraphs.

Obstruction to Left Ventricular Outflow.[7,8]   Midsystolic murmurs are characteristically found in patients with obstruction of the outflow tract. Combined phono- and echocardiographic studies are particularly useful in determining the underlying pathological condition in these cases, although conventional M-mode echocardiography alone may be of very limited value. Echophonocardiog-

raphy may also provide valuable guidelines when difficult decisions regarding the timing of invasive studies must be made. It may also be useful in serial observations of patients in whom the obstruction is not critical.

Congenital Valvular Aortic Stenosis (see also Chaps. 29 and 30).   This condition produces a characteristic midsystolic murmur best recorded from its position of maximal intensity in the second right interspace or aortic area (Fig. 4–4). In youthful subjects, this abnormality is almost invariably associated with an aortic ejection sound, which initiates the murmur. The ejection sound is widely transmitted over the precordium and can be recorded at the mitral area. Its identity can be established echophonocardiographically by its coincidence with the achievement of a maximally open position by the aortic valve (see Figure 3–11, p. 48). A_2 is well preserved in young individuals in whom the valve, although deformed, is capable of closing and being set into vibration at the onset of diastole.[9] With advancing age, the valve may become calcified and immobilized, with diminution or obliteration of both the ejection sound and A_2. The murmur itself is of little help in determining the severity of the valvular abnormality. There is a tendency for the murmur to peak later in systole with severe stenosis.[10] The loudness of the murmur is not proportional to the severity of the obstruction. A loud murmur may occur merely with sclerosis of the valve where there is no significant gradient across it. Conversely, in a moribund patient with the most severe stenosis, the murmur may become faint or disappear entirely as the left ventricular stroke volume declines. More useful information indicating a severe degree of stenosis may be provided as follows: (1) prolongation of left ventricular ejection time (LVET) may be determined from an accompanying carotid pulse tracing (Fig. 4–5)[10]; (2) paradoxical splitting of S_2 may appear, owing to a delay in A_2, associated with the long LVET (see Figure 3–9B, p. 46); (3) there may be evidence of concentric hypertrophy of the left ventricle, as manifest in the echocardiogram (Fig. 4–4); (4) the *a* wave

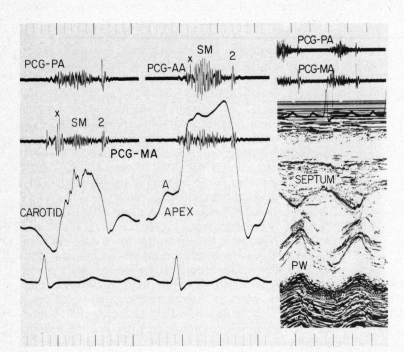

FIGURE 4–4   Congenital valvular aortic stenosis. An asymptomatic 10-year-old boy, successfully operated upon in infancy for coarctation of the aorta, had a residual murmur characteristic of valvular aortic stenosis presumably due to a bicuspid aortic valve. *Left,* Phonocardiogram at the cardiac apex (PCG-MA) shows a loud ejection sound (X) followed by a midsystolic murmur (SM) transmitted from the aortic area. The carotid pulse is shattered with coarse vibrations and peaks late in systole. *Center,* The "diamond shape" or prominent systolic murmur is best seen at the second right interspace (AA). The apexcardiogram is abnormal, with an exaggerated *a* wave followed by a systolic heave shown graphically by an upward slope. The findings are consistent with left ventricular hypertrophy. *Right,* Concentric hypertrophy of the left ventricle was verified by an echocardiogram which shows a small chamber but a thick septum and posterior wall (PW). The combined study indicated the presence of significant aortic stenosis despite absence of symptoms. At catheterization a systolic gradient of 80 mm Hg was demonstrated.

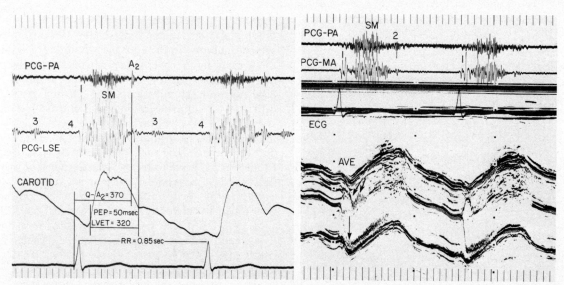

FIGURE 4-5   Subvalvular aortic stenosis. A 12-year-old boy with a loud midsystolic murmur maximal at the left sternal edge. *Left,* Phonocardiogram illustrating the murmur. The carotid pulse tracing is deformed by coarse vibrations coincident with the murmur. Left ventricular ejection time (LVET) is prolonged for the heart rate. Soft third and fourth heart sounds (S_3 and S_4) are also recorded. *Right,* Echophonocardiogram showing the auscultatory findings in conjunction with an aortic valve echo (AVE). The valve partially closes in early systole and vibrates at the time of the murmur (slanting arrows). The posterior cusp opens fully (vertical arrow), and there is no ejection sound, which, if present, would be manifest by discrete vibrations synchronous with full opening of the valve. Diagnosis of thick fibrous subvalvular aortic stenosis was confirmed by catheterization with a peak valve gradient of 75 mm Hg.

in the apexcardiogram may be exaggerated, and the appearance of its auscultatory counterpart, the S_4, may also provide an indirect indication of increased left ventricular mass and loss of compliance (Fig. 4–4)[11,12]; and (5) the jugular venous pulse may become abnormal in severe, longstanding aortic stenosis of any variety. One may note an unusually prominent *a* wave reflecting altered filling characteristics of the right ventricle, possibly due to encroachment by the hypertrophied interventricular septum—the so-called Bernheim syndrome.[13] A point system utilizing a combination of variables has recently been found useful by Nakamura et al.[14] in increasing the sensitivity and specificity of the noninvasive assessment of the severity of aortic stenosis.

Fibrous Subaortic Stenosis (see also p. 980).   This condition is congenital in origin and is associated with a murmur identical to that of valvular stenosis, although its focus of maximal intensity may be over the midprecordium rather than the aortic area. The carotid pulse is also similar to that in valvular stenosis. However, two observations are of value in differential diagnosis by echophonocardiographic methods: (1) the absence of an ejection sound at the time of full aortic valve opening in the patient with fibrous or diaphragmatic subaortic stenosis (Fig. 4–5),[15] and (2) partial closure and fluttering of the aortic valve in early systole (Fig. 4–5).[16] This curious behavior of the valve is not peculiar to fibrous subaortic stenosis but may occur in hypertrophic obstructive cardiomyopathy (HOCM) as well as, to a minor degree, in normal individuals. However, the combination of the midsystolic murmur, absence of an ejection sound, partial closure and fluttering of the aortic valve in early systole, and absence of poststenotic dilatation on the x-ray should permit a reasonably confident diagnosis of fibrous or diaphragmatic subaortic stenosis. An

early diastolic murmur of mild aortic regurgitation may be found in association with fibrous subvalvular stenosis. An estimate of severity may be provided by the same criteria as those listed above, under Congenital Valvular Aortic Stenosis.

Supravalvular Aortic Stenosis (see also Chap. 29).   The midsystolic murmur in this congenital abnormality is similar to that of valvular and subvalvular stenosis.[7,15] It is usually of great intensity over the aortic area, to the right of the upper sternum, and is well transmitted over the vessels of the neck. Graphic tracings can be used to display the murmur, but such records are of little value in localizing the obstruction or determining its severity. A simultaneous recording of both carotid pulses, however, may disclose an inequality in amplitude and slope, apparently resulting from the direction of the jet of blood that has traversed the stenotic area (Fig. 4–6). This usually leads to inequality of the carotid and brachial pulses, which are more prominent on the right side (p. 982). An ejection sound is usually not present in supravalvular aortic stenosis,[17] and aortic regurgitation is most unusual.

Valvular Aortic Stenosis of Rheumatic Origin (see also Chap. 32).   The findings here are similar to those found in the congenital variety, although the ejection sound is only rarely seen and, when present, is inconspicuous, especially later in the natural history, when the valve has calcified. The presence of associated valvular lesions may be helpful in establishing the etiology.

Atypical Presentation of Aortic Stenosis.   In older patients, particularly those suffering from complicating conditions such as emphysema, the presentation of aortic stenosis may differ markedly from that of congenital stenosis in childhood. In elderly patients, the murmur of valvular aortic stenosis, regardless of etiology, is some-

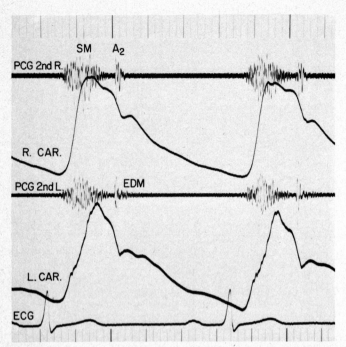

FIGURE 4–6 Supravalvular aortic stenosis. A loud midsystolic murmur was recorded in the right and left second intercostal spaces and was audible over the whole upper chest. Right and left carotid pulse tracings recorded simultaneously illustrate differences in their contours; note the more delayed upstroke in the left compared with the right carotid pulse. At catheterization a gradient of 95 mm Hg was recorded between left ventricle and aorta beyond the obstruction. The early diastolic murmur (EDM) of slight aortic regurgitation is unusual in this condition.

times heard best, if not exclusively, at the mitral area (Fig. 4–7).[18-20] Under these circumstances identification of the murmur as being ejection in character and presumably of aortic origin may be made by an experienced auscultator by noting the midsystolic peaking of the murmur and its termination before S_2. This latter sign may be obscured, however, by the faintness or absence of the second sound. The ejection sound is also faint or usually absent, because of the inevitable calcification of the valve. Clarification of this problem may be gained by noting the behavior of the murmur with an arrhythmia such as premature beats or atrial fibrillation, and confirmation by phonocardiography may be very helpful (Fig. 4–8). The ejection murmur of aortic stenosis fluctuates remarkably in intensity with the strength of left ventricular systole, whereas the murmur of mitral regurgitation is much less affected.[18] Other graphic records which may be helpful in differentiating aortic stenosis from mitral regurgitation include the carotid pulse tracing and systolic time intervals. The carotid upstroke is characteristically sharp in mitral regurgitation, but it is slow-rising and shattered in aortic stenosis (see Figure 3–22, p. 56, and Figure 4–4). PEP is prolonged in mitral regurgitation and LVET is shortened, giving an abnormally high PEP/LVET ratio. In aortic stenosis, the reverse is found—PEP is abbreviated and LVET is prolonged.[21]

Hypertrophic Obstructive Cardiomyopathy (HOCM) (see also p. 1409). The presence or absence of left ventricular outflow obstruction in patients with HOCM was an early

stimulus to the correlation of echo- and phonocardiographic abnormalities.[22,23] It is now well established that systolic anterior motion of the mitral valve impinging on the grossly hypertrophied septum results in obstruction to left ventricular outflow (Chap. 5) and produces a midsystolic murmur resembling that of valvular obstruction except that its location of maximal intensity is at the left sternal edge. The murmur may be augmented by an element of mitral regurgitation, which is a frequent additional physiological derangement. However, it is seldom possible to distinguish a separate holosystolic murmur at the cardiac apex. The midsystolic murmur suggests the presence of outflow tract obstruction[24] but may occur where there is concentric hypertrophy without obstruction.[25] Other features of HOCM that can be documented in a noninvasive assessment include the characteristic deformity of the carotid pulse—the spike-and-dome pattern, as described in Chapter 3—and the apexcardiogram with its exaggerated *a* wave and bifid or saddle-shaped appearance in systole (see Figure 3–30, p. 60). The cusps of the aortic valve can be seen, in an accompanying echo, to close partially at the time of the systolic anterior movement of the mitral leaflet and the onset of the murmur.[26] A combined study utilizing all these parameters with echocardiography is useful, therefore, in demonstrating the simultaneity and presumed physiological relationship of the systolic anterior movement of the mitral valve impinging on the hypertrophied septum and the dramatic array of auscultatory and pulsa-

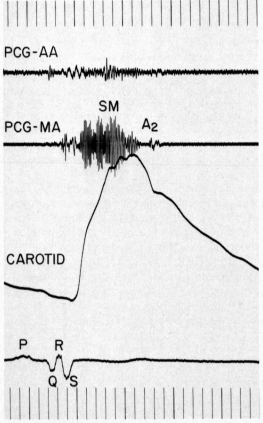

FIGURE 4–7 Aortic stenosis in an elderly man. The murmur is faint in the second right interspace (PCG-AA) but is prominent at the cardiac apex (MA). The carotid upstroke is delayed and demonstrates coarse vibrations.

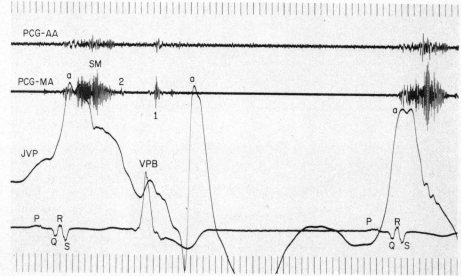

FIGURE 4–8 Aortic stenosis (same patient as in Figure 4–7). The weak ventricular premature beat (VPB) fails to produce a murmur, but the postextrasystolic beat results in accentuation of the murmur. The JVP demonstrates a prominent *a* wave in the conducted beats and a "cannon wave" with the VPB, owing to contraction of the right atrium against a closed tricuspid valve.

tile events that ensue (Fig. 4–9). In addition, the modifications in these signs produced by pharmacological and physical maueuvers, as described in Chapter 2, can be documented by echophonocardiography.

Ejection Through a Normal Valve into a Dilated Aortic Root. In hypertension, arteriosclerosis, and other conditions associated with aortic dilatation, a midsystolic murmur may be recorded over the aortic area. It is usually less intense than that associated with obstructive lesions and terminates earlier in systole. The upstroke of the carotid pulse is normal, and there is no prolongation of left ventricular systole manifest by lengthening of LVET and reversed splitting of S_2.

Obstruction to Right Ventricular Outflow (see also Chaps. 29 and 30). The physiological principles underlying the echophonocardiographic findings in obstruction to left ventricular outflow also apply to the right side of the heart. On the right side, however, the effect of inspiration in augmenting ventricular filling represents an additional factor.

Pulmonic Valve Stenosis. The murmur of pulmonic valvular stenosis is intense and of a harsh quality. It is maximal in the second left interspace and diminishes in all directions from this point. The murmur is midsystolic. However, more so than with the murmur of aortic stenosis, the timing of peak intensity can be used as an indicator of severity, being delayed in those patients with more severe obstruction. In the most severe cases, the murmur may peak late in systole and continue to or even *through* A_2, thus appearing to be holosystolic. Under these circumstances, however, since P_2 becomes further delayed with prolongation of right ventricular systole, the murmur remains *midsystolic* with respect to *right*-sided events of the cardiac cycle.[27] (See also Chap. 3.) The murmur is initiated by a pulmonary ejection sound which is also localized to the upper left sternal border and is loudest in *expiration* (Fig. 4–10).[28] Echophonocardiography can be very helpful in identifying an ejection sound by its exact coincidence with the achievement of a maximally open position by the pulmonary valve. The characteristic fluctuations of the sound with respiration can be readily documented. The phonocardiogram is also useful in displaying the increased separation of A_2-P_2, which is roughly proportional to the severity of the obstruction and the resultant rise in right ventricular systolic pressure.[27] The apexcardiographic transducer can be used to register the right ventricular heave, which marks the more severe examples of pulmonic valve stenosis.[29] The jugular venous pulse displays a prominent *a* wave in the presence of a thickened, hypertrophied, and noncompliant ventricle.

Subpulmonic (Infundibular) Stenosis. When this obstructive condition is found in isolation, i.e., without an as-

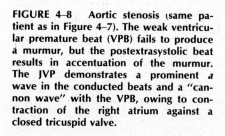

FIGURE 4–9 Hypertrophic obstructive cardiomyopathy (HOCM). *Left,* Carotid tracing illustrating a swift upstroke with a dip at the time of the midsystolic murmur, followed by a second hump during systole. *Right,* Echophonocardiogram showing the relationship between the murmur and the outflow tract obstruction resulting from the systolic anterior movement of the mitral valve (SAM), which appears to appose itself closely to the enormously hypertrophied septum.

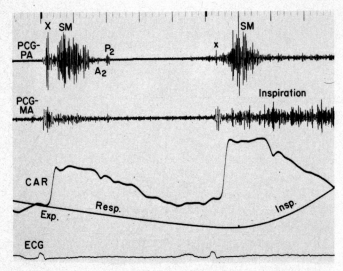

FIGURE 4-10 Valvular pulmonic stenosis. The first sound is not visible. The loud sound "X" at the beginning of systole is an ejection sound that is maximal in the second left interspace (PA). It is loud in expiration and diminishes with inspiration. The ejection sound is followed by a midsystolic murmur (SM). P_2 is diminutive and delayed.

sociated interventricular septal defect, the murmur is identical with that described earlier for valvular pulmonic stenosis,[30] although the location of its maximal intensity is lower along the left sternal border, in the third interspace. The ejection sound is lacking, however, as is the poststenotic dilatation on x-ray. Echocardiography reveals an early partial closing movement and fluttering of the pulmonary valve.[31] More often than in isolation, infundibular pulmonary stenosis occurs in conjunction with an interventricular septal defect, in which situation a whole spectrum of combinations of murmurs and heart sounds can be recorded as determined by the relative severity of the two major pathophysiological factors—the outflow obstruction and the interventricular defect.[32] At the one extreme, when the infundibular stenosis is mild, the physical signs as recorded phonocardiographically are dominated by the loud pansystolic murmur of the interventricular septal defect, upon which is superimposed the ejection murmur resulting from the stenosis. Frequently the silhouette of the murmur in the phonocardiogram taken low along the left sternal edge is holosystolic with a more or less constant intensity, whereas in the pulmonary area there is a definite midsystolic peak reflecting the obstructive lesion. There is no ejection sound. S_2 is widely split, as in valvular pulmonic stenosis, but P_2 is louder, probably reflecting the augmented flow through the pulmonary artery and higher pressures in the pulmonary artery as a result of the left-to-right shunt.

In cases in which the degree of infundibular stenosis is more severe, right-to-left shunting occurs through the ventricular septal defect, i.e., the classic tetralogy of Fallot. Under these circumstances the murmur from the ventricular defect disappears. The midsystolic murmur in the pulmonary area, however, can still be recorded, but its duration and intensity are lessened.[32] P_2 becomes inaudible and can rarely be recorded, even under ideal conditions. Thus the second sound (A_2) is single. An ejection sound of aortic origin is frequently audible and can be recorded widely over the precordium.

In the most extreme cases, when pulmonary atresia is present, the right-sided systolic murmur disappears, but there may be a short, early to midsystolic murmur resulting from ejection into a dilated aortic root. S_2 is single, and an aortic ejection sound can usually be recorded. Elsewhere over the thorax one can occasionally hear and record the continuous murmur from the bronchial collateral circulation.

Holosystolic Murmurs

Mitral Regurgitation[4,33,34] (see also Chap. 31). Combined echo- and phonocardiographic studies are particularly important in assessing patients with mitral regurgitation. Although the presence of the characteristic holosystolic murmur suggests the diagnosis by noninvasive means, neither the etiology nor the hemodynamic importance of the condition is usually apparent from the phonocardiographic findings alone. The echocardiographic features of mitral regurgitation are often nonspecific, but a useful index of the severity of the regurgitation is provided by the hyperdynamic left ventricular wall motion, left ventricular cavity dimensions, and left atrial enlargement (Chap. 5). Thus, whereas auscultation and phonocardiography establish the diagnosis, echocardiography is used to assess the severity of the regurgitation and, on occasion, its pathogenesis.

Mitral Regurgitation due to Rheumatic Heart Disease. The holosystolic murmur is best recorded at the cardiac apex (Fig. 4–11). It immediately follows S_1, which may be of reduced intensity unless there is a mixed lesion of stenosis and regurgitation. The murmur continues to or at times slightly beyond A_2. The second sound is normally split or may be more widely split than normal. However, variation with respiration is preserved. A third sound is a common accompaniment of moderate to severe mitral regurgitation,

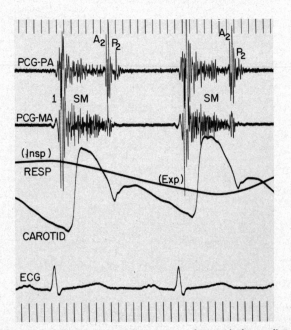

FIGURE 4-11 Mitral regurgitation due to rheumatic heart disease in a 25-year-old man with no symptoms and a small heart. The holosystolic murmur is most prominent at the cardiac apex (PCG-MA). S_1 is unusually loud, suggesting the possibility of early mitral stenosis, although there is no diastolic murmur.

and in the more severe cases a mid-diastolic rumble may be recorded in the mitral area.[35]

The echocardiographic appearance of rheumatic mitral regurgitation comprises a spectrum of mitral valve motion ranging from an apparently normal pattern to one in which the features of mitral stenosis are prominent. The combination of a holosystolic murmur and an echocardiogram consistent with mitral stenosis indicates the presence of mitral valvular disease with a rheumatic basis.

Mitral Regurgitation Secondary to Cardiomyopathy. Phonocardiography is of little help in the important differential diagnosis of severe diffuse cardiomyopathy as opposed to that of primary valvular disease. In cardiomyopathy, the murmur is holosystolic as in rheumatic heart disease, and there may be a prominent third sound that is also nonspecific, since it is a feature common to both cardiomyopathy and severe mitral regurgitation, regardless of pathogenesis. Systolic time intervals display similar abnormalities—prolongation of PEP and shortening of LVET, with a resulting increase in the PEP/LVET ratio (p. 54).[21] However, the echocardiogram may be most helpful in this differential diagnosis, since the dilated inert left ventricle of cardiomyopathy[36] contrasts sharply with

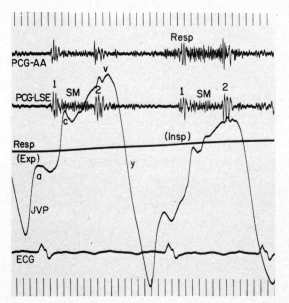

FIGURE 4–13 Tricuspid regurgitation, secondary to cor pulmonale resulting from thromboembolic disease. The phonocardiogram shows a holosystolic murmur at the left sternal edge (LSE). In this example the intensity of the murmur is not affected by inspiration. The accompanying JVP is abnormal with a very prominent cv plateau and y descent. The x' descent, which would normally follow the c wave, has been eliminated. Although the patient is in atrial flutter, there is an a wave in presystole which can be ascribed to atrial contraction.

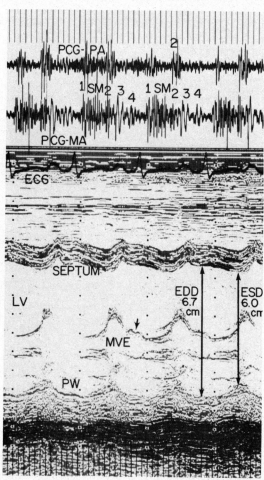

FIGURE 4–12 Systolic murmur with cardiomyopathy. The prominent holosystolic murmur at the cardiac apex (MA) is secondary to a severe diffuse alcoholic cardiomyopathy. There is very little difference between the left ventricular diameter in diastole (EDD) and that in systole (ESD). Additional phonocardiographic findings include gallop sounds (3 and 4). Arrow points to B notch on mitral valve echo, suggesting elevated left ventricular end-diastolic pressure. (Paper speed = 50 mm/sec.)

the hyperdynamic movements of the septum and posterior wall in severe mitral regurgitation of rheumatic origin (Fig. 4–12).

Tricuspid Regurgitation Secondary to Pulmonary Hypertension.[37] Although noninvasive methods are useful in the diagnosis of tricuspid regurgitation, the graphic registration of the murmur may be disappointing (Fig. 4–13). Even more than with mitral regurgitation, the intensity of the murmur fails to correlate with the severity of the hemodynamic abnormality.[38,39] It is often overshadowed by the murmurs of accompanying valvular disease, since tricuspid regurgitation is most often a complication of left-sided disease that has resulted in pulmonary hypertension. The murmur is classically recorded best at the left lower sternal edge. With dilatation of the right ventricle, its point of maximal intensity may be shifted toward the left to the usual location of mitral murmurs. This can lead to an erroneous impression of *mitral* regurgitation, when tricuspid insufficiency has developed as a late result of severe mitral stenosis with pulmonary hypertension. Accentuation of the murmur with inspiration (Carvallo's sign) is a well-known feature of tricuspid regurgitation[40] that can be documented phonocardiographically. An accompanying venous pulse tracing will illustrate the parallel accentuation of cv waves with inspiration. Carvallo's sign, however, is not invariably present[41] and can be abolished by the onset of right ventricular failure, which prevents the inspiratory augmentation of right ventricular stroke volume responsible for intensification of the murmur. A third sound and mid-diastolic flow rumble of right-sided origin are seen with the more severe cases of tricuspid regurgitation,[37] as in the analogous situation on the left side of the heart. Precordial movement at the left sternal edge consists

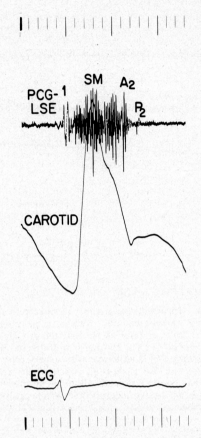

FIGURE 4–14 Ventricular septal defect with a large left-to-right shunt. A loud holosystolic murmur is seen, with accentuation in midsystole.

of a systolic heave of right ventricular hypertrophy when tricuspid regurgitation occurs as a consequence of right ventricular failure secondary to pulmonary hypertension.[42] The echocardiogram demonstrates a dilated right ventricular chamber and paradoxical movement of the interventricular septum (see Chap. 5). When tricuspid regurgitation occurs as a consequence of isolated damage to the valve itself rather than secondary to pulmonary hypertension, the physical signs and their graphic representation may be quite different (Chap. 31). The murmur may have a decrescendo configuration and be confined to early and midsystole.[43] This variant is discussed below, under Early Systolic Murmurs.

Ventricular Septal Defect (see also Chaps. 29 and 30). The murmur of a ventricular septal defect (VSD) is holosystolic, since in its typical expression (Roger's murmur)[44] it arises from the passage of blood throughout systole from the high-pressure left ventricle to the relatively low-pressure right ventricle through the defect. Thus the hemodynamic situation favors a holosystolic timing of the shunt as well as the murmur, which arises from the turbulence generated in the recipient chamber, the right ventricle. The murmur is quite intense and is located maximally in the third and fourth left interspaces, from which focus it diminishes centrifugally (Fig. 4–14).[45,46] The second heart sound is usually normal, although the degree of splitting may be somewhat exaggerated. However, respiratory variation is maintained.

In the smaller defects which characterize the classic Roger type of ventricular septal defect, the volume of the shunt is determined by the size of the septal aperture. The variations in hemodynamic patterns, which are conditioned by the size of the defect and the level of pulmonary arterial pressure, are roughly reflected in modifications in the graphic signs.[45] With larger shunts, the auscultatory and phonocardiographic signs of increased diastolic flow across the mitral valve may be manifest in an S_3 and mid-diastolic rumbling murmur. The apexcardiogram displays a hyperdynamic pattern—a systolic movement of normal shape but exaggerated amplitude and a prominent rapid filling wave. Although it is not usually possible to visualize the defect in the septum by M-mode echocardiography, one can detect indirect signs of the magnitude of the shunt in the size of the left-sided heart chambers and mobility of the left ventricular walls.

With pulmonary hypertension (the Eisenmenger type of VSD), the physical (Chap. 28) and graphic signs are remarkably altered (Fig. 4–15). The volume and direction of

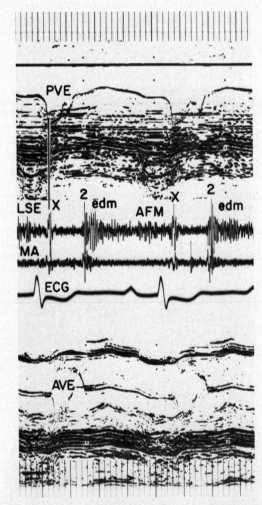

FIGURE 4–15 Dual echophonocardiogram in Eisenmenger's syndrome. A loud second sound (2) is followed by a high-frequency decrescendo diastolic murmur (edm) of pulmonary regurgitation. In the latter part of diastole, this merges with a lower frequency right-sided Austin Flint murmur (AFM). The loud ejection sound (X) is of pulmonary valve origin, as shown by the vertical line. The simultaneous echo of the aortic valve shows a tendency to closure in the latter half of systole, reflecting a dwindling stroke volume in this very ill patient.

shunting are now regulated by the relative resistances of the pulmonary and systemic circuits. As pressures in the two ventricles equilibrate in systole and as bidirectional shunting ensues owing to the large size of the defect, the systolic murmur resulting from the shunt disappears.[45] There remains a brief early to midsystolic ejection murmur resulting from flow into the dilated root of the pulmonary artery. This murmur is initiated by an ejection sound occurring at the time of full opening of the cusps of the pulmonic valve (Chap. 3). The timing of the ejection sound is delayed with pulmonary hypertension, owing to prolongation of the isovolumetric contraction time.[46] The second sound is very intense and is often palpable and results from the simultaneous closure of A_2 and an accentuated P_2. Accompanying murmurs that may be recorded in the more severe and longstanding cases of the Eisenmenger variant of ventricular septal defect include those of pulmonary regurgitation (Graham Steell), tricuspid regurgitation,[47] and, on occasion, a right-sided Austin Flint murmur.[48]

EARLY SYSTOLIC MURMURS

Acute Mitral Regurgitation (see also Chap. 32). Acute mitral regurgitation constitutes a syndrome that has been increasingly identified in recent years. Although less common than the chronic variety, acute mitral regurgitation is important because of its severity and reversibility in many instances, if it is accurately and promptly diagnosed. It occurs in association with rupture of the chordae tendineae or papillary muscle or with a severe damage to the valve itself, such as from trauma or infective endocarditis. Acute mitral regurgitation requires special consideration, since its auscultatory and phonocardiographic manifestations are unusual for mitral regurgitation—often resembling those of aortic stenosis. The murmur is usually pansystolic but tapers in intensity in late systole and in extreme cases may terminate before A_2.[49] The reason for the decrescendo character of the murmur is the unusual hemodynamic situation resulting from regurgitation of a large volume of blood during systole into a small, previously normal left atrium. The impact of the regurgitant bolus on a relatively noncompliant atrium results in an extraordinarily high v wave in late systole. Thus ventricular and atrial pressures (Fig. 4–16)[50,51] may equilibrate in late systole, with throttling of the regurgitant stream and suppression of the murmur. Despite its shortened duration, the murmur can be seen in a combined echophonocardiogram to be initiated at the time of mitral valve closure or well before the opening of the aortic valve, thus distinguishing it from a midsystolic murmur, which would also diminish in intensity in late systole but which would not start until after the aortic valve had opened. Other phonocardiographic signs include an S_3, as in the more usual types of mitral regurgitation. An S_4 may be recorded in acute mitral regurgitation[52] as well as its palpable counterpart, an a wave on the apexcardiogram. This is an important feature of the syndrome, which, like the unusual murmur described above, would not be expected in chronic mitral regurgitation. In the more severe cases a precordial heave that peaks in late systole can be recorded (Fig. 4–16). Its graphic configuration is qualitatively similar to the v wave of the left atrial pressure pulse, and it is thought to originate from the action of the whole heart being pushed

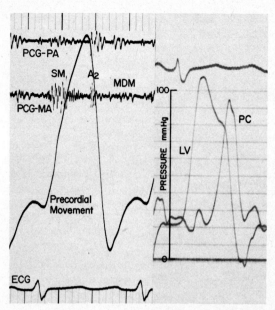

FIGURE 4–16 Acute mitral regurgitation in a young man with infective endocarditis. *Left,* Phonocardiogram at the cardiac apex (PCG-MA); an early systolic murmur (SM) begins with the onset of systole and terminates in mid- to late systole. *Right,* Pressure tracings from left ventricular (LV) and pulmonary capillary (PC) wedge positions. The high pressure (> 90 mm Hg) achieved in the left atrium in late systole results in equilibrium of pressures in LV and LA and termination of the systolic murmur. The unusual precordial movement pattern in the left-hand panel resembles the v wave in the PC wedge pressure and presumably reflects a forward thrust of the heart, resulting from massive left atrial expansion during systole. The mid-diastolic murmur (MDM) is a ventricular filling murmur or flow rumble.

against the chest wall, caused by sudden expansion during systole of the posteriorly located left atrium.[53]

Tricuspid Regurgitation due to Isolated Disease of the Valve (see also Chap. 32). When tricuspid regurgitation occurs owing to isolated disease of the valve itself rather than secondary to pulmonary hypertension, the phonocardiographic "silhouette" of the systolic murmur may be altered, so that it is decrescendo and terminates before the second heart sound. Isolated damage to the valve may occur from infective endocarditis or trauma. Under those circumstances, pressures in the right ventricle may be virtually normal. However, the high v wave generated in the right atrial pressure pulse by the regurgitant stream may lead to equalization of ventricular and atrial pressures in the latter part of systole, with diminution or suppression of the murmur. This occurs in a manner analogous to the alteration of the systolic murmur in acute mitral regurgitation, described above. Unfortunately, neither the timing nor the intensity of the murmur can be used to estimate the severity of the leak. Precordial movement in severe tricuspid regurgitation with normal right ventricular pressure may consist of an inward movement during systole and an expansion in diastole, reflecting massive volume changes in the underlying right ventricle.[54]

Congenital Heart Disease with Pulmonary Hypertension (see also Chaps. 29 and 30). Although the classic murmur of a ventricular septal defect is holosystolic, circumstances occur at both ends of the spectrum of severity of this condition that may drastically modify the physical signs and their graphic representation. The most minute of defects, resulting from a slitlike aperture through the muscular septum, may only momentarily provide a patent channel between the ventricles in early systole. Thus the murmur at the left sternal edge could terminate in midsystole. Physical examination is otherwise within normal limits, as are the electrocardiogram and chest roentgenogram. This type of minimal defect is likely to close spontaneously with the passage of time.

On the other hand, a very large defect results in free communication between the two ventricles, with equilibration of their peak systolic pressures at systemic levels. The direction of flow through the defect is determined by the relative resistance of the pulmonary and systemic vascular beds. Bidirectional shunting or predominantly right-to-left shunting may result (i.e., Eisenmenger complex). The systolic murmur becomes small in amplitude and is confined to early systole.[45] Accompanying signs of pulmonary hypertension include an ejection sound in the pulmonic area, a loud P_2, and, in severe cases, murmurs of regurgitation from the pulmonary and tricuspid valves.[47]

In similar fashion other shunts, such as in patent ductus arteriosus and atrial septal defect, may be altered significantly both hemodynamically and in their physical manifestations by the presence of pulmonary hypertension of severe degree. The characteristic continuous murmur of patent ductus, which will be described in more detail below, becomes abbreviated when there is an elevation of pressure in the pulmonary arterial system to the effect that the aortic and pulmonary pressures become equal in diastole. The murmur remains loud throughout systole and continues through the second sound but terminates in early diastole.[55] With even higher levels of pulmonary arterial pressure, shunting from right-to-left takes place through the ductus. Physical signs would then be indistinguishable from those of the Eisenmenger type of ventricular septal defect, with only a brief early systolic murmur, a pulmonary ejection sound, a loud P_2, and frequently a prominent decrescendo diastolic murmur of pulmonary regurgitation.[56] A similar alteration in physical signs and their graphic registration occurs with atrial septal defect complicated by severe pulmonary hypertension and right-to-left shunting, although in this circumstance, splitting of S_2 is preserved to a greater extent than in the Eisenmenger type of ventricular septal defect or patent ductus.[57]

LATE SYSTOLIC MURMURS

Mitral Valve Prolapse (see also Chap. 32). A wide spectrum of physical signs may be recorded in the mitral prolapse syndrome. In the milder cases the midsystolic click or clicks can be documented as well as alterations in their timing and intensity with various maneuvers. The click and late systolic murmur, the most characteristic features of the syndrome, can best be recorded at the cardiac apex. The click may coincide with prolapse of one or both cusps of the valve, as perceived in a simultaneous echocardiogram (see Figure 3–31, p. 61). The apexcardiogram in such cases may have an unusual configuration, with a notch at the time of the click and therefore a bifid configuration in systole. The murmur in most cases commences with the click and continues with increasing intensity to the second heart sound.[58] In some cases the murmur

may be of such intensity as to be audible to the patient and others in the room. Under these circumstances the quality of the murmur is musical and is aptly described as a whoop or honk. Its graphic repatient and others in the room. Under these circumstances the quality high-intensity vibrations of uniform frequency rather than the random frequencies which constitute most murmurs. Conversion of an ordinary late systolic murmur to a loud honk or whoop may occur transiently under the influence of changes of position.

In the presence of holosystolic prolapse (Fig. 4–17), the systolic murmur is also holosystolic and may achieve considerable intensity. A third heart sound and mid-diastolic flow rumble may be recorded as in mitral regurgitation of rheumatic origin; however, the first heart sound is intense, in contrast with its suppressed appearance in pure mitral regurgitation of rheumatic origin.[59] Prolapse of the mitral valve is thought to occur because of a redundancy of valve tissue with respect to the ring in which it is located.[60] Thus, maneuvers which decrease ventricular volume result in an earlier and more pronounced prolapse of the mitral valve. Phonocardiography in combination with echocardiography can be used to document the effects of pharmacological agents and postural changes that alter preload, afterload, and left ventricular contractility. For example, the effect of amyl nitrite is to decrease left ventricular volume at the onset of systole, causing the click to occur earlier in systole as well as increasing the intensity and duration of the murmur. Similar effects may be noted with standing or the Valsalva maneuvers (strain phase).[60] On the other hand, squatting or elevating the legs may cause the click to move later in systole and the murmur to become abbreviated and softer. A similar effect may be achieved with propranolol through the mechanism of increasing left ventricular volume.[60]

The diagnosis of mitral valve prolapse is relatively easy in the full-blown syndrome with characteristic auscultatory

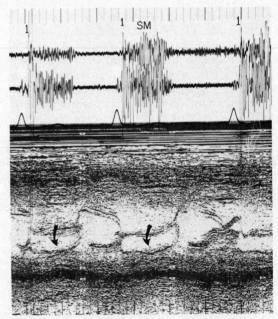

FIGURE 4–17   Mitral valve prolapse. Echophonocardiogram illustrating a holosystolic murmur associated with "hammock-shaped" prolapse of the valve of similar duration.

and echocardiographic findings. There are, however, borderline cases in which the manifestations are minimal or evanescent. In these cases, the echophonocardiographic technique emphasized in this chapter, specifically the parallel auscultatory and echocardiographic findings, combined with the pharmacological and physical maneuvers mentioned above, are extremely helpful.

DIASTOLIC MURMURS

VENTRICULAR FILLING MURMURS. These murmurs, which result from flow across the atrioventricular valves, are generally *mid-diastolic* in timing. Since they are dependent on flow across the mitral or tricuspid valve, they cannot begin until ventricular pressure has fallen below that in the atrium and the atrioventricular valve has opened. Thus there is inevitably a slight delay between the second heart sound (closure of semilunar valves) and the initiation of ventricular filling murmurs.[61] The term *"mid-diastolic"* serves to differentiate those murmurs from the *early* diastolic murmurs of semilunar valve regurgitation. Actually whether or not murmurs associated with ventricular filling do in fact occur in the first or the middle third of diastole depends to a major extent on the heart rate. At slow heart rates, with long diastoles, a "mid-diastolic" ventricular filling murmur may actually have run its course during the first third of diastole. The low pitch, which accounts for the rumbling character of ventricular filling murmurs, is the result of the relatively low pressure gradient that exists across the atrioventricular valve. By intracardiac phonocardiography the location of maximal intensity of these murmurs can be determined as being in the recipient chamber, the ventricle.[62]

The common denominator in the generation of diastolic murmurs that result from flow across atrioventricular valves is a disproportion between the volume of flow and the size of the orifice between the donor and recipient chambers. This can occur from three types of anatomical-physiological derangements:

1. *Stenosis of atrioventricular valves.* In mitral stenosis, which provides the classic example of murmurs of this type, the passage from atrium to ventricle is narrowed as a consequence of rheumatic fever or, rarely, a congenital defect. Tricuspid stenosis, although rarely diagnosed, is the right-sided analog.

2. *Increased flow across the valve.* Mitral and tricuspid regurgitation and shunts that result in increased flow across the atrioventricular valves cause rumbling murmurs, owing to excessive flow across nonobstructing valves.

3. *Normal volume of flow across a normal valve that closes prematurely.* The Austin Flint murmur can be so classified, since it results from premature partial closure of the mitral valve in diastole, owing to the aortic leak that leads to rising left ventricular diastolic pressure. Thus there is a normal volume of atrioventricular flow through a valvular orifice of diminishing size. These three categories of low-frequency diastolic murmurs will now be considered in further detail.

Stenosis of Atrioventricular Valves (See also Chap. 32)

Mitral Stenosis. The murmur of mitral stenosis is dependent on turbulence resulting from flow across the narrowed mitral orifice. Therefore the duration and intensity of the murmur are affected by the severity of the obstruction and the volume of flow across the valve.[63] Thus in situations characterized by very low flow across the valve, the murmur may be of minimal intensity, despite severe valvular disease.[64] Conversely, the intensity and duration of the murmur may be increased by exercise or other maneuvers that augment diastolic flow.[65]

Echophonocardiography can graphically demonstrate the opening of the mitral valve in early diastole and the coincident opening snap.[66,67] This event is followed by the diastolic murmur, which is often difficult to record away from its circumscribed zone of audibility. The patient should be tilted into a left lateral decubitus position, and the microphone should be placed at the point of the left ventricular apex impulse, as determined by palpation.[68] The early to mid-diastolic portion of the murmur occurs during the period of maximal ventricular filling. The duration of the murmur may be prolonged in the more severe cases, owing to persistence of a gradient across the mitral valve throughout a longer portion of diastole.[63]

Echophonocardiography has been very helpful in studies of the genesis of the presystolic crescendo phase of the diastolic murmur of mitral stenosis. This has traditionally been attributed to atrial systole.[69] In normal sinus rhythm, the characteristic crescendo murmur clearly follows the P wave in a multichannel graphic record and is initiated by atrial systole. However, it has been pointed out that the crescendo murmur may be found in cases in which the rhythm is atrial fibrillation, and consequently there is no effective atrial systole.[70,71] The suggestion has been made by Criley et al. that the final crescendo phase of the murmur is actually produced primarily by *ventricular* systole during the preisovolumetric phase of contraction.[72] Their studies based on phonocardiography and angiography indicate that the onset of the crescendo phase is at the time of the sharp closing movement of the valve apparatus by ventricular systole. Ventricular systole begins in the more severe cases while there is still antegrade flow across the valve orifice. Thus the rigid, scarred valve apparatus is thrust into the stream of blood that is still moving from atrium to ventricle, creating conditions for a high-velocity flow through a narrow orifice.[73] The presystolic crescendo murmur terminates with a loud first heart sound as the valve apparatus reaches the full extent of its move toward the atrium and is checked. The theory advanced by Criley et al. to explain this crescendo murmur has been supported by echophonocardiographic studies relating valve movements and the generation of the murmur in atrial fibrillation (Fig. 4–18) as well as in normal sinus rhythm.[74,75] The importance of ventricular systole in precipitating the swift closing movement of the mitral valve and the acoustic events dependent on this event can be demonstrated using noninvasive methods by combining an apexcardiogram with echo- and phonocardiographic tracings. The upstroke of the apexcardiogram signals precisely the time of left ventricular pressure rise; this provides a useful marker for analysis of those events of the cardiac cycle that are responsible for the characteristic galaxy of physical signs found in mitral stenosis at the beginning of systole (Fig. 4–19).

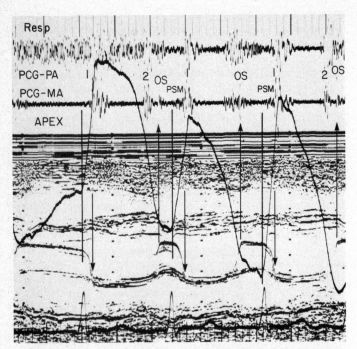

FIGURE 4–18   Mitral stenosis in atrial fibrillation. Echophonocardiogram illustrating a "presystolic" murmur (PSM) occurring only after the short diastoles. There is no PSM with the first cycle, which followed a longer diastole. The PSM is associated with the closing movement of the mitral valve (downward arrows). This, in turn, is initiated by ventricular systole, the onset of which is marked by the upstroke of the apex (heavy vertical lines). The relationship of the opening snap (OS) to opening of the mitral valve is shown by the upward arrows.

Tricuspid Stenosis. Tricuspid stenosis is a relatively rare condition occurring principally in association with far advanced rheumatic heart disease with mitral stenosis (p. 1115). Therefore the phonocardiographic signs may be overshadowed by those of the accompanying valvular disease.[76] Since most patients in the later stages of rheumatic heart disease will be in atrial fibrillation, the murmur of tricuspid stenosis will be found in early to mid-diastole, when there is a maximal gradient across the valve and a high velocity flow.[77] In normal sinus rhythm, the murmur may be confined to presystole and can be attributed to flow across the obstructing valve resulting from right atrial systole.[76] Maximal intensity of the murmur is at the left lower sternal edge.

Since the graphic signs described above could easily be confused with those of mitral stenosis, it is necessary to observe and record the effects of respiration on the intensity of the murmur.[78] A dramatic increase in intensity of the murmur with inspiration is very helpful, since this occurs with tricuspid but not with mitral stenosis. Simultaneous registration of the jugular venous pulse usually demonstrates enormous *a* waves in patients in normal sinus rhythm,[78] owing to retrograde flow in the venous system while the right atrium is contracting against a stenotic valve.[79] The echocardiogram may disclose alterations in the movements of the tricuspid valve in diastole similar to those of mitral stenosis. However, this valve is considerably more difficult to record by echo than is the mitral.

Left Atrial Myxoma (see also p. 1460). Murmurs associated with left atrial myxoma simulate those of mitral valve disease, but both the character and the intensity of

the murmurs may change profoundly on successive examinations or with alterations in position. The systolic murmur results from mitral regurgitation due to damage to the valve from trauma inflicted by the movable tumor mass[80] or from interference with apposition of the valve leaflets. A diastolic murmur is often present and is usually confined to late diastole or presystole. The pathogenesis of this murmur is probably analogous to that of the final crescendo phase of the presystolic murmur of mitral stenosis,[74] as can be demonstrated by combined echophonocardiographic observation (Fig. 4–20). Thus it can be shown that the "presystolic" crescendo actually occurs with the onset of ventricular systole at a time when the rising pressure in the ventricle is forcing the movable tumor back through the mitral orifice against the stream of blood that is still flowing from atrium to ventricle. The crescendo phase of the murmur culminates in the loud delayed first sound, related to the completed excursion of the tumor toward the atrium.[81]

Atrioventricular Flow Rumbles

Mitral Regurgitation Rapid flow across atrioventricular valves in early to mid-diastole often results in low-pitched rumbling murmurs simulating the physical sign of mitral stenosis. The most common example of this type of murmur is in mitral regurgitation, in which an increased volume of blood is moving from atrium to ventricle during passive ventricular filling. It is interesting that the flow rumble does not occur when the mitral valve has first

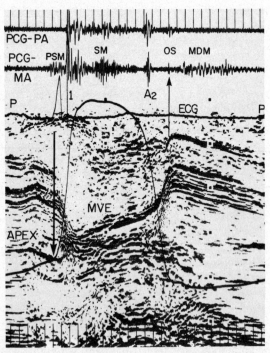

FIGURE 4–19   Mitral stenosis in a 49-year-old woman with a history of mitral commissurotomy 16 years previously with a good result. Sinus rhythm remains normal. An echophonocardiogram is combined with an apexcardiogram to show the relationship of the onset of LV systole to the presystolic crescendo murmur (PSM) (see text). The opening snap of the mitral valve (OS) occurs with full opening of the mitral valve (light arrow) and is followed by a mid-diastolic murmur (MDM). Mild accompanying aortic valve disease accounts for the crescendo-decrescendo systolic murmur transmitted to the mitral area (SM).

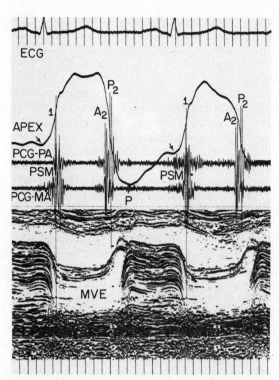

FIGURE 4–20 Left atrial myxoma. Echophonocardiogram illustrating the relationship between the presystolic murmur (PSM) and movement of the tumor mass through the mitral valve and into the atrium under the impact of ventricular systole. Timing of ventricular systole is provided by the apexcardiogram, the upstroke of which is indicated by an arrow.

opened and is most widely open with presumably maximal flow.[82,83] Rather it begins a few hundredths of a second later. Echophonocardiographic studies have clarified the relationship between valve motion and generation of the murmur.[74] These observations show that after opening widely in early diastole, the mitral valve makes a partial closing movement while presumably a high volume of blood is still moving antegrade across its closing orifice. This results, in effect, in a functional mitral stenosis, in which too large a volume of blood is moving across the valve for the dimensions of the aperture. A mid-diastolic pressure gradient may be demonstrated under these circumstances.[84,85]

Left-to-Right Shunts. A similar pathogenetic mechanism probably occurs in left-to-right shunts, such as patent ductus arteriosus or ventricular septal defect, in which there is augmented flow across a normal mitral valve.[86] On the right side of the heart, diastolic flow rumbles occur with atrial septal defect or anomalous pulmonary venous drainage in a manner analogous to the left-sided murmurs noted above. In atrial septal defect, a combined echophonocardiographic examination shows a closing movement of the tricuspid valve in early to mid-diastole at a time when a very large flow is taking place from atrium to ventricle (Fig. 4–21). The location of maximal intensity of the murmur by intracardiac phonocardiography is in the right ventricular inflow tract.[87]

Austin Flint Murmur. The apical rumbling diastolic murmur occurring in pure aortic regurgitation was first described by the renowned American clinician Austin Flint.[88] He attributed the murmur to functional mitral stenosis re-

sulting from impingement of the regurgitant stream on the anterior leaflet of the mitral valve. Although a number of alternative hypotheses to explain the genesis of the murmur have been advanced since Flint's time, modern studies combining echo- and phonocardiography support his original contention.[89] The mitral valve can be seen to effect a premature partial closing movement in early to mid-diastole and again following atrial systole while atrial contents are moving in an antegrade direction across the mitral orifice. Thus conditions exist for a functional type of mitral stenosis and the genesis of a murmur simulating organic obstruction. The murmur may be confined to late diastole (presystolic) in the milder cases, but in moderately severe aortic regurgitation there may be both mid-diastolic and late diastolic components, giving an hourglass configuration to the murmur on the phonocardiogram. The Flint murmur has been thought by some to be related to the vibrations of the anterior leaflet of the mitral valve, a characteristic echocardiographic feature of aortic regurgitation. These vibrations are the result, however, of the play on the leaflet of the regurgitating cascade of blood from the aortic root. The mitral valvular vibrations are therefore coincident in time with the early diastolic murmur of aortic regurgitation and *not* the Flint murmur, the timing of which is mid- and/or late diastolic.

In the most severe cases, such as in acute aortic insufficiency resulting from infective endocarditis, the Flint murmur may be confined to mid-diastole. This variant of the murmur is explained by the highly abnormal pressure relationships resulting from massive aortic regurgitation and generation of very high pressures in end diastole in the left

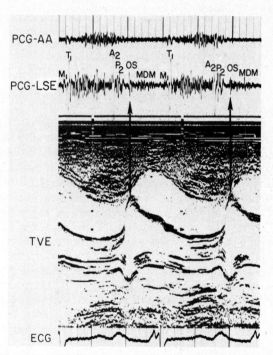

FIGURE 4–21 Mid-diastolic rumble in atrial septal defect. Echophonocardiogram demonstrating a mid-diastolic murmur (MDM) at the left sternal edge. The tricuspid valve is closing sharply during this phase of diastole while antegrade flow is occurring across it. Other phonocardiographic features of ASD include an accentuated T_1, an opening snap (OS) of tricuspid origin (arrow), and an ejection systolic murmur. The movements of the valve in systole are not well recorded.

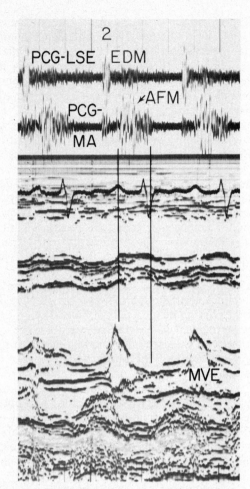

FIGURE 4–22   Austin Flint murmur in aortic regurgitation. An early diastolic murmur (EDM) is shown at top; in the lower phono channel, an Austin Flint murmur (AFM) is recorded at the cardiac apex (MA). It is associated with a rapid closing movement of the mitral valve, as seen in the echocardiogram (vertical arrows).

ventricle.[90,91] Thus, when the left ventricular end-diastolic pressure exceeds the pressure in the left atrium, the mitral valve closes prematurely in diastole, preventing further antegrade movement of blood across the valve (Fig. 4–22). Under these circumstances the Flint murmur is seen to arise during the mid-diastolic closing phase of mitral valve movement (Fig. 4–22). Accompanying features of this hemodynamic situation, as revealed in noninvasive studies, are the absence of M_1 due to premature mitral valve closure.[91,92] and the disappearance of the *a* wave in the apexcardiogram, since antegrade flow can no longer take place in response to atrial systole.[93] In summary, the ventricular filling murmurs, such as those associated with atrioventricular valvular regurgitation or the Flint murmur as well as the presystolic murmur of mitral stenosis, can all be shown by means of echophonocardiography to arise from antegrade flow across an orifice of diminished or diminishing size.[74,89]

SEMILUNAR VALVE REGURGITATION

Aortic Regurgitation (See also p. 1105)

Chronic Aortic Regurgitation. The early diastolic murmur of aortic regurgitation is the prototype of this class of

murmurs. It begins with the aortic component of the second heart sound and continues with decreasing intensity throughout most of diastole (Fig. 4–23).[94] Thus the murmur commences as the pressure within the left ventricle falls below that in the root of the aorta, allowing retrograde passage of blood across the incompetent valve, and it continues with lessening intensity as the volume and velocity of the regurgitant stream wane in the latter portion of diastole. By graphic techniques, the murmur of aortic regurgitation may be difficult to capture if it is faint because of its high frequency. Therefore phonocardiography is not useful as a means of determining the existence of a murmur that is doubtful on auscultation. The location of the murmur's maximal intensity should be determined by auscultation prior to application of the microphone for graphic registration. In *valvular* regurgitation, as with rheumatic heart disease, the location of maximal intensity is at the left sternal edge in the third or fourth interspace.[95] In aortic regurgitation associated with dilatation of the aortic root, the murmur may be maximal at the upper right sternal border.[95,96] In elderly or emphysematous individuals one may have to record the murmur from unusual locations, since it may be perceptible only at the cardiac apex or in the subxiphoid area.

Accompanying findings on noninvasive assessment include the alterations in the pulse contour noted on page 57. In the more severe cases the pulse may assume a bifid (bisferiens) shape during systole, its high amplitude reflecting the wide pulse pressure. The incisural notch in the carotid

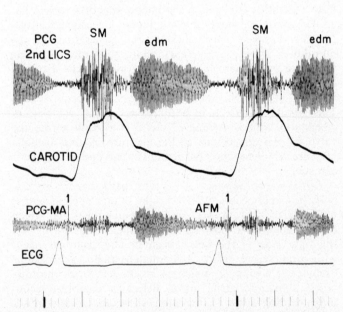

FIGURE 4–23   Aortic regurgitation. PCG at the second left intercostal space (2nd LICS) demonstrates a loud decrescendo diastolic murmur (edm) of unusual musical quality. There is a loud midsystolic murmur (SM) associated with the augmented stroke volume, although there was no stenosis of the aortic valve. At the cardiac apex (PCG-MA), the transmitted edm is seen, but in late diastole it merges with an Austin Flint murmur (AFM) of lower frequency. The incisural notch on the carotid tracing is poorly formed as a result of the valvular insufficiency.

tracing may disappear as the valve is unable to close and check the retrograde movement of blood at the onset of diastole (Fig. 4–23). Th e aortic component of S_2 is therefore diminished or absent.[97] The apexcardiogram verifies an increased amplitude representing hyperdynamic movements over the left ventricle associated with the increased stroke volume. The rapid filling wave is accentuated, and at the time of its peak, a third sound may be recorded as a result of the sudden massive filling of the left ventricle from two directions. In severe cases an exaggerated *a* wave is seen in the apexcardiogram,[98] reflecting a diminution in left ventricular compliance. Echocardiography completes the noninvasive assessment by supplying information regarding dilatation and hyperdynamic movements of the left ventricle, size of the aortic root, and vibrations of the anterior leaflet of the mitral valve. Despite the sophistication of these methods, however, it is worth emphasizing that the stethoscope remains the best tool for detecting aortic regurgitation.

Acute Aortic Regurgitation. In acute aortic regurgitation—an important syndrome that occurs with infective endocarditis, trauma, or aortic dissection—striking alterations in the graphic manifestations are found. In this situation the burden of massive regurgitation of sudden onset is placed on a ventricle that has not previously become dilated, as would be the case in the more common chronic form of aortic regurgitation. This results in dramatic elevations of left ventricular pressure in mid- to late diastole, so that left atrial pressure is exceeded and the mitral valve is closed prematurely in diastole. Equilibration of pressure in the left ventricle and aortic root occurs in mid- to late diastole in this situation,[99] and this results in sudden cessation of the regurgitant flow across the aortic valve and therefore truncation of the murmur in mid-diastole.[91]

Other accompanying features of this syndrome have been described above and include the confinement of the Austin Flint murmur to mid-diastole, absence of the mitral component of S_1, and disappearance of the *a* wave in the apexcardiogram as a result of inability of atrial systole to move blood into the left ventricle owing to the reversal of the atrioventricular pressure gradient.

Pulmonic Regurgitation. The murmur associated with regurgitation across the pulmonic valve occurs in two classes of physiological disturbances[100]:

1. When pulmonary hypertension results in dilatation of both the main pulmonary artery and the valve ring. As a result, the valve cusps become incapable of closing competently, and a regurgitant murmur ensues, known as the Graham Steell murmur.[47,101]

2. When the pressure in the pulmonary circuit is normal, but the valve is incompetent owing to a congenital malformation or surgical procedure.

These two pathogenetic mechanisms are manifest in different ways, as follows.

Pulmonary Hypertension (Graham Steell Murmur). The murmur associated with pulmonary hypertension (Graham Steell) is similar to that of aortic regurgitation, being high-pitched and decrescendo (Figs. 4–15 and 4–24), and follows the pulmonic component of S_2 in graphic records. It is unusual, however, to find a degree of separation of A_2-P_2 that will allow one to ascribe with confidence a decre-

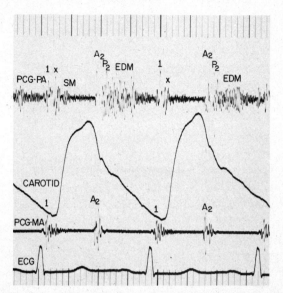

FIGURE 4–24   Patent ductus arteriosus, pulmonary hypertension, and pulmonary regurgitation in a 24-year-old woman known to have systemic pressure (140/70) in the pulmonary artery, with a bidirectional shunt. Phonocardiogram shows an ejection sound (X) in early systole and in the pulmonary area as well as a loud early diastolic murmur (EDM) of pulmonary regurgitation, which can be seen to follow immediately after P_2.

scendo, high-pitched murmur recorded at the upper left sternal edge to an aortic or pulmonic source on the basis of its inception with one or the other of the S_2 components. Rather, one must use the balance of clinical evidence to make this differential assessment.[102] The same problems in recording a high-pitched murmur exist with pulmonic as with aortic regurgitation, since most modern commercial phonocardiographic equipment is not particularly sensitive in the upper frequency range. Accompanying graphic signs often include an ejection sound of pulmonic origin, recordable in the second left intercostal space, and an accentuated P_2. The movements of the bulging pulmonary artery can often be recorded in the same location by application of the transducer used for apexcardiography over the palpable pulsation which precedes the vibrations of P_2.[103,104] Lower along the left sternal edge the heave of right ventricular hypertrophy can frequently be palpated and recorded, and there may be an associated *a* wave of right ventricular origin.[105] The venous pulse reflects the altered compliance of the right ventricle with exaggeration of the *a* wave. The echocardiogram, ideally performed in conjunction with the other graphic methods described above, can provide an estimate of right ventricular size and can confirm the presence of a pulmonic ejection sound by showing its coincidence with full opening of the pulmonic valve.[104,106] Finally, the echocardiogram can provide, especially in children, a measurement of right ventricular systolic time intervals, which may be of use in predicting the presence and severity of pulmonary hypertension.[107]

Pulmonic Regurgitation with Normal Pulmonary Arterial Pressures. The murmur of pulmonic regurgitation of valvular origin when pulmonary arterial pressure is normal differs from the Graham Steell murmur in that it is lower in pitch and located slightly later in diastole, so that its timing may be properly designated as mid-diastolic. These

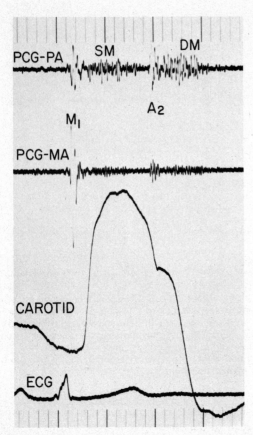

FIGURE 4–25 Pulmonary regurgitation due to organic valvular disease. Pulmonic valve stenosis had been relieved surgically, leaving a slight residual systolic murmur (SM) and a prominent early to mid-diastolic murmur of low frequency (DM). These murmurs are best seen in the second left interspace (PA).

differences reflect the later onset and reduced velocity of retrograde flow when pressure in the pulmonary artery is not high. Regurgitation begins after the pressure in the right ventricle has fallen below that in the pulmonary artery and a significant regurgitant movement of blood exists. The murmur therefore begins a perceptible distance after P_2, builds in intensity, and then fades away in mid- to late diastole (Fig. 4–25). It forms a crescendo-decrescendo silhouette made up of low-frequency vibrations, in contrast to the high-frequency, pennant-shaped graphic representation of the Graham Steell murmur, which follows immediately after P_2.

CONTINUOUS MURMURS[108]

DEFINITION OF CONTINUOUS MURMURS. Continuous murmurs may be defined as murmurs that begin in systole and persist without interruption through the second heart sound into diastole. They frequently terminate in the latter part of diastole and do not therefore necessarily continue throughout the cardiac cycle (Fig. 4–26). Graphic records may be useful in establishing the timing and duration of continuous murmurs, but the findings usually lack specificity.

CLASSIFICATION OF CONTINUOUS MURMURS. Continuous murmurs generally result from four classes of hemodynamic conditions: (1) connections between the aor-

ta and the pulmonary artery or its branches, (2) arteriovenous fistulas, (3) altered flow in arteries, and (4) altered flow in veins.

Aortopulmonary Connections

Patent Ductus Arteriosus. Patent ductus arteriosus is the classic example of this group of conditions.[109] Here, as in all fistulas, the magnitude, velocity, and duration of the abnormal flow and the resulting murmur are determined by the pressure relationships between the high-pressure aorta, which is the donor vessel, and the pulmonary artery or its branch, which is the recipient vessel. The murmur begins in systole when pressure in the aorta greatly exceeds that in the pulmonary artery and continues into diastole because of the persistence of a pressure gradient favoring the shunt. The peculiar quality and timing of the ductus murmur have been vividly described by Neill and Mounsey.[109]

...two opposing streams crash head-on within the pulmonary artery, one surging from the right ventricle upwards and backwards along its course, and the other, a narrower powerful jet, projected by the high aortic pressure through the ductus into the pulmonary artery, where it meets the on-coming stream from the right ventricle. Since the pulmonary orifice is larger than that of the ductus and since a different course is taken by the two streams, the greater flow into the pulmonary artery in early systole is from the right ventricle. Later as ventricular systole nears completion, the greater flow is from the ductus, and one may imagine turbulent eddies forming at the Waters meet of the main pulmonary artery until finally in diastole the flow is from the ductus alone. The typical patent ductus arteriosus murmur mirrors these events, since it continues and increases at end systole and beginning of diastole, and it is often punctuated by reverberations from beat to beat as eddies swirl within the pulmonary artery.

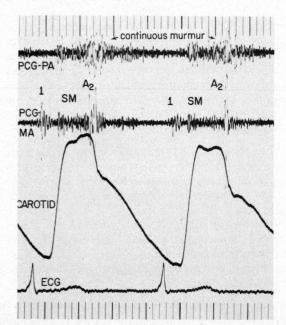

FIGURE 4–26 Patent ductus arteriosus. Phonocardiogram in the second left interspace (PA) demonstrates a prominent continuous murmur that is maximal at the time of S_2, obscuring the details of the latter. A_2 is well transmitted, however, to the cardiac apex (MA) and can be further identified by its position immediately before the incisural notch in the carotid tracing.

In graphic records the ductus murmur is usually best recorded at the upper left sternal border (Fig. 4–26). It is best to use two phonocardiographic microphones simultaneously, with the second one located at the cardiac apex.[3] The details of the second heart sound are usually obscured at the upper left sternal border, since the intensity of the murmur is maximal at the time of S_2. Since A_2 is usually widely transmitted, however, the second microphone can be used to appreciate A_2 in a location such as the cardiac apex, sufficiently removed from the main focus of intensity of the murmur. At the cardiac apex additional signs may be recorded that are of significance in estimating the volume of the shunt. These are S_3 and a mid-diastolic rumble.[86] The third sound is less helpful, since it is a normal finding in a child, but a mid-diastolic flow rumble indicates a substantially increased flow across the mitral valve and therefore a truly significant shunt. An additional noninvasive manifestation is echocardiographic evidence of dilatation of the left-sided heart chambers where the shunt is of large dimensions.

In patent ductus with high pulmonary vascular resistance, there is equilibration of pressures in diastole, which results in abbreviation and finally elimination of the diastolic phase of the murmur.[55] In more severe cases the systolic portion of the murmur may be confined to early systole. The murmur then ceases to be the major graphic manifestation of the abnormality and is replaced by the stigmata of pulmonary hypertension, as described on p. 83, including in some cases a loud murmur of pulmonary regurgitation (Fig. 4–24).[47,56]

An aortopulmonary window is associated with hemodynamic alterations similar to those of a patent ductus. Owing to the large size of the aperture between the great vessels, there is usually a significant degree of pulmonary hypertension, so that the murmur and other graphic findings are modified as in the case of patent ductus complicated by elevated pulmonary arterial pressure.

Systemic-Pulmonary Shunts Created Surgically. Operations designed to create fistulas between the aorta and the pulmonary artery or its branches (e.g., Blalock, Potts) result in murmurs resembling those of patent ductus arteriosus (PDA). The site of maximal intensity depends on the location of the shunt in the chest. Accompanying signs of increased flow (mid-diastolic rumble) or pulmonary hypertension, when the size of the communication has been larger than optimal, are identical with those of PDA.

Arteriovenous Connections. Shunts of this variety occur for a variety of reasons, both congenital and acquired. Examples include congenital or traumatically acquired arteriovenous fistulas and the shunts created surgically for purposes of hemodialysis. An example of a congenital connection of this type is a coronary arteriovenous fistula.[109,110] This anomaly consists of a tortuous, elongated arterial communication that drains, in most instances, into the right atrium, coronary sinus, or right ventricle. The physician's attention is attracted to the possibility of a coronary arteriovenous fistula by the discovery of a continuous murmur resembling that of a patent ductus arteriosus. The location of the murmur, however, is usually lower over the precordium than in patent ductus, with the exact location to the right or left of the sternum

being determined by the identity of the recipient chamber—right atrium or ventricle.

Traumatic fistulas may occur anywhere and must be discovered by searching with the stethoscope, especially in the region of scars from knife or bullet wounds.[111] Graphic records can serve to document the presence of such a murmur but seldom are of critical importance in making the diagnosis. The physiological consequences of the increase in systemic blood flow over a long period, however, may be manifest in echocardiograms showing dilatation and hyperdynamic movements of the left heart chambers.

Altered Flow in Arteries. When blood flow in major arteries—whether systemic or pulmonary—is altered by a significant constriction, a murmur may be generated. This is generally systolic in time—either exclusively or predominantly. However, when constriction has severely altered the pattern of blood flow, a continuous murmur may be produced. A systolic pressure gradient across the constricted segment is a prerequisite for the genesis of this type of continuous murmur.[112] In coarctation of the aorta, for instance, it has been shown that a very severe constriction (less than 2.5 mm in internal diameter) is required to produce the hemodynamic situation conducive to continuity of the murmur.[113] Lesser degrees of constriction result in a murmur confined to systole. An analogous situation may exist in the pulmonary arterial system with pulmonary branch stenosis[114,115] or occasionally with incomplete arterial occlusion by pulmonary embolism.[116]

Altered Flow in Veins. The most common continuous murmur is the venous hum. Its loudness and location (usually over the great veins at the lower part of the neck)[117] occasionally are confused with those of a patent ductus arteriosus. The venous hum, however, is truly a continuous murmur, existing through the cardiac cycle. Its intensity may increase in diastole. Graphic records can be used to demonstrate its presence, its cyclical silhouette, and, more importantly, its obliteration with recumbency or pressure over the great vein, from which it originates. Such documentation should not be necessary for the diagnosis of this ubiquitous and innocent physical sign.

SUMMARY

Not uncommonly, a well-planned noninvasive study may indicate the necessity for definitive invasive study. The timing of the hemodynamic or angiographic investigation and its objectives may be greatly clarified by the preliminary assessment in the graphics laboratory. Thus the protocol of the catheterization may be worked out in advance with greater precision and consequently greater safety as well as certainty that the data to be gathered will be appropriate to the patient's problem. Therefore the noninvasive techniques that have been described above are not to be considered competitive with cardiac catheterization (although occasionally they may render the latter unnecessary). Rather they permit the expensive and traumatic procedures to be used with greater sophistication in those situations in which precise answers to clearly thought-out questions are required for anatomical and physiological diagnosis.

References

1. Hinze, J. O.: Turbulence. 2nd ed. New York, McGraw-Hill Book Co., 1975, pp. 1–4 and 534–535.
2. Rushmer, R. F., and Morgan, C.: Meaning of murmurs. Am. J. Cardiol. *21*: 722, 1968.
3. Stein, P. D.: A physical and physiological basis for the interpretation of cardiac auscultation. Mount Kisco, N.Y., Futura Publishing Co., 1981, pp. 149–284.
4. Leatham, A.: Auscultation of the Heart and Phonocardiography. 2nd ed. New York, Churchill Livingstone, 1975.
5. Reddy, P. S., Shaver, J. A., and Leonard, J. J.: Cardiac systolic murmurs: Pathophysiology and differential diagnosis. Prog. Cardiovasc. Dis. *14*:1, 1971.
6. Castle, R. F.: Clinical recognition of innocent cardiac murmurs in children. J.A.M.A. *177*:1, 1961.
7. Perloff, J. K.: Clinical recognition of aortic stenosis; the physical signs and differential diagnosis of the various forms of obstruction to the left ventricular outflow. Prog. Cardiovasc. Dis. *10*:323, 1968.
8. Paley, H. W.: Left ventricular outflow tract obstruction. *In* Leon, D. F., and Shaver, J. A. (eds.): Physiologic Principles of Heart Sounds and Murmurs. New York, American Heart Association Monograph, No. 46, 1975, p. 107.
9. Stein, P. D., and Sabbah, H. N.: Origin of the second heart sound: clinical relevance of new observations. Am. J. Cardiol. *41*:108, 1978.
10. Bonner, A. J., Sacks, H. N., and Tavel, M. E.: Assessing the severity of aortic stenosis by phonocardiography and external pulse recordings. Circulation *48*: 247, 1973.
11. Goldblatt, A., Aygen, M. M., and Braunwald, E.: Hemodynamic-phonocardiographic correlations of the fourth heart sound in aortic stenosis. Circulation *26*: 92, 1962.
12. Gibson, T. C., Madry, R., Grossman, W., McLaurin, L. P., and Craige, E.: The A wave of the apexcardiogram and left ventricular diastolic stiffness. Circulation *49*:441, 1974.
13. Epstein, E. J., Doukas, N. G., Coulshed, N., and Brown, A. K.: Right ventricular systolic pressure gradients in aortic valve disease. Br. Heart J. *29*: 490, 1967.
14. Nakamura, T., Shettigar, U., Fowles, R. E., and Hultgren, H. N.: Noninvasive evaluation of severity of valvular aortic stenosis by a point score system. Circulation *66* (Suppl. 2):213, 1982.
15. Hancock, E. W.: Differentiation of valvar, subvalvar and supravalvar aortic stenosis. Guy's Hosp. Rep. *110*:1, 1961.
16. Davis, R. A., Feigenbaum, H., Chang, S., Konecke, L. L., and Dillon, J. C.: Echocardiographic manifestations of discrete subaortic stenosis. Am. J. Cardiol. *33*:277, 1974.
17. Vogel, J. H. K., and Blount, S. G., Jr.: Clinical evaluation in localizing level of obstruction to outflow from left ventricle. Importance of early systolic ejection click. Am. J. Cardiol. *15*:782, 1965.
18. Henke, R. P., March, H. W., and Hultgren, H. N.: An aid to identification of the murmur of aortic stenosis with atypical localization. Am. Heart J. *60*:354, 1960.
19. Burch, G. E., and Phillips, J. H.: Murmurs of aortic stenosis and mitral insufficiency masquerading as one another. Am. Heart J. *66*:439, 1963.
20. Roberts, W. C., Perloff, J. K., and Costantino, T.: Severe valvular aortic stenosis in patients over 65 years of age. Am. J. Cardiol. *27*:497, 1971.
21. Lewis, R. P., Rittgers, S. E., Forester, W. F., and Boudoulas, H.: A critical review of the systolic time intervals. Circulation *56*:146, 1977.
22. Shah, P. M., Gramiak, R., and Kramer, D. H.: Ultrasound localization of left ventricular outflow tract obstruction in hypertrophic obstructive cardiomyopathy. Circulation *40*:3, 1969.
23. Popp, R. L., and Harrison, D. C.: Ultrasound in the diagnosis and evaluation of therapy of idiopathic hypertrophic subaortic stenosis. Circulation *40*:905, 1969.
24. Sabbah, H. N., Marzilli, M., and Stein, P. D.: Intracardiac phonocardiography in experimental left ventricular cavity obstruction: Potential clinical applicability for the distinction of obliterating left ventricle from hypertrophic obstructive cardiomyopathy. Am. Heart J. *100*:77, 1980.
25. Come, P. C., Bulkley, B. H., Goodman, Z. D., Hutchins, G. M., Pitt, B., and Fortuin, N. J.: Hypercontractile cardiac states simulating hypertrophic cardiomyopathy. Circulation *55*:901, 1977.
26. Chahine, R. A., Raizner, A. E., Nelson, J., Winters, W. L., Miller, R. R., and Luchi, R. J.: Mid-systolic closure of the aortic valve in hypertrophic cardiomyopathy. Am. J. Cardiol. *43*:17, 1979.
27. Leatham, A., and Weitzman, D.: Auscultatory and phonocardiographic signs of pulmonary stenosis. Br. Heart J. *19*:303, 1957.
28. Hultgren, H. N., Reeve, R., Cohn, K., and McLeod, R.: The ejection click of valvular pulmonic stenosis. Circulation *40*:631, 1969.
29. Schmidt, R. E., and Craige, E.: Precordial movements over the right ventricle in children with pulmonary stenosis. Circulation *32*:241, 1965.
30. Vogelpoel, L., and Schrire, V.: Auscultatory and phonocardiographic assessment of pulmonary stenosis with intact ventricular septum. Circulation *22*:55, 1960.
31. Mills, P., Wolfe, C., Redwood, D., Leech, G., Craige, E., and Leatham, A.: Non-invasive diagnosis of subpulmonary outflow tract obstruction. Br. Heart J. *43*:276, 1980.
32. Vogelpoel, L., and Schrire, V.: Auscultatory and phonocardiographic assessment of Fallot's tetralogy. Circulation *22*:73, 1960.
33. Brigden, W., and Leatham, A.: Mitral incompetence. Br. Heart J. *15*:55, 1953.
34. Perloff, J. K., and Harvey, W. P.: Auscultatory and phonocardiographic manifestations of pure mitral regurgitation. Prog. Cardiovasc. Dis. *5*:172, 1962.
35. Nixon, P. G. F.: The third heart sound in mitral regurgitation. Br. Heart J. *23*: 677, 1961.
36. Corya, B. C., Feigenbaum, H., Rasmussen, S., and Black, M. J.: Echocardiographic features of congestive cardiomyopathy compared with normal subjects and patients with coronary artery disease. Circulation *49*:1153, 1974.
37. Wooley, C. F.: The spectrum of tricuspid regurgitation. *In* Leon, D. F., and Shaver, J. A.): Physiologic Principles of Heart Sounds and Murmurs. New York, American Heart Association Monograph, No. 46, 1975, p. 139.
38. Muller, O., and Shillingford, J.: Tricuspid incompetence. Br. Heart J. *16*:195, 1954.
39. Sepulveda, G., and Lukas, D. S.: The diagnosis of the tricuspid insufficiency — clinical features in 60 cases with associated mitral valve disease. Circulation *11*: 552, 1955.
40. Rivero-Carvallo, J. M.: Signo para el diagnóstico de las insuficiencias tricupídias. Arch. Inst. Cardiol. Méx. *16*:531, 1946.
41. Leon, D. F., Leonard, J. J., Lancaster, J. F., Kroetz, F. W., and Shaver, J. A.: Effect of respiration and pansystolic regurgitant murmurs as studied by biatrial intracardiac phonocardiography. Am. J. Med. *39*:429, 1965.
42. Mounsey, J. P. D.: Inspection and palpation of the cardiac impulse. Prog. Cardiovasc. Dis. *10*:187, 1967.
43. Rios, J. C., Massumi, R. A., Breesmen, W. T., and Sarin, R. K.: Auscultatory features of acute tricuspid regurgitation. Am. J. Cardiol. *23*:4, 1969.
44. Roger, H.: Recherches cliniques sur la communication congenitale des deux coeurs par inocclusion du septum interventriculaire. Bull. Acad. Méd. (Paris) *8*: 1074 and 1189, 1879.
45. Craige, E.: Phonocardiography in interventricular septal defects. Am. Heart J. *60*:51, 1960.
46. Leatham, A., and Segal, B. L.: Auscultatory and phonocardiographic findings in ventricular septal defect with left-to-right shunt. Circulation *25*:318, 1962.
47. Perloff, J. K.: Auscultatory and phonocardiographic manifestations of pulmonary hypertension. Prog. Cardiovasc. Dis. *9*:303, 1967.
48. Green, E. W., Arguss, N. S., and Adolph, R. J.: Right-sided Austin Flint murmur. Documentation by intracardiac phonocardiography, echocardiography and postmortem findings. Am. J. Cardiol. *32*:370, 1973.
49. Sanders, C. A., Scannell, J. G., Harthorne, J. W., and Austen, W. G.: Severe mitral regurgitation secondary to ruptured chordae tendineae. Circulation *31*: 506, 1965.
50. Raftery, E. B., Oakley, C. M., and Goodwin, J. F.: Acute subvalvar mitral incompetence. Lancet *2*:360, 1966.
51. Sutton, G. C., and Craige, E.: Clinical signs of acute severe mitral regurgitation. Am. J. Cardiol. *20*:141, 1967.
52. Cohen, L. S., Mason, D. T., and Braunwald, E.: Significance of an atrial gallop sound in mitral regurgitation: Clue to diagnosis of ruptured chordae tendineae. Circulation *35*:112, 1967.
53. Basta, L. L., Wolfson, P., Swain, L., Eckbert, D. L., and Abboud, F. M.: The value of left parasternal impulse recordings in the assessment of mitral regurgitation. Circulation *48*:1055, 1973.
54. Boicourt, O. W., Nagle, R. E., and Mounsey, J. P. D.: The clinical significance of systolic retraction of the apex impulse. Br. Heart J. *27*:379, 1965.
55. Myers, G. S., Scannell, J. G., Wyman, J. M., Dimond, E. G., and Hurst, J. W.: Atypical patent ductus arteriosus with absence of the usual aortic pressure gradient and the characteristic murmur. Am. Heart J. *41*:819, 1951.
56. Fishleder, B. L., Serra, C., Prati, P. L., and Friedland, C.: La persistencia del conducto arterial con hipertension pulmonar: Vareidad "diastolica ruda." Arch. Inst. Cardiol. Méx. *32*:610, 1962.
57. Sutton, G. C., Harris, A., and Leatham, A.: Second heart sound in pulmonary hypertension. Br. Heart J. *30*:743, 1968.
58. Barlow, J. B., Bosman, C. K., Pocock, W. A., and Marchand, P.: Late systolic murmur and non-ejection ('mid-late') systolic clicks.. Br. Heart J. *30*:203, 1968.
59. Dashkoff, N., Fortuin, N. J., and Hutchins, G. M.: Clinical features of severe mitral regurgitation due to floppy mitral valve. Circulation *50*(Suppl. III, Abst.):60, 1974.
60. Fontana, M. E., Kissel, G. L., and Criley, J. M.: Functional anatomy of mitral valve prolapse. *In* Leon, D. F., and Shaver, J. A. (eds.): Physiologic Principles of Heart Sounds and Murmurs. American Heart Association Monograph, No. 46, 1975, p. 126.
61. Nixon, P. G. F., and Wooler, G. H.: Left ventricular filling pressure gradient in mitral incompetence. Br. Heart J. *25*:382, 1963.
62. Esper, J., and Madoery, R. J.: Progresos en Auscultación y Fonomecanocardiografía. Buenos Aires, López Libreros, 1974, p. 301.
63. Wood, P.: An appreciation of mitral stenosis. Br. Med. J. *1*:1051 and 1113, 1954.
64. Ueda, H., Sakamoto, T., Kawai, N., Watanabe, H., Uozumi, Z., Okada, R., Kobayashi, T., and Kaito, G.: "Silent" mitral stenosis. Pathoanatomical basis of the absence of diastolic rumble. Jap. Heart J. *6*:206, 1965.
65. Ota, S.: Quantitative studies on the apical diastolic murmur in the mitral stenosis. Jap. Circ. J. *25*:410, 1961.
66. Joyner, C. R., Jr., and Dear, W. E.: The motion of the normal and abnormal mitral valve. A study of the opening snap. J. Clin. Invest. *45*:1029, 1966.
67. Craige, E.: Echocardiography in studies of the genesis of heart sounds and murmurs. *In* Yu, P. N., and Goodwin, J. F. (eds.): Progress in Cardiology. Philadelphia, Lea and Febiger, 1975.

68. Levine, S. A., and Harvey, W. P.: Clinical Auscultation of the Heart. Philadelphia, W. B. Saunders Co., 1959, p. 255.

69. Gairdner, W. T.: Further remarks on auricular systolic murmur. Med. Times Gaz. 2:460, 1864.

70. Constant, J.: Bedside Cardiology. Boston, Little, Brown and Co., 1976, p. 346.

71. Criley, J. M., and Hermer, A. J.: Crescendo presystolic murmur of mitral stenosis with atrial fibrillation. N. Engl. J. Med. 285:1284, 1971.

72. Criley, J. M., Feldman, J. M., and Meredith, T.: Mitral valve closure and the crescendo presystolic murmur. Am. J. Med. 51:456, 1971.

73. Lakier, J. B., Pocock, W. A., Gale, G. E., and Barlow, J. B.: Haemodynamic and sound events preceding first heart sound in mitral stenosis. Br. Heart J. 34: 1152, 1972.

74. Fortuin, N. J., and Craige, E.: Echocardiographic studies of genesis of mitral diastolic murmurs. Br. Heart J. 35:75, 1973.

75. Toutouzas, P., Koidakis, A., Velimezis, A., and Avgoustakis, D.: Mechanism of diastolic rumble and presystolic murmur in mitral stenosis. Br. Heart J. 36: 1096, 1974.

76. Bousvaros, G. A., and Stubington, D.: Some auscultatory and phonocardiographic features of tricuspid stenosis. Circulation 29:26, 1964.

77. Sanders, C. A., Hawthorne, J. W., DeSanctis, R. W., and Austen, W. G.: Tricuspid stenosis: A difficult diagnosis in the presence of atrial fibrillation. Circulation 33:26, 1966.

78. Perloff, J. K., and Harvey, W. P.: Clinical recognition of tricuspid stenosis. Circulation 22:346, 1960.

79. Sivaciyan, V., and Ranganathan, R.: Transcutaneous Doppler jugular venous flow velocity recording: Clinical and hemodynamic correlates. Circulation 57: 930, 1978.

80. Nasser, W. K., Davis, R. H., Dillon, J. C., Tavel, M. E., Helmen, C. H., Feigenbaum, H., and Fisch, C.: Atrial myxoma. I. Clinical and pathologic features in nine cases. Am. Heart J. 83:694, 1972.

81. Pitt, A., Pitt, B., Schaefer, J., and Criley, J. M.: Myxoma of the left atrium: Hemodynamic and phonocardiographic consequences of sudden tumor movement. Circulation 36:408, 1967.

82. Nixon, P. G. F.: The third heart sound in mitral regurgitation. Br. Heart J. 23: 677, 1961.

83. Silverman, B., and Fortuin, N.: Diastolic filling in cardiac disease. Clin. Res. 20(Abst.):398, 1972.

84. Hubbard, T. F., Dunn, F. L., and Neis, D. D.: A phonocardiographic study of the apical diastolic murmurs in pure mitral insufficiency. Am. Heart J. 57:223, 1959.

85. Nixon, P. G. F., and Wooler, G. H.: Left ventricular filling pressure gradient in mitral incompetence. Br. Heart J. 25:382, 1963.

86. Ravin, A., and Darley, W.: Apical diastolic murmurs in patent ductus arteriosus. Ann. Intern. Med. 33:903, 1950.

87. Wooley, C. F., Levin, H. S., Leighton, R. F., Goodwin, R. S., and Ryan, J. M.: Intracardiac sound and pressure events in man. Am. J. Med. 42:248, 1967.

88. Flint, A.: On cardiac murmurs. Am. J. Med. Sci. 44:29, 1862.

89. Fortuin, N. J., and Craige, E.: On the mechanism of the Austin Flint murmur. Circulation 45:558, 1972.

90. Reddy, P. S., Curtiss, E. I., Salerni, R., O'Toole, J. D., Griff, F. W., Leon, D. F., and Shaver, J. A.: Sound pressure correlates of the Austin Flint murmur: An intracardiac sound study. Circulation 53:210, 1976.

91. Mann, T., McLaurin, L., Grossman, W., and Craige, E.: Acute aortic regurgitation due to infective endocarditis. N. Engl. J. Med. 293:108, 1975.

92. Meadows, W. R., Van Praagh, S., Indreika, M., and Sharp, J. T.: Premature mitral valve closure. A hemodynamic explanation for absence of the first sound in aortic insufficiency. Circulation 28:251, 1963.

93. DiMattéo, J., LaFont, H., Hui Bon Hoa, F., et al.: La courbe méchanique ventriculaire dans l'insuffisance aortique. Arch. Mal. Coeur 60:1320, 1967.

94. Wells, B. G., Rappaport, M. B., and Sprague, H. B.: The graphic registration of basal diastolic murmurs. Am. Heart J. 37:586, 1949.

95. Harvey, W. P., and Perloff, J. K.: Some recent advances in clinical auscultation of the heart. Prog. Cardiovasc. Dis. 2:97, 1959.

96. Sakamoto, T., Kawai, N., Vozumi, Z., Yamada, T., Inoue, K., Chang, S. Y., and Ueda, H.: The point of maximum intensity of aortic diastolic regurgitant murmur with special reference to the right-sided aortic diastolic murmur. Jap. Heart J. 9:117, 1968.

97. Sabbah, H. N., Khaja, F., Anbe, D. T., and Stein, P. D.: The aortic closure sound in pure aortic insufficiency. Circulation 56:859, 1977.

98. Parker, E., Craige, E., and Hood, W. P., Jr.: The Austin Flint murmur and the A wave of the apexcardiogram in aortic regurgitation. Circulation 43:349, 1971.

99. Rees, J. R., Epstein, E. J., Criley, J. M., and Ross, R. S.: Hemodynamic effects of severe aortic regurgitation. Br. Heart J. 26:412, 1964.

100. Runco, V., and Levin, H. S.: The spectrum of pulmonic regurgitation. In Leon, D. F., and Shaver, J. A. (eds.): Physiologic Principles of Heart Sounds and Murmurs. New York, American Heart Association Monograph, No. 46, 1975, p. 175.

101. Steell, G.: The murmur of high pressure in the pulmonary artery. Med. Chron. 9:182, 1888.

102. Cohn, K. E., and Hultgren, H. N.: The Graham Steell murmur reevaluated. N. Engl. J. Med. 274:486, 1966.

103. Sakamoto, T., Matsuhisa, M., Inoue, K., Hayashi, T., and Ito, U.: Clinical and hemodynamic observation of indirect pulmonary artery pulse tracing. Cardiovasc. Sound Bull. 3:127, 1973.

104. Waider, W., and Craige, E.: First heart sound and ejection sounds. Am. J. Cardiol. 35:346, 1975.

105. Kesteloot, H., and Willems, J.: Relationship between the right apexcardiogram and the right ventricular dynamics. Acta Cardiol. 22:64, 1967.

106. Mills, P. G., Brodie, B., McLaurin, L., Schall, S., and Craige, E.: Echocardiographic and hemodynamic relationships of ejection sounds. Circulation 56:430, 1977.

107. Hirschfeld, S., Meyer, R., Schwartz, D. C., Korfhagen, J., and Kaplan, S.: The echocardiographic assessment of pulmonary artery pressure and pulmonary vascular resistance. Circulation 52:642, 1975.

108. Craige, E., and Millward, D. K.: Diastolic and continuous murmurs. Prog. Cardiovasc. Dis. 14:38, 1971.

109. Neill, C., and Mounsey, P.: Auscultation in patent ductus arteriosus, with a description of two fistulae simulating patent ductus. Br. Heart J. 20:61, 1958.

110. Gasul, B. M., Arcilla, R. A., Fell, E. H., Lynfield, J., Bicoff, J. P., and Luan, L. I.: Congenital coronary arteriovenous fistula. Pediatrics 25:531, 1960.

111. Muenster, J. J., Graettinger, J. S., and Campbell, J. A.: Correlation of clinical and hemodynamic findings in patients with systemic arteriovenous fistulas. Circulation: 20:1079, 1959.

112. Myers, J. D.: The mechanisms and significance of continuous murmurs. In Leon, D. F., and Shaver, J. A. (eds.): Physiologic Principles of Heart Sounds and Murmurs. New York, American Heart Association Monograph, No. 46, 1975, p. 201.

113. Spencer, M. P., Johnston, F. R., and Meredith, J. H.: The origin and interpretation of murmurs in coarctation of the aorta. Am. Heart J. 56:722, 1958.

114. Eldridge, F., Selzer, A., and Hultgren, H.: Stenosis of branch of pulmonary artery. An additional cause of continuous murmurs over the chest. Circulation 15:865, 1957.

115. Franch, R. H., and Gay, B. B., Jr.: Congenital stenosis of pulmonary artery branches. Am. J. Med. 35:512, 1963.

116. Levine, S. A., and Harvey, W. P.: Clinical Auscultation of the Heart. Philadelphia, W.B. Saunders Co., 1959, p. 613.

117. Palmer, R., and White, P. D.: Note on continuous humming murmur heard in supra- and infraclavicular fossae and over manubrium sterni in children. N. Engl. J. Med. 199:1297, 1928.

5

ECHOCARDIOGRAPHY
by Harvey Feigenbaum, M.D.

PRINCIPLES OF ECHOCARDIOGRAPHY
Creation of Image Using Pulsed Reflected Ultrasound

The term *echocardiography* refers to a group of tests that utilize ultrasound to examine the heart and record information in the form of echoes, i.e., reflected sonic waves. The upper limit for audible sound is 20,000 cycles/second, or 20 kiloHertz (kHz = 1000 cycles/second[1] The sonic frequency used for echocardiography ranges from 1 to 7 million cycles/second, or 1 to 7 megaHertz (MHz).[2] In adults the frequencies commonly employed are 2 to 3.5 MHz, while in children they are usually higher, ranging from 3.5 to 7.0 MHz. The *resolution* of the recording, which is the ability to distinguish two objects that are spatially close together, varies directly with the frequency and inversely with the wave length. High-frequency (short wave length) ultrasound can identify separate objects that are less than 1 mm apart. Beams having lower frequencies and longer wave lengths have poorer resolution. However, the degree of *penetration,* which is the ability to transmit sufficient ultrasonic energy into the chest to provide a satisfactory recording, is inversely proportional to the frequency of the signal. Since a high-frequency ultrasonic beam (i.e., 3 or 5 MHz) is unable to penetrate a thick chest wall, lower frequency ultrasonic beams are used in adults. While this permits penetration through the chest wall, it partially sacrifices resolution; however, even with a transducer producing a beam of 2.25 MHz, which is commonly used in adult echocardiography, it is still possible to resolve objects that are 1 to 2 mm apart.

Although diagnostic ultrasound, including echocardiography, is an imaging technique, there are many fundamental differences between ultrasound and other techniques used to create an image of an internal structure. Examinations that use ionizing radiation, whether in the form of an x-ray beam or a radioactive isotope, usually record the *shadow* of a structure, while ultrasound creates an image using *re-flected* energy. Visualization of a structure using light relies on the reflection of energy off the object in question and its capture in the eye or on photographic film; ultrasonic imaging utilizes the same basic principle. It should be recalled that imaging with both light and ultrasound is utilized in nature; indeed, several mammalian species, including bats, dolphins, and whales, rely on ultrasound instead of vision. The technology necessary to create ultrasonic images has been available for many years, and medical diagnostic ultrasound is an outgrowth of both industrial nondestructive testing of materials and naval sonar.[1–3]

The principles by which ultrasound creates an image are depicted in Figure 5–1. The transducer at the side of the beaker of water has a piezoelectric element that vibrates very rapidly and produces ultrasound when activated by an electrical field.[3] The original piezoelectric material used was quartz, but a variety of different ceramics are now used for this purpose. If a burst of electrical energy is imparted to the transducer, it will emit a burst of ultrasound, which travels through the beaker. As long as the medium through which the sound travels is homogeneous, the ultrasonic waves will travel in a straight line. When the ultrasound strikes an interface between two media which have different acoustical properties, the sound behaves according to the laws of reflection and refraction,[1,2] analogous to light. Whether or not ultrasound is reflected by an interface depends upon the difference in the acoustical impedances of the two media. Although acoustical impedance is the product of the density of the object and the velocity of sound through that object, for all practical purposes one can consider the acoustical impedance to be a function of density. Thus, if the interface is between a liquid and a solid, the ultrasonic wave will generally be reflected. If the interface is between two solids of different densities, the quantity of reflected ultrasound is usually less. Thus, the quantity of energy reflected is directly proportional to the difference in the acoustical impedances (or densities) of the object and its surrounding media and to the angle at which the

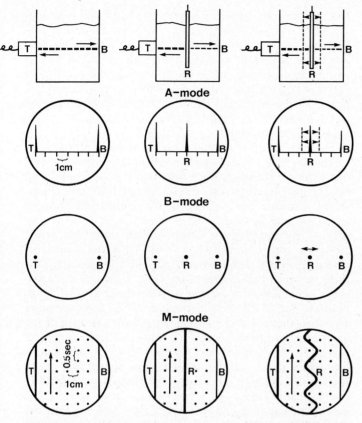

FIGURE 5-1 Diagrams illustrating the principles of acoustic imaging using pulsed reflected ultrasound (see text for details). T = transducer, B = beaker, R = rod. (Modified from Feigenbaum, H., and Zaky, A.: Use of diagnostic ultrasound in clinical cardiology. J. Indiana State Med. Assoc. *59*:140, 1966.)

beam strikes the object; i.e., the more perpendicular the beam is to the object, the lower the percentage of reflected energy.

The left panel of Figure 5-1 shows diagrammatically an ultrasonic beam, which consists of individual bursts of ultrasound that leave the transducer, travel through the fluid, strike the far side of the beaker, are reflected by this interface, retrace their original path, and again strike the transducer. The piezoelectric element in the transducer not only converts electrical energy into ultrasonic impulses but also converts ultrasound back to electrical energy. Thus, when the reflected ultrasound (echo) strikes the piezoelectric element in the transducer, an electrical signal is produced. If the time it takes for (a) the ultrasound to leave the transducer and return and (b) the velocity of sound through the medium are both known, the distance between the transducer and the reflected interface can be calculated. By calibrating the echograph (ultrasonoscope) for a velocity of sound in the medium under examination, the time that it takes for the ultrasound to leave and return as an echo can be automatically converted to distance. Thus, the far wall of the beaker is depicted on the oscilloscope as being 6 cm from the transducer.

If a rod is placed in the water so that it transects the ultrasonic beam, part of the energy will strike and be reflected by the rod before the beam strikes the far side of the beaker. Thus, the returning ultrasonic energy or echo from the rod will strike the transducer sooner than that returning from the far side of the beaker, and the corresponding electrical signal produced by the echo from the rod will be closer to the transducer than will that from the beaker. Also, since some of the ultrasonic energy is reflected by the rod, less energy will remain to strike the far wall of the beaker, and the magnitude of the echo (Fig. 5-1, center panel) will be reduced. There are adjustments in ultrasonic instrumentation which provide depth compensation and thereby correct for this loss of ultrasonic energy from distant or far objects. From examination of the A-mode echo ("A" refers to amplitude) in Figure 5-1 (center panel), one could deduce that the far wall of the beaker is 6 cm from the transducer and that an echo-reflecting object is present in the center of the beaker, 3 cm from the transducer.

If the rod were moving back and forth as in the right panel of Figure 5-1, the ultrasonic examination would differ. The transducer functions as a transmitter of ultrasound for a very short period of time, just over one μsec in commercial echocardiographs. During the remaining time the transducer functions as a receiver, waiting for echoes to be converted into electrical signals. The rapidity or the repetition rate with which the transducer fires the 1 μsec impulses varies depending upon the design of the instrument. Commercial M-mode instruments commonly pulse the transducer 1000 times/sec with 1 μsec impulses. Thus, the transducer functions as a receiver during approximately 999 μsec of each msec.

In the left and center panels of Figure 5-1, the wall of the beaker and the rod are not moving. All the ultrasonic impulses firing at a rate of 1000/sec take the same time to leave the transducer and return as echoes. Therefore, the signals or echoes seen on the oscilloscope are static. In the right panel, the object moves constantly and therefore the time required for the ultrasound to leave the transducer and return as an echo varies correspondingly and the echo signal on the oscilloscope moves. In the A-mode presentation the echo from the rod moves back and forth within the center of the beaker. To record the motion of the rod, one could make a movie or television recording of the moving echo on the oscilloscope. A more practical method of recording this echo motion is to convert the amplitude of the echo to brightness, which changes the display from the A-mode to the B-mode (the "B" refers to brightness), in which the returning echoes are displayed on the oscilloscope as dots rather than as spikes. Stronger signals are therefore taller on the A-mode and brighter on the B-mode presentation. Since the echoes are now dots instead of spikes, a dimension becomes available, and the element of time can be introduced by sweeping the oscilloscope. On the M-mode presentation ("M" refers to motion) displayed in Figure 5-1, the oscilloscope sweeps from bottom to top. In the left and center panels the structures are fixed, and therefore the M-mode presentation shows simply a series of parallel lines. In the right panel the rod moves back and forth in a regular manner, its echo inscribing a sinusoidal curve on the M-mode oscilloscope.

Thus, the M-mode presentation permits recording of amplitude and of the rate of motion of moving objects with great accuracy; the sampling rate is essentially 1000 pulses/second, the repetition rate of the transducer. Since electrocardiograms and other cardiac parameters are conventionally displayed on the oscilloscope together with the echocardiograph, the oscilloscope usually sweeps from left to right rather than from bottom to top; therefore, the transducer is generally displayed at the top of the oscilloscopic image rather than on the left side, as depicted in Figure 5-1.

M-Mode Echocardiography

Technique. The ultrasonic transducer is ordinarily placed on the surface of the chest, usually along the left sternal border (Fig. 5-2), and the ultrasonic beam is directed toward the part of the heart to be examined. In Figure 5-3 the ultrasound is depicted as passing through a small portion of the right ventricle, the interventricular septum, and the cavity and posterior wall of the left ventricle. This diagram is analogous to Figure 5-1 except that the transducer is now at the top rather than at the side. Therefore, on the echocardiogram, time is displayed on the abscissa and distance on the ordinate. The various structures which transect the ultrasonic beam produce echoes on the oscilloscope; the first object through which the beam travels is the chest wall, which produces a series of echoes. Since these echoes do not move with the cardiac cycle, they are displayed as a series of straight horizontal lines. The ultrasonic beam then strikes the anterior wall of the right ventricle, which may or may not be well imaged, depending upon the configuration of the patient's thoracic cage and the frequency of the beam; in this particular tracing the anterior wall of the right ventricle is indistinct.

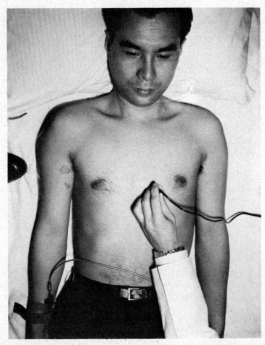

FIGURE 5-2 Placement of the ultrasonic echocardiographic transducer on the chest along the left sternal border. (From Feigenbaum, H., et al.: Left ventricular wall thickness measured by ultrasound. Arch. Intern. Med. *121*:391, 1968. Copyright 1968, American Medical Association.)

The next area recorded on the echocardiogram is a relatively echo-free space between the anterior right ventricular wall and the right side of the interventricular septum, which represents a portion of the right ventricular cavity. The echoes which make up the interventricular septum consist of echoes from the right and left sides of the septum. Posterior to the septal echoes is the relatively echo-free space of the left ventricular cavity. This cavity frequently has echoes from the mitral valve apparatus, only a

few of which are seen in Figure 5-3. The posterior boundary of the left ventricular cavity is the posterior left ventricular wall, which is made up of endocardial and epicardial echoes. The endocardial echo has the greater amplitude of motion, while the epicardial echo is more intense. Between these two echoes is the myocardium, which is more echo-producing than the intracavitary blood but less echo-producing than the epicardium and lung, which is posterior to the heart.

The M-Mode Tracing. An M-mode recording is sometimes called a one-dimensional or an "ice-pick" view of the heart. However, since time is the second dimension on M-mode tracings, this display is not truly one-dimensional. One can greatly augment the information provided by an isolated M-mode view of the heart, such as in Figure 5-3, by changing the direction of the ultrasonic beam, as in an arc or sector (Fig. 5-4). With the transducer placed along the left sternal border in approximately the third or fourth intercostal space (Fig. 5-2), the ultrasonic beam can be swept in a sector between the apex (Fig. 5-4*A*, position 1) and the base of the heart (Fig. 5-4*A*, position 4). When the transducer is pointed toward the apex of the heart, the ultrasonic beam traverses the left ventricular cavity at the level of the papillary muscles and passes through a small portion of the right ventricular cavity (Fig. 5-4*B*, position 1). Tilting the transducer superiorly and medially causes the ultrasonic beam to traverse the left ventricular cavity at the level of the edges of the mitral valve leaflets or the chordae (position 2). The beam again passes through a small portion of the right ventricle. By directing the transducer more superiorly and medially (position 3), more of the anterior leaflet of the mitral valve can be recorded and the beam may traverse part of the left atrial cavity. Further tilting of the transducer superiorly and medially (position 4) directs the beam through the root of the aorta, the leaflets of the aortic valve, and the body of the left atrium.

Figure 5-5 is a diagram of an echocardiographic record-

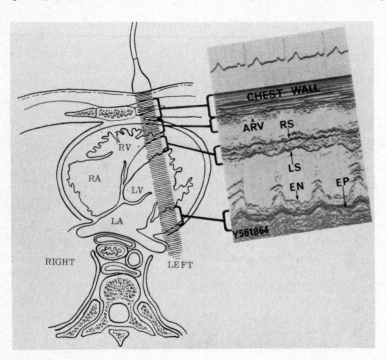

FIGURE 5-3 Diagrammatic cross-section of the heart and corresponding echocardiogram showing the cardiac structures transected by an ultrasonic beam directed toward the left ventricle. The ultrasound passes through the chest wall, the anterior right ventricular wall (ARV), a small portion of the right ventricular cavity, the interventricular septum, the cavity of the left ventricle, and the posterior left ventricular wall. RS = right side of interventricular septum, LS = left side of interventricular septum, EN = posterior left ventricular endocardium, EP = posterior left ventricular epicardium. (Modified from Popp, R. L., et al.: Estimation of right and left ventricular size by ultrasound. A study of the echoes from the interventricular septum. Am. J. Cardiol. *24*:523, 1969.)

FIGURE 5–4 Diagram demonstrating how the ultrasonic transducer is commonly directed in an arc or sector between the base of the heart and the apex (A). B, Cross-section of the heart parallel to the long axis of the left ventricle showing the structures through which the ultrasound beam passes as it is directed from the apex toward the base of the heart, as shown in A. T = transducer, S = sternum, ARV = anterior right ventricular wall, RV = right ventricular cavity, IVS = interventricular septum, LV = left ventricle, PPM = posterior papillary muscle, PLV = posterior left ventricular wall, AMV = anterior mitral valve, PMV = posterior mitral valve, AO = aorta, LA = left atrium, MV = mitral valve. (From Feigenbaum, H.: Clinical applications of echocardiography. Progr. Cardiovasc. Dis. 14:531, 1972, by permission of Grune and Stratton.)

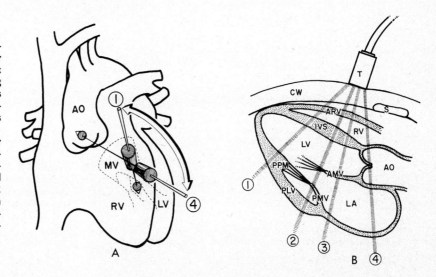

ing as the transducer is swept in a sector from the apex toward the base of the heart, the areas between the dotted lines in Figure 5–5 corresponding to the directions of the beam shown in Figure 5–4. An electrocardiogram helps to identify the events of the cardiac cycle. Beginning on the left side of Figure 5–5 (position 1), the chest wall echoes are recorded, followed by those of the anterior wall of the right ventricle. The right ventricular cavity is then recorded as an echo-free space. The next structure is the interventricular septum, with the right side of the septum frequently represented as a double or triple line and the left side as a single echo. Frequently, a mass of echoes originating from the posterior papillary muscle is evident posterior to the left ventricular cavity. Even further posterior is the posterior wall of the left ventricle. The intense echoes behind the heart originate from the lung. In transducer position 2 the principal change in the echogram is that parts of the mitral valve apparatus, either chordae or edges of the leaflets, are recorded within the left ventricular cavity. In this position the ultrasonic beam also traverses more of the body of the left ventricle, and the diameter of the left ventricular cavity, i.e., the distance between the left side of the interventricular septum and the posterior left ventricular endocardium, is greatest.

As the transducer is tilted slightly superiorly and medially, the anterior and posterior leaflets of the mitral valve are recorded. Tilting the transducer even further toward the base of the heart (position 3) causes the echoes produced by the posterior leaflet to drop out, and only the anterior leaflet of the mitral valve is recorded. The beam now passes through the posterior wall of the left atrium instead of that of the left ventricle. The posterior wall of the atrium moves posteriorly, i.e., away from the chest wall, during systole, while the posterior wall of the left ventricle moves anteriorly. When the transducer is directed toward the base of the heart (position 4), the beam passes through the anterior wall of the aorta (rather than the interventricular septum) and the posterior wall of the aortic root, which also constitutes the anterior wall of the left atrium (rather than the anterior leaflet of the mitral valve). Echoes from two or more leaflets of the aortic valve can frequently be recorded from between the two aortic walls.

FIGURE 5–5 Diagrammatic presentation of an M-mode echocardiogram as the transducer is directed from the apex (position 1) to the base of the heart (position 4). Areas between the dotted lines correspond to the transducer position, as depicted in Figure 5–4. EN = endocardium of the left ventricle, EP = epicardium of the left ventricle, PER = pericardium, PLA = posterior left atrial wall. Other abbreviations as in Figure 5–4. (From Feigenbaum, H.: Clinical applications of echocardiography. Progr. Cardiovasc. Dis. 14:531, 1972, by permission of Grune and Stratton.)

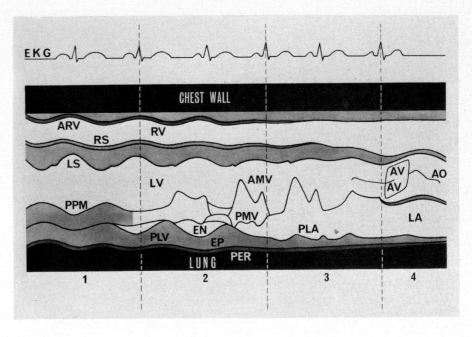

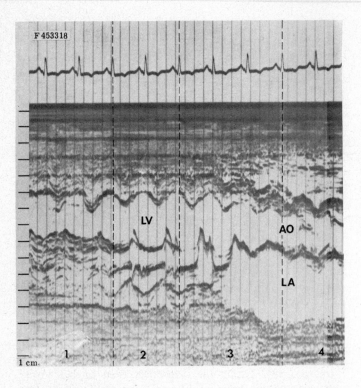

FIGURE 5–6   M-mode echocardiographic scan of the heart. Areas between the dotted lines correspond to those similarly designated in Figure 5–5. LV = left ventricular cavity, AO = aorta, LA = left atrium. (From Feigenbaum, H.: Clinical applications of echocardiography. Progr. Cardiovasc. Dis. *14*:531, 1972, by permission of Grune and Stratton.)

The leaflets separate and form a boxlike structure during systole and come together as a single line in diastole; the left atrial cavity lies behind the aorta.

Figure 5–6 is an actual M-mode scan on which many of the structures shown diagrammatically in Figure 5–5 can be recognized. However, the right ventricular cavity is not visible in positions 1 and 2; frequently, this cavity can be visualized only when the gain is turned down to record fewer echoes close to the transducer. In position 1, the posterior papillary muscle is recorded as a mass of somewhat ill-defined echoes approximately 2 to 3 cm from the

left side of the interventricular septum. In position 2, echoes having a pattern of motion characteristic of the leaflets of the mitral valve become apparent. This pattern is best noted by the rapid motion of the echoes in early diastole when the anterior leaflet moves anteriorly and the posterior leaflet posteriorly. A clearly defined endocardial echo behind the posterior leaflet of the mitral valve is recorded. In position 3, an echo from the anterior leaflet of the mitral valve is recorded, but the posterior leaflet has dropped out, and as the transducer is tilted further superiorly, the posterior wall of the left atrium replaces that of the left

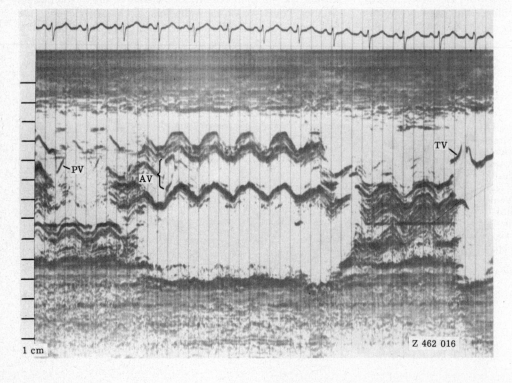

FIGURE 5–7   M-mode scan recording echoes from a pulmonic valve (PV), aortic valve (AV), and tricuspid valve (TV). (From Feigenbaum, H.: Echocardiography. 2nd ed. Philadelphia, Lea and Febiger, 1976.)

ventricle. In position 4, echoes from the aorta and the body of the left atrium are recorded, and echoes from the aortic valve leaflets are apparent in the last two cardiac cycles. These leaflets appear as thin echoes and form a boxlike configuration during ventricular systole.

Figure 5–7 shows echoes from the aorta and aortic valve; by tilting the transducer medially from the aortic valve, it is possible to record the anterior leaflet of the tricuspid valve, which is similar in appearance to the recording from the anterior leaflet of the mitral valve. When the transducer is directed superiorly and laterally from the aortic valve, a posterior leaflet of the pulmonary valve can be recorded (Fig. 5–7).

Two-Dimensional Echocardiography

M-mode echocardiography, the original ultrasonic technique developed for cardiac examination, has proved to be extremely valuable, especially in recording the motion of cardiac structures parallel to the ultrasonic beam. However, there are significant limitations to this method of examination; it does not permit effective evaluation of the shape of cardiac structures nor can it depict lateral motion, i.e., motion perpendicular to the ultrasonic beam. Real-time, cross-sectional, or two-dimensional echocardiography, officially designated two-dimensional echocardiography by the American Society of Echocardiography, has become popular because it provides information not available in M-mode echocardiography. By moving the ultrasonic beam very rapidly, two-dimensional echocardiography can depict cardiac shape and lateral motion, which are otherwise difficult or impossible to evaluate with M-mode echocardiography. Such recordings are displayed on movie film or videotape.

The principle of two-dimensional or cross-sectional echocardiography is depicted in Figure 5–8, in which the object of interest is a sphere on a wire which oscillates in a liquid medium. An M-mode examination of such an object would record the motion with great accuracy at a rapid sampling rate. However, as the ball moved upward it would leave the path of the stationary ultrasonic beam, and its image would therefore not be recorded during those instants. The M-mode tracing would record only that component of the motion that is parallel to the ultrasonic beam and obviously only while the ball is within the path of the beam. Thus, the full excursion would not be appreciated, and the shape of the object could not be recognized. However, if the ultrasonic beam were to move rapidly through an angle, a sector scan of the moving sphere would be obtained (Fig. 5–8B).

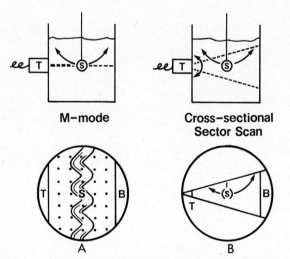

FIGURE 5–8 Diagrams demonstrating how the M-mode and cross-sectional examinations would record the motion of a moving sphere (S) in a beaker of water. The M-mode recording would show a series of wavy lines as the moving ball cuts across the ultrasonic beam (A). The cross-sectional recording would show a spatially correct spherical object moving within the pie-shaped sector image (B).

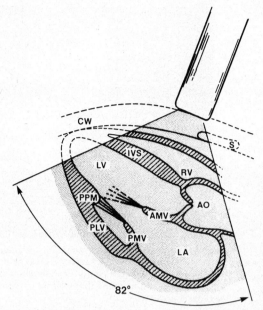

FIGURE 5–9 Diagram showing how to obtain a cross-sectional or two-dimensional image of the heart parallel to the long axis of the left ventricle. CW = chest wall. Other abbreviations as in Figure 5–4.

Each of the B-mode lines is laid down in a position on the oscilloscope which reflects the position of the ultrasonic beam. As the beam is directed upward, the echocardiographic B-mode lines would be laid down at a similar angle on the oscilloscope. Spatial orientation is now introduced into the recording and a reasonable facsimile of the spherical object becomes evident. In addition, almost the entire pendular motion of the ball can be appreciated by recording motion that is lateral as well as perpendicular to the ultrasonic beam. One disadvantage of this method is that the recording is on videotape, and the sampling rate therefore is usually reduced by 30 to 60 frames/second or less rather than the 1000 impulses/second recorded with the M-mode examination.

The type of examination diagrammed in Figure 5–8B is termed a "real-time, cross-sectional, or two-dimensional sector scan." The tip of the transducer is essentially stationary, and the beam can be moved in an arc, mechanically by oscillating a single transducer or by rotating a series of transducers.[4,5] The ultrasound can also be steered electronically using the so-called *phased array* principle, in which multiple ultrasonic elements are utilized to make up the beam and in which the firing sequence of the elements is controlled.[6] A computer or microprocessor is necessary to control the firing of the elements and the direction of the beam. There are many technical differences between a mechanical sector scanner and a phased array scanner.[2,7] The technology in two-dimensional echocardiography is still evolving, so the advantages and disadvantages of the two systems are constantly changing. Irrespective of which type of sector scanner one uses, the two-dimensional images are essentially similar. As might be anticipated, the phased-array scanners are generally more expensive than the mechanical scanners.

Since the patient is usually examined in the recumbent position, as with M-mode echocardiography, the standard orientation for two-dimensional echocardiography is for the transducer and anterior chest wall to be displayed at the top of the picture. Figure 5–9 shows a diagram of how a two-dimensional image of the heart might be obtained, and in Figure 5–10 are shown two individual frames representing stop-action sequences from a videotape recording of a normal heart in which the mitral and aortic valves and parts of the left ventricle, left atrium, and aorta are imaged. It must be recalled that all these structures do not lie in the same plane. For example, it is not ordinarily possible to include both the long axis of the apex and the aorta in a single picture; this is not the case with angiography. Since these two-dimensional echograms are displayed on videotape, they superficially resemble cineangiocardiograms. However, the latter display intracavitary contrast material, while the two-dimensional images represent individual "slices" of the heart.

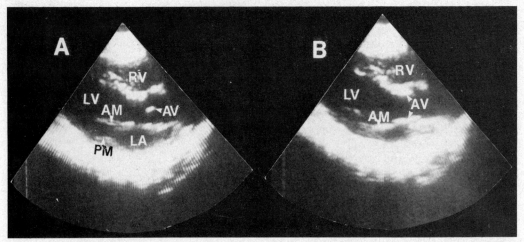

FIGURE 5-10   Long-axis cross-sectional echographic images of the left ventricle (LV), right ventricle (RV), mitral valve, aortic valve, and left atrium (LA) during diastole (A) and systole (B). During diastole the anterior (AM) and posterior (PM) mitral leaflets are apart and the aortic valve leaflets (AV) come together as a single echo in the midportion of the aorta (A). With systole, the mitral leaflets come together and the aortic valve leaflets separate (B).

Doppler Echocardiography

According to the Doppler principle, when an ultrasonic wave is reflected from a moving object, the frequency of the reflected ultrasound is altered and the difference in frequency between the ultrasound emitted and that received depends on the velocity of the reflecting interface and the angle at which the beam strikes the object. This change in frequency is often referred to as the *Doppler shift*. In order to calculate the actual velocity, the angle which the object in question makes with respect to the ultrasonic beam must be known. Although the moving target could be a cardiac valve or wall, Doppler ultrasound is used most often to examine the velocity of blood flow, the ultrasonic energy being reflected by the red blood cells. Since the frequency difference (Doppler shift) coming from the stream of moving blood is in the audible range, the frequency of which is related to the velocity of the moving object, the ultrasound energy is sent in a continuous wave and is therefore commonly called *continuous wave* or *CW Doppler*.

Doppler ultrasound has been used primarily to evaluate blood flow in superficial arteries and veins[8-11] and has proved to be useful in detecting obstructions in peripheral arteries[11] and venous thrombosis.[10] Recording the velocity of blood flow in the central aorta or major central arteries, such as the common carotid artery, has been used to reflect changes in aortic blood flow,[12-17] but *absolute* measurements of blood flow by this technique are quite difficult to accomplish. The pattern of blood flow in the central arteries is altered in conditions such as hypertrophic obstructive cardiomyopathy (HOCM)[18,19] and aortic regurgitation[20,21]; reverse flow during diastole has been noted in the latter, and it has been suggested that a semiquantitative estimate of the regurgitant fraction can be derived from a ratio of the reverse to the forward flow velocity on the Doppler recording.

Instrumentation has become available that combines the Doppler principle with standard pulsed ultrasound used for cardiac imaging.[22,23] By using pulsed instead of continuous wave ultrasound, it is now possible both to image the heart and to obtain a Doppler signal from some area within it.[24] Figure 5-11 demonstrates how a pulsed Doppler examination could be obtained from the root of the aorta. By gating the Doppler sample in the root of the aorta either on an M-mode or a two-dimensional echocardiogram, one will receive the Doppler signal from that area of the heart. There are three principal techniques for recording the resultant Doppler signal.[22] Since the returning sound is in the audible range, one will hear the Doppler shift during the examination. One can make the diagnosis by interpreting the sound generated from the Doppler examination either in real time during the actual examination or from an audio tape recording. There are also two methods of recording the Doppler signal on hard copy. The first technique utilizes the "time-interval histogram."[25,26] By using a zero-crossing technique to analyze the frequencies of the returning

sound, such a recording plots the frequencies of the sound against time. The direction of the flow is also indicated on the tracing; flow toward the transducer is plotted above the baseline and flow away from the transducer below the baseline. This particular technique is

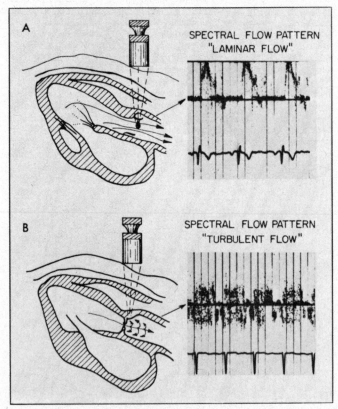

FIGURE 5-11   Illustration demonstrating the principle of how a time-interval histogram can distinguish "laminar flow" from "turbulent flow." With a Doppler sample in an area of laminar or normal flow, all dots that comprise the time interval histogram are close together, since all velocities at a given instant are relatively equal (A). With turbulent or disturbed flow (B) there are multiple velocities and directions of flow, and thus the Doppler signals are scattered above and below the baseline. (From Baker, D.W., Rubenstein, S.A., and Lorch, G.S.: Pulsed Doppler echocardiography: Principles and applications. Am. J. Med. *63*:69, 1977).

very useful in differentiating normal or "laminar flow" from abnormal or "turbulent or disturbed flow." Figure 5–11 demonstrates the time-interval histogram of laminar flow (A) and turbulent flow (B). If the sampling volume is recording an area of laminar blood flow, all returning frequencies are relatively homogeneous and the dots being plotted are close together. The recording would indicate that all the blood being sampled is moving in the same direction and at approximately the same frequencies. If the sampling volume is in an area of turbulent or disturbed flow, then a different time-interval histogram pattern is recorded. There will be multiple Doppler signals of differing frequencies and directions. Thus, on the time-interval histogram one sees multiple dots displayed, indicating variations in both frequency and direction. The ability to distinguish laminar from turbulent blood flow is one of the principal diagnostic uses for Doppler echocardiography.

Figure 5–12 is a Doppler echocardiographic recording of a patient with rheumatic mitral regurgitation. The M-mode echocardiogram is seen in the upper half of the recording. The site of the sample volume is indicated by a line on the M-mode tracing. The time-interval histogram is in the lower half of the recording. During systole the mitral regurgitant jet generates a turbulent signal with multiple frequencies, most of which are moving away from the transducer (arrow).

Because of the spatial orientation inherent in two-dimensional echocardiography, it is advantageous to obtain the Doppler signal by first placing the Doppler sampling volume on the two-dimensional echocardiogram.

There are many limitations to the time-interval histogram technique for recording the Doppler signal.[22,26] The principal advance has been to record a fast Fourier tracing of the Doppler signal. This method of analyzing the signal is far more accurate with regard to correct measurement of velocity recorded from the moving column of blood. All of the newer Doppler instruments have switched to some form of Fourier analysis of the Doppler signal. Figure 5–13 demonstrates a fast Fourier display of the Doppler signal from a patient with tricuspid regurgitation. The disturbed or turbulent flow (arrow) is recorded on this Doppler echocardiogram. The sampling volume (Doppler probe) is displayed on the M-mode echocardiogram posterior to the tricuspid valve (TV).

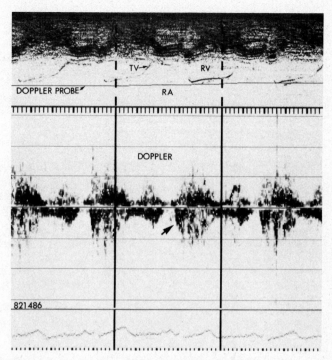

FIGURE 5–13 Doppler echocardiographic examination of a patient with tricuspid regurgitation using a fast Fourier recording of the Doppler signal. The disturbed or turbulent flow (arrow) is readily recognized. The Doppler probe is located within the right atrium (RA) posterior to the tricuspid valve (TV). RV = right ventricle.

Although the popularity of Doppler echocardiography has been increasing rapidly, there are still many difficulties with this type of examination.[22] Pulsed Doppler has a limitation in the maximum velocity that can be recorded with this technique. If the velocity is so great that the frequency of the returning sound wave is higher than the sampling rate of the pulsed Doppler, then "aliasing" will occur whereby the system will be unable to identify the frequency of the returning sound. Continuous-wave ultrasound does not have this problem, but it is difficult to localize the Doppler signal using continuous ultrasound. There are many continuing attempts to quantitate the Doppler signal both for blood flow and for quantitation of abnormal blood flow patterns, but all of these techniques still have their difficulties. It is possible to use multiple Doppler gates or sampling sites to display the blood flow patterns directly on the M-mode recording.[27] It is also theoretically possible that the Doppler blood flow patterns could be displayed on the two-dimensional echocardiogram.[28] However, these multiple gating Doppler techniques are still investigational.

Another limitation of pulsed Doppler echocardiography is that the depth of the examination is limited by the available frequency. With the frequency in the range of 3.0 to 3.5 MHz, it is difficult to obtain a Doppler signal from distances beyond 12 or 13 cm from the transducers. The pulse repetition rate must be reduced when examining distances this far from the transducer, and the ability to record high velocity flow is lost.

Contrast Echocardiography

Ultrasound is an extremely sensitive detector of intravascular bubbles. The injection of almost any liquid into the intravascular spaces will introduce many microbubbles that appear as a cloud of echoes on the echocardiogram. Figure 5–14 demonstrates an M-mode echocardiogram of a patient with a right-to-left shunt at the ventricular level. The contrast can be seen initially in the right ventricle. It then traverses the interventricular septum and appears in the left ventricle. As will be noted later, this technique is obviously a sensitive method of detecting right-to-left shunts. The contrast agents that have been used include the patient's blood, saline, dextrose in water, and indocyanine green dye.[29–31] In all cases the contrast effect originates from suspended microbubbles in the fluid. Injection of small quantities of carbon dioxide gas have also been used for contrast

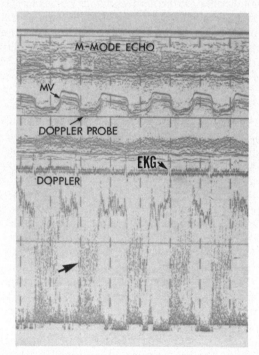

FIGURE 5–12 Doppler echocardiographic study of a patient with rheumatic mitral stenosis and insufficiency. The Doppler probe or sampling site is within the left atrium behind the mitral valve (MV). The Doppler signal generated by the regurgitant blood leaking into the left atrium can be seen as a band of downward displaced dots on the Doppler tracing (arrow). The line in the middle of the Doppler tracing is a baseline or zero reference.

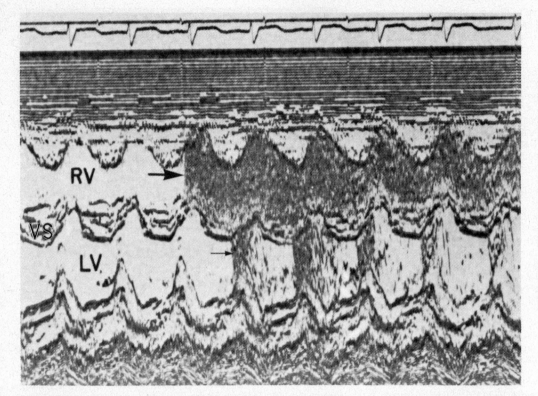

FIGURE 5–14 A contrast M-mode echocardiogram in a patient with a right-to-left shunt at the ventricular level. The dark mass of echoes from the injected contrast (large arrow) is initially seen in the right ventricular cavity (RV) and next is seen (small arrow) in the left ventricle (LV) above the mitral valve. Normally the contrast should not appear on the left side of the heart at all. If the shunt were at the atrial level, contrast would appear in the left and right ventricles simultaneously and would be seen posterior to the mitral valve. VS = ventricular septum. (From Seward, J. B., et al.: Echocardiographic contrast studies: Initial experience. Mayo Clin. Proc. *50*: 163, 1975.)

echocardiography.[32] Hydrogen peroxide will give a strong contrast effect by producing tiny intravascular bubbles of oxygen.[33] Commercially manufactured microbubbles may be available soon. The potential clinical uses for contrast echocardiography are numerous. There is much ongoing research in this area.

Technical Limitations

There are many technical difficulties inherent in ultrasound examinations of the heart. The principal problem is posed by the poor transmission of ultrasound through bony structures or through air-containing lungs, and the examiner must try to avoid these structures. A variety of techniques have been developed to circumvent this problem. The subxiphoid or subcostal examination was one of the first approaches shown to be useful, especially in patients with hyperinflated lungs and a low diaphragm.[34] Placing the transducer at the cardiac apex has also proved to be useful[35–37]; placing it into the suprasternal notch also avoids the lungs and bony thorax and allows imaging of the arch of the aorta, the left pulmonary artery, and the left atrium.[38] When this view is enlarged using the two-dimensional technique, a larger portion of the arch of the aorta, some of the arch vessels, and the descending aorta can be visualized.[39–40]

Despite improvements in echocardiographic techniques and instrumentation, there are still some patients in whom it is difficult to record satisfactory echocardiograms.[41] Patients with large, thick chest walls and small hearts represent the most difficult patients to examine, and chest deformities can occasionally be troublesome. The success rate for technically satisfactory echocardiograms is usually highest in younger patients. Another problem is that the echoes are recorded most effectively if the transducer is perpendicular or almost perpendicular to the structure in question. Small changes in angulation can decrease the quality of the recording. As a result, the examiner must be able to angle the probe as accurately as possible. Whether the heart is examined with a single-dimensional probe, as with M-mode echocardiography, or with two-dimensional device, proper direction of the ultrasonic beam is critical. Echocardiographic controls can also influence the image profoundly, and the operator must be skilled to make certain that artifacts and distortions are not introduced through improper use of the gain controls. Thus, although the echocardiographic examination is quite simple and painless for the patient, it can be extremely difficult to perform, so that a well-trained individual is required for both the examination and the interpretation of results.

EXAMINATION OF THE NORMAL HEART

M-Mode Echocardiogram

Echocardiograms can be extremely confusing to physicians not familiar with this technique. For example, many physicians are not aware of the fact that the mitral valve closes in mid-diastole, and thus the fact that the motion of its anterior leaflet resembles the letter "M" in diastole is not perfectly obvious. However, with a thorough knowledge of cardiac anatomy, physiology, and hemodynamics, it is not difficult to understand how an M-mode echocardiographic tracing is recorded and how the various structures should appear on such a recording. Figure 5–15 *A* shows an M-mode scan that encompasses the full length of the mitral valve apparatus. The echoes from this structure are striking and are readily identified. The anterior leaflet of the mitral valve shows a downward motion in mid-diastole, and the characteristic "M" pattern is recorded. The posterior mitral leaflet is essentially a mirror-image of the anterior leaflet, except the amplitude of its motion is less.

Figure 5–15*B* is an M-mode examination of a normal mitral valve. The end of systole, just prior to the opening of the valve, is designated "D." The maximum excursion of the anterior leaflets is designated "E" and the nadir of the initial diastolic closing wave "F." The diastolic closing rate, or the "E to F slope," is indicated by the line drawn on Figure 5–15*B*. This slope is frequently not straight but curved. With atrial systole, blood is propelled through the mitral orifice and the leaflets reopen. The peak of this reopening of the mitral valve is designated "A"; with atrial relaxation, the valve begins to close again. Ventricular systole begins during the downward slope of the mitral leaflet and may produce a slight interruption of the closure wave,

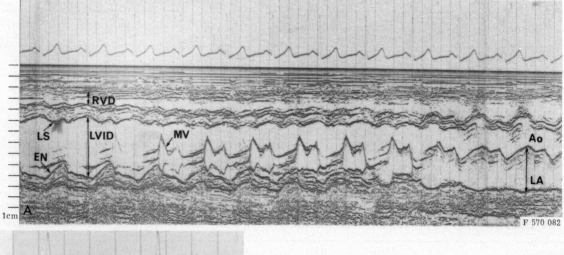

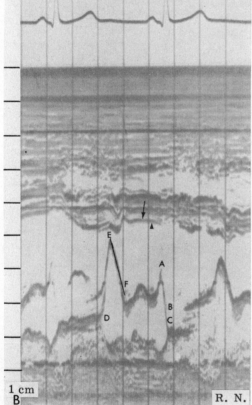

FIGURE 5–15 *A*, M-mode scan from the left ventricle to the aorta (AO) and left atrium (LA) in a normal subject. RVD = right ventricular dimension. LVID = left ventricular internal dimension, LS = left septal echoes, EN = posterior left ventricular endocardial echoes, MV = mitral valve. (From Chang, S.: M-mode Echocardiographic Techniques and Pattern Recognition. Philadelphia, Lea and Febiger, 1976.)

B, M-mode echocardiogram of a normal mitral valve. The letters A through F denote various portions of the anterior leaflet motion. The arrow indicates the leading edge of the echo from the left side of the interventricular septum; the arrowhead denotes the trailing edge of that echo (From Feigenbaum, H.: Echocardiography. 2nd ed. Philadelphia, Lea and Febiger, 1976.)

at point "B." (This is not always evident and is not so in Figure 5–15*B*.) Complete closure occurs following the onset of ventricular systole at "C."

The left ventricular cavity is bordered by the interventricular septum anteriorly and the posterior left ventricular wall posteriorly. Both walls move toward each other during systole, so that the diameter of the cavity decreases with systole. Both walls are approximately 1 cm thick in diastole, and the thickness increases during systole. A small portion of the right ventricular cavity lies anterior to the interventricular septum, and the anterior wall of the right ventricle is shown at the top of the tracing; the latter structure cannot always be imaged, especialy in adults.

As the ultrasonic beam is swept superiorly and medially toward the base of the heart, the posterior leaflet of the mitral valve drops out and the posterior left atrial wall is

seen to lie behind the anterior leaflet of the mitral valve. At the junction between the left atrium and ventricle the ultrasonic beam traverses both chambers during a given cardiac cycle. Because the atrioventricular junction moves in a superoinferior direction during each cycle, the stationary ultrasonic beam may record the left atrial wall during systole and the left ventricular wall during diastole. As the beam is directed more superiorly into the body of the left atrium, the relatively stationary posterior wall of the left atrium is imaged. The aorta, represented by two parallel moving echoes which move anteriorly during systole and posteriorly during diastole, lies anterior to the left atrium. The anterior wall of the aorta is in continuity with the echoes from the interventricular septum, and the posterior wall of the aorta is in continuity with the echoes of the anterior leaflet of the mitral valve. The aortic valve leaflets

TABLE 5–1   NORMAL VALUES OF ECHOCARDIOGRAPHIC MEASUREMENTS IN ADULTS

	RANGE (cm)	MEAN (cm)	NUMBER OF SUBJECTS
Age (years)	13 to 54	26	134
Body surface area (M²)	1.45 to 2.22	1.8	130
RVD—flat	0.7 to 2.3	1.5	84
RVD—left lateral	0.9 to 2.6	1.7	83
LVID—flat	3.7 to 5.6	4.7	82
LVID—left lateral	3.5 to 5.7	4.7	81
Posterior LV wall thickness	0.6 to 1.1	0.9	137
Posterior LV wall amplitude	0.9 to 1.4	1.2	48
IVS wall thickness	0.6 to 1.1	0.9	137
Mid IVS amplitude	0.3 to 0.8	0.5	10
Apical IVS amplitude	0.5 to 1.2	0.7	38
Left atrial dimension	1.9 to 4.0	2.9	133
Aortic root dimension	2.0 to 3.7	2.7	121
Aortic cusps' separation	1.5 to 2.6	1.9	93
Percentage of fractional shortening*	34% to 44%	36%	20%
Mean rate of circumferential shortening (Vcf),** or mean normalized shortening velocity	1.02 to 1.94 circ/sec	1.3 circ/sec	38

$$* \quad \frac{LVIDd - LVIDs}{LVIDd} \qquad ** \quad \frac{LVIDd - LVIDs}{LVIDd \times \text{Ejection time}}$$

RVD = Right ventricular dimension
LVID = Left ventricular internal dimension; d = end diastole; s = end systole
LV = Left ventricle
IVS = Interventricular septum

lie within the root of the aorta; only the anterior aortic valve leaflet is recorded in Figure 5–15, although both valve leaflets are better visualized in Figure 5–6. Two of the leaflets, probably the right coronary leaflet and the noncoronary leaflet, make up the boxlike configuration observed during systole as the aortic valve opens. As the leaflets come together in diastole a *single* echo is commonly recorded.

M-Mode Echocardiographic Measurements

Numerous measurements have been suggested for M-mode echocardiography. Figure 5–16 demonstrates some of the measurements that can be obtained from an M-mode echocardiogram. Most of these measurements involve the left ventricle, the aortic root, and the left atrium. The American Society of Echocardiography has standardized the common measurements used in M-mode echocardiography.[42] A key consideration in these measurements is that the leading edge of an echo, i.e., that portion of the echo closest to the transducer, is more readily identified and precisely measured than is the trailing edge. The arrow in Figure 5–15B denotes the leading edge of the echo from the left side of the interventricular septum, while the arrowhead in the same figure indicates the trailing edge. The precise location of the leading edge of an echo is easily accomplished and involves little error; however, the width of an individual echo, and therefore the identification of the trailing edge, varies depending on how the signal is processed in an individual instrument. Also, because of variations in instruments, the onset of the QRS complex in standard lead II is taken as denoting the end of diastole. The American Society of Echocardiography also recommends that the M-mode measurements be averaged from three or four cardiac cycles and preferably at end-expiration. The timing and location of the various measurements are indicated in Figure 5–16. The left ventricular dimension should be taken just beyond the mitral valve or at

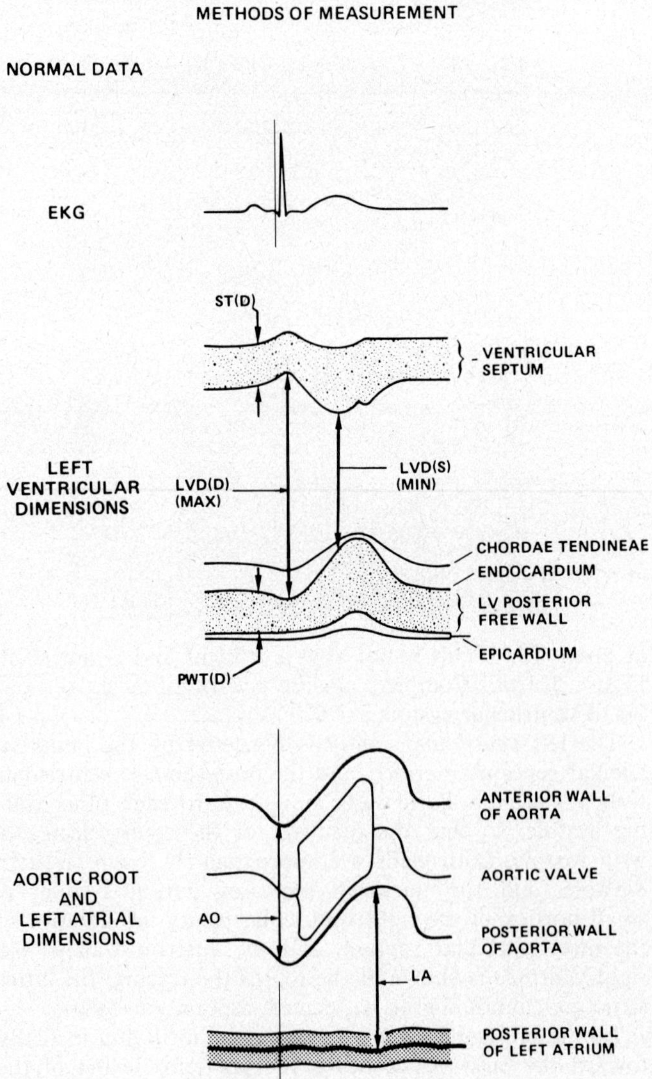

METHODS OF MEASUREMENT

FIGURE 5–16 Methods for obtaining M-mode echocardiographic measurements. ST(D) = diastolic septal thickness; LVD(D) and LVD(S) = diastolic and systolic left ventricular diameter; PWT(D) = diastolic posterior wall thickness; AO = aorta; LA = left atrium. (From Henry, W.L., Gardin, J.M., and Ware, J.H.: Echocardiographic measurements in normal subjects from infancy to old age. Circulation 62:1054, 1980.)

the chordae tendineae. In infants and young children, left ventricular dimensions are probably best recorded at the level of the mitral valve. The end-diastolic dimension is taken at the onset of the QRS complex, while end-systolic measurement is obtained at the instant of maximum posterior (downward) position of the interventricular septum, which usually precedes the peak anterior (upward) position of the posterior left ventricular wall. When septal motion is abnormal, the instant of peak upward position of the posterior ventricular endocardium may be taken at end-systole. A true right ventricular dimension can be obtained only when the anterior right ventricular wall is well delineated; otherwise, only an estimate of this dimension can be made.

Wall thickness is also measured from leading edge to leading edge, and the width of the interventricular septum is the distance from the anterior surface of the right to the anterior surface of the left septal echo. The thickness of the posterior left ventricular wall is measured from the anterior surface of the posterior left ventricular endocardial echo to that from the anterior surface of the posterior left ventricular epicardium.

Although mitral valve measurements have been made since the onset of echocardiography in the 1950's, these measurements are of limited value. The closing velocity or E to F slope is very non-specific and has relatively little diagnostic value. The amplitude of excursion of the mitral valve is still used for judging pliability of the valve. The American Society of Echocardiography decided that the D to E amplitude should be used to judge the excursion of the mitral valve rather than the C to E amplitude as recommended by some investigators (Fig. 5–15B).

Table 5–1 provides some normal values for commonly used M-mode echocardiographic measurements. These data represent approximations and do not conform in all instances to the criteria developed by the American Society of Echocardiography. Nor do they take into account that some changes in measurements occur during aging.[43] Normal values for children can be quite complex. The reader is encouraged to refer to some of the references, since more exhaustive normal values have been obtained.[2]

Two-Dimensional Echocardiographic Views

One could essentially obtain an infinite number of slices of the heart using two-dimensional echocardiography. In the early development of this technique investigators were utilizing many different approaches in examining the heart with this ultrasonic technique.[44] The American Society of Echocardiography has attempted to standardize and simplify the many two-dimensional examinations described.[45] The Society felt that all views could be categorized into three orthogonal planes, as illustrated in Figure 5–17. These planes are the long-axis, short-axis, and four-chamber. The long-axis plane is the imaging plane that transects the heart perpendicular to the dorsal and ventral surfaces of the body and parallel to the long axis of the heart. The plane transecting the heart perpendicular to the dorsal and ventral surfaces of the body, but perpendicular to the long axis of the heart, is defined as the short-axis plane. The plane that transects the heart approximately parallel to the dorsal and ventral surfaces of the body is referred to as the four-chamber plane. It should be emphasized that these views or planes are with reference to the heart and not to the thorax or body.

These ultrasonic planes or views can be obtained from more than one transducer location. Figure 5–18A demonstrates that one can obtain the long-axis view with the transducer in the apical position, in the parasternal position (left sternal border), or in the suprasternal notch. A short-axis view (Fig. 5–18B) cuts across the heart so that the left ventricle looks like a circle. The right ventricle can be seen curving around the left ventricle. Such an examination can be obtained with the transducer in the parasternal position or in the subcostal (subxiphoid) position. The four-chamber view is depicted in Figure 5–18C. Such a view permits the examination of all four cardiac chambers simultaneously. This type of examination can be obtained with the transducer over the cardiac apex or with the transducer in the subcostal position.

Table 5–2 lists the various two-dimensional echocardiographic examinations categorized according to the location of the transducer, the plane of the examination, and the cardiac structure being examined.

Figure 5–10 is an example of a parasternal long-axis examination

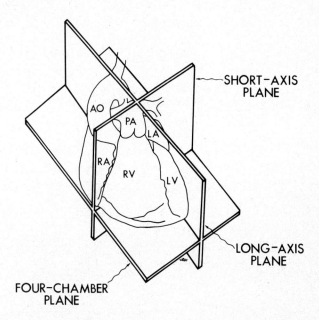

TWO-DIMENSIONAL ECHOCARDIOGRAPHIC IMAGING PLANES

FIGURE 5–17 Diagram demonstrating the three orthogonal planes for two-dimensional echocardiographic imaging. AO = aorta; PA = pulmonary artery; LA = left atrium; RA = right atrium; RV = right ventricle; LV = left ventricle. (From Henry, W.L., et al.: Report of the American Society of Echocardiography Nomenclature and Standards in Two-dimensional Echocardiography. Circulation *62*:212, 1980.)

through the left ventricle. The right ventricle, right atrium, and tricuspid valve can also be recorded with the transducer in the parasternal position (Fig. 5–19). The plane of the transducer does not exactly fit either the long axis or short axis. However, the plane is closer to that of the long axis than that of the short axis and thus is categorized as a long-axis study. Figure 5–20 shows the right ventricular inflow tract and right atrium by way of such a parasternal examination.

TABLE 5–2 TWO-DIMENSIONAL ECHOCARDIOGRAPHIC EXAMINATION

Parasternal Approach
  Long-axis plane
    Root of aorta: aortic valve, left atrium, left ventricular outflow tract
    Body of left ventricle, mitral valve
    Left ventricular apex
    Right ventricular inflow tract–tricuspid valve
  Short-axis plane
    Root of the aorta, aortic valve, pulmonary valve, tricuspid valve, right ventricular outflow tract, left atrium, pulmonary artery, coronary arteries
    Left ventricle, mitral valve
    Left ventricle, papillary muscles
    Left ventricle, apex
Apical Approach
  Four-chamber plane
    Four chamber
    Four chamber with aorta
  Long-axis plane
    Two chamber: left ventricle, left atrium
    Two chamber with aorta
Subcostal Approach
  Four-chamber plane
  Short-axis plane
    Left ventricle
    Right ventricle
    Inferior vena cava
Suprasternal Approach
  Four-chamber plane: arch of aorta–descending aorta
  Long-axis plane: arch of aorta–pulmonary artery, left atrium

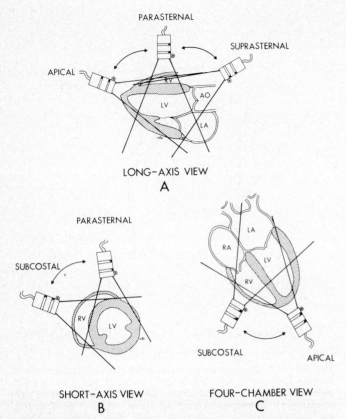

LONG-AXIS VIEW
A

SHORT-AXIS VIEW
B

FOUR-CHAMBER VIEW
C

FIGURE 5-18 Diagrams demonstrating how one can obtain the various orthogonal planes from different transducer positions. (From Henry, W.L., et al.: Report of the American Society of Echocardiography Nomenclature and Standards in Two-dimensional Echocardiography. Circulation _62_:212, 1980.)

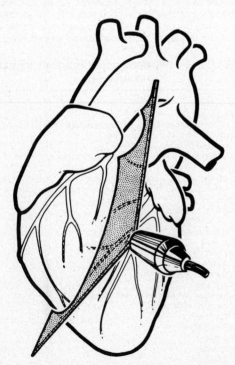

FIGURE 5-19 Transducer position for long-axis parasternal examination of the tricuspid valve, right atrium, and right ventricular inflow tract. (From Feigenbaum, H.: Echocardiography. 3rd ed. Philadelphia, Lea & Febiger, 1981.)

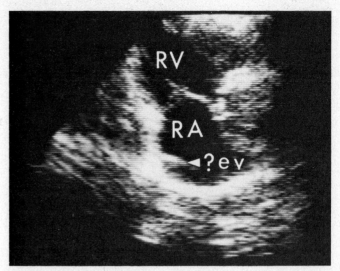

FIGURE 5-20 Two-dimensional echocardiogram of the right atrium (RA) and right ventricular inflow tract (RV). ev = eustachian valve. (From Feigenbaum, H.: Echocardiography. 3rd ed. Philadelphia, Lea & Febiger, 1981.)

Various short-axis examinations are diagrammatically illustrated in Figure 5-21. The short-axis views are commonly obtained at the level of the apex, the papillary muscles, the mitral valve, and the base of the heart. With slight variation in angulation the short-axis examination of the base of the heart can also record the pulmonary valve and the pulmonary artery with its bifurcation. It is also possible to use this examination to record the origins of the coronary arteries and the left atrial appendage.

Figure 5-22 diagrammatically illustrates the two commonly used two-dimensional echocardiographic views with the transducer placed at the cardiac apex. Plane 1 demonstrates the apical four-chamber view of the heart. Figure 5-23A shows an example of a four-chamber apical echocardiogram. It is possible to obtain an apical view of the long axis of the heart similar to that seen from the parasternal view. Such an examination would include portions of the right ventricle and the aorta. A more common examination is a so-called apical two-chamber view (Fig. 5-22, plane 2). This examination requires slight clockwise rotation of the transducer to avoid the right ventricle completely. Thus, one records only the left ventricle and the left atrium (Fig. 5-23B). This view can be considered a modification of an apical long-axis view.

The subcostal transducer location produces examinations roughly in the four-chamber and short-axis planes. The ultrasonic plane indicated in Figure 5-24A is similar to examining plane 1 in Figure 5-22. The resultant subcostal four-chamber echocardiogram appears in Figure 5-25A. Figures 5-24B and 5-25B show how the transducer can be rotated 90 degrees to provide a subcostal short-axis examination of the heart. The subcostal four-chamber view is particularly helpful in examining the interatrial and interventricular septa. By directing the transducer in a slightly modified short-axis examination, one can obtain an excellent view of the right side of the heart (Fig. 5-26A). The subcostal location also permits an opportunity to direct the ultrasonic beam through the inferior vena cava and hepatic vein[46] (Figs. 5-26B and 5-27).

The two examining planes with the transducer in the suprasternal notch are depicted in Figure 5-28. The ultrasonic view in Figure 5-28 A is roughly equivalent to that of a four-chamber plane, and the view in Figure 5-28B is somewhat comparable to that of the long-axis plane. However, it is probably best to orient the ultrasonic beam with regard to the arch of the aorta rather than to the heart, since one does not record much of the heart with the transducer in this position, especially in the adult. In addition, the planes are different than with the transducer at the apex or subcostal region. Thus, better terminology with regard to the examining plane from the suprasternal location would be parallel or perpendicular to the arch of the aorta. Figure 5-29 shows a suprasternal examination parallel to the arch of the aorta.

FIGURE 5–21 Diagrams showing how short-axis echographic cross-sectional images of the heart, which are perpendicular to the long axis of the left ventricle, are obtained. Diagram 1 shows a short-axis left ventricular echogram near the cardiac apex. Diagram 2 demonstrates part of the right ventricle (RV) and the circular left ventricular cavity (LV) at the level of the papillary muscles, which can be seen to bulge into the LV cavity. Diagram 3 is closer to the base of the heart and shows the left ventricle at the level of the mitral valve (MV). Diagram 4 shows a short-axis cross-section of the base of the heart with the aorta, aortic valve (AV), left atrium (LA), interatrial septum (IAS), right atrium (RA), tricuspid valve (TV), and right ventricular outflow tract (RV).

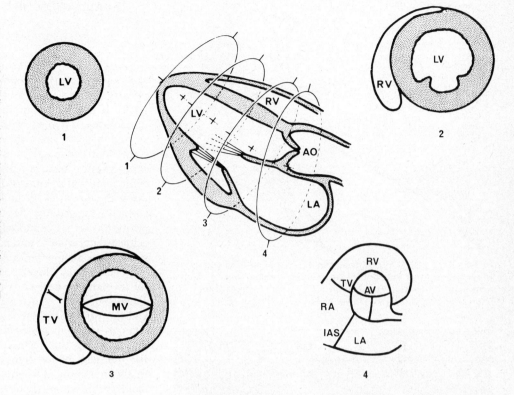

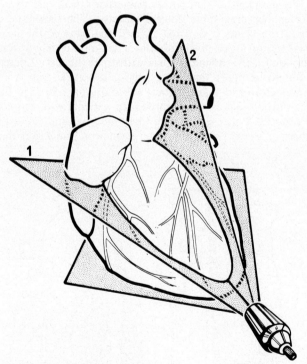

FIGURE 5–22 Transducer position and examining planes for apical two-dimensional echocardiograms. Plane 1 passes through the four chamber plane of the heart. Plane 2 represents the path of the ultrasonic beam for the two-chamber apical examination. (From Feigenbaum, H.: Echocardiography. 3rd ed. Philadelphia, Lea & Febiger, 1981.)

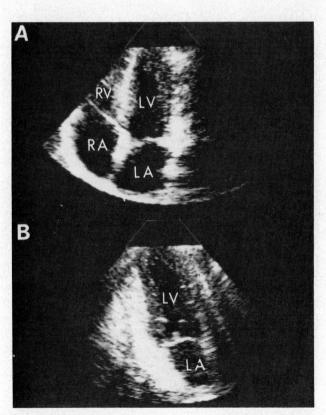

FIGURE 5–23 Four-chamber (A) and two-chamber (B) apical two-dimensional echocardiograms. RV = right ventricle; LV = left ventricle; RA = right atrium; and LA = left atrium. (From Feigenbaum, H.: Echocardiography. 3rd ed. Philadelphia, Lea & Febiger, 1981.)

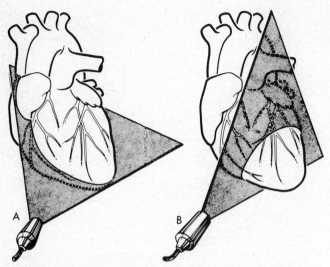

FIGURE 5–24 Diagrams showing the transducer position and examining planes for a subcostal four-chamber examination (A) and a subcostal short-axis examination (B). (From Feigenbaum, H.: Echocardiography. 3rd ed. Philadelphia, Lea & Febiger, 1981.)

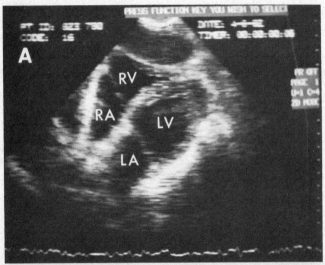

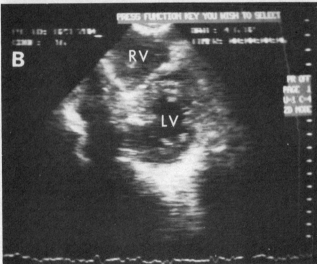

FIGURE 5–25 Two-dimensional echocardiograms obtained with the transducer in the subcostal position. Echogram A represents a four-chamber view and B is a short-axis examination. RV = right ventricle; RA = right atrium; LA = left atrium; LV = left ventricle.

EVALUATION OF CARDIAC PERFORMANCE

Assessment of Cardiac Chambers

As already noted, M-mode echocardiography provides the opportunity for examining the left ventricle, left atrium, root of the aorta, and a small portion of the right ventricle. It should be appreciated that the right ventricular dimensions obtained with the transducer along the left sternal boarder are subject to significant error, since the right ventricular cavity is irregular in shape and only a small portion of it is actually examined.[47] In addition, the right ventricular dimension varies significantly depending upon the direction of the ultrasonic beam and also the position of the patient. As the patient assumes a left lateral position, as is commonly done to obtain satisfactory echocardiographic examinations, right ventricular dimensions often change strikingly. As crude as measurement of right ventricular dimensions might be, it is still very helpful in many clinical situations in assessing the presence or absence of right ventricular dilatation[48] and hypoplasia.[49,50] On the other hand, it should be recognize d that subtle changes in right ventricular size can be missed or falsely suggested by this technique. Although, as already noted, the free wall of the right ventricle cannot be imaged routinely in adults, it is more accessible to measurement in children, in whom right ventricular hypertrophy is a common problem and in whom higher frequency transducers can be used. The subcostal approach has also recently been proposed for assessment of the right ventricular wall.[51]

Measurement of left atrial dimensions was one of the first echocardiographic determinations.[52] The technique in which the beam is directed toward the base of the heart provides an anteroposterior dimension of the left atrium. Although this examination has withstood the test of time,[53] it should be noted that the posterior left atrial wall is not always clear and that a variety of confusing echoes in this area of the heart can be recorded. In patients with thoracic deformities,[54] the left atrium may not assume its usual spherical shape,[55] and the anteroposterior dimension may

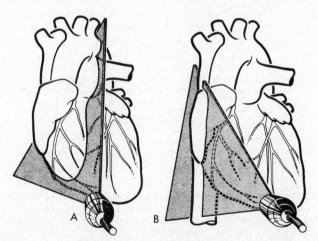

FIGURE 5–26 Diagram demonstrating the examining planes and transducer positions for the subcostal examination for the right side of the heart (A) and the inferior vena cava (B). (From Feigenbaum, H.: Echocardiography. 3rd ed. Philadelphia, Lea & Febiger, 1981.)

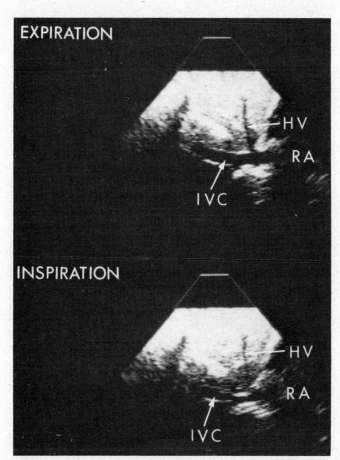

FIGURE 5–27 Subcostal two-dimensional echocardiogram of the inferior vena cava (IVC) and hepatic veins (HV). The inferior vena cava decreases in size with inspiration. RA = right atrium. (From Feigenbaum, H.: Echocardiography. 3rd ed. Philadelphia, Lea & Febiger, 1981.)

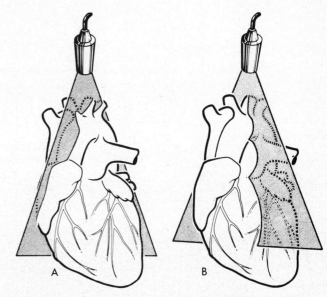

FIGURE 5–28 Transducer position in examining planes for the suprasternal examination parallel to the arch of the aorta (A) and perpendicular to the arch of the aorta (B). (From Feigenbaum, H.: Echocardiography. 3rd ed. Philadelphia, Lea & Febiger, 1981.)

be misleading in judging its overall size. In patients with pectus excavatum the superoinferior left atrial dimension, as obtained via the suprasternal approach, may more accurately reflect the true size of this chamber.[54] Recent experience suggests that two-dimensional echocardiographic examination may improve upon the echocardiographic assessment of left atrial size.[56,57] The location and shape of the interatrial septum as seen on two-dimensional echocardiography may help in assessing the state of the left atrium.[58]

The ability to evaluate the function of the left ventricle by means of echocardiography has been one of the principal factors in the increasing application of this technique. The standard M-mode technique may be used to record a dimension of the left ventricle between the left side of the interventricular septum and the endocardial surface of the posterior left ventricular wall.[59,60] Measurements of this dimension in end-diastole and end-systole may be made, and although these dimensions can be used to estimate ventricular volume, there are many potential errors in calculations,[61] since many assumptions that are not always valid are required to obtain the volume of a three-dimensional object from measurement of a single dimension. Irrespective of whether or not M-mode echocardiography can calculate true left ventricular volumes, simple dimensions of the left ventricle can provide an estimate of the overall size

and performance of the left ventricle in a large percentage of patients.[62]

The left ventricular internal dimension is usually measured at the level of the chordae tendineae or at the tips of the leaflets of the mitral valve (Fig. 5–30), where it provides a measure of the internal diameter at the upper third of the left ventricular cavity, probably including the outflow tract. The diastolic dimension correlates well with the overall size of the left ventricle and can be used to determine the presence of left ventricular dilation. The systolic dimension provides an indication of end-systolic size, and comparing systolic and diastolic dimensions provides an assessment of the myocardial shortening of the upper portion of the left ventricle. Fractional shortening, i.e., the difference between the end-diastolic and end-systolic dimensions divided by the end-diastolic dimension,[62] provides information analogous to the angiographic ejection

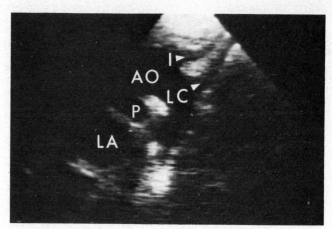

FIGURE 5–29 Suprasternal echocardiographic examination of the arch of the aorta (AO), pulmonary artery (P), and left atrium (LA). I = innominate artery; LC = left common carotid artery.

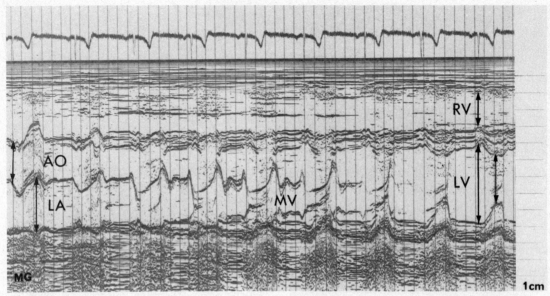

FIGURE 5–30   Normal M-mode echocardiogram showing some commonly used measurements. AO = aorta, LA = left atrium. MV = mitral valve, RV = right ventricle, LV = left ventricle.

fraction. The quotient of fractional shortening and ejection time provides the mean fractional or circumferential shortening.[63] While these measurements are useful in judging left ventricular performance, it must be appreciated that the ventricle must be contracting uniformly for them to reflect global function. These echocardiographic measurements assess the status of only the basal portion of the chamber and must be interpreted with caution in patients with segmentally diseased left ventricles.[64]

Another M-mode echocardiographic technique for assessing the status of the left ventricle is to measure the distance between the E point of the mitral valve and the left side of the interventricular septum.[65,66] Normally, the mitral E point and the left side of the septum are within a few millimeters of each other. The upper limits of normal of the mitral E point–septal separation (EPSS) is approximately 8 mm. As the left ventricular ejection fraction decreases, the EPSS increases. Although there are some limitations to the utility of this measurement, especially when there is regional left ventricular dysfunction, this measurement is useful and fairly popular. Even though the observation is principally empiric, there is some rationale behind the measurement. As the left ventricle dilates, the septum moves anteriorly. The opening of the mitral valve is largely dependent upon the volume of blood passing through that orifice. As the mitral valve flow or left ventricular stroke volume decreases, the amplitude of the E point is decreased. Thus, with a decreased stroke volume and/or left ventricular dilatation, the septum and anterior mitral leaflet would move in opposite directions. Therefore, with a decreased ejection fraction, which is stroke volume divided by diastolic volume, it is not unreasonable to expect an increase in the distance between the mitral valve E point and the interventricular septum. Naturally, if there is intrinsic valvular disease, such as mitral stenosis, then the excursion of the mitral valve is not a reliable indicator of flow through that orifice. In patients with aortic regurgitation, mitral valve flow is not an indicator of total left ventricular stroke volume, and one would not be able to provide an assessment of ejection fraction.

Most echocardiographic measurements of the cardiac chambers have been done with M-mode echocardiography. Such has been the case not only because M-mode echocardiography developed prior to two-dimensional echocardiography but also because of the convenience of having the recording on strip chart paper so that measurements can be made with simple calipers. Unfortunately, there are many theoretical limitations to the M-mode measurements. The lack of spatial orientation in the M-mode examination can distort the measurements in many individuals. This fact is true for all of the cardiac chambers.

Two Dimensional Echocardiography. The limited number of sampling sites for the M-mode dimension also curtails the clinical usefulness of these measurements. Thus, it is not surprising that there has been interest in using two-dimensional echocardiography for assessing the cardiac chambers. The hesitancy to use the two-dimensional approach has been partially because of the inconvenience associated with analyzing a recording made on videotape. With the advent of newer videotape and video disc systems, electronic calipers, bit pads, light pens, and computers, it is becoming more convenient to make the necessary measurements from the two-dimensional examination. It is hoped that the future computers will identify specific echoes and make measurements automatically.[67–69]

There have been a number of attempts to use two-dimensional echocardiography to calculate left ventricular volumes.[70–76] Several geometric formulas have been suggested.[71] These formulas include the area-length technique commonly used for angiographic volumes. The Simpson's rule formula is fairly attractive because it minimizes the effect of geometric shape for calculating volumes. An intriguing formula is that which describes the left ventricle as a bullet, which consists of a cylinder and a half of a prolate ellipse.[72] The formula for calculating left ventricular volume using the "bullet formula" is volume equals five-sixths the area of the left ventricle times the length of the left ventricle ($V = 5/6 AL$). This formula is attractive because of its simplicity and because the area of the left ventricle and the length of the left ventricle can be easily obtained with two-dimensional echocardiography. The accuracy and reproducibility of the various techniques for calculating left ventricular volumes have not been substantiated. Thus, the calculation of left ventricular volumes is not a routine part of the echocardiographic examination at the present time. There are limitations with any technique which attempts to calculate volume from an examination that is less than truly three-dimensional.

An interesting approach to calculating left ventricular ejection fraction eliminates some of the problems with the actual calculation of volumes.[77] By obtaining multiple diameters of the left ventricle one can transform the fractional shortening of these multiple diameters into ejection fraction either by measuring the fractional change of the length or by estimating fractional length change by a qualitative assessment of apical motion. This particular approach is attractive because of its simplicity and because it obviates some of the limitations of the two-dimensional calculations for volume.

Another simplified approach to assessing the left ventricle with two-dimensional echocardiography is merely to obtain minor axis measurements using the parasternal long-axis and short-axis views. It is possible to obtain a true minor dimension using the parasternal long-axis examination. One can also obtain a short-axis area at the level of the papillary muscles. Derived indices, such as fractional shortening or fractional area change, can be obtained with this approach. Figures 5–31 and 5–32 illustrate how one can obtain the minor dimension from the parasternal long-axis examination (Fig. 5–31) and how the short-axis area can be measured at the level of the papillary muscles (Fig. 5–32).

Attempts have also been made to use two-dimensional echocardiography for calculating right ventricular[78] and left atrial[56,57] volumes. There has also been an attempt at assessing the size of the right atrium using two-dimensional echocardiography.[78] As with the left ventricular measurements, none of the two-dimensional techniques has achieved wide acceptance. However, with the increasing interest in quantitative two-dimensional echocardiography one can anticipate that chamber assessment using the two-dimensional approach should become routine in the near future.

Although echocardiography has been used almost exclusively for evaluating the cardiac chambers at rest, there is increasing interest in performing the ultrasonic examination during or immediately after exercise.[79–81] Most of these studies have utilized supine bicycle exercise. However, in some cases, upright bicycle exercise or isometric exercise has been utilized.

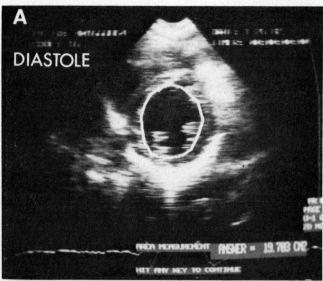

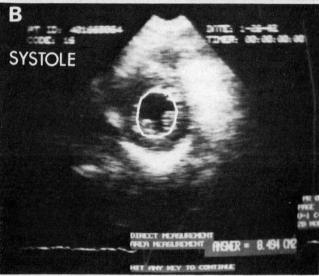

FIGURE 5–32 Short-axis two-dimensional echocardiograms demonstrating how the area of the left ventricle at the papillary muscle level can be measured in diastole and systole.

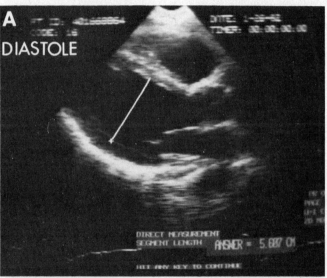

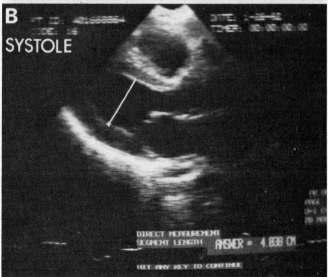

FIGURE 5–31 Parasternal long-axis examinations demonstrating how a minor dimension of the left ventricle can be measured in diastole and systole.

Echocardiography may also be employed to measure the thickness of the walls of the ventricle.[82–84] Although this measurement can also be made using angiography, many errors are inherent in this technique. For example, the presence of pericardial effusion invalidates the angiographic measurement of diastolic wall thickness. In addition, during systole much of the contrast material is squeezed out of the intertrabecular crevices, and the angiographically determined systolic thickness is probably too large. Echocardiography provides the opportunity for measuring left ventricular wall thickness more accurately, especially in systole. The absolute thickness of the ventricle is important in determining the presence of left ventricular hypertrophy (Fig. 5–33) and in estimating left ventricular mass.[84,85] Echocardiography also permits measurement of changes in left ventricular thickness during the cardiac cycle. Normally, the left ventricular wall thickens during systole, but in pathologic conditions this thickening decreases and actual systolic thinning has been noted in acute ischemia or myocardial infarction.[86,87]

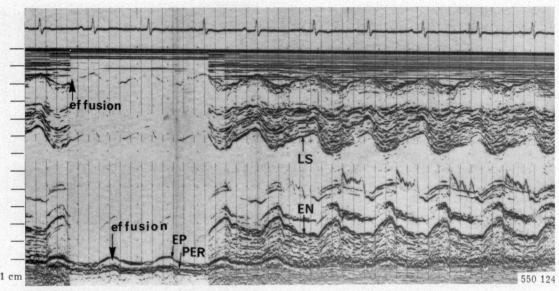

FIGURE 5–33 Left ventricular echocardiogram from a patient with left ventricular hypertrophy and a small pericardial effusion. The thickness of the interventricular septum and posterior left ventricular wall is markedly increased. LS = left septum, EN = posterior left ventricular endocardium, EP = posterior left ventricular epicardium, PER = posterior pericardium. (From Chang, S.: M-Mode Echocardiographic Techniques and Pattern Recognition. Philadelphia, Lea and Febiger, 1976.)

Hemodynamic Information

Since echocardiography has a sampling rate of 1000 impluses/second, the recording is virtually continuous and provides a very accurate assessment of cardiac motion. The motion of the valves has been examined primarily to detect abnormalities in anatomy; however, it also provides considerable physiologic information (Chaps. 3 and 4). The motion of a valve is influenced by the flow of blood through its orifice and by alterations in the relative pressure on its two sides.

There have been many studies correlating echocardiographic *mitral valve* motion with hemodynamics. Figure 5–34, for example, demonstrates simultaneous recording of left ventricular pressure and a mitral valve echogram in a patient with atrial fibrillation and severe aortic regurgitation; the latter is reflected in the fluttering of the anterior leaflet of the mitral valve,[88-90] and the for-

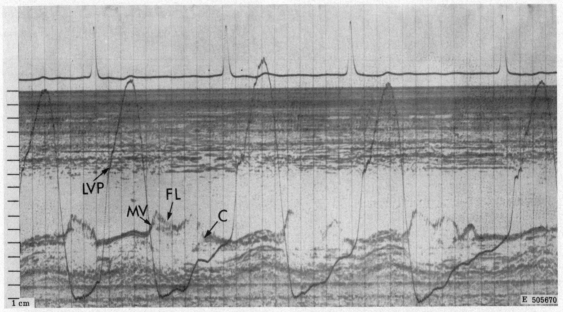

FIGURE 5–34 Simultaneous left ventricular pressure (LVP) and mitral valve echocardiogram (MV) from a patient with severe aortic regurgitation and atrial fibrillation. With a long diastolic internal pressure and a high left ventricular diastolic pressure, closure (C) of the valve occurs before the onset of electrical depolarization. Fluttering (FL) of the mitral valve can be noted. (From Feigenbaum, H.: Echocardiography. 2nd ed. Philadelphia, Lea and Febiger, 1976.)

mer is marked by variation in the duration of diastolic intervals and the left ventricular diastolic pressure. The first cardiac cycle has a low end-diastolic pressure, and the mitral valve closes with ventricular systole. The following diastolic intervals are longer, and the left ventricular diastolic pressure rises. With a high left ventricular diastolic pressure, as in the second cardiac cycle, the mitral valve is closed long before the onset of ventricular systole. Thus, in the setting of aortic regurgitation, premature closure of the mitral valve is a sign of a high left ventricular diastolic pressure.[91] This finding may be particularly helpful in the recognition of this hemodynamic abnormality in patients with acute aortic regurgitation secondary to bacterial endocarditis.[92,93]

Several investigators have demonstrated a relationship between mitral valve motion and blood flow through that orifice.[94,96-98] Figure 5-35 provides an example of how altered left ventricular hemodynamics influence mitral valve motion. The mitral valve echogram becomes distorted in patients who have tall and prominent *a* waves reflected in the left ventricular diastolic pressure.[99] Following atrial systole, closure of the valve is interrupted, and there is a plateau or notch between the A and C points just before

the onset of ventricular systole.[100] This type of abnormal motion of the mitral valve is commonly seen in patients with ischemic heart disease, aortic stenosis, hypertension, or cardiomyopathy and may be due to decreased left ventricular compliance (Fig. 5-35*B*). Ventricular pressure equals atrial pressure earlier than normal. Thus, the mitral valve commences its closure (A point) earlier than normal. Just prior to ventricular systole, the atrial and ventricular pressures equilibrate, and there is a plateau or notch between the A and C points. The mitral valve closes completely with ventricular systole but at a slightly delayed instant (C point). Although its exact mechanism is not understood, this delay in the C point might be a manifestation of a decreased rate of rise of left ventricular pressure. However, regardless of the mechanism responsible, in patients with a large atrial component to the left ventricular diastolic pressure, the onset of closure of the mitral valve with its A point occurs early, the C point is delayed, and a plateau or notch occurs between the A and C points. This echocardiographic abnormality can be measured by subtracting the A-C interval from the electrocardiographic P-R interval. Although this measurement does not correlate with left ventricular diastolic pressure,[100] it is helpful in

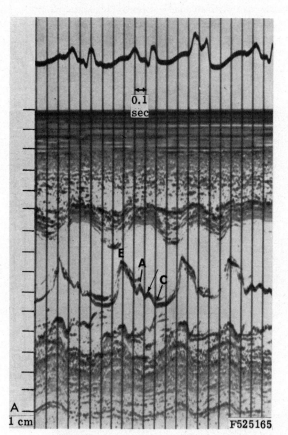

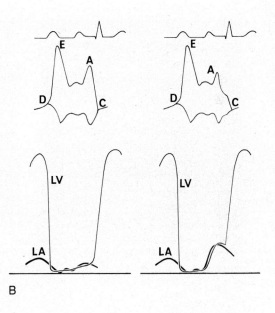

FIGURE 5-35   *A,* Mitral valve echocardiogram showing abnormal mitral valve closure in a patient with a high left ventricular end-diastolic pressure secondary to an elevated atrial component of the left ventricular pressure. Closure of the mitral valve (A to C) is prolonged and interrupted by a notch or plateau (arrow). (From Konecke, L. L., et al.: Abnormal mitral valve motion in patients with elevated left ventricular diastolic pressure. Circulation *47*:989, 1973, by permission of the American Heart Association, Inc.)

   B, Diagrams illustrating how the mitral valve echogram relates to changes in left ventricular and left atrial diastolic pressures. With normally low left-heart pressures (*left*) mitral valve closure, from A to C, is smooth and uninterrupted. With an elevated left ventricular end-diastolic pressure secondary to an elevated atrial component (*right*), there is commonly interruption in the closure of the mitral valve with prolongation of the A-C interval. (From Feigenbaum, H.: Echocardiography. Philadelphia, Lea and Febiger, 1972.)

identifying groups of patients with elevated left ventricular diastolic pressures.

A recent study has noted that the interval between the Q wave of the electrocardiogram and the mitral valve closure point or C point correlates with the left ventricular filling pressure or mean pulmonary capillary wedge pressure.[101] Also, there was an inverse relationship between these pressures and the time interval between closure of the aortic valve and opening of the mitral valve. The ratio Q=MVC/AVC=E correlated well with the mean pulmonary artery wedge pressure.

Although alterations in *tricuspid valve* flow appear to influence the tricuspid valve echogram, there has been little documentation of such a relationship. Abnormal (i.e., interrupted) closure of the tricuspid valve in patients with elevated right ventricular diastolic pressure has been noted,[2,102] and in patients with augmented flows through the tricuspid valve, as occurs with atrial septal defect, large tricuspid valves with augmented amplitudes of motion are frequently observed.[103]

Analysis of *aortic valve* motion also provides useful hemodynamic information. Thus, in patients with obstructive hypertrophic cardiomyopathy, or discrete subaortic stenosis, closure of the aortic valve occurs during midsystole as the subaortic obstruction suddenly becomes manifest (Fig. 5–36).[104–108] In patients with mitral regurgitation there may be gradual premature closure of the aortic valve late during systole as blood regurgitates into the left atrium and forward flow into the aorta diminishes.[2] This gradual late

systolic closure of the aortic valve may also be seen in low cardiac output states in which the left ventricle may not be capable of sustaining a continuous flow of blood across the aortic valve, and a correlation has been observed between the amplitude and duration of separation of the aortic leaflets and the left ventricular stroke volume.[111,112] In patients with severe aortic regurgitation and markedly elevated left ventricular diastolic pressure the aortic valve may open prior to ventricular systole.[109,110]

Echograms of the *pulmonary valve* have proved to be very useful in reflecting hemodynamic events as well. Although the pulmonary valve echogram is probably influenced in part by the movement of structures to which it is attached,[113] the pressure relationship between the right ventricle and the pulmonary artery also influences the motion of the pulmonary valve (Fig. 5–37). Normally, atrial systole produces a slight downward motion of the pulmonary valve.[114–116] Whether at least part of this motion is due wholly or in part to the posterior motion of the entire base of the heart with atrial systole is not clear. However, there is evidence to suggest that the normal rise in right ventricular pressure occurring during atrial contraction may affect the position of the pulmonary valve. In pulmonic stenosis, the right ventricular systolic and end-diastolic pressures rise without any similar elevation in pulmonary artery pressure, and the atrial contribution to right ventricular pressure is exaggerated and usually sufficient to open the pulmonary valve prior to ventricular systole (Fig. 5–37).[116] This exaggerated *a* wave in the pulmonary valve

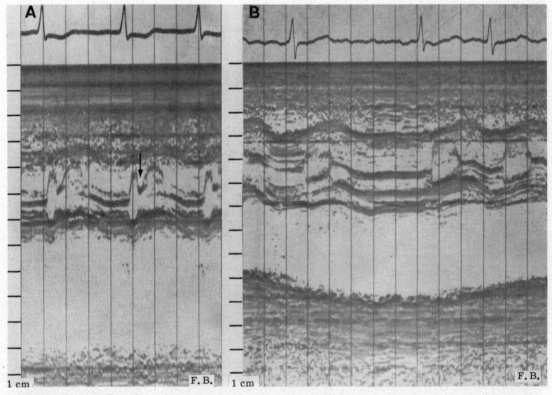

FIGURE 5–36 Aortic valve echocardiograms from a patient with hypertrophic obstructive cardiomyopathy before (*A*) and after (*B*) use of propranolol. With subvalvular obstruction here is closure of the aortic valve in early systole (arrow). This systolic closure disappears as the obstruction is relieved by the use of the beta-adrenergic blocking agent (*B*). (From Feigenbaum, H.: Clinical applications of echocardiography. Progr. Cardiovasc. Dis. *14*:531, 1972, by permission of Grune and Stratton.)

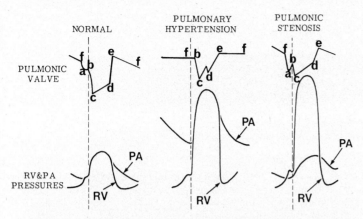

FIGURE 5-37 Diagrams demonstrating the relationship of the pulmonic valve echogram and right-heart pressure in the normal state, with pulmonary hypertension, and with pulmonic stenosis. PA = pulmonary artery pressure, RV = right ventricular pressure. (See text for details.) (From Feigenbaum, H.: Echocardiography. 2nd ed. Philadelphia, Lea and Febiger, 1976.)

echogram reflects the difference in pressures across the pulmonic valve at the end of ventricular diastole. In patients with elevated right ventricular diastolic pressure due to right ventricular failure, tricuspid regurgitation, constrictive pericarditis, or a communication between the aorta and right ventricle, the elevated pressure in the right ventricle in early diastole may cause opening of the pulmonic valve even prior to the onset of atrial systole.[117]

Pulmonary Hypertension. An increase in pulmonary artery pressure has been shown to influence pulmonary valve motion in several ways (Fig. 5-37).[118,119] One of the most consistent changes is the elimination of atrial systolic motion, and the absence or marked reduction of the pulmonary valve *a* wave is one of the echocardiographic signs of pulmonary hypertension. As might be expected, when right ventricular failure occurs in pulmonary hypertension, right ventricular diastolic pressure may rise sufficiently so that a small *a* wave may again be recorded.[2,118] Another sign of pulmonary hypertension is midsystolic closure of the pulmonary valve.[119] While this finding has not been explained, it is probably related to elevated pulmonary vascular resistance.[120] Several other less sensitive and specific signs of pulmonary hypertension have been reported using the pulmonary valve echogram. These include a flat diastolic (E-F) slope, delayed opening of the valve, and an increased velocity of opening of the valve.[118]

The pulmonary valve echogram has been used to calculate systolic time intervals (Chap. 3) of the right side of the heart,[121] and these intervals, in turn, have been used to estimate pulmonary artery pressure and the status of right ventricular performance.[122,123] The pre-ejection period is the time interval from the start of the electrocardiographic QRS to the onset of opening of the pulmonary valve, and the ejection time is the length of time that the pulmonary valve is open. The use of echocardiography for right-sided time intervals has been limited to children, primarily because in adults the closing of the pulmonary valve, which is necessary for measuring ejection time, is rarely recorded unless there is marked dilatation of the pulmonary artery.

With the two-dimensional echocardiographic examination of the inferior vena cava and hepatic vein, more information concerning right-sided hemodynamics is being

obtained. This particular examination can be helpful in assessing the central venous pressure by noting the size of the venous vessels.[124]

The *Doppler echocardiogram* records the pattern and velocity of blood flow within the heart and great vessels and thus would theoretically be an ideal tool for the noninvasive assessment of cardiac hemodynamics.[125] There have been numerous attempts to use Doppler echocardiography to measure left ventricular stroke volume.[13–16,126] Most techniques utilize the recording of Doppler flow from the thoracic aorta. The ultrasonic beam can be directed at either the ascending or the descending aorta. Theoretically, if one knew the velocity of the flow in the aorta together with the cross-sectional area of the aorta one could accurately calculate the flow. Unfortunately, this possibility has yet to be substantiated by multiple investigators. Since the flow is not laminar, the velocity in the center of the aorta is different from the velocity near the edge of the aorta. Theoretically, it is necessary to record the blood velocity profile across the aorta. In addition, the measurement of the cross-sectional area of the aorta has been difficult even with two-dimensional echocardiography. Despite these limitations the flow patterns can be assessed within the aorta using Doppler echocardiography and there is some evidence that it may be possible to follow sequential changes in blood flow in a given individual.[17,125] There is also a suggestion that by calculating blood flow acceleration in the aorta, which is the first derivative of the velocity, the functional state of the left ventricle can be assessed.[126]

As a general rule, the echocardiographic signs predicting altered hemodynamics, while relatively insensitive, are fairly reliable when present. They may be helpful in individual patients, especially when serial echograms are used and progressive changes are recorded.

ACQUIRED VALVULAR HEART DISEASE
(See also Chapter 32)

Rheumatic Mitral Valve Disease

MITRAL STENOSIS. The detection of mitral stenosis was the first clinical application of echocardiography[127–129] and remains an important technique in the evaluation of patients with suspected mitral valve disease since echocardiography can allow visualization of the mitral valve in a manner not possible with any other procedure. The M-mode examination provides a sensitive assessment of the motion and thickness of the valve leaflets,[105,130,131] while the two-dimensional technique provides a spatial image of the valve and allows direct measurement of the valve orifice.[132–134]

Figure 5-38 shows an M-mode echocardiogram of a patient with calcific mitral stenosis. The motion of the mitral valve is considerably altered from the normal pattern seen in Figure 5-15; the normal "M"-shaped configuration during diastole is no longer present, since the presence of a holodiastolic atrioventricular pressure gradient (diastasis) prevents rapid closure of the valve in mid-diastole. Although sinus rhythm was present, there was no reopening of the valve with atrial contraction and no *a* wave. Thus, the echocardiographic hallmark of mitral stenosis is the absence of valve closure in mid-diastole and of reopening

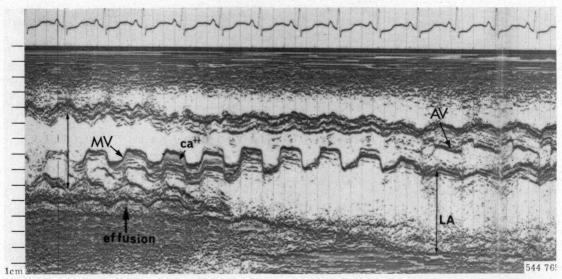

FIGURE 5–38 M-mode scan from a patient with mitral stenosis. The valve is calcified (ca++) and immobile. The left atrium (LA) is dilated and there is moderate posterior pericardial effusion. AV = aortic valve. (From Chang, S.: M-Mode Echocardiographic Techniques and Pattern Recognition. Philadelphia, Lea and Febiger, 1976.)

in late diastole. Although this decreased (flat) diastolic (E-F) slope is characteristic of mitral stenosis, it is not specific.[128,129] Other conditions such as decreased left ventricular compliance or a low cardiac output may also reduce the diastolic slope of mitral valve motion.[135–137]

In addition to the change in motion of the valve, the number of echoes originating from the valve is increased when the valve is fibrotic or calcified,[131] and the second echocardiographic sign of mitral stenosis is increased thickness of the valve leaflets. (Note that the quantity of echoes originating from the mitral valve in Figure 5–38 is considerably greater than in Figure 5–15.) The third sign is inadequate separation of the anterior and posterior leaflets of the valve during diastole.[137] Normally, the two leaflets move in opposite directions during diastole, but when fused, as in mitral stenosis, they do not separate widely and may actually appear to move in the same direction (Fig. 5–38). The echocardiographic findings of reduced diastolic slope, increased thickness, and decreased separation of the valve leaflets provide a sensitive and accurate method for detection of mitral stenosis. There are relatively few conditions that can be confused with hemodynamically significant mitral stenosis echocardiographically; these include reduced compliance of the left ventricle as well as a combination of mild rheumatic mitral stenosis and a markedly reduced cardiac output.

Besides establishing (or excluding) the diagnosis qualitatively, echocardiography can also provide some quantitation of the obstruction. The original criterion for judging the severity of mitral stenosis was the diastolic (E-F) slope[128,129]—the flatter the slope, the more severe the stenosis. More recent evaluation of this sign has shown it to be less accurate than was originally thought. Hemodynamic factors such as the rate of filling of the left ventricle and its compliance can influence the diastolic slope.[135,136] However, two-dimensional echocardiography provides an opportunity to visualize and measure the flow-restricting orifice of the stenotic mitral valve directly (Fig. 5–39). A

number of investigators have demonstrated that the two-dimensional quantitation of mitral stenosis is superior not only to the E-F slope on the M-mode echocardiogram,[134] but perhaps even to cardiac catheterization and Gorlin's formula in the presence of mitral regurgitation.[132]

Two-dimensional echocardiography also assists in the

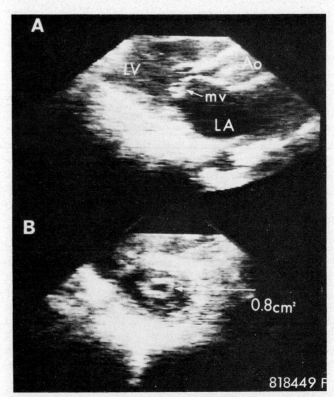

FIGURE 5–39 Two-dimensional echocardiograms of a patient with mitral stenosis. The domed mitral valve (mv) can be seen in the long-axis examination (*A*). The short-axis examination (*B*) demonstrates the orifice of the stenotic valve and provides the opportunity for determining the degree of stenosis.

qualitative diagnosis of mitral stenosis. By noting doming of the mitral leaflets (Fig. 5–39*A*) one can be assured of the valve's restricted motion. "Doming" of any valve on two-dimensional echocardiography is a characteristic sign of stenosis. The distortion in shape with opening of the valve indicates that the tips of the leaflets are restricted in their ability to open, whereas the bodies of the leaflets still wish to accommodate more blood flow. Thus the leaflets are curved or "domed." Doming is used to distinguish a valve that is truly stenotic from one that opens poorly because of low flow.

Echocardiography can also help determine whether or not a stenotic mitral valve is suitable for a commissurotomy by estimating its pliability[105,130] and degree of calcification.[131] The former is judged by measuring the greatest amplitude of motion of the mitral valve. If the anterior leaflet has an opening motion which exceeds 2 cm, the valve is considered to be pliable. Calcification or fibrosis of the valve is reflected by the number of echoes originating from the valve. Although echocardiographic evaluation is not absolutely specific for evaluating the mitral valve, it is probably more reliable than merely searching for an opening snap on auscultation or phonocardiography or for calcification on fluoroscopy.

Echocardiography is also useful for evaluating the effect of mitral stenosis on the cardiac chambers. The left atrium is almost always dilated (Fig. 5–38), and the left ventricular cavity is usually normal or reduced in size. A left atrial emptying index has been devised from the pattern of motion of the posterior aortic wall.[138,139] Normally the aortic wall echo, which is also the anterior wall of the left atrium, moves downward or posteriorly rapidly in early diastole. With mitral obstruction the early diastolic motion is reduced. The signs of pulmonary hypertension (described above) are commonly present on the pulmonary valve echogram in patients with mitral stenosis and sinus rhythm.

MITRAL REGURGITATION. Echocardiography is not as useful in the assessment of patients with rheumatic mitral regurgitation. None of the techniques using the mitral valve echogram, such as a rapid diastolic (E-F) slope[114,140,141] and wide separation of the leaflets during systole, for the detection of mitral regurgitation has proved to be reliable. Two-dimensional echocardiography, which images the regurgitant orifice in systole, has been proposed to solve this problem,[142] but its value has not yet been confirmed.

Doppler echocardiography offers a much better opportunity for the detection of mitral regurgitaton of any type.[143,144] Figure 5–12 demonstrates a Doppler examination in a patient with rheumatic mitral regurgitation. By placing the sampling gate in the left atrium behind the mitral valve, one can detect systolic turbulence indicative of the regurgitant jet. The Doppler technique appears to be reasonably sensitive; however, its ability to quantitate the degree of mitral regurgitation is still controversial.

Echocardiography is useful in evaluating the effect of regurgitation on the cardiac chambers. There is evidence of left ventricular diastolic overload, consisting of increased left ventricular end-diastolic dimensions and an augmented left ventricular stroke volume. The motion of the septum usually exceeds that of the posterior left ventricular wall;

left atrial dilatation is almost invariably present in chronic mitral regurgitation, and left atrial expansion during systole can occasionally be detected.[2,57] The echocardiographic differentiation between rheumatic and nonrheumatic mitral regurgitation is based on the thickening and restriction of motion which is present in patients with rheumatic valvular disease, even in those with essentially pure regurgitation. On the other hand, the leaflets are thin and delicate and move freely in the nonrheumatic forms.

Prolapsed and Flail Mitral Valve

PROLAPSE. Echocardiography is particularly useful in the diagnosis of prolapse of the mitral valve (p. 1089). Figure 5–40 demonstrates the principal M-mode finding in this condition—a fairly abrupt posterior (downward) motion of the mitral valve apparatus in mid- or late systo-

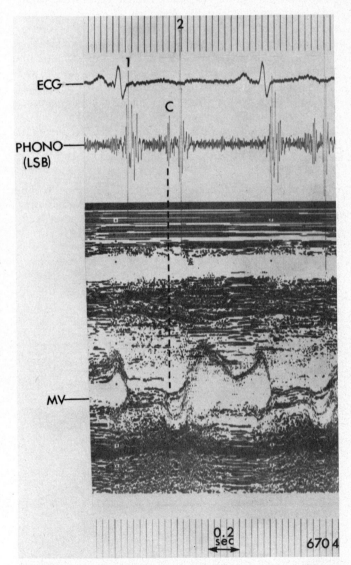

FIGURE 5–40 Phonocardiogram and M-mode echocardiogram from a patient with mitral valve prolapse. The late systolic click (C) on the phonocardiogram corresponds to late systolic posterior displacement of the mitral valve (MV). (From Tavel, M. E.: Clinical Phonocardiography and External Pulse Recordings, 3rd Ed. Chicago, Yearbook Medical Publishers, 1978.)

le.[145-147] This motion often commences simultaneously with the mid- or late systolic click (Fig. 5-40), a typical auscultatory and phonocardiographic finding in this condition (Chap. 4). Although this mid- or late systolic posterior motion of the mitral valve is a reasonably specific sign of mitral valve prolapse, it is not a very sensitive sign. Many patients with this lesion fail to show it, while in others the prolapse is a holosystolic event, i.e., there is posterior displacement of the valve throughout systole (Fig. 5-41).[148,149] Minor degrees of posterior displacement of the mitral valve can occur normally, and there is a troublesome "gray" zone in which it is difficult to determine whether the prolapse is normal or not.[150,151] Late or holosystolic prolapse, as in Figures 5-40 and 5-41, in which the leaflets move posteriorly by at least 5 mm (Fig. 5-41), is generally accepted as abnormal. However, when the holosystolic "hammocking" is less than 5 mm,[152] the diagnosis is not clear-cut.

Several findings on two-dimensional echocardiography have been suggested for the diagnosis of mitral valve prolapse,[153-155] including the recording of buckling of one or both mitral leaflets into the left atrium during systole. Figure 5-42 demonstrates a parasternal long-axis examination of a patient with mitral valve prolapse. Both leaflets can be seen buckling or herniating into the left atrium in late systole. Figure 5-43 demonstrates an apical four-chamber view of a patient with mitral valve prolapse. The level of the mitral valve annulus is noted by the dashed line. The anterior or septal mitral leaflet bulges well into the left atrium on this echocardiogram. Unfortunately, the amount of systolic prolapse noted on the two-dimensional echocardiograms also exhibits a continuum from normal to abnormal, and there may still be a problem in differentiating between prolapse and a normal variant with this technique.

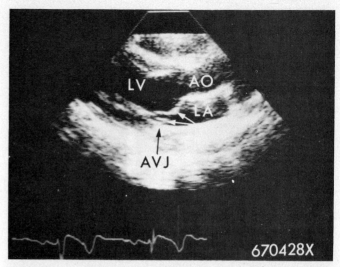

FIGURE 5-42 Two-dimensional long-axis echocardiogram of a patient with mitral valve prolapse. Both the anterior and posterior mitral leaflets (arrows) curve into the left atrium (LA). The posterior leaflet makes almost a hairpin turn as it moves to the atrial side of the atrioventricular junction (AVJ). LV = left ventricle; AO = aorta. (From Feigenbaum, H.: Echocardiography. 3rd ed. Philadelphia, Lea & Febiger, 1981.)

Secondary echocardiographic findings in patients with mitral valve prolapse include excessive amplitude of motion of the valve during diastole which can be appreciated in both M-mode and two-dimensional examinations. Some thickening of the leaflets is not uncommon and is presumably due to myxomatous degeneration; the latter is rarely confused with the thickening associated with mitral stenosis, but since valve motion is not restricted, it can be con-

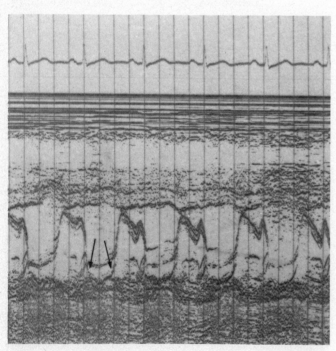

FIGURE 5-41 Mitral valve echocardiogram from a patient with holosystolic mitral prolapse (arrows). (From Feigenbaum, H.: Echocardiography. 2nd ed. Philadelphia, Lea and Febiger, 1976.)

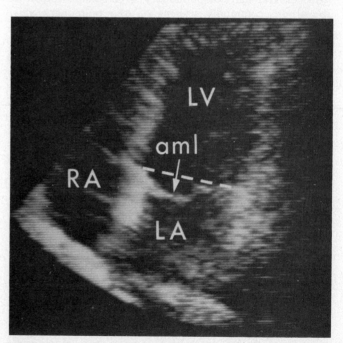

FIGURE 5-43 Apical four-chamber echocardiogram of a patient with mitral valve prolapse demonstrating a curved anterior mitral leaflet (aml) that extends beyond the plane of the mitral annulus (dashed line). LV = left ventricle; LA = left atrium; RA = right atrium. (From Feigenbaum, H.: Echocardiography. 3rd ed. Philadelphia, Lea & Febiger, 1981.)

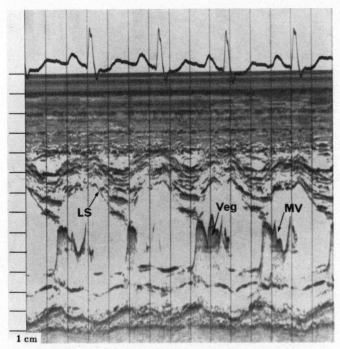

FIGURE 5–44 M-mode echocardiogram from a patient with torn chordae of the anterior mitral leaflet and vegetations (Veg) secondary to bacterial endocarditis. During diastole the anterior mitral leaflet (MV) exhibits chaotic coarse fluttering. LS = left septum. (From Feigenbaum, H.: Echocardiography. 2nd ed. Philadelphia, Lea and Febiger, 1976.)

fused with a vegetation.[156] Excessive motion of the atrioventricular ring, as determined by two-dimensional echocardiography, has been reported in patients with prolapse of the mitral valve. Also, the presence of an abnormal contraction pattern on the left ventricular echogram has been described in these patients[157,158]; the specificity and diagnostic usefulness of these findings remain to be defined.

FLAIL MITRAL VALVE. There are several reports in the literature describing the echocardiographic findings in patients with a flail mitral valve, i.e., with a leaflet that has lost its normal support and therefore flutters in the bloodstream. In many of these patients the mitral valve echogram presents an extreme form of mitral valve prolapse with marked posterior displacement of the mitral valve during systole.[2,159,160] In some patients flail valves are a consequence of infective endocarditis,[161] and vegetations can sometimes be imaged (Chap. 33). In Figure 5–44 a very coarsely fluttering anterior leaflet of the mitral valve is imaged, a motion which is characteristically chaotic, without a reproducible pattern from beat to beat.[159] This type of motion is suggestive of torn chordae tendineae inserting primarily into the anterior mitral leaflet. The principal finding in Figure 5–45, an echocardiogram of a patient with a flail mitral valve secondary to infective endocarditis, shows the echo of a structure, presumably a vegetation, attached to the mitral valve, which moves posteriorly into the left atrium during systole. Thus, the echocardiographic signs of a flail valve can be chaotic motion (as in Figure 5–44), excessive posterior motion during systole, or even recording of a portion of the mitral valve in the left atrium during systole (Fig. 5–45). These signs are all indicative of disruption of the valve but are not necessarily pathognomonic, since a vegetation without a flail valve may also be imaged in the left atrium.

Several studies of flail mitral valves have emphasized their fluttering motion during both diastole[162] and systole.[163] The systolic fluttering is probably a reliable sign of disruption of the mitral valve apparatus, but diastolic fluttering may not be specific, since other conditions such as aortic regurgitation and markedly increased flow across the mitral valve may cause the valve apparatus to flutter during diastole.

Utilizing two-dimensional echocardiography, it has also been noted in patients with ruptured chordae tendineae that a portion of the mitral valve apparatus prolapses or

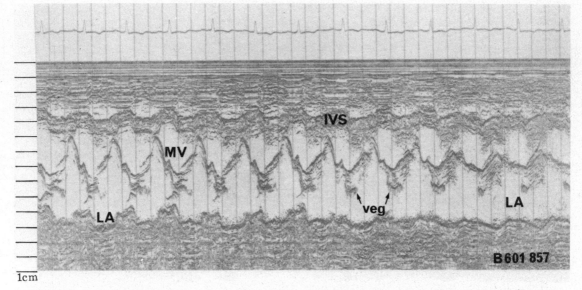

FIGURE 5–45 M-mode scan of a patient with infective endocarditis and vegetations (Veg) on the mitral valve. Echoes from the vegetations can be seen during systole within the left atrial cavity (LA). IVS = interventricular septum, MV = mitral valve. (From Chang, S.: M-Mode Echocardiographic Techniques and Pattern Recognition. Philadelphia, Lea and Febiger, 1976.)

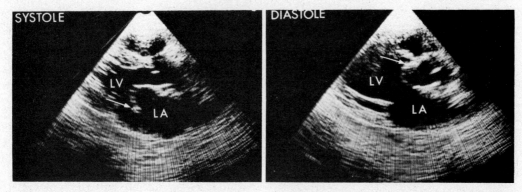

FIGURE 5–46   Long-axis echocardiogram demonstrating a mobile vegetation (arrows) on the anterior leaflet of a flail mitral valve. In systole the vegetation and leaflet protrude into the left atrium and in diastole the valve moves into the left ventricular outflow tract. LV = left ventricle, LA = left atrium. (From Feigenbaum, H.: Echocardiography. 3rd ed. Philadelphia, Lea & Febiger, 1981.)

herniates into the left atrium during systole (Fig. 5–46).[164] The differentiation between a prolapsing and a flail valve is that in the case of prolapse the body of the leaflet moves into the left atrium while the tips of the leaflets remain within the left ventricle, whereas with a flail valve the tips of the valve are displaced into the left atrium during systole.

Aortic Valve Disease

STENOSIS.   The echocardiographic hallmark of aortic stenosis is thickening of the leaflets with narrowing of the orifice.[165,166] Thus, the echocardiographic signs of aortic stenosis are similar to those of mitral stenosis but are not as reliable. Figure 5–47 compares a normal and a stenotic aortic valve. There are more echoes originating from the latter, and the leaflets do not open as widely. Assessment

of thickening of the valve is subjective, since even the normal valve sometimes appears to have excessive echoes, and assessing the motion of the leaflets can also be difficult at times. Thus, while standard M-mode echocardiography can be helpful in making the diagnosis of valvular aortic stenosis, both the sensitivity and the specificity of the technique leave much to be desired. For example, a noncalcified congenitally stenotic aortic valve may be totally unrecognized by M-mode echocardiography.[102] Furthermore, assessing the severity of aortic stenosis by measuring the separation of aortic valve leaflets on the M-mode tracing is quite imprecise.[166,167]

The severity of the stenosis, however, may be judged indirectly from determining any secondary effects on the left ventricle. Thus, the severity of the valvular obstruction[168–170,172] and the level of left ventricular systolic pressure[170,171] can be judged from the thickness of the left ven-

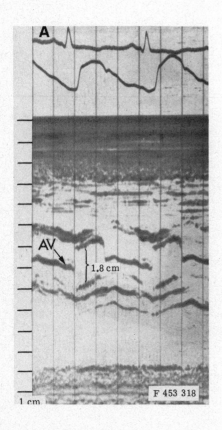

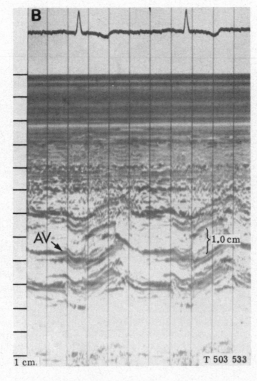

FIGURE 5–47 Aortic valve echocardiograms from a patient with a normal aortic valve (A) and from a patient with valvular aortic stenosis (B). The echoes are thinner and less echo-producing and separate more widely in the normal valve than in aortic stenosis. AV = aortic valve. (From Feigenbaum, H.: Echocardiography, 2nd ed. Philadelphia, Lea and Febiger, 1976.)

tricular wall. Unfortunately, the technique is not reliable in the presence of left ventricular dilatation. By obtaining a spatially correct image of the aortic valve using two-dimensional echocardiography, it is possible to appreciate its domed shape and to measure the diameter of the flow-restricting orifice (Fig. 5–48).[173,174] Thus, two-dimensional echocardiography has significantly improved the qualitative diagnosis of aortic stenosis, especially in the young patient. Unfortunately, there are still problems with attempting to quantitate the degree of aortic stenosis using two-dimensional echocardiography.[175] Although a diameter of the flow-restricting orifice can be obtained, its measurement has significant limitations. The diameter determined by echocardiography is probably more helpful in the young patient with a pliable aortic valve. Once the valve becomes rigid, the diameter no longer is a predictor of the orifice. Attempts at measuring the cross-sectional area of the stenotic aortic valve have not been nearly as successful as with the mitral valve. Thus, this technique is not practical. One can judge the pliability of the leaflets in short axis and gain further information concerning the severity of the stenosis.[176] Thus far, the two-dimensional technique, especially in the adult patient, can judge the extreme situations, but it is still difficult to distinguish between moderate and severe aortic stenosis.

Preliminary data suggest that Doppler echocardiography may be able to judge the pressure gradient across the aortic valve in patients with aortic stenosis, since, theoretically, at least, the velocity is a function of the pressure gradient.[177–179] These findings obviously must be confirmed before they can be used routinely in the clinical setting.

REGURGITATION. *Direct* echocardiographic examination of the aortic valve is of limited value in the detection of aortic regurgitation; however, several findings should be noted. When the aortic valve is disrupted or flail, it may flutter during diastole.[180–183] When present, this finding is quite reliable, but it is not sensitive and is rarely seen in patients with chronic aortic regurgitation. In patients with infective endocarditis and aortic regurgitation, echoes from a vegetation or a portion of the disrupted aortic valve prolapsing into the left ventricular outflow tract during diastole are commonly imaged.[180,182,184–186] However, the diagnosis of aortic regurgitation on the basis of diastolic separation of the aortic valve leaflets does not appear to be reliable.[187] The diagnosis of aortic valve prolapse with two-dimensional echocardiography has been reported.[155,188]

The most common echocardiographic finding in aortic regurgitation is fine fluttering of the anterior leaflet of the mitral valve during diastole (Fig. 5–34).[88–90] Rarely, the posterior mitral leaflet and even the left side of the interventricular septum also flutter.[189,190] These movements presumably are caused by the regurgitant jet flowing into the left ventricle. It is important to recognize that this finding is only of qualitative value in the detection of aortic regurgitation, and it is usually absent when aortic regurgitation coexists with rheumatic mitral stenosis, presumably because of the rigidity of the mitral valve under these circumstances.

Doppler echocardiography is able to detect aortic regurgitation in a high percentage of patients.[20,21,144,191] By placing the sampling volume in the left ventricular outflow tract, one can detect the high velocity turbulent flow during diastole. There is some confusion in differentiating aortic regurgitation from the turbulent diastolic flow with mitral stenosis. However, the abnormal flow from aortic regurgitation commences slightly before that from mitral stenosis, and one can help differentiate the valvular lesions by noting the onset of the turbulent flow and the opening of the mitral valve. There are also data indicating that one could judge the severity of the aortic regurgitation by the Doppler examination in the aorta.[20,21] The amount or per cent of diastolic reverse flow within the aorta has some relationship to the severity of aortic regurgitation.

Closure of the mitral valve in mid-diastole is consistent with severe, and usually acute, aortic regurgitation (Fig. 5–34).[91–93] Echocardiographic signs of left ventricular volume overload, with dilatation of the left ventricle and exaggerated motion of the interventricular septum, are helpful signs of moderate and severe aortic regurgitation. Echocardiography has been suggested as a useful method of assessing left ventricular function in patients with aortic regurgitation. A reduced fractional shortening and especially an enlarged end-systolic dimension on M-mode echocardiography have been suggested as indicators of reduced ventricular function and are useful in judging the timing for valvular surgery[192] (Chap. 32). Other investigators have suggested that exercise echocardiography can help assess left ventricular function in patients with aortic regurgitation.[193] The reliability of these techniques for timing valvular surgery for aortic regurgitation has yet to be determined.

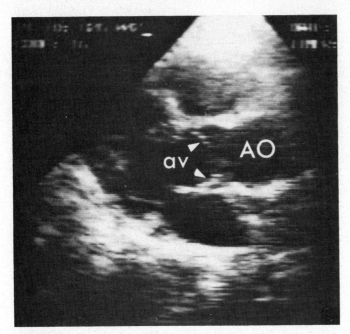

FIGURE 5-48 **Two-dimensional echocardiogram of a patient with valvular aortic stenosis. The domed aortic valve (av) can be easily recognized in this systolic frame. AO = aorta.**

Tricuspid Stenosis and Regurgitation

In *tricuspid stenosis,* the principal M-mode abnormality is a decrease in the diastolic slope of the anterior leaflet,[114,194] similar to that occurring in mitral stenosis. Again, as in the case of the mitral valve, a reduced diastolic slope occurs in, but is not specific for, tricuspid stenosis and may also be seen in the presence of a low cardiac output and reduced right ventricular compliance. However, a normal steep diastolic slope helps to exclude the presence of tricuspid stenosis. Thickening of the valve is not as prominent in tricuspid as it is in mitral stenosis, and this sign is not as valuable in diagnosing tricuspid valve disease. Also, since the posterior leaflet of the tricuspid valve cannot usually be imaged, reduced separation of the leaflets cannot be appreciated in the majority of patients with tricuspid stenosis.

Two-dimensional echocardiography offers a more reliable technique for the qualitative assessment of tricuspid stenosis.[195] By noting doming of the tricuspid valve the diagnosis of tricuspid stenosis can be made with fair reliability.

Aside from the diagnosis of tricuspid valve prolapse,[155,196] the M-mode and two-dimensional echocardiographic signs for *tricuspid regurgitation* are indirect. Both techniques detect a pattern indicative of a right ventricular volume overload. The M-mode echocardiogram reveals a dilated right ventricular dimension and anterior (rather than the normal posterior) motion of the interventricular septum during isovolumic contraction and sometimes during ejection.[47] Two-dimensional echocardiography notes an abnormal shape of the septum during diastole[197]; with increased diastolic flow through the tricuspid valve, as occurs in tricuspid regurgitation, atrial septal defect, and other conditions producing right ventricular volume overload, the augmented filling of the right ventricle indents the septum so that it bulges into the left ventricle during diastole.[197,198] During ejection the septum returns to its normal position, and the left ventricle again becomes spherical.

A more direct diagnosis of tricuspid regurgitation can be obtained with Doppler echocardiography or contrast echocardiography. Detecting a turbulent systolic jet in the right atrium with Doppler echocardiography is proving to be a very sensitive technique for detecting tricuspid regurgitation.[199] Because the right-sided chambers are close to the transducer, Doppler echocardiography is more reliable in detecting tricuspid regurgitation than mitral regurgitation. Contrast echocardiography is also useful in detecting tricuspid regurgitation.[200-202] With the injection of contrast into a peripheral arm vein in patients with tricuspid regurgitation, contrast echoes are recorded during systole in the inferior vena cava and hepatic veins. One can obtain some semiquantitative impression of the degree of tricuspid regurgitation using this technique.

Infective Endocarditis
(See also Chapter 33)

Echocardiography provides an opportunity for visualizing the vegetations of infective valvular endocarditis, which appear as echo-producing masses attached to the infected valve (Fig. 5–44).[184-186,203-205] Vegetations must be approximately 3 to 4 mm in diameter before they can be appreciated on the echocardiogram[203,206]; they are usually asymmetrical, commonly involving one leaflet more than another. If the vegetation is associated with destruction of

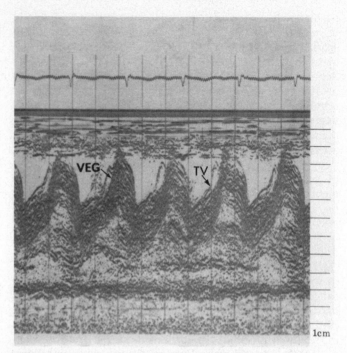

FIGURE 5–49   Echocardiogram demonstrating a large bacterial vegetation (VEG) on the tricuspid valve (TV). (From Feigenbaum, H.: Echocardiography, 2nd ed. Philadelphia, Lea and Febiger, 1976.)

the valve or if it is on a long "stalk," it can be readily imaged; its excessive motion can be appreciated on both M-mode (Fig. 5–45)[207,208] and two-dimensional echocardiography (Fig. 5–46).[209] Some very large vegetations have been described, and these seem often to involve the tricuspid valve (Fig. 5–49)[2,206,210,211] or may result from infection with *Candida albicans*.

Many patients with clinically proven infective endocarditis do not have recognizable vegetations on the echocardiogram,[212] especially if the involved valves remain competent.[206] In one study, only one-third of patients with proven endocarditis had vegetations that could be visualized on the echocardiogram.[212] Studies, especially using two-dimensional echocardiography,[213] have noted a much higher frequency of vegetations on the echocardiogram. However, the frequency is not 100 per cent,[214] so that a negative echocardiogram does not rule out endocarditis. When vegetations are evident, the valve frequently may be diseased to the point at which its function is significantly impaired[206] and surgical replacement may be necessary.[212,215] However, with more sensitive echocardiographic methods for detecting vegetations, principally two-dimensional echocardiography, the finding of vegetations is not as ominous as first thought.

Vegetations visualized echocardiographically need not be bacterial[216-218] or even infected.[219,220] Infected vegetations may be difficult to distinguish from myxomatous degeneration of the valve,[156,181,209,220] although this differentiation is usually readily accomplished clinically.

Prosthetic Valves

Despite extensive attention to this problem, there are still no sensitive and specific echocardiographic signs of prosthetic valve malfunction.[221-234] Most published reports of prosthetic valve malfunction represent isolated case studies, and the findings include large thrombi[229,235,236] and balls or discs that adhere to the cage intermittently or permanently.[223,225,226,231,237-243] Abnormal motion of a ball or disc usually results from thrombus[238] or ball variance.[231] A useful sign of a malfunctioning Björk-Shiley valve in the mitral position is a rounding of the E point on the M-mode echocardiogram.[245] An abnormal rocking motion of a prosthetic valve resulting from the sutures pulling loose from the annulus has been reported.[241,242] The significance of the "fine" intracavitary echoes originating from prosthetic valves in the mitral position is unclear.[243] Thickening of the porcine valve leaflets is useful in judging deterioration of this valve.[244]

An attempt has been made to assess the function of prosthetic mitral valves by noting that the motion of the prosthetic cage is reduced with obstruction. As with any other form of valvular regurgitation, when it occurs through a prosthetic valve there is evidence of ventricular volume overload. If regurgitation occurs through a prosthetic aortic valve, fluttering of the natural mitral valve may occur, just as is the case for regurgitation through the natural aortic valve. The motion of the interventricular septum is commonly abnormal for at least six months following open heart surgery.[246] Although the mechanism for this phenomenon has not been defined, if either the mitral or aortic prosthetic valve leaks significantly, the resultant left ventricular volume overload may prevent the occurrence of abnormal septal motion. Thus, *normal* septal motion in the first six months following aortic or mitral valve replacement is a sign of abnormality and suggests the presence of valvular regurgitation.[247-250] Doppler echocardi-

ography is probably the best echocardiographic technique for evaluating prosthetic valve regurgitation.[251]

Thus, while echocardiography can record the motion of a prosthetic valve, unfortunately it is not always possible to assess its function. Thrombi, vegetations, and malfunction can occur without specific echocardiographic change. Probably, a change in serial echocardiograms is more significant in judging deterioration of prosthetic valve function than is an isolated recording, and combining echocardiography with phonocardiography for determining the timing of valve opening and closing may be helpful in evaluating prosthetic valve function, especially in the mitral position.[235,252-256]

CALCIFIED MITRAL ANNULUS

Calcification of a mitral annulus can be readily demonstrated by echocardiography.[257-264] The principal finding is a band of dense echoes between the mitral valve and the posterior left ventricular wall (Fig. 5–50).

CONGENITAL HEART DISEASE
(See also Chapters 29 and 30)

Deductive Echocardiography

"Deductive echocardiography" refers to a technique useful in the diagnosis of congenital heart disease by which an attempt is made to deduce the anatomy of the heart by identifying the atria, atrioventricular valves, ventricles, semilunar valves, and great vessels.[265,266] The chest roentgenogram is useful in identification of the atria. The loca-

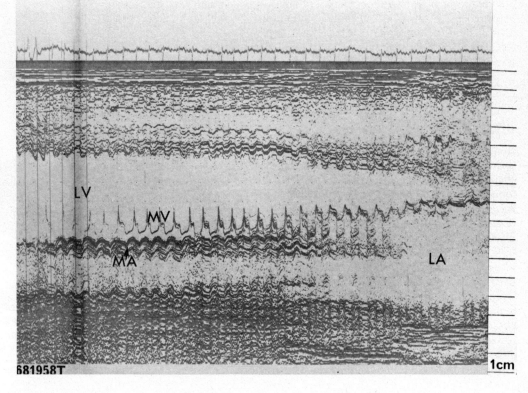

FIGURE 5–50 M-mode echocardiographic scan of a patient with a calcified mitral annulus (MA). The dark band of echoes from the annulus is posterior to the mitral valve (MV) and extends into the left ventricular cavity (LV). LA = left atrium.

681958T

1cm

tion of the trilobed lung or the stomach bubble can be used to decide whether or not the atria are in their normal position; the right atrium will be in its proper position if the lungs and the abdominal organs are also properly situated. The tricuspid valve is ordinarily in continuity with the "anatomic" right ventricle and the mitral valve with the left. Using M-mode echocardiography one can identify the mitral valve as that valve which is in direct continuity with a semilunar valve.[265,266] On the other hand, ventricular myocardium is usually interposed between the tricuspid and pulmonary valves. Thus, by using M-mode scanning to observe the relationship between an atrioventricular valve and the corresponding semilunar valve, it is possible to deduce whether it is a mitral or a tricuspid valve. Then, the anatomic ventricle to which it is connected can also be identified. Two-dimensional echocardiography is also useful for identifying the atrioventricular valves.[271] The tricuspid valve is attached to the interventricular septum closer to the apex than is the mitral valve.[267–269] The attachment of the two atrioventricular valves can be readily assessed using the apical four-chamber view.

The semilunar valves can be more difficult to differentiate, since they appear to be essentially identical on both M-mode and two-dimensional echocardiograms. Normally, the ejection time of the right ventricle exceeds that of the left, and this difference may be helpful in the differentiation of the semilunar valves. Unfortunately, the ejection time of the two valves may be similar in the presence of pulmonary hypertension. However, in such patients the administration of oxygen may lower the pulmonary artery pressure sufficiently to disclose a difference in ejection times and thereby assist in identification of the valves.[265] Two-dimensional echocardiography offers the opportunity of directly identifying the great vessels. It is possible to record the pulmonary artery bifurcation, which can be clearly differentiated from the nonbifurcating aorta.[270] It is also possible to record the arch of the aorta and its branches to help make a positive identification of that vessel. Having identified the individual valves and chambers, the echocardiographer then proceeds to localize these structures and determine their interrelationships.

Valvular Disease

The bicuspid aortic valve is probably the most common congenital anomaly (p. 976). Echocardiographic findings in this anomaly are based on the eccentric closure of the bicuspid aortic valve, so that the aortic valve echoes are no longer in the center of the aorta during diastole.[272,273] A useful though not totally reliable "eccentricity index" relates the width of the aortic lumen to the shortest distance between a cusp and the nearest margin of the aorta.[273] Two-dimensional echocardiography in patients with bicuspid aortic valves has also shown an eccentric position of the cusps in diastole.[274,275] Two-dimensional echocardiography can also identify the specific commissures in many patients. By identifying two rather than three commissures, one can make the echocardiographic diagnosis of bicuspid aortic valve.[275]

In aortic stenosis the echocardiographic findings are similar, if the valve is congenitally deformed or diseased as

a result of rheumatic fever. Figure 5–48 shows a two-dimensional echocardiogram obtained from a patient with a typically domed congenitally stenotic valve. The two-dimensional technique clearly improves on the diagnosis of congenital aortic stenosis,[173] since the M-mode examination can fail to appreciate the domed nature of the valve. Estimating the severity of aortic stenosis directly is very difficult to accomplish with the M-mode examination, but this can be done indirectly by measuring the extent of left ventricular hypertrophy.[168–172] Two-dimensional echocardiography offers the possibility of measuring the separation of the stenotic aortic leaflets. Some but not all echocardiographers feel that the separation is related to the severity of the aortic stenosis.[173,174]

The echocardiographic findings in congenital mitral stenosis resemble those in rheumatic mitral stenosis in older children and adults.[276–278] However, in the young child or infant the congenitally stenotic mitral valve is more mobile and is not nearly as thickened as a rheumatic valve and the diastolic slope is not as flat.

The echocardiographic findings in *valvular pulmonic stenosis* include an accentuation of the *a* wave on the pulmonary valve echogram as noted earlier in this chapter (Fig. 5–37 and p. 108).[116] The powerful right atrial contraction increases right ventricular end-diastolic pressure above the relatively low pulmonary artery diastolic pressure, so that transmission of the atrial contraction through the right ventricle leads to premature opening of the pulmonary valve. Normally, this wave rises to a maximum of approximately 5 mm with inspiration; in pulmonic stenosis it may increase to 10 mm. While the exaggerated

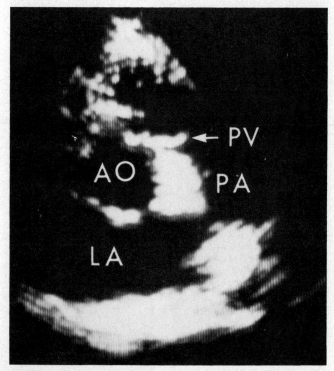

FIGURE 5–51 Two-dimensional echocardiogram of a patient with pulmonic stenosis. The domed, stenotic pulmonary valve (PV) curves into the pulmonary artery (PA) in the systolic frame. AO = aorta; LA = left atrium. (From Feigenbaum, H.: Echocardiography. 3rd ed. Philadelphia, Lea & Febiger, 1981.)

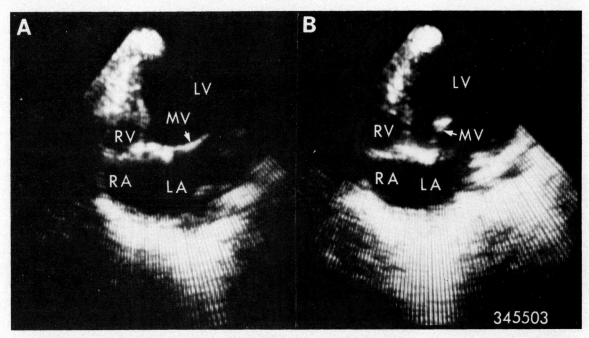

FIGURE 5–52 Apical four-chamber two-dimensional echocardiograms of a patient with tricuspid atresia. The mitral valve (MV) can be seen opening into a large left ventricular chamber (LV). The right ventricle (RV) is small and is separated from the right atrium (RA) by a dense band of linear echoes. No valvular structure could be identified in the region of the tricuspid valve. LA = left atrium. (From Feigenbaum, H.: Echocardiography. 3rd ed. Philadelphia, Lea & Febiger, 1981.)

a wave in pulmonic stenosis is a helpful sign, it must be appreciated that it is not specific, since it may also be present in patients with an elevated stroke volume, regardless of the cause.[54]

The domed stenotic pulmonary valve resembles the congenitally stenotic aortic valve on two-dimensional echocardiography.[279] Normally, the open leaflets are parallel to the wall of the pulmonary artery during systole, but when the valve is domed and stenotic, they curve away from the wall (Fig. 5–51). Though only a single leaflet of the pulmonary valve is ordinarily imaged, its domed appearance is sufficient to establish the diagnosis. The sensitivity and specificity of this technique still remain to be established.

The characteristic echocardiographic findings of *Ebstein's anomaly* of the tricuspid valve consist of increased motion, a position to the left of its usual location, varying diastolic slopes from beat to beat and, most reliably, delayed closure of the tricuspid valve.[280–282] Normally, and even in the presence of right bundle branch block, tricuspid follows mitral valve closure by less than 50 msec[283]; an interval between 50 and 70 msec should raise the suspicion of Ebstein's anomaly, and an interval greater than 70 msec strongly supports the diagnosis.

Two different approaches for the diagnosis of Ebstein's anomaly by means of two-dimensional echocardiography have been proposed:[284–286] the short-axis cross-sectional view of the tricuspid valve demonstrates the abnormally positioned tricuspid valve,[284] while with the apical approach, all four cardiac chambers can be imaged,[285,286] also allowing recognition of the malpositioned tricuspid valve.

VALVULAR ATRESIA. Atresia of cardiac valves is generally associated with hypoplasia of the ipsilateral ventricle (Chap. 29). Thus, aortic or mitral atresia is associated with a hypoplastic left ventricle,[287] while tricuspid or

pulmonary atresia is associated with hypoplasia of the right ventricle.[49,50] Diminutive ventricles have been noted on M-mode tracings in patients with valvular atresia, and the atretic valves have been imaged with both M-mode[287] and two-dimensional techniques (Fig. 5–52).[288,289]

SUBVALVULAR OBSTRUCTIONS. A variety of congenital subvalvular obstructions have been detected echocardiographically. Early systolic closure of the aortic valve has been observed in patients with both *discrete* (Fig. 5–53)[107–109] and *hypertrophic obstructive cardiomyopathy* (Fig. 5–36).[104–106] In addition, systolic fluttering of the aortic valve is often exaggerated, although some degree of aortic valve fluttering may be seen normally. Although midsystolic closure and fluttering of the aortic valve are not specific findings for subaortic stenosis, they can be very helpful in differentiating valvular from subvalvular obstruction, since they do not occur in the former condition. Narrowing of the left ventricular outflow tract can sometimes also be detected by the M-mode technique in patients with discrete subaortic stenosis,[290] but this area of the heart is difficult to image using this method.

Examination of the outflow tract is easier, however, with two-dimensional echocardiography, and the subvalvular obstruction can be more readily identified directly by this technique (Fig. 5–54).[291–293] Moreover, the two-dimensional technique also permits the classification of the types of discrete obstruction into the discrete membranous and the diffuse types.[291] The ability to distinguish between them may be of considerable clinical importance, since their management may differ. The membranous form is frequently situated just below the aortic valve and may therefore be difficult to recognize at catheterization, since the short subvalvular chamber can be missed on a pull-out pressure recording. Indeed, the thin membrane can even be

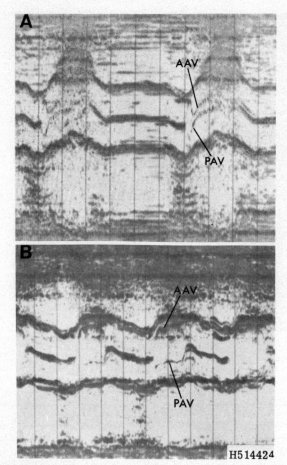

FIGURE 5-53 Aortic valve echograms from a patient with discrete subaortic stenosis before (A) and after (B) surgery for the subaortic obstruction. Prior to surgery the aortic valve anterior (AAV) and posterior (PAV) leaflets come together shortly after the onset of ventricular ejection and remain essentially closed throughout systole. This systolic closure of the valve leaflets is no longer present following surgery. (From Davis, R. A., et al.: Echocardiographic manifestations of discrete subaortic stenosis. Am. J. Cardiol. 33:277, 1974.)

missed on the angiogram, so that its recognition by two-dimensional echocardiography can be very helpful.

In *subpulmonic obstruction* the M-mode tracing exhibits coarse fluttering of the pulmonary valve.[294] The actual subpulmonic obstruction can be detected and its severity quantified in patients with tetralogy of Fallot by means of two-dimensional examination of the right ventricular outflow tract and subpulmonic area.[295]

Cardiac Shunts

Echocardiography can be helpful in the diagnosis of cardiac shunts by detecting the actual defect between the two sides of the heart, by evaluating the hemodynamic consequences of the shunted blood, and by visualizing the shunted blood using contrast and Doppler echocardiography. With M-mode echocardiography actual defects are rarely recognized. Large ventricular septal defects can occasionally be detected,[2] and the ventricular septal defects associated with tetralogy of Fallot are frequently appreciated by the recognition of an overriding aorta[296-298] in the

absence of continuity between the aorta and the ventricular septum. The lack of any identifiable interventricular septum can be helpful in making the diagnosis of a single ventricle.[49,299-301] The septal aneurysm often associated with a defect in the membranous ventricular septum can occasionally be detected by M-mode echocardiography[302,303] and more recently by two-dimensional echocardiography.[304]

Two-dimensional echocardiography is far more sensitive than the M-mode technique in the detection of intracardiac communications.[305-307] Figure 5-55 demonstrates a small ventricular septal defect, which could not be detected with M-mode echocardiography. Figure 5-56 demonstrates an apical four-chamber view in a patient with a single ventricle. The lack of an interventricular septum is striking and obvious on this recording.[308]

The two-dimensional echocardiographic examination, especially from the subcostal position, provides an opportunity for direct examination of the interatrial septum (Fig. 5-25A).[309] Figure 5-57 demonstrates findings in a patient with an ostium secundum atrial septal defect. A remnant of the interatrial septum can be seen attached to the ventricular septum. In contrast, Figure 5-58 demonstrates an atrial septal defect in a patient with an ostium primum defect. There is no residual septum attached to the ventricular septum. Thus, the two-dimensional technique not only helps identify the presence of an atrial septal defect, but is also an excellent means of differentiating a secundum from a primum type abnormality.[310,311] One can also identify more severe forms of endocardial cushion defect with a coexistent ventricular septal defect. A sinus venosus type atrial septal defect is the most difficult type of atrial septal defect to detect echocardiographically.[312]

The usual criteria for the identification of shunts by M-mode echocardiography are indirect and depend on their hemodynamic effects on the various cardiac chambers. In patients with left-to-right shunts distal to the atrioventricular valve (i.e., patent ductus arteriosus, ventricular septal defect, and aortopulmonary window), the left atrium is enlarged be-

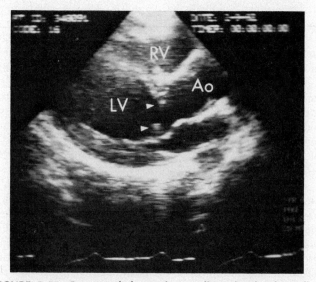

FIGURE 5-54 Parasternal, long-axis two-dimensional echocardiogram of a patient with a membranous discrete subaortic stenosis. The echoes from the subvalvular membrane (arrowheads) can be seen between the left ventricle (LV) and the aorta (AO). RV = right ventricle.

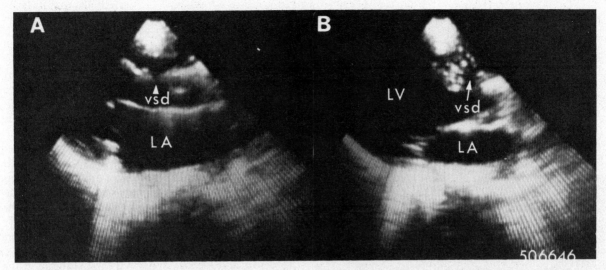

FIGURE 5-55   Two-dimensional long-axis echocardiograms of a patient with a membranous ventricular septal defect. *A*, The discontinuity of echoes from the ventricular septal defect (vsd) can be seen. *B,*A peripheral contrast injection fills the right ventricle, but an echo-free jet, i.e., negative contast, can be seen anterior to the ventricular septal defect. LV = left ventricle; LA = left atrium. (From Feigenbaum, H.: Echocardiography. 3rd ed. Philadelphia, Lea & Febiger, 1981.)

cause of the increased volume of blood flow that traverses it, and its dimension is the most critical measurement in judging the presence and severity of such a shunt.[54,303,313–315] It is useful to follow the size of the left atrium very closely in infants with known or suspected patent ductus arteriosus or ventricular septal defect, and management of such patients may be aided substantially by this measurement.[313,315] Left ventricular volume overload, as reflected in the combination of a dilated left ventricle and increased systolic motion of the ventricular septum which accompanies these left-to-right shunts, is also useful in confirming the pres-

ence and estimating the size of the shunt.[54,314,316,317] With left-to-right shunts at the atrial level (atrial septal defect or partial anomalous pulmonary venous return) the volume overload of the right ventricle is reflected in dilatation of the right ventricle and abnormal motion of the ventricular septum (Fig. 5–59)[47,48,318,319], the amplitude of tricuspid valve motion may also increase.[103] Small left-to-right shunts usually produce no abnormalities in the M-mode echocardiogram.

In *total anomalous pulmonary venous return* all four pulmonary veins empty into a common pulmonary venous

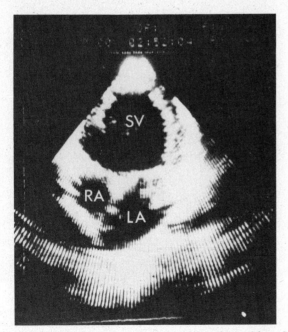

FIGURE 5-56   Cross-sectional echogram of a patient with a single ventricle (SV). The ultrasonic probe is placed at the apex of the heart, and the plane of the scan transects the interatrial septum so that all chambers can be seen simultaneously. This view is particularly helpful in demonstrating the absence of the interventricular septum. RA = right atrium, LA = left atrium.

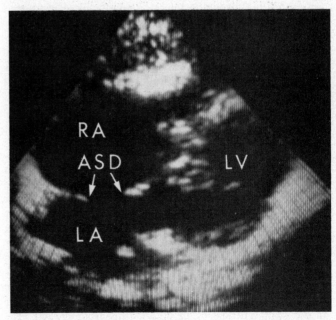

FIGURE 5-57   Subcostal two-dimensional echocardiogram of a patient with a secundum atrial septal defect. Remnants of the interatrial septum are visible on both sides of the defect (ASD). RA = right atrium; LA = left atrium; LV = left ventricle. (From Feigenbaum, H.: Echocardiography. 3rd ed. Philadelphia, Lea & Febiger, 1981.)

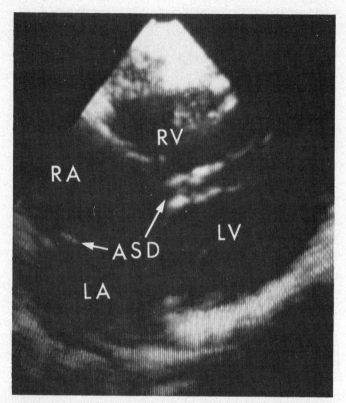

FIGURE 5–58 Subcostal two-dimensional echocardiogram of a patient with an ostium primum atrial septal defect. No residual septal tissue is apparent between the defect (ASD) and the interventricular septum. RA = right atrium; LA = left atrium; RV =right ventricle; LV = left ventricle. (From Feigenbaum, H.: Echocardiography. 3rd ed. Philadelphia, Lea & Febiger, 1981.)

chamber behind the left atrium which produces additional echoes posterior to the left atrium.[320] From an echocardiographic viewpoint the recording is similar to that in *cor triatriatum*, in which the additional echoes are imaged in the left atrium.[287,321,322]

Use of *contrast echocardiography* in the detection of circulatory shunts has recently increased. When injections are made into a peripheral vein, or through a central venous catheter, the echo-producing bubbles will traverse the right side of the heart. In the presence of a right-to-left shunt, however, some of these echoes will pass into and become apparent on the left side of the heart and aorta, the specific site depending on the location of the shunt (Fig. 5–14).[31,323–327] If the right-to-left shunt is at the atrial level, the bubbles will be visualized in the left atrium and behind the mitral valve in the inflow tract of the left ventricle. If the shunt is at the ventricular level, the echo-producing bubbles will be imaged in the left ventricular outflow tract above the mitral valve (Fig. 5–14). Although contrast echocardiography is very sensitive, it is not yet clear whether it can be used for quantification of shunts. *Negative contrast echocardiography* may be used for the detection of left-to-right shunts[328]; for example, in ventricular septal defect, contrast from a peripheral injection is diluted in the right ventricle by blood shunting from the left ventricle, producing a "negative jet" (Fig. 5–55). The negative contrast technique is clearly not as sensitive as the recording of right-to-left shunting. In the case of a left-to-right

shunt at the atrial level there is frequently some small right-to-left shunting so that even in patients with a predominant left-to-right shunt, one may record a small right-to-left shunt with contrast echocardiography.[329,330]

Although contrast echocardiography usually involves injection into a peripheral vein, a central vein, or the right side of the heart, it is possible, in the course of cardiac catheterization, to make the injection anywhere within the cardiovascular system,[324] and selective contrast echocardiography may be used to reduce the need for angiography, which may be especially helpful in infants. In addition, contrast echocardiography with retrograde injections through an arterial line may be used to detect blood shunting from the aorta to the pulmonary artery through a patent ductus arteriosus in critically ill infants.[331,332]

Doppler echocardiography is a very effective technique in the detection of intracardiac shunts[24] because of its ability to detect and localize abnormal flow patterns in the heart. It is particularly useful in the detection of ventricular septal defects[333] and patent ductus arteriosus,[334] anomalies which are rarely recognized using either M-mode or two-dimensional echocardiography. Left-to-right atrial shunts have also been detected with the Doppler technique.[26] An important use of Doppler echocardiography is the diagnosis of multiple shunts. Figure 5–60 demonstrates a Doppler echocardiographic study of a patient with a ventricular

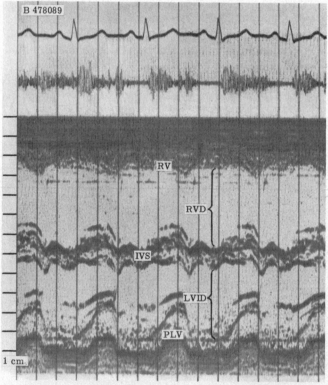

FIGURE 5–59 M-mode echocardiogram from a patient with atrial septal defect. The right ventricular dimension (RVD) is dilated and the right side of the interventricular septum (IVS) moves paradoxically. The left side of the interventricular septum shows a rapid upward motion with the onset of electrical depolarization and then flat motion during ventricular ejection. (From Feigenbaum, H.: Clinical applications of echocardiography. Progr. Cardiovasc. Dis. *14*:531, 1972, by permission of Grune and Stratton.)

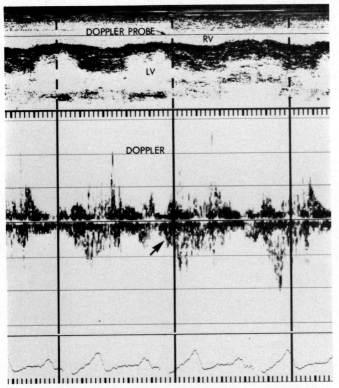

FIGURE 5-60 Doppler echocardiographic examination of a patient with a ventricular septal defect. Systolic turbulent flow (arrow) can be noted with a Doppler probe on the right ventricular side of the interventricular septum. RV = right ventricle; LV = left ventricle.

septal defect. The Doppler sample is obtained from the right ventricular side of the interventricular septum and demonstrates a turbulent systolic flow pattern in this area of the heart. This type of flow is altered in patients with pulmonary hypertension and ventricular septal defects.[27] Thus, the Doppler examination can help to identify those patients in whom the pulmonary artery pressure is significantly elevated in patients with ventricular septal defects.

Intracardiac shunts may be associated with other anomalies of the heart that can be recognized echocardiographically. For example, in patients with defects of the atrioventricular canal, many anomalies of the mitral and/or tricuspid valves in these defects can be appreciated on the echocardiogram.[335-338] On M-mode examination the mitral valve appears to be closer than normal to the interventricular septum (Fig. 5-61), a finding consistent with the abnormal insertion of the mitral leaflet in this anomaly. Also, the tricuspid valve echo appears to traverse the interventricular septum as a result of its abnormal position (Fig. 5-61).[335] The cleft in the mitral valve commonly present with ostium primum atrial septal defect may be detected using two-dimensional echocardiography.[311,339,340]

Another valvular anomaly that may be associated with an intracardiac shunt is a tricuspid valve that overrides the ventricular septum, which can pose major problems in the repair of a ventricular septal defect and which is therefore important to recognize preoperatively. The echocardiographic findings in this condition resemble those in atrioventricular canal defects in that the tricuspid valve is recorded to the left of the interventricular septum.[341-343]

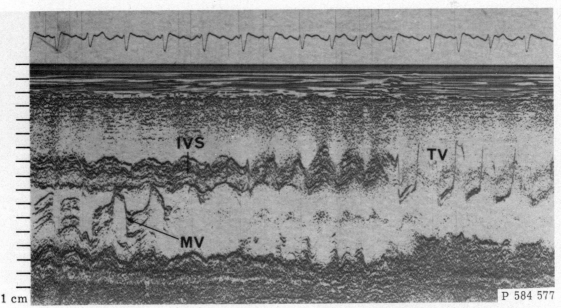

FIGURE 5-61 M-mode scan from a patient with ostium primum type endocardial cushion defect. In the vicinity of the left ventricle (left part of tracing), the right ventricle is dilated, and the intraventricular septal echoes (IVS) show abnormal movement consistent with a right ventricular volume overload. The systolic portion of the mitral valve (MV) is abnormally close to the interventricular septum. The tricuspid valve echoes (TV) seem to traverse the interventricular septum, and parts of the valve appear to lie within both ventricles. (From Feigenbaum, H.: Echocardiography, 2nd ed. Philadelphia, Lea and Febiger, 1976.)

Abnormalities of the Great Arteries

Although *supravalvular aortic stenosis* can be detected using an M-mode echocardiographic scan of the aorta,[344-346] the two-dimensional technique is superior.[288,347] The method of examination is similar to that used for the detection of valvular aortic stenosis, except that the scanning is carried out superior to the aortic valve. *Coarctation of the aorta* is detected with two-dimensional echocardiography by placing the probe in the suprasternal notch,[40,348] which allows imaging of both the narrowed segment of the aorta and the poststenotic dilatation and detection of the excessive pulsation of the aorta proximal to the coarctation.

Tetralogy of Fallot can be detected echocardiographically in a variety of ways. M-mode scanning usually demonstrates a dilated aorta with overriding of the right side with respect to the interventricular septum[296-298]; a defect between the interventricular septum and the anterior wall of the aorta and dilated right ventricle is also frequently visualized. M-mode examinations in *truncus* or *pseudotruncus arteriosus* are quite similar.[349,350] The trunk is usually larger than is the aorta in the tetralogy of Fallot, and the pulmonary valve cannot be imaged[351]; the left atrium is dilated in patients with truncus arteriosus and increased pulmonary blood flow.

Two-dimensional echocardiography has greatly improved the ultrasonic detection of anomalies of the great vessels.[295,352-355] Overriding of the septal defect by the aorta is detected more reliably by this technique (Fig. 5–62) than by M-mode echocardiography, since the latter is exquisitely sensitive to the position of the transducer.[2,102] In the diagnosis of truncus arteriosus, two-dimensional echocardiography helps to establish the number of great arteries leaving the heart. Normally, with a short-axis view of the great vessels, a circular aorta surrounded by a curved, tubular right ventricular outflow tract and pulmonary artery is recorded (Fig. 5–21, diagram 4); in truncus arteriosus only a single large circular vessel can be visualized.[352] In addition, a new technique has been devised by actually recording the branch of the truncus that supplies

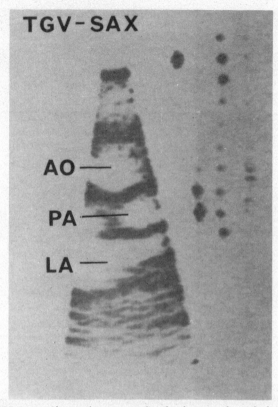

FIGURE 5–63　Short-axis cross-sectional echogram through the base of the heart in a patient with transposition of the great vessels. Instead of having a semicircular pulmonary artery and right ventricular outflow tract wrapped around a circular aorta (Fig. 5–21, diagram 4), one now records two circular great vessels with a more anterior aorta (AO) slightly to the right of the posterior pulmonary artery (PA). LA = left atrium. (From Feigenbaum, H.: Echocardiography. 2nd ed. Philadelphia, Lea and Febiger, 1976.)

the lungs in an effort to establish definitively the diagnosis of truncus arteriosus.[356]

Double-outlet right ventricle is another malformation to be considered in the differential diagnosis of tetralogy of Fallot. The echocardiogram can help to establish whether the left ventricle empties directly into a great artery,[271,357,358] and the M-mode tracing can be used to detect discontinuity between the mitral valve and the aorta, a useful sign in double-outlet right ventricle.[357-359] The tissue between the mitral valve and the aorta can be recognized using two-dimensional echocardiography,[2,354] and serial short-axis views of the heart permit elucidation of the relationship between the ventricles and great vessels.[271]

Transposition of the great arteries can be detected echocardiographically using both M-mode[360] and two-dimensional examinations. However, the M-mode technique has been totally replaced by the two-dimensional approach. The two-dimensional technique for the detection of transposition is based on determining the relationship between the two great arteries[295,362]; normally the pulmonary artery twists around the aorta as the latter passes posteriorly. With transposition of the great arteries, on the other hand, the two arteries run parallel to one another, and with a two-dimensional view parallel to the arteries it is possible to appreciate how the transposed arteries do not twist about each other.[361] A perpendicular or short-axis view of the great vessels demonstrates two circular struc-

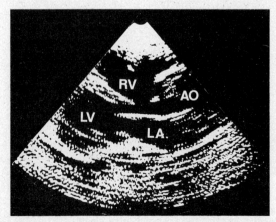

FIGURE 5–62　Cross-sectional echogram from a patient with tetralogy of Fallot. The overriding aorta (AO) is readily apparent in this spatially correct examination. The lack of continuity between the interventricular septum and the anterior wall of the aorta is also obvious. RV = right ventricle, LV = left ventricle, LA = left atrium.

tures (Fig. 5–63) rather than the pulmonary artery normally wrapping around the circular aorta (Fig. 5–21, diagram 4).[352]

Contrast echocardiography can also be useful in establishing the diagnosis of transposition.[363] With a peripheral venous injection, the majority of the echo-producing contrast usually appears in the aorta (which is situated posterior to the pulmonary artery), even though shunting of blood obviously occurs, and this results in *some* contrast appearing in the pulmonary artery.

CORONARY ARTERY DISEASE

ISCHEMIC MYOCARDIUM. The principal echocardiographic technique for identifying ischemic myocardium involves assessment of the motion of the various segments of the left ventricle.[364–368] The ischemic segment might be hypokinetic, akinetic, or dyskinetic. Figure 5–64 shows an M-mode scan from a patient with coronary artery disease; the base of the left ventricle adjacent to the aorta exhibits normal motion of both the left side of the septum and the posterior left ventricular endocardium. However, no septal motion is present in the vicinity of the papillary muscles near the apex. Similar changes may be present in the free wall of the left ventricle, depending on the location of ischemia or fibrosis in a given patient. While the frequent sampling rate of the M-mode echocardiogram allows the wall motion to be recorded accurately, the quantity of abnormally moving myocardium cannot be determined. In addition, many areas of the left ventricle, notably the apex and the inferior and lateral walls, are not accessible to the M-mode echocardiographic examination.

Fortunately, two-dimensional echocardiography can supply the information missing from the M-mode examination. Figure 5–65 shows a four-chamber echogram recorded in a patient with ischemic heart disease in whom the apex is akinetic but in whom the proximal left ventricular walls move normally. Two-dimensional echocardiography can provide an assessment of left ventricular function and thereby an estimation of the extent of ischemic damage of the myocardium.[369–373] Several observers suggest that two-dimensional echocardiography provides valuable diagnostic and prognostic information early after the onset of myocardial infarction.[374–375]

Because of the frequent serial tracings made possible by echocardiography, changes in wall motion can be detected as ischemia develops and disappears. The normal motion of the ventricle ceases in the presence of ischemia; since the stress of isometric exercise by means of forced handgrip[376–378] or of isotonic leg exercise[379–382] often precipitates ischemia, that segment of the left ventricle which ceases to move can be identified (Fig. 5–66).

Although there are many technical difficulties in obtaining echocardiograms during exercise, there has been increasing interest in this type of examination. There are many theoretical advantages to using echocardiography with stress. Two-dimensional echocardiography offers an excellent opportunity for judging regional wall motion changes with exercise. Many of the technical problems may be overcome by recording echocardiograms immediately *after* treadmill exercise.[383,384] Apparently the abnormal wall motion changes persist long enough for detection by echocardiography immediately after cessation of exercise.

Echocardiography also permits the measurement of changes in the thickness of the left ventricular wall.[87] The normal thickening of the left ventricle that occurs during contraction does not occur of course in fibrotic or ischemic tissue, and this finding[86,385,386] may prove to be more accurate in estimating ischemic damage than wall motion studies, which often overestimate it.[72,387,388] Systolic *thinning* of the ventricular wall may prove to be a finding specific for acute ischemia which could prove to be quite useful diagnostically.[87,389] Myocardial scars resulting from old infarcts tend to be thinner and denser (more echo-producing) than nonscarred muscle,[390] but they do not thicken during systole, as is the case for normal tissue, nor do they become thinner, as is the case for acutely ischemic myocardium.

VENTRICULAR ANEURYSMS. Since some alter-

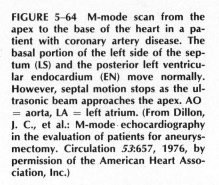

FIGURE 5–64 M-mode scan from the apex to the base of the heart in a patient with coronary artery disease. The basal portion of the left side of the septum (LS) and the posterior left ventricular endocardium (EN) move normally. However, septal motion stops as the ultrasonic beam approaches the apex. AO = aorta, LA = left atrium. (From Dillon, J. C., et al.: M-mode echocardiography in the evaluation of patients for aneurysmectomy. Circulation *53*:657, 1976, by permission of the American Heart Association, Inc.)

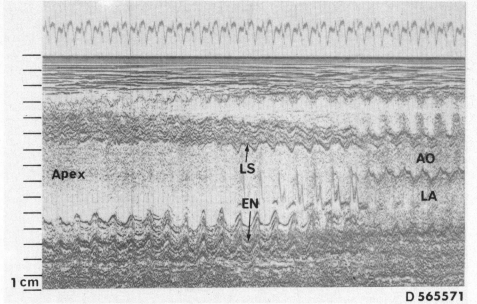

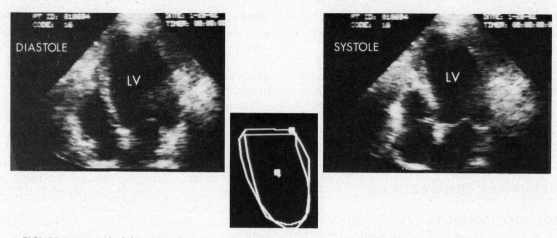

FIGURE 5–65 Apical four-chamber views of a patient with cornary artery disease. The apical half of the left ventricle (LV) is akinetic and in certain areas is dyskinetic. There is residual functioning muscle in the basal half of the septum and free wall.

ations in the shape of the left ventricle can be appreciated by M-mode echocardiography, the diagnosis of ventricular aneurysm is feasible.[391] In the presence of large apical aneurysms the distance between the septum and the posterior ventricular wall increases as the ultrasonic beam approaches the apex. However, since M-mode echocardiography is markedly affected by the position of the transducer, this technique is not very sensitive, and even moderate to large aneurysms may be missed. Two-dimensional echocardiography, on the other hand, with its greater ability to image the left ventricular apex, is proving to be both reliable and sensitive for detecting ventricular aneurysms (Fig. 5–67),[368,392–395] and the correlation with angiographic findings is excellent.[276]

When aneurysmectomy is considered, the evaluation of the function of the remaining myocardium is of critical importance (p. 1374), and echocardiography can often provide this important information. If the size of the left ventricle at its base, as determined by standard M-mode echocardiography, is markedly increased, the results of aneurysmectomy may be anticipated to be poorer than if this dimension is within normal limits or is only slightly increased.[391] Two-dimensional echocardiography is, of course, superior to M-mode examination because it permits an estimation of the amount of residual normally functioning myocardium.[396]

In pseudoaneurysm due to a contained rupture of the free wall following myocardial infarction, a large, relatively echo-free space is present, usually behind the posterior wall of the left ventricle.[397,398]

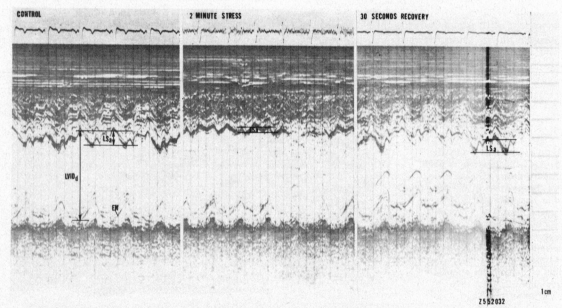

FIGURE 5–66 Serial M-mode echocardiograms from a patient with spasm of the left anterior descending coronary artery. At rest, the left septal echo amplitude (LS_a) is normal. During handgrip stress, the patient develops angina, and the amplitude of septal motion is markedly reduced. Following cessation of handgrip and the disappearance of pain, septal motion returns to normal. (From Widlansky, S., et al.: Coronary angiography, echocardiographic, and electrocardiographic studies on a patient with variant angina due to coronary artery spasm. Am. Heart J. *90*:631, 1975.)

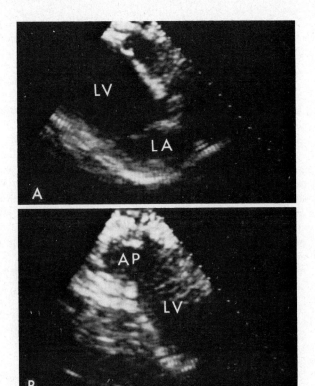

FIGURE 5-67 Parasternal long-axis two-dimensional echocardiograms of a patient with coronary artery disease, a scarred interventricular septum, and an apical aneurysm. *A* demonstrates the body of the left ventricle (LV) and left atrium (LA). Note the thin, relatively echo-dense septum. *B,* Apical examination reveals the aneurysm (AP). (From Feigenbaum, H.: Echocardiography. 3rd ed. Philadelphia, Lea & Febiger, 1981.)

Assessment of Ventricular Performance

Estimates of left ventricular ejection fraction by standard M-mode echocardiography, i.e., determination of the extent or rate of shortening, do not usually provide reliable information about left ventricular function in patients with coronary artery disease, since these calculations are based on the assumption that the two sampling sites imaged on the septum and posterior ventricular wall are representative of the entire ventricle. However, as noted in Figure 5-64, this may not be the case in ischemic heart disease, which frequently affects regions of the heart differently. On the other hand, when the diastolic diameter is increased by echocardiography it can be assumed that overall left ventricular function is severely impaired[366,391,399]— a poor prognostic sign in patients with acute myocardial infarction[366] and in patients with ischemic disease who may be candidates for bypass operation.[399] It has been suggested that an increase of the distance between the anterior mitral leaflet and the interventricular septum reflects abnormal left ventricular performance[65] in that both left ventricular dilatation and decreased amplitude of mitral valve motion due to reduced mitral valve flow, which are responsible for this separation, correlate inversely with the ejection fraction.

As discussed earlier (Fig. 5-35, p. 107) the motion of the mitral valve may be influenced by changes in left ventricular diastolic pressure. Abnormal or delayed closure of the mitral valve suggests an elevated left ventricular diastolic pressure and abnormal left ventricular performance (Fig. 5-35A). This finding can be added to other M-mode echocardiographic measurements to judge the overall status of the left ventricle.[366] Two-dimensional echocardiography, of course, can indicate the motion of individual wall segments, and the fraction of the left ventricle which moves abnormally can be estimated.[370-373]

Complications of Myocardial Infarction

Echocardiography is particularly useful in detecting complications of myocardial infarctions.[400] One of the most common, left ventricular aneurysm, has already been discussed. Another common problem following myocardial infarction is a mural thrombus.[401,402] Two-dimensional echocardiography is proving to be an excellent technique for detecting this complication. Most of these clots occur at the apex and always occur adjacent to akinetic or dyskinetic wall segments (Fig. 5-68).

Ventricular septal aneurysm and ventricular septal rupture have also been described using two-dimensional echocardiography.[403-406] There have been several echocardiographic findings in patients with papillary muscle dysfunction secondary to coronary artery disease. Earlier reports demonstrated the indirect M-mode findings of left ventricular volume overload in these patients.[407] Others have described a flail mitral leaflet and marked prolapse in these individuals.[410] A two-dimensional echocardiographic technique demonstrates incomplete closure of the mitral valve in the apical four-chamber view in patients with papillary muscle dysfunction (Fig. 5-68).[408] These patients also frequently have scarred, echo-dense papillary muscles. Right ventricular infarction has also been recognized with two-dimensional echocardiography,[409] which displays a dilated right ventricle and abnormal motion of the right ventricular free wall.

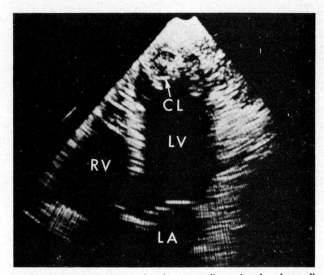

FIGURE 5-68 Apical four-chamber two-dimensional echocardiogram of a patient with an apical clot (CL). LV = left ventricle; RV = right ventricle; LA = left atrium. (From Feigenbaum, H.: Echocardiography. 3rd ed., Philadelphia, Lea & Febiger, 1981.)

Ultrasonic Examination of the Coronary Arteries

The principal value of echocardiography in patients with ischemic heart disease is determining the *consequences* of coronary obstruction, while the location of obstructions in the coronary arteries is predicted indirectly by assessing the motion of various segments of the left ventricle.[411,412] For example, abnormal motion of the interventricular septum suggests an obstruction of the proximal left anterior descending coronary artery.[412] Obviously, this is *indirect* evidence that is relatively insensitive, since the interventricular septum may move normally despite obstruction of the left anterior descending coronary artery.

Two-dimensional echocardiography can record the left main coronary artery and a small portion of the right coronary artery.[403] Obstructive lesions in the left main coronary artery have been demonstrated by several investigators.[414] Such obstructions are seen as masses of high intensity echoes in the vicinity of the left main coronary artery.[415,416] The echocardiographic technique for making this diagnosis is tedious and requires frame-by-frame analysis of the two-dimensional examination. This particular echocardiographic application has not achieved widespread acceptance, and its proper role in the management of patients has not been defined.

CARDIOMYOPATHIES
(See also Chapter 41)

Hypertrophic Obstructive Cardiomyopathy (HOCM)

Echocardiography is an important diagnostic tool in patients with HOCM and has enriched our understanding of this abnormality. The first echocardiographic abnormality to be noted was systolic anterior motion of the mitral valve (termed "SAM") (Fig. 5–69).[136,419–422] which appeared to be related to and was correlated with the presence of obstruction to left ventricular outflow.[104,423] The shorter the distance between the septum and the leaflet and the longer the duration of apposition between these two structures, the greater the degree of obstruction. This echocardiographic finding not only provided another diagnostic sign of HOCM but also demonstrated the critical importance of involvement of the mitral valve apparatus in the obstruction.[424] More recently SAM has been noted in a variety of patients, some of whom had no evidence of left ventricular hypertrophy[2,425–429]; it has been observed in patients with anemia and hypovolemia as well as in those with a hyperdynamic left ventricle.[427] It is possible that SAM is a nonspecific sign that occurs whenever the left ventricular systolic volume is reduced, either because of hypertrophy, as in HOCM, or in the presence of a hyperdynamic state.[429,430]

A second echocardiographic finding in patients with HOCM is midsystolic closure of the aortic valve (Fig. 5–36).[104–106] However, as noted earlier (p. 108), this sign is not specific for HOCM and is also present in patients with discrete subaortic stenosis. While not sensitive, this finding, when present, usually indicates a significant amount of obstruction.

Hypertrophy of the septum with abnormal organization of myocardial cells may be on e of the basic abnormalities of HOCM,[431,432] and key echocardiographic findings are disproportionate hypertrophy of the septum in relation to the posterior wall of the left ventricle, so that the ratio of thickness of septum to free wall exceeds 1.3 (Fig. 5–69),[433–435] and reduced motion of the hypertrophied septum.[436,437] It has also been shown that asymmetrical septal hypertrophy (ASH) is transmitted as an autosomal dominant trait and that there are patients with asymmetrical septal hypertrophy who do not show SAM and therefore do not have obstruction to left ventricular outflow (Fig. 5–70).[431,433,438,439] While the concept of recognizing ASH with or without obstruction to left ventricular outflow by echocardiography is an important one, there are limitations to its

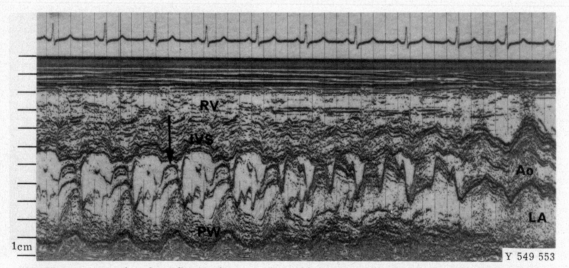

FIGURE 5–69   M-mode echocardiogram from a patient with hypertrophic subaortic stenosis demonstrating systolic anterior motion (arrow) of the mitral valve. RV = right ventricle, IVS = interventricular septum, PW = posterior left ventricular wall, Ao = aorta, LA = left atrium. (From Chang, S.: M-mode Echocardiographic Technique and Pattern Recognition. Philadelphia, Lea and Febiger, 1976.)

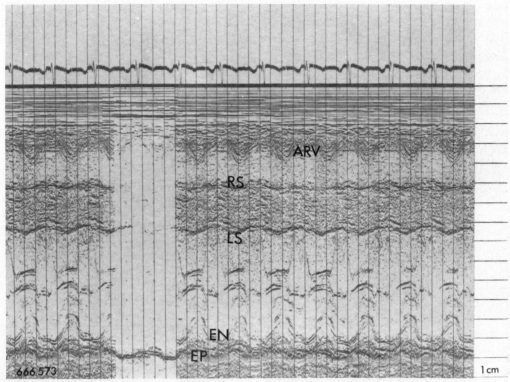

FIGURE 5–70 Echocardiogram from a patient with asymmetrical septal hypertrophy but no evidence of outflow obstruction. The distance between the right (RS) and left (LS) septal echoes is considerably greater than is the thickness of the posterior left ventricular myocardium between the endocardial (EN) and epicardial (EP) echoes.

echocardiographic diagnosis. First, the thickness of the septum may be difficult to measure echocardiographically; in Figure 5–69 the left side of the septum is clearly identified, but the right side is not as distinct and septal thickness cannot always be measured precisely. Second, it must be appreciated that ASH is not pathognomonic for HOCM and related myopathies[440,441] and can occur in a variety of other disease states (including right ventricular hypertrophy and coronary artery disease[440,442] and even in patients on chronic hemodialysis[443]) in a form which is indistinguishable echocardiographically from genetically determined ASH. In addition, some patients with HOCM may have concentric rather than asymmetrical hypertrophy, in which the septal and posterior left ventricular walls are equal in thickness.

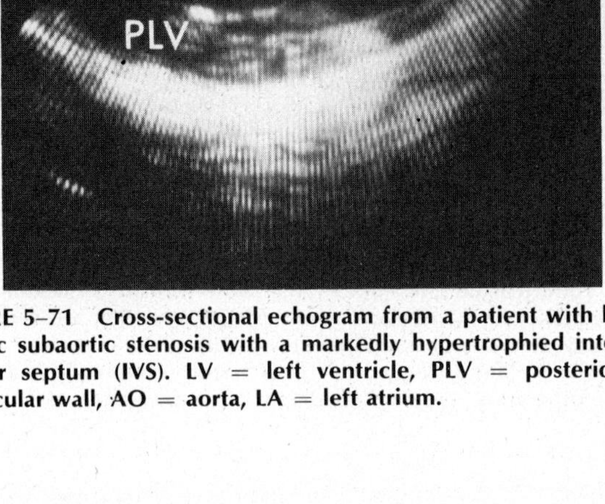

Two-dimensional echocardiography provides additional information by indicating the shape and location of the hypertrophied septum in patients with known or suspected HOCM (Fig. 5–71).[444–448] This technique can also be used to assess the effectiveness of myotomy and myectomy.[449] An intriguing but as yet unconfirmed observation is that the echoes from the diseased septum in HOCM are denser than those from the free posterior wall.

Congestive (Dilated) Cardiomyopathy

The echocardiogram characteristically reveals a dilated, poorly contracting left ventricle in patients with congestive cardiomyopathy (Fig. 5–72).[450,451] Signs of reduced cardiac output include a poorly moving aorta, reduced opening of the mitral valve, and slow closure of the aortic valve. The left atrium is dilated, and the abnormal closure of the mitral valve indicative of elevated left ventricular diastolic pressure is frequently noted. It must be appreciated that these findings are nonspecific and may occur in patients with coronary artery disease. However, at least one portion of the left ventricle, usually the posterior wall, contin-

FIGURE 5–71 Cross-sectional echogram from a patient with hypertrophic subaortic stenosis with a markedly hypertrophied interventricular septum (IVS). LV = left ventricle, PLV = posterior left ventricular wall, AO = aorta, LA = left atrium.

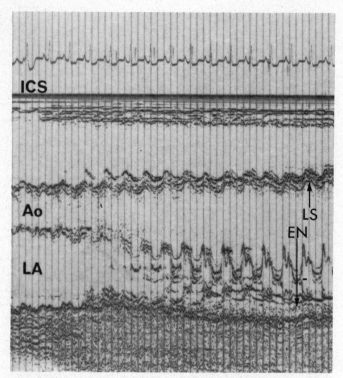

FIGURE 5–72 M-mode scan from a patient with congestive cardio-myopathy. The left atrium (LA) and left ventricle are markedly dilated. The motion of the left septum (LS) is reduced, and the posterior left ventricular endocardial (EN) motion is virtually absent. Motion of the aortic root (Ao) is diminished, and there is abnormal closure of the mitral valve.

ues to exhibit normal motion in most, though not all, patients with severe coronary artery disease.[451] In patients with cardiomyopathy the impairment of left ventricular wall motion is diffuse and includes the posterior wall. If mitral regurgitation develops in patients with cardiomyopathy, septal motion may increase slightly in keeping with the left ventricular volume overload (Fig. 5–72), although this increase in septal motion is certainly not as striking as that which occurs in primary mitral valve disease with secondary myocardial failure.

Restrictive (Infiltrative) Cardiomyopathy

The principal echocardiographic findings in patients with infiltrative cardiomyopathy are reduced wall motion and thickening of the left ventricular wall without dilatation[452,453]; these changes are usually uniform throughout the ventricle. Obviously, these findings are not specific for infiltrative cardiomyopathy and, like those obtained by means of electrocardiography, chest roentgenography, hemodynamics, and angiocardiography, must be interpreted in terms of the total clinical setting. There has been a fair amount of echocardiographic experience in examining patients with amyloid heart disease (Fig. 5–73).[454,455] Although the echocardiographic findings are usually nonspecific and show left ventricular hypertrophy, there are also frequently more specific findings in that the valves may be uniformly thickened in addition to the hypertrophy of the ventricular walls. The interatrial septum may

also be unusually thick, and one may note a peculiar speckled appearance of the myocardium, reflecting localized variations in echo density.

PERICARDIAL DISEASE
(See also Chapter 43)

Pericardial Effusion

The theory underlying the use of ultrasound in the recognition of pericardial effusion is relatively simple; since the acoustical properties of fluid differ significantly from those of cardiac muscle, the effusion surrounding the heart is less echo-producing than is the myocardium. Accordingly, the detection of effusion was one of the first and has remained one of the most useful applications of echocardiography.[456,457] Figure 5–33 shows the echocardiographic appearance of a relatively small pericardial effusion in a patient with left ventricular hypertrophy. There is a clear space between the posterior left ventricular epicar-

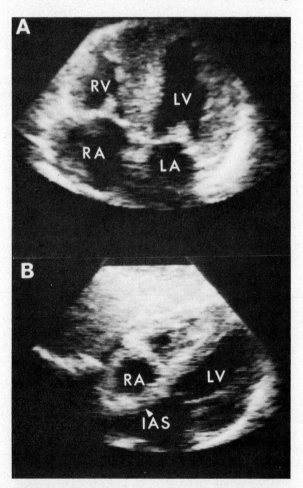

FIGURE 5–73 Four-chamber (A) and subcostal (B) two-dimensional echocardiograms of a patient with hereditary amyloidosis. The four-chamber view demonstrates markedly hypertrophied cardiac walls, especially the interventricular septum and free wall of the right ventricle. The tricuspid and mitral valve leaflets are also thickened. The left ventricle (LV) and right ventricle (RV) cavities are small. The subcostal examination demonstrates a thickened interatrial septum (IAS). RA = right atrium; LA = left atrium. (From Feigenbaum, H.: Echocardiography. 3rd ed. Philadelphia, Lea & Febiger, 1981.)

dial echo and the surrounding pericardium, and on close inspection there is also a small echo-free space between the anterior wall of the right ventricle and the chest wall. This figure demonstrates the sensitivity of echocardiography in detecting a small amount (as little as 20 ml) of pericardial fluid,[458] an amount which would easily be missed by other techniques.

A slightly larger quantity of fluid is apparent on the echogram shown in Figure 5–38. In this patient with mitral stenosis, a relatively echo-free space between the posterior wall of the left ventricle and the surrounding pericardium is present. This tracing points out that the pericardial effusion is not totally echo-free, but if the gain is increased sufficiently, this space can seemingly be obliterated. In fact, in Figure 5–38, the effusion is really apparent only when the gain setting is low enough for a fine differentiation between epicardial and pericardial echoes. On the right-hand portion of the tracing, where the gain was high enough for the myocardium to be imaged, a small effusion behind the left ventricle cannot be appreciated. Figure 5–38 also illustrates that an anterior pericardial effusion cannot be imaged in a large percentage of patients with pericardial effusion. It is possible that if the gain setting in the field near the transducer had been reduced, a small amount of effusion might have been detected. However, it is common for small- to moderate-sized effusions to be imaged only posteriorly.

Figure 5–74 is an echogram from a patient with a large pericardial effusion; although there is a potential space behind the left atrium, it rarely fills with pericardial fluid. When it does,[459,460] the quantity is considerably less than that behind the posterior wall of the left ventricle. There is a large echo-free space anteriorly, and during much of the cardiac cycle, the anterior and posterior cardiac walls move in the same direction, rather than in opposite directions, and the amplitude of motion of the anterior wall of the right ventricle is excessive. This type of cardiac motion has been referred to as a "swinging heart"[461,462]; as would be expected, the motion of all the cardiac structures is distorted by this excessive cardiac displacement, and any di-

agnosis based on this pattern of motion can be misleading. False-positive findings of prolapse of the mitral valve, of systolic anterior motion of the mitral valve, and of abnormal septal motion have all been reported in such patients.[463]

When the motion of the heart within the pericardial effusion is increased markedly and, in particular, when this is accompanied by tachycardia, the heart may not have returned to its previous position by the time the next cardiac cycle commences. Figure 5–75A demonstrates an echogram in such a patient; with each depolarization the heart is in a slightly different position, and the electrocardiographic QRS complex also varies[461,464] with alternating heights of R waves on the electrocardiogram, i.e., electrical alternans. When, in the same patient, the cardiac motion becomes regular, as reflected in the echogram in Figure 5–75B, electrical alternation ceases. Parenthetically it should be pointed out that the manner in which echocardiography helped to explain the mechanism for electrical alternans in patients with pericardial effusion is an excellent example of how this technique has elucidated cardiac physiological and pathophysiological phenomena.

Figure 5–74 also illustrates some of the difficulties inherent in attempting to measure the quantity of fluid by determining the separation between epicardial and pericardial echoes.[458] This is not an accurate technique, because this distance is a function of the direction of the transducer; for example, when the ultrasonic beam is directed toward the cardiac apex, the posterior echo-free space behind the left ventricle will be transected at an angle, and its thickness will be overestimated in comparison to the anterior space on M-mode echocardiography.[465,466] However, the quantity of fluid can be estimated as small (Fig. 5–33), moderate (Fig. 5–38), or large (Fig. 5–74).

Although some pericardial fluids are more echo-producing than others, the acoustic characteristics of fluid have not been shown to be of value in differential diagnosis. However, it has been the experience of most echocardiographers that large effusions that produce excessive cardiac motion, as illustrated in Figures 5–74 and 5–75, are often neoplastic in origin.[461]

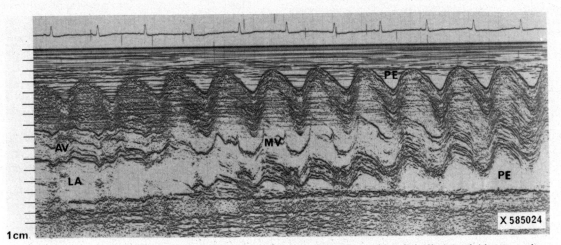

FIGURE 5–74 M-mode echocardiographic scan of a patient with a large pericardial effusion. Fluid (PE) can be seen both anteriorly and posteriorly. The entire heart is moving posteriorly during ventricular systole, producing distortion of all the echoes, including those from the mitral valve (MV). AV = aortic valve, LA = left atrium. (From Bonner, A. J., et al.: An unusual precordial pulse and sound associated with large pericardial effusion. Chest 68:829, 1975.)

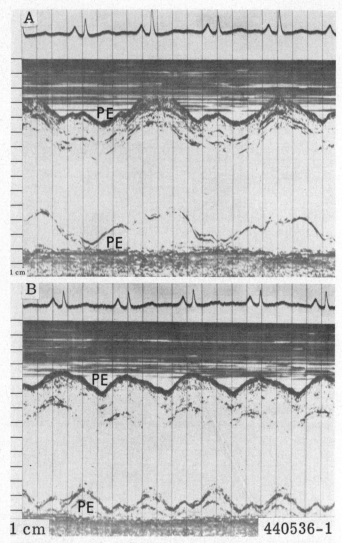

FIGURE 5–75 Echocardiograms from a patient with massive pericardial effusion (PE). *A*, Anterior right ventricular echo (ARV) and posterior left ventricular epicardial echoes move essentially in similar directions. The position of the heart differs slightly with each cardiac cycle. The corresponding electrocardiogram shows electrical alternation. Upon removal of some of the pericardial fluid (*B*), cardiac excursions are synchronous with each electrical depolarization, and electrical alternation is no longer present. (From Feigenbaum, H.: Echocardiography, 2nd ed. Philadelphia, Lea and Febiger, 1976.)

Although the diagnosis of pericardial effusion is one of the most common and important uses of echocardiography, it must be emphasized that there are technical difficulties associated with the application of this (as of every other) echocardiographic technique. Even when proper techniques are used, confusing situations can arise. For example, a retrocardiac pleural effusion can mimic a posterior pericardial effusion. However, the fact that there is usually significantly less pericardial effusion behind the left atrium than behind the ventricle can be a helpful sign. While a pleural effusion may also be less behind the left atrium, it decreases at the atrioventricular junction abruptly rather than gradually, as is the case with pericardial effusion; also, pleural effusions are not usually apparent anteriorly. Positioning the patient so that the pleural fluid no longer collects behind the heart will be helpful except where it is loculated.[467,468] A giant left atrium may produce an echo-free space behind the left ventricular wall and give the appearance of a large posterior pericardial effusion,[469] and even a retrograde hiatal hernia can present a confusing echogram.[470]

Although M-mode echocardiography is usually sufficient for the echocardiographic diagnosis of pericardial effusion, two-dimensional echocardiography also plays a role in this diagnosis. The two-dimensional approach is particularly helpful in patients with loculated effusions.[471] If there are adhesions to the point that the fluid is not evenly distributed within the pericardial cavity, then the two-dimensional approach will be superior to the M-mode examination, which might even be misleading. It is not surprising that two-dimensional echocardiography is more accurate in attempting to quantitate the degree of pericardial effusion, since this examination can record all of the fluid surrounding the heart (Fig. 5–76). The two-dimensional approach also can be helpful in distinguishing pleural from pericardial effusion. By identifying the descending aorta one can distinguish pericardial effusion, which separates the aorta from the heart, from pleural effusion, which collects posterior to the descending aorta.[472] Metastases to the pericardium have been detected with two-dimensional echocardiography as well.[473]

Once the diagnosis of pericardial effusion has been established, a number of echocardiographic criteria for the detection of cardiac tamponade have been suggested.[474-479]

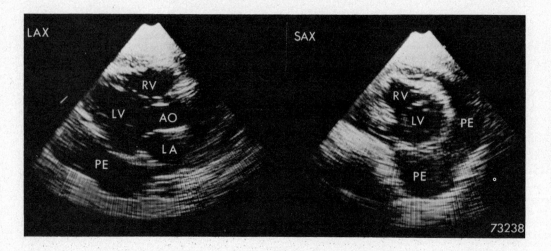

FIGURE 5–76 Long-axis (LAX) and short-axis (SAX) two-dimensional echocardiograms of a patient with a large pericardial effusion. The pericardial effusion (PE) can be seen accumulating posteriorly and laterally. RV = right ventricle; LV = left ventricle; AO = aorta; LA = left atrium. (From Feigenbaum, H.: Echocardiography. 3rd ed. Philadelphia, Lea & Febiger, 1981.)

The newest and possibly most reliable echocardiographic finding with tamponade is compression of the right ventricular free wall in early diastole. This finding is noted by a posterior displacement of the anterior free wall on the M-mode echocardiogram[477,478] (Fig. 5–77). The free wall then moves anteriorly following atrial systole. This observation has been confirmed with two-dimensional echocardiography by noting a collapse of the right ventricular free wall on the two-dimensional examination[478] (Fig. 5–78). Another study has noted a collapse of the right atrial free wall on the two-dimensional four-chamber view.[479] This right atrial sign is probably comparable to the right ventricular free wall collapse with tamponade. Both of these signs appear to be very sensitive for hemodynamic impairment secondary to the tamponade. The finding may antedate the clinical signs of tamponade. The other echocardiographic signs of tamponade, such as reduction of the size of the right ventricular cavity, flat diastolic motion of the left ventricular wall, and variations in the E to F slope of the mitral valve,[474–476] have not proved to be reliable.

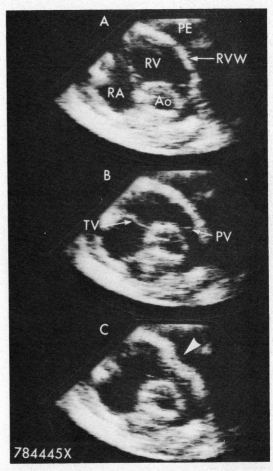

FIGURE 5–78 Parasternal short-axis two-dimensional echocardiograms in a patient with cardiac tamponade. *A* represents end-diastole. At end-systole (*B*), the right ventricle (RV) is smaller but normal in shape. Both the tricuspid valve (TV) and pulmonary valve (PV) are closed. With early diastole (*C*) the tricuspid valve has opened and the shape of the right ventricle has been distorted (large arrowhead) by collapse of the right ventricular wall (RVW). PE = pericardial effusion; RA = right atrium; AO = aorta. (From Armstrong, W.F., Schilt, B.F., Helper, D.J., Dillon, J.C., and Feigenbaum, H.: Diastolic collapse of the right ventricle with cardiac tamponade: An echocardiographic study. Circulation *65*:1491, 1982.)

Constrictive Pericarditis. Echocardiography can be of some value in the diagnosis of a thickened pericardium with constrictive pericarditis.[480–484] However, the reliability of the techniques is limited. Although a thickened pericardium can be detected in many patients,[2,480] particularly those who also have pericardial fluid, this finding by itself does not imply the presence of constriction. The echocardiographic signs of constriction include lack of diastolic motion, i.e., a flat diastolic slope of the posterior left ventricular wall,[2,487] abnormal motion of the interventricular septum,[485–487] and a very short and steep E to F slope of the mitral valve.[2] The echocardiographic signs of constriction are not very sensitive and are certainly not specific; at best they raise the suspicion of this condition.

CARDIAC TUMORS
(See also Chapter 42)

ATRIAL TUMORS. Left atrial myxoma is by far the most common cardiac tumor, and echocardiography has

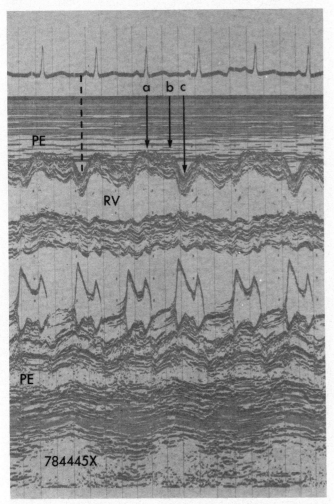

FIGURE 5–77 M-mode echocardiogram of a patient with pericardial effusion and clinical evidence of tamponade. The right ventricular free wall moves gradually posteriorly during systole (from a to b). In early diastole there is an abrupt downward or posterior motion of the right ventricular free wall (c and dashed line). PE = pericardial effusion; RV = right ventricle.

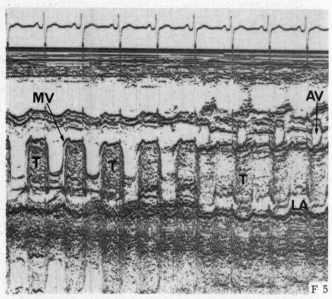

FIGURE 5–79 M-mode scan of a patient with a left atrial myxoma. The tumor echoes (T) can be seen behind the mitral valve (MV) during diastole and almost completely fill the left atrium (LA) during ventricular systole. RV = right ventricle, AV = aortic valve. (From Chang, S.: M-mode Echocardiographic Techniques in Pattern Recognition. Philadelphia, Lea and Febiger, 1976.)

proved to be an extremely important diagnostic technique for its recognition.[488–493] Figure 5–79 is from a patient with such a tumor in whom the clinical diagnosis was mitral stenosis, as is so commonly the case. The echocardiographic feature diagnostic of a left atrial tumor is the "mass" of extraneous echoes posterior to the mitral valve which almost fill the left atrial cavity during systole and which pass partly through the mitral orifice during diastole. The posterior leaflet of the mitral valve is virtually obscured by the echo-producing mass and only a faint trace of the anterior mitral leaflet can be imaged. An interesting echocardiographic sign in establishing the diagnosis of a mobile left atrial tumor is a slight echo-free gap between the anterior leaflet of the mitral valve and the extraneous echoes in early diastole,[489] a gap resulting from more rapid movement of the leaflets than of the tumor. However, it is difficult to distinguish left atrial tumor from thrombus. Although a large vegetation may also mimic a tumor, a vegetation is usually attached to the mitral valve

and a tumor is continuous with the left atrium. Occasionally a dense homogeneous tumor may produce only the echo of a leading edge with relatively few echoes from the body of the tumor (less than those illustrated in Figure 5–79).[2] Two-dimensional echocardiography is proving to be superior in the detection of cardiac masses, especially neoplasms.[494,495] Figure 5–80 demonstrates a two-dimensional echocardiogram of a patient with left atrial myxoma. The spatial orientation inherent in this examination provides additional useful information. The size and shape of the mass are more readily apparent. In addition, one can frequently detect the site of attachment of the mass to the cardiac structure. On rare occasion a two-dimensional echocardiogram might detect a myxoma missed on the M-mode tracing.

Thrombi are other space-occupying structures which have been identified[2,496,497] in the left atrium by means of echocardiography. However, since most of them are located in or near the left atrial appendage, an area which is not well visualized echocardiographically, this is not a sensitive technique for their detection. Two-dimensional echocardiography does improve on the M-mode technique in the detection of left atrial thrombi. However, the echocardiographic detection of clots in this chamber is still not as reliable as detecting masses in other areas of the heart.

Right atrial myxomas, which are not as common as the left atrial variety, have been detected echocardiographically.[489,498–501] Such tumors appear on echocardiograms as extraneous echoes behind the *tricuspid* valve in the right atrium during systole and in the right ventricle during diastole. As on the left side of the heart, a large vegetation involving the tricuspid valve can simulate a right atrial myxoma (Fig. 5–49). Bilateral atrial myxomas have also been detected echocardiographically.[502–504] One must be careful, however, in detecting masses within the right atrium. With the advent of two-dimensional echocardiography it is possible to detect various structures in the right atrium which are possibly normal variants. The so-called Chiari network may produce mobile echoes within the right atrium which may not be pathologic.[505] In addition, the eustachian valve may be prominent and simulate a pathologic mass.[500]

VENTRICULAR TUMORS. Myxomas can occur in the ventricles as well as in the atria[506–511] and have been imaged in both ventricles. When the tumors are mobile, they

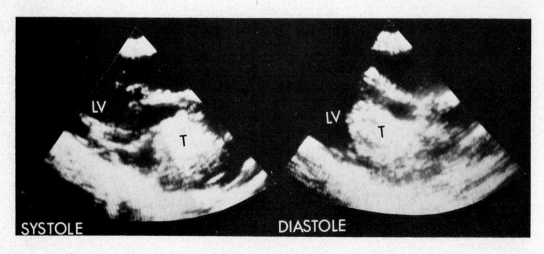

FIGURE 5–80 Long-axis two-dimensional echocardiogram of a patient with a left atrial myxoma. The tumor (*T*) is visible in the left atrium during systole and in the left ventricle (LV) during diastole. (From Feigenbaum, H.: Echocardiography. 3rd ed. Philadelphia, Lea & Febiger, 1981.)

can produce very dramatic echograms on both M-mode and two-dimensional examinations; they move above the mitral valve into the left ventricular outflow tract during systole.[512] Pedunculated right ventricular masses can prolapse into the pulmonary artery[513] or simulate pulmonic stenosis.[514] Rhabdomyomas[515,516] and fibromas[517] can also involve the ventricles and have been imaged successfully.[518]

The most common left ventricular mass is a thrombus. Such a mass usually is associated with an akinetic left ventricular wall[401,402] (Fig. 5–68).

INVASION AND METASTASIS TO THE HEART. Invasion of the walls of the heart[519,520] or compression of the heart[521–523] by neoplasms arising elsewhere has been imaged echocardiographically. Seeding of the pericardium with metastases and the production of pericardial effusion probably represent the most common types of cardiac involvement with malignant disease, and the detection of pericardial effusion has already been described[473] (p. 130). Occasionally, a massively thickened pericardium will be produced.[2] On echocardiogram the position and configuration of the heart may be distorted by a large tumor mass in the mediastinum. Echocardiography has also been shown to be helpful in distinguishing between cystic and solid tumors involving the heart.[524]

DISEASES OF THE AORTA
(See also Chapter 45)

DILATATION AND ANEURYSM. It is possible to examine almost the entire aorta using echocardiography. The root of the aorta and proximal portion of the ascending aorta are usually recorded with both M-mode and two-dimensional echocardiography. The two-dimensional technique utilizing the parasternal long-axis examination permits recording of the descending aorta posterior to the left atrium and left ventricle.[525,526] The suprasternal approach provides visualization of the arch of the aorta and the proximal portion of the descending aorta.[526] The abdominal aorta can then be viewed with the transducer in the subcostal position or over the abdomen itself.[527] In the adult it may still be difficult to record part of the ascending aorta because of the overlying sternum.

Supravalvular aortic stenosis can be detected echocardiographically using either ultrasonic technique.[344–347] As might be expected, dilatation of the aorta, such as occurs in the Marfan syndrome and cystic medial necrosis, is imaged relatively easily[528] (Fig. 5–81). The echocardiographic detection of coarctation of the aorta has already been discussed. Aneurysms of the abdominal aorta are routinely examined ultrasonically.[527]

AORTIC DISSECTION. The M-mode echocardiographic technique used for the recognition of dissection of the aortic root[529–531] is dependent on detecting a double echo in the vicinity of the wall of a dilated aorta; the extraneous echo is produced by the false channel.[532–534] Although these signs are useful in the diagnosis of dissection of the aortic root, it must be recognized that false positives result from double echoes[534,535] produced by the curvature of the sinuses of Valsalva and the artifacts inherent in the beam width in the ultrasonic examination (Fig. 5–47A).

Two-dimensional echocardiography has been used extensively for the detection of aortic dissection.[536,537] In addition

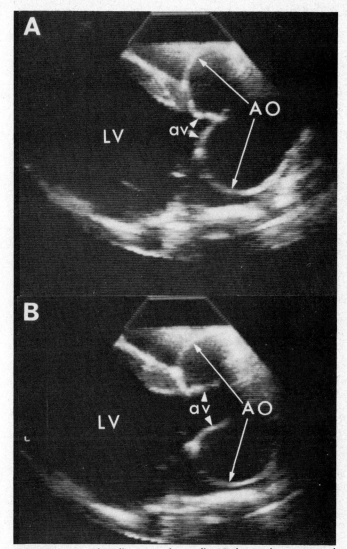

FIGURE 5–81 Diastolic (*A*) and systolic (*B*) long-axis, parasternal two-dimensional echocardiograms of a patient with Marfan syndrome. The aorta (AO) is markedly dilated. Note the marked discrepancy between the aortic valve (av) opening and the size of the aorta. LV = left ventricle. (From Feigenbaum, H.: Echocardiography. 3rd ed. Philadelphia, Lea & Febiger, 1981.)

to the usual transducer position one group of investigators has suggested using the right parasternal position for visualizing the ascending aorta.[538] This technique has been fairly successful in detecting dissection and noticing systolic fluttering of the intimal flap. The suprasternal notch has also been helpful in recording the torn intima, which separates away from the aortic wall.[539,540]

ANEURYSM OF THE SINUS OF VALSALVA. Since echocardiography allows examination of the root of the aorta, two-dimensional echocardiography has been used to image the sinuses of Valsalva, allowing detection of aneurysms of these sinuses. A bulging of the sinus, usually the anterior or right coronary sinus, into the right ventricular outflow tract, has been recorded. With rupture there is discontinuity of the anterior wall of the sinus and mid-systolic closure and coarse fluttering of the right coronary cusp of the aortic valve.[541–543] With rupture of the sinus of Valsalva into the right side of the heart, fluttering of the tricuspid valve as well as premature opening of the pulmonary valve have been reported.[117]

References

1. Carlsen, E. N.: Ultrasound physics for the physician: A brief review. J. Clin. Ultrasound 3:69, 1975.
2. Feigenbaum, H.: Echocardiography. 3rd ed. Philadelphia, Lea and Febiger, 1981.
3. Wells, P. N. T.: Ultrasonics in Clinical Diagnosis. 2nd ed. New York, Churchill Livingstone, 1977.
4. Griffith, J. M., and Henry, W. L.: A sector scanner for real-time two-dimensional echocardiography. Circulation 49:1147, 1974.
5. Eggleton, R. C., Feigenbaum, H., Johnston, K. W., Weyman, A. E., Dillon, J. C., and Chang, S.: Visualization of cardiac dynamics with real-time B-mode ultrasonic scanner. In White, D. (ed.): Ultrasound in Medicine. New York, Plenum Press, 1975, p. 385.
6. Von Ramm, O. T., and Thurstone, F. L.: Cardiac imaging using a phased array ultrasound system. Circulation 53:258, 1976.
7. Helak, J. W., Plappert, T., Muhammad, A., and Reichek, N.: Two dimensional echocardiographic imaging of the left ventricle: Comparison of mechanical and phased array systems in vitro. Am. J. Cardiol. 48:728, 1981.
8. Rushmer, R. F., Baker, D. W., and Stegall, H. F.: Transcutaneous Doppler flow detection as a non-destructive technique. J. Appl. Physiol. 21:554, 1966.
9. Lavenson, G. S., Rich, N. M., and Baugh, J. H.: Value of ultrasonic flow detection in the management of peripheral vascular disease. Am. J. Surg. 120:522, 1970.
10. Sigel, B., Popley, G. L., Boland, J., Wagner, D. K., and Mapp, E. M.: Augmentation of flow sounds in the ultrasonic detection of venous abnormalities. Invest. Radiol. 2:256, 1967.
11. Strandness, D. E., McCutcheon, E. P., and Rushmer, R. F.: Application of a transcutaneous Doppler flow meter in evaluation of occlusive arterial disease. Surg. Gynecol. Obstet. 122:1039, 1966.
12. Light, L. H.: Transcutaneous observation of blood velocity in the ascending aorta in man. Biol. Cardiol. 26:214, 1969.
13. Huntsman, L. L., Gams, E., Johnson, C. C., and Fairbanks, E.: Transcutaneous determination of aortic blood flow velocities in man. Am. Heart J. 89:605, 1975.
14. Sequeira, R. F., Light, L. H., Gross, G., and Raftery, E. B.: Transcutaneous aortovenography. A quantitative evaluation. Br. Heart J. 38:443, 1976.
15. Kolettis, M., Jenkins, B. S., and Webb-Peploe, M. M.: Assessment of left ventricular function by indices derived from aortic flow velocity. Br. Heart J. 38:18, 1976.
16. Colocousis, J. S., Huntsman, L. L., and Curreri, P. W.: Estimation of stroke volume changes by ultrasonic Doppler. Circulation 56:914, 1977.
17. Buchtal, A., Hanson, G. C., and Peisach, A. R.: Transcutaneous aortovenography. Potentially useful technique in management of critically ill patients. Br. Heart J. 38:451, 1976.
18. Joyner, C. R., Jr., Harrison, F. S., Jr., and Gruber, J. W.: Diagnosis of hypertrophic subaortic stenosis with a Doppler velocity flow detector. Ann. Intern. Med. 74:692, 1971.
19. Boughner, D. R., Schuld, R. L., and Persaud, J. A.: Hypertrophic obstructive cardiomyopathy. Assessment by echocardiographic and Doppler ultrasound techniques. Br. Heart J. 37:917, 1975.
20. Thompson, P. D., Mennel, R. G., MacVaugh, H., and Joyner, C. R.: The evaluation of aortic insufficiency in humans with a transcutaneous Doppler velocity probe. Ann. Intern. Med. 72:781, 1970.
21. Boughner, D. R.: Assessment of aortic insufficiency by transcutaneous Doppler ultrasound. Circulation 52:874, 1975.
22. Pearlman, A. S., Stevenson, J. G., and Baker, D. W.: Doppler echo-cardiography: Applications, limitations and future directions. Am. J. Cardiol. 46:1256, 1980.
23. Baker, D. W., Rubenstein, S. A., and Lorch, G. S.: Pulsed Doppler echocardiography: Principles and applications. Am. J. Med. 63:69, 1977.
24. Johnson, S. L., Baker, D. W., Lute, R. A., and Dodge, H. T.: Doppler echocardiography: The localization of cardiac murmurs. Circulation 48:810, 1973.
25. Lorch, G., Rubenstein, S., Baker, D., Dooley, T., and Dodge, H.: Doppler echocardiography. Use of a graphical display system. Circulation 56:576, 1977.
26. Goldberg, S. J., Areias, J. C., Spitaels, S. E. C., and deVilleneuve, V. H.: Use of time interval histographic output from echo-Doppler to detect left-to-right atrial shunts. Circulation 58:147, 1978.
27. Stevenson, G., Kawabori, I., and Brandestini, M.: Color-coded Doppler visualization of flow within ventricular septal defects: Implications for peak pulmonary artery disease. Am. J. Cardiol. 49:944, 1982.
28. Bommer, W. J., and Miller, L.: Real-time two-dimensional color-flow Doppler: Enhanced Doppler flow imaging in the diagnosis of cardiovascular disease. Am. J. Cardiol. 49:944, 1982 (Abstract).
29. Gramiak, R., Shah, P. M., and Kramer, D. H.: Ultrasound cardiography: Contrast studies in anatomy and function. Radiology 92:939, 1969.
30. Feigenbaum, H., Stone, J. M., Lee, D. A., Nasser, W. K., and Chang, S.: Identification of ultrasound echoes from the left ventricle using intracardiac injections of indocyanine green. Circulation 41:615, 1970.
31. Kerber, R. E., Kioschos, J. M., and Lauer, R. M.: Use of an ultrasonic contrast method in the diagnosis of valvular regurgitation and intracardiac shunts. Am. J. Cardiol. 34:722, 1974.
32. Meltzer, R. S., Serruys, P. W., Hugenholtz, P. G., and Roelandt, J.:

Intravenous carbon dioxide as an echocardiographic contrast agent. J. Clin. Ultrasound 9:127, 1981.
33. Gaffney, F. A., Lin, J-C., Peshock, R. M., and Buja, L. M.: Hydrogen peroxide: A new, reliable 2D echocardiographic contrast agent. Am. J. Cardiol. 49:955, 1982.
34. Chang, S., and Feigenbaum, H.: Subxiphoid echocardiography. J. Clin. Ultrasound 1:14, 1973.
35. Weyman, A. E., Peskoe, S. M., Williams, E. S., Dillion, J. C., and Feigenbaum, H.: Detection of left ventricular aneurysms by cross-sectional echocardiography. Circulation 54:936, 1976.
36. Silverman, N. H., and Schiller, N. B.: Apex echocardiography. A two-dimensional technique for evaluating congenital heart disease. Circulation 57:503, 1978.
37. Hickman, H. O., Weyman, A. E., Wann, L. S., Phillips, J. F., Dillion, J. C., Feigenbaum, H., and Marshall, J.: Cross-sectional echocardiography of the cardiac apex. Circulation 56:III-153 (Abstract), 1977.
38. Goldberg, B. B.: Suprasternal ultrasonography. J.A.M.A. 215:245, 1971.
39. Sahn, D. J., Goldberg, S. J., McDonald, G., and Allen, H. D.: Suprasternal notch real-time cross-sectional echocardiography for imaging the pulmonary artery, aortic arch, and decending aorta. Am. J. Cardiol. 39:266, 1977.
40. Snider, A. R., and Silverman, N. H.: Suprasternal notch echocardiography: A two-dimensional technique for evaluating congenital heart disease. Circulation 63:165, 1981.
41. Bansal, R. C., Tajik, A. J., Seward, J. B., and Offord, K. P.: Feasibility of two-dimensional echocardiographic examination in adults. Prospective study of 200 patients. Mayo Clin. Proc. 55:291, 1980.
42. Sahn, D. J., DeMaria, A., Kisslo, J., and Weyman, A.: Recommendations regarding quantitation in M-mode echocardiography: Results of a survey of echocardiographic measurements. Circulation 58:1072, 1978.
43. Henry, W. L., Gardin, J. M., and Ware, J.: Echocardiographic measurements in normal subjects from infancy to old age. Circulation 62:1054, 1980.
44. Tajik, A. J., Seward, J. B., Hagler, D. J., Mair, D. D., and Lee, J. T.: Two-dimensional real-time ultrasonic imaging of the heart and great vessels: Technique image orientation, structure identification, and validation. Mayo Clin. Proc. 53:271, 1978.
45. Henry, W. L., DeMaria, A., Gramiak, R., King, D. L., Kisslo, J. A., Popp, R. L., Sahn, D. J., Schiller, N. B., Tajik, A., Teichholz, L. E., and Weyman, A. E.: Report of the American Society of Echocardiography Nomenclature and Standards in Two-dimensional Echocardiography. Circulation 62:212, 1980.
46. Meltzer, R. S., McGhie, J., and Roelandt, J.: Inferior vena cava echo-cardiography. J. Clin. Ultrasound 10:47, 1982.
47. Popp, R. L., Wolfe, S. B., Hirata, T., and Feigenbaum, H.: Estimation of right and left ventricular size by ultrasound. A study of the echoes from the interventricular septum. Am. J. Cardiol. 24:523, 1969.
48. Diamond, M. A., Dillon, J. C., Haine, C. L., Chang, S., and Feigenbaum, H.: Echocardiographic features of atrial septal defect. Circulation 43:129, 1971.
49. Chestler, E., Jaffe, H. S., Vecht, R., Beck, W., and Schrire, V.: Ultrasound cardiography in single ventricle and the hypoplastic left and right heart syndromes. Circulation 42:123, 1970.
50. Meyer, R. A., and Kaplan, S.: Echocardiography in the diagnosis of hypoplasia of the left or right ventricle in the neonate. Circulation 46:55, 1972.
51. Matsukubo, H., Matsuura, T., Endo, N., Asayama, J., Watanabe, T., Furukawa, K., Kunishige, H., Katsume, H., and Ijichi, H.: Echocardiographic measurement of right ventricular wall thickness. A new application of subxiphoid echocardiography. Circulation 56:278, 1977.
52. Hirata, T., Wolfe, S. B., Popp, R. L., Helmen, C. H., and Feigenbaum, H.: Estimation of left atrial size using ultrasound. Am. Heart J. 78:43, 1969.
53. Yabek, S. M., Isabel-Jones, J., Bhatt, D. R., Nakazawa, M., Marks, R. A., and Jarmakani, J. M.: Echocardiographic determination of left atrial volumes in children with congenital heart disease. Circulation 53:268, 1976.
54. Goldberg, S. J., Allen, H. D., and Sahn, D. J.: In Pediatric and Adolescent Echocardiography. Chicago, Year Book Medical Publishers, 1975, pp. 34, 47, and 117.
55. Lemire, F., Tajik, A. J., and Hagler, D. J.: Asymmetric left atrial enlargement: An echocardiographic observation. Chest 69:779, 1976.
56. Schabelman, S., Schiller, N. B., Silverman, N. H., and Ports, T. A.: Left atrial volume estimation by two-dimensional echocardiography. Cathet. Cardiovasc. Diagn. 7:165, 1981.
57. Gehl, L. G., Mintz, G. S., Kotler, M. N., and Segal, B. L.: Left atrial volume overload in mitral regurgitation: A two dimensional echocardiographic study. Am. J. Cardiol. 49:33, 1982.
58. Dillon, J. C., Weyman, A. E., Feigenbaum, H., Eggleton, R. C., and Johnston, K. W.: Cross-sectional echocardiographic examination of the interatrial septum. Circulation 55:115, 1977.
59. Feigenbaum, H., Popp, R. L., Wolfe, S. B., Troy, B. L., Pombo, J. F., Haine, C. L., and Dodge, H. T.: Ultrasound measurements of the left ventricle: A correlative study with angiography. Arch. Intern. Med. 129:461, 1972.
60. Fortuin, N. J., Hood, W. P., Jr., and Craige, E.: Evaluation of left ventricular function by echocardiography. Circulation 46:26, 1972.
61. Teichholz, L. E., Kreulen, T., Herman, M. V., and Gorlin, R.: Problems in echocardiographic volume determinations: Echocardiographic-angiographic correlations in the presence or absence of asynergy. Am. J. Cardiol. 37:7, 1976.
62. McDonald, I. G., Feigenbaum, H., and Chang, S.: Analysis of left ventricular wall motion by reflected ultrasound: application to assessment of myocardial function. Circulation 46:14, 1972.

63. Quinones, M. A., Gaasch, W. H., and Alexander, J. K.: Echocardiographic assessment of left ventricular function: With special reference to normalized velocities. Circulation 50:42, 1974.

64. Feigenbaum, H.: Echocardiographic examination of the left ventricle. Circulation 51:1, 1975.

65. Massie, B. M., Schiller, N. B., Ratshin, R. A., and Parmley, W. W.: Mitral-septal separation: New echocardiographic index of left ventricular function. Am. J. Cardiol. 39:1008, 1977.

66. Child, J. S., Krivokapich, J., and Perloff, J. K.: Effect of left ventricular size on mitral E point to ventricular septal separation in assessment of cardiac performance. Am. Heart J. 101:797, 1981.

67. Skorton, D. J., McNary, C. A., Child, J. S., Newton, F. C., and Shah, P. M.: Digital image processing of two dimensional echocardiograms: Identification of the endocardium. Am. J. Cardiol. 48:479, 1981.

68. Garcia, E., Gueret, P., Bennett, M., Corday, E., Zwehl, W., Meerbaum, S., Corday, S., Swan, H. J., and Berman, D.: Real time computerization of two-dimensional echocardiography. Am. Heart J. 101:783, 1981.

69. Levy, R., Garcia, E., Zwehl, W., Murphy, F., Corday, S. R., Childs, W., Meerbaum, S., and Corday, E.: Objective echocardiographic quantitation of left ventricular volumes by use of automated computerized edge-detection analysis in canines and humans. Am. J. Cardiol. 49:897, 1982.

70. Schiller, N. B., Acquatella, H., Ports, T. A., Drew, D., Goerke, J., Ringertz, H., Silverman, N. H., Carlsson, E., and Parmley, W. W.: Left ventricular volume from paired biplane two-dimensional echocardiography. Circulation 60:547, 1979.

71. Folland, E. D., Parisi, A. F., Moynihan, P. F., Jones, D. R., Feldman, C. L., and Tow, D. E.: Assessment of left ventricular ejection fraction and volumes by real-time, two-dimensional echocardiography. Circulation 62:760, 1979.

72. Gueret, P., Meerbaum, S., Wyatt, S., Wyatt, H. L., Uchiyama, T., Lang, T. W., and Corday, E.: Two-dimensional echocardiographic quantitation of left ventricular volumes and ejection fraction. Importance of accounting for dyssynergy in short-axis reconstruction models. Circulation 62:1308, 1980.

73. Jacobs, L. E., Hall, J. D., Gubernick, I., Meister, S. G., and Barrett, M. J.: Axial versus lateral resolution: Inherent errors in two-dimensional echocardiography imaging. Am. J. Cardiol. 49:1020, 1982.

74. Kan, G., Visser, C. A., Lie, K. I., and Durrer, D.: Left ventricular volumes and ejection fraction by single plane two-dimensional apex echocardiography. Eur. Heart J. 2:339, 1981.

75. Starling, M. R., Crawford, M. H., Sorensen, S. G., Levi, B., Richards, K. L., and O'Rourke, R. A.: Comparative accuracy of apical biplane cross-sectional echocardiography and gated equilibrium radionuclide angiography for estimating left ventricular size and performance. Circulation 63:1075, 1981.

76. Barrett, M. J., Jacobs, L., Gomberg, J., Horton, L., Wolf, N. M., and Meister, S. G.: Simultaneous contrast imaging of the left ventricle by two-dimensional echocardiography and standard ventriculography. Clin. Cardiol. 5:208, 1982.

77. Quinones, M. A., Waggoner, A. D., Reduto, L. A., Nelson, J. G., Young, J. B., Winters, W. L., Jr., Ribeiro, L. G., and Miller, R. R.: A new, simplified and accurate method for determining ejection fraction with two-dimensional echocardiography. Circulation 64:744, 1981.

78. Watanabe, T., Katsume, H., Matsukubo, H., Furukawa, K., and Ijichi, H.,: Estimation of right ventricular volume with two dimensional echocardiography. Am. J. Cardiol. 49:1946, 1982.

79. Crawford, M. H., White, D. H., and Amon, K. W.: Echocardiographic evaluation of left ventricular size and performance during handgrip and supine and upright bicycle exercise. Circulation 59:1188, 1979.

80. Weiss, J. L., Weisfeldt, M. L., Mason, S. J., Garrison, J. B., Livengood, S. V., and Fortuin, N. J.: Evidence of Frank-Starling effect in man during severe semisupine exercise. Circulation 59:655, 1979.

81. Zwehl, W., Gueret, P., Meerbaum, S., Holt, D., and Corday, E.: Quantitative two dimensional echocardiography during bicycle exercise in normal subjects. Am. J. Cardiol. 47:866, 1981.

82. Feigenbaum, H., Popp, R. L., Chip, J. N., and Haine, C. L.: Left ventricular wall thickness measured by ultrasound. Arch. Intern. Med. 121:391, 1968.

83. Grossman, W., McLaurin, L. P., Moos, S. P., Stefadouros, M. A., and Young, D. T.: Wall thickness and diastolic properties of the left ventricle. Circulation 49:129, 1974.

84. Troy, B. L., Pombo, J., and Rackley, C. E.: Measurement of left ventricular wall thickness and mass by echocardiography. Circulation 45:602, 1972.

85. Devereux, R. B., and Reichek, N.: Echocardiographic determination of left ventricular mass in man. Anatomic validation of the method. Circulation 55:613, 1977.

86. Sasayama, S., Franklin, D., Ross, J., Kemper, W. S., and McKown, D.: Dynamic changes in left ventricular wall thickness and their use in analyzing cardiac function in the conscious dog. A study based on a modified ultrasonic technique. Am. J. Cardiol. 38:870, 1976.

87. Corya, B. C., Rasmussen, S., Feigenbaum, H., Knoebel, S. B., and Black, M. J.: Systolic thickening and thinning of the septum and posterior wall in patients with coronary artery disease, congestive cordiomyopathy, and atrial septal defect. Circulation 55:109, 1977.

88. Joyner, C. R., Dyrda, I., and Reid, M. M.: Behavior of the anterior leaflet of the mitral valve in patients with the Austin-Flint murmur. Clin. Res. 14:251 (Abstract), 1966.

89. Dillon, J. C., Haine, C. L., Chang, S., and Feigenbaum,. H.: Significance of mitral fluttering in patients with aortic insufficiency. Clin. Res. 18:304 (Abstract), 1970.

90. Winsberg, F., Gabor, G. E., and Hernberg, J. G.: Fluttering of the mitral valve in aortic insufficiency. Circulation 41:225 (Abstract), 1970.

91. Pridie, R. B., Beham, R., and Oakley, C. M.: Echocardiography of the mitral valve in aortic valve disease. Br. Heart J. 33:296, 1971.

92. Botvinick, E. H., Schiller, N. B., Wickramasekaran, R., Klausner, S. C., and Getz, E.: Echocardiographic demonstration of early mitral valve closure in severe aortic insufficiency. Its clinical implications. Circulation 51:836, 1975.

93. Mann, T., McLaurin, L., Grossman, W., and Craige, E.: Assessing the hemodynamic severity of acute aortic regurgitation due to infective endocarditis. N. Engl. J. Med. 293:108, 1975.

94. Laniado, S., Yellin, E., Kotler, M., Levy, L., Stadler, J., and Terdiman, R.: A study of the dynamic relations between the mitral valve echogram and phasic mitral flow. Circulation 51:104, 1975.

95. Layton, C., Gent, G., Pridie, R., McDonald, A., and Brigden, W.: Diastolic closure rate of normal mitral valve. Br. Heart J. 35:1066, 1973.

96. DeMaria, A. N., Lies, J. E., King, J. F., Miller, R. R., Amsterdam, E. A., and Mason, D. T.: Echographic assessment of atrial transport, mitral movement, and ventricular performance following electroversion of supraventricular arrhythmias. Circulation 51:273, 1975.

97. Lalani, A. V., and Lee, S. J. K.: Echocardiographic measurement of cardiac output using the mitral valve and aortic root echo. Circulation 54:738, 1976.

98. Rasmussen, S., Corya, B. C., Feigenbaum, H., Black, M. J., Lovelace, D. E., Phillips, J. F., Noble, R. J., and Knoebel, S. B.: Stroke volume calculated from the mitral valve echogram in patients with and without ventricular dyssynergy. Circulation 58:125, 1978.

99. Konecke, L. L., Feigenbaum, H., Chang, S., Corya, B. C., and Fischer, J. C.: Abnormal mitral valve motion in patients with elevated left ventricular diastolic pressures. Circulation 47:989, 1973.

100. Lewis, J. R., Parker, J. O., and Burggraf, G. W.: Mitral valve motion and changes in left ventricular end-diastolic pressures: A correlative study of the PR-AC interval. Am. J. Cardiol. 42:383, 1978.

101. Askenazi, J., Koenigsberg, D. I., Ziegler, J. H., and Lesch, M.: Echocardiographic estimates of pulmonary artery wedge pressure. N. Engl. J. Med. 305:1566, 1981.

102. Chang, S.: M-Mode Echocardiographic Techniques and Pattern Recognition. Philadelphia, Lea and Febiger, 1976.

103. Chiotellis, P., Lees, R., Goldblatt, A., Liberthson, R., and Myers, G.: New criteria for echocardiographic diagnosis of atrial septal defect. Circulation (Suppl. II) 52:134 (Abstract), 1975.

104. Shah, P. M., Gramiak, R., Adelman, A. G., and Wigle, E. D.: Role of echocardiography in diagnostic and hemodynamic assessment of hypertrophic subaortic stenosis. Circulation 44:891, 1971.

105. Feigenbaum, H.: Clinical applications of echocardiography. Progr. Cardiovasc. Dis. 14:531, 1972.

106. Sabbah, H. N., and Stein, P. D.: Mechanism of early systolic closure of the aortic valve in discrete membranous subaortic stenosis. Circulation 65:399, 1982.

107. Davis, R. A., Feigenbaum, H., Chang, S., Konecke, L. L., and Dillon, J. C.: Echocardiographic manifestations of discrete subaortic stenosis. Am. J. Cardiol. 33:277, 1974.

108. Wong, P., Cotter, L., and Gibson, D. G.: Early systolic closure of the aortic valve. Br. Heart J. 44:386, 1980.

109. Pietro, D. A., Parisi, A. F., Harrington, J. J., and Askenazi, J.: Premature opening of the aortic valve: An index of highly advanced aortic regurgitation. J. Clin. Ultrasound 6:170, 1978.

110. Nathan, M. P. R., Arora, R., and Rubenstein, H.: Mid-diastolic aortic valve opening in bacterial endocarditis of aortic valve. Clin. Cardiol. 5:294, 1982.

111. Yeh, H. C., Winsberg, F., and Mercer, E. M.: Echocardiographic aortic valve orifice dimension: Its use in evaluating aortic stenosis and cardiac output. J. Clin. Ultrasound 1:182, 1973.

112. Corya, B. C., Rasmussen, S., Phillips, J. F., and Black, M. J.: Forward stroke volume calculated from aortic valve echograms in normal subjects and patients with mitral regurgitation secondary to left ventricular dysfunction. Am. J. Cardiol. 47:1215, 1981.

113. Green, S. E., and Popp, R. L.: The relationship of pulmonary valve motion to the motion of surrounding cardiac structures: A two-dimensional and dual M-mode echocardiographic study. Circulation 64:107, 1981.

114. Edler, I., Gustafson, A., Karlefors, T., and Christensson, B.: Ultrasound cardiography. Acta Med. Scand. (Suppl.)370:68, 1961.

115. Gramiak, R., Nanda, N. C., and Shah, P. M.: Echocardiographic detection of pulmonary valve. Radiology 102:153, 1972.

116. Weyman, A. E., Dillon, J. C., Feigenbaum, H., and Chang, S.: Echocardiographic patterns of pulmonic valve motion in pulmonic stenosis. Am. J. Cardiol. 34:644, 1974.

117. Wann, L. S., Weyman, A. E., Dillon, J. C., and Feigenbaum, H.: Premature pulmonary valve opening. Circulation 55:128, 1977.

118. Nanda, N. C., Gramiak, R., Robinson, T. I., and Shah, P. M.: Echocardiographic evaluation of pulmonary hypertension. Circulation 50:575, 1974.

119. Weyman, A. E., Dillon, J. C., Feigenbaum, H., and Chang, S.: Echocardiographic patterns of pulmonary valve motion with pulmonary hypertension. Circulation 50:905, 1974.

120. Tahara, M., Tanaka, H., Nakao, S., Yoshimura, H., Sakurai, S., Tei, C., and Kashima, T.: Hemodynamic determinants of pulmonary valve motion during systole in experimental pulmonary hypertension. Circulation 64:1249, 1981.

121. Hirschfeld, S., Meyer, R., Schwartz, D. C., Korfhagen, J., and Kaplan, S.:

Measurement of right and left ventricular systolic time intervals by echocardiography. Circulation *51*:304, 1975.

122. Hirschfeld, S., Meyer, R., Schwartz, D. C., Korfhagen, J., and Kaplan, S.: The echocardiographic assessment of pulmonary artery pressure and pulmonary vascular resistance. Circulation *52*:642, 1975.

123. Mills, P., Amara, I., McLaurin, L. P., and Craige, E.: Noninvasive assessment of pulmonary hypertension from right ventricular isovolumic contraction time. Am. J. Cardiol. *46*:272, 1980.

124. Reeves, W. C., Leaman, D. M., Bounocore, E., Babb, J. D., Dash, H., Schwiter, E. J., Ciotola, T. J., and Hallahan, W.: Detection of tricuspid regurgitation and estimation of central venous pressure by two-dimensional contrast echocardiography of the right superior hepatic vein. Am. Heart J. *102*:374, 1981.

125. Magnin, P. A., Stewart, J. A., Myers, S., vonRamm, O., and Kisslo, J. A.: Combined Doppler and phased-array echocardiographic estimation of cardiac output. Circulation *63*:388, 1981.

126. Elkayam, U., Gardin, J. M., Berkley, R., Hughes, C., and Henry, W. L.: Use of Doppler blood flow velocity measurements to evaluate the response of systemic vascular resistance to vasodilators in patients with congestive heart failure. Am. J. Cardiol. *49*:943, 1982.

127. Edler, I.: Ultrasound cardiogram in mitral valve disease. Acta Chir. Scand. *111*:230, 1956.

128. Edler, I., and Gustafson, A.: Ultrasonic cardiogram in mitral stenosis. Acta Med. Scand. *159*:85, 1957.

129. Joyner, C. R., Reid, J. M., and Bond, J. P.: Reflected ultrasound in the assessment of mitral valve disease. Circulation *27*:506, 1963.

130. Effert, S.: Pre- and post-operative evaluation of mitral stenosis by ultrasound. Am. J. Cardiol. *19*:59, 1967.

131. Joyner, C. R., and Reid, J. M.: Ultrasound cardiogram in the selection of patients for mitral valve surgery. Ann. N.Y. Acad. Sci. *118*:512, 1965.

132. Henry, W. L., Griffith, J. M., Michaelis, L. L., McIntosh, C. L., Morrow, A. G., and Epstein, S. E.: Measurement of mitral orifice area in patients with mitral valve disease by real-time, two-dimensional echocardiography. Circulation *51*:827, 1975.

133. Nichol, P. M., Gilbert, B. W., and Kisslo, J. A.: Two-dimensional echocardiographic assessment of mitral stenosis. Circulation *55*:120, 1977.

134. Wann, L. S., Weyman, A. E., Dillon, J. C., and Feigenbaum, H.: Determination of mitral valve area by cross-sectional echocardiography. Ann. Intern. Med. *88*:337, 1978.

135. Zaky, A., Nasser, W. K., and Feigenbaum, H.: Study of mitral valve action recorded by reflected ultrasound and its application in the diagnosis of mitral stenosis. Circulation *37*:789, 1968.

136. Shah, P. M., Gramiak, R., and Kramer, D. H.: Ultrasound localization of left ventricular outflow obstruction in hypertrophic obstructive cardiomyopathy. Circulation *40*:3, 1969.

137. Duchak, J. M., Jr., Chang, S., and Feigenbaum, H.: The posterior mitral valve echo and the echocardiographic diagnosis of mitral stenosis. Am. J. Cardiol. *29*:628, 1972.

138. Strunk, B. L., London, E. J., Fitzgerald, J., Popp, R. L., and Barry, W. H.: The assessment of mitral stenosis and prosthetic mitral valve obstruction, using the posterior aortic wall echocardiogram. Circulation *55*:885, 1977.

139. Naccarelli, G. V., Moneir, A. M., Watts, L. E., and Zelis, R.: Echocardiographic assessment of mitral stenosis by the left atrial emptying index. Chest *76*:668, 1979.

140. Joyner, C. R., and Reid, J. M.: Application of ultrasound in cardiology and cardiovascular physiology. Progr. Cardiovasc. Dis. *5*:482, 1963.

141. Segal, B. L., Likoff, W., and Kingsley, B.: Echocardiography: Clinical application in mitral regurgitation. Am. J. Cardiol. *19*:50, 1967.

142. Wann, L. S., Feigenbaum, H., Weyman, A. E., and Dillon, J. C.: Detection of rheumatic mitral regurgitation using cross-sectional echocardiography. Am. J. Cardiol. *41*:1258, 1978.

143. Blanchard, D., Diebold, B., Peronneau, P., Foult, J. M., Nee, M., Guermonprez, J. L., and Maurice, P.: Non-invasive diagnosis of mitral regurgitation by Doppler echocardiography. Br. Heart J. *45*:589, 1981.

144. Quinones, M. A., Yung, J. B., Waggoner, A. D., Ostojic, M. C., Ribeiro, L. G. T., and Miller, R. R.: Assessment of pulsed Doppler echocardiography in detection and quantification of aortic and mitral regurgitation. Br. Heart J. *44*:612, 1980.

145. Dillon, J. C., Haine, C. L., Chang, S., and Feigenbaum, H.: Use of echocardiography in patients with prolapsed mitral valve. Am. J. Cardiol. *43*:503, 1971.

146. Kerber, R. E., Isaeff, D. M., and Hancock, E. W.: Echocardiographic patterns in patients with the syndrome of systolic click and late systolic murmur. N. Engl. J. Med. *284*:691, 1971.

147. Shah, P. M., and Gramiak, R.: Echocardiographic recognition of mitral valve prolapse. Circulation (Suppl. III) *42*:45 (Abstract), 1970.

148. Popp, R. L., Brown, O. R., Silverman, J. F., and Harrison, D. C.: Echocardiographic abnormalities in the mitral valve prolapse syndrome. Circulation *49*:428, 1974.

149. DeMaria, A. N., King, J. F., Bogren, H. G., Lies, J. E., and Mason, D. T.: The variable spectrum of echocardiographic manifestations of the mitral valve prolapse syndrome. Circulation *50*:33, 1974.

150. Sahn, D. J., Wood, J., Allen, H. D., Peoples, W., and Goldberg, S. J.: Echocardiographic spectrum of mitral valve motion in children with and without mitral valve prolapse: The nature of false positive diagnosis. Am. J. Cardiol. *39*:422, 1977.

151. Montella, S., Belli, C., Corallo, S., et al.: Variable aspects in mitral valve prolapse. Echocardiographic and phonocardiographic studies of 68 cases. G. Ital. Cardiol. *6*:601, 1976.

152. Markiewicz, W., Stoner, J., London, E., Hunt, S. A., and Popp, R. L.: Mitral valve prolapse in one hundred presumably healthy young females. Circulation *53*:464, 1976.

153. Sahn, D. J., Allen, H. D., Goldberg, S. J., and Friedman, W. F.: Mitral valve prolapse in children. A problem defined by real-time cross-sectional echocardiography. Circulation *53*:651, 1976.

154. Gilbert, B. W., Schatz, R. A., Von Ramm, O. T., Behar, V. S., and Kisslo, J. A.: Mitral valve prolapse. Two-dimensional echocardiographic and angiographic correlation. Circulation *54*:716, 1976.

155. Morganroth, J., Jones, R. H., Chen, C. C., and Naito, M.: Two dimensional echocardiography in mitral, aortic and tricuspid valve prolapse. The clinical problem, cardiac nuclear imaging considerations and a proposed standard for diagnosis. Am. J. Cardiol. *46*:1164, 1980.

156. Chandraratna, P. A. N., and Langevin, E.: Limitations of the echocardiogram in diagnosing valvular vegetations in patients with mitral valve prolapse, Circulation *56*:436, 1977.

157. Mathey, D. G., Decoodt, P. R., Allen, H. N., and Swan, H. J. C.: Abnormal left ventricular contraction pattern in the systolic click-late systolic murmur syndrome. Circulation *56*:311, 1977.

158. D'Cruz, I. A., Shah, S., Hirsch, L. J., and Goldberg, A. N.: Cross-sectional echocardiographic visualization of abnormal systolic motion of the left ventricle in mitral valve prolapse. Cathet. Cardiovasc. Diagn. *7*:35, 1981.

159. Duchak, J. M., Jr., Chang, S., and Feigenbaum, H.: Echocardiographic features of torn chordae tendineae. Am. J. Cardiol. *29*:260 (Abstract), 1972.

160. Sweatman, T., Selzer, A., Kamagaki, M., and Cohn, K.: Echocardiographic diagnosis of mitral regurgitation due to ruptured chordae tendineae. Circulation *46*:580, 1972.

161. Giles, T. D., Burch, G. E., and Martinez, E. C.: Value of exploratory "scanning" in the echocardiographic diagnosis of ruptured chordae tendineae. Circulation *49*:678, 1974.

162. Humphries, W. C., Hammer, W. J., McDonough, M. T., Lemole, G., McCurdy, R. R., and Spann, J. F., Jr.: Echocardiographic equivalents of a flail mitral leaflet. Am. J. Cardiol. *40*:802, 1977.

163. Meyer, J. F., Frank, M. J., Goldberg, S., and Cheng, T. O.: Systolic mitral flutter, an echocardiographic clue to the diagnosis of ruptured chordae tendineae. Am. Heart J. *94*:3, 1977.

164. Mintz, G. S., Kotler, M. N., Segal, B. L., and Parry, W. R.: Two-dimensional echocardiographic recognition of ruptured chordae tendineae. Circulation *57*:244, 1978.

165. Gramiak, R., and Shah, P. M.: Echocardiography of the normal and diseased aortic valve, Radiology *96*:1970.

166. Winsberg, F.: Aortic valve, *In* Gramiak, R., and Waag, R. C. (eds.): Cardiac Ultrasound. St. Louis, The C. V. Mosby Co., 1975, p. 74.

167. Chang, S., Clements, S., and Chang, J.: Aortic stenosis: Echocardiographic cusp separation and surgical description of aortic valve in 22 patients. Am. J. Cardiol. *39*:499, 1977.

168. Taleno, J., Frazin, L., Stephanides, L., Croke, R., Loeb, H., and Gunnar, R.: Echocardiographic index for estimating the severity of aortic stenosis. Circulation *54*:II-233 (Abstract), 1976.

169. Johnson, G. L., Meyer, R. A., Schwartz, D. C., Korfhagen, J., and Kaplan, S.: Echocardiographic evaluation of fixed left ventricular outlet obstruction in children. Circulation *56*:299, 1977.

170. Aziz, K. U., Van Grondelle, A., Paul, M. H., and Muster, A. J.: Echocardiographic assessment of the relation between left ventricular wall and cavity dimensions and peak systolic pressure in children with aortic stenosis. Am. J. Cardiol. *40*:775, 1977.

171. Reichek, N., and Devereux, R. B.: Reliable estimation of peak left ventricular systolic pressure by M-mode echographic-determined end-diastolic relative wall thickness: Identification of severe valvular aortic stenosis in adult patients. Am. Heart J. *103*:202, 1982.

172. Blackwood, R. A., Bloom, K. R., and Williams, C. M.: Aortic stenosis in children. Experience with echocardiographic predictions of severity. Circulation *57*:263, 1978.

173. Weyman, A. E., Feigenbaum, H., Dillon, J. C., and Chang, S.: Cross-sectional echocardiography in assessing the severity of valvular aortic stenosis. Circulation *52*:828, 1975.

174. Weyman, A. E., Feigenbaum, H., Hurwitz, R. A., Girod, D. A., and Dillon, J. C.: Cross-sectional echocardiographic assessment of the severity of aortic stenosis in children. Circulation *55*:773, 1977.

175. DeMaria, A. N., Bommer, J. W., Joye, J., Lee, G., Bouteller, J., and Mason, D. T.: Value and limitations of cross-sectional echocardiography of the aortic valve in the diagnosis and quantification of valvular aortic stenosis. Circulation *62*:304, 1980.

176. Godley, R. W., Green, D., Dillon, J. C., Rogers, E. W., Feigenbaum, H., and Weyman, A. E.: Reliability of two-dimensional echocardiography in assessing the severity of valvular aortic stenosis. Chest *79*:657, 1981.

177. Hatle, L., Angelsen, B. A., and Tromsdal, A.: Non-invasive assessment of aortic stenosis by Doppler ultrasound. Br. Heart J. *43*:284, 1980.

178. Stamm, R. B., and Martin, R. P.: Use of continuous wave Doppler for evaluation of stenotic aortic and mitral valves. Am. J. Cardiol. *49*:943, 1982.

179. Cannon, S. R., Richards, K. L., and Rollwitz, W. T.: Digital Fourier techniques in the diagnosis and quantification of aortic stenosis with pulsed-Doppler echocardiography. J. Clin. Ultrasound *10*:101, 1982.

180. Wray, R. M.: Echocardiographic manifestations of flail aortic valve leaflets in bacterial endocarditis. Circulation 51:832, 1975.

181. Estevez, C. N., Dillon, J. O., Walker, P. D., Feigenbaum, H., and Chang, S.: Echocardiographic manifestations of aortic cusp rupture in a case of myxomatous degeneration of the aortic valve. Chest 69:544, 1976.

182. Rolston, W. A., Hirschfeld, D. S., Emilson, B. B., and Cheitlin, M. D.: Echocardiographic appearance of ruptured aortic cusp. Am. J. Med. 62:133, 1977.

183. Fox, S., Kotler, M. N., Segal, B. L., and Parry, W.: Echocardiographic diagnosis of acute aortic valve endocarditis and its complications. Arch. Intern. Med. 137:85, 1977.

184. Sheikh, M. U., Covarrubias, E. A., Ali, N., Sheikh, N. M., Lee, W. R., and Roberts, W. C.: M-mode echocardiographic observations in active bacterial endocarditis limited to the aortic valve. Am. Heart J. 102:66, 1981.

185. Berger, M. Gallerstein, P. E., Benhuri, P., Balla, R., and Goldberg, E.: Evaluation of aortic valve endocarditis by two-dimensional echocardiography. Chest 80:61, 1981.

186. Martinez, E. C., Burch, G. E., and Giles, T. D.: Echocardiographic diagnosis of vegetative aortic bacterial endocarditis. Am. J. Cardiol. 34:845, 1974.

187. Feizi, O., Symons, C., and Yacoub, M.: Echocardiography of the aortic valve. I. Studies of normal aortic valve, aortic stenosis, aortic regurgitation and mixed aortic valve disease. Br. Heart J. 36:341, 1974.

188. Mardelli, R. J., Morganroth, J., Naito, M., and Chen, C. C.: Cross-sectional echocardiographic detection of aortic valve prolapse. Am. Heart J. 100:295, 1980.

189. Cope, G. D., Kisslo, J. A., Johnson, M. L., and Myers, S.: Diastolic vibration of the interventricular septum in aortic insufficiency. Circulation 51:589, 1975.

190. Friedewald, V. E., Jr., Futral, J. E., Kinard, S. A., and Phillips, B.: Oscillations of the interventricular septum in aortic insufficiency. J. Clin. Ultrasound 2:229 (Abstract), 1974.

191. Ciobanu, M., Abbasi, A. S., Allen, M., Hermer, A., and Spellberg, R.: Pulsed Doppler echocardiography in the diagnosis and estimation of severity of aortic insufficiency. Am. J. Cardiol. 49:339, 1982.

192. Henry, W. L., Bonow, R. O., Borer, J. S., Ware, J. H., Kent, K. M., Redwood, D. R., McIntosh, C. L., Morrow, A. G., and Epstein, S. E.: Observations on the optimum time for operative intervention for aortic regurgitation. I. Evaluation of the results of aortic valve replacement in symptomatic patients. Circulation 61:741, 1980.

193. Paulsen, W., Boughner, D. R., Persaud, J., and Devries, L.: Aortic regurgitation. Detection of left ventricular dysfunction by exercise echocardiography. Br. Heart J. 46:380, 1981.

194. Joyner, C. R., Hey, B. E., Jr., Johnson, J., and Reid, J. M.: Reflected ultrasound in the diagnosis of tricuspid stenosis. Am. J. Cardiol. 19:66, 1967.

195. Guyer, D., Gillam, L., Dinsmore, R., Clark, M. C., Block, P., Palacios, I., and Weyman, A. E.: Detection of tricuspid stenosis by two-dimensional echocardiography. Am. J. Cardiol. 49:1041 (Abstract), 1982.

196. Inoue, D., Furukawa, K., Matsukubo, H., Watanabe, T., and Katsume, H.: Subxiphoid two-dimensional echocardiographic detection of tricuspid valve prolapse. Chest 76:693, 1979.

197. Weyman, A. E., Wann, S., Feigenbaum, H., and Dillon, J. C.: Mechanism of abnormal septal motion in patients with right ventricular volume overload: A cross-sectional echocardiographic study. Circulation 54:179, 1976.

198. Tanaka, H., Tei, C., Nakao, S., Tahara, M., Sakurai, S., Kashima, T., and Kanehisa, T.: Diastolic bulging of the interventricular septum toward the left ventricle. Circulation 62:558, 1980.

199. Waggoner, A. D., Quinones, M. A., Young, J. B., Brandon, T. A., Shah, A. A., Verani, M. S., and Miller, R. R.: Pulsed Doppler echocardiographic detection of right-sided valve regurgitation. Experimental results and clinical significance. Am. J. Cardiol. 47:271, 1981.

200. Lieppe, W., Behar, V. S., Scallion, R., and Kisslo, J. A.: Detection of tricuspid regurgitation with two-dimensional echocardiography and peripheral vein injections. Circulation 57:128, 1978.

201. Wise, N. K., Myers, S., Fraker, T. D., Stewart, J. A., and Kisslo, J. A.: Contrast M-mode ultrasonography of the inferior vena cave. Circulation 63:1100, 1981.

202. Meltzer, R. S., vanHoogenhuyze, D., Serruys, P. W., Haalebos, M. M., Hugenholtz, P. G., and Roelandt, J.: Diagnosis of tricuspid regurgitation by contrast echocardiography. Circulation 63:1093, 1981.

203. Dillon, J. C., Feigenbaum, H., Konecke, L. L., Davis, R. H., and Chang, S.: Echocardiographic manifestations of valvular vegetations. Am. Heart J. 86:698, 1973.

204. Spangler, R. D., Johnson, M. D., Holmes, J. H., and Blount, S. G., Jr.: Echocardiographic demonstration of bacterial vegetations in active infective endocarditis. J. Clin. Ultrasound 1:126, 1973.

205. Sharma, S., Katdare, A. D., Munsi, S. C., and Kinare, S. G.: M-mode echocardiographic detection of pulmonic valve infective endocarditis. Am. Heart J. 102:131, 1981.

206. Andy, J. J., Sheikh, M. U., Ali, N., Barnes, B. O., Fox, L. M., Curry, C. L., and Roberts, W. C.: Echocardiographic observations in opiate addicts with active infective endocarditis. Am. J. Cardiol. 40:17, 1977.

207. Yoshikawa, J., Tanaka, K., Owaki, T., and Kato, H.: Cord-like aortic valve vegetation in bacterial endocarditis. Circulation 53:911, 1976.

208. Roy, P., Tajik, A. J., Giuliani, E. R., Schattenberg, T. T., Gau, G. T., and Frye, R. L.: Spectrum of echocardiographic findings in bacterial endocarditis. Circulation 53:474, 1976.

209. Gilbert, B. W., Haney, R. S., Crawford, F., McClellan, J., Gallis, H. A., Johnson, M. L., and Kisslo, J. A.: Two-dimensional echocardiographic assessment of vegetative endocarditis. Circulation 55:346, 1977.

210. Kisslo, J., Von Ramm, O. T., Haney, R., Jones, R., Juk, S. S., and Behar, V. S.: Echocardiographic evaluation of tricuspid valve endocarditis. An M-mode and two-dimensional study. Am. J. Cardiol. 38:502, 1976.

211. Berger, M., Delfin, L. A., Jelveh, M., and Goldberg, E.: Two-dimensional echocardiographic findings in right-sided infective endocarditis. Circulation 61:855, 1980.

212. Wann, L. S., Dillon, J. C., Weyman, A. E., and Feigenbaum, H.: Echocardiography in bacterial endocarditis. N. Engl. J. Med. 295:135, 1976.

213. Martin, R. P., Meltzer, R. S., Chia, B. L., Stinson, E. B., Rakowski, H., and Popp, R. L.: Clinical utility of two-dimensional echocardiography in infective endocarditis. Am. J. Cardiol. 46:379, 1980.

214. Hickey, A. J., Wolfers, J., and Wilcken, D. E. L.: Reliability and clinical relevance of detection of vegetations by echocardiography in bacterial endocarditis. Br. Heart J. 46:624, 1981.

215. Come, P. C., Isaacs, R. E., and Riley, M. F.: Diagnostic accuracy of M-mode echocardiography in active infective endocarditis and prognostic implications of ultrasound-detectable vegetations. Am. Heart J. 103:839, 1982.

216. Gottlieb, S., Khuddus, S. A., Balooki, H., Dominquez, A. E., and Myerburg, R. J.: Echocardiographic diagnosis or aortic valve vegetations in Candida endocarditis. Circulation 50:826, 1974.

217. Arvan, S., Cagin, N., Levitt, B., et al.: Echocardiographic findings in a patient with Candida endocarditis of the aortic valve. Chest 70:300, 1976.

218. Gomes, J. A., Calderon, J., Lajam, F., et al.: Echocardiographic detection of fungal vegetations in Candida parasilopsis endocarditis. Am. J. Med. 61:273, 1976.

219. Estevez, C. M., and Corya, B. C.: Serial echocardiographic abnormalities in nonbacterial thrombotic endocarditis of the mitral valve. Chest 69:801, 1976.

220. Fitchett, D. H., and Oakley, C. M.: Granulomatous mitral valve obstruction. Br. Heart J.38:112, 1976.

221. Winters, W. L., Gimenez, J. L., and Soloff, L.: Clinical applications of ultrasound in the analysis of prosthetic ball valve function. Am. J. Cardiol. 19:97, 1967.

222. Siggers, D. C., Srivongse, S. A., and Deuchar, D.: Analysis of dynamics of mitral Starr-Edwards valve prosthesis using reflected ultrasound. Br. Heart J. 33:401, 1971.

223. Johnson, M. L., Holmes, J. H., and Paton, B. C.: Echocardiographic determination of mitral disc valve excursion. Circulation 47:1274, 1973.

224. Douglas, J. E., and Williams, G. D.: Echocardiographic evaluation of the Björk-Shiley prosthetic valve. Circulation 50:52, 1974.

225. Chandraratna, P. A. N., Lopez, J. M., Hildner, F. J., Samet, P., Ben-Zvi, J., (with technical assistance of D. Gindlesperger): Diagnosis of Björk-Shiley aortic valve dysfunction by echocardiography. Am. Heart J. 91:318, 1976.

226. Bernal-Ramirez, J. A., and Phillips, J. H.: Echocardiographic study of malfunction of the Björk-Shiley prosthetic heart valve in the mitral position. Am. J. Cardiol. 40:449, 1977.

227. Smith, R. A., Kerber, R. E., and Snyder, J. W.: Noninvasive diagnostic evaluation of the normal Beall mitral prosthesis. Cathet. Cardiovasc. Diagn. 2:289, 1976.

228. Bomba, M. A., Capella, G., Pandolfini, E., and Rossi, P.: Morphology of the echoes of the Lillehei-Kaster prosthesis in aortic and mitral sites. Boll. Soc. Ital. Cardiol. 20:1775, 1975.

229. Bloch, W. N., Jr., Felner, J. M., Wickliffe, C., et al.: Echocardiographic diagnosis of thrombus on a heterograft aortic valve in the mitral position. Chest 70:399, 1976.

230. Bloch, W. N., Felner, J. M., Wickliffe, C., Symbas, P. N., and Schlant, R. C.: Echocardiogram of the porcine aortic bioprosthesis in the mitral position. Am. J. Cardiol. 38:293, 1976.

231. Wann, L. S., Pyhel, H. J., Judson, W. E., Tavel, M. E., and Feigenbaum, H.: Ball variance in a Harken mitral prosthesis. Echocardiographic and phonocardiographic features. Chest 72:785, 1977.

232. Bommer, W., Yoon, D., Grehl, T. M., Mason, D. T., Neumann, A., and DeMaria, A. N.: In vitro and in vivo evaluation of porcine bioprostheses by cross-sectional echocardiography. Am. J. Cardiol. 41:405 (Abstract), 1978.

233. Schapira, J. N., Martin, R. P., Fowles, R. E., Rakowski, H., Stinson, E. B., French, J. W., Shumway, N. E., and Popp, R. L.: Two-dimensional ultrasound sector scanning for assessment of patients with bioprosthetic valves. Am. J. Cardiol. 41:406 (Abstract), 1978.

234. Mintz, G. S., Carlson, E. B., and Kotler, M. N.: Comparison of noninvasive techniques in evaluation of the nontissue cardiac valve prosthesis. Am. J. Cardiol. 49:39, 1982.

235. Ben-Zvi, J., Hildner, F. J., Chandraratna, P. A., and Samet, P.: Thrombosis on Björk-Shiley aortic valve prosthesis: Clinical, arteriographic, echocardiographic, and therapeutic observations in seven cases. Am. J. Cardiol. 34:538, 1974.

236. Raj, M. V. J., Srinivas, V., and Evans, D. W.: Thrombotic jamming of a tricuspid prosthesis. Br. Heart J. 38:1355, 1976.

237. Kawai, N., Segal, B. L., and Linhart, J. W.: Delayed opening of Beall mitral prosthetic valve detected by echocardiography. Chest 67:239, 1975.

238. Oliva, P. B., Johnson, M. L., Pomerantz, M., and Levine, A.: Dysfunction of the Beall mitral prosthesis and its detection by cinefluoroscopy and echocardiography. Am. J. Cardiol. 31:393, 1973.

239. Pfeifer, J., Goldschlager, N., Sweatman, T., Gerbode, E., and Selzer, A.: Malfunction of mitral ball valve prosthesis due to thrombus. Am. J. Cardiol. 29:95, 1972.

240. Srivastava, T. N., Hussain, M., Gray, L. A., Jr., et al.: Echocardiographic diagnosis of a stuck Björk-Shiley aortic valve prosthesis. Chest 70:94, 1976.

241. Berndt, T. B., Goodman, D. J., and Popp, R. L.: Echocardiographic and phonocardiographic confirmation of suspected caged mitral valve malfunction. Chest 70:221, 1976.

242. Mehta, A., Kessler, K. M., Tamer, D., Pefkaros, K., Kessler, R. M., and Myerburg, R. J.: Two-dimensional echographic observations in major detachment of a prosthetic aortic valve. Am. Heart J. 101:231, 1981.

243. Schuchman, H., Feigenbaum, H., Dillon, J. C., and Chang, S.: Intracavitary echoes in patients with mitral prosthetic valves. J. Clin. Ultrasound 3:111, 1975.

244. Alam, M., Goldstein, S., and Lakier, J. B.: Echocardiographic changes in the thickness of porcine valves with time. Chest 79:663, 1981.

245. Assad-Morell, J. L., Tajik, A. J., Anderson, M. W., Tancredi, R. G., Wallace, R. B., and Giuliani, E. R.: Malfunctioning tricuspid valve prosthesis: Clinical phonocardiographic, echocardiographic and surgical findings. Mayo Clin. Proc. 42:443, 1974.

246. Burggraf, G. W., and Craige, E.: Echocardiographic studies of left ventricular wall motion and dimensions after valvular heart surgery. Am. J. Cardiol. 35:473, 1975.

247. Miller, H. C., Gibson, D. G., and Stephens, J. D.: Role of echocardiography and phonocardiography in the diagnosis of mitral paraprosthetic regurgitation with Starr-Edwards prostheses. Br. Heart J. 35:1217, 1973.

248. Miller, H. C., Stephens, J. D., and Gibson, D. G.: Echocardiographic features of mitral Starr-Edwards paraprosthetic regurgitation. Br. Heart J. 35:560, 1973.

249. Yoshikawa, J., Owaki, T., Kato, H., and Tanaka, K.: Abnormal motion of interventricular septum in patients with prosthetic valve. Cardiovasc. Sound Bull. 5:211, 1976.

250. Bourdillon, P. D. V., and Sharratt, G. P.: Malfunction of Björk-Shiley valve prosthesis in tricuspid position. Br. Heart J. 38:1149, 1976.

251. Veyrat, C., Cholot, N, Abitbol, G., and Kalmanson, D.: Non-invasive diagnosis and assessment of aortic valve disease and evaluation of aortic prosthesis function using echo pulsed Doppler velocimetry. Br. Heart J. 43:393, 1980.

252. Belenkie, I., Carr, M., Schlant, R. C., Nutter, D. O., and Symbas, P. N.: Malfunction of a Cutter-Smeloff mitral ball valve prosthesis: Diagnosis by phonocardiography and echocardiography. Am. Heart J. 86:339, 1974.

253. Brodie, B. R., Grossman, W., McLaurin, L., Starek, P. J. K., and Craige, E.: Diagnosis of prosthetic mitral valve malfunction with combined echophonocardiography. Circulation 53:93, 1976.

254. Gibson, T. C., Starek, J. K., Moos, S., and Craige, E.: Echocardiographic and phonocardiographic characteristics of the Lillehei-Kaster mitral valve prosthesis. Circulation 49:434, 1974.

255. Griffiths, B. F., Charles, R., and Coulshed, N.: Echophonocardiography in diagnosis of mitral paravalvular regurgitation with Björk-Shiley prosthetic valve. Br. Heart J. 43:325, 1980.

256. Waggoner, A. D., Quinones, M. A., Young, J. B., Nelson, J. G., Winters, W. L., Jr., Peterson, P. K., and Miller, R. R.: Echo-phonocardiographic evaluation of obstruction of prosthetic mitral valve. Chest 78:60, 1980.

257. Hirschfeld, D. S., and Emilson, B. B.: Echocardiogram in calcified mitral annulus. Am. J. Cardiol. 36:354, 1975.

258. Dashkoff, N., Karacuschansky, M., Come, P. C., and Fortuin, N. J.: Echocardiographic features of mitral annulus calcification. Am. Heart J. 94:585, 1977.

259. Gabor, G. E., Mohr, B. D., Goel, P. C., and Cohen, B.: Echocardiographic and clinical spectrum of mitral annular calcification. Am. J. Cardiol. 38:836, 1976.

260. Curati, W. L., Petitclerc, R., and Winsberg, F.: Ultrasonic features of mitral annulus calcification. A report of 21 cases. Radiology 122:215, 1977.

261. Schott, C. R., Kotler, M. N., Parry, W. R., and Segal B. L.: Mitral annular calcification. Clinical and echocardiographic correlations. Arch. Intern. Med. 137:1143, 1977.

262. D'Cruz, I. A., Cohen, H. C., Prabhu, R. Bisla, V., and Glick, G.: Clinical manifestations of mitral annulus calcification, with emphasis on its echocardiographic features. Am. Heart J. 94:367, 1977.

263. Meltzer, R. S., Martin, R. P., Robbins, B. S., and Popp, R. L.: Mitral annular calcification: Clinical and echocardiographic features. Acta Cardiol. 35:189, 1980.

264. Mellino, M., Salcedo, E. E., Lever, H. M., Vasudevan, G., and Kramer, J. R.,: Echographic-quantified severity of mitral annulus calcification: Prognostic correlation to related hemodynamic, valvular, rhythm and conduction abnormalities. Am. Heart J. 103:222, 1982.

265. Solinger, R., Elbl, F., and Minhas, K.: Deductive echocardiographic analysis in infants with congenital heart disease. Circulation 50:1072, 1974.

266. Meyer, R. A., Schwartz, D. C., Covitz, W., and Kaplan, S.: Echocardiographic assessment of cardiac malposition. Am. J. Cardiol. 33:896, 1974.

267. Foale, R., Stefanini, L., Rickards, A., and Somerville, J.: Left and right ventricular morphology in complex congenital heart disease defined by two dimensional echocardiography. Am. J. Cardiol. 49:93, 1982.

268. Hagler, D. J., Tajik, A. J., Seward, J. B., Edwards, W. D., Mair, D. D., and Ritter, D. G.: Atrioventricular and ventriculoarterial discordance (corrected transposition of the great arteries). Wide-angle two-dimensional echocardiographic assessment of ventricular morphology. Mayo Clin. Proc. 56:591, 1981.

269. Motro, M., Kishon, Y., Shem-Tov, A., and Neufeld, H. N.: Identification of a tricuspid valve in the mitral position in corrected tranposition of the great vessels by cross-sectional echocrdiography. Am. Heart J. 101:229, 1981.

270. Houston, A. V, Gregory, N. L., and Coleman, E. N.: Echocardiographic identification of aorta and main pulmonary artery in complete transposition. Br. Heart J. 40:377, 1978.

271. Henry, W. L., Maron, B. J., and Griffith, J. M.: Cross-sectional echocardiography in the diagnosis of congenital heart disease. Identification of the relation of the ventricles and great arteries. Circulation 56:267, 1977.

272. Nanda, N. C., Gramiak, R., Manning, J., Mahoney, E. B., Lipchik, E. O., and DeWeese, J. A.: Echocardiographic recognition of the congenital bicuspid aortic valve. Circulation 49:870, 1974.

273. Radford, D. J., Bloom, K. R., Izukawa, R., Moes, C. A. F., and Rowe, R. D.: Echocardiographic assessment of bicuspid aortic valves. Circulation 53:80, 1976.

274. Nanda, N. C., and Gramiak, R.: Evaluation of bicuspid aortic valves by two-dimensional echocardiography. Am. J. Cardiol. 41:372 (Abstract), 1978.

275. Brandenburg, R. O., Jr., Tajik, A. J., Edwards, W. D., Reeder, G. S., Shub, C., and Seward, J. B.: Accuracy of two-dimensional echocardiographic diagnosis of bicuspid aortic valve: Echocardiographic-anatomic correlative study in 115 patients. Am. J. Cardiol. 49:1040 (Abstract), 1982.

276. Lundstrom, N. R.: Echocardiography in the diagnosis of congenital mitral stenosis and an evaluation of the results of mitral valvulotomy. Circulation 46:44, 1972.

277. Driscoll, D. J., Gutgesell, H. P., and McNamara, D. G.: Echocardiographic features of congenital mitral stenosis. Am. J. Cardiol. 42:259, 1978.

278. Smallhorn, J., Tommasini, G., Deanfield, J., Doublas, J., Gibson, D., and Macartney, F.: Congenital mitral stenosis. Anatomical and functional assessment by echocardiography. Br. Heart J. 45:527, 1981.

279. Weyman, A. E., Hurwitz, R. A., Girod, D. A., Dillon, J. C., Feigenbaum, H., and Green, D.: Cross-sectional echocardiographic visualization of the stenotic pulmonary valve. Circulation 56:769, 1977.

280. Lundstrom, N. R.: Echocardiography in the diagnosis of Ebstein's anomaly of the tricuspid valve. Circulation 47:597, 1973.

281. Tajik, A. J., Gau, G. T., Giuliani, E. R., Ritter, D. G., and Schattenberg, T. T.: Echocardiogram in Ebstein's anomaly with Wolff-Parkinson-White pre-excitation syndrome, type B. Circulation 47:813, 1973.

282. Yuste, P., Minguez, I., Aza, V., Senor, J., Asin, E., and Martinezaabordiu, C.: Echocardiography in the diagnosis of Ebstein's anomaly. Chest 66:273, 1974.

283. Milner, S., Meyer, R. A., Venables, A. W., Korfhagen, J., and Kaplan, S.: Mitral and tricuspid valve closure in congenital heart disease. Circulation 53:513, 1976.

284. Henry, W.L, Sahn, D. J., Griffith, J. M., Goldberg, S. J., Maron, B. J., McAllister, H. A., Allen, H. D., and Epstein, S. E.: Evaluation of atrioventricular valve morphology in congenital heart disease by real-time cross-sectional echocardiography. Circulation (Suppl. II) 52:120 (Abstract), 1975.

285. Ports, T. A., Silverman, N. H., and Schiller, N. B.: Two-dimensional echocardiographic assessment of Ebstein's anomaly. Circulation 58:336, 1978.

286. Kambe, T., Ichimiya, S., Toguchi, M., Hibi, N., Fukui, Y., Nishimura, K., Sakamoto, N., and Hojo, Y.: Apex and subxiphoid approaches to Ebstein's anomaly using cross-sectional echocardiography. Am. Heart J. 100:53, 1980.

287. Lundstrom, N. R.: Ultrasound cardiographic studies of the mitral valve region in young infants with mitral atresia, mitral stenosis, hypoplasia of the left ventricle and cor triatriatum. Circulation 45:324, 1972.

288. Weyman, A. E., Caldwell, R. L., Hurwitz, R. A., Girod, D. A., Dillon, J. C., Feigenbaum, H., and Green, D.: Cross-sectional echocardiographic characterization of aortic obstruction. I. Supravalvular aortic stenosis and aortic hypoplasia. Circulation 57:491, 1978.

289. Rigby, M. L., Gibson, D. G., Joseph, M. C., Lincoln, J. C. R., Shinebourne, E. A., Shore, D. F., and Anderson, R. H.: Recognition of imperforate atrioventricular valves by two dimensional echocardiography. Br. Heart J. 47:329, 1982.

290. Popp, R. L., Silverman, J. F., French, J. W., Stinson, E. B., and Harrison, D. C.: Echocardiographic findings in discrete subvalvular aortic stenosis. Circulation 49:226, 1974.

291. Weyman, A. E., Feigenbaum, H., Dillon, J. C., Chang, S., Hurwitz, R. A., and Girod, D. A.: Cross-sectional echocardiography in the diagnosis of discrete subaortic stenosis. Am. J. Cardiol. 37:358, 1976.

292. DiSessa, T. G., Hagan, A. D., Isabel-Jones, J. B., Ti, C. C., Mercier, J. C., and Friedman, W. F.: Two-dimensional echocardiographic evaluation of discrete subaortic stenosis from the apical long axis view. Am. Heart J. 101:774, 1981.

293. Wilcox, W. D., Seward, J. B., Hagler, D. J., Mair, D. D., and Tajik, A. J.: Discrete subaortic stenosis. Two-dimensional echocardiographic features with angiographic and surgical correlation. Mayo Clin. Proc. 55:425, 1980.

294. Weyman, A. E., Dillon, J. C., Feigenbaum, H., and Chang, S.: Echocardiographic differentiation of infundibular from valvular pulmonary stenosis. Am. J. Cardiol. 36:21, 1975.

295. Caldwell, R. L., Weyman, A. G., Hurwitz, R. A., Girod, D. A., and Feigenbaum, H.: Right ventricular outflow tract assessment by cross-sectional echocardiography in tetralogy of Fallot. Circulation 59:395, 1979.

296. Chung, K. J., Nanda, N. C., Manning, J. A., and Gramiak, R.,: Echocardiographic findings in tetralogy of Fallot. Am. J. Cardiol. 31:126, 1973.

297. Tajik, A. J., Gau, G. T., Ritter, D. G., and Schattenberg, T. T.: Echocardiogram in tetralogy of Fallot. Chest 64:107, 1973.

298. Morris, D. C., Felner, J. M., Schlant, R. C., and Franch, R. H.: Echocardiographic diagnosis of tetralogy of Fallot. Am. J. Cardiol. 36:908, 1975.

299. Seward, J. B., Tajik, A. J., Hagler, D. J., Giuliani, E. R., Gau, G. T., and Ritter, D. G.: Echocardiogram in common (single) ventricle: Angiographic-anatomic correlation. Am. J. Cardiol. 39:217, 1977.

300. Bini, R. M., Bloom, K. R., Culham, J. A. G., Freedom, R. M., Williams, C. M., and Rowe, R. D.: The reliability and practicality of single crystal echocardiography in the evaluation of single ventricle, angiographic, and pathological correlates. Circulation 57:269, 1978.

301. Felner, J. W., Brewer, D. B., and Franch, R. H.: Echocardiographic manifestations of single ventricle. Am. J. Cardiol. 38:80, 1976.

302. Assad-Morell, J. L., Tajik, A. J., And Giuliani, E. R.: Aneurysm of membranous interventricular septum: Echocardiographic features. Mayo Clin. Proc. 49:164, 1974.

303. Fast, J. H., and Moene, R. J.: Echocardiographic diagnosis of an aneurysm of the membranous ventricular septum. Acta Paediatr. Scand. 66:521, 1977.

304. Canale, J. M., Sahn, D. J. Valdes-Cruz, L. M., Allen, H. D., Goldberg, S. J., and Ovitt, T. W.: Accuracy of two-dimensional echocardiography in the detection of aneurysms of the ventricular septum. Am. Heart J. 101:255, 1981.

305. Cheatham, J. P., Latson, L. A., and Gutgesell, H. P.: Ventricular septal defect in infancy: Detection with two dimensional echocardiography. Am. J. Cardiol. 47:85, 1981.

306. Piot, J. D., Lucet, P., Losay, J., Touchot, A., Petit, J., David, P., Piot, C., and Binet, J. P.: Diagnosis and localization of ventricular septal defects by two-dimensional echocardiography. 50 cases. Arch. Mal. Coeur. 74:1001, 1981.

307. Bierman, F. Z., Fellows, K., and Williams, R. G.: Prospective identification of ventricular septal defects in infancy using subxiphoid two-dimensional echocardiography. Circulation 62:807, 1980.

308. Rigby, M. L., Anderson, R. H., Gibson, D., Jones, O. D. H., Joseph, M. C., and Shinebourne, E. A.: Two dimensional echocardiographic categorisation of the univentricular heart. Br. Heart J. 46:603, 1981.

309. Smallhorn, J. F., Tommasini, G., Anderson, R. H., and Macartney, F. J.: Assessment of atrioventricular septal defects by two dimensional echocardiography. Br. Heart J. 47:109, 1982.

310. Dillon, J. C., Weyman, A. E., Feigenbaum, H., Eggleton, R. C., and Johnston, K. W.: Cross-sectional echocardiographic examination of the interatrial septum. Circulation 55:115, 1977.

311. Lieppe, W., Scallion, R., Behar, V. S., and Kisslo, J. A.: Two-dimensional echocardiographic findings in atrial septal defect. Circulation 56:447, 1977.

312. Nasser, F. N., Tajik, A. J., Seward, J. B., and Hagler, D. J.: Diagnosis of sinus venosus atrial septal defect by two-dimensional echocardiography. Mayo Clin. Proc. 56:568, 1981.

313. Goldberg, S. J., Allen, H. D., and Sahn, D. J.: Echocardiographic detection and management of patent ductus arteriosus in neonates with respiratory distress syndrome: A two-and-one-half year prospective study. J. Clin. Ultrasound 5:161, 1977.

314. Sahn, D. J., Vaucher, Y., Williams, D. E., Allen, H. D., Goldberg, S. J., and Friedman, W. F.: Echocardiographic detection of large left to right shunts and cardiomyopathies in infants and children. Am. J. Cardiol. 38:73, 1976.

315. Baylen, B. G., Meyer, R. A., Kaplan, S., Ringenburg, W. E., and Korfhagen, J.: The critically ill premature infant with patent ductus arteriosus and pulmonary disease—an echocardiographic assessment. J. Pediatr. 86:423, 1975.

316. Goldberg, S. J., Allen, H. D., Sahn, D. J., Friedman, W. F., and Harris, T.: A prospective 2½ year experience with echocardiographic evaluation of prematures with patent ductus arteriosus (PDA) and respiratory distress syndrome (RDS). Am. J. Cardiol. 35:139 (Abstract), 1975.

317. Baylen, B., Meyer, R. A., Korfhagen, J., Benzing, G., Bubb, M. E., and Kaplan, S.: Left ventricular performance in the critically ill premature infant with patent ductus arteriosus and pulmonary disease. Circulation 55:182, 1977.

318. McCann, W. D., Harbold, N. B., and Giuliani, B. R.: The echocardiogram in right ventricular overload. J.A.M.A. 221:1243, 1972.

319. Tajik, A. J.: Echocardiographic pattern of right ventricular diastolic volume overload in children. Circulation 46:36, 1972.

320. Paquet, M., and Gutgesell, H.: Echocardiographic features of total anomalous pulmonary venous connection. Circulation 51:599, 1975.

321. Canedo, M. I., Stefadouros, M. A., Frank, M. J., Moore, H. V., and Cundey, D. W.: Echocardiographic features of cor triatriatum. Am. J. Cardiol. 40:615, 1977.

322. Weindorf, S., Goldberg, H., Goldman, M., and Reitman, M.: Diagnosis of cor triatriatum by two-dimensional echocardiography. J. Clin. Ultrasound 9:97, 1981.

323. Duff, D. F., and Gutgesell, H. P.: The use of saline or blood for ultrasonic detection of a right-to-left intracardiac shunt in the early postoperative patient. Am. Heart J. 94:402, 1977.

324. Seward, J. B., Tajik, A. J., Spangler, J. G., and Ritter, D. G.: Echocardiographic contrast studies: Initial experience. Mayo Clin. Proc. 50:163, 1975.

325. Seward, J. B., Tajik, A. J., Hagler, D. J., and Ritter, D. G.: Peripheral venous contrast echocardiography. Am. J. Cardiol. 39:202, 1977.

326. Valdes-Cruz, L. M., Pieroni, D. R., Roland, A., and Varghese, P. J.: Echocardiographic detection of intracardiac right-to-left shunts following peripheral vein injections. Circulation 54:558, 1976.

327. Funabashi, T., Toshida, H., Nakaya, S., Maeda, T., and Taniguchi, N.: Echocardiographic visualization of ventricular septal defect in infants and assessment of hemodynamic status using a contrast technique. Circulation 64: 1025, 1981.

328. Weyman, A. E., Wann, L. S., Hurwitz, R.A., Dillon, J. C., and Feigenbaum, H.: Negative contrast echocardiography: A new technique for detecting left-to-right shunts. Circulation 56: II-89 (Abstract), 1977.

329. Kronik, G., and Mosslacher, H.: Positive contrast echocardiography in patients with patent foramen ovale and normal right hemodynamics. Am. J. Cardiol. 49:1806, 1982.

330. Bourdillon, P. D., Foale, R. A., and Rickards, A. F.: Identification of atrial septal defects by cross-sectional contrast echocardiography. Br. Heart J. 44:401, 1980.

331. Sahn, D. J., Allen, H. D., George, W., Mason, M., and Goldberg, S. J.: The utility of contrast echocardiographic techniques in the care of critically ill infants with cardiac and pulmonary disease. Circulation 56:959, 1977.

332. Sahn, D. J., Terry, R. W., O'Rourke, R., Leopold, G., and Friedman, W. F.: Multiple crystal echocardiographic evaluation of endocardial cushion defect. Circulation 50:25, 1974.

333. Stevenson, J. G., Kawabori, I., Dooley, T. K., and Guntheroth, W. G.: Diagnosis of ventricular septal defect by pulsed Doppler echocardiography—sensitivity, specificity, limitations. Circulation 58:322, 1978.

334. Stevenson, J. G., Kawabori, I., and Guntheroth, W.G.: Pulsed Doppler echocardiographic diagnosis of patent ductus arteriosus: Sensitivity, specificity, limitations, and technical features. Cathet. Cardiovasc. Diagn. 6:255, 1980.

335. Williams, R. G., and Rudd, M.: Echocardiographic features of endocardial cushion defects. Circulation 49:418, 1974.

336. Komatsu, Y., Nagai, Y., Shibuya, M., Takao, A., and Hirosawa, K.: Echocardiographic analysis of intracardiac anatomy in endocardial cushion defect. Am. Heart J. 91:210, 1976.

337. Yoshikawa, J., Owaki, T., Kato, H., Tomita, Y., and Baba, K.: Echocardiographic diagnosis of endocardial cushion defects. Jpn. Heart J. 16:1, 1975.

338. Beppu, S., Nimura, Y., Nagata, S., Tamai, M., Matsuo, H., Matsumoto, M., Kawashima, Y., Sakakibara, H., and Abe, H.: Diagnosis of endocardial cushion defect with cross-sectional and M-mode scanning of echocardiography. Differentiation from secundum atrial septal defect. Br. Heart J. 38:911, 1976.

339. Hagler, D. J., Tajik, A. J., Seward, J. B., and Ritter, D. G.: Real-time phased-array 80° sector echocardiography: Atrioventricular canal defects. Circulation 56:III-42 (Abstract), 1977.

340. Beppu, S., Nimura, Y., Sakakibara, H., Nagata, S., Park, Y-D., Baba, K., Naito, Y., Ohta, M., Kamiya, T., Koyanagi, H., and Fujita, T.: Mitral cleft in ostium primum atrial septal defect assessed by cross-sectional echocardiography. Circulation 62:1099, 1980.

341. LaCorte, M. A., Fellows, K. E., and Williams, R. G.: Overriding tricuspid valve: Echocardiographic and angiocardiographic features. Am. J. Cardiol. 37:911, 1976.

342. Seward, J. B., Tajik, A. J., Hagler, D. J., and Mair, D. D.: Straddling atrioventricular valve: Diagnostic two-dimensional echocardiographic features. Am. J. Cardiol. 41:354 (Abstract), 1978.

343. Smallhorn, J. F., Tommasini, G., and Macartney, F. J.: Detection and assessment of straddling and overriding atrioventricular valves by two-dimensional echocardiography. Br. Heart J. 46:254, 1981.

344. Usher, B. W., Goulden, D., and Murgo, J. P.: Echocardiographic detection of supravalvular aortic stenosis. Circulation 49:1257, 1974.

345. Bolen, J. L., Popp, R. L., and French, J. W.: Echocardiographic features of supravalvular aortic stenosis. Circulation 52:817, 1975.

346. Nasrallah, A. T., and Nihill, M.: Supravalvular aortic stenosis. Echocardiographic features. Br. Heart J. 37:662, 1975.

347. Weyman, A. E., Feigenbaum, H., Dillon, J. C., Chang, S., Hurwitz, R. A., and Girod, D. A.: Localization of left ventricular outflow obstruction by cross-sectional echocardiography. Am. J. Med. 60:33, 1976.

348. Sahn, D. J., Allen, H. D., McDonald, G., and Goldberg, S. J.: Real-time cross-sectional echocardiographic diagnosis of coarctation of the aorta. A prospective study of echocardiographic-angiographic correlations. Circulation 56:762, 1977.

349. Assad-Morell, J. L., Seward, J. B., Tajik, A. J., Hagler, D. J., Giuliani, E. R., and Ritter, D. G.: Echophonocardiographic and contrast studies in conditions associated with systemic arterial trunk overriding the ventricular septum. Circulation 53:663, 1976.

350. Chandraratna, P. A. N., Bhaduri, U., Littman, B. B., and Hildner, F. J.: Echocardiographic findings in persistent truncus arteriosus in a young adult. Br. Heart J. 36:732, 1974.

351. Chung, K. J., Alexson, C. G., Manning, J. A., and Gramiak, R.: Echocardiography in truncus arteriosus: The value of pulmonic valve detection. Circulation 48:281, 1973.

352. Henry, W. L., Maron, B. J., Griffith, J. M., Redwood, D. R., and Epstein, S. E.: Differential diagnosis of anomalies of the great arteries by real-time, two-dimensional echocardiography. Circulation 51:283, 1975.

353. Houston, A. B., Gregory, N. L., and Coleman, E. N.: Two-dimensional sector scanner echocardiography in cyanotic congenital heart disease. Br. Heart J. 39:1076, 1977.

354. Hagler, D. J., Tajik, A. J., Seward, J. B., Mair, D. D., and Titter, D. G.: Double-outlet right ventricle: Wide-angle two dimensional echocardiographic observations. Circulation 63:419, 1981.

355. Hagler, D. J., Tajik, A. J., Seward, J. B., Mair, D. D., and Ritter, D. G.:

Wide-angle two-dimensional echocardiographic profiles of conotruncal abnormalities. Mayo Clin. Proc. 55:73, 1980.

356. Rice, M. J., Seward, J. B., Hagler, D. J., Mair, D. D., and Tajik, A. J.: Definitive diagnosis of truncus arteriosus by two-dimensional echocardiography. Am. J. Cardiol. 49:1027 (Abstract), 1982.

357. Chestler, E., Jaffe, H. S., Beck, W., and Schrire, V.: Echocardiographic recognition of mitral-semilunar valve discontinuity: An aid to the diagnosis of origin of both great vessels from the right ventricle. Circulation 43:725, 1971.

358. Story, W. E., Felner, J. M., and Schlant, R. C.: Echocardiographic criteria for the diagnosis of mitral-semilunary valve continuity. Am. Heart J. 93:575, 1977.

359. Vaseenon, T., Zakheim, R. M., Park, M. K., et al.: Echocardiographic diagnosis of double-outlet right ventricle. Chest 70:362, 1976.

360. Gramiak, R., Chung, K. J., Nanda, N., and Manning, J.: Echocardiographic diagnosis of transposition of the great vessels. Radiology 106:187, 1973.

361. Sahn, D. J., Terry, R., O'Rourke, R., Leopold, G., and Friedman, W. F.: Multiple crystal cross-sectional echocardiography in the diagnosis of cyanotic congenital heart disease. Circulation 50:230, 1974.

362. King, D. L., Steeg, C. N., and Ellis, K.: Demonstration of transposition of the great arteries by cardiac ultrasonography. Radiology 107:181, 1973.

363. Mortera, C., Hunter, S., and Tynan, M.: Diagnosis of ventriculo-arterial discordance (transposition of the great arteries) by contrast echocardiography. Br. Heart J. 39:844, 1977.

364. Jacobs, J. J., Feigenbaum, H., Corya, B. C., and Phillips, J. F.: Detection of left ventricular asynergy by echocardiography. Circulation 48:263, 1973.

365. Corya, B. C., Feigenbaum, H., Rasmussen, S., and Black, M. J.: Anterior left ventricular wall echoes in coronary artery disease. Linear scanning with a single element transducer. Am. J. Cardiol. 34:652, 1974.

366. Corya, B. C., Rasmussen, S., Knoebel, S. B., and Feigenbaum, H.: Echocardiography in acute myocardial infarction. Am. J. Cardiol. 36:1, 1975.

367. Heikkil, J., and Nieminen, M.: Echoventriculographic detection, localization, and quantification of left ventricular asynergy in acute myocardial infarction. A correlative echo and electrocardiographic study. Br. Heart J. 37:46, 1975.

368. Feigenbaum, H., Corya, B. C., Dillon, J. C., Weyman, A. E., Rasmussen, S., Black, M. J., and Chang, S.: Role of echocardiography in patients with coronary artery disease. Am. J. Cardiol. 37:775, 1976.

369. Parisi, A. F., Moynihan, P. F., Folland, E. D., Strauss, W. E., Sharma, G. V., and Sasahara, A. A.: Echocardiography in acute and remote myocardial infarction. Am. J. Cardiol. 46:1205, 1980.

370. Wyatt, H. L., Meerbaum, S., Heng, M. K., Rit, J., Gueret, P., and Corday, E.: Experimental evaluation of the extent of myocardial dyssynergy and infarct size by two-dimensional echocardiography. Circulation 63:607, 1981.

371. Visser, C. A., Lie, K. I., Kan, G., Meltzer, R., and Durrer, D.: Detection and quantification of acute, isolated myocardial infarction by two dimensional echocardiography. Am. J. Cardiol. 47:1020, 1981.

372. Moynihan, P. F., Parisi, A. F., and Feldman, C. L.: Quantitative detection of regional left ventricular contraction abnormalities by two-dimensional echocardiography. I. Analysis of methods. Circulation 63:752, 1981.

373. Heger, J. J., Weyman, A. E., Wann, L. S., Rogers, E. W., Dillon, J. C., and Feigenbaum, H.: Cross-sectional echocardiographic analysis of the extent of left ventricular asynergy in acute myocardial infarction. Circulation 61:1113, 1980.

374. Horowitz, R. S., and Morganroth, J.: Immediate detection of early high-risk patients with acute myocardial infarction using two-dimensional echocardiographic evaluation of left ventricular regional wall motion abnormalities. Am. Heart J. 103:814, 1982.

375. Daly, K., Monaghan, M., Jackson, G., and Jewitt, D. E.: Cross-sectional echocardiography in the early detection of acute myocardial ischaemia and infarction. Br. Heart J. 45:610, 1981.

376. Widlansky, S., McHenry, P. L., Corya, B. C., and Phillips, J. F.: Coronary angiography, echocardiographic and electrocardiographic studies on a patient with variant angina due to coronary artery spasm. Am. Heart J. 90:631, 1975.

377. Paulsen, W. J., Boughner, D. R., Friesen, A., and Persaud, J. A.: Ventricular response to isometric and isotonic exercise: Echocardiographic assessment. Br. Heart J. 42:738, 1976.

378. Mitamura, H., Ogawa, S., Hori, S., Yamazaki, H., Handa, S., and Nakamura, Y.: Two dimensional echocardiographic analysis of wall motion abnormalities during handgrip exercise in patients with coronary artery disease. Am. J. Cardiol. 48:711, 1981.

379. Wann, L. S., Faris, J. V., Childress, R. H., Dillon, J. C., Weyman, A. E., and Feigenbaum, H.: Exercise cross-sectional echocardiography in ischemic heart disease. Circulation 60:1300, 1979.

380. Amon, K. W., and Crawford, M. H.: Upright congestive echocardiography. J. Clin. Ultrasound 7:373, 1979.

381. Mason, S. J., Weiss, J. L., Weisfeldt, M. L., Garrison, J. B., and Fortuin, N. J.: Exercise echocardiography: Detection of wall motion abnormalities during ischemia. Circulation 59:50, 1979.

382. Morganroth, J., Chen, C. C., David, D., Sawin, H. S., Parrotto, C., and Meixell, L.: Exercise cross-sectional echocardiographic diagnosis of coronary artery disease. Am. J. Cardiol. 47:20, 1981.

383. Maurer, G., and Nanda, N. C.: Two dimensional echocardiographic evaluation of exercise-induced left and right ventricular asynergy: Correlation with thallium scanning. Am. J. Cardiol. 48:720, 1981.

384. Limacher, M. C., Quinones, M. A., Poliner, L. R., Waggoner, A. D., Nelson, J. G., and Miller, R. R.: Detection of coronary artery disease with exercise two-dimensional echocardiography: Description of a clinically applicable and accurate method. Circulation 64:IV-94 (Abstract), 1981.

385. Kerber, R. E., Marcus, M. L., Ehrhard, J., Wilson, R., and Abboud, F. M.: Correlation between echocardiographically demonstrated segmental dyskinesis and regional myocardial perfusion. Circulation 52:1097, 1975.

386. Lieberman, A. N., Weiss, J. L., Jugdutt, B. I., Becker, L. C., Bulkley, P. H., Garrison, J. G., Hutchins, G. M., Kallman, C. A., and Weisfeldt, M. L.: Two-dimensional echocardiography and infarct size: Relationship of regional wall motion and thickening to the extent of myocardial infarction in the dog. Circulation 63:739, 1981.

387. Weyman, A. E., Franklin, T. D., Egenes, K. M., and Green, D.: Correlation between extent of abnormal regional wall motion and myocardial infarct size in chronically infarcted dogs. Circulation 56:III-72 (Abstract), 1977.

388. Gallagher, K. P., Kumada, T., Koziol, J. A., McKown, M. D., Kemper, W. S., and Ross, J.: Significance of regional wall thickening abnormalities relative to transmural myocardial perfusion in anesthetized dogs. Circulation 62:1266, 1980.

389. Weiss, J. L., Bulkley, B. H., Hutchins, G. M., and Mason, S. J.: Two-dimensional echocardiographic recognition of myocardial injury in man: Comparison with postmortem studies. Circulation 63:401, 1981.

390. Rasmussen, S., Corya, B. C., Feigenbaum, H., and Knoebel, S. B.: Detection of myocardial scar tissue by M-mode echocardiography. Circulation 57:230, 1978.

391. Dillon, J. C., Feigenbaum, H., Weyman, A. E., Corya, B. C., Peskoe, S., and Chang, S.: M-mode echocardiography in the evaluation of patients for aneurysmectomy. Circulation 53:657, 1976.

392. Teichholz, L. E., Cohen, M. V., Sonnenblick, B. M., and Gorlin, R.: Study of left ventricular geometry and function by B-scan ultrasonography in patients with and without asynergy. N. Engl. J. Med. 291:1220, 1974.

393. Weyman, A. E., Peskoe, S. M., Williams, E. S., Dillon, J. C., and Feigenbaum, H.: Detection of left ventricular aneurysms by cross-sectional echocardiography. Circulation 54:936, 1976.

394. Rakowski, H., Martin, R. P., Schapira, J. N., Wexler, L., Silverman, J. F., Cipriano, P. R., Guthaner, D. F., and Popp, R. L.: Left ventricular aneurysm: Detection and determination of resectability by two-dimensional ultrasound. Circulation 56:III-153 (Abstract), 1977.

395. Barrett, M. J., Charuzi, Y., and Corday, E.: Ventricular aneurysm: Cross-sectional echocardiographic approach. Am. J. Cardiol. 46:1133, 1980.

396. Barrett, M., Charuzi, Y., Davidson, R. M., Silverberg, R., Heng, M. K., Swan, H. J. C., and Corday, E.: Two-dimensional echo assessment of residual myocardial function in left ventricular aneurysm. Am. J. Cardiol. 41:406 (Abstract), 1978.

397. Gatewood, R. P., Jr., and Nanda, N. C.: Differentiation of left ventricular pseudoaneurysm from true aneurysm with two dimenstional echocardiography. Am. J. Cardiol. 46:869, 1980.

398. Catherwood, E., Mintz, G. S., Kotler, M. N., Parry, W. R., and Segal, B. L.: Two-dimensional echocardiographic recognition of left ventricular pseudoaneurysm. Circulation 62:294, 1980.

399. Corya, B. C., Rasmussen, S., Knoebel, S. B., and Feigenbaum, H.: M-mode echocardiography in evaluating left ventricular function and surgical risk in patients with coronary artery disease. Chest 72:181, 1977.

400. Mintz, G. S., Victor, M. F., Kotler, M. N., Parry, W. R., and Segal, B. L.: Two-dimensional echocardiographic identification of surgically correctable complications of acute myocardial infarction. Circulation 64:91, 1981.

401. Asinger, R. W., Mikell, F. L., Elsperger, J., and Hodges, M.: Incidence of left-ventricular thrombosis after acute transmural myocardial infarction. Serial evaluation by two-dimensional echocardiography. N. Engl. J. Med. 305:297, 1981.

402. Reeder, G. S., Tajik, A. J., and Seward, J. B.: Left ventricular mural thrombus. Two-dimensional echocardiographic diagnosis. Mayo Clin. Proc. 56:82, 1981.

403. Scanlan, J. G., Seward, J. B., and Tajik, A. J.: Visualization of ventricular septal rupture utilizing wide-angle two-dimensional echocardiography. Mayo Clin. Proc. 54:381, 1979.

404. Rogers, E. W., Glassman, R. D., Feigenbaum, H., Weyman, A. E., and Godley, R. W.: Aneurysms of the posterior interventricular septum with postinfarction ventricular septal defect. Echocardiographic identification. Chest 78:741, 1980.

405. Dabrowski, R. C., Troup, P. J., Olinger, G. N., and Wann, L. S.: Ventricular septal rupture detected by cross-sectional echocardiography. Clin. Cardiol. 4:39, 1981.

406. Stephens, J. D., Giles, M. R., and Banim, S. O.: Ruptured postinfarction ventricular septal aneurysm causing chronic congestive cardiac failure. Detection by two-dimensional echocardiography. Br. Heart J. 46:216, 1981.

407. Tallury, V. K., DePasquale, N. P., and Burch, G. E.: The echocardiogram in papillary muscle dysfunction. Am. Heart J. 83:12, 1972.

408. Godley, R. W., Wann, L. S., Rogers, E. W., Feigenbaum, H., and Weyman, A. E.: Incomplete mitral leaflet closure in patients with papillary muscle dysfunction. Circulation 63:565, 1981.

409. D'Arcy, B., and Nanda, N. C.: Two-dimensional echocardiographic features of right ventricular infarction. Circulation 65:167, 1982.

410. Corya, B. C.: Applications of echocardiography in acute myocardial infarction. In Brest, A. N. (ed.): Cardiovascular Clinics. Philadelphia, F. A. Davis Co., 1975, pp. 113–127.

411. Dortimer, A. C., DeJoseph, R. L., Shiroff, R. A., Liedtke, A. J., and Zelis, R.: Distribution of coronary artery disease. Prediction by echocardiography. Circulation 54:724, 1976.

412. Kolibash, A. J., Beaver, B. M., Fulkerson, P. K., Khullar, S., and Leighton,

R. F.: The relationship between abnormal echocardiographic septal motion and myocardial perfusion in patients with significant obstruction of the left anterior descending artery. Circulation 56:780, 1977.

413. Weyman, A. E., Feigenbaum, H., Dillon, J. C., Johnston, K. W., and Eggleton, R. C.: Non-invasive visualization of the left main coronary artery by cross-sectional echocardiography. Circulation 54:169, 1976.

414. Rink, L. D., Feigenbaum, H., Godley, R. W., Weyman, A. E., Dillon, J. C., Phillips, J. F., and Marshall, J. E.: Echocardiographic detection of left main coronary artery obstruction. Circulation 65:719, 1982.

415. Rogers, E. W., Feigenbaum, H., Weyman, A. E., Godley, R. W., Johnston, K. W., and Eggleton, R. C.: Possible detection of atherosclerotic coronary calcification by two-dimensional echocardiography. Circulation 62:1046, 1980.

416. Friedman, M. J., Sahn, D. J., Goldman, S., Eisner, D. R., Gittinger, N. C., Lederman, F. L., Puckette, C. M., and Tiemann, J. J.: High predictive accuracy for detection of left main coronary artery disease by antilog signal processing of two-dimensional echocardiographic images. Am. Heart J. 103:194, 1982.

417. Gould, K. L., Mozersky, D. J., Hokanson, D. E., Baker, D. W., Kennedy, J. W., Sumner, D. S., and Strandness, D. E., Jr.: A noninvasive technic for determining patency of saphenous vein coronary bypass grafts. Circulation 46:595, 1972.

418. Pisko-Dubienski, Z. A., Baird, R. J., and Wilson, D. R.: Noninvasive assessment of aorta-coronary saphenous vein bypass graft patency using directional Doppler. Circulation (Suppl. I) 51:188, 1975.

419. Pridie, R. B., and Oakley, C. M.: Mechanism of mitral regurgitation in hypertrophic obstructive cardiomyopathy. Br. Heart J. 32:203, 1970.

420. Popp, R. L., and Harrison, D. C.: Ultrasound in the diagnosis and evaluation of therapy of idiopathic hypertrophic subaortic stenosis. Circulation 40:905, 1969.

421. King, J. F., DeMaria, A. N., Reis, R. L., Bolton, M. R., Dunn, M. I., and Mason, D. T.: Echocardiographic assessment of idiopathic hypertrophic subaortic stenosis. Chest 64:723, 1973.

422. Shah, P. M., Taylor, R. D., and Wong, M.: Abnormal mitral valve coaptation in hypertrophic obstructive cardiomyopathy: Proposed role in systolic anterior motion of mitral valve. Am. J. Cardiol. 48:258, 1981.

423. Henry, W. L., Clark, C. E., Glancy, D. L., and Epstein, S. E.: Echocardiographic measurement of the left ventricular outflow gradient in idiopathic hypertrophic subaortic stenosis. N. Engl. J. Med. 288:989, 1973.

424. Henry, W. L., Clark, C. E., Griffith, J. M., and Epstein, S. E.: Mechanism of left ventricular outflow obstruction in patients with obstructive asymmetric septal hypertrophy (idiopathic hypertrophic subaortic stenosis). Am. J. Cardiol. 35:337, 1975.

425. Buckley, B. H., and Fortuin, N. J.: Systolic anterior motion of the mitral valve without asymmetric septal hypertrophy. Chest 69:694, 1976.

426. Levisman, J. A.: Systolic anterior motion of the mitral valve due to hypovolemia and anemia. Chest 70:687, 1976.

427. Mintz, G. S., Kotler, M. N., Segal, B. L., and Parry, W. R.: Systolic anterior motion of the mitral valve in the absence of asymmetric septal hypertrophy. Circulation 57:256, 1978.

428. Crawford, M., Groves, B., and Horwitz, L.: Mitral valve systolic anterior motion producing dynamic subaortic stenosis without asymmetric septal hypertrophy. Circulation 56:III-69 (Abstract), 1977.

429. Gardin, J. M., Talano, J. V., Stephanides, L., Fizzano, J., and Lesch, M.: Systolic anterior motion in the absence of asymmetric septal hypertrophy. A buckling phenomenon of the chordae tendineae. Circulation 63:181, 1981.

430. Maron, B. J., Gottdiener, J. S., and Perry, L. W.: Specificity of systolic anterior motion of anterior mitral leaflet for hypertrophic cardiomyopathy. Br. Heart J. 45:206, 1981.

431. Henry, W. L., Clark, C. E., Roberts, W. C., Morrow, A. G., and Epstein, S. E.: Difference in distribution of myocardial abnormalities in patients with obstructive and non-obstructive asymmetric septal hypertrophy (ASH): Echocardiographic and gross anatomic findings. Circulation 50:447, 1974.

432. Henry, W. L., Clark, C. E., and Epstein, S. E.: Asymmetric septal hypertrophy: the unifying link in the IHSS disease spectrum: observations regarding its pathogenesis, pathophysiology, and course. Circulation 47:827, 1973.

433. Abbasi, A. S., MacAlpin, R. N., Eber, L. M., and Pearce, M. L.: Echocardiographic diagnosis of idiopathic hypertrophic cardiomyopathy without outflow obstruction. Circulation 46:897, 1972.

434. Henry, W. L., Clark, C. E., and Epstein, S. E.: Asymmetric septal hypertrophy (ASH). Echocardiographic identification of the pathognomonic anatomic abnormality of IHSS. Circulation 47:225, 1973.

435. Sayaya, J., Longo, M. R., and Schlant, R. C.: Echocardiographic interventricular septal wall motion and thickness: A study in health and disease. Am. Heart J. 87:681, 1974.

436. Cohen, M. V., Cooperman, L. B., and Rosenblum, R.: Regional myocardial function in idiopathic hypertrophic subaortic stenosis: An echocardiographic study. Circulation 52:842, 1975.

437. TenCate, F. J., Hugenholtz, P. G., and Roelandt, J.: Ultrasound study of dynamic behaviour of left ventricle in genetic asymmetric septal hypertrophy. Br. Heart J. 39:627, 1977.

438. Clark, C. E., Henry, W. L., and Epstein, S. E.: Familial prevalence and genetic transmission of idiopathic hypertrophic subaortic stenosis. N. Engl. J. Med. 289:709, 1973.

439. Feizi, O., and Emanuel, R.: Echocardiographic spectrum of hypertrophic cardiomyopathy. Br. Heart J. 37:1286, 1975.

440. Maron, B. J., Savage, D. D., Clark, C. E., Henry, W. L., Vlodaver, Z., Edwards, J. E., and Epstein, S. E.: Prevalence and characteristics of disproportionate ventricular septal thickening in patients with coronary artery disease. Circulation 57:250, 1978.

441. Maron, B. J., Henry, W. L., Roberts, W. C., and Epstein, S. E.: Comparison of echocardiographic and necropsy measurements of ventricular wall thicknesses in patients with and without disproportionate septal thickening. Circulation 55:341, 1977.

442. Henning, H., Roeske, W., Karliner, J., Crawford, M., and O'Rourke, R.: Inferior myocardial infarction (IMI): A common cause of asymmetric septal hypertrophy (ASH). Circulation 54:II-191 (Abstract), 1976.

443. Abbasi, A.S., Slaughter, J. C., and Allen, M. W.: Asymmetric septal hypertrophy in chronic hemodialysis patients. Circulation 54:II-190 (Abstract), 1976.

444. Cohen, M. V., Teichholz, L. E., and Gorlin, R.: B-scan ultrasonography in idiopathic hypertrophic subaortic stenosis. Study of left ventricular outflow tract and mechanism of obstruction. Br. Heart J. 38:595, 1976.

445. Martin, R. P., French, J. W., Pittman, M. M., and Popp, R. L.: Analysis of idiopathic hypertrophic subaortic stenosis by wide angle phased array echocardiography. Circulation 54:II-191 (Abstract), 1976.

446. Tajik, A. J., Seward, J. B., Hagler, D. J., and Mair, D. D.: Experience with real-time two-dimensional sector angiography. Am. J. Cardiol. 41:353 (Abstract), 1978.

447. Maron, B. J., Gottdiener, J. S., Bonow, R. O., and Epstein, S. E.: Hypertrophic cardiomyopathy with unusual locations of left ventricular hypertrophy undetectable by M-mode echocardiography. Identification by wide-angle two-dimensional echocardiography. Circulation 63:409, 1981.

448. Maron, B. J., Gottdiener, J. S., and Epstein, S. E.: Patterns and significance of distribution of left ventricular hypertrophy in hypertrophic cardiomyopathy. A wide angle, two-dimensional echocardiographic study of 125 patients. Am. J. Cardiol. 48:418, 1981.

449. Schapiro, J. N., Stemple, D. R., Martin, R. P., Rakowski, H., Stinson, E. B., and Popp, R. L.: Single and two-dimensional echocardiographic visualization of the effects of septal myectomy in idiopathic hypertrophic subaortic stenosis. Circulation 58:850, 1978.

450. Abbasi, A. S., Chahine, R. A., MacAlpin, R. N., and Kattus, A. A.: Ultrasound in the diagnosis of primary congestive cardiomyopathy. Chest 63:937, 1973.

451. Corya, B. C., Feigenbaum, H., Rasmussen, S., and Black, M. J.: Echocardiographic features of congestive cardiomyopathy compared with normal subjects and patients with coronary artery disease. Circulation 49:1153, 1974.

452. Child, J. S., Levisman, J. A., Abbasi, A. S., and MacAlpin, R. N.: Echocardiographic manifestation of infiltrative cardiomyopathy. A report of seven cases due to amyloid. Chest 70:726, 1976.

453. Borer, J. S., Henry, W. L., and Epstein, S. E.: Echocardiographic observations in patients with systemic infiltrative disease involving the heart. Am. J. Cardiol. 39:184, 1977.

454. Siqueira-Filho, A. G., Cunha, C. L., Tajik, A. J., Seward, J. B., Schattenberg, T. T., and Giuliani, E. R.: M-mode and two-dimensional echocardiographic features in cardiac amyloidosis. Circulation 63:188, 1981.

455. Nomeir, A. M., and Watts, L. E.: Amyloid heart disease. South Med. J. 74:1412, 1981.

456. Edler, I.: Diagnostic use of ultrasound in heart disease. Acta Med. Scand. 308:32, 1955.

457. Feigenbaum, H., Waldhausen, J. A., and Hyde, L. P.: Ultrasound diagnosis of pericardial effusion. J.A.M.A. 191:107, 1965.

458. Horowitz, M. S., Schultz, C. S., Stinson, E. B., Harrison, D. C., and Popp, R. L.: Sensitivity and specificity of echocardographic diagnosis of pericardial effusion. Circulation 50:239, 1974.

459. Lemire, F., Tajik, A. J., Giuliani, E. R., Gau, G. T., and Schattenberg, T. T.: Further echocardiographic observations in pericardial effusion. Mayo Clin. Proc. 51:13, 1976.

460. Nanda, N. C., Reeves, W., and Gramiak, R.: Echocardiographic demonstration of pericardial effusion behind the left atrium. Clin. Res. 24:232A, 1976.

461. Feigenbaum, H., Zaky, A., and Grabhorn, L.: Cardiac motion in patients with pericardial effusion: a study using ultrasound cardiography. Circulation 34:611, 1966.

462. Krueger, S. K., Zucker, R. P., Dzindzio, B. S., and Forker, A. D.: Swinging heart syndrome with predominant anterior pericardial effusion. J. Clin. Ultrasound 4:113, 1976.

463. Nanda, N. C., Gramiak, R., and Gross, C. M.: Echocardiography of cardiac valves in pericardial effusion. Circulation 54:500, 1976.

464. Gabor, G. E., Winsberg, F., and Bloom, H. S.: Electrical and mechanical alternation in pericardial effusion. Chest 59:341, 1971.

465. Prakash, R., Moorthy, K., DelVicario, M., and Aronow, W. S.: Reliability of echocardiography in quantitating pericardial effusion. A prospective study. Clin. Res. 24:236A, 1976.

466. D'Cruz, I., Prabhu, R., Cohen, H. C., and Glick, G.: Potential pitfalls in quantification of pericardial effusions by echocardiography. Br. Heart J. 39:529, 1977.

467. Feigenbaum, H., Zaky, Z., and Waldhausen, J. A.: Use of reflected ultrasound in detecting pericardial effusion. Am. J. Cardiol. 19:84, 1967.

468. Abbasi, A. S., Ellis, N., and Flynn, J. U.: Echocardiographic M-scan technique in the diagnosis of pericardial effusion. J. Clin. Ultrasound 1:300, 1973.

469. Ratshin, R. A., Smith, M. K., and Hood, W. P., Jr.: Possible false-positive diagnosis of pericardial effusion by echocardiography in presence of large left atrium. Chest 65:112, 1974.

470. Popp, R. L., and Harrison, D. C.: Echocardiography. In Weissler, A. M. (ed.): Noninvasive Cardiology. New York, Grune and Stratton, 1974.

471. Martin, R. P., Rakowski, H., French, J., and Popp, R. L.: Localization of pericardial effusion with wide angle phased array echocardiography. Am. J. Cardiol. 42:904, 1978.

472. Haaz, W. S., Mintz, G. S., Kotler, M. N., Parry, W., and Segal, B. L.: Two dimensional echocardiographic recognition of the descending thoracic aorta: Value in differentiating pericardial from pleural effusions. Am. J. Cardiol. 46:739, 1980.

473. Chandraratna, P. A., and Aronow, W. S.: Detection of pericardial metastases by cross-section echocardiography. Circulation 63:197, 1981.

474. D'Cruz, I. A., Cohen, H. C., Prabhu, R., and Glick, G.: Diagnosis of cardiac tamponade by echocardiography: Changes in mitral valve motion and ventricular dimensions: with special reference to paradoxical pulse. Circulation 52:460, 1975.

475. Settle, H. P., Adolph, R. J., Fowler, N. O., Engel, P., Agruss, N. S., and Levenson, N. I.: Echocardiographic study of cardiac tamponade. Circulation 56:951, 1977.

476. Schiller, N. B., and Botvinick, E. H.: Right ventricular compression as a sign of cardiac tamponade. An analysis of echocardiographic ventricular dimensions and their clinical implications. Circulation 56:774, 1977.

477. Shina, S., Yaginuma, T., Kondo, K., Kawai, N., and Hosoda, S.: Echo-cardiographic evaluation of impending cardiac tamponade. J. Cardiogr. 9:555, 1979.

478. Armstrong, W. F., Schilt, B. F., Helper, D. J., Dillon, J. C., and Feigenbaum, H.: Diastolic collapse of the right ventricle with cardiac tamponade: An echocardiographic study. Circulation 65:1491, 1982.

479. Gillam, L. D., Guyer, D., King, M. E., Marshall, J., and Weyman, A. E.: Hydrodynamic compression of the right atrial free wall, a new highly-sensitive echocardiographic sign of cardiac tamponade. Am. J. Cardiol. 49:1010, 1982.

480. Schnittger, I., Bowden, R. E., Abrams, J., and Popp, R. L.: Echo-cardiography: Pericardial thickening and constrictive pericarditis. Am. J. Cardiol. 42:388, 1978.

481. Lewis, B. S.: Real time two dimensional echocardiography in constrictive pericarditis. Am. J. Cardiol. 49:1789, 1982.

482. Pandian, N., Skorton, D., Kieso, R., Pai, A. L., and Kerber, R.: Characterization of left ventricular diastolic filling in constrictive pericarditis by two-dimensional echocardiography: Experimental and clinical studies. Circulation 64:IV-204, 1981.

483. Elkayam, U., Kotler, M. N., Segal, B., and Parry, W.: Echocardiographic findings in constrictive pericarditis: A case report. Isr. J. Med. Sci. 12:1308, 1976.

484. Chandraratna, P. A. N., and Imaizumi, T.: Echocardiographic diagnosis of thickened pericardium. Cardiovasc. Med. 3:1279, 1978.

485. Gibson, T. C., Grossman, W., McLaurin, L. P., Moos, S., and Craige, E.: An echocardiographic study of the interventricular system in constrictive pericarditis. Br. Heart J. 38:738, 1976.

486. Pool, P. E., Seagren, S. C., Abbasi, A. S., Gharuzi, Y., and Kraus, R.: Echocardiographic manifestations of constrictive pericarditis: Abnormal septal motion. Chest 68:684, 1975.

487. Voelkel, A. G., Pietro, D. A., Folland, E. D., Fisher, M. C., and Parisi, A. F.: Echocardiographic features of constrictive pericarditis. Circulation 58:871, 1978.

488. Effert, S., and Domanig, E.: The diagnosis of intra-atrial tumor and thrombi by the ultrasonic echo method. Germ. Med. Meth. 4:1, 1959.

489. Wolfe, S. B., Popp, R. L., and Feigenbaum, H.: Diagnosis of atrial tumors by ultrasound. Circulation 39:615, 1969.

490. Finegan, R. E., and Harrison, D. C.: Diagnosis of left atrial myxoma by echocardiography. N. Engl. J. Med. 282:1022, 1970.

491. Schattenberg, T. T.: Echocardiographic diagnosis of left atrial myxoma. Mayo Clin. Proc. 43:620, 1968.

492. Kostis, J. B., and Moghadam, A. N.: Echocardiographic diagnosis of left atrial myxoma. Chest 58:550, 1970.

493. Abdulla, A. M., Stefadouros, M. A., Mucha, E., Moore, H. V., and O'Malley, G. A.: Left atrial myxoma: Echocardiographic diagnosis and determination of size. J.A.M.A. 238:510, 1977.

494. Perry, L. S., King, J. F., Zeft, H. J., Manley, J. C., Gross, C. M., and Wann, L. S.: Two-dimensional echocardiography in the diagnosis of left atrial myxoma. Br. Heart J. 45:667, 1981.

495. Tway, K. P., Shah, A. A., and Rahimtoola, S. H.: Multiple bilateral myxomas demonstrated by two-dimensional echocardiography. Am. J. Med. 71:896, 1981.

496. Furukawa, K., Katsume, H., Matsukubo, H., and Inoue, D.: Echo-cardiographic findings of floating thrombus in left atrium. Br. Heart J. 44:599, 1980.

497. Schweizer, P., Bardos, P., Erbel, R., Meyer, J., Merx, W., Messmer, B. J., and Effert, S.: Detection of left atrial thrombi by echocardiography. Br. Heart J. 45:148, 1981.

498. Farooki, Z. Q., Green, E. W., and Arciniegas, E.: Echocardiographic pattern of right atrial tumour motion. Br. Heart J. 38:580, 1976.

499. Atsuchi, Y., Nagai, Y., Nakamura, K., et al.: Echocardiographic diagnosis of prolapsing right atrial myxoma. Jpn. Heart J. 17:798, 1976.

500. Riggs, T., Paul, M. H., DeLeon, S., and Ilbawi, M.: Two dimensional echocardiography in evaluation of right atrial masses: Five cases in pediatric patients. Am. J. Cardiol. 48:961, 1981.

501. Howard, R. J., Pollick, C., Rambihar, V., Drobac, M., Martin, R. P., Popp, R. L., and Rakowski, H.: Two-dimensional echocardiographic detection of right atrial tumors. Am. J. Cardiol. 49:1041 (Abstract), 1982.

502. Nicholson, K. G., Prior, A. L., Norman, A. G., Naik, D. R., and Kennedy, A.: Bilateral atrial myxomas diagnosed preoperatively and successfully removed. Br. Heart J. 2:440, 1977.

503. Fitterer, J. D., Spicer, M. J., and Nelson, W. P.: Echocardiographic demonstration of bilateral atrial myxomas. Chest 70:282, 1976.

504. Gustafson, A. G., Edler, I. G., and Dahlback, O. K.: Bilateral atrial myxomas diagnosed by echocardiography. Acta Med. Scand. 201:391, 1977.

505. Werner, J. A., Cheitlin, M. D., Gross, B. W., Speck, S. M., and Ivey, T. D.: Echocardiographic appearance of the Chiari network: Differentiation from right-heart pathology. Circulation 63:1104, 1981.

506. Morgan, D. L., Palazola, J., Reed, W., Bell, H. H., Kindred, L. H., and Beauchamp, G. D.: Left heart myxomas. Am. J. Cardiol. 40:611, 1977.

507. Meller, J., Teichholz, L. E., Pichard, A. O., Matta, R., Litwak, R., Herman, M. V., and Massie, K. F.: Left ventricular myxoma. Echocardiographic diagnosis and review of the literature. Am. J. Med. 63:816, 1977.

508. Roelandt, J., Bletter, W. B., Leuftink, E. W., vanDorp, W. G., tenCate, F., and Nauta, J.: Ultrasonic demonstration of right ventricular myxoma. J. Clin. Ultrasound 5:191, 1977.

509. Asayama, J., Kunishige, H., Katsume, H., Watanabe, T., Matsukubo, H., Endo, N., Matsuura, T., Ijichi, H., Onouchi, Z., Tomizawa, M., Goto, M., and Nakata, K.: The ultrasound cardiographic findings of myxoma in the right ventricular wall. Cardiovasc. Sound Bull. 5:129, 1975.

510. Roelandt, J., Bletter, W. B., Leuftink, E. W., vanDorp, W. G., tenCate, F., and Nauta, J.: Ultrasonic demonstration of right ventricular myxoma. J. Clin. Ultrasound 5:191, 1977.

511. Krivokapich, J., Warren, S. E., Child, J. S., Kaufman, J. A., Vieweg, W. V., and Hagan, A. D.: M-mode and cross-sectional echocardiographic diagnosis of right ventricular cavity mass. J. Clin. Ultrasound 9:5, 1981.

512. Levisman, J. A., MacAlpin, R. N., Abbasi, A. S., Ellis, N., and Eber, L. M.: Echocardiographic diagnosis of a mobile, pedunculated tumor in the left ventricular cavity. Am. J. Cardiol. 36:957, 1975.

513. Nanda, N. C., Barold, S. S., Gramiak, R., Ong, L. S., and Heinle, R. A.: Echocardiographic features of right ventricular outflow tumor prolapsing into the pulmonary artery. Am. J. Cardiol. 40:272, 1977.

514. Chandraratha, P. A. N., Pedro, S. S., Elkins, R. C., and Grantham, N.: Echocardiographic, angiocardiographic, and surgical correlations in right ventricular myxoma simulating valvar pulmonic stenosis. Circulation 55:619, 1977.

515. Farooki, Z. Q., Henry, J. G., Arciniegas, E., and Green, E. W.: Ultrasonic pattern of ventricular rhabdomyoma in two infants. Am. J. Cardiol. 34:842, 1974.

516. Milner, S., Abramowitz, J. A., and Levin, S. E.: Rhabdomyoma of the heart in a newborn infant. Diagnosis by echocardiography. Br. Heart J. 43:623, 1980.

517. Yabek, S. M., Isabel-Jones, J., Gyepes, M. T., and Jarmakani, J. M.: Cardiac fibroma in a neonate present with severe congestive heart failure. J. Pediatr. 91:310, 1977.

518. Ports, T. A., Schiller, N. B., and Strunk, B. L.: Echocardiography of right ventricular tumors. Circulation 56:439, 1977.

519. Bluschke, V., Köhler, E., Ruppert, C., and Böcker, K.: Diagnosis of a cardiac metastasis of a fibrosarcoma by two-dimensional echocardiography (author's transl.). Z. Kardiol. 70:492, 1981.

520. Koiwaya, Y., Kawachi, Y., Orita, Y., Nakamura, M., Hirata, T., Yamamota, K., and Omae, T.: Echocardiographic detection of metastatic cardiac mural tumor. J. Clin. Ultrasound 8:443, 1980.

521. Canedo, M. I., Otken, L., and Stefadouros, M. A.: Echocardiographic features of cardiac compression by a thymoma simulating cardiac tamponade and obstruction of the superior vena cava. Br. Heart J. 39:1038, 1977.

522. Baduini, G., Paolillo, V., and Di Summa, M.: Echocardiographic findings in a case of acquired pulmonic stenosis from extrinsic compression by a mediastinal cyst. Chest 80:507, 1981.

523. Shah, A., and Schwartz, H.: Echocardiographic features of cardiac compression by mediastinal pancreatic pseudocyst. Chest 77:440, 1980.

524. Farooki, Z. Q., Adelman, S., and Green, E. W.: Echocardiographic differentiation of a cystic and a solid tumor of the heart. Am. J. Cardiol. 39:107, 1977.

525. Mintz, G. S., Kotler, M. N., Segal, B. L., and Parry, W. R.: Two dimensional echocardiographic recognition of the descending thoracic aorta. Am. J. Cardiol. 44:232, 1979.

526. Come, P. C., Sacks, B., Vine, H., McArdle, C., Koretsky, S., and Weintraub, R.: Ultrasonic visualization of the posterior thoracic aorta in long axis: Diagnosis of a saccular mycotic aneurysm. Chest 79:470, 1981.

527. Goldberg, B. B.: Aortosonography. Int. Surg. 62:294, 1977.

528. Lababidi, Z., and Monzon, C.: Early cardiac manifestations of Marfan's syndrome in the newborn. Am. J. Cardiol. 102:943, 1981.

529. Nanda, N. C., Gramiak, R., and Shah, P. M.: Diagnosis of aortic root dissection by echocardiography. Circulation 48:506, 1973.

530. Millward, D. K., Robinson, N. J., and Craige, E.: Dissecting aortic aneurysm diagnosed by echocardiography in a patient with rupture of the aneurysm into the right atrium. Am. J. Cardiol. 30:427, 1972.

531. Moothart, R. W., Spangler, R. D., and Blout, S. G., Jr.: Echocardiography in aortic root dissection and dilatation. Am. J. Cardiol. *36*:11, 1975.

532. Kronzon, I., and Mehta, S. S.: Illustrative echocardiogram: Aortic root dissection. Chest *65*:88, 1974.

533. Yuste, P., Aza, V., Minguez, I., Cerezo, L., and Martinez-Bardiu, C.: Dissecting aortic aneurysm diagnosed by echocardiography. Br. Heart J. *36*: 111, 1974.

534. Brown, O. R., Popp, R. L., and Kloster, F. E.: Echocardiographic criteria for aortic root dissection. Am. J. Cardiol. *36*:17, 1975.

535. Krueger, S. K., Starke, H., Forker, A. D., and Eliot, R. S.: Echocardiographic mimics of aortic root dissection. Chest *67*:441, 1975.

536. Victor, M. F., Mintz, G. S., Kotler, M. N., Wilson A. R., and Segal, B. L.: Two dimensional echocardiographic diagnosis of aortic dissection. Am. J. Cardiol. *48*:1155, 1981.

537. Smuckler, A. L., Nomeir, A. M., Watts, L. E., and Hackshaw, B. T.: Echocardiographic diagnosis of aortic root dissection by M-mode and two-dimensional techniques. Am. Heart J. *103*:897, 1982.

538. D'Cruz, I. A., Jain, M., Campbell, C., and Goldberg, A. N.: Ultrasound visualization of aortic dissection by right parasternal scanning, including systolic flutter of the intimal flap. Chest *80*:239, 1981.

539. Nicholson, W. J., and Cobbs, B. W., Jr.: Echocardiographic oscillating flap in aortic root dissecting aneurysm, Chest *70*:305, 1976.

540. Krueger, S. K., Wilson, C. S, Weaver, W. F., Reese, H. E., Caudill, C. C., and Rourke, T.: Aortic root dissection: Echocardiographic demonstration of torn intimal flap. J. Clin. Ultrasound *4*:35, 1976.

541. Matsumoto, M., Matsuo, H., Beppu, S., Yoshioka, Y., Kawashima, Y., Nimura, Y., and Abe, H.: Echocardiographic diagnosis of ruptured aneurysms of sinus of Valsalva. Report of two cases. Circulation *53*:382, 1976.

542. Rothbaum, D. A., Dillon, J. C., Chang, S., and Feigenbaum, H.: Echocardiographic manifestation of right sinus of Valsalva aneurysm. Circulation *49*:768, 1974.

543. Engle, P. J., Held, J. S., van der Bel-Kahn, J., and Spitz, H.: Echocardiographic diagnosis of congenital sinus of Valsalva aneurysm with dissection of the interventricular septum. Circulation *63*:705, 1981.

6

RADIOLOGICAL AND ANGIOGRAPHIC EXAMINATION OF THE HEART

by Murray G. Baron, M.D.

The radiological examination of the heart provides detailed information regarding cardiac structure and function that cannot be duplicated with a similar degree of accuracy by any other diagnostic method. The appearance of the heart and lungs on ordinary chest roentgenograms often indicates the presence of heart disease and, at times, is diagnostic of a specific cardiac abnormality. Correct interpretation of the cardiac shadow in the frontal view is particularly important, because a chest roentgenogram in this projection is included as part of most routine medical examinations and provides a convenient survey method for the detection of otherwise unsuspected heart disease. In those patients with a known cardiac condition, the chest roentgenogram is of use in assessing its severity, in documenting the progress of the disease, in evaluating the presence and severity of secondary complications, and as an indicator of the efficacy of treatment. *Fluoroscopy* is of value in the detection of intracardiac and coronary arterial calcification and in the diagnosis of conditions such as pericardial effusion or atrial septal defect. Aside from such

specific indications, fluoroscopy is of limited usefulness. Of all the imaging techniques, *angiocardiography* is the most comprehensive method for studying the intracardiac anatomy. Although it is an "invasive procedure" in that it is usually carried out in conjunction with cardiac catheterization (Chap. 9) (digital radiographic examinations can be carried out with intravenous injection of contrast medium [p. 191]), the risk to the patient is usually minimal, while the anatomical and hemodynamic information derived from angiocardiograms is often essential for establishing a correct diagnosis and planning a logical therapeutic approach. A special form of angiography, that of the coronary arteries (i.e., coronary arteriography), is considered in Chapter 10.

THE CARDIAC SERIES

The heart appears relatively homogeneous on a chest film because the myocardium, valves, and other cardiac structures have essentially the same radiodensity as blood, and their shadows blend imperceptibly with one another. Intracardiac lesions cannot be visualized unless they are calcified. The contours of the cardiac silhouette are clearly outlined because they contrast with the adjacent radiolucent air-containing lungs. Only those chambers and vessels that form a border on any particular view can be evaluated. However, the heart is a three-dimensional structure, and therefore multiple views are required in order to bring each of the chambers and great vessels into profile. Even then, the posterior border of the heart cannot be clearly identified unless the esophagus is filled with radiopaque material. A complete plain film study of the heart comprises four views of the chest: frontal, lateral, 60-degree right anterior oblique, and 45-degree left anterior oblique. On the first three views the patient swallows barium in order to opacify the esophagus.

Except in the more severe congenital anomalies, such as the transposition complexes or hypoplasia of the left ventricle, the chambers of the heart and great vessels always occupy the same relative position within the cardiac silhouette. *Dilatation* of each structure affects the contours of the heart in a fairly characteristic manner that is similar from case to case. However, this is not true with concentric cardiac *hypertrophy*. As the ventricular wall thickens, it tends to encroach on the cavity and may not increase the outer diameter of the chamber. Considerable myocardial hypertrophy can be present without causing a significant change in the shape of the cardiac silhouette. Even when the hypertrophy does result in cardiac enlargement, the appearance of the heart is often nonspecific.

Frontal View (Fig. 6–1)

In this view, the upper half of the right cardiac border is formed by the superior vena cava and the lower half by the right atrium. The caval portion is relatively straight, while the lateral margin of the atrium forms a gentle, con-

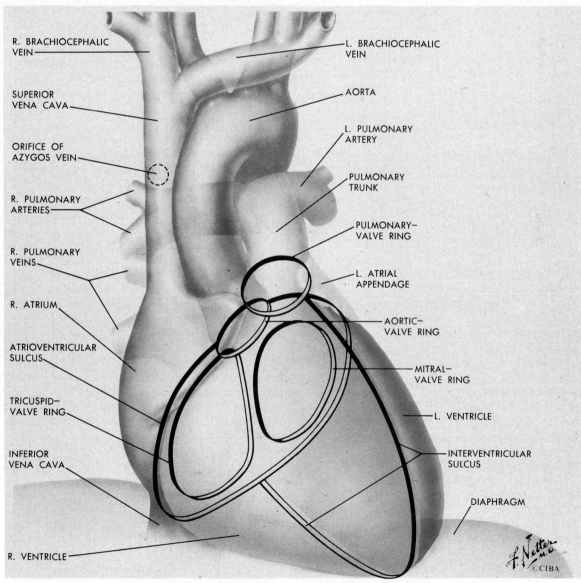

FIGURE 6–1   Frontal projection of the heart. (Reproduced with permission from The CIBA Collection of Medical Illustrations by Frank H. Netter, M.D. Vol. 5, The Heart, edited by F. Y. Yonkman. Copyright 1969, CIBA Pharmaceutical Co., Division of CIBA-GEIGY Corp. All rights reserved.)

vex curve that extends to the diaphragm. The junction of the two structures is usually indicated by a shallow angle, where their contours meet. If the patient can take a sufficiently deep inspiration, a small portion of the inferior vena cava may become visible as a triangular shadow between the diaphragm and the border of the right atrium.

The left cardiac border is composed of three distinct curvatures: The uppermost bulge is formed by the aortic knob, below which is the curve of the main pulmonary artery and sometimes a portion of the left pulmonary artery; most of the remainder of the left cardiac contour represents the anterolateral margin of the left ventricle. The left atrial appendage reaches the left border of the heart and is seen in profile as a short, straight segment between the pulmonary artery and the left ventricle. If the atrium is not enlarged, this segment cannot be delimited on plain films; however, it is identifiable fluoroscopically, because its pulsations are not in phase with those of the ventricle.

THE ATRIA. Enlargement of the *right atrium* causes broadening of the cardiac silhouette to the right, with accentuation of the curvature of the atrial contour (Fig. 6–2). Normally, the *right ventricle* does not form a border in the frontal projection and cannot be viewed directly. As the ventricle dilates, it tends to push the left ventricle laterally and posteriorly, causing widening of the cardiac shadow to the left. Especially with congenital lesions, such as tetralogy of Fallot, the enlarged right ventricle may extend beyond the left ventricle and form the left cardiac border. The cardiac apex is then elevated and rounded (see Figure 6–37, p. 172).

As the *left atrium* increases in size, its appendage bulges from the left cardiac contour, the border of the atrium may form a second contour within the right part of the cardiac shadow, and the left bronchus may be displaced upward. The last two signs, although accurate, are relatively insensitive and are not present unless there is considerable dilatation of the atrium. Even then, they may be absent.

When the left atrium enlarges, it tends to project backward beyond the remainder of the heart. This localized increase in the thickness of the heart causes the central portion of the cardiac silhouette to be abnormally dense. The increased density ends suddenly at the margins of the left atrium, and its right border can be visualized as a distinct contour through the cardiac silhouette (Fig. 6–2). However, if the atrium distends from side to side more than posteriorly, so that it does not form a localized bulge, its shadow blends in with the rest of the heart, and its borders may not be visualized. Furthermore, when the right atrium enlarges, it may also extend posteriorly, alongside the left atrium, obliterating the latter's right border. A double contour, even when present, is often difficult to visualize on standard films. Because the roentgen technique used for chest films is adjusted so that the exposure provides an optimal picture of the lungs, an enlarged heart is usually underpenetrated. The dense cardiac shadow then obscures the contour of the left atrium, although it may be quite obvious on an overexposed film or one made with a Bucky grid.

Occasionally, the confluence of the *right pulmonary veins* is visible through the right portion of the cardiac silhouette and can resemble the double density caused by left

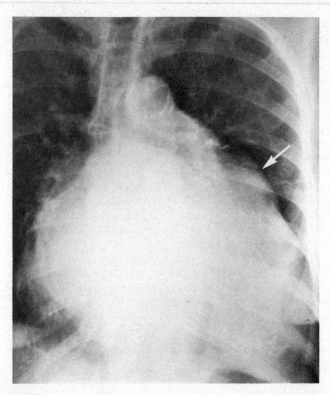

FIGURE 6–2 Enlargement of the atria, frontal view. The enlargement of the right portion of the cardiac silhouette and the increased curvature of its border are caused by dilatation of the right atrium. The left atrial appendage is dilated and forms a localized bulge (arrow) on the left cardiac border. The double contour on the right side, the increased density of the central portion of the heart, and the elevation of the left main bronchus are all signs of left atrial enlargement. The widening of the heart to the left indicates ventricular enlargement, in this case involving both ventricles. The patient had severe mitral valve disease with pulmonary hypertension and tricuspid regurgitation.

atrial enlargement. However, the lateral border of the venous shadow is relatively straight and not convex as is the contour of an enlarged left atrium. In addition, when the left atrium is enlarged, the entire central portion of the cardiac silhouette is abnormally dense. A giant left atrium can extend beyond the right atrium and form part, or all, of the right cardiac border, in which case the margin of the right atrium is seen within the cardiac silhouette. Elevation of the left main bronchus has some drawbacks as a sign of left atrial enlargement. Often, the bronchus is hidden by the hilar and mediastinal shadows. When the bronchus can be identified, it is difficult to be certain whether its course is normal or not if the displacement is not marked. Displacement of the bronchus must be interpreted with caution if the film was not made during full inspiration or if the patient was supine rather than erect. In both situations, the carinal angle is widened and the left bronchus elevated.

Abnormal prominence of the left atrial appendage is the most sensitive sign of left atrial enlargement in the frontal view. The appendage dilates along with the body of the atrium, and its segment on the left heart border, which is normally flat, becomes convex. As the appendage becomes larger, it forms a well-defined bulge immediately beneath the pulmonary artery segment. An aneurysm of the antero-

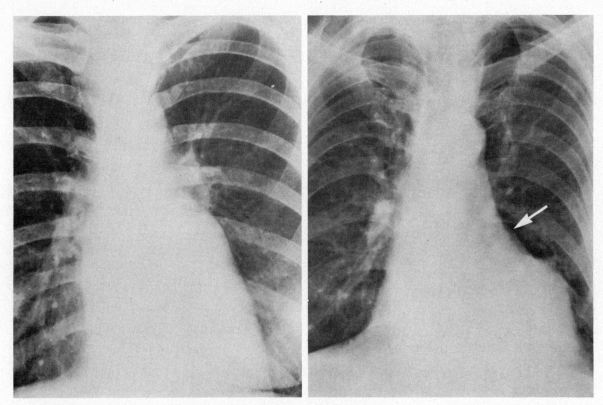

FIGURE 6–3 Dilatation of the left atrial appendage—differential diagnosis. *A*, Mitral stenosis. The only sign of left atrial enlargement is dilatation of its appendage, which forms a bulge on the left cardiac contour immediately beneath the pulmonary artery segment. *B*, Ventricular aneurysm. In this case, the bulge on the left cardiac contour is separated from the pulmonary artery segment. The intervening portion of the heart border is formed by the left atrial appendage (arrow) and the basal portion of the anterolateral left ventricular wall.

lateral wall of the left ventricle can cause a similar bulge but at a lower level on the cardiac contour, some distance below the pulmonary artery (Fig. 6–3).

THE LEFT VENTRICLE. The shape of an enlarged *left ventricle* depends, to some extent, on the underlying cause. When the dilatation results from a diastolic overload, particularly in aortic regurgitation, the chamber enlarges mainly along its long axis. The cardiac apex is displaced downward and to the left (Fig. 6–4*A*). Although this axis of the ventricle is elongated when the dilatation is due to myocardial disease, the width of the chamber is also significantly increased, so that the dilated ventricle assumes a more globular shape (Fig. 6–4*B*).

As the left ventricle enlarges, it becomes more difficult to evaluate the size of the left atrium on the frontal film. Widening of the cardiac silhouette to the left tends to minimize, or even mask, the prominence of a dilated left atrial appendage (see Figures 6–8 and 6–11). In order to judge the size of the two chambers properly, it is usually necessary to obtain other views of the heart, particularly the left oblique projection (see Figure 6–14*C*). When both the left atrium and the left ventricle are enlarged, the relative degrees of dilatation of the chambers have diagnostic importance. Left atrial enlargement does not necessarily indicate disease of the mitral valve but can occur in response to elevation of the left ventricular end-diastolic pressure. In the latter case, the degree of enlargement of the left atrium will be less than that of the left ventricle, while the oppo-

site is usually true when the chambers are dilated because of mitral valve disease.

CARDIAC VALVES. The frontal view is of limited usefulness for the detection of *valve calcification*. The aortic valve is projected over the left border of the spine, and calcific deposits on the valve cusps are usually obscured by the vertebral bodies. The mitral valve lies below and to the left of the aortic valve within the densest portion of the cardiac shadow, and only relatively coarse calcific deposits can be visualized. Valve calcifications are easier to recognize by means of fluoroscopy. As the heart beats, the mitral valve describes a shallow, elliptical trajectory, with its long axis oriented to the left and slightly downward, while the aortic valve moves in a vertical direction.

Lateral View (Fig. 6–5)

The anterior border of the cardiac shadow is formed by the body and the outflow tract of the right ventricle, the supravalvular portion of the main pulmonary artery, and the aorta. The normal ventricle abuts the lower third of the sternum. Because lung is interposed between the sternum and the cardiac structures, the upper retrosternal space is radiolucent. As the right ventricle dilates, its outflow portion extends anteriorly toward the sternum and encroaches on the retrosternal clear space. However, this is not always a reliable sign of right ventricular enlargement,

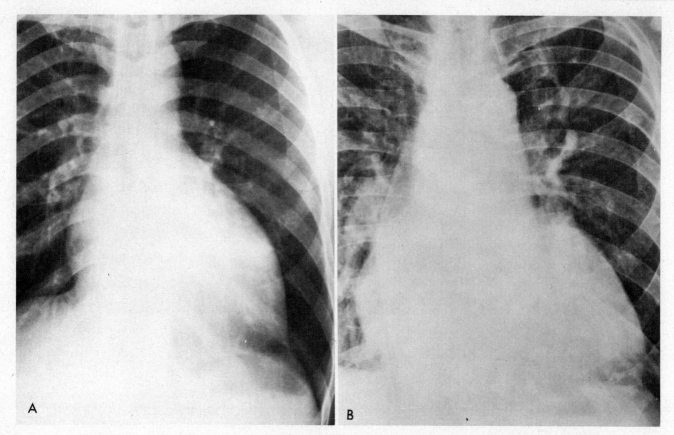

FIGURE 6–4 Enlargement of the left ventricle, frontal view. *A*, Aortic regurgitation. Enlargement of the left ventricle has occurred mainly along its long axis, so that the cardiac apex is displaced downward and to the left. This shape of the cardiac silhouette is characteristic of the type of ventricular dilatation associated with regurgitation of the aortic valve. (From Donoso, E., and Gorlin, R. [eds.]: Current Cardiovascular Topics. Vol. 3, Angina Pectoris. New York, Stratton Intercontinental Medical Book Co., 1977.) *B*, Ischemic heart disease with significant impairment of myocardial function. The long and short axes of the ventricle are more or less evenly elongated, causing the chamber to have a globular shape.

because it depends upon the shape of the chest as well as upon the size of the heart. In a patient with a narrow chest, as in the "straight back" syndrome, the retrosternal space is often obliterated by a normal-sized heart simply because there is no space for it in the thorax. Conversely, in a patient with pulmonary emphysema and a barrel-shaped chest, the heart can be considerably enlarged and still barely reach the sternum.

The posterior border of the heart is formed by the posterior aspect of the left atrium and the left ventricle. On a film made during deep inspiration, the supradiaphragmatic portion of the inferior vena cava and a small part of the right atrium may be uncovered. The ventricular border is usually clearly seen as it is outlined by adjacent air-containing lung. However, the left atrial component of the posterior cardiac border merges with the shadow of the mediastinum and is not well delineated. The esophagus lies directly behind the heart and, when filled with opaque material, can be used to evaluate left atrial size. The normal atrium, in the erect position, does not affect the esophagus, but as it enlarges, it indents the anterior wall of the esophagus and displaces it posteriorly (Fig. 6–6*A*). The indentation caused by an enlarged atrium begins immediately below the carina and involves the midportion of the esophagus. The lower esophagus lies below the atrium and is adjacent to the left ventricle. When only the atrium is

enlarged, the supradiaphragmatic portion of the esophagus remains in its normal postion and shows no indentation.

The portion of the esophagus immediately above the diaphragm may be indented by an enlarged left ventricle (Fig. 6–6*B*). More commonly, the dilated ventricle extends laterally as well as posteriorly and bypasses the esophagus (Fig. 6–7). When both the left atrium and the left ventricle are dilated, the esophagus is usually displaced posteriorly in one continuous sweep, beginning just below the carina and continuing down to the diaphragm (Fig. 6–8).

On occasion, the appearance of the esophagus in the lateral view can be misleading. If there are tertiary contractions of the esophagus or if it is not well distended with barium, no indentation or displacement will be seen even though the left atrium is of considerable size. Furthermore, because the esophagus is not fixed to the heart, it may slide medially as the heart enlarges and will not appear displaced when viewed from the side. On the other hand, the esophagus is loosely attached to the descending aorta and can be pulled backward when this vessel is tortuous, the displacement being almost identical to that caused by an enlarged atrium. The correct cause of the displacement can be recognized because the curve of the esophagus exactly parallels that of the aorta.

The relationship between the shadow of the inferior vena cava and the posterior border of the heart in the lat-

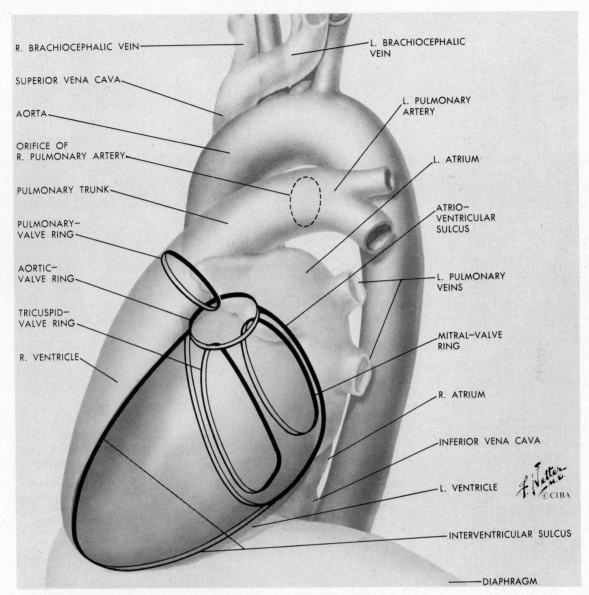

FIGURE 6–5 Lateral projection of the heart. (Reproduced with permission from The CIBA Collection of Medical Illustrations by Frank H. Netter, M.D. Vol. 5, The Heart, edited by F. Y. Yonkman. Copyright 1969, CIBA Pharmaceutical Co., Division of CIBA-GEIGY Corp. All rights reserved.)

eral projection provides a fairly accurate indicator of left ventricular size. The cava can usually be identified as a curvilinear shadow that extends upward and forward from the right diaphragm (see Figure 6–5). The lower part of the cardiac border is formed by the left ventricle and, as it curves forward, it crosses the posterior margin of the caval shadow about 2 cm above the left leaf of the diaphragm. As the left ventricle dilates, the apex of the chamber extends downward, and the point of intersection between the border of the ventricle and the cava moves closer to a diaphragm (Fig. 6–8).[1] However, the accuracy of this sign is considerably diminished if the patient is rotated slightly to either side and the film is not a true lateral projection.[2]

When valvular calcification is identified in the lateral view, fluoroscopy is usually not needed to determine whether the leaflets of the aortic valve or the mitral valve are involved. The two valves can be separated by a line drawn from the origin of the left main bronchus to the anterior costophrenic sulcus. (The bronchus can be recognized because it is projected on end and casts a round, lucent shadow at the lower end of the trachea.) The mitral valve almost always lies below this line, while the aortic valve lies more anteriorly, above the line (Figs. 6–7 and 6–9).[3]

RIGHT ANTERIOR OBLIQUE VIEW (Fig. 6–10). If the patient is properly positioned, the cardiac silhouette will be projected completely to the left of the shadow of the spine. The upper half of the right heart border is formed by the posterolateral wall of the left atrium and its lower half by the back of the right atrium. As in the lateral view, the left atrial contour cannot be satisfactorily delineated unless the esophagus is filled with barium. The ascending aorta forms the relatively straight, upper portion of the left cardiac contour. Beneath this segment,

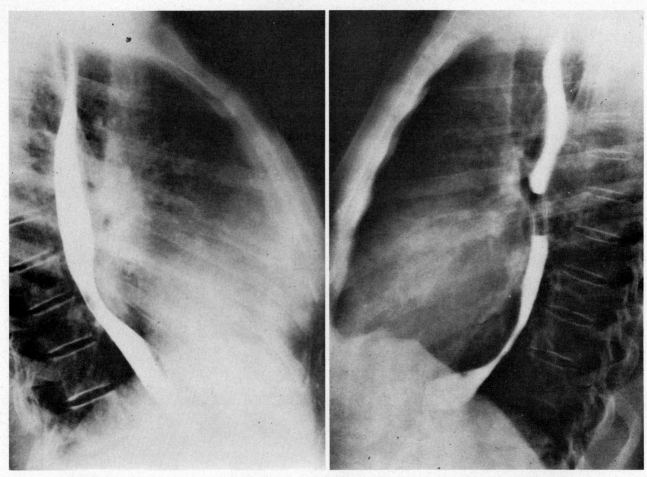

FIGURE 6–6   Indentation of the esophagus by the left cardiac chambers. *A*, Enlarged left atrium. The indentation on the anterior esophageal wall begins just below the level of the carina and involves only the midportion of the esophagus. The lower esophagus is in its normal position and shows no indentation. *B*, Enlarged left ventricle. The dilated ventricle extends posteriorly and impinges on the lowermost portion of the esophagus. The esophageal indentation continues to the diaphragm.

the cardiac border slopes downward and to the left in a shallow curve formed by the margins of the outflow tract of the right ventricle and the main pulmonary artery. The inferior continuation of the curve represents the anterior border of the left ventricle.

The information provided by this view regarding left atrial size is essentially the same as that gained from the lateral projection. When the atrium is large, it indents or displaces the barium-filled esophagus. The lowermost portion of the esophagus will not be affected if the left ventricle is normal in size. When the ventricle is also enlarged, the esophagus is displaced backward in a continuous curve that extends from the carina to the diaphragm.

Dilatation of the outflow tract of the right ventricle and the main pulmonary artery produces a bulge on the left cardiac contour just beneath the straight aortic segment. This is a common finding when there is a sizable left-to-right shunt through an atrial or ventricular septal defect. In mitral valve disease, abnormal prominence of the right ventricular outflow tract usually signifies the presence of pulmonary hypertension (Fig. 6–11).

The right anterior oblique view is the best for detection of mitral valve calcification. The valve is seen within the midportion of the cardiac silhouette, free of the shadow of the spine (Fig. 6–11), and because it is projected tangentially, it exhibits its maximal range of motion between systole and diastole. The valve can be located fluoroscopically because it is aligned with the atrioventricular sulcus in this view. In adults, the sulcus usually contains an accumulation of fat and casts a lucent, vertical, linear shadow that moves from side to side with the heartbeat. If no calcific densities are identified in relation to the sulcus, one can assume that the mitral valve is free of significant calcification. The aortic valve is situated above and slightly to the right of the mitral valve and moves in a vertical direction.

LEFT ANTERIOR OBLIQUE VIEW (Fig. 6–12). This is the only projection of the cardiac series in which the body of the left atrium can be visualized directly. The posterior atrial wall forms the upper third of the left cardiac contour, just beneath the left main bronchus. The lower two-thirds of this contour are formed by the left ventricle. The right border of the cardiac shadow represents mostly right atrium except for a short segment just above the diaphragm, where the right ventricle comes into profile. The arch of the aorta parallels the plane of the film in this view and is projected with a minimum of foreshortening. The

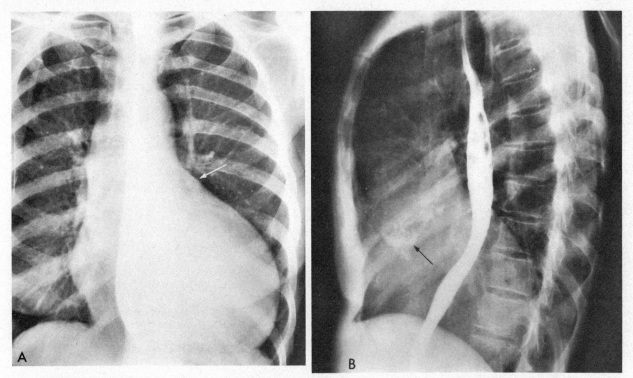

FIGURE 6-7   Dilatation of the left ventricle in aortic valve disease. *A*, Frontal view. The cardiac silhouette is elongated downward and to the left, indicating left ventricular enlargement. There is slight prominence of the left atrial appendage (arrow). The esophagus is displaced medially. *B*, Lateral view. The left ventricle is markedly enlarged and extends posterior to the esophagus. The aortic valve is densely calcified (arrow). The indentation on the anterior wall of the midesophagus is caused by the moderately dilated left atrium. There was no evidence of mitral valve disease.

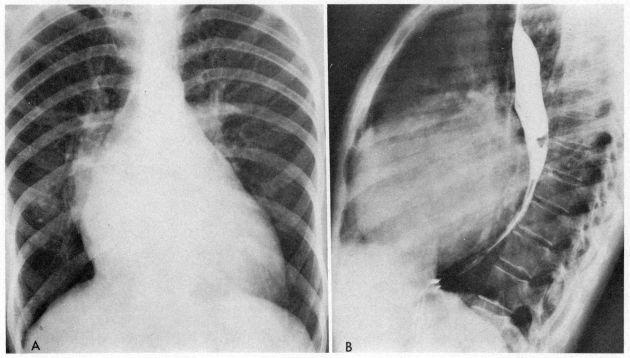

FIGURE 6-8   Enlargement of the left atrium and left ventricle. *A*, Frontal view. The abnormal density of the central portion of the cardiac silhouette and the double contour on the right side indicate enlargement of the left atrium. The bulge of the atrial appendage on the left cardiac border is less prominent than would be expected, considering the size of the atrium, because the widening of the cardiac shadow. The displacement of the apex of the heart downward and to the left is caused by enlargement of the left ventricle. The increased size of the pulmonary vessels in the upper lungs and the narrowed vessels at the bases as well as the Kerley B lines in the costophrenic sulci reflect the presence of pulmonary venous hypertension. *B*, Lateral view. The esophagus is displaced backward in a continuous curve from the carina to the diaphragm. The posterior border of the heart crosses the shadow of the inferior vena cava almost at the level of the diaphragm, confirming the presence of left ventricular enlargement.

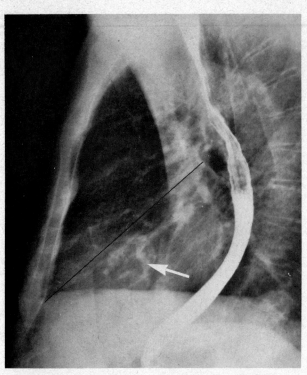

FIGURE 6-9 Mitral valve calcification, lateral view. The valvular calcification (arrow) lies below the line drawn from the left main bronchus to the anterior costophrenic sinus, localizing it to the mitral valve. The aortic valve, in this view, lies more anteriorly, above the line.

FIGURE 6-10 Right anterior oblique projection of the heart. (Reproduced with permission from The CIBA Collection of Medical Illustrations by Frank H. Netter, M.D. Vol. 5, The Heart, edited by F. Y. Yonkman. Copyright 1969, CIBA Pharmaceutical Co., Division of CIBA-GEIGY Corp. All rights reserved.)

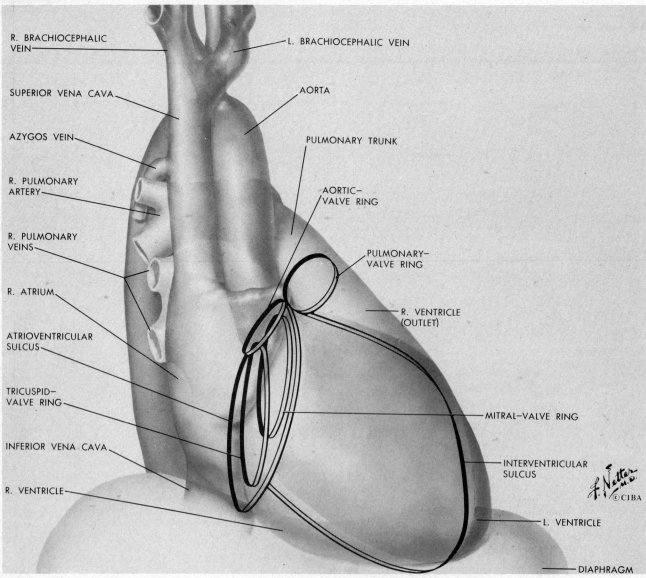

FIGURE 6–11 Mitral valve disease. Right anterior oblique view. The outflow tract of the right ventricle is dilated, indicating elevation of pulmonary artery pressure. The calcified mitral valve (arrow) is clearly visible within the midportion of the cardiac silhouette. The size of the left atrium cannot be evaluated because of esophageal spasm.

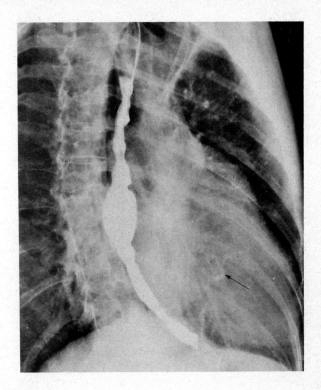

FIGURE 6–12 Left anterior oblique projection of the heart. (Reproduced with permission from The CIBA Collection of Medical Illustrations by Frank H. Netter, M.D. Vol. 5, The Heart, edited, by F. Y. Yonkman. Copyright 1969, CIBA Pharmaceutical Co., Division of CIBA-GEIGY Corp. All rights reserved.)

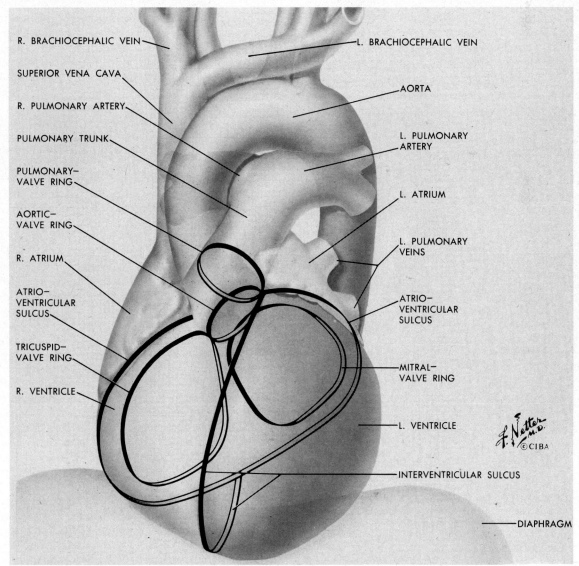

R. BRACHIOCEPHALIC VEIN

SUPERIOR VENA CAVA

R. PULMONARY ARTERY

PULMONARY TRUNK

PULMONARY-VALVE RING

AORTIC-VALVE RING

R. ATRIUM

ATRIO-VENTRICULAR SULCUS

TRICUSPID-VALVE RING

R. VENTRICLE

L. BRACHIOCEPHALIC VEIN

AORTA

L. PULMONARY ARTERY

L. ATRIUM

L. PULMONARY VEINS

ATRIO-VENTRICULAR SULCUS

MITRAL-VALVE RING

L. VENTRICLE

INTERVENTRICULAR SULCUS

DIAPHRAGM

origins of the great vessels are maximally separated. The atrioventricular valves are projected *en face* so that calcification of the mitral valve is more difficult to detect than in the right oblique view. The aortic valve is projected almost tangentially, and calcification of its cusps is easily seen.

Enlargement of the *right atrium* causes widening of the cardiac silhouette to the right and an increase in the curvature of the right cardiac contour (Fig. 6–13). In some instances, it may not be possible to separate the atrial and ventricular components of this border on plain films. This can be resolved by fluoroscopy, because the borders of the chambers move in opposite directions during the cardiac cycle.

Normally, the segment of the left cardiac contour formed by the left atrium is straight or slightly concave. As the chamber increases in size, this border becomes convex (Fig. 6–13) and encroaches on the "aortic window," the clear space beneath the aortic arch. Upward displacement of the left main bronchus is often better seen in this view than in the frontal projection. Because the barium-filled esophagus is often projected over the border of the heart, it may obscure the left atrial contour. The left anterior oblique view, therefore, should be obtained first when filming a cardiac series, before the patient is given barium to swallow.

When the left ventricle dilates, its long axis elongates in a posterior direction as well as downward and laterally. The ventricle is thus foreshortened in the frontal view, and its size can easily be underestimated. However, when the

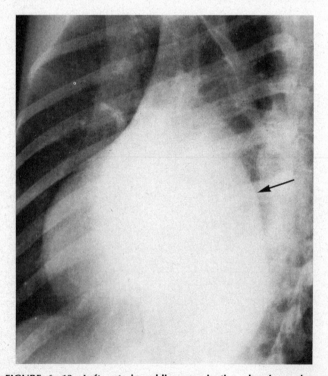

FIGURE 6–13 Left anterior oblique projection showing enlargement of both atria in mitral valve disease. The right side of the cardiac silhouette is enlarged and its curvature increased because of dilatation of the right atrium. The convexity of the upper left cardiac border (arrow) just beneath the left main bronchus indicates that the left atrium is also enlarged. (From Baron, M. G.: Left anterior oblique view for evaluation of left atrial size. Circulation *44*:926, 1971, by permission of the American Heart Association, Inc.)

patient is in the left oblique position, the long axis of the ventricle is aligned parallel to the film. For this reason, this view is essential, in addition to the frontal view, for proper evaluation of left ventricular size (Fig. 6–14). Whether the ventricle is elongated (Fig. 6–15) is of considerably greater diagnostic significance than whether the cardiac silhouette is projected clear of the shadow of the spine or not. The latter sign depends to a large extent on the position of the patient.[4] The steeper the oblique angle, the more likely that the shadow of the ventricle—regardless of its size—will not overlap the spine. Even with a standard degree of obliquity, the ventricle that is elongated mainly to the left will tend to clear the spine, whereas the same size ventricle extending more posteriorly will not. In addition, this sign may be falsely positive if the right ventricle is significantly enlarged. An increase in the size of this chamber displaces the left ventricle to the left and posteriorly, and the heart may not clear the shadow of the spine in the left oblique view, even though the left ventricle is normal in size.

Heart Size

Although heart disease can certainly be present without causing cardiomegaly, the converse is not true. Enlargement of the heart is indicative of cardiac disease and, at times, may be its first overt manifestation. When a patient is known to have heart disease, changes in cardiac size over a period of time can be used to evaluate the progress of the disease or the results of treatment.

Even though an experienced observer can estimate cardiac size with an acceptable degree of accuracy from the appearance of the cardiac silhouette, a more objective method of measurement is often desirable. A simple measurement of one or more diameters of the cardiac silhouette has little meaning, because normal heart size varies considerably with sex and body habitus. The *cardiothoracic ratio* was designed to compensate for these factors and uses the width of the chest as an indicator of body build. A vertical reference line is drawn on the frontal chest film through the spinous processes of the vertebrae. The sum of the maximum distances from this line to the right and to the left borders of the cardiac silhouette constitutes the transverse cardiac diameter (Fig. 6–16). This value is then divided by the greatest width of the thorax as measured from the inner margins of the ribs to give the cardiothoracic ratio. A value of 0.5 is generally considered to indicate the upper limit of normal heart size, but a figure of 0.6 is preferable, since it will decrease the number of false-positive results.[5,6] Unfortunately, the maximum width of the chest is not a particularly accurate index of body build, and its use introduces a second variable that is independent of the presence or absence of cardiac disease. The transverse cardiac diameter alone is a better measure of heart size if it is compared with standard tables of cardiac diameters in adults of different height and weight.[7]

A more accurate determination of cardiac size can be achieved by calculating the relative cardiac volume.[8,9] Three measurements are required: the long axis of the heart (L) is measured on the frontal film from the break in the right cardiac contour, where the superior vena cava

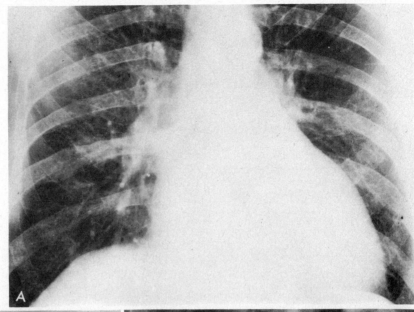

FIGURE 6-14 Left atrial and left ventricular enlargement. *A*, Frontal view. The heart is elongated and has a configuration most suggestive of aortic regurgitation. There is no evidence of left atrial enlargement. *B*, Lateral view. Although the esophagus appears to be displaced backward to some extent, this is difficult to evaluate because it is not well distended. *C*, Left anterior oblique view. The double bulge of the left cardiac contour reflects the considerable increase in size of the left atrium as well as of the left ventricle. Elevation of the left main bronchus is well visualized in this projection. The patient has both aortic and mitral valve disease.

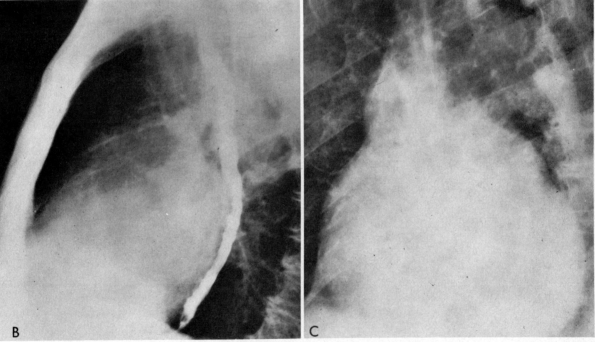

joins the right atrium, to the cardiac apex; the short axis (S) is measured from the right cardiophrenic angle to the junction of the pulmonary artery and left atrial segments on the left heart border; the third dimension (D) represents the greatest anteroposterior diameter of the heart and is measured on the lateral chest film (Fig. 6–17). The final calculation is made from the formula

$$\frac{L \times S \times D \times K}{\text{Body surface area}} = \text{Relative cardiac volume}$$

K is a constant that is related to the distance between the x-ray tube and the film. For the usual 6-foot chest film, K equals 0.42. Figures for body surface area are obtained from the DuBois standards.[10]

A volume of less than 450 cc/m² for women and 500 cc/m² for men is considered to be normal. Values over 490 cc/m² for women and 540 cc/m² for men are definitely abnormal. Aside from the inherent mathematical accuracy of this method, it is of particular value because it is not significantly affected by the phase of the cardiac cycle. Even in patients with large stroke volumes and a considerable change in the apparent size of the heart between systole and diastole, the relative cardiac volume varies little because it is determined from the volumes of all four cardiac chambers. When the ventricles contract during systole, the atria become larger as they fill with blood, whereas in diastole the atria decrease in size and the ventricles distend. The measurement has definite prognostic significance in

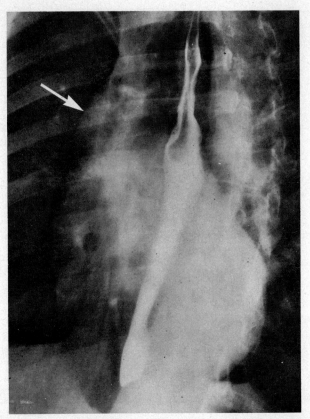

FIGURE 6-15 Left ventricular enlargement, left anterior oblique view. The cardiac silhouette is enlarged downward, to the left, and posteriorly, indicating dilatation of the left ventricle. The ascending aorta is widened (arrow).

ischemic heart disease[11] but not in the presence of aortic regurgitation or mitral valve disease. The measurement will obviously be grossly incorrect if enlargement of the cardiac silhouette is due to a pericardial effusion.

In most instances, calculation of cardiac volume, or even measurement of the transverse cardiac diameter, is too time-consuming to be a routine procedure. A visual estimate of heart size from the frontal film is generally adequate for most clinical purposes. However, several possible pitfalls must be recognized if gross errors are to be avoided.

First, the degree of inspiration is the single factor with the greatest effect on the apparent size of the heart. During a maximal inspiratory effort, a patient should be able to lower his or her diaphragm at least to the level of the tenth rib posteriorly. If the diaphragm is at a higher level, the long axis of the heart lies more horizontally, and its transverse diameter is increased (Fig. 6-18). In addition, because lung volume is decreased, the heart, which does not change in size, occupies a relatively greater portion of the available thoracic space.

Second, because chest films are exposed at random, some are made during diastole and others during systole. In the great majority of patients, the difference in the transverse cardiac diameter between the two phases of the cardiac cycle is relatively small.[12] However, in patients with a slow heart rate and a large stroke volume, such as a trained athlete or a patient with complete atrioventricular block, the change in transverse diameter between systole

and diastole may be as much as 2 cm. When two films of such a patient are compared, the differences in heart size can be misinterpreted to indicate an important change in the cardiac status. This error can be avoided by calculation of the relative cardiac volume.

Third, visualization of more of the cardiac apex than is usually seen can cause the heart to appear abnormally large. The heart lies anteriorly and is situated below the highest point of the curve of the diaphragm. In the frontal projection, the cardiac silhouette appears to end at the diaphragm because its lowermost portion is obscured by the shadows of the abdominal viscera. However, when there is a moderate quantity of air in the stomach, the "infradiaphragmatic portion" of the heart may be seen through the gastric air bubble. This causes the cardiac silhouette to appear larger than it really is. Mistakes can be avoided if the area beneath the left diaphragm is simply covered before the size of the heart is assessed (Fig. 6-19).

Fourth, when the anteroposterior diameter of the chest is abnormally narrow because of loss of the thoracic kyphotic curvature, or pectus excavatum, the heart may be compressed between the sternum and the spine and splayed to one or both sides. The transverse cardiac diameter is then abnormally large. The cause of the apparent cardiomegaly is obvious if a lateral film is available. However, the chest deformity can usually be recognized from the appearance of the ribs on the frontal film. The course of the posterior ribs tends to be horizontal or angled upward, while the downward slope of the anterior ends of

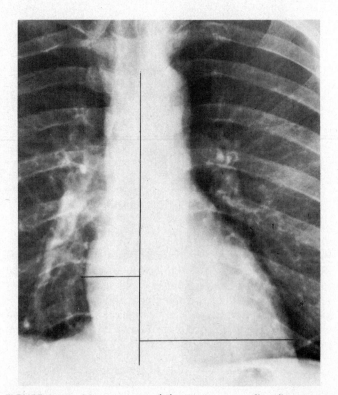

FIGURE 6-16 Measurement of the transverse cardiac diameter. A vertical reference line is first drawn through the spinous processes of the vertebrae. The greatest distances from this line to the right and to the left margins of the cardiac silhouette are then measured. Their sum constitutes the transverse cardiac diameter.

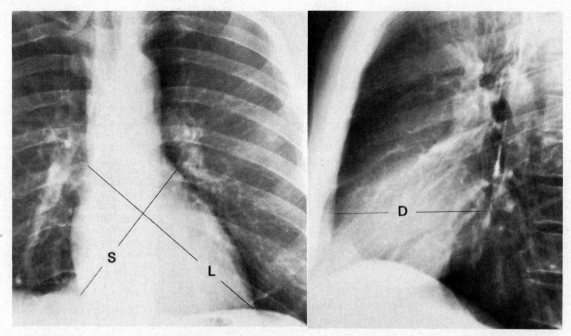

FIGURE 6-17   Measurement of relative cardiac volume. *A,* Frontal projection. The long axis of the heart (L) is measured from the break in the right cardiac contour, where the superior vena cava joins the right atrium, to the apex of the heart. The short diameter (S) extends from the right cardiophrenic angle to the junction of the left atrial and pulmonary artery segments. This line is roughly perpendicular to the long axis. *B,* Lateral view. The widest anteroposterior dimension of the cardiac silhouette constitutes the depth of the heart (D). If the posterior border of the heart cannot be clearly identified, the anterior margin of the barium-filled esophagus can be used as the boundary for this measurement.

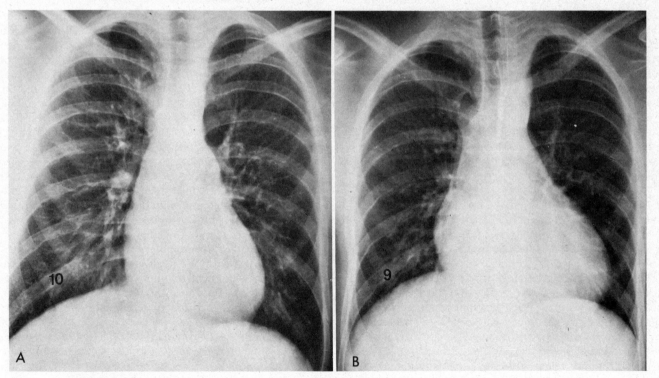

FIGURE 6-18   The effect of respiration on heart size in a patient with coarctation of the aorta. *A,* Deep inspiration. The aortic knob is obscured, and ribs 5 to 9 on the right side and 8 on the left show notching of the undersurface—an appearance pathognomonic of coarctation. The patient has taken a deep inspiration, lowering the diaphragm to the 10th posterior interspace. Although the heart is normal in size, elongation of its long axis indicates some enlargement of the left ventricle. *B,* With a lesser inspiratory effort, the diaphragm is at the level of the 9th posterior interspace. The long axis of the heart is displaced toward the horizontal, increasing the transverse cardiac diameter. The heart appears larger than in *A.*

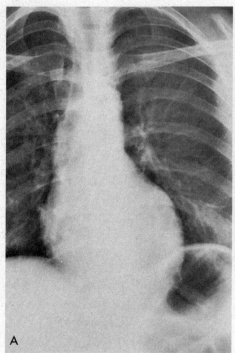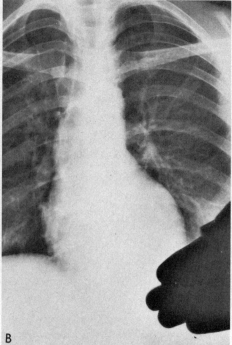

FIGURE 6–19 The "infradiaphragmatic" portion of the cardiac silhouette. *A*, A portion of the apical and diaphragmatic aspects of the heart, usually hidden by the diaphragm and the abdominal organs, is seen through the gastric air bubble. Visualization of this additional area of the heart causes the cardiac shadow to appear enlarged. *B*, Same film. Evaluation of heart size is simplified if the area beneath the diaphragm is covered. The heart is normal.

the ribs is much steeper than normal. In addition, the cardiac silhouette is not as dense as expected for a heart with such a large transverse diameter, and the ribs and vascular markings in the left lower lobe are easily visible through it.

Finally, the size of the cardiac shadow is also determined by the degree to which the heart is magnified on the film. The farther the heart is from the film, or the nearer the x-ray tube to the film, the larger the cardiac silhouette. Most bedside examinations are made with a tube-to-film distance of three feet, with the cassette behind the patient. The shadow of the heart is therefore more magnified and appears larger than on a standard chest film made at a distance of six feet, with the patient facing the cassette. Thus it is extremely difficult to compare the size of the heart on a portable film with that on a standard chest film with any degree of accuracy.

ACQUIRED HEART DISEASE

Coronary Artery Disease (See also Chapter 39)

There is no direct relationship between the appearance of the heart and the presence or severity of coronary artery disease. So long as myocardial function is not significantly impaired, the heart size is normal, even in a patient who may be totally incapacitated by angina. Similarly, if sufficient functioning muscle remains after a myocardial infarction, the heart can retain its normal configuration. On the other hand, the finding of an enlarged heart may at times be the first indication of coronary artery disease.[13,14]

Ischemic heart disease, from a practical standpoint, is a disease of the left ventricle. Enlargement of the heart implies significant impairment of left ventricular function, and the degree of dilatation is roughly related to the de-

gree of limitation of ventricular contractility. Since the size of the heart is an indicator of cardiac decompensation, the chest film is a simple means of following the course of ischemic heart disease.

Deterioration of left ventricular function results in an increase in left ventricular end-diastolic pressure. This, in turn, interferes with left atrial emptying, and the atrium tends to dilate. The appearance of the heart at this stage of left ventricular failure may be similar to that of mitral valve disease (Fig. 6–20). With further progression, the right heart chambers also enlarge, and the cardiac silhouette becomes rounded. The appearance may also resemble that caused by a pericardial effusion; the cardiac pulsations are markedly diminished in both conditions. The two can usually be differentiated by the appearance of the hilar vessels. Cardiac enlargement of this extent is associated with some degree of congestive failure, and the hilar vessels become engorged and unduly prominent. On the other hand, the dilated cardiac silhouette caused by a pericardial effusion tends to obscure the hilar vessels (see Fig. 6–43).[15]

A myocardial infarct cannot be identified on plain films unless it is calcified or forms an aneurysm. In some cases, the abnormal motion of the infarcted segment of the ventricular wall can be noted on fluoroscopic examination, but because the septal and diaphragmatic aspects of the ventricle are not adequately visualized, a large number of infarcts cannot be detected. When calcium is deposited within an infarct, it produces a fine shell that is seen as a dense, curvilinear line when viewed tangentially. However, when projected *en face* or obliquely, the calcific layer is often too thin to cast a recognizable shadow. Both the thinning of the ventricular wall and the calcification, if present, are more easily detected by computed tomography (p. 189).

A calcified infarct is almost always transmural in extent.

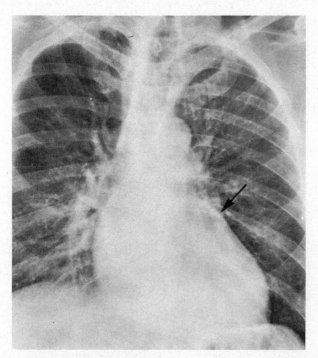

FIGURE 6–20 Mitral configuration in ischemic heart disease. The left ventricle is dilated because of myocardial ischemia. Ventricular end-diastolic pressure is elevated and is the cause of the left atrial dilatation (arrow).

Because the fibrotic scar is thin, the calcific rim lies close to, and parallels, the outer border of the heart (Fig. 6–21). The infarcts visualized in the frontal projection involve the anterolateral wall of the left ventricle or its apex, although on a well-penetrated film it may be possible to detect a calcified infarct of the interventricular septum. Because of its proximity to the outer border of the heart, the calcific rim of an infarct can be confused with calcification of the pericardium. However, calcific deposits on the pericardium are usually coarser and more irregular. In addition, they tend to accumulate over the atrioventricular sulci and the interventricular groove to a greater extent than over the free wall of the left ventricle (Fig. 6–22).

An *aneurysm* that is not calcified can be detected when it projects beyond the normal cardiac contour. Even when the left ventricle is markedly enlarged, the border of the chamber is made up of a single smooth curve. A localized bulge in this curve is presumptive evidence of a ventricular aneurysm (see Figure 6–3B). However, some aneurysms project from the cardiac contour only during systole and blend in with the curve of the distended ventricle during diastole. This type of aneurysm may be recognizable by means of fluoroscopy, but as a rule, fluoroscopy is not a very effective method for detection of a ventricular aneurysm. Considerably more than half of all aneurysms will be hidden within the cardiac silhouette and cannot be detected by fluoroscopy.[16] In the occasional case when an aneurysm is so large that it forms most of the left cardiac contour, the appearance of the heart can be almost identical to that of a failing ventricle due to diffuse as opposed to localized myocardial fibrosis (Fig. 6–23). Fluoroscopic examination is useful in this instance to determine the need for angiocardiography. In most cases, an aneurysm of this

size will pulsate paradoxically, whereas the pulsations of a dilated, flabby ventricle will be in proper phase, although grossly diminished in amplitude.

Calcific deposits within the coronary arteries are usually thin and their shadows are not very dense. Because of the blurring caused by motion of the heart, they are almost never seen on plain films, and a careful fluoroscopic examination is required for their detection. Most commonly, calcification occurs first in the proximal portions of the coronary arteries near the base of the heart. When the calcification is more extensive, it may be seen more distally in the vessels in the atrioventricular sulci or the interventricular groove. Calcific plaques are too fine to be visible when viewed *en face* and are seen only where they are projected tangentially. Thus, coronary calcification appears as a single, sharp, linear shadow or, if the entire circumference of the vessel is involved, as two parallel linear densities. When the calcified vessel is projected on end, it casts a fine, ring-shaped shadow.

Coronary artery calcification is very common in patients with ischemic heart disease.[17,18] However, it does not always indicate the presence of ischemic heart disease. The significance of calcification of the coronary arteries varies with the age of the patient, the incidence of coronary artery calcification not associated with stenosis increasing with age. It has little importance as an indicator of significant coronary artery narrowing in patients older than 65 or 70.[18,19] On the other hand, there is an extremely high

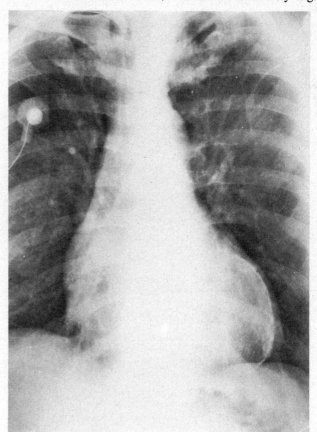

FIGURE 6–21 Calcified myocardial infarct. The rim of calcium paralleling the lateral border of the heart outlines an old infarct of the anterolateral left ventricular wall. Although the calcification extends around to the anterior and posterior surfaces of the ventricle, it is well visualized only where it is projected tangentially.

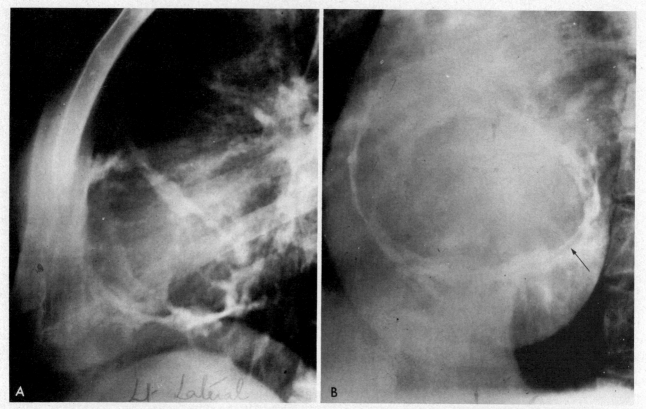

FIGURE 6–22   Pericardial calcification. *A,* Lateral chest film of a young woman showing dense, calcific patches distributed along the course of the atrioventricular sulcus and over the anterior portion of the right ventricle. *B,* Left anterior oblique view. The lucent line within the calcified sulcus (arrow) most likely represents the circumflex branch of the left coronary artery, which is not calcified. (Courtesy of Dr. S. Bharati.)

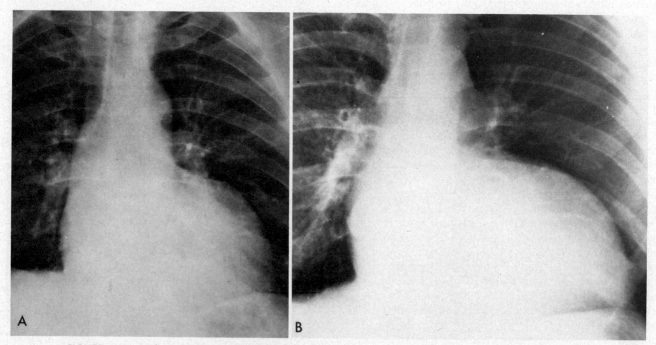

FIGURE 6–23   Left ventricular aneurysm. *A,* The aneurysm is so large that it forms almost the entire lateral profile of the left ventricle. (From Donoso, E., and Gorlin, R. [eds.]: Current Cardiovascular Topics. Vol. 3, Angina Pectoris. New York, Stratton Intercontinental Medical Book Co., 1977.) *B,* An almost identical appearance can be caused by the dilated, failing ventricle that results from diffuse ischemic disease. The two can be distinguished by fluoroscopy, because an aneurysm of this size will show paradoxical pulsations.

correlation between coronary artery calcification and coronary artery disease in patients under the age of 50. Because the search for coronary artery calcification is time-consuming and involves moderate radiation exposure, it is not a suitable screening procedure. There is little point in searching for such calcification in patients who have other evidence of coronary atherosclerosis or who are in the older age group. From a practical standpoint, such a study is best limited to younger patients who have chest pain of unknown etiology.[20]

Mitral Valve Disease (See also Chapter 32)

Disease of the mitral valve, whether it causes stenosis or regurgitation, results in dilatation of the left atrium. When *mitral stenosis* predominates, the heart is usually normal in size, and the left atrium may be the only chamber that is enlarged. There is a poor correlation between the size of the left atrium and the severity of the mitral stenosis, but moderate to marked left atrial enlargement occurs more commonly in patients with atrial fibrillation than in those with normal sinus rhythm.[21,22] In *mitral regurgitation,* diastolic overloading of the left ventricle causes the chamber to enlarge together with the left atrium. In practice, it is difficult to determine which of the two lesions is predominant.

Longstanding, moderate, or severe mitral stenosis is commonly associated with pulmonary arterial hypertension and dilatation of the right ventricle. As a result, the transverse diameter of the heart is widened, and the cardiac apex is displaced to the left. Dilatation of the left ventricle also widens the cardiac silhouette to the left, so that in many cases it is difficult to be sure whether the cardiac enlargement is due to the right ventricle alone or to both ventricles. This is further complicated by the fact that rheumatic heart disease often involves both the aortic and mitral valves. The combination of aortic regurgitation and mitral stenosis can produce a cardiac shape indistinguishable from that associated with mitral regurgitation. Conversely, a marked degree of mitral regurgitation may be present in the absence of significant enlargement of the left ventricle. This is most commonly seen following rupture of a papillary muscle or a chorda tendineae, when regurgitation, although severe, is of recent onset.[23]

Calcification of the mitral valve (Fig. 6–9) is indicative of stenosis (although there may be some accompanying regurgitation). The calcium is usually deposited in clumps on the valve leaflets but may also involve the commissures.[24] Extensive calcification may be visible on chest films, but fluoroscopy is required to detect smaller deposits. Valvular calcification must be distinguished from *calcification of the mitral annulus.* The latter occurs in older patients, particularly women,[25] and as long as the calcification does not extend onto the valve leaflets, it does not signify the presence of mitral valve disease.[26] The calcified annulus appears as a broad, curved shadow that may form a complete ring or, if the entire annulus is not involved, a U-shaped or J-shaped density. The curve of a calcified annulus has a larger diameter than that of a calcified valve, and it tends to appear as one continuous deposit rather than as separate calcific clumps (Fig. 6–24).

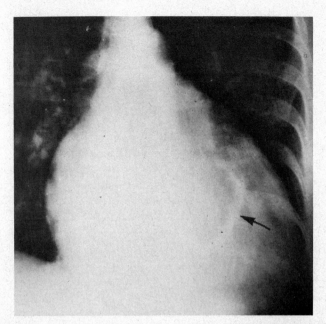

FIGURE 6–24 Calcification of the mitral annulus. The broad, curved density (arrow) in the mitral region represents calcification of the valve annulus. The arc of the calcific shadow is larger than that of the mitral orifice, distinguishing it from calcification of the leaflets, and it is too small for the calcium to be within the atrioventricular sulcus.

Except for its rare occurrence in metabolic calcinosis, calcification of the left atrium signifies mitral stenosis. The calcification may appear as a thin shell completely outlining the atrial wall or as a curvilinear shadow involving only one portion of the atrial circumference. The posterior atrial wall is the area most commonly involved and is best seen in the lateral view, below the carina and just in front of the esophagus (Fig. 6–25). If the atrial appendage is calcified, it presents as a short, arcuate density along the left border of the heart below the pulmonary segment in the frontal view and within the midportion of the cardiac silhouette in the lateral view. In the great majority of cases, a mural thrombus is present when the left atrium is calcified.[27] The calcium is usually deposited within the wall of the atrium but on occasion is present only within the thrombus.[28]

Narrowing of the mitral orifice results in elevation of left atrial and pulmonary venous pressures. Eventually, pulmonary hypertension may result. These changes are associated with a sequence of alterations in the appearance of the lungs and especially of the pulmonary vascular pattern. The resultant pictures are not specific for mitral stenosis but occur with any disease that causes an elevation of left atrial pressure (p. 172). *Pulmonary hemosiderosis* and pulmonary ossifications, however, are rarely encountered with any form of heart disease other than mitral stenosis.

Because of the chronic pulmonary congestion and elevated capillary pressure caused by mitral stenosis, small intraalveolar hemorrhages are common. Hemosiderin from the broken-down red cells is picked up by phagocytes, and clusters of these iron-laden cells form small nodules that can be seen on the chest film.[29,30] Their appearance is almost identical to that seen in idiopathic hemosiderosis or

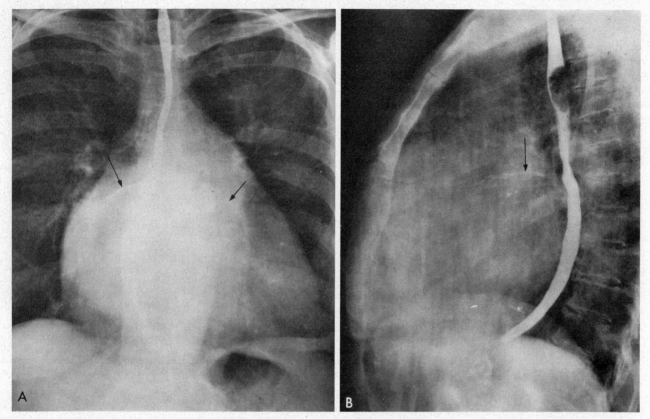

FIGURE 6-25 Calcification of the left atrium in rheumatic mitral disease. *A,* Frontal view. The left atrium is enlarged, its upper margin outlined by a fine rim of calcium (arrows). The right atrium is dilated, and there is biventricular enlargement. *B,* Lateral view. The calcified superior wall of the atrium is visualized (arrow) just below the level of the carina. The esophagus is displaced backward in a continuous curve that extends to the diaphragm, indicating dilatation of both left atrium and left ventricle.

in some of the miliary lung diseases (Fig. 6–26*A*). Although in mitral stenosis the nodules are distributed mainly in the mid and lower lung fields, rather than evenly throughout the lungs, the main differential point is the association with a cardiac shadow that has a mitral configuration.

Pulmonary ossifications are probably also the result of intraalveolar hemorrhage. The nodules of bone lie within the alveoli, mostly in the lower portions of the lungs. They are larger and more dense than hemosiderotic nodules and are fewer in number (Fig. 6–26*B*). The nodules vary considerably in size and often have an irregular shape. This, together with their distribution, serves to differentiate them from other calcific nodules in the lungs, such as those caused by histoplasmosis or chickenpox pneumonia.[31] Both pulmonary hemosiderosis and ossifications occur in patients with longstanding mitral disease, often with pulmonary hypertension. However, the two are unrelated, and it is not uncommon for one to be present without the other. The bony nodules are pathognomonic of mitral stenosis but can occur when the valve is partially occluded by a myxoma of the left atrium.[32]

Aortic Valve Disease (See also Chapter 32)

Aortic regurgitation causes elongation and dilatation of the left ventricle. The cardiac apex is displaced downward, to the left, and posteriorly (Fig. 6–4*A*). Often the entire ascending aorta is dilated, and fluoroscopic examination reveals an increase in the amplitude of its pulsations.

Aortic stenosis is more difficult to recognize on chest films. The heart is usually normal in size or only slightly enlarged, even with severe narrowing of the valve. However, the shape of the heart is often abnormal. Concentric hypertrophy of the left ventricle causes an increase in the curvature of the lower left cardiac contour and blunting of the cardiac apex (Fig. 6–27). Elongation of the long ventricular axis occurs occasionally in pure aortic stenosis but is never marked. Significant dilatation of the left ventricle in the absence of aortic regurgitation indicates failure of the myocardium and heralds the end stage of the disease.

Calcification of the aortic valve is common in congenital as well as acquired stenosis.[33,34] Poststenotic dilatation involving the ascending aorta at the junction of its proximal and middle thirds also occurs with both types of aortic stenosis. The poststenotic bulge may protrude from the right side of the mediastinum in the frontal view but is best seen on the left anterior oblique projection.[35] There is no correlation between the degree of poststenotic dilatation and the severity of the stenosis.[36] A similar localized dilatation of the ascending aorta can occur when the stenosis is due to a membranous web in the subvalvular region, but it is not associated with the hypertrophic form of subaortic stenosis.

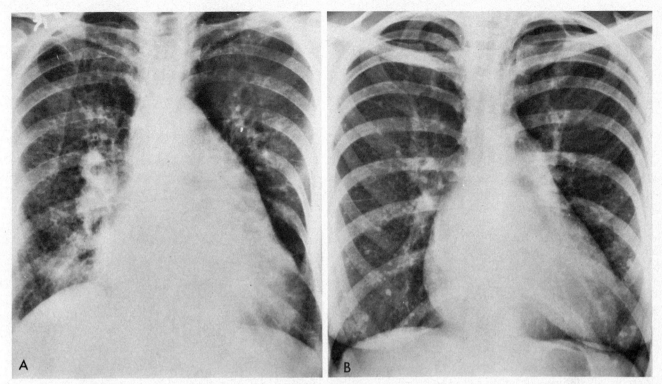

FIGURE 6-26 Lung changes in mitral stenosis. *A,* Pulmonary hemosiderosis. The lower lungs are studded with small nodules of moderate radiodensity. The left atrium and left ventricle are enlarged. Kerley B lines are present in the lateral basal portions of the lungs. *B,* Pulmonary ossifications. Scattered calcific nodules of differing size and shape are present in the lower lungs. They represent foci of organized bone within the alveoli. The left atrium is enlarged, and a double contour can be seen through the right side of the cardiac silhouette. The left atrial appendage is obscured by the dilated left ventricle.

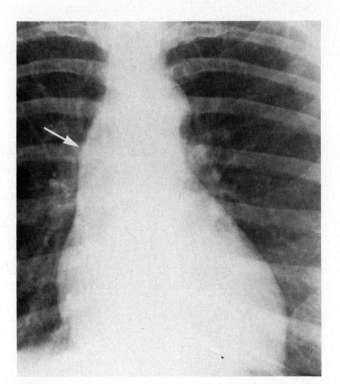

FIGURE 6-27 Aortic stenosis. The transverse diameter of the heart is slightly enlarged, and the curvature of the left cardiac contour is accentuated, suggesting left ventricular hypertrophy. The prominence of the midascending aorta (arrow) is due to poststenotic dilatation. A gradient of 90 mm Hg was measured across the aortic valve.

PRIMARY MYOCARDIAL DISEASE (See also Chapter 41)

The roentgen manifestations depend on whether the main effect of the disease is impairment of myocardial contractility, as in congestive (dilated) cardiomyopathy, or thickening of the ventricular wall, as in restrictive or hypertrophic cardiomyopathy. In either case, the heart may appear normal in the early stages or when the disease is of limited severity. More extensive involvement usually results in cardiac enlargement.

Diminution of ventricular function is reflected in an increase in the size of the ventricles. The cardiac silhouette is enlarged and tends to have a globular shape. The transverse cardiac diameter is widened, the curves of the heart border are accentuated, and cardiac pulsations are diminished. The hilar vessels are often prominent because of elevated left ventricular end-diastolic pressure, and the overall appearance of the heart may be similar to that seen with extensive ischemic disease of the myocardium.

In general, the degree of cardiac dilatation is proportional to the impairment of myocardial function. This relationship does not hold with myocardial hypertrophy. Severe and incapacitating degrees of hypertrophy may be present with only minimal or moderate cardiac enlargement. Most commonly, only the left ventricle is hypertrophied, but both ventricles may be involved. As the wall of the left ventricle thickens, the transverse cardiac diameter increases and the curvature of the left heart border becomes accentuated. This configuration is suggestive of myocardial hypertrophy, but as a rule the chest film is of little value in establishing a definite diagnosis or in evaluating the extent of the disease.

Congenital Heart Disease
(See also Chapters 29 and 30)

As a general rule, the younger the patient with congenital heart disease, the more difficult it is to make an accurate diagnosis from films of the chest. Although some congenital lesions seen in infants are associated with a fairly characteristic cardiac silhouette, e.g., the egg-shaped heart of complete transposition of the great arteries (see Figure 29–57, p. 1000), or the "snowman" heart of total anomalous pulmonary venous drainage; in a significant number of cases these same lesions produce nonspecific changes. Furthermore, infants who attract clinical attention because of heart disease often have complex abnormalities that involve multiple lesions, each one producing some distortion of the cardiac silhouette and thus compounding the diagnostic difficulties. An additional problem is the inability to see the heart clearly in infants because it is obscured by the overlapping shadow of the thymus. Perhaps the most important information regarding the nature of heart disease in young children is gained from the appearance of the pulmonary vessels. A decrease in the vasculature indicates a right-to-left shunt, while an increase usually indicates a left-to-right shunt.

Actually, in the symptomatic child, the radiological appearance of the heart is not of major diagnostic importance, because these children will usually require further study with other imaging modalities such as echocardiography or angiocardiography in order to delineate the specific cardiac abnormalities accurately. Once the correct diagnosis is established, the course of the disease or the results of surgical correction can be followed with serial chest films. For these purposes, the pertinent parameters are changes in cardiac size and shape and the pulmonary vascular pattern. The routine chest film is considerably more important in the *detection* of congenital cardiac lesions that were overlooked in childhood.

ATRIAL SEPTAL DEFECT (See also pp. 960 and 1031). With the exception of the bicuspid aortic valve, the secundum type of atrial septal defect is the most common congenital cardiac lesion of adult life.[37–39] A significant number of these patients are first recognized as having heart disease because of an abnormal chest film, while others have been considered to have rheumatic mitral stenosis.[40,41] The characteristic picture of an atrial septal defect shows a generalized increase in pulmonary vascularity, dilatation of the main pulmonary artery, and enlargement of the right ventricle (Fig. 6–28). These findings are present in almost every case in which there is a significant shunt. The right atrium is often dilated, particularly in older patients. Enlargement of the left atrium is not uncommon and occurs in more than half of patients over the age of 40.[40,42] Enlargement of the left atrium may be related to the presence of atrial fibrillation or, in older patients, can represent one of the effects of coronary artery disease. In other cases, the size of the atrium is referable to the regurgitation of left ventricular blood because of prolapse of the mitral valve during systole. There is a statistically significant association between mitral valve prolapse and atrial septal defect[43,44] (p. 1090).

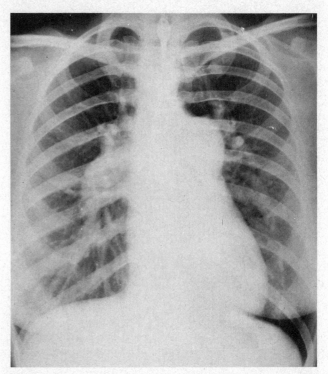

FIGURE 6–28   Atrial septal defect. The transverse diameter of the heart in this 25-year-old woman is within normal limits. The main pulmonary artery is greatly dilated, and the pulmonary vessels throughout the lungs are widened, indicating a left-to-right shunt. Right ventricular pressure was 87/5 mm Hg.

There is little correlation between the appearance of the heart and lungs and the size of the atrial shunt or the pulmonary arterial pressure. Heart size seems to be related more to the age of the patient than to any other single factor. As a general rule, for any given set of hemodynamic parameters, the older the patient, the larger the heart.[42,45]

The left-to-right shunt through the atrial septal defect increases pulmonary blood flow and causes the vessels in the lungs to dilate. Although the pulmonary pressure may be considerably elevated because of the increased flow, it usually declines after the defect is closed. However, when the pulmonary hypertension is due to an elevation of vascular resistance rather than of pulmonary blood flow,[46] it usually remains the same or may even progress following surgical correction. The two causes of pulmonary hypertension cannot always be differentiated from the chest film. Although in many cases the typical changes of elevated pulmonary resistance are reflected in a marked disparity between the dilated central pulmonary arteries and the constricted peripheral vessels (Fig. 6–29), severe elevation of vascular resistance can be present while the peripheral pulmonary vessels still appear engorged.

Differentiation of an atrial septal defect from other left-to-right shunts is often possible if there is marked pulmonary plethora. The peripheral pulmonary vessels are usually constricted when there is a large ventricular septal defect, and a patent ductus arteriosus rarely causes such marked vascular dilatation. Distinction between a secundum type of atrial septal defect and an ostium primum lesion is usually not possible. In general, the heart tends to be larger with the latter defect, and because of the pres-

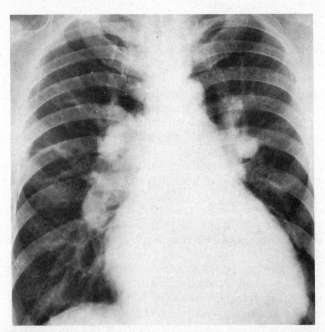

FIGURE 6–29 Atrial septal defect, with elevated pulmonary vascular resistance. Secundum atrial septal defect. There is a marked disparity between the size of the hilar arteries and the peripheral pulmonary vessels, indicating an increase in pulmonary vascular resistance. The right ventricular pressure was almost at systemic levels.

ence of mitral regurgitation, dilatation of the left atrium is more common. A secundum atrial septal defect in which the left atrium is enlarged can present a cardiac configuration almost identical to that seen with mitral valve disease. The distinction between the two conditions can be made from the appearance of the pulmonary vessels. In mitral stenosis, there is a redistribution of pulmonary blood flow with constriction of the vessels at the lung bases and dilatation of the vessels in the upper lobes. When there is significant shunting through an atrial septal defect, all the pulmonary vessels, at the bases as well as at the apices, are dilated (Fig. 6–30*A*). However, once the characteristic vascular pattern of elevated pulmonary resistance appears, it often is not possible to differentiate an atrial septal defect from other causes of pulmonary hypertension.

PATENT DUCTUS ARTERIOSUS (See also pp. 967 and 1038). A small or moderate shunt through a patent ductus often produces no abnormalities in the radiological appearance of the heart or lungs. When the ductal flow is large, the pulmonary vessels become dilated, and the left atrium and left ventricle enlarge. The aorta is usually prominent in contrast to the rather diminutive aorta often seen with an atrial or a ventricular septal defect. However, this is not a strong differential point, particularly in adults. It is difficult to make an accurate diagnosis of a patent ductus from plain films unless the duct is calcified.

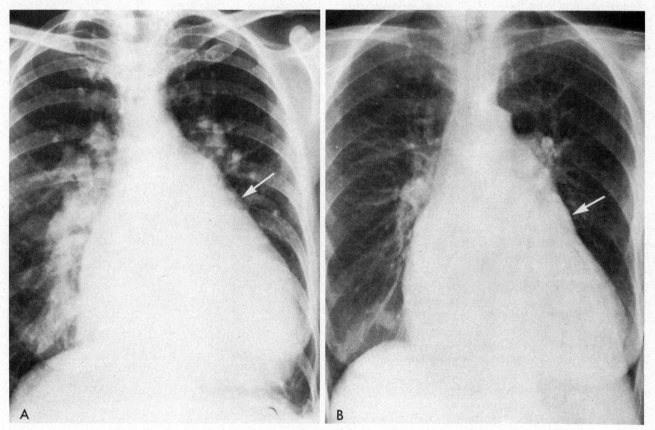

FIGURE 6–30 The diagnostic value of the pulmonary vascular pattern. *A*, Secundum atrial septal defect. The heart is large because of dilatation of the ventricles and the right atrium. The left atrium is also enlarged (arrow). Because of the left-to-right shunt, the pulmonary vessels throughout the lungs are dilated. *B*, Mitral stenosis. The shape of the heart is almost the same as in *A*. Both ventricles as well as the right atrium are dilated. The left atrium is enlarged (arrow) and extends to the right beyond the border of the right atrium. Pulmonary vessels in the lung bases are constricted, while vessels in the upper lobe are distended. The redistribution of pulmonary blood flow is characteristic of postcapillary pulmonary hypertension; this does not occur with a left-to-right shunt.

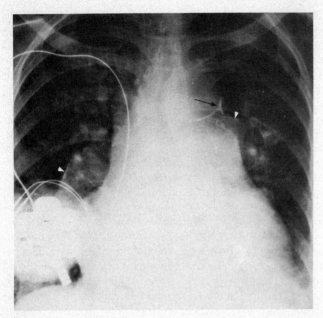

FIGURE 6-31 Calcification of the ductus arteriosus. The inverted Y-shaped calcific deposit (black arrow) is diagnostic of a patent ductus arteriosus. The calcified duct forms the vertical portion of the shadow, while the lower limbs represent calcification in the roof of the main pulmonary artery. Calcium has also been deposited in the walls of the hilar pulmonary arteries (white arrowheads). These vessels are markedly dilated, but the peripheral vessels are constricted, indicating the presence of elevated pulmonary resistance.

Calcification of the ductus is relatively uncommon, but when present it provides a pathognomonic x-ray picture. The calcified ductus is seen as a curvilinear density within the aortic shadow below the arotic knob,[47] slanting downward and to the right. It does not parallel the outer border of the descending aorta, which differentiates it from a calcific atheromatous plaque on the aortic wall. The ductus calcification often has an inverted Y-shape, with the lower limbs representing extension of the calcification onto the main pulmonary artery (Fig. 6–31). Although calcification of the ligamentum arteriosum has been observed on rare occasions at autopsy, it can be assumed that when a calcified ductus is identified on a chest film, it is patent. In most cases, the pulmonary artery pressure is elevated and there is reversal of the shunt.

PULMONIC VALVE STENOSIS (See also pp. 986 and 1037). Because of the increased resistance to ventricular emptying, stenosis of the pulmonic valve is accompanied by hypertrophy of the right ventricle. This has little effect on the configuration of the cardiac silhouette, and significant enlargement of the heart is uncommon. Nevertheless, the heart often has a characteristic appearance because of poststenotic dilatation of the pulmonary artery. Dilatation of the main pulmonary artery is related to distortion of the pressure vectors within the vessel caused by the high-velocity jet of blood spurting through the stenotic valve.[48] Because the jet is usually directed toward the left, the left pulmonary artery tends to be dilated. In addition, the artery protrudes farther laterally than normal. In the frontal view, the shadow of the main pulmonary artery is increased in height and width and often is considerably larger than the normal-sized aortic knob. The left pulmonary artery, which usually courses almost directly posteri-

orly and is largely hidden by the main pulmonary artery, is abnormally prominent because it projects outward from the hilum (Fig. 6–32). These changes may not be evident in infants or young children.

The roentgen diagnosis of pulmonic valve stenosis is based on dilatation of the main pulmonary artery and prominence of the left pulmonary artery. If the latter is not dilated or displaced laterally, the diagnosis is much less certain. Dilatation of only the main pulmonary artery can be seen with pulmonic valve stenosis but also occurs with idiopathic dilatation of the pulmonary artery and in some cases of patent ductus. Prominence of the left pulmonary artery without dilatation of the main pulmonary artery is of little significance and most commonly is due to elevation of the hilum secondary to partial shrinkage of the left upper lobe because of previous inflammatory disease.

The cardiac output is usually within normal limits in isolated pulmonic stenosis. In the absence of an atrial or ventricular septal defect, all the blood ejected by the right ventricle must flow through the pulmonary circulation. The vascularity of the lungs is therefore not decreased, no matter how tight the valvular stenosis. However, in the end stages of the disease, once the right ventricle fails, pulmonary blood flow may decrease considerably, and this is associated with marked dilatation of the right ventricle and right atrium (Fig. 6–33).

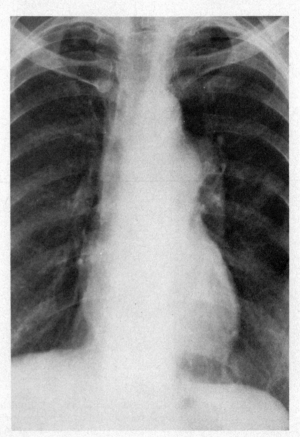

FIGURE 6-32 Pulmonic valvular stenosis. The heart is normal in size, but the main pulmonary artery is dilated. The left pulmonary artery is considerably wider than the right and protrudes outward from the cardiac shadow. The peripheral pulmonary vasculature is within the limits of normal.

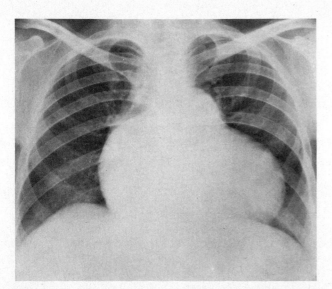

FIGURE 6–33 Pulmonic valvular stenosis with right heart failure. Congenital stenosis of the pulmonic valve in a 38-year-old woman. The shadow of the heart is widened to the left, and the cardiac apex is rounded and elevated because of dilatation of the right ventricle. The tricuspid valve was regurgitant, and the right atrium is markedly enlarged. The main pulmonary artery is dilated, and there is decreased vascularity of the lungs.

COARCTATION OF THE AORTA (See also pp. 973 and 1038).

In most cases, the diagnosis of coarctation of the aorta can be made from the frontal chest film.[49] The aortic knob and the uppermost portion of the descending aorta have a rather constant abnormal contour. Classically, this is described as having a "figure-three" configuration (Fig. 6–34). The upper convex arc is formed by the aortic knob and the left subclavian artery, while the lower arc represents the dilated portion of the aorta immediately beyond the stenotic area.[50] The indentation on the lateral aortic contour, between the two bulges, marks the site of the coarctation. The aorta also produces a double indentation on the left margin of the barium-filled esophagus, the curves being a mirror image of those on the lateral border of the aorta. In many cases, however, this pathognomonic appearance is not present. Obliteration of the aortic knob, although less specific, is a more constant sign of coarctation.

The aortic knob is not a discrete anatomical structure. It represents the most posterior portion of the aortic arch, distal to the origin of the left subclavian artery as it turns downward to become the descending aorta. Where the curve of the aorta is parallel to the x-ray beam, it is viewed on end and is projected as a circular shadow. The right portion of the shadow cannot be seen as it blends in with the mediastinum, but the remainder of the shadow forms a localized bulge on the left side of the mediastinum—the aortic knob.

When there is coarctation of the aorta, the aortic arch appears to be foreshortened,[51] and the left subclavian artery arises from its descending limb, near the coarcted segment and beyond the aortic knob (see Figure 29–26, p. 975). The subclavian artery is usually dilated and comes into profile along the left side of the mediastinum, thus overlying and obscuring the medial portion, or all, of the aortic knob (Figs. 6–18 and 6–35).[52] Although obscuration

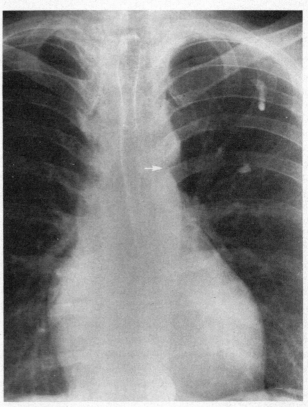

FIGURE 6–34 Coarctation of the aorta. The lateral border of the proximal descending aorta is composed of two arcs separated by a sharp indentation (arrow). The latter represents the site of coarctation. The upper bulge is formed by the dilated left subclavian artery, which obscures the aortic knob, and the lower bulge is caused by poststenotic dilatation of the aorta. The two bulges also indent the barium-coated esophagus. (From Baron, M. G.: Obscuration of the aortic knob in coarctation of the aorta. Circulation *43*:311, 1971, by permission of the American Heart Association, Inc.)

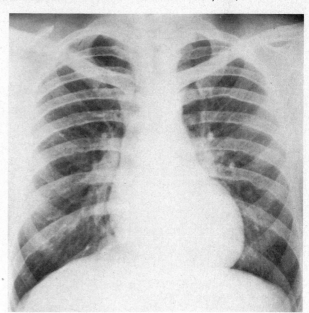

FIGURE 6–35 Coarctation of the aorta. The size of the heart in this young boy is within the limits of normal, but the rounding of the cardiac apex suggests left ventricular hypertrophy. The aortic knob is obscured, and there is notching of the ribs. Each indentation on the undersurface of a rib is outlined by a rim of sclerotic bone, characteristic of the notches that result from pressure atrophy of bone.

of the knob is suggestive of coarctation, a similar appearance can be caused by enlargement of the supraaortic lymph nodes or by obliteration of the pulmonary recess above the aorta, usually as a result of pleuritis.

Because of the increased resistance to blood flow offered by the coarcted segment, a collateral circulation usually develops between the internal mammary arteries, which arise above the coarctation and the intercostal arteries that join the aorta below the coarcted segment. The intercostal arteries become dilated and tortuous, and the amplitude of their pulsations increases. The constant pounding of the arteries on the undersurfaces of the ribs causes localized erosions of the bone and produces multiple, discrete notches. True rib notches can be distinguished from the normal irregularities of the inferior rib margins because each notch is outlined by a rim of sclerotic bone (Fig. 6–35).

Notching of the ribs, together with obscuration of the aortic knob, is diagnostic of coarctation of the aorta. Absence of rib notching, however, does not exclude the diagnosis, since this occurs in almost one-fourth of all adults with coarctation.[53] On the other hand, rib notching alone is not a specific finding. Although coarctation of the aorta is the most common cause, notching does occur in a number of other conditions.[54]

INDICATORS OF CONGENITAL HEART DISEASE

Certain extracardiac abnormalities are commonly associated with anomalies of the heart. Some of these are evident on the chest film and, although it may not be possible to deduce the presence of a specific cardiac lesion from their presence, they do indicate the likelihood of coexisting congenital heart disease.

ABNORMALITIES OF SITUS. Normally, the apex of the heart is on the same side as the left atrium. Thus, the apex is on the left in situs solitus and on the right in situs inversus. However, in certain anomalies, the cardiac apex may lie on the opposite side and cannot be used as an indicator of situs. Nevertheless, the situs can usually be determined from the chest film. If the aortic knob and the stomach bubble are on the same side, the left atrium will also be on that side.[55] The position of the left atrium indicates the situs of the heart.

Discordance between the cardiac apex and the gastric air bubble—regardless of which side each is on and regardless of the situs of the patient—almost always signifies the presence of ventricular inversion or polysplenia. This does not hold if the abnormal position of the heart is secondary to pulmonary disease. Occasionally, the

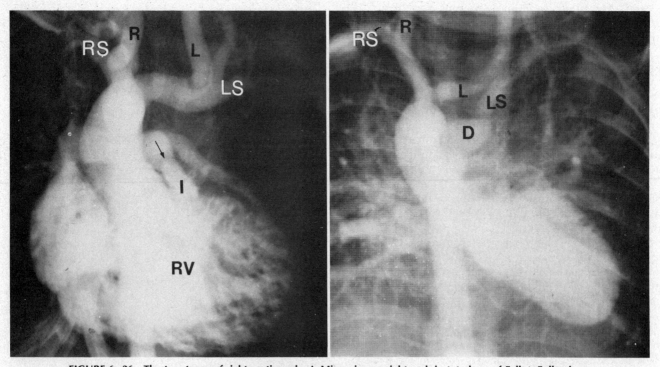

FIGURE 6–36   The two types of right aortic arch. *A,* Mirror-image right arch in tetralogy of Fallot. Following a venous injection of contrast material, the aorta and pulmonary artery become opacified simultaneously. The right ventricle (RV) extends to the left border of the heart and obscures the left ventricle. The infundibulum (I) is narrowed. The pulmonic valve is stenotic (arrow). The first branch to arise from the right aortic arch is the left innominate artery, which gives rise to the left common carotid (L) and the left subclavian artery (LS). The second branch is the right common carotid artery (R) and, lastly, the right subclavian artery (RS). *B,* Right arch with posterior diverticulum. Levocardiogram phase of a venous angiogram. The first branch to arise from the right aortic arch is the left common carotid artery (L), followed by the right common carotid artery (R) and the right subclavian artery (RS). A large diverticulum (D) extends from the distal aortic arch to the left and gives rise to the left subclavian artery (LS). (*B* from Baron, M. G.: Right aortic arch. Circulation *44*:1137, 1971, by permission of the American Heart Association, Inc.)

situs of the patient is indeterminate. The cardiac silhouette is usually abnormal, the apex often cannot be identified, the stomach may be on either side, and the liver shadow extends across the upper abdomen. This picture is diagnostic of asplenia, a syndrome associated with multiple, profound cardiac anomalies.[56-58]

RIGHT AORTIC ARCH. There are two major types of right aortic arch. In the first, the pattern of origin of the great vessels is a mirror image of the pattern found when there is a normal left arch. The first branch to arise from the proximal portion of the arch is a left innominate artery, which divides into the left common carotid artery and the left subclavian artery. The next branch is the right common carotid artery and, lastly, the right subclavian artery (Fig. 6–36A). All the vessels lie anterior to the trachea. In the second type of right arch, there is no innominate artery. The first vessel arising from the aorta is the left common carotid artery, followed by the right common carotid and then the right subclavian artery. The left subclavian arises independently as a fourth branch from the aorta. Actually, it does not come directly from the aorta but originates from a diverticulum of the distal arch, which extends to the left behind the esophagus (Fig. 6–36B). This last type of right arch is the one most commonly encountered in adults and is not associated with an increased incidence of congenital heart disease. On the other hand, a cardiac anomaly, most often tetralogy of Fallot, is present in over 90 per cent of those cases with a mirror-image type of right arch.[59,60]

Both types of right aortic arch appear the same on the frontal chest film. The aortic knob is situated on the right side of the mediastinum and displaces the trachea to the left. If the esophagus is opacified, the aortic indentation is seen on its right border. Differentiation between the two types of right arch can be made from the appearance of the barium-filled esophagus in the lateral view. The posterior diverticulum commonly present in the "benign" type of right arch produces a marked, localized anterior bowing of the upper esophagus.[61] With a mirror-image right arch, all the great vessels course in front of the trachea, and the esophagus appears normal in the lateral view.

AZYGOS CONTINUATION OF THE INFERIOR VENA CAVA. When the suprarenal portion of the inferior vena cava fails to develop, blood from the lower extremities, the kidneys, and the retroperitoneum returns to the heart by way of the azygos venous system. Although this may exist as an isolated anomaly, it is often associated with congenital heart disease, particularly the polysplenia syndrome. Because of the increased blood flow, the azygos vein is dilated and appears as a rounded mass in the right tracheobronchial angle. The true nature of the mass can often be recognized by means of fluoroscopic examination, since the vein will diminish in size when the patient performs the Valsalva maneuver. In addition, the upper portion of the dilated azygos trunk may be visible on adequately penetrated films along the right side of the vertebral bodies.[62]

Dilatation of the azygos vein does not necessarily signify an abnormality of the inferior vena cava. The vein may be enlarged as a result of congestive failure or portal hypertension. However, in the absence of a known cause for azygos vein dilatation, a femoral venogram may be required to determine whether there is an interruption of the inferior vena cava.

THE PULMONARY VASCULATURE

Almost all the linear shadows within the lung field are cast by the pulmonary arteries and veins. The normal vessels radiate outward from the hila and exhibit an orderly branching pattern as they extend peripherally. The vessels taper gradually, becoming progressively smaller with each successive division. An abrupt change in the caliber of a vessel is abnormal. Vessels at the lung bases are normally larger than those at the apices because they serve a greater volume of lung (Chap. 17). The terminal branches of the arteries and veins, in the outer third of the lungs, are so small that most cannot be visualized as individual structures. Nevertheless, the summation of their shadows imparts a slight overall density to the pulmonary fields. It is often possible to distinguish pulmonary veins from pulmonary arteries because the veins course toward the left atrium and converge to enter the cardiac silhouette at a lower level than do the arteries. In the upper lobes, the vessels follow parallel courses with the vein lateral to the artery.[63]

DECREASED PULMONARY BLOOD FLOW. The size of the pulmonary vessels conforms to the volume of blood within them. When flow is diminished, the vessels become narrow, and many of the small branches are no longer visible. Because of the paucity of vascular shadows in the peripheral pulmonary fields, the background density of the lung decreases and the lungs appear abnormally radiolucent.

A regional decrease in perfusion, which can involve as much as an entire lung, is commonly produced by an embolus of a pulmonary artery or one of its branches[64] (p. 1586). A similar change can result from partial obstruction of a vessel because of vasoconstriction or extrinsic compression. In any case, the increase in local vascular resistance causes a redistribution of blood flow to other portions of the lung, and the affected area becomes oligemic.

Diffuse diminution of pulmonary vascularity involving both lungs can occur with right heart failure or in the presence of a right-to-left shunt. In the former instance, the decreased blood flow reflects an abnormally low cardiac output, and the right heart chambers are dilated. When there is a right-to-left shunt, the lungs are oligemic because some of the blood from the right heart bypasses the pulmonary circulation (see Figure 29–43, p. 991). In almost all instances, the main pulmonary artery is small, and its segment on the left cardiac contour may lose its normal convexity or, as in the boot-shaped heart of the tetralogy of Fallot, become concave (Fig. 6–37).

A marked decrease in pulmonary blood flow is usually accompanied by an increase in the bronchial collateral circulation. Although it is possible for the bronchial vessels to become so prominent that the vascularity of the lung actually appears to be increased, the resulting vascular pattern is abnormal. Bronchial arteries arise from the descending aorta and do not radiate out from the pulmonary hilum. Because of the decreased pulmonary arterial flow, the hilar shadows are small. The bronchial vessels do not branch in a regular fashion, and there is little difference between their caliber in the central portions of the lung

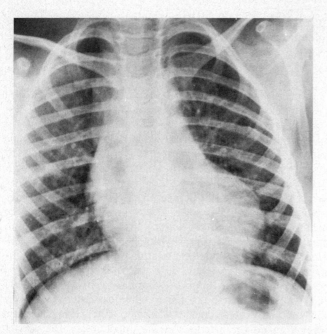

FIGURE 6–37 Bronchial collateral circulation in tetralogy of Fallot. The heart is slightly widened, the apex is rounded and elevated, the prominence of the normal main pulmonary artery is absent, and there is a right aortic arch. These findings are typical of tetralogy of Fallot. Although the pulmonary vasculature does not appear decreased, its pattern is definitely abnormal. The vessels do not radiate from the hilum, do not branch in an orderly fashion, and do not taper as they progress outward into the lungs. This pattern is characteristic of bronchial collateral vessels.

and in the periphery (Fig. 6–37). This imparts a reticular appearance to the peripheral pulmonary field. Frequently, as the large bronchial arteries leave the aorta, they produce one or more indentations on the anterior border of the barium-filled esophagus.

INCREASED PULMONARY BLOOD FLOW. As pulmonary blood flow increases, the vessels in the lungs become enlarged and abnormally prominent. Lesser degrees of overcirculation produce no apparent change in the pulmonary vasculature, and small left-to-right shunts usually cannot be detected on plain films. A moderate increase in pulmonary vascularity can be seen in high-output states such as severe anemia, hyperthyroidism, or pregnancy and with left-to-right shunts. More marked pulmonary plethora is almost always due to a large shunt.

Overcirculation of blood results in dilatation and increasing tortuosity of the pulmonary arteries and veins. The vessels in the periphery of the lungs as well as those at the hila are affected (Fig. 6–28). All the vessels are enlarged, so that the normal gradation in size between the vessels at the lung bases and those at the apices is maintained. There is nothing specific about the appearance of the pulmonary vessels or their pattern to indicate the cause of the increased blood flow. However, if the patient is cyanotic, the presence of an increased circulation strongly suggests the diagnosis of a persistent truncus arteriosus, transposition of the great arteries (see Figure 29–57, p. 1000), or total anomalous venous drainage.

PULMONARY HYPERTENSION (See also Chapter 25). A significant increase in pulmonary blood flow causes the pressure within the pulmonary arteries to rise. The roentgen picture reflects the overcirculation of blood through the lungs rather than the degree of elevation of

the arterial pressure. On the other hand, when the hypertension results from an increase in pulmonary vascular resistance, the appearance of the lung parenchyma and the pulmonary vessels can provide a rather accurate indicator of pulmonary arterial and venous pressures.[65]

The pattern of vascular changes seen on the x-ray in pulmonary hypertension due to increased vascular resistance depends on the severity of the hypertension and the location of the lesions that impede blood flow through the lungs.[66,67] Lesions downstream in relation to the pulmonary capillary bed, such as mitral stenosis, or left ventricular failure cause elevation of pulmonary venous pressure. This affects all the pulmonary veins equally. However, the pressure in the veins at the bases of the lungs is higher than that at the apices in the erect man, because hydrostatic pressure is greatest in the dependent portions of the lungs. With relatively, slight increases in venous pressure, the veins tend to dilate, but as the venous pressure increases further, the veins constrict. Venoconstriction occurs first in the higher pressured veins of the lower lungs,[68–70] causing an elevation in local vascular resistance. The pulmonary blood flow is then redistributed to the areas of lesser resistance, the upper portions of the lungs. Radiologically, this is manifested by a reversal of the relative sizes of the pulmonary vessels. The shadows of the vessels at the lung bases become attenuated, while the upper lobe vessels dilate (Fig. 6–30B). Further elevation of pulmonary venous pressure usually results in interstitial pulmonary edema and, eventually, alveolar edema.

Narrowing of the small pulmonary arteries, from spasm of their muscular coat or thickening of the medial and intimal layers of their walls, results in precapillary pulmonary hypertension (Chap. 25). Many of the terminal arterial branches are often occluded. The peripheral vessels that remain decrease in size and no longer appear as individual shadows on the film. The outer portions of the lungs then appear more radiolucent than normal, and vascular markings are hardly visible at all.[71] Because of the generalized increase in the peripheral arterial resistance, pressure in the central vessels is elevated, and their elastic walls stretch. Thus, the main pulmonary artery, the right and left pulmonary arteries, and their first- and sometimes second-order branches become dilated. The decrease in the caliber of the vessels beyond this point is abrupt, and many of the branches appear to be amputated (Fig. 6–29).

Although precapillary pulmonary hypertension often occurs without abnormalities on the venous side of the circuit, as in primary pulmonary hypertension (Chap. 25) or pulmonary embolization (Chap. 46), it can also develop as a response to longstanding elevation of pulmonary venous pressure. This is commonly seen with stenosis of the mitral valve. Initially, there is a redistribution of pulmonary blood flow and evidence of interstitial edema, but over a period of time the typical picture of precapillary hypertension develops (Chap. 25). Hypertrophy and dilatation of the right atrium and ventricle occur in response to the elevation of pulmonary arterial pressure.

Pulmonary Edema (See also Chapter 17)

In the normal lung, there is a constant transudation of fluid from the pulmonary capillaries into the interstitial tissues. The fluid is drained by an extensive network of pulmonary lymphatics and eventually returns to the bloodstream. If fluid pours into the interstitium faster than it can be removed, the fluid content of the tissue increases. Although the patient may be severely tachypneic during this stage of interstitial edema, there are few, if any, abnormal auscultatory findings. Continued outpouring of fluid so overloads the interstitial tissues that the fluid leaks through the alveolar walls into the pulmonary air spaces.[72] As the alveoli fill, the characteristic bubbly rales of pulmonary edema appear, and the diagnosis becomes clinically obvious. However, the edematous thickening of the interstitial tissues that precedes the stage of alveolar edema produces changes in the roentgen appearance of the lungs that can be detected on the ordinary chest film. These films are a sensitive indicator of the development of pulmonary congestion.

INTERSTITIAL EDEMA. The interstitial connective tissues invest the bronchi and bronchioles as well as the pulmonary vessels, lymphatics, and nerves. They support the alveolar air spaces and form the septa that delimit the pulmonary lobules. This reticular interstitial network is too fine to cast recognizable individual shadows on the chest film, but the summation of all their superimposed shadows does contribute an overall, faint homogeneous density to the pulmonary fields.

Even when the interstitial tissues are thickened by edema, most are still too thin to cast discrete shadows. However, their summation now produces numerous, small linear shadows that are randomly distributed throughout the lungs. These overlap and distort the shadows of the pulmonary vessels so that they can no longer be clearly visualized (Fig. 6–38). In addition, where the vessels can be seen, their outlines are indistinct because of the edema of

the connective tissue that surrounds them.[73] Convergence of the pulmonary septa in the region of the lung roots causes an accentuation of the background density in this region, producing a perihilar haze (Fig. 6–39).[74]

Where the thickened interlobular septa are viewed on end, they may cast discrete shadows. This occurs most commonly in the outer portions of the lung bases. The edematous septa cast short, horizontal linear shadows that are parallel to each other and perpendicular to the pleural surface and are called Kerley B lines (Fig. 6–40).[75,76] Kerley A lines also appear when the interstitial tissues are swollen.[77,78] They are longer than B lines, measuring as much as 4 to 6 cm in length, and are not limited to the basal areas of the lungs. They are situated deep within the lungs and do not extend to the pleural surface (Fig. 6–39).

Edema of the subpleural connective tissue causes an increase in the thickness and density of the interlobar fissures, and often their shadows first become visible with the onset of congestive failure.[79] However, from a practical standpoint this sign is of little value. If the x-ray tube is not aligned perpendicular to the patient, even a thickened fissure will not be visualized because it is projected obliquely rather than on end. Films in an intensive care unit are usually made with portable equipment, and the orientation of the x-ray tube and the patient is determined visually by the technologist. The appearance or disappearance of a pleural fissure most often represents an artifact of positioning rather than the presence or absence of pulmonary congestion (Fig. 6–41).

The appearance of peribronchial cuffing is caused by edematous swelling of the bronchial walls and the connective tissue around the bronchi.[80] At least one of the bronchi is usually projected on end near the upper part of the

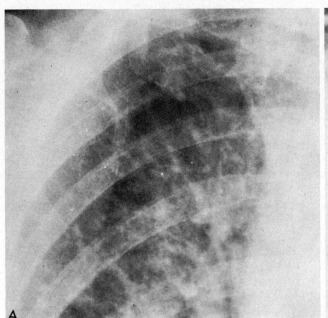
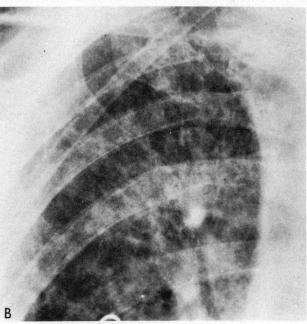

FIGURE 6–38 Interstitial pulmonary edema. *A,* Portable film made shortly after admission for an acute myocardial infarction. The vessels in the right upper lung are prominent and congested. However, their shadows can be delineated. At this time the patient was relatively asymptomatic. *B,* The following day the patient became tachypneic. The portable film shows an increase in the random shadows within the lung, obscuring the outlines of the pulmonary vessels. (From Rabin, C. B., and Baron, M. G.: Radiology of the Chest. Baltimore, Williams and Wilkins Co., 1979.)

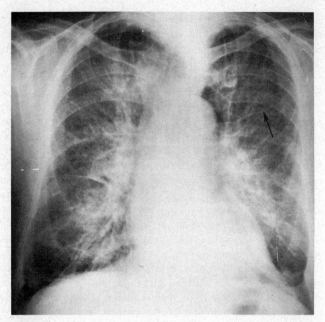

FIGURE 6-39 Interstitial pulmonary edema. There is an indistinct haze in the perihilar regions, and vascular shadows cannot be identified in the peripheral portions of the lungs. The short fissure on the right side is thickened because of subpleural edema, and the linear shadow in the left upper lobe (arrow) is a Kerley A line. (From Rabin, C. B., and Baron, M. G.: Radiology of the Chest. Baltimore, Williams and Wilkins Co., 1979.)

hilum and casts a thin, sharply outlined ring shadow. In the presence of interstitial edema, this shadow becomes broader and indistinct (Fig. 6-41). Vascular congestion is reflected by an increase in the thickness of the artery that accompanies the bronchus, but this is difficult to appreciate unless the diameter of the artery is accurately measured and compared with the diameter of the same vessel on previous films.

The roentgen picture of interstitial edema is not unique, and thickening of the interstitial tissues from almost any cause can produce a similar appearance. However, when thickening is due to fibrosis or lymphangitic carcinomatosis, for example, the shadows tend to be sharply outlined, whereas they are less distinct when due to edema. Preliminary work has indicated that nuclear magnetic resonance (NMR) imaging (Chap. 11B) will provide the most accurate measure of the amount of lung water and its distribution, independent of perfusion and ventilation abnormalities.[81]

ALVEOLAR EDEMA. The shadows of alveolar edema appear when the air in the alveoli is replaced by fluid. The appearance differs from other causes of pulmonary consolidation mainly in the distribution of the opacities and in the rapidity with which their pattern can change. It is uncommon for all the alveoli in any area to be completely filled with fluid. The intermingling of alveoli partially filled with air and fluid-filled alveoli results in a less dense shadow than in many forms of pneumonia, in which the regional involvement tends to be more uniform. The confluent, patchy densities of pulmonary edema tend to involve the inner two-thirds of the lungs and create the appearance of wings extending outward from the mediastinum (Fig. 6-42).[82] Most often, both lungs are equally affected, but on occasion only one lung appears edema-

tous.[83] This usually represents a transitory state, and within a day or two the typical hazy patchy shadows appear in the opposite lung.

Oxygen toxicity, shock lung, or bronchopneumonia can produce a roentgen picture similar to that of pulmonary edema. In general, however, the shadows in these conditions are more stable, whereas those of pulmonary edema tend to change rapidly, clearing in one area and appearing in another. Such evanescent shadows are also characteristic of eosinophilic pneumonia, but this is asssociated with a peripheral eosinophilia not present in pulmonary edema.

THE PERICARDIUM (See also Chapter 43)

The pericardium is a closed, invaginated sac that completely surrounds the heart except for a small area on its posterior surface where the pulmonary veins enter the left atrium. The visceral layer of pericardium is intimately applied to the heart and to the great arteries and veins. It is reflected from these vessels and doubles back to form the outer wall of the sac, the parietal pericardium. A small amount of fluid, 20 to 30 ml, is usually contained within the pericardial cavity.

PERICARDIAL EFFUSION. As fluid collects in the pericardial space, the parietal pericardium is pushed outward, increasing the size of the cardiac silhouette. The flu-

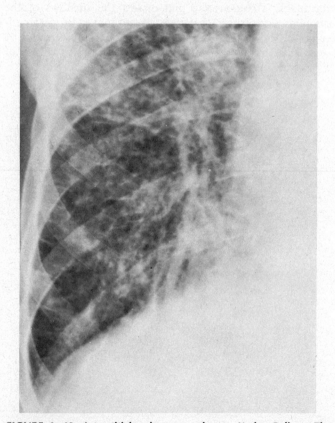

FIGURE 6-40 Interstitial pulmonary edema—Kerley B lines. The short, horizontal linear shadows in the periphery of the right lower lobe represent edematous interlobular septa projected on end. (From Rabin, C. B., and Baron, M. G.: Radiology of the Chest. Baltimore, Williams and Wilkins Co., 1979.)

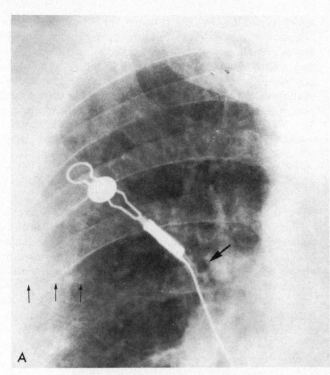

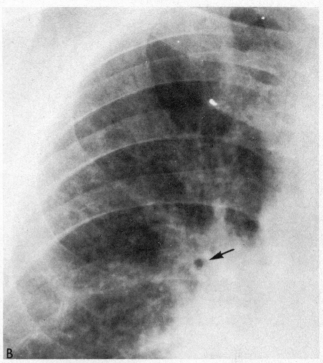

FIGURE 6-41 Interstitial pulmonary edema—peribronchial cuffing. *A,* At the time of this film, the patient was not in congestive heart failure. The vessels in the right upper lung are clearly outlined. The thin circular shadow (oblique arrow) represents a bronchus viewed on end. The outer part of the short fissure (vertical arrows) can be visualized. *B,* Several days later the patient became tachypneic. The pulmonary vessels are now poorly outlined because of edema of the interstitial tissues. The wall of the anterior segmental bronchus (arrow) is thick and hazy as a result of peribronchial edema. The short fissure cannot be identified even though the patient is in failure. This "disappearance" of the fissure is due to a change in the angulation of the x-ray tube in relation to the patient. (From Rabin, C. B., and Baron, M. G.: Radiology of the Chest. Baltimore, Williams and Wilkins Co., 1979.)

id fills in all the recesses between the cardiac structures and smoothes out the normal bulges and indentations of the cardiac contours. The end result is a smoothly distended, flask-shaped cardiac shadow. Even though there may be no tamponade, cardiac pulsations are diminished because of the damping effect of the fluid. These characteristics of a pericardial effusion are not specific, and almost identical findings can be caused by a failing heart with generalized dilatation of the cardiac chambers and decreased myocardial contractility.

The two conditions usually can be distinguished by the appearance of the pulmonary hila. The pericardial sac extends to the level of the bifurcation of the main pulmonary artery, or slightly above. Therefore, as it distends laterally, it tends to cover up the shadows of the hilar vessels.[15] On the other hand, the failing heart is associated with pulmonary congestion and abnormally prominent vessels. This distinction can be made from the frontal chest film and does not require fluoroscopy (Fig. 6-43).

A second, and pathognomonic, sign of a pericardial effusion is displacement of the epicardial fat line. A variable amount of fat is usually present beneath the epicardium, particularly around the coronary vessels in the atrioventricular and interventricular sulci. With increasing age, the accumulation of fatty tissue tends to increase and spreads between the epicardium and the walls of the ventricles. The layer of fat over the anterior surface of the heart is projected on end in the lateral view and appears as a relatively radiolucent band abutting the retrosternal soft tis-

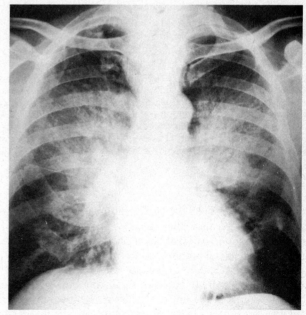

FIGURE 6-42 Pulmonary edema. A film made shortly after myocardial infarction shows hazy areas of increased density in the central portion of each lung. Air-filled bronchi are visualized within the density, indicating that it represents consolidation of lung. The appearance and pattern are characteristic of alveolar pulmonary edema. Because air-filled alveoli are intermingled with fluid-filled ones, the shadows are only moderately dense and are not homogeneous. (From Rabin, C. B., and Baron, M. G.: Radiology of the Chest. Baltimore, Williams and Wilkins Co., 1979.)

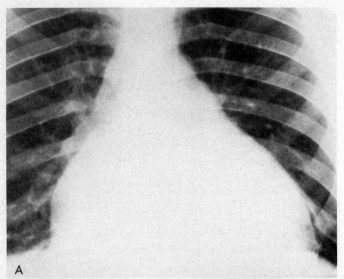

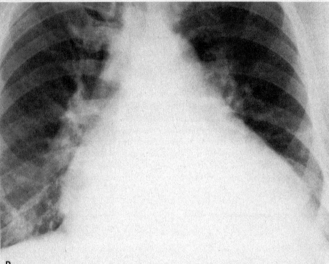

FIGURE 6–43 Differentiation between pericardial effusion and a dilated heart. *A,* Pericardial effusion. The cardiac silhouette is markedly enlarged, and its contours are smoothed out. Most of the right hilum and all of the left hilum are obscured by the shadow of the heart. *B,* Cardiac failure. The cardiac silhouette is enlarged, and its contours are smoothed out. However, in this case the hilar vessels are dilated, and both hilar shadows are abnormally prominent.

sues. The shadows of the pericardium and epicardium are not discrete, because they blend imperceptibly with the shadow of the retrosternal soft tissues. When the latter tissues contain a fair amount of fat, they form a second lucent band, immediately behind the sternum. The two layers of pericardium and the small amount of fluid can then be seen as a fine linear soft tissue shadow between the two bands (Fig. 6–44*B*). Their combined shadow is normally no thicker than 2 mm. The pericardial shadow can be identified in about 40 per cent of routine lateral chest films.[84]

As fluid collects between the layers of pericardium, the pericardial soft tissue stripe becomes progressively wider and displaces the epicardial fat line away from the sternum into the cardiac silhouette (Fig. 6–44*C*). This line is more

easily identified by fluoroscopy than on plain films.[85] Absence of an identifiable fat line has no significance. Relatively small amounts of pericardial effusion can be detected by computed tomography. In addition to indicating the volume of the effusion, the scan also provides an indication of the nature of the fluid. For example, a hemopericardium casts a denser shadow and therefore has a higher CT number than a simple serous effusion.[86]

CONSTRICTIVE PERICARDITIS. In most cases of constrictive pericarditis the appearance of the heart is nonspecific. The heart is often small or normal in size but may be enlarged.[87] Cardiac pulsations are usually diminished but can be normal. Calcification of the pericardium (Fig. 6–22) is the one finding that is suggestive of constrictive pericarditis. It is usually a sequel to tuberculous pericardial infection (Fig. 6–44*A*). Since this is a relatively rare cause of pericarditis at present, pericardial calcification is absent in almost 90 per cent of cases of constrictive pericarditis.[88] Conversely, the presence of pericardial calcification is not diagnostic of constrictive pericarditis and can occur without any evidence of restriction of the heart. A diagnosis of pericarditis can be made, in the absence of pericardial calcification, by computed tomography which demonstrates the thickening of the pericardium.[89,90]

CONGENITAL ABSENCE OF THE PERICARDIUM

The most common form of this anomaly is absence of the left pericardium. This is almost always associated with a defect in the mediastinal portion of the left parietal pleura, so that the pericardial space and the pleural space communicate with each other. The appearance of the heart on the frontal chest film is characteristic.[91] Although the trachea remains in the midline, the cardiac shadow is shifted into the left hemithorax. The pulmonary artery segment is abnormally prominent and is sharply demarcated from the shadow of the aortic knob. The left ventricle is elongated and has a broad area of contact with the diaphragm (Fig. 6–45). Fluoroscopic findings are unique. The mobility of the heart is markedly increased, and it appears to bounce around wildly with each beat. A similar type of hyperactivity may be seen with a pneumopericardium. Here, too, the restraining effect of the pericardium is absent. However, with a pneumopericardium, the heart is not displaced from its normal position. If necessary, the diagnosis of absent left pericardium can be confirmed by inducing a left pneumothorax. Because the pleural and pericardial spaces are no longer separated, the injected air will appear between the diaphragm and the heart and beneath the intact right pericardium.

Partial absence of the pericardium is rare. It can occur on either side but is more common on the left. In some cases, the appearance of the heart is entirely normal, and the defect is found incidentally at surgery or at autopsy. If the left atrial appendage herniates through the defect, it will bulge from the left cardiac border,[92] and distinction from a mediastinal tumor or mitral valvular disease may be difficult on plain films. Fluoroscopy usually shows increased pulsation of the appendage if the pericardium is absent. A similar bulge on the right side of the heart can be caused by herniation of the right atrial appendage.[93]

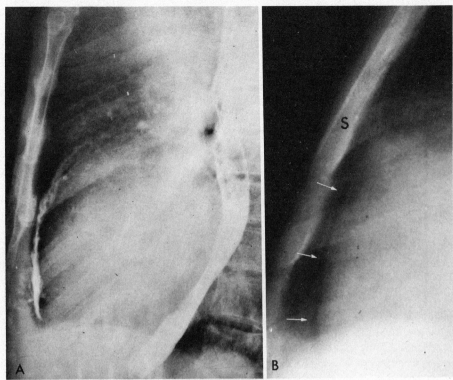

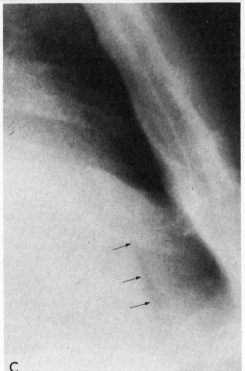

FIGURE 6–44 Pericardial shadows. *A*, Pericardial calcification. The calcified pericardium casts a linear shadow behind the lucency of the retrosternal fat and in front of the lucency of the epicardial fat. The patient had tuberculous pericarditis many years previously. *B*, Routine lateral chest film of another patient shows a considerable accumulation of fat in the retrosternal region. The fine linear soft tissue density (arrows) represents the two layers of pericardium and the small amount of fluid normally between them. The lucency between the pericardium and the cardiac silhouette is caused by fat beneath the epicardium. S = sternum. *C*, Right lateral chest film. The epicardial fat line (arrows) is displaced backward. The broad band of density between the epicardial fat and the retrosternal fat represents the two layers of pericardium and a collection of fluid between them. (From Baron, M. G.: Interlobar effusion. Circulation *44*: 475, 1971, by permission of the American Heart Association, Inc.)

ANGIOCARDIOGRAPHY

In order to visualize the internal anatomy of the heart, the radiodensity of the blood must be increased so that it will contrast with the cardiac soft tissue structures. Rapid serial films are required to record the passage of the opacified blood through the heart and provide information regarding the function of the cardiac chambers and the pattern of blood flow within the heart and great vessels.

TECHNIQUE. Opacification of the blood is accom-

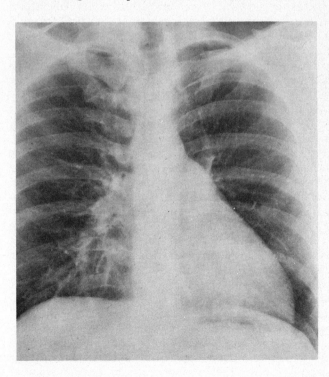

FIGURE 6–45 Congenital absence of left pericardium. The heart has shifted into the left hemithorax and no longer overlaps the right border of the spine. Despite the cardiac displacement, the trachea is in its normal position. The main pulmonary artery is prominent and is sharply demarcated from the aortic knob.

plished by the intravascular injection of a radiopaque contrast material. All the angiographic media used currently are solutions of water-soluble organic iodine compounds. The amount of iodine delivered per unit time and the volume of blood into which it is delivered determine the degree of opacification of the blood on the angiocardiogram. This in turn depends on the concentration of the contrast material and the speed with which it is injected. As the concentration of iodine in the contrast agent is increased, the viscosity also increases, and it becomes more difficult to inject. Thus, a contrast material that is moderately concentrated but more liquid is usually preferable to a denser but thicker one. In order to minimize dilution of the radiopaque bolus by nonopacified blood, the contrast material must be introduced rapidly and as close to the point of interest as possible. This requires selective catheterization of the vessel or chamber and the use of a pressure injector[94] or the use of digital angiography.

The radiological equipment used for angiocardiography must be able to provide sharply detailed pictures in rapid sequence. The image on the output screen of the image intensifier is photographed by a 35-mm cine camera, usually at the rate of 30 or 60 frames per second or on 100- to 105-mm film at a rate of 6 to 12 frames per second. As the images are recorded on the film, they can also be seen on the television monitor, so that the entire procedure is carried out under fluoroscopic control.

The internal structure of the heart is complex, and multiple views are usually needed in order to delineate the pertinent anatomy adequately. If only a single changer or image intensifier is available, a separate injection of contrast material is required for each view. Because the amount of contrast material that can be given safely to a patient is limited, it is difficult, especially in children, to obtain a complete study during one catheterization without biplane equipment. Stereoscopic filming has been attempted in the past but has not proved to be particularly effective or practical. A cardiac catheterization laboratory, unless designed solely for coronary arteriography, should have the capability of obtaining simultaneous biplane films.[95]

There is no one set of optimal views for all of angiocardiography. Projections are chosen depending on the nature of the cardiac lesion and the area of the heart to be visualized. Thus, frontal and lateral views will effectively demonstrate infundibular narrowing, ventricular septal defect, and stenosis of the pulmonic valve associated with a tetralogy of Fallot. But, in order to visualize adequately the supravalvular region of the pulmonary artery in the same patient, it is necessary to angle the equipment or prop up the patient, so that the frontal x-ray beam is oriented toward the patient's head, anteriorly. Evaluation of left ventricular contractility is best accomplished from films made in the left and right oblique projections. Complex angled views, in which the x-ray tube is tilted in relation to the coronal, sagittal, and cross-sectional planes of the patient, were first used for delineation of the coronary arteries but have proved to be of extreme value in the study of congenital cardiac lesions.[96–98] These angled views can be obtained by turning the patient and propping him or her partially upright, by rotating the patient and angling the x-ray tube, or by rotating and angling the x-ray tube while the patient remains supine. Each method requires specific types of

equipment and has its own advantages and disadvantages. No one technique is clearly superior to all others.

Complications

The hazards of selective angiocardiography fall into two major groups: those due to mechanical trauma from the catheter and from the force of the injected stream of contrast material, and those due to the pharmacological effects of the contrast media.

Mechanical trauma can result in perforation of the heart or dissection of the contrast material into the myocardium. Perforation of a ventricle usually has no serious sequelae.[99] The muscular wall contracts around the puncture site once the catheter is removed, and there is only minor leakage of blood into the pericardium. The perforation should be recognized before injection of the main bolus of contrast material if a small test injection is routinely made to confirm the position of the catheter. Contrast material injected into the pericardium causes considerable pain, but this can be controlled with medication and usually abates within a day or so. Although the amount of contrast material injected is usually not enough to produce cardiac tamponade, the solution is hypertonic and will increase in volume as it draws fluid into the pericardial cavity. Most of the contrast material can be withdrawn by pericardiocentesis, so that thoracotomy is usually not required.

Perforation of the atrium is a more serious consequence of catheterization. The thinner atrial wall does not seal off the puncture site as well as does the ventricular wall, and a greater outpouring of blood into the pericardium usually accompanies atrial perforation. Although this may cause cardiac tamponade, the bleeding often ceases spontaneously. Therefore, it is not necessary to rush the patient to the operating room once the perforation is discovered. The catheter should be removed and the patient's vital signs carefully monitored. Accumulation of blood in the pericardium can be detected and measured by echocardiography or CT scanning.

Intramural deposition of contrast material usually results when the catheter tip is trapped by muscular trabeculae and cannot recoil during the injection. The full force of the fluid jet issuing from the catheter is thus applied to the endocardium. Small intramural dissections are usually of no consequence; however, if a critical portion of the conduction system is involved, significant arrhythmias can result. A large intramural deposit is more serious because of the volume of myocardium that is injured. Rarely, a myocardial infarct results. The intramural location of the contrast material is easily recognized because it appears denser than the opacified blood within the cardiac lumen and because it persists for some time after the opacified blood is cleared from the heart.

Even though there is no evidence of intramural injection, the force of the jet of contrast material impinging on the ventricular wall can cause an arrhythmia. Most often, this is simply a self-limited short run of extrasystoles. However, heart block or ventricular tachycardia is encountered on rare occasions and may require medication or cardioversion. The jet effect can be largely avoided through careful technique and proper catheter design. The velocity of the jet exiting from the tip of the catheter can be decreased if there are side holes near the tip.[100] Recently, the use of balloon-tipped catheters has almost completely solved this problem, since contrast material exiting from holes in the side of the catheter is kept away from the wall of the heart by means of the balloon at the catheter tip.

The angiocardiographic media commonly used are combinations of meglumine and sodium salts of organic iodine compounds. They all cause similar hemodynamic effects and alterations in cardiac function. Newer non-ionic contrast materials appear to have less of a hemodynamic effect.[101-103] The exact mechanism of each of the changes is not completely understood but is probably the result of multiple factors: the volume of contrast material injected, its hypertonicity, the pharmacological effect of the iodine and sodium, and the myocardial toxicity of the agents.

Within one or two minutes of the intravascular injection of contrast material, a definite peripheral vasodilation occurs that results in systemic hypotension. At the same time, there is a significant, transient expansion in plasma volume.[104,105] After the first three or four cardiac cycles, the left ventricular end-diastolic pressure and volume increase,[106,107] as do the pressures in the left atrium and pulmonary artery. There is a concomitant increase in left ventricular function. Several beats later, hemodynamic evidence indicating some depression of myocardial contractility begins to appear. These changes gradually revert to normal over a period of 10 to 20 minutes. Cardiac reaction to the injection of contrast material in normal patients is different from that in patients with coronary artery disease and may be used as an approximate test of ventricular function.[108,109]

All the contrast agents have a slight but definite toxicity, primarily toward the kidneys[110] and central nervous system. Some patients exhibit a mild allergic reaction, usually in the form of hives, but anaphylactic reactions are extremely rare. Sensitivity testing is of no value in identifying those patients who will react adversely to the contrast material.[111] Patients with a previous allergic history are more prone to develop a reaction, but this does not constitute an absolute contraindication to angiocardiography. Most reactions can be avoided by premedication with antihistaminics and/or steroids. Contrast material is not well tolerated, and may prove fatal, in patients with pulmonary hypertension. Those patients with a right ventricular end-diastolic pressure of over 20 mm Hg are at the greatest risk. The cause of the reaction is not known but seems to be related to the osmolality of the contrast material.[99]

Hives and other minor allergic reactions can be successfully managed with antihistaminics. More severe reactions, namely respiratory arrest or cardiac arrest, usually require intubation and assisted ventilation as well as vasopressor agents to maintain blood pressure. Convulsive seizures tend to be self-limited and can be controlled with barbiturates or Valium. Because iodine compounds are excreted by the kidneys, mostly through glomerular filtration, the hypertonic effects of the contrast material can be increased and prolonged by dehydration, especially in the presence of renal disease. Therefore, patients should be well hydrated before an angiographic study.[112]

INTERPRETATION OF THE ANGIOCARDIOGRAM

The multiple films of an angiocardiographic sequence contain considerable information regarding cardiac anatomy and function. Rather than attempting to comprehend everything at once, it is preferable to review the films in a systematic fashion. Films should be scanned several times, with a different aspect of the study being evaluated at each reading. Such an orderly approach lessens the chances of overlooking significant findings and simplifies their correct interpretation. Eventually, this structured type of approach becomes a habit, no longer requiring a conscious effort.

PATTERN OF BLOOD FLOW

Except for the occasional artifact due to a ventricular arrhythmia or interference of a catheter with closure of a valve, the flow of the radiopaque bolus on an angiocardiogram can be assumed to represent the true pattern of blood flow in that heart. Normally, blood flows through the heart in only one direction, and the sequence of opacification of the cardiac chambers is always the same. Only those chambers and vessels downstream in relation to the site of injection of the contrast material will be visualized. The angiocardiogram is completed once the opacified blood flows through the major systemic arteries. The flow rate of blood through the various organs varies greatly, and the original bolus of contrast material returns to the great veins over a period of time and is too diluted to allow revisualization of the cardiac chambers. The occasional exception is seen in infants and young children in whom the right atrium and ventricle may be reopacified by the venous return from the cerebral circulation. In older children and adults such revisualization is almost never seen except in the presence of a large, peripheral arteriovenous fistula. Deviations from the normal pattern of blood flow fall into two groups: (1) opacification of a chamber or vessel before its proper turn, indicating that the direction of blood flow is normal but that one or more of the intermediate structures is bypassed; and (2) the direction of blood flow is reversed, and a chamber or vessel upstream to the point of injection becomes opacified.

Premature visualization of a chamber or vessel is the result of a right-to-left shunt and indicates the presence of an abnormal communication between the two sides of the heart. However, pressures in the left cardiac chambers are normally higher than those on the right side, so that the flow through an uncomplicated atrial septal defect, for example, should be from left to right. In order for the flow to travel in the opposite direction, there must be a reversal of the pressure differential between the two sides of the heart, and this implies the presence of a second lesion. Most often, the pressures on the right side are abnormally high because of either increased resistance to emptying, as in tricuspid atresia (Figure 29–51, p. 995, and Figure 6–46) or pulmonic stenosis, or diastolic overloading, as in total anomalous pulmonary venous drainage. Less commonly, the pressures in the left heart and aorta are lower than normal because of an upstream obstruction, as in mitral atresia or preductal coarctation of the aorta.

In either case, the obstruction must lie beyond the chamber from which the shunt originates but upstream in relation to the recipient chamber or vessel. Thus, if there is a right-to-left shunt through an atrial septal defect, and there is no diastolic overloading of the atrium, the cause of the increased resistance to flow can be present anywhere from the tricuspid valve to the point of entry of the pulmonary veins into the left atrium. Although a lesion beyond the left atrium, such as mitral or aortic stenosis, can

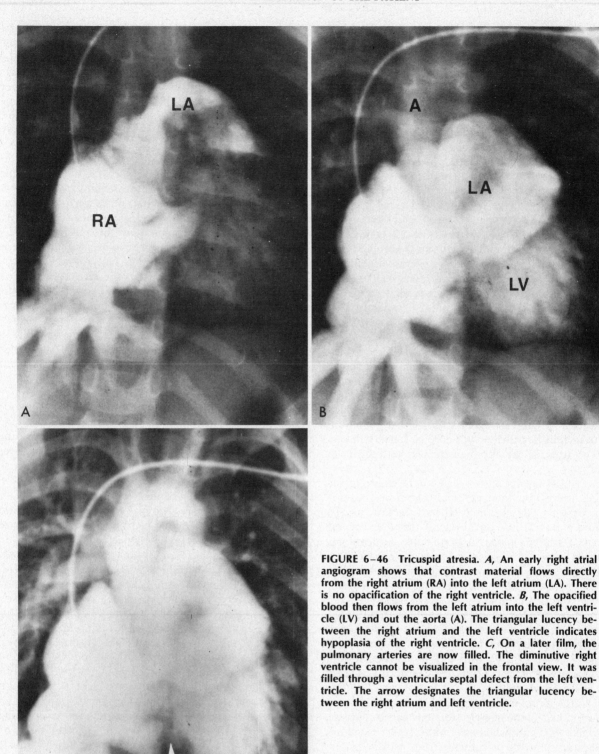

FIGURE 6–46 Tricuspid atresia. *A,* An early right atrial angiogram shows that contrast material flows directly from the right atrium (RA) into the left atrium (LA). There is no opacification of the right ventricle. *B,* The opacified blood then flows from the left atrium into the left ventricle (LV) and out the aorta (A). The triangular lucency between the right atrium and the left ventricle indicates hypoplasia of the right ventricle. *C,* On a later film, the pulmonary arteries are now filled. The diminutive right ventricle cannot be visualized in the frontal view. It was filled through a ventricular septal defect from the left ventricle. The arrow designates the triangular lucency between the right atrium and left ventricle.

result in elevation of the right atrial pressure, it causes an even greater elevation of left atrial pressure, so that the shunt would still be from left to right.

At times, two lesions can be localized from the sequence of opacification of the cardiac chambers. If contrast material injected into the right atrium first opacifies the left atrium, then the left ventricle, and finally the right ventricle, the presumptive diagnosis is tricuspid atresia with a right-to-left shunt through the atrial septum and a left-to-right shunt through a ventricular septal defect (Fig. 6–46).[113,114] More often, the abnormal flow pattern simply indicates the general location of the lesions, and a definitive diagnosis depends upon identification of specific anatomical abnormalities. If the opacified blood flows from the right atrium into the right ventricle as well as into the left atrium, a second injection of contrast material into the right ventricle is usually required in order to study the infundibular region of the right ventricle, the pulmonic valve, and the pulmonary circulation (see Figures 29–36, p. 986, 29–37, p. 987, 29–38, p. 988, and 29–46, p. 992).

Premature visualization of the descending aorta from an injection on the right side of the heart indicates reversed flow through a patent ductus arteriosus. This is most often due to preductal coarctation of the aorta.[115] The ascending aorta and the subclavian and carotid arteries are not visualized because they are filled by antegrade flow of nonopacified blood from the left ventricle. However, if the entire aorta is opacified through the ductus, the pressure in the ascending aorta must be similar to that in the descending aorta, and the possibility of a coarctation is excluded (Fig. 6–47). Usually, this pattern of flow is seen with hypoplasia of the left heart[116,117] but is rarely caused by severe pulmonary hypertension.[118]

Rare exceptions to the rule that two lesions are needed to produce a right-to-left shunt are a pulmonary arteriovenous fistula and anomalous drainage of a systemic vein (such as a persistent left superior vena cava) into the left atrium.[119]

Opacification of a chamber or vessel upstream in relation to the site of injection of the contrast material results from a left-to-right shunt or when a cardiac valve is incompetent. Some retrograde filling of the inferior or superior vena cava from the right atrium or of the pulmonary

veins from the left atrium is not abnormal because the orifices of these vessels are not guarded by valves.

Backward visualization of a structure not contiguous to the one in which the contrast material is injected signifies a left-to-right shunt. Accurate localization of the lesion is usually possible when the jet of opacified blood crossing the defect between the two sides of the heart can be identified.[120,121] This usually requires selective injection of contrast material into the chamber from which the shunt arises. If the shunt itself is not visualized, it may be possible to establish the diagnosis by correlating the appearance of the opacified blood on the right side of the heart with the filling of the left-heart structures. For example, if, following a supraaortic injection of contrast material, the pulmonary artery does not become opacified until the proximal descending aorta is filled, a patent ductus is most likely. However, filling of the pulmonary artery when only the ascending aorta is opacified is indicative of an aorticopulmonary window.

In some instances, the defect cannot be localized with certainty without two or more selective angiograms. If the right atrium becomes opacified during the levocardiogram phase of a right ventriculogram, the presence of an atrial septal defect is statistically most likely. However, the shunt could have originated in the left ventricle (atrioventricular septal defect) or in the aorta (ruptured sinus of Valsalva aneurysm). A left ventricular injection, and possibly an aortogram, is required to exclude these lesions. A similar picture can be caused by anomalous drainage of a pulmonary vein into the right atrium. Usually, this need not be excluded, since it will become evident at the time of

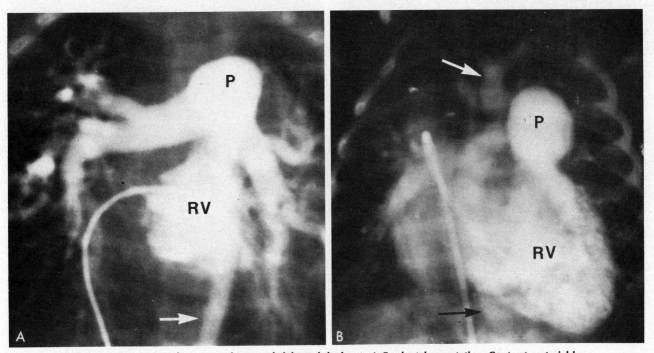

FIGURE 6–47 Patent ductus arteriosus and right-to-left shunt. *A,* Preductal coarctation. Contrast material has been injected selectively into the right ventricle (RV). The descending aorta (arrow) is filled through a patent ductus from the pulmonary artery (P). The ascending aorta and great vessels are not opacified. *B,* Hypoplastic left heart syndrome and interruption of the inferior vena cava. A catheter inserted into the femoral vein reaches the heart by way of the azygos vein, and contrast material is injected selectively into the right ventricle (RV). Both the ascending aorta (white arrow) and the descending aorta (black arrow) are filled from the pulmonary artery (P) by way of a patent ductus arteriosus.

operative repair of the atrial defect. However, if important, the abnormal venous connection can be demonstrated by selective injections into the right and left pulmonary arteries. When there is more than one left-to-right shunt, only the most proximal one that is opacified can be identified with certainty. For example, opacification of the right ventricle from a left ventricular injection indicates the presence of a ventricular septal defect. Forward flow of the opacified blood from the right ventricle rapidly fills the pulmonary artery, and it is usually not possible to recognize the presence of an associated patent ductus arteriosus. A second injection above the aortic valve is needed to evaluate this possibility (Fig. 6–48).

Cardiac Chambers

The size of a cardiac chamber may reflect an abnormal pattern of blood flow and has little diagnostic specificity. Although a chamber may be small because of malseptation, more commonly this is the result of a decreased volume load because of an anomaly that allows blood to bypass the chamber during embryonic life. Thus, tricuspid atresia or pulmonary valve atresia with an intact ventricular septum is associated with a diminutive right ventricle. A small left ventricle is often associated with a double-outlet right ventricle, and when the aortic or mitral valve is atretic, the ventricle may be represented only by an endocardium-lined slit.

When estimating chamber size from the angiogram, it is important to consider the size of the other cardiac chambers, a possible source of distortion. Enlargement of the right ventricle causes posterior displacement of the ventricular septum and the left ventricle. The left ventricle may be rotated medially, so that its lateral projection resembles that normally seen in the left anterior oblique view. The shadow of the ventricle is thus foreshortened, and the chamber, although normal in size, can appear small.

Dilatation of a chamber usually results from a volume overload, as in valvular regurgitation or a shunt, or from a decrease in the functional capacity of the myocardium. The underlying cause of such dilatation can be determined from a properly designed angiographic study. A right-sided angiocardiogram is usually inadequate when the cause of left ventricular enlargement is sought. A selective left ventriculogram is required in order to study contractility of the ventricular wall and to demonstrate regurgitation of the mitral valve. An aortogram is needed to evaluate the competency of the aortic valve and the possibility of

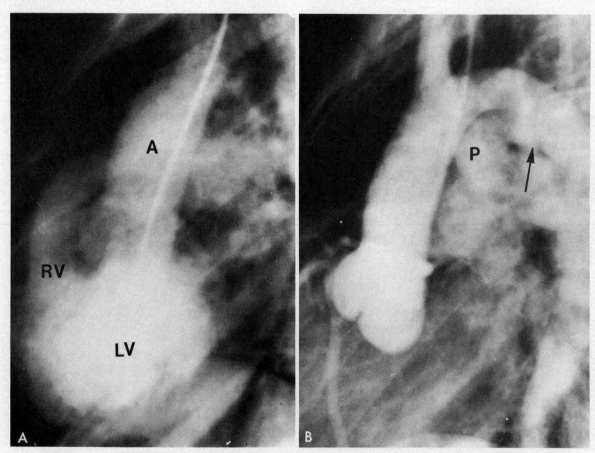

FIGURE 6–48   Multiple left-to-right shunts. *A*, Left ventriculogram, lateral view. Contrast material injected into the left ventricle (LV) flows rapidly across a large ventricular septal defect into the right ventricle (RV). The pulmonary artery is opacified by antegrade flow from the right ventricle. Although the aorta (A) is well opacified, it is not possible to identify a patent ductus arteriosus. *B*, The catheter was withdrawn into the ascending aorta, and a second injection was made. This time the pulmonary artery (P) is opacified by way of a patent ductus arteriosus (arrow). (From Angrissola, A. B., and Puddu, V. [eds.]: Cardiologia D'Oggia. Torino, C. B. Edizion Scientifiche, 1976.)

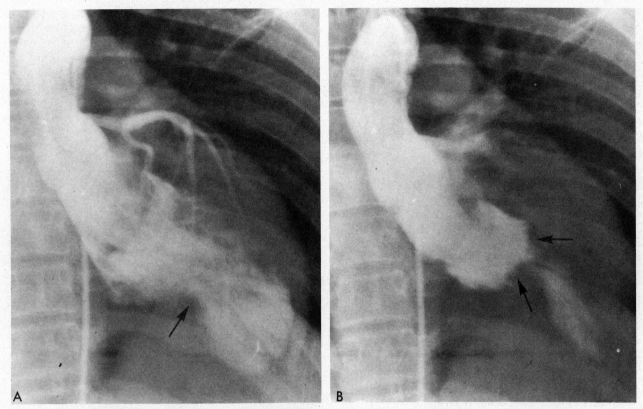

FIGURE 6–49   Left ventriculogram in hypertrophic obstructive cardiomyopathy. *A*, Diastole. The left ventricular wall is abnormally thickened because of muscular hypertrophy. The indentation on the medial aspect of the chamber (arrow) is caused by hypertrophy of the interventricular septum and the medial papillary muscle. *B*, Systole. As the heart contracts, the papillary muscles (arrows) constrict the midbody of the ventricle and sequester the apical region.

an anomalous left coronary artery (see Figure 29–22, p. 972).

Myocardial hypertrophy can be detected on the angiocardiogram. The distance between the edge of an opacified cardiac chamber and the outer border of the heart represents the combined thickness of the cardiac wall and the pericardium. A significant increase in this distance on an angiocardiogram can be due to hypertrophy of the myocardium or a pericardial effusion; however, hypertrophy rarely causes the thickness of the atrial wall to increase by more than a few millimeters. Atrial wall thickness of 8 mm or more is diagnostic of pericardial disease, almost always an effusion.[122]

Filling defects within the opacified atrium that occur early in the angiographic sequence, when contrast material is first injected into the chamber, usually result from incomplete mixing of the contrast material with the incoming nonopaque venous blood. The defects disappear after one or two cardiac cycles. A persistent defect that appears essentially the same from film to film indicates the presence of an intraluminal mass, either a thrombus or a tumor. A local dilution defect, such as that caused by nonopaque blood shunted through an atrial septal defect, can mimic the appearance of a mass. However, these dilution defects are never sharply outlined, and their appearance constantly changes during the cardiac cycle.

Ventricular filling defects are almost always due to hypertrophied musculature. In the right ventricle, the thickened myocardial bands and trabeculae cause scalloped indentations on the margins of the opacified chamber or round filling defects within it. Hypertrophy of the crista supraventricularis and the septal and parietal bands produce a narrowing of the infundibulum. Hypertrophic papillary muscles in the left ventricle are best seen in the frontal projection, since they encroach on the superior and inferior aspects of the ventricular cavity, narrowing the midbody of the chamber (Fig. 6–49). When the interventricular septum hypertrophies, it assumes a fusiform shape and bulges into the adjacent portions of both ventricular cavities.[123,124]

A thin, lucent line stretching across the outflow portion of the left ventricle is usually due to a subaortic membrane. This lesion may be difficult to demonstrate, and multiple views of the opacified ventricle are often required. The subaortic membrane can be delineated without equivocation, if contrast material is injected selectively into the space between the membrane and the aortic valve.[125] A more jagged, V-shaped lucent line seen in the outflow portion of the left ventricle in the frontal view is characteristic of hypertrophic obstructive cardiomyopathy[126] (Fig. 41–13, p. 1417). The linear defect is present only in late systole, when the anterior mitral leaflet swings forward and makes contact with the ventricular septum.

If the minor intrusions of the muscular trabeculae are ignored, the overall shape of the ventricular cavities is regular. Local outpocketings of the lumen are abnormal. On the left side, they usually represent postmyocardial infarction aneurysm (Figure 39–16, p. 1364) or, rarely, a con-

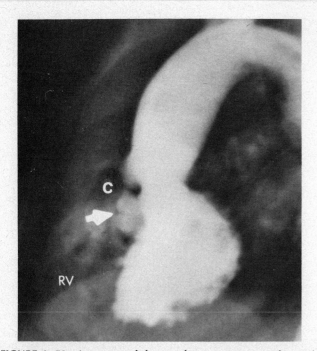

FIGURE 6–50 Aneurysm of the membranous septum. Left ventricular angiocardiogram, lateral view. The scalloped protrusion of the left ventricle (arrow) arises from the region of the membranous septum and extends anteriorly into the right ventricle beneath the crista supraventricularis (C). The right ventricle (RV) is opacified because of a small shunt through a defect in the aneurysm.

genital aneurysm or ventricular diverticulum. As the ventricle contracts, the aneurysm remains unchanged or bulges outward, and the contrast material pools within it. The opacified blood persists in the aneurysm, while it is washed away from the rest of the chamber. Aneurysms of the right ventricle are rare and are usually related to previous surgery.

An aneurysm of the membranous septum communicates with the left ventricular cavity and arises immediately beneath the commissure between the right coronary and noncoronary aortic cusps. The aneurysm usually has a trabeculated contour and extends anteriorly into the outflow tract of the right ventricle (Fig. 6–50). It is likely that most membranous septal aneurysms are misnamed and actually are formed by a portion of the tricuspid valve that has adhered to the margins of a membranous ventricular septal defect.[127,128]

Cineangiocardiography is required for a detailed study of ventricular function. End-diastolic and end-systolic volumes can be calculated from the size of the opacified ventricle in one or two projections and can be used to derive stroke volume, ejection fraction, and other measurements of myocardial performance (Chap. 14). It is also possible to divide the ventricular wall into segments and measure the shortening of each one during systole to disclose abnormalities in regional wall motion that may not be apparent from simple observation of the contracting chamber.[129,130]

Hypercontractility of the musculature is usually associated with hypertrophy and results in abnormal constriction of the ventricular lumen in end systole. In the right ventricle, this is most easily seen in the infundibular region. Normally, this area narrows slightly during systole.

However, when the muscular contraction is abnormally forceful, the caliber of the infundibulum may be decreased by 80 per cent or more. Such systolic narrowing of the infundibulum is commonly seen with pulmonic valve stenosis.[131] If the infundibulum distends normally during diastole, the systolic narrowing was caused by hypercontraction of the musculature (Fig. 6–51). However, if the infundibulum is fibrotic, the narrowing is fixed, and it appears essentially the same in systole and diastole.

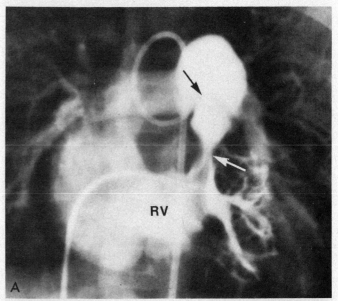

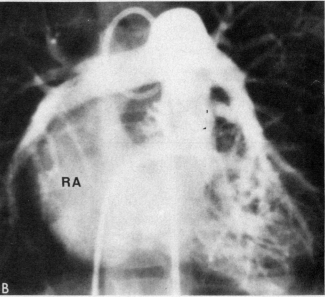

FIGURE 6–51 Pulmonary stenosis with hypercontraction of the infundibulum. *A,* Systole. A catheter has been advanced through the inferior vena cava to the right ventricle (RV). The stenotic pulmonic valve forms a dome (black arrow) bulging away from the ventricle. The infundibulum is markedly narrowed (white arrow). The multiple filling defects within the apical regions of the right ventricle are caused by hypertrophied trabeculae. The second catheter is positioned in the arch of the aorta. *B,* Diastole. The infundibulum appears of normal caliber, indicating that the narrowing was due to muscular contraction and does not represent fixed infundibular stenosis. The right atrium (RA) is opacified because of tricuspid regurgitation. (From Angrissola, A. B., and Puddu, V. [eds.]: Cardiologia D'Oggia. Torino, C. B. Edizion Scientifiche, 1976.)

Hypercontraction of the left ventricle is manifested mainly in the body of the chamber. When there is a diffuse increase in contractility of the ventricular wall, the end-systolic volume of the chamber is decreased, and the cavity of the ventricle, except for its outflow portion, may be completely effaced. This can represent a response to obstruction in the aortic valve or the subaortic region but also occurs without known cause.[132] Eccentric hypertrophy and hypercontractility of the ventricle usually involves the septum and the papillary muscles and produces a pinching of the body of the ventricle that sequesters the apical region from the rest of the chamber (Fig. 6–49).[126,133]

Cardiac Valves

Angiocardiography is probably the best single method for evaluation of the structure of cardiac valves. It is an accurate and sensitive technique for the detection of stenosis of the aortic and pulmonic valves and, to a lesser extent, of the mitral valve. It is not very effective for evaluation of tricuspid stenosis. Regurgitation of all four valves, even of the slightest degree, can be routinely demonstrated.

When the blood on both sides of the valve is opacified, and the valve is viewed tangentially, the cusps normally appear as thin, smooth, curvilinear lucencies. If the valve is projected obliquely or *en face*, the cusps usually cannot be identified. However, because the cusps are sheetlike structures, it is not necessary to visualize both surfaces in order to study their function. For example, on a supravalvular aortogram, the line of demarcation between the opacified blood in the aorta and the radiolucent blood in the ventricle actually represents the aortic surface of the valve cusps. The cusps are more easily seen on this type of examination, and in many instances their motion can be studied in greater detail (Fig. 6–52).

STENOSIS.[134] The cusps of the normal aortic and pulmonic valves are rarely identified during systole because of their rapid motion. Even in the fully opened position, the cusps are not still, since their free margins are unsupported and tend to vibrate in the rapidly flowing arterial stream. However, during diastole, the cusps coapt and support each other so that they are relatively immobile for a considerable part of the cardiac cycle.

When the valve is stenotic, the cusps cannot separate from each other, and they form a membrane with a narrow orifice. During systole, the membrane, stretched taut by the stream of blood ejected from the ventricle, is relatively motionless. A dome-shaped curvilinear lucency, bulging away from the contracting chamber, is the angiographic hallmark of valvular stenosis (Figs. 6–52 and 6–53).[135,136] If the cusps cannot be seen during systole, it may be assumed that the valve is not stenotic. The aortic

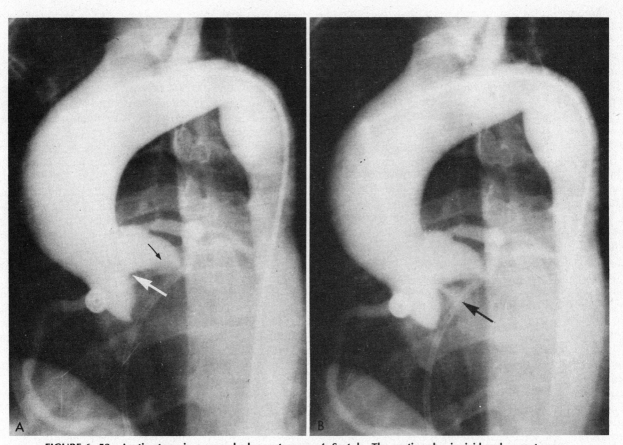

FIGURE 6–52 Aortic stenosis, supravalvular aortogram. *A,* Systole. The aortic valve is rigid and cannot open. The narrow dilution defect (white arrow) represents radiolucent blood ejected from the left ventricle and indicates the diameter of the valve orifice. The irregularity of the left coronary cusp (black arrow) is caused by a vegetation on the valve. There is poststenotic dilatation of the ascending aorta. *B,* Diastole. The valve hardly moves at all, and there is a fine jet of aortic regurgitation (arrow).

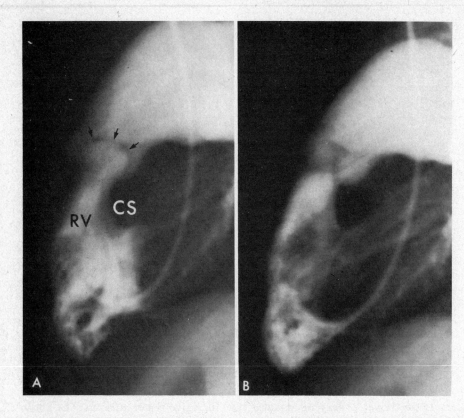

FIGURE 6–53 Pulmonic valve stenosis. Right ventriculogram, lateral view. *A*, Systole. The pulmonic valve (arrows) forms a dome, bulging away from the right ventricle (RV). The crista supraventricularis (CS) is hypertrophied. *B*, Diastole. The three cusps of the valve can be identified and appear normal. (From Baron, M. G.: The angiocardiographic diagnosis of valvular stenosis. Circulation *44*:143, 1971, by permission of the American Heart Association, Inc.)

and pulmonic valves are so well visualized that mild degrees of stenosis may be detected on the angiogram before a pressure gradient is demonstrable. On the other hand, when a gradient across either valve is due to increased blood flow, the angiographic appearance of the valve will be normal. It should be noted that so long as the cusps are pliable, the valve will appear normal during diastole, no matter how narrow its orifice (Fig. 6–53). A dysplastic valve is usually considerably thicker than a simple stenotic valve and has an irregular, nodular contour. Valve motion tends to be markedly limited.

Both the mitral and tricuspid valves are best studied in the right anterior oblique projection. The mitral valve can be adequately delineated on a selective left ventriculogram. The interface between the opacified ventricle and the nonopacified left atrium represents the ventricular surface of the mitral leaflets. During systole, this interface is normally washed away by the incoming atrial blood. However, if the valve is stenotic, the interface persists and assumes a dome-shaped contour, convex toward the ventricle (Fig. 6–54). If the valve is fibrotic and rigid, the interface will be somewhat irregular and will move only slightly between systole and diastole.[137] The same information can be obtained from a selective pulmonary arteriogram. In this case, the valve leaflets will be seen as linear lucencies, separating the opacified left atrium from the opacified left ventricle.

The tricuspid valve is more difficult to visualize. On a selective right atrial injection, it may be seen as a curved interface between the opacified atrium and the radiolucent right ventricle. However, after a few cardiac cycles, when the ventricle becomes opacified, it is difficult to identify the valve. As a general rule, pressure measurements across

the tricuspid valve are more accurate for the detection of stenosis than is the angiocardiogram.

The angiocardiographic diagnosis of valvular atresia is made from the course of the blood flow and the associated anatomical abnormalities. When the tricuspid valve is atretic, blood flows directly from the right atrium into the left atrium. The right ventricle is abnormally small and fills through an interventricular communication.[138] A similar appearance can be seen with atresia of the pulmonic valve when the ventricular septum is intact. In this case, however, the diminutive right ventricle is opacified directly from the right atrium (see Figure 29–40, p. 989).[139] Aortic and mitral atresia is generally associated with hypoplasia of the left heart chambers. The ascending aorta is often no larger than a major visceral artery and fills from the right side of the heart through the ductus. The appearance of the aorta is so characteristic that the general diagnosis of hypoplasia of the left heart can often be made from a retrograde aortogram (see Figure 29–34, p. 983).

REGURGITATION.[140] In order to evaluate valvular competency, contrast material should be injected selectively into the chamber or vessel just beyond the valve. With normal flow, only those structures downstream in relation to the point of injection will be opacified. If the valve is incompetent, the contrast material will reflux into the upstream chamber. When studying the mitral and tricuspid valves, the patient should be placed in the right anterior oblique position. In this view, the valves are seen on end, separating the atrium from the ventricle, and there is no overlapping of the shadows of the two chambers.

Catheter position creates a possible source of error in evaluating insufficiency of the tricuspid and pulmonic valves. In order to reach their downstream side, the cathe-

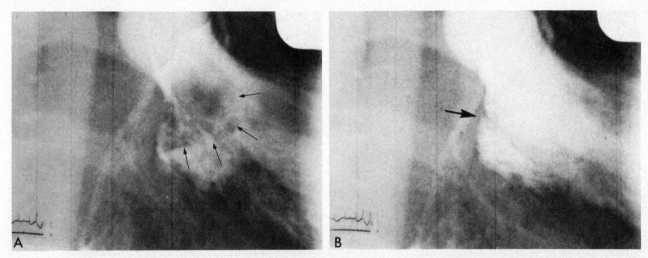

FIGURE 6–54 Mitral stenosis. Left ventricular angiogram, right anterior oblique view. *A*, Diastole. The mitral valve cannot open completely and forms a dome (arrows) that bulges into the left ventricle during atrial contraction. The leaflets are outlined by contrast material within the left ventricle and radiolucent blood in the atrium. *B*, Systole. The mitral valve (arrow) is closed. The wide excursion of the leaflets between the two phases of the cardiac cycle indicates that they are pliable.

ter must be passed through the valve. Most often, the catheter will lie in a commissure between the cusps and does not interfere with valve closure. Nevertheless, small amounts of regurgitation, probably due to the catheter, are sometimes seen. On occasion, the artifactual regurgitation may be of moderate degree,[141] but even then, it is rarely great enough to be of clinical importance. Free reflux of opacified blood is indicative of true valvular regurgitation. If there is any question as to the cause of the reflux, the catheter should be repositioned, and a second angiogram should be performed. It is unlikely that an artifact will be exactly duplicated.

Catheter position is of less concern with the left-sided cardiac valves, because the catheter can be passed retrograde through the aorta and reach the downstream chamber without traversing the valve. If the catheter is not positioned in the valve orifice, artifactual regurgitation is extremely rare unless the pressure injection triggers a run of extrasystoles. When the regurgitation is the result of a cardiac arrhythmia, the recipient chamber rapidly clears of contrast material once normal sinus rhythm has been restored. In true regurgitation, opacification of the chamber persists. A minimal amount of regurgitation may occur through the normal aortic valve, but this never opacifies more than a portion of the outflow tract of the left ventricle.

It is possible to gauge visually the severity of mitral valve regurgitation from a left ventriculogram by means of the relative densities of the left atrium and the aorta.[142] Equal opacification of the two structures indicates wide-open regurgitation, while a slight degree of reflux will produce only a minimum increase in the density of the left atrium. However, the size of the atrium must be taken into consideration. When the left atrium is very large, the regurgitant contrast material becomes so diluted by the blood already in the chamber that the amount of regurgitation will usually be underestimated.

The same principle can be used to measure aortic regur-

gitation. However, because of the rapid forward flow of blood within the aorta, the position of the catheter is very important. If the catheter tip is not adjacent to the valve, much of the contrast material will be washed away as it is injected, and the severity of the valvular regurgitation as judged by the opacity of the left ventricle will appear to be less than it actually is and may be overlooked completely.

SPECIFIC VALVULAR ABNORMALITIES. In the right anterior oblique projection, the subaortic portion of the right margin of the left ventricle is formed by the mitral valve. On a selective left ventriculogram, during systole, the mitral valve sharply delimits the opacified ventricle from the nonopacified left atrium. The line of demarcation is rather straight and almost vertical, extending from the aortic valve to the posteroinferior free wall of the ventricle. Protrusion of a portion of the valve beyond this line into the left atrium is indicative of *mitral prolapse*.[143,144] Usually, the angiocardiographic diagnosis is substantiated by echocardiography. However, the reverse is not true. In many instances, when the echocardiogram is positive, the roentgen appearance of the valve is normal. Whether this is because the echocardiographic criteria are not sufficiently specific or because the angiocardiogram is too gross a technique for detecting this abnormality is not certain.[145]

Ebstein's malformation of the tricuspid valve is best demonstrated on a right atrial angiogram in the frontal projection. The tricuspid valve normally overlies the shadow of the spine or is projected slightly to the left of it. Because the valve is attached to the fibrous skeleton of the heart, its position is not affected by the size of the right atrium. Significant leftward displacement of the tricuspid valve into the right ventricle is diagnostic of Ebstein's anomaly.[146] The septal and posterior leaflets of the valve can often be seen as linear lucencies within the opacified right ventricle.

A cleft in the anterior leaflet of the mitral valve is the common denominator in all forms of *endocardial cushion defects of the atrioventricular canal type*. The mitral orifice,

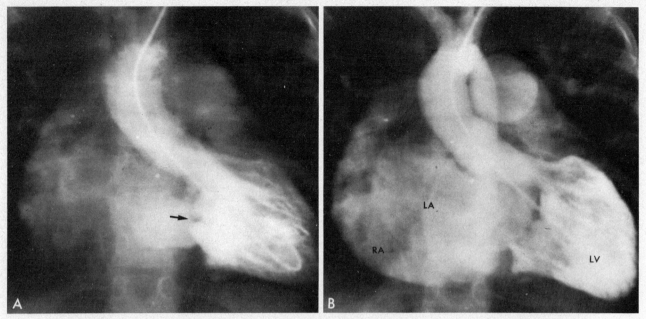

FIGURE 6-55   Endocardial cushion defect. Left ventriculogram, frontal view. *A*, Systole. The right border of the left ventricle is scalloped. The lucent niche (arrow) indicates a cleft in the anterior mitral valve leaflet. The valve is regurgitant, and contrast material refluxes into the left atrium. *B*, Diastole. The upper segment of the anterior mitral valve leaflet has swung into the outflow portion of the left ventricle, producing an apparent narrowing (arrow). This has been termed the "gooseneck" deformity. Contrast material has refluxed from the left ventricle (LV) into the left atrium (LA) and across the ostium primum defect into the right atrium (RA). Antegrade flow from the right atrium has filled the right ventricle and pulmonary artery. (From Baron, M. G., et al.: Endocardial cushion defects: Specific diagnosis by angiocardiography. Am. J. Cardiol. *13*:162, 1964.)

in these conditions, is rotated, so that the anterior mitral valve leaflet forms the right border of the left ventricle in the frontal projection. During systole, this border is scalloped rather than straight because of the abnormal valve tissue. During diastole, the two segments of the anterior leaflet swing open in different directions, causing an apparent narrowing of the outflow portion of the left ventricle (gooseneck deformity), and outline the upper margin of the defective ventricular septum (Fig. 6-55).[147] The angiocardiographic manifestations of an endocardial cushion defect are so specific that the angiocardiogram is the most accurate means for establishing this diagnosis.

Spatial Relationships

The heart is composed of three pairs of structures: the atria, the ventricles, and the great vessels. In all normal hearts, the two members of each pair have a constant positional relationship to each other and to the other cardiac structures. Although minor variations can result from dilatation of one or more of the chambers, a definite reversal of position is always due to a developmental fault.

Normally, the right atrium is situated to the right of the left atrium and slightly anteriorly. When the left atrium becomes very large, as it can in mitral disease, it may extend to the right, beyond the right atrium. However, the mitral valve and the left atrial appendage remain in their normal position to the left of the midline. The right ventricle lies anterior to and partly to the right of the left ventri-

cle. When the right ventricle dilates, it may extend to the left, beyond the border of the left ventricle. Nevertheless, the tricuspid valve maintains its normal position, and part of the right ventricle still lies on the right side of the left ventricle. The pulmonic valve and main pulmonary artery are positioned to the left of the root of the aorta and in front of it. Although the pulmonary artery may be projected to the right of the aorta in a steep left anterior view, it is not possible to project the aortic valve in front of the pulmonic valve in any view.[148] When the aorta is large and overrides the ventricular septum, as in tetralogy of Fallot, it may extend farther anteriorly than the pulmonary artery, but its posterior margin, which is in contact with the mitral valve, is still behind the pulmonary artery.

In general, when the side-to-side relationship of one pair of cardiac structures is reversed, the downstream pairs will be similarly affected. If the right atrium is situated on the left side of the heart, the ventricles and the great vessels will also be reversed—a condition called situs inversus. When the ventricles are inverted, the atria are usually in their normal position, but the great vessels are transposed—a condition called ventricular inversion (corrected transposition) (p. 1003). In isolated transposition of the great vessels, the atria and ventricles are positioned normally.

Identification of a cardiac chamber is usually based largely on its position and its relationship to the other chambers. In the presence of a rotational anomaly, this criterion is no longer valid. In general, the side-to-side relationship of the atria is concordant with the situs of the body. The right atrium usually receives the two venae cavae and the coronary sinus, while the pulmonary veins empty into the left atrium. On rare occasions, a left superior vena cava can enter the left atrium, or the inferior venae cava may be absent. However, anomalous drainage of the pulmonary veins is considerably more common. Pulmonary veins are therefore a less reliable indicator of atrial situs than are systemic veins. None of these is of any value in the asplenia syndrome because of the symmetrical development of the body and the indeterminate cardiac situs.

The ventricles can usually be identified because of their internal structure. The left ventricle tends to be oval in shape, while the right ventricle is trapezoidal. The trabeculation of the left ventricular wall is finer than that on the right, and the papillary muscles are often seen in the frontal view as two finger-like lucent defects within the opacified chamber. Of greater importance is the relationship between the inflow and outflow valves of each ventricle. In the left ventricle, the mitral valve and the aortic valves are in fibrous continuity. In contrast, the tricuspid valve and the pulmonic valve are separated by the muscular infundibulum of the right ventricle. This distinction does not hold when both great vessels arise from the right ventricle, because in this anomaly the mitral and aortic valves are also separated by a band of myocardium. The great vessels are identified primarily by the organs to which their branches are distributed.

The angiocardiogram of the heart in situs inversus in the frontal projection is a mirror image of the normal presentation. The right atrium and right ventricle lie on the left side of the heart. The aorta ascends along the left side of the mediastinum, and the aortic knob is on the right side. The anatomy of the bronchial tree is the reverse of normal, and there is almost always situs inversus of the abdominal viscera.

When the ventricles are inverted, the two atria are in normal position. The right ventricle, the one with the muscular infundibulum, lies on the left side of the anatomical left ventricle. The aorta arises from the right ventricle, to the left of the pulmonary artery, and its ascending limb forms the left margin of the superior mediastinum. The arch of the aorta extends posteriorly and to the right, so that the aortic knob is completely hidden within the mediastinal shadow. The main pulmonary artery arises from the left ventricle within the cardiac silhouette and divides almost symmetrically into right and left main branches. The aorta and pulmonary artery often lie side by side and are superimposed on each other in the lateral view. The abnormal position of the pulmonary artery can be identified in the lateral view because it is set back on the ventricle and does not arise flush with its anterior wall (see Figure 29–63, p. 1006). The appearance of a step between the ventricle and the pulmonary artery has not been encountered in any other cardiac anomaly.

In transposition of the great arteries, the aorta arises from the infundibular portion of the right ventricle. Usually, the aorta lies directly in front of the main pulmonary artery (see Figure 29–59, p. 1002), but in a small percentage of cases the vessels lie alongside each other.[148,149] The relationship of the great arteries therefore cannot be used as the sole criterion for differentiating transposition from ventricular inversion.[150,151]

COMPUTED TOMOGRAPHY (CT)

The development of computed tomographic equipment with rapid scan times (in the range of 1 to 4 seconds) and the capability of performing multiple scans in rapid sequence (dynamic scanning) has made the CT scanner a valuable tool for the study of heart disease and the evaluation of cardiac function. Not only does the scan provide cross-sectional images of the heart and vessels, but the sensitivity to small differences in x-ray absorption is so great that it is possible to differentiate various types of soft tissue and to detect small concentrations of contrast material within the blood stream. As a result, adequate opacification of the cardiac chambers and vessels can usually be obtained from a rapid intravenous bolus of contrast material or even from a prolonged intravenous infusion.

Despite the short scan times, the image of the heart represents the summation of several cardiac cycles. The image is essentially that of the heart in full diastole. For most diagnostic purposes, this has proven to be adequate. Sharper images of the heart, at specific points in the cardiac cycle, can be obtained by gating the scanner with the EKG. As a result, the effective scan time is reduced to about 0.1 second and images of the heart during the isovolumetric phases of end systole and end diastole are obtained.[152]

The myocardium cannot be adequately distinguished from the blood in the cardiac cavities on scans made without contrast enhancement. However, the pericardium can usually be identified, as it is set off by the subepicardial fat,[89] and the diagnosis of constrictive pericarditis and pericardial effusion (Fig. 43–6, p. 1479) can be made.[152a] The CT scan is also a sensitive detector of coronary artery calcifications[153] (Fig. 6–56A). The cross-sectional view is optimal for the recognition of anomalies of the aortic arch, the great vessels, and the venae cavae and the demonstration of the anatomic relationships of the vessels to other thoracic structures.[154]

Following the intravenous injection of contrast material, the cardiac chambers are clearly visualized as the blood becomes more radiodense than the surrounding myocardium. (Fig. 6–56B and C) Chamber size and shape can be accurately determined even on nongated scans.[155] Left ventricular aneurysms are easily detected. Filling defects within the chambers stand out prominently as localized areas of radiolucency, making the CT scan a sensitive method for the identification of cardiac tumors (Fig. 42–4, p. 1465)[156,157] and thrombi.[158,159,159a]

The interatrial and interventricular septae are visible as lucent bands between the opacified chambers, while the free cardiac wall is delimited between the chambers and the air-containing lung surrounding the heart. (Fig. 6–56C) Thus, the thickness of the myocardium can be measured and the degree and distribution of myocardial hypertrophy plotted.[160] Regional wall motion can be evaluated from gated scans as the difference between the contour of the ventricle in end systole and end diastole.[159,161] An accurate determination of the ejection fraction can be determined from measurements of the chamber volumes from the scans.

The potential of computed tomography for the evaluation and sizing[161a] of acute myocardial infarcts is not fully

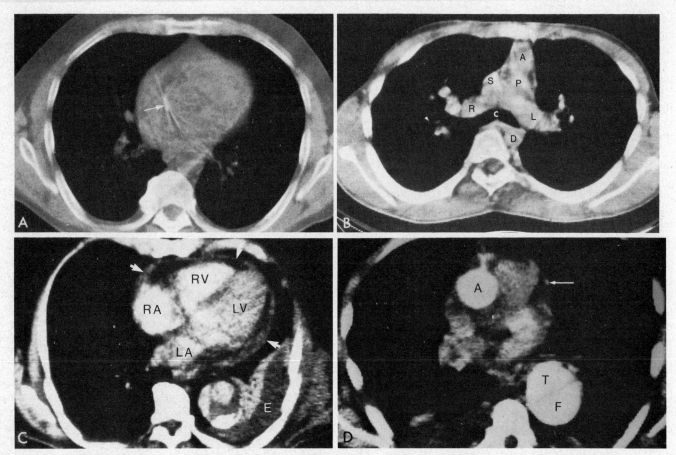

FIGURE 6–56 Computerized tomograms of cardiovascular disease. *A,* Coronary artery calcification. Nonenhanced scan through base of heart, just below aortic valve. The dense, radiopaque shadow (arrow) represents a calcific plaque in the right coronary artery. A section 1 cm higher showed a similar plaque in the left anterior descending coronary artery. Neither was identified on a routine chest film. (Courtesy of Dr. David Naidich, New York, New York.) *B,* Complete transposition of the great arteries, section at the level of the carina (C). The vascular pedicle of the heart is narrow because the aorta (A) lies directly in front of the pulmonary artery (P). Contrast material has been injected intravenously and opacifies the superior vena cava (S). R—Right pulmonary artery; L—left pulmonary artery D—descending aorta. (Courtesy of Dr. David Naidich, New York, New York.) *C,* Cardiac chambers, contrast-enhanced scan. The patient has recently had a repair of an aortic dissection. The interatrial septum is seen as a lucent line between the right atrium (RA) and the left atrium (LA). This is continuous anteriorly with the interventricular septum. LV—left ventricle; RV—right ventricle. The pericardium (arrows) is thickened. There is a left pleural effusion (E) with a band of atelectatic lung immediately in front of it. The descending aorta is visualized to the left of the spine, just medial to the effusion. Two opacified channels are present. The non-opacified region represents clot. (Courtesy of Dr. Diana F. Guthaner, Stanford, California.) *D,* Status following repair of aortic dissection, contrast-enhanced scan. A graft was placed in the ascending aorta (A). There is still flow in the true (T) and false (F) channels in the descending aorta. They are separated by a radiolucent band representing the dissected intima and part of the media. The opaque structure (arrow) to the left of the heart represents a patent bypass graft, to the left anterior descending coronary artery filled with contrast material. (Courtesy of Dr. Diana F. Guthaner, Stanford, California.)

known. Old infarcts of significant size can usually be identified as areas of thinning of the cardiac wall, but this is not seen with a fresh infarct. However, a diffuse blush of the ventricular myocardium can be demonstrated by performing a CT scan of the heart utilizing a bolus of contrast material. Following occlusion of a coronary artery, the contrast material does not reach the involved myocardium, and a perfusion defect is seen in the myocardial blush. It is likely that the nonperfused wall segment represents not only the infarct but the surrounding zone of injury as well.[152]

A more accurate picture of the ischemic area is seen on scans performed 24 hours after the infarction. The ischemically damaged myocardial cell reacts differently to intravascular contrast material than does the intact cell or the dead cell.[162] If an intravenous infusion of contrast material is administered, an area of enhanced blush will appear around the central nonopacified region. This border is thought to represent a zone of ischemically damaged, but friable, myocardium surrounding the central zone of myocardial necrosis.[152]

Opacification of the aorta and its major branches is usually adequate on a contrast-enhanced scan for the detection of aortic aneurysm (Fig. 43–4, p. 1544) and dissection[153,154] (Fig. 6–56C and D). When there is flow within the false channel, the dissected intima is clearly visualized as a radiolucent septum separating the two channels. Utilizing sections at various levels and sagittal reconstruction of the image, it is often possible to delimit accurately the extent of the dissection (p. 1551).

CT scanning is also of value in determining patency of a coronary bypass graft.[162a] On a transverse section below the level of the aortic valve, the grafts are seen in cross section as small, round shadows (Fig. 6–56D). Following the intravenous injection of contrast material, these shadows should become more radiopaque if the graft is patent.[165]

DIGITAL SUBTRACTION ANGIOGRAPHY

In order for vessels or cardiac chambers to be visualized by x-ray, the radiodensity of the blood within them must be significantly increased over that of the surrounding structures. This is accomplished by the rapid intravascular injection of relatively large volumes of contrast material. Digital processing of the fluoroscopic image, however, can intensify small differences in radiodensity so that the concentration of contrast material required for adequate opacification is significantly decreased.

Digital radiography is essentially a form of subtraction imaging.[165a] A TV image obtained prior to the injection of contrast material is converted to digital form. The picture is divided into a matrix of as many as one million picture

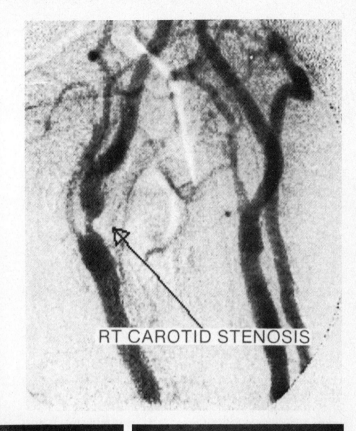

FIGURE 6–57 Digital subtraction angiogram, 70-degree right posterior oblique projection of a 58-year-old patient with hypertension and asymptomatic carotid bruits. There is moderate to marked stenosis of the right internal carotid artery at its origin and moderate stenosis of left external carotid artery at its origin. (Reproduced with permission from Weinstein, M. A., Modic, M. T., Buonocore, E., and Meaney, T. F.: Digital subtraction angiography. Clinical experience at The Cleveland Clinic Foundation. Vasc. Diag. Therap. *3*:19, 1982.)

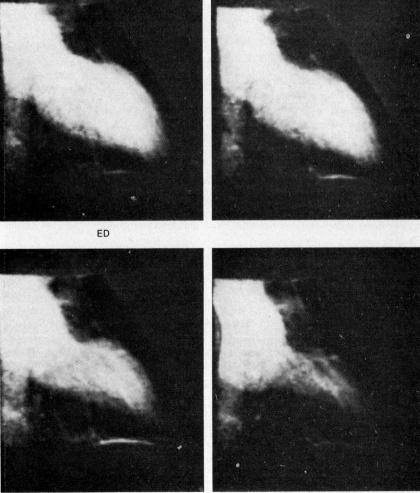

FIGURE 6–58 A series of mask mode images obtained by digital subtraction angiography from a patient with occlusion of the left anterior descending artery. The study was obtained after central intravenous injection of 40 ml of Renografin-76. These mask mode images in the right anterior oblique projection reveal hypokinesis of the anterolateral wall. ED = end-diastole; ES = end-systole. (Reproduced with permission from Higgins, C. B., Norris, S. L., Gerber, K. H., Slutsky, R. A., Ashburn, W. L., and Baily, N.: Quantitation of left ventricular dimensions and function by digital video substraction angiography. Radiology *144*: 461, 1982.)

elements (pixels). The density of each of these pixels is determined and assigned a numerical value. A second image, following the injection of contrast material is processed in the same manner and one is subtracted from the other. Thus, each pixel whose density has not changed between the two frames is canceled out, while those representing the opacified blood vessels remain. This image is electronically intensified and converted back to an analog picture.[166,166a,166b,166c]

In the last few years, digital angiography has become a standard means for studying diseases of peripheral vessels, especially the aorta, carotid, renal, and iliac arteries[167,168,168a] (Fig. 6–57). Application of the technique to cardiac imaging has been slow because of the problems imposed by motion of the heart. These have been overcome, to some extent, by gating techniques and by newer methodologies that allow real time subtraction with frame rates of 30 per second or greater.[169] As a result, ventricular volumes and ejection fractions can be accurately determined and segmental wall motion studied[170,170a,170b,170c,170d] (Fig. 6–58).

Although intravenous studies have the advantage of being relatively "non-invasive," the combination of digital radiography with ventricular or aortic injections provides images with significantly greater anatomic detail. This is especially true for the study of the coronary arteries. It is likely that, in the near future, diagnostically adequate coronary angiograms will be possible from a mid-stream aortic root injection. Similarly, the amount of contrast material required for ventriculography may be decreased so that it will not produce significant alteration of cardiac hemodynamics.

One other major potential of digital fluoroscopy is the measurement of blood flow. If a cursor is positioned over a vessel and each frame is subtracted from the previous one, a histogram is produced that depicts the increase in density of the vessel as the opacified blood reaches it, thus providing a measurement of the rate of blood flow.

References

1. Hoffman, R. B., and Rigler, L. G.: Evaluation of left ventricular enlargement in the lateral projection of the chest. Radiology 85:93, 1965.
2. Bachman, D. M., Ellis, K., and Austin, J. H. M.: The effects of minor degrees of obliquity on the lateral chest radiograph. Radiol. Clin. North Am. 16:465, 1978.
3. McGinnis, K. D., Eyler, W. R., and Alvarez, H., Jr.: Cardiac laminagraphy. Radiology 77:553, 1961.
4. Ravin, A., and Nice, C. M.: The angle of clearance of the left ventricle. Ann. Intern. Med. 36:1413, 1952.
5. Glover, L., Baxley, W. A., and Dodge, H. T.: A quantitative evaluation of heart size measurements from chest roentgenograms. Circulation 47:1289, 1973.
6. Nickol, K., and Wade, A. J.: Radiographic heart size and cardiothoracic ratio in three ethnic groups: A basis for a simple screening test for cardiac enlargement in men. Br. J. Radiol. 55:399, 1982.
7. Ungerleider, H. E., and Clark, C. P.: A study of the transverse diameter of the heart silhouette with prediction table based on the teleroentgenogram. Trans. Life Insur. Med. Dir. Am. 25:84, 1938.
8. Jonsell, S.: A method for determination of heart size by teleroentgenography (a heart volume index). Acta Radiol. 20:325, 1939.
9. Keats, T. E., and Enge, I. P.: Cardiac mensuration by the cardiac volume method. Radiology 85:850, 1965.
10. DuBois, E. F.: Basal Metabolism in Health and Disease. 2nd ed. Philadelphia, Lea & Febiger, 1931, p. 119.
11. Oberman, A., Jones, W. B., Riley, C. P., Reeves, T. J., Sheffield, L. T., and Turner, M. E.: Natural history of coronary artery disease. Bull. N.Y. Acad. Med. 48:1109, 1972.
12. Gammill, S. L., Krebs, C., Meyers, P., Nice, C. M., Jr., and Becker, H. C.: Cardiac measurements in systole and diastole. Radiology 94:115, 1970.
13. Kannel, W. B., Castelli, W. P., and McNamara, P. M.: The coronary profile: 12-year follow-up in the Framingham study. J. Occup. Med. 9:613, 1967.
14. Sherman, R. S., Bertrand, C. A., and Duffy, J. C.: Roentgenographic detection of cardiomegaly in employees with normal electrocardiograms. Am. J. Roentgenol. 119:493, 1973.
15. Felson, B.: More chest roentgen signs and how to teach them. Radiology 90:429, 1968.
16. Sos, T. A., Levin, D. C., Sniderman, K. W., and Beckmann, C. F.: Cinefluoroscopy in evaluating left ventricular contractility and aneurysms. Circulation 56 (Suppl.):III-18, 1977.
17. Bartel, A. G., Chen, J. T., Peter, R. H., Behar, V. S., Yihong, K., and Lester, R. G.: The significance of coronary calcification detected by fluoroscopy. A report of 360 patients. Circulation 49:1247, 1974.
18. Hamby, R. I., Tabrah, F., Wisoff, B. G., and Hartenstein, M. L.: Coronary artery calcification: clinical implications and angiographic correlates. Am. Heart J. 87:565, 1974.
19. Frink, R. J., Achor, R. W. P., Brown, A. L., Jr., Kincaid, O. W., and Brandenburg, R. O.: Significance of calcification of the coronary arteries. Am. J. Cardiol. 26:241, 1970.
20. Oliver, M. F.: The diagnostic value of detecting coronary calcification (Editorial). Circulation 42:981, 1970.
21. Chen, J. T. T., Behar, V. S., Morris, J. J., Jr., McIntosh, H. D., and Lester, R. G.: Correlation of roentgen findings with hemodynamic data in pure mitral stenosis. Am. J. Roentgenol. 102:280, 1968.
22. Probst, P., Goldschlager, N., and Selzer, A.: Left atrial size and atrial fibrillation in mitral stenosis. Factors influencing their relationship. Circulation 48:1282, 1973.
23. Raphael, M. J., Steiner, R. E., and Raftery, E. B.: Acute mitral incompetence. Clin. Radiol. 18:126, 1967.
24. Edwards, J. E.: An Atlas of Acquired Diseases of the Heart and Great Vessels. Philadelphia, W. B. Saunders Co., 1961, pp. 22–66.
25. Korn, D., Desanctis, R. W., and Sell, S.: Massive calcification of the mitral annulus: a clinical pathological study of 14 cases. N. Engl. J. Med. 267:900, 1962.
26. Hemley, S. D.: Mitral annulus calcification. Radiology 83:464, 1964.
27. Seltzer, R. A., Harthorne, J. W., and Austen, W. G.: The appearance and significance of left atrial calcification. Am. J. Roentgenol. 100:307, 1967.
28. Leonard, J. J., Katz, S., and Nelson, D.: Calcification of the left atrium: its anatomic location, diagnostic significance and roentgenologic demonstration. N. Engl. J. Med. 256:629, 1957.
29. Lendrum, A. C., Scott, L. D. W., and Park, S. D. S.: Pulmonary changes due to cardiac disease with special reference to hemosiderosis. Q. J. Med. 19:249, 1950.
30. Taylor, H. E., and Strong, G. F.: Pulmonary hemosiderosis in mitral stenosis. Ann. Intern. Med. 42:26, 1965.
31. Kerley, P.: Lung changes in acquired heart disease. Am. J. Roentgenol. 80:256, 1958.
32. Galloway, R. W., Epstein, E. J., and Coulshed, N.: Pulmonary ossific nodules in mitral valve disease. Br. Heart J. 23:297, 1961.
33. Lehman, J. S., Florence, H., Schimert, A. P., and Evans, G. C.: Acquired aortic valvular stenosis. Its diagnosis by conventional radiological study. Radiology 81:24, 1963.
34. Spindolo-Franco, H., Fish, B. G., Dachman, A., Grose, R., and Attai, L.: Recognition of bicuspid aortic valve by plain film calcification. Am. J. Roentgenol. 139:867, 1982.
35. Jarchow, B. H., and Kincaid, O. W.: Poststenotic dilatation of the ascending aorta: its occurrence and significance as a roentgenologic sign of aortic stenosis. Proc. Mayo Clin. 36:23, 1961.
36. Rockoff, S. D., and Austen, W. G.: The hemodynamic significance of the radiologic changes in acquired aortic stenosis. Am. Heart J. 65:458, 1963.
37. Cooley, D. A., Hallman, G. L., and Hammam, A. S.: Congenital cardiovascular anomalies in adults: results of surgical treatment in 167 patients over the age of 35. Am. J. Cardiol. 17:303, 1966.
38. Mark, H., and Young, D.: Congenital heart disease in the adult. Am. J. Cardiol. 15:293, 1965.
39. Fisher, J. M., Wilson, J. R., and Theilen, E. O.: Recognition of congenital heart disease in the fifth to eighth decades of life. Diagnostic criteria and natural history. Circulation 25:831, 1962.
40. Novack, P., Segal, B., Kasparian, H., and Likoff, W.: Atrial septal defect in patients over 40. Geriatrics 18:421, 1963.
41. Kuzman, W. J., and Yuskis, A. S.: Atrial septal defects in the older patient simulating acquired valvular heart disease. Am. J. Cardiol. 15:303, 1965.
42. Siltanen, P.: Atrial septal defect of secundum type in adults. Clinical and hemodynamic studies of 129 cases before and after surgical correction under cardiopulmonary bypass. Acta Med. Scand. (Suppl.) 497, 1968.
43. Betriu, A., Wigle, E. D., Felderhof, C. H., and McLoughlin, M. J.: Prolapse of the posterior leaflet of the mitral valve associated with secundum atrial septal defect. Am. J. Cardiol. 35:363, 1975.
44. Rippe, J. M., Sloss, L. J., Angoff, G., and Alpert, J. S.: Mitral valve prolapse in adults with congenital heart disease. Am. Heart J. 97:561, 1979.
45. Markman, P., Hawitt, G., and Wade, E. G.: Atrial septal defect in the middle-aged and elderly. Q. J. Med. 34:409, 1968.
46. Edwards, J. E.: The pathology of atrial septal defect. Semin. Roentgenol. 1:24, 1966.
47. Ruskin, H., and Samuel, E.: Calcification in the patent ductus arteriosus. Br. J. Radiol. 23:710, 1950.
48. Holman, E.: On circumscribed dilatation of an artery immediately distal to a partially occluding band: poststenotic dilatation. Surgery 36:3, 1954.
49. Martin, E. C., Stratford, M. A., and Gersony, W. M.: Initial detection of co-

arctation of the aorta: An opportunity for the radiologist. Am. J. Roentgenol. *137*:1015, 1981.

50. Figley, M. M.: Accessory roentgen signs of coarctation of the aorta. Radiology *62*:671, 1954.

51. Gladnikoff, H.: The roentgenological picture of coarctation of the aorta and its anatomical basis. Acta Radiol. *27*:8, 1946.

52. Baron, M. G.: Obscuration of the aortic knob in coarctation of the aorta. Circulation *43*:311, 1971.

53. Sloan, R. D., and Cooley, R. N.: Coarctation of the aorta. Radiology *61*:701,1953.

54. Boone, M. L., Swenson, B. E., and Felson, B.: Rib notching: its many causes. Am. J. Roentgenol. *91*:1075, 1964.

55. Elliott, L. P., and Schiebler, G. L.: X-ray Diagnosis of Congenital Cardiac Disease. Springfield, Ill., Charles C Thomas, 1968.

56. Ivemark, B. I.: Implication of agenesis of the spleen on the pathogenesis of conotruncus anomalies in childhood—An analysis of heart malformations in the splenic agenesis syndrome, with 14 new cases. Acta Paediatr. Upps. *44* (Suppl. 104):7, 1955.

57. Van Mierop, L. H. S., Patterson, P. R., and Reynolds, R. W.: Two cases of congenital asplenia with isomerism of the cardiac atria and the sinoatrial nodes. Am. J. Cardiol. *13*:407, 1964.

58. Ruttenberg, H. D., Neufeld, H. N., Lucas, R. V., Jr., Carey, L. S., Adams, P., Jr., Anderson, R. C., and Edwards, J. E.: Syndrome of congenital cardiac disease with asplenia. Distinction from other forms of congenital cyanotic cardiac disease. Am. J. Cardiol. *13*:387, 1964.

59. Stewart, J. R., Kincaid, O. W., and Titus, J. L.: Right aortic arch: Plain film diagnosis and significance. Am. J. Roentgenol. *97*:377, 1966.

60. Felson, B., and Palayew, M. J.: The two types of right aortic arch. Radiology *81*:745, 1963.

61. Baron, M. G.: Right aortic arch. Circulation *44*:1137, 1971.

62. Berdon, W. E., and Baker, D. H.: Plain film findings in azygos continuation of the inferior vena cava. Am. J. Roentgenol. *104*:452, 1968.

63. Michelson, E., and Salik, J. O.: Vascular pattern of lung as seen on routine and tomographic studies. Radiology *73*:511, 1959.

64. Westermark, N.: On the roentgen diagnosis of lung embolism. Acta Radiol. *19*: 357, 1938.

65. Milne, E. N. C.: Physiological interpretation of the plain radiograph in mitral stenosis, including a review of criteria for the radiological estimation of pulmonary arterial and venous pressures. Br. J. Radiol. *36*:902, 1963.

66. Simon, M.:The pulmonary vessels: their hemodynamic evaluation using routine radiographs. Radiol. Clin. North Am. *1*:363, 1963.

67. Steiner, R. E.: Radiology of pulmonary circulation. Chamberlain Lecture, 1963. Am. J. Roentgenol. *91*:249, 1964.

68. Simon, M.: The pulmonary veins in mitral stenosis. J. Fac. Radiol. *9*:25, 1958.

69. West, J. B., Dollery, C. T., and Heard, B. E.: Increased pulmonary vascular resistance in the dependent zone of the isolated dog lung caused by perivascular edema. Circ. Res. *17*:191, 1965.

70. Hughes, J. M. B., Glazier, J. B., Maloney, J. E., and West, J. B.: Effect of interstitial pressure on pulmonary blood flow. Lancet *1*:192, 1967.

71. Doyle, A. E., Goodwin, J. F., Harrison, C. V., and Steiner, R. E.: Pulmonary vascular patterns in pulmonary hypertension. Br. Heart J. *19*:353, 1957.

72. Fishman, A. P., and Renkin, E. M. (eds.): Pulmonary Edema. Bethesda, American Physiological Society, 1979, 261 pp.

73. Harrison, M. O., Conte, P. J., and Heitzman, E. R.: Radiological detection of clinically occult cardiac failure following myocardial infarction. Br. J. Radiol. *44*:265, 1971.

74. Chait, A.: Interstitial pulmonary edema. Circulation *45*:1323, 1972.

75. Kerley, P. J.: Radiology in heart disease. Br. Med. J. *2*:594, 1933.

76. Fleischner, F. G., and Reiner, L.: Linear x-ray shadows in acquired pulmonary hemosiderosis and congestion. N. Engl. J. Med. *250*:900, 1954.

77. Grainger, R. G.: Interstitial pulmonary oedema and its radiological diagnosis. A sign of pulmonary venous and capillary hypertension. Br. J. Radiol. *31*:201, 1958.

78. Trapnell, D. H.: The peripheral lymphatics of the lung. Br. J. Radiol. *36*:660, 1963.

79. Meszaros, W. T.: Lung changes in left heart failure. Circulation *47*:859, 1973.

80. Don, C., and Johnson, R.: The nature and significance of peribronchial cuffing in pulmonary edema. Radiology *125*:577, 1977.

81. Hayes, C. E., Case, T. A., Ailion, D. C., Morris, A. H., Cutillo, A., Blackburn, C. W., Durney, C. H., and Johnson, S. A.: Lung water quantitation by nuclear magnetic resonance imaging. Science *216*:1313, 1982.

82. Fleischner, F. G.: The butterfly pattern of acute pulmonary edema. Am. J. Cardiol. *20*:39, 1967.

83. Richman, S. M., and Godar, T. J.: Unilateral pulmonary edema. N. Engl. J. Med. *264*:1148, 1961.

84. Lane, E. J., Jr., and Carsky, E. W.: Epicardial fat: lateral plain film analysis in normals and in pericardial effusion. Radiology *91*:1, 1968.

85. Jorgens, J., Kundel, R., and Lieber, A.: The cinefluorographic approach to the diagnosis of pericardial effusion. Am. J. Roentgenol. *87*:911, 1962.

86. Tomoda, H., Hoshiai, M., Furuya, H., Matsumoto, S., Tanabe, T., Tamachi, H., Sasamoto, H., Koide, S., Kuribayashi, S., and Matsuyama, S.: Evaluation of pericardial effusion with computed tomography. Am. Heart J. *99*:701, 1980.

87. Heinz, M., and Abrams, H. L.: Radiologic aspects of operable heart disease. IV. The variable appearance of constrictive pericarditis. Radiology *69*:54, 1957.

88. Shanks, S. C., and Kerley, P. (eds.): A Textbook of X-ray Diagnosis. 4th ed. Philadelphia, W. B. Saunders Co., 1972, p. 353.

89. Moncada, R., Baker, M., Salinas, M., Demos, T. C., Churchill, R., Love, L.,

90. Reynes, C., Hale, D., Cardoso, M., Pifarre, R., and Gunnar, R.: Diagnostic role of computed tomography in pericardial heart disease: Congenital defects, thickening, neoplasms and effusions. Am. Heart J. *103*:263, 1982.

90. Doppman, J. L., Rienmuller, R., Lissner, J., Cyran, J., Bolte, H. D., Strauer, B. E., and Hellwig, H.: Computed tomography in constrictive pericardial disease. J. Comput. Assist. Tomogr. *5*:1, 1981.

91. Ellis, K., Leeds, N. E., and Himmelstein, A.: Congenital deficiencies in the parietal pericardium. A review with 2 new cases including successful diagnosis by plain roentgenography. Am. J. Roentgenol. *82*:125, 1959.

92. Chang, C. H., and Leigh, T. F.: Congenital partial defect of the pericardium associated with herniation of the left atrial appendage. Am. J. Roentgenol. *86*: 517, 1961.

93. Chang, C. H., and Amory, H. I.: Congenital partial right pericardial defect associated with herniation of the right atrial appendage. Radiology *84*:660, 1965.

94. Williamson, D. E.: Experimental determination of flow equation in catheters for cardiology. Am. J. Roentgenol. *94*:704, 1965.

95. Inter-Society Commission for Heart Disease Resources: Optimal resources for examination of the chest and cardiovascular system. Catheterization—angiographic laboratories. Circulation *53*:A-1, 1976.

96. Bargeron, L. M., Jr., Elliott, L. P., Soto, B., Bream, P. R., and Curry, G. C.: Axial cineangiography in congenital heart disease. I. Concept, technical and anatomic considerations. Circulation *56*:1075, 1977.

97. Elliott, L. P., Bargeron, L. M., Jr., Bream, P. R., Soto, B., and Curry, G. C.: Axial cineangiography in congenital heart disease. II. Specific lesions. Circulation *56*:1048, 1977.

98. Elliott, L. P., Green, C. E., Rogers, W. J., Hood, W. P., Mantle, J. A., and Papapietro, S. E.: Advantages of the caudo-cranial left anterior oblique left ventriculogram in adult heart disease. Am. J. Cardiol. *49*:369, 1982.

99. Mills, S. R., Jackson, D. C., Older, R. A., Heaston, D. K., and Moore, A. V.: The incidence, etiologies and avoidance of complications of pulmonary angiography in a large series. Radiology *136*:295, 1980.

100. Susman, N., and Diboll, W. B., Jr.: Fluid dynamics in the tip of the multiholed angiographic catheter. Radiology *92*:843, 1969.

101. Bettmann, M. A.: Angiographic contrast agents: Conventional and new media compared. Am. J. Roentgenol. *139*:787, 1982.

102. Stake, G., Bjornstad, P. G., Nordshus, T., and Sorland, S. J.: Metrizamide and Metrizoate for cardioangiography in infants and children. Acta Radiol. [Diagn.] *22*:359, 1981.

103. Cumberland, D. C.: Amipaque in coronary angiography and left ventriculography. Br. J. Radiol. *54*:203, 1981.

104. Mullins, C. B., Leshin, S. J., Mierzwiak, D. S., Alsobrook, H. D., and Mitchell, J. H.: Changes in left ventricular function produced by the injection of contrast media. Am. Heart J. *83*:373, 1972.

105. Iseri, L. T., Kaplan, M. A., Evans, M. J., and Nickel, E. D.: Effect of concentrated contrast media during angiography on plasma volume and plasma osmolality. Am. Heart J. *69*:154, 1965.

106. Hammermeister, K. E., and Warbasse, J. R.: The immediate hemodynamic effects of cardiac angiography in man. Am. J. Cardiol. *31*:307, 1973.

107. Carleton, R. A.: Change in left ventricular volume during angiocardiography. Am. J. Cardiol. *27*:460, 1971.

108. Cohn, P. F., Horn, H. R., Teichholz, L. E., Kreulen, T. H., Herman, M. V., and Gorlin, R.: Effects of angiographic contrast medium on left ventricular function in coronary artery disease. Comparison with static and dynamic exercise. Am. J. Cardiol. *32*:21, 1973.

109. Brundage, D. H., and Cheitin, M. D.: Left ventricular angiography as a function test. Chest *64*:70, 1973.

110. D'Elia, J. A., Gleason, R. E., Alday, M., Malarick, C., Godley, K., Warram, J., Kaldany, A., and Weinrauch, L. A.: Nephrotoxicity from angiographic contrast material. A prospective study. Am. J. Med. *72*:719, 1982.

111. Pendergrass, H. P., Tondreau, R. L., Pendergrass, E. P., Ritchie, D. J., Hildreth, E. A., and Askovitz, S. I.: Reactions associated with intravenous urography: historical and statistical review. Radiology *71*:1, 1958.

112. Giammona, S. T., Lurie, P. R., and Segar, W. E.: Hypertonicity following selective angiocardiography. Circulation *28*:1096, 1963.

113. Ellis, K., Griffiths, S. P., Bordiuk, J. M., Burris, J. O., and Baker, D. H.: Some congenital anomalies of the tricuspid valve: angiocardiographic considerations. Radiol. Clin. North Am. *6*:383, 1968.

114. Kieffer, S. A., and Carey, L. S.: Tricuspic atresia with normal aortic root: roentgen-anatomic correlation. Radiology *80*:605, 1963.

115. Chesler, E., Moller, J. H., and Edwards, J. E.: The congenital cardiovascular anomalies underlying "reversed coarctation." Am. Heart J. *75*:34, 1968.

116. Eliot, R. S., Shone, J. D., Kanjuh, V. I., Ruttenberg, H. B., Carey, L. S., and Edwards, J. E.: Mitral atresia. Am. Heart J. *75*:325, 1968.

117. Miller, G. A. H.: Aortic atresia. Diagnostic cardiac catheterization in first week of life. Br. Heart J. *33*:367, 1971.

118. Rudolph, A. M.: The changes in circulation after birth. Their importance in congenital heart disease. Circulation *41*:343, 1970.

119. Shumacker, H. B., Jr., King, H., and Waldhausen, J. A.: The persistent left superior vena cava. Ann. Surg. *155*:797, 1967.

120. Baron, M. G., Wolf, B. S., Steinfeld, L., and Gordon, A.: Left ventricular angiocardiography in the study of ventricular septal defects. Radiology *81*:223, 1963.

121. Baron, M. G., Wolf, B. S., Steinfeld, L., and Van Mierop, L. H. S.: Angiocardiographic diagnosis of subpulmonic ventricular septal defect. Am. J. Roentgenol. *103*:93, 1968.

122. Figley, M. M., and Bagshaw, M. A.: Angiocardiographic aspects of constrictive pericarditis. Radiology *69*:46, 1957.

123. Adelman, A. G., McLoughlin, M. J., Marquis, Y., Auger, P., and Wigle, E. D.: Left ventricular cineangiocardiographic observations in muscular subaortic stenosis. Am. J. Cardiol. 24:689, 1969.

124. Bourdarias, J. P., Ourbak, P., Ferrane, J., Sozutek, Y., Scebat, L., and Lenegre, J.: Obstructive cardiomyopathy. Cineangiographic study of 50 cases. Am. J. Roentgenol. 102:853, 1968.

125. Schaffer, A. I., Kania, H., Cucci, C. E., and DePasquale, N. P.: New technique for angiographic visualization of membranous subaortic stenosis. Br. Heart J. 34:742, 1972.

126. Simon, A. L.: Angiographic diagnosis of idiopathic hypertrophic subaortic stenosis. Radiol. Clin. North Am. 6:423, 1968.

127. Baron, M. G., Wolf, B. S., Grishman, A., and Van Mierop, L. H. S.: Aneurysm of the membranous septum. Am. J. Roentgenol. 191:1303, 1964.

128. Freedom, R. M., White, R. D., Pieroni, D. R., Varghese, P. J., Krovetz, L. J., and Rowe, R. R.: The natural history of the so-called aneurysm of the membranous ventricular septum in childhood. Circulation 49:375, 1974.

129. Herman, M. V., Heinle, R. A., Klein, M. D., and Gorlin, R.: Localized disorders in myocardial contraction. Asynergy and its role in congestive heart failure. N. Engl. J. Med. 277:222, 1967.

130. Sniderman, A. D., Marpole, D., and Fallen, E. L.: Regional contraction patterns in normal and ischemic left ventricle in man. Am. J. Cardiol. 31:484, 1973.

131. Lester, R. G., Osteen, R. T., and Robinson, A. F.: Infundibular obstruction secondary to pulmonary valvular stenosis. Am. J. Roentgenol. 94:78, 1965.

132. Criley, J. M., Lewis, K. B., White, R. I., Jr., and Ross, R. S.: Pressure gradients without obstruction: a new concept of "hypertrophic subaortic stenosis." Circulation 32:88, 1965.

133. Braunwald, E., Morrow, A. G., Cornell, W. P., Aygen, M. M., and Hilbish, T. F.: Idiopathic hypertrophic subaortic stenosis: clinical, hemodynamic and angiographic manifestations. Am. J. Med. 29:924, 1960.

134. Baron, M. G.: The angiocardiographic diagnosis of valvular stenosis. Circulation 44:143, 1971.

135. Takekawa, S. D., Kincaid, O. W., Titus, J. L., and DuShane, J. W.: Congenital aortic stenosis. Am. J. Roentgenol. 98:800, 1966.

136. Rudhe, U.: Angiocardiography in pulmonic stenosis. Radiol. Clin. North Am. 2:395, 1964.

137. Demany, M. A., Kay, E. B., and Zimmerman, H. A.: An angiocardiographic sign for the evaluation of the stenotic mitral valve. Am. J. Cardiol. 18:843, 1966.

138. Kieffer, S. A., and Carey, L. S.: Tricuspid atresia with normal aortic root: roentgen-anatomic correlation. Radiology 80:605, 1963.

139. Desilets, D. T., Marcano, B. A., Emmanouilides, G. C., and Gyepes, M. T.: Severe pulmonary valve stenosis and atresia. Radiol. Clin. North Am. 6:367, 1968.

140. Baron, M. G.: Angiocardiographic evaluation of valvular insufficiency. Circulation 43:599, 1971.

141. Cairns, K. B., Kloster, F. E., Bristow, J. D., Lees, M. H., and Griswold, H. E.: Problems in the hemodynamic diagnosis of tricuspid insufficiency. Am. Heart J. 75:173, 1968.

142. Björk, V. O., Lodin, H., and Malers, E.: The evaluation of the degree of mitral insufficiency by selective left ventricular angiocardiography. Am. Heart J. 60:691, 1960.

143. Criley, J. M., Lewis, K. B., Humphries, J. O., and Ross, R. S.: Prolapse of the mitral valve: clinical and cine-angiocardiographic findings. Br. Heart J. 28:488, 1966.

144. Kittredge, R. D., Shimomura, S., Cameron, A., and Bell, A. L. L., Jr.: Prolapsing mitral leaflets. Cineangiographic determination. Am. J. Roentgenol. 109:84, 1970.

145. Perloff, J. K.: Evolving concepts of mitral-valve prolapse. N. Engl. J. Med. 307:369, 1982.

146. Ellis, K., Griffiths, S. P., Burris, J. O., Ramsay, G. C., and Fleming, R. J.: Ebstein's anomaly of the tricuspid valve, angiocardiographic considerations. Am. J. Roentgenol. 92:1338, 1964.

147. Baron, M. G.: Endocardial cushion defects. Radiol. Clin. North Am. 6:343, 1968.

148. Beuren, A.: Differential diagnosis of the Taussig-Bing heart from complete transposition of the great vessels with a posteriorly overriding pulmonary artery. Circulation 21:1071, 1960.

149. Barcia, A., Kincaid, O. W., Davis, G. D., Kirklin, J. W., and Ongley, P. A.: Transposition of the great arteries. An angiocardiographic study. Am. J. Roentgenol. 100:249, 1967.

150. Jackson, H.: The transposition complexes and other cardiovascular malalignments. Br. J. Radiol. 42:721, 1969.

151. Anselmi, G., Munoz, S., Blanco, P., Machado, I., and de la Cruz, M. V.: Systematization and clinical study of dextroversion, mirror-image dextrocardia, and laevoversion. Br. Heart J. 34:1085, 1972.

152. Doherty, P. W., Lipton, M. J., Berninger, W. H., Skioldebrand, C. G., Carlsson, E., and Redington, R. W.: Detection and quantification of myocardial infarction in vivo using transmission computed tomography. Circulation 63:597, 1981.

152a. Riemuller, R., Doppman, J. L., Reichardt, B., and Strauer, B. E.: Diagnostic signs of constrictive pericardial diseases by computed tomography. J. Am. Coll. Cardiol. 1:737, 1983.

153. Masuda, Y., Yoshida, H., Morooka, N., Takahashi, O., Watanabe, S., Inagaki, Y., Uchiyama, G., and Tateno, Y.: ECG synchronized computed tomography in clinical evaluation of total and regional cardiac motion: Comparison of post–myocardial infarction to normal hearts by rapid sequential imaging. Am. Heart J. 103:230, 1982.

154. Webb, W. R., Gamsu, G., Speckman, J. M., Kaiser, J. A., Federle, M. P., and Lipton, M. J.: CT demonstration of mediastinal aortic arch anomalies. J. Comput. Assist. Tomogr. 6:445, 1982.

155. Ringertz, H. G., Skioldebrand, C. G., Refsum, H., Tyberg, J. V., Napel, S. A., and Lipton, M. J.: A comparison between the information in gated and nongated computed cardiac CT images. J. Comput. Assist. Tomogr. 6:933, 1982.

156. Sutton, D., Al-Kutoubi, M. A., and Lipkin, D. B.: Left atrial myxoma diagnosed by computerized tomography. Br. J. Radiol. 55:80, 1982.

157. Godwin, J. D., Axel, L., Adams, J. R., Schiller, N. B., Simpson, P. C., Jr., and Gertz, E. W.: Computed tomography: A new method for diagnosing tumor of the heart. Circulation 63:448, 1981.

158. Godwin, J. D., Hertkens, R. J., Skioldebrand, C. G., Brundage, B. H., Schiller, N. B., and Lipton, M. J.: Detection of intraventricular thrombi by computed tomography. Radiology 138:717, 1981.

159. Watanabe, S.: Diagnostic CT imaging of the heart and aorta in health and disease. Japan. Cir. J. 45:1030, 1981.

159a. Tomoda, H., Hashiai, M., Furuya, H., Kuribayashi, S., Ootaki, M., Matsuyama, S., Koide, S., Kawada, S., and Shotsu, A.: Evalation of intracardiac thrombus with computed tomography. Am. J. Cardiol. 51:843, 1983.

160. Lackner, K., and Thurn, P.: Computed tomography of the heart: ECG-gated and continuous scans. Radiology 140:413, 1981.

161. Mattrey, R. F., and Higgins, C.: Detection of regional myocardial dysfunction during ischemia with computerized tomography: Documentation and physiologic basis. Invest. Radiol. 17:329, 1982.

161a. Slutsky, R. A., Mattery, R. F., Long, S. A., and Higgins, C. B.: In vivo estimation of myocardial infarct size and left ventricular function by prospectively gated computerized transmission tomography. Circulation 67:759, 1983.

162. Newell, J. D., Higgins, C. B., and Abraham, J. L.: Uptake of iodinated contrast material by the ischemically damaged myocardial cell. Invest. Radiol. 17:61, 1982.

162a. Daniel, W. G., Dohring, W., Stender, H-S., and Lichtlen, P. R.: Value and limitations of computed tomography in assessing aortocoronary bypass graft patency. Circulation 67:983, 1983.

163. Hedberg, E., Wolverson, M., Sundaram, M., Connors, J., and Susman, N.: CT findings in thoracic aortic dissection. Am. J. Roentgenol. 136:13, 1981.

164. Godwin, J. D., Turley, K., Herkens, R. J., and Lipton, M. J.: Computed tomography for follow up of chronic aortic dissections. Radiology 139:655, 1981.

165. Guthaner, D. F., Brody, W. R., Ricci, M., et al.: The use of computed tomography in the diagnosis of coronary artery bypass graft patency. Cardiovasc. Intervent. Radiol. 3:3, 1980.

165a. Crummy, A. B., Stieghorst, M. F., VanLysel, M. S., and Dobbins, J. T.: Applying digital subtraction arteriography. J. Cardiovasc. Med. 8:345, 1983.

166. Harrington, D. P., Boxt, L. M., and Murray, P. D.: Digital subtraction angiography: Over-view of technical principles. Am. J. Roentgenol. 139:781, 1982.

166a. Engels, P. H. C., Ludwig, J. W., and Verhoeven, L. A. J.: Left ventricle evaluation by digital video subtraction angiocardiography. Radiology 144:471, 1982.

166b. Higgins, C. B., Norris, S. L., Gerber, K. H., Slutsky, R. A., Ashburn, W. L., and Baily, N.: Quantitation of left ventricular dimensions and function by digital video subtraction angiography. Radiology 144:461, 1982.

166c. Weinstein, M. A., Modic, M. T., Buonocore, E., and Meaney, T. F.: Digital subtraction angiography. Clinical experience at The Cleveland Clinic Foundation. Vasc. Dis. Therapy. 3:19, 1982.

167. Crummy, A., Strother, C. M., Sackett, J. F., Ergun, D. L., Shaw, C. G., Kruger, R. A., Misretta, C. A., Turnipseed, W. D., Lieberman, R. T., Myerowitz, P. D., and Ruzicka, F. F.: Computerized fluoroscopy: Digital subtraction for intravenous angiocardiography and arteriography. Am. J. Roentgenol. 135:1131, 1980.

168. Meaney, T. F., Weinstein, M. A., Buonocore, E., Pavlicek, W., Borkowski, G. P., Gallagher, J. P., Sufka, B., and MacIntyre, W. J.: Digital subtraction angiography of the human cardiovascular system. Am. J. Roentgenol. 135:1153, 1980.

168a. .0.5 Brody, W. R., Enzmann, D. R., Miller, D. C., Guthaner, D. F., Pelc, N. J., Keys, G. S., and Riederer, S. J.: Intravenous arteriography using digital subtraction techniques. JAMA 248:671, 1982.

169. Kruger, A., Miller, F. J., Jr., Nelson, J. A., Liu, P. Y., and Bateman, W.: Digital subtraction angiography using a temporal bandpass filter: Associated patient motion properties. Radiology 145:315, 1982.

170. Vas, R., Diamond, G. A., Forrester, J. S., Whiting, J. S., Pfaff, M. J., Levisman, J. A., Nakano, F. S., and Swan, H. J. C.: Computer enchanced digital angiography: Correlation of left ventricular ejection fraction and regional wall motion. Am. Heart J. 104:732, 1982.

170a. Gerber, K. H., Slutsky, R. A., Bhargava, V., Ashburn, W. L., and Higgins, C. B.: Detection and assessment of severity of regional ischemic left ventricular dysfunction by digital fluoroscopy. Am. Heart J. 104:27, 1982.

170b. Tobis, J., Nalcioglu, O., Johnston, W. D., Seibert, A., Iseri, L. T., Roeck, W., Grad, E., and Henry, W. L.: Digital angiography in assessment of ventricular function and wall motion during pacing in patients with coronary artery disease. Am. J. Cardiol. 51:668, 1983.

170c. Kroenberg, M. W., Price, R. R., Smith, C. W., Robertson, R. M., Perry, J. M., Pickens, D. R., Domanski, M. J., Partain, C. L., and Friesinger, G. C.: Evaluation of left ventricular performance using digital subtraction angiography. Am. J. Cardiol. 51:837, 1983.

170d. Goldberg, H. L., Borer, J. S., Moses, J. W., Fisher, J., Cohen, B., and Skelly, N. T.: Digital subtraction intravenous left ventricular angiography: Comparison with conventional intraventricular angiography. J. Am. Coll. Cardiol. 1:858, 1983.

7
ELECTROCARDIOGRAPHY AND VECTORCARDIOGRAPHY

by Charles Fisch, M.D.

The clinical electrocardiogram (ECG) records changing potential of an electrical field imparted by a generator, i.e., the heart or, more appropriately, at any moment an aggregate of cardiac cells. It does not record directly the electrical activity of the source itself. Such activity is registered only when an electrode is in immediate contact with the tissue generating the current and at the moment when the electrode senses the edge of the wave of activation or recovery. At all other times, whether in vitro or in vivo, only potential differences in an electrical field are registered. It is important to appreciate that the ECG, while recording the changes of an electrical field, may fail to reflect accurately the activity of the source itself and often

provides only an approximation of the voltage generated by the heart. Efforts to predict surface potentials from the knowledge of behavior of the cardiac generator—the so-called electrocardiographic forward problem—or to predict the electrical behavior of the cardiac generator from the body surface potentials—the so-called electrocardiographic inverse problem—have to date been unsuccessful.[1]

Despite this basic limitation, the ECG has evolved into an extremely useful clinical laboratory tool and is the only practical means of recording the electrical behavior of the heart. Its usefulness as a diagnostic methodology is the result of careful, often purely deductive analysis of innumerable patient records and of studies correlating the ECG with basic electrophysiological properties of the heart; with clinical and laboratory findings; and with anatomical, pathological; and experimental observations.[2] The result has been that electrocardiography can be used, within limits, to identify anatomical, metabolic, ionic, and hemodynamic changes. It is often an independent marker of myocardial disease and occasionally the only indicator of a pathological process.[3-11]

Electrocardiography serves as a gold standard for the diagnosis of arrhythmias. Arrhythmias have been studied by a variety of methods for centuries, but none of the diverse methods has approached the levels of sensitivity and specificity offered by the ECG. Free of the assumptions required for interpreting the electrocardiographic P, QRS, ST, or T waveforms, arrhythmias recorded from the surface of the body, with rare exceptions, accurately reflect intracardiac events. However, even in the area of rhythm analysis, certain limitations must be appreciated. While most arrhythmias are due to disordered impulse formation or conduction (or both) of the specialized tissue, the ECG reflects the electrical behavior of the myocardium and not of the specialized tissue. For simple arrhythmias, this dichotomy poses no problem; however, in complex arrhythmias, when recognition and interpretation of the behavior of specialized tissue is critical, such information must be derived by deductive reasoning. In addition, intracardiac ECG studies have demonstrated that small changes in the speed of conduction, or cycle length, may be a critical determinant of rhythm behavior, but such small changes may not be appreciated in a tracing inscribed with standard direct writing equipment. Furthermore, on rare occasion, arrhythmias induce voltage changes too small to register in the ECG. These limitations, once appreciated as inherent in the ECG, rarely interfere with proper analysis of even the most complex arrhythmias.

The contribution of electrocardiography to the diagnosis and management of patients with heart disease is equaled, if not exceeded, by its impact on clinical and basic electrophysiological research. The clinical ECG continues to stimulate an exchange of ideas between the clinical electrocardiographer and the basic and clinical investigator. Numerous electrophysiological concepts derived through deductive analysis of the ECG have ultimately been confirmed in the laboratory. Similarly, concepts first developed in an animal laboratory have been identified in man by clinical electrocardiographers. As a result of such interaction, electrocardiography, at first a largely empirical body of knowledge, is gradually acquiring firm experimental bases.

As with any other laboratory procedure, the sensitivity and specificity of the ECG and of its individual components are critical determinants of its clinical usefulness. This is far more complex for the ECG than for other laboratory techniques developed for a single purpose, since its multiple waveforms may be identically or differentially influenced by a wide spectrum of physiological, pathophysiological, or anatomical changes. Thus, it may be difficult— if not impossible—to identify a singular cause for an ECG abnormality. Sensitivity and specificity can be enhanced through the examiner's careful formulation of the question the ECG is expected to answer, attention to the intra- and extracellular environment present at the time of the recording, use of proper recording technique, and assessment of

serial tracings, all coupled with skillful interpretation of the ECG findings.[12]

THEORETICAL CONSIDERATIONS

Essential to an understanding of the derivation and interpretation of the clinical ECG is information about (1) the physical and electrophysiological events responsible for the electrical potential, recorded as the transmembrane action potential, and the spread of excitation; (2) the role of the volume conductor; and (3) the theoretical basis of the lead systems.

ELECTRICAL BASES AND THEORY (THE DIPOLE, VOLUME CONDUCTOR, MAGNITUDE OF POTENTIAL, AND POLARITY OF THE ELECTRICAL FIELD)

At any moment in time, the cardiac generator can be viewed as a dipole or doublet consisting of a positive and a negative charge separated by a small distance. Since the dipole generates a force that has magnitude and direction, it can be expressed as a vector. By convention the arrowhead of the vector indicates the positive pole. When such a dipole is immersed in a volume conductor, an electrical field is generated.[13,14] In a homogeneous volume conductor, the field is symmetrically distributed. The lines of the electrical field are symmetrical in relation to a line that is perpendicular to and transects the dipole at its midpoint.

At any moment in time, the magnitude of the potential at a given point (P) in the volume conductor can be estimated using the solid-angle concept, or the concept relating the potential to an angle formed by a line drawn from P to the midpoint of the dipole axis and the dipole axis itself (Fig. 7–1).

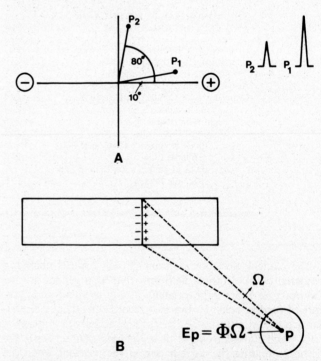

FIGURE 7–1   *A,* The potentials at points P₁ and P₂ are inversely proportional to the square of the distance from the source and proportional to the cosine of angle formed by a line drawn from point P to the midpoint of the dipole axis and the axis itself. *B,* The potential E is proportional to the solid angle Ω and the strength of the charged surface subtending the angle Φ. (Modified from Wolff, L.: Electrocardiography: Fundamentals and Clinical Application. 3rd ed. Philadelphia, W. B. Saunders Co., 1962, p. 15.)

The electrical surface with its boundary projected to P results in a cone and defines the solid angle subtended by the area in question. The segment of a sphere inscribed by a radius of unity drawn about point P, with P as the center of the sphere, and its border delineated by the cone, is proportional to the area of electrical activity. With variables such as tissue resistance and geometry being constant, the voltage at P can be expressed as $Ep = \phi \cdot \Omega$, where ϕ is voltage per unit of the solid angle and Ω is the solid angle.[15,16]

An alternative and perhaps clinically more applicable approach to estimating Ep considers the distance (r) of P from the source, the strength of the source (m), and the cosine of the angle formed by a line drawn from P to the midpoint of the dipole axis and the dipole axis (Θ), with the magnitude of the angle estimated in reference to the positive pole of the dipole. This relationship can be expressed as $Ep = \dfrac{m \cos \Theta}{\gamma^2}$. According to this formula, when the angle is 90°, the line drawn from P is perpendicular to the dipole axis and the Ep is zero. In the ECG the inscription would be isoelectric or equiphasic. On the other hand, with the angle becoming smaller, the P is closer to the positive pole of the dipole and the voltage becomes greater.[9,15,16]

Assuming that the volume conductor is homogeneous and infinite and has a uniform boundary and that the generator is located in the center of the volume conductor, both approaches for estimation of Ep at P are correct. Such assumptions, however, are not valid in man (see below).

The influence of polarity of the dipole, the distance from the dipole, and the strength of the electrical field on waveform are critical for proper analysis and interpretation of the ECG. These relationships can be studied using a hypothetical experimental dipole or cardiac tissue immersed in a homogeneous volume conductor. An exploring electrode placed in a line with the axis of the dipole and gradually moved from left (negative pole) to right (positive pole) records a negative-positive deflection. A remote electrode, located outside the electrical field, fails to record a potential. However, when the electrode is moved into the negative field, it encounters and records a gradually increasing negativity. As the electrode nears and passes the negative pole of the dipole and finds itself halfway between the two poles, a sharp reversal of polarity is registered (intrinsicoid deflection) and the electrode enters the field of positivity. The positive voltage declines gradually as the electrode moves away from the positive pole. Finally, the electrode moves out of the electrical field and a potential is no longer registered.

A similar sequence of events is registered with the electrode stationary and the electrical field moving relative to the electrode. When the positive field moves toward the electrode, a positive potential is recorded; when the electrode finds itself in the negative field, a negative potential is recorded.

Electrophysiological Bases and Theory

Transmembrane ionic fluxes are responsible for voltage differences between activated and resting tissue. These ionic fluxes are reflected as the transmembrane action potential, the cellular counterpart of the clinical ECG. The ECG counterparts of the TAP phases 0, 1, 2, 3, and 4 are the QRS complex, the ST segment, the T wave, and the isoelectric baseline, respectively (see Chapter 19).

DEPOLARIZATION AND REPOLARIZATION. To progress logically toward an understanding of the ECG, we will review the effect of a muscle strip immersed in a homo volume conductor on the electrical field generated by the muscle strip and on the electrode immersed in the field. A muscle strip, when uniformly positive on the outside, is in a resting or polarized state. Because it exhibits no difference of potential and fails to impart an electrical field, an electrode immersed in the volume conductor registers an isoelectric line. Stimulation of the muscle strip at any given point increases membrane permeability, and positive charges enter the cell. The result is depolarized (relatively negative) muscle in apposition to polarized (relatively positive) muscle, with a potential difference across a boundary. In the surrounding medium the current flows from the positively (source) to the negatively (sink) charged muscle. The moving boundary between the polarized (positive) and the depolarized (negative) muscle can be represented by a dipole or vector. This dipole or vector moves along the muscle fiber from the point of excitation, leaving in its wake tissue that is electrically negative (depolarized) in relation to the still polarized (resting) muscle. When the wave of depolarization reaches the end of the muscle strip, the surface becomes uniformly negative and the strip is now completely depolarized. Since a difference of potential no longer exists, an isoelectric baseline is inscribed. The most intense difference of potential exists at the boundary between depolarized and resting tissue, and the recorded voltage changes reflect the events taking place at this boundary.[13,14]

Restitution of membrane polarity, or *repolarization*, can be viewed as a "wave" of positivity enveloping the cells or tissue. As a result, the outside of the cell is again uniformly positive. Since the boundary moves in the direction of the depolarized, negative muscle, an electrode located at the point of origin of repolarization records a positive potential. An electrode placed at the opposite end records a negative potential. In an isolated preparation of myocardial tissue, the direction of repolarization is the same as that of depolarization but is preceded by the negative pole of the dipole. The repolarization inscribes an area equal to that inscribed by depolarization but of opposite polarity.

EFFECT OF THE BOUNDARY OF DEPOLARIZATION AND REPOLARIZATION ON POLARITY OF THE RECORDED POTENTIAL. Three electrodes placed on a muscle strip will illustrate the effect of a boundary potential, which can be represented as a dipole or vector, on the recording electrode[9] (Fig. 7–2). Electrode A is located at the point of excitation, electrode B at the midpoint of the muscle strip, and electrode C at the end of the muscle strip. Immediately after excitation, electrode A finds itself in the most intensively negative field. As the dipole moves away, the potential becomes less negative, and at the end of depolarization the inscription returns to the baseline. Thus, the electrode at point A inscribes a negative deflection. At the moment of excitation, electrode B is located in the positive field of the dipole. As the dipole moves toward the recording electrode, the latter registers a gradually increasing positivity and records an upright deflection. When the dipole passes the electrode, there is a sudden reversal of polarity, and the electrode finds itself in a strongly negative field. A downward, negative deflection is recorded. With the dipole moving away, the electrode at point B registers a less negative potential, and finally, when the strip is completely depolarized, an isoelectric baseline is recorded. Thus, the electrode at point B registers a positive-negative deflection. Electrode C is located in the positive field throughout the entire process of depolarization. As the dipole approaches the electrode, the field becomes more intensively positive, with the most intense positivity at the moment immediately prior to completion of depolarization. Thus, the electrode at point C records an upright deflection.

SEQUENCE OF ACTIVATION OF THE HEART. For a proper analysis of the ECG, recognition of the se-

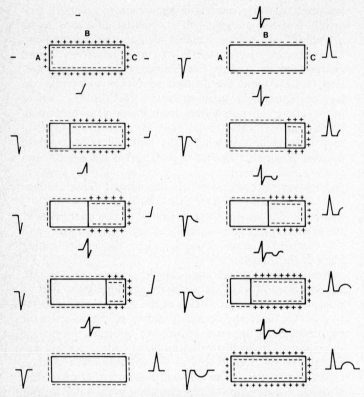

FIGURE 7–2   Potential generated during depolarization (*left vertical sequence of panels*) and repolarization (*right vertical sequence of panels*) recorded with an exploring electrode located at the endocardium (A), epicardium (C), and midway between the two (B). (Modified from Barker, J. M.: The Unipolar Electrocardiogram: A Clinical Interpretation. New York, Appleton-Century-Crofts, Inc., 1952.)

resembling a wavefront seen when a pebble is thrown into water. The sinoatrial node is located in the right atrium and initially activates the right atrium in a right and anterior direction, followed by excitation of the left atrium in a left and posterior direction. It has been suggested that preferential internodal pathways connect the sinoatrial node and the atrioventricular (AV) junctional tissue and that these specialized internodal pathways are capable of conducting an impulse in the face of a quiescent atrium.[18] The concept has attracted considerable interest and is the subject of continued investigation.[19]

The impulse arrives at the AV node, where it is delayed, most likely owing to decremental conduction (p. 624).[20] Study of the sequence of ventricular activation in the dog reveals an early (0 to 5 msec) and almost simultaneous activation of the central left side of the septum and the high anterior and apical posterior paraseptal areas of the left ventricle. At 5 to 10 msec after the onset of ventricular activation, the wave of activation envel left and right ventricular walls and the remainder of the septum; the latter is completely activated at 12 msec. The earliest epicardial breakthrough occurs at the anterior right epicardial surface near the apex, followed by anterior and posterior paraseptal areas of the left ventricle. At 18 msec, activation of the central portion of the two ventricles is complete. Excitation continues along the lateral and basal aspect of the left ventricle, with the basal portion of the septum last to depolarize.[15]

Studies of perfused human heart indicate that its path of activation closely follows that of the canine heart (Fig. 7–3). The results obtained in the resuscitated human heart were validated by comparing the process of activation with that of a perfused and in situ dog heart. The only difference was that the activation proceeded more rapidly in the perfused dog preparation.[17] By means of intracardiac mapping during surgery it has also been shown that epicardial breakthrough occurred in the right ventricle followed by activation of the anterior and inferior left ventricle.[21]

In contrast to the reasonably accurate information regarding the process of activation, knowledge of the sequence of *repolarization* in an intact heart is incomplete and difficult to define. For one thing, the experimental design itself may alter the sequence of repolarization. Simi-

quence of cardiac activation is as important as the understanding of the physical and electrophysiological bases of the cardiac current. The sequence of activation of the heart has been studied in animals, primarily in the dog and in the isolated perfused human heart.[17] The normal impulse originates in the sinoatrial node and traverses the atria in a wavelike front with a velocity of approximately 1000 mm/sec. The wave of atrial activation is described as one

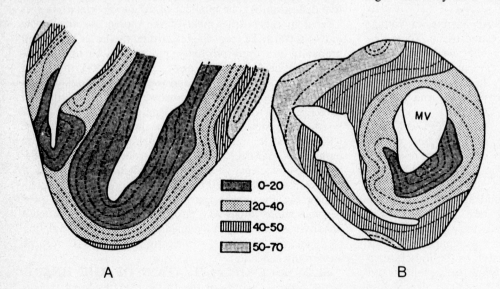

0–20
20–40
40–50
50–70

A   B

FIGURE 7–3 Sequence of ventricular activation of an isolated human heart. *A* and *B* represent sagittal and coronal sections, respectively. The dotted lines denote 5-msec sequences, while changes in pattern represent 20-msec intervals. (Durrer, D., et al.: Total excitation of the isolated human heart. Circulation *41*:899, 1970, by permission of the American Heart Association, Inc.)

larly, electrodes used to plot the wave of repolarization may induce a current of injury and interfere with the recording of meaningful data. Human studies indicate that atrial repolarization follows approximately the same path as atrial depolarization, with the polarity of repolarization opposite to that of depolarization. Ventricular repolarization proceeds in a direction *opposite* to that of depolarization, and its polarity is therefore the *same* as that of depolarization. The process of repolarization recorded directly from the epicardium indicates that in the intact ventricle repolarization begins at the epicardium—a sequence opposite to that observed in isolated muscle strip. The reason for the in vivo reversal of the order of repolarization is not entirely clear. The presence of a transmural pressure gradient may be an important factor, since it prolongs the duration of the excited state of the endocardium and, consequently, recovery begins at the epicardium.

VENTRICULAR GRADIENT. The concept of ventricular gradient (G), introduced by Wilson, is a method for describing the relationships between depolarization (QRS) and repolarization (T).[22] As stated above, in the isolated muscle strip depolarization and repolarization are equal in duration and follow the same path. The net areas of the QRS complex (AQRS) and the T wave (AT) are equal but of opposite polarity, so that their sum is zero and there is no gradient. In the intact heart, on the other hand, repolarization proceeds from the epicardium to endocardium, in a direction opposite to that of depolarization; the algebraic sum of their respective areas is no longer zero; and a gradient is said to exist. AQRS, AT, and G can be expressed as a vectorial quantity from any two of the three bipolar limb leads of the ECG. AQRS and AT are expressed in the form of vectors and are plotted using the Einthoven triangle or Bayley triaxial reference system. A parallelogram of the AQRS and the AT is constructed, with the resultant diagonal vector being the manifest AQRST vector or gradient (G). The G vector and the mean QRS vector are located in about the same plane. The G forms an angle of approximately 30° with the mean spatial QRS vector.

G is an index of variation in duration of the excited state and thus of the local rate of repolarization. Although it is of theoretical value in the study of T-wave abnormalities, the variations between individuals and in the same individual and the tedious calculations required, especially when small changes may prove important, limit its clinical usefulness. The electrocardiographer intuitively evaluates the ventricular gradient whenever reading the cardiogram.[11]

THEORETICAL BASES OF SURFACE LEADS. At any instant the surface leads reflect projection of the electrical current of the equivalent or "net" dipole expressed as the mean instantaneous spatial vector. Orientation of a lead axis is defined as one that records a maximal voltage when its axis is parallel to that of the axis or vector of the equivalent dipole. The voltage registered in any lead, having magnitude and direction, can be expressed as a vector (lead vector), with the amplitude of deflection in any lead paralleling the magnitude of the vector. Since more than one dipole may exist at any instant, the net potential and consequently the resultant lead vector reflect the contribution of all such dipoles. Furthermore, because dipole vectors may vary in magnitude and direction, the equivalent or "net" dipole is an approximation of these forces and consequently its expression on a lead axis is also an approximation.

THE NORMAL ELECTROCARDIOGRAM AND VECTORCARDIOGRAM

Leads

Bipolar limb leads introduced by Einthoven register the direction, magnitude, and duration of voltage changes in the frontal plane. The three bipolar leads—I, II, and III—record the difference in potential between left arm (LA) and right arm (RA), left leg (LF) and RA, and LF and LA, respectively.

Unipolar limb leads are constructed by connecting all three extremities to a "central terminal" (Fig. 7–4B). Although in reality the central terminal registers a small voltage, for practical purposes it is considered to have a zero potential and serves as the *indifferent* or *reference electrode*. The potential differences recorded by the positive terminal, the *exploring electrode*, are dominated by local electrical events. When placed on the right arm, left arm, or left foot, the exploring electrode registers the potential from the respective limb. The letter V identifies a unipolar lead and the letters r, l, and f the respective extremities. If one disconnects the central terminal from the extremity from which the potential is being recorded, the amplitude registered by the respective unipolar limb lead is augmented; such leads are designated as aV_r, aV_l, and aV_f.

Locations of the exploring electrode for the *precordial leads* are as follows: V_1—fourth interspace to the right of the sternum; V_2—fourth interspace to the left of the sternum; V_3—midway between leads V_2 and V_4; V_4—fifth interspace at the midclavicular line; V_5—anterior axillary line at the level of lead V_4; and V_6—midaxillary line at the level of lead V_4.[23] (Fig. 7–4B).

Of the six precordial leads, it is assumed that leads V_1 and V_2, V_3 and V_4, and V_5 and V_6 face the right side of the septum, the septum itself, and the left side of the septum, respectively, and are referred to as right ventricular, septal or transitional, and left ventricular leads, respectively.

THE NORMAL ELECTROCARDIOGRAM

THE P WAVE

The cardiac impulse originating in the sinoatrial node activates the right and left atria in the general direction

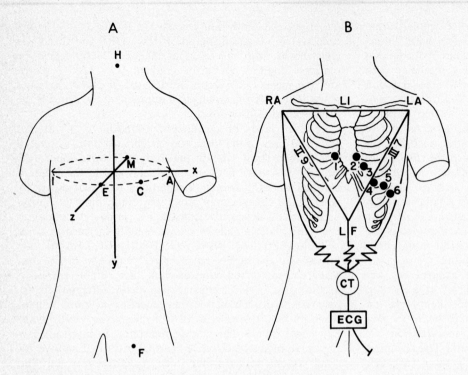

FIGURE 7-4 *A,* Frank electrode system. Five horizontal electrodes are placed at the level where the fifth intercostal space intersects the sternal line. Specific locations include fifth intercostal space and sternum (E), the midaxillary line (A-I), and the vertebral column (M). Electrode C is located halfway between points E and A, while electrodes H and F are on the back of the neck and left lower extremity, respectively. *B,* ECG lead system. Leads I, II, and III are formed by connecting RA-LA, RA-LF, and LA-LF, respectively. The indifferent electrode of the unipolar system is obtained by connecting RA, LA, and LF through 50,000-ohm resistance into a central terminal (CT). (For details about positioning of the exploring unipolar electrode, see p. 199.)

from right to left atrium, inferiorly and posteriorly. Initial activation of the right atrium, an anterior chamber, is directed anteriorly and inferiorly and is followed by activation of the left or posterior atrium, directed to the left, posteriorly, and inferiorly.

The P wave is rounded with a notch corresponding to the separation between right and left atrial activation. Amplitude of the P wave is normally less than 2.5 mm (0.25 mV) with a duration less than 0.12 sec (Table 7-1). The P wave and the *Ta segment,* or atrial repolarization, define atrial electrical systole. The P vector varies from $-50°$ to $+60°$. In the precordial leads the P wave is positive except in lead V_1, where the P wave may be upright, biphasic, or negative.

The Ta segment is inscribed during the QRS complex and the early part of the ST segment. It is best seen in the

TABLE 7-1

A. P WAVE: HEIGHT AND DURATION IN NORMAL ADULTS

	LEAD I	LEAD II	LEAD III	LEAD V_1*
P height (mV)				
Mean	0.49	1.03	0.69	0.40
Range	0.2 to 1.0	0.3 to 2.0	0 to 2.0	0.05 to 0.80
P duration (sec)				
Mean	0.08	0.09	0.07	0.05
Range	0.05 to 0.12	0.05 to 0.12	0.02 to 0.13	0 to 0.08
R-R interval (sec)				
Mean	0.16	0.16	0.16	
Range	0.12 to 0.20	0.12 to 0.20	0.12 to 0.20	

B. AMPLITUDE OF Q, R, S, AND T WAVES ON SCALAR ECG OF 100 NORMAL ADULTS†

	I	II	III	aV_r	aV_l	aV_f	V_1	V_5	V_6
Patients with									
Q wave	38%	41%	50%	—	38%	40%	0%	60%	75%
Q amplitude									
Mean	0.4	0.6	0.9	—	0.4	0.7	0	0.3	0.3
Range	0 to 1.0	0 to 1.6	0 to 2.3	—	0 to 1.1	0 to 1.7	0	0 to 1.8	0 to 1.8
R amplitude									
Mean	5.6	8.9	4.5	1.3	3.4	6.0	1.9	12.6	10.2
Range	1.0 to 10.0	2.0 to 16.9	1.0 to 12.1	0 to 2.9	0 to 8.2	0 to 13.8	1.0 to 6.0	7.0 to 21.0	5.0 to 18.0
S amplitude									
Mean	2.0	2.1	2.4	7.0	2.6	—	8.0	2.5	1.3
Range	0 to 5.0	0 to 3.7	0 to 6.4	2.2 to 11.8	0 to 5.8	—	3.0 to 13.0	0 to 5.0	0 to 2.0
T amplitude									
Mean	1.9	2.3	1.0	—	0.3	1.7	1.0	3.3	1.0
Range	1.0 to 3.0	1.0 to 4.0	−2.0 to 2.0	—	−1.0 to 2.0	0 to 4.0	−2.0 to 2.0	2.0 to 7.0	1.0 to 4.0

*Twenty-five per cent of the series had a small terminal negative deflection of the P wave in lead V_1.

†Values of Q, R, S and T amplitudes are in millimeters (1 mm = 0.1 mv).

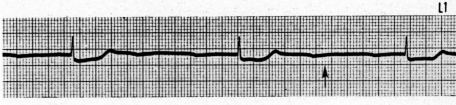

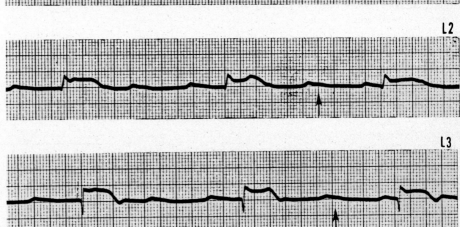

FIGURE 7–5   Atrial infarction. The tracing illustrates sinus rhythm, complete AV block, and an acute inferior myocardial infarction. The Ta segment indicative of atrial infarction is elevated in leads II and III (arrows) and depressed in lead I (arrow).

presence of AV block (Fig. 7–5).[24] Duration of the Ta segment varies from 0.15 to 0.45 sec, and its amplitude is low, reaching 0.08 mV. The magnitude of the Ta is directionally related to the area of the P wave and thus the heart rate. The vector of the Ta is opposite to that of the P vector and is oriented superiorly, to the right, and somewhat posteriorly. Similarly, the P wave and the Ta areas are equal and opposite in direction, and the resultant gradient is zero. In the presence of atrial enlargement, the Ta segment may result in displacement of the ST segment.

THE P-R INTERVAL. The P-R interval includes the intraatrial, AV nodal, and His-Purkinje conduction, and its duration varies from 0.12 to 0.20 or 0.22 sec (Table 7–1). AV conduction is discussed in Chapter 19.

The QRS Complex

Familiarity with the sequence of ventricular activation is a prerequisite for proper analysis of the normal and abnormal QRS complex. As stated above, ventricular activation proceeds more or less symmetrically about the septum and from the endocardium to the epicardium. Consequently, much of its voltage is canceled; in fact, only 10 to 15 per cent of the potential generated by the heart is ultimately recorded on the surface ECG.

The QRS complex can be described by four vectors[11] (Fig. 7–6): (1) initial septal activation from left to right, anteriorly, inferiorly, or superiorly, followed by further septal activation from left to right (0.01 sec); (2) an overlapping wave of excitation involving both ventricles, with the vector directed inferiorly and slightly to the left (0.02 sec); (3) unopposed activation of the apical and central portions of the left ventricle, the thin right ventricular wall having been depolarized, with a resultant vector directed posteriorly, inferiorly, and to the left (0.04 sec); and, finally, (4) activation of the posterior basal portion of the left ventricle and septum, with a vector directed superiorly and posteriorly (0.06 sec).

FIGURE 7–6 Correlation between the order of ventricular activation (A), scalar ECG (B), and vectorcardiogram (C). A, The sequence of ventricular activation is represented by four instantaneous frontal plane vectors. B, The four vectors plotted on leads I and III at the appropriate time during inscription of the QRS. C, Using the method of construction of vectors described in Figure 7–7, one can derive each of the four vectors in the frontal plane. A line joining the ends of the vectors results in a frontal plane QRS loop. The same method can be used to derive the orthogonal X, Y, and Z leads from the frontal, transverse, or sagittal planes. (Times given are in seconds.)

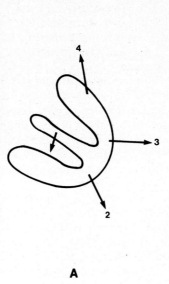

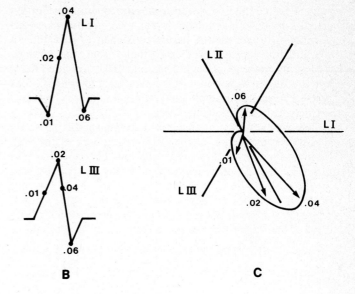

Septal activation from left to right and anteriorly results in an initial Q wave in leads I, II, III, V_5, and V_6 and an R wave in the right precordial and septal leads V_1 to V_4. Lead aV_f registers an R or Q wave depending on whether the septal vector is directed superiorly or inferiorly. The ventricular vector directed inferiorly and to the left is reflected by an R wave in leads II and III and in the transitional or septal leads V_3 and V_4. The third vector, that of the unopposed force directed to the left, posteriorly, and somewhat inferiorly, gives rise to an R wave in leads I, II, III, aV_1, aV_f, V_5, V_6, and occasionally V_4, with an S wave in leads aV_r, V_1, V_2, V_3, and at times V_4. The terminal force directed superiorly and posteriorly and perhaps to the right may result in a terminal S wave in leads I, V_5, and V_6. A lead positioned in the right fourth interspace in the midclavicular line (V_{4r}) may record a terminal R wave (R′), which may also occasionally be recorded in lead V_1.[23] The interrelationship of the order of ventricular activation, inscription of the scalar ECG, and the vectorcardiogram are illustrated in Figure 7–6.

The magnitude of the Q, R, and S waves is given in Table 7–1.

THE QRS AXIS, POSITION, AND ROTATION.

The electrical position of the heart can be described by the QRS axis and the rotation of the heart on the anteroposterior and longitudinal (apex-to-base) axes. As the *order* of activation can be viewed as a sequence of instantaneous dipoles or vectors, *total* cardiac activation can be presented as a mean QRS vector. When such a vector is placed within the triangle formed by leads I, II, and III, which define the frontal plane, and assuming that this triangle is equilateral, that the heart is located in its center, and that the thorax is a homogeneous volume conductor with a uniform boundary, projection of the vector on the respective leads permits an estimate of the magnitude of voltage recorded in each lead. Similarly, if one knows the voltage in each of the leads, the mean QRS vector can be reconstructed and the axis deviation of the QRS complex can be estimated (Fig. 7–7).

The preceding assumptions—the Einthoven postulates—are applicable in the experimental setting. In the human, however, the heart is a large organ; it is not a point generator nor is it centrally located, and the thorax is not a homogeneous conductor within a uniform boundary. Burger, using a model of a human torso, with nonhomogeneous conduction to reflect the nature of human organs and an eccentrically located generator, found that the triangle formed by the axes of leads I, II, and III is not equilateral but is scalene, with lead I being shortest and lead III longest.[25] The scalene triangle configuration is more consistent with clinical electrocardiography.

The most accurate method for determining the QRS axis is based on estimation of the QRS area in each of the limb leads and a plot of these as vectors on the respective lead axis of a triaxial reference system. From the positive end of the vector, lines perpendicular to the lead axis are dropped. A vector is drawn from the center of the triaxial reference system to the point where the perpendicular lines cross. This vector defines the direction and magnitude of the mean QRS vector ($\overset{\Delta}{\text{AQRS}}$). The same method is used to estimate the T vector ($\overset{\Delta}{\text{AT}}$). Normally, the angle be-

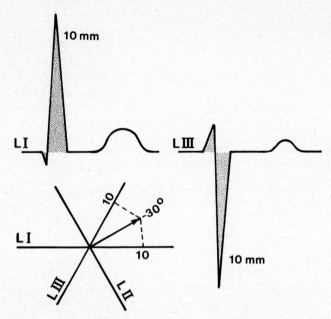

FIGURE 7–7 Electrical axis plotted on leads I and II of the Einthoven triangle. Peak amplitudes of the R wave in lead I and of the S wave in lead III—in this instance each measuring 10 mm—are plotted on their respective leads. Perpendicular lines are dropped and the point at which these cross is identified. A line drawn from the point where leads I, II, and III cross to the point where the two "perpendicular" lines intersect identifies the electrical axis of the QRS (30°). The same approach is used for plotting the P and T axes.

When the P, QRS, or T wave area is plotted on the respective lead, the mean P, QRS, or T vector is identified. The latter represents the mean magnitude, direction, and polarity of the entire period of depolarization. This is a more accurate but impractical method of estimating the electrical axis. Although the direction of the QRS axis and of the mean QRS vector differ, as a rule both lie in the same quadrant.

tween $\overset{\Delta}{\text{AQRS}}$ and $\overset{\Delta}{\text{AT}}$ does not exceed 30°. For practical purposes, however, the assumption that the magnitude of the force projected on a given lead axis is directionally related to the cosine of the angle subtended by the lead vector and lead axis allows a rapid and reasonably accurate estimate of the QRS axis. Thus, if the mean QRS vector is perpendicular to a given lead axis, the angle between the two is 90°, the cosine of the angle is zero, and the QRS will be isoelectric, very small, or equiphasic. On the other hand, when the mean QRS vector is parallel to a lead axis, the angle between the two is zero, the cosine of the angle is one, and the amplitude of the QRS will be greatest in that lead.

Plotted on a hexaxial reference system, axes of 0° to +90°, 0° to −90°, and +90° to −90° are in the range of normal, left, and right, respectively (Fig. 7–8). These values are arbitrary because the ranges vary among investigators. Other values suggested for the left axis include +30° to −120°[8] and −30° to −90°.[11] Similarly, the definition of right axis includes ranges from +60° to +180°[9] and from +60 to −120°.[8]

"Abnormal" or "marked left-axis deviation," diagnosed by an axis shift of −30° or greater, should not be considered synonymous with left-axis deviation. The former rarely, if ever, reflects positional change alone and is probably due to left anterior divisional block.

An *anteroposterior axis* allows the apex to face either the

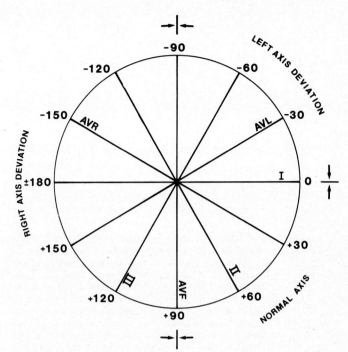

FIGURE 7-8 The frontal plane hexaxial reference system and the respective ranges of axis deviation.

left arm or the left foot or to assume a position between the two. Thus, when a QRS complex in aV_l resembles that in leads V_5 and V_6, the position is horizontal. On the other hand, when the QRS complex in aV_f reflects that in leads V_5 and V_6, the position is vertical. Similarly, in the horizontal position the QRS complex in aV_f and in the vertical position the QRS complex in aV_r resemble the QRS complex in lead V_1. When the apex is approximately equidistant from the two extremities, both aV_l and aV_f exhibit QRS complexes resembling those in leads V_5 and V_6, and the position is said to be intermediate. If the position shifts more toward the left arm or the left foot, the position is said to be semihorizontal and semivertical, respectively. In the semihorizontal position, the QRS complex in lead aV_l resembles that of leads V_5 and V_6, while the QRS complex in lead aV_f is small. In the semivertical position, the QRS complex in lead aV_f resembles that of leads V_5 and V_6, while the QRS complex in aV_l is small.

Clockwise and counterclockwise rotation along the *longitudinal, apex-to-base axis* can be recognized by analysis of the precordial leads. The direction of rotation is described by viewing the heart from a position below the diaphragmatic surface. *Clockwise rotation* results in a shift of the right ventricle and thus the right ventricular QRS complex (rS) is further to the left and occasionally may be registered in all the precordial positions. Similarly, *counterclockwise rotation* results in a more anterior shift of the left ventricle and a more posterior displacement of the right ventricle. Consequently, the left precordial QRS pattern (qR) is shifted further to the right and may be registered, for example, in the V_3 position.

THE ST SEGMENT

The ST segment reflects phase 2 of the transmembrane action potential. Since during phase 2 there is little change in this potential, the ST segment is usually isoelectric.

THE T WAVE

The mechanism and sequence of ventricular repolarization were described earlier. In the adult, the unipolar leads inscribe an upright T wave in all leads except in aV_r and occasionally V_1. Rarely, persistence of a juvenile T wave pattern results in inverted T waves in leads V_1, V_2, and V_3. The amplitude of the T wave is given in Table 7-1.

THE U WAVE

The U wave is a diastolic event and its genesis not clear. It has been suggested that the U wave represents a surface reflection of a negative afterpotential.[26,27] The two prevailing concepts of the mechanism of the U wave include repolarization of the Purkinje fibers[20,28] and a mechanical event, probably diastolic relaxation of the myocardium.[29,30]

The U wave is upright and its amplitude is 5 to 50 per cent that of the T wave. The tallest U wave is recorded in leads V_2 and V_3, where its amplitude may reach 2 mm (Fig. 7-9). Ordinarily the U wave is clearly separated from the T wave. However, under conditions in which the U wave appears early, such as with foreshortened ventricular filling and ejection or when the Q-T interval is prolonged (as with hypocalcemia or after administration of drugs such as quinidine), the U wave may be difficult to separate from the T wave; on the other hand, when the Q-T interval is foreshortened, as with digitalis or hypercalcemia, the U wave is easily identifiable.[31]

THE Q-T INTERVAL

The Q-T interval, measured from the beginning of the QRS complex to the end of the T wave, reflects, within certain limitations, the duration of depolarization and repolarization. Importantly, the Q-T interval may not always accurately reflect the recovery time of the heart. In some parts of the heart repolarization is complete before the end of the Q-T interval, while in other areas repolarization may continue after the end of the Q-T interval, but because of the small magnitude of the potential or because of cancellation, it cannot be identified in the surface tracing. In addition, because the onset of the QRS complex or the end of the T wave or both may be difficult to define, one cannot always obtain an accurate measurement of the Q-T interval. The point at which the line of maximal downslope of the T wave crosses the baseline helps to identify the end of the T wave.

Duration of the Q-T interval varies with the cycle length, and numerous formulas have been suggested to correct for heart rate. Bazett proposed a formula for estimating the Q-T interval corrected for heart rate,[32] or the *Q-Tc interval:* $\dfrac{Q\text{-}T}{k\sqrt{R\text{-}R}}$ where constant k is 0.37 for men and 0.40 for women. The upper limit of the Q-Tc interval is 0.39 sec for men and 0.44 sec for women. Because of the variability of measurements and potential influences other than heart rate, different ranges of normalcy are accepted by different investigators. For practical purposes, there-

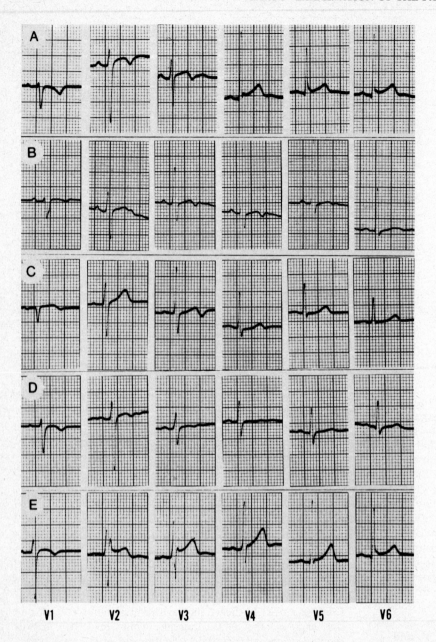

V1   V2   V3   V4   V5   V6

FIGURE 7–9 Abnormal ECG in absence of clinical heart disease. *A,* Persistence of juvenile T-wave inversion in leads V_1, V_2, and V_3 and ST-segment elevation in leads V_4, V_5, and V_6 due to early repolarization recorded in a 21-year-old man. *B,* Notched T waves and isolated T-wave inversion in leads V_3, V_4, and V_5 recorded in a 19-year-old man. *C,* Isolated midprecordial T-wave negativity recorded in a 24-year-old man. *D,* Abnormal T waves in leads V_1 to V_4 recorded in a 45-year-old woman. *E,* RR' pattern in leads V_2 and V_3 and ST-segment elevation in leads V_2 to V_6 due to early repolarization recorded in a 32-year-old man. A normal U wave follows the T wave.

fore, minor deviations from the expected Q-Tc interval should be disregarded as being of questionable clinical significance.

DERIVATION OF NORMAL ELECTROCARDIOGRAPHIC VALUES

Ideally, ranges of normalcy for ECG components should be based on an analysis of randomly selected, preferably consecutive, routine cardiograms recorded in young individuals free of cardiovascular disease. If such data are to be useful as a frame of reference for recognizing abnormal ECG values, only unequivocal ECG changes should be considered. Inclusion of measurements such as QRS or T-wave amplitude, for example, is nonproductive. Although statistical differences may exist among groups of individuals, in any one subject the significance of a given amplitude and of minor changes from tracing to tracing is difficult to assess, because variations often reflect a normal curve of distribution. Similarly, there is a lack of agreement as to when a given absolute value becomes abnormal.

In a study of 776 consecutive patients 18 to 25 years of age who were hospitalized because of mental illness and were free of cardiovascular disease, the prevalence of abnormal cardiograms was extremely low. Results showed left-axis deviation in excess of $-30°$, right-axis deviation (RAD) greater than $+120°$, first-degree AV block, right bundle branch block (RBBB), nonspecific intraventricular conduction defect (IVCD), left ventricular hypertrophy (LVH), prevalence of atrial premature complexes (APC) and ventricular premature complexes (VPC) greater than 6 per minute, and Wolff-Parkinson-White syndrome (WPW) was noted in 1.4, 2.1, 0.3, 0.3, 0.1, 0.1, 0.7, 0.8, and 0.3 per cent, respectively.[33] Similar findings were recorded in a group of 5000 male members of the Canadian Air Force.[34] Significantly, in neither series were abnormalities of the ST segment, left bundle branch block (LBBB), or atrial fibrillation encountered.

Much of the criticism leveled against electrocardiography regarding the lack of uniform criteria and intra- and interreader discrepancy can be ascribed to preoccupation with such minor changes. For example, while bundle branch block (BBB) or inversion of T waves should be read with a high degree of consistency, minor changes in the T wave, QRS amplitude, or ST segment may not be interpreted uniformly by the same reader or different readers. However, such minor discrepancies are often clinically unimportant. The normal and inescapable biological range in ECG values is particularly frustrating to those who attempt to develop accurate "stand-alone" computer programs for interpretation of the ECG.

THE NORMAL VECTORCARDIOGRAM

Vectorcardiography can be defined as registration of the time course of mean instantaneous spatial cardiac vectors.[11,35-38] The concept of vectorcardiography was introduced in 1920 by Mann.[35,39] By plotting on a triaxial reference system a number of vectors derived simultaneously from leads I and III, and by connecting the ends of the derived vectors, Mann recorded a loop, which he termed a monocardiogram (Fig. 7–6C); the term vectorcardiogram (VCG) was coined by Wilson in 1938.[40] The advent of the cathode-ray oscilloscope allowed direct recording of the loop. The cathode-ray tube has two sets of plates controlling the horizontal and vertical displacement of an electronic beam. The *X (transverse) lead* is connected to the right and left plates, the *Y (vertical) lead* to the superior and inferior plates. The anterior and posterior connections of the *Z (sagittal) lead* are connected to the lower and upper plates. The X, Y, and Z leads constitute the *orthogonal lead system.*

The positive orientation indicated by the arrows is to the left for the X lead, to the foot (or inferior) for the Y lead, and to the back (or posterior) for the Z lead. A vector directed to the left, inferiorly, and posteriorly will inscribe a positive deflection in leads X, Y, and Z, respectively (Fig. 7–10).

VCG loops are recorded in three planes: frontal, transverse, and sagittal. The left sagittal view is recommended by the American Heart Association Committee on Electrocardiography, although both right and left views are in use. Any two of the three leads of the orthogonal system will define a plane and will inscribe a loop in a given plane. The combination of X and Y, X and Z, or Y and Z will register the VCG loop in the frontal, transverse, or sagittal planes, respectively. To correct for nonuniformity of the conducting medium, eccentricity of the heart as a source, presence of a number of dipoles, and variation in vectorial expression of the magnitude of an electrical signal, and to assure that the three leads are perpendicular, a number of corrected orthogonal leads have been devised.[36,41-44] Although none is ideal, the Frank system, because of its relative simplicity, is most widely used.[41] The values and recordings included in this chapter were derived using the Frank system (Fig. 7–4A).

The VCG differs from the ECG only in the method of display of the electrical field generated by the heart. While the ECG reflects best the changes in time and amplitude, the VCG adds the important dimension of recognition of direction in *time.* Despite the corrected nature of the orthogonal leads, the assumptions and limitations implicit in

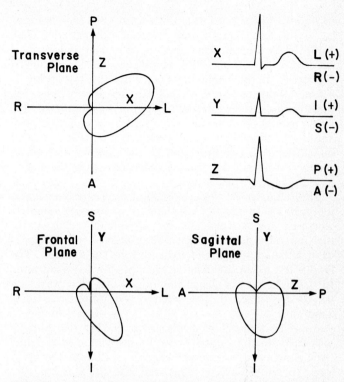

FIGURE 7–10 The transverse, frontal, and sagittal planes and the respective orthogonal leads XZ, XY, and YZ that define the planes. The arrow indicates the positive pole. Normal transverse, frontal, and right sagittal loops are diagrammed.

The right upper panel diagrams the orthogonal X, Y, and Z leads. When the vector points to the left (L), inferiorly (I), or posteriorly (P), a positive or upright deflection is recorded. Similarly, if the current flows to the right (R), superiorly (S), and anteriorly (A), a negative or downward deflection is recorded. In this instance the mean vector is oriented to the left, inferiorly, and posteriorly.

the ECG are also applicable to the VCG. The less than optimal sensitivity and specificity add a certain degree of empiricism, so that the findings on VCG must be correlated with clinical and laboratory information for proper interpretation.

Whether because of the relative complexity of recording with VCG compared with the ECG or because of its failure to add information to that gained from the ECG, thus making routine use of VCG a questionable practice in terms of cost versus benefit, the fact remains that the technique of vectorcardiography is not widely used. Unquestionably, the spatial VCG is without equal as a teaching tool, and an understanding of the VCG is essential for an intelligent appreciation of the ECG. In selected cases, the VCG may provide clinically useful information not otherwise obtainable. Because of differences of opinion, it is difficult to list the specific clinical or pathological conditions in which the VCG is superior to the ECG. It has been suggested that the VCG is particularly useful in detecting right ventricular hypertrophy (RVH), atrial enlargement, and myocardial infarction. While in myocardial infarction the VCG is perhaps more sensitive than the ECG, its specificity is not greater.[37]

The order of activation and repolarization of the heart and the vectorial presentation—the basis of the clinical VCG—were described earlier. In a three-dimensional projection the major portion of the normal QRS loop is located in the left, inferior, and posterior octant[38,41,45-47] (Fig. 7-10). In the frontal plane, the loop is narrow and elongated, and in about one-third of subjects the inscription is clockwise; in the remaining two-thirds the inscription is counterclockwise or a figure-of-eight. The loop is most frequently located in the left inferior quadrant. In the transverse plane, the loop is inscribed counterclockwise and is oval in appearance, and the major portion is located in the left posterior quadrant. In the right sagittal plane, the loop is inscribed clockwise and is located in the anterior and posterior quadrants.

The P loop of the VCG normally requires magnification for analysis. In the frontal plane, it is inscribed counterclockwise and is located in the left inferior quadrant. In the transverse plane, the usual inscription is counterclockwise, although a figure-of-eight may be encountered. The loop is located in the anterior and posterior left quadrants. In the right sagittal plane, the loop is inscribed clockwise and is positioned in the anterior and posterior inferior quadrants.

Analysis of the T loop also requires that the loop be magnified. In the frontal plane, its inscription is variable, with a maximal orientation similar to that of the QRS loop. In the transverse plane, the inscription is counterclockwise and the maximal T vector is located in the left anterior quadrant. In the right sagittal plane, the loop is inscribed clockwise and its maximal vector is located in the anterior and inferior quadrants.

The loops illustrated in this chapter are interrupted every 2.5 msec, each dot representing a 2.5-msec interval. The dot or line is comma shaped, with the thin end indicating the direction of the loop. The spacing of the dots reflects the speed of conduction, i.e., the closer the dots, the slower the conduction.

The VCG is most useful in analysis of the QRS complex. Although the QRS loop is routinely inscribed in the three orthogonal planes, with few exceptions, the characteristic patterns can be recognized in the transverse plane.

TABLE 7–2   DIRECTION AND MAGNITUDE OF MAXIMUM P VECTOR IN NORMAL SUBJECTS

PLANE	DIRECTION (DEGREES) Mean	95% range	MAGNITUDE (MV) Mean	95% range
Transverse	−5	−50 to 60	0.07	0.04 to 0.10
Right sagittal	85	50 to 110	0.12	0.04 to 0.18
Frontal	65	15 to 90	0.12	0.06 to 0.20

From Chou, T.-C., et al.: Clinical Vectorcardiography. 2nd ed. New York, Grune and Stratton, 1974, p. 50.

Patterns with a superior or inferior orientation require frontal projection for analysis. Of these, the most commonly encountered abnormalities include block of the divisions of the left bundle and inferior myocardial infarction.

Normal values for the VCG are given in Tables 7–2 to 7–4.

BODY SURFACE POTENTIAL MAPPING

Body surface potential mapping may contribute information not available from the 12-lead ECG or the VCG, i.e., it provides regional electrophysiological information that cannot be extracted using these methods.[48] Analysis of

TABLE 7–3   DIRECTION AND MAGNITUDE OF MAXIMUM T VECTOR IN NORMAL SUBJECTS (200)

PLANE	DIRECTION (DEGREES) Mean	95% range	MAGNITUDE (MV) Mean	95% range
Transverse	35	0 to 65	0.5	0.25 to 0.75
Right sagittal	45	20 to 90	0.4	0.20 to 0.70
Frontal	35	20 to 55	0.5	0.25 to 0.75

From Chou, T.-C., et al.: Clinical Vectorcardiography. 2nd ed. New York, Grune and Stratton, 1974, p. 67.

TABLE 7–4   SOME CHARACTERISTICS OF THE NORMAL QRSsÊ LOOP

CHARACTERISTIC	TRANSVERSE PLANE Mean	95% range	RIGHT SAGITTAL PLANE Mean	95% range	FRONTAL PLANE Mean	95% range
Max QRS vector						
Direction (degrees)	−10	−80 to 20.0	100	50 to 165	35	10 to 65
Magnitude (mV)	1.30	0.85 to 1.95	1.00	0.3 to 1.9	1.50	0.9 to 2.2
0.02-sec vector						
Direction	55	0 to 120.0	15	−30 to 75	20	Widely scattered
Magnitude	0.40	0.15 to 0.75	0.30	0.10 to 0.55	0.25	0.05 to 0.7
0.04-sec vector						
Direction	−20	−90 to 25.0	110	60 to 170	35	−10 to 70
Magnitude	1.15	0.55 to 1.90	0.90	0.25 to 1.80	1.25	0.4 to 2.2
0.06-sec vector						
Direction	−90	−125 to −35	160	115 to 220	85	Widely scattered
Magnitude	0.45	0 to 0.9	0.55	0.1 to 1.0	0.25	0 to 0.6
Time of occurrence of max QRS vector (msec)	38	30 to 48	Same		Same	
Direction of inscription	Counterclockwise		Clockwise		Clockwise 65% Figure-of-eight 25% Counterclockwise 10%	

From Chou, T.-C., et al.: Clinical Vectorcardiography. 2nd ed. New York, Grune and Stratton, 1974, p. 60.

surface potentials has been applied to the diagnosis of old inferior myocardial infarction,[49] localization of the bypass pathway in the Wolff-Parkinson-White syndrome,[50,51] recognition of ventricular hypertrophy,[52] estimation of the size of a myocardial infarction, and the effects of different interventions designed to reduce infarct size.[53,54] The limiting factor at present is the complexity of the recording and

analysis, which requires 100 or more electrodes, sophisticated instrumentation, and dedicated personnel. Initial efforts toward reducing the number of electrodes without loss of pertinent information are promising.[55] Once the technical obstacles have been overcome, large numbers of patients can be studied and the ultimate utility of this procedure can be evaluated.

THE ABNORMAL ELECTROCARDIOGRAM AND VECTORCARDIOGRAM

Any discussion of the normal ECG would be incomplete without consideration of the abnormal ECG in the "absence" of heart disease and the role of the ECG in the diagnosis of heart disease in the aged as models for appreciation of the *limitations of "normalcy" of the ECG* and therefore the limitation involved in establishing criteria for electrocardiographic abnormalities.

Implicit in a consideration of the *abnormal ECG in a normal heart* is recognition of the fact that the presence of anatomical and functional disorders has been excluded on the basis of clinical and other laboratory evaluation. Since the ECG may on occasion be a more sensitive marker of a myocardial abnormality than either the clinical or the laboratory evaluation being used as the gold standard for normalcy, the ECG is being put to an inappropriate test. For example, RBBB is nearly always an acquired lesion indicative of anatomical abnormality, despite the fact that it is frequently recorded in the absence of clinically evident heart disease and is often associated with a favorable long-term prognosis. It would be difficult to suggest that RBBB is a false-positive abnormality, since the lack of clinical evidence for organic heart disease and a favorable prognosis do not necessarily assure that the heart is normal. ECG findings in the aged (discussed below) may be a further indication that this method is a more sensitive and independent marker of organic heart disease, in certain instances, than are the other "reference" tests. Despite these reservations about our ability to rule out heart disease, abnormal tracings may be recorded in patients with unequivocally normal hearts, and the ECG changes may be those of the QRS complex, the ST segment, and the T wave.

Abnormalities of the QRS include a QS complex in lead aV_1, a QS or QR complex in leads III and aV_f, a QS complex in leads V_1 and V_2, a tall R wave in lead V_1, an R' wave in leads V_1 and V_2, and high voltage of the R wave over the left ventricle.

A frequent "normal" alteration of the ST segment is an elevation, the so-called early repolarization, which can be recorded in the inferior, left precordial, and rarely right precordial leads.

Abnormal T waves include persistence of juvenile T-wave inversion over the right precordium, isolated mid-precordial T-wave inversion (Fig. 7–9),[56] terminal T-wave inversion associated with ST-segment elevation due to early repolarization, and right precordial T-wave inversion in middle-aged women (Fig. 7–9). A variety of physiological influences alter the T wave in the normal heart, and these

are discussed in the section dealing with ST-segment and T-wave changes.

Further consideration of the problem of establishing criteria of normalcy is aided by analysis of the ECG in individuals over the age of 70. There is considerable evidence that ECG abnormalities present in the aged are acquired, and a number of these abnormalities are independent markers of organic heart disease.[33,57] The occurrence of left-axis deviation, right-axis deviation, first-degree AV block, RBBB, LBBB, ST-segment and T-wave changes, atrial fibrillation, and WPW in the aged is 51, 1, 9, 5, 3, 16, 8, and 0.3 per cent, respectively. As indicated earlier, the prevalence of these same abnormalities in a group of individuals 18 to 25 years of age is in most cases much lower (see p. 204). This difference in prevalence of ECG abnormalities between the two age groups, coupled with a parallel increase in ECG abnormalities with age and the development of heart disease and a high degree of correlation of some of the ECG abnormalities with clinical heart disease, favors the ECG as an independent marker of heart disease. Specific abnormalities that correlate significantly with clinical heart disease are LBBB, IVCD, ST-segment and T-wave changes, and atrial fibrillation.[32] While ECG findings such as myocardial infarction, acquired left anterior divisional block, and RBBB do not correlate statistically with evidence of clinical heart disease, they are obvious *markers* of heart disease. This dichotomy may result from the fact that the pathological process itself may not interfere with cardiac function or that signs and symptoms of heart disease may be difficult to elicit in the aged, or both.

With the above considerations in mind, a discussion of accepted criteria for abnormalcy of ECG components follows.

ABNORMAL P WAVE AND THE Ta SEGMENT

Although an atrial abnormality usually implies atrial enlargement or hypertrophy, P-wave changes may reflect altered intraatrial pressure, volume, or conduction. Furthermore, shift of the site of origin of the P wave with an intraatrial conduction disturbance may simulate a pathological state.

As stated earlier, initial atrial activation occurs in the right atrium and is directed anteriorly and inferiorly. As a result, enlargement or preponderance of the right atrium is manifest by an atrial vector that is increased in magnitude and shifted to the right. The P wave is normal in duration, low or isoelectric in lead I, and tall—but more importantly, peaked or pointed—in leads II, III, and aV$_f$ (Fig. 7–11B). P waves in leads V$_{4r}$, V$_1$, and V$_2$ may be upright and increased in amplitude. A P-wave axis greater than +90° with an isoelectric P wave in lead I is rarely, if ever, a normal finding (Fig. 7–11). In the adult the most common cause of right atrial abnormality is chronic obstructive lung disease. Nonspecificity of P pulmonale is suggested by the presence of the P pulmonale pattern in the absence of right atrial enlargement. Such P waves, termed "pseudo-P pulmonale," have been found in association with a variety of disorders of the left heart, including coronary artery disease with angina pectoris, and less often in the absence of heart disease. It has been suggested that in the presence of left heart disease, "pseudo-P pulmonale" reflects an increase of the left atrial component of the P waves.[58]

Left atrial abnormality is manifest by prolongation of the P wave, shortening or absence of the P-R segment, and a shift of the P vector to the left and posteriorly (Fig. 7–11 A). The duration of the P wave is 0.12 sec or longer, the wave is notched, and its axis is shifted to the left. Because the vector is increased in magnitude and oriented posteriorly, lead V$_1$ registers a prominent negative P wave. A negative P wave in lead V$_1$, 0.04 sec in duration and 1 mm in depth, is consistent with left atrial preponderance,[59] the so-called P mitrale. Although this abnormality is common in mitral valve disease, the most frequent cause is left ventricular disease, with the increased left ventricular end-diastolic pressure reflected in the atrium.

In *biatrial* enlargement, both anterior and posterior forces are increased. The abnormality includes a prominent initial part of the P wave coupled with the left axis of the terminal portion of the P wave and a biphasic P wave in leads V$_1$ and occasionally in V$_2$ (Fig. 7–11C).

In the presence of atrial fibrillation, atrial disease can occasionally be suspected from an analysis of the QRS complex. With severe tricuspid regurgitation, right atrial enlargement displaces the tricuspid valve down and to the left. As a result, lead V$_1$ (and sometimes V$_2$), normally subtended by the right ventricle, now reflects the intracavitary (qR) right atrial potential as indicated by QR, qR, or qrS complexes in leads V$_1$ or V$_1$ and V$_2$ followed by a normal progression of R-wave amplitude from leads V$_2$ or V$_3$ to V$_6$ (Fig. 7–12).[10]

Atrial enlargement can also be suspected when coarse, relatively large fibrillatory waves are present, especially in lead V$_1$. This is in contrast to atrial fibrillation complicating arteriosclerotic and hypertensive heart disease, in which the fibrillatory waves are fine and frequently unidentifiable.

In the VCG, the P loop parallels the changing direction of the maximal P vector.[37,38,60] In the transverse plane, *right atrial enlargement* is recognized when a major portion of the loop is displaced anteriorly. The inscription is counterclockwise. In the right sagittal plane, the loop is inscribed counterclockwise and is displaced anteriorly and inferiorly; the posteriorly located component remains unaltered. In the frontal plane, the loop is narrow and has a vertical orientation.

In the transverse plane, *left atrial enlargement* is inscribed in a counterclockwise direction or in the form of a figure-of-eight. With the exception of an initial component located anteriorly, the loop is shifted posteriorly and to the left. In the right sagittal plane, the loop is located more superiorly than normal and the major portion of the loop is located posteriorly; the inscription is clockwise. In the frontal plane, the loop is shifted to the left.

In *biatrial enlargement*, the horizontal plane loop inscribes both the increased early anterior and the late posterior components of the loop.

Intraatrial conduction abnormalities can result in enlargement of the loop in the absence of dilatation or hypertrophy. The loop displays localized conduction and anatomical abnormalities, the latter in the form of "notches" and "bites."[61]

Alteration of atrial repolarization (Ta), recognized by deviation from the T-P segment, can be either secondary or primary (Figs. 7–5 and 7–13). The usual pathological causes of secondary Ta-segment depression, which may exceed 1 mm (0.1 mV), include atrial dilation, hypertrophy, or intraatrial block. In chronic obstructive lung disease, for example, depression of the Ta segment may be exaggerated and mistaken for ST-segment displacement.

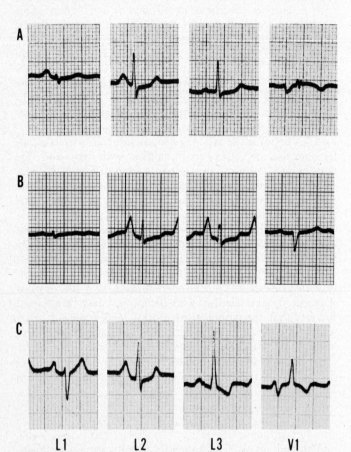

L1   L2   L3   V1

FIGURE 7–11 Atrial hypertrophy, *A*, Recording from a patient with mitral stenosis showing left atrial enlargement characterized by prolonged duration of the P wave, loss of the P-R segment, left-axis deviation of the F wave, and a negative orientation in lead V$_1$. A common feature not clearly visible in this tracing is notching of the P wave. *B*, Recording from a patient with chronic obstructive lung disease showing right atrial enlargement manifest by right-axis deviation of the P wave and a tall, peaked P wave in leads II and III. *C*, Recording from a patient with mitral stenosis showing biatrial enlargement manifest by a tall P wave in lead II, a notched P wave with left-axis deviation of the terminal component in lead III, and a pronounced large biphasic P wave in lead V$_1$.

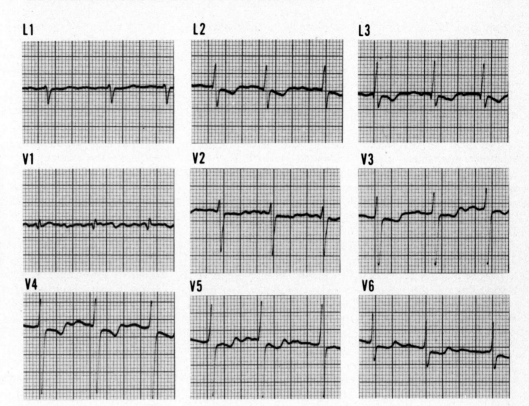

FIGURE 7–12 Rheumatic valvular heart disease with tricuspid regurgitation. The basic rhythm is atrial fibrillation. The right-axis deviation, "squatty" QRS in lead V_1, and clockwise rotation are consistent with mitral valve disease. The QR pattern in V_1 reflects the right atrial intracavitary potential and indicates a regurgitant tricuspid valve.

The usual causes of *primary* Ta-segment changes are pericarditis, atrial infarction, and atrial injury due to penetrating wounds. *Pericarditis* exaggerates the normally negative Ta-segment, and Ta-segment depression is recorded in all leads except aVR, in which it is elevated (Fig. 7–13).[24,62,63] Occasionally, a Ta-segment abnormality may be the only convincing evidence of acute pericarditis.

The incidence of *atrial infarction* in myocardial infarction is variously reported as 1 to 42 per cent.[62,63] Isolated atrial infarction in the absence of ventricular infarction is a most unlikely event. The manifestations of infarction may include elevation of the Ta segment in leads I, II, III, V_5, or V_6 or a depression that may exceed 1.5 mm in precordial leads and 1.0 mm in leads I, II, and III. Reciprocal Ta-segment changes may be present[64] (Fig. 7–5). Attempts to localize the site of atrial infarction electrocardiographically

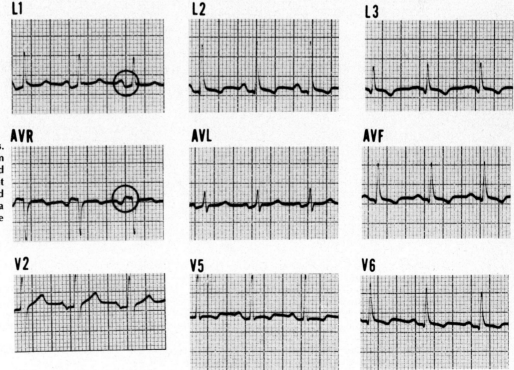

FIGURE 7–13 Acute pericarditis. The tracing shows sinus rhythm with nonspecific ST-segment and T-wave changes. The Ta segment is depressed in leads I, II, V_2, and V_5 and is elevated in lead aV_r. Ta displacement is the only change diagnostic of acute pericarditis.

have been unsuccessful.[65] Supraventricular arrhythmias frequently accompany atrial infarction. The ECG changes that occur in atrial infarction have been reproduced in experimental animal.[5,66]

Penetrating injury of the atria due to gunshot wounds or perforation in the course of cardiac catheterization may be associated with diagnostic Ta-segment depression. Ta-segment displacement is also frequently observed following open heart surgery, and whether or not the displacement reflects mechanical injury, associated pericarditis, hemopericardium, or a combination of these factors is still unclear.

VENTRICULAR HYPERTROPHY

LEFT VENTRICULAR HYPERTROPHY (LVH)

ECG manifestations of LVH include an increase in voltage; shift of the mean QRS axis posteriorly, superiorly, and to the left; prolongation of depolarization (delayed intrinsicoid deflection); and gradual shift of the ST segment and T wave in a direction opposite to that of the QRS complex (Fig. 7–14). The exact mechanism of the voltage increase is not clear. In addition to the muscle mass, other factors may play a role, such as intracavitary blood volume,[67,68] proximity to the chest wall, conducting properties of intrathoracic organs, location of the heart within the thorax, intraventricular and transmural pressures, and perhaps unopposed inscription of a portion of the QRS complex due to delayed activation.

The left superior and posterior orientation of the mean QRS vector in LVH is most likely related to hypertrophy of the basal portion of the left ventricle with delayed, and at times unopposed, activation. Variables that may be responsible for delayed depolarization include increased muscle mass, increased Purkinje activation, and localized intraventricular conduction delays. Marked superior orientation is noted in association with left anterior divisional block.

Prolongation of the excited state through the myocardium and prolongation of activation result in a change in the order of repolarization, which proceeds from endocardium to epicardium, resulting in a reversal of T-wave polarity. Of the mechanisms responsible for reversal of repolarization, increased muscle mass without a concomitant increase in the capillary bed—so-called relative coronary insufficiency—may be an important factor. It is also possible that as the muscle mass outgrows the Purkinje fiber mass, more of the activation proceeds through the myocardium, and this can contribute to a change in the T-wave

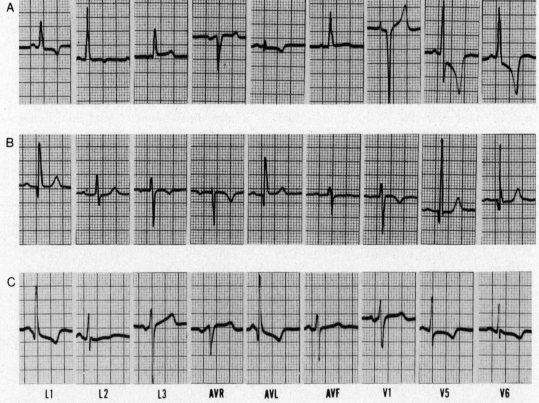

| | L1 | L2 | L3 | AVR | AVL | AVF | V1 | V5 | V6 |

FIGURE 7–14   Left ventricular hypertrophy (LVH). *A*, Tracing from a 23-year-old patient with severe aortic stenosis. The precordial leads were obtained at one-half standard. The voltage and characteristic ST-T changes of LVH are evident. *B*, Tracing from a patient with acute aortic regurgitation due to endocarditis showing a prominent Q wave in leads I, aV$_I$, and V$_5$ and a prominent R wave in leads V$_5$ and V$_6$. Voltage criteria are consistent with LVH. Prominent Q waves reflect the diastolic overload. *C*, Tracing from a 37-year-old patient with aortic regurgitation demonstrates voltage and ST-T changes consistent with LVH as well as prominent Q waves in leads I and aV$_I$ and a prominent R wave in lead V$_1$. These changes indicate a diastolic overload component of the LVH. Although prominent septal forces in the presence of LVH nearly always indicate a diastolic overload, absence of such Q waves does not rule out LVH of this type.

vector. ST-segment depression may be due to the onset of repolarization prior to the completion of depolarization.

The mean QRS vector, increased in magnitude and oriented toward the left, posteriorly and superiorly, results in a positive deflection in leads I, II, V_5, and V_6 and a positive or negative deflection in leads III and aV_f. The precordial transitional zone is shifted to the left. Leads V_1 and V_2 record an rS pattern, but in some instances the initial R wave may be absent for reasons that may remain obscure. Lack of the initial R wave may be erroneously interpreted as an anteroseptal myocardial infarction.

QRS voltage criteria for LVH include $R_I + S_{III} \geq 25$ mm, R in $aV_1 > 12$ mm, R in $aV_f > 20$ mm, S in $V_1 \geq 24$ mm, R in V_5 or $V_6 > 26$ mm, R in V_5 or $V_6 + S$ in $V_1 > 35$ mm.[11,69] The following point system for diagnosing LVH has been suggested:[11,70]Amplitude of R or S wave in limb leads ≥ 20 mm *or* S_1 in V_1 or $V_2 \geq 30$ mm *or* R wave in V_5 or $V_6 \geq 30$ mm = 3 points. ST-segment changes with or without digitalis = 1 or 2 points, respectively. Left atrial enlargement = 3 points. Left-axis deviation $-30°$ or more = 2 points. QRS duration ≥ 0.09 sec and intrinsicoid deflection in V_5 and $V_6 \geq 0.05$ sec = 1 point each. Left ventricular hypertrophy is considered to be likely if the points total 4 and to be present if the total is 5 or more. The diagnosis of LVH is strengthened by a delayed intrinsicoid deflection in lead V_5 or V_6, measuring more than 0.05 sec in the adult. The ST segment and T wave are directed opposite to the QRS complex. Characteristically, the T wave is negative and asymmetrical, its ascending limb being steeper, with occasional terminal positive inscription (Fig. 7–14). The J point and the ST segment are depressed in leads I, aV_1, V_5, and V_6. T-wave inversion is greater in lead V_6 than in V_4. In the presence of a vertical position, the above changes are recorded in leads II, III, and aV_f. Left atrial preponderance is found frequently in LVH.

The shortcomings of the ECG in terms of sensitivity and specificity in the diagnosis of LVH have long been recognized.[71] This is true for both the voltage and the point systems. On the one hand, autopsy data indicate that voltage consistent with LVH can be present in patients without myocardial hypertrophy,[72] while on the other hand, normal ECG values were recorded in about 40 to 50 per cent of patients with LVH, based on echocardiographic findings.[71] This is not surprising, since the ECG reflects an electrical current and only indirectly an anatomical change, and the magnitude of this current is subject to a variety of influences discussed earlier. Furthermore, it is often difficult to differentiate between a delayed intrinsicoid deflection and conduction abnormalities due to focal delays and blocks. Left-axis deviation of less than $-30°$ is of little help in the diagnosis of LVH. Similarly, an axis greater than $-30°$ is often due to intraventricular conduction manifest because of left anterior divisional block and may not be related to LVH. The sensitivity and specificity of the ECG criteria for LVH improve when more than one criterion is applied. An ECG diagnosis of LVH in patients with cardiac disorders that are likely to result in such hypertrophy is secure when the abnormal QRS voltage is accompanied by ST-segment and T-wave changes in the absence of abnormalities that alone may induce these changes.

The concept of *diastolic overload* is found by the author to be clinically useful at times.[73] It may point to such lesions as patent ductus arteriosus, ventricular septal defect, or aortic or mitral valve regurgitation. The ECG pattern is one of LVH but with a prominent Q wave in the leads facing the left side of the septum, namely, I, aV_1, V_5, and V_6, and a reciprocal, prominent R wave in the leads facing the right side of the septum, namely, V_1 and V_2. As a rule, the Q wave is narrow, measuring 0.025 sec or less, and its depth is 2 mm or greater. The concept of systolic or "pressure" overload, characterized by high-amplitude R waves and ST-segment and T-wave changes in the left ventricular leads and present in disorders with an increased resistance to left ventricular outflow, is of limited usefulness (Fig. 7–14).

The VCG changes in LVH are due to an increase in and rotation of the forces further to the left and posteriorly. These events are best reflected in the transverse plane. The VCG loop is increased in magnitude, elongated, inscribed counterclockwise as a rule, and shifted posteriorly. The occasional posterior orientation of the initial part of the loop simulates anteroseptal myocardial infarction. The termination of the loop is anterior, to the right, and superior to the origin of the loop. The loop is therefore open, and this displacement accounts for the ST-segment shift. Secondary T-wave changes shift the T loop to a direction opposite to that of the QRS loop, namely, anteriorly, to the right, and superiorly.[38,74,75]

RIGHT VENTRICULAR HYPERTROPHY (RVH)

In contrast to LVH, RVH is not simply an exaggeration of the normal. For RVH to become manifest, the right ventricular mass must be sufficiently large to overcome the left ventricular forces. For this reason, the specificity of the ECG pattern of RVH is much greater but the sensitivity is relatively low, varying from 25 to 40 per cent depending on the criteria used.[76] While the ECG changes of RVH result largely from the chamber's anatomical dominance, the etiology of the heart disease and associated hemodynamic alterations often contribute to the abnormal ECG pattern. At times, the etiology of the cardiac disorder and the severity of right ventricular pressure can be estimated from an analysis of the ECG.

In RVH the axis shifts to the right, the degree of axis deviation varying with the clinical disorder, and this is accompanied by vertical position and clockwise rotation. Based on the QRS pattern in lead V_1, RVH can generally be separated into three groups, namely, a dominant R wave (R, qR rR, rsR') (Fig. 7–15), RS (Rs, Rsr'), and rS or rsr' complex. The different QRS patterns may provide a clue to the degree of elevation in right ventricular pressure. In general a qR complex, a prominent R wave with a slur on the upstroke, or an rsr' complex (incomplete RBBB) suggest that right ventricular pressure exceeds, is equal to, or is lower than left ventricular pressure, respectively. Examples include severe pulmonary stenosis or primary pulmonary hypertension, tetralogy of Fallot or Eisenmenger complex and atrial septal defect, respectively. In the latter, hypertrophy of the outflow tract of the right ventricle is responsible for the r' wave.

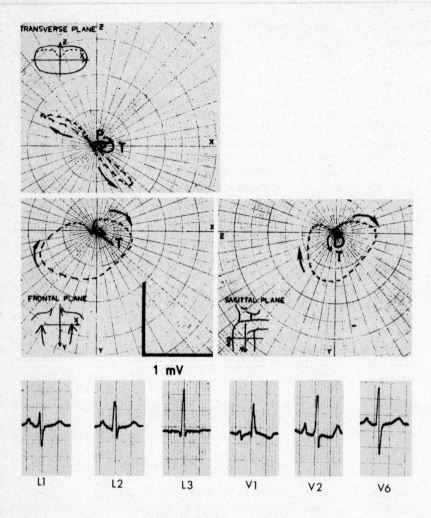

1 mV

L1   L2   L3   V1   V2   V6

FIGURE 7–15   Right ventricular hypertrophy (RVH). In the transverse plane of the VCG, anterior and rightward displacement of the mid and late portions of the QRS loop with a figure-of-eight inscription can be seen. In the frontal plane, the QRS loop is inscribed clockwise and displaced to the right. In the sagittal plane, the loop is inscribed clockwise and displaced anteriorly. The T-wave loop is inscribed counterclockwise. The time scale is the same for all VCG. The loop is interrupted every 2.5 msec, as indicated by each dot or comma. The ECG illustrates the classic pattern of moderately severe to severe RVH (see text).

In the presence of RVH the delay of ventricular activation results in earlier recovery of the endocardium, and repolarization proceeds from endocardium to epicardium. The ST segment is thereby depressed and the T wave inverted in lead V_1 and occasionally in V_2. Significant ST-segment depression and T-wave inversion is, as a rule, indicative of moderate or severe hypertension.

In the adult with acquired RVH the most commonly encountered ECG changes include right-axis deviation and an R/S ratio $\geq$ 1 in V_1, with an R wave 5 mm or greater. Isolated right-axis deviation in excess of $+100°$ to $-90°$ is considered by some to be indicative of RVH,[77] but this criterion alone is less sensitive. The R/S ratio in lead V_1 alone is not diagnostic of RVH, since it may be recorded in patients with a posterior infarction or occasionally in the absence of heart disease. In the normal subject, an R/S ratio greater than 1 in lead V_1 may also be accompanied by right-axis deviation.

ECG changes due to acute pulmonary embolus with pulmonary hypertension (acute cor pulmonale) and chronic obstructive lung disease often differ from the classic pattern seen in RVH and will be discussed separately.

ACUTE PULMONARY EMBOLUS (ACUTE COR PULMONALE) (see also p. 1578).   The most characteristic ECG feature of this disorder is probably the transient nature of the changes (Fig. 7–16). The ECG changes are most likely related to acute pulmonary hypertension with right atrial and ventricular dilatation, hypoxia, and per-

haps myocardial ischemia. From time to time, the changes include P pulmonale; right-axis deviation with clockwise rotation; an S1, S2, or S3 pattern; complete or incomplete RBBB; or T-wave inversion in the right precordial and inferior leads. T-wave changes may last a few days, while the axis deviation, clockwise rotation, and RBBB may persist as long as 1 to 3 weeks. The acute atrial dilatation coupled with myocardial ischemia is probably responsible for the frequent atrial arrhythmias. Sensitivity and specificity of the ECG in diagnosis of acute cor pulmonale is relatively low; this test is diagnostic in about 25 per cent of patients. Both transient T-wave alterations and the RBBB, although nonspecific and frequently seen in a variety of chronic cardiac disorders, are of diagnostic value when accompanied by a clinical picture suggestive of acute cor pulmonale.

CHRONIC OBSTRUCTIVE LUNG DISEASE (COLD) AND COR PULMONALE (see also p. 1592). The ECG pattern of COLD and COLD with pulmonary hypertension (cor pulmonale) can be ascribed to a combination of positional changes, increased lung volume, and RVH. ECG changes include right-axis deviation of the P wave, increased amplitude and "peaked" appearance of the P wave in the limb leads, and "peaked" and biphasic morphology wave in lead V_1 (Fig. 7–11, p. 208). A P-wave axis of $+90°$ is highly suggestive of COLD. Because of the large P-wave area, the Ta segment is exaggerated and occasionally interpreted as ST-segment depression. Right-axis deviation and clockwise rotation are characteristic find-

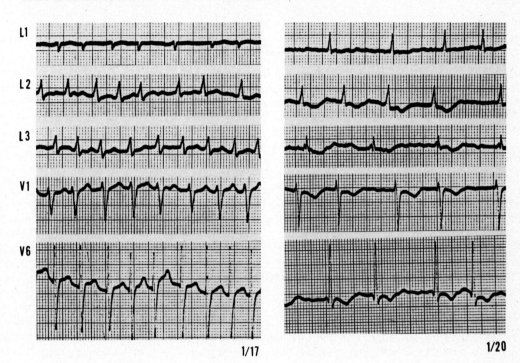

FIGURE 7–16 Acute pulmonary embolus. The basic rhythm is atrial fibrillation. On 1/17 the ventricular rate was about 150 bpm, with the axis shifted to the right and an RS pattern in lead V_6. On 1/20 this rate slowed to about 75 to 100 bpm. The axis and QRS complex in V_6 are both normal.

ings. Occasionally, an S1, S2, S3 pattern may be present. Amplitude of the precordial R wave is reduced in leads V_5 and V_6, often measuring less than 7 mm. When the clockwise rotation is marked, absence of the R wave in precordial leads simulates an anterior myocardial infarction. With progression to pulmonary hypertension and RVH, prominent R waves may appear in leads V_1 and V_2. These changes are probably due to unopposed late activation of the crista terminalis and right ventricular free wall. Right atrial dilatation is probably responsible for the QR pattern in V_1, with the Q wave reflecting right atrial intracavitary potential (as occurs also in tricuspid regurgitation (Fig. 7–12, p. 209). As indicated, the sensitivity of the ECG for cor pulmonale is relatively low, the test being diagnostic in about 25 to 40 per cent of patients with confirmed RVH.[76]

In *biventricular hypertrophy*, the LV forces are dominant and often obscure the RVH.

In RVH, the characteristic VCG changes of the QRS loop are recorded in the transverse plane, with three general patterns recognized (Fig. 7–17). In type A, the loop is inscribed clockwise, occasionally in a figure-of-eight (Fig. 7–15), and is positioned in the right and left anterior quadrants. In type B, the loop is inscribed clockwise, or counterclockwise, is often figure-of-eight, and is located primarily in the left anterior and to a lesser extent in the left and right posterior quadrants. In type C, the loop is inscribed counterclockwise, with 50 per cent of the loop located in posterior left and right quadrants. Of the three, type A usually reflects severe RVH, while type B is most often encountered in patients with atrial septal defect and mitral stenosis. Type C can be recorded with chronic obstructive lung disease.[78,79]

VENTRICULAR HYPERTROPHY IN THE PRESENCE OF CONDUCTION DEFECTS. The diagnosis of ventricular hypertrophy in the presence of BBB is difficult, if not impossible, owing in part to the fact that a por-

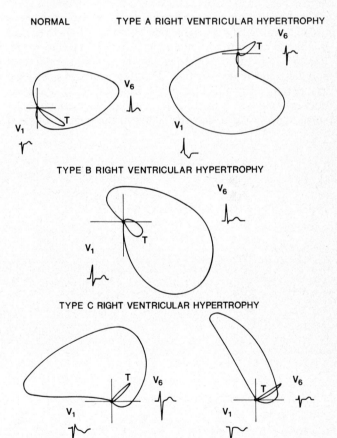

FIGURE 7–17 Diagrammatic representation of the three common, but not exclusive, VCG patterns of right ventricular hypertrophy recorded in the horizontal plane. When compared with the normal, the QRS loops are located in the right and left anterior quadrants in Type A and in the left anterior and to a lesser extent left and right posterior quadrants in Type B; a major portion of the loop is located in the left and right posterior quadrants in Type C. (Modified from Chou, T. C., Helm, R. A., and Kaplan, S.: Clinical Vectorcardiography. 2nd ed. New York, Grune and Stratton, 1974, pp. 87, 99, and 102.)

tion of cardiac activation may be unopposed for a period of time, resulting in misleading voltage changes. It has been suggested that in the presence of RBBB, an R' greater than 10 to 15 mm indicates associated RVH.[80] However, it is not unusual to record preoperatively a normal QRS complex in lead V_1, only to register postoperatively an RBBB with an R' wave greater than 10 or 15 mm, indicating that this criterion of RVH may not be valid in the presence of RBBB. LBBB makes a diagnosis of RVH and LVH essentially impossible. In the presence of RBBB, LVH may be suspected when one sees a deep S wave in lead V_1 and tall R wave in lead V_6. However, such an interpretation is subject to the limitations imposed by the relatively low sensitivity and specificity of the voltage criteria.

INTRAVENTRICULAR CONDUCTION DEFECTS

The bundle of His bifurcates into right and left bundles (see Fig. 19–2, p. 607). The right bundle, wirelike, descends subendocardially on the right side of the septum. At the base of the right ventricular anterior papillary muscle, it breaks up and supplies fibers to the free right ventricular wall and the right side of the septum. The left bundle divides into an anterior division (LAD) and posterior division (LPD), which supply the left ventricular wall and left side of the septum. Discrete anatomical lesions, asynchrony of conduction in the bundles or its branches, nonuniformity of refractoriness, changes in membrane responsiveness, and a decrease in the magnitude of phase 4

may, singly or in combination, cause block of conduction in the bundle branches (BBB) and the divisions of the left bundle. However, most commonly BBB is due to an anatomical lesion. In transient BBB, the specific underlying electrophysiological mechanism may be difficult to define.

In this section the emphasis is primarily on fixed nonrate-related blocks. Rate-dependent conduction abnormalities are included in the discussion of aberration (p. 244).

Left Bundle Branch Block

Interruption of LBB results in early activation of the right side of the septum and of the right ventricular myocardium. Transseptal activation from right to left is transmyocardial and thus slow, and probably a major cause of the prolonged ventricular activation.[81–83] Initial activation of the ventricles proceeds from right to left, inferiorly, and more often anteriorly than posteriorly. This is followed by continued activation of the septum and of the adjacent free left ventricular wall, with the activation proceeding to the left, posteriorly, and inferiorly. This phase of activation is rapid, presumably because the impulse enters the Purkinje system below the site of the BBB. Last to be activated are the lateral wall and basal aspect of the left ventricle, with a vector oriented posteriorly, superiorly, and, less frequently, inferiorly.

In complete LBBB, the QRS complex is prolonged, measuring 0.12 to 0.18 sec (Fig. 7–18). An upright notched or slurred R wave reflecting the right-to-left myocardial activation is recorded in leads I and V_6. A small R wave followed by an S wave is present in aV_f, the R wave

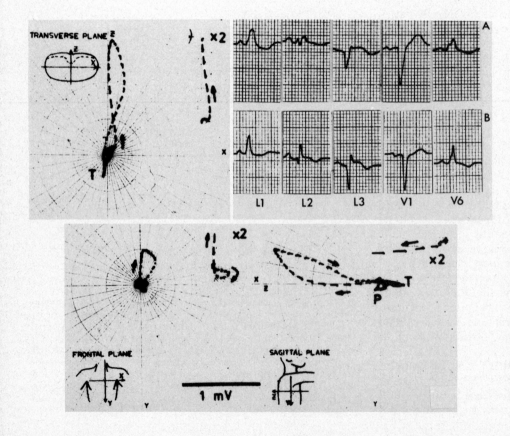

FIGURE 7–18 The ECG illustrates an intermittent LBBB (panel A) and an inferior myocardial infarction and normal intraventricular conduction in panel B. The VCG was recorded when LBBB was present. In the transverse plane, the initial anteriorly oriented portion of the QRS loop is decreased, and the entire loop shows a figure-of-eight inscription and is displaced posteriorly. There is a generalized slowing of inscription indicated by close spacing of the dots. This is particularly evident in the midportion of the QRS loop. (The duration of the loop is 120 msec.) A narrow T loop is directed anteriorly and slightly to the right. In the frontal plane, the QRS loop is displaced superiorly with the initial force directed inferiorly and to the left. The initial inscription is counterclockwise but clockwise during the remainder of the loop. A general slowing of inscription is present and is most pronounced in the midportion of the QRS loop. In the sagittal plane, there is posterior displacement of the QRS loop with a significant decrease of the initial anterior force. There is general slowing of inscription, which is most pronounced in the midportion of the QRS loop. The narrow T loop is directed opposite to the direction of the QRS loop. The initial portion of the QRS loop is displayed two times the standard ($\times$ 2).

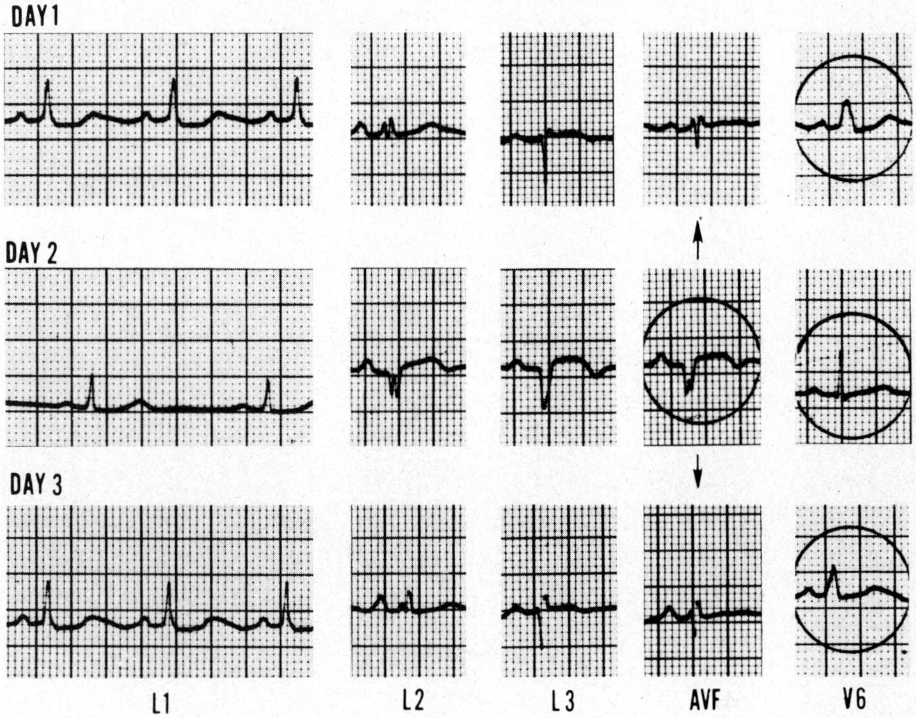

DAY 1

DAY 2

DAY 3

L1   L2   L3   AVF   V6

FIGURE 7–19 Inferior myocardial infarction obscured by incomplete LBBB due to acceleration of the heart rate. On day 1, the heart rate is 83 bpm and incomplete LBBB is registered (circle). On day 2, the heart rate slowed to 60 bpm and incomplete LBBB is no longer evident (circle). Features of inferior myocardial infarction are now recorded in leads II, III, and aV$_f$ (circle). On day 3, the heart rate accelerated to 88 bpm, and incomplete LBBB recurred, masking the inferior myocardial infarction (arrows).

and the S wave reflect, respectively, the initial septal activation directed inferiorly and the superior orientation of the final vector. An rS or a QS complex, depending on whether the initial activation is oriented anteriorly or posteriorly, is recorded in lead V$_1$, with the S wave reflecting activation of the left ventricle from right to left. An initial R wave in lead V$_1$ is present in about 45 per cent of cases of LBBB.[81] One clinically important feature of LBBB is an absence of a septal Q, owing to the initial right-to-left septal activation. Similarly, a Q wave fails to register when either myocardial infarction complicates preexisting LBBB or when LBBB complicates an acute myocardial infarction. The frontal axis in LBBB may be either normal or directed to the left (−30° to −90°), the prevalence of the two being about equal.[84] Although it has been accepted that an abnormal left axis in excess of −45° is nearly always due to a left anterior divisional block, LBBB per se may also result in pronounced left-axis deviation. The precordial leads V$_1$ to V$_4$ may exhibit a small R wave, with the R waves in the midprecordial leads occasionally lower in amplitude than those in the right precordial leads.

The direction of the ST-segment and T-wave vectors is opposite to that of the QRS vector in LBBB. In the presence of an upright QRS complex in leads I, aV$_l$, and V$_6$ the ST segment is depressed and the T waves are inverted. The opposite is true in leads V$_1$, V$_2$, and V$_3$, where a predominantly negative QRS complex is recorded. The ST-segment and T-wave changes are secondary, and the magnitude of the change parallels the magnitude of the QRS aberration. Occasionally LBBB is associated with an isoelectric ST segment and a T-wave vector concordant with the QRS vector. Such primary T-wave changes suggest a myocardial abnormality independent of the LBBB, which may be due, for example, to accompanying myocardial ischemia. However, this is not always a reliable sign of a primary myo-

cardial disorder, as is evidenced by the return of normal T waves when left bundle conduction normalizes.

Incomplete LBBB implies a greater delay of conduction in the left than in the right bundle, with initial right-to-left septal activation and loss of the septal Q wave.[83,85] However, in contrast to complete LBBB, the left bundle ultimately contributes to activation of the septum and left ventricular wall. ECG criteria for incomplete LBBB include a QRS complex of 0.10 to 0.12 sec, loss of the initial septal Q wave, slurring or notching (Fig. 7–19), and often high voltage of the QRS complex.

In the transverse plane of the VCG, the QRS loop of LBBB is oriented to the left and posteriorly. The initial portion of the loop reflects septal activation and is inscribed slowly from right to left and anteriorly. The remainder of the loop is inscribed clockwise with slow inscription of the midportion, most likely reflecting slow intramyocardial conduction through the left ventricular wall. The T loop points in a direction opposite to that of the QRS (Fig. 7–18).[86]

Right Bundle Branch Block

In the presence of RBBB the septum is activated normally, i.e., from left to right. While the left ventricle is activated normally, right ventricular depolarization is delayed, the right ventricle being last to be activated, and this terminal activation is unopposed. Prolongation of the QRS complex is largely due to delayed activation of the septum and right ventricular wall. The initial dominant septal force is directed from left to right, anteriorly and superiorly, followed by a vector dominated by the left ventricle, oriented to the left, inferiorly, and either somewhat anteriorly or posteriorly. The final vector representing acti-

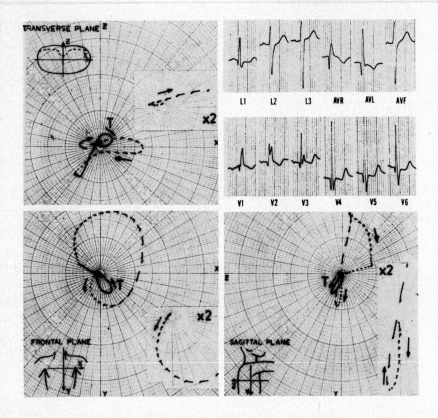

FIGURE 7–20 The ECG illustrates an anterior myocardial infarction, RBBB, and left anterior divisional block (LADB). In the transverse plane, the VCG displays an initial QRS force directed to the right and slightly anteriorly with a clockwise inscription. The decrease in the anteriorly directed initial QRS force is due to the infarction. A delayed terminal QRS loop exhibiting a figure-of-eight inscription is displaced anteriorly. The terminal, anteriorly directed, slowly inscribed part of the loop is due to RBBB. The clockwise-inscribed T-wave loop is oriented in a direction opposite to that of the main QRS force. In the frontal plane, the initial QRS is directed to the right and inferiorly. The loop is inscribed counterclockwise and is displaced superiorly and to the left. The superior and leftward displacement of the loop is due to LADB. The delayed terminal QRS forces are shifted superiorly and to the right. In the sagittal plane, the initial QRS loop is directed inferiorly and slightly anteriorly, with a decrease of the initial anteriorly directed QRS force. The delayed terminal loop is displaced anteriorly and superiorly. The initial portion of the QRS loop is displayed at two times the standard ($\times$ 2).

vation of the right ventricle is directed to the right, anteriorly, and either superiorly, inferiorly, or horizontally.

The characteristic ECG changes of RBBB are recorded in lead V_1. The initial normal septal activation inscribes an R wave, followed by an S wave reflecting left ventricular activation and a final R' wave due to depolarization of the right ventricle from left to right and anteriorly. The depth of the S wave in lead V_1 will vary depending on whether the left ventricular activation generates a more posteriorly or anteriorly oriented vector. In the former, a prominent S wave will separate the R wave from R' wave, while in the

latter, the S wave may be shallow or a slur or, indeed, may be absent. Leads facing the left side of the septum, namely, I, aV_1, V_5, and V_6, record an initial Q wave followed by an R wave of normal duration and a prolonged, relatively shallow S wave. The latter reflects delayed activation of the right ventricle (Figs. 7–20 to 7–22).

The T wave is usually inverted in lead V_1 and occasionally in V_2, while it is upright in the remaining precordial and limb leads.

The characteristic VCG feature is evident in the transverse plane and consists of a slowly inscribed termi-

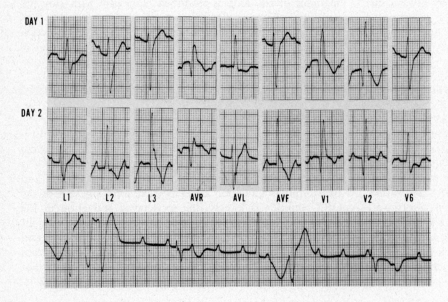

FIGURE 7–21 Acute anterior myocardial infarction complicated by RBBB, LADB, left posterior divisional block (LPDB), and complete AV block. On day 1, the ECG records a sinus rhythm; LADB in leads I, II, and III; RBBB in leads V_1 and V_2; and anterior myocardial infarction manifest by a deep Q wave in leads V_1 and V_2. On day 2, the RBBB and anterior infarction are again noted, but with LPDB recorded in leads I, II, and III. The LPDB is indicated by shift of axis to the right, as estimated on the basis of the initial 0.08 sec of the QRS and the appearance of Q waves and tall R waves in leads II, III, and aV_f. Complete AV block, ventricular premature beats, prolonged Q-T interval, and deeply inverted T waves are recorded in row 3.

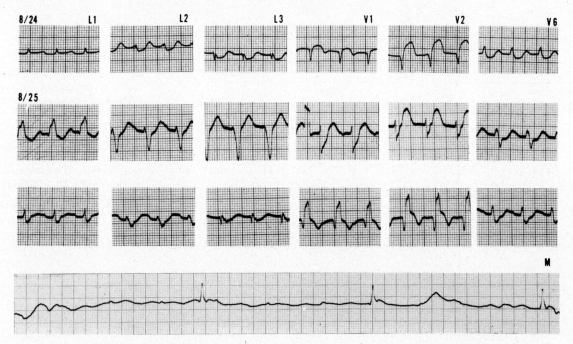

FIGURE 7–22 Acute anterior myocardial infarction complicated by alternating bundle branch block. On 8/24, the acute anterior myocardial infarction is manifest by a QS pattern with elevation of the ST segment in leads V_1 and V_2 and reciprocal ST-segment depression in leads II, III, and V_6. On 8/25, row 2, the pattern is that of LBBB, which obscures the myocardial infarction; in row 3, RBBB and acute anterior myocardial infarction are present. This is followed by complete AV block with an idioventricular rate of about 25 bpm. (M=monitor lead.)

nal appendage directed to the right and anteriorly. The initial septal and left ventricular portion of the loop is normal (Fig. 7–20).[87,88]

Divisional (Fascicular) Blocks

The ventricular conduction system, including the right bundle branch and the two divisions of the left bundle, can be considered for purposes of clinical electrocardiography to consist of three divisions (fascicles) (Fig. 7–23). Some accept the existence of the midseptal "branch" and thus a four-divisional system. However, only patterns consistent with left anterior divisional and left posterior divisional block are recognizable in the ECG. Divisional blocks are, with rare exception, acquired.[33]

According to some investigators, evidence for the existence of anatomically discrete divisions of the left bundle branch is not convincing. However, experimental data tend to support a functional divisional conduction system.[89,90] Furthermore, synchronous endocardial activation at three sites, namely, the middle anterior, and posterior paraseptal areas, is consistent with the concept of existence of functional divisions of the left bundle. This concept is also supported by distinctive and predictable ECG patterns. Thus, from the ECG standpoint, the concept of divisions of the left bundle is a useful one.[91,92]

BLOCK OF ANTERIOR DIVISION OF THE LEFT BUNDLE BRANCH (ANTERIOR FASCICULAR BLOCK). In the presence of left anterior divisional block, the initial septal activation proceeds inferiorly, anteriorly, to the right, and occasionally to the left. This is followed by activation of inferior and apical areas with the vector oriented inferiorly, to the left, and anteriorly. Final

activation is that of the anterolateral and posterobasal left ventricular wall, the vector oriented superiorly, posteriorly, and to the left.

The resultant ECG pattern is characteristic (Fig. 7–23). Lead I records a dominant R wave, with or without an initial Q wave. The presence or absence of a Q wave depends on whether the initial septal activation is directed to the right or to the left. Since the initial activation is directed inferiorly, leads II, III, and aV_f inscribe an R wave followed by a deep S wave reflecting activation of the anterolateral and posterobasal segments of the left ventricle. The QRS axis varies from $-30°$ to $-90°$ (Figs. 7–20, 7–21, 7–24, and 7–25).

The precordial transitional zone is frequently displaced to the left. The amplitude of the R wave is diminished, with a prominent S wave in V_5 and V_6 reflecting the superior orientation of the mean left ventricular vector. The S wave is exaggerated when the final order of activation is directed to the right. Because of the inferior orientation of the initial vector, the midprecordial leads may register an initial Q wave. Such patterns could be mistaken for anteroseptal myocardial infarction[93] were it not for the fact that an R wave is recorded when the leads are placed an interspace lower. The T waves are normally upright except in lead aV_r and occasionally in leads aV_1 and V_1.

Of the three VCG planes, the frontal is the most useful for visualization of left anterior divisional block (Fig. 7–26). The inscription of the loop is counterclockwise, initially directed to the right and inferiorly, with the major and remaining portion of the loop displaced superiorly. The superior orientation reflects activation of the anterior and lateral left ventricular wall.[38,92–95] Left anterior divisional block is nearly always an acquired abnormality and thus a

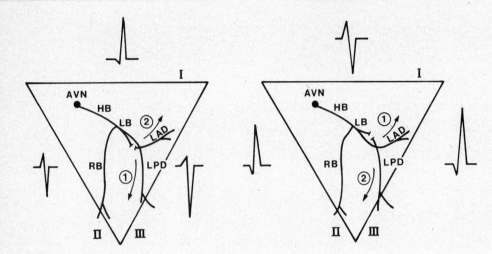

FIGURE 7–23 Diagrammatic representation of the conduction system. Interruption of the LAD (*left*) results in an initial inferior (*1*) followed by a dominant superior (*2*) direction of activation; interruption of the LPD (*right*) results in an initial superior (*1*) followed by a dominant inferior (*2*) direction of activation. AVN = atrioventricular node; HB = His bundle; LB = left bundle; RB = right bundle; LAD = left anterior division; LPD = left posterior division.

marker of organic disease. Often, however, it is present without clinical evidence of heart disease, but the prognosis depends on the underlying disease.

BLOCK OF POSTERIOR DIVISION OF THE LEFT BUNDLE BRANCH (POSTERIOR FASCICULAR BLOCK).   Left posterior divisional block is a rare finding and its pattern is nonspecific. It can be recorded in asthenic individuals and patients with emphysema, RVH, and extensive lateral infarction.[91] Diagnosis is secure only if a normal ECG is recorded prior to appearance of the block.

In the presence of left posterior divisional block, activation begins in the midseptal and paraseptal areas, with the vector directed to the left, anteriorly, and superiorly. This is followed by activation of the left ventricular anterior and anterolateral walls, with the vector directed to the left and anteriorly. Final activation is of the inferior and posterior walls with the vector directed inferiorly, posteriorly, and to the right. In the limb leads, the initial superior and left orientation of septal vectors is reflected as an R wave in lead I and a narrow, 0.025-msec Q wave in leads II, III, and aV$_f$. The R wave in lead I is small and is followed by a deep S wave reflecting the inferior, posterior, and right orientation of the wave of activation (Figs. 7–21 and 7–23). The initial superior force and final inferior force result in a QR complex in leads II, III, and aV$_f$. The frontal axis varies from about +90° to +120°, or perhaps +80° to +140°. The T wave is usually normal.

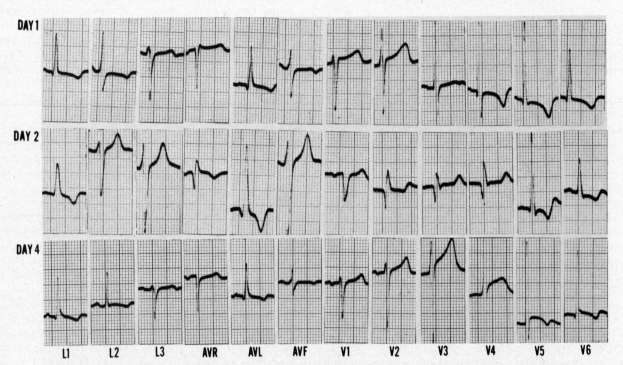

FIGURE 7–24   Transient Q waves and left anterior divisional block (LADB) recorded after aortic valve surgery. On day 1, nonspecific ST-segment and T-wave changes and voltage consistent with LVH are recorded. On day 2, LADB and prolongation of the QRS are accompanied by a Q wave in leads V$_1$ to V$_4$. On day 4, the QRS duration is normal, and LADB and Q waves are no longer present.

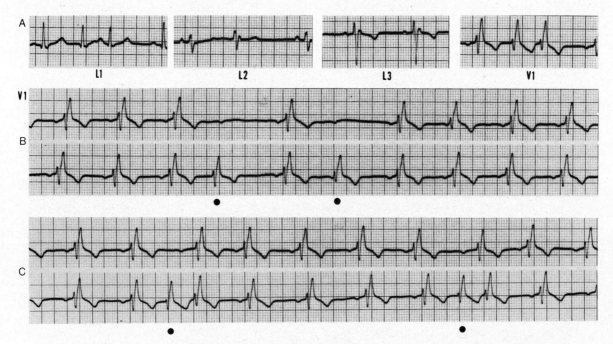

FIGURE 7–25   Concealed junctional discharge manifest as Mobitz (Type II) AV block and intermittent prolongation of the P-R interval. *A,* Normal sinus rhythm interrupted by supraventricular premature complexes, left anterior divisional block, and RBBB. *B,* Mobitz (Type II) AV block due to concealed junctional discharge. The mechanism is supported by the presence of manifest junctional prematures in the second tracing (solid circles). *C,* Isolated, unexpected P-R prolongation (upper tracing) is due to concealed junctional discharge, as suggested by manifest interpolated premature junctional complexes with similar prolongation of the P-R interval in the lower tracing. (Solid circles = manifest junctional impulses.)

In the frontal plane of the VCG, the inscription is clockwise, initially superior and to the left, but with the major portion of the loop located in the right inferior quadrant.[92,96]

RIGHT BUNDLE BRANCH BLOCK AND DIVISIONAL BLOCKS. RBBB with left anterior divisional block is the most common combination of the left divisional and bundle branch blocks. The activation during the first 0.08 sec determines the axis and identifies the left anterior divisional block. The delay of depolarization due to RBBB results in a final activation of the right ventricle to the right and anteriorly (Figs. 7–21 and 7–25).

RBBB with left posterior divisional block is a rare combination. The initial 0.08 sec defines the axis and divisional block while the final delayed activation, oriented to the right and anteriorly, reflects RBBB (Fig. 7–21).

Block of the right bundle and both divisions of the left bundle (trifascicular block) can be entertained in the presence of RBBB with alternating left anterior and posterior divisional blocks. Such patterns are usually associated with Mobitz (type II) AV block. It has been suggested that RBBB with either of these hemiblocks and a prolonged P-R interval may be a manifestation of trifascicular block. Although the prolonged P-R interval may be due to delayed conduction in the remaining division, the delay may also reflect AV nodal delay.[97]

The VCG records the characteristic terminal portion of the RBBB loop in the transverse plane, while the left anterior divisional block[94,98] and left posterior hemiblock[98,99] are best visualized in the frontal plane. The characteristic features of RBBB and left anterior divisional block with and without RBBB are shown in Figures 7–20 and 7–26. An initial inferior with rapid upward displacement of the loop or an initial superior with rapid inferior displacement in the frontal plane is recorded with left anterior or left posterior divisional block, respectively. A terminal and delayed activation to the right and anteriorly in the transverse plane is the characteristic finding in RBBB.

NONSPECIFIC INTRAVENTRICULAR CONDUCTION DEFECT (IVCD). The QRS complex may be abnormally prolonged but without the characteristic pattern of either RBBB or LBBB. Such conduction delays are referred to as "nonspecific" IVCD. These often resemble LBBB or LBBB with an abnormal left-axis deviation, a combination suggesting left anterior hemiblock with peripheral conduction delay. Presence of a normal Q wave supports peripheral delay as the cause of QRS prolongation. Although such a nonspecific prolongation may be due to drugs or electrolyte abnormalities, it is most often due to organic heart disease.

BILATERAL BUNDLE BRANCH BLOCK. This diagnosis can be entertained when alternating RBBB and LBBB are present. Any other combination of conduction delays cannot be differentiated from block in the AV junction. For example, block in both bundles results in complete AV block. Similarly, intermittent delay or block in one bundle and complete block of conduction in the contralateral bundle will manifest either as bundle branch block with a prolonged P-R interval or intermittent AV block. In the presence of BBB, a superimposed AV block due to failure of conduction in the contralateral bundle branch cannot be differentiated from block in the AV junction (Fig. 7–22).[100]

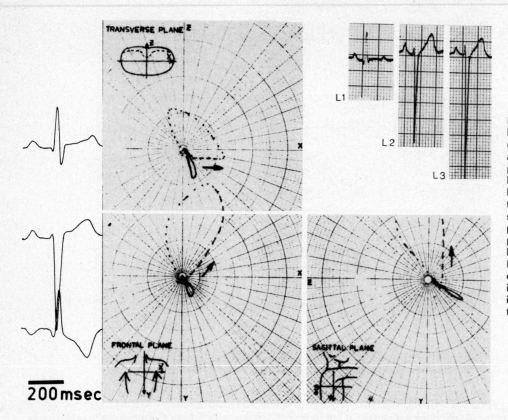

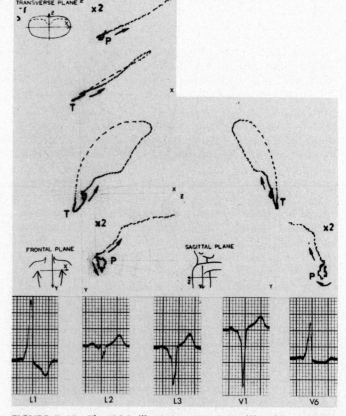

FIGURE 7–26 Left anterior divisional block and left ventricular hypertrophy (LVH). The ECG pattern of qR in lead I and rS in leads II and III indicates presence of left anterior divisional block. The diagnostic VCG features of left anterior divisional block are an initial small inferior deflection with rapid superior and counterclockwise displacement of the loop in the frontal plane, and the major area of the loop located in the left upper quadrant. LVH is suggested on ECG by the ST-T changes in lead I and the QRS voltage in leads II and III. On the VCG, LVH is indicated by posterior displacement of the loop in the horizontal plane.

Wolff-Parkinson-White (WPW) Syndrome
(See also pp. 628 and 712)

WPW, or preexcitation,[101,102] is an electrocardiographic syndrome characterized by a short P-R (≤ 0.12 sec) interval, prolonged QRS (≥ 0.12 sec) complex, a slur on the upstroke of the QRS (delta wave), and (as a rule) a normal P-J interval (Figs. 7–27, 7–28). Secondary ST-segment and T-wave changes are nearly always present. Ectopic atrial tachycardia is recorded in about 50 per cent of patients with WPW. The characteristic pattern of WPW can be altered by abnormalities of AV and intraventricular conduction. The prevalence of WPW in the general population is approximately 3 per thousand; the fact that this figure is identical for both the young and the aged supports a congenital origin for WPW.[33]

Although Wilson is credited with the initial report of WPW,[103] it was Cohn who brought the electrocardiograph to America and first described an ECG pattern to become known as WPW. His patient was described in 1913, and suffered from a supraventricular tachycardia.[104] In 1930, this pattern was recognized as a discrete ECG syndrome.[101] Shortly thereafter the bypass concept of WPW was proposed, and this concept has stood the test of time.[105] It is of interest to note that over the years a variety of mechanisms have been proposed to explain the ECG pattern of WPW, including an excitable focus within the ventricle mechanically triggered by contraction of the atrium, accelerated conduction over a segment of the normal AV pathway, and, most recently, AV nodal bypass coupled with conduction through the Mahaim fibers.[106]

In WPW the QRS complex is a fusion between the impulse traversing the bypass and the normal AV junction. The bypass component of the QRS complex, or *delta wave*,

FIGURE 7–27 The ECG illustrates type B Wolff-Parkinson-White syndrome and simulates an inferior myocardial infarction. The VCG displays a delayed initial QRS force, indicated by close spacing of the dots. This initial force is directed to the left, posteriorly, and superiorly. The T-wave loop is oriented in a direction opposite to that of the initial QRS force. The initial portion of the QRS loop is also recorded at twice the standard ($\times$ 2).

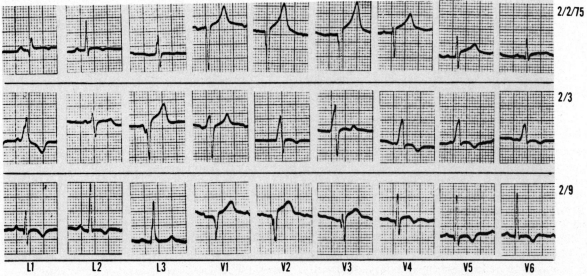

FIGURE 7–28 Anterior myocardial infarction obscured by type A Wolff-Parkinson-White syndrome. On 2/2/75, a Q wave in leads V_1 to V_4 indicates an anterior myocardial infarction. On 2/3, WPW Type A obscures the myocardial infarction. On 2/9, AV conduction is normal, WPW is no longer present, and the anterior myocardial infarction with evolutionary ST-segment and T-wave changes is evident.

varies depending on the size of the ventricular muscle mass activated through the bypass. In some instances, especially in the presence of AV conduction delay, the entire ventricular mass may be activated by the impulse propagated through the bypass, and the entire QRS complex becomes a delta wave.[107]

Traditionally, WPW has been classified into types A and B. *Type A* is characterized by a prominent positive initial QRS deflection in leads V_1 and V_2 (Fig. 7–28) and *type B* by a predominantly negative deflection in leads V_1 and V_2 (Fig. 7–27).[108] In type A, the initial inscription of the QRS complex, the delta wave, reflects early activation of the posterior left ventricle and, in type B, early activation of the anterior superior right ventricle. *Type C WPW*, characterized by a negative delta wave in the left lateral leads, has also been described. Presence of more than one QRS pattern suggests the possibility of multiple bypass tracts. A short P-R interval with a normal QRS complex accompanied by atrial tachycardia (the Lown-Ganong-Levine syndrome) has been suggested as a variant of WPW.[109]

First-, second-, and third-degree AV block have been reported with WPW. The mechanisms that could explain the coexistence of WPW and AV block are many, but in any one patient the exact cause is usually unclear.[107] Right and left BBB have been described in association with WPW. In the presence of a BBB, an ipsilateral bypass, by preexciting the ventricle normally activated by the blocked bundle branch, will obscure the BBB.[110] Both supernormal and concealed conduction have been invoked to explain unexpected patterns of behavior of bypass conduction.[111]

WPW often complicates ECG interpretation because it may obscure or simulate a variety of patterns. It may mask (Fig. 7–28) or may simulate myocardial infarction. When the QRS vector is directed toward the left ventricular cavity, the cavity becomes initially positive and a Q wave will not be recorded. A diagnosis of ventricular hypertrophy in the presence of WPW (as in BBB) may be

difficult, if not impossible. WPW has been mistaken for RBBB, LBBB, and RVH. Supraventricular arrhythmias with aberration, resulting from conduction through the bypass, have been mistaken for ventricular tachycardia. Aberration due to WPW should be suspected when the ventricular rate is rapid, often approaching 300 bpm, or when the QRS morphology of the bizarre complexes is upright in leads V_1 and V_2 as well as in V_5 and V_6.

The characteristic VCG feature of WPW syndrome is a slowly inscribed initial portion of the loop, the delta wave of the ECG, which is best seen in the horizontal plane.[37,38,112] The delta is defined as that portion of the loop which begins at point E, the resting or isoelectric point of the electronic beam, and ends with resumption of normal conduction speed. The direction of this initial portion of the loop classifies the WPW into type A, B, or C. Normally, the duration of the slow inscription varies from 0.02 to 0.08 sec, depending on how much of the ventricle is activated through the anomalous pathway.

In *type A WPW*, the slow portion of the loop is directed to the left and anteriorly. The remainder of the QRS loop, usually inscribed counterclockwise, maintains the same direction as the delta wave and is located in the left anterior quadrant. In about 20 per cent of cases, the maximal vector of the loop points in the direction of the left posterior quadrant. In the ECG these changes are manifest by an upright QRS complex in leads V_1 and V_6.

Type B WPW is recognized by an initial slow inscription oriented to the left and posteriorly or slightly anteriorly. The major portion of the loop is located in the left posterior quadrant. In the ECG these are reflected as a QS complex in leads V_1 and V_2 and an R wave in leads V_5 and V_6 (Fig. 7–27).

Type C WPW is a rarely encountered variant characterized by a Q wave in leads V_5 and V_6. The slowly inscribed initial portion of the loop is directed anteriorly to the right, with the remainder of the loop inscribed normally.

MYOCARDIAL INFARCTION

Myocardial damage manifest by elevation of the ST segment was first observed in the dog with injection of silver nitrate[113] and shortly thereafter with ligation of a coronary artery.[114] In 1920, the ECG of myocardial infarction was described in man.[115]

The ECG changes of myocardial infarction are those of ischemia, injury, and cellular death and are, within limits, reflected by T-wave changes, ST-segment displacement, and the appearance of Q waves, respectively. Such a clear-cut differentiation, although clinically useful, may be overly simplistic and artificial. For example, T-wave changes may be due to ischemia, injury, or death of muscle. Similarly, a Q wave may be due to impairment of transmembrane ionic fluxes and not necessarily cellular death. However, for the purpose of this discussion, T-wave changes, ST-segment displacement, and appearance of a Q wave are assumed to reflect ischemia, injury, and cell death, respectively.

ISCHEMIA

In the dog, the earliest change following ligation of a coronary artery is the almost immediate appearance of a primary T-wave change. (For a definition of primary and secondary T-wave changes, see page 232.) After 60 to 90 seconds, there is a maximal shift of the ST segment. The T wave is now positive and peaked, and the change is as a rule a primary change.[116–118] In man, unless an ECG is recorded at the moment of occlusion, the initial T-w ave stage is usually missed. Occasionally, a giant R wave is recorded early during the ischemic episode. This is seen in experimental animals[119,120] and in man.[121,122] Such changes in the QRS could contribute to the T-wave abnormality, and the T-wave alteration would reflect both primary and secondary changes in repolarization.

Normally the process of repolarization proceeds from the epicardium to the endocardium, and an upright T wave is recorded. Ischemia prolongs the regional duration of recovery, with the ischemic area being last to repolarize. If the ischemia is subendocardial, the direction of repolarization remains unchanged and the polarity of the T wave remains upright. In the presence of subepicardial ischemia, the duration of the excited state is longer in the epicardium; the normal order of repolarization is reversed, proceeding from endocardium to epicardium; and an inverted T wave is inscribed. Because of local prolongation of recovery, the late phase of repolarization may be unopposed, and a large and prolonged T wave may be registered.[123]

INJURY

Two concepts based on systolic and diastolic phenomena have been suggested to explain the ST-segment displacement. One postulates local reduction or loss of resting potential, resulting in a *diastolic current of injury*. The second concept assumes an unopposed current flowing from the injured area during the isoelectric ST segment, resulting in a *systolic current of injury*. These systolic and diastolic phenomena cannot be differentiated with the ordinary clinical alternating-current (AC) electrocardiograph but can be recorded experimentally with direct-current (DC) equipment (Fig. 7–29).

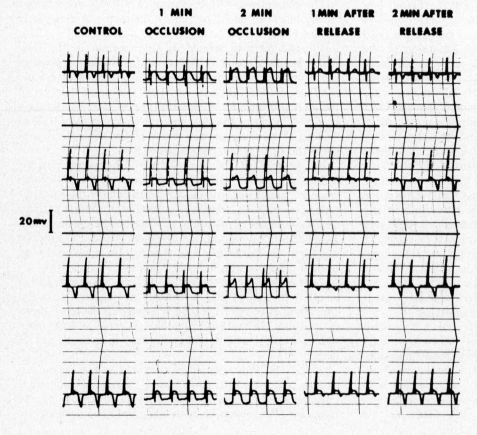

CONTROL | 1 MIN OCCLUSION | 2 MIN OCCLUSION | 1 MIN AFTER RELEASE | 2 MIN AFTER RELEASE

20mv

FIGURE 7–29 Simultaneous epicardial electrograms recorded from four sites. The electrodes were distributed randomly in the ischemic area, with some closer to the center of the ischemic area than others. After one minute of occlusion, TQ-segment depression is apparent in all recordings. After two minutes of occlusion, TQ-segment depression has increased. The ST-segment takeoff is slightly elevated or isoelectric in all recordings. The polarity of the T wave is changed from a negative during the control period to positive. These recordings emphasize that major changes in action potential downstroke, shape, and timing can occur without significant alteration of phase 2 and of the action potential. Similarly, T-wave changes can occur without a significant shift of the true ST segment. True TQ-segment depression appears to be the major cause of ST-segment displacement and the true ST-segment shift of lesser magnitude and variable. T waveform is markedly altered with occlusion. (From Vincent, G. M., et al.: Mechanisms of ischemic ST-segment displacement. Circulation 56:559, 1977, by permission of the American Heart Association, Inc.)

The concept of *diastolic current* proposes that localized injury is associated with a flow of current from the uninjured to the injured area. As a result, the T-Q segment is displaced downward but is automatically shifted to control level by the capacitor-coupled amplifier of the ECG. When the entire heart (including the injured area) is depolarized, the ST segment is elevated with respect to the depressed but rectified (isoelectric) diastolic T-Q segment (Fig. 7–30).

The concept of *systolic current* proposes that during the ST segment, the normal heart is depolarized but the injured area undergoes early repolarization. The result is a current flow from the more positive injured area to a more negative or uninjured area. The result is true elevation of the ST segment. Similarly, if, rather than repolarizing early, the injured area fails to depolarize with the normal myocardium, a current of injury would exist and an elevated ST segment would be recorded (Fig. 7–30). Earlier experimental studies indicate that during injury both systolic and diastolic currents are present,[124] and at times the systolic precedes the diastolic current of injury. A more recent study suggests that the diastolic current predominates while the systolic current plays a lesser role and that the magnitude of the current is modified by the heart rate[125] (Fig. 7–29). As indicated, the clinical ECG does not differentiate between systolic and diastolic currents of injury. Furthermore, unless the onset of the injury is recorded, even a DC coupled ECG would not identify the mechanism of the ST-segment shift.

For reasons outlined earlier, an electrode facing subendocardial injury registers an elevated ST segment, while an epicardial electrode subtended by the normal myocardium registers ST-segment depression. Similarly, an electrode facing epicardial injury registers elevation of the ST segment, while the endocardial electrode inscribes ST-segment depression.

INFARCTION

Infarction implies necrosis and an electrically inert myocardium. The diagnostic feature of infarction is the *Q wave*. Two concepts have been invoked to explain the appearance of the Q wave. The theory of proximity, the "window" theory, suggests that the electrically inert myocardium allows an electrode to record the intracavitary negativity.[126,127] There is ample evidence, however, to suggest that a Q wave can be recorded in the absence of a transmural infarction.[128] Heterogeneity of electrophysiological changes associated with the dynamic events of ischemia and subsequent healing, with intermingling of fibrous and viable tissue, has been suggested as an explanation.[127,129–131]

According to the vectorial concept, the electrically inert myocardium fails to contribute to the normal electrical forces and the result is a vector that points away from the area of infarction, reflected by a Q wave. Theoretically, the infarction vector represents the force that alters the normal vector. It is equal to but opposite in direction from the vector generated by the infarcted myocardium prior to infarction.[37] If the net vector is directed normally but is reduced in magnitude, a Q wave will not be recorded, but the amplitude of the QRS complex will be reduced, indicating loss of myocardium. However, the specificity of such a change for infarction is low.

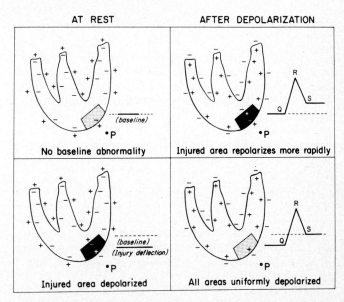

FIGURE 7–30 Systolic (*upper row*) and diastolic (*lower row*) currents of injury. *Upper row,* The ischemic area (shaded) is electrically identical to the nonischemic heart at rest, and there is no shift of the baseline potential. During repolarization, however, the ischemic area (black) has repolarized early and is positive relative to the depolarized heart, the baseline is shifted upward (positive), and the ECG records an elevated ST segment. Similarly, if the ischemic area fails to depolarize with the remainder of the heart, it would be positive relative to the remainder of the heart and a positive ST segment would be recorded. This latter mechanism may also be operative.

Lower row, The ischemic area (black) is depolarized at rest, thus negative relative to the remainder of the heart, and the baseline is shifted down (negative). This shift is not recognizable on ECG. However, with completion of depolarization the injured area is also depolarized; its potential becomes identical to that of the rest of the heart; and the ST segment, although isoelectric, is elevated relative to the depressed baseline, so that an elevated ST segment is registered.

These two mechanisms cannot be differentiated with the ECG, and although both contribute to the current of injury, the systolic is thought to dominate (Fig. 7–29). (From Scher, A. M.: Electrocardiogram. *In* Ruch, I. C., and Patton, H. D. (eds.): Physiology and Biophysics. Philadelphia, W. B. Saunders Co., 1974.)

DIAGNOSIS OF MYOCARDIAL INFARCTION
(See also p. 1283)

One of the most valuable contributions of the ECG is in the diagnosis of myocardial infarction. Usually it is the first laboratory test performed; the technique is reliable and reproducible, can be applied serially, and when properly interpreted is the cornerstone of the laboratory diagnosis of myocardial infarction. In 1933 Wilson and his associates clearly defined the role of the electrocardiogram in the diagnosis of myocardial infarction (at that time referred to as "coronary occlusion"):

In general we found the electrocardiogram far more helpful in the diagnosis of coronary occlusion than the physical findings, but of less value than the clinical history. There are many cases in which characteristic electrocardiographic changes are absent, although electrocardiograms that are within normal limits in every respect are relatively rare, especially during the period immediately following the vascular accident. Since the most distinctive of the electrocardiographic signs of infarction occur at this time and are transient, a series of curves taken at frequent intervals during the first month are far more likely to give important information than a single curve.[132]

It is difficult and perhaps inappropriate to discuss the sensitivity, specificity, and diagnostic power of the ECG in myocardial infarction without first acknowledging the fact that the ECG changes differ significantly depending on the stage and size of the infarction. Similarly, recognition of, and attention to, subtle and atypical changes, realization of the great importance of serial tracings, and an appreciation of the effect of coexisting conduction defects will enhance the diagnostic value of the ECG.

The discussion of the ECG in diagnosis of myocardial infarction will include (a) the earliest change in suspected myocardial infarction, the "first ECG"; (b) the classic pattern of myocardial infarction and its evolution; (c) the minor, subtle, atypical, and nonspecific changes; (d) diagnosis of old infarction; and (e) the effect of conduction defects on the diagnosis.

THE FIRST ECG. The first ECG is "diagnostic" of acute infarction in slightly more than half the patients. This statement should be accepted with the reservation that a single ECG may never be "diagnostic" (see p. 226). However, a pattern of ST-segment displacement, especially with associated Q-wave and T-wave changes, and a clinical history suggestive of ischemic heart disease is highly suggestive—if not diagnostic3 of acute myocardial infarction. In a study of all patients admitted to an emergency room and subsequently proven to have myocardial infarction, 65 per cent had an initial diagnostic ECG and 20 per cent were said to have a normal tracing.[133] In another study of 198 patients, the ECG recorded on the first day was diagnostic of infarction in 72 per cent of men and 61 per cent of the women. Serial tracing increased the sensitivity to 93 per cent.[134] In a series of 449 patients, the initial ECG was interpreted as diagnostic of myocardial infarction in 229 (51 per cent), probable myocardial infarction in 120 (27 per cent), doubtful in 30 (7 per cent), and no evidence of infarction in 70 (16 per cent). Serial cardiograms increased the accuracy to 83 per cent.[135]

In 150 patients with "slight or subacute infarction" treated at home, a pattern diagnostic of myocardial infarction was seen in 27 patients (18 per cent). Seventy-two patients showed significant but not diagnostic abnormalities. LVH was present in 10 patients and minor, 0.5-mm ST-segment depression and lowering of T waves were present in 24 patients. The ECG was borderline in seven and normal in 10 patients.[136]

CLASSIC PATTERN AND EVOLUTION OF INFARCTION. The sequence of ECG evolution of myocardial infarction in man is, in many respects, similar to that recorded in the experimental animal. If the ECG is inscribed at the onset of myocardial infarction, the characteristic early change—namely, an abnormal T wave—is often recorded. The T wave may be prolonged, increased in magnitude, and either upright or inverted.[122,137] This is followed by ST-segment elevation in leads facing the area of injury, with reciprocal depression in the "opposite leads." The upright T wave may exhibit terminal inversion at a time when the ST segment is still elevated. A Q wave may be present in the first ECG or may not appear for hours or sometimes days. The amplitude of the QRS complex may diminish and may be replaced by a QS pattern.

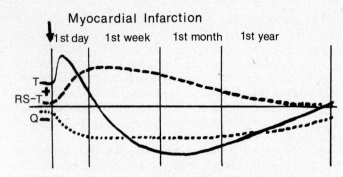

FIGURE 7–31 Evolution of the T wave, ST segment, and Q wave after myocardial infarction. (From Lepeschkin, E.: Modern Electrocardiography. Baltimore, Williams and Wilkins Co., 1951.)

As the ST segment returns to the baseline, symmetrically inverted T waves evolve.[115] The time of appearance and the magnitude of the changes vary from patient to patient.[138,139] Representative time sequences and magnitudes of the T wave, ST segment, and Q wave are illustrated in Figure 7–31.

The classic evolution of acute myocardial infarction is documented in approximately one-half to two-thirds of the patients (Fig. 7–32). In a prospective study of 230 patients, 66 per cent showed diagnostic changes characterized by typical evolution of ST segment and T waves with the appearance of Q waves, while in 34 per cent the infarct was manifest by ST-segment and T-wave changes only (Fig. 7–33).[140]

SUBTLE, ATYPICAL, NONSPECIFIC PATTERNS OF INFARCTION. Atypical features and characteristics of early infarction seen in about 40 to 50 per cent of the first ECG's include a normal ECG; subtle ST-segment and T-wave changes: isolated T-wave abnormality; transient normalization of the ST segment, T wave, or QRS complex (Fig. 7–33); involvement of electrically "silent" areas (Fig. 7–34); or the masking effect of conduction defects (Figs. 7–19, 7–22, and 7–28). Awareness and recognition of the early, nondiagnostic, "atypical" or subtle abnormalities will improve the diagnostic sensitivity of the ECG.

Although ECG changes can be documented within seconds after experimental myocardial infarction,[116] such changes may be delayed in man. A normal initial ECG in a patient with evolving clinical acute myocardial infarction may be due to absence of ischemia at the time of the initial tracing, a delay in evolution of the characteristic pattern, an initially small infarct that produces diagnostic ECG changes only after extension, transient normalization of the ECG in the course of evolution of acute myocardial infarction (Fig. 7–33), or infarction in an electrocardiographically silent area of the myocardium (Fig. 7–34).[135,136]

Evolution of the characteristic ST-segment and T-wave changes coupled with appearance of Q waves is highly specific for acute myocardial infarction. In the first ECG, the sensitivity and specificity of the ST-segment change alone, especially when marked, is high. At times, however, *evolving* changes in the ST segment need to be demonstrated,[136] since conditions such as pericarditis, early repolarization, hyperkalemia, or ventricular aneurysm and Prinzmetal's angina may also manifest ST-segment elevation. Subtle, "minor" ST-segment elevation can be easily overlooked but is a relatively common, isolated early finding.

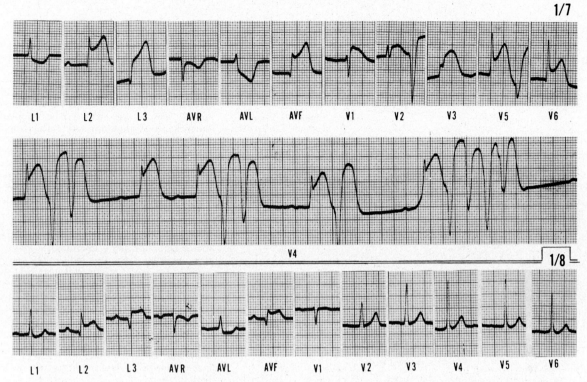

FIGURE 7–32 Acute inferior myocardial infarction and transient extensive anterior injury. Tracing on 1/7 shows elevation of the ST segment in leads II, III, and aV$_f$. V$_1$ through V$_6$ with reciprocal depression of the ST segment in leads I and aV$_l$. In the second row the acute injury is accompanied by ventricular premature complexes (isolated and couplets) and a short run of ventricular tachycardia. On 1/8, the anterior current of injury is no longer present, and the residual pattern is that of an acute inferior myocardial infarction manifest by a Q wave and ST-segment elevation in leads II, III, and aV$_f$.

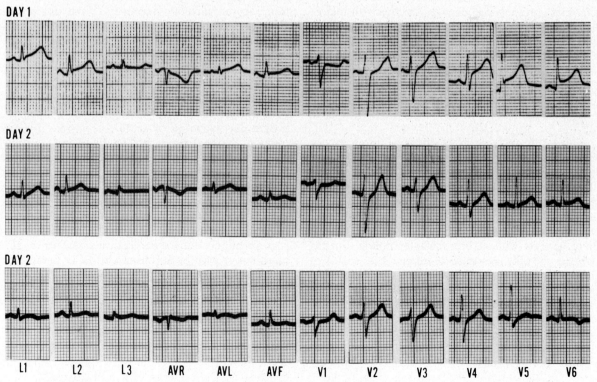

FIGURE 7–33 Normalization of the ECG in the course of evolution of an acute myocardial infarction ultimately manifest by T-wave changes only. Day 1, current of injury in leads I, II, aV$_l$, V$_4$, V$_5$, and V$_6$. Day 2, row 2, ECG is normal. Day 2, row 3, T waves are inverted in leads I, aV$_l$, V$_5$, and V$_6$. Inversion of the T wave is the only evidence of infarction.

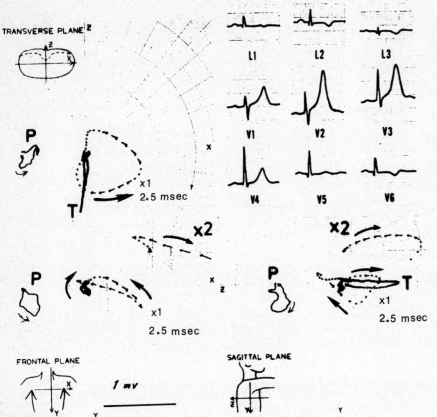

FIGURE 7–34 The ECG illustrates an inferior and posterior infarction. In the transverse plane, the VCG displays anterior displacement of the QRS loop with the anteriorly displaced area about 70 per cent of the entire loop owing to the posterior infarction. The large but narrow T loop is directed anteriorly and to the right and is inscribed counterclockwise at a uniform rate. In the frontal plane, the initial QRS force is directed superiorly and is inscribed clockwise with an inscription of 20 msec located superiorly. The initial leftward QRS magnitude, along the 0 to 180° axis, is 0.25 mV. In the sagittal plane, the initial QRS force is directed superiorly and anteriorly and is inscribed clockwise with a portion displaced superiorly. The entire QRS loop is also shifted anteriorly consistent with a posterior infarction. The large but narrow T-wave loop is directed anteriorly and is inscribed clockwise at an almost uniform rate. The initial QRS force in the frontal and sagittal planes, is displayed at two times the standard ($\times$ 2), while the P-wave loop is displayed at four times the standard in each of the three planes. The Q waves in leads II, III, and V_6 and T-wave changes in leads I, II, III, V_5, and V_6 indicate an inferior apical infarction, while the tall R waves in leads V_1, V_2, and V_3 reflect the posterior infarction. The tall T waves in leads V_1, V_2, and V_3 may be due to the inferior or posterior infarction or both.

ST-segment depression may reflect subendocardial ischemia, infarction, or reciprocal changes secondary to infarction at an "opposite" site. It has also been suggested that depression of the ST segment in leads V_1 to V_4 in the presence of an inferior infarction may be due to associated ischemia caused by significant obstruction of the left anterior descending coronary artery.[141] Minor subtle ST-segment depression is a common early finding of acute myocardial infarction and should be viewed with suspicion.[134,142]

Tall, peaked T waves seen in experimental coronary occlusion[116] are occasionally recorded in man and are thought to represent subendocardial ischemia.[122,137] More often, the initial T wave may be isoelectric, negative, or biphasic. This frequently subtle and nonspecific T-wave change is often the earliest recorded sign of infarction and is probably indicative of subepicardial ischemia. In about 20 to 30 per cent of patients with myocardial infarction, a T-wave abnormality is the only sign of acute infarction.

An *abnormal U wave* is a frequent marker of ischemic heart disease. Negative or biphasic U waves have been reported in up to 30 per cent of patients with chronic angina pectoris, either as a persistent finding or as a transient manifestation during an episode of angina. It is most often recorded in leads I, II, and V_4 to V_6. Appearance of a negative U wave during exercise-induced ischemia has been appreciated for some time[31,143,144] and has recently been found to be highly specific for disease of the left anterior descending coronary artery.[145,146] A negative U wave is seen in 10 to 60 per cent of patients with anterior infarction

and in up to 30 per cent of patients with inferior infarction.[31] Appearance of a negative U wave may precede other ECG changes of infarction by several hours (Fig. 7–35).[147]

An abnormal QRS complex, ST segment, and T wave may normalize transiently in the course of evolution of acute myocardial infarction (Fig. 7–33). Such normalization, termed the "intermediate phase," may be due to reversible ischemia or injury or conduction defects.[148,149] Frequently, however, it represents a phase during progressive evolution of acute, irreversible myocardial infarction. Normalization of the ECG may be misleading and may suggest regression of the acute process or absence of myocardial infarction. Normalization and subsequent reappearance of ST-segment displacement alone in the presence of other unequivocal ECG signs of infarction may be a manifestation of "reelevation"—a frequent finding in acute infarction.[150]

A premature ventricular contraction with a qR or QR morphology even in the absence of ECG findings of infarction suggests the presence of myocardial infarction.[151] This finding may prove particularly useful when the myocardial infarction is masked, for example, by LBBB or WPW.

OLD INFARCTION (THE Q WAVE). ECG diagnosis of an old infarction is often difficult and frequently impossible without the availability of tracings documenting the acute episode. A definitive diagnosis of old infarction depends on the presence of a pathological Q wave. Only rarely can it be based on T-wave changes alone. While a Q wave may be absent in transmural infarction[152] and present in nontransmural infarction,[130,131,153] in essence, the sensitivity and specificity of the ECG for diagnosis of an old myocardial infarction still depend on the Q wave. The specificity of the Q wave is relatively high; its sensitivity is quite low. Within 6 to 12 months after an acute myocardial infarction, about 30 per cent of the tracings, although abnormal, are no longer diagnostic of infarction.[154] Similarly, by the end of 10 years, or sooner, some 6 to 10 per cent of the cardiograms revert to normal.[155]

In a series of 1184 tracings correlating myocardial infarction with postmortem findings, the specificity and sensitivity of the Q wave were 89 and 61 per cent, respectively, and varied with location of the infarction. Anteriorly located Q waves (leads V_1 to V_4) and inferiorly located Q waves (leads II, III, and aV_f) were falsely positive in 46 per cent, while only 4 per cent of Q waves greater than 0.03 sec present in the lateral leads (V_5 and V_6) or in a combination of anterior and inferior leads with another lead proved to be falsely positive. The sensitivity of the Q wave was lowest for infarction located in the lateral basal portion of the left ventricle.[156] This anatomical area is usually reflected in leads I and aV_l.

In another study, a Q wave of 0.04 sec or more in lead aV_f indicated the presence of coronary artery disease and asynergy of the inferior wall in 94 and 76 per cent of cases, respectively.[157]

MYOCARDIAL INFARCTION AND CONDUCTION DELAYS. Conduction defects may not interfere

with, may mask, or may falsely suggest the diagnosis of myocardial infarction. In RBBB, the initial order of activation is normal and thus the pattern of infarction is unaltered (Figs. 7–20 to 7–22). In LBBB the sequence of early activation is altered, with the initial septal vector directed from right to left. As a result the earliest left ventricular intracavitary potential is positive. In keeping with the "window" concept of infarction, a Q wave cannot be registered except when there is extensive septal infarction. Restated in terms of the dipole or vector concept, since the free wall infarct is inscribed during the latter part of the QRS complex after the septal activation is complete, the direction of initial activation expressed as a dipole or vector is unaltered by the infarction, and the infarct is masked (Figs. 7–18, 7–19, and 7–22).

Numerous studies have been designed in an attempt to define diagnostic criteria for myocardial infarction in the presence of LBBB. None of the criteria has proved to be of significant help, and these criteria rarely correlate with autopsy findings.[158,159] In a study of 52 patients with LBBB and autopsy findings of myocardial infarction, the following ECG findings were thought to correlate with myocardial infarction: (1) a Q wave 0.04 sec or greater in leads I, aV_l, V_5, or V_6; (2) rapid serial ST-segment and T-wave changes; (3) acute ST-segment elevation disproportionate to the area of the QRS complex; and (4) a Q wave of any size in lead V_6. Others suggest that a deep S wave in leads

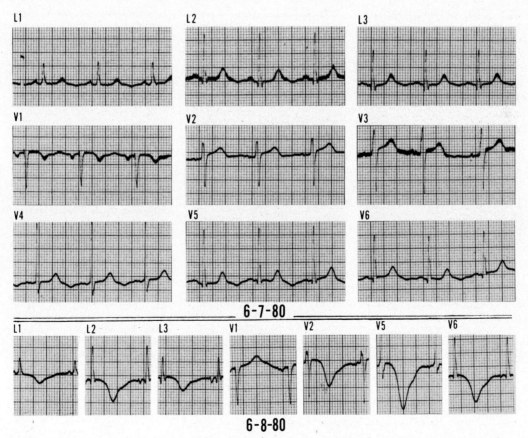

FIGURE 7–35 Negative U wave as the only marker of an acute ischemic episode. On 6/7/80 a negative U wave was recorded in leads I, II, III, and V_4 to V_6 and an upright, reciprocal U wave was present in lead V_1. On 6/8/80 a prolonged Q-T interval and deeply inverted T waves are present in all the leads—evolutionary changes consistent with an acute myocardial infarction. At necropsy the infarction proved to be subendocardial.

V_5 and V_6, a qRs complex with a slurred S wave in leads V_5 and V_6, loss of the R wave in the precordial leads, or a Q wave in leads II, III, and aV_f is consistent with myocardial infarction complicating LBBB. However, in another study of patients with LBBB, the significance of Q waves, broad R waves, notched mid and left precordial S waves, rsR' complexes, ST-segment elevation, and T-wave changes was addressed and found to lack significant correlation with myocardial infarction.[159] A somewhat better correlation was noted between an ECG suggestive of acute inferior myocardial infarction and postmortem findings.

Studies of patients with intermittent LBBB and myocardial infarction provide additional evidence that LBBB masks myocardial infarction (Fig. 7–19).[160] It should be noted, however, that occasionally when acute infarction is evident during normal intraventricular conduction, acute changes are also recognizable in the presence of LBBB. Primary T waves in the presence of LBBB may be indicative of an associated myocardial disorder, including ischemia (see T-Wave Abnormalities, p. 222). It is reasonable to conclude, however, that in face of fixed LBBB, a diagnosis of myocardial infarction is difficult and frequently impossible.[161]

Block of divisions of the LBB may simulate[93] or obscure myocardial infarction.[91,162,163] In addition, in WPW as in LBBB, the initial vector may be directed from right to left, precluding the appearance of a Q wave (Fig. 7–28). The ECG pattern of infarction masked by WPW is recognizable during normalization of intraventricular conduction[164,165] and may also be suggested when conduction occurs across the bypass tract by changes in ST segments and T waves.[165]

LOCALIZATION OF INFARCTION

ECG localization of myocardial infarction other than differentiation of anterior from inferior and posterior is at best an approximation of its true anatomical location.[166,167] Accuracy is affected, for example, by the distance of the electrode from the heart, a common variable. The area subtending a precordial electrode varies with the anteroposterior (AP) diameter of the chest, which is greater in individuals with an increased diameter. Consequently, the same size infarct would be reflected in more leads than in individuals with a normal AP diameter.

Acknowledging the limitations of localization and using the Q wave as a marker of infarction, one can identify an infarct as *septal* when a Q wave is present in leads V_1 and V_2; *anterior* when it is present in leads V_3 and V_4 (Fig. 7–20); *anteroseptal* if present in V_1 to V_4 (Fig. 7–28); *lateral* when present in leads I, aV_l, V_5, and V_6; *anterolateral* when present in leads I, aV_l, and V_3 to V_6; *extensive anterior* when present in leads I, aV_l, and V_1 to V_6 (Fig. 7–32); *high lateral* when present in leads I and aV_l; *inferior* when present in leads II, III, and aV_f (Figs. 7–5, 7–18, 7–19, 7–32, and 7–34); *anteroinferior, transseptal,* or *apical* when present in leads II, III, and aV_f and in one or more of leads V_1 to V_4 (Fig. 7–36). A *posterior* infarct is recognized by a prominent R wave in V_1 or V_2 and a *posterolateral* infarct by a Q wave in leads I and aV_l and a prominent R wave in lead V_1 or V_2 (Fig. 7–34). A *right ventricular infarction* can be suspected when an elevated right ventricular ST segment, especially in lead V_{4r}, complicates a transmural inferior left ventricular septal infarction.[168,169]

Subendocardial infarction is suggested by a depressed ST

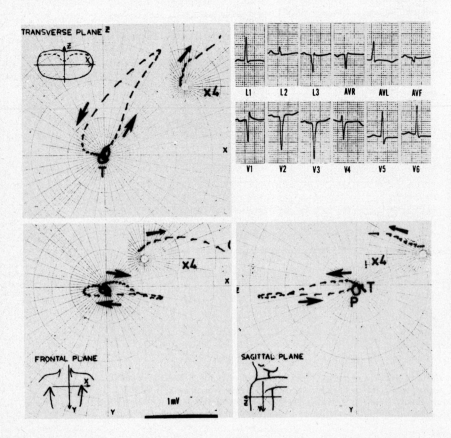

FIGURE 7–36 The ECG illustrates an anteroseptal and inferior myocardial infarction. On VCG, the transverse plane displays an initial QRS force directed to the left and posteriorly, with the entire QRS loop displaced posteriorly. The small oval T loop is situated anteriorly and to the right. In the frontal plane, the initial QRS force is directed to the right and superiorly and is inscribed clockwise. The duration of the superiorly displaced initial force is 22.5 msec and the amplitude of the superiorly displaced and leftward directed force along the 0 to 180° axis is 0.3 mV. In the sagittal plane, the initial QRS force is directed posteriorly and superiorly, with posterior displacement of the QRS loop. The small T-wave loop is located anteriorly. The initial QRS force is displayed four times the standard ($\times$ 4).

segment, a normal T wave, and a QRS complex with an occasionally decreased R-wave amplitude. The infarct usually involves the anterior wall, and changes are reflected in leads I, II, aV_1, and V_2 to V_6. Less frequently, subendocardial infarction involves the inferior wall. Isolated, symmetrically inverted precordial T waves, 5 mm or greater in amplitude, with the T waves deeper on the right side than on the left, are often associated with subendocardial infarction (Fig. 7–35).[170] Differentiation between a subendocardial and transmural infarction based on the presence or absence of a Q wave is not always reliable.[130,131] Autopsy studies indicate that while subendocardial lesions may be accompanied by a Q wave, the Q wave may be absent in transmural infarction. It has been suggested that as many as 50 per cent of subendocardial myocardial infarctions manifest Q waves, making definitive differentiation of subendocardial and transmural infarction based on the Q wave highly tenuous.[142,171–174] Such an estimate requires confirmation.

Infarction isolated to the posterior left ventricular wall is rarely detected. This area, the last to be depolarized, is inscribed during the terminal 0.04 to 0.06 sec of the QRS complex. Theoretically, therefore, it cannot be expressed as an initial positive wave in leads V_1 and V_2. In keeping with the dipole concept, however, the S wave may become smaller—a sign that lacks any degree of specificity. In a small number of patients, posterior myocardial infarction may be suspected when there is ST-segment depression in lead V_1 or V_2 (or both), an R wave in lead V_1 of 0.04 sec, and an R/S ratio greater than 1.[175,176] The exact mechanism of the change in the initial QRS forces in leads V_1 and V_2 is not clear.[177] Some have suggested that posterior myocardial infarction is not manifest on ECG and that the findings in lead V_1 or V_2 or both reflect an associated lateral

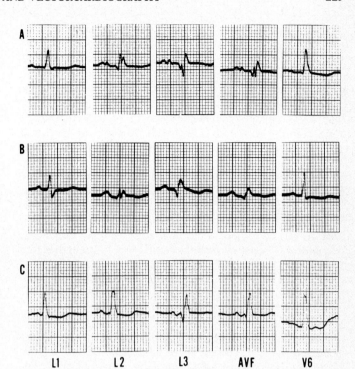

L1 L2 L3 AVF V6

FIGURE 7–37 Inferior myocardial infarction with periinfarction block. These ECGs recorded from three different patients (A, B, and C) all illustrate inferior myocardial infarction with intraventricular conduction delay. S waves in leads I and V_6 and the positive terminal portion of the QRS complex in leads II, III, and aV_f indicate late unopposed activation of the inferior wall. Although in these tracings, particularly A and B, the inferior infarction is easily recognizable, periinfarction block is helpful in detecting inferior infarction when Q- and T-wave changes are not "diagnostic." For example, in C, diagnosis of inferior infarction is strengthened by the periinfarction block. (For VCG showing periinfarction, see Figure 7–38.)

FIGURE 7–38 Inferior myocardial infarction and periinfarction block. Q waves in leads II, III, and aV_f coupled with T-wave changes are indicative of inferior myocardial infarction. QRS duration is 0.10 sec. S waves in leads I and V_6 suggest inferior periinfarction block (see Figure 7–37).

In the VCG, superior displacement of the initial forces with clockwise rotation indicates an inferior myocardial infarction. In the sagittal plane, the superior displacement and clockwise rotation of the increased initial forces are consistent with inferior myocardial infarction. In the frontal plane terminal delay of the forces located inferiorly and to the right of the E point is indicated by close spacing of the dots and identifies periinfarction block. Total duration of the QRS is 10 msec. Slowing of conduction is also recorded in the transverse and sagittal planes.

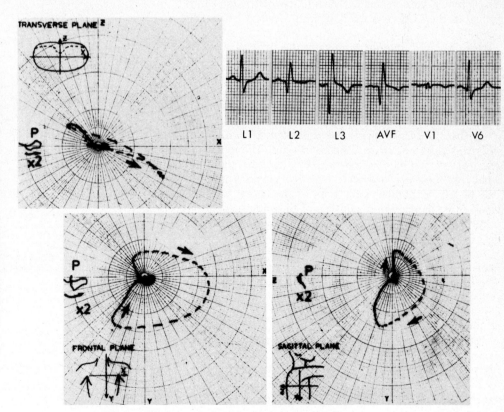

TRANSVERSE PLANE

LI L2 L3 AVF V1 V6

FRONTAL PLANE   SAGITTAL PLANE

infarction. In patients with an inferior or lateral myocardial infarction, an R wave of increased amplitude, 0.04 sec in duration in leads V_1 and V_2, suggests concomitant posterior wall involvement (Fig. 7–34).

Periinfarction block, as originally defined, is a specific conduction abnormality due to myocardial infarction.[178] The ECG changes include a Q wave of 0.04 sec and a QRS complex in the limb leads of 0.10 sec, with a slurred prolonged terminal component facing the site of infarction. Periinfarction block is not synonymous with left anterior divisional block. In our experience periinfarction block may be of help in the diagnosis of old inferior infarction when the characteristic changes are no longer evident. Presence of terminal, somewhat delayed activation facing lead II, III, or aV_f and a terminal negative wave in leads I, V_5, and V_6—signs of periinfarction block—strengthen the diagnosis of myocardial infarction (Figs. 7–37 and 7–38).

THE VCG IN MYOCARDIAL INFARCTION

The appearance of the loop in myocardial infarction depends on the site and size of the infarction. Deviation from normal reflects loss of forces normally generated by the infarcted area and resultant dominance of the noninfarcted myocardium. Anterior myocardial infarction is best visualized in the transverse plane, while an inferior infarction is best displayed in the frontal or sagittal plane.

Anteroseptal myocardial infarction[179] is recognized in the transverse plane by loss of the first 10- to 20-msec forces, with the initial position of the loop oriented posteriorly and to the left. The entire loop is displaced posteriorly with loss of the anterior convexity. In the vast majority of cases, the loop is inscribed in a counterclockwise direction. The initial posterior and left orientation of the loop is reflected in the ECG as a QS complex in leads V_1 to V_4 (Fig. 7–36).

In a *localized anterior infarction*, the transverse loop is similar in appearance to that present in anteroseptal myocardial infarction except for a normally inscribed initial force in a left and anterior direction. This initial inscription is displayed in the ECG as an R wave in lead V_1 and at times in V_2 (Fig. 7–20).

In the transverse plane, an *anterolateral infarction* is inscribed clockwise or as a figure-of-eight. The initial normal part of the loop is followed by posterior and somewhat rightward displacement, reflecting the more extensive loss of left ventricular wall. Loss of the lateral wall may result in an increase in magnitude of the initial left-to-right portion of the loop, reflected in the ECG as a tall R wave inscribed in the right precordial leads.

In an *extensive anterior infarction*, the transverse loop reflects loss of both the septal and free left ventricular walls. The initial normal anteriorly inscribed portion of the loop is lost, and the loop is shifted posteriorly and inscribed clockwise. The ECG shows a loss of R wave, at times, in all precordial leads.

Inferior myocardial infarction is best displayed in the frontal and sagittal planes (Figs. 7–34 and 7–36).[180] In the frontal plane, the loop is most often inscribed in a clockwise direction. The initial portion of the loop is directed superiorly, the superior displacement exceeding 25 to 30

msec. The loop crosses the X axis at 0.30 msec to the left of the point of origin.[180] It has been suggested that when the above diagnostic findings are absent, a shift to the left of the QRS loop combined with clockwise rotation is strongly indicative of an inferior infarction.[181] Occasionally, when the inferior septum is spared, the initial loop may have a normal orientation, that is, to the right and inferiorly. This is followed by clockwise inscription and superior displacement of the remainder of the loop. In such instances the ECG will record a small initial R wave in leads II, III, and aV_f.

In a *posterior myocardial infarction*,[177,182] the initial forces are normal in the transverse plane, but more than half the loop is ultimately displaced anteriorly. In the majority of cases, inscription of the loop is counterclockwise. The anterior displacement of the loop is reflected in the ECG by a prominent R wave in lead V_1 or V_2 that may exceed 0.04 sec in duration (Fig. 7–34).

A summary of VCG criteria for myocardial infarction is presented in Table 7–5.

NONINFARCTION Q WAVES

While the vast majority of abnormal Q waves are due to myocardial infarction, a significant number have other causes, including positional changes, congenital electrophysiological and anatomical abnormalities of the septum, loss of electrical activity without cellular death,[149] replacement of the myocardium by a variety of pathological processes, alteration of the initial vector due to conduction defects or hypertrophy, and other less commonly observed disorders.

Noninfarction Q waves may be transient or permanent.

TABLE 7–5 SUMMARY OF VECTORCARDIOGRAPHIC CRITERIA FOR DIAGNOSIS OF MYOCARDIAL INFARCTION (MI)

Anteroseptal MI (1 and 2)*
  1. Initial anterior QRS forces absent
  2. 0.02-sec QRS vector directed posteriorly
Localized Anterior MI (1,2, and 3)
  1. Initial anterior septal forces present
  2. 0.02-sec QRS vector directed posteriorly
  3. Voltage criteria for left ventricular hypertrophy absent
Anterolateral MI (1,2, and 3)
  1. Initial anterior septal forces normal
  2. Initial rightward QRS forces > 0.022 sec
  3. Efferent limb of transverse plane QRS loop inscribed clockwise
  4. Initial rightward QRS forces > 0.16 mV
  5. Maximum frontal plane QRS vector > 40°, QRS loop inscribed counterclockwise
Extensive Anterior MI (1 and 2)
  1. Initial anterior QRS forces absent
  2. Transverse plane QRS loop inscribed clockwise
Inferior MI (1 or more)
  1. Initial superior QRS forces > 0.025 sec
  2. Initial superior QRS forces ≥ 0.020 sec, maximum left superior force ≥ 0.25 mV
  3. Maximum frontal plane QRS vector < 10°, efferent limb of frontal QRS loop inscribed clockwise
  4. Bites in afferent limb of frontal QRS loop
Inferolateral MI (1 and 2)
  1. Initial rightward QRS forces > 0.022 sec
  2. Initial superior QRS forces > 0.025 sec

*Numbers in parentheses after each type of infarction indicate the minimum requirements for the diagnosis.

From Chou, T.-C., et al.: Clinical Vectorcardiography. 2nd ed. New York, Grune and Stratton, 1974, p. 229.

Transient Q waves have been produced experimentally in animals[153] and observed in patients during anginal attacks.[183,184] Such Q waves have been explained by a transient loss of electrophysiological function, the phenomenon referred to by some as "myocardial concussion."[185] Q waves have been recorded with severe metabolic disturbances accompanying shock or pancreatitis.[186,187] Similarly, transient Q waves have been noted during cardiac surgery and ascribed variously to transient ischemia and hypoxia, spasm, localized metabolic and electrolyte disturbances, and possible hypothermia (Fig. 7–24).[188] Rarely a transient Q wave may result from tachycardia.[189] The author has recorded transient Q waves and ST-segment and T-wave changes due to air embolism of the coronary artery complicating induction of a therapeutic pneumothorax.

The largest group of noninfarction Q waves is that comprising a variety of pathological processes that affect the myocardium,[190] including myocarditis, cardiac amyloidosis, neuromuscular disorders such as progressive muscular dystrophy, myotonia atrophica, Friedreich's ataxia,[191] scleroderma, postpartum myopathy, myocardial replacement by tumor, sarcoidosis, idiopathic cardiomyopathy, and anomalous coronary artery.

Noninfarction Q waves commonly accompany hypertrophic cardiomyopathy[192] and may simulate anterior or inferior myocardial infarction (Fig. 7–39). The exact mechanism of the Q wave in this condition is unclear. Increased septal mass or abnormal depolarization because of anomalous architecture of the septal myocardium, or both, has been proposed as the cause.[193] A recent study suggests that the electrophysiological characteristics of septal muscle may differ from normal. For example, the refractory period of the myocardium responsible for the Q wave exceeds the refractory period of the junctional tissue. This relationship may be altered by tachycardia with disappearance of the Q wave.[194]

A Q wave can be due to COLD with or without cor pulmonale, pulmonary embolism, and pneumothorax. In COLD, findings in the precordial leads frequently simulate anterior myocardial infarction.[195] The mechanism responsible for the QS complex is clockwise rotation and downward displacement of the diaphragm and of the heart. As a result, the electrodes are located superior to the initial vector; when this vector is directed inferiorly, a QS pattern results. By placing the electrode one interspace lower, it is often possible to record an R wave and thus provide strong evidence against myocardial infarction. Occasionally in COLD the Q wave may simulate an inferior myocardial infarction.[196] The positional origin of the anterior or inferior Q waves may be suspected when the Q wave is accompanied by other ECG findings of COLD. However, since both COLD and myocardial infarction frequently coexist, differential diagnosis may at times be difficult or impossible.

Abnormal Q waves, especially in lead III and rarely in lead aV$_F$, with an S wave in lead I, can be recorded in acute cor pulmonale due to *pulmonary embolism* (see Fig. 7–16, p. 213). Clockwise rotation with superior orientation of the initial vector is most likely reponsible for the Q wave in lead III. A Q wave in lead II is rarely recorded. Occasionally acute pulmonary embolus may simulate anterior myocardial infarction

Spontaneous pneumothorax, particularly on the left, may result in a pattern simulating anterior myocardial infarction with occasional absence of the R wave in all the precordial leads.[198]

In LBBB the initial forces are directed from right to left and either superiorly or inferiorly. When the inferiorly directed forces dominate, a QS complex may be recorded in the precordial leads, simulating an anterior myocardial infarction.[199,200] If the initial vector is oriented to the left and superiorly, a QS complex may be registered in the inferior leads, suggesting inferior myocardial infarction.[200]

With left anterior divisional block, the transitional zone is shifted to the left, and an initial Q wave may appear in the right precordial leads. Loss of the forces normally contributed by the left anterior division results in a vector directed inferiorly, posteriorly, and to the right. Con-

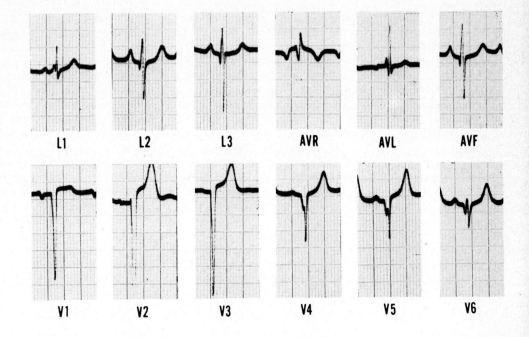

FIGURE 7–39   Noninfarction Q waves due to hypertrophic cardiomyopathy. This tracing recorded in a 16-year-old girl shows left axis deviation and Q waves in leads V$_3$ to V$_6$.

L1   L2   L3   AVR   AVL   AVF

V1   V2   V3   V4   V5   V6

sequently, right precordial leads may register a qrS complex suggestive of an anteroseptal infarction. By placing the electrodes one interspace lower, an rS complex can be recorded attesting to the positional nature of the Q wave.[91,93]

Noninfarction Q waves are frequent in WPW (p. 220). WPW type B, with the initial forces directed from right to left, registers a QS complex in the right precordial leads and may be mistaken for anteroseptal or anterior myocardial infarction. Rarely, preexcitation of the left lateral wall, with the vector oriented anteriorly and to the right, simulates lateral infarction.[201] Most often, however, WPW simulates inferior infarction (Fig. 7–27). The Q waves recorded in leads II, III, and aV_f are due to superior orientation of the initial vector and may be seen with either type A or type B WPW.[202]

In LVH, failure to record an R wave in leads V_1 to V_4 may suggest an anteroseptal myocardial infarction.[195] Similarly, reciprocal elevation of the ST segments in these leads may contribute to an erroneous diagnosis of myocardial infarction. The exact mechanism of the initial negative deflection of the QRS is not clear, but it may be related to posterior rotation or inferior orientation of the initial vector.[195,199]

ST-SEGMENT AND T-WAVE CHANGES

ST-SEGMENT ELEVATION. Most of the causes of ST-segment elevation have been discussed in connection with a specific mechanism or etiology. In addition to the three most common organic causes—namely, acute myocardial infarction, pericarditis, and Prinzmetal's angina—ST-segment elevation is occasionally observed in acute cor pulmonale,[203] hypothermia(?), hyperkalemia, cerebrovascular accidents, LVH, LBBB, hypertrophic cardiomyopathy, and invasion of the heart by neoplastic tissue.[204] Elevation of the ST segment may also be an artifact caused by excessive inertia of the stylus of the electrocardiograph. In the normal heart the most common cause of ST-segment elevation is so-called *early repolarization*, a normal variant (see Fig. 7–9E, p. 204).

T-WAVE ABNORMALITIES. A *primary T-wave change* indicates a regional alteration in the duration of the depolarized state. Some common clinical conditions associated with primary T-wave changes include myocardial ischemia, electrolyte abnormalities, effects of drugs, and a variety of primary myocardial and extracardiac disorders such as myocarditis and subarachnoid hemorrhage, respectively.

Giant negative or, at times, upright T waves, usually associated with a prolonged Q-T interval have been described with subarachoid hemorrhage, complete heart block with marked bradycardia (Fig. 7–21), in myocardial ischemia (Fig. 7–35), and following cardiac resuscitation.

Secondary T-wave changes result from alterations of the timing or sequencing of depolarization, or both, with an obligatory change of the order of repolarization. For example, in LBBB, left ventricular epicardial activation is delayed because of slow conduction through the ventricular myocardium. As a result, repolarization begins in the subendocardium and an inverted T wave is recorded in the epicardial leads (Fig. 7–22). The change in the area of the QRS complex and T waves is identical but opposite in direction. Occasionally LBBB is associated with an upright T wave in the left ventricular leads, suggesting that in addition to altered activation due to LBBB, regional abnormalities of repolarization contribute to the T-wave morphology.

Intermittent LBBB is an ideal model for evaluating the significance of primary T-wave changes in the presence of LBBB.[161] In a study of 13 patients with primary T-wave changes over the anteroseptal and anterior wall recorded during normal intraventricular conduction, primary T-wave changes were also present after the appearance of LBBB in nine of the 13. On the other hand, two of 14 patients with normal T waves during normal intraventricular conduction exhibited primary ST-segment and T-wave changes with LBBB.[161] Such data suggest that primary T-wave change in the presence of LBBB may be a useful sign of myocardial abnormality. Occasionally, however, normal T waves are recorded during normal intraventricular conduction in patients manifesting primary T waves with LBBB.

Rate-Related T-Wave Changes. Postextrasystolic T-wave change was first described in 1915.[205] Since then, a number of mechanisms have been proposed to explain this observation, including an abnormal pathway of repolarization, prolonged diastolic filling time,[206] and an abrupt change in the cycle length.

Minor T-wave changes may be present following an abrupt cycle change or after an interpolated ventricular premature complex. Each is a physiological phenomenon and in keeping with in vitro studies of normal cardiac tissue. However, more pronounced T-wave alterations suggest a myocardial disorder.[207,208]

T-wave inversion is occasionally noted following supraventricular or ventricular tachycardia. The magnitude of the T-wave inversion varies, and when extreme, it may resemble the T-wave changes seen with cerebrovascular accidents or myocardial ischemia.[209] The exact mechanism of the posttachycardia T wave is obscure.

T Wave Alternans. Isolated T wave alternans, i.e., without a change in either the QRS complex or the P wave, was first noted in the cat papillary muscle.[210] It is relatively rare and its mechanism not clear.[211] Alternans of phases 2 and 3 of the action potential of the T wave has been recorded without any demonstrable change in phase 0, supporting the concept that isolated alternation of repolarization reflected in the T wave is possible. T wave alternans of the type mentioned above is most often present during tachycardia or during a sudden change in cycle length. Isolated T wave alternans, independent of tachycardia or premature systole, is nearly always associated with advanced heart disease or severe electrolyte disturbance (Fig. 7–40)[212] or may follow cardiac resuscitation.

Notched, Bifid T Waves. Notched, bifid T waves are relatively common in the absence of heart disease, especially in the young.[213] They may also be present in congenital organic heart disease, the prolonged Q-T syndrome (Fig. 7–41), central nervous system disorders,[214] and alcoholic cardiomyopathy or following the administration of drugs, especially the phenothiazines.[215] The mechanism of the bifid or notched T wave is unclear. It has been suggested that in some instances it is due to nonuniform repolarization

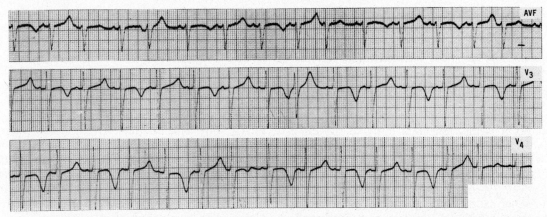

FIGURE 7–40   Isolated alternation of the T wave. The rhythm is sinus with occasional supraventricular premature complexes, probably atrial in origin. The QRS is normal in duration, with alternation of polarity of the T wave.

secondary to differential innervation of the anterior and posterior ventricular walls.[214,216] It has also been proposed that it may reflect regional delay of repolarization secondary to delayed depolarization.

NONSPECIFIC ST-SEGMENT AND T-WAVE CHANGES. Although the ST segment and T wave represent different electrophysiological events and their respective changes may have different clinical connotations, the widespread practice among electrocardiographers is to refer to either one or both as *ST-T changes*. While it is more appropriate to discuss the two separately—and whenever feasible, this will be attempted—it should be recognized that abnormalities of the ST segment and T wave frequently coexist.

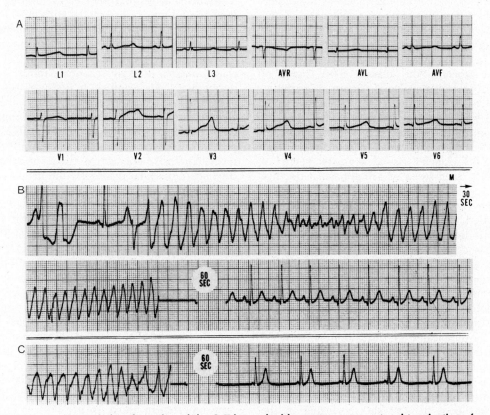

FIGURE 7–41   Congenital prolongation of the Q-T interval with spontaneous onset and termination of ventricular tachycardia and fibrillation. *A,* The rhythm is sinus with a rate of 55 bpm, the Q-T interval measures approximately 0.56 sec, and the T wave is notched. The notched T wave is best seen in leads V₂ to V₄. *B,* The tracing is continuous and illustrates spontaneous onset and termination of a ventricular tachycardia and fibrillation lasting about 90 sec. *C,* Spontaneous termination of an episode of ventricular tachycardia and flutter lasting about 90 msec. Both the Q-T interval and the T-wave morphology normalize after termination of ventricular arrhythmia. In addition to normalization of the Q-T interval and the T wave, the P-R interval is foreshortened. A possible mechanism that could explain the normalization of repolarization and shortening of the P-R interval is an increase in the level of catecholamines in response to the ventricular arrhythmia. The morphology of the T waves in *C* also suggests hyperkalemia.

Nondiagnostic ST-segment and T-wave changes are the most common ECG abnormality and account for about 50 per cent of the abnormal tracings recorded in a general medical hospital.[217] It has been estimated that nondiagnostic T-wave changes comprise 2.4 per cent[217] and 4.5 per cent[218] of all routine cardiograms. An abnormal T wave is extremely common because the wave is highly sensitive to a variety of abnormalities and interventions, and of all the ECG changes it is therefore least likely to suggest a specific diagnosis. This fact has been recognized since 1925, when Wilson first recorded inversion of the T wave following the ingestion of cold water.[219]

Although statistically an abnormal T wave suggests the presence of an abnormal or, more appropriately, an altered state,[220] it is recorded with relative frequency in the absence of any disorder (see Fig. 7–9, p. 204) as a reflection of a physiological event.[221] For these reasons, any T-wave change must be interpreted with extreme caution and must *always* be correlated with all available clinical and laboratory information. Misinterpretation of the significance of a T-wave abnormality is the most common cause of "iatrogenic ECG heart disease." Attempts to identify the etiology of an abnormal ST segment, T wave, or ST-T segment in isolation from clinical and other laboratory findings often fail.

The accepted "classic" ST-T changes, such as those seen with LVH, digitalis administration, and ischemic heart disease, are of relatively low specificity. For example, a negative wave reflecting persistence of a juvenile pattern cannot be differentiated from the symmetrically inverted T wave due to myocardial ischemia. The "classic" ST-T change of LVH may be due to ischemic heart disease or digitalis, while the marked ST-segment depression due to ischemia or subendocardial infarction may be simulated by the administration of digitalis in the presence of moderate or severe disease. When correlated with clinical and other laboratory data, ST-T changes assume a greater degree of diagnostic specificity. In a series of 410 abnormal tracings analyzed without regard to clinical data, 70 per cent could be interpreted only as "nonspecific ST-T change." This number was reduced to 10 per cent when such changes were correlated with available clinical information.[217]

The nonspecific and labile nature of the ST segment and the T wave, especially the latter, should not be unexpected. Repolarization is a much more diverse process than depolarization. Depolarization, i.e., activation, is rapid, with a reasonably uniform potential difference across the boundary of activation and is reflected in the rate of rise of phase 0 and the amplitude of the action potential.[222] Repolarization, displayed as the ST segment and T wave, reflects phases 2 and 3 of the action potential, is considerably longer and is nonuniform, with many simultaneous boundaries and with differing potentials across various boundaries.[223] It has been shown that shortening of the monophasic action potential by as little as 12 to 18 msec will alter the morphology of the T wave, and importantly, the change can be seen with involvement of 10 per cent or less of the myocardial mass. The magnitude of the T-wave changes, unlike that of the QRS complex, is not related to the mass of the myocardium. This condition has been ascribed to cancellation of repolarization voltages and to uneven contributions from the different regions of repolarization to the genesis of the T wave.[224] Such experimental findings explain, at least partially, the nonspecific character of ST-segment and T-wave changes.

Thus, a variety of clinical conditions could alter the ST segment and the T wave.[225] Abnormalities associated with clinically normal hearts were discussed above. Other ST-segment and T-wave changes can be grouped as being due to (1) physiological interventions, (2) pharmacological agents, (3) extracardiac disorders without obvious anatomical abnormality of the heart, (4) myocardial changes due to primary myocardial disease, (5) myocardial disorders secondary to systemic disease, and (6) disorders resulting from coronary artery disease. The last is discussed in connection with myocardial infarction.

Some of the more common *physiological phenomena* responsible for abnormalities of the ST segment and T wave include a change in position and a resultant abnormal ST segment and T wave in leads II, III, and aV_F; effects of cold, hyperventilation, anxiety, food, and especially glucose; and tachycardia and sympathetic and parasympathetic influences. *Pharmacological agents* causing such changes include digitalis, antiarrhythmic drugs, and drugs used in psychophysiological disorders such as phenothiazines, tricyclics, and lithium. In addition to altering the direction of the ST-T segment, drugs may shorten or prolong the Q-T or Q-U interval and may be associated with bifid T waves and often a prominent U wave. *Extracardiac disorders* that alter the ST segment and T wave include, among others, electrolyte abnormalities, cerebrovascular events,[226] shock and hemorrhage, anemia, allergic reactions, infections, endocrine abnormalities (especially hypothyroidism), and acute abdominal disorders. Primary and secondary *diseases of the myocardium* include, among others, congestive cardiomyopathy of unknown etiology, hypertrophic cardiomyopathy, postpartum myocardiopathy, myocarditis, amyloidosis, hemochromatosis, connective tissue abnormalities, sarcoidosis, neuromuscular disorders, and neoplasm.

U-WAVE ABNORMALITY. An abnormal U wave may be increased in amplitude, inverted or prolonged. A negative U wave is documented in about 1 per cent of cardiograms recorded in a general hospital.[227] An exaggerated upright U wave may be due to hypokalemia, a variety of drugs (particularly digitalis), and some of the antiarrhythmic agents (e.g., amiodarone).

The most common causes of a *negative U wave* are hypertension, aortic and mitral valve disease, RVH, and myocardial ischemia (Fig. 7–35). The last was discussed in conjunction with myocardial infarction (p. 226). A negative U wave can occasionally be found in other metabolic or organic diseases. In hypertension, a negative U wave may be the earliest sign of myocardial involvement, appearing long before any change in the T wave, and has been reported in about 16 per cent of ECG's with an upright T wave and 45 per cent with negative T waves. It may revert to normal with control of the hypertension.[31] The majority of patients with aortic regurgitation and about 10 per cent of patients with aortic stenosis manifest a negative U wave. Approximately 5 and 80 per cent of patients with systolic and diastolic overload of the right ventricle, respectively, manifest a negative U wave in leads

II, III, V_1, and V_2.[31] In essence, a negative U wave, even as an isolated finding in an otherwise normal ECG, is strongly indicative of a pathophysiological state.

Q-T INTERVAL ABNORMALITY (see also p. 203). *Shortening of the Q-T interval* may be recorded with hyperkalemia, digitalis, hypercalcemia, and acidosis. *Prolongation of the Q-T interval* may be primary and independent of the QRS, or it may reflect secondary changes of repolarization due to abnormal depolarization, or a combination of the two. Prolongation of the Q-T interval, independent of QRS duration, can be congenital (Fig. 7–41) or acquired.[228,229] Acquired disorders include ischemic heart disease, hypothermia, cardiomyopathy, mitral valve prolapse, complete heart block, a condition following cardiac resuscitation, electrolyte changes, and administration of drugs (p. 243). Q-T interval prolongation is a relatively frequent complication of acquired cerebral lesions, especially subarachnoid hemorrhage, and can also be present during and following neurosurgical procedures.

ELECTRICAL ALTERNANS. This discussion deals only with alternation in amplitude and direction. Alternation of the QRS complex was noted in the experimental animal and man as early as 1908 and 1910, respectively,[230,231] followed by documentation of alternation of the P wave, ST segment, and T wave (Fig. 7–40).

Isolated *alternation of the P wave* is seen frequently in the experimental setting but is rare in man. Most often it accompanies alternation of the QRS complex and occasionally the QRS complex and the T wave. The latter situation is referred to as *total alternans* and suggests pericardial effusion usually due to malignancy and frequently associated with tamponade or impending tamponade.

Although pericardial effusion is the most common cause of alternation of the QRS complex, *QRS alternans* is also seen with myocardial ischemia and myocardial disease due to causes other than ischemia or drugs.[232] Two mechanisms of QRS alternans have been proposed, namely, positional oscillation and aberrancy of intraventricular conduction. The early suggestion that oscillation or alternation of position is the mechanism of alternans of the QRS complex[233] was proved with the advent of echocardiography[234] (see Fig. 5–75, p. 132). The concept of oscillation also explains the fact that P wave alternans is seen predominantly with massive pericardial effusion.

ST segment alternans has been described in dogs after ligation of the coronary artery, in severely ill infants with congenital heart disease, and in patients with Prinzmetal's angina.[232] For a discussion of *T wave alternans*, see page 232. *U wave alternans* is least common. In the few cases described, the difficulty of separating the T wave and U wave as well as differentiation from a bifid T wave makes a definitive diagnosis most difficult.

The mechanism of alternans in severe myocardial disorders but in the absence of pericardial effusion is obscure. It has been ascribed to uneven duration of the excited state or to two alternating foci of impulse formation. However, the fact that alternation of depolarization, activation, and repolarization can be recorded in a single cell suggests that the mechanism is probably related to transmembrane ionic fluxes.[235] Alternans of a human atrial monophasic action potential[236] adds further credence to the primary role of transmembrane ionic events.

THE OSBORNE WAVE. An Osborne wave, seen in hypothermia, is a deflection inscribed between the QRS complex and the beginning of the ST segment (Fig. 7–42).[237] It has been variously suggested that this wave reflects delay of depolarization, a current of injury, or early repolarization.[238] In the left ventricular leads the polarity of the wave is positive and its amplitude is inversely related

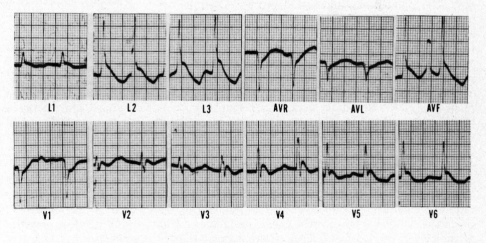

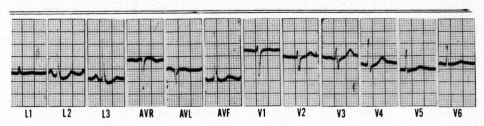

FIGURE 7–42 Osborne wave. *Upper panel*, Recorded during hypothermia, the P-R interval is 0.28 sec; the QRS complex measures 0.10 sec and is followed by a wave (the Osborne wave) that merges with the ST segment; and the T wave is inverted in leads I, II, III, aV$_f$, V$_5$, and V$_6$. It is difficult to separate the Osborne wave from the initial part of the ST segment. *Bottom panel*, Recorded after the temperature returned to normal. The tracing is normal.

to body temperature. The electrophysiological mechanism of the Osborne wave remains unclear.

THE ECG AND ELECTROLYTE ABNORMALITIES

Potassium

HYPERKALEMIA. In experimental hyperkalemia there is a good correlation between plasma K and the surface ECG.[239] The earliest ECG change, at a plasma level of about 5.7 mEq/liter, is a tall, peaked, most often symmetrical T wave with a narrow base and a normal or decreased Q-Tc interval. The QRS complex widens uniformly at a level of 9 to 11 mEq/liter and an occasional acute current of injury resembling myocardial infarction may be present.[240] Reduction in P-wave amplitude, intraatrial conduction delay, and P-R interval prolongation are recorded at a plasma level of about 7.0 mEq/liter. At plasma K levels of about 8.4 mEq/liter or higher, the P wave is no longer recognizable. When the plasma concentration exceeds 12 mEq/liter, either ventricular fibrillation or arrest follows. Sinoatrial node fibers, being more resistant to the depressive action of K than is atrial myocardium, continue to generate impulses that are now delayed in their exit or may fail to propagate because of depressed intraatrial conduction. The result may be Wenckebach (type I) or Mobitz (type II) sinoatrial (SA) block. Junctional escape and junctional rhythm are relatively common in experimental hyperkalemia.[241]

In clinical hyperkalemia, abnormalities of impulse formation and conduction appear at K levels lower than those observed in the experimental animal, and the correlation between plasma K and the ECG is less reliable. A tall, peaked, symmetrical T wave with a narrow base, the so-called "tented" T wave, is the earliest ECG abnormality.[242] The pointed, symmetrical appearance and narrow base of the T wave help to differentiate the effect of hyperkalemia from other causes of tall T waves, often a normal variant. The tented appearance and the narrow base are probably more characteristic of hyperkalemia than is the amplitude of the T wave. T waves suggestive of hyperkalemia are found in about 20 per cent of patients with elevated plasma K levels and are usually best seen in leads II, III, V_2, V_3, and V_4. A decrease in amplitude of the R wave, appearance of a prominent S wave, widening of the QRS complex, depression of the ST segment, and an occasional elevation of the ST segment evolve as plasma K continues to rise and approaches 8 to 9 mEq/liter (Fig. 7–43).[240] A decrease in amplitude and prolongation of the P wave and lengthening of the P-R interval followed by disappearance of the P wave often makes recognition of arrhythmias in hyperkalemia difficult, if not impossible.[243]

With hyperkalemia, depression of intraventricular conduction is characteristically diffuse and fairly uniform and results in prolongation of both the initial and terminal parts of the QRS complex. The resulting pattern may resemble RBBB, LBBB, left anterior or posterior divisional block, or a combination of the four. When the ECG resembles RBBB, the initial phase of the QRS complex is prolonged, in contrast to the conventional RBBB, in which only the terminal portion of the QRS complex is delayed.

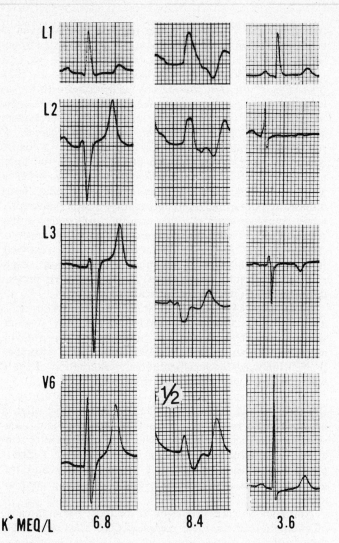

FIGURE 7–43 ECG changes of hyperkalemia. After treatment with potassium (K+ level = 3.6 mEq/liter), the P-R interval, QRS, and T waves are normal. At a K+ level of 6.8 mEq/liter the P-R interval and QRS complex are prolonged, with shift of the QRS axis to the left. The T waves are symmetrical, narrow based, and tall—the so-called tented T wave. At a K+ level of 8.4 mEq/liter, there is further prolongation of the P-R interval, the P wave is difficult to identify, the QRS complex is prolonged to 0.20 sec, and the QRS axis is normal. Prolongation of both initial and terminal portions of the QRS complex, characteristic of K+-induced intraventricular conduction, is best illustrated in lead V6. (From Fisch, C.: Electrolytes and the heart. *In* Hurst, J. W. (ed.): The Heart. New York, McGraw-Hill Book Co., 1982, p. 1599.)

Similarly, when the ECG simulates LBBB, an S wave indicates slowing of the terminal portion of the QRS (Fig. 7–43). In conventional LBBB, on the other hand, prolongation involves only the initial component of the QRS complex.

In man, as in animals, SA block (p. 691), either Wenckebach (type I) or Mobitz (type II), passive or accelerated junctional or ventricular escape rhythms may be present. Potassium may normalize physiologically or functionally inverted T waves, but as a rule it has no effect on T-wave inversion due to organic disorders or drugs.[244]

HYPOKALEMIA. Patients treated for diabetic coma have been found to have a prolonged Q-T interval, abnormal T waves, occasionally a depressed ST segment—

changes proved to be due to hypokalemia.[245] There is a reasonable correlation between ECG changes and K concentrations below 2.3 or 3.0 mEq/liter.[246–248] The hypokalemia is characterized by an exaggerated U wave without a significant change in Q-T duration (Fig. 7–44). Depression of the ST segment and its gradual fusion with the U wave, less commonly inversion of the T wave, and an increase in amplitude of the QRS complex may also be present. Prominent U waves with ST-segment and T-wave changes are not specific for hypokalemia, however. Such abnormalities can be the result of digitalis and other drugs, ventricular hypertrophy, and bradycardia.

CALCIUM

The effects of calcium on the ECG were recognized in 1922.[249] In general, the ECG changes due to alteration in Ca levels correlate with the effect of Ca ion on the transmembrane action potential. Changes in duration of phase 2 parallel the altered duration of the ST segment and the Q-T interval.

Hypocalcemia prolongs phase 2, reflected by prolongation of the ST segment and Q-T interval (Fig. 7–45). The Q-aT (Q to the apex of the T wave) and Q-T intervals are prolonged, but the Q-Tc interval rarely exceeds 140 per cent of the normal. If longer, the U wave is likely to be included in the measurement. Hypocalcemia does not affect phase 3 of the action potential or the T wave.[248] Hypocalcemia with hyperkalemia, most often seen in patients with chronic renal disease, results in a prolonged ST segment and a "tented" T wave (Fig. 7–45). Hypocalcemia and hypokalemia exhibit a prolonged ST segment and a prominent terminal wave that includes both T and U waves.[246]

Hypercalcemia shortens phase 2 of the action potential and the ST segment. Occasionally the ST segment is depressed and the Q-T interval shortened (Fig. 7–45).

The correlation between the Q-T interval and serum Ca concentration is unpredictable, largely because the Q-T duration is affected by factors other than calcium levels, such as age, sex, heart rate, myocardial disease, drugs, and other electrolytes. It has been suggested that when one eliminates factors known to alter the Q-T interval, a reasonably good correlation is found between the ECG and calcium levels. This assumption is supported by the fact that Ca levels in pure hypocalcemia induced by EDTA show a reasonably good correlation with the Q-T interval. Of the three intervals—Q-T, Q-oT (Q to the onset of the T wave), and Q-aT—the Q-aT interval can be measured with greatest accuracy and correlates best with the Ca level.[250]

MAGNESIUM

Administration of magnesium may result in a statistically significant shortening of the Q-T interval. As a rule, however, abnormalities of the ST segment due to hypermagnesemia cannot be identified on the ECG because the changes are dominated by calcium.[251] Hypomagnesemia cannot be recognized on the ECG.

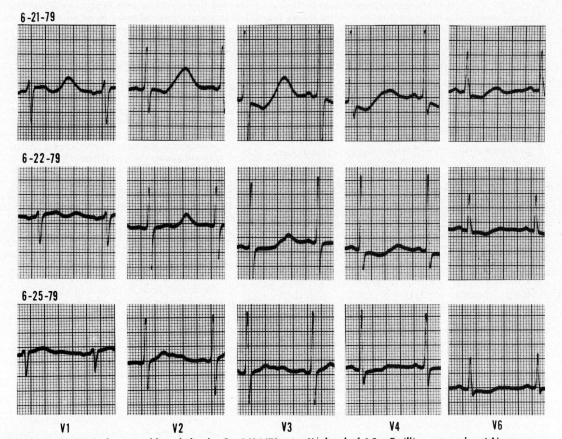

FIGURE 7–44 ECG changes of hypokalemia. On 9/21/79, at a K+ level of 1.3 mEq/liter, a prominent U wave with a prolonged Q-U interval is present. On 6/22/79, after potassium replacement, the U wave is less prominent, and on 6/25/79, at a K+ of 3.9 mEq/liter the Q-T interval and the U wave are normal. (From Fisch, C.: Electrolytes and the heart. *In* Hurst, J. W. (ed.): The Heart. New York, McGraw-Hill Book Co., 1982, p. 1599.)

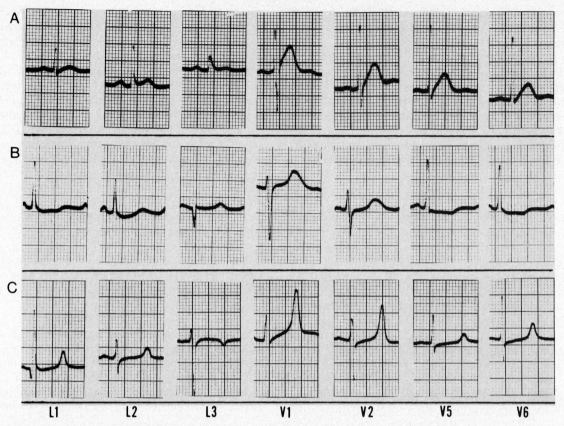

FIGURE 7–45   ECG changes of hypercalcemia, hypocalcemia, and hypocalcemia with hyperkalemia. *A*, Tracing recorded at a Ca^{++} level of 17.0 mg/dl shows short ST segment of hypercalcemia. *B*, At a Ca^{++} level of 5.9 mg/dl the Q-T interval is prolonged characteristic of hypocalcemia. *C*, Tracing recorded at a K$^+$ level of 6.2 mEq/liter, Ca^{++} of 5.3 mg/dl, and phosphorus of 12.2 mg/dl. The prolonged Q-T interval and the tented T wave reflect hypocalcemia and hyperkalemia seen in chronic renal disease. (Fisch, C.: Electrolytes and the heart. *In* Hurst, J. W. (ed.): The Heart. New York, McGraw-Hill Book Co., 1982, p. 1599.)

EFFECTS OF DRUGS ON THE ECG

DIGITALIS (See also p. 523)

The cardiac glycosides differ little with regard to their effect on the ECG. Alterations of the ST segment and T wave are the earliest recognizable changes due to digitalis. The T-wave amplitude is lowered, and the ST segment is depressed and shortened, with occasional appearance of a prominent U wave.[252] While the "characteristic" digitalis-induced ST segment is described as sagging, it is often difficult if not impossible to differentiate it from ST-segment depression of other causes. When the ST segment is also shortened, digitalis is the likely cause of the depression. ST-segment displacement due to digitalis may be greatly exaggerated by myocardial disease, tachycardia, and high-amplitude QRS complexes. Rarely, digitalis causes symmetrical inversion of the T wave similar to that in pericarditis and ischemia, but there is usually associated shortening of the Q-T interval. A peaked, "tented" T wave, probably due to concomitant hyperkalemia, can also be present.

Digitalis has no significant effect on depolarization of the atrium or ventricle. Consequently, prolongation of intraatrial and intraventricular conduction is rare.[253]

Classification of Digitalis-Induced Arrhythmias. Digitalis has been known to induce nearly every known arrhythmia, and a comprehensive discussion of the subject is beyond the scope of this review.[254–256] The following general classification, based on the electrophysiological effects of the cardiac glycoside and less so on the ECG morphology or site of origin of the arrhythmia, encompasses most of the digitalis-induced arrhythmias. The classification is enlarged upon in Table 7–6 and is discussed in terms of clinical relevance below.

1. Ectopic rhythms due to enhanced automaticity or reentry or both

and, perhaps, to delayed diastolic afterdepolarizations (p. 620) (Fig. 7–46): atrial tachycardia with block (see Fig. 21–13, p. 701), atrial fibrillation and flutter, nonparoxysmal junctional tachycardia, (Fig. 21–19, p. 705), ventricular premature contractions, ventricular tachycardia (Fig. 7–46), ventricular flutter and fibrillation, multiple ectopic rhythms, bidirectional ventricular tachycardia (Fig. 7–47), or accelerated escape.

2. Depression of pacemaker: Sinoatrial node arrest (p. 691).

3. Depression of conduction: SA block, AV block, exit block, or reciprocation.

4. AV dissociation: Suppression of the dominant pacemaker with passive escape of the lower junctional focus or inappropriate acceleration of a subsidiary pacemaker, or, rarely, dissociation within the AV junction (double junctional tachycardia).

Therapeutic and Toxic Effects. Appearance of ectopic rhythms in the course of digitalis administration is nearly always a sign of toxicity. On the other hand, depression of AV conduction may at times be a desirable therapeutic endpoint. Acknowledging that some degree of overlap is unavoidable and that the clinical significance of an arrhythmia may differ depending on the setting, we can divide the effects of digitalis on the ECG into three general groups—therapeutic, excessive and/or toxic, and unequivocally toxic.

Clinically acceptable effects of digitalis include some prolongation of the P-R interval; slowing of the ventricular response in atrial flutter and fibrillation: and in atrial fibrillation, the appearance of isolated AV junctional escape impulses. Conversion of atrial arrhythmias to sinus rhythm, either directly or indirectly, is another desirable effect of the drug.

Excessive or toxic effects, or both, are heralded by the appearance of atrial tachycardia with block, nonparoxysmal junctional tachycardia (Fig. 7–48), AV dissociation, second- and third-degree AV block, SA

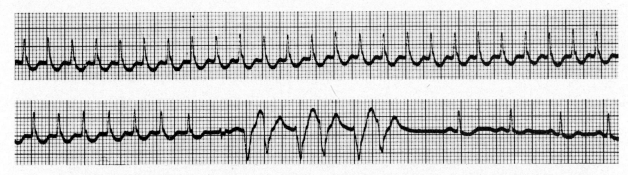

FIGURE 7–46 Supraventricular tachycardia treated with large doses of digitalis terminating with ventricular tachycardia and 3:2 Wenckebach (type I) exit block. Atrial tachycardia at a rate of 230 bpm is followed by a bigeminal rhythm, with ventricular complexes all of similar morphology. The longer cycles are less than twice the shorter cycle, suggesting a ventricular tachycardia with a 3:2 Wenckebach exit block. The interectopic ventricular cycle length is 0.22 sec. One possible mechanism of the ventricular tachycardia is delayed afterdepolarization, or "triggered" automaticity.

block, AV junctional rhythm, and reciprocating rhythm. Ventricular arrhythmias due to digitalis are an unequivocal sign of toxicity. This group includes isolated ventricular premature contractions (VPC), ventricular bigeminy, multifocal or multiform VPC, ventricular tachycardia, and "bidirectional" ventricular tachycardia, flutter, and fibrillation.

A *diagnosis of digitalis toxicity* is seldom based on the ECG alone. Pharmacodynamics of the glycoside and extracardiac and cardiac factors that alter tolerance to the drug must be considered.[256] The numerous arrhythmias ascribed to digitalis and summarized in Table 7–6 represent a composite of a number of studies of digitalis toxicity reported over a period of 21 years. The data should be viewed in light of the retrospective nature of the studies and the fact that interpretation and recognition of arrhythmias were subject to changes in our knowledge about electrophysiology and electrocardiography during the interim between studies. For example, atrial tachycardia with block and nonparoxysmal junctional tachycardia were noted in only a small number of early studies but were increasingly recognized as analysis of arrhythmias became more sophisticated. In addition, a serious limitation of any such study is the low specificity of many of the arrhythmias for digitalis toxicity.[257]

The wide spectrum of arrhythmias induced by digitalis and the coexistence of a number of different arrhythmias in the same tracing can be explained by the effects of the interplay of digitalis and myocardial and extracardiac factors on the electrophysiological properties of cardiac tissues. The magnitude of the effect of the drug on specialized tissue, the SA node, specialized atrial tissue, AV junctional tissue, and the Purkinje fibers varies and, in fact, may have an opposite effect on cells with the same functional properties. Furthermore,

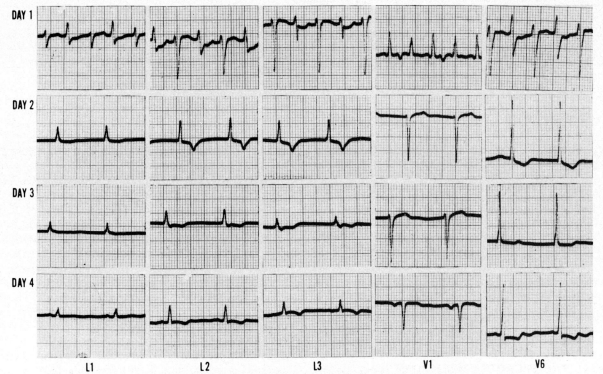

FIGURE 7–47 Bidirectional ventricular tachycardia and junctional tachycardia due to digitalis. On day 1, the ECG shows bidirectional ventricular tachycardia with alternation of the axis and RBBB. The divisions of the left bundle are the site of the tachycardia. On day 2, the rhythm is junctional at a rate of 83 bpm, with retrograde P waves in leads II and III and an R-P interval of about 0.20 sec. On day 3, the junctional rate is 68 and retrograde P waves follow the R wave by an interval of about 0.08 sec. On day 4, normal sinus rhythm is accompanied by nonspecific T-wave changes in leads II, III, and V$_6$ and negative U waves in lead V6.

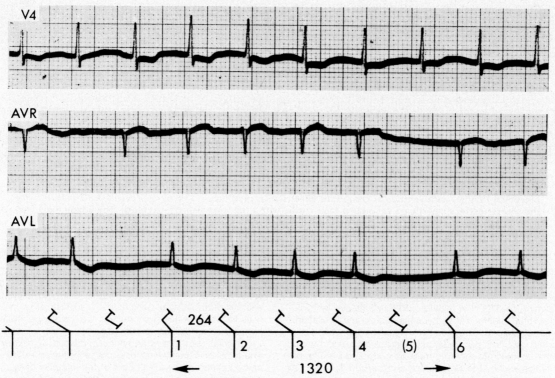

FIGURE 7-48 Atrial fibrillation and nonparoxysmal junctional tachycardia with Wenckebach (type I) exit block due to digitalis intoxication. Lead V₄ illustrates a regular ventricular rhythm at a rate of 107 bpm, characteristic of this arrhythmia. In leads aV_r and aV_l the R-R cycle foreshortens gradually and the long pause is shorter than the length of two of the preceding R-R cycles. This is characteristic of a Wenckebach structure and identifies Wenckebach (type I) exit block from the junctional focus. Although at first glance leads aV_r and aV_l suggest atrial fibrillation, the repetitive Wenckebach structure indicates that there is, in addition, a regular junctional rhythm with a Wenckebach (type I) exit block.

The actual interectopic junctional interval and delay of conduction from the pacemaker to surrounding tissue can be calculated from the ECG with the aid of the Lewis diagram (bottom). The number of *manifest* QRS cycles of the Wenckebach sequence (QRS1 to QRS6) is four. To this number is added one additional pacemaker cycle to take into account the cycle that fails to manifest a QRS(5). The duration of the sequence from QRS1 to QRS6 is 1320 msec. The latter is divided by the five cycles, and the actual interectopic interval of the junctional pacemaker is calculated to be 264 msec. The increased distance between the junctional pacemaker and the manifest QRS is a measure of delay of conduction from the pacemaker to the myocardium. The same method is used to calculate the sinoatrial node (SAN) rate and conduction time to the atrium in the presence of Wenckebach type I exit block. The SAN and P wave are substituted for the junctional pacemaker and QRS, respectively.

the electrocardiographic expression of electrophysiological effects of digitalis is a net result of altered automaticity, refractoriness, excitability, and conduction. Also, digitalis may act directly on the specialized tissue or its action may be mediated through the sympathetic or parasympathetic system or both.[258,259] In addition, the sensitivity of the tissues to digitalis may be altered by factors such as a changing acid-base balance, plasma and intracellular electrolyte levels, oxygen saturation, and mechanical stretch. Similarly, improvement of cardiac function with treatment may alter the variables affecting the electrophysiological properties of the cardiac tissue and consequently the tissue's response to digitalis.

Arrhythmias identical to those due to digitalis toxicity can be caused by heart disease, drugs other than digitalis, and a variety of extracardiac factors.[260]

Selected arrhythmias due to digitalis have been singled out for discussion here because of their frequency and relatively high specificity for digitalis toxicity.

ATRIAL TACHYCARDIA WITH BLOCK (see also p. 701).

The cause of this arrhythmia can be ascribed almost equally to severe heart disease and to digitalis toxicity.[260-263] The diagnosis of atrial tachycardia with block may occasionally be difficult. At rapid rates it resembles atrial flutter. The amplitude of the atrial deflections may be low,

and only careful attention to lead V₁ may disclose the true nature of the arrhythmia.

NONPAROXYSMAL JUNCTIONAL TACHYCARDIA (see also p. 704). In the proper setting, this arrhythmia is highly specific for digitalis excess or toxicity.[264] Other less common causes of nonparoxysmal junctional tachycardia, namely, acute myocardial infarction, open heart surgery, myocarditis, and general anesthesia, must be ruled out. Nonparoxysmal junctional tachycardia differs from paroxysmal junctional or supraventricular tachycardia. It appears and disappears gradually and, when repetitive, the coupling, or relation of the first ectopic complex, to the dominant impulse varies. The rate is 70 to 130 bpm. AV dissociation resulting from acceleration of the AV junctional pacemaker is recorded in 85 per cent of the cases. The ectopic junctional focus activates both atria and ventricles in the remaining 15 per cent of cases. Rarely, two junctional foci coexist, one controlling the atria and the other the ventricles, resulting in a double junctional tachycardia.[265]

In the absence of exit block, the rhythm in non-

TABLE 7–6   CARDIAC ARRHYTHMIAS DUE TO DIGITALIS (10 STUDIES, 661 PATIENTS)

	NO. OF SERIES	NO. OF ARRHYTHMIAS		
Ventricular Arrhythmias		470 (71%)		
Ventricular premature contractions			420	
Bigeminy	9			150
Multifocal	4			121
Not specified	4			79
Other (frequent, unifocal, occasional, etc.)	3			70
Ventricular tachycardia	7		50	
AV Block		194 (29%)		
First-degree	7		87	
Second-degree	10		58	
Wenckebach	3			4
Third-degree	6		37	
Unspecified	2		12	
Atrial Arrhythmias		177 (26%)		
Atrial fibrillation	9		80	
with slow rate	2			21
PAT with block	7		59	
Atrial premature beats	4		27	
Atrial flutter	4		11	
Sinoatrial Node Arrhythmias		85 (13%)		
Sinus tachycardia	3		29	
Sinus bradycardia	4		27	
with nodal escape	1			11
Sinus arrest	2		11	
SA block	3		7	
Wandering pacemaker	3		11	
AV Dissociation	4	65 (9.8%)		
AV Nodal Arryhthmias		47 (7%)		
Nodal tachycardia	4		32	
Nodal rhythm	2		11	
Nodal premature beats	1		4	

From Knoebel, S.B., and Fisch, C.: Recognition and therapy of digitalis toxicity. Progr. Cardiovasc. Dis. *13*:71, 1970.

paroxysmal junctional tachycardia is generally perfectly regular and the diagnosis usually simple. Recognition becomes more difficult in the presence of exit block.[266] A high degree of exit block may suggest a slow junctional rhythm or AV block. If the exit block is Mobitz (type II), with 3:2 exit block, a bigeminal rhythm appears, with longer cycles exact multiples of shorter cycles. If the exit block is Wenckebach (type I), the gradually shortening R-R interval and lack of the expected relationship of the long pause to the shorter cycles (i.e., the pause is not a multiple of the shorter cycle), atrial fibrillation may be suggested (Fig. 7–48). Only a careful search for the Wenckebach structure will reveal the true nature of the arrhythmia. Nonparoxysmal junctional tachycardia with an irregular ventricular response without conforming to the Wenckebach (type I) or Mobitz (type II) structure precludes the diagnosis, and nonparoxysmal junctional tachycardia cannot be differentiated from atrial fibrillation. Occasionally, this arrhythmia is masked and becomes evident with slowing of the dominant rhythm; it may appear as nonparoxysmal junctional tachycardia or as a single accelerated escape impulse.[267]

Differentiation of nonparoxysmal junctional tachycardia with aberrant intraventricular conduction from ventricular tachycardia may be difficult, if not impossible. A rapid heart rate, a bizarre QRS complex, and AV dissociation are common to both arrhythmias. In the presence of WPW, nonparoxysmal junctional tachycardia may be associated with fusion and capture complexes.[107]

VENTRICULAR ARRHYTHMIAS. Ventricular premature contractions (VPC) are the most common manifestation of digitalis toxicity but, at the same time, are the least specific as a sign of glycoside toxicity.[268] None of the morphological features of the QRS complex helps to differentiate VPC due to digitalis from those of other causes. The exception is ventricular bigeminy, with accurate coupling but varying morphology—a criterion that is suggestive of digitalis toxicity.

The problems of recognition associated with digitalis-induced VPC are also applicable to ventricular tachycardia. Ventricular tachycardia with exit block (Fig. 7–46) and bidirectional ventricular tachycardia (Fig. 7–47) strongly suggest digitalis intoxication. A bidirectional tachycardia of supraventricular origin is extremely rare. When the ventricular tachycardia originates in the divisions of the left bundle branch, the QRS complex may be normal in duration,[269] and the diagnosis rests on the presence of ventricular capture and fusion complexes. Studies in animals and man confirm that narrow QRS complex tachycardias may be ventricular in origin.

Digitalis-induced ventricular fibrillation is seldom recorded in man. It is rarely, if ever, the initial manifestation of digitalis toxicity but is usually preceded by other digitalis-induced arrhythmias.

In rare instances, ventricular parasystole is due to digitalis. This is particularly the case when parasystole is accompanied by other arrhythmias known to be due to digitalis intoxication.

The presence of diverse ectopic rhythms, either simultaneously or serially, is strongly suggestive of digitalis toxicity as is the appearance of ectopic rhythms and AV conduction.[253]

AV DISSOCIATION (see also p. 735). AV dissociation appearing in the course of digitalis administration is strongly indicative of digitalis overdosage or intoxication.[270]

AV CONDUCTION DELAY. Depression of AV conduction may be due to a vagal effect of the glycoside and can be reversed with atropine or catecholamines released during normal activities or during exercise. Such depression may also be due to a "direct" extravagal effect of the drug on the cell.[258,259,271]

In contrast to ectopy, depression of conduction may be either a desirable therapeutic effect or a manifestation of digitalis toxicity. The differentiation of the two is a clinical decision. For example, in atrial fibrillation and atrial flutter depression of AV conduction is desirable. In the presence of sinus rhythm, however, AV delay, other than simple prolongation of the P-R interval, is, with rare exception, evidence of digitalis overdose. Although AV block in the presence of sinus rhythm is frequently mentioned as a sign of digitalis intoxication, third-degree AV block is a relatively rare manifestation of glycoside toxicity.

ACCELERATED JUNCTIONAL ESCAPE. This arrhythmia is an interesting manifestation of digitalis intoxication. It is seen in the same clinical conditions as is nonparoxysmal junctional tachycardia and its clinical significance is probably the same in both.[267] Accelerated junctional escape follows the rules set for cardiac arrhythmias induced by delayed afterdepolarization[272] and may be the clinical counterpart of the arrhythmias induced in the Purkinje fiber and the intact animal.

"MASKED" (SUPPRESSED) DIGITALIS TOXICITY. Toxic effects of glycosides, especially enhanced junctional or Purkinje automaticity, may be suppressed by a more rapidly discharging, higher pacemaker. Slowing of the dominant rhythm may unmask the toxic ectopic rhythm, manifesting in the form of a single complex or an ectopic tachycardia. Sinus bradycardia, SA block, AV block, a compensatory pause following a spontaneous ectopic impulse,[267,273] and carotid sinus stimulation may be the mechanisms of slowing of the dominant rhythm and unmasking of toxicity.

The possibility of masked digitalis toxicity should be considered when digitalis is administered to patients with atrial fibrillation in clinical states in which slowing of the ventricular rate by digitalis is difficult or impossible. These include thyrotoxicosis, infection, pulmonary embolism, "high-output" failure, and occasionally intractable and perhaps far advanced heart failure.[257]

Other Drugs

QUINIDINE (see also p. 656). The ECG manifestations of quinidine are secondary to depression of conduction, automaticity, and excitability. At the level of the SA and AV nodes, the effect may be sinus bradycardia, sinus arrest, SA block, P-R interval prolongation, or rarely, a higher degree of AV block. Quinidine prolongs the P wave; slows intraatrial conduction and the rate of atrial flutter and fibrillation; and converts atrial fibrillation to atrial flutter, atrial flutter to fibrillation, and both—ultimately—to sinus rhythm. The combination of a slower flutter rate and acceleration of AV conduction due to the antivagal atropine-like effect of quinidine may result in an atrial flutter with 1:1 AV conduction (Fig. 7–49). Similar-

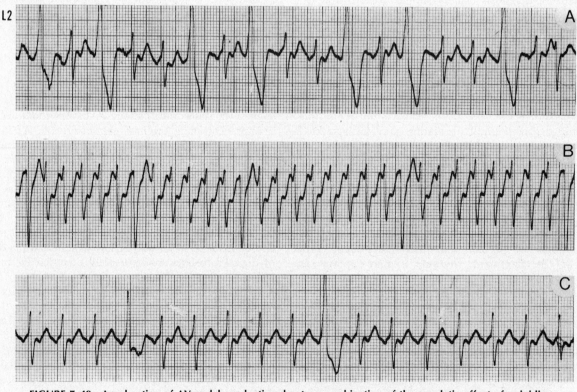

FIGURE 7–49 Acceleration of AV nodal conduction due to a combination of the vagolytic effect of quinidine and slowing of the rate of flutter by the drug. *A,* Atrial flutter with an f-f interval of 0.20 sec, 2:1 AV conduction, and ventricular premature systoles. *B,* Recording after administration of 900 mg of quinidine. The f-f interval is increased to 0.23 sec. Coupled with the vagolytic effect of quinidine on the AV node, this results in 1:1 AV conduction. *C,* Recording after administration of 10 mg of Tensilon shows that 2:1 AV conduction has been reestablished.

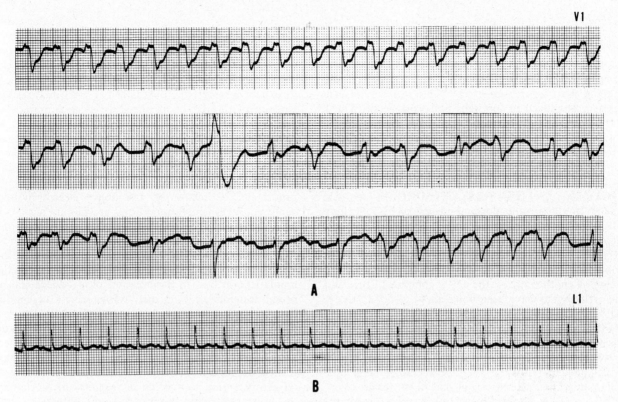

FIGURE 7-50 Intraventricular aberration due to quinidine and acceleration of the heart rate. In panel *B*, a control tracing, the ECG is normal with a sinus rate of 130 bpm. After administration of quinidine (panel *A*), heart rate is 120 bpm and the QRS widened to 0.20 sec. In row 2, AV conduction changed to a 3:2 Wenckebach (type I) block interrupted by one VPC. P-wave duration is prolonged and the P-R interval measures 0.28 sec. The QRS complex following the longer pause is somewhat narrower, probably owing to a longer period of recovery. In row 3, 1:1 AV conduction is interrupted by 2:1 AV conduction. P waves measure 0.20 sec in duration, the P-R interval is 0.40 sec, and the QRS complexes are foreshortened to 0.16 sec. The intraventricular delay to 0.16 sec is caused by quinidine, while the much wider QRS complexes of 0.20 sec in the presence of 1:1 AV conduction reflect both the effect of quinidine and the accelerated heart rate.

ly, an acceleration of sinus rate and ventricular rate in atrial fibrillation can occur following the administration of quinidine.

At high plasma drug levels, the QRS complex is prolonged, and this usually affects the entire complex (Fig. 7–50).[274] The durations of the T wave and the Q-T interval are also prolonged (Fig. 7–48). Depending on the effect of the drug on the QRS complex, the T-wave change may be secondary, primary, or a combination of the two. An upright T wave may lose amplitude or may become notched or inverted, while an inverted T wave may become more deeply inverted. The ST segment remains isoelectric and the U-wave amplitude is increased.[8] The T-wave changes are indistinguishable from a variety of other abnormal T waves. It has been suggested that the combination of a prolonged QRS complex, an abnormal T wave, and a dominant U wave is fairly specific for quinidine effect. However, similar changes may be seen with other drugs. Digitalis in combination with quinidine causes elongation and depression of the ST segment and a decrease in T-wave amplitude. With appearance of a prominent U wave, the pattern is indistinguishable from that of hypopotassemia.[246]

Quinidine toxicity can be dose-dependent or dose-independent. Widening of the QRS complex, AV block, and pronounced bradycardia are usually produced by high levels of quinidine.[274] On the other hand, ventricular arrhythmias including the torsades de pointes variant of ventricular tachycardia and ventricular fibrillation (p. 725) may appear with low plasma levels of quinidine.[275]

PROCAINAMIDE (see also p. 657). The effect of procainamide on the ECG is the same as that of quinidine but quantitatively less pronounced, so that ECG abnormalities are less often encountered. The P wave and P-R intervals may be prolonged, the T wave lower and notched, and the U-wave amplitude increased.[276] As with quinidine, procainamide administered with digitalis results in an ECG pattern indistinguishable from that in hypopotassemia.

DISOPYRAMIDE (see also p. 659). The electrophysiological effects of disopyramide are similar to those of quinidine[277–279] and consist of slowing of the upstroke of phase 0 and prolongation of the transmembrane action potential. In the ECG, depression of conduction is manifest by lengthening of the P-R interval, the P wave, and the QRS complex. The Q-T interval may be prolonged and the T wave lowered and at times notched. Ventricular tachycardia, including torsades de pointes similar to that seen with quinidine, and ventricular fibrillation have been observed with disopyramide.[280]

PHENOTHIAZINES (see also p. 1840). ECG changes due to phenothiazine derivatives reflect the effect of these drugs on ventricular repolarization. Changes are most commonly seen with thioridazine and are less pronounced with chlorpromazine and trifluoperazine[215,281,282] and include prolongation of the Q-T interval and widening and notching of the T wave. The U-wave amplitude may be increased, but the ST segment usually remains unchanged. At higher levels the T wave decreases in amplitude and may become inverted.[283] These effects are usually most pronounced in the right precordial leads. The P wave and the QRS complex are not altered. Large doses of phenothiazines have been observed to induce ventricular arrhythmias and probably are the mechanism of occasional sudden death following ingestion of large amounts of these drugs.

TRICYCLIC ANTIDEPRESSANT DRUGS (see also p. 1838). In therapeutic doses these drugs may prolong the P-R interval, QRS complex, and Q-T interval; alter the ST segment and T wave; and induce atrial and ventricular arrhythmias. Toxic doses of the drugs may, in addition to the above listed effects, result in second- and third-degree AV block. Lengthening of the QRS complex, BBB, and cardiac arrhythmias have been noted in 44 to 50, 15 to 17, and 11 to 17 per cent, respectively.[284]

LITHIUM (see also p. 1841). Lithium affects cardiac repolarization and the sinoatrial node. The most common ECG abnormalities due to lithium are T-wave changes.[285] However, dysfunction of the SA node, including sinus bradycardia, sinoatrial node arrest, or exit block (either Wenckebach [type I] or Mobitz [type II]), is more characteristic of lithium toxicity. Interestingly, the ECG changes occur often at therapeutic levels of the salt. Lithium has no recognizable effects on the P-R interval or the QRS complex. A normal A-H interval with only slight prolongation of the H-V interval has been documented,[286] suggesting a selective action of lithium on the sinoatrial node.

MECHANISMS OF ARRHYTHMIAS DERIVED FROM ECG ANALYSIS

The ECG diagnosis of specific arrhythmias is discussed in Chapter 22, so that only selected mechanisms will be included here. These have been singled out because, in contrast to the arrhythmias discussed in Chapter 22, which can usually be diagnosed clinically, the concepts included in this section can as a rule (1) be inferred only from analysis of the ECG; (2) represent general principles, in that they apply to arrhythmias originating from different sites; (3) are clinically important; and (4) serve as ECG models of basic electrophysiological phenomena.[5,287-290]

ABERRATION

Intraventricular aberration, a term introduced and defined by Lewis, describes a supraventricular impulse with abnormal, bizarre intraventricular conduction (Fig. 7–51).[291] It refers to intraventricular conduction abnormalities related to changing heart rate or other functional alterations in electrophysiological properties, anomalous AV conduction, metabolic and electrolyte abnormalities, and toxic effects of drugs. The term aberration, as used currently, does not include fixed organic conduction defects.

The speed of conduction generally depends on the magnitude of the transmembrane resting potential (phase 4),

the rate of rise of depolarization (dV/dt of phase 0), and the amplitude of the action potential. The relation of the dV/dt of phase 0 to the magnitude of the resting potential can be expressed as membrane responsiveness.[292] Excitation prior to completion of repolarization or in the presence of a reduced resting potential, as in hyperkalemia, results in a slowing of the dV/dt of phase 0, lower amplitude of the action potential, and slower conduction. Similarly, a shift of membrane responsiveness to the right, as, for example, with antiarrhythmic drugs such as quinidine, procainamide, or disopyramide, is associated with slowing of conduction.[293] The numerous ECG manifestations of aberration can be related to the above electrophysiological changes. When these alterations are nonuniform, conduction of the specialized tissue may also become nonuniform and aberration results.[294]

More specifically, the mechanisms for aberration include from time to time (1) excitation prior to completion of repolarization (i.e., in the presence of a reduced transmembrane potential), (2) unequal refractoriness of conducting tissue resulting in local delay or block of conduction, (3) prolongation of the action potential due to prolongation of the preceding cycle length and thus voltage-dependent refractoriness, (4) failure of restitution of transmembrane electrolyte concentration during diastole, (5) failure of the refractory period to shorten in response to acceleration of the heart rate, (6) a reduced take-off potential secondary to diastole depolarization, (7) concealed transseptal conduction with delay or block of bundle branch conduction, (8) diffuse depression of intraventricular conduction including that of specialized as well as myocardial tissue, (9) anomalous ventricular activation due to congenital anatomical abnormalities such as the bundle of Kent and Mahaim and James fibers, and (10) "predestination" of intraventricular conduction secondary to altered intraatrial conduction.[18]

QRS aberration may result when any of the above mechanisms alter conduction in the bundle branches or the divisions of the left bundle branch (or a combination of the two), the Purkinje fibers, or the myocardium. RBBB is the most common form of aberrancy and is frequently associated with left anterior divisional block. Aberrancy due to LBBB is much less common and in our experience nearly always due to heart disease, although the heart disease may not be clinically evident.[295] An abnormality of intraventricular conduction due to diffuse depression of conduction in the Purkinje system and in the myocardium should be suspected when both the initial and terminal portions of the QRS complex are abnormal.

Of the numerous mechanisms and manifestations of aberration, nine will be considered in further detail: (1) premature excitation, (2) the Ashman phenomenon, (3) acceleration-dependent aberrancy, (4) deceleration-dependent aberrancy, (5) concealed conduction, (6) diffuse myocardial depression of conduction, (7) abnormal anatomical pathways, (8) postextrasystolic aberrancy, and (9) electrical (QRS) alternans.

Premature Excitation. Conduction will fail or be delayed if the stimulus falls during the effective or the relative refractory period of recovery.[5] When the impulse falls during the relative refractory period of a single bundle branch, the unilateral delay results in a bundle branch block. The duration of the refractory period may equal that of

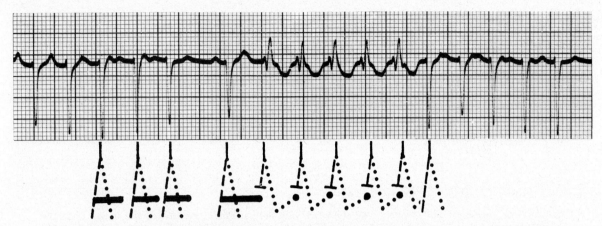

FIGURE 7–51 Atrial tachycardia with Wenckebach (type I) AV block, ventricular aberration due to the Ashman phenomenon, and probably concealed transseptal conduction. The long pause of the atrial tachycardia is followed by five QRS complexes with RBBB morphology. The RBBB of the first QRS reflects the Ashman phenomenon. The aberration is perpetuated by concealed transseptal activation from the left bundle into the right bundle with block of the anterograde conduction of the subsequent sinus impulse in the right bundle. Foreshortening of the R-R cycle, a manifestation of the Wenckebach structure, disturbs the relationship between transseptal and anterograde sinus conduction, and RBB conduction is normalized. In the diagram, the dashes indicate the RBB and the dots the LBB, while the solid bar denotes the refractory period. Following the long pause, the refractory period of the RBB is prolonged and is responsible for the RBBB of the first QRS. The impulse conducted along the LBB is propagated across the septum, engages the RBB, and blocks anterograde conduction of the sinus impulse.

the transmembrane action potential, so-called voltage-dependent refractoriness, or it may exceed it, so-called time-dependent refractoriness. Duration of the refractory period depends to a great extent on the basic heart rate and on the duration of the immediately preceding cycle(s). Normally, the refractory period shortens with acceleration of the heart rate and lengthens with slowing of the heart rate. It is possible, therefore, to maintain fixed coupling of a premature excitation to the dominant impulse but, by prolonging the preceding cycle, to lengthen the refractory period sufficiently to induce aberration.[296]

With all variables affecting conduction being constant, the degree of aberration is largely a function of prematurity of excitation. On rare occasions, however, the opposite may be noted, namely, a shorter R-P interval may be followed by a normal QRS complex while a longer R-P interval will exhibit an abnormal QRS complex (see Gap Phenomenon, p. 252).

The site of conduction depression and thus the morphology of the aberrant QRS complex is determined by the length of the refractory period of the AV node, the bundle of His, and the bundle system itself. Normally, at slow heart rates, the right bundle branch has the longest refractory period, with the left bundle and the AV node somewhat shorter and the bundle of His the shortest. Only at very rapid rates may the duration of the refractory period of the left bundle exceed that of the right bundle.[297]

Effect of Changing Cycle Length on Refractoriness (Ashman Phenomenon). This form of aberrancy, also a function of premature excitation, differs little electrophysiologically from that due to early excitation described above. The difference is that the abnormal conduction is a function of an altered duration of the refractory period rather than of changing prematurity of stimulation. Since the duration of the refractory period is a function of the immediately preceding cycle length, the longer the preceding cycle, the longer the refractory period that follows. Consequently, with a fixed stimulus interval, sudden prolongation of the immediately preceding cycle length may result in aberration. This relationship of aberrancy to changes in the preceding cycle length is known as the Ashman phenomenon.[296] It has been demonstrated that aberrancy so initiated may persist for a number of cycles (Fig. 7–51). With rare exception, aberrancy due to the Ashman phenomenon exhibits the RBBB morphology. The RBBB may be associated with left anterior or rarely with left posterior divisional block.

In the presence of irregular supraventricular rhythms, such as atrial fibrillation, repetitive atrial tachycardia, or atrial tachycardia with Wenckebach (type I) AV block (Fig. 7–51), aberration due to the Ashman phenomenon is suggested by the following: (1) a relatively long cycle immediately preceding the cycle terminated by the aberrant QRS

complex, (2) RBBB aberrancy with normal orientation of the initial QRS vector, (3) irregular coupling of the aberrant QRS complex, and (4) lack of a compensatory pause following the aberrant QRS complex.

Acceleration-dependent aberrancy (tachycardia-dependent aberrancy, phase 3 aberrancy). This form of aberration has been recognized since 1913.[298] At certain critical heart rates, impaired intraventricular conduction results in aberrancy (Figs. 7–50 and 7–52). This phenomenon has been described using a variety of terms. The one most commonly used is tachycardia-dependent aberrancy or phase 3 aberrancy; however, neither term is entirely appropriate. Aberration often appears at relatively slow rates, frequently below 75 bpm; similarly, because of the slow rate at which the conduction fails, one would have to postulate an extremely long transmembrane action potential in order to accept excitation during phase 3 as the cause of the impaired conduction. Finally, conduction will also fail with excitation during phase 2 of the action potential. The term *acceleration-dependent aberrancy* appears most appropriate.

The appearance and disappearance of aberration often depends on very small changes in cycle length, a change frequently difficult if not impossible to detect in the ECG. Assuming that a reasonably long recording is available, a comparison of the earliest available cycle length terminated by a normal QRS complex with the cycle length terminated by the first aberrant QRS complex will aid in the diagnosis of acceleration-dependent aberrancy. The difference in the duration of two such cycles is often less than 0.04 sec. The importance of such a minimal foreshortening of the cycle length for this diagnosis can be demonstrated with atrial pacing in which a 10-msec or shorter decrease in cycle length may result in aberrant conduction. In some instances, as in paroxysmal atrial tachycardia, there may be no demonstrable change in cycle length preceding the onset of aberrant conduction. Such aberration is probably a function of the duration of the tachycardia and perhaps due to a failure of restitution of the ionic gradient during diastole (time-dependent refractoriness).[295]

Acceleration-dependent aberrancy differs in a number of respects from the physiological aberrancy observed in a normal heart. Differences include (1) appearance of aberrancy at relatively slow heart rates, (2) predominance of LBBB morphology, (3) independence from the immediately preceding cycle length, (4) occasional appearance with no, or only slight change in cycle length, and (5) association with heart disease.

QRS aberrancy may persist at an R-R interval considerably longer than the interval that initiated the aberrancy (Fig. 7–52). Three mechanisms have been suggested to explain this paradox: (1) concealed

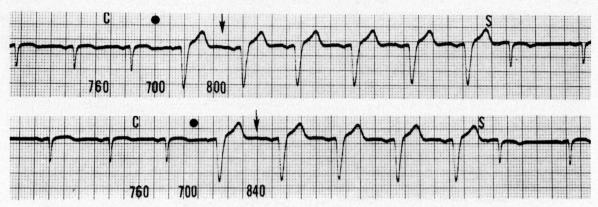

FIGURE 7–52 Acceleration-dependent QRS aberrancy with the paradox of persistence at a longer cycle and normalization at a shorter cycle than that which initiated the aberrancy. LBBB appears at a cycle length of 700 msec and is perpetuated at cycle lengths of 800 and 840 msec; conduction normalizes after a cycle length of 600 msec (S). Perpetuation of LBBB at a cycle length of 800 and 840 msec is probably due to transseptal concealment, similar to that described in Figure 7–51. Unexpected normalization of the QRS (S) following the atrial premature contraction is probably due to equalization of conduction in the two bundles; however, supernormal conduction in the left bundle cannot be excluded. (From Fisch, C., et al.: Rate dependent aberrancy. Circulation *48*:714, 1973, by permission of the American Heart Association, Inc.)

transseptal activation blocking conduction in the contralateral bundle; (2) "fatigue" of the bundle; and (3) concealed transseptal conduction coupled with suppression of conduction due to the increased heart rate, somewhat analogous to suppression of pacemakers by an ectopic tachycardia. A discrepancy of as much as 210 msec between the cycles initiating and terminating the aberration suggests that concealed transseptal conduction may not be the sole factor responsible for the unexpected persistence of aberrancy at the longer cycle lengths. The difference cannot be explained solely on the basis of time consumed by conduction along the contralateral bundle and across the septum.[299] Normal transseptal activation in the human heart is about 60 to 70 msec; in the diseased heart, it may be prolonged to 115 msec.[300] It is likely, therefore, that a combination of mechanisms is operative.

One mechanism that would explain the unexpected delay in normalization of intraventricular conduction is "fatigue."[295] The term "fatigue" is a descriptive one and may reflect failure of restitution of transmembrane ionic gradients and lowering of the transmembrane resting potential and/or a shift of the membrane responsiveness to the right. A different mechanism, namely, concealed conduction, may explain the delayed normalization of bundle branch conduction in patients with atrial fibrillation. Concealed conduction of atrial fibrillatory impulses into the blocked bundle may result in a true bundle-to-bundle interval that is considerably shorter than the manifest QRS interval.

Occasionally, paradoxical normalization of the QRS complex without a change in heart rate—or, in fact, with acceleration of the heart rate—has been documented (Fig. 7–52). Mechanisms that may explain this phenomenon include physiological shortening of the refractory period in response to acceleration of the heart rate, equalization of conduction in the two bundles, conduction during the supernormal period, and the gap phenomenon (p. 252).

Deceleration-dependent aberrancy (bradycardia-dependent aberrancy, phase 4 aberrancy). A prolonged cycle may be terminated by an aberrant QRS and foreshortening of the cycle may normalize the QRS (Fig. 7–53).[103,301] It has been suggested that this form of aberrancy is due to a gradual loss of transmembrane resting potential during a prolonged diastole with excitation from a less negative take-off potential.[302] Because a small change in resting potential may have a pronounced effect on the rate of rise of phase 0 of the action potential, deceleration aberrancy may be seen with a relatively small prolongation of the cycle length.[303] In order to exclude ventricular escape as the cause for the apparent aberrancy, two or more consecutive aberrant QRS complexes must be recorded and all must be preceded by the same P-R interval. In atrial fibrillation, deceleration-dependent aberrancy cannot be considered because an idioventricular escape rhythm is likely. Similarly, concealed conduction (p. 246) into the bundle with a shorter bundle-to-bundle interval cannot be excluded with certainty. Concealed conduction may also be operative in pa-

tients with sinus rhythm and Wenckebach (type I) AV block, with the blocked P wave concealing the bundle and resulting in a short bundle-to-bundle interval and thus in aberrancy of the QRS complex following the Wenckebach pause. In such cases, the bundle-to-bundle interval may be considerably shorter than the manifest QRS cycle and may be even shorter than the QRS cycle during 1:1 AV conduction. Consequently, acceleration-dependent QRS aberrancy, rather than deceleration-dependent QRS aberrancy, may be present. Because both deceleration- and acceleration-dependent aberrancy reflect disordered electrophysiological function, the two often coexist.

Concealed Conduction. Bundle branch conduction may be impaired by concealed penetration of a supraventricular impulse or by transseptal activation from the contralateral bundle (Fig. 7–51). In atrial fibrillation, concealed conduction into a bundle branch can be considered when acceleration-dependent aberrancy persists at a QRS cycle that is longer than a cycle terminated by a normal QRS. Transseptal concealed conduction into a bundle branch from the contralateral bundle should be suspected if aberrancy, once initiated, persists at rates slower than the rate that initiated the aberrancy (Fig. 7–52).

Diffuse Myocardial Depression. Drugs and metabolic and electrolyte disorders are frequent causes of QRS aberrancy (Figs. 7–43 and 7–50). The severity of depression of conduction varies, and the QRS may exhibit RBBB or LBBB, divisional block, or the two combined. As indicated previously, aberrancy can be differentiated from ordinary BBB by the presence of distortion in the initial and terminal components of the QRS complex.

Anomalous AV Conduction. Activation of the ventricle over an abnormal AV pathway results in intraventricular aberration. The pathways of conduction resulting in QRS aberrancy include the Mahaim fibers, the bundle of Kent, and probably a combination of Mahaim and James fibers[18] (see also Fig. 21–26, p. 714).

The Mahaim fibers leave the AV node or the bundle of His and preexcite different areas of the interventricular septum. This mechanism has been invoked to explain aberrant junctional escape complexes when the QRS complex measures less than 0.12 sec. However, similar complexes may originate in the divisions of the left bundle branch, and the two sites of origin cannot be differentiated with certainty.

An AV nodal bypass tract may preferentially activate different parts of the His bundle and result in QRS aberrancy. It has been suggested that a tract bypassing the AV node, as manifested by a short P-R interval, when associated with distal conduction over Mahaim fibers may result in a QRS indistinguishable from WPW. Altered intraatrial conduction or conduction over the internodal pathways with preferential activation of segments of the AV junction, His bundle, or ventricular septum may theoretically result in QRS aberrancy.[18]

Postextrasystolic Aberration. Aberrant intraventricular conduction of a sinus impulse terminating a compensatory pause is rare and

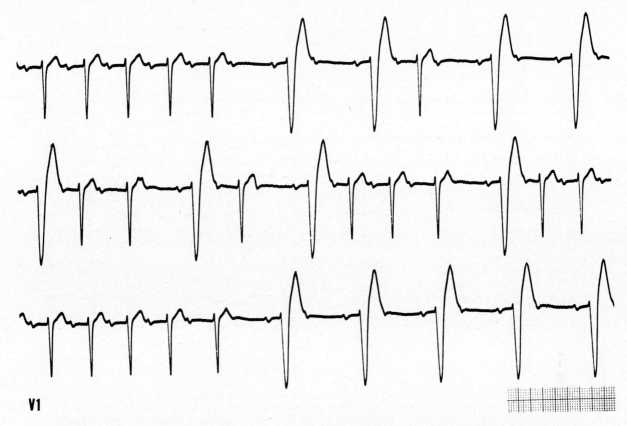

V1

FIGURE 7–53 Deceleration-dependent aberrancy. The basic rhythm is sinus with Wenckebach (type I) AV block. With 1:1 AV conduction, the QRS complexes are normal in duration; with 2:1 AV block or after the longer pause of a Wenckebach sequence, LBBB appears. Slow diastolic depolarization (phase 4 of the transmembrane action potential) during the prolonged cycle is implicated as the cause of the LBBB.

must be differentiated from an aberrant escape complex. The exact mechanism of the postpausal aberrancy is not clear. It may be due to slow diastolic depolarization, unequal recovery of conducting or myocardial tissue, or increased diastolic volume.

Electrical (QRS) Alternans. The exact mechanism of QRS alternans is obscure and may differ from one case to another (p. 132). In supraventricular tachycardia with bidirectional "ventricular" complexes, the alternation is probably a result of alternate conduction over the two divisions of the left bundle with or without accompanying RBBB. In severe myocardial disease or digitalis intoxication, QRS alternans probably reflects nonuniform recovery of the ventricles and the basic mechanism may be related to altered ionic fluxes as suggested by the phenomenon of alternation of the transmembrane action potential. The QRS alternans in cardiac tamponade, as indicated earlier, is due to rotation of the heart.

CONCEALED CONDUCTION

Concealed conduction (CC) is a common manifestation of normal and diseased cardiac tissue, so that an understanding of this concept is prerequisite for analysis of all but the most simple cardiac arrhythmias. To understand CC is to appreciate the fact that the analysis of complex arrhythmias is one of deductive reasoning, since, as stated earlier, the surface ECG reflects electrical activity of myocardial tissue while the genesis of arrhythmias is related to abnormal function of the specialized tissues.

CC was observed and defined by Englemann in the course of studying an isolated heart preparation, some years before Einthoven introduced the electrocardiograph. In 1887, Englemann wrote, "Every effective atrial stimulation, even if it does not elicit a ventricular systole, prolongs the subsequent AV interval."[304] Thirty-eight years later this phenomenon was recorded in the AV node of the dog with the aid of the ECG.[305] Further studies in the intact animal,[299,306] in isolated cardiac cells,[307] and in man using His bundle electrography[308] validated the concept that had been derived by careful deductive analysis of the ECG,[309] i.e., that an incompletely conducted impulse can affect the behavior of subsequent AV conduction.

The concept of CC has been gradually extended to conduction within the sinoatrial node, perinodal tissue, atrium,[310] AV node, ventricular septum, and bundle branches[299] (Fig. 7–54). The concealing impulse may be normal, ectopic, automatic, or reentrant, and its conduction may be antegrade or retrograde.

A number of classifications of CC and its ECG manifestations have been proposed. Consideration of three variables—namely, the site of origin of the impulse which is concealed, the site of concealment, and the ECG manifestation—will define most all forms of CC. Concealed conduction can be grouped according to its effect on impulse formation, conduction, or both. More specifically, the effects include delay of conduction, block of conduction (Fig. 7–25), repetitive concealment, enhancement of conduction, reentrant rhythm, and premature resetting of a pacemaker. ECG manifestations of these six major categories are numerous, and each represents an interesting ECG model of basic electrophysiological phenomena.[290,309,311]

FUSION

A fusion complex, either atrial or ventricular, results from simultaneous activation of the atria or ventricles by impulses originating at two different sites. The resultant fusion complex frequently represents a spectrum of P waves or QRS complexes, their morphology depending on the relative contribution of the two impulses. The timing of the two impulses contributing to the fusion complex must be such that simultaneous excitation of the chambers is possible. For example, in the case of fusion between a sinus and ventricular impulse, the P-R interval must be sufficiently long for the sinus impulse to have reached the ventricle.

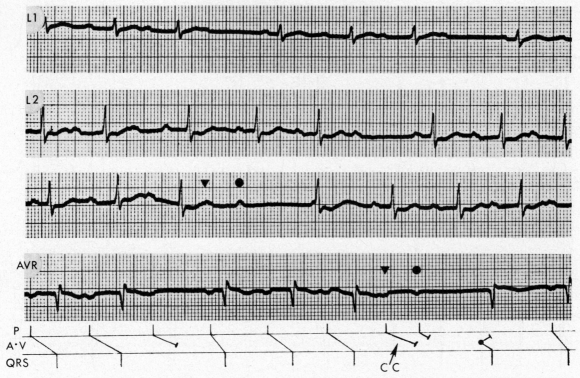

FIGURE 7–54 Block of atrial premature complex (APC) due to concealed conduction. The basic rhythm is sinus with a Wenckebach type I AV block. Two of the blocked sinus P waves of the Wenckebach sequence (▼) are followed by blocked APC (●), in spite of the fact that the APC is sufficiently distant from the preceding QRS (R-P interval) to allow for its conduction. Failure of the APC to conduct results from refractoriness of the AV node secondary to penetration of the preceding blocked sinus P wave (▼) into the AV node (↑CC). The result is unexpected block of the APC. Conduction of the blocked sinus P wave (▼) to the level of the AV node is not recorded in the surface ECG and thus concealed, recognized only by its effect on the subsequent APC, i.e., unexpected block.

Atrial fusions are relatively rare because the unprotected sinoatrial node is discharged by the ectopic impulse, thus eliminating the opportunity for dual excitation of the atria. In addition, because of the low amplitude of the P wave and a frequent lack of morphological detail, atrial fusions may be difficult to recognize. Atrial fusion is usually seen in atrial parasystole or during the interplay of sinoatrial and junctional impulses. Theoretically, it may also result from fusion of two atrial ectopic impulses.

Ventricular fusions are common and clinically important because, with rare exception, their presence confirms the ventricular origin of an arrhythmia. The mechanism of ventricular fusion varies.[312] In AV dissociation, a fusion complex may result from fusion of junctional and ventricular impulses. The ventricular contribution may be that of a single late diastolic VPC, idioventricular rhythm, ventricular parasystole, ventricular tachycardia, or paced ventricular rhythm. Although the supraventricular impulse that fuses with a ventricular complex is usually of sinoatrial origin, it may arise within the atrium or in the AV junction. Rarely a ventricular fusion may be the result of two or more ventricular rhythms.

By definition, a ventricular fusion differs in morphology from the normal, supraventricular QRS complex. However, the aberration may be extremely subtle, and in such instances a careful analysis of the T wave in search of secondary T-wave changes may prove useful. In the presence of BBB, fusion of the supraventricular impulse and an ipsilateral VPC may result in a QRS complex that is normal in appearance.

In WPW, the QRS complex is a fusion, a result of a supraventricular impulse, usually from the sinoatrial node, activating the ventricle through two pathways. The degree of QRS aberrancy depends on a relative contribution of the impulse conducting through the two pathways. Fusion between a supraventricular impulse conducting through an anomalous pathway and an impulse originating in the ventricle or AV junction has also been described.[107]

CAPTURE (See also Fig. 21–48, p. 735)

Capture implies activation of the ventricle by an atrial impulse in the presence of AV dissociation. The timing of the P wave is such that the impulse arrives in the AV junction when the latter is no longer refractory and conduction of the atrial impulse is possible.

In the presence of an idioventricular rhythm, the QRS complex resulting from activation by an atrial impulse (capture) may be normal, aberrant, or a ventricular fusion. The ventricular focus may be discharged and reset by the capture, or it may remain unaffected. If the supraventricular impulse reaches the ventricular pacemaker at the moment it discharges or shortly thereafter, the pacemaker will fail to reset. Similarly, in partial capture, a fusion will fail to discharge the pacemaker. Failure of the early impulse to discharge the pacemaker is due to physiological refractoriness and is an example of *interference*.

In the presence of a dominant junctional rhythm, a concealed penetration, capture of the junctional pacemaker by an atrial impulse will reset and prolong the return cycle length of the junctional focus (see Concealed Conduction p. 247).

PARASYSTOLE (See also p. 622)

Parasystole is most likely an automatic rhythm of an independent and protected focus. The protection is manifest by the inability of an extraneous impulse—be it sinus or ectopic—to alter the rhythmicity of the parasystolic impulse. Parasystolic protection must be demonstrated by activation of the chamber, the site of the parasystolic rhythm, at a time when the extraneous impulse should reset the parasystolic focus yet fails to do so. Functional unidirectional protection of the parasystolic focus, i.e., *entrance block*, is the characteristic feature of parasystole, although the existence of unidirectional protection or block as an absolute prerequisite has been questioned. It has been suggested that the parasystolic rate is more rapid than the manifest rate, and that the slower manifest rate is a manifestation of an exit block.[313] If such is the case, the protection is one of interference between two foci, and a unidirectional block need not be invoked.

Although one of the characteristic features of parasystole is its regularity, spontaneous variations of parasystolic cycle length were recognized as early as 1920.[314] In some instances, the changing rate is probably related to a changing slope of diastolic depolarization of the automatic fibers or to conduction delay from the focus. It has been suggested that a parasystolic rhythm can be altered in a predictable manner by electrotonus generated[315,316] by nonparasystolic impulses. The role of electrotonus in clinical parasystole must await further study.

Parasystole may be continuous or intermittent.[317] Intermittency appears to be due to failure of protection, allowing the extraneous impulse to discharge and to reset the parasystolic pacemaker. In sinus rhythm with intermittent parasystole, for example, the first impulse of each parasystolic sequence exhibits fixed coupling, a relationship which strongly suggests that the parasystolic focus was discharged and reset by the sinus impulse.[318]

Exit block, first described in conjunction with parasystole, explains the occasional failure of a parasystolic impulse to become manifest at a time when the atrium or ventricle is no longer refractory (see p. 251).

Parasystole may originate in the sinoatrial node, atrium, AV junction, and ventricle. Coexistence of an atrial and a ventricular and two or more ventricular parasystolic rhythms has been observed. The ECG manifestations of parasystole include (1) varying coupling of the parasystolic impulse to the dominant impulse; (2) a common denominator of the manifest interectopic intervals, the longer interectopic intervals being multiples of the common denominator, with a variation of 0.04 sec per cycle from the established common denominator acceptable;[288] (3) fusions; and (4) manifestation of the parasystolic impulse whenever the ventricle or the atrium is not in a refractory state.

Atrial parasystole differs from AV nodal or ventricular parasystole in that both the parasystolic and sinus rhythms originate in the same chamber. Because an atrial parasystole discharges the unprotected sinus node and thus is manifest as atrial begeminy, the parasystolic nature of the rhythm is frequently unrecognized. The sinoatrial node is discharged by each parasystolic impulse, and consequently the sinus impulse is entrained to the parasystolic impulse by a fixed interval, i.e., the sinus rate. As a result, a bigeminal relationship exists between the sinoatrial node and the parasystolic rhythms, the sequence being sinus P, parasystolic P–sinus P, parasystolic P. Atrial parasystole is identifiable only when the parasystolic impulse fails to influence the sinus node and the two discharge independently.

An automatic ventricular parasystole discharging rapidly may have to be differentiated from ventricular tachycardia, a nonprotected and most often a reentrant rhythm. Demonstration of protection of the ectopic focus will identify a parasystolic ventricular tachycardia. Protection of a parasystolic focus is present when an extraneous impulse arrives at a moment when the cardiac tissue surrounding the ectopic focus responsible for the tachycardia is no longer refractory but fails to disturb its rhythmicity. This type of protection has to be differentiated from protection due to interference between the tachycardia and the extraneous impulse, the interference due to a physiological refractory state of the surrounding tissue induced by the rapidly discharging ventricular focus. It follows that the parasystolic nature of a tachycardia can be proved only when the rate of the tachycardia is sufficiently slow for the heart, including the pacemaker, to recover its excitability. Clinically the combination of a sufficiently slow rate of the parasystolic tachycardia and presence of an appropriately timed extraneous impulse is rare, so that proof of parasystolic nature of a tachycardia may be difficult. The concept of protection of a pacemaker due to physiological interference is illustrated in Figure 7–55.

Occasionally parasystolic ventricular tachycardia is associated with exit block and a slow manifest heart rate. In such cases the presence of an underlying regular rapid parasystolic focus is suggested when long cycles are multiples of the shortest manifest cycle.

Sinus parasystole has been reported, but such observations are infrequent because the sinus node is rarely protected.[289]

SUPERNORMAL CONDUCTION AND EXCITATION

Supernormal conduction[319] should be differentiated from supernormality of excitability. The latter indicates that a

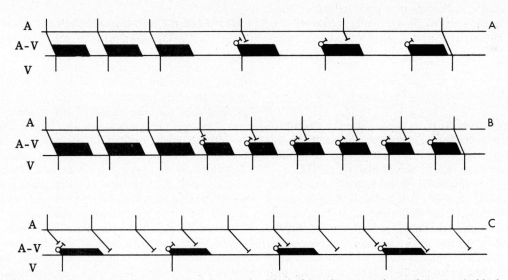

FIGURE 7–55 Diagram of AV dissociation due to physiological interference and complete organic block. *A*, Slowing of the sinus rate is associated with AV junctional escape rhythm. The escape impulse induces a physiological refractoriness that blocks atrial conduction. Dissociation is thus due to physiological interference. *B*, Junctional tachycardia interrupts the sinus rhythm. Each junctional impulse induces a refractory period during which atrial impulses fail to reach the ventricle, resulting in AV dissociation due to physiological refractoriness. In *A* and *B*, absence of organic block is evident by normal AV conduction when the atrial impulse "clears" the refractory period. Refractoriness also protects the junctional pacemaker from being affected by the atrial impulse. *C*, The ventricular rate is regular and slow and the atrial rate exceeds the ventricular rate, a finding not present in *A* and *B*. Because of the slow rate, AV conduction has ample opportunity to recover and conduct but fails to do so, indicating presence of complete organic AV block. A = atrium, AV = AV nodal (junctional) conduction; V = ventricle; black bar = AV nodal refractory period.

subthreshold stimulus falling within the supernormal period of recovery elicits a propagated response—in other words, its stimulus strength becomes threshold. The phenomenon is commonly seen in the presence of malfunctioning artificial cardiac pacemakers. Pacemaker stimuli that otherwise fail to elicit a propagated response may do so when falling on the downstroke of the T wave, the supernormal period of cardiac recovery, and elicit a propagated ventricular response.

Since supernormality of conduction is a manifestation of depressed tissue and while conduction is slower than normal but more rapid than would be expected under the circumstances, the term *relative supernormality* is more appropriate.[320] Supernormality of conduction has been invoked to explain more rapid AV conduction than expected or conduction when AV block is expected. Similarly, supernormal conduction has been suggested as a mechanism of alternation of the P-R interval with a paradoxical R-P/P-R relationship.

Supernormality of intraventricular conduction is suspected when unexpected normalization of intraventricular conduction occurs at a cycle length shorter than that of the prolonged QRS complexes (Fig. 7–52).[321] In WPW, supernormality of conduction of the anomalous pathway has been reported.[111]

While existence of supernormality of intraventricular conduction is accepted,[322] supernormality of AV conduction is questioned on both experimental and clinical grounds. In a comprehensive review of the subject, a variety of mechanisms have been proposed that could explain paradoxical improvement of conduction without invoking supernormality of conduction. Some of the mechanisms suggested include ventricular fusion, equalization of conduction in both bundles (Fig. 7–52), the gap phenomenon (Fig. 7–55), retrograde excitation of a nonconducting bundle by a PVC, "peeling back" of AV nodal refractories, a vagal effect on conduction, and dual AV nodal conduction.[323]

WENCKEBACH STRUCTURE (See also p. 730)

The Wenckebach (type I) block was originally described as a form of AV conduction abnormality characterized by a gradual prolongation of the P-R interval leading to failure of atrial conduction and a ventricular pause (Fig. 7–50).[324] While the P-R interval is progressively longer, the increment is gradually smaller, so that the R-R cycle gradually shortens. Return of the P-R interval to its control state following the long pause, coupled with the longest P-R interval immediately prior to the blocked P wave, cause the long R-R cycle to be shorter than the two preceding ventricular cycles. Similarly, the R-R cycle preceding the blocked P wave is shorter than the R-R cycle immediately following the pause. This R-R structure is not essential for the diagnosis of AV nodal Wenckebach, because the gradual prolongation of P-R is evident in the ECG. However, Wenckebach block can be a manifestation of conduction of an impulse originating anywhere in the heart, and the delayed conduction, the exit delay per se, may not be evident on the surface ECG. It can be recognized only by the Wenckebach structure of the manifest waves, either P or

QRS. Wenckebach block has been described in conjunction with impulses originating in the sinoatrial nodal,[325] ectopic atrial,[326] AV nodal (Fig. 7–48),[254] Purkinje (Fig. 7–46), and perhaps ventricular myocardial foci[327] and impulses generated by artificial pacing.[328]

Wenckebach-type conduction delay has been described in the bundle branches and the divisions of the left bundle.[329] In the former, the block is identified by a sequence of gradual prolongations of bundle branch duration, beginning with a normal QRS complex and ending with a complete BBB.

In the presence of Wenckebach exit from a sinoatrial, AV junctional, or ventricular pacemaker, the true basic interectopic interval of the pacemaker itself is estimated by measuring the interval from the wave initiating the Wenckebach sequence (P-P for exit from sinoatrial pacemaker and R-R for exit from the AV nodal junctional or ventricular pacemaker) to the wave terminating the long pause. This interval is divided by the number of manifest P-P or R-R cycles, adding one in order to account for cycle lost because of the block of an impulse. Having identified and plotted the interectopic intervals, and the manifest P or QRS and by joining the two (Lewis diagram), conduction time from the ectopic focus to the manifest P wave or QRS complex can be estimated. This method is applicable provided that the ectopic rhythm is regular and the exit delay follows the classic Wenckebach pattern. The method of estimating the interectopic interval and conduction time to the surrounding tissue is shown in Figure 7–48.

The precise mechanism responsible for the Wenckebach block is unclear. Decremental conduction, inhomogeneity of the wavefront, concealed reentry, and concealed conduction have all been invoked.

INTERFERENCE AND DISSOCIATION BETWEEN PACEMAKERS (INTERFERENCE DISSOCIATION) (See also p. 735)

Interference between two impulses results from a fortuitous, temporally related discharge of two pacemakers. When the interference is between atrial and ventricular pacemakers and the point of interference is in the AV junction, AV dissociation results (Fig. 7–56). The currently accepted definition of interference is one of failure of conduction because of physiological refractoriness. This definition is in keeping with known electrophysiological mechanisms of conduction or refractoriness or both.[330] Dissociation due to physiological refractoriness (interference) should be differentiated from that due to organic block. Dissociation due to physiological interference may involve isolated impulses or a train of impulses lasting for varying periods of time. AV dissociation due to physiological refractoriness of the AV node is illustrated diagrammatically in Figure 7–55. Although dissociation due to interference usually refers to AV dissociation, interference between two impulses originating within a single chamber and between impulses originating in either cardiac chamber and the AV junction are occasionally encountered.

In the atrium, an early atrial premature complex (APC) reaching the sinoatrial node when the nodal or perinodal tissue is refractory, results in interference between the sinoatrial node and the APC, and an interpolated APC is re-

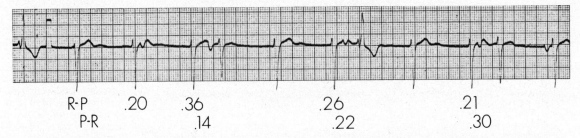

R-P .20 .36 .26 .21
P-R .14 .22 .30

FIGURE 7–56 Gap phenomenon. The tracing shows sinus bradycardia with AV dissociation and occasional ventricular capture. A P wave with an R-P interval of 0.21 sec is followed by a normal QRS, while a P wave with an R-P interval of 0.26 sec results in a QRS complex with RBBB. This paradox is explained by the fact that the P wave that follows the shorter R-P interval is delayed in the AV junction, the P-R interval prolonged to 0.30 sec allowing the RBB to recover. On the other hand, the P wave preceded by a longer R-P interval, measuring 0.26 sec, conducts more rapidly, with a P-R interval of 0.22 sec, and reaches the RBB before it had a chance to recover, so that RBBB results.

corded. Similarly, intraatrial interference is noted when a junctional impulse activates the atrium simultaneously with a sinus impulse. The result is an atrial fusion.

Interference between atrial impulses and a more rapid junctional rhythm due either to inappropriate acceleration of the junctional pacemaker or to slowing of the sinus rate results in AV dissociation.[330–332] Rarely, AV dissociation results from interference between two junctional impulses, a double junctional rhythm.[265] All forms of ventricular rhythm, VPC, ventricular tachycardia, fascicular tachycardia, and accelerated idioventricular rhythm may lead to AV dissociation because of interference between the retrograde ventricular and antegrade conduction of an atrial or junctional impulse. An atrial or junctional impulse may reach the ventricle only to find parts of the ventricle refractory because of activation by an ectopic ventricular impulse, resulting in QRS fusion. Dissociated atrial and junctional foci may synchronize[331] their rates and rhythms and maintain this entrainment for a prolonged period of time. The mechanism of such synchronization is not clear.[333] AV dissociation due to physiological interference may be enhanced by a simultaneous delay of AV conduction. The latter is suggested by failure of P waves to conduct when such conduction would normally be expected. Although both the refractoriness and delayed conduction contribute to the AV dissociation, the relative contribution of each is difficult, if not impossible, to quantitate from the ECG.

VENTRICULOATRIAL AND UNIDIRECTIONAL CONDUCTION
(See also p. 623)

Retrograde conduction in the presence of normal antegrade conduction is a common phenomenon and frequently accompanies VPC[334] and ventricular tachycardia.[335] One-to-one retrograde ventriculoatrial conduction in ventricular tachycardia makes differentiation of supraventricular arrhythmia with aberrancy and ventricular tachycardia from the surface ECG practically impossible.

Unidirectional conduction has been documented experimentally[336,337] and clinically. Retrograde AV conduction in the presence of complete antegrade block is an electrocardiographic example of unidirectional conduction (Fig. 7–57). A number of mechanisms have been proposed to explain this observation,[336] including mechanical stimulation

of the atrium by ventricular contraction, stimulation by ventricular contraction of a latent ectopic pacemaker located above the site of AV block, and retrograde conduction along an anomalous or normal AV pathway. Retrograde conduction over a normal AV pathway is the mechanism most widely accepted and supported by clinical and experimental observations. Retrograde conduction with an R-P interval of 0.10 to 0.11 sec may be recorded in the presence of complete anterograde block, supporting the early experimental observation that normal unidirectional conduction can coexist with complete block in an opposite direction. Unidirectional retrograde conduction has been documented following VPC, idioventricular rhythm, and ventricular pacing.[338]

EXIT BLOCK. Exit block is defined as failure of an ectopic impulse to propagate. The most commonly recognized example is sinoatrial exit block (p. 691). Experimental[327,339] and clinical observations suggest that exit block is due largely to delay or failure of impulse propagation and not to abnormal impulse formation. The concept of exit block was first proposed to explain failure of a parasystolic impulse to manifest when the heart was not refractory.[314] It has subsequently been shown to be a property of all spontaneous and artificial pacemaker–induced rhythms.[340,341]

Exit block can manifest the Wenckebach (type I) (Figs. 7–46 and 7–48) or Mobitz (type II) structure. The Wenckebach structure may be identified by the P-P or R-R interval. Type II exit block is suggested by a long pause that is a multiple of the basic cycle length. Even in type II block, however, the long cycle may be slightly shorter than a multiple of the basic cycle length, since conduction from the focus terminating the long cycle may be slightly more rapid than that preceding the exit block. Exit block may fail to conform to either type I or type II block. If the basic P-P or R-R cycles are irregular, a diagnosis of exit block is impossible.

By definition, the diagnosis of exit block can be entertained only when failure of conduction occurs at a time when the surrounding myocardium is not refractory; otherwise, failure of propagation is a manifestation of interference.

ENTRANCE BLOCK. Entrance block is present when an impulse fails to reach and discharge, suppress, or reset a pacemaker. Such an entrance block is, for example, an integral component of parasystole and of some cases inter-

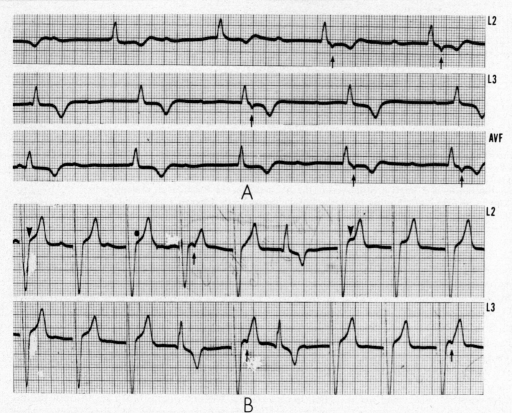

FIGURE 7–57   Unidirectional block. A, Complete antegrade AV block with an occasional negative retrograde P wave (↑) and a normal R-P interval. A similar relationship is seen in B, recorded from the same patient, in which the pacemaker-activated QRS is followed by a retrograde P wave (↑) with normal conduction measured from the pacemaker artifact to the retrograde P. Failure to record a retrograde P wave may be due to failure of retrograde conduction, antegrade conduction of a sinus P with resultant refractoriness of the AV node, or absolute refractoriness of the atrium following a sinus P wave. Although it may be impossible to differentiate between the three mechanisms, on the basis of the temporal P-QRS relationship, one may postulate antegrade activation of the AV node with refractoriness of the AV node (●) and similarly absolute refractoriness of the atrium (▼).

polated APC. Failure to affect a pacemaker early in the cycle when the area surrounding the pacemaker is still refractory is an expected and physiological phenomenon. Such a protective mechanism is not true entrance block but interference between two foci due to physiological refractoriness. Failure to discharge a focus after the latter recovers, however, denotes true entrance block. The impulse is most likely blocked in the tissue surrounding the site of impulse formation.

GAP PHENOMENON. This phenomenon is recognized by the paradox of improved distal conduction associated with earlier excitation (Fig. 7–56). The more premature the impulse, the longer the proximal delay allowing the distal tissue to recover more fully with improvement or normalization of distal conduction. The gap phenomenon has been documented in the dog and in man.[299,342] Type I gap is present with a proximal delay in the AV node, which allows the His and infra-His tissues to recover. Type II gap is present when the delay occurs in the proximal His system, allowing the more distal His-Purkinje system to recover.[343] It has been suggested that the gap phenomenon can occur between any two tissues of the conducting system provided that (1) the effective refractory period of the distal tissue is longer than the functional refractory period of the proximal tissue and (2) the relative refractory period of the proximal tissue allows for sufficient delay for the distal tissue to recover.

The two types of gap cannot be differentiated with certainty on the ECG. It has been suggested that a normal QRS complex is in keeping with type I gap,[343] although equal delay in both bundles cannot be ruled out. An abnormal QRS complex is consistent with either type I or type II gap.

Conduction of APC may be associated with the gap phenomenon. As the APC becomes progressively more premature, AV conduction may be blocked, only to resume at a shorter coupling interval (type I gap). Similarly, a gradual shortening of the coupling may result in BBB, usually on the right, and the QRS complex may normalize with further shortening of the coupling interval (Fig. 7–56).

Paradoxical improvement of conduction with shorter coupling intervals has also been ascribed to supernormality of AV conduction. Assuming that supernormality of AV conduction exists, a differential diagnosis between the gap phenomenon and true supernormality of AV conduction is impossible on the basis of ECG findings.[344]

We wish to acknowledge the advice and counsel of Dr. Marvin Dunn, Chief of Cardiology, University of Kansas School of Medicine, in the preparation of this chapter.

References

1. Scher, A. M., and Spach, M. S.: Cardiac depolarization and repolarization and the electrocardiogram. In Berne, R. M., Sperelakis, N., and Geiger, S. R. (eds.): Handbook of Physiology, The Cardiovascular System. Vol. I., Sect. 2. Bethesda, Md., American Physiological Society, 1979, pp. 357–392.
2. Burch, G. E., and DePasquale, N. P.: A History of Electrocardiography. Chicago, Year Book Medical Publishers, 1964.
3. Waller, A. D.: A demonstration on man of electromotive changes accompanying the heart's beat. J. Physiol. 8:229, 1887.
4. Einthoven, W.: Selected Papers on Electrocardiography. Edited by A. Snellen. Leiden, University Press, 1977.
5. Lewis, T.: The Mechanism and Graphic Registration of the Heart Beat. London, Shaw and Sons, Ltd., 1920, p. 228.
6. Wilson, F. N.: Selected Papers. Edited by F. D. Johnston and E. Lepeschkin. Ann Arbor, Mich., Edward Brothers, Inc., 1954.
7. Pardee, H. E. B.: Clinical Aspects of the Electrocardiogram. New York, Paul B. Hoeber, Inc., 1924.

8. Lepeschkin, E.: Modern Electrocardiography. Baltimore, Md., Williams and Wilkins Co., 1951.
9. Barker, J. M.: The Unipolar Electrocardiogram: A Clinical Interpretation. New York, Appleton-Century-Crofts, Inc., 1952.
10. Sodi-Pallares, D.: New Bases of Electrocardiography. St. Louis, The C. V. Mosby Co., 1956.
11. Cooksey, J. D., Dunn, M., and Massie, E.: Clinical Vectorcardiography and Electrocardiography. 2nd ed. Chicago, Year Book Medical Publishers, 1977.
12. Fisch, C.: The clinical electrocardiogram: A classic. American Heart Association. Lewis A. Connor Memorial Lecture. Circulation 62 (Suppl. III):1, 1980.
13. Craib, W. H.: A study of the electrical field surrounding active heart muscle. Heart 14:71, 1927.
14. Wilson, F. N., MacLeod, A. G., and Barker, P. S.: The distribution of the action currents produced by the heart muscle and other excitable tissues immersed in extensive conducting media. J. Gen. Physiol. 16:423, 1933.
15. Scher, A. M.: Electrocardiogram. In Ruch, T. C., and Patton, H. D. (eds.): Physiology and Biophysics. 20th ed. Philadelphia, W. B. Saunders Co., 1974, pp. 67–68.
16. Wolff, L.: Electrocardiography: Fundamentals and Clinical Application. 3rd ed. Philadelphia, W. B. Saunders Co., 1962, p. 15.
17. Durrer, D., VanDam, R. T., Freud, G. E., Janse, M. J., Meijler, F. L., and Arzbaecher, R. C.: Total excitation of the isolated human heart. Circulation 41:899, 1970.
18. James, T. N., and Sherf, L.: Specialized tissues and preferential conduction in the atria of the heart. Am. J. Cardiol. 28:414, 1971.
19. Spach, M. S., Miller, W. T., III, Dolber, P. D., Kootsey, J. M., Sommer, J. R., and Mosher, C. E., Jr.: The functional role of structural complexities in the propagation of depolarization in the atrium of the dog: Cardiac conduction disturbances due to discontinuities of effective atrial resistivity. Circ. Res. 50:175, 1982.
20. Hoffman, B. F., and Cranefield, P. F.: Electrophysiology of the Heart. New York, McGraw-Hill Book Co., 1960.
21. Wyndham, C. R., Meeran, M. K., Smith, T., Sazena, A., Engelman, R. M., Levitsky, S., and Rosen, K. M.: Epicardial activation of the intact human heart without conduction defect. Circulation 59:161, 1979.
22. Wilson, F. N., MacLeod, A. G., Barker, P. S., and Johnston, F. D.: The determination and the significance of the areas of the ventricular deflections of the electrocardiogram. Am. Heart J. 10:46, 1934.
23. Wilson, F. N., Johnston, F. D., Rosenbaum, F. F., Erlanger, H., Kossmann, C. E., Hecht, H., Cotrim, N., de Oliveira, R. M., Scarsi, R., and Barker, P. S.: The precordial electrocardiogram. Am. Heart J. 27:19, 1944.
24. Tranchesi, J., Adelardi, V., and de Oliveira, J. M.: Atrial repolarization—Its importance in clinical electrocardiography. Circulation 22:635, 1960.
25. Burger, H. C., and Van Milaan, J. B.: Heart—Vector and leads. Br. Heart J. 9:154, 1947.
26. Lepeschkin, E.: U wave of the electrocardiogram. Arch. Intern. Med. 96:600, 1955.
27. Lepeschkin, E., Katz, L. N., Schaefer, H., Shanes, A. M., and Weidmann, S.: The U wave and afterpotentials in cardiac muscle: Panel discussion. Ann. NY Acad. Sci. 65:942, 1957.
28. Watanabe, Y.: Purkinje repolarization as a possible cause of U wave in the electrocardiogram. Circulation 51:1030, 1975.
29. Lepeschkin, E.: Physiological basis of the U wave. In Schlant, R. C., and Hurst, J. W. (eds.): Advances in Electrocardiography. New York, Grune and Stratton, 1972, pp. 431–477.
30. Kishida, H., Cole, J. S., and Surawicz, B.: Negative U wave: A highly specific but poorly understood sign of heart disease. Am. J. Cardiol. 49:2030, 1982.
31. Lepeschkin, E.: The U wave of the electrocardiogram. Mod. Concepts Cardiovasc. Dis. 38:39, 1969.
32. Bazett, H. C.: An analysis of the time-relations of electrocardiograms. Heart 7:353, 1920.
33. Fisch, C.: The electrocardiogram in the aged. Cardiovasc. Clin. 12:65, 1981.
34. Manning, G. W.: Electrocardiography in selection of Royal Canadian Air Force crew. Circulation 10:401, 1954.
35. Burch, G. E., Abildskov, J. A., and Cronvich, J. A.: Spatial Vectorcardiography. Philadelphia, Lea and Febiger, 1953.
36. Grishman, A., and Scherlis, L.: Spatial Vectorcardiography. Philadelphia, W. B. Saunders Co., 1953.
37. Chou, T. C., Helm, R. A., and Kaplan, S.: Clinical Vectorcardiography. 2nd ed. New York, Grune and Stratton, 1974.
38. Benchimol, A.: Vectorcardiography. 2nd ed. New York, Robert E. Krieger Publishing Co., 1975.
39. Mann, H.: A method of analyzing the electrocardiogram. Arch. Intern. Med. 25:283, 1920.
40. Wilson, F. N., and Johnston, F. D.: The vectorcardiogram. Am. Heart J. 16:14, 1938.
41. Frank, E.: An accurate clinically practical system for spatial vectorcardiography. Circulation 13:737, 1956.
42. Helm, R. A.: An accurate lead system for spatial vectorcardiography. Am. Heart J. 53:415, 1957.
43. McFee, R., and Parungao, A.: An orthogonal lead system for clinical electrocardiography. Am. Heart J. 62:93, 1961.
44. Duchosal, P. W., and Grosgurin, J. R.: The spatial vectorcardiogram obtained by the use of trihedron and its scalar comparisons. Circulation 5:237, 1952.

45. McCall, B. W., Wallace, A. G., and Estes, E. H., Jr.: Characteristics of the normal vectorcardiogram recorded with the Frank lead system. Am. J. Cardiol. 10:514, 1962.
46. Draper, H. W., Peffer, C. J., Stallman, F. W., Littmann, D., and Pipberger, H. V.: The corrected orthogonal electrocardiogram and vectorcardiogram in 510 normal men (Frank lead system). Circulation 30:853, 1964.
47. Pipberger, H. V., Goldman, M. J., Littmann, D., Murphy, G. P., Cosma, J., and Snyder, J. R.: Correlations of the orthogonal electrocardiogram and vectorcardiogram with constitutional variables in 518 normal men. Circulation 35:536, 1967.
48. Abildskov, J. A., Burgess, M. J., Urie, P. M., Lux, R. L., and Wyatt, R. F.: The unidentified information content of the electrocardiogram. Circ. Res. 40:3, 1977.
49. Vincent, G. M., Abildskov, J. A., Burgess, M. J., Millar, K., Lux, R. L., and Wyatt, R. F.: Diagnosis of old inferior myocardial infarction by body surface isopotential mapping. Am. J. Cardiol. 39:510, 1977.
50. De Ambroggi, L., Taccardi, B., and Macchi, E.: Body surface maps of heart potentials. Tentative localization of pre-exited areas in 42 Wolff-Parkinson-White patients. Circulation 54:251, 1976.
51. Iwa, T., and Magara, T.: Correlation between localization of accessory conduction pathway and body surface maps in Wolff-Parkinson-White syndrome. Jap. Circ. J. 45:1192, 1981.
52. Holt, J. H., Barnard, A. C. L., and Lynn, M. S.: A study of human heart as a multiple dipole electrical source. II. Diagnosis and quantitation of left ventricular hypertrophy; III. Diagnosis and quantitation of right ventricular hypertrophy. Circulation 40:697, 1969.
53. Maroko, P. R., Libby, P., Lovell, J. W., Sobel, B. E., Moss, J., and Braunwald, E.: Precordial S-T segment elevation mapping: An atraumatic method for assessing alterations in the extent of myocardial ischemic injury. Am. J. Cardiol. 29:223, 1972.
54. Muller, J. E., Maroko, P. R., and Braunwald, E.: Precordial electrocardiographic mapping. A technique to assess the efficacy of intervention designed to limit infarct size. Circulation 57:1, 1978.
55. Lux, R. L., Burgess, M. J., Wyatt, R. F., Evans, A. K., Vincent, G. M., and Abildskov, J. A.: Clinically practical lead systems for improved electrocardiography: Comparison with precordial grids and conventional lead systems. Circulation 59:356, 1979.
56. Grant, R. P.: Clinical Electrocardiography: The Spatial Vector Approach. New York, McGraw-Hill Book Co., Blakiston Division, 1957, p. 47.
57. Fisch, C.: The electrocardiogram in the aged: An independent marker of heart disease? Am. J. Med. 70:4, 1981.
58. Chou, T. C., and Helm, R. A.: The pseudo P pulmonale. Circulation 32:96, 1965.
59. Morris, J. J., Estes, E. H., Whalen, R. E., Thompson, H. K., and McIntosh, H. D.: P wave analysis in valvular heart disease. Circulation 29:242, 1964.
60. Haywood, L. J., and Selvester, R. H.: Analysis of right and left atrial vectorcardiograms. Circulation 33:577, 1966.
61. Zoneraich, O., and Zoneraich, S.: Intraatrial conduction disturbances: Vectorcardiographic patterns. Am. J. Cardiol. 37:736, 1976.
62. Spodick, D. H.: Diagnostic electrocardiographic sequences in acute pericarditis. Significance of PR segment and PR vector changes. Circulation 48:575, 1973.
63. Zimmerman, H. A., Bersano, E., and Dicosky, C.: The Auricular Electrocardiogram. Springfield, Ill., Charles C Thomas, 1968.
64. Cushing, E. H., Feil, H. S., Stanton, E. J., and Wartman, W. B.: Infarction of the cardiac auricles (atria): Clinical, pathological and experimental studies. Br. Heart J. 4:17, 1942.
65. Gardin, J. M., and Singer, D. H.: Atrial infarction. Importance, diagnosis and localization. Arch. Intern. Med. 141:1345, 1981.
66. Sanders, A.: Experimental localized auricular necrosis: An electrocardiographic study. Am. J. Med. Sci. 198:690, 1939.
67. Brody, D. A.: A theoretical analysis of intracavitary blood mass influence on the heart–lead relationship. Circ. Res. 4:731, 1956.
68. Battler, A., Froelicher, V. F., Gallagher, K. P., Kumada, T., McKown, D., Kemper, W. S., and Ross, J., Jr.: Effects of changes in ventricular size on regional and surface QRS amplitudes in the conscious dog. Circulation 62:174, 1980.
69. Sokolow, M., and Lyon, T. P.: The ventricular complex in left ventricular hypertrophy as obtained by unipolar precordial and limb leads. Am. Heart J. 37:161, 1949.
70. Romhilt, D. W., Bove, K. E., and Norris, R. J.: A critical appraisal of the electrocardiographic criteria for the diagnosis of left ventricular hypertrophy. Circulation 40:185, 1969.
71. Reichek, N., and Devereux, R. B.: Left ventricular hypertrophy: Relationship of anatomic, echocardiographic and electrocardiographic findings. Circulation 63:1391, 1981.
72. Cumming, G. R., and Proudfit, W. L.: High-voltage QRS complexes in the absence of left ventricular hypertrophy. Circulation 19:406, 1959.
73. Cabrera, E., and Gaxiola, A.: A critical re-evaluation of systolic and diastolic overloading patterns. Progr. Cardiovasc. Dis. 2:219, 1959.
74. Wallace, A. G., McCall, B. W., and Estes, E. H., Jr.: The vectorcardiogram in left ventricular hypertrophy; a study of the Frank lead system. Am. Heart J. 63:466, 1962.
75. Abbott-Smith, C. W., and Chou, T.-C.: Vectorcardiographic criteria for the diagnosis of left ventricular hypertrophy. Am. Heart J. 79:361, 1970.

76. Scott, R. C.: The electrocardiographic diagnosis of right ventricular hypertrophy: correlation with anatomic findings. Am. Heart J. 60:659, 1960.

77. Burch, G. E., and DePasquale, N. P.: Electrocardiography in the Diagnosis of Congenital Heart Disease. Philadelphia, Lea and Febiger, 1967.

78. Benchimol, A., and Tio, S.: Early involuntary vectorcardiographic signs of right ventricular hypertrophy. Am. Heart J. 80:19, 1970.

79. Hugenholtz, P. G., and Gamboa, R.: Effect of chronically increased ventricular pressure on electrical forces of the heart. Circulation 30:511, 1964.

80. Dodge, H. T., and Grant, R. P.: Mechanisms of QRS complex prolongation in man. Right ventricular conduction defects. Am. J. Med. 21:534, 1956.

81. Grant, R. P., and Dodge, H. T.: Mechanisms of QRS complex prolongation in man: Left ventricular conduction disturbances. Am. J. Med. 20:834, 1956.

82. Becker, R. A., Scher, A. N., and Erickson, R. V.: Ventricular excitation in experimental left bundle branch block. Am. Heart J. 55:547, 1958.

83. Rodriguez, M. I., and Sodi-Pallares, D.: The mechanism of complete and incomplete bundle branch block. Am. Heart J. 44:715, 1952.

84. Haft, J. I., Herman, M. V., and Gorlin, R.: Left bundle branch block. Etiologic, hemodynamic and ventriculographic considerations. Circulation 43:279, 1971.

85. Sodi-Pallares, D., Bisteni, A., Testelli, M. R., and Medrano, G. A.: Ventricular activation and the vectorcardiogram in bundle-branch blocks: Clinical and experimental studies with a critical appraisal of the vectorcardiographic methods of Frank and Grishman. Circ. Res. 9:1098, 1961.

86. Wallace, A. G., Estes, E. F., and McCall, B. W.: The vectorcardiographic findings in left bundle branch block: A study using the Frank lead system. Am. Heart J. 63:508, 1962.

87. Baydar, I. D., Walsh, T. J., and Massie, E.: A vectorcardiographic study of right bundle branch block with the Frank lead system: Clinical correlation in ventricular hypertrophy and chronic pulmonary disease. Am. J. Cardiol. 15:185, 1965.

88. Penaloza, D., Gamboa, R., and Sime, F.: Experimental right bundle branch block in the normal human heart: Electrocardiographic, vectorcardiographic and hemodynamic observations. Am. J. Cardiol. 8:767, 1961.

89. Watt, T. B., Murao, S., and Pruitt, R. D.: Left axis deviation induced experimentally in a primate heart. Am. Heart J. 70:381, 1965.

90. Watt, T. B., Jr., Freud, G. E., Durrer, D., and Pruitt, R. D.: Left anterior arborization block combined with right bundle branch block in canine and primate hearts. An electrocardiographic study. Circ. Res. 22:57, 1968.

91. Rosenbaum, M. B., Elizari, M. V., and Lazzari, J. O.: The Hemiblocks: New Concepts of Intraventricular Conduction Based on Human Anatomical, Physiological and Clinical Studies. Oldsmar, Fla., Tampa Tracings, 1970.

92. Rosenbaum, M. B.: The hemiblocks: Diagnostic criteria and clinical significance. Mod. Concepts Cardiovasc. Dis. 39:141, 1970.

93. McHenry, P. L., Phillips, J. F., Fisch, C., and Corya, B. R.: Right precordial qrS pattern due to left anterior hemiblock. Am. Heart J. 81:498, 1971.

94. Kulbertus, H., Collignon, P., and Humblet, L.: Vectorcardiographic study of QRS loop in patients with left superior axis deviation and right bundle branch block. Br. Heart J. 32:386, 1971.

95. Lemberg, L., Castellanos, A., Jr., and Arcebal, A. G.: The vectorcardiogram in acute left anterior hemiblock. Am. J. Cardiol. 28:483, 1971.

96. Benchimol, A., and Desser, K. B.: The Frank vectorcardiogram in left posterior hemiblock. J. Electrocardiol. 4:129, 1971.

97. Rosenbaum, M. B., Elizari, M. V., Lazzari, J. O., Nau, G. J., Levi, R. J., and Halpern, M. S.: Intraventricular trifascicular blocks. The syndrome of right bundle branch block with intermittent left anterior and posterior hemiblock. Am. Heart J. 78:306, 1969.

98. Medrano, G. A., Brenes, C. P., De Micheli, A., and Sodi-Pallares, D.: Clinical electrocardiographic and vectorcardiographic diagnosis of left anterior subdivision block isolated or associated with RBBB. Am. Heart J. 83:447, 1972.

99. Varriale, P., and Kennedy, R. J.: Right bundle branch block and left posterior fascicular block: Vectorcardiographic and clinical features. Am. J. Cardiol. 29:459, 1972.

100. Lepeschkin, E.: The electrocardiographic diagnosis of bilateral bundle branch block in relation to heart block. Progr. Cardiovasc. Dis. 6:445, 1964.

101. Wolff, L., Parkinson, J., and White, P. D.: Bundle-branch block with short P-R interval in healthy young people prone to paroxysmal tachycardia. Am. Heart J. 5:685, 1930.

102. Oehnell, R. F.: Pre-excitation, a cardiac abnormality. Acta Med. Scand. (Suppl.) 152:1, 1944.

103. Wilson, F. N.: A case in which the vagus influenced the form of the ventricular complex of the electrocardiogram. Arch. Intern. Med. 16:1008, 1915.

104. Cohn, A. E., and Fraser, F. R.: Paroxysmal tachycardia and the effect of stimulation of the vagus nerves by pressure. Heart 5:93, 1913.

105. Holzmann, N., and Scherf, D.: Ueber Elektrokardiogramme mit verkuerzter Vorhof-Kammer-Distanz und positiven P-Zacken. Z. Klin. Med. 121:404, 1932.

106. Lev, M., Fox, S. M., Bharati, S., and Greenfield, S. L., Jr.: Mahaim and James fibers as a basis for a unique variety of ventricular preexcitation. Am. J. Cardiol. 36:880, 1975.

107. Fisch, C., Pinsky, S. T., and Shields, J. P.: Wolff-Parkinson-White syndrome. Report of a case associated with wandering pacemaker, atrial tachycardia, atrial fibrillation and incomplete A-V dissociation with interference. Circulation 16:1004, 1957.

108. Rosenbaum, F. F., Hecht, H. H., Wilson, F. N., and Johnston, F. D.: The

109. Lown, B., Ganong, W. F., and Levine, S. A.: The syndrome of short P-R interval, normal QRS complex and paroxysmal rapid heart action. Circulation 5:693, 1952.

tential variations of the thorax and the esophagus in anomalous atrioventricular excitation (Wolff-Parkinson-White syndrome). Am. Heart J. 29:281, 1945.

110. Pick, A., and Fisch, C.: Ventricular preexcitation (WPW) in presence of bundle branch block. Am. Heart J. 55:504, 1958.

111. McHenry, P. L., Knoebel, S. B., and Fisch, C.: The Wolff-Parkinson-White (WPW) syndrome with supernormal conduction through the anomalous bypass. Circulation 34:734, 1966.

112. Tonkin, A. M., Wagner, G. S., Gallagher, J. J., and Lope, G. D.: Initial forces of ventricular depolarization in the Wolff-Parkinson-White syndrome. Analysis based upon localization of the accessory pathway by epicardial mapping. Circulation 52:1030, 1975.

113. Eppinger, H., and Rothberger, J.: Ueber die folgender Durchschneidung der Tawaraschen Schenkel des Reizleitungssystems. Ztschr. f. Klin. Med. 19:1, 1910.

114. Smith, F. N.: The ligation of coronary arteries with electrocardiographic study. Arch. Intern. Med. 22:8, 1918.

115. Pardee, H. E. B.: An electrocardiographic sign of coronary artery obstruction. Arch. Intern. Med. 26:244, 1920.

116. Bayley, R. H., LaDue, J. S., and York, D. J.: Electrocardiographic changes (local ventricular ischemia and injury) produced in the dog by temporary occlusion of a coronary artery, showing a new state in the evaluation of myocardial infarction. Am. Heart J. 27:164, 1944.

117. Bayley, R. H., LaDue, J. S., and York, D. J.: Further observations on the ischemia-injury pattern produced in the dog by temporary occlusion of a coronary artery. Incomplete T division patterns, theophylline T reversion, and theophylline conversion of the negative T pattern. Am. Heart J. 27:657, 1944.

118. Bayley, R. H., and LaDue, J. S.: Electrocardiographic changes of impending infarction, and the ischemia-injury pattern produced in the dog by total and subtotal occlusion of a coronary artery. Am. Heart J. 28:54, 1944.

119. Ekmekci, A., Toyoshima, H., Kwocyznski, J. K., Nagaya, T., and Prinzmetal, M.: Angina pectoris. V. Giant R and receding S wave in myocardial ischemia and certain nonischemic conditions. Am. J. Cardiol. 7:521, 1961.

120. Holland, R. P., and Brooks, H.: Precordial and epicardial surface potentials during myocardial ischemia in the pig. A theoretical and experimental analysis of the TQ and ST segments. Circ. Res. 37:471, 1975.

121. Maseri, A., L'Abbate, A., Baroldi, G., Chierchia, S., Marzilli, M., Ballestra, A. M., Severi, S., Parodi, O., Biagini, A., Distante, A., and Pesola, A.: Coronary vasospasm as a possible cause of myocardial infarction. A conclusion derived from the study of "preinfarction" angina. N. Engl. J. Med. 299:1271, 1978.

122. Madias, J. E.: The earliest electrocardiographic sign of acute transmural myocardial infarction. J. Electrocardiol. 10:193, 1977.

123. Surawicz, B.: The pathogenesis and clinical significance of primary T-wave abnormalities. In Schlant, R. C., and Hurst, J. W. (eds.): Advances in Electrocardiography. New York, Grune and Stratton, 1972, pp. 377–421.

124. Samson, W. E., and Scher, A. N.: Mechanism of S-T segment alteration during acute myocardial injury. Circ. Res. 8:780, 1960.

125. Vincent, G. M., Abildskov, J. A., and Burgess, M. J.: Mechanisms of ischemic ST-segment displacement. Evaluation by direct current recordings. Circulation 56:559, 1977.

126. Wilson, F. N., Hill, I. G. W., and Johnston, F. D.: The form of the electrocardiogram in experimental myocardial infarction. III. The later effects produced by ligation of the anterior descending branch of the left coronary artery. Am. Heart J. 10:903, 1935.

127. Wilson, F. N., Johnston, F. D., and Hill, I. G. W.: The form of the electrocardiogram in experimental myocardial infarction. IV. Additional observations on the later effects produced by ligation of the anterior descending branch of the left coronary artery. Am. Heart J. 10:1025, 1935.

128. Kossman, C. E., and de la Chapelle, C. E.: The precordial electrocardiogram in myocardial infarction. Am. Heart J. 15:700, 1938.

129. Prinzmetal, M., Kennamar, R., and Maxwell, M.: Studies on the mechanism of ventricular activity. VIII. The genesis of the coronary QS wave in through-and-through infarction. Am. J. Med. 17:610, 1954.

130. Cook, R. W., Edwards, J. E., and Pruitt, R. D.: Electrocardiographic changes in acute subendocardial infarction. I. Large subendocardial and large nontransmural infarcts. Circulation 18:603, 1958.

131. Cook, R. W., Edwards, J. E., and Pruitt, R. D.: Electrocardiographic changes in acute subendocardial infarction. II. Small subendocardial infarcts. Circulation 18:613, 1958.

132. Wilson, F. N., MacLeod, A. G., Barker, P. S., Johnston, F. D., and Klostermeyer, L. L.: The electrocardiogram in myocardial infarction with particular reference to the initial deflection of the ventricular complex. Heart 16:155, 1933.

133. Behar, S., Schor, S., Kariv, I., Barell, V., and Modan, B.: Evaluation of electrocardiogram in emergency room as a decision-making tool. Chest 71:486, 1977.

134. Gunraj, D. R., and Rajapakse, D. A.: Daily ECG confirmation in acute myocardial infarction. Practitioner 213:361, 1974.

135. McGuinness, J. B., Begg, T. B., and Semple, T.: First electrocardiogram in recent myocardial infarction. Br. Med. J. 2:449, 1976.

136. Short, D.: The earliest electrocardiographic evidence of myocardial infarction. Br. Heart J. 32:6, 1970.

137. Dressler, W., and Roesler, H.: High T waves in the earliest stage of myocardial infarction. Am. Heart J. 34:627, 1947.

138. Mills, R. M., Jr., Young, E., Gorlin, R., and Lesch, M.: Natural history of S-T segment elevation after acute myocardial infarction. Am. J. Cardiol. 35:609, 1975.

139. Thygesen, K., Horder, M., Lyager Nielsen, B., and Hyltoft Petersen, P.: Evolution of ST segment and Q and R waves during early phase of inferior myocardial infarction. Acta Med. Scand. 205:25, 1979.

140. Abbott, J. A., and Scheinman, M. M.: Nondiagnostic electrocardiogram in patients with acute myocardial infarction: Clinical and anatomic correlations. Am. J. Med. 55:608, 1973.

141. Salcedo, J. R., Baird, M. G., Chambers, R. D., and Beanlands, D. S.: Significance of reciprocal ST segment depression in anterior precordial leads in acute inferior myocardial infarction: Concomitant left anterior descending coronary artery disease? Am. J. Cardiol. 48:1003, 1981.

142. Raunio, H., Rissanen, V., Romppanen, T., Jokinen, Y., Rehnberg, S., Helin, M., and Pyörälä, K.: Changes in the QRS complex and ST segment in transmural and subendocardial myocardial infarctions. A clinicopathologic study. Am. Heart J. 98:176, 1979.

143. Morris, S. N., and McHenry, P. L.: Role of exercise stress testing in healthy subjects and patients with coronary heart disease. Am. J. Cardiol. 42:659, 1978.

144. Lepeschkin, E., and Surawicz, B.: Characteristics of true-positive and false-positive results of electrocardiographic master, two-step exercise tests. N. Engl. J. Med. 258:511, 1958.

145. Gerson, M. C., Phillips, J. F., Morris, S. N., and McHenry, P. L.: Exercise-induced U wave inversion as a marker of stenosis of the left anterior descending coronary artery. Circulation 60:1014, 1979.

146. Gerson, M. C., and McHenry, P. L.: Resting U wave inversion as a marker of stenosis of the left anterior descending coronary artery. Am. J. Med. 69:545, 1980.

147. Duke, M.: Isolated U wave inversion in acute myocardial infarction. Cardiology, 60:220, 1975.

148. Solomon, R. B., and Shapiro, H. H.: The electrocardiographic "intermediate phase" of an acute myocardial infarction. Am. Heart J. 71:582, 1966.

149. Hasset, M. A., Williams, R. R., and Wagner, G. S.: Transient QRS simulating myocardial infarction. Circulation 62:975, 1980.

150. Nakagaki, O., Yano, H., Mitsutake, A., Kikuchi, Y., Takeshita, A., Kanaide, H., and Nakamura, M.: Reelevation of ST segment on precordial mapping in natural time course following acute anterior myocardial infarction. Jap. Circ. J. 45:562, 1981.

151. Benchimol, A., Lasry, J. E., and Carvalho, F. R.: The ventricular premature contraction. Its place in the diagnosis of ischemic heart disease. Am. Heart J. 65:334, 1963.

152. Durrer, D., Van Lier, A. A. W., and Böller, J.: Epicardial and intramural excitation in chronic myocardial infarction. Am. Heart J. 68:765, 1964.

153. Gross, H., Rubin, I. L., Laufer, H., and Bloomberg, A. E.: Transient abnormal Q waves in the dog without myocardial infarction. Am. J. Cardiol. 14:669, 1964.

154. Kaplan, B. M., and Berkson, D. M.: Serial electrocardiograms after myocardial infarction. Ann. Intern. Med. 60:430, 1964.

155. Kalbfleisch, J. M., Shadaksharappa, K. S., Conrad, L. L., and Sarkar, N. K.: Disappearance of the Q-deflection following myocardial infarction. Am. Heart J. 76:193, 1968.

156. Horan, L. G., Flowers, N. C., and Johnson, J. C.: Significance of the diagnostic Q wave of myocardial infarction. Circulation 43:428, 1971.

157. Helfant, R. H.: Q waves in coronary heart disease: Newer understanding of their clinical implications (editorial). Am. J. Cardiol. 38:662, 1976.

158. Scott, R. C.: Current concepts of ventricular activation in the normal heart, in left bundle branch block, and in left bundle branch block with myocardial infarction. Am. Heart J. 64:696, 1962.

159. Horan, L. G., Flowers, N. C., Tolleson, W. J., and Thomas, J. R.: The significance of diagnostic Q waves in the presence of bundle branch block. Chest 58:214, 1970.

160. Luy, G., Bahl, O. P., and Massie, E.: Intermittent left bundle branch block. A study of the effects of left bundle branch block on the electrocardiographic patterns of myocardial infarction and ischemia. Am. Heart J. 85:332, 1973.

161. Rosenbaum, F. F., Erlanger, H., Cotrim, N. C., Johnston, F. D., and Wilson, F. N.: The effects of anterior infarction complicated by bundle branch block upon the form of the QRS complex of the canine electrocardiogram. Am. Heart J. 27:783, 1944.

162. Altieri, P., and Schaal, S. F.: Inferior and anteroseptal myocardial infarction concealed by transient left anterior hemiblock. J. Electrocardiol. 6:257, 1973.

163. Dhingra, R. C., Wyndham, C., Ehsani, A. A., and Rosen, K. M.: Left anterior hemiblock concealing diaphragmatic infarction and simulating anteroseptal infarction. Chest 67:716, 1975.

164. Wolff, L., and Richman, J. L.: The diagnosis of myocardial infarction in patients with anomalous atrioventricular excitation (Wolff-Parkinson-White syndrome). Am. Heart J. 45:545, 1953.

165. Brackbill, T. S., Dove, J. T., Murphy, G. W., and Barold, S. S.: The diagnosis of myocardial infarction in the Wolff-Parkinson-White syndrome. Chest 65:493, 1974.

166. Hellerstedt, N., Jonasson, R., and Orinius, E.: Electrocardiographic diagnosis of ventricular infarction. Acta Med. Scand. 208:213, 1980.

167. Sullivan, W., Vlodaver, Z., Tuna, N., Long, L., and Edwards, J. E.: Correlation of electrocardiographic and pathologic findings in healed myocardial infarction. Am. J. Cardiol. 42:724, 1978.

168. Candell-Riera, J., Figueras, J., Valle, V., Alvarez, A., Gutierrez, L., Cortadellas, J., Cinca, J., Salas, A., and Rius, J.: Right ventricular infarction: Relationships between ST segment elevation in V_{4R} and hemodynamic, scintigraphic, and echocardiographic findings in patients with acute inferior myocardial infarction. Am. Heart J. 101:281, 1981.

169. Chou, T.-C., Van Der Bel-Kahn, J., Allen, J., Brockmeier, L., and Fowler, N. O.: Electrocardiographic diagnosis of right ventricular infarction. Am. J. Med. 70:1175, 1981.

170. Pruitt, R. D., Klakeg, C. W., and Chapin, L. E.: Certain clinical states and pathologic changes associated with deeply inverted T wave in the precordial electrocardiogram. Circulation 11:517, 1955.

171. Pipberger, H. V., and Lopez, E. A.: "Silent" subendocardial infarcts: Fact of fiction? Am. Heart J. 100:597, 1980.

172. Savage, R. N., Wagner, G. S., Ideker, R. E., Podolsky, S. A., and Hackel, D. B.: Correlation of postmortem anatomic findings with electrocardiographic changes in patients with myocardial infarction: Retrospective study of patients with typical anterior and posterior infarcts. Circulation 55:279, 1977.

173. Levine, H. D., and Phillips, E.: Appraisal of newer electrocardiography correlations in 150 consecutive autopsied cases. N. Engl. J. Med. 245:833, 1951.

174. Uromov, G., and Gocheva, A.: Comparison of the electrocardiographic and pathoanatomic data in 110 fresh myocardial infarct patients. Vutr. Boles. 20:67, 1981.

175. Perloff, J. K.: The recognition of strictly posterior myocardial infarction by conventional scalar electrocardiography. Circulation 30:706, 1964.

176. Benchimol, A., and Desser, K. B.: The electrovector-cardiographic diagnosis of posterior wall myocardial infarction. In Fisch, C. (ed.): Complex Electrocardiography. Philadelphia, F. A. Davis Co., 1973, pp. 182–197.

177. Tranchesi, J., Teixeira, V., Ebaid, M., Bocalandro, I., Bocanegra, J., and Pilleggi, F.: The vectorcardiogram in dorsal or posterior myocardial infarction. Am. J. Cardiol. 7:505, 1961.

178. First, S. R., Bayley, R. H., and Bedford, D. R.: Peri-infarction block; electrocardiographic abnormality occasionally resembling bundle branch block and local ventricular block of other types. Circulation 2:31, 1950.

179. Starr, J. W., Wagner, G. S., Draffin, R. M., Reed, J. B., Walston, A., II, and Behar, V. S.: Vectorcardiographic criteria for the diagnosis of anterior myocardial infarction. Circulation 53:229, 1976.

180. Starr, J. W., Wagner, G. S., Behar, V. S., Walston, A., II, and Greenfield, J. C., Jr.: Vectorcardiographic criteria for the diagnosis of inferior myocardial infarction. Circulation 49:829, 1974.

181. Young, E., and Williams, C.: The frontal plane vectorcardiogram in old inferior myocardial infarction; criteria for diagnosis and electrocardiographic correlation. Circulation 37:604, 1968.

182. Toutouzas, P., Hubner, P., Sainani, G., and Shillingford, J.: Value of vectorcardiogram in diagnosis of posterior and inferior myocardial infarctions. Br. Heart J. 31:629, 1969.

183. Rubin, I. L., Gross, H., and Vigliano, E. M.: Transient abnormal Q waves during coronary insufficiency. Am. Heart J. 71:254, 1966.

184. Meller, J., Conde, C. A., Donoso, E., and Dack, S.: Transient Q waves in Prinzmetal's angina. Am. J. Cardiol. 35:691, 1975.

185. DePasquale, N. P., Burch, G. E., and Phillips, J. H.: Electrocardiographic alterations associated with electrically "silent" areas of myocardium. Am. Heart J. 68:697, 1964.

186. Mamlin, J. J., Weber, E. L., and Fisch, C.: Electrocardiographic pattern of massive myocardial infarction without pathologic confirmation. Circulation 30:539, 1964.

187. Shugoll, G. I.: Transient QRS changes simulating myocardial infarction associated with shock and severe metabolic stress. Am. Heart J. 74:402, 1967.

188. Klein, H. O., Gross, H., and Rubin, I. L.: Transient electrocardiographic changes simulating myocardial infarction during open-heart surgery. Am. Heart J. 79:463, 1970.

189. Rubin, I. L., Gross, H., and Arbeit, S. R.: Transitory abnormal Q waves during bouts of tachycardia. Am. J. Cardiol. 11:659, 1963.

190. Goldberger, A. L.: Myocardial Infarction. Electrocardiographic Differential Diagnosis. St. Louis, The C. V. Mosby Co., 1979.

191. Hewer, R. L.: The heart in Friedreich's ataxia. Br. Heart J. 31:5, 1969.

192. Frank, S., and Braunwald, E.: Idiopathic hypertrophic subaortic stenosis: Clinical analysis of 126 patients with emphasis on the natural history. Circulation 37:759, 1968.

193. Coyne, J. J.: New concepts of intramural myocardial conduction in hypertrophic obstructive cardiomyopathy. Br. Heart J. 30:546, 1968.

194. Cosio, F. G., Moro, C., Alonso, M., de la Calzada, C. S., and Llovet, A.: The Q waves of hypertrophic cardiomyopathy. An electrophysiologic study. N. Engl. J. Med. 302:96, 1980.

195. Surawicz, B., Van Horne, R. G., Urbach, J. R., and Bellet, S.: QS and QR pattern in leads V_3 and V_4 in absence of myocardial infarction. Electrocardiographic and vectorcardiographic study. Circulation 12:391, 1955.

196. Littman, D.: The electrocardiographic findings in pulmonary emphysema. Am. J. Cardiol. 5:339, 1960.

197. Romhilt, D., Susilavorn, B., and Chou, T.-C.: Unusual electrocardiographic manifestation of pulmonary embolism. Am. Heart J. 80:237, 1970.

198. Diamond, J. R., and Estes, M. N.: ECG changes associated with iatrogenic left pneumothorax simulating anterior myocardial infarction. Am. Heart J. 103:303, 1982.

199. Chou, T. C.: Pseudo infarction (noninfarction Q waves). In Fisch, C. (ed.): Cardiovascular Clinics, Complex Electrocardiography. Vol. 6. Philadelphia, F. A. Davis Co., 1973, p. 200.

200. Myers, G. B.: QRS-T patterns in multiple precordial leads that may be mistaken for myocardial infarction. III. Bundle branch block. Circulation 2:60, 1950.

201. Kennedy, R. J., Varriale, P., and Alfenito, J. C.: Textbook of Vectorcardiography. New York, Harper and Row, 1970.

202. Kariv, I.: Wolff-Parkinson-White syndrome simulating myocardial infarction. Am. Heart J. 55:406, 1958.

203. Spodick, D. H.: Electrocardiographic response to pulmonary embolism. Mechanisms and sources of variability. Am. J. Cardiol. 30:695, 1972.

204. Harris, T. R., Copeland, G. D., and Brody, D. A.: Progressive injury current with metastatic tumor of the heart. Case report and review of the literature. Am. Heart J. 69:392, 1965.

205. White, P. D.: Alternation of the pulse: A common clinical condition. Am. J. Med. Sci. 150:82, 1915.

206. Edmands, R. E., Greenspan, K., and Fisch, C.: Effect of cycle-length alteration upon the configuration of the canine ventricular action potential. Circ. Res. 9:602, 1966.

207. Scherf, D.: Alterations in the form of the T waves with changes in heart rate. Am. Heart J. 28:332, 1944.

208. Ashman, R., Ferguson, F. P., and Gremillion, A.: The effect of cycle-length changes upon the form and amplitude of the T deflection of the electrocardiogram. Am. J. Physiol. 143:453, 1945.

209. Currie, G. M.: Transient inverted T waves after paroxysmal tachycardia. Br. Heart J. 4:149, 1942.

210. Taussig, H. B.: Electrograms taken from isolated strips of mammalian ventricular cardiac muscle. Bull. Johns Hopkins Hosp. 43:81, 1928.

211. Fisch, C., Edmands, R. E., and Greenspan, K.: T wave alternans: An association with abrupt rate change. Am. Heart J. 81:817, 1971.

212. Wellens, H. J. J.: Isolated electrical alternans of the T wave. Chest 62:319, 1972.

213. Awa, S., Linde, L. M., Oshima, M., Okuni, M., Momma, K., and Nakamura, N.: The significance of late phased dart T wave in the electrocardiogram of children. Am. Heart J. 8:619, 1970.

214. Millar, K., and Abildskov, J. A.: Notched T waves in young persons with central nervous system lesions. Circulation 37:597, 1968.

215. Surawicz, B., and Lasseter, K. C.: Effect of drugs on the electrocardiogram. Progr. Cardiovasc. Dis. 13:26, 1970.

216. Abildskov, J. A.: Central nervous system influence upon electrocardiographic waveforms. In Schlant, R. C., and Hurst, J. W. (eds.): Advances in Electrocardiography. New York, Grune and Stratton, 1976.

217. Friedberg, C. K., and Zager, A.: "Nonspecific" ST and T-wave changes. Circulation 23:655, 1961.

218. Sleeper, J. C., and Orgain, E. S.: Differentiation of benign from pathologic T waves in the electrocardiogram. Am. J. Cardiol. 11:338, 1963.

219. Wilson, F. N., and Finch, R.: The effect of drinking iced-water upon the form of the T deflection of the electrocardiogram. Heart 10:275, 1923.

220. Ostrander, L. D., Jr.: The relation of "silent" T wave inversion to cardiovascular disease in an epidemiologic study. Am. J. Cardiol. 25:325, 1970.

221. Wasserburger, R. H.: The riddle of the labile T wave. Am. J. Cardiol. 2:179, 1958.

222. Burgess, M. J., and Lux, R. L.: Physiologic basis of the T wave. In Schlant, R. C., and Hurst, J. W. (eds.): Advances in Electrocardiography. New York, Grune and Stratton, 1976, pp. 327–337.

223. Abildskov, J. H.: Nonspecificity of ST-T changes. In Fisch, C. (ed.): Cardiovascular Clinics, Complex Arrhythmias. Vol. 6. Philadelphia, F. A. Davis Co., 1973, pp. 170–177.

224. Autenrieth, G., Surawicz, B., Kuo, C. S., and Arita, M.: Primary T wave abnormalities caused by uniform and regional shortening of ventricular monophasic action potential in dog. Circulation 51:668, 1975.

225. Marriott, J. L. H.: Coronary mimicry: Normal variants, and physiologic pharmacologic and pathologic influences that simulate coronary patterns in the electrocardiogram. Ann. Intern. Med. 52:411, 1960.

226. Abildskov, J. A.: Electrocardiographic wave form and the nervous system (editorial). Circulation 41:371, 1970.

227. Palmer, J. H.: Isolated U wave negativity. Circulation 7:205, 1953.

228. Ward, O. C.: New familial cardiac syndrome in children. J. Ir. Med. Assoc. 54:103, 1964.

229. Abildskov, J. A.: The prolonged QT interval. Ann. Rev. Med. 30:171, 1979.

230. Hering, H. E.: Experimentalle Studien an Saugetieren uber das Electrocardiogramme. Z. Exp. Pathol. Ther. 7:363, 1909.

231. Lewis, T.: Notes upon alternation of the heart. Quart. J. Med. 4:141, 1910.

232. Williams, R. R., Wagner, G. S., and Peter, R. H.: ST-segment alternans in Prinzmetal's angina. A report of two cases. Ann. Intern. Med. 81:51, 1974.

233. McGregor, M., and Baskind, E.: Electric alternans in pericardial effusion. Circulation 11:837, 1955.

234. Feigenbaum, H., Zaky, A., and Grabhorn, L. L.: Cardiac motion in patients with pericardial effusion. A study using reflected ultrasound. Circulation 34:611, 1966.

235. Kleinfeld, M., and Stein, E.: Electrical alternans of components of action potential. Am. Heart J. 75:528, 1968.

236. Pop, T., and Fleischmann, D.: Alternans in human atrial monophasic action potential. Br. Heart J. 39:1273, 1977.

237. Osborn, J. J.: Experimental hypothermia. Respiratory and blood pH changes in relation to cardiac function. Am. J. Physiol. 175:389, 1953.

238. Santos, E. M., and Kittle, C. F.: Electrocardiographic changes in the dog during hypothermia. Am. Heart J. 55:415, 1958.

239. Winkler, A. W., Hoff, H. E., and Smith, P. K.: Electrocardiographic changes and concentration of potassium in serum following intravenous injection of potassium chloride. Am. J. Physiol. 124:478, 1948.

240. Levine, H. D., Wanzer, S. H., and Merrill, J. P.: Dialyzable currents of injury in potassium intoxication resembling acute myocardial infarction of pericarditis. Circulation 13:29, 1956.

241. Fisch, C., Martz, B. L., and Priebe, F. H.: Enhancement of potassium-induced atrioventricular block by toxic doses of digitalis drugs. J. Clin. Invest. 39:1885, 1960.

242. Levine, H. D., Vasifdar, J. P., Lown, B., and Merrill, J. P.: "Tent-shaped" T waves of normal amplitude in potassium intoxication. Am. Heart J. 43:437, 1952.

243. Fisch, C.: Electrolytes and the heart. In Hurst, J. W. (ed.): The Heart. New York, McGraw-Hill Book Co., 1982, p. 1599.

244. Wasserburger, R. H., and Corliss, R. J.: Value of oral potassium salts in differentiation of functional and organic T wave changes. Am. J. Cardiol. 10:673, 1962.

245. Bellet, S., and Dyer, W. W.: The electrocardiogram during and after emergence from diabetic coma. Am. Heart J. 13:72, 1937.

246. Surawicz, B., and Lepeschkin, E.: The electrocardiographic pattern of hypopotassemia with and without hypocalcemia. Circulation 8:801, 1953.

247. Surawicz, B., Braun, H. A., Crum, W. B., Kemp, R. L., Wagner, S., and Bellet, S.: Quantitative analysis of the electrocardiographic pattern of hypopotassemia. Circulation 16:750, 1957.

248. Surawicz, B.: Relationship between electrocardiogram and electrolytes. Am. Heart J. 73:814, 1967.

249. Carter, E. P., and Andrus, E. C.: Q-T interval in human electrocardiogram in absence of cardiac disease. JAMA 78:1922, 1922.

250. Nierenberg, D. W., and Ransil, B. J.: Q-at$_c$ interval as a clinical indicator of hypercalcemia. Am. J. Cardiol. 44:243, 1979.

251. Kleeman, C., and Singh, B. N.: Serum electrolytes and the heart. In Maxwell, M. H., and Kleeman, C. R. (eds.): Clinical Disorders of Fluid and Electrolyte Metabolism. New York, McGraw-Hill Book Co., 1979, p. 145.

252. Cohn, A. E., Fraser, F. R., and Jamieson, A.: The influence of digitalis on the T wave of the human electrocardiogram. J. Exp. Med. 21:593, 1915.

253. Fisch, C., Greenspan, K., Knoebel, S. B., and Feigenbaum, H.: Effect of digitalis on conduction of the heart. Progr. Cardiovasc. Dis. 6:343, 1964.

254. Fisch, C., and Knoebel, S. B.: Recognition and therapy of digitalis toxicity. Progr. Cardiovasc. Dis. 13:71, 1970.

255. Smith, W. T., and Haber, E.: Digitalis. N. Engl. J. Med. 289:945, 1010, 1063, and 1125; 1973.

256. Fisch, C., Zipes, D. P., and Noble, R. J.: Digitalis toxicity: Mechanism and recognition. In Yu, P., and Goodwin, R. (eds.): Progress in Cardiology. Philadelphia, Lea and Febiger, 1975, pp. 37–70.

257. Surawicz, B., and Mortelmans, S.: Factors affecting individual tolerance to digitalis. In Fisch, C., and Surawicz, B. (eds.): Digitalis. New York, Grune and Stratton, 1969.

258. Gold, H., Kwit, N. T., Otto, H., and Fox, T.: On vagal and extravagal factors in cardiac slowing by digitalis in patients with auricular fibrillation. J. Clin. Invest. 18:429, 1939.

259. Mendéz, C., Aceves, J., and Mendéz, R. J.: The anti-adrenergic action of digitalis on the refractory period of the A-V transmission system. J. Pharmacol. Exp. Ther. 131:199, 1961.

260. Barker, P. S., Wilson, F. N., Johnston, F. D., and Wishart, S. W.: Auricular paroxysmal tachycardia with auriculoventricular block. Am. Heart J. 25:765, 1943.

261. Lewis, T.: Paroxysmal tachycardia. Heart 1:43, 1909.

262. Lown, B., and Levine, H. D.: Atrial Arrhythmias, Digitalis and Potassium. New York, Landsberger Medical Books, 1958.

263. Morgan, W. L., and Breneman, G. M.: Atrial tachycardia with block treated with digitalis. Circulation 25:787, 1962.

264. Pick, A., and Dominquez, P.: Nonparoxysmal A-V nodal tachycardia. Circulation 16:1022, 1957.

265. Chevalier, R. B., and Fisch, C.: Dissociation of pacemakers located within the atrioventricular node. Am. J. Cardiol. 5:654, 1960.

266. Pick, A., Langendorf, R., and Katz, L. N.: A-V nodal tachycardia with block. Circulation 24:12, 1961.

267. Knoebel, S. B., and Fisch, C.: Accelerated junctional escape. A clinical and electrocardiographic study. Circulation 50:151, 1974.

268. Friedberg, C. K., and Donoso, E.: Arrhythmias and conduction disturbances due to digitalis. Progr. Cardiovasc. Dis. 2:408, 1959.

269. Cohen, H. C., Gozo, E. G., Jr., and Pick, A.: Ventricular tachycardia with narrow QRS complexes (left posterior fascicular tachycardia). Circulation 45:1035, 1972.

270. Jacob, D. R., Donoso, E., and Friedberg, C. K.: A-V dissociation—A relatively frequent arrhythmia. Analysis of 30 cases with detailed discussion of the etiologic significance of digitalis, physiologic mechanisms, and differential diagnosis. Medicine 40:101, 1961.

271. Hoffman, B. F., and Singer, D. H.: Effects of digitalis on electrical activity of cardiac fibers. Progr. Cardiovasc. Dis. 7:226, 1964.

272. Rosen, M. R., Fisch, C., Hoffman, B. F., Danilo, P., Jr., Lovelace, D. E., and Knoebel, S. B.: Can accelerated atrioventricular junctional escape rhythms be explained by delayed afterdepolarization? Am. J. Cardiol. 45:1272, 1980.

273. Castellanos, A., Jr., Lemberg, L., Centurion, M. J., and Berkovits, B. V.: Concealed digitalis-induced arrhythmias unmasked by electrical stimulation of the heart. Am. Heart J. 73:484, 1967.

274. Gold, H., Otto, H. L., and Satchwell, H.: The use of quinidine in ambulatory patients for the prevention of paroxysms of auricular flutter and fibrillation; with especial reference to dosage and the effects of intraventricular conduction. Am. Heart J. 9:219, 1933.

275. Selzer, A., and Wray, H. W.: Quinidine syncope: Paroxysmal ventricular fibrillation occurring during treatment of chronic atrial arrhythmias. Circulation 30:17, 1964.

276. Kayden, H. J., Brodie, B. B., and Steele, J. M.: Procaine amide. A review. Circulation 15:118, 1957.

277. Kus, T., and Sasyniuk, B.: Electrophysiological action of disopyramide phosphate on canine ventricular muscle and Purkinje fibers. Circ. Res. 37:844, 1975.

278. Befeler, B., Castellanos, A., Jr., Wells, D. E., Vagueiro, M. C., and Yeh, B. K.: Electrophysiologic effects of the antiarrhythmic agent, disopyramide phosphate. Am. J. Cardiol. 35:282, 1975.

279. LaBarre, A., Strauss, H. C., Scheinman, M. M., Evans, G. T., Bashore, T., Tiedeman, J. J., and Wallace, A. G.: Electrophysiologic effects of disopyramide phosphate on sinus node function in patients with sinus node dysfunction. Circulation 59:226, 1979.

280. Wald, R. W., Waxman, M. B., and Colman, J. M.: Torsades de pointes ventricular tachycardia. A complication of disopyramide shared with quinidine. J. Electrocardiol. 14:301, 1981.

281. Kelly, H. G., Fay, J. E., and Laverty, S. G.: Thioridazine hydrochloride (Mellaril): Its effect on the ECG and a report of two fatalities with ECG abnormalities. Canad. Med. Assoc. J. 89:546, 1963.

282. Ban, T. A. and St. Jean, A.: The effect of phenothiazines on the electrocardiogram. Canad. Med. Assoc. J. 91:537, 1964.

283. Wendkos, M. H.: The significance of electrocardiographic changes produced by thioridazine. J. New Drugs 4:322, 1964.

284. Marshall, J. B., and Forker, A. D.: Cardiovascular effects of tricyclic antidepressant drugs: Therapeutic usage, overdose, and management of complications. Am. Heart J. 103:401, 1982.

285. Rector, W. G., Jr., Jarzobski, J. A., and Levin, H. S.: Sinus node dysfunction associated with lithium therapy: Report of a case and a review of the literature. Nebr. Med. J. 64:193, 1979.

286. Wellens, H. J. J., Cats, V. M., and Duren, D. R.: Symptomatic sinus node abnormalities following lithium carbonate therapy. Am. J. Med. 59:285, 1975.

287. Katz, L. N., and Pick, A.: Clinical Electrocardiography. Philadelphia, Lea and Febiger, 1956.

288. Scherf, D., and Schott, A.: Extrasystoles and Allied Arrhythmias. Chicago, Year Book Medical Publishers, 1973.

289. Schamroth, L.: The Disorders of Cardiac Rhythm. Oxford, Blackwell Scientific Publications, 1979.

290. Pick, A., and Langendorf, R.: Interpretation of Complex Arrhythmias. Philadelphia, Lea and Febiger, 1979.

291. Lewis, T.: Observations upon disorders of the heart's action. Heart 3:279, 1912.

292. Weidmann, S.: Effect of the cardiac membrane potential on the rapid availability of the sodium carrying system. J. Physiol. 127:213, 1955.

293. Gettes, L. S.: The electrophysiologic effects of antiarrhythmic drugs. Am. J. Cardiol. 28:526, 1971.

294. Singer, D. H., and Ten Eick, R. E.: Aberrancy: Electrophysiologic aspects. Am. J. Cardiol. 28:381, 1971.

295. Fisch, C., Zipes, D. P., and McHenry, P. L.: Rate dependent aberrancy. Circulation 48:714, 1973.

296. Gouaux, J. L., and Ashman, R.: Auricular fibrillation with aberration simulating ventricular paroxysmal tachycardia. Am. Heart J. 34:366, 1947.

297. Mendez, C., Gruhzit, C. C., and Moe, G. K.: Influence of cycle length upon refractory period of auricles, ventricles and A-V in the dog. Am. J. Physiol. 184:287, 1956.

298. Lewis, T.: Certain physical signs of myocardial involvement. Br. Med. J. 1:484, 1913.

299. Moe, G. K., Mendez, C., and Han, J.: Aberrant A-V impulse propagation in the dog heart: A study of functional bundle branch block. Circ. Res. 16:261, 1965.

300. Katz, A., and Pick, A.: The transseptal conduction time in the human heart. Circulation 27:1061, 1963.

301. Dressler, W.: Transient bundle branch block occurring during slowing of the heart beat and following gagging. Am. Heart J. 58:760, 1959.

302. Singer, D. H., Lazarra, R., and Hoffman, B. F.: Interrelationship between automaticity and conduction in Purkinje fibers. Circ. Res. 21:537, 1967.

303. Fisch, C., and Miles, W. M.: Deceleration ("bradycardia") dependent left bundle branch block: A spectrum of bundle branch conduction delay. Circulation 65:1029, 1982.

304. Engelmann, T. W.: Beobachtungen und Versuche am suspendieren Herzen. Pfluegers Arch. 56:149, 1894.

305. Lewis, T. and Master, A. M.: Observations upon conduction in the mammalian heart. A-V conduction. Heart 12:209, 1925.

306. Moe, G. K., Abildskov, J. A., and Mendéz, C.: An experimental study of concealed conduction. Am. Heart J. 67:338, 1964.

307. Hoffman, B. F., Cranefield, P. R., and Stuckey, J. H.: Concealed conduction. Circ. Res. 9:194, 1961.

308. Rosen, K. M., Rahimtoola, S. H., and Gunnar, R. M.: Pseudo A-V block secondary to premature nonpropagated His bundle depolarization. Documentation by His bundle electrocardiography. Circulation 42:367, 1970.

309. Langendorf, R.: Newer aspects of concealed conduction of the cardiac impulse. In Wellens, H. J. J., Lie, K. I., and Janse, M. J. (eds.): The Conduction System of the Heart: Structure, Function and Clinical Implications. Philadelphia, Lea and Febiger, 1976.

310. Sung, R. J., Myerburg, R. J., and Castellanos, A.: Electrophysiological demonstration of concealed conduction in the human atrium. Circulation 58: 940, 1978.

311. Fisch, C., Zipes, D. P., and McHenry, P. L.: Electrocardiographic manifestations of concealed junctional ectopic impulses. Circulation 53:217, 1976.

312. Malinow, M. R., and Langendorf, R.: Different mechanisms of fusion beats. Am. Heart J. 62:320, 1961.

313. Scherf, D., and Bornemann, C.: Parasystole with a rapid ventricular center. Am. Heart J. 62:320, 1961.

314. Kaufman, R., and Rothberger, C. J.: Beitrage zur Entstehungsweise der extrasystolischer Allorhythmien. Z. ges. exper. Med. 11:40, 1920.

315. Moe, G. D., Jalife, J., and Mueller, W. J.: Reciprocation between pacemaker sites: Reentrant parasystole? In Kulbertus, H. E. (ed.): Reentrant Arrhythmias. Mechanisms and Treatment. Baltimore, Md., University Park Press, 1977, p. 271.

316. Jalife, J., and Moe, G. K.: Effect of electrotonic potentials on pacemaker activity of canine Purkinje fibers in relation to parasystole. Circ. Res. 39:801, 1976.

317. Fisch, C., and Chevalier, R. B.: Intermittent atrial parasystole. Circulation 22:1149, 1960.

318. Steffens, T. G.: Intermittent ventricular parasystole due to entrance block failure. Circulation 44:442, 1971.

319. Adrian, E. D., and Lucas, K.: On the summation of propagated disturbances in the nerve and muscle. J. Physiol. 44:68, 1912.

320. Adrian, E. D.: The recovery process of excitable tissues. J. Physiol. 54:1, 1920.

321. Lewis, T., and Master, A. M.: Supernormal recovery phase, illustrated by two clinical cases of heart block. Heart 11:371, 1924.

322. Mihalick, M. J., and Fisch, C.: Supernormal conduction of the right bundle branch. Chest 57:395, 1970.

323. Moe, G. K., Childers, R. W., and Merideth, J.: An appraisal of "supernormal" A-V conduction. Circulation 38:5, 1968.

324. Wenckebach, K. F.: Zur Analyse des unregelmössigen Pulses. II. Uber den regelmössig intermillierenden Pulse. Zschr. Klin. Med. 37:475, 1899.

325. Schamroth, L., and Dove, E.: The Wenckebach phenomenon in sino-atrial block. Br. Heart J. 28:350, 1966.

326. Omori, Y.: Repetitive multifocal paroxysmal atrial tachycardia: With cyclic Wenckebach phenomenon under observation for 13 years. Am. Heart J. 82:527, 1971.

327. Greenspan, K., Anderson, G. J., and Fisch, C.: Electrophysiologic correlate of exit block. Am. J. Cardiol. 28:197, 1971.

328. Mehta, J., and Khan, A. H.: Pacemaker Wenckebach phenomenon due to antiarrhythmic drug toxicity. Cardiology 61:189, 1976.

329. Cerqueira-Gomes, M., and Teixeira, A. V.: Wenckebach phenomenon in the posterior division of the left branch. Am. Heart J. 82:377, 1971.

330. Pick, A.: A-V dissociation. A proposal for comprehensive classification and consistent terminology (editorial). Am. Heart J. 66:147, 1963.

331. Segers, M., LeQuime, J., and Denolin, H.: Synchronization of auricular and ventricular beats during complete heart block. Am. Heart J. 33:685, 1947.

332. Fisch, C., and Knoebel, S. B.: Junctional rhythms. Progr. Cardiovasc. Dis. 13:141, 1970.

333. Levy, M. N., and Edelstein, J.: The mechanism of synchronization in isorhythmic A-V dissociation. II. Clinical studies. Circulation 42:689, 1970.

334. Kistin, A. D., and Landowne, M.: Retrograde conduction from premature ventricular contractions, a common occurrence in the human heart. Circulation 3:738, 1951.

335. Kistin, A. D.: Retrograde conduction to the atria in ventricular tachycardia. Circulation 24:236, 1961.

336. Winternitz, M., and Langendorf, R.: Auriculoventricular block with ventriculoauricular response. Report of six cases and critical review of the literature. Am. Heart J. 27:301, 1944.

337. Ashman, R., and Hafkesbring, R.: Unidirectional block in heart muscle. Am. J. Physiol. 91:65, 1929.

338. Castillo, C., and Samet, P.: Retrograde conduction in complete heart block. Br. Heart J. 29:553, 1967.

339. Anderson, G. J., Greenspan, K., and Fisch, C.: Electrophysiologic studies on Wenckebach structures below the atrioventricular junction. Am. J. Cardiol. 30:232, 1972.

340. Pick, A., Langendorf, R., and Jedlicka, J.: Exit block. In Fisch, C. (ed.): Complex Electrocardiography. Cardiovascular Clinics. Vol. 5. Philadelphia, F. A. Davis Co., 1973, pp. 113–133.

341. Parkinson, J., and Papp, C.: Repetitive paroxysmal tachycardia. Br. Heart J. 9:241, 1947.

342. Durrer, D.: Electrical aspects of human cardiac activity: A clinical-physiological approach to excitation and stimulation. Cardiovasc. Res. 2:1, 1968.

343. Gallagher, J. J., Damato, A. N., Caracta, A. R., Varghese, P. J., Josephson, M. E., and Lau, S. H.: Gap in A-V conduction in man: Types I and II. Am. Heart J. 85:78, 1973.

344. Agha, A. S., Castellanos, A., Jr., Wells, D., Ross, M. D., Befeler, B., and Myerburg, R. J.: Type I, type II and type III gaps in bundle branch conduction. Circulation 47:325, 1973.

8

EXERCISE STRESS TESTING

by L. Thomas Sheffield, M.D.

EXERCISE TESTING FOR CORONARY ARTERY DISEASE*

Coronary artery disease is a frequent cause of episodic chest discomfort in adults. Unless the description of the episodes (precipitating factors, time course, quality, location, and alleviating factors) is typical of angina pectoris, the physician will usually seek additional information. Diagnosis would be aided if the physician were able to observe the patient during an attack of chest discomfort to determine exactly what degree of stimulus was required to provoke the attack and were able to record an electrocardiogram during the episode. This was the rationale of Goldhammer and Scherf when they introduced exercise stress testing for coronary artery disease in 1933.[1] Their test was individualized to the patient, but Master adapted the electrocardiographic recording to his two-step fitness test and made it a standardized procedure. The two-step test was not very stressful to most subjects, and the notion grew that more vigorous testing might detect disease at an earlier stage.[2] Treadmills and bicycles were found to be better suited for providing patients with strenuous exercise, and with these innovations maximal exercise tests became feasible.[3]

Indications for Noninvasive Exercise Stress Testing. Dynamic exercise testing such as performed on treadmill or bicycle, and hereafter called simply exercise stress testing, has various specific purposes in the diagnosis and treatment of heart disease. It is used to aid in the diagnosis of chest pain in adults, especially when the clinical description is not entirely typical of angina pectoris (Table 8–1). Even when the diagnosis is certain, stress testing is fre-

quently used to determine the approach to therapy, since the results of the test may provide information concerning the risk of complications. Those patients shown to be at high risk should have prompt definitive and often surgical therapy, whereas those with least risk might be best treated more conservatively (Chap. 39). Exercise testing is also useful in evaluating the degree of benefit from vasodilator, beta-blocking, or antiarrhythmic therapy or combinations of these. Among postinfarction patients, it has helped to identify the low-risk subjects who can proceed rapidly toward rehabilitation (Chaps. 38 and 40) and those who should proceed more slowly and perhaps be studied by coronary arteriography because of decreased myocardial reserve, angina, or arrhythmias (pp. 265 and 1293).

Stress testing is generally recommended to minimize the risk among middle-aged persons contemplating a physical fitness program and who are unaccustomed to exercise. Exercise testing has also proved useful in measuring the degree of benefit derived from surgical procedures such as coronary bypass, correction of congenital heart malformations,[4] aortic valve replacement, or iliofemoral bypass. Some controversy attends the use of exercise screening of professionals, such as commercial airline pilots, whose sudden incapacitation could cause great harm to others. This is because the number of false-positive results in asymptomatic individuals is rather high. Those favoring this ap-

TABLE 8–1 **INDICATIONS FOR NONINVASIVE EXERCISE STRESS TESTING**

To aid in diagnosis of chest pain
To evaluate the prognostic severity of coronary heart disease
To evaluate therapy of known coronary heart disease
To guide rehabilitation following myocardial infarction
To evaluate the benefit of surgical procedures
To provide a safety checkup prior to a fitness program
To screen high-risk professionals
To assess, in part, the risk factor in asymptomatic persons

---

*The use of radionuclide techniques for the study of the response of the ventricle and of the coronary circulation to exercise is discussed in Chapter 11.

plication argue that the disadvantage of false-positive results is more than offset by the consideration of public safety.

Finally and most controversial is the use of exercise stress testing in the asymptomatic general public. Because the prevalence of coronary artery disease is low in this group, an ischemic type of response in this setting would much more likely be a false-positive than a true one. For that reason the test probably should not be used to seek out unexpected coronary heart disease diagnosis in the asymptomatic public, but it can be used effectively in its proper role as part of a risk factor assessment program in which serum cholesterol, triglyceride, high-density lipoprotein, blood glucose, blood pressure, smoking history, age, and sex are combined with the exercise test in order to give an accurate assessment of an asymptomatic individual's risk of developing coronary heart disease in the future. Considered as a risk factor, the abnormal test result offers an otherwise unavailable opportunity to prevent disease. When positive, it is far more predictive of a coronary event than are the "classical" risk factors (Fig. 8–1).

Controversies Concerning the Application of Stress Testing. Recent issues and concerns in this field have been (1) that the correlation between exercise electrocardiograms and coronary angiograms has been poorer than expected in spite of the good agreement between exercise tests and clinical follow-up[5]; an important reason for this discrepancy has been the wide range of methodological variation among the reported studies[6]; (2) that epidemiological concepts have been introduced to explain why the test cannot be as accurate in screening asymptomatic subjects as it is in adults with chest pain; and (3) that the exercise test has been extended to include heart rate, blood pressure, and endurance observations in addition to the electrocardiogram. These issues are discussed below.

PHYSIOLOGY OF EXERCISE TESTING

CORONARY ARTERIAL RESERVE. The human body incorporates reserve capability in every organ system to permit either performance of function at levels much higher than those required in the resting state or continuation of normal function at moderate levels of performance even though disease processes may have incapacitated a considerable fraction of the total organ function. The heart and blood vessels are no exception, and most measurements of cardiovascular function during the resting state are poor predictors of circulatory performance during vigorous exercise. During exercise, intracardiac shunts that, at rest, are from left to right may reverse and become predominantly right to left. Pulmonary artery pressures and pressure differences across cardiac valves that are unimpressive at rest may become critical during heavy exercise. Left ventricular wall motion in a certain region that is normal at rest may become feeble during vigorous work, simulating an aneurysm. Finally, we have learned that advanced degrees of coronary arterial obstruction may exist without myocardial ischemia, owing to the remarkable physical flow properties of fluids in restricted tubes. Exercise is, at present, the safest and most convenient means of stimulating the myocardium to demand maximal or near maximal blood flow and is the only way of stimulating such a rigorous demand for oxygen delivery that even moderate impairment of coronary blood flow capacity becomes detectable.

CARDIAC OUTPUT INCREASES IN EXERCISE. As an adult exercises maximally, cardiac output may rise from 5 to 25 liters per minute.[7] Vasodilation in the skeletal muscular bed helps permit this increase in flow to take place, but in addition an increase in mean arterial pressure occurs. Pressure increases of 50 per cent are typical, dictating corresponding increases in the contractile force of myocardial fibers, a major determinant of myocardial oxygen consumption. There is typically a slight increase in stroke volume with exercise, although most changes in stroke volume represent adaptation to varying body attitudes, which change the inflow pressure of the returning venous blood.[8] Since adaptation of stroke volume to increasing cardiac output demand is limited, the principal mechanism of increasing cardiac output is that of raising heart rate. With an increasing heart rate, the duration of systolic ejection per beat diminishes. Attainment of normal

FIGURE 8–1 Graph of the relative capacity to predict coronary events among the various risk factors used in the Framingham Study compared with the stress test. (Reproduced with permission from Ellestad, M. H.: Stress Testing: Principles and Practice. 2nd ed. Philadelphia, F. A. Davis Co., 1980, p. 100.)

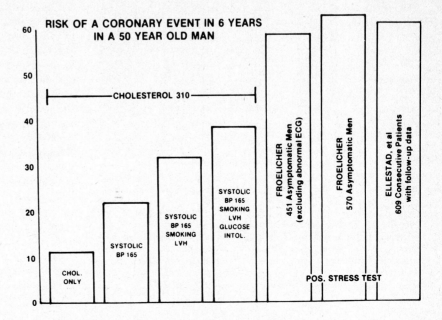

systolic emptying in shorter and shorter periods requires increasing the rate of tension development in the myocardial fibers, a valuable adaptive mechanism that parallels increases in contractility but also exacts a price—increasing the oxygen consumption with each contraction.

MYOCARDIAL OXYGEN CONSUMPTION IN EXERCISE. Myocardial oxygen consumption per contraction is determined principally by the tension developed by the myofibrils and the inotropic (contractile) state and is reflected in the rapidity with which tension is generated and shortening occurs[9] (Chap. 36). Both these determinants of myocardial oxygen consumption are greatly increased by exercise, resulting in a net increase in oxygen consumption per contraction during exercise. Myocardial oxygen consumption per minute is a function of heart rate, which increases in proportion to the intensity of exercise; in the normotensive person the increase in heart rate accounts for the greatest increment in coronary blood flow during exercise (Fig. 8–2). Measurements of contractility and heart wall tension are not practical in the intact human; fortunately, there is excellent correlation between myocardial oxygen consumption and the product of heart rate and systolic blood pressure.[10] The rate-pressure product is a reliable index of the myocardial perfusion requirement in patients with coronary artery disease as well as in normal people,[10] and persons with stable angina pectoris tend to experience chest pain at a repeatable rate-pressure product.[11]

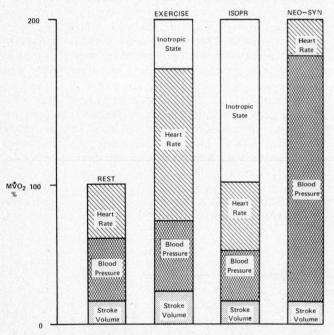

RELATIVE INFLUENCE OF FACTORS AFFECTING MV̇O₂ IN THE NORMAL HEART

Basal and activation O₂ consumption not shown

FIGURE 8–2 Myocardial oxygen consumption first in the resting state (V̇O₂ max = 100%) and then as it is increased under various circulatory conditions. The relative contributions of systolic pressure development by the ventricle (blood pressure), the heart rate, and the increase in the inotropic state are shown during mild muscular exercise, infusion of isoproterenol (ISOPR), and infusion of the pressor agent Neo-Synephrine (NEO-SYN). (From Ross, J., Jr.: Factors regulating the oxygen consumption of the heart. *In* Russek, H. I., and Zohman, B. L. (eds.): Changing Concepts in Cardiovascular Disease. Baltimore, Williams and Wilkins Co., 1972, pp. 20–31.)

Because of these changes involved in vigorous exercise, the oxygen consumption per contraction increases from about 1.2×10^{-3} ml/100 gm to about 1.9×10^{-3} ml/100 gm per beat. At normal oxygen content of about 19 ml/dl, and when the fraction of oxygen taken up by the myocardium is essentially unchanged, coronary blood flow must increase from about 60 ml/100 gm at rest to about 240 ml/100 gm during vigorous aerobic exercise.[12] It is apparent that this degree of coronary flow increase may not take place if there is severe or moderately severe obstructive disease of principal coronary arteries, and regions of the heart that are adequately perfused at rest therefore become ischemic during exercise. Exercise stress testing is based on the premise that exercise-induced ischemia may be detected by both subjective and objective means and can be used to make diagnostic inferences.

In view of the high incidence of coronary atherosclerosis as the cause of myocardial ischemia, it is easy to overlook other potential causes. Theoretically, pulmonary insufficiency, by inadequately oxygenating the blood, can cause myocardial ischemia. However, the remarkable vasodilating capability of the normal coronary circulation allows precapillary resistance to drop as a means of compensation. The resulting increase in coronary flow and the high myocardial capacity for oxygen extraction compared with other tissues explain why this is rarely, if ever, a clinical problem.[13] Reduced oxygen transport capacity of the blood, due either to anemia or to carbon monoxide exposure, may occasionally cause myocardial ischemia. More frequently, a marked chronic increase in cardiac loading and secondary hypertrophy of the heart, as in aortic valve stenosis, may result in oxygen requirements that exceed the perfusion capacity of even a normal coronary vasculature. Although none of these conditions is common compared with coronary atherosclerosis, frequently the degree of myocardial hypoperfusion from one of these causes is aggravated by coexisting coronary atherosclerosis.

Although earlier it was thought that maximal exercise might provoke myocardial ischemia in persons with normal coronary arteries,[14] the advent of high-performance exercise testing and angiographic correlation has led to a consensus that the coronary vasculature is not the limiting factor in cardiac performance. In near maximal or maximal exercise, at least as performed in currently employed exercise protocols, myocardial ischemia does not result if the heart and its coronary arteries are normal and if there is no disorder of oxygen transport.[15] However, these exercise protocols employ progressively increasing levels of exercise, so that each level serves as a warm-up period for the level to come. There is some evidence that normal individuals engaging in sprint-type exercise without adequate warm-up may indeed develop myocardial ischemia.[16] If this finding is confirmed, it would suggest that adaptations to vigorous exercise take place in the myocardium and its vessels in the course of vigorous exercise, permitting high levels of coronary blood flow, and without adaptation there may indeed be insufficient myocardial perfusion to serve the heart adequately during bursts of intense exercise. On the other hand, when exercise intensity is increased gradually, not only does the large degree of coronary reserve prevent the development of ischemia when these vessels are normal, but this reserve probably also prevents ischemia when mild or moderate degrees of atherosclerotic obstruction are present. In most studies, correlations of exercise tests with angiograms show that there is a moderately severe or far-advanced degree of coronary atherosclerosis when exertional ischemia is demonstrated.[17–20]

MYOCARDIAL ISCHEMIA DUE TO INSUFFICIENT CORONARY BLOOD FLOW INCREASE. Unfortunately, it is not now known to what extent the coronary blood flow rate appropriate for a given level of myocardial work must be reduced in order to produce evidence of ischemia, measured either by deterioration of some work function or by the electrocardiogram. It is unlikely that a small percentage of reduction, such as 5 per cent below optimal, would be perceptible in the relatively brief exercise tests currently employed.[21,22] On the other hand, tests of longer duration, i.e., 20 or 30 minutes instead of the typical 6 to 9 minutes, would be susceptible to complicating factors such as musculoskeletal conditioning or variations in pulmonary function. In spite of this we do have a basis for roughly estimating the threshold change required to produce ischemia. Patients with uncomplicated angina pectoris undertaking threadmill tests usually make the transition from normal function to ischemia in the course of an increase of one stage in the exercise protocol. Since these stages usually produce an increase in the rate-pressure product of approximately 40 per cent, the threshold for manifestation of detectable ischemia probably lies in this range as well.[23] This phenomenon has definite practical implications with regard to the design of exercise stress protocols, since the incorporation of greater increases in work from one stage to the next would tend to reduce the precision with which one can estimate the ischemic threshold. The importance of accurate estimation of the threshold of ischemia in a given subject is now becoming appreciated and is discussed later in this chapter.

Relationship Between Degree of Coronary Atherosclerosis and Degree of Blood Flow Restriction. With continued refinement of coronary angiography and the widespread availability of coronary revascularization surgery, it is now especially important to know the degree of coronary artery stenosis that corresponds to clinical heart disease as well as the degree of atherosclerosis that is compatible with normal health and therefore unlikely to be responsible for symptoms at present or in the near future. Gould and colleagues studied the degree of reactive hyperemic blood flow that was possible following temporary vascular occlusion with various degrees of external compression of coronary arteries in dogs.[24] They found that in the basal state, over 80 per cent occlusion was necessary before a significant drop in coronary blood flow occurred. Although a measurable reduction in maximal hyperemic flow took place with 40 to 60 per cent occlusion, in order to produce a 50 per cent reduction in hyperemic flow, about 70 per cent occlusion was required. Logan reported similar findings when examining the flow rates possible in diseased coronary arteries removed post mortem and perfused with blood under controlled hydrostatic pressure.[25] In the most common type of stenosis, with the lumen tapering to a minimum diameter and then gradually widening, the degree of dynamic resistance corresponds to the minimum lumen area. On the other hand, if the length

of the stenotic segment is increased, the actual resistance will be greater than that predicted by lumen area.[26]

Thus both clinical and laboratory studies confirm the high degree of reserve in normal coronary artery blood flow capacity. They indicate that although degrees of coronary atherosclerosis that obstruct the lumen up to 50 per cent represent a distinct warning, in the sense of indicating the presence of a potentially dangerous atherosclerotic process, such stenosis is unlikely to be responsible for ischemia, even during ordinary exertion. The relative insensitivity of physiological tests such as the exercise test for detecting moderate coronary atherosclerosis makes it all the more important to enhance test sensitivity in any way possible. This requires that the degree of exercise stress be of a very high order, either maximal or nearly so, and that the means of detecting ischemia be enhanced by the use of multiple modes of observation and multiple high-quality electrocardiographic leads.

Interestingly, exercise tests for ischemia, insensitive as they are for predicting exact coronary anatomy, correspond well with follow-up observations of actual coronary heart disease.[27] In a follow-up study of 2700 patients, Ellestad and colleagues found that 1067 normal responders had only a 7 per cent incidence of progression to angina, myocardial infarction, or death in 4 years, whereas 609 patients with abnormal ("positive") responses had a 46 per cent incidence of combined events in the same period.[27] McNeer and colleagues, combining observations of ST segment, exercise endurance, and maximal heart rate from exercise testing of 1472 patients, were able to define 876 patients with chest pain at low risk who had a 7 per cent mortality during 4 years of observation, whereas 134 patients who were classified to be at high risk according to the exercise test demonstrated a 37 per cent mortality during the same interval.[28]

CONSEQUENCES OF MYOCARDIAL ISCHEMIA

Chest Discomfort. Current experience suggests that chest discomfort is not as sensitive an indicator of myocardial ischemia as some of the objective indices used,[29,30] since it occurs only about half as frequently as ST-segment depression.[18,31] However, when angina pectoris does occur during testing, it is a valuable finding and increases the likelihood that significant coronary artery disease is present.

Accurate differentiation of angina pectoris from chest pain of other origin depends upon careful evaluation of the symptom.[32] True angina is a deep visceral discomfort (pp. 5 and 1335). Patients frequently use the terms "pressure," "squeezing sensation," or "a bursting feeling." They may deny that the sensation is actual pain, preferring to call it an unpleasant or disagreeable feeling. Conversely, a sharp, clearly painful sensation is unlikely to be angina pectoris, especially if it is superficial in location. The classic locations of spontaneous angina pectoris—substernal, interscapular, and anterior cervical—are encountered when ischemia is induced by stress testing. Radiation of discomfort to the shoulders, medial aspects of the arms, elbows, and, less commonly, forearms and hands and up the neck into the mandible is also found in stress testing. Nonanginal pain is usually located elsewhere, in the right hemithorax or in the left midclavicular line at the level of the 4th through the 6th interspaces without any central component. The time-intensity course of discomfort helps in its identification. Angina that occurs during diagnostic exercise testing with progressively increasing workload will increase in severity until termination of exercise. "Walk-through angina" may occur with steady mild exercise but is most unlikely during stress testing. Nonanginal chest pain frequently fails to crescendo and may even improve or disappear with continued exercise. Hot, or sometimes cold, discomfort in a bandlike pattern accross the sternum is likely to be an angina-equivalent if the time-intensity characteristic is appropriate. A full description of any chest discomfort and its distinguishing characteristics should be recorded and evaluated as part of every exercise test.

ST-Segment Displacement. Occurrence and disappearance of negative displacement of a flat or downward-sloping ST segment corresponding to the application and termination of exercise stress has been a hallmark of ischemia since introduction of the exercise test (pp. 267 to 269). Positive, or upward, displacement of the ST segment occurs less commonly. Negative ST-segment displacement is probably the result of subendocardial ischemia (p. 222), and ST elevation is probably due to subepicardial or transmural ischemia (p. 223). In both cases the ST-segment phenomenon has a vectorial or directional quality in contrast with the ST-segment elevation of pericarditis, which is found in most leads of the electrocardiogram and is present at rest and usually not altered by exercise. It is well known, but sometimes overlooked, that coronary atherosclerosis is not the only cause of subendocardial ischemia. Poor oxygen delivery by the blood for any reason, coronary arterial spasm (p. 1360), and high left ventricular pressure from any cause may also result in myocardial ischemia and displacement of the ST segment. Nearly all these causes may be readily detected. Unfortunately, displacement of the ST segment sometimes occurs in the absence of any known cause of ischemia and behaves equivocally when certain drugs such as digitalis are present.[33]

Arrhythmias. An additional diagnostic problem is the interpretation of cardiac arrhythmias, particularly ventricular extrasystoles, which occur or increase with exercise. Ischemia is one cause of arrhythmias, yet the nonspecific nature of this finding, if it occurs without any clear evidence of ischemia, has as yet made the presence or absence of exertional arrhythmias almost useless in diagnostic stress testing. It is true that the statistical probability of developing coronary heart disease is some three times greater in otherwise healthy men with exertional ventricular arrhythmias, but how this should affect management of the individual patient is by no means clear.[34] On the other hand, ventricular arrhythmias accompanying ST-segment depression or in the postinfarction patient carry a much more serious prognosis than ST-segment depression occurring alone.[35]

Reduction in Maximal Cardiac Pump Function. In patients without valvular heart disease, myocarditis, or cardiomyopathy, the inability to sustain a normal peak level of cardiac work, as reflected in the heart rate–systolic blood pressure product, suggests significant coronary ar-

tery obstruction.[36]Also, patients who develop transient pump failure, as reflected in an actual drop in blood pressure without cessation or reduction of exercise, usually have advanced coronary obstruction.[37] Lastly, inability to continue the progressively increasing exercise of a graded treadmill or bicycle test protocol for a normal time is an important sign of myocardial ischemia when other possible causes have been excluded.[28]

One might think that any measure of the heart's function would therefore deteriorate when myocardial ischemia occurs, either spontaneously or when provoked by exercise stress. This is esentially true when the ischemia is "global," i.e., when the entire left ventricle or a large portion of it becomes ischemic as a result of widespread coronary atherosclerosis. But the issue becomes complex when ischemia is regional and affects primarily a single portion of the left ventricle. In this case, other less affected portions of myocardium may have both the strength and the blood supply to compensate for local deterioration of function, and external measurement of blood pressure and heart rate, the electrocardiogram, or degree of work endurance may not reflect the abnormality. This may occur in the intact myocardium when there is localized stenosis of a minority of the coronary vessels and branches and may also occur in the presence of localized and well-healed infarctions.

TYPES OF EXERCISE TESTS

Exercise tests are used in two distinctly different settings: the noninvasive cardiovascular laboratory in the hospital or physician's office and the cardiac catheterization laboratory. The requirements of these two facilities differ considerably, as can be seen from Table 8–2.

In the *noninvasive laboratory*, generally, the electrocardiographic data assume more importance than in the catheterization laboratory. There is need for higher intensity of exercise, with the aim of detecting maximal coronary reserve. It is necessary to employ a familiar form of exercise in order to secure the greatest possible degree of subject cooperation.

In the *catheterization laboratory*, a major constraint is the necessity of having the subject lie on an x-ray-equipped catheterization table. Surgical draping and other

---

TABLE 8–2 Uses of Exercise Testing

IN THE NONINVASIVE LABORATORY
To detect and evaluate ischemia by electrocardiogram and other means
To evaluate left ventricular performance in exercise by kinetocardiogram or apexcardiogram
To detect ischemia in exercise by thallium-201 scintigraphy
To measure left ventricular performance in exercise by gated blood pool scintigraphy
To measure functional capacity as a guide to timing surgical replacement of diseased valves
To evaluate effects of surgical treatment of congenital heart disease and coronary artery disease
To measure physical fitness and effects of athletic training in normal individuals and patients with coronary artery disease

IN THE CATHETERIZATION LABORATORY
To evaluate valve gradients at high flow rates
To measure shunts and pressures in response to exercise
To measure left ventricular function in exercise
To measure coronary blood flow in response to exercise
To study myocardial metabolism during exercise

practical considerations usually prohibit use of the arms for exercise, leaving leg-pedaling ergometer exercise as the most practical means of stressing the circulation. Circulatory stress is proportional to the mass of exercising muscle, so use of the legs, involving the large hamstring and quadriceps femoris muscle groups, is desirable. On the other hand, maximal gross oxygen consumption and cardiac output in the recumbent position are less than that attainable in the erect position.[38] Although absence of the restraint of gravity on venous return improves venous inflow to the heart and results in larger stroke volumes than in the erect position, high-volume ventilation is less efficient because the diaphragm is more cephalad in the recumbent position. Fortunately most research and diagnostic studies that employ exercise in the catheterization laboratory do not require maximal or near maximal exercise. Measurements made at rest and at two or more progressive levels of exercise allow the construction of a work-response relationship. Whether this involves regulation of coronary blood flow or the hydrodynamic resistance of a valve, useful and usually satisfactory information can be obtained at submaximal exercise levels.

ISOMETRIC EXERCISE. In addition to dynamic exercise, static exercise has received considerable attention recently. In the general population, static exercise has been the subject of books and systems for (usually cosmetic) muscle building and strength improvement. Because of its popularity, investigators have studied the effects of static or isometric exercise on patients with ischemic heart disease.[39,40] The effect of moderate isometric exercise (approximately one-half maximal effort) is to raise the systemic vascular resistance, causing about a one-third increase in mean arterial pressure as well as a moderate (typically 20 per cent) increase in heart rate. Since both these changes contribute to an increase in cardiac work reflected in the rate-pressure product, isometric exercise in the form of a firm, sustained handgrip has been used to provoke either clinical angina pectoris or ventricular dysfunction manifested by a ventricular filling sound or mitral incompetence.[39,41] These occur readily in a patient with a very low anginal threshold, but since the increase in the rate-pressure product caused by this maneuver is only modest, such a clinical test, though useful at the bedside, does not rival a high-performance dynamic exercise test.

RELATIONSHIP OF WORKING MUSCLE MASS TO CIRCULATORY STRESS. The distribution of work among skeletal muscles affects hemodynamic performance. Any specified amount of work is done most efficiently when the largest muscle mass is employed. Thus 300 kpm/min of pedaling work can be performed with the least rise in the rate-pressure product when it is performed by both legs. If performed by a single leg, the rate-pressure product will be higher, and the progressive rise is continued when the work is performed by both arms or a single arm.[38] This relationship also holds true for isometric work. The lowest rate-pressure product is obtained when a weight is carried on the back, and the greatest rise in rate-pressure product occurs when the same weight is carried in one hand.[42]

CHOICE OF EXERCISE MODE. Factors determining the choice of exercise mode are therefore the type of data to be collected, the group of subjects to be studied, the familiarity of the subjects with various exercise devices,

and the intensity of exercise intended. When measurement of maximal exercise capacity is intended, possible choices include the motor-driven treadmill and the upright bicycle ergometer.

Treadmill. The motor-driven treadmill permits the highest oxygen consumption rate of any common exercise device, involving as it does both legs, the torso, and both arms. In contrast to electronically controlled bicycle ergometers, treadmills can be calibrated without resort to any special instrumentation. External control of the work rate is attained with a minimum of subject cooperation— either the subject maintains his position on the treadmill without grasping the support rails or he does not. Conversely, the work rate in the step test and with the mechanical bicycle ergometer is controlled entirely by the subject. When the subject becomes tired, adherence to a standard work rate with these devices becomes progressively more difficult. Although the controlled bicycle ergometer maintains work rate by increasing its resistance in proportion to decreasing pedal velocity, this may produce a surprising and threatening aspect to the subject, who may thus discontinue exercise short of the work rate attainable with a more familiar device.

The treadmill provides exercise most familiar to North Americans, and both active and sedentary persons can attain their maximal oxygen consumptions even with untrained legs and knees. The principal disadvantages of the treadmill are that it is expensive, the noisiest of exercise devices, and most demanding of space. Electrocardiographic recordings during treadmill exercise are moderately distorted, owing to both myographic artifact and the bouncing effect of soft tissues with each footstep. Finally, treadmill exercise is not suitable for studies requiring a relatively immobile thorax, such as those involving indwelling vascular catheters or sensitive precordial detectors such as echocardiographs or scintillation cameras.

Bicycle. The upright bicycle excels in providing undistorted electrocardiograms, and it is possible for the subject to maintain the thorax immobile long enough for sensitive precordial measurements, even phonocardiograms, to be recorded during exercise. Intravascular catheters may be kept in place, expired air may be collected easily, and with perseverance both echocardiographic and scintigraphic observations may be made. Mechanical bicycle ergometers cost much less than do electronically regulated ones. All types are quieter than treadmills and require only one-third to one-half the space needed for a treadmill. Their main disadvantages are that they are unfamiliar to many North American adults, a situation which seems now to be improving, and that they depend upon complete subject cooperation in order to maintain a constant work rate in following a specific protocol.

Variable Step. The variable step is the simplest and lowest cost device for attaining maximal exercise in a relatively stationary position.[43] Well suited for athletically trained individuals, it has not proved as acceptable to older or sedentary subjects because of the concentration of stress in the knees and thighs. Step exercise produces the greatest distortion in the electrocardiogram of these three work forms. Because of the vertical motion involved, use of sensitive precordial detectors is impossible, and the employment of intravascular catheters would be least practical with this form of exercise.

TIME COURSE OF EXERCISE INTENSITY. The pattern of exercise intensity should be determined by the purpose of testing and the characteristics of the population to be tested. If the testing is to determine minimal qualification standards for some activity, such as participation in a school sports program or qualification for a certain industrial operation, the test may be limited to a fixed duration of exercise, with the intensity chosen appropriately. The Master two-step test is a popular example of a test of fixed duration with exercise intensity chosen individually for the subject.[29] In a fixed length of time, originally 11/2 minutes and later 3 minutes, a certain number of ascents of a two-step stair are performed, the number being determined by the sex, age, and weight of the subject.

Single-level vs. Multilevel Tests. If the group to be tested is fairly homogeneous in exercise capacity, the exercise test may consist of a single level of exercise suitable for that group. In selecting an exercise test suitable for a wide range of subjects—from sedentary elderly subjects to vigorous younger ones—it is apparent that no single level of exercise would provide suitable stress in each case. For this reason exercise test protocols are dominated by graded or progressive increases in work rate with time. The initial work rate is low enough for the least powerful subject, and the progression continues until work rates suitable for the strongest subject have been reached (Fig. 8–3). In such a progressive test the highest stage completed gives an indication of that subject's functional capacity. The duration of each interval depends upon whether it is intended that the subject reach circulatory steady state in each stage before going on to the next. This requires about 5 or 6 minutes for most subjects. Since exercise tests that last longer than about 20 minutes introduce the possibility of fatigue and internal heat burden, thereby complicating the measurement of functional capacity, the use of stages 6 minutes long would permit only three or four different levels of exercise. A practical compromise involves using stages of 3 minutes' duration, permitting five different exercise intensity levels which may be spaced more closely in terms of work rate and thus may be more precise in measuring maximal functional capacity. The Bruce treadmill protocol is an example of such a test.[44]

Another approach is to employ small increases in work intensity in stages so brief that the rate of work increase is virtually continuous, and the concept of circulatory steady state is set aside entirely.[43] Although such protocols are not well adapted for time-consuming measurements such as oxygen consumption or cardiac output, they can offer a precise measurement of maximal functional capacity. The Balke-Ware test, with stages only 1 minute in duration, is an example of this approach.[45]

An exercise test consisting of individual periods of exercise progressively increasing in intensity and separated by rest periods will permit time-consuming physiological studies during each stage of exercise after steady state has been attained, yet the intervening rest periods will avoid the pitfall of cumulative fatigue from earlier stages. Such tests typically consist of 6-minute exercise periods, 5 to 10 minutes of rest, the next higher exercise level for 6 minutes, and so on, with the progression sometimes carried out over the space of several days.[46] Owing to their precision, such test patterns are favored by work physiologists. On

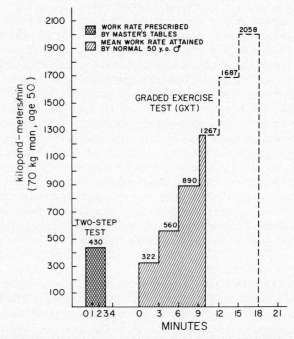

EXTERNAL WORK INVOLVED IN A SINGLE–STAGE AND IN A MULTIPLE–STAGE EXERCISE TEST

FIGURE 8–3 Rate of energy output in kilopond-meters/minute developed by a 50-year-old, 70-kg man performing a single-stage test (Master two-step); the *rate* of work, i.e., the number of ascents per minute, is the same in the single and double tests. The calculation is as follows:

70 kg (body weight) × 0.46 (height of steps in meters) × 20 (number of ascents) ÷ 1.5 (duration of test in minutes) = 430 (kpm/min). The work rate involved in the GXT (shaded area) is that performed by a normal 50-year-old, 70-kg man who walks 10 minutes on the treadmill while attaining his target heart rate (90% of age-predicted maximal exercise heart rate; see Table 8–3). The external work rate (equivalent rate of climb × body weight) 113 m/min (treadmill speed) × 16% (treadmill grade) × 70 kg (body weight), or 1267 kpm/min. The dotted line outlines the work rates involved in the higher stages for the same body weight. (From Sheffield, L. T., and Roitman, D.: Stress testing methodology. Prog. Cardiovasc. Dis. **19**:33, 1976, by permission of Grune and Stratton.)

the other hand, because of the protracted nature of such testing, this pattern is not ordinarily well suited for purposes of disease diagnosis.

Termination of Exercise: Open-ended vs. Closed-ended Tests. Regardless of which exercise protocol is used, exercise should always be terminated upon recognition of any evidence that further exercise may be harmful to the subject. This would include certain arrhythmias and other electrocardiographic changes, a drop in blood pressure, or incoordination of gait. These and other safety considerations will be elaborated later. Tests that are terminated, usually by the subject, before arriving at a scheduled endpoint or before manifesting diagnostic evidence of disease should be termed incomplete or nondiagnostic. For terminating exercise, tests may be considered open-ended or close-ended. In open-ended tests, the duration of the test is determined by the reaction of the subject to exercise, and work is continued until a certain degree of reaction has taken place. Closed-ended tests, generally milder in intensity, are continued for a certain fixed period (for example, the 3-minute double two-step test). Of the open-ended tests, four distinct choices are available for termination of exercise: (1) exercise to a fixed heart rate, such as 150 beats/min[47]; (2) exercise to a variable heart rate, such as 90 per cent of predicted maximal[48]; (3) exercise to symptom-limited maximum tolerance[44]; and (4) exercise to physiologically documented maximal aerobic capacity.[49]

Exercise to a Fixed Heart Rate. Exercise to a fixed heart rate is popular in Europe, especially in Scandinavian countries. It has a physiological basis, since weaker subjects will perform less work in reaching a heart rate of 150 beats/min than will robust subjects who should be stressed harder. Nomograms have been developed that enable one to predict maximal aerobic capacity on the basis of the work level required to attain a heart rate of 150 beats/min.[49] Although such estimates have a variance of 10 to 15 per cent, they provide clinically useful information. The principal disadvantage of this method of testing is that it stresses subjects of different ages unequally. A heart rate of 150 beats/min (or any other chosen value) will be attained at a much smaller fraction of maximal exercise capacity in the younger person than in the older one, for some of whom it may represent a nearly maximal rate. Therefore such a test finds its greatest usefulness in testing groups of persons in approximately the same age range.

Exercise to an Individualized Heart Rate. Exercise to 90 per cent (or some other relatively high percentage) of estimated maximal heart rate has the advantage of avoiding the discomfort of all-out maximal exercise, while retaining test sensitivity by presenting nearly maximal stress to persons of all ages. The highest heart rate anyone can attain during exercise gradually decreases with age. There is a moderate amount of individual variation, one standard deviation of maximal heart rate being ±10 beats/min.[50,51] Additionally, it has been found that persons actively engaged in athletics have maximal heart rates that are about 7 beats/min lower than physically untrained subjects of the same age.[50] Finally, the regression of maximal heart rate with age differs slightly between the sexes.[51] Thus by taking age, sex, and physical training into account, it is possible to arrive at a target heart rate that is approximately 90 per cent of maximal for that subject.

Post Infarction Exercise Testing. Exercise testing is frequently performed just before the discharge from the hospital of acute myocardial infarction patients, in order to identify those who are at increased risk and thus who may need additional treatment. Such testing can also identify low-risk patients who may safely follow an accelerated convalescence and early return to work. Early testing is indicated when this information can be applied beneficially to the patient's management. Such testing would probably

not be indicated in the case of the elderly patient, already retired and not intending to resume an active life, especially if the patient was expected to be under regular medical observation after discharge. Predischarge exercise testing is *contraindicated* in the patient with persistent ventricular arrhythmias, any evidence of cardiac failure, or recurrent chest pain.

In the recent postinfarct patient, the modified treadmill stages zero and one-half (or similarly low work levels in other protocols) are employed, and exercise is usually terminated at 70 or 75 per cent of predicted maximal heart rate or at the onset of effort intolerance. Test interpretation is based upon evidence of ischemia and degree of exercise tolerance. The very low-risk category consists of patients able to exercise to the specified heart rate or to the point of normal fatigue and breathlessness without manifesting either ST-segment depression or angina pectoris. Intermediate-risk patients are those demonstrating transient ischemia but normal exercise tolerance; poor-risk patients are those showing evidence of ischemia at a low heart rate or exercise level.

Subjective Maximal Exercise. Subjective maximal exercise testing is easiest to define. The subject simply exercises in a standardized work pattern until unable to continue because of intolerable fatigue, dyspnea, or pain. The high level of circulatory stress provided by maximal exercise makes it possible to demonstrate exertional cardiac ischemia in some cases where lower levels of exercise would have been insufficient to expose it. At any unaccustomed level of exercise there is some slight theoretical danger of precipitating circulatory arrest or myocardial infarction. On the basis of reported instances, however, the frequency of this complication is reassuringly very low.

The subjective nature of the endpoint for this test naturally raises the question of whether all subjects stress themselves to the same degree or whether the more timid ones may tolerate appreciably less fatigue or discomfort than more aggressive subjects. However, proponents of subjective maximal testing report that subjective variability with this test is low.[52] This variability may be reduced by comparing the subject's maximum test heart rate with the predicted target heart rate (Table 8–3). If the attained heart rate is more than 10 beats/min below the target heart rate, if the test is otherwise negative, and if there is no obvious cause of blunted heart rate response, the test may be classified as incomplete and nondiagnostic.

DOCUMENTED MAXIMAL AEROBIC CAPACITY. Exercise to physiologically documented maximal aerobic capacity is a highly valuable investigative tool in work physiology. Typically, interrupted tests of fixed duration are employed with measurement of oxygen uptake at each stage. A level of work will finally be found at which the

TABLE 8–3 GRADED EXERCISE TEST—TARGET HEART RATES

Age (years)	30	35	40	45	50	55	60	65
Predicted maximal heart rate—men	193	191	189	187	184	182	180	178
Target heart rate—men (90% of maximal)	173	172	170	168	166	164	162	160
Predicted maximal heart rate—women	190	185	181	177	172	168	163	159
Target heart rate—women (90% of maximal)	171	167	163	159	155	151	147	143

oxygen uptake reaches a plateau, and the least amount of exercise that clearly demonstrates such a plateau represents maximal aerobic exercise. Any exercise greater than this represents supramaximal or sprint-type exercise, which can be supported only briefly on an anaerobic basis. This type of testing, ideal for studies of normal physiology and the quantitation of training effect, is not well suited for the clinical diagnostic laboratory because of the physical discomfort involved at this level of exercise, the possible hazards, and the large amounts of time involved in interrupted testing.

SPECIFIC EXERCISE TESTS: THE BRUCE, NAUGHTON, AND SHEFFIELD PROTOCOLS. These three tests share the following characteristics: (1) For each subject an appropriate cardiovascular history and examination should be performed prior to the exercise test. (2) The subject should be tested either after an overnight fast or no earlier than 2 hours after a light meal. The patient should be informed of the indications for the test, the details of its procedure, and the potential hazards of testing and should then execute written informed consent. A 12-lead conventional resting electrocardiogram must be recorded and examined for possible exercise contraindications, and the interpretation should be recorded prior to exercise.

During and after exercise, a bipolar CM_5 lead (Naughton test),[53] a CB_5 lead (Bruce test),[54] or Wilson leads V_2 and V_5 and limb lead aV_f (Sheffield test)[48] (Fig. 8–4) should be continuously displayed on an oscilloscope and then recorded on paper at least once per exercise stage and at each minute post exercise. Blood pressure should be measured before exercise, at least once during each exercise stage, and every 2 minutes post exercise until stable.

Exercise is carried out on a motor-driven treadmill according to stages defined in Table 8–4. Exercise is contin-

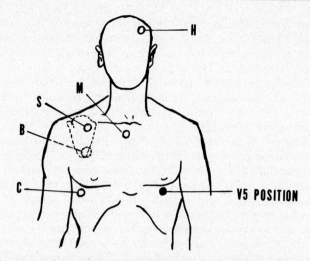

FIGURE 8–4 Locations of electrodes for some commonly used bipolar electrocardiographic leads. These leads are designated "C(*)$_5$," where * is replaced by the letter denoting the negative or reference electrode (e.g., CH_5 indicates that the active electrode is at V_5 and the reference electrode is on the head).

ued by the subject until terminated because of the appearance and progression of symptoms, exhaustion, or the development of ventricular arrhythmia (all tests). Negative tests are classified "incomplete" if the subject did not come within 10 beats/min of target heart rate (Table 8–3); positive tests are valid at any heart rate (Sheffield test).

In the postexercise period, a complete 12-lead electrocardiogram should be recorded immediately and at 2 and 4 minutes post exercise in addition to any other leads. The sitting position is employed because of the discomfort often caused by lying supine and still after near maximal exercise. Brief pulmonary auscultation for rales and wheezes

TABLE 8–4 THREE TREADMILL EXERCISE TEST PROTOCOLS

	STAGE	SPEED (MPH)	ELEVATION (% GRADE)	DURATION (MIN)	APPROXIMATE VO$_2$/KG/MIN (ML)
Bruce test	1	1.7	10.0	3	18.0
	2	2.5	12.0	3	25.0
	3	3.4	14.0	3	34.0
	4	4.2	16.0	3	46.0
	5	5.0	18.0	3	55.0
	6	5.5	20.0	3	—
	7	6.0	22.0	3	—
Modified Naughton test	1	2.0	0.0	3	7.0
	2	2.0	3.5	3	10.5
	3	2.0	7.0	3	14.0
	4	2.0	10.5	3	17.5
	5	2.0	14.0	3	21.0
	6	2.0	17.5	3	24.5
	7	3.0	12.5	3	28.0
	8	3.0	15.0	3	31.5
	9	3.0	17.5	3	35.0
	10	3.0	20.0	3	38.5
	11	3.0	22.5	3	42.0
	12	3.4	20.0	3	45.5
	13	3.4	22.0	3	49.0
	14	3.4	24.0	3	52.5
	15	3.4	26.0	3	56.0
Sheffield test* (GXT)	0	1.7	0.0	3	8.0
	½	1.7	5.0	3	12.0
	1	1.7	10.0	3	18.0

*Stages 2 through 7 of the Sheffield test are identical to those of the Bruce test.

is also worthwhile. Cardiac auscultation should be carried out as quickly as possible in order to detect exercise-induced mitral regurgitation or atrial or ventricular gallops. Postexercise observation should continue for 6 minutes or until all exercise-induced abnormalities have disappeared. Exercise testing should be supervised by a physician trained in the procedure, and the exercise laboratory should be equipped and organized for patient safety measures, as described later in this chapter.

EXERCISE ELECTROCARDIOGRAPHY

TYPES OF ST-SEGMENT DISPLACEMENT. When during exercise myocardial perfusion is inadequate to meet increased oxygen requirements, it is the subendocardium that becomes ischemic, since its perfusion is most precarious. As a consequence, a diastolic injury potential characterized by a vector that is opposite in direction to the major QRS vector is produced; hence there is ST-segment depression in leads with dominant R waves. The ST-segment ischemic displacement phenomenon in exercise stress testing, like that produced by angina at rest, is generally of three types.[55-57] The most common type is a displacement beginning at the QRS-ST junction which is downward or negative in polarity and which is followed by an initially upsloping ST segment as it merges into the T wave. As exercise progresses and presumably as ischemia also progresses, the degree of J-point depression increases and the ST segment becomes less and less upsloping. In its most characteristic form the ST segment becomes entirely flat for the first 80 msec of its duration and with further change may actually become negative or downsloping.

As an interpretive criterion, 0.10 mv (1 mm) or more of flat ST-segment displacement in a standard electrocardiographic lead is commonly considered indicative of ischemia. This is a conservative balance between *sensitivity* to detect ischemia and *specificity* to avoid false-positive results. At one time 0.05 mv (0.5 mm) ST displacement was used as a criterion of ischemia, and although the number of patients with obstructive coronary artery disease who were missed was small, the number of normal persons who shared this response was excessive, i.e., there were few false-negatives but many false-positives (high sensitivity, low specificity). Others have required 0.20 mv (2 mm) ST displacement for an ischemic response; this reduces the number of patients with positive tests who do not have ischemic heart disease but misses many patients with documented coronary obstruction; there were few false-positives but many false-negatives (high specificity, low sensitivity).

Other types of electrocardiographic leads (bipolar leads or Frank leads) have sensitivities different from the standard leads, warranting different criteria of ischemia. ST displacement of 0.20 mv (2 mm) is a logical and frequently used criterion for bipolar leads. The corresponding value for Frank leads would lie between 0.05 and 0.10 mv (0.5 to 1 mm) and in practice has not been adequately defined.

When we realize that the spectrum of ischemic ST-segment displacement varies from zero to nearly the amplitude of the QRS in some patients, it is apparent that any criterion we use is arbitrary, dictated partly by the recording format and partly by the desire for an optimal compromise between ability to detect disease and to reject nondisease.

An important feature of this type of response is its prompt improvement as soon as exercise is terminated and remarkably quick disappearance early in the postexercise period (Fig. 8–5, Type I). The brevity of this response makes it almost impossible to detect unless electrocardiographic recording and display are carried out *during* exercise and continued without interruption into the immediate postexercise period.

The second most frequent ST-displacement response begins as in the first example, but instead of immediate improvement with termination of exercise, the response becomes progressively more abnormal for several seconds or minutes following exercise (Fig. 8–5, Type II). In the postexercise period there is additional negative displacement of the flat or downsloping ST, which is frequently, but not always, associated with chest discomfort. In most cases this protracted response shows an evolutionary pattern in the course of returning to normal, developing a downsloping ST segment with upward convexity and merging into an inverted T wave. Usually from 5 to 20 minutes is required for the T wave to become fully upright thereafter and for the ST segment to return fully to its preexercise isoelectric contour. It is thought that the degree of ST-segment shift reflects the severity of myocardial ischemia, whereas the degree of coronary obstruction responsible for ischemia is inversely related to the amount of exercise stress required to provoke ischemia and directly related to the duration of ST-segment depression after exercise, once ischemia is provoked. Thus transient ST

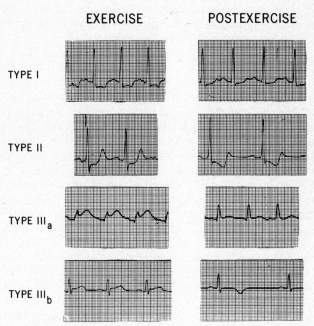

EXERCISE   POSTEXERCISE

TYPE I

TYPE II

TYPE III_a

TYPE III_b

FIGURE 8–5 Types of exertional ST-segment displacement:
I: Transient depression during exercise that has virtually disappeared 1 minute after exercise.
II: Depression during exercise that becomes more pronounced after exercise before belatedly returning to normal.
IIIa: ST elevation characteristic of Prinzmetal's angina.
IIIb: ST elevation of modest degree usually caused by dyskinesis or scarring of the left ventricle.

depression (Type I) occurring only with vigorous exercise would represent minor prognostic abnormality, whereas protracted ST depression (Type II) provoked only by mild exercise would constitute a major prognostic abnormality, such as usually caused by severe multivessel or left main coronary artery disease.

The least common ST-segment response, occurring in only 3 to 5 per cent of most series, consists of ST-segment *elevation* rather than depression. At least two mechanisms can be responsible for ST-segment elevation. Intense, localized transmural ischemia may be produced in Prinzmetal's variant angina by spastic occlusion of a single major coronary vessel. Although episodes of transmural ischemia caused by coronary spasm characteristically occur at rest, there is now substantial evidence that it can be provoked by exercise as well[58] (p. 1242). Similar intense localized ischemia may be provoked by exercise (Fig. 8–5, Type IIIa). This type of response, when severe, usually distorts the QRS complex as well, causing the QRS-T configuration to resemble temporarily a directly recorded monophasic action potential. This response usually goes through a phase of T-wave inversion in the process of disappearing.

A second kind of ST-segment elevation response has been described (Fig. 8–5, Type IIIb). This is most frequently found in the longitudinal leads, reflecting the diaphragmatic surface of the left ventricle. This type of ST-segment elevation does not distort the QRS complex, is not followed by the evolutionary pattern of T-wave inversion in its improvement and disappearance, and has been related to the presence of scarring or dyskinesia due to preexisting disease, rather than to temporary ischemia of otherwise normal myocardium.[59,60] Alternatively, it is possible that during exercise, as a greater quantity of myocardium becomes ischemic and akinetic, the larger noncontractile mass of myocardium behaves like a ventricular aneurysm, producing ST-segment elevation.

Depression of the QRS-ST junction (J) during exercise occurs in normal persons, although usually not more than 0.20 mv (2 mm). When this occurs, an upsloping depression of the ST segment results. Unfortunately, the ischemic ST-segment response goes through this phase in the process of approaching flat or downsloping ST-segment depression. In order to differentiate this reaction from normal, the exercise should, if possible, be continued to a higher level so a clearly ischemic response may evolve in the abnormal while the ST segment remains steeply upsloping in the normal. Thus with respect to ST-segment slope in exercise there are three zones of prognostic significance: a steeply upsloping ST segment (normal), a gently upsloping one (probably abnormal), and a flat or downsloping ST segment (definitely abnormal).[61] As with ST-displacement criteria, any division between zones will be arbitrary, but we have found it useful to consider slopes greater than 1 mv/sec (40 per cent slope when paper speed is 25 mm/sec) normal and those 0 to 1 mv/sec probably abnormal. Another useful rule of thumb is that an upsloping ST segment may be considered abnormal when the degree of depression at 0.06 sec from the J-point is depressed by 1.5 mm or more.[62]

There is renewed interest in R-wave amplitude change as a sign of exertional ischemia.[63,64] The *Brody effect* is an augmentation of the radially directed electrocardiographic

signal due to the highly conductive intracavitary blood.[65] Further increase in this blood pool due to ischemic dysfunction might augment the electrocardiographic signal still more. Conversely, animal studies have shown reduction of electrocardiographic signal in response to increase in intraventricular pressure.[66] However, at present there are not enough published data on ischemic QRS-amplitude changes to develop a reliable perspective.[66] Although T-wave changes—specifically T-wave inversions—during exercise are quite uncommon in normal subjects, they are nonspecific and occur not only in patients with coronary artery disease but also in those with hypertension and cardiomyopathy.

Recording Electrocardiographic Effects of Ischemia. As discussed on p. 222, subendocardial ischemia ordinarily produces not ST-segment depression, but rather T-P-QRS elevation.[59,67,68] Since clinical electrocardiographs are not direct-coupled and thus are insensitive to direct-current voltages, it is not possible to distinguish between true depression of one portion of the electrocardiogram, such as the ST segment, and true elevation of every other portion of the electrocardiogram, such as the T-P-Q segment (See Figure 7–29 p. 222). It is only by means of direct-coupled recorders connected to the exposed heart that the true nature of an ST displacement can be established. Although it is helpful to understand the true electrical alteration caused by ischemia, it continues to be impractical (if not impossible) to record and measure *true* shifts in the T-P-Q segment "baseline" by body surface recordings with conventional instruments. *Ischemic ST-segment depression* is a term widely used in this chapter even though it may be technically incorrect or only partially correct.

The Electrode-skin Interface. It has long been recognized by electrocardiographers[69] and electroencephalographers that a nonmetallic electrolyte interface must be interposed between the skin and the metal recording electrode in order to minimize recording artifacts.[70]

In 1959 Shackel described a quick, painless, and effective means of reducing skin impedance for recording purposes.[71] Our adaptation of his method involves the use of a No. 6 spherical dental burr inserted into a variable-speed hobby grinding tool.* When rotating at an intermediate speed and touched lightly to the skin (2 to 5 gm pressure) for 1 second, a pinhead-sized area of cornified epithelium is abraded without pain or bleeding. An exercise electrocardiographic electrode applied over this spot, or alternately over an area prepared by lightly rubbing with fine sandpaper and scrubbing with acetone, will have a contact impedance of 1 to 5 kilohms instead of the 10 to 50 kilohms usually obtained without any kind of dermabrasion.

Silver–silver chloride electrodes are best, but stainless steel electrodes are satisfactory if the active surface is maintained properly. Burnishing the surface with a coarse pencil-shaped typewriter eraser is effective. In either case the metallic electrode should be recessed within a cup-shaped plastic housing filled with electrolyte paste. The more viscous the paste, the more satisfactory the resultant electrocardiograms, and therefore electrolyte cream has not proved satisfactory for this purpose. The electrode is then adhered to the skin with ring-shaped plastic seals which are coated on both sides with adhesive. Recessed, adhesive, disposable exercise electrocardiographic electrodes were developed by Mason and Likar and are now commercially available from numerous sources.[72] The cable that connects the electrodes to the recorder should be shielded, preferably all the way to the electrode, to reduce power-line artifact. The cable should be thin, light, and compliant and should introduce no electrical potential of its own when flexed or agitated. Some exercise electrocardiographic systems contain preamplifier circuits located at the patient end of the cable. This virtually eliminates the problem of power-line artifact while only slightly increasing the bulk of the cable system carried by the subject.

Electrocardiographic Leads for Detection of Ischemia. There is not uniform agreement on the number of electrocardiographic leads required for optimal exercise electrocardiography. Some investigators use only a single bipolar lead, requiring application of only two

---

*Such as a Dremel Moto-tool, model #380.

or three electrodes, whereas Blackburn et al.,[73] Mason and Likar,[74] and Phibbs and Buckels[75] have shown that some ischemic type of electrocardiographic responses will be missed if only a single lead is recorded. The range of positive yield from a single V_5-like lead has varied from as low as 60 per cent to over 90 per cent of the yield possible when 12 conventional leads are recorded. Blackburn has reported that the positive yield of the 12-lead series can be virtually retained by using the 6 leads V_3 through V_6 and limb leads II and a V_f.[73] Although this appears to be a 50 per cent reduction in the number of leads required, in practice all 4 torso electrodes must be applied in order to record any limb leads or Wilson precordial leads, and therefore to record these 6 leads, 8 electrodes must be applied instead of the 10 electrodes required for all 12 leads. Another practical consideration is that the ready availability of automatic three-channel electrocardiographs makes it easier to record a 12-lead sequence than it would be to select any 6 leads individually. Tubau and coworkers find that a combination of 12 conventional leads and 2 bipolar leads gives greater sensitivity than 1, 2, or 3 leads.[76]

Bipolar electrocardiographic leads were popularized during the era when it was thought that radiotelemetry was necessary to overcome the technical problems of recording the exercise electrocardiogram.[77] The miniature radio transmitters used for this purpose could accept only a bipolar input signal, so this was derived by placing an active electrode over the V_5 position, where the electrocardiographic signal is strongest, and a reference electrode somewhere on the right side of the chest. Various positions for the reference electrode became standardized (Fig. 8–4). On the basis of current evidence the recommended choice of exercise electrocardiographic leads is the conventional 12-lead set using torso (Mason-Likar) locations for limb leads. This procedure is easy to follow using an unmodified automatic three-channel electrocardiographic recorder, and the same leads used during and after exercise may be used for the resting control electrocardiogram.

BIOLOGICAL AND PHARMACOLOGICAL EFFECTS.
Ischemic heart disease is one of several causes of ST-segment depression. The subendocardial region is the most distal tissue perfused by the coronary vasculature, and thus perfusion pressure is lowest here. Yet it is this tissue which is subjected to direct ventricular pressure and thus has the greatest intramural force resisting coronary flow. Therefore any disparity between perfusion requirement and supply, short of total arterial occlusion, will affect the subendocardium first and most profoundly and will spread outward with increasingly severe underperfusion.

Pressure Overload. Pressure overload of the left ventricle due to either arterial hypertension or obstruction of ventricular outflow may thus be expected to interfere with subendocardial perfusion, even in the absence of atherosclerosis. Lepeschkin showed that young college students with hypertension may show ST-segment depression with exercise,[78] and it is now generally accepted that ventricular overload may result in a false-positive exercise electrocardiogram.[18]

Another relationship between hypertension and exercise electrocardiography is that diuretics administered as antihypertensive therapy may lower the serum potassium concentration sufficiently to cause equivocal changes in the exercise electrocardiogram. The ability of hypokalemia to confound interpretation of the exercise electrocardiogram has been established,[79] and therefore when conducting an exercise test, one should assure that the potassium concentration is normal or should at least exclude possible causes of hypokalemia.

The mechanism producing the various manifestations of prolapse of the mitral valve (p. 1089) is not understood, be they premature beats, chest discomfort, or ST-segment changes. It is known, however, that these patients develop exertional ST-segment depression in the absence of coronary atherosclerosis.[80]

Abnormal Activation Sequence of Ventricles. Abnormal activation sequence of the ventricles, especially the left, alters repolarization and prohibits interpretation of ST-segment changes.[81] This includes not only left bundle branch block but also the Wolff-Parkinson-White syndrome (a subtle source of false-"positive" reaction if it occurs only during exercise (Fig. 8–6). It has also been claimed that patients with short P-R intervals but no delta waves may have false-positive exercise electrocardiographic responses,[82] but this has not been substantiated. It is generally supposed that left ventricular ischemia may be recognized in the lateral electrocardiographic leads when right bundle branch block is present, though perhaps with somewhat less sensitivity.[83,84]

Digitalis Effect. Digitalis is notorious for its obfuscating effect on the ST segment.[85-87] Even when digitalis effect is not apparent in the resting electrocardiogram, it still may be responsible for exertional ST-segment depression.[78] This effect persists longer than the half-life of the glycoside in the blood would suggest.[85] Therefore a conservative policy would be to discontinue digoxin therapy a week before exercise electrocardiography. If glycoside therapy is necessary for its inotropic effect, one should question seriously whether an exercise test is even indicated. It would be convenient if digitalis caused only a limited degree of ST-segment displacement, e.g., not more than 0.20 mv, for then greater displacement could be attributed to ischemia. Although this is thought to be true in the case of marked ST-segment depression (i.e., ≥ 0.40 mv), no dependable upper limit of digitalis-caused ST-segment displacement has been defined. On the other hand, digitalis is not accused of causing falsely negative ECG responses. The absence of ST-segment deviation at peak exercise or thereafter may be considered a valid negative response.

Psychoactive Drugs. Tricyclic and other antidepressant drugs are said to cause false-positive and false-negative responses, especially in women.[88] This effect is by no means understood and needs additional study. Women have been said to manifest more false-positive and false-negative exercise electrocardiographic responses than men,[89] but Linhart et al. do not confirm this if drug effects are taken into account.[88] We have found that asymptomatic women show exertional ST depression with the same frequency as do asymptomatic men.[50]

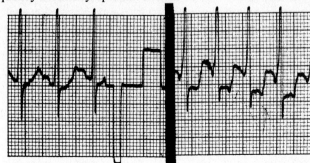

FIGURE 8–6 **Wolff-Parkinson-White syndrome conduction disturbance developing during exercise and mimicking ischemic type of ST depression.** *Left panel,* Recording immediately prior to disturbance. (Courtesy of I. Martin Grais, M.D.)

Antihypertensives and Vasodilators.   Most antihypertensive drugs are not known to have any effect on the exercise electrocardiogram, although one study implicated methyldopa,[88] and the effect of kaliuretic diuretics has already been mentioned (p. 236). Nitroglycerin, nifedipine, and other effective vasodilating drugs will permit a higher level of exercise performance before the effects of ischemia become apparent. For this reason exercise testing is an objective means of assessing the degree of benefit of a therapeutic regimen. However, drugs will rarely prevent ischemia altogether in a progressive exercise test, and thus they are not a significant source of false-negative exercise electrocardiographic results.

Beta-adrenergic Blockers.   These agents, which are at once antiarrhythmic, antianginal, and antihypertensive, act to prevent angina by reducing two principal components of the myocardial oxygen requirement: heart rate and contractility. A compensatory increase in stroke volume, a more "oxygen-efficient" means of achieving an increase in cardiac output, a reduction in systemic vascular resistance, and an increase in peripheral oxygen extraction combine to permit an increased level of exercise performance in the patient with angina pectoris. Beta blockers will blunt the heart rate increase at any level of exercise, and therefore the target heart rate concept does not apply here. Instead, exercise should be continued until evidence of ischemia or exercise intolerance develops. As in the case of nitrate therapy, exercise testing is useful to measure the beneficial effect of therapy. If, on the other hand, the diagnosis of angina pectoris is in doubt, consideration should be given to tapering and discontinuing propranolol and substituting short-acting antianginal therapy if necessary until the patient ceases propranolol ingestion for about 2 days. The possible hazards of this maneuver, insofar as precipitating acute myocardial infarction is concerned, are discussed on p. 1350.

EVALUATION OF ELECTROCARDIOGRAPHIC DATA

Conventional Criteria of Ischemia.   Three important developments complicate clinical interpretation of the electrocardiogram: the time course of ST-segment changes, the effect of lead choice, and the work threshold of ischemia.

Time Course of ST-Segment Changes.   The accumulated experience in interpreting the postexercise electrocardiogram indicating that 0.10 mv of ST-segment depression is a critical index of ischemia does not necessarily apply to tracings recorded during exercise. J-point depression, with an upsloping ST segment, is a normal response to exercise,[90] and the area overlying the J-ST segment increases in proportion to the tachycardia.[91] However, it has been shown that, in exercise, upsloping ST-segment depression of sufficient degree indicates ischemia.[92] Lozner and Morganroth find the specificity of exercise electrocardiograms much improved if one requires that 0.20 mv ST depression, appearing in exercise, must persist for at least 1 minute post exercise in order to qualify as an ischemic response.[93] Thus a Type I ST-segment response (Fig. 8–5) with depression that persists less than 1 minute after exercise is relatively less specific for coronary artery disease—and when disease is present, it is more likely to be single-vessel or mild two-vessel disease—than a Type II segment

with depression that persists for 20 minutes. These findings suggest that 0.10 mv of ST-segment depression may be a sufficient criterion of ischemia *after* exercise, but a larger degree of change, proportional to the heart rate, should be required for tracings recorded *during* exercise.

Effect of Electrocardiographic Lead Choice.   Different electrocardiographic leads, which have differing amplitude sensitivity for the electrocardiographic waveform, require appropriately different amplitude criteria of ST-segment change.[94,95] Bipolar leads, e.g., CM_5, show greater QRS amplitude, greater T amplitude, and greater ST-shift amplitude than is found in Wilson lead V_5. Conversely, Frank lead X shows slightly lower waveform amplitude than V_5. These differences in "scale factor," or amplitude sensitivity, should be taken into account in the interpretation. Investigators thus usually use a 0.20 mv ST-segment shift criterion for bipolar leads. The corresponding ST-segment criterion for Frank lead X would be about 0.08 mv, a difficult measurement to make visually.

Work Threshold of Ischemia.   Finally, the *intensity* of cardiac work at which ischemia occurs is even more important than its presence.[28,96] In subjects in whom the ischemia occurs only at normal peak exercise levels, the coronary blood flow is adequate at rest and during most levels of submaximal stress and becomes inadequate only when maximal or near maximal exercise is undertaken. This high work threshold of ischemia usually corresponds with moderate coronary atherosclerotic obstruction; however, ischemia (or any cardiovascular incapacitation) at a low level of exercise is a very grave finding, corresponding usually with far advanced coronary obstructive disease.

Sex Differences in Electrocardiographic Response.   Exercise electrocardiographic responses in men correspond more closely than in women with the presence or absence of coronary artery disease.[89] The influence of tranquilizers and other psychoactive drugs in women was mentioned earlier. Perhaps the most important factor explaining the sex difference in test accuracy is the different prevalence of

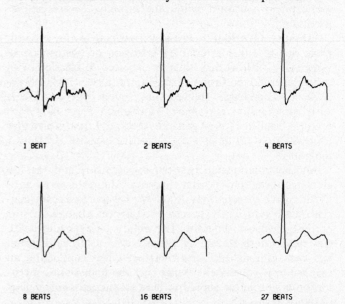

1 BEAT   2 BEATS   4 BEATS

8 BEATS   16 BEATS   27 BEATS

FIGURE 8–7 Reduction of distortion generated by exercise through averaging multiple electrocardiographic complexes by computer. Increasing the number of beats averaged decreases the amount of distortion.

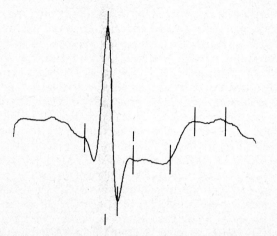

FIGURE 8–8 Computer-processed V₅ lead recorded at peak of exercise. Note absence of myographic artifact. Vertical recognition lines, from left to right, indicate QRS onset, R peak, S nadir, J point, J point +80 msec, T peak, and predicted end of T wave.

coronary disease in men and women. It is well recognized that the accuracy of any less than perfect test is lower in test populations having lower disease prevalence, but too often we forget that men and women constitute separately identifiable "test populations." Classic documentation of this effect has come forth from the Coronary Artery Surgery Study, involving tests on 3153 patients.[97] They found that when allowance was made for disease prevalence, men and women demonstrated the same rate of false-positive and false-negative responses.

Computer Analysis. Development of ST-segment criteria other than exactly one or two divisions of the chart paper and problems with exercise artifact distortion of the electrocardiogram have set the stage for computer enhancement of electrocardiogram interpretation. By computerized averaging of electrocardiographic complexes, myographic and other artifacts are eliminated or reduced (Fig. 8–7). Recognition algorithms identify the points on the electrocardiogram to be measured (Fig. 8–8). Measurements made by computer have the capacity of much greater precision than is possible by visual measurement of conventionally recorded electrocardiograms, and they adapt readily to variations in diagnostic criteria, depending on the phase of the test (control, exercise, or postexercise) and the leads being employed. Several investigators have developed exercise electrocardiographic computer systems,[98–101] and commercial adaptations of these systems are now available.

NONELECTROCARDIOGRAPHIC OBSERVATIONS

Nonelectrocardiographic events in the course of exercise stress testing have been increasingly recognized as equal to, if not more important than, ST-segment changes.[102] Reeves considers the exercise test to be an intensive extension of the history and physical examination.[103] By this he means that the supervising physician has a distinctive opportunity to watch the reactions of the patient to symptoms produced by exercise and to question the patient about the essential qualities of these symptoms while they are present.

BLOOD PRESSURE. The normal blood pressure response to exercise is a progressive rise in systolic pressure with increase in exercise intensity and very little change in the diastolic pressure. Froelicher finds the systolic range at peak exercise to range from 162 to 216 mm Hg. In younger individuals the diastolic pressure may fall slightly, whereas in middle-aged and older adults it is likely to rise.[104] Any rise or fall of diastolic pressure in normal persons is not likely to exceed 10 mm Hg. The resultant rise in mean blood pressure with exercise reflects the fact that fall of the systemic resistance with exercise is insufficient in itself to allow for the rise in cardiac output. In most exercise protocols the systolic blood pressure rises about 8 to 10 mm Hg per stage (Fig. 8–9). Although in the interest of safety it is common to specify a level of resting blood pressure, such as 180/110 mm Hg, over which exercise testing will not be carried out, in fact there are no reported instances of stroke or other hypertensive complication during diagnostic exercise testing. A pathological fall in blood pressure during exercise is encountered occasionally, and although an insensitive sign, it is claimed to be highly specific for severe coronary artery disease.[36,105,106]

Fundamentally, failure of arterial pressure to rise during exercise reflects an inadequate elevation of cardiac output in the face of vasodilation in exercising muscle. Any condition that severely limits the normal exercise-induced rise in cardiac output—cardiomyopathy, valvular heart disease, or coronary artery disease—is the most common cause of failure of cardiac output, and therefore of arterial pressure, to rise during exercise. In patients with coronary artery disease, a large portion of the left ventricle must exhibit impaired function, due to ischemia or infarction or both, for arterial pressure to decline. In the absence of old infarction, this finding often denotes the development of widespread ischemia during exercise, as in patients with disease of the left main coronary artery, a left main equivalent lesion, or three-vessel disease.

HEART RATE. After an initial overreaction to the beginning of exercise and subsequent stabilization requir-

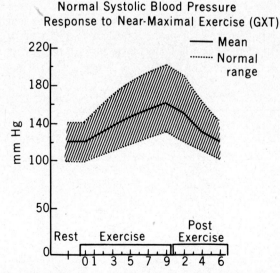

FIGURE 8–9 Mean and normal ranges of systolic blood pressure measured indirectly during and after exercise. (From Sheffield, L. T.: Electrocardiographic stress testing. *In* Chung, E. K. (ed.): Non-invasive Cardiac Diagnosis. Philadelphia, Lea & Febiger, 1976, p. 86.)

ject becomes unable to maintain the set pedaling speed. If there are any limitations to maximal exercise capacity other than cardiovascular ones, these should be carefully noted, since psychological, musculoskeletal, or other noncardiovascular limitations do not have the prognostic implications mentioned above.

EFFORT ANGINA. Although numerous kinds of chest discomfort are encountered during exercise testing, the finding of symptoms distinguished clearly as anginal may improve the sensitivity of exercise electrocardiographic testing considerably. Cole and Ellestad report that whereas ST-segment changes alone detect 64 per cent of patients with significant coronary artery disease, when characteristic chest discomfort was also considered a positive finding, the detection rate rose to 85 per cent.[115]

INTERPRETATION OF STRESS TESTS
(See also p. 1340)

Few diseases manifest a wider spectrum of morbidity and length of survival than coronary artery disease. Therefore we need to know not just whether or not a patient has the disease, but also how severely it is likely to affect his future. Exercise stress testing can help determine this, but in order to make the best use of this procedure the dimensions of the test results should be familiar. Terms used in evaluating stress test results are found in Table 8–5.

Figures-of-merit for Evaluating Tests. *Sensitivity* gives an index of the capability of a test to detect abnormality. The value is given as a percentage or decimal fraction. Although one would wish every test to have a sensitivity of 100 per cent, in the medical realm tests with high sensitivity frequently have the disadvantage of yielding some abnormal results erroneously. The sensitivity of near maximal and maximal exercise tests for coronary artery disease is generally between 60 and 70 per cent when only the ST-segment behavior is considered; however, when combined with other exercise test observations, test sensitivity increases to over 90 per cent.[18,115,116]

Specificity indicates the ability of a test to recognize a normal subject. This is a very important characteristic because of the potential harm should diagnosis of a serious disease be applied to a subject in error. Because of this concern, tests are not usually considered for clinical application unless they have high specificity. Specificity of the near maximal exercise electrocardiographic test usually ranges from 90 to 95 per cent.[18,115,116]

Accuracy is the measure of the capability of a test to yield correct results. It gives a general or overall figure-of-merit for a test, since it includes the ability of the test to recognize true-positives as well as true-negatives.

True-positive is the most clinically useful test result because of the avenue it opens for primary or secondary prevention of overt disease. In a predictive sense the true-positive result would identify the individual who, although healthy at present, is destined to manifest angina pectoris, myocardial infarction, or sudden death in the foreseeable future. *False-positive*, *true-negative*, and *false-negative* results do not require elaboration.

Predictive value indicates the clinical significance of a positive test result. It is the percentage of likelihood that a positive result is true. This term takes into consideration the prevalence of the disease in the population tested. If the prevalence is high, such as the prevalence of coronary atherosclerosis in a population of adults consulting a physician for chest pain, the number of true-positive results will be high and the number of false-positive results will be low, yielding a high predictive value. On the other hand, if the same test is conducted in the population at large in which the prevalence of coronary artery disease is probably between 1 and 2 per cent, the yield of true-positives will be overwhelmed by the large number of false-positives, and the predictive value will be quite low.

Relative risk indicates how a subject's statistical prognosis is changed by virtue of his having undergone a test. Most studies have shown very close agreement on relative risk, finding that persons with abnormal test results have about 13 times greater incidence of coronary disease than those with a negative test result.

When exercise test results are thought of in terms of relative risk instead of clinical diagnosis, justification can be seen for screening selected asymptomatic subjects. Those giving abnormal responses qualify for special attention to reduce risk factors, not to diagnose a disease. Kattus showed the value of this approach in screening 309 asymptomatic executives.[117] Half of those with abnormal responses then participated in a remedial exercise program; all improved their functional capacity, and in one-third electrocardiographic responses converted to normal compared with one-seventh of the nonexercising controls.

Bayes' Theorem (see also Fig. 39–2, p. 1340). In 1763 the English philosopher Thomas Bayes demonstrated the way in which the predictive value of a test is influenced not only by the sensitivity of the test but most especially by the "prior probability" that an individual has the disease tested for (i.e., the prevalence of the disease in

---

TABLE 8–5 TERMS USEFUL IN EVALUATION OF TEST RESULTS

Sensitivity	=	$\dfrac{\text{Number of true-positive detections}}{\text{Total number of positives in the group tested}}$
Specificity	=	$\dfrac{\text{Number of true normals detected}}{\text{Total number of normals in the group tested}}$
Accuracy	=	$\dfrac{\text{Number of true test results (true-positives + true-negatives)}}{\text{Total number of tests performed}}$
True-positive	=	Abnormal test result in individual who has (or will have) the disease*
False-positive	=	Abnormal test result in one who does not (and will not) have the disease
True-negative	=	Normal test result in one who does not (and will not) have the disease
False-negative	=	Normal test result in one who has (or will have) the disease
Predictive value	=	$\dfrac{\text{True-positives}}{\text{True-positives + false-positives}}$
Relative risk (risk ratio)	=	$\dfrac{\text{Disease rate** in persons with a positive test result}}{\text{Disease rate in persons with a negative test result}}$

*Whatever disease the test aims to detect.
**This may be in terms of current prevalence, future incidence, or both and should be specified when the term is used.

the population being tested). This relationship is described by the following formula:

$$P[C/A] = \frac{P[A/C]}{P[A]} = \frac{P[A/C] \cdot P[C]}{P[A/C] \cdot P[C] + P[A_i/C_i] \cdot P[C_i]}$$

where

$P[C/A]$ = probability that a person with a positive test has the disease tested for
C = sensitivity of test
C_i = 1 − specificity of test
A = prevalance of disease
A_i = rarity of disease (complement of A)

Applying this formula to some realistic approximations and assuming that exercise test sensitivity for ischemic heart disease is 80 per cent, that specificity is 90 per cent, and that in a population of North American adults complaining of chest pain the prevalance of ischemic heart disease is 50 per cent, Bayes' theorem would then determine that a patient with a positive exercise test would have an 89 per cent probability of having ischemic heart disease.

If sensitivity = 0.80, specificity = 0.90, and prevalence = 0.50

$$P = \frac{0.50 \times 0.80}{(0.50 \times 0.80) + (0.50 \times 0.10)} = 0.89$$

On the other hand, if the test with unchanged sensitivity and specificity is applied to a group of asymptomatic adults with a disease prevalance of 3 per cent, the probability that an individual with a positive test has ischemic heart disease is only 20 per cent! Of 100 such positive tests, 80 of them would be false-positives.

If sensitivity = 0.80, specificity = 0.90, and prevalence = 0.03

$$P = \frac{0.03 \times 0.80}{(0.03 \times 0.80) + (0.97 \times 0.10)} = 0.20$$

Thus in assessing the meaning of an exercise test result, Bayes' theorem emphasizes the importance of considering the identifiable risk group from which an individual comes.[118] The patient with typical chest pain and positive exercise electrocardiogram, who has an 89 per cent likelihood of having significant coronary artery disease, presents justification for accepting this diagnosis and commencing treatment. However, a patient with atypical chest pain, and thus only about a 20 per cent pretest likelihood of having coronary artery disease, after being tested and found positive will have a 67 per cent probability of coronary disease. That is, there is one chance in three that he does not. In such a case one would like to have additional evidence for the presence of disease before embarking on a potentially dangerous or difficult course of treatment. In the asymptomatic person whose positive test raises his disease probability from 3 to 20 per cent (Fig. 8–1), only moderate preventive measures that would be unlikely to be harmful or burdensome to anyone are justified, although they could be expected to reduce the likelihood of future coronary events.

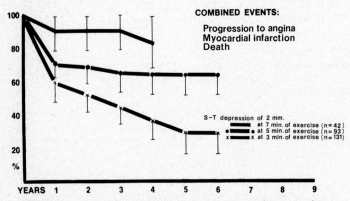

FIGURE 8–11   Continued survival without progression to angina or myocardial infarction with ST depression after 7 minutes (————), 5 minutes (•————•), and 3 minutes (x————x) of exercise. Healthy survival is proportional to exercise capacity. (From Ellestad, M. H.: Stress Testing: Principles and Practice. Philadelphia, F. A. Davis Co., 1975, p. 167.)

PROGNOSTIC SIGNIFICANCE OF EXERCISE TEST RESULTS.

The foregoing should have suggested that the exercise test result should be considered as a quantitative risk factor rather than as a simple disease/no disease classification. Persons without clinical evidence of coronary artery disease who manifest ST-segment depression after only mild exercise have a greater than 50 per cent likelihood of progression of coronary heart disease, as reflected in the development of angina or a myocardial infarction, in the succeeding 4 years, those who develop ischemia only after moderate exercise have a less than 50 per cent likelihood of progression, and patients with ischemia only after strenuous exercise have less than 20 per cent likelihood of progression of disease in the next 4 years (Fig. 8–11).[96] The prognostic value of the treadmill test prevails also in survivors of myocardial infarction; 4 years after testing, patients with abnormal treadmill responses had 30 per cent greater progression of coronary disease than did survivors with a normal test response.[96] Limited stress testing 3 weeks after myocardial infarction (p. 1293) identified patients with more than twice the risk of additional coronary events in the next 4 years than those with normal responses.[119]

McNeer and colleagues found that in patients with angiographically significant coronary artery disease, those with exercise-induced ST-segment depression have over three times greater mortality during 4 years of observation than those without.[28] This landmark study utilized the Duke University computerized data bank. Results from 2290 patients were involved. They employed 12-lead electrocardiograms throughout exercise testing and used a conventional criterion of ≥0.10 mv flat or downsloping (or elevated) ST-segment deviation from baseline. The Bruce treadmill stages were used. Negative tests required attainment of ≥85 per cent of predicted maximal heart rate. Follow-ups occurred at 6 months, 1 year, 2 years, 3 years, and 4 years and were 99.5 per cent complete. They also noted the importance of maximum achieved heart rate during testing. Those whose heart rates did not reach 120 beats/min showed less than 75 per cent survival over 4 years, those reaching heart rates of 120 to 159 beats/min showed over 85 per cent survival, and those with exercise heart rates 160 beats/min or greater had 95 per cent survival. By taking into account ST-segment response, exercise duration, and heart rate, it is possible to identify a low-risk group of patients who, even though afflicted with coronary artery disease, may be expected to show over 90 per cent survival in 4 years. On the other hand, it is also possible to identify a high-risk subgroup based on these observations who can expect only 60 per cent survival over the same interval (Fig. 8–12).

Goldschlager and colleagues found that the Type II ST-segment depression (i.e., ST-segment depression which, instead of improving immediately upon cessation of exercise, becomes more pronounced before improvement begins) is useful in predicting severe coronary artery obstruction (Fig. 8–5, Type II).[120] From 86 to 91 per cent of their patients with this finding had advanced two-vessel, three-vessel, or left main coronary disease. Blumenthal and colleagues reported similar findings. The occurrence of a strongly positive exercise stress test had a 57 per cent predictive accuracy for the presence of left main coronary artery disease.[121] The

ALL CHEST PAIN PATIENTS

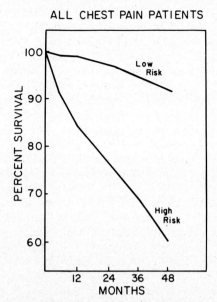

FIGURE 8-12 Prediction of survival on basis of exercise test. "Low-risk" patients had normal ST-segment, heart rate, and exercise duration responses, whereas "high-risk" patients did not. (From McNeer, J. F., et al.: The role of the exercise test in the evaluation of patients for ischemic heart disease. Circulation 57:64, 1978, by permission of the American Heart Association, Inc.)

use of exercise test data makes it possible to separate those patients whose unfavorable risk indicates prompt consideration for coronary arteriography for bypass surgery while also identifying patients who are good candidates for medical, physical, and dietary therapy.[28]

SAFETY OF EXERCISE TESTING

The primary requirements of any elective test are that it be as safe as possible and that the ratio of benefit to risk be favorable. Exercise stress testing enjoys an excellent safety record. Maintenance of a high order of patient safety in testing depends on continual attention to three important factors: contraindications to testing, indications for terminating exercise, and incidence and management of complications.

CONTRAINDICATIONS TO TESTING. It is necessary that the subject considered for exercise stress testing understand the nature of the procedure, the importance of cooperation with the supervising physician, the necessity for reporting all symptoms promptly, and the realization of the very slight but definite risk which the procedure entails in an individual with preexisting cardiovascular disease. Although informed consent may be given verbally to the supervising physician after a discussion of the procedure, use of written and signed informed consent is more likely to avoid omission of important details, will emphasize the importance of the procedure to the subject, and will communicate to the subject the concern which the supervising physician, his coworkers, and his institution have for his well-being.

True contraindications to testing are conditions that are likely to be aggravated by vigorous exercise (Table 8-6). Naturally such a list is headed by unhealed myocardial infarction. Breach of this contraindication has been known to be due to misinterpretation or omission of the resting control 12-lead electrocardiogram. This emphasizes that the supervising physician must be expert in the interpretation of symptoms of coronary heart disease and of resting and exercise electrocardiograms.

Another important contraindication is unstable angina pectoris (p. 1355), variably called preinfarctional angina or intermediate coronary syndrome and defined as "angina pectoris which is newly developed or has definitely become worse in frequency, ease of provocation, and severity (including rest angina) in the last 4 weeks."

Exercise may safely be conducted in the presence of mild to moderate aortic stenosis, with careful attention to blood pressure, the patient's symptoms, and electrocardiogram. Only severe aortic stenosis with palpably prolonged left ventricular ejection time and with clear-cut electrocardiographic left ventricular hypertrophy is a contraindication. The other contraindications are self-explanatory. The AMA Council on Scientific Affairs has recently reported on indications and contraindications for exercise testing, and they are essentially identical with those proposed herein.[122] *Relative* contraindications include known left main coronary disease or the equivalent, severe hypertension, and hypertrophic obstructive cardiomyopathy.

In addition to clinical contraindications, there are conditions which do not compromise safety but which in one way or another limit the usefulness of test results. These include confusing variables such as left ventricular hypertrophy, left bundle branch block, digitalis effect, and others. These were detailed in the preceding section on electrocardiography. When one or more of these conditions are present, one should reconsider whether the expected benefit of the test fully justifies its use.

TERMINATION OF EXERCISE. Termination of exercise has two aspects. Technically, it is determined by whether the test is (1) a subjective maximal one, in which uncomplicated termination is determined by the subject; or (2) a near maximal test, in which an objective endpoint, such as a target heart rate, would be reached and the test then terminated. The aspect of termination most important here is the one of patient safety. In this light items 1 through 11 in Table 8-7 are applicable. These are specific expressions of the general conviction that exercise testing should cease whenever any important sign of work intolerance is recognized or when any condition appears that is more than likely to contribute to morbidity or mortality. Chest pain should convincingly simulate angina pectoris and should be tolerated until it is clear that it is definitely progressing and not stabilizing or regressing in the face of

TABLE 8-6 CONTRAINDICATIONS TO EXERCISE TESTING

Myocardial infarction—impending, acute, or healing
Unstable angina pectoris
Acute myocarditis or pericarditis
Known ominous coronary artery disease pattern
Severe aortic stenosis
Congestive heart failure
Severe hypertension
Uncontrolled cardiac arrhythmias
Intracardiac conduction block greater than first-degree
Acute systemic illness
Unwillingness to give informed consent

TABLE 8–7   INDICATIONS FOR TERMINATING GRADED EXERCISE TESTING

1. Angina-like pain that is progressive during exercise
2. Excessive degree (≥ 0.4 mv) of ischemic type of ST-segment depression or elevation during exercise
3. Ectopic supraventricular tachycardia (regular or irregular)
4. Ventricular premature beats aggravated by exercise or precipitated by exercise (over 25% of beats)
5. Electrocardiogram consistent with ventricular tachycardia
6. *Any* recognized type of intracardiac block precipitated by exercise
7. Signs of peripheral circulatory insufficiency (pallor, diminished pulse, clammy skin, exhaustion, staggering gait)
8. Drop in systolic blood pressure during mild or moderate exercise (e.g., below Stage 3 of Bruce test)
9. Excessive fatigue or dyspnea
10. Failure of monitoring equipment
11. Subject wishes to stop exercise

increasing exercise. The "diagnostic degree" of ST-segment depression should be quite pronounced, more than an estimated 2 mm, since ST-segment depression is frequently overestimated during the quick scrutiny possible during exercise, especially when evaluated by means of an oscilloscope.

INCIDENCE OF COMPLICATIONS.   The safety of exercise stress testing is well documented. Reports from nine groups, ranging from 500 to 170,000 tests, represent a cumulative experience of about 260,000 tests from about 80 medical centers. The largest single reported experience (170,000 tests) resulted from Rochmis and Blackburn's questionnaire survey of 73 medical centers.[123] They found that 16 deaths were associated with exercise testing and that an additional 40 patients required hospitalization for nonfatal complications such as prolonged chest pain or cardiac arrhythmias. This amounts to a mortality rate of 10 per 100,000 tests and a morbidity rate of 24 per 100,000. Eight of the reports include a total of greater than 90,000 tests, among which there were 13 nonfatal infarctions and 3 deaths.[3,124–130] This yields a mortality rate of 3.3 per 100,000 while maintaining a complication rate comparable to that found in the larger survey.

It is not possible to anticipate and prevent the rare instance when a small coronary arterial plaque—insufficient to provoke detectable ischemia during even maximal exercise—may be the site of subintimal hemorrhage, resulting in dislodgment, occlusion of the vessel, and infarction or death. Such an occurrence is far less likely than the risks patients face every day. The more common risks of exercise testing can be detected by careful, attentive search for contraindications prior to testing; meticulous observation of the patient during exercise with monitoring of the electrocardiogram and the blood pressure as well as the subject's symptoms and appearance; and close attention to the patient after exercise, including auscultation and palpation of the heart and inspection of the cervical veins, skin, and general appearance.

TABLE 8–8   EQUIPMENT AND SUPPLIES FOR MANAGEMENT OF COMPLICATIONS

1. Direct-current defibrillator with full tube of electrode paste
2. Assorted airways, ventilation bag, oxygen, and laryngoscope
3. Intravenous fluid (5% dextrose) with tubing, needles, and assorted syringes
4. Assorted drugs, including lidocaine, quinidine, disopyramide, procainamide, phenytoin, propranolol, atropine, isoproterenol, norepinephrine, metaraminol, furosemide, digoxin, dopamine

MANAGEMENT OF COMPLICATIONS.   Appropriate management of exercise test complications depends primarily on the prior establishment of a protocol to be followed by everyone involved in the testing. This includes knowledge of what persons or services to employ immediately, such as anesthesia/airway therapy, emergency patient transport service, and so on, depending on the local setting. A preselected set of equipment and medications in a specific location and arranged in an established pattern is necessary (see Table 8–8). A previously specified treatment routine is essential and should include arranging for transfer of the patient and admission to a coronary care unit.

Rare complications of exercise stress testing include supraventricular tachycardias, such as paroxysmal atrial tachycardia or atrial fibrillation, and ominous multifocal ventricular premature complexes with excessively close coupling to preceding beats or occurring repetitively. Established ventricular tachycardia occurs infrequently, and in our experience has always been self-limiting upon cessation of exercise except when paroxysmal ventricular tachycardia was a preexisting problem in the patient tested. We have not encountered an episode of primary ventricular fibrillation in the course of approximately 25,000 exercise tests. Other complications include atrioventricular block; vasovagal syncope that has progressed through sinus bradycardia to several seconds of complete cardiac arrest before reverting to completely normal, uncomplicated cardiovascular function; prolonged postexercise angina pectoris; and rare instances of myocardial infarction.

References

1. Goldhammer, S., and Scherf, D.: Elektrokardiographische Untersuchungen bei Kranker mit Angina Pectoris ("ambulatorischer Typus"). Zschr. klin. Med. *122*:134, 1933.
2. Rowell, L. B., Taylor, H. L., Simonson, E., and Carlson, W. S.: The physiologic fallacy of adjusting for body weight in performance of the Master two-step test. Am. Heart J. *70*:461, 1965.
3. Blomqvist, C. G.: Use of exercise testing for diagnostic and functional evaluation of patients with arteriosclerotic heart disease. Circulation *44*:1120, 1971.
3a. Froelicher, V. F.: Exercise testing and training: Clinicial applications. J. Am. Coll., Cardial. *1*:114, 1983.
4. James, F. W., Kaplan, S., Schwartz, D. C., Chou, T., Sandker, M. J., and Naylor, V.: Response to exercise in patients after total surgical correction of tetralogy of Fallot. Circulation *54*:671, 1976.
5. Borer, J. S., Brensike, J. F., Redwood, D. R., Itscoitz, S. B., Passamani, E. R., Stone, N. J., Richardson, J. M., Levy, R. I., and Epstein, S. E.: Limitations of the electrocardiographic response to exercise in predicting coronary-artery disease. N. Engl. J. Med. *293*:367, 1975.
6. Philbrick, J. T., Horwitz, R. I., and Feinstein, A. R.: Methodologic problems of exercise testing for coronary artery disease: Groups, analysis and bias. Am. J. Cardiol. *46*:807, 1980.
7. Epstein, S. E., Beiser, G. D., Stampfer, M., Robinson, B. F., and Braunwald E.: Characterization of the circulatory response to maximal upright exercise in normal subjects and patients with heart disease. Circulation *35*:1049, 1967.
8. Astrand, P., and Rodahl, K.: Evaluation of physical work capacity on the basis of tests. *In* Textbook of Work Physiology. New York, McGraw-Hill Book Co., 1970, Chapter 11.
9. Braunwald, E., Ross, J., Jr., and Sonnenblick, E. S.: Mechanism of Contraction of the Normal and Failing Heart. 2nd ed. Boston, Little, Brown and Co., 1976, pp. 166–200.
10. Gobel, F. L., Nordstrom, L. A., Nelson, R. R., Jorgensen, C. R., and Wang, Y.: The rate-pressure product as an index of myocardial oxygen consumption during exercise in patients with angina pectoris. Circulation *57*:549, 1978.
11. Robinson, B. F.: Relation of heart rate and systolic blood pressure to the onset of pain in angina pectoris. Circulation *35*:1073, 1967.
12. Cannon, P. J., Weiss, M. B., and Sciacca, R. R.: Myocardial blood flow in coronary artery disease: Studies at rest and during stress with inert gas washout techniques. Prog. Cardiovasc. Dis. *22*:95, 1977.
13. Hillis, L. D., and Braunwald, E.: Myocardial ischemia. N. Engl. J. Med. *296*: 971, 1977.

14. Harrison, T. R., and Reeves, T. J.: Less common and rare causes of ischemic heart disease. *In* Principles and Problems of Ischemic Heart Disease. Chicago, Year Book Medical Publishers, 1968, Chapter 5.

15. Froelicher, V. F., Jr.: Use of the exercise electrocardiogram to identify latent coronary atherosclerotic heart disease. *In* Amsterdam, E. A., Wilmore, J. H., and DeMaria, A. N. (eds.): Exercise in Cardiovascular Health and Disease. New York, Yorke Medical Books, 1977, Chapter 13.

16. Barnard, R. J., MacAlpin, R., Kattus, A. A., and Buckberg, G. D.: Ischemic response to sudden strenuous exercise in healthy men. Circulation *48*:936, 1973.

17. Mason, R. E., Likar, I., Biern, R. O., and Ross, R. S.: Multiple-lead exercise electrocardiography. Experience in 107 normal subjects and 67 patients with angina pectoris, and comparison with coronary cinearteriography in 84 patients. Circulation *36*:517, 1967.

18. Roitman, D., Jones, W. B., and Sheffield, L. T.: Comparison of submaximal exercise ECG test with coronary cineangiocardiogram. Ann. Intern. Med. *72*: 641, 1970.

19. Ascoop, C. A., Simoons, M. L., Egmond, W. E., and Bruschke, A. V. G.: Exercise test, history, and serum lipid levels in patients with chest pain and normal electrocardiogram at rest: Comparison to findings at coronary arteriography. Am. Heart J. *82*:609, 1971.

20. Bartel, A. G., Behar, V. S., Peter, R. H., Orgain, E. S., and Kong, Y.: Graded exercise stress tests in angiographically documented coronary artery disease. Circulation *49*:348, 1974.

21. Wyatt, H. L., Forrester, J. S., Tyberg, J. V., Goldner, S., Logan, S. E., Parmley, W. W., and Swan, H. J. C.: Effect of graded reductions in regional coronary perfusion on regional and total cardiac function. Am. J. Cardiol. *36*: 185, 1975.

22. Waters, D. D., Da Luz, P., Wyatt, H. L., Swan, H. J. C., and Forrester, J. S.: Early changes in regional and global left ventricular function induced by graded reduction in regional coronary perfusion. Am. J. Cardiol. *39*:537, 1977.

23. Sheffield, L. T., and Roitman, D.: Systolic blood pressure, heart rate, and treadmill work at anginal threshold. Chest *63*:327, 1973.

24. Gould, K. L., Hamilton, G. W., Lipscomb, K., Ritchie, J. L., and Kennedy, J. W.: Method for assessing stress-induced regional malperfusion during coronary arteriography. Experimental validation and clinical application. Am. J. Cardiol. *34*:557, 1974.

25. Logan, S. E.: On the fluid mechanics of human coronary artery stenosis. IEEE Trans. Biomed. Eng. *22*:327, 1975.

26. Feldman, R. L., Nichols, W. W., and Pepine, C. J.: What is the coronary hemodynamic significance of the length of a coronary artery obstruction? Clin. Res. *24*:216A, 1976.

27. Ellestad, M. H.: Stress Testing Principles and Practice. Philadelphia, F. A. Davis Co., 1975, p. 175.

28. McNeer, J. F., Margolis, J. R., Lee, K. L., Kisslo, J. A., Peter, R. H., Kong, Y., Behar, V. S., Wallace, A. G., McCants, C. B., and Rosati, R. A.: The role of the exercise test in the evaluation of patients for ischemic heart disease. Circulation *57*:64, 1978.

29. Master, A. M., Friedman, R., and Dack, S.: The electrocardiogram after standard exercise as a functional test of the heart. Am. Heart J. *24*:777, 1942.

30. Ellestad, M. H., Allen, W., Wan, M. C. K., and Kemp, G. L.: Maximal treadmill stress testing for cardiovascular evaluation. Circulation *39*:517, 1969.

31. Weiner, D. A., McCabe, C., Hueter, D., Hood, W. B., Jr., and Ryan, T.: The predictive value of chest pain as an indicator of coronary disease during exercise testing. Circulation *54* (Suppl. II):II-10, 1976.

32. Harrison, T. R., and Reeves, T. J.: Analysis of symptoms. *In* Principles and Problems of Ischemic Heart Disease. Chicago, Year Book Medical Publishers, 1968, Chapter 6.

33. Varnauskas, E.: The ECG and exercise testing. *In* Julian, D. G. (ed.): Angina Pectoris. New York, Churchill Livingstone, 1977, Chapter 7.

34. Koppes, G., McKiernan, T., Bassan, M., and Froelicher, V. F.: Treadmill exercise testing. Part II. Curr. Prob. Cardiol. *7*:1, 1977.

35. Udall, J. A., and Ellestad, M. H.: Predictive implications of ventricular premature contractions associated with treadmill stress testing. Circulation *56*: 985, 1977.

36. Robinson, B. F.: Relation of heart rate and systolic blood pressure to the onset of pain in angina pectoris. Circulation *35*:1073, 1967.

37. Thomson, P. D., and Kelleman, M. H.: Hypotension accompanying the onset of exertional angina. Circulation *52*:28, 1975.

38. Astrand, P., and Saltin, B.: Maximal oxygen uptake and heart rate in various types of muscular activity. J. Appl. Physiol. *16*:977, 1961.

39. Nutter, D. O., Schlant, R. C., and Hurst, J. W.: Isometric exercise and the cardiovascular system. Mod. Concepts Cardiovasc. Dis. *41*:11, 1972.

40. Lowe, D. K., Rothbaum, D. A., McHenry, P. L., Corya, B. C., and Knoebel, S. B.: Myocardial blood flow response to isometric (handgrip) and treadmill exercise in coronary artery disease. Circulation *51*:126, 1975.

41. Helfant, R. H., deVilla, M. A., and Meister, S. G.: Effect of sustained isometric handgrip exercise on left ventricular performance. Circulation *44*:982, 1971.

42. Jackson, D. H., Reeves, T. J., Sheffield, L. T., and Burdeshaw, J.: Isometric effects on treadmill exercise response in healthy young men. Am. J. Cardiol. *31*: 344, 1973.

43. Nagle, F. J., Balke, B., and Naughton, J. P.: Gradational step tests for assessing work capacity. J. Appl. Physiol. *20*:745, 1965.

44. Bruce, R. A., Blackmon, J. R., Jones, J. W., and Strait, G.: Exercising testing in adult normal subjects and cardiac patients. Pediatrics *32*:742, 1963.

45. Balke, B., and Ware, R. W.: An experimental study of "physical fitness" of Air Force Personnel. U.S. Armed Forces Med. J. *10*:675, 1959.

46. Hellerstein, H. K., Hornsten, T. R., Baker, R. A., and Hoppes, W. L.: Cardiac performance during postprandial lipemia and heparin-induced lipolysis. Am. J. Cardiol. *20*:525, 1967.

47. Astrand, P., and Rhyming, I.: A nomogram for calculation of aerobic capacity (physical fitness) from pulse rate during submaximal work. J. Appl. Physiol. *7*: 218, 1954.

48. Sheffield, L. T.: Graded exercise test (GXT) for isochemic heart disease. A submaximal test to a target heart rate. *In* Exercise Testing and Training of Apparently Healthy Individuals: A Handbook for Physicians. American Heart Association Committee on Exercise, 1972, pp. 35-38.

49. Astrand, I.: Aerobic work capacity in men and women with special reference to age. Acta Physiol. Scand. *49* (Suppl. 169):1, 1960.

50. Lester, F. M., Sheffield, L. T., and Reeves, T. J.: Electrocardiographic changes in clinically normal older men following near maximal and maximal exercise. Circulation *36*:5, 1967.

51. Sheffield, L. T., Maloof, J. A., Sawyer, J. A., and Roitman, D.: Maximal heart rate and treadmill performance of healthy women in relation to age. Circulation *57*:79, 1978.

52. Bruce, R. A., Gey, G. O., Cooper, M. N., Fisher, L. D., and Peterson, D. R.: Seattle heart watch: Initial clinical, circulatory and electrocardiographic responses to maximal exercise. Am. J. Cardiol. *33*:459, 1974.

53. Patterson, J. A., Naughton, J., Pietras, R. J., and Gunnar, R. M.: Treadmill exercise in assessment of the functional capacity of patients with cardiac disease. Am. J. Cardiol. *30*:757, 1972.

54. Bruce, R. A., and Hornsten, T. R.: Exercise stress testing in evaluation of patients with ischemic heart disease. Prog. Cardiovasc. Dis. *11*:371, 1969.

55. Feil, H., and Siegel, M. L.: Electrocardiographic changes during attacks of angina pectoris. Am. J. Med. Sci. *175*:255, 1928.

56. Wood, F. C., and Wolferth, C. C.: Angina pectoris. The clinical and electrocardiographic phenomena of the attack and their comparison with the effects of experimental temporary coronary occlusion. Arch. Intern. Med. *47*: 339, 1931.

57. Wilson, F. N., and Johnston, F. D.: The occurrence in angina pectoris of electrocardiographic changes similar in magnitude and kind to those produced by myocardial infarction. Am. Heart J. *22*:64, 1941.

58. Prinzmetal, M., Kennamer, R., Merliss, R., Wada, T., and Bor, N.: Angina pectoris. I. A variant form of angina pectoris. Am. J. Med. *27*:375, 1959.

59. Chahine, R. A., Raizner, A. E., and Ishimori, T.: The clinical significance of exercise-induced ST-segment elevation. Circulation *54*:209, 1976.

60. Fortuin, N. J., and Friesinger, G. C.: Exercise-induced ST segment elevation: Clinical, electrocardiographic and arteriographic studies in twelve patients. Am. J. Med. *49*:459, 1970.

61. Rijneke, R. D., Ascoop, C. A., and Talmon, J. L.: Clinical significance of upsloping ST segments in exercise electrocardiography. Circulation *61*:671, 1980.

62. Ellestad, M. H.: Stress Testing. 2nd ed. Philadelphia, F. A. Davis Co., 1980.

63. Berman, J. L., Wynne, J., and Cohn, P. F.: Multiple-lead QRS changes with exercise testing. Diagnostic value and hemodynamic implications. Circulation *61*:53, 1980.

64. Baron, D. W., Ilsley, C., Sheiban, I., Poole-Wilson, P. A., and Rickards, A. F.: R wave amplitude during exercise. Relation to left ventricular function and coronary artery disease. Br. Heart J. *44*:512, 1980.

65. Brody, D. A.: A theoretical analysis of intracavitary blood mass influence on the heart-lead relationship. Circ. Res. *4*:731, 1956.

66. Lekven, J., Chatterjee, K., Tyberg, J. V., Stowe, D. F., Mathey, D. G., and Parmley, W. W.: Pronounced dependence of ventricular endocardial QRS potentials on ventricular volume. Br. Heart J. *40*:891, 1978.

67. Vincent, G. M., Abildskov, J. A., and Burgess, M. J.: Mechanisms of ischemic ST-segment displacement. Evaluation by direct current recordings. Circulation *56*:559, 1977.

68. Samson, W. E., and Scher, A. M.: Mechanism of S-T segment alteration during acute myocardial injury. Circ. Res. *8*:780, 1960.

69. Einthoven, W.: Weiteres über das Elektrokardiogramm. Arch. ges. Physiol. *122*:517, 1908.

70. Abarquez, R. F., Freiman, A. H., Reichel, F., and LaDue, J. S.: The precordial electrocardiogram during exercise. Circulation *22*:1060, 1960.

71. Shackel, B.: Skin-drilling. A Method of diminishing galvanic skin-potentials. Am. J. Psychol. *72*:114, 1959.

72. Mason, R. E., and Likar, I.: A new system of multiple-lead exercise electrocardiography. Am. Heart J. *71*:196, 1966.

73. Blackburn, H., Katigbak, R., Mitchell, P., and Imbimbo, B.: What electrocardiographic leads to take after exercise? Am. Heart J. *67*:184, 1964.

74. Mason, R. E., and Likar, I.: A new approach to stress tests in the diagnosis of myocardial ischemia. Trans. Am. Clin. Climatol. Assoc. *76*:40, 1964.

75. Phibbs, B. P., and Buckels, L. J.: Comparative yield of ECG leads in multistage stress testing. Am. Heart J. *90*:275, 1975.

76. Tubau, J. F., Chaitman, B. R., Bourassa, M. G., and Waters, D. D.: Detection of multivessel coronary disease after myocardial infarction using exercise stress testing and multiple ECG lead systems. Circulation *61*:44, 1980.

77. Bellet, S., Deliyiannis, S., and Eliakim, M.: The electrocardiogram during exercise as recorded by radioelectrocardiography. Comparison with postexercise electrocardiogram (Master two-step test). Am. J. Cardiol. *8*:385, 1961.

78. Lepeschkin, E., and Surawicz, B.: Characteristics of true-positive and false-

positive results of electrocardiographic Master two-step exercise tests. N. Engl. J. Med. *258*:511, 1958.

79. Riley, C. P., Oberman, A., and Sheffield, L. T.: Electrocardiographic effects of glucose ingestion. Arch. Intern. Med. *130*:703, 1972.

80. Greenspan, M., Iskandrian, A. S., Mintz, G. S., Croll, M. N., Segal, B. L., Kimbiris, D., and Bemis, C. E.: Exercise myocardial scintigraphy with[201] thallium. Chest *77*:47, 1980.

81. Whinnery, J. E., Froelicher, V. F., Jr., Stewart, A. J., Longo, M. R., Jr., Triebwasser, J. H., and Lancaster, M. C.: The electrocardiographic response to maximal treadmill exercise of asymptomatic men with left bundle branch block. Am. Heart J. *94*:316, 1977.

82. Astrand, I., Blomqvist, G., and Orinius, E.: ST changes at exercise in patients with short P-R interval. Acta Med. Scand. *185*:205, 1969.

83. Whinnery, J. E., Froelicher, V. F., Jr., Stewart, A. J., Longo, M. R., Jr., and Triebwasser, J. H.: The electrocardiographic response to maximal treadmill exercise of asymptomatic men with right bundle branch block. Chest *71*:335, 1977.

84. Johnson, S., O'Connel, J., Becker, P., Moran, J. F., and Gunnar, R.: The diagnostic accuracy of exercise ECG testing in the presence of complete right bundle branch block. Circulation *52*(Suppl. II):II–48, 1975.

85. Kawai, C., and Hultgren, H. N.: The effect of digitalis upon the exercise electrocardiogram. Am. Heart J. *68*:409, 1964.

86. Liebow, I. M., and Feil, H.: Digitalis and the normal work electrocardiogram. Am. Heart J. *22*:683, 1941.

87. Yu, P. N. G., Lovejoy, F. W., Hulfish, B., Howell, M. M., Joos, H. A., Tenney, S. M., Haroutunian, L. M., and Evans, H. W.: Cardiorespiratory responses and electrocardiographic changes during exercise before and after intravenous digoxin in normal subjects. Am. J. Med. Sci. *224*:146, 1952.

88. Linhart, J. W., Laws, J. G., and Satinsky, J. D.: Maximum treadmill exercise electrocardiography in female patients. Circulation *50*:1173, 1974.

89. Cumming, G. R., Dufresne, C., Kich, L., and Samm, J.: Exercise electrocardiogram patterns in normal women. Br. Heart J. *35*:1055, 1973.

90. Robb, G. P., and Marks, H. H.: Latent coronary artery disease: Determination of its presence and severity by the exercise electrocardiogram. Am. J. Cardiol. *13*:603, 1964.

91. Sheffield, L. T., Holt, J. H., Lester, F. M., Conroy, D. V., and Reeves, T. J.: On-line analysis of the exercise electrocardiogram. Circulation *40*:935, 1969.

92. Kurita, A., Chaitman, B. R., and Bourassa, M. G.: Significance of exercise-induced junctional S-T depression in evaluation of coronary artery disease. Am. J. Cardiol. *40*:492, 1977.

93. Lozner, E. C., and Morganroth, J.: New criteria for evaluating "positive" exercise tests in asymptomatic patients. Am. J. Cardiol. *39*:288, 1977.

94. Blackburn, H., Taylor, H. L., Okamoto, N., Rautaharju, P., Mitchell, P. L., and Kerkhof, A. C.: Standardization at the exercise electrocardiogram. A systematic comparison of chest lead configurations employed for monitoring during exercise. *In* Karvonen, M. J., and Barry, A. J. (eds.): Physical Activity and the Heart. Springfield, Ill., Charles C Thomas, 1967, Chapter 9.

95. Froelicher, V. F., Jr., Wolthius, R., Keiser, N., Stewart, A., Fischer, J., Longo, M. R., Jr., Triebwasser, J. H., and Lancaster, M. C.: A comparison of two bipolar exercise electrocardiographic leads to lead V_5. Chest *70*:611, 1976.

96. Ellestad, M. H., and Wan, M. K. C.: Predictive implications of stress testing. Follow-up of 2700 subjects after maximum treadmill stress testing. Circulation *51*:363, 1975.

97. Weiner, D. A., McCabe, C. H., Fisher, L. D., Chaitman, B. R., and Ryan, T. J.: Similiar rates of false positive and false negative exercise tests in matched males and females (CASS). Circulation *58*(Suppl. II):II–140, 1978.

98. Sheffield, L. T.: The use of the computer in exercise electrocardiography. Prac. Cardiol. *4*:101, 1978.

99. Blomqvist, G.: The Frank lead exercise electrocardiogram. A quantitative study based on averaging technic and digital computer analysis. Acta Med. Scand. *178*(Suppl. 440):5, 1965.

100. McHenry, P. L., Stowe, D. E., and Lancaster, M. C.: Computer quantitation of the the ST segment response during maximal treadmill exercise. Circulation *38*:691, 1968.

101. Simoons, M. L., Boom, H. B. K., and Smallenburg, E.: On-line processing of orthogonal exercise electrocardiogram. Comput. Biomed. Res. *8*:105, 1975.

102. Sheffield, L.T.: The meaning of exercise test findings. *In* Fox, S. M., III (ed.): Coronary Heart Disease. Prevention, Detection, Rehabilitation with Emphasis on Exercise Testing. Denver, Department of Professional Education International Medical Corp., 1974, Chapter 9.

103. Harrison, T. R., and Reeves, T. J.: The exertional electrocardiogram. *In*

Principles and Problems of Ischemic Heart Disease. Chicago, Year Book Medical Publishers, 1968, Chapter 25.

104. Wolthuis, R. A., Froelicher, V. F., Jr., Fischer, J., and Triebwasser, J. H.: The response of healthy men to treadmill exercise. Circulation *55*:153, 1977.

105. Morris, S. N., Phillips, J. F., Jordan, J. W., and McHenry, P. L.: Incidence and significance of decreases in systolic blood pressure during graded treadmill exercise testing. Am. J. Cardiol. *41*:221, 1978.

106. Baker, T., Levites, R., and Anderson, G. J.: The significance of hypotension during treadmill exercise testing. Circulation *54*(Suppl. II):II–11, 1976.

107. Andersen, K. L.: The cardiovascular system in exercise. *In* Falls, H. B. (ed.): Exercise Physiology. New York, Academic Press, 1968, Chapter 3.

108. Berman, J. L., Wynne, J., and Cohn, P. F.: Value of a multivariate approach for interpreting treadmill exercise tests in coronary artery disease. Am. J. Cardiol. *41*:375, 1978.

109. Lewis, R. P., Boudoulas, H., Welch, T. G., and Forester, W. F.: Usefulness of systolic time intervals in coronary artery disease. Am. J. Cardiol. *37*:787, 1976.

110. Lance, V. Q., and Spodick, D. H.: Systolic time intervals utilizing ear densitography. Advantages and reliability for stress testing. Am. Heart J. *94*:62, 1977.

111. Bruce, R. A.: Exercise testing of patients with coronary heart disease. Principles and normal standards for evaluation. Ann. Clin. Res. *3*:323, 1971.

112. Froelicher, V. F., Thompson, A. J., Longo, M. R., Triebwasser, J. H., and Lancaster, M. C.: Value of exercise testing for screening asymptomatic men for latent coronary artery disease. Prog. Cardiovasc. Dis. *18*:265, 1976.

113. Froelicher, V. F., and Lancaster, M. C.: The prediction of maximal oxygen consumption from a continuous exercise treadmill protocol. Am. Heart J. *87*:445, 1974.

114. Ellestad, M. H.: Stress Testing. Principles and Practice. Philadelphia, F. A. Davis Co., 1975, Chapter 8.

115. Cole, J. P., and Ellestad, M. H.: Significance of chest pain during treadmill exercise: Correlation with coronary events. Am. J. Cardiol. *41*:227, 1978.

116. Aronow, W. S., and Cassidy, J.: Five year follow-up of double Master's test, maximal treadmill stress test, and resting and postexercise apexcardiogram in asymptomatic persons. Circulation *52*:616, 1975.

117. Kattus, A. A., Jorgensen, C. R., Worden, R. E., and Alvaro, A. B.: ST segment depression with near-maximal exercise: Its modification by physical conditioning. Chest *62*:678, 1972.

118. Melin, J. A., Piret, L. J., Vanbutsele, R. J. M., Rousseau, M. F., Cosyns, J., Brasseur, L. A., Beckers, C., and Detry, J. M. R.: Diagnostic value of exercise electrocardiography and thallium myocardial scintigraphy in patients without previous myocardial infarction: A bayesian approach. Circulation *63*:1019, 1981.

119. DeBusk, R. F., Davidson, D. M., Houston, N., and Fitzgerald, J.: Serial ambulatory electrocardiography and treadmill exercise testing after uncomplicated myocardial infarction. Am. J. Cardiol. *45*:547, 1980.

120. Goldschlager, N., Selzer, A., and Cohn, K.: Treadmill stress tests as indicators of presence and severity of coronary artery disease. Ann. Intern. Med. *85*:277, 1976.

121. Blumenthal, D. S., Weiss, J. L., Mellits, E. D., and Gerstenblith, G.: The predictive value of a strongly positive stress test in patients with minimal symptoms. Am. J. Med. *70*:1005, 1981.

122. Council on Scientific Affairs, American Medical Association: Indications and contraindications for exercise testing. J.A.M.A. *246*:1015, 1981.

123. Rochmis, P., and Blackburn, H.: Exercise tests. A survey of procedures, safety and litigation experience in approximately 170,000 tests. J.A.M.A. *217*:1061, 1971.

124. Doyle, J. T., and Kinch, S. H.: The prognosis of an abnormal electrocardiographic stress test. Circulation *41*:545, 1970.

125. Bruce, R. A., Hornsten, T. R., and Blackmon, J. R.: Myocardial infarction after normal responses to maximal exercise. Circulation *38*:552,1968.

126. Jelinek, M. V., and Lown, B.: Exercise stress testing for exposure of cardiac arrhythmia. Prog. Cardiovasc. Dis. *16*:497, 1974.

127. Sheffield, L. T., and Reeves, T. J.: Graded exercise in the diagnosis of angina pectoris. Mod. Conc. Cardiovasc. Dis. *34*:1, 1965.

128. Kattus, A. S., Hanafee, W. N., Lingmise, W. P., Jr., MacAlpin, R. N., and Rivin, A. U.: Diagnosis, medical and surgical management of coronary insufficiency. Ann. Intern. Med. *69*:115, 1968.

129. McHenry, P. L., Morris, S. N., and Jordan, J. W.: Stress testing in coronary heart disease. Heart and Lung *3*:83, 1974.

130. Atterhog, J. H., Jonsson, B., and Samuelsson, R.: Exercise testing: A prospective study of complication rates. Am. Heart J. *98*:572, 1979.

9

CARDIAC CATHETERIZATION

by William H. Barry, M.D., and William Grossman, M.D.

TECHNICAL ASPECTS

Historical Review. According to André Cournand, cardiac catheterization was first performed (and so named) in 1844 by Claude Bernard,[1] who catheterized both the right and the left ventricles of a horse by means of a retrograde approach from the jugular vein and carotid artery. There followed an era of investigation of cardiovascular physiology in animals that resulted in the development of many important techniques and principles—including pressure manometry and the application of the Fick principle for measuring cardiac output—subsequently applied to the study of patients with heart disease.

Although others had previously passed catheters into the great veins, Werner Forssmann is generally credited as the first to pass a catheter into the heart of a living human being.[2] At age 25, he exposed a vein in his own left arm, introduced a ureteral catheter into the venous system, and advanced it under fluoroscopic control into the right atrium. He then walked to the Radiology Department, where the catheter position was documented by a chest x-ray. During the next 2 years, Forssmann continued to perform catheterization studies, including six additional attempts to catheterize himself.

The potential of Forssmann's technique was appreciated by other investigators. In 1930, Klein reported on catheterization of the right ventricle in 11 patients and measurement of cardiac output using the Fick principle.[3] The cardiac outputs were 4.5 and 5.6 liter/min in two patients without heart disease.[1] Except for these and several other studies, application of cardiac catheterization to evaluate the circulation in normal and disease states was limited and fragmentary until the work of Cournand and Richards, who in 1941 began a remarkable series of investigations of right-heart physiology in humans.[4–6] In 1947, Dexter and his colleagues at the Peter Bent Brigham Hospital reported their studies of congenital heart disease and mentioned some observations on "the oxygen saturation and source of pulmonary capillary blood" obtained from a catheter in the pulmonary artery "wedge" position.[7] Subsequent work from Dexter's laboratory[8] and by Lagerlof and Werkö[9] showed that the pressure measured in the pulmonary artery "wedge" position was an accurate estimate of pulmonary venous and left atrial pressure. During this exciting early period, catheterization was used to investigate problems in cardiovascular physiology by McMichael in England,[10] Lenegre in Paris,[11,12] and Cournand, Warren, Stead, Bing, Dexter, Burchell, Wood, and their respective coworkers in this country.[13–22]

Further developments came rapidly. Some of the highlights include the following: Retrograde left-heart catheterization was first introduced by Zimmerman[23] and Limon Lason[24] and their respective coworkers in 1950. The percutaneous technique developed by Seldinger in 1953 was soon applied to cardiac catheterization of both the left and right heart chambers.[25] Transseptal left-heart catheterization was developed[26] and applied clinically by Ross, Braunwald, and Morrow,[27] and it quickly became accepted as a standard technique. Selective coronary arteriography was developed by Sones et al. in 1959[28,29] and was perfected in the ensuing years. In 1970, a practical balloon-tipped flow-guided catheter technique was introduced by Swan, Ganz, and their collaborators, making possible the applicability of catheterization outside the conventional catheterization laboratory.[30] Many other landmark events could be mentioned and the contributions of many individuals could be recognized, but these have been detailed elsewhere.[31]

In this chapter, we discuss current methods of cardiac catheterization, including technical aspects important for optimal use of these methods and accurate interpretation of the data obtained. The development of these techniques and their application to the study of normal and abnormal human cardiac physiology have played a decisive role in improving the diagnosis and treatment of patients with cardiac disease.

Fluoroscopy and Image Intensification. A modern cardiac fluoroscopy unit is a central component of any cardiac catheterization facility. Such a unit[32] consists of three components: an x-ray generating system; an image intensifier; and an image recording system, usually a video camera and monitor and a 35-mm cine camera. The cine camera is used almost exclusively for cardiac angiography.

X-ray Source. An x-ray tube consists of a glass container evacuated of air, containing a cathode, which is the electron source, and an anode, toward which flow the negatively charged electrons emitted from the cathode. The number of electrons flowing from the cathode to the anode per unit of time (current in mA) is largely controlled by the temperature of the cathode. The energy of the electrons is controlled by the potential difference (kv) between the cathode and the anode. When electrons strike the anode, a few pass close to nuclei of the atoms of the anode material and produce "Bremsstrahlung" or "braking radiation" x-ray photons. The radiation spectra thus produced can be filtered (normally with aluminum) to remove lower energy photons that cannot penetrate a human torso but can increase radiation exposure. In operation, the control system for the x-ray tube produces and adjusts the direct-current high voltage (kv), adjusts the x-ray tube current (mA), provides for selection of anode focal spot size, and controls exposure time (pulse width in msec). A small focal spot yields better resolution but produces higher heating, which can shorten the life of the anode.

A portion of the x-ray photons thus produced is allowed to pass upward through an adjustable lead-shielded exit port (cone) and thence through the patient. The interaction of an x-ray photon with body tissue results in attenuation of an x-ray beam, which is influenced by x-ray photon energy. Subject contrast range is determined by minimum and maximum penetration values of the body section and is thus influenced by the energy spectrum of the x-ray photon.

Intensifying Screens. Imaging intensifier screens convert x-ray photons into lower energy photons in the visible light spectrum and amplify the image obtained. The most commonly used input phosphor screen is of the cesium-iodide type, which typically absorbs 50 per cent or more of incident radiation. In this layer, incident x-ray photons are converted into light. In direct contact with the input phosphor is a second layer, the photocathode, which converts the light image into an electron image. The electrons emitted from the photocathode are electrically focused on a smaller output screen, where electrons are absorbed and produce another light image. Input phosphor screens vary from 5 to 12 inches in diameter, and many intensifier systems have two or three interchangeable screens or "tubes" of different sizes that may be selected by the operator when differing degrees of magnification are required. The typical output screen is slightly less than 1 inch in diameter.

Gain in light intensity occurs because of acceleration of electrons between the photocathode and the output screen and because the output screen is smaller in area than is the input screen. Modern image intensifier tubes have a gain of 5000× or more and thus markedly diminish radiation exposure to the patient and operator.

Radiation Hazards. Radiation exposure during cardiac catheterization and angiography ranges from 21 to 39 mrad for the primary operator and from 12 to 20 mrad for the assistant (1 rad = 100 ergs/gm in any tissue).[33] Approximately one-half this exposure occurs during fluoroscopy and one-half during cine operation. On the basis of a recommended maximum dose of 100 mrad/week to the lens of the eye for occupational workers, it is advised that an operator be limited to five procedures per week. Exposure of catheterization personnel should be monitored by means of film badges worn at the collar level. Radiation exposures to patients during cardiac catheterization are significant and range to 28 rad.

The following guidelines help reduce radiation exposure to patients and operators:

1. The smallest x-ray beam possible should be used.
2. Fluoroscopy and cineangiography times should be kept to a minimum.
3. Personnel should remain as far as possible from the patient and should wear lead aprons.
4. Personnel should be shielded during cineangiography if this is practical.

CARDIAC CATHETERIZATION

Catheter Insertion. Of the various approaches to cardiac catheterization, certain ones are of historical interest only (i.e., transbronchial approach, posterior transthoracic left atrial puncture, and suprasternal puncture of the left atrium). The majority of catheterizations performed currently utilize either of two approaches: catheterization by direct exposure of an artery and a vein (including umbilical vessels in neonates) and catheterization by the percutaneous approach (including transseptal catheterization). Each method has its advantages and disadvantages, its adherents and detractors. In reality, the methods are not mutually exclusive but rather complementary, and it is our belief that the physician performing cardiac catheterization should be well versed in both techniques. The methods employed in the authors' laboratories are described below.

Brachial Approach. This approach involves surgical exposure of the brachial artery and basilic vein in the antecubital fossa and insertion of the catheters directly following vessel incision. The percutaneous approach of Seldinger may also be used in adults via the brachial vessels if catheters of small size (No. 5 French) are used.[25] The brachial approach is utilized in patients with obstructive and/or thrombotic arterial disease involving the abdominal aorta, iliac artery, or femoral artery; suspected thrombosis of the femoral vein or inferior vena cava; or coarctation of the aorta. It may also be advantageous in obese patients, in whom the percutaneous femoral technique may be technically quite difficult and in whom bleeding may be hard to control after removal of the catheter.

Procedure. After the brachial artery is localized by means of palpation in the right antecubital fossa, local anesthesia is induced with 5 to 15 ml of 1 to 2 per cent lidocaine, and a single transverse incision is made just proximal to the flexor crease. Tissues are separated by blunt dissection, and a medial vein is isolated and encircled proximally and distally with 3-0 or 4-0 silk. The brachial artery is isolated from adjacent nerves and fascia and is encircled proximally and distally with moistened umbilical tape or silicone Elastomer surgical tape.

Right-heart catheterization is accomplished by means of antegrade passage of an appropriate catheter (e.g., Cournand, Goodale-Lubin, Swan-Ganz) via the basilic or brachial vein to the right atrium, right ventricle, pulmonary artery, and pulmonary capillary "wedge" positions under fluoroscopic guidance. In the wedge position, the catheter occludes the distal pulmonary artery segment, and thus the catheter tip is exposed to only the pulmonary venous pressure. Pressure recorded from the wedge position is accepted as a true wedge pressure only if a characteristic left atrial waveform is exhibited and if completely oxygenated blood (>95 per cent oxygen saturation) can be aspirated from the catheter.[31] Left-heart catheterization is then accomplished by means of retrograde passage of an appropriate catheter (e.g., Eppendorf, Lehman angiographic, Sones, NIH) through a transverse brachial arteriotomy to the ascending aorta and left ventricle.

Systemic administration of heparin (5000 units) at the time of left-heart catheterization and coronary arteriography is indicated to prevent thrombotic complications. In case of difficulty in passing catheters from the brachial artery around the shoulder, an end-hole catheter with a flexible guidewire protruding beyond the tip may be useful. As catheters with or without the aid of guidewires are advanced in the vascular system, their passage should be monitored fluoroscopically; if progress of the catheter is difficult, or if the patient complains of pain, caution should be exercised to avoid dissection or perforation of the vessel wall. Occasionally, spasm of the vessel around the catheter may occur, owing to the relatively small size of vessels in the upper extremities. In this case administration of small amounts of morphine should promptly facilitate catheter manipulation; if not, a catheter of smaller diameter should be used.

Following completion of hemodynamic and angiographic studies, the catheters are withdrawn, and the artery is repaired. In our laboratory, a Fogarty balloon catheter is routinely passed proximally and distally to remove any thrombi that may have formed within the arterial lumen during the catheterization. After proximal and distal flow is deemed adequate, 15 ml of heparinized solution (1500 units in 15 ml of 5 per cent dextrose in water) are infused into the artery proximally and distally through a small polyethylene catheter. The artery is immediately occluded with vascular clamps proximal and distal to the

arteriotomy site. A stay suture is placed at each end of the arteriotomy, which is then closed using a continuous stitch of 6–0 Tevdek. It
is important not to raise an intimal flap nor to penetrate the posterior
intima with the needle. After suturing, first the distal and then the
proximal clamp is removed. Minor leaks usually respond to gentle
pressure applied directly with a finger over the site of the arteriotomy
repair. The radial pulse should be palpable and as strong as it was
prior to catheterization. If it is absent or markedly reduced, the artery
should be reopened, a Forgarty balloon catheter passed again, and
the vessel repaired. If this does not result in return of the pulse, an
experienced vascular surgeon should be consulted. The vein may be
tied off or repaired directly.

The wound is then flushed with sterile saline and a 1 per cent povidone-iodine solution, and the skin incision is closed with 3–0 to 4–0
nylon, which should be removed within 7 to 10 days. Alternatively, an
absorbable material may be used, so that suture removal is unnecessary. Antibiotic ointment (10 per cent povidone-iodine) is applied to
the suture line, and the area should be covered with a dressing.

Postcatheterization orders should include the following:

1. Resume all previous medications.
2. Measure blood pressure and pulse and inspect dressing every
15 minutes for 1 hour, every hour for 4 hours, then every 4 hours for
24 hours.
3. Call a house officer or attending physician *and* a member of the
catheterization laboratory staff in the event of bleeding, loss of pulse,
hypotension, or chest pain.
4. Encourage oral fluid intake of 2 to 3 liters over 6 to 8 hours (if
an angiographic contrast agent has been administered).
5. Administer analgesic medication, as needed.

Femoral Approach. Right- and left-heart catheterization via the femoral approach is usually performed from
the right groin, although the left groin may be used if necessary. The major landmarks of the femoral area are the
anterior superior iliac spine, the pubic tubercle, and the inguinal ligament running between them. The femoral nerve,
artery, and vein are located in the femoral triangle below
the inguinal ligament. Proceeding from lateral to medial,
the relationship of these structures may be remembered
with the aid of the mnemonic NAVY (*n*erve, *a*rtery, *v*ein,
empt*y* space).

Procedure. The femoral artery is located by means of palpation
at a point approximately two fingerbreadths below the inguinal ligament. The skin and subcutaneous tissue over the artery are
anesthetized with 10 to 15 ml of 1 per cent lidocaine. The anesthetic
must be given carefully and must not be injected directly into a vessel. It is important that percutaneous puncture of the femoral vessels
be a correct distance below the inguinal ligament; if it is too high, hemostasis may be impaired, owing to the posterior course of the vessels in the pelvic cavity; if it is too low, the vein may run behind the
artery, and the artery may be entered after it bifurcates into the pro-
funda and superficial femoral branches. Although the inguinal crease
is usually just below the inguinal ligament, this relationship is not constant, and the use of the inguinal ligament as the primary landmark is
therefore advised.

When performing right-heart and left-heart catheterization via the
femoral approach, we prefer to enter the femoral vein first. This is accomplished using an 18-gauge Seldinger needle, which consists of a
blunt, tapered external cannula with a sharp obturator. After a ¼-inch
skin incision has been made at the correct distance below the inguinal ligament and medial to the arterial pulse, the needle and obturator are inserted with a smooth motion at a 45-degree angle. If the
patient has discomfort as the needle penetrates the deeper femoral
tissues, additional lidocaine can be infiltrated through the needle, after removing the obturator and ascertaining that the needle is extravascular. A small syringe is then attached to the needle, which is
slowly withdrawn while continuous gentle aspiration is performed.
When the vein is entered, blood is easily aspirated. The syringe is removed without moving the needle, and a Teflon-coated guidewire
(preferably a J tip) is inserted into the needle and is advanced into
the vein (Fig. 9–1). The guidewire should pass easily, with its course
checked fluoroscopically. The needle is then withdrawn over the

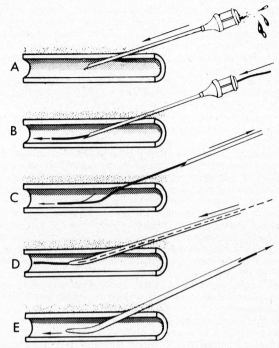

**FIGURE 9–1 The Seldinger technique. The Seldinger needle is in-
serted through the vessel at an angle no steeper than 45 degrees.
The needle obturator is withdrawn, and the needle is slowly pulled
out until the tip is within the lumen of the vessel (*A*). A flexible
tipped guidewire is then inserted into the vessel through the needle
(*B*), and the needle is withdrawn (*C*). A catheter (or sheath with obturator) is then inserted into the vessel over the guidewire (*D*). The
guidewire is then removed, leaving the catheter (or sheath) in the
vessel lumen (*E*). (From Kory, R. C., et al.: A Primer of Cardiac Catheterization. Springfield, Ill. Courtesy of Charles C Thomas, 1965.)**

guide, and a venous sheath of appropriate size with obturator is
placed into the vein over the guidewire. The sheath should be inserted with a twisting, forward pressure. The obturator and guidewire are
then removed, and the sheath is flushed via a stopcock.

Catheter Insertions. The femoral artery may then be punctured at
a 45-degree angle with the Seldinger needle, once a skin incision ¼-
inch long and deep has been made directly over the arterial pulse.
The obturator is removed, and the needle is slowly withdrawn until
the tip enters the artery lumen and a pulsatile flow of arterial blood
exits from the needle hub. A Teflon-coated J guidewire is inserted
into the needle and advanced into the artery. The guidewire should
advance easily, with its position observed on fluoroscopy as it passes
into the abdominal aorta. The needle is then withdrawn over the
guidewire, and the artery is compressed firmly at the puncture site. A
No. 8 French arterial sheath with a proximal hemostasis valve and a
side-port extension tube is inserted into the artery over the guidewire.
The sheath obturator and guidewire are removed, and the sheath is
flushed via the side-arm extension tube, which is connected to a
pressure transducer for continuous monitoring of femoral arterial
pressure. It is, of course, possible to insert an end-hole catheter into
the artery directly over the guidewire without use of a sheath. This
would be appropriate if only one arterial catheter were to be used.
However, use of the arterial sheath greatly facilitates catheter changes, permits use of a greater variety of catheters, and allows continuous monitoring of femoral artery pressure during left-heart
catheterization.[34] With sheaths in the femoral artery vein, and the
femoral artery pressure recorded for monitoring purposes, it is possible to proceed to right- and left-heart catheterization.

Right-heart Catheterization. The right-heart catheters used with
the femoral approach are the same as those described for the brachial approach (i.e., Cournand, Goodale-Lubin, or Swan-Ganz) (Fig.
9–2). The first two of these catheters have an elbow bend, which facilitates passage from the right ventricle into the pulmonary artery. As
the catheter is advanced through the sheath and into the inferior
vena cava, its motion should be observed on fluoroscopy. The move-

ment of the catheter should be gentle and the passage effortless; catheter advancement should never be forced. While the right-heart catheter is passed from the groin, it frequently enters the renal or hepatic veins. If this occurs, the catheter should be withdrawn and rotated before it is advanced farther. A guidewire may be used if a tortuous venous system makes catheter passage difficult.

Once the right atrium has been entered, a pressure tracing from this chamber should be recorded, and a sample of blood should be obtained for measurement of oxygen saturation. The catheter is then advanced through the right ventricle and into the pulmonary artery. Blood pressure and oxygen saturation should then be measured in the pulmonary artery. A difference between right atrial (or superior vena caval) and pulmonary artery oxygen saturation of greater than 5 per cent should indicate the possibility of a left-to-right shunt. Occasionally it is difficult to maneuver a Cournand or a Goodale-Lubin catheter from the right ventricle to the pulmonary artery from the groin, in which case it is best to remove the right-heart catheter and use a balloon-tipped, flow-directed catheter for the right-heart study. In addition, in patients with left bundle branch block, a balloon catheter is preferred because of the reduced likelihood of trauma to the right bundle branch during right-heart catheterization with this type of catheter. Catheter-induced right bundle branch block in a patient with complete left bundle branch block results in complete heart block and can cause asystole. A Gorlin or Cournand right-heart pacing catheter may also be used in this situation to initiate emergency pacing, if necessary.

The right-heart catheter is then used to record pulmonary artery wedge pressure; it is advanced under fluoroscopic guidance into a peripheral pulmonary artery branch during a deep inspiration. To record a wedge pressure with a balloon-type catheter, the balloon is inflated while the catheter tip is in a proximal pulmonary artery. The catheter is then advanced until the pressure configuration changes to that of a wedge pressure. Deflation of the balloon at this point should result in reappearance of pulmonary artery pressure. To re-obtain wedge pressure, the balloon is *slowly* inflated while catheter pressure is monitored until the pressure waveform changes to a wedge contour. Overinflation of the balloon, or inflation of the balloon in a distal vessel, carries the risk of pulmonary artery rupture. Also, to reduce the likelihood of pulmonary infarction and/or pulmonary artery rupture, the balloon should not be left inflated for longer than the time required to record pressure and obtain a sample of blood to determine oxygen saturation. Positioning of the Cournand or balloon-tipped catheter during right-heart catheterization may be facilitated by the use of guidewires, but catheters should not be advanced into the wedge position with a guidewire protruding beyond the catheter tip.

Left-heart Catheterization. When using a right femoral artery sheath, this procedure may be performed with a variety of catheters (Fig. 9–2). Closed end-hole catheters (Lehman angiographic, Eppendorf) similar to those used in the direct brachial approach may be introduced through the sheath and advanced into the aorta and left ventricle. However, passage of catheters through the frequently tortuous iliofemoral system is facilitated by the use of end-hole catheters with J guidewires. In our laboratory the most commonly used catheter for this purpose is the "pigtail" catheter, which has multiple side holes and an end hole and can be used for angiography as well as pressure measurement. After introduction of the left-heart catheter, 5000 units of heparin are administered intravenously for anticoagulation.

When preformed catheters are used (pigtail, Judkins, or Amplatz), a J-shaped guidewire is inserted into the catheter prior to introducing the catheter into the sheath. Then, when the catheter tip is within the sheath, the J guide is advanced beyond the tip and into the femoral artery for several centimeters. Under fluoroscopic observation, the catheter is then advanced into the aorta, with the guidewire tip preceding it. Again, the catheter passage should be effortless. When the catheter is in the abdominal aorta, the guidewire is removed, and the catheter and sheath are flushed with heparinized saline. The catheter and sheath should be flushed every 5 minutes after heparin administration and every 2 minutes if heparin is not used.

The catheter is advanced carefully around the aortic arch to avoid inadvertently entering the aortic arch vessels. The pressure just above the aortic valve is recorded along with simultaneous femoral artery pressure via the side arm of the sheath. As will be discussed later, the peak femoral artery pressure is frequently slightly higher than the peak central aortic pressure; however, mean systolic pressures are usually identical. The catheter is then passed across the aortic valve into the left ventricle. If the aortic valve is abnormal, a guidewire may be required to stiffen the catheter to permit crossing of the aortic valve. In aortic stenosis, crossing the valve with a pigtail catheter may not be possible, in which case a right Judkins coronary catheter is usually employed. The valve is traversed with a straight-tip guidewire, and the catheter is then advanced over the wire into the ventricle for pressure measurement. Other catheters, such as the Sones, left Judkins, and Gensini, may be preferable in selected patients. Not more than 15 minutes or so should be expended in attempting to cross an aortic valve with a single type of catheter before trying another.

When the catheter enters the left ventricle, the left ventricular and femoral artery pressures are recorded to evaluate aortic valve function, and the left ventricular and pulmonary artery wedge pressures are recorded to evaluate mitral valve function. Cardiac output is measured, and a right-heart pullback is performed to evaluate the pulmonic and tricuspid valves by recording, in close time sequence, pulmonary artery, right ventricular, and right atrial pressures. If left ventricular angiography is planned, and the aortic valve was not crossed with a pigtail or other catheter suitable for ventricular angiography, an exchange guidewire may be introduced into the left ventricle, the catheter may be removed over the guidewire, and a pigtail catheter may be advanced over the exchange guidewire back into the left ventricle.

Termination of the Procedure. Following completion of the hemodynamic and angiographic studies, the catheters are removed. Preformed arterial catheters should be withdrawn from the artery into the sheath with several centimeters of guidewire protruding from the catheter tip to avoid trauma to the arterial intima. Following administration of protamine to reverse the heparin effect, the arterial and venous sheaths are removed, and the vessels are firmly compressed by hand or a mechanical compressor for 15 to 20 minutes, with control of bleeding during this time. With this technique significant hematoma formation occurs in fewer than 2 per cent of patients. In patients with hypertension, or wide pulse pressure (aortic regurgitation), longer groin compression times may be required to achieve hemostasis.

Postcatheterization orders should include the following:

1. Bed rest until the morning after the procedure, with a sandbag applied to the groin for the first 6 hours.
2. Resume all previous medications.
3. Check vital signs every 15 minutes for 1 hour, every hour for 4 hours, and every 4 hours thereafter for 24 hours.
4. Check right (or left, depending on entry site) groin and pedal pulse at above schedule. Call a house officer or attending physician *and* a member of the catheterization laboratory staff in the event of bleeding, loss of pulse, hypotension, or chest pain.
5. Encourage oral fluid 2 to 3 liters over 6 to 8 hours (if angiographic contrast agent has been administered).

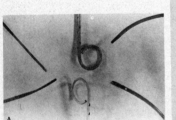
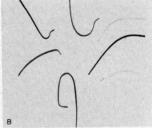

FIGURE 9–2 *A*, Examples of injection catheters in current use. Beginning at top and proceeding clockwise: pigtail, No. 8.2 French (Cook); Gensini, No. 7 French; NIH, No. 8 French; pigtail, No. 8 French (Cordis); Lehman ventriculography, No. 8 French; and Sones, No. 7.5 French tapering to No. 5.5 French. *B*, Different types of catheters currently in wide use for selective coronary angiography. At the bottom, center, is the left coronary Judkins catheter. Proceeding clockwise from this catheter are the right coronary Judkins catheter, the right (R2) and the left (L3) Amplatz catheters, the Schoonmaker multipurpose catheter, the standard Sones catheter (woven dacron, USCI), and the polyurethane Sones-type catheter (Cordis). (Reproduced with permission from Grossman, W. F.: Cardiac Catheterization and Angiography. 2nd ed. Philadelphia, Lea and Febiger, 1980.)

6. Administer analgesic medication, as needed. The patient is always seen on rounds by the catheterization team several hours after and the day following catheterization, or more often, if complications develop.

Transseptal Catheterization. When the aortic valve cannot be crossed by the retrograde approach from either the brachial or the femoral artery, and it is essential that the left ventricular pressure be measured, transseptal catheterization of the left ventricle may be performed. In our experience, approximately 5 per cent of severely stenotic valves cannot be crossed in a retrograde manner within a reasonable period of time, and these patients, as well as those with tilting-disc prosthetic aortic valves, are candidates for this procedure. Patients with porcine heterograft valves and ball-cage prosthetic aortic valves can safely undergo retrograde left ventricular catheterization.[35] Transseptal left-heart catheterization is also indicated in patients with suspected mitral valve obstruction in whom a pulmonary artery wedge pressure cannot be measured.

Procedure. Transseptal catheterization is performed in our laboratory using the Teflon 70-cm No. 8 French catheter developed by Brockenbrough and Braunwald.[36] Prior to insertion of the catheter into the right femoral vein, a Brockenbrough needle is inserted into the catheter, with a Bing stylet protruding 1 cm or so beyond the needle tip to prevent penetration of the catheter wall by the needle (Fig. 9–3). The distance (in millimeters) between the catheter butt and the direction indicator on the needle should be measured with the stylet just inside the catheter tip (measurement No. 1), with the needle tip just inside the catheter tip (measurement No. 2), and with the needle tip 1 cm beyond the catheter tip (measurement No. 3). Measurement No. 1 minus measurement No. 2 should equal the distance that the stylet protrudes beyond the needle tip. If the catheter is matched to

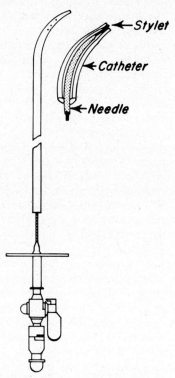

FIGURE 9–3 The Brockenbrough transseptal needle, catheter, and stylet. Use of the stylet prevents inadvertent puncture of the catheter by the needle tip during insertion of the needle into the catheter. The wide flange near the needle hub is pointed on one side to indicate the direction of the needle tip. (From Grossman, W.: Cardiac Catheterization and Angiography. 2nd ed. Philadelphia, Lea and Febiger, 1980.)

the needle, the needle tip should not protrude more than 12 mm beyond the catheter tip when the needle is fully advanced. These measurements are written on a blackboard by a technician for easy reference.

With the patient positioned for a straight frontal projection, the Brockenbrough catheter is advanced to the junction of the right atrium and the superior vena cava by means of a guidewire. The guidewire is removed, the catheter is flushed, and right atrial pressure is recorded. The transseptal needle with its stylet is inserted and then gently advanced through the transseptal catheter under fluoroscopic observation. It is important to allow free rotation of the needle as it is advanced by holding the needle itself (not the direction indicator) between the fingertips. When the tip of the stylet is near the tip of the catheter, the stylet is removed, and the needle is advanced until the needle tip is just within the catheter. The needle is firmly held in this position, with the direction indicator pointing up, to prevent inadvertent extension of the needle tip out of the catheter. The needle is flushed and connected to a pressure transducer, so that a phasic right atrial pressure and a mean pressure can be recorded through the needle and can be verified as similar to that recorded through the catheter prior to insertion of the needle. It is important not to use soft or excessively long lengths of connecting tubing for this purpose, since it is possible to overdamp the pressure recorded through the 21-gauge needle tip.

Puncture of Atrial Septum. After right atrial pressure has been recorded, the direction indicator is rotated clockwise to the 4 o'clock position with fluoroscopic and pressure monitoring. The catheter and needle as a unit are then pulled inferiorly. The catheter will move over the aortic root in a sudden leftward motion; further inferior pull will usually result in a second, smaller leftward motion, as the catheter tip enters the fossa ovalis. Right atrial phasic pressure should be monitored during this time. The catheter and needle (with the needle tip still within the catheter) are then advanced, and the catheter tip will move superiorly, sliding up the interatrial septum. It will usually "hang up" on the lip of the fossa ovalis, at the level of or slightly superior to the plane of the aortic valve. Occasionally, the catheter will pass easily into the left atrium through a patent foramen ovale and will be manifest as leftward motion of the catheter tip and by the appearance of a left atrial phasic waveform. If this occurs, the oxygen saturation of blood aspirated through the needle should be checked and the pressure recorded to document entry into the left atrium. The catheter is then gently advanced 1 or 2 cm over the needle, and the needle is removed. More commonly, the foramen ovale is not patent and must be punctured with the needle tip. This is done during pressure and fluoroscopic monitoring by advancing the needle 1 cm beyond the catheter tip, when the tip is firmly wedged in the fossa ovalis.

After the needle penetrates the interatrial septum, a left atrial pressure waveform (usually a higher mean pressure than in the right atrium) will be evident. Entry into the left atrium should be confirmed by measurement of oxygen saturation. The needle and catheter are then slowly advanced into the left atrium, with the needle position indicator maintained in the 4 o'clock position. Resistance is usually encountered as the catheter tip punctures the septum, and it is important to stabilize the catheter position by holding the catheter in the groin with the left hand while advancing the catheter and needle with the right hand. When the catheter traverses the septum and enters the left atrium (a 1- to 2-cm leftward motion), the needle is withdrawn, the catheter is flushed, left atrial pressure is recorded, and blood is withdrawn for measurement of oxygen saturation through the catheter. Passage of the catheter from the left atrium into the left ventricle is achieved by advancing the catheter tip through the mitral valve. The transseptal catheter may enter a pulmonary vein or left atrial appendage. In this case, the left ventricle may be entered by withdrawing the catheter slowly while rotating it counterclockwise and/or by inserting a coiled-tip occluder to increase the bend in the catheter tip.

It is important to emphasize that transseptal catheterization—as indeed all cardiac catheterization procedures—should be done only by or under the supervision of physicians experienced in the technique. The transseptal needle may perforate the right atrial wall, enter the coronary sinus or the aorta, or perforate the left atrial wall. The small needle tip itself (21-gauge) is not likely to cause a major problem unless an atrial wall is torn; however, passage of the catheter through these structures may result in tamponade and death. Thus, the emphasis placed on pressure monitoring through the needle is important.

Pediatric Cardiac Catheterization. The methods described above are broadly applicable to the cardiac catheterization of children, but *special considerations for the newborn* should be emphasized. In such patients, meticulous attention must be given to maintenance of body temperature by means of heating pads, an infared lamp, or other devices designed for this purpose. In addition, precise attention must be paid to fluid balance, with care being taken to replace exactly the volume of fluid and blood removed, so as to cause neither hypovolemia and hypotension nor hypervolemia with pulmonary edema. In the newborn, the umbilical artery and vein may be used for catheterization for about 72 hours after birth. Of course, catheters should be of small diameters and lengths in procedures involving neonates, infants, and children. The reader is referred to texts and reviews detailing special technical considerations in cardiac catheterization of newborns.[31,37–39]

Catheter Sizes and Construction. In addition to the above-mentioned considerations, it is important that individuals involved in cardiac catheterization understand the sizing of catheters, needles, and guidewires and that they have a knowledge of different methods and materials used in their construction. Cardiac catheters differ in size, length, shape, and material of construction. The last factor determines the friction coefficient, hardness, curve retention, moisture absorption, and autoclavability. In addition, it is clear that different catheter materials have varying degrees of thrombogenicity.[40] Cardiac catheters are usually constructed of woven Dacron, polyethylene, or polyurethane. Some catheter walls are reinforced with stainless steel braids to increase torque control and to enable the catheter to withstand high intraluminal pressures during the injection of angiographic contrast material. In addition, the walls of most cardiac catheters are impregnated with lead or barium salts to render them radiopaque.

The outside diameter (OD) of a catheter is indicated in French units: one French (F) unit = 0.33 mm (0.013 inches). Thus a No. 7 French (7F) catheter has an OD of 2.33 mm. The internal diameter (ID) of a catheter is always, of course, less than the OD, the exact relationship between OD and ID depending on the thickness of the catheter wall. The ID of the catheter determines the thickness of the guidewire that can be passed through the catheter. The guidewire must in turn be small enough to fit through the lumen of the needle used for vessel puncture in percutaneous catheterization techniques. The diameter of the guidewire is usually expressed in inches (0.032, 0.035, 0.038, and so on), whereas needle size is expressed in "gauge," indicating the OD of the needle. An 18-gauge thin-walled needle has an OD of 0.086 inches. The cardiologist beginning to use these techniques must be familiar with these units. In addition, it is wise to check that catheter, guidewire, and needle are all compatible in size and length before the vessel is punctured.

MEASUREMENT OF HEMODYNAMIC PARAMETERS

Pressure Measurement

Theoretical Considerations. Myocardial contractile force is transmitted through the fluid medium of blood as a pressure wave. An important objective of the cardiac catheterization procedure is to assess accurately the forces, and therefore the pressure waves, generated by various cardiac chambers. *A pressure wave may be considered a complex periodic fluctuation in force per unit area*, with one cycle consisting of the time interval from the onset of one wave to the onset of the next. The number of cycles within 1 second is termed the *fundamental frequency* of the waveform. Thus, for a left ventricular pressure waveform at a heart rate of 120 beats/min, the fundamental frequency would be 2 sec^{-1}, or 2 Hz.

Considered as a complex periodic waveform, the pressure wave may be subjected to a type of analysis developed by the French physicist Fourier, whereby any complex waveform may be considered to be the mathematical summation of a series of simple sine waves of differing frequencies and amplitudes.[41–43] The practical consequence

of this analysis is that in order to record pressure accurately a system must respond in such a way that output amplitude is directly proportional to input throughout the range of frequencies contained within the pressure wave. If components in a given frequency range are either suppressed or exaggerated by the transducer system, the recorded signal will be a grossly distorted version of the original physiological waveform. For example, the incisura of the aortic pressure wave contains frequencies above 10 cycles/sec; if the pressure measurement system were unable to respond to these, the incisura would be slurred or absent.

The *frequency response* of a pressure measurement system may be defined as the ratio of output amplitude/input amplitude over a range of frequencies of the input or pressure wave. An ideal pressure measurement system would have an output/input ratio of one over an infinite range of input frequencies. In practice this is never the case, and the frequency response characteristics reflect the interaction of the *natural frequency* of the system and the degree of *damping*. If the sensing membrane in the pressure measurement system were shock-excited, in the absence of friction it would oscillate for an indefinite period of time in simple harmonic motion. The frequency of this motion would be the *natural frequency* of the system. The amplitude of the output signal tends to be augmented as the frequency of that signal approaches the natural frequency of the system (Fig. 9–4A). Optimal damping dissipates the energy of the oscillating system gradually, thereby maintaining the nearly flat frequency response curve (constant input/output ratio) as it approaches the region of the pressure measurement system's natural frequency. An extensive literature on the question of what frequency response is desirable and on the testing, construction, and evaluation of different pressure measurement systems is available.[31,44]

Fluid-filled Catheter Systems. With fluid-filled catheters, an external pressure transducer is used to detect changes in pressure at the catheter tip that are transmitted to the transducer by the fluid column in the catheter. A pressure transducer consists basically of a diaphragm that is deformed in a linear fashion by the application of pressure within the physiological range. Deformation of the diaphragm produces a proportional change in electrical resistance within the transducer. By use of a Wheatstone bridge-type circuit, this change in transducer resistance is converted into an electrical potential, which is then amplified and recorded as an analog signal that represents pressure applied to the transducer. Operation of the bridge requires an excitation voltage, usually supplied by the pressure amplifier. A variable resistance control, by means of which the electrical potential can be adjusted to zero when no pressure is applied, permits balancing of the transducer. Calibration of the system is performed by applying known pressures to the transducer by means of a mercury manometer and observing the analog voltage output. The sensitivity of the amplifiers used in pressure recording systems is adjustable, so that a given pressure may be made to correspond to a precise deflection of the recorder.

Because movement of the transducer diaphragm is necessary to produce a voltage output for a given pressure, a certain volume of fluid must move through the catheter-connector tubing system to the transducer to produce a

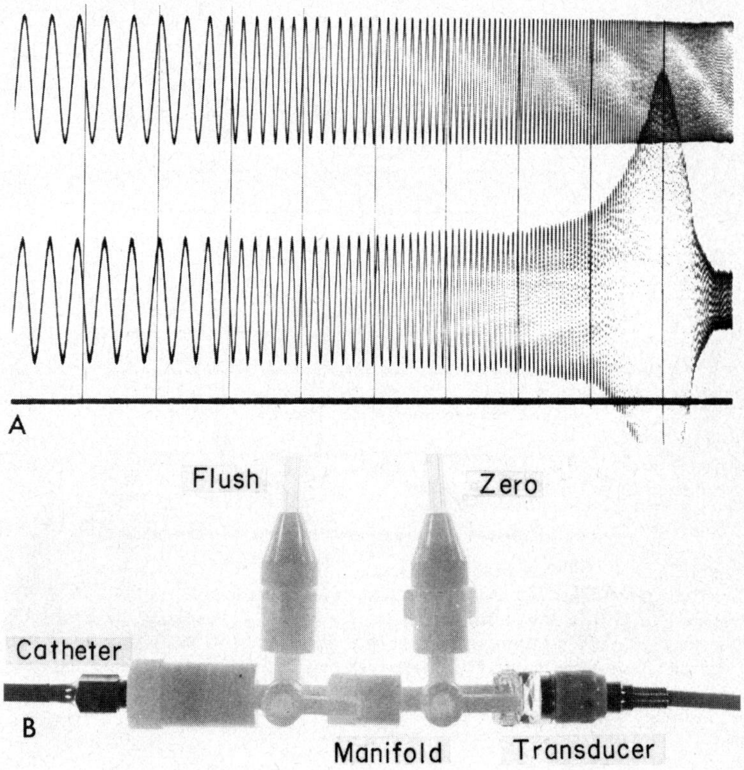

FIGURE 9–4 Recording of phasic pressures with a fluid-filled catheter system.

A, The upper trace shows a "true" phasic pressure of 20 mm Hg (sine wave of increasing frequency) generated within a closed chamber. The lower trace shows the same, pressure recorded with a fluid-filled 110-cm catheter–external transducer system. Note that the pressures are equal in amplitude up to a frequency of about 15 Hz. As the frequency of the pressure sine wave increases above this point, an increase in amplitude occurs owing to resonance in the catheter-transducer system. The "resonant frequency" is about 40 Hz, and above this frequency, the amplitude of the signal falls rapidly. In this case, since the resonant frequency is well above most frequencies contained in the intracardiac pressure waveforms, little distortion of intracardiac pressure by the catheter-transducer recording system will be present. (The vertical lines are 1 sec apart.)

B, The system used to record the pressure in A. A small volume-displacement transducer is attached directly to the back end of a two–side-arm manifold. Fluid-filled tubings are attached to the side arms for "zero" pressure reference and catheter flushing, and the front end of the manifold is connected directly to the catheter. Care must be taken during filling of the transducer and manifold to remove all air bubbles, which can markedly lower the resonant frequency of the system.

pressure recording. This tends to cause low-frequency resonance in the system. The resonant frequency of a fluid-filled system should be above the frequencies contained in intracardiac pressure waveforms (see above). For usual clinical purposes, a system with frequency response that is flat to 10 or 12 Hz with a resonant frequency above this level is adequate. This can be achieved most easily by use of small volume-displacement transducers, with imposition of as few stopcocks and connecting tubings as possible between the catheter hub and the transducer. The system used in our cardiac catheterization laboratories is shown in Figure 9–4B.

With an aqueous fluid–filled catheter attached to a transducer, the transducer will indicate zero pressure when the catheter tip is at the same height as the transducer. If the catheter tip is elevated above the transducer, a positive pressure of 1 mm Hg will be indicated for every 1.36 cm of height difference; if the catheter tip is below the transducer level, a negative pressure of the same magnitude will be indicated. These effects are due simply to gravitational force acting on the fluid column in the catheter and the specific gravity of mercury of 13.6. The transducer is therefore positioned at a level approximately the same as that of the heart, usually the midchest. If the transducer is placed at a different height, attaching a second fluid-filled catheter to the transducer and positioning the tip of that catheter at the zero (midchest) level permit proper zeroing of the transducer relative to the catheter tip position within the heart (Fig. 9–4B). It is important to note that pressures measured inside the heart chambers do not necessarily equal the true transmural pressures, because of the normal intrathoracic negative pressure, which ranges between 0 and −8 mm Hg during normal respiration.

Even when a pressure measurement system has a high degree of sensitivity, uniform frequency response, and optimal damping and is properly zeroed and balanced, distortions and inaccuracies in the pressure waveform may occur. Motion of the catheter within the heart and great vessels accelerates the fluid contained within the catheter, and such *catheter whip* artifacts may produce superimposed waves of ± 10 mm Hg. Catheter whip artifacts are particularly common in tracings from the pulmonary arteries and are difficult to avoid.

Manometer-tipped Catheters. In order to minimize artifacts associated with low resonant frequency systems, catheter whip, and excessive damping, many laboratories employ micromanometer-tipped catheters, with which the pressure transducer is actually placed in the cardiac chamber in which pressure is being measured. As is evident in Figure 9–5, there may be a distinct difference in waveform between "true" left ventricular pressure (as recorded using an intracardiac micromanometer) and that recorded through a standard fluid-filled catheter system. Low resonant frequency and inadequate damping of the fluid-filled system in this example resulted in exaggeration of the high-frequency components in the left ventricular pressure rise and fall, with corresponding artifactual overshoot of the pressures in early diastole and early systole. More optimal damping and natural frequency characteristics of the fluid-filled system can minimize these artifacts but cannot eliminate them. In addition, a 30- to 40-msec delay in the pressure waveform occurs with fluid-filled catheter systems, necessitating the use of manometer-tipped catheters in situations in which recording of simultaneous pressure and angiographic volume, echocardiographic, phonocardiographic, or electrocardiographic data is required. The high-frequency response of manometer-tipped catheter transducers (resonant frequency = 25 to 40 kHz) permits their application for the detection and recording of intracardiac sounds.

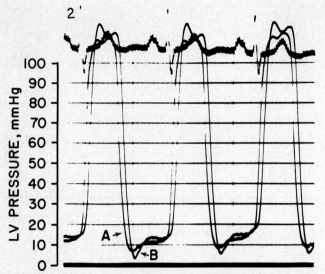

FIGURE 9–5   Left ventricular pressures recorded with a manome-ter-tipped catheter (A) and a fluid-filled catheter–external transduc-er system with a low resonant frequency (B). Note undershoot of pressure in early diastole, overshoot of pressure in early systole, and delay of fluid-filled catheter pressure relative to the "true" pressure. (From Grossman, W.: Cardiac Catheterization and Angiography. 2nd ed. Philadelphia, Lea and Febiger, 1980.)

Most manometer-tipped catheters do not have an end-hold and must therefore be inserted via arteriotomy or a vascular sheath. Millar* manufactures a No. 8 French end-hole manometer-tipped angiocatheter that can be used with a guidewire. Since the zero level of the manometer-tipped catheter may drift, it is most useful to have a fluid-filled lumen in the catheter by means of which a true zero pressure reference level can be established.

Representative Pressure Tracings.   In evaluating pressure tracings, specific phasic and mean pressure values should be measured, the phasic pressure waveform contours not-ed, and pressures in different chambers compared. Analy-sis of these data, interpreted in the light of cardiac output and angiographic measurement, permits detection and quantitation of valvular, myocardial, and pericardial ab-normalities.

NORMAL PRESSURE WAVEFORMS.   An understanding of pressure waveforms, both under normal conditions and in various disease states, is predicated on a thorough compre-hension of the events of the cardiac cycle (Fig. 12–25, p. 431). Shown in Figure 9–6 are normal pressure waveforms obtained with fluid-filled catheters.

_____

*Millar Instruments, Inc., P.O. Box 18227, Houston, Texas 77023.

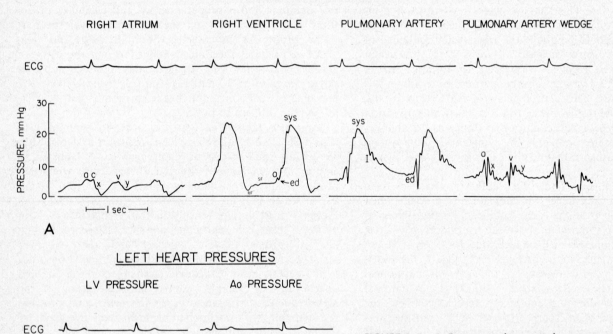

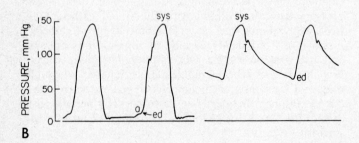

FIGURE 9–6   A, Representative normal pressure tracings from the right side of the heart; sys = systolic, ed = end-diastolic. B, Repre-sentative normal pressures from the left ventricle (LV) and aorta (Ao).

The *right atrial pressure waveform* consists of two major positive deflections—the *a* and *v* waves. The *a* wave is due to atrial systole and follows the P wave of the electrocardiogram. As the pressure declines from the peak of the *a* wave (the *x* decent), a small positive deflection, the *c* wave, occurs concomitant with tricuspid valve closure. After the "*c*" wave, right atrial pressure continues to fall (*x* descent) even though the atrium is filling with blood (the tricuspid valve is closed), owing to atrial relaxation. After full atrial relaxation occurs, at the nadir of the *x* descent, the pressure in the atrium starts to rise as atrial filling continues from peripheral venous return. This rise in the right atrial pressure during right ventricular systole is termed the *v* wave, and it reaches a peak just before the opening of the tricuspid valve. Following opening of the tricuspid valve, the right atrium empties into the right ventricle, and pressure in the atrium falls, constituting the *y* descent. Following the *y* descent, pressure in the atrium is equal to ventricular diastolic pressure and slowly increases as the ventricle fills. Peak *a* and *v* wave pressures are measured, and the mean pressure is obtained electronically. Normal values are shown in Table 9–1.

The *diastolic phase of the right ventricular pressure pulse* consists of an early rapid filling wave, during which approximately 60 per cent of ventricular filling ocurs; a slow filling period, accounting for approximately 25 per cent of ventricular filling; and an atrial systolic wave *(a)*, accounting for approximately 15 per cent of ventricular filling. During diastole, right atrial and right ventricular pressures are nearly equal, because of the low resistance to flow across the tricuspid valve. Two pressures are usually measured: the peak systolic right ventricular pressure and the end-diastolic right ventricular pressure immediately following the *a* wave. The normal range of values for the pressures is shown in Table 9–1.

The *pulmonary artery pressure waveform* contains a systolic pressure owing to flow of blood into the pulmonary artery from the right ventricle. As right ventricular ejection ends, pressure in the pulmonary artery falls, and when right ventricular pressure drops below the pulmonary pressure, the pulmonary valve closes, resulting in the incisura on the pressure waveform. Pressure in the pulmonary artery then falls gradually as blood flows through the pulmonary arteries and veins into the left atrium and ventricle. The nadir of this pressure in late diastole is termed the end-diastolic pulmonary artery pressure. This

pressure, the peak systolic pressure, and the mean pulmonary artery pressure are the parameters usually measured. It is not unusual to observe a small (≤ 5 mm Hg) gradient in peak systolic pressure between the right ventricle and the pulmonary artery.

The *pulmonary artery wedge pressure* has a waveform similar to that of the left atrial pressure but is both damped and delayed by transmission through the capillary vessels. A normal wedge pressure should show *a* and *v* waves, which reflect, respectively, left atrial systole and left atrial filling during left ventricular systole (see discussion of right atrial pressure above). However, *c* waves may not be apparent on the wedge pressure tracing. The *x* and *y* descents should be distinct in a wedge pressure tracing if it is not overdamped. The peak *a* and *v* wave pressures are usually measured, as in the mean wedge pressure. In a normal pulmonary circulation of low vascular resistance, the pulmonary artery flow is diminished at end diastole, so that end-diastolic pulmonary artery and mean pulmonary artery wedge pressures are approximately equal. Mean pulmonary artery pressure is always higher than mean wedge pressure. Normal values for pulmonary artery wedge pressure are presented in Table 9–1.

Normal left heart pressure waveforms are shown in Figure 9–6. The *left atrial pressure waveform* was discussed in the description of the pulmonary artery wedge pressure. Unless a transseptal catheterization is performed, pulmonary artery wedge pressure is recorded as an acceptable substitute for the actual left atrial pressure. It is important to recognize that this can be a source of error, unless a properly damped wedge pressure is observed and confirmed by determination of oxygen saturation.

The components of the *left ventricular waveform* are similar to those already described for that of the right ventricle. The pressures in the left ventricle in diastole (as well as systole) are normally higher than those in the right ventricle, owing in part to the greater wall thickness of the left ventricle, which results in greater chamber stiffness.

The *central aortic pressure tracing* consists of a systolic wave, followed by the incisura, which denotes closure of the aortic valve, and then a gradual fall in pressure as the blood flows from the aorta through the peripheral arterial capillary and venous vessels. Pressure is normally measured at peak systole and at end diastole, and the mean pressure is determined electronically.

The *peripheral arterial pressure*, commonly measured

TABLE 9–1 RANGE OF NORMAL RESTING HEMODYNAMIC VALUES

	a WAVE	*v* WAVE	MEAN	SYSTOLIC	END-DIASTOLIC	MEAN
Pressures						
Right atrium	2–10	2–10	0–8			
Right ventricle				15–30	0–8	
Pulmonary artery				15–30	3–12	9–16
Pulmonary artery wedge and left atrium	3–15	3–12	1–10			
Left ventricle				100–140	3–12	
Systemic arteries				100–140	60–90	70–105
Oxygen consumption index (ml/min/m²)		110–150				
Arteriovenous oxygen difference (ml/l)		30–50				
Cardiac output index (l/min/m²)		2.5–4.2				
Resistances (dynes-sec-cm⁻⁵)						
Pulmonary vascular		20–120				
Systemic vascular		770–1500				

during cardiac catheterization in the brachial or femoral artery, has a waveform similar to that described for the central aorta. However, because of resonance within the arterial system, the peripheral arterial pressure may show a wider pulse pressure with a higher peak systolic pressure than that seen in the central aorta. The mean pressure is usually identical to or up to 5 mm Hg lower than the central aortic pressure. Thus, the peak systolic pressure gradients measured between the left ventricle and the systemic arterial system may vary depending on whether the central aortic pressure or a peripheral arterial pressure is measured. However, mean systolic gradients are not usually significantly different.

ABNORMAL PRESSURE TRACINGS.   As discussed in greater detail in subsequent chapters, pressure tracings may be virtually diagnostic of certain conditions. In *valvular aortic stenosis* (p. 1095), there is a pressure gradient between the left ventricle and the aorta; however, in addition, the rise in aortic pressure is slow and delayed compared with that of the left ventricle (Fig. 9–7). In contrast, hypertrophic obstructive cardiomyopathy (p. 1409) may also result in a large systolic pressure gradient but will show near identity of the slopes and timing of the left ventricular and aortic pressure increases. Both conditions are associated with increased ventricular stiffness and therefore may show prominent atrial systolic waves transmitted into the left ventricular pressure tracing in late diastole.[45] *Aortic regurgitation* is characterized by near equalization of aortic and left ventricular pressures at end diastole, marked widening of the aortic pulse pressure, and slurring of the aortic incisura. *Mitral stenosis* is associated with a diastolic pressure gradient (pulmonary artery wedge or left atrium vs. left ventricle) across the mitral valve, which increases substantially with exercise (Fig. 9–8). If the patient is in sinus rhythm, a marked discrepancy will be seen between the large left atrial systolic wave (*a* wave) and the small or absent *a* wave in the left ventricular tracing.

A large *v* wave in the pulmonary artery wedge tracing may be present in patients with *mitral regurgitation* (p. 1081). The amplitude of the *v* wave is increased because the left atrium is being filled during systole not only with blood entering from the pulmonary veins but also

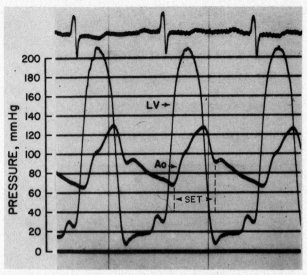

FIGURE 9–7   Left Ventricular (LV) and aortic (Ao) pressure tracings in aortic stenosis. During systole, there is a large pressure gradient between LV and Ao, and the rate of rise of the aortic pressure is slow. The systolic ejection time (SET) is the period of time in each cycle during which blood is being ejected from the left ventricle into the aorta. The vertical time lines are 1 sec apart. (From Grossman, W.: Cardiac Catheterization and Angiography. 2nd ed. Philadelphia, Lea and Febiger, 1980.)

with blood leaking across the mitral valve. It should be emphasized that accurate evaluation of mitral valve function by measuring simultaneous pulmonary artery wedge and left ventricular pressure is based on the assumption that the wedge pressure accurately reflects both phasic and mean left atrial pressure. This is shown in Figure 9–9, in which simultaneous wedge and left atrial pressures were recorded. If the wedge pressure is overdamped, it is possible to overestimate the severity of mitral stenosis and underestimate the severity of mitral regurgitation.

Detection of *stenosis and regurgitation of the tricuspid* (p. 1117) *and pulmonic valves* (p. 1121) during right-heart catheterization is usually assessed by rapid pullback of the catheters from the pulmonary artery to the right ventricle to the right atrium. However, more precise measurement

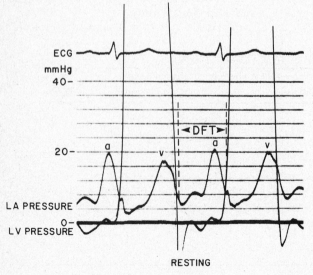

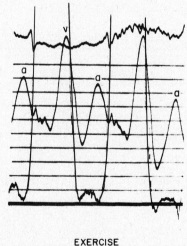

RESTING   EXERCISE

FIGURE 9–8 Left atrial (LA) and left ventricular (LV) pressures in a patient with mitral stenosis at rest (*left*) and during exercise (*right*). During diastole, there is a gradient of pressure between LA and LV. The diastolic filling time (DFT) is the period of time in each cycle when the mitral valve is open. The gradient is greater during exercise as flow across the stenotic valvular orifice increases. (From Grossman, W.: Cardiac Catheterization and Angiography. 2nd ed. Philadelphia, Lea and Febiger, 1980.)

SIMULTANEOUS PULMONARY ARTERY WEDGE (PAW) AND LEFT ATRIAL (LA) PRESSURES

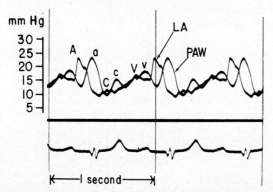

FIGURE 9–9 Simultaneous pulmonary artery wedge (PAW) and left atrial (LA) pressures. *A, C,* and *V* refer to the PAW and *a, c,* and *v* to the LA pressure pulses, respectively. The PAW pressure wave is delayed relative to the LA pressure because of the time required for retrograde propagation of the pressure wave through the pulmonary capillary bed. (From Kory, R. C., et al.: A Primer of Cardiac Catheterization. Springfield, Ill. Courtesy of Charles C Thomas, 1965.)

of simultaneous pressures can be performed using a double-lumen right-heart catheter, in which the lumen tips are separated at the end of the catheter by a distance sufficient to permit monitoring pressures on opposite sides of the tricuspid valve or pulmonary outflow tract and valve.

Measurement of Cardiac Output

Fick Oxygen Method. Of the numerous techniques devised over the years to measure cardiac output,[46] two have won general acceptance in cardiac catheterization laboratories: the Fick oxygen method and the indicator-dilution technique. These methods resemble each other in that they are based on the theoretical principle enunciated by Adolph Fick in 1870.[47] The principle, which was never actually applied by Fick, states that total uptake or release of any substance by an organ is the product of blood flow to the organ and the arteriovenous concentration difference of the substance. For the lungs, the substance released to the blood is oxygen, and the pulmonary blood flow can be determined by measurement of the *arteriovenous differences of oxygen* across the lungs and the *oxygen consumption* per minute. If there is no intracardiac shunt, and pulmonary blood flow is equal to systemic blood flow, this application of the Fick principle also provides a measure of systemic blood flow.

Oxygen consumption is commonly estimated by measurement of oxygen extracted by the lungs over a given time period. A "steady state" is required in which oxygen consumption and cardiac output are constant over the time period of measurement. Oxygen consumption is measured by collecting all the air expired by the patient over a 3-minute time period.

O_2 content of room air (ml O_2/liter of air) =

$$\frac{pO_2 \text{ room air}}{\text{Corrected barometric pressure}} \times 1000$$

O_2 content of expired air (ml O_2/liter) =

$$\frac{pO_2 \text{ expired air}}{\text{Corrected barometric pressure}} \times 1000$$

The ml O_2 consumed/liter of expired air is calculated as the difference between these two values. The minute ventilation is calculated by dividing the total volume of air expired by the number of minutes of collection and is calculated as liters of air per minute. Oxygen consumption is then calculated as

(ml O_2 consumed/liter of expired air) $\times$ (liter of expired air/min of collection) = ml O_2 consumed/min

For clinical application, it is acceptable to neglect the small error introduced by the fact that the volume of CO_2 expired is not identical to the volume of O_2 consumed, since the respiratory quotient is approximately 0.8. Many other considerations are important in the measurement of oxygen consumption by this method.[31] The O_2 consumption in ml/min is usually divided by body surface area to correct for differences in O_2 consumption rate due to differences in size among patients. The normal basal oxygen consumption index is between 110 and 150 ml O_2/min/m² body surface area. It may be underestimated if expired air collection is incomplete owing to an imperfectly fitted mouthpiece or a perforated eardrum.

The arteriovenous oxygen difference across the lungs is determined as the difference between the oxygen content of pulmonary artery blood and that of left ventricular or systemic arterial blood, since pulmonary venous blood is not generally sampled. Actually, because of bronchial venous and thebesian venous drainage, the oxygen content of systemic arterial blood is commonly 2 to 5 ml/liter lower than that of pulmonary venous blood as it leaves the alveoli, and a small overestimation of cardiac output, of little clinical significance, results.

The pulmonary arterial blood is used for determination of mixed venous blood oxygen content, which can be measured by a variety of methods. The standard method is the manometric technique of Van Slyke and Neill.[48] This measurement takes 20 to 45 minutes and has generally been supplanted by methods that measure the O_2 saturation of hemoglobin by reflectance oximetry. Oxygen content (ml O_2/liter blood) is then calculated by multiplying the fraction of O_2 saturation by the theoretical oxygen-carrying capacity ([hemoglobin, gm/100 ml] $\times$ 1.36 [ml O_2/gm Hb]) $\times$ 10. The arteriovenous oxygen content difference is then simply calculated as the arterial minus the venous blood O_2 content.

Cardiac output/m² (cardiac index) is calculated as

$$\frac{O_2 \text{ consumption (ml/min/m}^2)}{\text{Arteriovenous } O_2 \text{ difference (ml/liter)}} = \text{liters/min/m}^2$$

The normal range is 2.5 to 4.2 liters/min/m². The average error in determining oxygen consumption is approximately 6 per cent. The error for arteriovenous oxygen difference determination is approximately 5 per cent, and the total error in measurement of cardiac output by this method is probably about 10 per cent.[46,49–52] The Fick oxygen method is most accurate in patients with low cardiac output, in whom the arteriovenous oxygen difference is wide.

Indicator-dilution Method.   The Fick method is merely a specific application of the indicator-dilution method, in which O_2 being continuously infused by the lungs is the indicator and is diluted in the pulmonary blood flow. Stewart was the first to use a dye indicator-dilution method to measure cardiac output; he used the continuous infusion technique and reported his first studies in 1897.[53] Numerous indicators have since been successfully employed.[46] Indocyanine green dye has gained the widest acceptance in clinical practice, although recently thermodilution (in which cold saline is the indicator) has become widely used.[54–59] When indocyanine green dye is used, a bolus is rapidly injected into the pulmonary artery, and its appearance and concentration in arterial blood are recorded from a peripheral systemic artery (e.g., brachial, femoral, or radial). A time-concentration curve is thus recorded that exhibits a rapid rise to a peak and then a gradual decline in concentration that is interrupted by a secondary rise due to recirculation of the dye (Fig. 9–10, *top*). The problem of isolating those data that relate only to the first pass of the indicator has been approached by several investigators, but the method originally proposed by Kinsman, Moore, and Hamilton[60] is the one still used most widely today. Kinsman and coworkers showed mathematically that the true "first-pass" curve will be given by plotting the concentration decline on semilogarithmic paper and extrapolating the early linear part of the plot.

The cardiac output (CO) is then calculated as CO $=$ $i/(\overline{c} \times t)$, where i is the quantity of indicator injected, $\overline{c}$ is the average concentration of the indicator during its first pass, and t is the total duration of the curve. The product of $\overline{c}$ and t is easily measured as the area under the first-pass curve, as determined by planimetry. This may be further simplified by the use of any number of available computer methods in which the semilogarithmic replotting, area computation, and cardiac output calculation are all accomplished electronically. More precise methodological details, as well as a discussion of sources of error, can be found elsewhere.[31,46] Most laboratories,[54,61–63] but not all,[57] have found there to be excellent agreement between the indicator-dilution methods and independent methods for measuring cardiac output, particularly when the cardiac output is normal or elevated. The error of the indicator-dilution method is greatest in patients with extremely low outputs, severe mitral or aortic regurgitation, or intracardiac shunts. Therefore it complements the Fick method of cardiac output determination, in which the accuracy is greatest in patients having low cardiac output with wide arteriovenous oxygen differences.

It is important to note that indocyanine green dye can cause interference when oxygen content is determined by spectrophotometric methods. Therefore, if cardiac output is to be determined by both the Fick and the indocyanine green dye indicator-dilution methods *in the same patient*, the former measurement should be done first. Not only does the use of cold saline (thermodilution) as an indicator avoid this problem, but also this technique can be performed repeatedly without buildup of indicator or recirculation problems. For these reasons, the thermo-

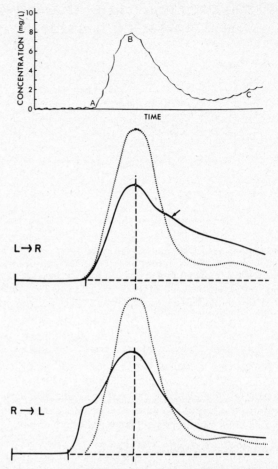

FIGURE 9–10   Time-concentration curves generated by injecting indocyanine green dye into the right heart and sampling in the brachial artery. *Top*, Normal curve showing appearance of the dye in arterial blood (A) and the peak concentration (B), followed by an exponential disappearance and then recirculation of the dye (C). *Center*, The solid line is a schematic drawing of the time-concentration curve in a patient with a left-to-right shunt. There is an early recirculation "bump" (arrow) on the downslope of the curve due to the dye that is shunted from left to right and then reappears in the left circulation. The dotted line represents a normal dye concentration curve. *Bottom*, Time-concentration curve in the presence of a right-to-left shunt, showing early appearance of the dye in the brachial artery. The early appearing dye passes through the shunt and thus does not traverse the pulmonary circulation. The dotted line represents a normal dye concentration curve. (Top panel from Grossman, W.: Cardiac Catheterization and Angiography. 2nd ed. Philadelphia, Lea and Febiger, 1980. Center and lower panels from Kory, R. C., et al.: A Primer of Cardiac Catheterization. Springfield, Ill. Courtesy of Charles C Thomas, 1965.)

dilution method has become the most commonly used indicator-dilution technique for measuring cardiac output.

Angiographic Measurement of Cardiac Output.   Measurement of left ventricular end-diastolic and end-systolic volumes by quantitative left ventricular angiography, described on p. 470, permits calculation of left ventricular stroke volume. In the absence of atrial fibrillation or significant mitral or aortic regurgitation, systemic cardiac output may be estimated by multiplying the stroke volume by the heart rate during the angiogram. This method is a less accurate method of measuring cardiac output than either the indicator-dilution or the Fick method.

Regional Blood Flows.   The principles discussed above may be applied to measure regional blood flows. Three common examples are intracardiac shunt flow as measured by the Fick principle, coronary sinus flow by thermodilution, and regurgitant valve flow by a combination of angiographic and Fick measurements of cardiac output.

INTRACARDIAC SHUNTS. Detection, localization, and quantification of intracardiac shunts can generally be accomplished with precision at cardiac catheterization. Although intracardiac shunts are usually suspected prior to catheterization, this is not always the case. Therefore, the operator must always be alert to the possibility of an intracardiac shunt and must search for one when unexpected arterial oxygen desaturation is detected or an inappropriately high mixed venous (i.e., pulmonary artery) oxygen saturation is observed.

Detection and Localization of Shunts. In a patient with a *left-to-right shunt* (atrial septal defect, ventricular septal defect, patent ductus arteriosus) pulmonary blood flow is higher than systemic blood flow, and the pulmonary artery oxygen saturation is greater than the true mixed venous blood saturation. The anatomical location of the shunt is determined by obtaining multiple samples for oxygen saturation. In the traditional oximetry run duplicate samples are drawn in rapid succession from the left, right, and main pulmonary arteries[7,64,65]; the outflow tract, body, and inflow area of the right ventricle; the low, mid, and high right atrium; the low and high superior vena cava; and the inferior vena cava at the level of the diaphragm. Oxygen content of blood from these locations normally shows variability due to streaming of up to 20 ml/liter in the right atrium, 10 ml/liter in the right ventricle, and 5 ml/liter in the pulmonary artery.[7,64] Variations above these values generally indicate the entrance of oxygenated blood into the right heart through an abnormal communication. The level of the "oxygen step-up" generally locates the anatomical position of the left-to-right shunt. If, for example, oxygen content of right atrial blood samples is 148, 152, and 156 ml/liter (average 152 ml/liter), that of right ventricular blood samples is 151, 152, and 153 ml/liter (average 152 ml/liter), but that of pulmonary artery blood is 180, 182, and 178 ml/liter (average 180 ml/liter), there is a significant oxygen step-up in the pulmonary artery (+28 ml/liter) indicative of a left-to-right shunt at that level (e.g., patent ductus arteriosus or aortopulmonary window).

One limitation of the oxygen method of detecting intracardiac shunts is its low degree of sensitivity. Small shunts ($\dot{Q}_p/\dot{Q}_s \leq 1.3$) at the level of the pulmonary artery or right ventricle and shunts at the atrial level with $\dot{Q}_p/\dot{Q}_s < 1.5$ are not consistently detected by this technique alone because of the normal variability in O_2 saturation described above.[65] A more sensitive technique for the detection of small left-to-right intracardiac shunts involves detection of the early appearance of hydrogen in the right heart after inhalation of hydrogen gas using a right-heart hydrogen-sensitive platinum-tipped electrode catheter to measure direct-current voltage changes. In addition, in the presence of a left-to-right shunt, injection of indocyanine green dye into the pulmonary artery with sampling from the femoral artery will demonstrate early recirculation on the downslope of the dye curve.[64,66–68] These techniques are easily performed and can sometimes detect left-to-right shunts too small to be detected by the oxygen step-up method (Fig. 9–10, *center*).

In *right-to-left shunts*, arterial blood is unsaturated, and cyanosis is frequently noted. Clinically, the site of entry of a right-to-left cardiac shunt may be localized by noting which of the left-heart chambers is the first to show desaturation. However, it is usually difficult to enter the pulmonary vein and left atrium in the adult, as discussed previously. Small right-to-left shunts may be detected by injecting indocyanine dye into a vena cava and detecting the early appearance of the dye in arterial blood prior to the primary peak (Fig. 9–10, *bottom*). The site of origin of the shunt can then be localized by injecting dye at a more distal site in the right heart until its early appearance disappears.

It should be remembered that an abnormal catheter position can also be useful in detecting an abnormal communication. This is particularly true for atrial septal defects and for anomalous pulmonary veins emptying into the right atrium. In addition, angiographic methods may be used to detect and localize intracardiac shunts (Chap. 10).

Shunt Quantification. The usefulness of the oximetry run method of shunt detection is enhanced by the fact that the data obtained are also used in quantification of the shunt. When the shunt is unidirectional (e.g., left-to-right), its magnitude is simply calculated as the difference between the pulmonary and systemic blood flows. Pulmonary blood flow ($\dot{Q}_p$) in liters/min is given as:

$$\dot{Q}_p = \frac{O_2 \text{ consumption (ml/min)}}{\underset{\text{(ml/liter)}}{PV\ O_2 \text{ content}} - \underset{\text{(ml/liter)}}{PA\ O_2 \text{ content}}}$$

where PV and PA refer to pulmonary venous and pulmonary arterial blood, respectively. If a pulmonary vein has not been entered, systemic arterial oxygen content may be used in lieu of PV O_2 content, as long as the systemic arterial oxygen saturation is 95 per cent or more. If systemic oxygen saturation is less than 95 per cent, one must determine whether a right-to-left shunt is present. If such a shunt exists, then a value of PV O_2 content is calculated from the assumption that it is 98 per cent of blood oxygen capacity, and this is used in calculated $\dot{Q}_p$. If arterial desaturation is present but is not due to a right-to-left intracardiac shunt, the observed systemic arterial oxygen content is used to calculate $\dot{Q}_p$.

Systemic blood flow ($\dot{Q}_s$) in liters/min is calculated as

$$\dot{Q}_s = \frac{\dot{Q}_2 \text{ consumption (ml/min)}}{\left[\begin{array}{c}\text{Systemic arterial}\\O_2 \text{ content (ml/liter)}\end{array}\right] - \left[\begin{array}{c}\text{Mixed venous}\\O_2 \text{ content (ml/liter)}\end{array}\right]}$$

Mixed venous oxygen content is obtained as the average oxygen content of blood in the chamber immediately upstream in relation to the shunt, as defined by the level of the O_2 step-up in the oximetry run. The formula used to calculate mixed venous oxygen content when the shunt is at the level of the right atrium as in atrial septal defect was derived by Flamm and coworkers.[69] They found that $\dot{Q}_s$ calculated from mixed venous oxygen content derived as

$$\frac{3\ \text{SVC } O_2 \text{ content} + 1\ \text{IVC } O_2 \text{ content}}{4}$$

most closely approximated $\dot{Q}_s$ measured by left ventricular to brachial artery indicator-dilution curves in patients with atrial septal defect.

Calculation of the shunt flow itself is then given as $\dot{Q}_p - \dot{Q}_s$. If the shunt is wholly left-to-right, this value is positive, whereas a negative value is observed in patients with pure right-to-left shunts (e.g., tetralogy of Fallot). When there is *bidirectional shunting*, the more complicated formula at the bottom of the page must be used.[31]

REGURGITANT FLOWS. In aortic or mitral valve regurgitation, left ventricular stroke volume measured angiographically is greater than the forward stroke volume (calculated by dividing the Fick cardiac output by the heart rate), and the difference is the volume of regurgitant blood that leaks across the abnormal valve(s) during each cardiac cycle. Calculation of this regurgitant flow from data obtained during cardiac catheterization can be helpful in evaluating the severity of regurgitant lesions. The regurgitant fraction (RF) is defined as

$$RF = \frac{\begin{bmatrix} \text{Angiographic} \\ \text{stroke volume} \end{bmatrix} - \begin{bmatrix} \text{Fick stroke} \\ \text{volume} \end{bmatrix}}{\text{Angiographic stroke volume}}$$

As a general rule, regurgitant fractions exceeding 30 to 40 per cent are considered hemodynamically important. However, because of potential errors of measurement of both the angiographic and Fick stroke volume, this measurement must be interpreted in light of other hemodynamic, angiographic, and clinical data.

CORONARY SINUS FLOW. Coronary sinus blood flow may be measured during cardiac catheterization by the thermodilution technique.[70] A themodilution catheter is inserted into the coronary sinus via a right antecubital vein. Saline at room temperature is continuously infused, and the temperature of the blood-saline mixture downstream in the coronary sinus is monitored by an external thermistor on the catheter. The temperature of the injected saline is monitored by an internal thermistor near the catheter injection orifice. The relationship is

$$F_B = F_I \times 1.19 \times \left(\frac{T_B - T_I}{T_B - T_M} - 1 \right) \text{ml/min}$$

where F_B = coronary sinus blood flow
  F_I = flow of room temperature saline injectate (ml/min)
  T_B = body temperature (°C)
  T_I = injectate temperature (°C)
  T_M = temperature of blood-injectate mixture (°C)

F_I must be great enough (usually 40 ml/min) to insure adequate turbulence for blood-injectate mixing in the coro-

nary sinus. This method allows continuous and repeated measurements of coronary sinus blood flow, approximating 95 per cent of coronary arterial flow.[70]

Other techniques may also be used to estimate coronary blood flow.[31] For example, a small amount of the inert gas isotope xenon-133 may be injected selectively into a coronary artery, and the initial washout of radioactivity from the heart can be recorded with a scintillation camera (Chap. 11). The regional myocardial blood flow in the distribution of that coronary artery can be estimated from the rate constant (k) derived from a semilogarithmic plot of the radioactivity washout curve, the partition coefficient of the tracer in myocardial tissue. (λ), and the specific gravity of myocardial tissue (ρ). The formula used is

Myocardial blood flow $(\text{cm}^3/100 \text{ gm tissue} \times \text{min})$ =

$$\frac{k \ (\text{min}^{-1}) \ \lambda \ 100}{\rho \ (\text{gm/cm}^3)}$$

Inaccuracies in the measurement of coronary blood flow with this method may occur because of recirculation of the isotope, deposition of xenon in myocardial fat, and local inhomogeneity of flow.

Measurement of Vascular Resistance

Theoretical Considerations. Hydraulic resistance (R) is defined by analogy to Ohm's law as the ratio of the mean pressure drop (ΔP) to flow (Q) between two points in a liquid flowing in a tube. The applicability of this simple equation to pulsatile flow in vascular beds is dubious. Nevertheless, vascular resistance calculated in this fashion has become standard practice in hemodynamic laboratories, and the calculated resistances so obtained often yield important clinical information. Poiseuille's studies of laminar steady-state flow in rigid glass tubes showed that

$$Q = \frac{\pi (\Delta P) r^4}{8 \eta l}$$

where r = radius of the tube, l = length of the tube, and η = viscosity of the fluid.[43] By rearrangement, it can be seen that resistance (R) is given by

$$R = \frac{\Delta P}{Q} = \frac{8 \eta l}{\pi r^4}$$

Thus, under the ideal conditions of laminar fluid flow in rigid tubes, resistance is directly proportional to the length of the tube and to the viscosity of the fluid and *inversely proportional to the fourth power of the tube's radius*. It is clear from this that reduction in cross-sectional area of a vessel lumen is the most powerful determinant of resis-

---

$$L \rightarrow R = \frac{\text{PBF (PA O}_2 \text{ content} - \text{Mixed venous O}_2 \text{ content)}}{\text{(PV* O}_2 \text{ content} - \text{Mixed venous O}_2 \text{ content)}}$$

$$R \rightarrow L = \frac{\text{PBF (PV* O}_2 \text{ content} - \text{BA O}_2 \text{ content) (PV* O}_2 \text{ content} - \text{PA O}_2 \text{ content)}}{\text{(Ba O}_2 \text{ content} - \text{Mixed venous O}_2 \text{ content) (PV* O}_2 \text{ content} - \text{Mixed venous O}_2 \text{ content)}}$$

---

*If actual PV is not measured, assume 98 per cent blood O_2 capacity in a patient whose pulmonary function is normal or presumed to be so.

tance to flow. It was observed by Reynolds in 1883 that the pressure drop across a length of tubing exceeded that predicted by the Poiseuille equation at a critical flow rate, dependent on the diameter of the tube and the viscosity of the fluid. He defined the Reynold's number (R_e) as being equal to $\dfrac{\overline{V}D\rho}{\mu}$, where $\overline{V}=$ average velocity of flow, $D =$ diameter of the tube, $\rho=$ density of the fluid, and $\mu =$ its viscosity.[43] When this number is exceeded, flow becomes turbulent, and the pressure drop exceeds that predicted by the Poiseuille equation, which assumes laminar flows. For blood, $R_e = 2000$, and it appears likely that during normal blood flow in arteries, R_e is not exceeded and that flow remains laminar. However, across severely stenotic valves or in areas of severe luminal arterial narrowing, this may not be the case. This will be considered further in the subsequent discussion of calculation of stenotic valve areas.

Calculations of Vascular Resistance. Vascular resistance for the systemic and pulmonary vascular beds. (SVR and PVR, respectively) is usually calculated as

$$SVR = \frac{80\,(AO_m - RA_m)}{Q_s}$$

and

$$PVR = \frac{80\,(PA_m - LA_m)}{Q_p}$$

where AO_m, RA_m, PA_m, and LA_m are the aortic, right atrial, pulmonary artery, and left atrial mean pressures in mm Hg; Q_s and Q_p are the systemic and pulmonary blood flows in liters/min (which are equal to the cardiac output in the absence of a shunt); and 80 is the factor used to convert resistance from "hybrid" units (mm Hg/liter/min) to metric units (dynes-sec-cm^{-5}). (See also Chap. 25.) These values can be corrected for body size by multiplying (not dividing) them by body surface area—an important factor in evaluating vascular resistance in infants and adolescents.

Cardiac output, usually measured by the Fick or indicator-dilution method, is used in the calculation of blood flow. It is important to appreciate that in the presence of an intracardiac shunt, in which pulmonary and systemic blood flows are not equal, the respective blood flows through each circuit must be measured and used in the calculation of resistance. Often, the mean pulmonary artery wedge pressure is used as an approximation of mean left atrial pressure, since there is ample evidence that these two measurements, when properly obtained, closely approximate each other.[71,72]

The normal value for systemic vascular resistance has been reported to be 1130 ± 178 dynes-sec-cm^{-5} (mean $\pm$ standard deviation).[73] Thus values for systemic vascular resistance less than 1500 dynes-sec-cm^{-5} are probably normal. The normal pulmonary vascular resistance has been reported as 67 ± 23 dynes-sec-cm^{-5},[73] and therefore values of pulmonary vascular resistance less than 120 dynes-sec-cm^{-5} are probably normal.

Abnormal increases of systemic and pulmonary vascular resistance may be seen in a variety of conditions (Chaps. 25 and 26). It may be important to determine whether the increased resistance is fixed (i.e., due to chronic anatomical and pathological changes) or functional (i.e., due to increased tone in small muscular arteries and arterioles), since this finding can have important clinical implications. For example, in the systemic bed, major elevations in vascular resistance may lead to a low cardiac output and left ventricular failure, particularly in the presence of mitral regurgitation. Lowering systemic resistance with specific agents (e.g., nitroprusside, hydralazine, prazosin, erythrityl tetranitrate) at the time of cardiac catheterization may yield important information about the potential therapeutic usefulness of such reduction of afterload in chronic therapy (Chap. 16).[74-83] Marked fixed increases in pulmonary vascular resistance in patients with congenital heart disease and abnormal communication between the pulmonary and systemic circuits (e.g., ventricular septal defect, atrial septal defect, patent ductus arteriosus) may contraindicate corrective surgery. Therefore, a demonstration that the increased resistance is not fixed may be of considerable importance in the individual patient. In the catheterization laboratory various agents and manipulations have been utilized to assess the reversibility of high vascular resistance, including oxygen inhalation, infusions of acetylcholine, infusions of tolazoline hydrochloride (Chap. 25), and exercise.[84-93]

Since blood flow is pulsatile, and the vascular beds have nonlinear elastic and capacitative properties, the concept of *vascular impedance* has been employed. Resistance varies continuously with pressure, and blood flow is influenced by many factors, such as inertia, reflected waves, and the phase angle between pulse and flow velocities.[43,94,95] The impedance modulus is calculated to express the spectrum of impedance versus the frequency of a pressure wave.[43]

Stenotic Valves: Calculations of Orifice Area. The evaluation of valvular stenosis in the catheterization laboratory includes a calculation of orifice size based on measurement of the pressure gradient and flow across a valve. The equations used for the aortic and mitral valves were derived and validated by Gorlin.[31,96,97]

The following equations are used when valvular gradients are measured directly:

$$\text{Aortic valve area (cm}^2) = \frac{F}{44.5\,\sqrt{\Delta P}}$$

$$\text{Mitral valve area (cm}^2) = \frac{F}{38.0\,\sqrt{\Delta P}}$$

where $F =$ flow across the orifice in ml/sec and $\Delta P =$ mean pressure gradient in mm Hg across the orifice. A pressure drop across a stenotic valve occurs because of viscous resistance to flow (Poiseuille) and turbulent flow (Reynolds). The empirical constants 44.5 and 38.0 relate these factors to valve area and differ between aortic and mitral valves because of variations in flow pattern.

For specific application to cardiac valves, F is derived as:

$$\text{Flow (F) (ml/sec)} = \frac{\text{Cardiac output (ml/min)}}{\text{DFP (sec/min) or SEP (sec/min)}}$$

The diastolic filling period (DFP) and systolic ejection period (SEP) are derived by measuring the diastolic filling time (mitral valve opening to closure, Fig. 9–8) or systolic ejection time (aortic valve opening to closure, Fig. 9–7) per beat and multiplying by the heart rate.

In a typical patient, cardiac output might be 4300 ml/min, mean transmitral diastolic pressure gradient = 14 mm Hg, diastolic filling time per beat directly measured from the pressure tracings = 0.42 sec/beat, and heart rate = 72 beats/min. Thus, the mitral valve area will be

$$\frac{(4300\ ml/min) \div (0.42\ sec/beat \times 72\ beats/min)}{38\ \sqrt{14\ mm\ Hg}} = 1.0\ cm^2$$

It is important to remember that variations in flow patterns may alter the relationship between orifice area and pressure gradient. In addition, stiff valve leaflets may be more widely opened at high flow velocities (and higher pressure gradients). Therefore, estimation of valve areas, particularly at low flow rates, may be in error and should be considered measurements of functional orifice size. In addition, the presence of valvular regurgitation will result in a falsely low valve area calculation, since the actual valve flow per beat is greater than the flow calculated from the systemic cardiac output. Stenotic valve areas calculated in patients with regurgitation across the stenotic valve should therefore be considered to be the lower limits of the true valve area. In general, errors in estimation of valve flow cause greater inaccuracies in calculations of valve area than do errors in measurement of the pressure gradient across the valve. Nevertheless, hemodynamic measurement of valve area, corrected for body surface area (valve area index), has proved very useful in the clinical management of patients.

Exercise.   In many patients with heart disease, hemodynamics may be only slightly disturbed or normal at rest but become markedly abnormal during the stress of exercise. Exercise of a patient during cardiac catheterization (p. 262) can therefore provide very important information regarding the cause of symptoms that are exercise-related. Most commonly, bicycle ergometry in the supine position is used during catheterization; upright bicycle exercise, upper extremity exercise, or straight leg-raising may also be used, if appropriate.

In supine bicycle ergometry, the patient's feet are attached by straps to the pedals of the bicycle ergometer which is attached to the catheterization table or suspended from the ceiling. The workload may be adjusted by varying the speed of and resistance to turning of the pedals. When the subject's feet are upon the pedals, intracardiac pressures normally increase slightly (i.e., by 2 to 4 mm Hg), owing to increased venous return by gravity from the legs and elevation of the diaphragm. As the exercise load is increased, oxygen consumption is increased. Exercise level is frequently expressed as metabolic equivalents of resting O_2 consumption (METS), a level of 2 METS corresponding to a doubling of O_2 consumption and usually achieved at a workload of about 75 kg-meter/min. During exercise, increased O_2 consumption by skeletal muscles is supplied by increased cardiac output and a widened arteriovenous O_2 content difference. When exercise is carried out in the supine position, cardiac output is normally increased mainly by an increase in heart rate, with only slight increases in stroke volume.[98] Patients with cardiac disease may be unable to increase cardiac output normally

with exercise because of their inability to maintain stroke volume with increased heart rate and thus will supply most of the increased O_2 required by exercising tissue by means of an increase in the arteriovenous O_2 difference. The "exercise factor" expressed as $\triangle CO$ during exercise (ml/min)/$\triangle O_2$ consumption (ml/min) is a measure of this response. It is normally greater than or equal to 6.0, since cardiac output normally increases linearly with increasing O_2 consumption. If the exercise factor is less than 6.0, the increase in cardiac output in response to exercise is impaired.

Changes in intracardiac pressures during exercise are also important. The left ventricular end-diastolic pressure does not normally increase above 16 mm Hg during exercise, but in ischemic, myocardial, and valvular disease it may rise to considerably higher levels. In some patients, exercise may exacerbate mitral or tricuspid regurgitation and usually markedly increases the left atrial–left ventricular pressure gradient in mitral stenosis (Fig. 9–8) (Chap. 32). Thus, an abnormal increase in pressures, an inadequate rise in the cardiac ouput, or both in response to the stress provided by mild to moderate exercise in the supine position can be a very important finding at catheterization (p. 483). In practice, it is important to maintain a given exercise load for at least 3 to 4 minutes before measuring cardiac output and pressures in order to assure a steady state of O_2 consumption and cardiac output. Pressures and the electrocardiogram, as well as the patient's symptoms, should be carefully monitored during exercise to avoid complications.

APPLICATIONS OF CARDIAC CATHETERIZATION

Indications.   As with any diagnostic procedure, the decision to perform cardiac catheterization must be based upon a careful balance between the risk of the procedure and the anticipated value of the information obtained. Cardiac catheterization is generally recommended when there is a need to confirm the presence of a clinically suspected condition, define its anatomical and physiological severity, and determine the presence or absence or associated conditions. This need most commonly arises when clinical assessment suggests that the patient may benefit from a *cardiac operation*. Cardiac catheterization is usually coupled with angiographic and/or arteriographic examination and may yield information that will be crucial in defining the need for cardiac operation as well as its risks and anticipated benefit for a given patient.

Although few would disagree that consideration of heart surgery is an adequate reason for performance of catheterization, there are differences of opinion about whether *all* patients being considered for such procedures should undergo preoperative cardiac catheterization.[99,100] In this regard, it should be emphasized that the risks of catheterization are small compared with those of operation in patients in whom (1) an incorrect diagnosis was made, (2) the presence of an unsuspected additional condition prolongs and complicates the planned surgical approach, or (3) the hemodynamic assessment by clinical means was inaccurate. The operating room is not a good place for surprises; preoperative cardiac catheterization can provide the surgical team with a precise and complete road map of the course ahead and thereby permit a carefully reasoned and maximally efficient operative procedure. Futhermore, information obtained by cardiac catheterization may be invaluable in the assessment of the crucial determinants of prognosis, such as left ventricular function and patency of the coronary arteries. For these reasons, we recommend that cardiac catheterization be carried out on almost all adult patients for whom a cardiac operation is contemplated. Of course, it is possible that in time noninvasive techniques may be further perfected and shown to be acceptable substitutes for catheterization data.[101] Following operation, catheterization may be necessary to evaluate the results of operation (graft patency, prosthetic valve function, and so forth).

A second broad indication for performing cardiac catheterization combined with coronary arteriography (Chap. 10) is to clarify the diagnosis in patients with *chest pain of uncertain etiology*, in whom there is confusion regarding the presence of obstructive coronary disease. The data obtained will help relieve the anxiety of the patient and aid the physician in advising the patient concerning the appropriateness of his or her future personal or professional plans. Another example within this category might be the symptomatic patient with a suspected *cardiomyopathy*. Although some may be satisfied with a clinical diagnosis of this condition, the implications of such a diagnosis in terms of therapy and prognosis are so important that cardiac catheterization is usually recommended in such patients in order to rule out potentially correctible conditions (e.g., occult valvular or pericardial disease), even though the likelihood of their presence may appear remote on clinical grounds.

A third important indication for cardiac catheterization is the need to define the response of a patient to *specific pharmacological therapy*. This may be necessary during treatment of an unstable patient (e.g., following acute myocardial infarction) or in an intensive care unit setting, when monitoring of right and left atrial pressures, systemic pressures, and cardiac output is essential to patient management. In addition, the response of patients with chronic heart failure to afterload reduction or to changes in ventricular preload may be most precisely determined by cardiac catheterization. Pharmacological intervention with vasodilators in the treatment of pulmonary hypertension,[102] or with anticoagulation in suspected acute pulmonary embolism (Chap. 46), might well be considered of sufficient potential risk to warrant cardiac catheterization and/or angiography.

Contraindications. If it is important to consider the *indications* for cardiac catheterization in each patient, it is equally important to ascertain whether there are any *contraindications*. Over the past several years, our concept of contraindications has been modified, because patients previously considered too ill for this procedure with serious conditions such as acute myocardial infarction, intractable ventricular tachycardia, and cardiogenic shock have tolerated catheterization and coronary arteriography surprisingly well.[103–105] A long list of relative contraindications must be kept in mind, however, and these include all intercurrent conditions that can be corrected and whose correction would improve the safety of the procedure. Ventricular irritability may greatly increase the risk of left-heart

catheterization and can interfere with the interpretation of ventriculography. Hypertension should be controlled prior to and during cardiac catheterization. Other conditions that should be corrected prior to elective cardiac catheterization if at all possible include febrile illness, decompensated left-heart failure, anemia, digitalis toxicity, and electrolyte disturbance. Infective endocarditis and pregnancy are relative though not absolute contraindications to cardiac catheterization.

Anticoagulant therapy is a more controversial contraindication. Some experienced physicians in this field have cautioned against catheterization in patients receiving anticoagulants, particularly when the percutaneous approach is used,[106–108] whereas others suggest that anticoagulation in such patients may be safe or even desirable.[109,110] It is our policy to maintain the prothrombin time less than 18 seconds and to avoid heparin administration for 4 to 6 hours prior to the procedure. If anticoagulant therapy cannot be interrupted, we prefer heparin because it can be easily and immediately reversed by intravenous administration of protamine sulfate should uncontrollable bleeding or cardiac perforation occur in the course of catheterization. If transseptal catheterization is planned, it is mandatory that coagulation be normal.

Design of Catheterization Protocol. Every cardiac catheterization should have a protocol, that is, a carefully reasoned sequential plan designed specifically for the individual patient being studied. Although this protocol may exist only in the mind of the operator, it is our practice to prepare a written protocol and post it prominently in the laboratory so that all personnel are made award of exactly what is planned and thus may be reasonably expected to anticipate the needs of the operator. Certain general principles should be considered in the design of a protocol. First, hemodynamic measurements should precede angiographic studies, so that the physiological state may be as basal as possible at the time of pressure and flow measurements. Second, pressure and blood oxygen saturation should be measured and recorded for each chamber immediately after entry and before passing on to the next chamber. If problems should develop during the later stages of a catheterization procedure (atrial fibrillation or other arrhythmia, pyrogen reaction, hypotension, or reaction to contrast material), the physician will wish that pressures and saturations had been measured initially rather than waiting for the time the catheter is being withdrawn. A third principle is that pressure and cardiac output measurements should be made simultaneously insofar as this is possible. Beyond these general guidelines, the protocol will reflect individual differences from patient to patient. With regard to angiography, it is important to sequence the contrast injections, so that the most important diagnostic study is performed first in a given patient.

Preparation and Premedication of the Patient. The emotional as well as the "medical" preparation of the patient for cardiac catheterization is the responsibility of the operator. It is good practice always to inform the patient and his or her family that there is some risk involved, although unless there are special circumstances they may be reasonably reassured that special problems are unlikely. The discomfort and duration of the procedure should, however, not be understated.

Usually patients scheduled for catheterization are admitted to the hospital 24 to 48 hours prior to the procedure. However, some centers are now performing cardiac catheterization on an outpatient basis for selected stable patients.[111,112] The degree to which this practice will become widely adopted is uncertain at present.

The question of administering prophylactic antibiotics is frequently raised, and some laboratories routinely administer them prior to catheterization,[113] although there are essentially no studies to support their use,[114] and we do not routinely use prophylactic antibiotics in our laboratories.

A wide variety of sedatives has been employed for premedication. We routinely use diazepam (Valium), 5 to 10 mg orally, and diphenhydramine (Benadryl), 25 to 50 mg orally, 1/2 hour prior to starting the procedure. When coronary arteriography is to be part of the procedure, some operators favor the addition of 0.4 mg atropine subcutaneously in order to avoid excessive bradycardia.[115] It is our practice to have the patient fasting (except for oral medications) after midnight. We allow a light breakfast if the patient is not scheduled for catheterization until late in the morning or afternoon.

Prior to catheterization the skin overlying the vessels to be entered (femoral areas or antecubital fossa) should be prepared by shaving and thorough cleansing with iodine or Zephiran chloride solution. This procedure as well as careful sterile technique during the catheterization procedure minimizes the incidence of infection.

Complications of Cardiac Catheterization: Incidence Prevention, and Treatment

There is an extensive literature describing a wide array of complications associated with cardiac catheterization.[107,108,115–144] The incidence of various complications has been reported by the Registry of the Society for Cardiac Angiography.[145] A total of 53,581 patients underwent catheterization and angiography in 66 laboratories over a period of 14 months, beginning in October 1979. There were 75 deaths (0.14 per cent), 40 myocardial infarctions (0.07 per cent), and 35 cerebrovascular accidents (0.07 per cent). The incidence of deaths was greater in patients under 1 year of age (1.75 per cent) and over age 60 (0.25 per cent) than in patients between 1 and 60. In patients undergoing coronary angiography, the mortality ranged from 0.86 per cent in patients with significant left main coronary artery disease to 0 per cent in patients with normal coronary arteries or only minimal coronary disease. Vascular complications occurred in 291 patients (0.57 per cent), the majority (62 per cent) in patients undergoing catheterization via the brachial approach. However, there was no difference between the brachial and femoral techniques in the incidence of serious complications, in contrast to another report.[146]

These data indicate that the incidence of complications of cardiac catheterization as currently practiced is low, although careful attention to detail and meticulous technique are required to achieve this standard of performance.

The problem of *arterial thrombosis* deserves special attention.[113,116–118,122,124,132] Sones has reported 2 to 3 per cent segmental occlusion at the site of arteriotomy.[113] It is generally acknowledged that the incidence of thrombosis is re-

lated to the duration of the procedure, the number of catheters used, the presence of underlying arterial disease, and the technique of arterial repair.[31] With regard to the percutaneous femoral approach, local complications include thrombosis, distal embolization, false aneurysm, and delayed hemorrhage.[120,127,128,135,136,142] Serious complications involving the femoral artery are usually related to the presence of preexisting iliofemoral disease, and in such patients it is preferable to avoid a percutaneous femoral approach.

Perforation of the heart or intrathoracic great vessels can occur with any approach but most commonly involves the right ventricular outflow tract and apex.[107] These areas are subject to perforation during right ventricular angiography or pacemaker placement. Perforations of the aorta, iliac artery, subclavian artery, or great veins have all been reported and are generally associated with excessive catheter manipulation. In many such instances, catheter manipulation was continued despite resistance to passage or complaints by the patient of pain related to the catheter passage. Since transseptal left-heart catheterization entails controlled perforation of the interatrial septum, perforation of the heart is its main hazard. Unintentional perforation of the aorta, atrial wall, coronary sinus, or right atrial appendage may occur, leading to cardiac tamponade.

Vagal reactions are common and may be quite serious. They are frequently, but not always, incited by pain in a tense, anxious patient and consist of nausea, hypotension, and bradycardia. In older patients, the entire picture of a vagal reaction may be present without bradycardia. If promptly recognized, vagal reactions usually respond dramatically to cessation of catheter manipulation, intravenous atropine (0.5 to 1.0 mg), and elevation of the legs to increase venous return. If the hypotension and bradycardia persist for any period of time, serious arrhythmias and/or irreversible shock may develop, particularly in patients with ischemic heart disease or aortic stenosis.

Myocardial infarction may complicate cardiac catheterization but rarely occurs unless left ventriculography or coronary arteriography is part of the procedure.[115,122,129–131] Documentation of myocardial infarction, when less than transmural in extent, may be difficult in such patients, since intramuscular injections and soft tissue trauma during the catheterization procedure may lead to increases in serum enzymes (LDH, GOT, and CK) that are often used to diagnose the presence of infarction.[143,144] However, following uncomplicated cardiac catheterization, it was shown that although total CK was increased in nearly all patients, none had elevation of CK-MB activity.[134]

Electrical hazards have been reported in association with cardiac catheterization.[138–141] Currents of only a few microamperes transmitted to a small area of myocardium by the wires of electrode catheters, catheters filled with saline, thermistor catheters, or manometer-tipped catheters may produce ventricular fibrillation. This occurrence is now rare, because of the use of common grounding of all electrical equipment, transformer isolation of electrical equipment from the power line by means of current-limiting devices, and establishment of an equal potential environment.[147]

Contamination of catheters or fluids administered during cardiac catheterization with sterile bacterial products or other foreign substances can result in a *pyrogen reac-*

tion, characterized by rigors followed by temperature elevation. If this occurs during catheterization, catheters and fluids should be set aside for subsequent culture; the reaction itself usually responds to small amounts of morphine sulfate (2 mg) administered intravenously. Pyrogen reactions are best treated by prevention. Careful cleaning and sterilization of catheters are essential in this regard.

Other Procedures Involving Cardiac Catheterization

Cardiac catheterization techniques are now being employed in an increasing number of procedures for purposes other than hemodynamic or angiographic study. In many instances the approaches and catheters used and the indications and complications for these procedures differ, and they will therefore be discussed separately.

INTRACARDIAC ELECTROCARDIOGRAPHY AND PACING. Electrodes mounted on the tips of cardiac catheters can be used to record intracardiac electrical activity and to stimulate the heart at selected sites. This technique is of great value in elucidating the mechanism and treating a variety of arrhythmias, as discussed in Chapters 19, 20, and 21. Both acute and chronic pacing are also carried out, most commonly, through pacing catheters, as described in Chapter 22.

Transvenous Endomyocardial Biopsy. Nonoperative cardiac biopsy was initially developed as a needle biopsy technique similar to needle biopsy of the kidney or liver.[148-150] In 1962, Japanese workers reported a method for transvenous endomyocardial biopsy of the right ventricle[151]; this has subsequently been modified and applied to endomyocardial biopsy of both right and left ventricles by a number of investigators.[152-157] This method is illustrated in Figure 9–11. A No. 9 French venous sheath is placed in

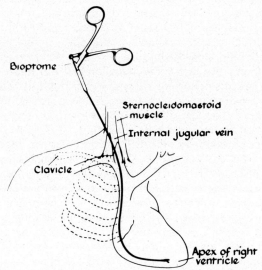

FIGURE 9–11 Endomyocardial biopsy. The biotome is introduced via the right internal jugular vein and is passed across the tricuspid valve into the right ventricle. With the biotome a small segment of right ventricular endocardium is removed from the interventricular septum for microscopic examination. (From Mason, J. W., et al.: Myocardial biopsy. *In* Willerson, J. T., and Sanders, C.A. (eds.): Clinical Cardiology. New York, Grune and Stratton, 1977.)

the internal jugular vein via a percutaneous approach. The bioptome is inserted into the sheath and advanced to the right atrium and across the tricuspid valve. After positioning of the end of the bioptome against the endocardium of the interventricular septum, by fluoroscopy, the bioptome is opened, gently advanced against the endocardium, and then closed. On withdrawal of the bioptome, a small (1 to 2 mm in diameter) portion of right ventricular myocardium with attached endocardium is obtained. This maneuver is repeated three times, and specimens are processed for light and electron microscopic study. This technique is useful in the diagnoses of hypertrophic and congestive cardiomyopathies (Chap. 41), amyloid and other infiltrative cardiomyopathies (p. 1422), and immunological rejection in cardiac transplant recipients (p. 1445).[152,153,155,158] Serial endomyocardial biopsies have been used to evaluate cardiac toxicity in patients receiving high-dose systemic adriamycin therapy for carcinoma (p. 1690).[159] A particularly promising application of this technique may be in detection of inflammatory myocarditis. In a recent report by Nippoldt et al.[160] of clinicopathological correlates in 100 consecutive patients undergoing right ventricular endomyocardial biopsy at the Mayo Clinic, myocarditis was detected in 15 per cent of patients with unexplained congestive heart failure and in 15 per cent of patients with unexplained dysrhythmia or syncope. In some cases, inflammatory myocarditis and associated congestive heart failure may respond to immunosuppressive drugs.[161] Complications, which have been rare, include cardiac perforation and tamponade, pericarditis, and atrial and ventricular tachyarrhythmias.

CORONARY ANGIOPLASTY. Over the past several years, transluminal coronary angioplasty has become an accepted method of treating selected patients with angina pectoris due to atheromatous coronary artery disease (p. 1353). This technique was developed by Grüntzig[162,163] and was an outgrowth of his previous extensive work on transluminal dilation of peripheral arterial stenoses.[162-167] For performance of transluminal dilation of coronary artery stenoses, a small (No. 3 French) dilating catheter is passed down a coronary artery, via a large guiding catheter, placed from the femoral or brachial artery in the coronary artery ostium. Recently, Simpson et al.[168] have developed a dilation catheter that has an independently movable, flexible-tipped guidewire within the dilation catheter, to facilitate passage of the dilation catheter down the appropriate coronary artery branch and crossing of the stenosis (Fig. 9–12). When the stenosis is passed with the dilating catheter, a polyvinyl chloride balloon on the dilating catheter is inflated, compressing and splitting the atheroma (Fig. 9–13).

Results of coronary angioplasty have been encouraging. A report from the Registry of the National Heart, Lung, and Blood Institute[169] indicated that this procedure was successful in 59 per cent of 631 patients, with an average decrease in the degree of stenosis from 83 to 31 per cent. Emergency bypass graft surgery was required in 6 per cent of patients, and the mortality was less than 1 per cent. The majority of patients undergoing the procedure had single-vessel disease (80 per cent), and the success rate appears greatest in lesions of the left anterior descending coronary artery. This technique also appears to be suitable for se-

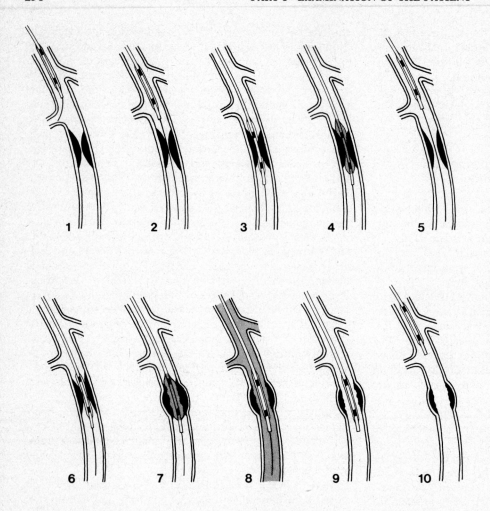

FIGURE 9–12 Schematic diagram of the dilation process: (1) A curved guidewire has been used to direct the balloon catheter away from the most proximal side branch, but it is not suitable for crossing the stenosis. (2) With the dilation catheter maintained beyond the origin of the first branch vessel, the guidewire is withdrawn, straightened, and advanced across the stenosis. (3) The deflated balloon is advanced over the guidewire and into the stenosis. (4) Initial inflation shows a persistent central indentation in the contrast-filled balloon due to incomplete dilation of the stenosis. (5) If myocardial ischemia develops before effective dilation, the guidewire may be advanced as the balloon is withdrawn from the stenosis, permitted reperfusion of the distal vessel. (6) After reperfusion, the balloon is readvanced into the stenosis. (7) Repeated inflation results in elimination of residual balloon deformity. (8) Contrast injection through the guiding catheter demonstrates brisk flow around the deflated balloon. (9) Removal of the guidewire from the dilation catheter permits measurement of the residual transstenotic pressure gradient. (10) Withdrawal of the balloon from the stenosis permits recording of the pullback gradient. (Reproduced with permission from Simpson, J. B. et al.: New catheter system for coronary angioplasty. Am. J. Cardiol. *49*: 1219, 1982.)

lected patients with unstable angina,[170] and improvement in exercise capacity soon after coronary angioplasty has been documented.[161,170,171] This improvement seems to be sustained in approximately 80 per cent of patients for 1 year,[169] whereas 15 to 20 per cent of patients experienced a recurrence of stenosis.

Further improvement in results with continuing development of catheter design and operator experience is to be anticipated, and this technique may eventually be more widely utilized in treating patients with multivessel disease.

Intracoronary Thrombolysis (see also p. 1324). In 1981 Rentrop and colleagues[172] reported on their initial experience with 29 patients with acute myocardial infarction, in whom selective infusion of streptokinase into an obstructed coronary artery was performed. Streptokinase, a plasmin-activating enzyme, was infused directly into the obstructed coronary artery via a standard coronary angiographic catheter at a rate of 2000 units/min, after a bolus of 10,000 to 20,000 units, to an average total dose of 128,000 units. Opening of the occluded vessel occurred within 15 to 90 minutes of initiation of streptokinase infusion in 22 of the 29 patients. An example of the efficacy of intracoronary streptokinase is shown in Figure 9–14. Reports by Ganz[173] and Mathey[174] have confirmed that in 70 to 90 per cent of patients with acute myocardial infarction, recanalization of an occluded artery may be achieved with this technique. Ganz and colleagues[173] have utilized a small selective catheter passed through the coronary angiograph-

ic catheter for infusion of a mixture of streptokinase and plasminogen in the immediate vicinity of the coronary thrombosis.

Whether or not reperfusion of coronary arteries with this method reduces the size of myocardial infarction is not yet established. Markis et al.[175] have reported improved myocardial uptake of thallium-201 after coronary artery thrombolysis, and Reduto el al.[176] and Rentrop et al.[177] have found that left ventricular function has improved in some patients following successful streptokinase infusion. These results suggest that intracoronary thrombolysis can indeed salvage jeopardized myocardium, although much work remains to be done in this area.

Percutaneous Intraaortic Balloon Pump Insertion. Intraaortic balloon pump (IABP) counterpulsation provides mechanical circulatory assistance by lowering aortic pressure in systole and increasing aortic pressure in diastole. Cardiac output is increased and left ventricular filling pressure is decreased by the reduction in afterload; myocardial ischemia is alleviated by reduction in oxygen demand while oxygen supply is increased. Therefore, this technique can have a dramatic beneficial effect in patients with cardiogenic shock (p. 1317) and severe, acute myocardial ischemia (p. 1359). It has become a well-accepted method of providing temporary circulatory support for critically ill patients, tiding them over during a stressful procedure, such as cardiac catheterization and angiography, and/or until cardiac surgery can be performed.[178] In

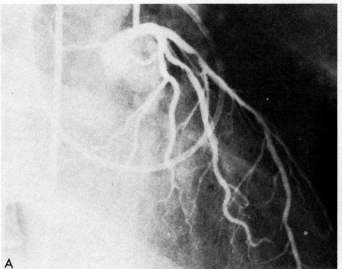

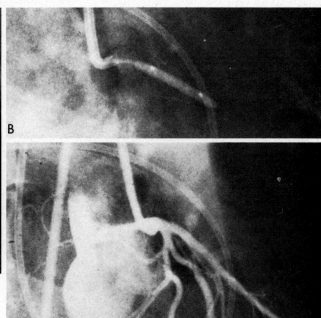

FIGURE 9–13 Balloon dilation of coronary artery. Coronary arteriography cine frames obtained in the right anterior oblique projection before balloon dilation of proximal left anterior descending coronary artery stenosis (*top*), during inflation of the contrast-filled balloon on the dilation catheter, which has been passed across the stenosis over a 0.018-inch guidewire (*middle*), and after balloon dilation of the stenotic region (*bottom*). There is significant relief of stenosis following the dilation procedure. The stenosis was not altered by the intracoronary administration of nitroglycerin. (From Barry, W. H., and Levin, D. unpublished data.)

the past, IABP catheters have been inserted via a direct surgical approach, requiring a cutdown on the femoral artery and surgical repair of the artery after the balloon pump has been removed. With this method, however, the incidence of complications was not inconsiderable. For example, in the series reported by Pace et al.[179] from the Brigham and Women's Hospital, thrombotic or embolic occlusion of the femoral artery occurred in 29 per cent of the patients, and there was a significant incidence of more severe problems, including dissection of the aorta or iliac artery, contributing to an overall mortality associated with the use of the balloon pump of 4.8 per cent.

Because of the widespread applicability of IABP, there has been great interest in developing techniques for percutaneous insertion and removal of the balloon catheter, in hopes of reducing the complication rate. The method that has been developed involves insertion of an IABP catheter through a No. 12 French sheath placed percutaneously in the femoral artery. The catheter is advanced into the central aorta under fluoroscopic control. Passage of the catheter past a tortuous iliac artery is facilitated by use of a 15-inch sheath that allows advancement of the sheath introducer into the abdominal aorta, leading with a guidewire.[180] More recently, an IABP catheter with a central lumen has been developed, and this also allows use of a guidewire during placement of the catheter in the central aorta,[181] as well as monitoring of central aortic pressure during counterpulsation. For removal, the catheter and

sheath are withdrawn simultaneously, and the artery is compressed until hemostasis is achieved.

With these methods, successful insertion can be achieved in over 90 per cent of patients. The reported incidence of complications of this technique varies from 0 to 26 per cent[180–183] and is undoubtedly influenced in part by the population of patients in which it is employed. However, the incidence of severe complications, such as aortic or iliac dissection, appears lower with the percutaneous method, especially when the long sheath technique or the central lumen guidewire catheter is employed and fluoroscopy is utilized. The risk of ischemic limb complications remains significant, particularly in persons with atherosclerotic peripheral vascular disease and in women; in these patients the No. 12 French sheath may cause arterial obstruction. Therefore, use of IABP is usually restricted to those patients who are primarily Class IV with refractory myocardial ischemia, congestive heart failure, or cardiogenic shock.

Miscellaneous Therapeutic Procedures. The technique of *balloon atrial septostomy*, developed by Rashkind, has become a standard procedure to improve mixing between systemic and pulmonary circulations in neonates with transposition of the great arteries and in patients with intact atrial septum or inadequate interatrial communication (Chap. 29).[184,185,185a]

There has been extensive experience primarily in Japan and Germany with *nonoperative closure of a patent ductus*

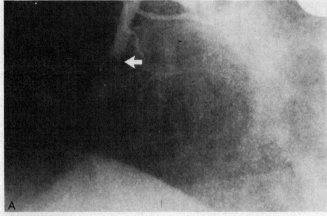

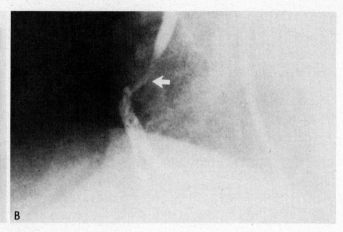

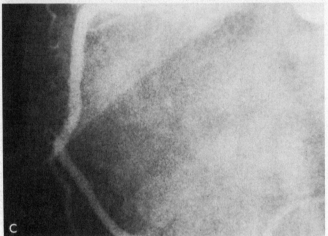

FIGURE 9–14   Effect of administering intracoronary streptokinase in a patient presenting with acute inferior myocardial infarction. The initial contrast injection into the right coronary artery (*A*) demonstrated complete proximal occlusion (arrow); *B*, The appearance after 20 minutes of streptokinase infusion; patency of the vessel was achieved, but there was definite residual thrombus (arrow). *C*, The artery two weeks later. Note the complete clearing of all residual thrombus. (Courtesy of Dr. John Markis, Beth Israel Hospital, Boston, Mass.)

arteriosus (Chap. 30).[185a,186-188] This has been accomplished by insertion of a plug, mounted on the tip of a catheter, into the patent ductus. Extension of this technique to *closure of an atrial septal defect* using a transvenous umbrella technique has bee reported.[185a,189,190]

A technique for *transvenous pulmonary embolectomy* has been devised that utilizes a catheter with a suction-cupped tip.[191,192] This catheter is advanced to the pulmonary artery, and its tip is manipulated by externally controlled, braided wires within its wall until the suction cup makes contact with the embolus. The application of suction by syringe produces adherence of the end of the embolus to the suction cup, and the catheter and suction cup are then withdrawn together with the embolus.

In another interesting therapeutic application of cardiac catheterization, Taylor and colleagues have reported therapeutic *embolization of the pulmonary artery* in pulmonary arteriovenous fistulas.[193]

Special "snare" catheters have been designed to *retrieve from within the heart catheter fragments* introduced iatrogenically.[194,195] Use of these techniques can obviate thoracotomy and cardiotomy.

This is by no means an exhaustive description of all the therapeutic uses of cardiac catheterization but should serve to illustrate how techniques originally developed to perform hemodynamic measurements have evolved into the therapeutic procedures. Thus, it is clear that cardiac catheterization can no longer be considered solely a diagnostic procedure.

References

1. Cournand, A.: Cardiac catheterization. Development of the technique, its contributions to experimental medicine, and its initial application in man. Acta Med. Scand. *579* (Suppl.):1, 1975.
2. Forssmann, W.: Die Sondierung des rechten Herzens. Klin. Wschr. *8*:2085, 1929.
3. Klein, O.: Zur Bestimmung des zirkulatorischen Minutensvolumen nach dem Fickschen Prinzip, Münch. Med. Wschr. *77*:1311, 1930.
4. Cournand, A. F., and Ranges, H. S.: Catheterization of the right auricle in man. Proc. Soc. Exp. Biol. Med. *46*:462, 1941.
5. Richards, D. W.: Cardiac output by the catheterization technique in various clinical conditions. Fed. Proc. *4*:215, 1945.
6. Cournand, A. F., Riley, R. L., Breed, E. S., Baldwin, E. F., and Richards, D. W.: Measurement of cardiac output in man using the technique of catheterization of the right auricle. J. Clin. Invest. *24*:106, 1945.
7. Dexter, L., Haynes, F. W., Burwell, C. S., Eppinger, E. C., Sagerson, R. P., and Evans, J. M.: Studies of congenital heart disease. II. The pressure and oxygen content of blood in the right auricle, right ventricle, and pulmonary artery in control patients, with observations on the oxygen saturation and source of pulmonary "capillary" blood. J. Clin. Invest. *26*:554, 1947.
8. Hellems, H. K., Haynes, F. W., and Dexter, L.: Pulmonary "capillary" pressure in man. J. Appl. Physiol. *2*:24, 1949.
9. Lagerlof, H., and Werkö, L.: Studies on circulation of blood in man. Scand. J. Clin. Lab. Invest. *7*:147, 1949.
10. McMichael, J., and Sharpey-Schafer, E. P.: The action of intravenous digoxin in man. Qt. J. Med. *13*:1123, 1944.
11. Lenegre, J., and Maurice, P.: Premiers recherches sur la pression ventriculaire droite. Bull. Mem. Soc. Med. Hop. Paris *80*:239, 1944.
12. Lenegre, J., and Maurice, P.: La derivation directe intracavitaire des courants electrique de l'oreillette et du ventriculaire droite. Paris Med. *35*:23, 1945.

13. Stead, E. A., Jr., and Warren, J. V.: Cardiac output in man: Analysis of mechanisms varying cardiac output based on recent clinical studies. Arch. Intern. Med. 80:237, 1947.

14. Stead, E. A., Jr., Warren, J. V., and Brannon, E. S.: Cardiac output in congestive heart failure: Analysis of reasons for lack of close correlation between symptoms of heart failure and resting cardiac output. Am. Heart J. 35: 529, 1948.

15. Bing, R. J., Hammond, M. M., Handelsman, J. C., Powers, S. R., Spencer, F. C., Eckenhoff, J. E., Goodale, W. T., Italkenschiel, J. H., and Kety, S. S.: Catheterization of coronary sinus and middle cardiac vein in man. Proc. Soc. Exp. Biol. Med. 66:239, 1947.

16. Bing, R. J., Vandam, L. D., Gregoire, F., Handelsman, J. C., Goodale, W. T., and Echenhoff, J. E.: Measurement of coronary blood flow, oxygen consumption and efficiency of the left ventricle in man. Am. Heart J. 38:1, 1949.

17. Vandam, L. D., Bing, R. J., and Gray, F. D., Jr.: Physiological studies in congenital heart disease. IV. Measurements of circulation in 5 selected cases. Bull. John Hopkins Hosp. 81:192, 1947.

18. Bing, R. J., Vandam, L. D., and Gray, F. D., Jr.: Physiological studies in congenital heart disease. I. Procedures. Bull. Johns Hopkins Hosp. 80:107, 1947.

19. Burchell, H. B.: Cardiac catheterization in diagnosis of various cardiac malformations and diseases. Proc. Mayo Clin. 23:481, 1948.

20. Wood, E. H., Geraci, J. E., Pollack, A. A., Groom, D., Taylor, B. D., Pender, J. W., and Puch, D. G.: General and special techniques in cardiac catheterization. Proc. Mayo Clin. 23:494, 1948.

21. Burwell, C. S., and Dexter, L.: Beri-beri heart disease. Trans. Assoc. Am. Physicians 60:59, 1947.

22. Harvey, R. M., Ferrer, M. I., Cathcart, R. T., Richards, D. W., Jr., and Cournand, A.: Some effects of digoxin upon heart and circulation in man: Digoxin in left ventricular failure. Am. J. Med. 7:439, 1949.

23. Zimmerman, H. A., Scott, R. W., and Becker, N. D.: Catheterization of the left side of the heart in man. Circulation 1:357, 1950.

24. Limon Lason, R., and Bouchard, A.: El cateterismo intracardico; cateterization de las cavidades izquierdas en el hombre. Registro simultaneo de presion y electrocardiograma intracavetarios. Arch. Inst. Cardiol. Mexico 21:271, 1950.

25. Seldinger, S. I.: Catheter replacement of the needle in percutaneous arteriography: A new technique. Acta Radiol. 39:368, 1953.

26. Ross, J., Jr.: Transseptal left heart catheterization: A new method of left atrial puncture. Ann. Surg. 149:395, 1959.

27. Ross, J., Jr., Braunwald, E., and Morrow, A. G.: Transseptal left atrial puncture: A new method for the measurement of left atrial pressure in man. Am. J. Cardiol. 3:653, 1959.

28. Sones, F. M., Jr., Shirey, E. K., Proudfit, W. L., and Westcott, R. N.: Cine coronary arteriography. Circulation 20:773, 1959.

29. Sones, F. M., Jr., and Shirey, E. K.: Cine coronary arteriography. Mod. Concepts Cardiovasc. Dis. 31:735, 1962.

30. Swan, H. J. C., Ganz, W., Forrester, J., Marcus, H., Diamond, G., and Chonette, D.: Catheterization of the heart in man with use of a flow directed balloon-tipped catheter. N. Engl. J. Med. 283:447, 1970.

31. Grossman, W.: Cardiac Catheterization and Angiography. 2nd ed. Philadelphia, Lea and Febiger, 1980.

32. Sprawls, P., Jr.: The Physical Principles of Diagnostic Radiology. Baltimore, University Park Press, 1977, pp. 1–166.

33. Reuter, F. G.: Physician and patient exposure during cardiac catheterization. Circulation 58:134, 1978.

34. Barry, W. H., Levin, D. C., Green, L. H., Bettman, M. A., Mudge, G. H., Jr., and Phillips, D.: Left heart catheterization and angiography via the percutaneous femoral approach using an arterial sheath. Cathet. Cardiovasc. Diagn. 5:401, 1979.

35. Karsh, D. L., Michaelson, S. P., Langon, R. A., Cohen, L. S., and Wolfson, S.: Retrograde left ventricular catheterization in patients with an aortic valve prosthesis. Am. J. Cardiol. 41:893, 1978.

36. Brockenbrough, E. C., and Braunwald, E.: A new technique for left ventricular angiocardiography and transseptal left heart catheterization. Am. J. Cardiol. 6: 1062, 1960.

37. Keane, J. F., Freed, M. D., Fellows, K. E., and Fyler, D. C.: Pediatric cardiac angiocardiography using a 4 French catheter. Cathet. Cardiovasc. Diagn. 3: 313, 1977.

38. Lees, M. H., Bristow, J. D., Way, C., and Brown, M.: Cardiac output by Fick principle in infants and young children. Am. J. Dis. Child. 114:144, 1967.

39. Jarmakani, J. M.: Cardiac catheterization in heart disease in infants, children, and adolescents. In Moss, A. J., Adams, F. H., and Emmanouilides, G. C. (eds.): Heart Disease in Infants and Children. Baltimore, Williams and Wilkins Co., 1977.

40. Nachnani, G. H., Lessin, L. S., Motomiya, T., and Leusen, W. N.: Scanning electron microscopy of thrombogenesis on vascular catheter surfaces. N. Engl. J. Med. 286:139, 1972.

41. Fry, D. L.: Physiologic recording by modern instruments with particular reference to pressure recording. Physiol. Rev. 40:753, 1960.

42. Noble, F. W.: Electrical Methods of Blood Pressure Recording. Springfield, Ill., Charles C. Thomas, 1953.

43. McDonald, D. A.: Blood flow in Arteries. 2nd ed. Baltimore, Williams and Wilkins Co., 1974.

44. Wood, E. H., Leusen, I. R., Warner, H. R., and Wright, J. L.: Measurement of pressures in man by cardiac catheters. Circ. Res. 2:294, 1954.

45. Grossman, W., McLaurin, L. P., and Stefadouros, M. A.: Left ventricular stiffness associated with chronic pressure and volume overloads in man. Circ. Res. 35:793, 1974.

46. Guyton, A. C., Jones, C. E., and Coleman, T. G.: Circulatory Physiology: Cardiac Output and Its Regulation. 2nd ed. Philadelphia, W. B. Saunders Co., 1973.

47. Fick, A.: Über die Messung des Blutquantums in den Herzventrikeln. Sitz der Physik. Med. Ges. Wurzburg 1870, p. 16.

48. Van Slyke, D. D., and Neill, J. M.: The determination of gases in blood and other solutions by vacuum extraction and manometric measurements. J. Biol. Chem. 8:654, 1962.

49. Barratt-Boyes, B. G., and Wood, E. H.: The oxygen saturation of blood in the venae cavae, right heart chambers, and pulmonary vessels of healthy subjects. J. Lab. Clin. Med. 50:93, 1957.

50. Selzer, A., and Sudrann, R. B.: Reliability of the determination of cardiac output in man by means of the Fick principle. Circ. Res. 6:485, 1958.

51. Thomassen, B.: Cardiac output in normal subjects under standard conditions. The repeatability of measurements by the Fick method. Scand. J. Clin. Lab. Invest. 9:365, 1957.

52. Visscher, M. B., and Johnson, J. A.: The Fick principle: Analysis of potential errors and its conventional application. J. Appl. Physiol. 5:635, 1953.

53. Stewart, G. N.: Researches on the circulation time and on the influences which affect it. IV. The output of the heart. J. Physiol. 22:159, 1897.

54. Hamilton, W. F., Riley, R. L., Attyah, A. M., Cournand, A., Fowell, D. M., Himmelstein, A., Noble, R. P., Remington, J. W., Richards, D. W., Wheeler, N. C., and Witham, A. C.: Comparison of Fick and dye injection methods of measuring cardiac output in man. Am. J. Physiol. 153:309, 1948.

55. Rahimtoola, S. H., and Swan, H. J. C.: Calculation of cardiac output from indicator dilution curves in the presence of mitral regurgitation. Circulation 31: 711, 1965.

56. Shepherd, R. L., Higgs, L. M., and Glancy, D. L.: Comparison of left ventricular and pulmonary arterial injection sites in determination of cardiac output by the indicator dilution technique. Chest 62:175, 1972.

57. Reddy, P. S., Curtiss, E. I., Bell, B., O'Toole, J. D., Salerni, R., Leon, D. F., and Shaver, J. A.: Determinants of variation between Fick and indicator dilution estimates of cardiac output during diagnostic catheterization. Fick vs. dye outputs. J. Lab. Clin. Med. 87:568, 1976.

58. Branthwaite, M. A., and Bradley, R. D.: Measurement of cardiac output by thermodilution in man. J. Appl. Physiol. 24:434, 1968.

59. Ganz, W., Donoso, R., Marcus, H. S., Forrester, J. S., and Swan, H. J. C.: A new technique for measurements of cardiac output by thermodilution in man. Am. J. Cardiol. 27:392, 1971.

60. Kinsman, J. M., Moore, J. W., and Hamilton, W. F.: Studies on the circulation. I. Injection method. Physical and mathematical considerations. Am. J. Physiol. 89:322, 1929.

61. Moore, J. W., Kinsman, J. M., Hamilton, W. G., and Spurling R. G.: Studies on the circulation. II. Cardiac output determinations; comparison of the injection method with the direct Fick procedure. Am. J. Physiol. 89:331, 1929.

62. Doyle, J. T., Wilson, J. S., Lepine, C., and Warren, J. V.: An evaluation of the measurement of the cardiac output and of the so-called pulmonary blood volume by the dye-dilution method. J. Lab. Clin. Med. 41:29, 1953.

63. Eliasch, H., Lagerlof, H., Bucht, H., Ek, J., Eriksson, K., Bergstrom, J., and Werkö, L.: Comparison of the dye dilution and the direct Fick methods for the measurement of cardiac output in man. Scand. J. Lab. Clin. Invest. 7 (Suppl. 20):73, 1955.

64. Dalen, J. E.: Shunt detection and measurement. In Grossman, W. (ed.): Cardiac Catheterization and Angiography. Philadelphia, Lea and Febiger, 1974, p. 96.

65. Dexter, L., Haynes, F. W., Burwell, C. S., Springer, E. C., Seibel, R. E., and Evans, J. M.: Studies of congenital heart disease. I. Technique of venous catheterization as a diagnostic procedure. J. Clin. Invest. 26:547, 1947.

66. Hyman, A. L., Myers, W., Hyatt, K., DeGraff, A. C., Jr., and Quiroy, A. C.: A comparison study of the detection of cardiovascular shunts by oxygen analysis and indicator dilution methods. Ann. Intern. Med. 56:535, 1962.

67. Swan, H. J. C., and Wood, E. H.: Localization of cardiac defects by dye dilution curves recorded after injection of T-1824 at multiple sites in the heart and great vessels during cardiac catheterization. Proc. Staff Meet. Mayo Clin. 28: 95, 1953.

68. Castillo, C. A., Kyle, J. C., Gilson, W. E., and Rowe, G. G.: Simulated shunt curves. Am. J. Cardiol. 17:691, 1966.

69. Flamm, M. D., Cohn, K. E., and Hancock, E. W.: Measurement of systemic cardiac output at rest and exercise in patients with atrial septal defect. Am. J. Cardiol. 23:258, 1969.

70. Ganz, W., Tamura, K., Marcus, H. S., Donose, R., Yoshida, S., and Swan, H. J. C.: Measurement of coronary sinus blood flow by continuous thermo-dilution in man. Circulation 44:181, 1971.

71. Rapaport, E., and Dexter, L.: Pulmonary "capillary" pressure. In Methods in Medical Research. Chicago, Year Book Medical Publishers, 7:85, 1958.

72. Connolly, D. C., Kirklin, J. W., and Wood, E. H.: The relationship between pulmonary artery pressure and left atrial pressure in man. Circ. Res. 2:434, 1954.

73. Barratt-Boyes, B. G., and Wood, E. H.: Cardiac output and related

measurements and pressure values in the right heart and associated vessels, together with an analysis of the hemodynamic response to the inhalation of high oxygen mixtures in healthy subjects. J. Lab. Clin. Med. 51:72, 1958.

74. Goldberg, S., Grossman, W., and Mann, J. T.: Vasodilator therapy of heart failure in the setting of valvular heart disease: Determinants of increased cardiac output. Am. J. Med. 65:161, 1978.

75. Cohn, J. N.: Vasodilator therapy for heart failure. The influence of impedance on left ventricular performance. Circulation 48:5, 1973.

76. Chatterjee, K.: Vasodilator therapy for heart failure. Ann. Intern. Med. 83: 421, 1975.

77. Braunwald, E., Welch, G. H., Jr., and Morrow, A. G.: The effects of acutely increased systemic resistance on the left atrial pressure pulse: A method for the clinical detection of mitral insufficiency. J. Clin. Invest. 37:35, 1958.

78. Grossman, W., Harshaw, C. W., Munro, A. B., Becker, L., and McLaurin, L. P.: Lowered aortic impedance as therapy for severe mitral regurgitation. J. A. M. A. 230:1101, 1974.

79. Harshaw, C. W., Munro, A. B., McLaurin, L. P., and Grossman, W.: Reduced systemic vascular resistance as therapy for severe mitral regurgitation of valvular origin. Ann. Intern. Med. 83:312, 1976.

80. Bolen, J. L., and Alderman, E. L.: Hemodynamic consequences of afterload reduction in patients with chronic aortic regurgitation. Circulation 53:879, 1976.

81. Goodman, D. J., Rossen, R. M., Holloway, E. L., Alderman, E. L., and Harrison, D. C.: Effect of nitroprusside on left ventricular dynamics in mitral regurgitation, Circulation 50:1025, 1974.

82. Chatterjee, K., Parmley, W. W., Massie, B., Greenberg, B., Werner, J., Klausner, S., and Norman A.: Oral hydralazine therapy for chronic refractory heart failure. Circulation 54:879, 1976.

83. Miller, R. R., Vismara, L. A., Zelis, R., Amsterdam, E. A., and Mason, D. T.: Clinical use of sodium nitroprusside in chronic ischemic heart disease. Effects on peripheral vascular resistance, venous tone, and on ventricular volume, pump, and mechanical performance. Circulation 51:328, 1975.

84. Fritts, H. W., Harris, P., Clauss, R. H., Odell, J. E., and Cournand, A.: The effect of acetylcholine on the human pulmonary circulation under normal and hypoxic conditions. J. Clin. Invest. 37:99, 1958.

85. Wood, P., Besterman, E. M., Towers, M. K., and McIlroy, M. B.: The effect of acetylcholine on pulmonary vascular resistance and left atrial pressure in mitral stenosis. Br. Heart J. 19:279, 1957.

86. Dresdale, D. T., Michton, R. J., and Schultz, M.: Recent studies in primary pulmonary hypertension including pharmacodynamic observations on pulmonary vascular resistance. Bull. N. Y. Acad. Med. 30:195, 1954.

87. Rudolph, A. M., Paul, M. H., Sommer, L. S., and Nadas, A. S.: Effects of tolazoline hydrochloride (Priscoline) on circulatory dynamics of patients with pulmonary hypertension. Am. Heart J. 55:424, 1958.

88. Vogel, J. H. K., Grover, R. F., Jamieson, G., and Blount, S. G., Jr.: Long term physiologic observations in patients with ventricular septal defect and increased pulmonary vascular resistance. Adv. Cardiol. 11:108, 1974.

89. Grover, R. F., Reeves, T. J., and Blount, S. G., Jr.: Tolazoline hydrochloride (Priscoline): An effective pulmonary vasodilator. Am. Heart J. 61:5, 1961.

90. Brammel, H. L., Vogel, J. H. K., Pryor, R., and Blount, S. G., Jr.: The Eisenmenger syndrome. Am. J. Cardiol. 28:679, 1971.

91. Moret, P., Covarrubias, E., Condert, J., and Duchosall, F.: Cardiocirculatory adaptation to chronic hypoxia. Acta Cardiol. (Brux.) 27:596, 1972.

92. Penazola, D., Sime, F., Banchero, N., Gamboa, R., Cruz, J., and Marticorena, E.: Pulmonary hypertension in healthy men born and living at high altitudes. Am. J. Cardiol. 11:150, 1963.

93. Vogel, J. H. K., Weaver, W. F., Rose, R. L., Blount, S. G., Jr., and Grover, R. F.: Pulmonary hypertension on exertion in normal men living at 10,150 feet (Leadville, Colorado). Med. Thorac. 19:461, 1962.

94. Milnor, W. R.: Pulsatile blood flow. N. Engl. J. Med. 287:27, 1972.

95. Nichols, W. W., Conti, C. R., Walker, W. E., and Milnor, W. R.: Input impedance of the systemic circulation in man. Circ. Res. 40:421, 1977.

96. Gorlin, R., and Gorlin, G.: Hydraulic formula for calculation of area of stenotic mitral valve, other valves, and central circulatory shunts. Am. Heart J. 41:1, 1951.

97. Cohen, M. V., and Gorlin, R.: Modified orifice equation for the calculation of mitral valve area. Am. Heart J. 84:839, 1972.

98. Marshall, R. J., and Shepherd, J. J.: Cardiac function in health and disease. Philadelphia, W. B. Saunders Co., 1968.

99. St. John Sutton, M. G., St. John Sutton, M., Aldershaw, P., Sacchetti, R., Paneth, M., Lennox, S. C., Gibson, R. V., and Gibson, D. G.: Valve replacement without preoperative cardiac catheterization. N. Eng. J. Med. 305: 1233, 1981.

100. Roberts, W. C.: No cardiac catheterization before cardiac valve replacement— a mistake. Am. Heart J. 103:930, 1982.

101. Alpert, J. S., Sloss, L. J., Cohn, P. F., and Grossman, W.: The diagnostic accuracy of combined clinical and noninvasive cardiac evaluation: Comparison with findings at cardiac catheterization. Cathet. Cardiovasc. Diagn. 6:359, 1980.

102. Lupi-Herrera, E., Sandoval, J., Seoane, M., and Bialostozky, D.: The role of hydralazine therapy for pulmonary arterial hypertension of unknown cause. Circulation 65:648, 1982.

103. Diamond, G., Marcus, H., McHugh, T., Swan, H. J. C., and Forrester, J.: Catheterization of the left ventricle in acutely ill patients. Br. Heart J. 33:489, 1971.

104. Gold, H. K., Keinbach, R. C., Sanders, C. A., Buckley, M. J., Mundth, E. D., and Austen, W. G.: Intraaortic balloon pumping for ventricular septal defect or mitral regurgitation complicating acute myocardial infarction. Circulation 47:1191, 1973.

105. Gold, H. K., Leinbach, R. C., Sanders, C. A., Buckley, M. J., Mundth, E. D., and Austen, W. G.: Intraaortic balloon pumping for control of recurrent myocardial ischemia. Circulation 47:1197, 1973.

106. O'Brien, K. P., Glancy, D. L., and Brandt, P. W. T.: Cardiac catheterization: indications, current techniques, and complications. Ausralast. Radiol. 14:378, 1970.

107. Braunwald, E., and Swan, H. J. C. (eds.): Cooperative study on cardiac catheterization. Circulation 37 (Suppl. 111):1, 1968.

108. Mortensen, J. D.: Clinical sequelae from arterial needle puncture, cannulation, and incision. Circulation 35:1118, 1967.

109. Kloster, F. E., Bristow, J. D., and Seaman, A. J.: Cardiac catheterization during anticoagulant therapy. Am. J. Cardiol. 28:675, 1971.

110. Walker, W. J., Mundall, S. L., Broderick, H. G., Prasad, B., Kin, J., and Ravi, J. M.: Systemic heparinization for femoral percutaneous angiography. N. Engl. J. Med. 288:826, 1973.

111. Mahrer, P. R., and Eshoo, N.: Outpatient cardiac catheterization and coronary angiography. Cathet. Cardiovasc. Diagn. 7:355, 1981.

112. Perrigo, E. S., Kuehne, M. L., and Michienzi, F.: Twenty month experience in outpatient cardiac catheterization. Circulation 62: (Supp. 111):216, 1980.

113. Sones, J. M., Jr.: Cine coronary arteriography. In Hurst, J. W., and Logue, R. B. (eds.): The Heart. 2nd ed. New York, McGraw-Hill Book Co., 1970, p. 377.

114. Sande, M. A., Levinson, M. E., Lukas, D. S., and Kaye, D.: Bacteremia associated with cardiac catheterization. N. Engl. J. Med. 281:1104, 1969.

115. Green, G. S., McKinnon, C. M., Rosch, J., and Judkins, M. P.: Complications of selective percutaneous transfemoral coronary arteriography and their prevention. Circulation 45:552, 1972.

116. Campion, B. C., Frye, R. L., Pluth, J. R., Fairbairn, J. F., and Davis, G. D.: Arterial complications of retrograde brachial arterial catheterization. Mayo Clin. Proc. 46:589, 1971.

117. Jeresaty, R. M., and Liss, J. P.: Effects of artery catheterization on arterial pulse and blood pressure in 203 patients. Am. Heart J. 76:481, 1968.

118. Machleder, H. I., Sweeney, J. P., and Barker, J. F.: Pulseless arm after brachial artery catheterization. Lancet 1:407, 1972.

119. Bristow, J. D., Seaman, A. J., Kloster, F. E., Herr, R. H., and Griswold, H. E.: Late, heparin-induced bleeding after retrograde arterial catheterization. Circulation 37:393, 1968.

120. Kloster, F. E., Bristow, J. D., and Griswold, H. E.: Femoral artery occlusion following percutaneous catheterization. Am. Heart J. 79:175, 1970.

121. Gupta, P. K., and Haft, J. I.: Complete heart block complicating cardiac catheterization. Chest 61:185, 1972.

122. Chahine, R. A., Herman, M. V., and Gorlin, R.: Complications of coronary arteriography: Comparison of the brachial to the femoral approach. Ann. Intern. Med. 76:862, 1972.

123. Eshagy, B., Loeb, H. S., Miller, S. E., Scanlon, P. J., Towne, W. D., and Gunnar, R. M.: Mediastinal and retropharyngeal hemorrhage: A complication of cardiac catheterization. J. A. M. A. 226:427, 1973.

124. Brener, B. J., and Couch, N. P.: Peripheral arterial complications of left heart catheterization and their management, Am. J. Surg. 125:521, 1973.

125. Hey, E. G., Jr., Dyrda, I., and Joyner, C. R.: Entanglement of a cardiac catheter on a heart valve prosthesis. N. Engl. J. Med. 275:434, 1966.

126. Goodman, D. J., Rider, A. K., Billingham, M. E., and Schroeder, J. S.: Thromboembolic complications with the indwelling balloon tipped pulmonary arterial catheter. N. Engl. J. Med. 291:777, 1974.

127. Stanger, P., Heymann, M. A., Tarnoff, H., Hoffman, J. I. E., and Rudolph, A. M.: Complications of cardiac catheterization of neonates, infants and children. Circulation 50:595, 1974.

128. Murphy, T. O., Piper, C. A., and Anderson, C. L.: Complications of left heart catheterization. Am. Surgeon 37:472, 1971.

129. Price, H. P., and Takaro, T.: Unusual coronary emboli associated with coronary arteriography. Chest 63:698, 1973.

130. Walson, W. J., Lee, G. B., and Amplatz, K.: Biplane selective coronary arteriography via percutaneous transfemoral approach. Am. J. Roentgenol. 100 : 332, 1967.

131. Takaro, T., Pifarre, R., and Wuerflein, R. D.: Acute coronary occlusion following coronary arteriography: Mechanisms and surgical relief. Surgery 72: 1018, 1972.

132. Nicholas, G. G., and DeMuth, W. E.: Long term results of brachial thrombectomy following cardiac catheterization. Ann. Surg. 183:436, 1976.

133. Smith, W. R., Glauser, F. L., and Jemison, P.: Ruptured chordae of the tricuspid valve: The consequence of flow directed Swan-Ganz catheterization. Chest 70:790, 1976.

134. Roberts, R., Ludbrook, P. A., Weiss, E. S., and Sobel, B. E.: Serum CPK isoenzymes after cardiac catheterization. Br. Heart J. 37:1144, 1975.

135. Takahashi, O., Zakheim, R., Park, M. K., Mattioli, L., and Diehl, A. M.: The effects of transfemoral cardiac catheterization on limb blood flow in children. Chest 71:159, 1977.

136. Rosengart, R., Nelson, R. J., and Emmanoulides, G. C.: Anterior tibial compartment syndrome in a child: An unusual complication of cardiac catheterization. Pediatrics 58:456, 1967.

137. Dawson, D. M., and Fisher, E. G.: Neurologic complications of cardiac catheterization. Neurology 27:496, 1977.

138. Bousvaros, G. A., Conway, D., and Hopps, J. A.: An electrical hazard of selective angiocardiography. Can. Med. Assoc. J. 87:286, 1962.
139. Starmer, C. F., Whalen, R. E., and McIntosh, H. D.: Hazards of electric shock in cardiology. Am. J. Cardiol. 14:537, 1964.
140. Mody, S. M., and Richings, M.: Ventricular fibrillation resulting from electrocution during cardiac catheterization. Lancet 2:698, 1962.
141. Starmer, C. F., McIntosh, H. D., and Whalen, R. E.: Electrical hazards and cardiovascular function. N. Engl. J. Med. 284:181, 1971.
142. Lang, E. K.: A survey of a complications of percutaneous retrograde arteriography, Seldinger technique. Radiology 81:257, 1963.
143. Adrouny, Z. A., Stephenson, M. J., Straube, K. R., Dotter, C. T., and Griswold, H. E.: Effect of cardiac catheterization and angiocardiography on the serum glutamic oxalozcetic transminase. Circulation 27:565, 1963.
144. Burckhardt, D., Vera, C. A., LaDue, J. S., and Steinberg, I.: Enzyme activity following angiography. Am. J. Roentgenol. 102:406, 1968.
145. Kennedy, J. W.: Complications associated with cardiac catheterization and angiography. Cathet. Cardiovasc. Diagn. 8:5, 1982.
146. Davis, K., Kennedy, J. W., Kemp, H. G., Jr., Judkins, M. P., Gosselin, A. F., and Killip, T.: Complications of coronary arteriography. Circulation 59:1105, 1979.
147. Shabetai, R., and Adolph, R. J.: Principles of cardiac catheterization In Fowler, H. O. (ed.): Cardiac Diagnosis and Treatment. 2nd ed. Hagerstown, Md., Harper and Row, p. 86.
148. Sutton, D. C., and Sutton, G. C.: Needle biopsy of the human ventricular myocardium. Review of 54 consecutive cases. Am. Heart J. 60:364, 1960.
149. Bulloch, R. T., Murphy, M. L., Pearce, M. B.: Intracardiac needle biopsy of the ventricular septum. Am. J. Cardiol. 16:227, 1965.
150. Hirose, T., and Bailey, C. P.: New myocardial biopsy needle. Angiology 16: 288, 1965.
151. Sakakibara, S., and Konno, S.: Endomyocardial biopsy. Jap. Heart J. 3:537, 1962.
152. Caves, P., Billingham, M. B., Coltart, J., Rider, A., and Stinson, E.: Transvenous endomyocardial biopsy—application of a method for diagnosing heart disease. Postgrad. Med. J. 51:286, 1975.
153. Hess, O. M., Schneider, J., Turina, M., Heeb, S., Grob, P., and Krayenbuehl, K. P.: Die transvenose Endomyokardbiopsie in der Bewiteilung der kongestivan Kardiomyopathie. Schweiz. Med. Wschr. 109:293, 1977.
154. Mason, J. W.: Technique for right and left ventricular endomyocardial biopsy. Am. J. Cardiol. 41:887, 1978.
155. Olsen, E. G. J.: Results of endomyocardial biopsy—histological, histochemical and ultrastructural analysis. Postgrad Med. J. 51:295, 1975.
156. Peters, T. J., Brooksby, I. A. B., Webb-Peploe, M. M., Wells, G., Jenkins, B. S., and Coltart, D. J.: Enzymic analysis of cardiac biopsy material from patients with valvular heart disease. Lancet 1:269, 1976.
157. Kawai, C., and Kitaura, Y.: New endomyocardial biopsy catheter for the left ventricle. Am J. Cardiol. 40:63, 1977.
158. Colucci, W. S., Lorell, B. H., Schoen, F. J., Warhol, M. J., and Grossman, W.: Hypertrophic obstruction due to Fabry's disease, N. Engl. J. Med. 307:926, 1982.
159. Bristow, M. R., Mason, J. W., Billingham, M. E., and Daniels, J. R.: Doxorubicin cardiomyopathy: Evaluation by phonocardiography, endomyocardial biopsy, and cardiac catherization. Ann. Intern. Med. 88: 168, 1978
160. Nippoldt, T. B., Edwards, W. D., Holmes, D. R., Relder, G. S., Hartzler, G. O., and Smith, H. C.: Right ventricular endomyocardial biopsy. Clinicopathologic correlates in 100 consecutive patients. Mayo Clin. Proc. 57: 407, 1982.
161. Mason, J. W., Billingham, M. E., and Ricci, D. R.: Treatment of acute inflammatory myocarditis assisted by endomyocardial biopsy. Am. J. Cardiol. 45: 1037, 1980.
162. Grüntzig, A. R., Jenning, A., and Siegenthaler, W. E.: Non-operative dilation of coronary artery stenosis. N. Eng. J. Med. 301:61, 1979.
163. Grüntzig, A.: Transluminal dilatation of coronary artery stenosis. Lancet 1:263, 1978.
164. Grüntzig, A.: Perkutane Dilatation von Koronarstenosen—Beschreibung eines neuen Kathetersystems. Klin. Wschr. 54:543, 1976.
165. Grüntzig, A., Schneider, H. J.: Die perkutane dilatation chronischer Koronarstenosen—Experiment und Morphologie. Schweiz. Med. Wschr. 107: 1588, 1977.
166. Grüntzig, A., Myler, R. K., Hamma, E. S., and Turina, M. I.: Coronary transluminal angioplasty. Circulation 56 (Suppl. 11):316, 1977.
167. Grüntzig, A., and Hepff, H.: Perkuntane Rekanalization chronischer arterieller Verschlusse mitg einen neuen Dilatationkatheter. Deutsch. Med. Wschr. 99: 2502, 1974.
168. Simpson, J. B., Baim, D. S. Robert, E. W., and Harrison, D. C.: A new catheter system for coronary angioplasty. Am. J. Cardiol. 49:1216, 1982.
169. Kent, K. M., et al.: Percutaneous transluminal coronary angioplasty: Report from the Registry of the National Heart, Lung, and Blood Institute. Am. J. Cardiol. 49: 2011, 1982.
170. Williams, D. O., Riley, R. S., Singh, A. K., Gervertz, H., and Most, A. H.: Evaluation of the role of coronary angioplasty in patients with unstable angina pecrotis. Am. Heart J. 102:1, 1981.
171. Crowley, M. J., Vetorovee, G. W., and Wolfgang, T. C.: Efficacy of percutaneous transluminal coronary angioplasty: Technique, patient selection, laboratory results, limitations, and complications. Am. Heart J. 101:272, 1981.
172. Rentrop, P., Blanke, H., Karsch, K. R., Daiser, H. Kostering, H, and Leitz, K.: Selective intracoronary thrombolysis in acute myocardial infarction and unstable angina pectoris. Circulation 63:307, 1981.
173. Ganz, W., Buchburder, N., Marcus, H., Mondkar, A., Maddahi, J., Charuzi, Y., O'Connor, L., Shell, W., Fishbein, M., Kass, R., Miyamoto, A., and Swan, H. J. C.: Intracoronary thrombolysis in evolving myocardial infarction. Am. Heart J. 101:4, 1981.
174. Mathey, D. G., Kuch, K. H., Tilsner, V., Krebber, H. J., and Bleifeld, W.: Nonsurgical coronary artery recanalization in acute transmural myocardial infarction. Circulation 63:489–497, 1981.
175. Markis, J. E., Malagold, M., Parker, J. A., Silverman, K. J., Barry, W. H., Als, A. V., Paulin, S., Grossman, W., and Braunwald, E.: Myocardial salvage after intracoronary thrombolysis with streptokinase in acute myocardial infarction. N. Engl. J. Med. 305:777, 1981.
176. Reduto, L. A., Smalling, R. W., Freund, G. C., and Gould, K. L.: Intracoronary infusion of streptokinase in patients with acute myocardial infarction: Effects of reperfusion on left ventricular performance. Am. J. Cardiol. 48:403, 1981.
177. Rentrop, P., Blouke, H., and Karsch, K. R.: Effects of non-surgical coronary reperfusion on the left ventricle in human subjects compared with conventional treatment. Am. J. Cardiol. 49:1, 1982.
178. Levine, F. H., Gold, H. K., Leinbach, R. G., Daggett, W. M., Austen, W. G., and Buckley, M. J.: Management of actute myocardial ischemia with intra-aortic balloon pumping and coronary bypass surgery. Circulation 58:1, 1978.
179. Pace, P. D., Tilney, N. L., Lesch, M., and Couch, N. P.: Peripheral arterial complications of intra-aortic balloon counterpulsation. Surgery 88:685, 1977.
180. Vignola, P. A., Swaye, P. S., Gosselin, A. F.: Guidelines for effective and safe intraaortic balloon pump insertion and removal. Am. J. Cardiol. 48:660, 1981.
181. Leinbach, R. C., Goldstein, J., Gold, H. K., Moses, J. W., Collins, M. B., and Subramanian, V.: Percutaneous wire-guided balloon pumping. Am. J. Cardiol. 49:1707, 1982.
182. Harvey, J. C., Goldstein, J. E., McCabe, J. C., Hoover, E. L., Gay, W. A., Jr., and Subramanian, V. A.: Complications of percutaneous intraaortic balloon pumping. Circulation 64 (Suppl. 11), 114, 1981.
183. Bregman, D., Nichols, A. B., Weiss, M. B., Powers, E. R., Martin, E. C., and Casarella, W. J.: Percutaneous intraaortic balloon insertion. Am. J. Cardiol. 46:261, 1980.
184. Rashkind, W. J., and Miller, W. W.: Creation of an atrial septal defect without thoracotomy: A pallative approach to complete transposition of the great vessels. J.A.M.A. 196:991, 1966.
185. Rashkind, W. J., and Miller, W. W.: Transposition of the great arteries: Results of palliation by balloon atrial septostomy in 31 patients. Circulation 38:453, 1968.
185a.Rashkind, W. J.: Transcathetler treatment of congenital heart disease, Circulation 67:711, 1983.
186. Portsmann, W., Wierny, L., and Warnke, H.: Der Verschluss des Ductus Arteriosus Persistens ohne Thorakotomie. Fortschr. Roentgenstr. 109:133, 1968.
187. Portsmann, W., Wierny, L., Warnke, H., Gertsberger, G., and Romaniuk, P. A.: Catheter closure of patent ductus arteriosus: 62 cases treated without thoracotomy. Radiol. Clin. North Am. 9:203, 1971.
188. Sato, K., Fiyino, M., Kozuka, T., Naito, Y., Kitamura, S., Nakano, S., Ohyama, C., and Kawashima, Y.: Transfemoral plug closure of patent ductus arteriosus: Experience in 61 consecutive cases treated without thoracotomy. Circulation 51:337, 1975.
189. Mills, N. L., and King, T. D.: Nonoperative closure of left to right shunts. J. Thorac. Cardiovasc. Surg. 72:371, 1976.
190. King, T. D., Thompson, S. L., Steiner, C., and Mills, N. L.: Secundum atrial septal defect. Nonoperative closure during cardiac catheterization. J.A.M.A. 235:2506, 1976.
191. Scoggins, W. G., and Greenfield, L. J.: Transvenous pulmonary embolectomy for acute massive pulmonary embolism. Chest 71:213, 1977.
192. Greenfield, L. J., Reif, M., and Guenter, C. A.: Hemodynamic and respiratory response to transvenous pulmonary embolectomy. J. Thorac. Cardiovasc. Surg. 62:890, 1971.
193. Taylor, B. G., Cockerill, E. M., Manfredi, F., and Klatte, E.: Therapeutic embolization of the pulmonary artery in pulmonary arterio-venous fistula. Ann. J. Med. 64:360, 1978.
194. Massumi, R. A., and Ross, A. M.: Atraumatic non-surgical techniques for removal of broken catheters from cardiac cavities. N. Engl. J. Med. 277:195, 1967.
195. Bloomfield, A.: Techniques of non-surgical retrieval of iatrogenic foreign bodies from the heart. Ann. J. Cardiol. 27:538, 1971.

10

CORONARY ARTERIOGRAPHY

by Goffredo G. Gensini, M.D.

Radner was the first to outline the coronary arteries in living man in 1945.[1] The earliest studies consisted of incidental opacifications of the coronary arteries at the time of retrograde aortography. Later, methods that would permit intentional, satisfactory visualization of the human coronary arteries were tested by many investigators. These methods included random injections, acetylcholine arrest, intrabronchial pressure elevation, occlusion aortography, and differential opacification of the aortic stream. These methods are of historical interest only. Extensive bibliographic references may be found in an earlier work on this subject.[2]

In May, 1959, Sones reported a straightforward approach to achieve opacification of the coronary arteries, i.e., the deliberate, selective catheterization of each vessel with a special catheter, designed by Sones himself.[3,4] He demonstrated that the human coronary arteries can be individually and selectively catheterized with safety, in both health and disease, provided that appropriate instrumentation and methods are used. In this light, all current methods of coronary arteriography may be considered as more or less successful modifications of Sones' original idea. Entire "families" of preshaped catheters have been developed by numerous investigators.[5-9] Generally speaking, these preshaped catheters make possible quick entry into the coronary arteries. In expert hands, both the Judkins' femoral approach[4] and Sones' brachial cutdown method have been shown to provide a high degree of safety and reliability.

TECHNIQUE

REQUISITES FOR SUCCESS. The requisites for successful catheterization of the coronary arteries are few: a properly designed catheter, a first-class imaging system, and an expert hand. A flawless cine camera and good filming techniques are necessary to insure appropriate recording of coronary opacifications. For the safety of the patient, a relatively nontoxic contrast agent, continuous electrocardiographic monitoring, frequent pressure monitoring, and a DC-defibrillator are necessary.

The ingredients for maintenance of efficiency in a cardiovascular laboratory are the quality, experience, and dedication of the personnel. In the author's opinion, selective coronary arteriography should be performed full time by physicians with a solid background in *cardiology*. No amount of elaborate radiological and electronic apparatus can take the place of the trained and experienced operator. On the other hand, in cine coronary arteriography, the appropriate selection and flawless performance of the equipment rank closely in importance to the skill and knowledge of the physician and technical personnel using the equipment.[2]

PATIENT TEACHING AND PREPARATION. The instruction and psychological preparation of the patient scheduled to undergo coronary arteriography should begin as soon as he or she arrives in the hospital. Physicians and nursing personnel caring for patients undergoing cardiovascular diagnostic procedures should be familiar with these tests and should be able to answer intelligently any of the patients' questions. Patients need to feel that the staff is competent and efficient. It is the duty of the cardiovascular team and of all personnel caring for these patients to gain their confidence and dispel doubts and unnecessary fears. The relative benefits and risks of coronary arteriography and what will be expected of the patient and what the patient should expect must be explained beforehand.

In certain x-ray projections, the diaphragm covers the distal portion of the coronary vessels and obscures some important areas of perfusion. During the procedure, therefore, the operator occasionally asks the patient to take a deep breath, hold it, and at the same time avoid bearing down, which would produce a Valsalva effect and elevate the diaphragm.

If signs of bradycardia appear following injection of contrast material into a coronary artery, the patient is instructed to cough. The patient should be told that a strong, immediate cough is expected in response to this directive. Bradycardia is an expected phenomenon in this setting, but if prolonged, it may be followed by extrasystoles and, eventually, ventricular fibrillation. As soon as the operator observes that a patient's heart rate is slowing, the catheter tip should be withdrawn from the coronary ostium, and the patient should be told to cough. Coughing clears the contrast agent from the vessel and acts as a mechanical stimulus to the heart. The instruction to cough should be given only by the physician manipulating the catheter.

I believe that it is desirable for patients to express their feelings about coming to the hospital and the performance of these tests. We encourage them to ask questions, even during the examination. One thing is certain: Patients who are relaxed and confident require less medication and are less likely to experience complications, such as peripheral arterial spasm and nausea, during coronary arteriography.

PREPARATION OF THE PATIENT

Although hospitalization is required for patients whose condition is unstable, and although in many laboratories hospitalization is required for all patients who undergo coronary arteriography, it is the author's practice to carry out coronary arteriography on an outpatient basis in elective, ambulatory cases. We admit such patients to the laboratory on the morning of the examination and discharge them several hours after the procedure, if their condition is stable. In our opinion, the clinical status of the patient and the suspected underlying pathology, rather than the arteriography itself, should dictate the mode of admission and the length of stay in the hospital, that is, which patient should be admitted as an inpatient before the procedure or, having come as an outpatient, should remain in the hospital after the procedure.

The author's facility for outpatient catheterization includes a large room immediately adjacent to the cardiac laboratory. This room is staffed by a nurse and it is furnished with five comfortable Barcaloungers. Privacy, when needed, is achieved using ceiling-mounted curtains that can effectively screen one easy chair from the others. A bed is also provided as a temporary alternative to the easy chair. Upon arrival in the outpatient facility, or upon admission to the hospital, the patient is visited by two members of the cardiovascular laboratory team and given a complete explanation of the procedure before being asked to sign a consent form. The possible risks of coronary arteriography are explained in simple, readily understandable terms. All of this information is also summarized in a booklet that is given to the patient and to his family at the time the appointment for the procedure is arranged.

For a patient with a history of valvular heart disease, ampicillin is ordered or, if he or she is allergic to penicillin, erythromycin. The patient should receive no solid food after midnight on the day of the examination but is encouraged to drink juices and water up to one hour prior to the procedure. One hour before the procedure, an electrocardiogram is recorded. Secobarbital, 100 mg, and diazepam (Valium), 5 mg, are given orally unless congestive heart failure is present, in which case secobarbital is omitted. If a patient takes digitalis daily, he or she should be given this medication before going to the laboratory. We recommend that patients who have been receiving propranolol be instructed to taper the dosage at least three days before any left-heart studies. High doses of propranolol depress myocardial contractility and produce hemodynamic changes that may result in increased left ventricular end-diastolic pressure and decreased ejection fraction.

Before each procedure, cardiovascular technicians specially trained to assist the physician during cardiac catheterization procedures prepare the necessary sterile instruments and pressure gauges. A pressurized drip containing 5000 units of heparin in 500 ml of 5 per cent dextrose and water rather than continuous pressure monitoring is used intraarterially to maintain catheter patency throughout the procedure. (Many laboratories utilize continuous pressure monitoring using a three-stopcock manifold.) Having prepared the pressurized drip, the technicians should make certain that the DC-defibrillator, located in the procedure room, is turned on and available, with paddles already spread with conductive paste for immediate use if necessary.

Upon arrival in the laboratory, the patient reclines on the Cardiodiagnost* unit. Monitoring type electrocardiographic leads† are applied. The technician places surgical drapes on the patient, and the operator performs a cut-down on the right brachial artery under local anesthesia. We never administer general anesthesia, since it adds to the risk, nor do we use prophylactic cardiac pacing or atropine unless they are indicated for reasons independent of the coronary arteriogram and left heart studies. The use of any drug not medically indicated for the treatment of preexisting conditions (except mild sedatives) should be discouraged prior to coronary arteriography. Bradycardia associated with the injection of a contrast agent into a coronary artery is promptly treated by having the patient cough at the appropriate time. In the several thousand procedures we have performed using the Sones' technique, atropine was never used prior to coronary arteriography (unless medically indicated for reasons other than the arteriography), nor was it ever needed during the procedure. Furthermore, published reports[10-12] indicate that atropine may actually be harmful in eurhythmic patients with severe ischemic heart disease in normal sinus rhythm.

THE TRANSBRACHIAL APPROACH (SONES' METHOD)[2-4]

The vessel is isolated by blunt dissection (Fig. 10–1A), and a 1-mm vertical incision is made in the vessel with the tip of a No. 11 blade (Fig. 10–1B). Bleeding is controlled proximally and distally with umbilical tapes or silicone loops. The Sones catheter, 7, 7½, or 8 French, 80 cm long, is introduced into the distal segment of the brachial artery, and 3 ml of saline solution containing 2500 units of heparin (Panheparin, 5000 units/ml) is injected to prevent clotting from distal arterial stasis during the procedure. The catheter is withdrawn, reintroduced proximally in the same incision (Fig. 10–1C), and advanced under fluoroscopic visualization until the tip is at the level of the left ventricle. Baseline pressure measurements, which include left ventricular pressure and dp/dt, are then recorded. While pressures are still being recorded, the catheter is withdrawn from the left ventricle to the ascending aorta to determine if a pressure gradient is present within the left ventricle or between the left ventricle and the aorta.

The Sones catheter is then replaced by a Lehman or Eppendorf thin-walled ventriculography catheter,** 7 or 8 French, 100 cm long, with the tip directed into the left ventricle. An automatic injector delivers 35 ml of contrast material, an agent containing diatrizoate

---

*Cordis Corporation, Box 370428, Miami, Florida 33137.

†Red Dot monitoring electrodes, 3M Center, Medical Product Division, St. Paul, Minnesota 55101.

**United States Catheter and Instrument Co., a division of C.R. Bard, Inc., Billerica, Massachusetts 01821.

meglumine, 66 per cent, and diatrizoate sodium, 10 per cent (Renografin-76), into the left ventricle. A 35-mm cine camera records the diastolic and systolic phases of the ventricular cycles at a rate of 40 frames each second. Routinely, we take this cine left ventriculogram in the right anterior oblique (RAO) projection. In almost all cases and particularly whenever the presence of a lesion of the interventricular septum is suspected, an additional left ventricular injection is performed and recorded with 30 degrees cranial angulation in a 60-degree left anterior oblique projection.[13]

Whenever contraction abnormalities,[14,15] elevation of left ventricular end-diastolic pressure,[16] or enlargement of the left ventricle is detected, nitroglycerin is injected into the left ventricle in doses of 0.6 mg in 1.5 ml of distilled water. The left ventriculogram is then repeated as soon as the left ventricular end-diastolic pressure has reached its lowest value or 3 minutes later, whichever occurs first.

The ventriculography catheter is then removed, the Sones catheter is reintroduced, and both the right and left coronary arteries are catheterized in both the left anterior oblique and right anterior oblique views. We also routinely take cranial angulation of the left and right coronary artery in anterior oblique views and caudal angulation of the left coronary artery in left anterior oblique views.

The catheter is then removed, and forceful bleeding is allowed to occur for a second or two. The tip of the catheter is reinserted into the distal segment of the brachial artery, and aspiration with a syringe is undertaken until a forceful arterial backflow is obtained. A second dose of 2500 units of heparin is injected into the distal arterial segment, the catheter is removed, and the artery is closed with a 6-0 Polydek* Lock-stitch suture (Fig. 10–1D).

---
*Deknatel, Queens Village, New York.

An inexpensive but highly effective and practical tool that is most helpful for suturing of the vessel is a pair of magnifying goggles.* The skin is sutured with 3-0 silk. A sterile pressure dressing is applied to the .wound, and the patient is returned to his or her room. The average laboratory stay per patient is 45 minutes; often, especially in young patients without tortuous brachiocephalic vessels, a procedure may be completed in 30 minutes.

THE PERCUTANEOUS FEMORAL APPROACH (JUDKINS' METHOD)[6]

The percutaneous insertion of a catheter into a peripheral artery was first described by Seldinger in 1953,[26] and this procedure was extensively utilized in Europe in the 1950's. Dotter and Gensini reported on percutaneous transfemoral retrograde catheterization of the left ventricle and systemic arteries of man in 1960; in closing they stated, "In providing a means for direct catheterization of the coronary orifice, it . . . makes possible detailed coronary artery visualization in vivo."[27]

The percutaneous transfemoral approach to coronary arteriography became truly practical when Judkins designed a series of special catheters** made of polyurethane, preformed into curves suitable for the right or left coronary arteries, thereby achieving a "coronary artery–seeking" tip configuration. Each catheter, 100 cm in length, is

---
*optiVISOR DA-5 (3+), Bowen and Company, Inc., Rockville, Maryland 30852.
**Cordis Corporation, Box 370428, Miami, Florida.

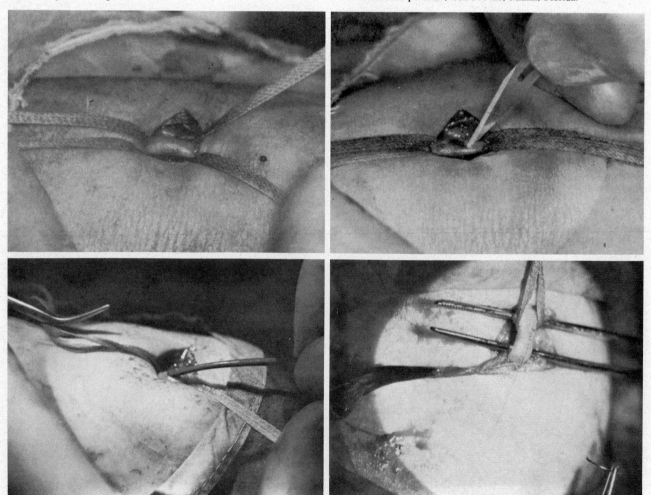

FIGURE 10–1   *A,* The brachial artery has been isolated, and bleeding is controlled by pulling on proximal and distal umbilical tapes. *B,* A 1-mm incision is made with a No. 11 blade. *C,* A Sones catheter is introduced into the proximal segment of the artery. *D,* Sutured brachial artery. (From Gensini, G. G.: Coronary Arteriography. Mount Kisco, N.Y., Futura Publishing Co., 1975.)

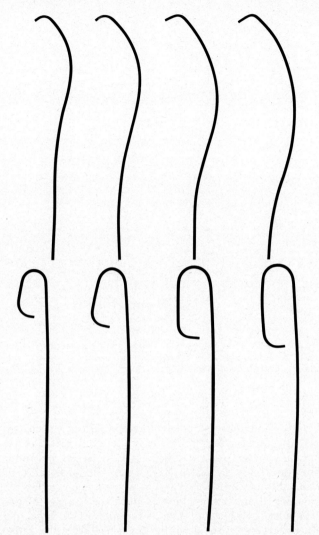

FIGURE 10–2 Judkins' catheters. *Top,* **Right coronary tip curves.** *Bottom,* **Left coronary tip curves. (Courtesy of Cordis Corporation, Miami, Florida.)**

phy catheter is withdrawn and the left coronary catheter is then introduced. If one observes the protruding wire and/or the catheter entering one of the branches of the aortic arch, the catheter should be drawn back and the guide drawn back into the catheter. The natural curvature present on the catheter can then be used to direct it over the arch and into the ascending aorta. Once in the ascending aorta, the guide is withdrawn and the catheter is advanced while its concavity follows that of the aortic arch (Fig. 10–3A). The left-sided catheter naturally seeks the left coronary artery and, therefore, the arteriographer should be very careful in identifying the entrance of the catheter into the left coronary ostium the moment that this takes place. Prior to injecting the contrast agent, the angiographer should be certain that the catheter is not wedged into the left main coronary artery; this can be accomplished by a small test injection of contrast or by monitoring the pressure recorded from the tip of the catheter.

After completion of the visualization of the left coronary artery in multiple views, the left coronary catheter is withdrawn, and the right coronary artery catheter is inserted over the same wire. This catheter is usually manipulated with ease into the ascending aorta by drawing the guidewire back from the tip and advancing the catheter with the angled tip pointed to the inner aspect of the curve of the aortic arch. Once in the root of the aorta, the catheter is rotated so that the tip projects forward and slightly to the right of the patient (Fig. 10–3B). This is best accomplished by viewing the patient in the left anterior oblique projection. In this view, one can usually detect whether or not the catheter is approaching the right coronary artery. After the right coronary artery has been successfully visualized, the catheter is withdrawn, and pressure is applied over the inguinal area until adequate hemostasis is achieved. Usually the patient is released from the laboratory with a pressure bandage in place.

After coronary arteriography, the nurse checks the dressing for bleeding and records the patient's blood pressure and right radial pulse rate every 15 minutes for two hours. The pressure bandage is removed 30 minutes after the patient's return to the room, and the wound is re-dressed. The patient rests in bed for two hours and resumes the usual diet.

Later on the same day, the patient is visited by the physician who performed the examination, is told about the results of the procedure, and is advised on the further management of his or her problems.

now available in sizes 7 or 8 French, with four sizes of the terminal curve. They should be inserted using Teflon-coated guidewires. A catheter introducer may also be utilized in order to avoid damage or kinking of the catheter during its first pass into the artery. The four sizes of the terminal curve are designed to suit different aortic diameters. The appropriate size should be selected according to an assessment made prior to catheterization, based on patient size and the appearance of the aorta on a plain chest x-ray (Fig. 10–2).

From a procedural point of view, the technique of transfemoral coronary arteriography and left ventriculography is simple: The appropriate site of puncture overlying the femoral artery is identified and a small stab wound is made with a No. 11 blade; the opening is enlarged in the direction of the artery with straight, fine forceps. A left ventriculography catheter, either a Gensini*[28] or a pigtail,† is usually introduced first in order to measure the aortic and left ventricular pressures and to perform left ventriculography. With all types of catheters, the soft pliable end of the spring guidewire should protrude for at least an inch to find its way along the aorta and minimize the possibility of vascular trauma. Many investigators use a safety-tip J-shaped wire, so that the possibility of vascular trauma will be further diminished. After left ventriculography is performed, the ventriculogra-

---

*United States Catheter and Instrument Co., a division of C. R. Bard, Inc., Billerica, Massachusetts 01821.

†Cordis Corporation, Box 370428, Miami, Florida 33137.

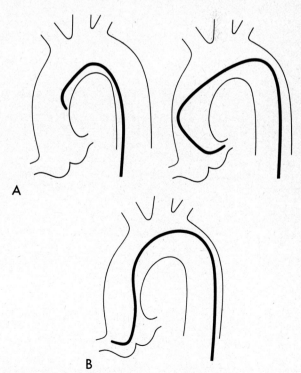

A

B

FIGURE 10–3 Judkins' technique of entering the left coronary artery (A) and the right coronary artery (B).

MULTIPLE VIEWS

One of the major problems in interpreting coronary arteriograms has been the considerable overlap and foreshortening of the main left coronary artery, of the proximal branches of the left anterior descending artery, and of the branches of the right coronary artery at the crux. Occasionally, despite the many projections obtained utilizing conventional angulation of the x-ray beam (i.e., perpendicular to the long axis of the patient), doubts may linger as to the integrity of these segments. Consequently, several authors, beginning with Bunnell, Greene, and others in 1973,[17] have described additional views in multiple obliquity, utilizing cranial and caudal angulation of the x-ray beam.[13,17–22,43,47–51]

Throughout this chapter we shall use the terminology proposed by Paulin and illustrated in Figures 10–4 through 10–7.

The most important problem areas are the main left coronary artery and its proximal branches, notably the bifurcation; the initial course of the left anterior descending and circumflex arteries; and the bifurcation between the left anterior descending and its major diagonal branch. In general, whenever there is a reason to question the integrity of these areas, the right anterior oblique projection with caudal angulation is employed. When heart size is normal or almost so, the left anterior oblique with cranial angulation is employed as well; in the presence of cardiomegaly the left anterior oblique projection with caudal angulation is employed.

Cranial angulation is possible with the simple technique of elevating the chest (utilizing a radiolucent wedge) and

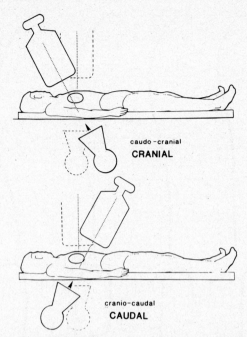

FIGURE 10–5 Terminology for radiographic projections. (From Paulin, S.: Terminology for radiographic projections in cardiac angiography. Cathet. Cardiovasc. Diagn. *7*:341, 1981, with permission.)

rotating the patient to achieve the desired degree of obliquity. In practice, this technique is extremely cumbersome, especially when using a cradle and the Sones technique. However, these problems have been alleviated with the availability of various types of x-ray equipment capable of longitudinal angulation, such as the U or C arm, the parallelogram, or elevation of the x-ray table. This angulation is achieved by either elevating the table (Spectrum table), angling the table and the U arm (Cardiodiagnost*), or angling the x-ray tube and image intensifier (parallelogram, LAD† system).

Like many other technical or procedural refinements, these special views may, at times, be most valuable; however, caution is advised against their overutilization, which could lead to unwarranted prolongation of the study and, consequently, to greater risk for the patient.

COMPLICATIONS

Coronary arteriography is routinely performed in approximately 1000 laboratories of this nation. A report from the National Center for Health Care Technology[29] suggests that nearly 300,000 coronary arteriograms were performed in 1980. In the state of New York alone over 25,000 coronary arteriograms were performed in 1981.[30]

Any diagnostic intervention that is potentially hazardous must be reserved for patients in whom the benefits derived from the procedure outweigh the risks. If the incidence and severity of complications vary from one in-

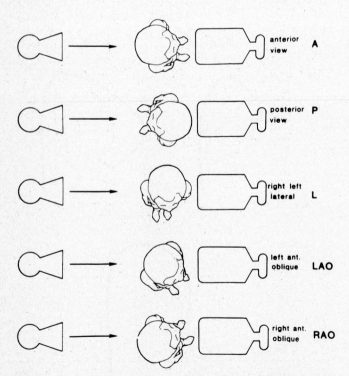

anterior view **A**

posterior view **P**

right left lateral **L**

left ant. oblique **LAO**

right ant. oblique **RAO**

FIGURE 10–4 Terminology for radiographic projections. (From Paulin, S.: Terminology for radiographic projections in cardiac angiography. Cathet. Cardiovasc. Diagn. *7*:341, 1981, with permission.)

---

*North American Philips, United X-Ray Corporation, Fall River, Massachusetts 02723.
†General Electric Medical Division, Westwood, Massachusetts 02090.

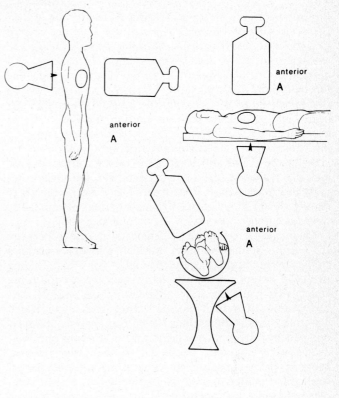

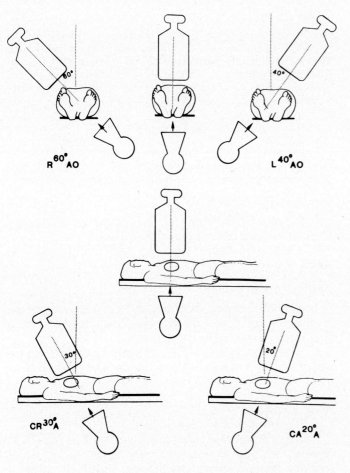

FIGURE 10–6 Terminology for radiographic projections. (From Paulin, S.: Terminology for radiographic projections in cardiac angiography. Cathet. Cardiovasc. Diagn. 7:341, 1981, with permission.)

FIGURE 10–7 Terminology for radiographic projections. (From Paulin, S.: Terminology for radiographic projections in cardiac angiography. Cathet. Cardiovasc. Diagn. 7:341, 1981, with permission.)

stitution to another, rules that may be valid in one setting may not apply in another. Earlier nationwide surveys demonstrated that this is indeed the case for coronary arteriography, i.e., that the incidence of serious complications could vary widely. In fact, reports of the mortality of coronary arteriography ranged from 0.05 to 2.37 per cent.[31,32]

The most authoritative and recent reports on mortality and complications related to cardiac catheterization and angiography are those by the Registry Committee of the Society for Cardiac Angiography.[33,34] These reports are based on 53,581 patients studied over a period of 14 months and describe significant complications in 950 patients (1.8 per cent) (Table 10–1). Catheterization-related mortality for the purpose of inclusion in the Society's reports was defined as death that (1) occurred during the procedure, (2) occurred within 24 hours after the proce-

dure and was not attributable to any non–catheterization-related cause, or (3) occurred several days after the procedure but was clearly precipitated by an event occurring during the procedure. An example of the latter is a myocardial infarction occurring during the procedure and resulting in death four days later. There were 75 deaths overall in these 53,581 patients, a mortality rate of 0.14 per cent. However, eight of these deaths occurred among the 457 patients studied under the age of one year (mortality rate in this group = 1.7 per cent). There were 24 deaths in patients between one and 60 years of age, resulting in a mortality rate of 0.07 per cent, and 43 deaths in those over 60 years of age, with a mortality rate of 0.25 per cent. Overall the mortality rate was 0.12 per cent for males and 0.18 per cent for females. Mortality was, as expected, closely related to the patient's functional class.

Patients who were in Class IV had a mortality rate of 0.67 per cent, whereas the mortality rate was 0.02 per cent in Class I and Class II patients. Mortality was also related to the extent of left ventricular dysfunction. In patients with an ejection fraction equal to or better than 50 per cent, the mortality was 0.05 per cent; for those with an ejection fraction of 30 to 49 per cent, the mortality was 0.23 per cent; and for patients with an ejection fraction < 30 per cent, mortality was 0.76 per cent. As anticipated, mortality during or following coronary arteriography was closely related to the extent and severity of coronary artery disease and was highest in the 2,452 patients with left main coronary artery disease—0.86 per cent. There was no mortality among the 11,418 patients who had normal or minimally diseased coronary arteries at the time of angiography.

There was no significant difference in mortality between the patients studied with the brachial technique and those studies by the femoral artery technique. The events leading to the 75 deaths were closely scrutinized and the following conclusions could be drawn: Three of these patients died several days after their catheterization from an unrelated cause and should be excluded from the analysis. Twenty-one patients arrived at the laboratory in extremis and their deaths were expected, irrespective of the catheterization. Most of these patients were either suffering from recent myocardial infarction and cardiogenic shock, or had complex congenital malformations. Thus there were a total of 51 unexpected deaths which were considered to be causally related to the procedure, reducing the mortality rate to 0.10 per cent. In conclusion, according to this authoritative study, catheterization-related mortality occurs mostly in patients with far-advanced cardiac disease. Nearly one third of the unexpected deaths occurred suddenly after a seemingly uneventful procedure. Many of the patients dying unexpectedly had 90 per cent or more obstruction of the left main coronary artery or 90 per cent or more obstruction of all three major vessels.

As shown on Table 10–1, the other major complications were myocardial infarction (0.7 per cent), cerebrovascular accident (0.07 per cent), arrhythmia (0.56 per cent), vascular complications (0.57 per cent), and other unspecified complications (0.41 per cent). An interesting finding concerning indications for and hazards of coronary arteriography is a higher incidence of death within the 24 hours before than within the 24 hours after the tests.[35,36] Fear seems to play a major part in causing death in some of these patients.

The author's belief in the relative safety of properly performed selective coronary arteriography therefore rests on the basis of his experience as well as that of many other institutions where mortality related to the technique is maintained at or below 0.1 per cent. The author shares the opinion expressed by Judkins and Gander[37] that in institutions where the mortality exceeds 0.1 per cent, the entire coronary arteriography program should be reevaluated, and that in those where the rate exceeds 0.3 per cent, these studies should be discontinued.

Sones precisely defined the problem and expressed the sentiment shared by many angiographers[38]:

The safe performance of consistently superior studies demands a high level of technical competence. At present, it appears that at least two years of special training are required to provide a

TABLE 10–1 MAJOR COMPLICATIONS ASSOCIATED WITH CARDIAC CATHETERIZATION AND ANGIOGRAPHY*

	NUMBER	PER CENT OF TOTAL
Death	75	0.14
MI	40	0 .07
CVA	35	0.07
Arrhythmia	287	0.56
Vascular	291	0.57
Other	222	0.41
Total	950	1.82

From Kennedy, W. J., et al.: Complications associated with cardiac catheterization and angiography. Cathet. Cardiovasc. Diagn. 8:8, 1982.

cardiologist or radiologist with enough experience to perform such studies independently. This responsibility should not be entrusted to enthusiastic but inadequately trained individuals. The risk of mortality attributable to this study in the classes of patients for whom it is indicated should be lower than one per thousand. When significantly higher rates are encountered, inept performance, poor judgment, or both, must be assumed.

INDICATIONS*

In the author's opinion,[39] when the associated mortality is below 0.1 per cent, the indications for selective cine coronary arteriography and left-heart studies are as follows:

Symptomatic Patients

1. Presence of chest pain in adults in whom a diagnosis of ischemic heart disease cannot be excluded.
2. Cardiac problems requiring open-heart surgery in adults.

Asymptomatic Patients

1. Abnormal resting ECG in persons whose occupations involve the safety of other persons (truck or bus drivers, aircraft pilots, air traffic controllers).
2. Abnormal exercise ECG, or thallium studies consistent with myocardial ischemia, in persons with one or more additional risk factors.
3. Myocardial infarction (studies should be done 4 to 8 weeks afterward).
4. Successful cardiac resuscitation.

Evolving acute myocardial infarction, cardiogenic shock, repeated episodes of ventricular fibrillation, other uncontrollable life-threatening arrhythmias, threat of extension of myocardial infarction, and uncontrollable heart failure such as occurs with septal perforation or papillary muscle rupture are, under certain circumstances, indications for emergency coronary arteriography. It should be understood, however, that these are heroic measures performed in highly specialized centers and that the higher mortality rate associated with these types of patients cannot and should not be confused with or added to the incidence of complications of elective coronary arteriography.

CONTRAINDICATIONS

Coronary arteriography and left-heart studies are usually not performed under the following circumstances:

*Editor's Note: There is considerable variability in currently accepted indications for coronary arteriography. Other discussions of this subject are found in Chapters 38 and 39.

1. If acute myocardial infarction is well established (the patient is asymptomatic) and infarction has been present for longer than 6 hours and for less than 3 weeks.

2. When coronary revascularization must be deferred or is considered to be contraindicated because of other debilitating conditions, including massive obesity.

3. A laboratory incapable of producing films of consistent diagnostic quality or with mortality greater than 3 per 1000 related to arteriography in uncomplicated patients. Such a laboratory should suspend its activity, investigate, identify, and eliminate the causes of its inadequacy.

GOALS OF CORONARY ARTERIOGRAPHY

The primary goal of coronary arteriography is the identification, localization, and assessment of obstructive lesions present within the arteries of the heart. Combined with contrast and hemodynamic studies of the left ventricle, it remains the most important method of defining the presence and severity of coronary atherosclerosis and the adequacy of myocardial function.

An important distinction must be made between arteriography employed in part or entirely for research purposes and that performed strictly for the care of patients. Techniques, methods, and protocols that may be considered acceptable and necessary in selected groups of consenting and informed volunteers for the purpose of conducting needed research studies are not the subject of this chapter, which will deal exclusively with well-established routine techniques of coronary arteriography, utilized in the daily care of patients with known or suspected coronary artery disease. Coronary arteriography is performed for the primary purpose of determining the presence (or the absence), extent, and severity of coronary artery disease and the adequacy of left ventricular function and not specifically for the purpose of determining whether or not a patient is a candidate for coronary bypass surgery.

The knowledge gained through coronary arteriography, left-heart catheterization, and left ventriculography often help in the management of the patient with known or suspected coronary artery disease, regardless of whether or not that particular patient happens to be a possible surgical candidate. To state that coronary arteriography should be performed only to decide on the possibility of coronary bypass surgery would seem to be akin to stating that an electrocardiogram should be performed only to decide whether or not a patient should be admitted to a coronary care unit.

NORMAL CORONARY ARTERY ANATOMY

Strict anatomical descriptions of the coronary arteries are available from standard textbooks of anatomy, and excellent monographs on this subject have been written by James[40] and McAlpine.[41] However, most of the descriptions contained in these works are based on views and perspectives obtained from anatomical specimens. The arteriographer, instead, uses an entirely different set of reference points and is less inclined to emphasize landmarks that are visible on the specimen but which may not be readily recognized on the radiographic image. Since our description is based on selective cine coronary arteriograms and is directed to physicians interested in interpreting them, we shall

follow, whenever possible, the point of view of the arteriographer.

DIMENSIONS OF THE CORONARY ARTERIES. Coronary arteriography accurately depicts the origin, distribution, and appearance of the coronary arteries in living intact subjects.[2] *Quantitative* coronary arteriography[23] can actually define the *exact dimensions* of the coronary arteries in living man and their changes during physiological, pharmacological, or surgical interventions. MacAlpin et al. applied this method to calculate the size of human coronary arteries in living patients without coronary artery disease.[42]

On the basis of vessel size, the left coronary artery system is almost always more important than the right coronary artery system in the blood supply to the left ventricle, even in cases classified anatomically as having "right coronary artery preponderance" (see p. 320).

(see p. 320)

Dimensions of coronary ostia[41] (mm)
Right: $3.7 \pm 1.1 \times 2.4 \pm 0.9$ (Range = 0.5 to 7.0)
Left: $4.7 \pm 1.2 \times 3.2 \pm 1.1$ (Range = 1.0 to 8.5)

THE REGION OF THE CORONARY OSTIA. In the left anterior oblique view, the major axis of the outflow tract of the left ventricle and ascending aorta tips slightly to the left of the observer. Schematically, the outflow tract of the left ventricle and aorta may be regarded as a nearly cylindrical structure with a bulge in the middle, owing to the presence of the aortic sinuses. A line drawn along the *upper* edge of this bulge marks the area of the aortic ring or the plane dividing the aortic sinus from the ascending aorta. A line drawn along the *lower* edge of this bulge divides the floor of the aortic cusps from the outflow tract of the ventricle (the aortoventricular plane).

These landmarks are easily identifiable on an aortogram, and the origin of the two coronary arteries can readily be described in relation to them. Figure 10–8 shows the opacification of the aorta, both in diastole (*A*) and in systole (*B*) in the left anterior oblique view. The plane of the aortic ring and the aortoventricular plane are identified as 1 and 2, respectively. The right sinus of Valsalva (rsv), the left sinus of Valsalva (lsv), and the posterior sinus of Valsalva (psv) are shown in Figure 10–8*A*. In Figure 10–8*B*, R, L, and P identify the semi-open right, left, and posterior cusps, respectively. The origin of the right coronary artery is seen to the left and immediately above the right sinus of Valsalva in *A*. The position of the right coronary artery ostium in relation to the described landmarks may vary. In over 90 per cent of our patients, it was located high in the right sinus of Valsalva, immediately below the level of the ring. Occasionally it was found close to the aortoventricular plane and, in a few cases (1 to 2 per cent), above the ring. The left coronary artery originates from the left sinus of Valsalva. The ostium of the left coronary artery is usually located at the level of the aortic ring, and can often be seen as a small protuberance at this level, directly coinciding with the left edge of the broken line under 1.

A *horizontal section drawn at the level of the aortic valve* shows the relationship of the tip of the catheter as it would approach this valve (Fig. 10–9*A*). In the right anterior oblique view, the noncoronary sinus of Valsalva lies to the left and below the tip of the catheter. The left sinus is above and to the right of it. The right sinus is anterior to

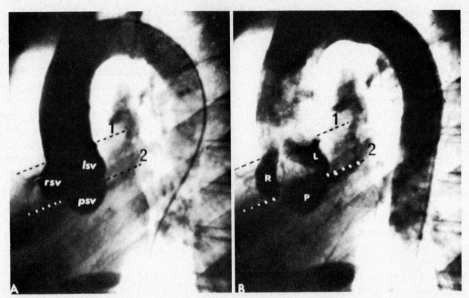

FIGURE 10–8 Left anterior oblique projections showing opacification of the aorta during diastole (*A*) and systole (*B*). See text for explanation. (From Gensini, G. G.: Coronary Arteriography. Mount Kisco, N.Y., Futura Publishing Co., 1975.)

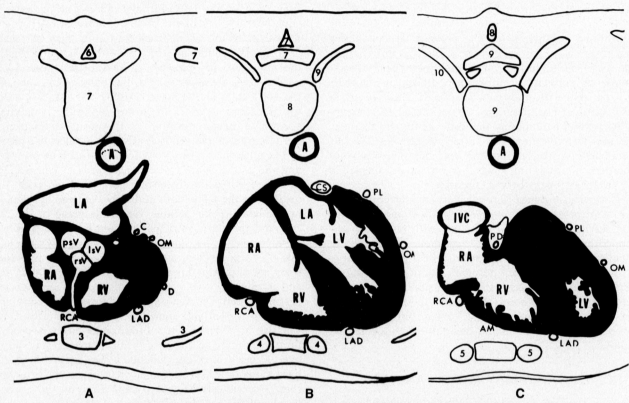

A **B** **C**

FIGURE 10–9 *A*, Horizontal body section drawn at the level of the aortic valve and seventh thoracic vertebra.
B, Horizontal body section drawn at the level of the eighth thoracic vertebra.
C, Horizontal body section drawn at the level of the ninth thoracic vertebra.
(From Gensini, G. G.: Coronary Arteriography. Mount Kisco, N.Y., Futura Publishing Co., 1975.)

(3)	Third rib or vertebra	(LA)	Left atrium	(CS)	Coronary sinus
(4)	Fourth rib or vertebra	(SC)	Scapula	(PL)	Posterolateral branch
(5)	Fifth rib or vertebra	(RA)	Right atrium	(LV)	Left ventricle
(6)	Sixth rib or vertebra	(RV)	Right ventricle	(LAD)	Left anterior descending branch
(7)	Seventh rib or vertebra	(psV)	Posterior sinus of Valsalva	(RCA)	Right coronary artery
(8)	Eighth rib or vertebra	(OM)	Obtuse marginal branch	(PD)	Posterior descending branch
(9)	Ninth rib or vertebra	(C)	Circumflex	(AM)	Acute marginal branch
(10)	Tenth rib	(lsV)	Left sinus of Valsalva	(IVC)	Inferior vena cava
(A)	Descending aorta	(D)	Diagonal branch	(rsV)	Right sinus of Valsalva

the catheter and is located at a level between the left and the posterior sinuses. The right sinus overlaps the left sinus by two thirds of its area and the posterior sinus by only one third. At this level, the right atrium is to the left of the catheter and the right ventricle is to the right and inferior to it. The left atrium is located posteriorly and to the left. The left ventricle does not yet appear at this level. The right coronary artery is directly anterior to the catheter, whereas the main left coronary artery is above, to the right, and slightly posterior to it. If the patient is positioned for the left anterior oblique projection, the right sinus of Valsalva will appear on the left and the left sinus will be on the right and at a slightly higher level. The noncoronary sinus is posterior and below the other two sinuses. The right atrium will be to the left, whereas the right ventricle will be in front of and to the left of the catheter. The left atrium is on the right and is, in this view, one of the most posterior structures. The coronary arteries will bear the same relationship to the catheter as the one described for their respective sinuses of Valsalva, i.e., the right coronary is to the left and the left coronary to the right of the catheter.

A *horizontal section drawn at the level of the eighth vertebral body* transects all four chambers of the heart (Fig. 10–9B). This section is useful to gain an appreciation of the topographical anatomy of the ventricular and atrial septa and the relationship between the major coronary branches, the ventricles, and the atria. In the right anterior oblique view, the main stem of the right coronary artery is anterior and to the left; the left anterior descending branch is anterior and to the right. The obtuse marginal branch is located posteriorly, partially overlapped by the left anterior descending branch. The posterolateral branch of the circumflex is the most posterior one and appears to be located between the right coronary artery and the left anterior descending branch. The posterior descending branch is below this section and thus does not appear at this level. The right atrium and ventricle are the most anterior structures, the atrium on the left and the ventricle on the right. The projection of the edges of the vertebral bodies appears to touch the leftmost border of the right atrium. The descending aorta, which is anterior to and to the side of the spine, is behind the body of the left atrium. The right or anterior atrioventricular groove, along which the right coronary artery runs, overlaps the base of the tricuspid valve. The interventricular and interatrial septa form a wall which, in a 30-degree right anterior oblique projection, is perpendicular to the line of sight of an outside observer looking in. Therefore, the septa are seen together as a curtain that separates the right atrium and ventricle, which are in front of it, and from the left atrium and ventricle, which are behind it. The left or posterior atrioventricular groove and the base of the mitral valve divide the left atrium from the left ventricle. The observer sees the left atrium to the left and the left ventricle to the right.

In the left anterior oblique view, both ventricles are anterior and both atria are posterior to the observer; the right cavities are seen on the left and the left cavities on the right. The major axis of the interventricular septum points directly to the observer when the patient is in a 30-degree left anterior oblique position. When using steeper degrees of obliquity, such as the 45- and 60-degree left anterior oblique views, the anterior aspect of the interven-

tricular septum is slightly to the left of the observer and the posterior aspect tips slightly to the right. The border of the heart shadow, which is to the right of the observer, is the posterolateral wall of the left ventricle. The one on the left is the right anterior atrioventricular groove. The projection of the aorta and of the spine partially overlaps the posterolateral wall of the left ventricle in both the 30- and 45-degree left anterior oblique projection but is distinct from it in the 60-degree left anterior oblique view. The obtuse marginal and posterolateral branches also overlap one another and are superimposed with the edge of the spine and the full width of the descending aorta in shallower left anterior oblique projections (30 and 45 degrees). Therefore, the 60-degree left anterior oblique projection is especially useful to separate these vessels and visualize them apart from the confusing shadows of the vertebral column.

A final *horizontal section drawn at the level of the ninth vertebral body* (Fig. 10–9C), has many points in common with the section just described. At this level, however, the left atrium is no longer present and only the apex of the left ventricle appears. A new structure that is visible here is the distal segment of the right coronary artery, which runs directly posterior to the lower segment of the anterior aspect of this artery, so that these two structures appear to be superimposed.

In order to define better the relationship of the coronary arteries to the mass of the heart and to major landmarks of the thorax, it may be useful to utilize an imaginary horizontal projection (Fig. 10–10). In this projection the thorax is transected at the level of the eighth thoracic

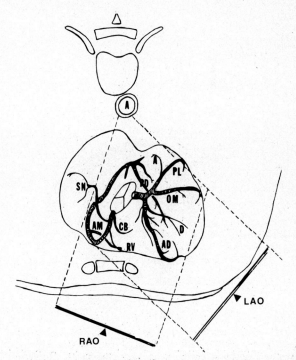

FIGURE 10–10 Horizontal projection of the heart demonstrating the relationship of the coronary arteries to the major landmarks of the thorax. The position of the input screen of the image intensifier over the chest is shown for both the left anterior oblique and the right anterior oblique projections. See text for details. Labels are as described in the legend of Figure 10–11. (From Gensini, G. G.: Coronary Arteriography. Mount Kisco, N.Y., Futura Publishing Co., 1975.)

vertebra, and the coronary arteries are visualized in their entirety, from the sinuses of Valsalva to their terminal branches, as if they were draped over a transparent heart. In this illustration, the input screen of the image intensifier is shown for a 20-degree right anterior oblique and a 45-degree left anterior oblique projection; the outlines of the heart shadow (actually its girth) are drawn as they appear at the level of the eighth vertebral body. The plane of the aortic valve, which is above this section and is steeply inclined from top to bottom, from left to right, and from front to back, appears as an ellipse, owing to its projection on the plane of the section utilized.

In the right anterior oblique projection (Fig. 10–11), the right coronary artery courses along the right atrioventricular groove, at first directed toward the input screen of the image intensifier and then away from it. The considerable foreshortening of the initial and terminal segments of the right coronary artery, which occurs in the right anterior oblique projection, can be adequately appreciated from this illustration. Conversely, these two segments of the right coronary artery are obviously well delineated in the left anterior oblique projection, which instead tends to foreshorten the posterior descending and, to a lesser extent, the right ventricular branches. When visualized in the right anterior oblique projection, the ventricular branches of the right coronary artery are generally directed toward the right border of the screen, whereas the atrial branches (of which only the sinus node branch is illustrated) are directed toward the left border of the screen.

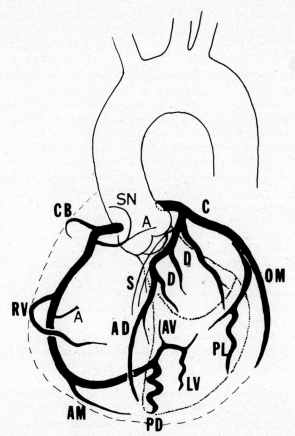

FIGURE 10–12 Diagram of right and left coronary arteries as viewed in the left anterior oblique projection. (Labels as in Figure 10–11; AV = atrioventricular node branch.) (From Gensini, G. G.: Coronary Arteriography. Mount Kisco, N.Y., Futura Publishing Co., 1975.)

The main left coronary artery is only moderately inclined in relationship to the plane of the section displayed in this view. The left anterior descending branch and atrioventricular segment of the circumflex, respectively, are directed toward both the right and left anterior oblique projections, and away from the plane of the image intensifier and are thus foreshortened in these views. In order to visualize the left anterior descending artery without foreshortening, the best view is the left lateral projection.

An overview of the entire coronary arterial system and its relationship to the left ventricle and the aorta is demonstrated in the right anterior oblique (RAO) projection in Figure 10–11 and in the left anterior oblique (LAO) projection in Figure 10–12. [The outlines of the left ventricle, the mitral valve, and the diaphragm are shown with dotted or dashed lines.] These illustrations are based on representative coronary arteriograms of healthy individuals and, *when taken as broad outlines*, represent the general appearance and distribution of coronary arteries in the majority of the human population. More as well as less common normal anatomical variations are illustrated and discussed later in the text.

Right Coronary Artery (Table 10–2)

The right coronary artery originates from the right sinus of Valsalva (usually its right half) and is best seen in the left anterior oblique view. In this view, the right coronary

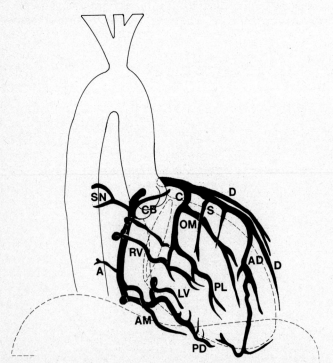

FIGURE 10–11 Diagram of right and left coronary arteries as viewed in the right anterior oblique projection. The abbreviations shown here and utilized throughout the chapter are as follows: CB = conus branch; SN = sinus node branch; RV = right ventricular branch; AM = acute marginal branch; A = atrial branch; PD = posterior descending branch; LV = left ventricular branch; C or C$_x$ = circumflex; OM = obtuse marginal branch; PL = posterolateral branch; S = septal branch; D = diagonal branch; AD or LAD = left anterior descending branch (preferably LAD). (From Gensini, G. G.: Coronary Arteriography. Mount Kisco, N.Y., Futura Publishing Co., 1975.)

TABLE 10–2 RIGHT CORONARY ARTERY—ANATOMICAL CONSIDERATIONS

Branch of Right Coronary Artery (Abbreviation)	International Anatomical Classification	Percentage of Time from RCA	Other Sites of Origin and Time Present	Area Perfused	Best Angiographic View*	Site of Origin and Route if Comes from RCA	Role in Collateral Blood Supply (Usual)
Right coronary artery (RCA)	Arteria coronaria dextra			RA and part of LA, RV, posterosuperior IV septum, SN, and AV node	L⁶⁰°AO	Right sinus of Valsalva; anteriorly and inferiorly along right AV groove	
Conus branch (CB)	Ramus coni arteriosi	60%	As separate vessel (1 mm from RCA ostium), 40%	Outflow tract, right ventricle	R³⁰°AO	Within first 2 cm; runs centrally to left of pulmonic valve	When LAD or RCA is occluded, acts as anastomotic ring of Vieussens
Sinus node (SN(R))	Ramus nodi sinoatrialis dexter	59%	C, 39%; C and RCA, 2%	Right and left atria, sinus node	R³⁰°AO	Within first 3 cm (occasionally from mid, rarely from distal portion of RCA); runs cranially, dorsally, and to right base of SVC (opposite direction of CB)	Atrial branches connect with distal portion of RCA or C
Right ventricular (RV)	Ramus ventricularis dexter anterior	100%	Additional RV branches of LAD infrequently seen in angiocardiography	Right ventricle	R³⁰°AO	Mid anterior portion of RCA; over anterior surface of right ventricle	Connects with branches of LAD; may connect with more distal RVB or AM
Atrial (A)	Ramus atrialis	100%	None	Right atrium	R³⁰°AO	Above or at level of AM directed cranially, posteriorly, and to right	May join branches from SN artery
Acute marginal (AM)	Ramus marginalis dexter	100%	None	Inferior and diaphragmatic surface of RV— occasionally posteroapical IV septum	RAO, LAO CR³⁰°R³⁰°AO CR³⁰°L⁶⁰°AO	At or about acute margin along or close to AM, toward apex	Connects with anterior or posterior descending
AV node (AVN(R))	Ramus nodi atrioventricularis	87.9%	C, 11.9%; RCA and C, 0.2%	AVN, lower portion of IA septum	CR³⁰°L⁶⁰°AO	Originates proximal to or at top of U curve at crux cordis; runs cranially and toward center of heart	May join septal branch of anterior descending
Posterior descending (PD)	Ramus interventricularis	86%	C, 14%; RCA and C, 4%	Posterior and diaphragmatic area of septum	CR³⁰°L⁶⁰°AO CR³⁰°L³⁰°AO	When present, most important terminal branch of RCA; level of crux cordis; posterior IV sulcus	Joins septal and terminal branches of anterior descending
Left ventricular branch (LVB)	Rami posterolaterales dextri (proximales)	80%	C, 20%	Diaphragmatic aspect of LV	CR³⁰°L⁷⁵°AO	Beyond crux cordis, runs centrally in angle formed by left posterior AV groove and posterior IV sulcus; if LV branches are large and numerous, PL branch of C may not be present	Joins branches of C, especially AC and PL branches
Posterolateral (PL)	Rami posterolaterales dextri (distales)	20%	C, 80%	Posterior and diaphragmatic LV wall	CR³⁰°L⁷⁵°AO	Most terminal branch of RCA, when present (See above, LVB)	(See above, LVB)

*The terminology for radiographic projections in cardiac angiography recommended by Paulin[22] has been utilized throughout this chapter. See also Refs. 13, 17–21, 43, 47–51.

Modified from Kelly, A. E., and Gensini, G. G.: Coronary arteriography and left heart studies. Heart Lung 4:85, 1975.

C = circumflex branch.

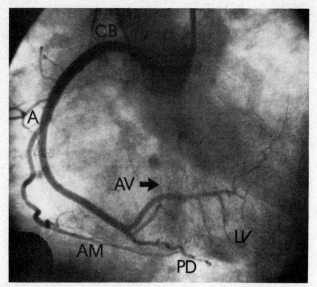

FIGURE 10–13 Right coronary artery, left anterior oblique view. (Labels as in Figure 10–11.)

and left ventricular branches. In 12 per cent of cases, the right coronary artery may not even reach the crux cordis but essentially ends with the branch to the acute margin. In the remaining 4 per cent of cases, two posterior descending branches are present, one from the right and one from the circumflex. A normal right coronary artery is usually of rather generous dimension, especially in its first and second segments. Its lumen diameter usually exceeds 2.5 mm.

From a surgical standpoint, the main stem of the right coronary artery is divided into three segments: the proximal, from the ostium to the main right ventricular branch; the mid segment, from the right ventricular branch to the acute margin; and the distal portion, from the acute margin of the heart to the origin of the posterior descending branch. The posterior descending branch (PD) is considered the fourth and final segment of the right coronary artery (Fig. 10–15).

In order of origin, the most important branches of the right coronary artery are the following: conus branch, sinus node branch, right ventricular branches, atrial branch, acute marginal branch, AV node branch, posterior descending, and left ventricular and left atrial branches.

In about 60 per cent of patients, the first branch of the right coronary artery is the *conus branch*. In the remaining 40 per cent, this branch originates as a separate vessel approximately 1 mm from the ostium of the main right coronary artery, in which case the conus artery is either not opacified or only poorly opacified by selective injection of the right coronary artery. Since its ostium is small, catheterization is usually difficult, although not impossible. Regardless of its origin, the conus branch is a fairly small vessel that curves away from the main right coronary artery and proceeds ventrally, encircling the outflow tract of the right ventricle at about the level of the pulmonic valve. In the left anterior oblique projection, the conus branch

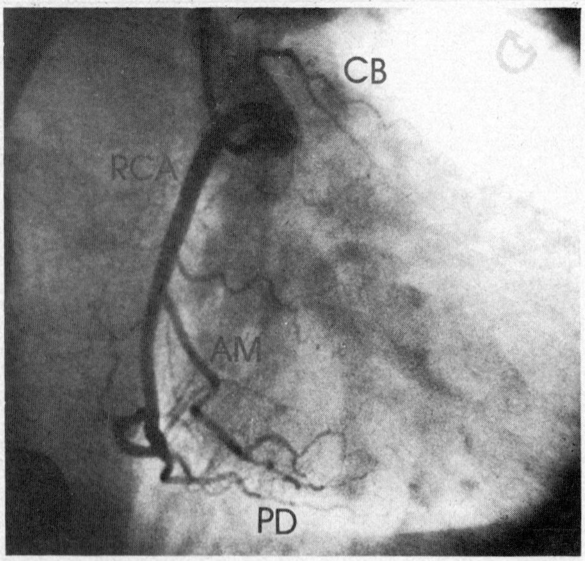

artery veers sharply to the left of the observer, is directed (at least for the first few millimeters) toward the sternum, and then curves downward, actually following the right atrioventricular groove in the general direction of the acute margin of the heart and the diaphragm (Fig. 10–13). When the right coronary artery reaches the acute margin of the heart, it curves posteriorly and follows the atrioventricular groove toward the crux cordis. In the left anterior oblique view, this change of direction is seen as a rather shallow and smooth angle, occasionally highlighted by the origin of the acute marginal branch. However, in the right anterior oblique view, this angle is more acute, and the posterior and anterior sides of this angle may be superimposed (Fig. 10–14).

In 84 per cent of cases, the right coronary artery reaches the level of the crux cordis and at that point gives rise to the posterior descending, left atrial, atrioventricular node,

FIGURE 10–14 Right coronary artery, right anterior oblique view. (Labels as in Figure 10–11.)

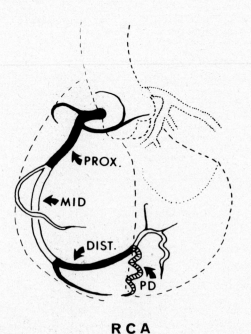

RCA

FIGURE 10–15 Principal segments of the right coronary artery. (From Gensini, G. G.: Coronary Arteriography. Mount Kisco, N.Y., Futura Publishing Co., 1975.)

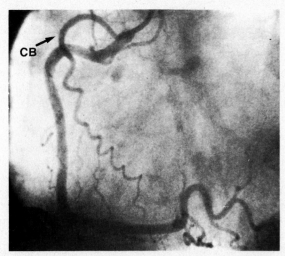

FIGURE 10–16 Right coronary artery, left anterior oblique view. CB = conus branch.

The second branch of the right coronary artery—or the first, when the conus artery is of independent origin—is also of great importance. This is the *sinus node branch*, which arises from the right coronary artery in 59 per cent of cases and from the left circumflex in 39 per cent. In a small percentage of cases (2 per cent), two sinus node branches are present, one originating from the right coronary artery and the other from the circumflex. When the sinus node artery is a branch of the right coronary artery, it usually originates from the initial portion of this vessel and runs in the opposite direction to the conus branch, i.e., cranially, dorsally, and to the right. Actually, the sinus node branch divides into two distinct rami, which are usually quite constant and have a relatively fixed configuration and distribution (Fig. 10–17). One points upward and acquires a recurrent course and is the artery that actually supplies blood to the sinus node; the other, which runs posteriorly, is essentially a left atrial branch.

In the left anterior oblique projection, the sinus node artery is directed toward the right of the frame. When the sinus node branch is viewed at the appropriate angle, these two divisions appear to form a wide Y, acquiring the shape of a ram's horns (Fig. 10–17). The horn to the left of the observer encircles the superior vena cava and runs through the sinus node, whereas the one to the right pro-

seems to continue directly past the catheter tip, toward the sternum, often making an upward swing in the general direction of the upper left corner of the film (Fig. 10–16). In most cases this vessel doubles up on itself and runs for a short segment inferiorly and to the right of the observer.

FIGURE 10–17 *Top,* right coronary artery, left anterior oblique projection. The sinus node branch (SNB) is identified. It has a small atrial branch, directed inferiorly and to the right of the observer (K). It then turns upward and divides into two major branches, the sinus node branch proper (SN), directed to the left and toward the upper edge of frame, and a left atrial branch (A), directed to the observer's right. These major divisions resemble the horns of a ram. *Bottom,* Right coronary artery, right anterior oblique projection. The conus branch (CB) and the sinus node branch (SN) are visualized.

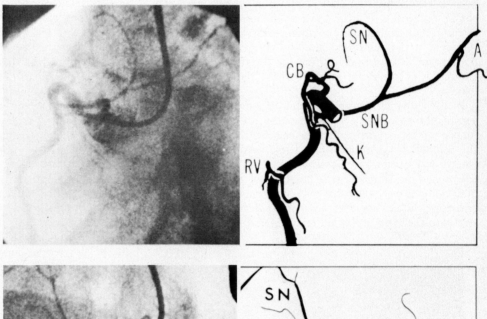

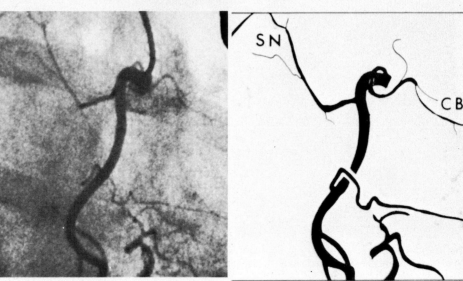

vides the blood supply to the superior and posterior walls of the left atrium. The conus branch is also shown in this figure. It can be readily appreciated that this vessel runs in the opposite direction to the sinus node artery, i.e., to the left of the observer, toward the outflow tract of the right ventricle and pulmonary artery.

The sinus node branch is well demonstrated in the right anterior oblique view and appears to be directed toward the upper left corner of the field (Figs. 10–17, *bottom*, and 10–18). The branch runs toward the ostium of the superior vena cava and encircles this vessel in a clockwise direction. As already indicated, branches to the right and left atria originate from this vessel; the importance of these fine branches becomes apparent following occlusion of the right and/or circumflex coronary arteries, since they are the sources of collateral blood supply to the circumflex or to the more distal segments of the right coronary artery.

When the sinus node branch originates from the left coronary artery, it often arises from the proximal portion of the circumflex artery (see page 327). It then ascends to the right, beneath the left atrial appendage and behind the aorta, crossing the posterior aspect of the left atrium to reach the interatrial septum. It terminates near the base of the superior vena cava in a pattern similar to the one described when this branch originates from the right coronary artery. When the sinus node artery arises from the circumflex artery, it may serve as an important route of intercoronary collateral circulation in cases of occlusion of the right or left coronary artery. Occasionally, the sinus node branch may originate from the distal segment of the circumflex or the distal segment of the right coronary artery.

In its course along the anterolateral aspect of the atrioventricular groove, the right coronary artery gives origin to one or more ventricular branches with distribution to the wall of the right ventricle. These vessels may vary in length and number. Often they reach the interventricular sulcus and anastomose with branches of the left anterior descending artery when this vessel is occluded. In the right anterior oblique view, they are seen to arise almost at right angles to the main artery (Figs. 10–11, 10–14, and 10–18).

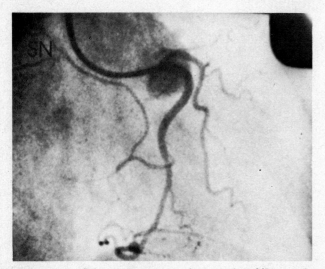

FIGURE 10–18 Right coronary artery, right anterior oblique projection. In this view the sinus node branch appears to be directed toward the upper left corner of the frame.

They appear to be directed toward the sternum in the left anterior oblique view (Fig. 10–12) but toward the apex in the right anterior oblique view. In the left anterior oblique view they are greatly foreshortened but are well displayed in the R$^{30°}$AO and CR$^{30°}$R$^{30°}$AO views. The *acute marginal branch* is a relatively large and constant vessel that arises from the right coronary artery at about the level of the lower aspect of the right atrium just before or at the acute margin of the heart (Figs. 10–11 and 10–14). The ramus is directed toward the apex. The *anterior right ventricular branches*, including the conus and acute marginal arteries, may vary from a minimum of two to a maximum of seven, but usually number from three to five.

The right atrial artery originates at about the level of the acute marginal branch but travels in the opposite direction, cranially, and toward the right heart border (i.e., toward the right of the observer in the left anterior oblique view and toward the left in right anterior oblique). This vessel often receives branches that originate from the sinus node artery and bypass obstructions located in the anterior segment of the right coronary artery.

In its posterior portion, between the acute margin and the crux cordis, the right coronary artery also gives rise to small branches to the posterior ventricular wall; these are much less important than the acute marginal or the anterior ventricular branches and are often difficult to identify. Rarely, one can see one or two branches directed to the atrial wall.

James[40] has called attention to a characteristic inverted U curve formed by the right coronary artery at the level of the interventricular sulcus as it passes beneath the posterior interventricular vein (Fig. 10–19). This curve may often be identified in cine arteriograms in the anteroposterior and left anterior oblique views, although it may also be visible in the right anterior oblique view. When the right coronary artery is viewed in the left anterior oblique projection, past the acute margin of the heart, it is apparent that this vessel continues in its gentle sweep toward that posterior area of the heart logically called the crux (i.e., the cross) of the heart, since this is where the atrial and ventricular septa meet the atrioventricular plane at a 90-degree angle. There, the right coronary artery makes a sharp, inverted U curve and terminates in several important branches: the AV node, posterior descending, left ventricular, and left atrial branches.

The *AV node branch*, characteristically a slender and very straight vessel which appears to run almost vertically in the left anterior oblique view, is directed toward the center of the heart shadow (Fig. 10–19). This vessel, like many other posterior right coronary branches, is not as readily demonstrated in the right anterior oblique view owing to the superimposition of other much larger branches such as the main stem of the right coronary artery itself or the left atrial branches. This area of the right coronary artery is a key landmark because it is easy to identify and can be utilized as a point of reference to define the relative participation of the right coronary artery to the blood supply of the posterior interventricular septum and the posterior wall of the left ventricle.

The most important branch of the right coronary artery has its origin at, or very close to, this area of the crux cordis, often proximally to the inverted U curve. This is the

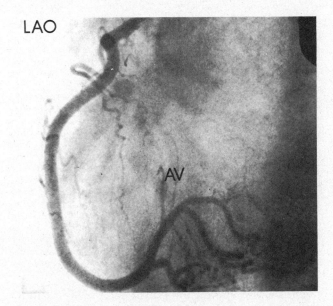

LAO

AV

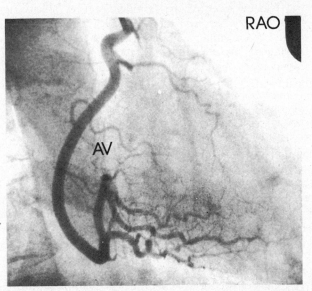

RAO

AV

FIGURE 10–19 Right coronary artery. *Top,* Left anterior oblique view. *Bottom,* Right anterior oblique view. Characteristic upside-down U-curve of distal right coronary artery with origin of AV node branch.

posterior descending branch of the right coronary artery, which, with its septal arteries, is the only source of blood supply to the posterosuperior wedge of the interventricular septum. The posterior descending branch is considerably foreshortened in the left anterior oblique view owing to the fact that its axis is directed both inferiorly and toward the observer (Fig. 10–15). The right anterior oblique view provides a better way of visualizing the posterior descending branch (Fig. 10–20). In this view, while there may be some confusion due to the superimposition of the acute marginal branches and of the more distal left ventricular branches, it can be distinguished from these other branches because several short septal branches leave the posterior descending artery at a 90-degree angle directed toward the posterosuperior portion of the interventricular septum. The best view to display the posterior descending branch for all its length and to separate it from the left ventricular and posterolateral branches (when present) is the $CR^{30°}R^{30°}AO$ view (Fig. 10–21).

A useful technique to help define that area of interventricular septum supplied by the posterior descending branch of the right coronary artery is to continue filming past the arterial phase, during the parenchymal phase of the injection. Often, that portion of the interventricular septum supplied by the posterior descending branch will stand out, in the right anterior oblique view, as a triangle with its longest side along the diaphragm, its shortest side toward the spine, and its hypotenuse located superiorly, in contact with that portion of the septum supplied by the anterior descending branch (Fig. 10–22).

In 70 per cent of cases, the posterior descending branch does not reach the apex of the heart but continues only for approximately two thirds of the posterior interventricular sulcus; the portion of the posterior interventricular septum close to the apex is supplied by the recurrent branch of the anterior descending. Occasionally, the posterior descending branch is a much shorter vessel that supplies only the extreme posterosuperior segment of the septum. In these cases, the remaining portion of the posterior interventricular septum is supplied by a similar branch of the circumflex coronary artery or, less frequently, by the terminal segment of the acute marginal branch.

Occasionally, two vessels may run in a roughly parallel fashion along the posterior interventricular sulcus. Some-

FIGURE 10–20 Right coronary artery, right anterior oblique view. The posterior descending branch can be distinguished from the other right coronary artery branches by the several short septals that leave this vessel at a 90-degree angle, directed toward the thickness of the posterosuperior wedge of the interventricular septum. (From Gensini, G. G.: Coronary Arteriography. Mount Kisco, N.Y., Futura Publishing Co., 1975.)

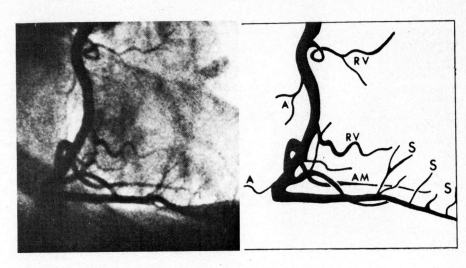

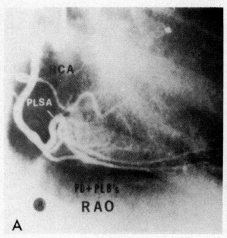

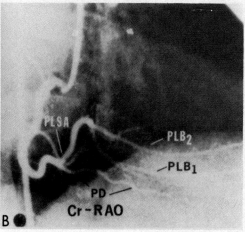

FIGURE 10–21 Selective right coronary arteriogram. *A*, Nonangled right anterior oblique (RAO) view. Note the superimposition of the posterior descending (PD) and posterolateral (PLB's) branches. *B*, Cranial–right anterior oblique (Cr-RAO) view results in a "stair-step" effect of the distal branches. There is separation of the posterior descending branch from the first and second posterolateral branches. Note the improved visualization of the posterolateral segment artery (PLSA). RCA = right coronary artery. (From Elliott, L. P., Green, C. E., Roger, W. J., Mantle, J. A., Papapietro S. E., Hood, W. P., and Russell, R. O.: Advantage of the cranial–right anterior oblique view in diagnosing mid left anterior descending and distal right coronary artery disease. Am. J. Cardiol. *48*:754, 1981.)

times one of these branches originates midway between the acute margin and the posterior interventricular sulcus. In such cases, the posterosuperior portion of the posterior interventricular septum and the AV node are supplied by the most distal posterior descending branch, whereas the posteroinferior portion is supplied by the more proximal posterior descending branch.

In a small percentage of cases (3 per cent), the main stem of the right coronary artery divides even before it reaches the acute margin, runs along the atrioventricular groove, reaches the posterior aspect of the heart, and gives origin to the posterior descending branch. The inferior ramus, on the other hand, runs diagonally along the anterior surface of the right ventricle to the acute margin in order to reach—again, with an oblique path—the posterior aspect of the right ventricle. In such cases, the more proximal ramus of the coronary artery provides the blood supply to the inferior and posterior walls of the right ventricle, whereas the branch running along the posterior atrioventricular groove gives origin to the posterior descending artery.

The most distal branch of the right coronary artery is usually a left atrial branch, which, when present, runs along the posterior-left atrioventricular groove and then curves upward from the crux cordis, superiorly, posteriorly, and away from the right coronary artery. This branch

appears to curve upward toward the spine, pointing to the upper right corner of the frame in the left anterior oblique view. The behavior of the terminal portion of the right coronary artery has been the source of a great deal of controversy and misunderstanding. Bianchi,[44] Spalteholz,[45] and Schlesinger,[46] divided the coronary circulation into "right preponderant" and "left preponderant," depending on which artery crossed the crux. When both arteries reached the crux without crossing it, the circulation was considered to be "balanced." Actually, in 84 per cent of our patients the posterior descending is a branch of the right coronary artery and in 70 per cent it runs along the posterior interventricular sulcus up to its mid portion and even farther, toward the direction of the apex. According to these anatomical definitions, the right coronary artery could therefore be considered the preponderant artery in 84 per cent of the population. In reality, as has been demonstrated by many anatomists and as is clearly visible in the majority of coronary arteriograms, the left coronary artery gives rise to the greatest number of ramifications directed toward the thickest part of the left ventricular wall, toward the largest portion of the interventricular septum, toward the largest part of the atria, and toward the smallest portion of the right ventricle. It is therefore evident that the left coronary artery is, by far, the predominant artery in man. The right coronary artery, instead, gives origin to the

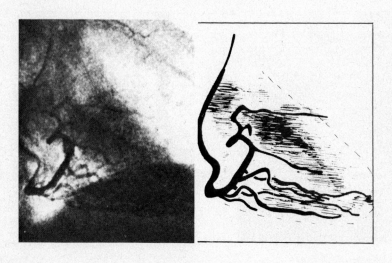

FIGURE 10–22 Definition of the area of the interventricular septum supplied by the posterior descending, obtained by filming past the arterial phase, during the parenchymal phase of the injection. That portion of the interventricular septum supplied by the posterior descending stands out, in the RAO view, as a triangle. (From Gensini, G. G.: Coronary Arteriography. Mount Kisco, N.Y., Futura Publishing Co., 1975.)

branch of the sinus node and to the branch of the AV node in approximately 60 per cent of cases and appears to be more often involved in perfusion of areas of specialized autonomic tissue.

In patients with so-called right preponderant coronary anatomy, the right coronary artery does not terminate with the posterior descending branch, even though this is its most important branch. Instead, the right coronary artery continues beyond the origin of the posterior descending branch and beyond the crux, passing along the diaphragmatic aspect of the left ventricle. In this area it gives off a variable number of posterolateral branches (sometimes referred to as posterior left ventricular branches). These branches can sometimes be quite large, even larger than the posterior descending branch itself. They supply blood to the diaphragmatic aspect of the left ventricle and can be seen best in a 45-degree left anterior oblique projection. In this view, the entire sweep of the right coronary artery resembles a sickle, the blade being formed by the main stem of the right coronary artery and the handle being formed by the posterior descending and posterior left ventricular branches (Fig. 10–13).

From a surgical standpoint, the main question that needs to be resolved is whether or not the right coronary artery gives rise to the posterior descending and, eventually, to important left ventricular branches. Whenever the right coronary artery provides such a branch or branches in patients who are being subjected to coronary artery revascularization, clinically significant obstructions or occlusions of this artery should be bypassed with a graft, placed downstream with respect to the most distal lesion. If the right coronary artery does not give rise to the posterior descending branch, any right-sided lesion is considered surgically insignificant.

Left Coronary Artery (Table 10–3)

The left coronary artery, usually the largest and shortest coronary artery, originates from the left sinus of Valsalva. The ostium of the left coronary artery is usually located at the level of the aortic ring and often can be found immediately above it (Fig. 10–8). Owing to the inclination of the aortic valvular plane over the sagittal, frontal, and horizontal planes, the position of the ostium of the left coronary artery appears to be located at a higher level than the right coronary artery orifice. Often the left coronary ostium appears as much as 1 cm higher than the right. This is true in all the common projections used in coronary arteriography. The axis of the ostium of the left coronary artery is located from 20 to 50 degrees (average = 30 to 40 degrees) posterior to the frontal plane.

Main Stem of the Left Coronary Artery. This vessel is directed anteriorly, to the left, and downward. The path of its axis in the horizontal plane varies from about 30 degrees anteriorly to 20 degrees posteriorly to the frontal plane. This means that the ostium of the left coronary artery is located posterior to the axis of this artery. This anatomical detail is a highly significant arteriographic finding, since it indicates that the catheterization of the main left coronary artery is best approached in a 30-degree right anterior oblique view, but the course of this artery is best

outlined by a far shallower view. Owing to its path in the frontal plane, it is not easily identifiable in the left oblique view over 45 degrees, since the artery is then seen almost on end and appears to be greatly foreshortened, being almost perpendicular to the plane of the image intensifier. Because of its position within the chest, the main left coronary artery would be seen best in the anteroposterior view if it were not for the occasional superimposition of the spinal column. An excellent compromise is to film the main left coronary artery in a very shallow (10-degree) right anterior oblique projection, just enough to shift the spine slightly away from this vessel. The main left coronary artery may also be reasonably well visualized in the standard 30-degree right anterior oblique view (Fig. 10–23, top) or in a shallow (40- to 45-degree) left anterior oblique view (Fig. 10–23, bottom).

Bunnell et al.[17] were the first to introduce the "tilted"[13] or angulated[47–51] views in coronary angiography, primarily

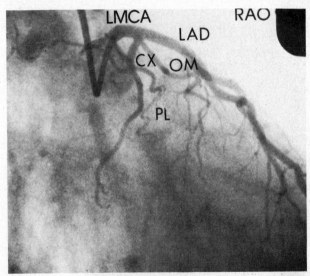

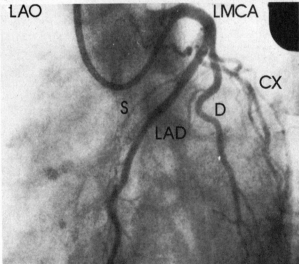

FIGURE 10–23 Left coronary artery. *Top,* Right anterior oblique view. *Bottom,* Left anterior oblique view. (Same patient as in Figures 10–13 and 10–14.) LMCA = left main coronary artery; LAD = left anterior descending artery; CX = circumflex coronary artery; OM = obtuse marginal branch; S = septal branch; D = diagonal branch; PL = posterolateral branch.

TABLE 10–3   LEFT CORONARY ARTERY—ANATOMICAL CONSIDERATIONS

Branch of Left Coronary Artery	Abbreviation	International Anatomical Classification	Number of Vessels	Percentage of Time From LCA
Left main	MLCA	Arteria coronaria sinistra	Absent if C and LAD have separate ostia	
Anterior descending (proximal and mid portion)	LAD	Ramus interventricularis anterior (pars proximalis)	1, rarely 2	98%
First diagonal	1°D	Ramus diagonalis (proximalis)	1	100%
First septal	1°S	Ramus septalis anterior (proximalis)	1	99.8%
Septals (minor)	S	Rami septales anteriores (distales)	Several	100%
Apical portion (interventricular)	IV	Ramus interventricularis anterior (pars distalis)	1	100%
Second diagonal	2°D	Ramus diagonalis (distalis)	1 or 3	100%
Circumflex	C or Cx	Ramus circumflexus	1	97%
Obtuse margin	OM	Ramus marginalis sinister	1 or 2	97%
Sinus node	SN (L)	Ramus nodi sinoatrialis sinister	0 or 1	C, 39%
Atrial circumflex	AC	Ramus atrialis sinister	1	98%
Posterolateral	PL	Rami posterolaterales sinistri	1 or 2	80%
Posterior descending	PD	Ramus inter ventricularis posterior	1	18%
AV node	AVN (L)	Ramus nodi atrioventricularis	1	11.9%

Modified from Kelly, A. E., and Gensini, G. G.: Coronary arteriography and left heart studies. Heart Lung 4:85, 1975.

OTHER SITES OF ORIGIN AND TIME PRESENT	AREA PERFUSED	BEST ANGIOGRAPHIC VIEW	SITE OF ORIGIN AND ROUTE IF COMES FROM LCA	ROLE IN COLLATERAL BLOOD SUPPLY (USUAL)
2% absent; from RCA, 0.1%	Entire LV, LA except the posterior portion of IV septum and adjacent area when PD is branch of RCA	$CR^{30}R^{20}AO$ AP $CR^{30}L^{45-60}AO$ $CA^{20}L^{60}AO$	LF sinus of Valsalva; runs behind pulmonary artery	None
Left sinus of Valsalva, separate ostium, 2%	Anterior 2/3 of IV septum, anterior portion of LV	$R^{20-30}AO$ $L^{60}AO$ $CR^{30}L^{60}AO$ $CR^{30}R^{30}$ $CA^{20}R^{30}AO$	Beneath left auricular appendage and pulmonary artery; runs along IV sulcus	Joins PD through its terminal branches
None	High lateral wall of LV	$CR^{30}L^{45-60}AO$	AD; runs in high lateral aspect of LV free wall	Joins lateral branch of C
RCA, 0.2%	Superior and anterior portion of IV septum	(lacks motion) $R^{20}AO$ $CR^{30}R^{20-30}AO$	AD, 90° angle; runs in anterior and superior half of IV septum	Joins posterior septals
None	Inferior and anterior 1/3 of septum	(lacks motion) $CR^{30}R^{20-30}AO$	AD, 90° angle; runs in anterior and inferior half of IV septum	Joins posterior septals
	Anterior aspect of apex	$CR^{30}R^{20-30}AO$ $L^{60}AO$	Continuation of AD. Route: Lower IV groove and apex	Joins posterior descending lateral branch of C
	Lower lateral aspect of LV free wall	$L^{60}AO$ $CR^{30}L^{45}AO$	Distal 2/3 of AD. Route: Diagonally along LV free wall	Joins lateral branch of C
RCA, right sinus of Valsalva, 1%; left sinus of Valsalva, separate ostium, 2%	Obtuse margin of heart and its entire posterior wall, post-IV septum when PD is branch of C, left atrium	$R^{30}AO$ $L^{60}AO$ $CA^{20}R^{30}AO$	Main LCA at level of anterior left AV sulcus beneath left auricular appendage. Route: Along left AV sulcus beneath left auricular appendage and below left pulmonary vein	Joins AD and/or RCA through its terminal branch
RCA, 3%	Obtuse margin of heart and adjacent posterior LV	$R^{30}AO$ $CA^{20}R^{30}AO$	Within first 5 cm C. Route: Laterally and posteriorly along OM of heart	May connect with D, AD, PL, PD
RCA, 59%, RCA and C, 2%	Sinus node, right and left atria	$R^{30}AO$ $L^{60}AO$	Initial C, few millimeters beyond origin. Route: Runs cranially, dorsally, to right, to base of SVC	Atrial branches connect with proximal portion of RCA
RCA, 2%	Left atrial wall	$R^{30}AO$ $L^{60}AO$	First 4 cm C runs along posterior left AV groove	Joins terminal RCA, terminal C
RCA, 20%	Posterior and diaphragmatic LV wall	$R^{30}AO$	Terminal C; posterior aspect of left AV groove. Route: Caudally and to left on post-LV	Joins with terminal branches of RCA, with lateral branch of C
RCA, 78%; RCA and C, 4%	Posterior IV septum and diaphragmatic LV	$CR^{30}R^{30}AO$ $L^{60}AO$	Terminal C; to left of crux cordis	Joins septal and terminal branch of C
RCA, 87.9%; RCA and C, 0.2%	AV node, lower portion of IA septum	$L^{60}AO$	Level of U curve at crux cordis. Route: Runs cranially and to center of heart	Joins septal branch of AD

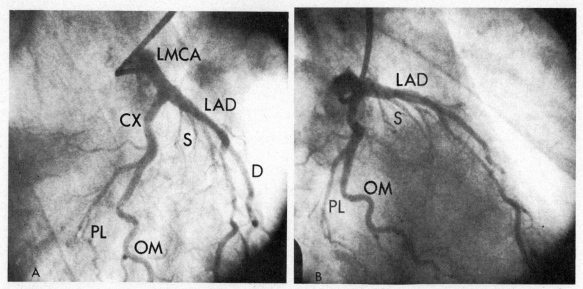

FIGURE 10–24   Left coronary artery. *A*, Hemiaxial left anterior oblique view. Excellent demonstration of main left coronary artery. *B*, Conventional left anterior oblique view. The main left coronary artery is highly foreshortened.

to improve the visualization of the proximal left coronary artery. This most important vessel is particularly well seen CR³⁰°L⁶⁰°AO and CR³⁰°R³⁰°AO (Fig. 10–24*A*). Occasionally, among patients with horizontal hearts and/or cephalad-directed proximal left coronary artery, a CA³⁰°L⁶⁰°AO may be quite useful[21,47] (Fig. 10–25*A* and *B*).

The main stem of the left coronary artery is usually the largest of the main trunks, often exceeding 4.5 mm in diameter. It is also one of the shortest among the important vessels of the body. We have observed many left coronary arteries of only 1 or 2 mm in length. Sometimes the main left coronary artery may actually be missing, with the left coronary ostium appearing like a shallow funnel with two separate openings—the left anterior descending and the circumflex. When it is short, visualization of the main left

coronary artery may be difficult and could be missed in many frames. In these cases the tip of the catheter appears to be in direct contact with the bifurcation between the left anterior descending and the circumflex branches.

The main left coronary artery divides into its two branches, the anterior descending and the circumflex, while still in the space between the aorta and pulmonary artery. Occasionally, however, its mode of termination may not be a straightforward bifurcation. Indeed, in approximately one fifth of our cases, there were more than two branches. In such patients, in the left anterior oblique view, the branch arching away from the left coronary artery and running in the direction of the crux of the heart is the circumflex branch; the one forming a wide arch and descending vertically toward the apex is the anterior de-

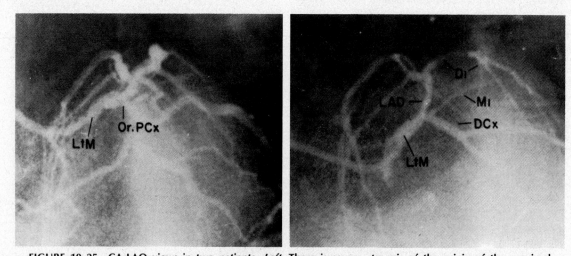

FIGURE 10–25   CA-LAO views in two patients. *Left,* There is severe stenosis of the origin of the proximal circumflex (Or.PCx). This area was unmasked by this view. *Right,* The entire proximal left anterior descending artery (LAD) was narrowed. There is an early-arising first marginal (M¹) which on other views could not be distinguished from a ramus intermedius or first diagonal. The origin of the first diagonal (D¹) is nicely seen. LtM = left main artery; D-LAD=distal left anterior descending artery; DCx=distal circumflex artery. (From Elliot, L. P., Bream, P. R., Soto, B., Russell, R. O., Rogers, W. J., Mantle, J. A., and Hood, W. P.: Significance of caudal left anterior oblique view in analyzing the left main coronary artery and its major branches. Radiology *139*:39, 1981.)

scending branch. The other branches, located between the anterior descending and circumflex and distributing to the free wall of the left ventricle, run in a lateral and caudal direction toward the apex and are named diagonal branches of the left ventricle. The best projection to observe the division of the left main stem into its branches is the CR[30°] L[60°]AO,[52] but a standard left anterior oblique may be adequate in most cases (Fig. 20–23, *bottom*). In this projection the two principal rami, the circumflex and the anterior descending, run along opposite borders of the cardiac shadow, whereas the diagonal branches occur in the angle subtended by these vessels. When all these branches are particularly evident and tortuous, the ensemble takes on the appearance, in the left oblique projection, of an octopus whose head is represented by the main stem and whose tentacles are represented by the left coronary branches, which seem to wave and contract with each cardiac cycle. In approximately 0.5 per cent of cases, the only artery arising from the left sinus of Valsalva is the anterior descending, since the circumflex is, in those cases, a branch of the right coronary artery.

In patients with high diaphragms, with horizontal hearts, and with horizontal or cephalad-directed left coronary arteries, a "weeping willow" view (CA[30°]L[60°]AO) may improve the visualization of the division of the left main stem into its branches[47] (Fig. 10–25A and *B*).

Left Anterior Descending Coronary Artery. This is the vessel in the human heart with the most constant origin, course, and distribution. Generally, it begins as a continuation of the main left coronary artery, passes to the left of the pulmonic valve, and runs along the anterior interventricular sulcus.

The size, length, and distribution of the left anterior descending are key factors in the balance of the perfusion to the interventricular septum, the lateral wall, and the apex of the left ventricle. Thus, according to D. B. Effler (personal communication), it should be classified arteriographically into Types I, II, and III depending on its length and the amount of myocardium it perfuses. The Type I left anterior descending is a small-caliber vessel that reaches only two thirds of the way from the base of the heart to the apex and that seems to be more prevalent in women. The Type II left anterior descending is a vessel of larger caliber and, by definition, reaches the apex of the left ventricle. The Type III left anterior descending extends from the base of the heart to the apex and around to the diaphragmatic aspect of the left ventricle, where it augments the normal perfusion pattern of the posterior descending artery. Anastomoses with the posterior descending branch are often visualized following occlusion of the right coronary artery.

The left anterior descending coronary artery can be well visualized in all projections. In the right anterior oblique view, it approaches the left border of the cardiac shadow (Fig. 10–11); in the anteroposterior view, it appears as the branch of the left coronary artery that runs caudally, with a more or less vertical course, separating the right from the left ventricle; in the L[60°]AO, left lateral, and CR[30°]L[60°] AO views, it is represented by the branch of the left coronary artery that is directed more ventrally than any of the other branches (Fig. 10–23, *bottom*). Sometimes, in both the right anterior oblique and the anteroposterior views, it

may be difficult to distinguish the anterior descending from the many left ventricular branches of the circumflex. However, this task can be simplified by observing the film in motion. In so doing, all the anteriorly located vessels (the anterior descending, the septal, and the diagonal branches) appear to move in a direction opposite to the posteriorly located arteries (i.e., the ventricular branches of the circumflex, such as the obtuse and the posterolateral branches). Another cine angiographic feature typical of the left anterior descending (and especially of its septal branches) is their relative lack of motion, when compared to the behavior of the circumflex and of the right coronary artery.

The branches of the left anterior descending artery are, in order of origin, the first diagonal, the first septal, the right ventricular (infrequently demonstrated), the minor septals, the second diagonal, and the apical. From a surgical standpoint, it is helpful to divide the left anterior descending artery into proximal, mid, and apical segments (Fig. 10–26). The most important landmark along the course of this artery is the origin of the major (and usually first) septal branch. That portion of the anterior descending artery located between its origin from the main left coronary artery and the first septal branch is the proximal third. The middle third runs from the origin of the main septal branch to the origin of the second diagonal branch. Distal to that vessel we find the terminal (or apical) segment of the anterior descending, which usually reaches the apex, encircles it, and often runs for a short distance along the posterior interventricular groove (Type III LAD).

In most cases, the first branch of the anterior descending is a rather large vessel that distributes to the free wall of the left ventricle, roughly midway between the anterior interventricular groove and the obtuse margin of the heart. Owing to their diagonal course along the free wall of the left ventricle, this vessel and any other branch of the anterior descending artery with distribution to the same general area of the myocardium are called "diagonals." The first diagonal often originates quite close to the bifurcation of the main left coronary artery and in more than 10 per cent of cases has a separate origin from the main stem, so that the left coronary artery ends in a trifurcation rather than a bifurcation.

The best projections to observe the origin and course of the diagonal branches are the left anterior oblique (Fig. 20–23, *bottom*) and the CR[30°]R[30°]AO views (Fig. 10–24A). In the right anterior oblique view, the first diagonal is often superimposed on the left anterior descending artery, and it may be quite difficult to separate the two vessels, at least along their more proximal segments. The more distal two thirds of the first diagonal, however, are well visualized in the right anterior oblique view. Here the diagonal appears to run along the border of the left heart shadow roughly parallel to the shadow of the ribs (Figs. 10–20 to 10–23, *top*; Fig. 10–24; and Fig. 10–25A and *B*).

Although there may be several small "diagonal" branches, one of these is referred to as the second diagonal branch and serves to separate the apical third of the left anterior descending artery from its middle third. This vessel branches off at an acute angle from the left anterior descending artery and distributes to the lateral portion of the apex.

The septal branches, which vary in number, arise from the left anterior descending artery at about a 90-degree angle. They run along the septum from front to back and in a caudal direction, with distribution to about two thirds of the upper portion of the septum and perfusing almost the entire septum in its inferior third (Figs. 10–24 and 10–25*A* and *B*). The more posterior and superior third of the septum receives its blood supply through the short branches derived from the posterior descending branch. Therefore, in a large percentage of cases, the septum is another important area of anastomosis between the right and left coronary arteries. On the other hand, when the posterior descending branch originates from the circumflex, the left coronary artery is the sole source of blood supply for the entire interventricular septum.

The largest (and usually the first) septal branch is of extreme importance because of its prominent role in supplying blood to the septum and its consistency of origin, course, and distribution. For these reasons, the first septal branch represents a major landmark in the identification and description of the left anterior descending artery, both in health and, especially, in disease. As indicated, its origin serves to separate the first third of the anterior descending artery from its middle third. Any lesions of the anterior descending artery are usually classified in relation to this branch, i.e., as proximal or distal to it. The first septal artery is seen in the right anterior oblique view as that vessel which originates at a clear-cut 90-degree angle from its parent vessel, running vertically toward the diaphragm, in the middle of the heart shadow (Fig. 10–25*A* and *B*). The first septal is seen in an entirely different perspective in the left anterior oblique view, in which it appears to run above the left anterior descending artery, inclining from right to left and from top to bottom, with a course parallel to the left anterior descending artery (Fig. 10–25*C*).

The more cranial septal branches are better demonstrated angiographically than the lower septal branches, since they are of greater length and caliber. Their characteristic branching from the left anterior descending artery and their straight course, lacking the slight tortuosity of the other branches, make them easy to identify (Fig. 10–25*A* and *B*) and, in turn, help to distinguish the anterior descending artery from the large diagonal branches, with which it could be confused in the right anterior oblique view. Another cineangiographic feature, typical of the left anterior descending and septal branches, is their relative lack of motion. This is especially evident when the left coronary artery is viewed against the background of the circumflex in the right anterior oblique view (Fig. 10–25*A* and *B*).

In its course, the left anterior descending artery gives off one or more *branches to the right ventricle*. The highest of these runs toward the conus branch of the right coronary artery, at the level of the pulmonic valve, forming, as a consequence of obstructions or occlusions of either the right coronary or left anterior descending artery, the anastomotic ring of Vieussens[52]; the other branches run obliquely over the right ventricular surface, anastomosing with similar branches of the right coronary artery. These branches are seldom angiographically identifiable in normal subjects; however, they become more readily appreciable in cases of occlusion of the parent vessel, thus acquiring great importance as collateral channels.

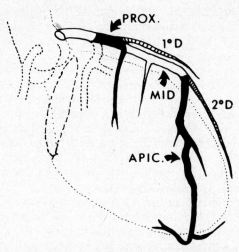

FIGURE 10–26   Diagram of left anterior descending branch in right anterior oblique projection showing its division into proximal, mid, and apical segments. The first and second diagonal branches are also shown. (From Gensini, G. G.: Coronary Arteriography. Mount Kisco, N.Y., Futura Publishing Co., 1975.)

The terminal branches of the Type III left anterior descending artery are the apical branches (Figs. 10–26 to 10–28). They distribute to both the anterior and the diaphragmatic aspects of the apex. Usually at least two branches can be seen (especially in the right anterior oblique view): the recurrent posterior and the recurrent lateral apical branches, the former turning around the apex and supplying its diaphragmatic portion (Figs. 10–26 and 10–27) and the latter supplying the lateral aspect of the apex.

Left Circumflex Artery.   This vessel usually departs at a rather sharp angle from the main left coronary artery to run posteriorly along the atrioventricular groove, toward the crux cordis, which, however, it reaches in only 16 per cent of cases. In 84 per cent of cases, the circumflex ends distal to the obtuse margin without reaching the posterior interventricular sulcus. When the circumflex reaches and passes beyond this region, it gives origin to the posterior descending branch (Fig. 10–29); in such cases, the left coronary artery not only is the sole source of blood supply to the entire interventricular septum but also gives origin to the branch supplying the atrioventricular node.

In the anteroposterior and right anterior oblique views, the left circumflex artery usually appears as the vessel first

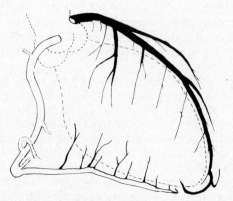

FIGURE 10–27   Diagram of blood supply to interventricular septum from right coronary artery and left anterior descending branch. (From Gensini, G. G.: Coronary Arteriography. Mount Kisco, N.Y., Futura Publishing Co., 1975.)

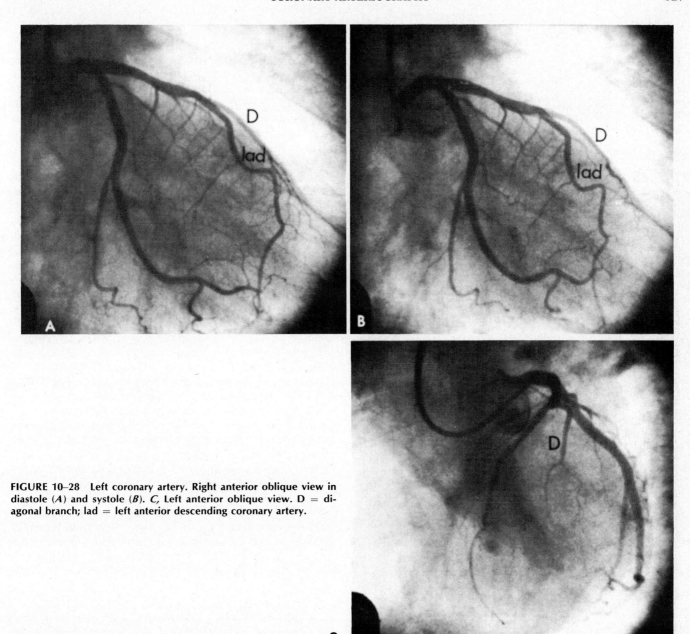

FIGURE 10–28 Left coronary artery. Right anterior oblique view in diastole (A) and systole (B). C, Left anterior oblique view. D = diagonal branch; lad = left anterior descending coronary artery.

to depart from the general direction taken by the left coronary artery (Figs. 10–24B and 10–28A and B). It forms a circle directed first caudally and then toward the center of the heart, coursing along the left atrioventricular groove. In the left anterior oblique view (Fig. 10–30), it appears to take the course directly opposite to that of the anterior descending artery, moving caudally and posteriorly toward the vertebral column, occasionally encircling the posterior border of the heart shadow (Figs. 10–23, top, and 10–30).

Soon after its origin, the circumflex not infrequently divides into two parallel branches, which are occasionally of nearly equal caliber. The lower, and usually the larger, of the two gives origin to the ventricular branches. The superior one, called the *atrial circumflex*, gives origin to branches for the atrial wall. More commonly, however, the atrial circumflex is a relatively slender branch that runs opposite to the ventricular branches.

In the 41 per cent of cases in which the *sinus node artery* is a branch of the left coronary artery, this vessel usu-

ally originates from the initial portion of the circumflex, a few millimeters beyond the origin of the latter. Less frequently, it takes off from the mid portion of the circumflex and rarely from its distal segment.

The largest and most constant branch (or branches) of the circumflex is the *branch* (or branches) *to the obtuse margin*. This vessel (or vessels) arises from the circumflex and runs along the ventricular wall, somewhat posteriorly and in the direction of the apex. Very often one of these branches acquires a special importance and appears as the very large branch which, in the left anterior oblique view, runs along the posterior edge of the left ventricular border (Fig. 10–28C). It maintains a path which, in the right anterior oblique view, is slightly inclined in relation to the course of the left anterior descending coronary artery (Fig. 10–28A and B).

The proximal portions of the obtuse marginal, anterior descending, and diagonal branches may be closely superimposed on one another when the origin of the obtuse

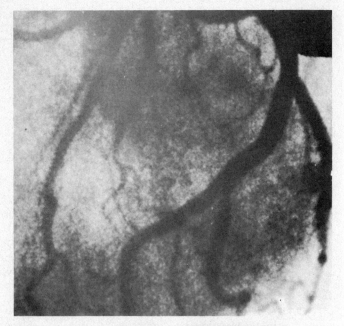

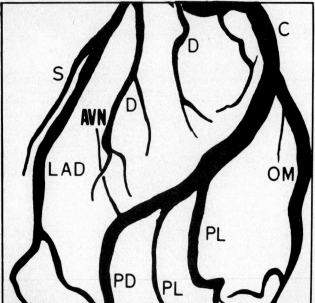

marginal is along the initial segment of the circumflex. This bunching up of several vessels may make it difficult to recognize minor (and sometimes even major) lesions of any one of these branches in either the right or the left anterior oblique view (Figs. 10–23*B* and 10–30). In such cases, the CA$^{20°}$R$^{30°}$AO view may be necessary to separate the various branches adequately.

There is considerable variation in the anatomy of the obtuse marginal branches of the left circumflex artery. Anywhere from one to four of these branches may be present, and they vary in size from quite large (as large as the left anterior descending artery) to quite small. They supply the lateral wall of the left ventricle above its diaphragmatic surface. After giving rise to the obtuse marginal branches, the circumflex artery continues along the left atrioventricular groove for a variable distance toward the crux of the heart. Because of its close relationship to the atrioventricular groove (and mitral valve ring), this portion of the circumflex artery moves widely with systole and diastole, i.e., toward the apex in systole and away from it in diastole. This motion is especially evident in the right anterior oblique projection. In over 80 per cent of cases, the circumflex artery does not reach the crux of the heart but terminates along the left atrioventricular groove after giving rise to the obtuse marginal branches. In 14 per cent of cases, the so-called left preponderant coronary anatomy exists (Fig. 10–29). In these patients, the posterior descending and posterolateral branches do not arise from the right coronary artery but instead arise from the left circumflex.

After giving rise to the obtuse marginal branches, the left circumflex artery continues all the way around the left atrioventricular groove. As it passes along this groove and reaches the diaphragm, it gives rise to the posterolateral branches, and when it reaches the crux of the heart, it turns forward to continue along the posterior interventric-

FIGURE 10–29 Left coronary artery, left anterior oblique view. Origin of posterior descending branch (PD) and AV node branch (AVN) from circumflex. (From Gensini, G. G.: Coronary Arteriography. Mount Kisco, N.Y., Futura Publishing Co., 1975.)

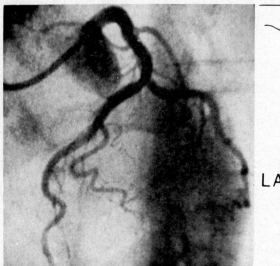

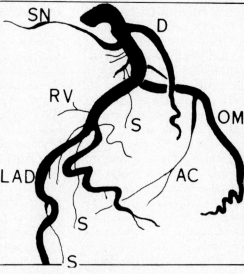

FIGURE 10–30 Left coronary artery, left anterior oblique view. (From Gensini, G. G.: Coronary Arteriography. Mount Kisco, N.Y., Futura Publishing Co., 1975.)

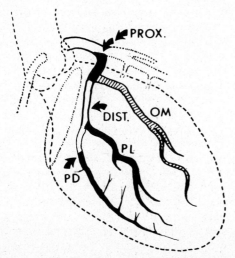

FIGURE 10–31 Diagram of circumflex in right anterior oblique view, showing its division into four segments (or into five segments when the posterior descending is a branch of the circumflex). (From Gensini, G. G.: Coronary Arteriography. Mount Kisco, N.Y., Futura Publishing Co., 1975.)

ular groove as the posterior descending artery. Regardless of its origin—whether it is a branch of the right coronary artery or of the circumflex—the posterior descending coronary artery follows the same course along the posterior interventricular groove and supplies the same portion of the posterior interventricular septum (p. 319). Its origin from the circumflex is best seen in the left anterior oblique view (Fig. 10–29), although it soon becomes foreshortened. For this reason, the best means of observing its middle and distal portions, as well as the posterior septal arteries that issue from it, is by using the right anterior oblique projection. The AV node branch, which originates from the distal segment of the circumflex in 12 per cent of cases, is also well visualized in the left anterior oblique view (Fig. 10–29). It appears as a slender and straight vessel departing from the circumflex at a 90-degree angle in a direction opposite to the posterior descending artery.

From a surgical standpoint, the circumflex is divided into four or five segments (Fig. 10–31).

Tables 10–2 and 10–3 summarize the nomenclature, abbreviations, and course of all the coronary arteries and their major branches.

ANATOMY OF CORONARY ARTERIES IN DISEASE

AGING OF THE CORONARY ARTERIES. Aging of the arterial wall is associated with gradual distention caused by progressive deterioration of the elastic tissue that results in dilatation of the lumen. During the average life span, the cross-sectional area of the arteries increases six or seven times.[53] Degeneration of the elastic fibers in the media may be accompanied by calcification, which can occur without atheroma.[54] Two of these three changes typical of aging, i.e., dilatation of the lumen and calcification of the wall, may occasionally be seen during coronary arteriography in the elderly. This pattern has been noted in a few healthy octogenarians with atypical chest pain or valvular heart disease.

CORONARY ATHEROSCLEROSIS. Coronary atherosclerosis may begin at a relatively young age, i.e., in the twenties or thirties, in patients at high risk and, in the majority of these patients, progresses rapidly[55,56]; on the other hand, if an individual has reached age 50 to 60 with normal coronary arteries, chances are that he or she will remain free of coronary artery disease throughout the entire life span.[55,57]

Postmortem studies have repeatedly demonstrated that the incidence of coronary atherosclerosis peaks at about age 60[58] and declines in the very old, presumably because patients with severe lesions succumb to the disease before they reach an advanced age. Thus, coronary atherosclerosis is not a manifestation of age; on the contrary, longevity and severe coronary atherosclerosis are usually mutually exclusive. However, the changes typical of aging arteries may occasionally coexist with the truly pathological changes of atherosclerosis.[59]

MICROSCOPIC CHANGES

1. *Alterations of the elastic lamina:* There is no obvious arteriographic counterpart of this stage of the atherosclerotic process.

2. *Early deposition of lipid material:* Separation of the elastic fibers and elevation of the surface of the intima occur. These changes appear in the arteriogram as minute nickings and are generally smooth "regular irregularities" (Fig. 10–32).

3. *Fibrous plaques and atheromatous foci:* These fibrolipid plaques may become thick and encroach grossly upon the lumen of the artery, possibly leading to severe obstruction. The lesions are identifiable on the coronary arteriogram as fairly regular reductions in lumen diameter that may, upon serial studies, become progressively more severe in a stepwise fashion (Fig. 10–33).

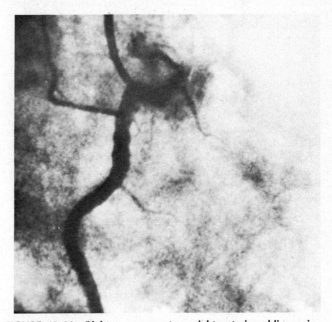

FIGURE 10–32 Right coronary artery, right anterior oblique view. Minute irregularities are observed at several points and resemble minute nickings or scallopings of the wall. (From Gensini, G. G.: Coronary Arteriography. Mount Kisco, N.Y., Futura Publishing Co., 1975.)

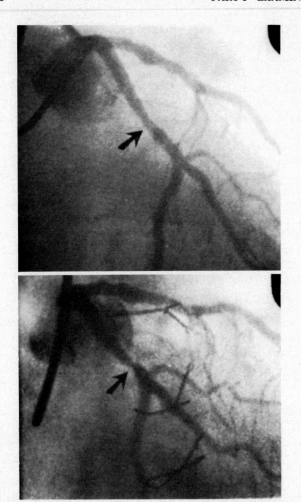

FIGURE 10-33 Left coronary artery, left anterior oblique view. The circumflex showed a relatively minor irregularity (*top*), which became considerably more severe at the time of a later arteriogram (*bottom*). (From Gensini, G. G., and Kelly, A. E.: Incidence and progression of coronary artery disease. An angiographic correlation in 1263 patients. Arch. Intern. Med. *129*:22, 1972, copyright 1972, American Medical Association.)

4. *Vascularization, hemorrhage, rupture, and ulceration:* Hemorrhage into a plaque, probably associated with superimposed, localized spasm is a logical explanation for the sudden appearance of unstable angina (whether it be "de novo," with a changing pattern, or new rest angina). The rapid swelling of an existing plaque, especially when associated with superimposed spasm, would transform a functionally unimportant lesion into a subocclusive one, encroaching markedly upon the lumen of the vessel, severely reducing blood flow to a segment of the myocardium, and resulting in ischemia and pain (Fig. 10-34). Patients with such lesions may hover for days and even weeks in a state of episodic or continuous pain, without reaching the point of widespread necrosis (p. 1355). In some, the spasm and swelling may regress, leading to a reduction in the severity of the stenosis, an increase in blood flow to the ischemic region, a return of the angina to its stable pattern, or even disappearance of angina. Others will instead experience infarction, usually through the superimposition of a thrombus. A large percentage of severe atheromatous lesions appear highly irregular in shape and show no consistent pattern, except that they are "irregularly irregular" (Fig. 10-35). These stenoses probably have had the most complex life history (and are possibly the oldest). They are produced by atherosclerotic lesions in which many or perhaps all of the stages described are intermingled or have occurred in chaotic succession, i.e., accumulation of hemorrhages, ulceration, thrombosis, calcium deposits, further ulceration, healing, and so on.

5. *Thrombosis:* Usually the presence of a thrombus in a coronary artery is associated with well-established atherosclerotic lesions (rarely with less than a 25 per cent reduction in lumen diameter.)[60] Once an occlusion has been produced by a thrombus, recanalization may occur as a result of three different mechanisms[61]:

1. The thrombus may undergo lysis.[62]

2. Organization of the thrombus may occur, with retraction of its core.[61]

3. Finally (and perhaps more frequently), organization of the thrombus may occur with growth of capillaries into its base.[63]

A *fresh* thrombus is usually associated with a distinct angiographic appearance that differs from ordinary atherosclerotic narrowing, in which there is usually gradual, funnel-like tapering or irregular, craggy narrowing of the lumen. In contrast, the hallmark of a fresh thrombus is abrupt interruption of the contrast-filled lumen, which has a fairly distinct rim or lip at the edges. It may be difficult or impossible to differentiate a recanalized thrombus from severe atherosclerotic stenosis by arteriography; both lesions can appear as localized irregular narrowings, despite the striking difference in the clinical history.

INCIDENCE OF CORONARY ARTERY DISEASE IN PATIENTS REFERRED FOR INVASIVE DIAGNOSTIC STUDIES

Eighty-nine per cent of patients in our laboratory are studied by coronary arteriography because the diagnosis of

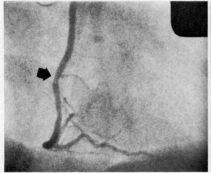
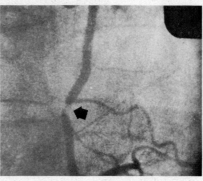

FIGURE 10-34 Right coronary artery, right anterior oblique projection. A functionally unimportant lesion can be seen at the time of the first coronary arteriogram (arrow, left panel). Two years later (arrow, right panel) a slightly magnified view of same vessel showed severe progression of the disease to an occlusive lesion. (From Gensini, G. G., and Kelly, A. E.: Incidence and progression of coronary artery disease. An angiographic correlation in 1263 patients. Arch. Intern. Med. *129*:22, 1972, copyright 1972, American Medical Association.)

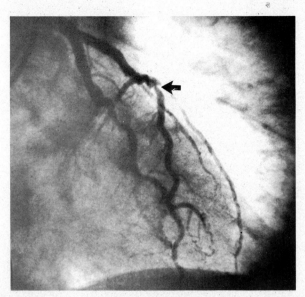

FIGURE 10–35 Left coronary artery, right anterior oblique view. Examples of highly irregular stenotic lesions, one of which is indicated by the arrow.

coronary artery disease was made or could not be ruled out by the referring physician; the remaining 11 per cent are adults with a clinical diagnosis of valvular or congenital heart disease with no symptoms or signs suggestive of coronary artery disease. Males predominate in the first group (suspected coronary artery disease) in a ratio of 3 to 1, whereas among the patients with valvular or congenital heart disease the sex incidence is more equally divided (55 per cent are males). Eighty-one per cent of patients referred with a clinical diagnosis of coronary artery disease are found to have angiographically detectable arterial lesions, and 77 per cent have *significant* involvement, defined as 50 per cent reduction of the diameter of the main left coronary artery or 75 per cent or more reduction of the diameter of the lumen in the right coronary artery, left anterior descending artery, or circumflex or in their major branches, i.e., posterior descending, major septal, major diagonal, lateral, obtuse marginal, or posterolateral. Among males, significant coronary artery disease is generally found in more than 80 per cent of those referred with this suspected diagnosis; in females this rate drops to nearly 50 per cent.

About 25 per cent of the adults referred with a clinical diagnosis of valvular or congenital heart disease (but without symptoms of myocardial ischemia) are found to have some atherosclerotic involvement. Unexpected, *significant* lesions are detected in less than 14 per cent of the patients in this "noncoronary" group.

SINGLE- VS. MULTIPLE-VESSEL DISEASE. Among patients with *significant* coronary artery disease, single-vessel involvement is found in 24 per cent (7.4 per cent in the right coronary artery, 12.2 per cent in the left anterior descending artery, and 4.4 per cent in the circumflex). In another 27 per cent of these patients, two vessels are involved. In the remaining 49 per cent the disease affects the three main vessels, i.e., the right coronary artery, the anterior descending artery, the circumflex, and/or their major branches. Within this last group we include a smaller subset (10 per cent) in which there is 50 per cent or greater reduction in lumen diameter of the main left coronary artery.

OCCLUSIVE AND SUBOCCLUSIVE LESIONS. In nearly two thirds of patients with significant coronary artery disease there is complete occlusion of one or more vessels. Of these occlusions, 40 per cent involve the right coronary artery, 33 per cent the left anterior descending artery, and 27 per cent the circumflex. If we add to the patients with complete occlusion of one or more branches those patients with one or more *almost* complete (99 per cent) obstructions, the number of patients with significant lesions of the occlusive type would approach 75 per cent of the population with significant coronary artery disease who are studied. If lesions of the secondary branches are disregarded and only the major coronary arteries of patients with significant coronary artery disease are analyzed, we find that two thirds of the significant obstructive lesions are found at the level of these large branches. Only 5 per cent of those patients with complete occlusion of one vessel demonstrate apparent normalcy of the other two main arteries. In the remaining 95 per cent, either one or both main vessels are seriously affected by the obstructive atherosclerotic process (Fig. 10–36). Most patients with 99 per cent obstruction are also found to have lesions of lesser degree in at least one of the other arteries. Narrowing resulting in a 75 per cent reduction in lumen diameter is occasionally found to be an isolated lesion.

SEGMENTAL LOCALIZATION OF OCCLUSIONS. In patients with completely occluded *right coronary arteries,* 53 per cent of the lesions are situated in the proximal third, 38 per cent are in the middle third, 10 per cent are in the distal third, and 7 per cent are in the posterior descending branch or the posterior left ventricular branches of the right coronary artery. The occlusions of the *left anterior descending artery* are localized as follows: 39 per cent are proximal to the first septal; 47 per cent are in the mid segment, distal to the first septal; 25 per cent involve the major diagonal branch; and 5 per cent involve the apical segment of the left anterior descending branch. The majority of the occlusions of the *circumflex* artery are located either within the first few millimeters of this vessel, in the initial portion of the obtuse marginal branch, or immedi-

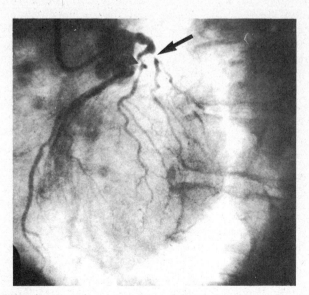

FIGURE 10–36 Left coronary artery, left anterior oblique view. Severe atherosclerotic involvement of left anterior descending branch and circumflex (small and large arrows, respectively).

ately distal to it. Only 10 per cent of the lesions are at the level of the posterolateral branches.

THE CORONARY COLLATERALS[64] (see also p. 1267). The clinical course of coronary artery disease in man is complex and often unpredictable. Coronary arteriography has shown that the same anatomical degree of obstruction in any one vascular segment may be associated with very different clinical manifestations in different individuals, ranging from absent or minimal symptoms to transmural infarctions and death. Blood flow to the myocardium, and thus the viability and function of the myocardial cells, is influenced, on the one hand, by the rate at which the coronary obstructive lesions progress (and sometimes regress) and, on the other, by the rate at which the anastomotic vessels develop into functioning and sizable collateral channels capable of replacing at least a portion of that blood flow no longer reaching the ischemic area through its primary route.

Our direct experience, based on several thousand selective coronary arteriograms performed in normal dogs and in patients clinically free of coronary artery disease, indicates that functioning, *angiographically demonstrable arterial collaterals are not present in normal hearts.* Coronary arteriography performed during life, as opposed to injection of contrast into postmortem specimens, depends upon, and thus reveals, the function of the vessel being visualized. Contrast material is not forced into the coronary arteries but is mixed with the flow of blood as blood enters the coronary ostium from the aorta. Consequently, only vessels within the resolving power of the system (100 μ or more in diameter) and carrying functionally significant blood flow receive enough contrast agent to become individually detectable, in the beating heart, by current cine radiographic techniques. Hence, we must assume that in hearts with normal coronary arteries, blood flow through the anastomotic channels is, at best, minimal, and we may therefore conclude that, although coronary collaterals are anatomically present, they are functionally inoperative in the normal heart.

Whenever coronary occlusion is produced in an experimental animal, a massive and lasting pressure gradient develops between the healthy and the occluded vascular segment. In those animals surviving the initial insult, this pressure gradient produces a manifold increase in the collateral blood flow, thereby stimulating a rapid increment in the size of the available anastomoses. A similar process occurs when an atherosclerotic plaque begins to obstruct the lumen; the pressure beyond the obstruction falls, generating a pressure gradient between the segment of coronary artery proximal to the obstruction and the segment beyond the site of obstruction. By the same token, a gradient of pressure is established between a nearby coronary artery and the segment of the diseased artery distal to the obstruction. The gradient generates blood flow across preexisting anastomotic channels and thus enlarges them. The flow of blood across the now functioning anastomoses sets the stage for their opacification with contrast agent and their visualization during arteriography.

Coronary atherosclerosis affects many points within the coronary arterial tree. The severity of the obstruction, however, is not the same at all levels. It is conceivable that pressure gradients of variable magnitude develop between various points within the coronary arterial system, thus

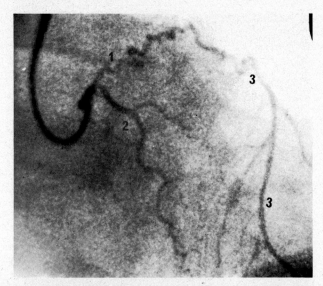

FIGURE 10–37 Right coronary artery, right anterior oblique view. The left anterior descending branch (3) is opacified by way of the conus branch (1). The right coronary artery is occluded after the right ventricular branch (2). (From Gensini, G. G.: Coronary Arteriography. Mount Kisco, N.Y., Futura Publishing Co., 1975.)

gradually producing different degrees of flow across anastomoses and a complex and variable pattern of collateral networks. We have never observed coronary collaterals in patients with less than 90 per cent reduction in lumen diameter. This fact is now so universally accepted that the demonstration of coronary collaterals is considered one of the most reliable signs that a perfusion deficit exists in the arterial segment under scrutiny.

A coronary anastomosis may be described as either intercoronary or homocoronary (i.e., intersegmental). An *intercoronary anastomosis* joins one of the three principal arteries to one another: (1) RCA to LAD (Figs. 10–37 and 10–38) or vice versa, (2) RCA to circumflex (Figs. 10–39 and 10–40) or vice versa, (3) LAD to circumflex or vice versa. A *homocoronary (or intersegmental) anastomosis* joins two points along the same artery. This type of collateral network may either be similar to the intercoronary type, such as when a well-defined branch proximal to an obstruction connects to another easily identifiable distal branch, or it may have a different origin, such as is the case for the "bridge collaterals," which grow out of vasa vasorum or minute, unnamed branches.

INTERVENTIONAL CORONARY ARTERIOGRAPHY

An important advance contributing to the diagnostic yield of coronary arteriography, as well as to our understanding of the pathophysiology of coronary artery disease, is the concept of acute intervention during coronary arteriography. The most common interventions during arteriography are the injection of vasodilators, of vasoconstrictors, and of thrombolytic agents and the mechanical dilatation of the atherosclerotic narrowings.

Coronary Spasm and Vasodilators
(See also pp. 1336 and 1360)

Observation on the effect of nitrates on the coronary arteries have been made since the early years of coronary ar-

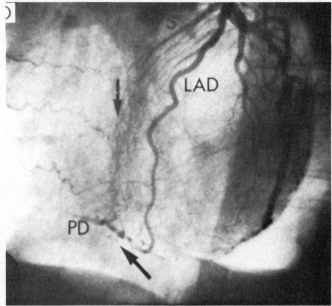

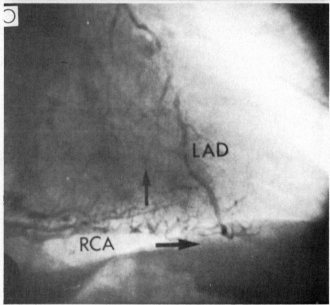

FIGURE 10–38 *Top,* Left coronary artery, left anterior oblique view. Opacification of right coronary artery by collateral from left anterior descending branch. *Bottom,* Right coronary artery, right anterior oblique view. Opacification of left anterior descending by collateral from right coronary artery.

teriography. A more recent technique is the use of ergonovine maleate as a test for the provocation of spasm.[65,66] Many other substances have also been utilized, usually in specific research protocols, and include, among others, morphine, alpha and beta stimulants and blockers, cholinergic and anticholinergic agents, and calcium channel blockers. In January, 1960, a few months after Prinzmetal's published report,[67] we were able to document the appearance of spontaneously occurring coronary spasm associated with chest pain in a patient with angina pectoris and mild coronary artery disease as well as the resolution of this spasm and disappearance of the pain with the administration of a sublingual nitrate; this provided the first reported clinical case in which the presence of spasm and its resolution were documented by means of coronary arteriography[24] (Fig. 10–41). Shortly thereafter we reported on

the use of Pitressin for the pharmacological *provocation* of spasm in dogs[42] and its resolution with administration of isosorbide dinitrate.[68]

The concept of vasomotion as a cause of ischemia was initially controversial, since angina pectoris was thought to be consistently associated with either fixed coronary atherosclerotic obstruction or other organic disease in which the demand could outstrip the capacity of the coronary vascular bed. The problem of symptomatic coronary artery spasm remained dormant for almost a decade. In 1975, Maseri provided for the first time the missing correlation between the clinical, echocardiographic, hemodynamic, and angiographic characteristics of spontaneous or primary angina.[69] Two developments appear to be responsible for this rediscovery of the clinical role of coronary spasm in ischemic heart disease: First, coronary arteriography was often performed following administration of nitroglycerin or atropine or both; the former is known to produce vasodilation and thus to prevent or resolve spasm, and the latter may prevent coronary spasm by a different mechanism. When arteriographers became aware of the existence of spasm-induced angina, they began to alter their protocol to increase the diagnostic yield of coronary arteriography. Second, the availability of coronary bypass surgery led to a dramatic increase in the utilization of coronary arteriography and extended the indication of this diagnostic procedure to patients with unstable angina, a group which may very well include patients with Prinzmetal's angina or with spasm superimposed on existing organic lesions.

There are two additional reasons why spontaneously occurring coronary spasm was not identified during coronary arteriography: (1) most arteriographers used to refrain from injecting the coronary arteries, or even exploring these vessels with a catheter, during episodes of pain, hypertension, severe arrhythmias, or other alarming electrocardiographic changes—all phenomena associated with Prinzmetal's angina; and (2) Prinzmetal's angina tends to occur at night or in the early morning, an inconvenient time for most arteriographers and their staff to perform coronary arteriography.

The study initiated by the Cleveland Clinic group in 1972 and reported by Heupler and others in 1978 on the use of ergonovine maleate represents a complete reversal of this attitude.[65] This agent, first recommended by Stein in 1949 for the diagnosis of angina pectoris, is now widely accepted and utilized in aggressive cardiac laboratories as the provocative test for documentation of coronary arterial spasm.[70]

As Helfant wrote, "After being moribund for some two decades, the role of coronary artery spasm in ischemic heart disease has been resuscitated, revived, and resurrected."[71]

There are four major types of coronary spasm:

1. Iatrogenically induced, i.e., caused by catheter manipulation inside a coronary artery or branch.

2. Due to nitrate withdrawal in factory workers.

3. Spontaneously occurring (primary angina, formerly called variant or Prinzmetal's angina) (Figs. 10–41 and 10–42).

4. Superimposed on well-defined coronary obstructions.

The latter two types are clinically important phenomena and may justify a provocative test such as that utilizing ergonovine maleate.

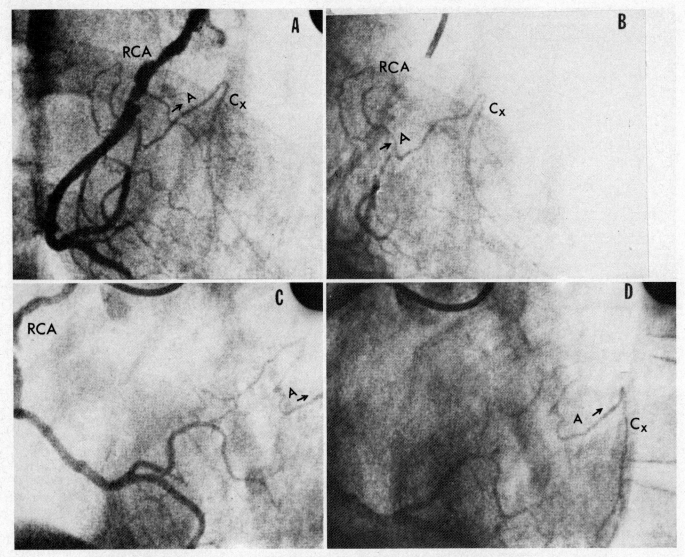

FIGURE 10–39   Early (*A*) and late (*B*) opacification of right coronary artery (RCA) in the right anterior oblique view. Early (*C*) and late (*D*) opacification of right coronary artery in left anterior oblique view. Collateral circulation is evident between the terminal branches of the right coronary artery and the atrial branch (A) of the circumflex (C_x). (From Gensini, G. G.: Coronary Arteriography. Mount Kisco, N.Y., Futura Publishing Co., 1975.)

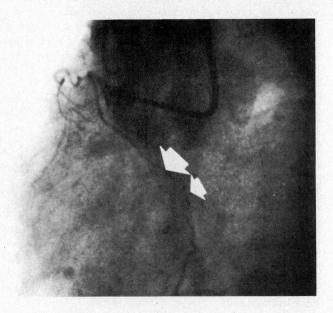

FIGURE 10–40   Right coronary artery injection, left anterior oblique view. Example of Kugel's artery (arrows), which connects atrial branches arising from the proximal right coronary artery, to atrial branches arising from the distal right coronary. The proximal right coronary artery is completely occluded and the distal artery fills through these atrial branches and Kugel's artery.

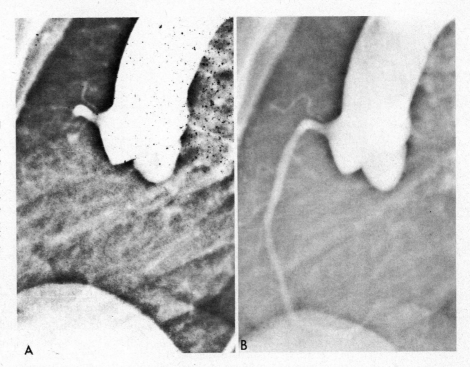

FIGURE 10–41 Right coronary artery, lateral view. *A,* Baseline coronary arteriogram. *B,* Coronary arteriogram 3.5 minutes after administration of 5 mg of sublingual isosorbide dinitrate. (From Gensini, G. G., et al.: Arteriographic demonstration of coronary artery spasm and its relief after the use of a vasodilator in the case of angina pectoris and in the experimental animal. Angiology *13*:550, 1962, with the permission of the copyright owner, The Angiology Research Foundation, Inc., all rights reserved.)

Besides its role in the provocation of "primary" angina pectoris in patients with no or insignificant coronary artery disease, coronary spasm is often superimposed on clinically significant organic obstructions and contributes to the development of myocardial ischemia (Fig. 10–43). A significant body of evidence is accumulating on the role of coronary spasm as an important factor associated in a subset of patients (possibly a large one) with myocardial infarction.[72] Autopsies of patients who died suddenly and coronary arteriograms of those who were resuscitated after ventricular fibrillation have shown the existence of a significant subset of patients with no or mild obstructive lesions. These lesions would have been, in themselves, inadequate to cause the profound and sudden ischemia leading to the terminal event without the superimposition of spasm.

The use of provocative pharmacological testing for coronary spasm is associated with potential risk.[73] Ergonovine maleate, in progressive doses of 0.1 to 0.3 mg, is a sensitive, specific, and reasonably safe means of provoking spasm. However, its end-point must be recognized and documented without delay, and specific treatment must be at hand to be initiated immediately. In our opinion, to terminate the effect of ergonovine, there is no substitute for

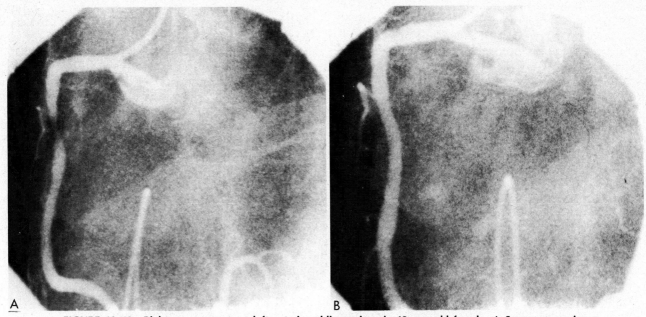

FIGURE 10–42 Right coronary artery, left anterior oblique view, in 48-year-old female. *A,* Severe narrowing of right coronary artery during an episode of Prinzmetal's angina. *B,* Spasm has disappeared 3 minutes after sublingual administration of 0.4 nitroglycerin. (From Gensini, G. G.: Coronary Arteriography. Mount Kisco, N.Y., Futura Publishing Co., 1975.)

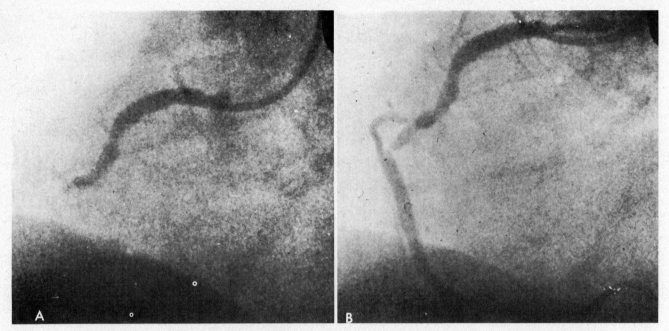

FIGURE 10–43   Right coronary artery, left anterior oblique view, in 49-year-old male. *A*, Apparent total occlusion. No contrast agent progressed beyond the point shown at any time during or after injection. *B*, Five minutes after administration of 5 mg of chewable isosorbide dinitrate (Sorbitrate [Stuart Pharmaceuticals, Division of ICI America, Inc., Wilmington, Delaware]). (From Gensini, G. G.: Coronary Arteriography. Mount Kisco, N.Y., Futura Publishing Co., 1975.)

parenteral nitroglycerin, which should be *injected* into the left ventricle (or intravenously) in doses of 0.4 mg as soon as the ergonovine test is terminated (Fig. 10–44) or at the first sign of an adverse effect such as arrhythmia; reduction in contractility, especially associated with hypotension; a marked rise in left ventricular end-diastolic pressure; coronary artery occlusion; or severe ischemic pain. In refractory spasm nitroglycerin (in boluses of 0.2 mg) may also be injected into the involved coronary artery.

The effect of injection of nitroglycerin is a most rewarding and impressive pharmacodynamic event. Injected as a single 0.4-mg bolus into the left ventricle, it instantly reduces elevated left ventricular end-diastolic pressure, often with simultaneous improvement in the indices of contractility, and it induces moderate reductions in the systolic left ventricular pressure and a minimal increase in the pulse rate.[25] Coronary spasm, if present, promptly disappears; the patient becomes more comfortable, with alleviation of any chest pain or dyspnea; and left ventricular hypokinetic segments begin contracting vigorously.[15]

In over 2500 coronary arteriograms performed we have never observed a serious adverse or deleterious effect arising from administration of nitroglycerin. Most misconceptions and lost therapeutic opportunities appear to have been due to the occasional patient (2 to 3 per cent) who responds with excessive peripheral vasodilatation to the administration of nitroglycerin. This in no way impairs the function of the heart as a pump but warrants prompt treatment with simple elevation of the lower extremities and with intravenous fluids. Theoretically, a pure alpha adrenergic stimulant, such as phenylephrine, should be administered if simple physical measures prove inadequate, but we have never found this to be necessary.

Coronary Occlusion and Thrombolysis

An impressive body of knowledge on the pathophysiology and therapy of myocardial infarction has been accumulated during the last few years, since Rentrop's[74–76] demonstration of the safety and usefulness of coronary arteriography during the acute phases of myocardial infarction. These findings demonstrated that the direct cause of acute myocardial infarction in the majority of patients with symptoms of chest pain and ST-segment elevation is acute intraluminal coronary thrombosis, generally superimposed on an obstructive atherosclerotic lesion.[77,78] Either rupture of the plaque, spasm of the wall or both may precede the final thrombotic occlusion in most patients. Chazov, who first suggested the use of fibrinolytic agents for the treatment of thromboembolism and infarction,[79,80] was also the first to report in 1976[81,82] on the successful intracoronary administration of fibrinolysin in acute myocardial infarction. Mazur[83] earlier had reported on the use of parenteral streptokinase in patients with this condition. Dotter[84] in 1974 described his success with selective intra-arterial perfusion of streptokinase in thrombotic occlusion of peripheral arteries.

The experiences of Rentrop and associates,[74–76] followed by the reports of Ganz et al.,[85] gave the real impetus to this technique, which is now widely applied in many cardiac laboratories including the author's. Recanalization of an occluded coronary artery can be achieved in nearly 80 per cent of patients during the evolving stage of myocardial infarction.[86] However, the quality of the late results appears to be inversely related to the duration of ischemia.[87] It follows that early recognition of the syndrome and prompt catheterization of the affected artery are the key to the

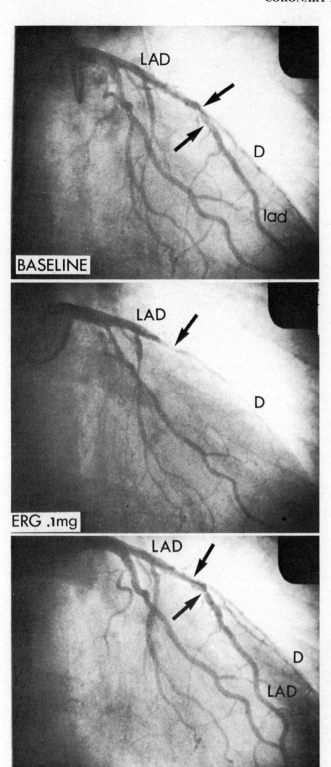

FIGURE 10–44 Left coronary artery, right oblique view. *Top,* Baseline injection. Arrows point to area of 50 to 75 per cent narrowing along left anterior descending branch. *Center,* After administration of 0.1 mg ergonovine in left ventricle. There is complete occlusion of left anterior descending, with total lack of filling of its mid and apical segments. The small *branch* seen is a diagonal branch and not the LAD proper. *Bottom,* Resolution of occluding spasm one minute after injection of 0.4 mg of nitroglycerin into the left ventricle.

successful application of this technique. Our protocol, which has been applied in 100 patients during the last 14 months, is designed with the safety of the patient well in mind and emphasizes simplicity and promptness of action.

PROCEDURE. The St. Joseph's Hospital Emergency Room is usually alerted by the Advance Life Support Unit about the impending arrival of a suspected myocardial infarction patient. As soon as the patient enters the emergency room, he or she is seen by the emergency room physician; if the diagnosis of myocardial infarction is confirmed by the presence of persistent ST-segment elevation, a blood sample for routine and coagulation studies is obtained, an I.V. nitroglycerin drip is started at 30 to 60 μg/min unless severe hypotension (systolic pressure below 80 mm Hg) is present. A lidocaine drip may also be started if frequent extrasystoles are present. If the ST-segment elevation does not disappear within five minutes from the beginning of the administration of nitroglycerin, the cardiovascular laboratory physician and the attending physician are immediately notified, while the patient and/or the family is advised of the availability of the myocardial infarction intervention protocol. If permission is obtained from the patient and the referring physician, the cardiovascular team is summoned and the patient is taken to the cardiovascular laboratory.

A team composed of an experienced cardiac angiographer, two laboratory nurses, and one laboratory technician is available at all times, less than 20 minutes away from the cardiovascular laboratory.

The Sones technique described previously is used; only the Sones catheter is employed for all functions and the left ventriculogram is delayed until the end of the procedure. As soon as the affected artery (or its parent) is entered, an injection of Renografin 76 is made to ascertain the status and level of the occluding lesions. Intracoronary nitroglycerin, 0.4 mg, is given, followed two minutes later by a second opacification of the artery. If the occlusion is persistent, an intracoronary bolus of 10,000 units of streptokinase is given. The streptokinase drip is then begun at 4000 units/min and continued for 30 minutes. Arteriograms are performed at 10, 20, and 30 minutes. A few ventricular premature beats occur at the time of the reopening of the artery. The drip is diminished to 3000 units/min and continued for an additional 30 minutes, again filming every 10 minutes. Generally the infusion is discontinued after 60 minutes.

A left ventriculogram is performed in the RAO view using 25 ml or less of Renografin 76 and the procedure is discontinued. Following the procedure the patient is treated with intravenous heparin (1000 units/hr in patients weighing between 150 and 200 lbs).

IDENTIFICATION AND ASSESSMENT OF JEOPARDIZED MYOCARDIUM

Both an expert and a novice arteriographer can benefit from a *systematic* approach to the analysis of coronary and left ventricular contrast studies. The following are suggested steps for an orderly analysis of a coronary arteriogram and left ventriculogram.

1. *Are the coronary arteries free of atherosclerotic lesions?*

A normal artery has smooth walls, tapers toward the periphery, is free of isolated areas of radiolucency, and possesses all expected important branches unless these originate from another vessel. Nicking and scalloping of an arterial border usually indicate early atherosclerotic changes. With regard to possible anatomical variations, the following three principles should be kept in mind:

a. Coronary artery disease is far more frequent than are unusual anatomical variations.

b. There are thousands of collaterals for any one variant, aberrant, or anomalous vessel.

c. Before an unusual vessel is accepted as a variant, an occlusion or a large collateral channel should be suspected. Conversely, systolic narrowing that disappears during diastole is pathognomonic of "myocardial

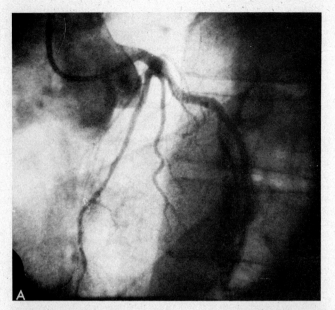

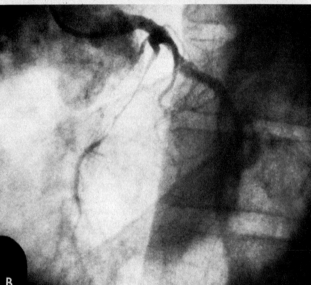

bridging" (Fig. 10–45), i.e., the intramyocardial course of an epicardial artery, and should not be confused with a permanent obstruction.

2. *Is the ventricle normal in size, shape, vigor, and symmetry of contraction?*

The normal pattern of left ventricular contraction as seen on cine ventriculography is a uniform, almost concentric inward motion of all points along the inner surface during systolic ejection. This pattern depends on the coordinated and sequential contraction of the myocardial mass, which is intended to produce maximum effective work at minimum cost (myocardial synergy).[88,89]

The normal outline of the human left ventricular cavity, as seen in the right anterior oblique projection during diastole, is that of an ellipsoid, with the tip inclined downward 45 degrees. During systole, the concentric inward motion of the anterior and posterior walls (and to a lesser extent of the apex) squeezes the sides and tips of the ellipsoid toward the center without changing the dimension of the base (mitral valve). At the peak of systolic ejection, the outline of the left ventricular cavity often resembles a pear core or an ice cream cone. When this outline enlarges or loses this characteristic appearance, left ventricular enlargement or asynergy should be suspected (Fig. 10–46).

The distribution of the coronary arteries to the left ventricular myocardium follows a broad outline that allows division of the ventricular mass into a number of segments according to the areas perfused by the major myocardial branches. We have found that division of the left ventricular silhouette into five major segments in the right anterior oblique projection and into two major segments in the left anterior oblique projection is adequate for the description of abnormalities of wall motion (Fig. 10–47). Depending on the degree of motion impairment, each segment can be

FIGURE 10–45 Left coronary artery, left anterior oblique view. In diastole (A) there is slight nicking and scalloping of the left anterior descending coronary artery. During systole (B) there is severe systolic narrowing (myocardial bridging) of the left anterior descending coronary artery, which is almost totally obliterated.

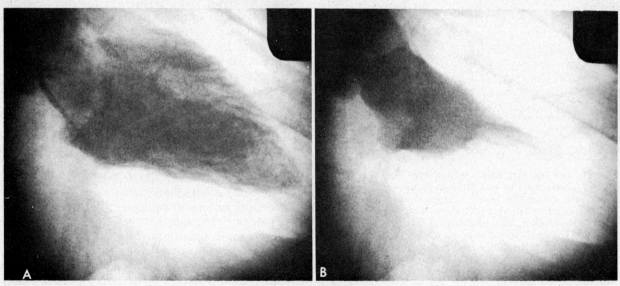

FIGURE 10–46   Normal left ventricle, right anterior oblique view, in diastole (A) and systole (B).

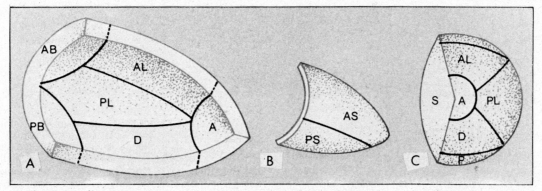

FIGURE 10–47 Schematic division of left ventricular wall, including septum, into seven segments.

A, Shell of free wall of ventricle as seen from front right after removal of interventricular septum. Segments are designated apical (A), anterobasal (AB), anterolateral (AL), diaphragmatic (D), posterobasal (PB), and posterolateral (PL).

B, Shell of interventricular septum as seen in the same projection, with division into portions supplied by anterior septal (AS) and posterior septal (PS) branches.

C, Apical view of left ventricle. S = septum. (From Gensini, G. G.: Coronary arteriography. Role in myocardial revascularization. Postgrad. Med. *63:*121, 1978.)

described as normal, hypokinetic (reduced motion), akinetic (absent motion), dyskinetic (systolic bulging), or aneurysmal (Fig. 10–48).

A useful means of quantifying ventricular performance is the ejection fraction (stroke volume/end-diastolic volume), usually calculated from the right anterior oblique images (Chap. 14). If a ventricle appears not to be enlarged in systole or diastole, if the silhouette conforms with the normal description and exhibits vigorous and symmetrical contraction of all segments, and if the ejection fraction is 55 per cent or greater, the left ventriculogram can be said to be normal. At this point, a patient found to have normal coronary arteries and a normal ventriculogram can be classified as having no evidence of ischemic heart disease caused by obstructive atherosclerosis of the coronary arteries and to have good left ventricular function. He or she should be suitably reassured, and another

cause for chest pain should be sought. In our experience, the three most common causes of chest pain or discomfort in patients with normal coronary arteries are reflux esophagitis, cervical arthritis, and psychoneurosis.

3. *If the coronary arteries are not free of disease, is there any lesion that has resulted in a 75 per cent or greater reduction in luminal diameter?*

Experimental studies in animals have shown that stenosis up to 70 or 80 per cent may not impair resting coronary flow, although constrictions of 50 to 60 per cent may cause ischemia during exercise. For this reason, a lesion causing a 75 per cent or greater reduction in luminal diameter (i.e., a reduction to one fourth its original size) is considered capable of producing a perfusion deficit.[90,91] Multiple projections are necessary for accurate assessment of a lesion, because of the possibility of underestimation of slit- or crescent-shaped narrowings.

FIGURE 10–48 Localized and generalized abnormalities of cardiac contraction. Arrows represent motion from end-diastole to end-systole. (From Herman, M. V., and Gorlin, R.: Implications of left ventricular asynergy. Am. J. Cardiol. *23:*538, 1969.)

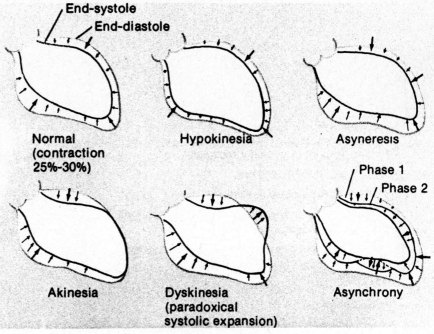

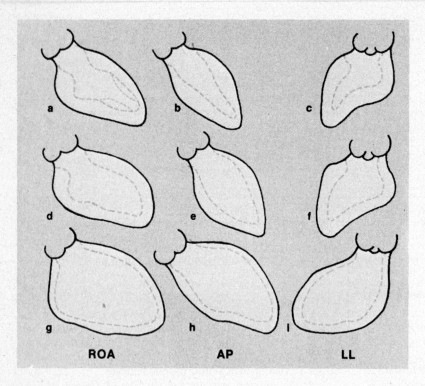

FIGURE 10–49 Diagrams of left ventricular cavity in diastole (solid lines) and systole (dashed lines) as seen in right oblique anterior (ROA), anteroposterior (AP), and left lateral (LL) projections. *a, b,* and *c,* Normal left ventricle (inner dashed lines in *a* denote imprint of papillary muscles). *d, e,* and *f,* Mild left ventricular enlargement, mainly at expense of an increased left ventricular end-systolic volume. *g, h,* and *i,* Severe left ventricular enlargement and hypokinesia. (From Gensini, G. G.: Coronary arteriography. Role in myocardial revascularization. Postgrad. Med. *63*:121, 1978.)

4. *If the ventricle is not normal, describe any abnormalities in terms of alteration of size, vigor, shape, or synergy of contraction.*

Abnormalities observed on the left ventriculogram may involve the entire ventricle or may be localized to a segment. They result in a change of shape and volume or in alterations in the contraction pattern. Additional abnormalities of the left ventriculogram are seen with certain valvular defects, such as mitral regurgitation, mitral stenosis, and aortic stenosis, or with septal perforation.

Table 10–4 summarizes the common abnormalities of the left ventriculogram. Diagrams of a normal ventricle as well as two different degrees of left ventricular enlarge-

ment are included in Figure 10–49. Figures 10–50 and 10–51 give additional examples.

5. *Is the luminal narrowing sufficiently proximal to jeopardize a sizable myocardial segment?*

Atherosclerosis is a diffuse process and can be found at all levels along the epicardial course of a coronary artery. Although multiple bypass grafts are now commonplace and are often made to relatively small branches, there is general agreement that a relationship exists between blood flow through the graft (and the size of the anastomosis), on the one hand, and the likelihood of graft patency, on the other. If narrowing involves a small branch or is located at the periphery of a vessel, or if the involved artery

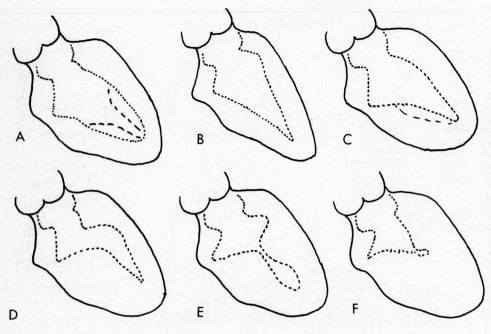

FIGURE 10–50 Diagrammatic representation of the left ventricular cavity in diastole (solid line) and systole (dotted line) as seen in RAO view. *A,* Normal ventricle, with pear-core configuration in systole due to the imprint of the papillary muscles (dashed line). *B,* Normal ventricle, ice cream cone configuration. *C,* Normal ventricle, pointed boot configuration. Only the posterior papillary muscle (dashed line) can be seen faintly. *D,* Ballerina foot configuration due to localized hyperkinesis of the diaphragmatic segment and mild hypokinesis of the anterior segment. *E,* Hourglass configuration due to hypertrophy of the anterior and posterior walls. *F,* Cavity obliteration. (From Gensini, G. G.: Coronary Arteriography. Mount Kisco, N.Y., Futura Publishing Co., 1975.)

TABLE 10-4 THE ABNORMAL LEFT VENTRICULOGRAM

Diffuse Abnormalities
Abnormalities of volume
  Enlargement
    End-systolic
    End-diastolic
  Reduction
    End-diastolic
    End-systolic (cavity obliteration)
Abnormalities in rate of volume change
  Hypokinesia
    Mild
    Moderate
    "Quivering" ventricle
  Hyperkinesia
    Mild
    Moderate
    Severe
Segmental Abnormalities (Asynergy)
Decreased function
  Hypokinesia (asyneresis)
  Asynchrony
  Akinesia
  Dyskinesia
Increased function
  Hyperkinesia
    (Asymmetrical hypertrophy?)
Segmental early relaxation phenomenon (SERP)
Filling Defects
Valvular Involvement
Mitral stenosis
Mitral regurgitation
Aortic stenosis
Septal Perforation (Acquired Ventricular Septal Defect)

From Gensini, G. G.: Coronary Arteriography. Mount Kisco, N.Y., Futura Publishing Co., 1975.

perfuses a myocardial segment of trivial magnitude, there is little justification for performing or extending surgery for that lesion.

6. *Does the narrowed coronary artery perfuse a viable myocardial segment?*

This is a crucial and often difficult decision to make. Clearly, there is no point in trying to revascularize a scar. Furthermore, reperfusion of a freshly necrotic segment may be undesirable. Many infarctions seen postoperatively may be due to reperfusion of an already necrotic segment rather than to failure of a properly placed graft.[92]

Viability of a myocardial segment is best assessed by the combination of pre- and postintervention ventriculography (p. 1369). If the myocardial segment perfused by an obstructed or occluded artery is either normally contracting or mildly hypokinetic, there should be little doubt as to its viability. Conversely, if it is aneurysmal or clearly dyskinetic, there is no point in considering a bypass to its parent vessel. The difficult part of the decision-making concerns a segment that is severely hypokinetic or akinetic, in which case the segment's behavior must be examined before and after the performance of maneuvers that potentiate contractility. The contractions of the segment should be critically examined during a normally conducted beat and during a postextrasystolic beat (Fig. 10-52) as well as before and after the administration of nitroglycerin (Fig. 10-53).[14,15] If improvement is apparent, the segment may be assumed to be viable and its revascularization is of potential benefit.

7. *Is the distal coronary segment both identifiable (by antegrade flow or through collaterals) and suitable for bypass graft surgery?*

Unless an artery can be positively identified and its course, diameter, branching, and lumen correctly assessed, it should not be chosen as a target for a bypass graft. For example, an arterial segment (distal to an occlusion) that fills incompletely or not at all may be diffusely diseased, may have virtually no lumen, or may be too small for successful anastomosis. If it is the only segment in need of repair, the cardiologist and surgeon would be ill advised in

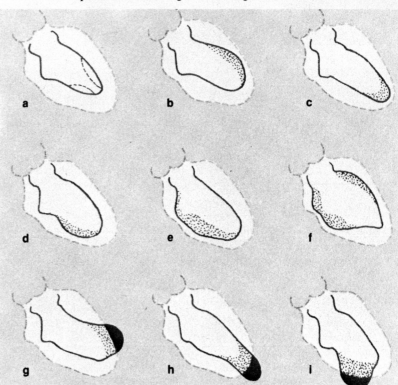

FIGURE 10-51 Selected examples of frequently observed segmental left ventricular contraction abnormalities. Diastole is represented by dashed lines and systole by solid lines; akinetic segments are represented by dotted areas and dyskinetic segments by dotted and black areas; normal end-systolic contour is represented by the white area within the solid line. (Dashed lines within solid line in *a* denote imprint of papillary muscles.) *a*, Normal ventricle. *b*, Anterolateral akinesia. *c*, Apical akinesia. When mild, or simply hypokinetic, pattern is often described as "lazy apex." *d*, Diaphragmatic akinesia, soupspoon configuration. *e*, Posterobasal and diaphragmatic akinesia. *f*, Anterobasal, anterolateral, diaphragmatic, and posterobasal akinesia. *g*, Anterolateral dyskinesia. *h*, Apical dyskinesia. *i*, Diaphragmatic dyskinesia. (From Gensini, G. G.: Coronary arteriography. Role in myocardial revascularization. Postgrad. Med. *63*:121, 1978.)

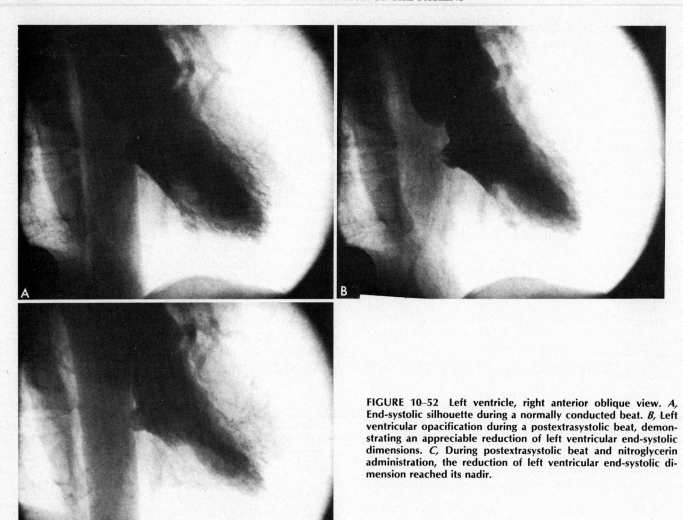

FIGURE 10–52 Left ventricle, right anterior oblique view. *A,* End-systolic silhouette during a normally conducted beat. *B,* Left ventricular opacification during a postextrasystolic beat, demonstrating an appreciable reduction of left ventricular end-systolic dimensions. *C,* During postextrasystolic beat and nitroglycerin administration, the reduction of left ventricular end-systolic dimension reached its nadir.

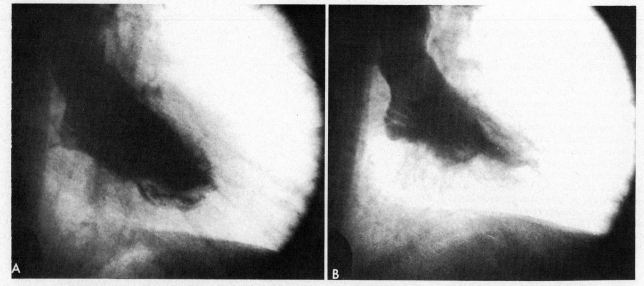

FIGURE 10–53 Left ventricle, end-systolic silhouette, right anterior oblique view. Before (*A*) and after (*B*) administration of 0.4 mg of nitroglycerin in the left ventricle demonstrating a striking improvement of left ventricular synergy, with nearly complete disappearance of diaphragmatic hypokinesis and marked improvement of ejection fraction.

respectively referring and accepting the patient. An exception to this rule is a nonfilling anterior descending coronary artery *in the presence of unimpaired motion of the anterolateral wall.* Should operation be indicated because of the involvement of another artery that could clearly be the target for bypass, exploration of the inadequately identified segment distal to a complete occlusion should be performed in any case in the hope that it might be suitable for a graft. This is frequently the case in occlusions of the left anterior descending artery, when the patency of that segment is maintained by collaterals originating from a conus artery that is inadequately opacified because of its separate ostium in the right sinus of Valsalva.

When the arterial segment beyond a stenosis is adequately opacified, its suitability for a bypass is a function of size, distribution, and the degree of peripheral involvement, as follows:

   a. *Size* (diameter of vessel at site of intended anastomosis): A vessel is totally unsuitable if the size is 0.7 mm or less, poor if 0.8 to 1.0 mm, acceptable for internal mammary anastomosis if 1.1 to 1.4 mm, and good for any type of graft if 1.5 mm or larger.
   b. *Distribution*: Length of a segment and number of branches beyond the stenosis are expressions of size and importance of the myocardial segment perfused and broadly correlate with flow requirement. Clearly, the larger the segment, the better would be the long-term patency and clinical usefulness of a graft. The necessity of evaluating the distribution pattern of a vessel when considering coronary artery bypass surgery is exemplified by the different size and length of the left anterior descending coronary artery. Classification of this vessel into its three types (see p. 325) is helpful in assessing the prognosis in disease of the left anterior descending artery. Total occlusion of a Type I left anterior descending artery may be associated with little muscle damage, because it perfuses a limited area of the anteroseptal portion of the left ventricle. In contrast, the Type III vessel is usually of a larger caliber and perfuses the anterior two thirds of the interventricular septum, the anteroapical portion of the left ventricle, and even a portion of the diaphragmatic surface of the left ventricle; total occlusion of this vessel may be lethal, and those who do survive usually present with a postinfarction ventricular aneurysm.
   c. *Peripheral involvement*: An artery free of disease distal to the intended site of anastomosis is ideal for grafting. Peripheral lesions up to 50 per cent reduction in the lumen may be acceptable, but the expected long-term patency of the graft, or its potential for long-term effectiveness, is diminished.

8. *Is overall myocardial function acceptable for revascularization surgery?*

A few investigators have reported dramatic results with bypass grafts in patients with poor left ventricular function. However, these cases are the exceptions rather than the rule (p. 1368). There is a relatively high surgical mortality among these patients, but in some instances the long-term clinical results have been encouraging.[93]

STRATIFICATION OF CORONARY ARTERY DISEASE: GRADING THE SEVERITY OF OBSTRUCTIVE LESIONS

The universally accepted method of identifying an obstructive lesion on a coronary arteriogram is subjective examination by a trained arteriographer who reviews the film with an experienced but unaided eye. Computer-assisted methods (quantitative angiography)[23] may be utilized for experimental research or for special projects but are still impractical for use on a routine basis.

A grading method that disregards the limitations of the human eye (however well trained it might be) is unrealistic and doomed to failure. The system employed by the author is based on the demonstration that a trained observer can easily distinguish reductions in lumen diameter to one-fourth, one-half, or three-fourths the original size.[2] Obviously it is easy to identify both complete occlusion and lesions that cause almost complete occlusion, classified as "99 per cent" obstructions. Once these fundamental "benchmarks" are established, only one questionable situation remains, i.e., stenosis of 90 per cent, in which the lumen is narrowed by more than three fourths but is not quite reduced to an almost invisible thread (and appears to be about one tenth the size of the original lumen).

A number of approaches and methods for defining the severity of an obstructive lesion have been proposed by various authors. Our classification, adopted by the Ad Hoc Committee on Grading of Coronary Arterial Disease of the American Heart Association, is as follows (Fig. 10–54)[94]:

Normal—Lumen appears perfectly smooth and even; no restriction, indentation, loss of density, or sudden bulging.
25%—Lumen diameter is reduced *by* one fourth its former width.
50%—Lumen diameter is reduced *to* one half its former width.
75%—Lumen diameter is reduced *to* one fourth its former width.
90%—Lumen appears to be reduced to about one tenth its former diameter.
"99%"*—Lumen appears to be almost totally obliterated but some contrast still passes through the obstruction.
Occlusion—Total obstruction of a vessel without any filling of the distal segment from the proximal portion.

The current method of classifying patients with coronary artery disease as having single-, double-, and triple-vessel involvement does not anticipate changes in the natural history of the disease that may occur spontaneously or that could be achieved with a different treatment modality, such as with medical or surgical therapy. The profound difference that exists between 99 per cent obstruction of the proximal left anterior descending artery and 75 per cent obstruction of its apical segment is indisputable, yet both lesions are included in the category of single-vessel disease. Therefore, it is widely recognized that a method that assigns a different severity score depending on the degree of luminal narrowing and the geographical importance of its location would be desirable. A scoring technique which received some recognition was that of Friesinger et al., in which each of the three main coronary trunks was given a score from zero to five, depending on whether the vessel was normal or showed progressively severe changes.[95] Unfortunately, Freisinger's score did not distinguish between proximal and distal lesions or between a lesion of a branch and that of its parent vessel.

_____

*"99%," as used here to describe a degree of luminal narrowing, merely indicates the greatest reduction in lumen diameter detectable with our image intensifier short of vessel separation and is not intended to be mathematically accurate. A simple calculation would show that even when starting with a very large lumen (e.g., 4 mm in diameter), the narrowest segment still identifiable (100 μ) with a cesium iodide image intensifier and 35-mm film would be equivalent to a 97.5 per cent diameter reduction. Thus, "99 per cent" is written in quotes.

Several years ago, recognizing these shortcomings, the author devised a system that takes into consideration the geometrically increasing severity of lesions, the cumulative effects of multiple obstructions, the significance of their locations, the modifying influence of the collaterals, the size and quality of the distal vessel, and the importance of the status of myocardial function.[9] This system requires no additional effort or calculation on the part of the arteriographer, once the location and the severity of each lesion, the presence of collaterals, and the suitability of a graft have been properly scored on a computer card or with the aid of a small keyboard. The fundamental concept forming the basis of this system is the hypothesis that the severity of coronary artery disease must be regarded as a consequence of the functional significance of the vascular narrowing and the extent of the area perfused by the involved vessel or vessels; the presence of an effective coronary collateral circulation may, on the other hand, modify the functional significance of a severe obstruction or occlusion.

The percentage of reduction in lumen diameter (from 0 to 100 per cent) is assigned a degree of severity (called ischemia numerical grade, or ING) from 1 to 32 (Fig. 10–54), each grade being twice as large as the previous one. Using this method, the ING of a "99 per cent" obstruction, for example, is 16 times greater than the one corresponding to a 25 per cent reduction of lumen diameter, a fact in keeping with Poiseuille's law as well as with clinical observation. Just as it is only too obvious that a 90 per cent obstruction is far more severe than a 25 per cent one, it would similarly be illogical to give to 90 per cent stenosis of the main left coronary artery the same "weight" as that assigned to 90 per cent obstruction of the terminal segment of the circumflex coronary artery. Accordingly, the left ventricular myocardium is divided into nine myocardial perfusion areas (MAP's), each receiving its blood supply from a well-defined coronary branch. MAP's are assigned a numerical value of either 0.5 or 1.0, depending on size. Each MAP thus becomes a multiplying factor to be used in the final equation. The value of this multiplying factor and the distribution of the nine MAP's are shown in Figure 10–55. The severity of coronary artery disease equals the MAP multiplied by ING (MAP per ING, or MAPpING). A proximal lesion involves all dependent MAP's. If multiple lesions are present in the same vessel, the ING's are added to a maximum of 32. When collateral circulation (CC) is present, a lower ING is used; in other words, the computer utilizes a formula that takes into consideration the contribution of col-

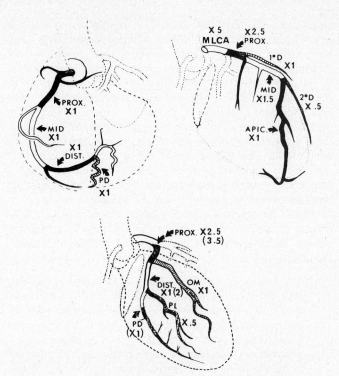

FIGURE 10–55 The principal vascular segments (from left to right) of the right coronary artery, left anterior descending branch, and circumflex. Each segment is followed by a multiplying factor (e.g., X1, X2.5, etc.) to indicate the functional significance of the area supplied by that segment. The numbers shown are based on an "average" coronary circulation but may differ depending on the relative quantities of myocardium perfused by the vessel in question. PROX = proximal segment; MID = midsegment; DIST = distal segment; PD = posterior descending branch; MLCA = main left coronary artery; 1°D = first diagonal; 2°D = second diagonal; APIC = apical; OM = obtuse marginal branch; PL = posterolateral. (From Gensini, G. G.: Coronary Arteriography. Mount Kisco, N.Y., Futura Publishing Co., 1975.)

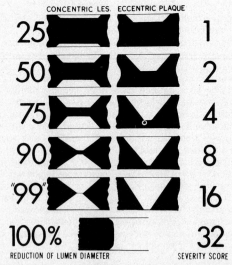

CONCENTRIC LES.   ECCENTRIC PLAQUE

25   1
50   2
75   4
90   8
"99"   16
100%   32

REDUCTION OF LUMEN DIAMETER   SEVERITY SCORE

FIGURE 10–54 The roentgenographic appearance of concentric lesions and eccentric plaques resulting in 25, 50, 75, 90, and "99" per cent obstruction as well as complete (100 per cent) occlusion. The column on the right indicates the relative severity of these lesions using a score of 1 for the 25 per cent obstruction and doubling that number as the severity of these obstructions progresses according to the reduction of lumen diameter (left column). (From Gensini, G. G.: Coronary Arteriography. Mount Kisco, N.Y., Futura Publishing Co., 1975.)

lateral blood flow to a myocardial perfusion area beyond a severe obstruction or occlusion. This formula proportionally reduces the score of an occlusion or of a severe obstruction according to the quality of reopacification achieved by the collateral channels and the integrity of the distal segment.

After the scores for each segment of the arteries have been calculated, they are added together to produce a severity score per artery; these scores are then added to obtain a total score for the entire coronary system. The final score is obtained by leaving the arterial score unchanged when the ejection fraction (EF) is normal or by adding a progressively larger number (from 20 to 80) for progressively more severe reductions of ejection fraction.[9]

Although this method may not be ideal, it provides more useful information than the simple division of patients into single-, double-, and triple-vessel disease. The advantages of this scoring method are as follows:

1. It provides an accurate stratification of patients according to the functional significance of their disease.[96]
2. It lends itself to computer elaboration, storage, retrieval, and analysis.
3. It provides an opportunity to match patients with similar degrees of coronary artery disease but who are receiving different forms of treatment.
4. It allows for continuous, microprocessor-assisted studies of interobserver and intraobserver variability. Computer hardware and software to elaborate and store this type of information are readily available and are inexpensive.

PITFALLS OF CORONARY ARTERIOGRAPHY

Judkins has properly called attention to "an unheralded complication of coronary arteriography that is frequently overlooked but equal in importance to the most severe . . . the incomplete or nondiagnostic study."[37] Another similarly unheralded "complication" of coronary arteriography is the misinterpretation of the arteriogram,[96a,96b] whether the result of inadequate training, inadequate views, honest mistakes, or limitations of the technique itself.

The following list presents some of the most common problems leading to inappropriate conclusions in the evaluation of coronary arteriograms.

Operator-Related Sources of Error

Iatrogenically Induced Coronary Spasm. The presence of an obstruction immediately distal to the tip of the catheter should suggest the possibility of catheter-induced spasm, especially if the catheter was pushed deeply into a main vessel or became wedged in a small branch vessel. Opacification should be repeated after the vessel in question is not entered for at least 15 minutes and nitroglycerin or isosorbide dinitrate[24,25] has been administered to the patient. In questionable cases, opacification may have to be repeated during an adequate sinus flush injection to exclude the effect of additional catheter manipulation on a potentially hyperactive area of the vessel.

Iatrogenically induced spasm appears more frequently (3 per cent of all cases studied in our laboratory) during catheterization of the right coronary artery, probably because deep penetration by the catheter occurs more easily in this artery. A similar phenomenon involving the main left coronary artery is very rare; we have seen it only once in over 3000 coronary arteriograms.

The following features are typical of iatrogenically induced spasm:
— localization to the initial segment of the right coronary artery, at or within a few millimeters from the catheter
— no apparent hindrance to blood flow
— no association with pain or with ST-segment changes
— tendency to disappear spontaneously within 10 to 20 minutes, provided that the catheter is removed from the coronary artery; spasm may disappear more rapidly with nitroglycerin or isosorbide dinitrate, even though dilatation of the unaffected segment may occur prior to disappearance of the constricting area
— negative ergonovine test

Inadequate Force of Injection. Weak, hesitant injections should be avoided; they provide little information and may lead to misinterpretation. Slow, laminar flow into the injected vessel may result in incomplete mixing and layering[97] of contrast agent and blood. The separation between the two streams may then give the false appearance of luminal narrowing when, in fact, no narrowing exists. If flow into the injected vessel is too rapid, the trickle of contrast agent dripping out of the catheter is quickly swept away with each heart cycle, never *fully* opacifying the vessel under study and occasionally even *failing* to opacify some important branches.

Fixed Number and/or Angle of Projection. The use of fixed anteroposterior and lateral views in coronary arteriography is inappropriate; multiple projections, including hemiaxial views (see p. 308), are necessary to eliminate (or at least minimize) confusion arising because of superimposition, foreshortening, and doubling-up of vessels. During the course of the procedure, the operator should be aware of the specific requirements of the individual set of arteries under study and must vary the number of injections and the angle of obliquity accordingly. Careful attention must be paid to the following segments of vessels: main left coronary artery, initial segment of the left anterior descending artery (Fig. 10–56), the initial segment of the circumflex artery, the first diagonal branch, and the initial segment of the obtuse marginal branch.

Superimposition of The Diaphragm (and Underexposure of the Corresponding Area of Myocardium). This combination results in inadequate visualization of the distal segment and branches of the right coronary artery (and/or of the circumflex) (Fig. 10–57). Severe narrowings may be easily missed, with dire consequences for the patient.

Superselective Catheterization of Branches of Either Left or Right Coronary Artery. In a small number of cases, the main left coronary artery is very short and quickly divides into the anterior descending and the circumflex branches. In a few cases, the main stem is totally missing, and the two arteries originate either from a very short funnel or directly from two separate ostia. These anatomical variations almost invariably lead to the superselective catheterization of either the anterior descending or the circumflex branch. This problem may occur even with main left coronary arteries of normal length. Sometimes the catheter may slip into a secondary branch, such as the obtuse marginal or the diagonal. On the right side, it is possible to enter a conus branch that has a separate ostium or a right ventricular branch, thereby inadvertently preventing opacification of the main stem. Superselective catheterization of branches may be performed intentionally for special reasons, but the unnecessary use of this technique is dangerous for two reasons: first, it may lead to ventricular fibrillation if the amount of contrast agent injected is too large relative to vessel size and flow, and, second, an undetected superselective injection may be mistakenly interpreted as an occlusion of the other branch or branches (Fig. 10–58).

Mistaking a Vein for a Coronary Artery (and Vice Versa).[98] This should be an extremely rare situation. Two conditions, however, may create some confusion: one condition is the forceful injection of the contrast agent through a catheter wedged into a branch (see Superselective Catheterization above), so that the vein draining that segment will be promptly filled; the second condition is encountered when an occluded coronary artery is filled late by collateral circulation, while a normally perfused, adjoining segment is draining the contrast agent in the venous system. In the first situation, a vein may appear to be an artery, whereas in the second, an artery may be mistaken for a vein.

Artifactual Demonstration of Collateral Channels. This is another possible pitfall stemming from forceful injection with the catheter in a wedged position.[97,99]

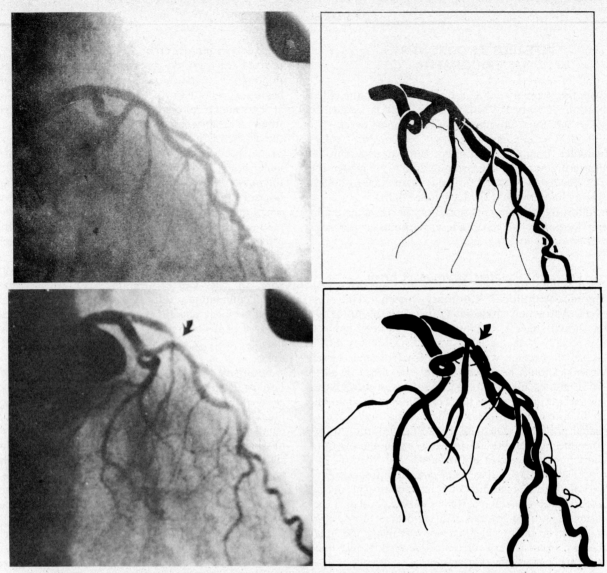

FIGURE 10–56 *Top,* RAO view of left coronary artery shows superimposition of left anterior descending and obtuse marginal branch of circumflex. *Bottom,* Slightly different view uncovers severe narrowing of left anterior descending at level of first septal branch (arrow). (From Gensini, G. G.: Coronary Arteriography. Mount Kisco, N.Y., Futura Publishing Co., 1975.)

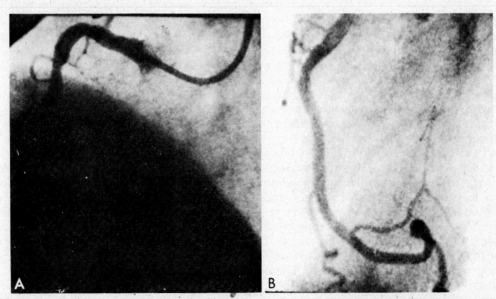

FIGURE 10–57 *A,* Superimposition of diaphragm. *B,* Clear view of obscured vessels obtained with deep inspiration. (From Gensini, G. G.: Coronary Arteriography. Mount Kisco, N.Y., Futura Publishing Co., 1975.)

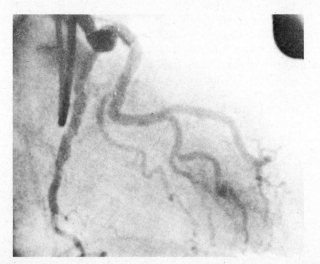

FIGURE 10–58 Left coronary artery, right anterior oblique view. Apparent total occlusion of left anterior descending branch resulting from superselective injection into the circumflex artery. (From Gensini, G. G.: Coronary Arteriography. Mount Kisco, N.Y., Futura Publishing Co., 1975.)

Patient-Related Sources of Error

MYOCARDIAL BRIDGES.[98,100–107] Casual analysis of the arteriogram may lead to the erroneous diagnosis of organic narrowing if the rhythmic changes of the vessel dimensions are overlooked. This error is not likely to occur with cine techniques, especially when the differences between the systolic and the diastolic appearance of the vessel (and therefore the presumed organic lesion) are most pronounced (Fig. 10–45).

Anomalous Origin of a Coronary Artery.[97,102] An anomaly occurring in slightly less than 1 per cent of cases is the origin of the circumflex coronary artery from either the right coronary artery (Fig. 10–59) or the right sinus of Valsalva. Failure to opacify such an anomalous vessel is more likely to occur when there is a separate ostium in the right sinus of Valsalva. However, even when the circumflex is a branch of the right coronary artery, its point of origin is very close to the ostium, and thus slightly deeper penetration of the catheter into the main trunk may lead to failure of visualization (or poor visualization) of the anomalous branch. Overlooking the existence of the right-sided circumflex may then lead to the incorrect diagnosis of occlusion of this artery.

Another relatively common anomaly is the high origin of either the right or the left coronary arteries. In these cases, exploration of the respective sinuses with the catheter will fail to opacify the displaced ostium, since it lies well above the sinuses. Rarer anomalies include (1) origin of the main left coronary artery from either the right sinus of Valsalva or the right coronary artery; (2) origin of the left anterior descending coronary artery from the right sinus of Valsalva; (3) origin of all three coronary arteries from either the right or left sinus of Valsalva via two or three distinct ostia; and (4) a single coronary artery. A variety of anatomical arrangements is possible with the latter anomaly, but the most important clinically is the type in which the left coronary artery originates from either the right sinus of Valsalva or the proximal portion of the right

coronary artery and passes between the right ventricular outflow tract and the aorta to reach the left atrioventricular groove. This anomaly may be associated with sudden death.

Unusual Predominance of Right or Left Coronary Artery. Perhaps one of the most common variations is the total preponderance of the left coronary artery. In such cases, the right coronary artery provides only the most proximal atrial and right ventricular branches and sometimes does not even reach the acute margin of the heart. This anatomical variation should not be confused with the results of coronary occlusion.

A slightly more confusing anomaly is the overwhelming predominance of the right coronary artery, extending either over the apex and anterior surface of the left ventricle or over the lateral wall or both. In the first instance, the posterior descending artery continues well beyond its usual area of distribution along the posterior interventricular groove, encircles the apex, and distributes along the inferior third of the anterior interventricular groove. In these cases, an occlusion of the posterior descending artery will affect a much larger area of the interventricular septum

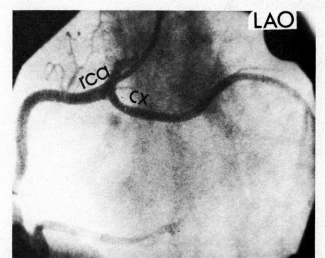

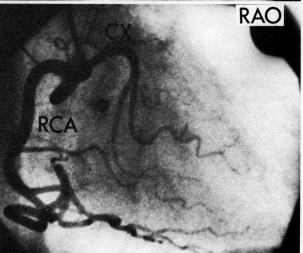

FIGURE 10–59 Left anterior oblique view (*top*) and right anterior oblique view (*bottom*) of right coronary artery (RCA) giving origin to anomalous circumflex (CX).

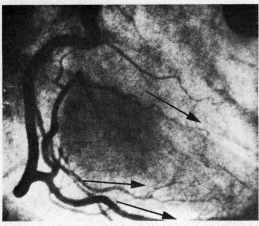

FIGURE 10–60 Right anterior oblique view showing exceptional predominance of right coronary artery sending branches to entire posterolateral and left marginal surface of left ventricle (arrows). (From Gensini, G. G.: Coronary Arteriography. Mount Kisco, N.Y., Futura Publishing Co., 1975.)

and *may* be accompanied by electrocardiographic evidence of diaphragmatic *and* apical infarction or ischemia (and possibly even anterior infarction or ischemia). Misinterpretation of this pattern may conceivably lead to a fruitless search for a possible site for an anterior descending graft, whereas a right-sided graft would be the only one needed. In the second instance, the right coronary artery continues well beyond the left ventricular segments adjoining the posterior interventricular septum and supplies the entire posterolateral and left marginal surface of the left ventricle (Fig. 10–60). Thus, in these patients the left circumflex is expected to be quite small or absent. Absent or incomplete visualization of these branches would be the consequence of a lesion of the right coronary artery rather than of the circumflex branch.

Unrecognized Total "Amputation" of a Coronary Branch. According to Paulin, "the most difficult situation for angiographic assessment is the complete amputation of a coronary branch exactly at the site of its origin and in the absence of any collateral filling of its distal extension. We have seen this occur with regard to the left anterior descending artery: casual scrutiny of the films may lead to misinterpretation, and both a large septal artery and a large side branch to the anterolateral aspect of the left ventricular wall may be confused with it. Do not accept an artery which does not show the typical curve at the apex of the heart as being the left anterior descending before visualization of the corresponding increased extension of the posterior branches indicates the presence of variation."[97] Similar situations may occur with one of the diagonal branches of the left anterior descending artery, with the marginal and posterolateral branches of the circumflex, and with the right or the left ventricular branches of the right coronary artery. Unexplained gaps between their areas of distribution must be critically questioned and repeatedly inspected. Occasionally, minute collateral channels will be identified upon repeated and careful scrutiny; at other times, identification of abnormal segmental wall motion in the area of the gap may be more than adequate "circumstantial" evidence to suspect such a flush occlusion. Other possible causes of error in coronary arteriography include:[109]

1. Absence or early bifurcation of the main left coronary artery, leading to nonvisualization of one of its branches.

2. Superimposition of the main left coronary artery branches masking a proximal lesion.

3. Injection beyond a stenosis of the main left coronary artery, thereby overlooking that lesion.

4. Eccentricity of and/or crescent-shaped stenoses, leading to underestimation of their severity.

5. Separate origin of the conus artery, leading to underestimation of the collateral supply and failure to recognize the distal patency of an occluded left anterior descending artery.

6. Partial recanalization of an occluding thrombus, thereby interpreting as stenosis a chronically or acutely recanalized thrombus.

Anomalies of the coronary arteries can be divided into those affecting myocardial perfusion and those that do not affect perfusion. Among those that affect coronary perfusion are:

1. Coronary artery fistulas. These anomalies, from a coronary artery to any of the four cardiac chambers or the pulmonary artery, may range in size from insignificant to large.

2. Origin of left coronary artery from pulmonary artery.

3. Congenital coronary atresia.

4. Origin of left coronary artery from the right sinus of Valsalva.

Anomalies usually not altering myocardial perfusion include:

1. Origin of the circumflex coronary artery from the right sinus of Valsalva.

2. Origin of the left anterior descending artery from the right sinus of Valsalva (rare).

3. Single coronary artery.

4. Origin of all coronary arteries from one sinus of Valsalva.

5. "Horseshoe coronary artery" with ostia in the left and right sinus of Valsalva.[111]

6. Origin of one or both coronary arteries from above the sinuses of Valsalva.

References

1. Radner, S.: Attempt at roentgenologic visualization of coronary blood vessels in man. Acta Radiol. 26:497, 1945.
2. Gensini, G. G.: Coronary Arteriography. Mount Kisco, N.Y., Futura Publishing Co., 1975, p. 261.
3. Sones, F. M., Jr.: Acquired heart disease: Symposium on present and future of cineangiocardiography. Am. J. Cardiol. 3:710, 1959.
4. Sones, F. M., Jr., and Shirey, E. K.: Cine coronary arteriography. Mod. Concepts Cardiovasc. Dis. 31:735, 1962.
5. Ricketts, H. J., and Abrams, H. L.: Percutaneous selective coronary cine arteriography. J.A.M.A. 181:620, 1962.
6. Judkins, M. P.: Selective coronary arteriography: A percutaneous transfemoral technic. Radiology 89:815, 1967.
7. Amplatz, K., Formanek, G., Stanger, P., and Wilson, W.: Mechanics of selective coronary artery catheterization via femoral approach. Radiology 89:1040, 1967.
8. Bourassa, M. G., Lesperance, J., and Campeau, L.: Selective coronary arteriography by the percutaneous femoral artery approach. Am. J. Roentgenol. 107:377, 1969.
9. Wells, D. E., Befeler, B., Winkler, J. B., Myerburg, R. J., Castellanos, A., and Castillo, C. A.: A simplified method for left heart catheterization including coronary arteriography. Chest 63:959, 1973.
10. Goldstein, R. E., Karsh, R. B., Smith, E. R., Orland, M., Norman, D., Farnham, G., Redwood, D. R., and Epstein, S. E.: Influence of atropine and of vagally mediated bradycardia on the occurrence of ventricular arrhythmias following acute coronary occlusion in closed-chest dogs. Circulation 47:1180, 1973.

11. Massumi, R. A., Mason, D. T., Amsterdam, E. A., DeMaria, A., Miller, R. R., Scheinman, M. M., and Zelis, R.: Ventricular fibrillation and tachycardia after intravenous atropine for treatment of bradycardias. N. Engl. J. Med. *287*: 336, 1972.

12. Webb, S. W., Adgey, A. A. J., and Pantridge, J. F.: Autonomic disturbance at onset of acute myocardial infarction. Br. Med. J. *3*:89, 1972.

13. Paulin, S.: Tilted view in cardiac angiography. Medicamundi *24*:2, 1979.

14. Gensini, G. G.: Patterns of ventricular contractions and myocardial contractility in the intact animal and man: Effects of ISDN. *In* Gensini, G. G.: The Study of the Systemic, Coronary and Myocardial Effects of Nitrates. Springfield, Ill., Charles C Thomas, 1972.

15. Helfant, R. H., Pine, R., Meister, S. G., Feldman, M. S., Trout, R. G., and Banka, V. S.: Nitroglycerin to unmask reversible asynergy: Correlation with post coronary bypass ventriculography. Circulation *50*:694, 1974.

16. Gensini, G. G., Dubiel, J., Huntington, P. P., and Kelly, A. E.: Left ventricular end-diastolic pressure before and after coronary arteriography. Am. J. Cardiol. *27*:453, 1971.

17. Bunnell, I. L., Greene, D. G., Tandon, R. N., and Arani, D. T.: The half-axial projection: A new look at the proximal left coronary artery. Circulation *48*: 1151, 1972.

18. Sos, T. A., Lee, J. G., Levin, D. C., and Baltaxe, H. A.: New lordotic projection for improved visualization of the left coronary artery and its branches. Am. J. Roentgenol. *121*:575, 1974.

19. Lesperance, J., Saltiel, J., Petitclerc, R., and Bourassa, M. G.: Angulated views in the sagittal plane for improved accuracy of cinecoronary angiography. Am. J. Roentgenol. *121*:565, 1974.

20. Aldridge, H. E., McLoughlin, M. J., and Taylor, K. W.: Improved diagnosis in coronary cinearteriography with routine use of 110° oblique views and cranial and caudal angulations: Comparison with standard oblique views in 100 patients. Am. J. Cardiol. *36*:568, 1975.

21. Arani, D. T., Bunnell, I. L., and Green, D. G.: Lordotic right posterior oblique projection of the left coronary artery. A special view for special anatomy. Circulation *52*:504, 1975.

22. Paulin, S.: Terminology for radiographic projection in cardiac angiography. Cathet. Cardiovasc. Diagn. *7*:341, 1981.

23. Gensini, G. G., Kelly, A. E., DaCosta, B. C. B., and Huntington, P. P.: Quantitative angiography: The measurement of coronary vasomobility in the intact animal and man. Chest *60*:522, 1971.

24. Gensini, G. G., DiGiorgi, S., Murad-Netto, S., and Black, A.: Arteriographic demonstration of coronary artery spasm and its release after the use of a vasodilator in a case of angina pectoris and in the experimental animal. Angiology *13*:550, 1962.

25. Esente, P., Giambartolomei, A., and Gensini, G. G.: The use of injectable nitroglycerin in the cardiac catheterization laboratory. Angiology *33*:319, 1982.

26. Seldinger, S. I.: Catheter replacement of the needle in percutaneous arteriography: A new technique. Acta Radiol. *39*:368, 1953.

27. Dotter, C. T., and Gensini, G. G.: Percutaneous retrograde catheterization of left ventricular and systemic arteries of man. Radiology *75*:885, 1960.

28. Gensini, G. G.: A new Teflon catheter for percutaneous catheterization and contrast material injection. Radiology *81*:939, 1963.

29. Coronary Artery Bypass Surgery: NCHCT Technology Assessment Forum. J.A.M.A. *246*:1645, 1981.

30. N.Y. State Dept. of Health, Cardiac Diagnostic Center, 1981.

31. Adams, D. F., and Abrams, H. L.: Complications of coronary arteriography: A follow-up report. Cardiovasc. Radiol. *2*:89, 1979.

32. Erikson, V., Helmius, G., and Savada, S.: Complications of coronary arteriography. Acta Radiol. [Diagn.] (Stockh.) *22*(5):535, 1981.

33. Kennedy, J. W., et al.: Complications associated with cardiac catheterization and angiography. Cathet. Cardiovasc. Diagn. *8*:5, 1982.

34. Kennedy, J. W., et al.: Mortality related to cardiac catheterization and angiography. Cathet. Cardiovasc. Diagn. *8*:323, 1982.

35. Schlant, R. C., Abrams, H. L., Gensini, G. G., and Mullins, C. B.: Indications for and hazards of coronary arteriography (Panel). Am. J. Cardiol. *29*:139, 1973.

36. Hildner, F. J., Javier, R. P., Ranaswany, K., and Samet, P.: Pseudo complications of cardiac catheterization. Chest *63*:15, 1973.

37. Judkins, M. P., and Gander, M. P.: Prevention of complications of coronary arteriography (Editorial). Circulation *49*:599, 1974.

38. Sones, F. M., Jr.: Indications and value of coronary arteriography. *In* Halonen, P., and Louhija, A. (eds.): Advances in Cardiology. Early Diagnosis of Coronary Heart Disease. Basel, S. Karger, 1973.

39. Gensini, G. G.: Indications for cardiac catheterization, angiography and coronary arteriography. Geriatrics *30*:63, 1975.

40. James, T. N.: Anatomy of the Coronary Arteries. New York, Paul B. Hoeber, 1961.

41. McAlpine, W.: Heart and Coronary Arteries. New York, Springer-Verlag, 1975.

42. MacAlpin, R. N., Abassi, A. S., Grollman, J. H., and Eber, L.: Human coronary artery size during life. Circulation *46*(Suppl. II):6, 1972.

43. Elliott, L. P., Green, C. E., Rogers, W. J., Mantle, J. A., Papapietro, S. E., Hood, W. P., and Russell, R. O.: Advantage of cranial-right anterior oblique view in diagnosing mid left anterior descending and distal right coronary artery disease. Am. J. Cardiol. *48*:754, 1981.

44. Bianchi, A.: Morfologia dellearteriae coronariae cordis. Arch. Ital. Anat. Embriol. *3*:87, 1904.

45. Spalteholz, W.: Die Arterien der Herzwand. Leipzig, Hirzel, 1924.

46. Schlesinger, M. J.: Relation of anatomic pattern to pathologic conditions of the coronary arteries. Arch. Pathol. *30*:403, 1940.

47. Elliott, L. P., Bream, P. R., Soto, B., Russell, R. O., Rogers, W. J., Mantle, J. A., and Hood, W. P.: Significance of caudal left-anterior-oblique view in analyzing the left main coronary artery and its major branches. Radiology *139*: 39, 1981.

48. Miller, R. A., Warkentin, D. L., Felix, W. G., Hashemian, M., and Leighton, R.: Angulated views in coronary angiography. Am. J. Roentgenol. *134*:407, 1980.

49. Aldridge, H. E.: Special projections. Cleveland Clin. Q. *47*:145, 1980.

50. Guthaner, D., and Wexler, L.: New aspects of coronary angiography. Radiol. Clin. North Am. *18*:501, 1980.

51. Elliott, L. P., Green, C. E., Rogers, W. J., Mantle, J. A., Papapietro, S., and Hood, W. P.: The importance of angled right oblique views in improving visualization of the coronary arteries. Part I: Caudocranial view. Radiology *142*:631, 1982. Part II: Craniocaudal view. Radiology *142*:637, 1982.

52. Vieussens, R.: Nouvelles decouvertes sur le coeur. Paris, 1706.

53. Gould, S. E. (ed.): Pathology of the Heart. 2nd ed. Springfield, Ill., Charles C Thomas, 1960, p. 559.

54. Lansing, A. I.: Experimental studies on arteriosclerosis. *In* Symposium on Atherosclerosis. Publication No. 338. Washington, D.C., National Academy of Sciences, National Research Council, 1954, p. 50.

55. Gensini, G. G., and Kelly, A. E.: Incidence and progression of coronary artery disease. An angiographic correlation in 1,263 patients. Arch. Intern. Med. *129*: 814, 1972.

56. Kimbiris, D., Lavine, P., VanDenBroek, H., Najmi, M., and Likoff, W.: Devolutionary pattern of coronary atherosclerosis in patients with angina pectoris. Coronary arteriographic studies. Am. J. Cardiol. *33*:7, 1974.

57. Marchandise, B., et al.: Angiographic evaluation of natural history of normal coronary arteries and mild coronary atherosclerosis. Am. J. Cardiol. *41*:216, 1978.

58. Baroldi, G., and Scomazzoni, G.: Coronary circulation in the normal and the pathologic heart. Washington, D.C., Office of the Surgeon General, Department of the Army, 1967.

59. Classification of atherosclerotic lesions. Report of a study group. Definition of terms. W.H.O. Tech. Rep. Ser. *143*:4, 1958.

60. Vlodaver, A., and Edwards, J. E.: Pathology of coronary atherosclerosis. Progr. Cardiovasc. Dis. *14*:256, 1971.

61. Roberts, W. C.: Coronary arteries in fatal acute myocardial infarction. Circulation *45*:215, 1972.

62. Esente, P., Gensini, G. G., Huntington, P. P., Kelly, A. E., and Black, A.: Left ventricular aneurysm without coronary artery obstruction or occlusion. Am. J. Cardiol. *34*:658, 1974.

63. Roberts, W. C.: Does thrombosis play a major role in the development of symptom-producing atherosclerotic plaques? Circulation *48*:1161, 1973.

64. Gensini, G. G., and DaCosta, B. C. B.: The coronary collateral circulation in living man. Am. J. Cardiol. *24*:393, 1969.

65. Heupler, F. A., Proudfit, W. L., Razavi, M., Shirey, E. K., Greenstreet, R., and Sheldon, W. C.: Ergonovine maleate provocative test for coronary arterial spasm. Am. J. Cardiol. *41*:631, 1978.

66. Heupler, F. A.: Provocative testing for coronary arterial spasm: Risk, method and rationale (Editorial). Am. J. Cardiol. *46*:335, 1980.

67. Prinzmetal, M., et al.: Angina pectoris: I. A variant form of angina pectoris: Preliminary report. Am. J. Med. *27*:375, 1959.

68. Gensini, G. G., et al.: The coronary circulation: An experimental and clinical study. Proc. IV Congreso Mundial de Cardiologia. Mexico City, 1963, p. 325.

69. Maseri, A., Mimmo, R., Chierchia, S., Marchesi, C., Pesola, A., and L'Abbate, A.: Coronary artery spasm as a cause of acute myocardial ischemia in man. Chest *68*:625, 1975.

70. Stein, I.: Observations on the action of ergonovine on the coronary circulation and its use in the diagnosis of coronary artery insufficiency. Am. Heart J. *37*: 36, 1949.

71. Helfant, R. H.: Coronary arterial spasm and provocative testing in ischemic heart disease. Am. J. Cardiol. *41*:787, 1978.

72. Maseri, A., L'Abbate, A., Barold, G., Chierchia, S., Marzilli, M., Ballestra, A. M., Severi, S., Parodi, O., Biagini, A., Distante, A., and Pesola, A.: Coronary vasospasm as a possible cause of myocardial infarction. A conclusion derived from the study of "preinfarction" angina. N. Engl. J. Med. *299*:1271, 1978.

73. Buxton, A., Goldberg, S., Hirshfeld, J. W. et al.: Refractory ergonovine-induced coronary vasospasm: Importance of intracoronary nitroglycerin. Am. J. Cardiol. *46*:329, 1980.

74. Rentrop, P., Blanke, H., and Wiegand, K. R.: Wiedereroffnung verschossener Kranzgefasse im akuten Infarkt mit Hilfe von Kathetern (Transluminale Rekanalisation). Dtsch. Med. Wochenschr. *104*:1401, 1979.

75. Rentrop, P., Blanke, H., and Kostering, K.: Acute myocardial infarction: Intracoronary application of nitroglycerin and streptokinase in combination with transluminal recanalization. Clin. Cardiol. *2*:534, 1979.

76. Rentrop, P., Blanke, H., and Karsch, K. R.: Selective intracoronary thrombolysis in acute myocardial infarction. Circulation *63*:307, 1981.

77. DeWood, M. A., Spores, J., and Notske, R.: Prevalence of total coronary occlusion during the early hours of transmural M.I. N. Engl. J. Med. *303*:897, 1980.

78. Leinbach, R. C., and Gold, H. K.: Coronary angiography during acute myocardial infarction: A search for spasm. Am. Heart J. *103*:768, 1982.

79. Chazov, E. I., and Andreyenko, G. V.: A pilot study of thrombosis therapy with soviet-made fibrinolysin. Kardiologia *4*:59, 1962 (see Ref. #82).

80. Chazov, E. I.: Actual problems and prospect of therapy of M.I. and its complications. Kardiologia 5:3, 1965.

81. Chazov, E. I., Matveeva, L. S., Mazaev, A. V., et al.: Intracoronary administration of fibrinolysin in acute M.I. Ter. Arkh. 4:8, 1976 (see Ref. # 82).

82. Chazov, E. I., and Lakin, K. M.: Anticoagulants and fibrinolytics. Chicago, Yearbook Medical Publisher, 1980.

83. Mazur, N. A.: The use of streptokinase in patients with M.I. Ter. Arkh. 38:93, 1966 (see Ref. #82).

84. Dotter, C. T., Rosch, J., and Seaman, A. J.: Selective clot lysis with low-dose streptokinase. Radiology 111:31, 1974.

85. Ganz, W., Buchbinder, H., and Marcus, H.: Intracoronary thrombolysis in evolving myocardial infarction. Am. Heart J. 101:4, 1981.

86. Rentrop, P.: Mortality and functional changes after intracoronary streptokinase infusion. Circulation 66:II-335, 1982.

87. Schwarz, F., Schuler, G., and Katus, H.: Intracoronary thrombolysis in myocardial infarction: Duration of ischemia as a major determinant of late results after recanalization. Am. J. Cardiol. 50:933, 1982.

88. Herman, M. V., Gorlin, R., and Sonnenblick, E. H.: Ventricular motion studies in coronary artery disease. In Gensini, G. G. (ed.): The Study of the Systemic, Coronary and Myocardial Effects of Nitrates. Springfield, Ill., Charles C Thomas, 1972.

89. Herman, M. V., and Gorlin, R.: Implications of left ventricular asynergy. Am. J. Cardiol. 23:538, 1969.

90. Gould, K. L., and Lipscomb, K.: Effects of coronary stenoses on coronary flow reserve and resistance. Am. J. Cardiol. 34:48, 1974.

91. Gould, K. L., Lipscomb, K., and Hamilton, G. W.: Physiologic basis for assessing critical coronary stenosis: Instantaneous flow response and regional distribution during coronary hyperemia as measures of coronary flow reserve. Am. J. Cardiol. 33:87, 1974.

92. Bulkley, B. H., and Hutchins, G. M.: Myocardial consequences of coronary artery bypass surgery: A clinicopathological study of 53 patients. Am. J. Cardiol. 39:268, 1977.

93. Pigott, J. D., Kouchoukos, N. T., and Oberman, G.: Late results of medical and surgical therapy for patients with coronary artery disease and depressed ejection fraction. Circulation. 66:II-220, 1982.

94. American Heart Association Committee Report: A reporting system on patients evaluated for coronary artery disease. Circulation 51:7, 1975.

95. Friesinger, G. C., Humphries, J. O., and Ross, R. C.: Prognostic significance of coronary arteriography. In Kaltembach, M., Lichtlen, P., and Friesinger, G. C. (eds.): Coronary Heart Disease. Stuttgart, George Thieme Verlag, 1973.

96. Gensini, G. G., Giambartolomei, A., Esente, P., Archambault, T., and Shaw, C.: Natural history of coronary artery disease. Angiographic findings in 830 patients: Importance and significance of the angiographic coronary score. Circulation 66:II-369, 1982.

96a. Meier, B., Gruentzig, A. R., Goebel, N., Pyle, R., von Gosslar, W., and Schlumpf, M.: Assessment of stenoses in coronary angioplasty. Inter- and intraobserver variability. Int. J. Cardiol. 3:159, 1983.

96b. Zir, L. M.: Editorial Note: Observer variability in coronary angiography. Int. J. Cardiol. 3:171, 1983.

97. Paulin, S., and Schlossman, D.: Coronary angiography: Technique and normal anatomy. Crit. Rev. Clin. Radiol. Nucl. Med. 4:333, 1973.

98. Baltaxe, H. A., Amplatz, K., and Levin, D. C.: Coronary Angiography. Springfield, Ill., Charles C Thomas, 1973.

99. Sheldon, W. C.: On the significance of coronary collaterals. Am. J. Cardiol. 24:303, 1969.

100. Crainicianu, A.: Anatomische Studien uber die Coronararterien und experimentelle Untersuchunger uber ihre Durchgangigkeit. Virchows Arch. Pathol. Anat. 238:1, 1922.

101. Amplatz, K., and Anderson, R.: Angiographic appearance of myocardial bridging of the coronary artery. Invest. Radiol. 3:213, 1968.

102. Black, H. A., Manion, W. C., Mattingly, T. W., and Baroldi, G.: Coronary artery anomalies. Circulation 30:927, 1964.

103. Vladover, R. Z., Neufeld, H. N., and Edwards, J. E.: Pathology of coronary disease. Semin. Roentgenol. 7:4, 1952.

104. Edwards, J. E., Burnshides, C., Swarm, R. L., and Lansing, A. I.: Arteriosclerosis in the intramural and extramural portions of coronary arteries in the human heart. Circulation 13:235, 1956.

105. Geiringer, E.: The mural coronary. Am. Heart J. 41:359, 1951.

106. Polacek, P.: Relation of myocardial bridges and loops on the coronary arteries to coronary occlusions. Am. Heart J. 61:44, 1961.

107. Bloor, C. M., and Lowman, R. M.: Myocardial bridges in coronary angiography. Am. Heart J. 65:195, 1963.

108. Levin, D.: Pitfalls in coronary arteriography. In Abrams, H. L. (ed.): Coronary Arteriography. A Practical Approach. Boston, Little, Brown and Company, 1983.

109. Levin, D.: Anomalies and anatomic variations of the coronary arteries. In Abrams, H. L. (ed.): Coronary Arteriography. A Practical Approach. Boston, Little, Brown and Company, 1983.

110. Esente, P., Gensini, G., Giambartolomei, A., and Bernstein, D.: Bidirectional blood flow in angiographically normal coronary artery. Am. J. Cardiol., in press.

11

CARDIAC IMAGING

A—Nuclear Cardiology

by B. Leonard Holman, M.D.

GLOSSARY

Absorbed dose   The energy absorbed by the patient from the decay of the **radionuclide**; expressed in rads or millirads (1 rad = 100 ergs/g).

Algorithm   An explicitly defined process made up of a number of discrete steps or instructions; these instructions are frequently coded into computer languages (computer program, software).

Analog-to-digital conversion (ADC)   Conversion of continuous analog signals (voltages) to discrete digital information.

Annihilation photons   The two 511-kev **photons** emitted during **positron** decay; these photons are released in opposite directions (180-degree angle between photons).

Background   Any radiation coming from an undesired location, including radioactivity emanating from structures surrounding the organ of interest (target organ).

Beta rays   Nonpenetrating radiation (electrons) emitted during beta decay; ³H is a **radionuclide** that undergoes beta decay.

Characteristic x-rays   Low-energy photons released after electron capture (a type of radioactive decay); thallium-201 is an example of a **radionuclide** that decays by electron capture, and its characteristic x-rays are used for scintigraphic imaging.

Coincidence detection   Simultaneous detection of the two **annihilation photons** emitted during positron decay.

Collimator   The lens of the imaging system, absorbing photons traveling in inappropriate directions and originating from parts of the body other than the region under investigation; collimators are usually made of lead with holes to allow desired photons to pass through to the **crystal**.

(a) **Parallel-hole**   Collimator with thousands of holes in a lead-absorbing sheet. The holes are parallel to each other and perpendicular to the crystal (straight-bore) or at some other angle to the crystal (for example, at a 30-degree slant). Standard high-sensitivity and high-resolution collimators are types of parallel-hole collimators.

(b) **High-sensitivity**   A collimator designed to achieve high count rates by using large, short holes.

(c) **High-resolution**   A collimator designed to maximize spatial resolution by using small, long holes; as a result, sensitivity is reduced.

(d) **Pinhole**   Single-hole (2 to 8 mm in diameter) collimator in which the magnification and resolution increase with decreasing distance between patient and collimator; allows for high resolution but offers poor sensitivity.

(e) Converging A multihole collimator with holes that converge toward the center of the collimator; the field of view is compressed to encompass a small organ on a large crystal; allows for high resolution and high sensitivity.

(f) Cylindrical (single-bore) A central hole in a large mass of lead; used only with the scintillation probe.

(g) Multiple pinhole A collimator with multiple holes for acquiring tomographic images.

Compton scatter A change in the direction of travel of a photon due to an interaction between the photon and matter (the patient or the crystal); a major cause of loss of spatial resolution; presents most difficulty at lower photon energies.

Count(s) The disintegrations that the detector records. Counts/disintegrations represents the efficiency of the detector.

Count rate The number of counts recorded per unit of time (counts/min).

Crystal (sodium iodide scintillation) A high-density photon absorber that converts the energy of the incident photon to a number of light photons.

Cycle-length window The range of cardiac cycle times (R-R interval times) that will be accepted in a gated radionuclide ventriculogram.

Dead time The time required for the camera-computer system to recover after an interaction between a photon and the crystal; counts will not be recorded during this time (~ 5 μsec); the dead time determines the maximum count rate that can be accurately recorded.

Disintegration The radioactive decay of one atom.

Disintegration rate Number of disintegrations per unit of time (disintegrations/sec). The standard units are the curie (2.22×10^{12} disintegrations/min) and the millicurie (1 Ci = 1000 mCi).

Electron volts The unit of energy for the photon; usually expressed in thousands (kev) or millions (Mev) of electron volts (1 Mev = 1.6×10^{-6} erg).

Electronic cursor An electronic device for selecting a **region-of-interest** by manually defining the region on an oscilloscope or video display; light pens and joysticks are examples.

Emission tomography See **Tomography, emission**.

Frames The division of a dynamic study into discrete temporal units; for example, a radionuclide angiocardiogram can be collected at a rate of 20 frames per second.

Functional image, Parametric image An image in which intensity reflects a physiological parameter rather than activity; for example, intensity may be proportional to blood flow or to ejection fraction.

Gamma rays Electromagnetic waves with short wavelengths that originate from nuclear transitions; made up of photons capable of giving up energy in discrete interactions with matter.

Gating (physiological) Acquisition of data only during some physiological event. In cardiovascular applications, acquisition is usually gated to the cardiac cycle. Data may be acquired from the entire cardiac cycle by dividing the R-R interval into frames that represent counts acquired at preset time intervals after the R wave; prospective selection of frame intervals is termed **matrix mode**; retrospective selection is termed **list mode**.

Generator, radionuclide A device (usually an inorganic resin) through which a short-lived nuclide (the daughter) can be eluted (separated) from a long-lived parent (^{99}Mo$\rightarrow$^{99m}Tc, ^{113}Sn$\rightarrow$^{113m}In).

Half-life

(a) Physical The time necessary for the activity of a nuclide to decay to one-half its original activity (^{99m}Tc = 6 hours, ^{201}Tl = 73.1 hours).

(b) Biological The time necessary for the concentration of the tracer to fall to one-half its original concentration.

Isotope Different nuclides of the same element, having the same proton number but different mass numbers; for example, $^{11}_{6}$C, $^{12}_{6}$C, $^{13}_{6}$C, $^{14}_{6}$C are isotopes of carbon.

kev See **Electron volts**.

List mode **Acquisition of data from a dynamic study** in the form of a sequence of individual scintillation events which can then be re-formatted retrospectively into a variable number of **frames**.

Matrix The two-dimensional array into which positional data from the gamma camera are pigeonholed (32×32, 64×64, 128×128).

Matrix (histogram) mode Acquisition of data from a dynamic study such as a radionuclide angiocardiogram which can be re-formatted into a predefined number of **frames** and framing rate.

Mev See **Electron volts**.

Parametric image See **Functional image**.

Photon A packet of energy associated with electromagnetic radiation (gamma rays, x-rays, or light); the energy units are **electron volts** or kiloelectron volts (kev).

Photopeak The energy of the predominant photons released during decay of the **radionuclide** (^{99m}Tc = 140 kev, ^{201}Tl = 69 to 83 kev).

Pixel A single picture element in a digitized image; one of the **matrix** elements.

Positron A positively charged electron released during positron decay of a nucleus; interacts with an electron, transforming the mass of the electron and the positron into two 511-kev **annihilation photons**.

Pulse-height analyzer An electronic discriminator that selects those pulses arising from photons with energies approximating that of the **photopeak** and rejects pulses due to scattered radiation above and below the **photopeak**; the range of energies that are accepted constitutes the "window" of the analyzer.

Radionuclide An atom or species of atom with an unstable nucleus that will spontaneously decay to a more stable form, emitting radiation in the process; examples include thallium-201 (^{201}Tl), tantalum-178 (^{178}Ta), and technetium-99m (^{99m}Tc, where "Tc" is the abbreviation for the element technetium, "99" is its atomic mass, and "m" indicates the metastable state).

Reformat To rearrange retrospectively the parameters of a study; to convert **list mode** data to **matrix mode** data.

Region-of-interest The **pixels** or matrix elements of a digitized image (or series of images in a dynamic study) that outline a desired structure, organ, or region within the image; may be defined manually with an **electronic cursor**.

Resolution

(a) Spatial The ability of the detector to separate adjacent sources of activity.

(b) Temporal The maximum combination of framing rate and number of **frames** that can be acquired.

(c) Energy The ability of the detector to discriminate between photons of adjacent energies.

Scintigram An image of the distribution of radioactivity obtained with a **scintillation camera** after the internal administration of a **radionuclide**.

Scintigraphy The process of acquiring a **scintigram**.

Scintillation camera

(a) Single-crystal, Anger-type An imaging device with a single sodium iodide crystal with a 10- to 15-inch diameter and ¼- to ½-inch thickness; the detector records the spatial distribution of the internally administered radiotracer.

(b) Multicrystal An imaging with multiple crystals and a high count rate capability.

Scintillation probe A device that records radioactivity but does not provide positional or spatial information.

Time-activity curve A histogram (in the **matrix mode**) of the change in the count rate as a function of time.

Tomography, emission

(a) Transaxial Transverse-section reconstruction of the radionuclide distribution obtained by acquiring images or "slices" (about 1 to 2 cm in thickness) of the head or body; uses **coincidence detection** (positrons) or **single-photon detection** (nuclides such as ^{99m}Tc or ^{201}Tl).

(b) Limited angle Images obtained by focusing at varying depths within the organ of interest; the images maintain the same spatial orientation as do conventional images (the two-dimensional image is oriented parallel to the detector); can be obtained with standard **scintillation cameras** and specially designed **collimators**.

Radionuclide methods provide a safe, relatively atraumatic, often quantitative approach to assessing a variety of cardiac functions.[1] Their recent popularity can be attributed to the fact that they can be applied during exercise and other physiological and pharmacological interventions; they can be applied to very ill patients; they can provide a direct measure of cardiac function, myocardial blood flow, and metabolism; and they can provide quantitative landmarks to help evaluate the temporal progress of cardiac disease.

In this chapter, we will describe these methods, discussing first the required instrumentation and then the techniques used to assess cardiac wall motion and hemodynamics, myocardial perfusion, myocardial metabolism, and acute infarction and to detect pulmonary emboli.

INSTRUMENTATION

THE SCINTILLATION (ANGER, GAMMA) CAMERA

The scintillation camera provides a pictorial representation of the distribution of radioactivity. This device consists of a collimator, a position-sensitive detector (a large, flat sodium iodide crystal), and 37 to 91 photomultiplier tubes closely packed against the crystal. When gamma rays interact with the crystal, a portion of the gamma-ray energy is converted to light. The light is then converted into an electrical signal by the photomultiplier tubes. Electronically, the detector then calculates the position of the interaction and the energy of the gamma rays.

The *collimator* is analogous to a lens (Fig. 11–1). It is made from material that readily absorbs gamma rays, usually lead. The gamma rays can reach the crystal only by passing through the holes or channels of the collimator. The most common collimator is the *parallel-hole* collimator. Only gamma rays emitted from the patient in a direction perpendicular to the crystal can enter the detector. The diameter and length of the channels (holes) strongly affect the spatial resolution and sensitivity of the system. *High-resolution* parallel-hole collimators result in high spatial resolution at the expense of sensitivity, while *high-sensitivity* collimators result in an increase in count rate by a factor of two or three over high-resolution collimators but with a loss of resolution of about 25 per cent. A *general-purpose* collimator represents a compromise with regard to both resolution and sensitivity.

Multiple-hole collimators that diverge toward the patient are sometimes used to increase the field of view of the system (*diverging* collimators). Conversely, holes that converge toward the camera increase sensitivity with a smaller field of view (*converging* collimators). In a *slant-hole* collimator the holes are angled with respect to the detector, and the camera can obtain an oblique view with the detector flat against the chest.

A pinhole collimator can be used to magnify the image. It is considerably less sensitive than a parallel-hole collimator and is therefore used for imaging small organs. A collimator with several pinholes can be used to image an organ from several slightly different angles simultaneously to produce tomographic images.

For nuclear cardiology, a *general-purpose* collimator is used for time-dependent studies such as exercise thallium-201 and gated blood pool imaging. *High-resolution* collimators are generally used for studies obtained at rest. Recently a high-resolution, square-hole collimator has been introduced with increased sensitivity so that it may be used in time-dependent studies, such as during or after exercise. *High-sensitivity* collimators are used when the photon number is limited, as in first-pass radionuclide angiocardiography. *Slant-hole* collimators are used to maximize separation between atria and ventricles and to permit imaging along the long axis of the ventricles. *Seven-pinhole* collimators have been used for limited-angle tomography but offer no significant advantages.

The important performance parameters of the Anger scintillation camera are sensitivity, spatial resolution, field uniformity, energy resolution, and count-rate linearity. *Sensitivity* is defined as the number of recorded counts per gamma ray emitted from a radioactive tracer. The sensitivity of a gamma camera will depend on three principal factors: the gamma ray energy, the thickness of the crystal, and the collimator employed. *Spatial resolution* is a measure of the imaging system's ability to resolve small structural details in an object. One measure of resolution is the camera's response to a line source, expressed as the line spread function. Spatial resolution can be described in terms of the full-width at half-maximum, the width of the line spread function at 50 per cent of the maximum value.

The characteristics of the Anger camera, such as the thickness of the sodium iodide crystal, represent a compromise between sensitivity and spatial resolution. For example, a 12-mm (½ inch-thick) crystal will absorb 98 per cent of the 140 kev photons of technetium-99m and 100 per cent of the 68 to 82 kev photons of thallium-201. A 6-mm (¼ inch-thick) crystal will absorb 84 per cent of the 140 kev photons of technetium-99m and 100 per cent of the 68 to 82 kev photons of thallium-201. The intrinsic resolution of thallium-201 is better with a thinner crystal, although the improvement in resolution drops with distance from the collimator. A ⅜-inch thick crystal is therefore a good compromise if both thallium-201 and technetium-99m are to be imaged with the same camera.

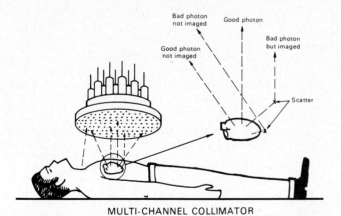

MULTI-CHANNEL COLLIMATOR

FIGURE 11–1 The multi-channel collimator acts as a lens for photon detection. (From Budinger, T. F., and Rollo, F. D.: Physics and instrumentation. Progr. Cardiovasc. Dis. *20*:19, 1977, by permission of Grune and Stratton, Inc.)

The *standard field of view* of most mobile cameras is 25 cm. Smaller diameters are used on some special-purpose cameras. The diameter should be large enough to encompass the entire heart within the field of view using parallel-hole collimators (20 cm for circular fields of view). Detectors with a large field of view (35 to 50 cm) are useful for pulmonary scintigraphy (see later).

Count-rate linearity refers to a linear increase in the detected count rate as the activity increases. The count-rate loss should be less than 10 per cent of count rates at 50,000 counts per second, but this loss increases rapidly at higher counting rates. Other effects may also be seen at higher counting rates. For example, spurious counts can be recorded due to the coincidence of two low-energy photons. Finally, the uniformity of the camera can change at higher count rates. Recent improvements in camera design based on digital electronics have substantially increased the range of count-rate linearity.

THE MULTICRYSTAL CAMERA

The multicrystal scintillation camera has 294 separate sodium iodide scintillation crystals arranged in a matrix of 14 × 21 crystals. The crystals are 9.5 mm square and 2.5 mm thick. There are 35 photomultiplier tubes connected to the crystal array. An event is located in a particular crystal through detection of the simultaneous pulse from both a row and a column photomultiplier tube. A digital computer, which is an integral part of the camera, accumulates the image in its memory for display and processing.

The camera has good sensitivity, even at energies above 200 kev, because of its thick crystals. The constant picture element size means that, except for the effects of scattered radiation, image resolution is constant over the full energy range of 50 to 500 kev. The electronics have been designed for very fast processing of scintillation events leading to a short resolving time and a maximum count rate of 400,000 to 500,000 events per second—three to four times faster than the Anger camera. This is an advantage for rapid, dynamic studies, such as first-transit radionuclide angiocardiography.

Disadvantages of the matrix detector are related mainly to the light lost in the complex light guides and the coarse nature of the matrix itself. Approximately 50 per cent of the light from the crystals is lost in the light pipe arrangement. The energy resolution for technetium-99m is therefore about 50 per cent full-width at half-maximum compared to the Anger camera's resolution of 13 per cent. This means that in imaging studies with thick sources at energies from 50 to 200 kev, significant scattered radiation will lead to loss of image contrast. The coarse spatial resolution is determined by the size of the individual crystals (9.5 mm × 9.5 mm).

THE SINGLE-PROBE DETECTOR

The scintillation probe offers the advantage of portability and enables the measurement of cardiac function in settings where it might be difficult to bring in an Anger scintillation camera (such as the operating room, the recovery room, and the intensive care unit). While cardiac studies performed with the scintillation probe provide reasonably accurate measurements of left ventricular ejection fraction and other measures of global left ventricular function, they do require considerable training to perform and are of limited use in patients with very poor function, when it may be difficult to determine the edge of the ventricle and to determine background.

The standard sodium iodide scintillation probe is 1 to 3 inches in diameter and between 1 and 2 inches in depth. The crystal may be housed in a cylindrical collimator, a parallel-hole collimator similar to the low-resolution/high-efficiency collimators used with scintillation cameras, or a converging collimator. The sodium iodide crystal is used with a high temporal resolution rate meter (10 to 50 msec). Information is acquired after the intravenous injection of an intravascular tracer, such as technetium-99m–labeled red blood cells, and the studies are gated to the patient's electrocardiogram as in the equilibrium radionuclide angiocardiogram (see below). Although the data can be displayed directly on a strip chart recorder, most systems now use a microprocessor for data acquisition and analysis. The time-activity curves are displayed on an oscilloscope, and the processed data are read out through a teleprinter or a console.

More recently, substantially smaller probes have been constructed using *cadmium telluride* crystals. With these smaller systems, it may be possible to monitor patients sequentially over prolonged periods with a probe permanently positioned to the patient's chest. Sequential monitoring may be particularly useful in patients with acute myocardial infarction and other patients in the intensive care setting.

TOMOGRAPHIC IMAGING SYSTEMS

Tomography is used in an attempt to solve one of the major constraints of standard two-dimensional imaging: the overlap of adjacent structures and background on the organ or tissue of interest. Both single-photon and positron-emission tomography are now in use.

Two techniques for performing tomography are *limited-angle* and *transaxial*. The seven-pinhole and rotating slant-hole collimators are examples of limited-angle tomography that are adaptable to standard Anger cameras and single-photon tracers. Because of the limited angle, depth resolution is poor. While the instrumentation is relatively inexpensive, requiring only the purchase of the collimator and reconstruction software, the future of this technique remains uncertain.

Transaxial tomography provides improved depth resolution and is the most promising approach to the quantification of in vivo distribution of radiotracers. *Positron-transaxial tomography* systems are, in fact, being used to quantify regional myocardial metabolism and perfusion (p. 1251). Prototype single-photon transaxial tomographic instruments have been limited either by poor sensitivity (rotating gamma cameras) or poor resolution (ring detector systems). It is anticipated that further improvements in design will overcome these limitations and that tomography may play an increasingly important role by improving the accuracy of current scintigraphic methodologies and by more accurately reflecting the extent of altered myocardial perfusion, wall motion abnormalities, and global ventricular function.

THE COMPUTER

A computer is necessary for nearly all procedures in nuclear cardiology. It may be an integral part of the imaging system or may be separate from the scintillation camera as either a mobile or stationary system. The computer should be adequate for first-pass and equilibrium (gated) radionuclide angiocardiography; this requires high temporal resolution (a minimum of 30 to 40 frames per second) and a matrix capability of at least 64 × 64 picture elements (pixels). Two basic types of computers are used in nuclear medicine: general-purpose (programmable) and special-purpose (hard-wire) units. The general-purpose systems are more flexible and programs can be developed and changed by the users. Special-purpose systems have fixed programs and are more limited in capability. The size and configuration of the computer system will vary with the types of procedures to be performed and local factors in a given department.

EXERCISE TESTING

An exercise table and bicycle are used for supine exercise testing during radionuclide angiocardiography. This equipment must not move during the study. The patient should be well-stabilized on the table and the table itself must not move while the patient is exercising. The bicycle should permit the application of variable workloads, variable positions for the pedals to facilitate patient comfort, and variable positions for the patient. Some prefer a 45-degree angle for the patient's upper body. With equilibrium angiocardiography, exercise testing in the 45-degree upright position is particularly helpful for patients with pulmonary disease or heart failure and is used routinely in many departments. Equipment for upright exercise should also be available, since this is commonly used for first-pass radionuclide angiocardiography and thallium exercise studies. The most common method for upright exercise with ^{201}Tl-imaging is treadmill ergometry, which is superior to the bicycle because it is more likely to stress the patient maximally.

CARDIAC PERFORMANCE

Cardiac performance is a prime factor in determining appropriate medical and surgical management for patients with coronary heart disease.[2-5] Ventricular ejection fraction and regional wall motion are directly related to clinical prognosis in patients with chronic coronary heart disease[2-4] and after myocardial infarction.[6,7] Although invasive techniques involving left ventricular catheterization and radiocontrast angiography provide reliable measurements of ejection fraction and regional wall motion[8] (p. 473), they have limited application in critically ill patients. Radionuclide techniques are noninvasive, requiring only a peripheral intravenous injection, and thus offer distinct advantages over more conventional, invasive methods. The radionuclide techniques are safe and repeatable and do not induce measurable hemodynamic alterations.[9,10] In addition, cardiac performance can be studied during a variety of physiological or pharmaceutical interventions.

RADIOPHARMACEUTICALS

The primary requirement of a radiopharmaceutical for first-pass radionuclide angiocardiography (p. 356) is that it remain intravascular during its first passage through the right and left heart phases. The secondary requirement is that the physical properties of the radionuclide be satisfactory with respect to the instrumentation being used.

The radionuclide that is used for virtually all phases of radionuclide angiocardiography is technetium-99m. It has a 6-hour half-life, a photon energy of 140 kev, and minimal nonpenetrating radiation, and it effectively labels a large number of pharmaceuticals—a requirement that is particularly important for equilibrium studies. While pertechnetate leaks out rapidly into the extracellular space with an intravascular half-life of approximately one hour, it does remain intravascular during the first intravascular transit. Because the tracer must remain intravascular only during its first transit, technetium-99m pertechnetate can be used for first-pass studies. Since ^{99m}Tc-pertechnetate (^{99m}TcO$_4^-$) is the chemical form of ^{99m}Tc after elution from the ^{99}Mo* → ^{99m}Tc generator, it is the most readily available and the least expensive of the technetium-99m pharmaceuticals.

The major disadvantage of ^{99m}Tc is its long half-life relative to the duration of the procedure. After intravenous injection, the material persists in the intravascular and extracellular space, precluding serial studies, and only two or three first-pass studies are possible within a 6-hour period. As a result, evaluation in multiple projections or after multiple physiological or pharmacological interventions is not possible.

One approach to increasing the number of serial studies is the use of ^{99m}Tc-sulfur colloid, a radiopharmaceutical extracted by the reticuloendothelial system, thereby radically shortening the biological half-life. The pharmaceutical is extracted primarily by the liver and spleen within several minutes after intravenous injection.[11] The disadvantage of

this approach is the relatively high radiation dose to the bone marrow. Approximately 5 per cent of the dose is sequestered by the bone marrow, the most radiosensitive of the body's tissues. ^{99m}Tc-pyrophosphate is an attractive alternative in the coronary care unit. Acute infarct scintigraphy can be performed three hours after the initial first-pass study. Thus, two studies can be performed after the injection of a single radiopharmaceutical. ^{99m}Tc-DTPA (diethylenetriaminepentaacetic acid) has also been suggested for first-pass studies, since clearance of this radiopharmaceutical from the blood is more rapid than that of ^{99m}Tc-pertechnetate, reducing the whole-body radiation dose and, more importantly, shortening the time between sequential studies.[9]

The development of ultrashort-lived nuclides should increase the flexibility of this technique. Gold-195m has a 30-second half-life and an acceptable gamma energy of 262 kev for use with multicrystal cameras and with Anger cameras using medium-energy collimators and adequate shielding.[12] It is obtained from a ^{195}Hg→^{195m}Au generator system. Its parent, mercury-195m, has a sufficiently long half-life (41.6 hours) so that each generator will last up to three or four days.

The advantages of gold-195m are that multiple views can be obtained and serial responses to exercise or drug interventions can be studied by repeating the injection at frequent intervals without build-up of significant background activity and with minimal patient radiation dose. Also, because of the reduced patient dose relative to ^{99m}Tc, larger doses can be injected, taking full advantage of the higher count-rate capacities of multicrystal cameras and digital Anger cameras. Limitations of this tracer are that the parent, ^{195m}Hg, may be present as a contaminant in the injected dose; the half-life of the tracer is too short to permit measurement of the parent prior to each injection; high-energy photons result in scattered radiation; and the high cost of the generator will make it practical only in hospitals that carry out a large number of first-pass studies.

Other ultrashort half-life tracers have been introduced, including tantalum-178, with a half-life of 9 minutes,[13] and iridium-191m, with a half-life of 4.9 seconds.[14] Tantalum-178 is used with low-energy imaging systems such as the multiwire proportional camera. Iridium-191m is used for children, in whom the 4.9-second half-life is tolerable. Both tracers are obtained from long-lived parents by elution through generator systems.

The radiopharmaceutical for equilibrium (ECG-gated) studies (p. 360) must remain within the intravascular space throughout the course of the study. If continual monitoring is anticipated, the radiopharmaceutical must remain within the intravascular space for at least one or two half-lives. ^{99m}Tc–human serum albumin (HSA) and ^{99m}Tc-tagged red blood cells (RBCs) have been advocated for this purpose. ^{99m}Tc-HSA is less satisfactory for gated studies because (1) there is proportionately more activity in the liver, since the liver albumin space is larger than the intravascular space; and (2) the blood clearance of ^{99m}Tc-HSA is fairly rapid, precluding prolonged monitoring and repeat studies.

Once the initial equilibration of the tracer has been reached, ^{99m}Tc-RBCs are cleared from the blood very slowly. The red cells can be tagged in vivo by injecting 300 to 400 μg of stannous iron intravenously and injecting ^{99m}Tc-pertechnetate 15 minutes later. Approximately 60 to 80 per cent of the pertechnetate attaches to and labels the red blood cells; the remainder is excreted through the kidneys or labels iodine traps, such as the kidney and stomach. Equilibration is reached after 5 minutes. Since rapid renal clearance is a precondition for optimal studies, this technique is less satisfactory in patients with poor renal clearance and results in high background activity and poor target-to-background ratios. The primary advantage of this technique is the ease with which the red cells can be labeled. Recently, kits have been developed for in vitro labeling of the patient's own red cells. The major advantage of this approach is the high labeling efficiency (greater than or equal to 98 per cent). This technique does take more time than in vivo labeling, but with the newly developed kits, labeling can be performed in 15 to 30 minutes.

---

*Mo = molybdenum.

TECHNIQUE

Radionuclide angiocardiography can be used to measure (1) left and right ventricular *ejection fraction*; (2) indices of *regional ventricular performance*; (3) left ventricular *cardiac output*; (4) end-diastolic and end-systolic *ventricular volumes*; (5) indices of early *systolic* and *diastolic function*; (6) indices of aortic, mitral, and tricuspid *regurgitation*; (7) indices of *asynchrony*; (8) *transit times* within the central circulation; and (9) *intracardiac shunts*. In addition, visual assessment of the cardiac chambers and the great vessels is also a routine part of the examination. All these indices can be assessed with either first-pass or equilibrium studies except for transit time measurements and shunt detection, which can be achieved only with first-pass methods.

FIRST-PASS STUDIES

First-pass radionuclide angiocardiography measures indices of cardiac performance from the initial transit of the radiotracer through the heart. For accurate quantitation of first-pass studies, it is important that the radiopharmaceutical be injected in as small a volume as possible, that it be injected rapidly, and that it not be delayed in the venous structures. While in some validation studies a central venous catheter[15] or a Swan-Ganz catheter[16] was used to administer the radiopharmaceutical, satisfactory results have been obtained using a 19-gauge butterfly-type needle inserted into a prominent medial antecubital vein[9] or, in children, into an external jugular vein.[17] Approximately 20 mCi of the radiopharmaceutical (or correspondingly less if several studies are going to be obtained in rapid sequence) should be injected rapidly in a volume of less than 1 ml and flushed immediately. Several techniques have been suggested for intravenous delivery.[18-20]

Data Collection. The manner in which data are collected during the first transit of the tracer through the central circulation depends on the purpose of the investigation. If the data are to be used in conjunction with an equilibrium study to define general anatomy, images of one frame per second over approximately 60 to 90 seconds can be obtained. If the data are to be used to determine the ejection fraction from the cyclic changes in activity over the right or left ventricle, a framing rate of at least 25 frames per second will be needed. If cardiac output is to be measured, a blood sample will be needed after the isotope has reached equilibrium. Collection can be done in list mode, in which case each event is collected sequentially and formatting is done after acquisition; otherwise, data may be collected within frames of predetermined duration. The former method is more flexible but requires more expensive data processing equipment (see Gating, p. 361).

Transit Times. By placing regions of interest over several different structures, the transit times between these structures can be measured. For example, in the modified left anterior oblique projection, the transit time from the right ventricle to the left ventricle can be obtained from regions over these two structures using the formula

$$\bar{t} = \frac{\int tA_L(t)dt}{\int A_L(t)dt} - \frac{\int tA_R(t)dt}{\int A_R(t)dt} \qquad (1)$$

where $\bar{t}$ is the mean transit time, $A_R(t)$ is the first-transit time-activity curve from the right ventricle, and $A_L(t)$ is the first-transit time-activity curve from the left ventricle. Because of interference ("cross-talk") between the regions due to recirculation of activity, it is often difficult to obtain a first-transit curve that accurately represents activity from a single structure. For this reason, the mean transit time is often approximated by the time between peak activities obtained from two separate structures, such as the right and left ventricles.

Pulmonary blood volume can be calculated from the formula

$$\bar{t} = V/F \qquad (2)$$

where $\bar{t}$ is the mean transit time, F equals flow, and V equals volume. A number of techniques have been suggested for the quantitation of pulmonary transit time.[21] These techniques work reasonably well in patients with normal or moderately altered pulmonary vascular flow or volume, but serious errors can occur in patients with cardiopulmonary collapse.[22-24] Measurements of pulmonary transit time have not met with wide clinical acceptance.

Cardiac Output. Measurement of cardiac output by the indicator dilution technique, i.e., the Stewart-Hamilton principle (p. 290), requires knowledge of the time-activity (or concentration) profile of the tracer after its injection into the bloodstream. The profile can be obtained by direct arterial sampling or by external monitoring. In both cases, flow (F) is calculated from the equation

$$F = \frac{I}{\int_0^T C(t)dt} \qquad (3)$$

where I (isotope) is the initial quantity of tracer injected and the denominator is the area under the time-activity curve corrected for recirculation of the tracer. Knowledge of the initial quantity of material injected is required to calculate cardiac output using Equation 3; measurement of the denominator of Equation 3 is less straightforward because of the recirculation peak superimposed on the tail of the dilution curve. Several techniques have been proposed to correct for recirculation. The most common method involves a semilogarithmic extrapolation of the tail of the first curve.[25,26] The area of the resulting curve can be obtained numerically or planimetrically. Another technique involves a least-squares analysis of the upslope of the curve and a portion of the downslope. This technique is based on the "gamma variate" function, which is related to the gamma function.[27-29]

Determination of the time-activity profile for measurement of cardiac output by external monitoring of radioactivity requires algebraic manipulation of Equation 3. Because the numerator (I) represents the total quantity of isotope injected (in counts per minute [cpm]), it is equal to the equilibrium concentration of isotope (C_{eq}) times the blood volume (BV):

$$I \text{ (cpm)} = C_{eq}(cpm/ml) \times BV \text{ (ml)} \qquad (4)$$

Equation 3 now becomes

$$F = \frac{C_{eq} \bullet BV}{\int_0^T C(t)dt} \qquad (5)$$

The area monitored by an external probe can, in theory, be any part of the circulatory system. Generally, precordial count rates are obtained because a relatively large blood pool can be monitored, increasing the statistical accuracy of the data. Although the external monitor senses only a small fraction of the total blood volume, the same fraction of it is involved in the assessment of both C_{eq} and the area of the time-activity curve; as a result, the fraction of the blood volume observed does not appear in Equation 5. The only other variable needed for measurement of cardiac output is the blood volume, which must be determined independently.

Some additional constraints are involved in the measurement of cardiac output. The assumption that the volume of blood during the first transit is equal to that at equilibrium further limits the accuracy of this technique. Lung and chest wall blood volumes contain more tracer during equilibrium than during first-pass, and Compton scatter from adjacent blood pools is greater at equilibrium. This error results in an overestimation of cardiac output, and no method for its correction has been generally accepted. In addition, this technique measures forward flow. In the presence of valvular regurgitation, in which both backward and forward flow occur, only the net forward flow is measured.

VENTRICULAR PERFORMANCE. The most frequent application of radionuclide angiocardiography is to evaluate ventricular performance, both subjectively and quantitatively.

Anatomy. By observing the passage of the bolus during the first transit, it is possible to make a subjective analysis of cardiac anatomy. This is particularly useful for detecting intracardiac shunts but may also be of use in evaluating patients with valvular and congenital abnormalities (see p. 359). Gross changes can be observed, such as the large left atrium and the small, normally functioning left ventricle of mitral stenosis; the large left atrium and ventricle of mitral or aortic regurgitation; or the greatly enlarged right atrium of tricuspid regurgitation. Knowledge of the fine anatomy required for defining valvular lesions cannot be obtained with this technique, and thus its clinical application is not widespread.

Much more useful has been the definition of segmental wall motion. A radionuclide angiocardiogram with high temporal resolution is constructed from the left ventricular time-activity curve corrected for background. Each of two to four successive cardiac cycles is divided into 16 frames, and the corresponding frames of each cycle are added together to yield one summed or composite cardiac cycle.[30] The composite image is played back repetitively, producing a cine display for subjective analysis of regional wall motion abnormalities. Quantitative measurements of hemiaxis shortening can be determined from the superimposed end-diastolic and end-systolic images.

Quantitative Measurements. When the entire heart is considered to be the region of interest, a time-activity curve of combined right and left ventricular activity is generated (Fig. 11-2). To obtain meaningful hemodynamic information, the activity of the left ventricle must be isolated from that of the surrounding anatomical structures. Separation between the two ventricles is achieved temporally, since the activity enters the left ventricle after it has been cleared from the right ventricle. Frames corresponding to the left ventricular phase are determined and summed. From the composite image of the left ventricular blood pool, the contour of the left ventricle can be determined using either an electronic cursor or an edge-detection algorithm.

Background Correction. Even when the left ventricle is accurately delineated, the resultant activity is not entirely due to blood in its cavity. Background activity emanates from lung tissue behind and adjacent to the heart and from scattered radioactivity from other structures. A second region must be assigned for the correction of background. The ejection fraction can be underestimated by as much as 25 per cent if background correction is not made.

Best results are obtained when a semiannular background region is placed around the left ventricle but not overlying the aorta.[11] An alternative approach to background correction determines the count rate occurring from the left ventricle just prior to the left ventricular phase and uses this activity for background correction.[15]

Left Ventricular Ejection Fraction. Time-activity curves of left ventricular and background activity are generated. The curve is made up of a series of oscillations with the greatest amplitude of these oscillations occurring at the greatest height of the curve itself. The count rates at the peaks in the oscillation are proportional to end-diastolic volume. If ejection fraction were determined from only one oscillation, the statistical reliability of the information would be poor; therefore, at least three or, if possible, five cardiac cycles should be averaged, beginning at the peak of the left ventricular time-activity curve (Fig. 11-3). The difference in count rate between end diastole and end systole is proportional to stroke volume. Ejection fraction (EF) is obtained by dividing that number by the end-diastolic

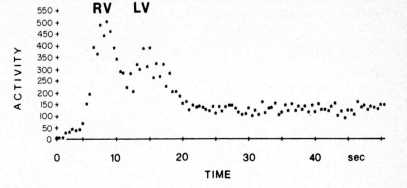

FIGURE 11-2 Time-activity curve resulting from the first transit of the radiotracer through the right ventricle (RV) and left ventricle (LV). (From Ashburn, W. L., et al.: Left ventricular ejection fraction—a review of several radionuclide angiographic approaches using the scintillation camera. Progr. Cardiovasc. Dis. *20*:267, 1978, by permission of Grune and Stratton, Inc.)

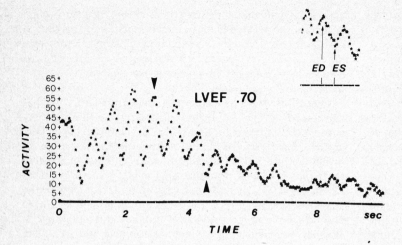

FIGURE 11–3 Time-activity curve from left ventricular region. Each point represents total counts for 40 msec. The highest value (peak) for each cycle corresponds to end-diastole (ED) and the subsequent low value (valley) to end systole (ES). An average left ventricular ejection fraction (LVEF) of 0.70 was calculated for the three cycles between the arrows. (From Ashburn, W. L., et al.: Left ventricular ejection fraction—a review of several radionuclide angiographic approaches using the scintillation camera. Progr. Cardiovasc. Dis. *20*:267, 1978, by permission of Grune and Stratton, Inc.)

count rate minus background:

$$EF = \frac{\text{Diastolic counts} - \text{Systolic counts}}{\text{Diastolic counts} - \text{Background counts}} \quad (6)$$

When multicrystal cameras are used, the counting rate is sufficiently high to allow calculation of the ejection fraction from the maxima and minima of the oscillations on the left ventricular time-activity curve. With single-crystal cameras, the sensitivity, and hence the counting rate, is lower. If only the maximum and minimum counting rates are used for each oscillation, the statistical reliability of the data is compromised.

These techniques for determining ejection fraction have been validated by comparison with values obtained using single-plane and biplane contrast ventriculography. Correlation coefficients ranging from r = 0.94 to r = 0.97 have been reported by a number of groups who have compared the two techniques.[11,15,16]

Left Ventricular Ejection-Phase Indices. A number of ejection-phase performance indices (p. 480) can be measured from the left ventricular time-activity curve. *Left ventricular ejection rate* can be measured from either the equilibrium or the first-pass radionuclide angiocardiogram. A weighted least-squares analysis can be used to fit the ejection phase data (four to nine data points per ejection phase) to a straight line.[11] The slope of this line, representing the change in counts with time, *dC/dT*, is determined and normalized to the average number of counts over the ejection phase ($dC/dT/C_{ave}$). This measurement, unlike the left ventricular ejection fraction, appears to be sensitive to changes in the inotropic state in patients with cardiac disease. The normal value for the normalized left ventricular ejection rate is 3.40 ± 0.17 $dC/dT/C_{ave}$. In patients who have coronary artery disease, this value is 1.22 ± 0.11 $dC/dT/C_{ave}$.

Indices of diastolic function are more sensitive for detecting the effects of myocardial ischemia than are systolic indices such as ejection fraction[31] (p. 1247). These changes in the diastolic properties of the ventricle are seen in acute myocardial ischemia and may be present even at rest in patients with coronary artery disease.[32,33] Both first-pass and equilibrium methods can be used to derive indices of diastolic function (as well as the other phase indices described in this section) from the left ventricular volume curve. The *peak diastolic filling rate* expresses diastolic filling as a fraction of the end-diastolic volume per second. It is calculated from the diastolic portion of the left ventricular volume curve by fitting a third-order polynomial to the first 400 msec of diastole.[34] The point of maximum filling is determined by setting the second derivative of the polynomial to zero. The third-order polynomial is then differentiated to yield the maximum filling rate, which is normalized to the total end-diastolic counts. With this method, the peak diastolic filling rate has been found to be 2.14 ± 0.63 end-diastolic volume/sec in normals and is reduced in about 90 per cent of patients with previous myocardial infarction when they are studied at rest. Patients with coronary artery disease but without previous infarction may also have abnormal filling rates at rest, but the incidence of this abnormality remains controversial (56 to 85 per cent).[34,35]

Right Ventricular Ejection Fraction. Right ventricular performance is difficult to quantitate, since the geometry of the right ventricle is complex, making calculation of the right ventricular ejection fraction by standard geometrical methods extremely difficult. A radionuclide method for this measurement has been developed and is similar in many respects to that for left ventricular ejection fraction.[36] The radiotracer is injected intravenously, through either a large medial antecubital vein or the jugular vein, in a volume of less than 2 ml. The first pass of the radioactive bolus through the central circulation is recorded in the 30-degree right anterior oblique projection. The ejection fraction is measured from the time-activity curve derived from the right ventricular blood pool. A region of interest is assigned to this pool, carefully excluding the right atrium and the pulmonary artery. A second semiannular region of interest is placed outside the right ventricle adjacent to the apical anterior and inferior walls. A high-frequency time-activity curve (25 frames/sec) is generated from both the right ventricular and the background regions of interest. Right ventricular ejection fraction is calculated by dividing the difference in counts between end-diastole and end-systole by the number of counts at end diastole after correcting for background. Three to five beats from the downslope of the right ventricular time-activity curve are used for the calculation.

Background correction of the right ventricular ejection fraction measurement appears necessary only when serial studies are performed, since background activity alters right ventricular ejection fraction by less than 5 per cent.[36]

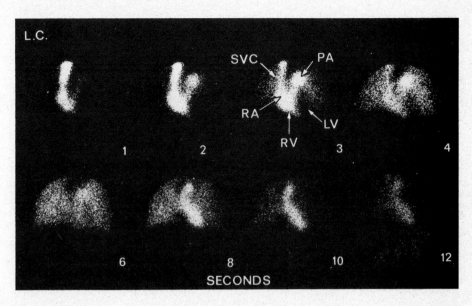

FIGURE 11–4 First-transit radionuclide angiogram. At one second, the tracer is in the superior vena cava, right atrium, and right ventricle. By three seconds, the radioactivity is entering the lungs through the pulmonary arteries. By eight seconds, the radioactivity has returned to the left side of the heart. The left ventricle and aorta are clearly seen, and the lung background is rapidly diminishing. Numbers represent time of frames in seconds following the injection. (SVC = superior vena cava; RA = right atrium; RV = right ventricle; LV = left ventricle; PA = pulmonary artery.)

Because the activity is high and the background is low during transit through the right ventricle, single-crystal cameras can be used for this purpose, although multicrystal cameras provide significantly higher counting rates and therefore improve the statistical reliability of the measurement.[37] Using the first-pass method, investigators have found the mean right ventricular ejection fraction normally to be between 0.52 and 0.57.[36-38]

End-Diastolic Volume. End-diastolic volume can be approximated from a first-pass radionuclide angiocardiogram with high temporal resolution using geometrical techniques. After the time-activity curve has been obtained, those frames representing end-diastolic volume are summed. The left ventricular contour is determined by means of an electronic cursor or an edge-detection algorithm. A grid of known dimensions is then placed between the radioactive source and the detector for size correction, and the volume is determined using the technique of Sandler and Dodge.[39] Since the ventricular edges are not as well defined with first-pass radionuclide angiocardiography as with contrast left ventriculography, and because only

one projection is usually obtained, it would not be expected that the resultant measurement would be the most precise, although recent studies have shown a reasonable correlation between the two methods.

SHUNT DETECTION. In normal patients, the lung time-activity curve has a characteristic appearance after intravenous injection of a first-pass tracer. There is an early peak due to the appearance of radiotracer in the lungs. This is followed by rapid clearance as the tracer moves into the systemic circulation. Eventually some recirculation will occur as the tracer returns from the systemic circulation to the right side of the heart and the lungs (Fig. 11–4). In patients with *left-to-right shunts*, tracer passes from the left to the right side of the heart, short-circuiting the systemic circulation and resulting in rapid recirculation to the lungs. On first-pass radionuclide angiocardiography, the three distinct phases (right heart, lungs, and left heart) merge owing to rapid recirculation, and a clear definition of the left ventricle is not possible because of the high level of radioactivity in the lungs (Fig. 11–5).

Several indices have been suggested for quantifying left-

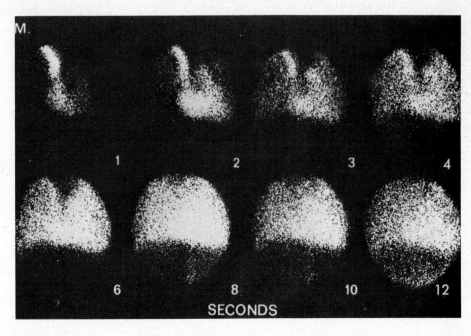

FIGURE 11–5 Left-to-right shunt at atrial level. Recirculation of radioactivity is seen in the lungs. In addition, radioactivity reappears in the right atrium, right ventricle, and pulmonary artery at 8, 10, and 12 seconds (bottom right). (From Treves, S., et al.: Intracardiac shunts. *In* James, A. E., et al. (eds.): Pediatric Nuclear Medicine. Philadelphia. W. B. Saunders Co., 1974, p. 231.)

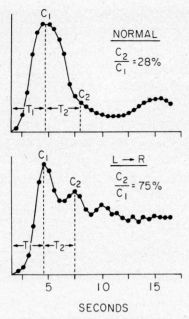

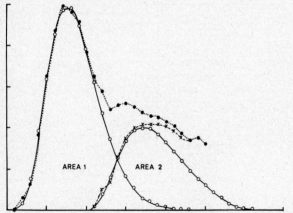

FIGURE 11–6　C_2/C_1 ratios for detection of left-to-right shunts. C_1 is peak activity, T_1 is the time between the first appearance of activity and the peak, T_2 is equal to T_1 but begins at the end of T_1, and C_2 is the degree of activity at the end of T_2. (From Treves, S., et al.: Intracardiac shunts. *In* James, A. E., et al. (eds.): Pediatric Nuclear Medicine. Philadelphia, W. B. Saunders Co., 1974, p. 231.)

to-right shunts. The C_2/C_1 index[40,41] is the ratio between peak activity (C_1) at time T and the activity at a time equal to T following peak activity (C_2), which is equal to that from the first appearance of the tracer to peak activity (Fig. 11–6). While this approach has been useful for the detection of left-to-right shunts, it has been less satisfactory for reproducible quantification.[42]

At the present time, the most satisfactory method for quantification of left-to-right shunts is to calculate the ratio of pulmonary flow to systemic flow ($\dot{Q}_p/\dot{Q}_s$).[43] ^{99m}Tc-pertechnetate is injected intravenously as a bolus (200 μCi/kg or 2 mCi, whichever is greater) into the right external jugular vein to ensure that the tracer enters the right side

FIGURE 11–7　Quantitation of the left-to-right shunt by gamma variate analysis. For details, see the text. (From Maltz, D. L., et al.: Quantitative radionuclide angiocardiography: Determination of Q_p:Q_s in children. Circulation *47*:1049, 1973, by permission of the American Heart Association, Inc.)

of the heart as a discrete bolus. The degree to which the bolus disperses can be assessed by obtaining a time-activity curve over the superior vena cava; its duration should be 2 seconds or less. The patient is positioned to obtain an anterior view, so that the right lung can be separated from the heart. Recording is begun immediately after injection and continued for 30 to 60 seconds. Since high temporal resolution is not required for evaluation of the pulmonary dilution curve, frames of 0.5-second duration can be used.

The time-activity curve is generated by creating a region of interest over the right lung (Fig. 11–7). The component of the washout curve due to recirculation (Area 2 in Figure 11–7) is extracted from the curve using gamma variate analysis. After extracting the systemic flow component and determining its area, the portion of the curve due to pulmonary blood flow ($\dot{Q}_p$) (Area 1 in Figure 11–7) is extracted, and its area is measured. The size of the left-to-right shunt can then be determined from the formula

$$\dot{Q}_p/\dot{Q}_s = \frac{\text{Area 1}}{\text{Area 1} - \text{Area 2}} \qquad (7)$$

More sophisticated algorithms have been suggested using deconvolution analysis to correct for variations in the rate of injection. Using either gamma variate or deconvolution analysis, the correlation with oximetric measurement of the pulmonary-to-systemic flow ratio has been excellent.[43] However, the technique cannot distinguish between poor ventricular performance and left-to-right shunting and should be used only when left ventricular performance is adequate.

Right-to-left shunts can be detected from inspection of the radionuclide angiocardiogram and by early visualization of either the left heart chambers or the aorta.[44,45] An alternative approach is intravenous injection of a radioactive inert gas (xenon-133 or krypton-81m). Since the inert gas is extracted with very high efficiency from the lungs, significant systemic activity indicates a right-to-left shunt.[46,47]

EQUILIBRIUM STUDIES

First-pass dynamic radionuclide studies are limited to the counts acquired during a few cardiac cycles. To increase the total number of counts and, hence, the resolution of the radionuclide angiocardiogram, a tracer that remains in the intravascular system can be imaged at equilibrium. To achieve high temporal resolution, count acquisition is gated to a physiological marker, usually the R wave of the electrocardiogram.

Unlike the first-pass study, the radionuclide must reach equilibration within the intravascular space prior to imaging. This means that all four cardiac chambers as well as the great vessels and surrounding organs, such as liver and spleen, will be visualized at the same time. As a result, special attention must be paid to separation of the right from the left side of the heart and separation of the surrounding organs from the heart. This can be accomplished by obtaining views in multiple projections and with specially designed collimators, since imaging is not restricted to one or two positions as in first-pass studies.

Since a large number of counts can be obtained by constructing one average cardiac cycle as a composite of many cycles, a high-resolution collimator can be used. The most informative projection is the modified left anterior oblique (MLAO), with the detector angled so that the right and left ventricles are completely separated. This usually occurs between 35 and 45 degrees in the left anterior oblique (LAO) projection. An additional 30-degree caudal tilt is required to separate the left atrium from the left ventricle and to enable imaging parallel to the long axis of the left ventricle. Since caudal angulation of this magnitude is difficult to achieve with standard collimators, the angulation should be built into the collimator. The 30-degree slant-hole collimator can then be placed flat against the patient's chest.

While global left ventricular hemodynamic information and much information concerning regional wall motion can be obtained from the modified left anterior oblique projection, other views—particularly the shallow (30-degree) right anterior oblique (RAO), anterior, and 70-degree left anterior oblique projections—are useful for providing information concerning the anterior, inferior, and lateral walls of the left ventricle, which are not imaged tangentially in the MLAO projection.

Gating. In gated studies, a "gate" is opened by a control signal. When the gate is closed, the signals are not passed on, and it appears that there are no scintillations. The control signal is usually based on some cyclic physiological process, such as the cardiac cycle. Two general methods are used for collecting all phases of the cardiac cycle simultaneously—*in-memory gating* and *gated list mode* collection. When in-memory gating is used, the main memory is divided into a large number of image matrices (Fig. 11-8). With the occurrence of the R wave, which is the control signal, the scintillation data are directed to the first frame. After a predefined time, usually 25 msec, the data are directed to the second frame. After each subsequent 25 msec, data are directed sequentially to each of the remaining frames until the next R wave, when data are redirected to the first frame. Each matrix is a map of the two-dimensional distribution of the tracer during a specific portion of the cardiac cycle.

With this technique, the data can be viewed while being acquired, so that one can determine immediately whether the data collection is adequate. In-memory gating requires a constant heart rate and cannot be applied effectively in the presence of an arrhythmia. It also requires considerable main computer memory if adequate temporal and spatial resolution is to be achieved.

In the gated list mode, scintigraphic data are collected in a list mode along with samples of the electrocardiogram. In other words, the data are recorded as a list or table as they are received by the computer. After the collection period is over, the data are reformatted by sorting the list. With this method, the number of frames per second and the size of the image matrix can be determined *after* the data have been collected. Also, frames having a predefined R-R interval time can be analyzed, so that patients with arrhythmia can be studied.[48,49] This method uses a very large amount of auxiliary memory. Reformatting times may be long without the aid of array processors or large computers.

Data Collection. Between 2 million and 10 million counts are collected in 30 to 60 frames of 64 × 64 elements. More counts are collected when the patient is at rest and high resolution studies are required; fewer counts are collected during transient periods of steady-state heart rate, such as during exercise. For measurements of ejection fraction, a temporal resolution of 50 msec (20 frames per second) is necessary at rest and 40 msec (25 frames per second) with exercise. To obtain peak ejection rates and peak filling rates, 40 msec per frame at rest and 20 msec with exercise are required.[50]

Radionuclide Cineangiocardiography. The cinematic display is an endless loop of the sequential frames that make up the equilibrium study. Data from the angiocardiogram can be interpolated to produce a continuous, flicker-free cinematic display. Overall anatomy, such as size and position of the great vessels, can be evaluated subjectively as can global and regional left and right ventricular size and function (Fig. 11-9). Criteria for the subjective interpretation of regional ventricular performance are de-

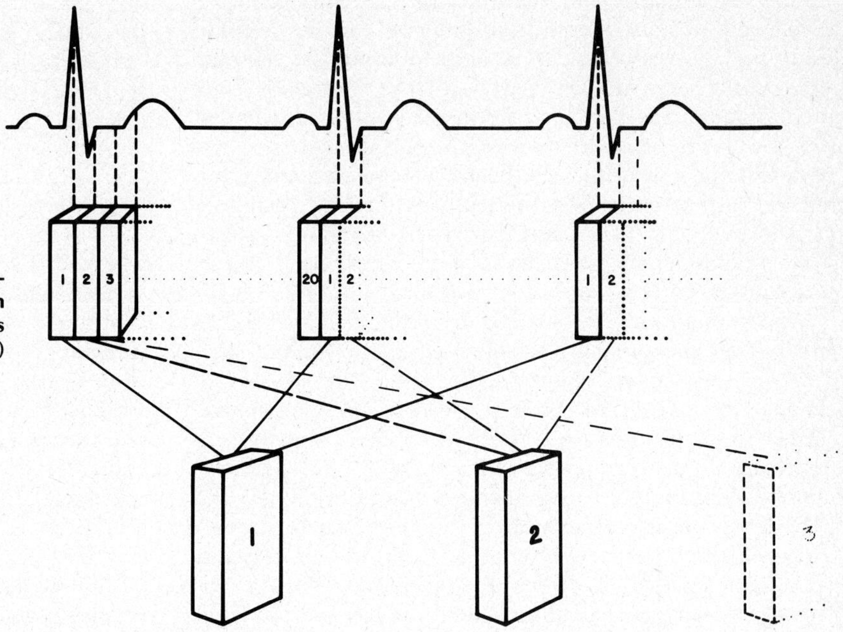

FIGURE 11-8 Camera acquisition is gated to the patient's electrocardiogram. Counts are stored in frames, where frame 1 represents the total counts obtained during the first portion (twentieth second) of all cardiac cycles recorded.

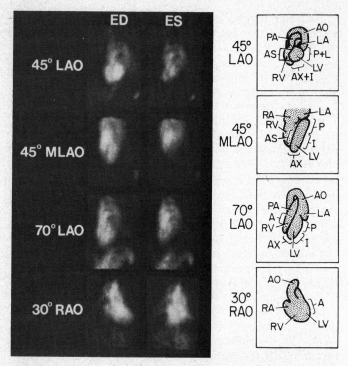

FIGURE 11–9 Normal equilibrium (gated) radionuclide angio-cardiogram. LAO = left anterior oblique projection; MLAO = modified left anterior oblique; RAO = right anterior oblique; ED = end diastole; ES = end systole; PA = pulmonary artery; AS = anteroseptal; RV = right ventricle; AX = apex; I = inferior; LV = left ventricle; P = posterior; L = lateral; LA = left atrium; AO = aorta; RA = right atrium.

rived from contrast ventriculography. The left ventricle is divided into anatomical segments, usually the anterior wall (best seen on the 30-degree RAO and 70-degree LAO views), anteroseptum (best seen on the 45-degree LAO or MLAO view), apex (seen on all views), and inferoposterior wall (best seen on the 45-degree MLAO and 70-degree LAO views). Each segment is assigned a score: 3 = normokinesis, 2 = mild hypokinesis, 1 = severe hypokinesis, 0 = akinesis, and −1 = dyskinesis.

Numerical Analysis. Quantitative measurements of global and regional ventricular function can be obtained from the time-activity curves derived from the left and right ventricles and from regions of the ventricles. Since the radiopharmaceutical is uniformly mixed in the blood at equilibrium, a time-activity curve over the ventricles will represent the changes in ventricular volume occurring during the cardiac cycle. However, because activity is distributed throughout the intravascular space, including tissue in front of and behind the heart, accurate background correction is essential.

Wall motion can be assessed by radionuclide methods either from the geometrical approaches used in the standard contrast angiographic method or from analysis of changes in count rate. Background-corrected activity recorded from the region of the left ventricle is directly proportional to this chamber's blood volume. Although the radionuclide method provides limited spatial resolution and edge definition, it does offer an accurate measure of the activity viewed by the detector or a region of the detector. Therefore, assessment of global and regional ventricular function based on changing count rates has two inherent advantages over the geometrical approaches borrowed from

contrast angiography: (1) The geometrical approaches assess only that part of the ventricular wall which is tangential to the detector. Techniques based on left ventricular activity assess the three-dimensional space viewed by the corresponding region of the detector, assessing ventricular function regardless of its orientation to the detector. Techniques based on activity do not require assumptions concerning left ventricular shape—a consideration that is particularly important in patients with asynergy, in whom such geometrical assumptions may not be valid. (2) The need to define the margins of the left ventricle during end-systole is eliminated with the count-rate method. During end-systole, the difference between ventricular and background activity may be small and edge resolution particularly poor.

Background Correction. The left ventricular time-activity curve is generated after the left ventricular outline has been defined using a light pen or an electronic cursor and after subtraction of background. As with first-pass probe studies, background correction is critical, since approximately 33 to 50 per cent of the activity emanating from the area of the left ventricle is due to background. The background regions, usually representing areas just lateral and inferior to the heart and including a portion of the interventricular septum, can be defined manually or automatically using predefined computer algorithms.

Several general approaches have been suggested for background correction: (1) fixed ventricular and background regions can be defined from the end-diastolic frame; and (2) a variable left ventricular region, shrinking during systole and expanding during diastole, can be defined. Background regions may be continuous or interrupted and may extend into the septum. Background regions never abut the base of the ventricle. However, each of these approaches can result in accurate measures of ejection fraction if applied carefully and if adequately controlled comparisons are made regularly with measurements derived at cardiac catheterization.

Left Ventricular Ejection Fraction. Once background activity is known with reasonable accuracy, ejection fraction can be determined from changes in count rate rather than from geometrical analysis,[50–53] since changes in left ventricular activity are directly proportional to changes in ventricular blood volume. Ejection fraction is calculated from the formula

$$\text{LVEF} = \frac{\text{EDC} - \text{SC}}{\text{EDC} - \text{BC}} \tag{8}$$

where LVEF is left ventricular ejection fraction; EDC, or "end-diastolic counts," represents the activity emanating from the region of the left ventricle during the frame corresponding to end diastole; and ESC, or "end-systolic counts," represents left ventricular activity during the end-systolic frame; BC stands for background counts. These two frames can be determined from the time-activity curve and correspond to the maximum and minimum points, respectively. Ejection fraction obtained using this algorithm correlates very well with ejection fractions derived by means of contrast ventriculography (r = 0.92).[50]

Ventricular Volume and Cardiac Output. Left ventricular volume can be measured using geometrical or count-rate principles. The count-rate method compares the background-corrected left ventricular activity with the activity in a known volume of the patient's blood.[54] To obtain volumes in milliliters and output in liters/min, attenuation corrections must be introduced.[55] This is the most difficult of the numerical analyses to measure accurately because of the varying attenuation among patients, particularly between men and women, and the careful attention to detail that is required.

Functional Images. It is important for the physician who is accustomed to using contrast ventriculography to keep in mind the differences between contrast and radionuclide studies. The contrast ventriculogram represents volume information relatively poorly because mixing of the contrast is not complete and because there are difficulties with film linearity. However, because it has excellent resolution, it defines the edges of the ventricle well; therefore, volume can be calculated from the two-dimensional silhouette of the ventricle, and edge motion is used to evaluate wall motion. By comparison, the radionuclide angiocardiogram has poor spatial resolution, but the image data are directly proportional to ventricular volume after background correction. For this reason, techniques such as functional imaging have been very useful aids in the interpretation of the radionuclide angiocardiogram. Subjective assessment of the cineangiocardiogram must rely on catching the wall motion abnormality on target, hence the need for multiple views. With function-imaging techniques, we take advantage of the count-rate changes that occur throughout the ventricle and result in intensity changes in the image rather than alterations on the edges of the image.

Functional images are physiological maps. After certain arithmetic operations have been performed on a group of images, the resultant image or images are no longer representative of the basic activity distribution but are representative of some physiological function, such as regional ejection fraction or onset of contraction. In such an image the intensities are proportional to a function rather than to the original activity distributions.

Ejection-Fraction Image. The ejection-fraction image makes use of the proportionality between background-corrected left ventricular count rate and blood volume. By subtracting the end-systolic image from the end-diastolic image, an image of regional stroke volume can be obtained. The stroke-volume image is divided by the background-corrected end-diastolic image to produce an ejection-fraction image, a map of regional ejection fractions throughout the left ventricle.[56]

In the ejection-fraction image, the intensity of each of the matrix areas is directly proportional to the regional ejection fraction. The normal ejection-fraction image is characterized by a peripheral ejection shell comprising matrices with greater than 50 per cent ejection—i.e., a reduction in blood volume of 50 per cent between diastole and systole in any given matrix area within the end-diastolic perimeter of the left ventricle. The width of the normal ejection shell exceeds one-third of the left ventricular transverse diameter throughout its inferoposterior and apical extent. Thinning of the ejection shell corresponds to hypokinesis, and absence of the shell corresponds to akinesis (Fig. 11–10). The accuracy of this technique compares favorably with contrast ventriculography for the detection of ventricular asynergy.[56]

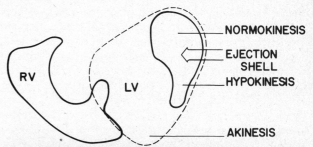

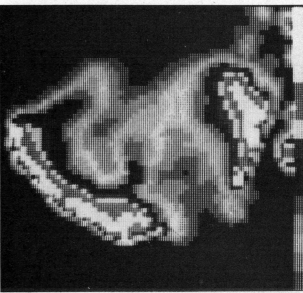

FIGURE 11–10 *A*, Schematic representation of left ventricular ejection shell with thinning (hypokinesis) and fracture (akinesis). *B*, Corresponding ejection fraction image in a patient with a large akinetic segment (apical) and adjacent hypokinesis. (From Maddox, D. E., et al.: The ejection fraction image: A noninvasive index of regional left ventricular wall motion. Am. J. Cardiol. *41*:1230, 1978.)

Paradox Image. If the end-diastolic frame is subtracted from the end-systolic frame, the resultant image will show areas of left ventricular paradox. The presence and extent of paradox in each picture element is determined from the end-diastolic (ED) and end-systolic (ES) counts within that picture element according to the equation

$$\text{Paradox} = \text{ES} - \text{ED} \qquad (9)$$

The extent of paradox may be determined in terms of both the number of picture elements (pixels) within the left ventricle demonstrating paradox and the number of counts within those pixels. Both the number of pixels and the number of counts are normalized by dividing the number of pixels demonstrating paradox by the number of picture elements within the entire left ventricle during end diastole and the number of counts within the left ventricle during end diastole, respectively. There is an excellent correlation between this technique and contrast ventriculography for detecting dyskinetic wall motion.[57]

Phase Images. The radionuclide angiocardiogram can be used to assess regional ventricular performance quantitatively at different intervals during the cardiac cycle and to characterize regional asynchrony. For example, the most sensitive components of the cardiac cycle may be during early systole and during relaxation rather than at end systole. Furthermore, delayed regional contraction and early systolic paradox characterize ventricular contraction in zones bordering on previous infarction.[58] Assessment of regional asynchrony is also useful to detect the foci of ventricular activation in patients with altered patterns of contraction due to pacemakers and to arrhythmias.[59]

Phase images pictorially describe the pattern of cardiac contraction. The first Fourier harmonic is used to fit a cosine wave to the time-activity curve for each pixel in the image. This approach therefore assumes that the ventricular volume curve is similar to one cycle or period of a cosine wave. Each pixel in the image is then coded to a color or gray scale to reflect the phase angle or regional phase delay. In normal patients, the onset of contraction is fairly homogeneous throughout the right and left ventricles and begins soon after the R wave. Contraction begins at the base of the interventricular septum and spreads to the body of the septum, the apex, and then laterally throughout the ventricles. In patients with foci of premature ventricular activation, the focus corresponds to the region with an abnormally early onset of ventricular contraction on the phase image.[59]

While phase imaging is imperfect owing to the assumptions necessary in fitting harmonic waves to the ventricular volume curve and to superimposition of normally contracting myocardium on regions of asynchrony, it does provide useful information regarding sequential electrical events from a sequential assessment of mechanical events.

Regional Ejection Fraction. Several methods have been suggested for measuring regional ejection fraction. Basically, one method divides the ventricle into radial sectors while the other divides it into rectangular segments bordering the major and minor axes of the left ventricle.[60,61] Background is subtracted regionally, using areas adjacent to the various regions. Regional ejection fraction is then calculated from the count-rate changes in each segment using Equation 8 (p. 362). Both methods yield similar results. With the rectangular method, normal regional ejection fraction is 0.66 ± 0.13 in the anteroseptum, 0.85 ± 0.12 in the apex, and 0.74 ± 0.16 in the inferoposterior segment.

This method is not as sensitive as functional imaging because normal and abnormal ventricular segments are mixed in the much larger region of interest that must be used for quantification. On the other hand, regional ejection fraction measurements are reproducible and useful in studies that require quantitative measures of wall motion, such as before and during drug therapy.

Right Ventricular Ejection Fraction. Although equilibrium (ECG-gated) radionuclide ventriculography can be used for the sequential assessment of global and regional left ventricular performance, there are anatomical differences between the left and right sides of the heart that make assessment of right ventricular ejection fraction using count-rate techniques and the equilibrium radionuclide angiocardiogram more difficult. The right atrium lies behind the right ventricle to a greater extent than the left atrium overlies the left ventricle. This interference is solved in first-pass radionuclide angiocardiography by imaging in the right anterior oblique projection, thus spatially separating the right atrium from the right ventricle. This

cannot be done easily using equilibrium radionuclide ventriculography because the right ventricle is superimposed on the left in that projection. Thus, initial attempts at measuring the ejection fraction by equilibrium methods have necessitated the use of either multiple regions of interest in an effort to define the right ventricular perimeter throughout the cardiac cycle[62] or a background region of interest extending into the right atrium and pulmonary outflow tract.[63]

An alternative method for assessing right ventricular ejection fraction from the equilibrium radionuclide angiocardiogram involves use of the slant-hole collimator, which provides a 30-degree caudal tilt that more effectively separates the right atrium from the right ventricle.[64] A fixed background correction region is defined in the usual manner for measurement of the global left ventricular ejection fraction. The same regions are also used for the right ventricle. Background is then subtracted from each pixel of the end-diastolic and end-systolic frames. The end-diastolic right ventricular perimeter is defined manually from the ejection fraction image and the end-diastolic frame. The ejection fraction image separates the right atrium from the right ventricle since the atrium moves paradoxically in relation to the right ventricle. Time-activity curves are then generated from the right ventricular region of interest to determine the frames corresponding to right ventricular end systole and end diastole.

Right ventricular ejection fraction is then calculated from the formula

$$RVEF = \frac{EDC - ESC}{EDC - BC} \qquad (10)$$

where RVEF is right ventricular ejection fraction, EDC represents the counts within the right ventricular region of interest in the frame corresponding to right ventricular end-diastole, ESC represents the counts within the right ventricular region of interest in the right ventricular end-systolic frame, and BC represents the background counts.

With this method, right ventricular ejection fraction in patients without cardiopulmonary disease averages 0.59 ± 0.08 (SD). The correlation between right ventricular ejection fraction measured by both first-pass and equilibrium techniques is excellent.[64]

Valvular Regurgitation. The severity of aortic and mitral regurgitation can be measured from the radionuclide angiocardiogram.[65-67] While first-pass techniques have been described for assessing left-sided regurgitation, the greatest experience has been derived from equilibrium (gated) studies. Radionuclide angiocardiography is performed as described above. Regions of interest are drawn over the left and right ventricles by visual inspection, taking care to include the entire right ventricular or left ventricular area, while excluding as much of the atria, pulmonary artery, and aorta as possible. This is best accomplished with the 30-degree slant-hole collimator and the stroke-volume image for outlining the ventricles. Changes in the counts in each ventricular area between systole and diastole are then determined. Since the same regions of interest are used for both systole and diastole, and since only the absolute change in counts is recorded, background activity is not subtracted. The results are expressed as a ratio of the change in counts in the left ventricular area over the change in counts in the right ventricular area (LV/RV stroke-index ratio).

In patients without aortic or mitral regurgitation, the left-to-right ventricular stroke-index is 1.15 ± 0.15. The ratio is greater than one in normal patients because the right ventricular stroke volume is underestimated owing to overlapping of the right atrium on the right ventricle. In patients with mitral or aortic regurgitation, the ratio is greater than 1.35. There is good agreement between the stroke-volume index and qualitative angiographic estimates of regurgitation.

Some constraints that must be considered when applying this technique are that (1) right-sided regurgitation should not be present, (2) global left ventricular ejection fraction should be greater than 0.30, and (3) there should be good separation of the right atrium from the right ventricle. There is always some overlap of the right atrium on the right ventricle, even with a slant-hole collimator, and this problem may be more severe with significant right atrial enlargement.

Tricuspid regurgitation can be diagnosed and assessed by evaluating the change in liver blood volume during the cardiac cycle.[68] Normally there is no change in liver blood volume; however, with tricuspid regurgitation, liver blood volume increases by 1 per cent or more soon after ventricular end-systole.

EXERCISE

The advantage of radionuclide angiocardiography over other methods for assessing ventricular performance is that it can be performed during physiological stresses and during pharmacological interventions. This is particularly helpful in the evaluation of patients with suspected cardiopulmonary disease because diagnostic and management decisions often cannot be based on resting ventricular performance alone but require additional information about coronary and cardiac reserves.

Exercise is the most frequently applied stress and is particularly useful in evaluating patients suspected of having coronary artery disease[69,70] (p. 366). With equilibrium radionuclide angiocardiography, a resting study is performed with the patient in the same position as will be used later during exercise. This is usually the 45-degree left anterior oblique projection, so that the right and left ventricles can be viewed separately, and with the patient supine or 45 degrees upright. The 45-degree upright position increases the likelihood that the patient will achieve an adequate exercise level but requires an appropriately designed table and camera mount. A high-sensitivity collimator is used because the acquisition time is short. A restraining harness is used to minimize patient motion under the camera during exercise. The imaging table should be secure, with minimal motion. Exercise loads are increased stepwise by 25-watt increments at 3-minute intervals until the patient experiences symptoms of angina, dyspnea, or fatigue of sufficient severity to limit further exercise or until the patient develops hypertension, arrhythmia, or marked ST-segment changes. Electrocardiographic leads are recorded and monitored continuously throughout the study. Multigated blood pool imaging is performed during the final 2 minutes of each exercise period.

This technique requires patient cooperation, since significant movement during the exercise test will substantially reduce spatial resolution and because the patient must maintain his maximal level of exercise for at least two minutes so that adequate counting statistics can be acquired. This may be particularly difficult for many patients who are not accustomed to supine bicycle exercising or who have peripheral vascular disease. As a result, many patients will become fatigued well below their maximum predicted heart rate response.

Exercise radionuclide angiocardiography can also be performed with the first-pass technique. Only resting and peak exercise studies are obtained with ^{99m}Tc tracers; studies can be obtained at each stage of exercise with ^{195m}Au. This method has several advantages in that upright bicycle exercising can be employed. As a result, more patients will achieve maximum levels of stress. The first-pass study also requires that the patient maintain his maximum exercise level for a considerably shorter time than with equilibrium radionuclide angiocardiography and does not require a steady-state heart rate for as long a period as equilibrium imaging.

Other forms of stress, such as isometric hand-grip, atrial pacing, and the cold pressor test, have been suggested as alternative methods, particularly for patients who cannot use the bicycle ergometer.[71,72] With *isometric hand-grip*, an abnormal response in patients with coronary artery disease is based on impaired regional left ventricular performance. The global ejection fraction response alone does not identify patients with coronary artery disease. While some reports have suggested that regional dysfunction occurs in most patients with coronary artery disease,[71] this method is not as sensitive as dynamic exercise.[73] The *cold pressor test* is performed by having the patient place his hand in a bucket of ice water for several minutes. This response to cold results in systemic vasoconstriction mediated through alpha-adrenergic receptors.[74] The increase in the pressure-rate double product may be used to stress patients with coronary disease, resulting in a depression in left ventricular performance.[72] This test appears to be fairly sensitive for the detection of coronary artery disease, provided that the patient is not receiving beta-adrenergic blocker therapy.[74]

Comparison of First-Pass and Equilibrium Angiocardiography

Both the first-pass and equilibrium radionuclide angiocardiogram provide accurate measurement of global left ventricular ejection fraction. Correlation between the two methods is high ($r = 0.87$[75] and $r = 0.89$[9]). Other hemodynamic indices (such as the peak ejection rate) that depend on high temporal resolution of the left ventricular time-activity curve cannot be obtained as accurately from first-pass studies; they require the high counts obtained with gated studies. Regional wall motion can be assessed with either method, although, again, the high counting rate obtained with the gated studies provides superior spatial resolution and improved accuracy, particularly when indices of regional wall motion, such as regional ejection fraction, are measured.

Background is a greater problem with equilibrium studies than with first-pass studies and accounts for as much as half the activity from the left ventricular region-of-interest with the former method. As a result, it may be easier to detect the edges of the left ventricle with first-pass studies despite the lower intrinsic resolution. However, equilibrium studies are superior for patient monitoring and for sequential studies. Imaging can be continued for up to four hours after injection of the radiopharmaceutical, allowing imaging in multiple projections and during physiological or pharmacological interventions. With first-pass studies, a radiopharmaceutical must be administered each time imaging is to be performed. Background activity precludes more than two or three studies during the effective half-life of the tracer, thus limiting the number of sequential studies possible with ^{99m}Tc, for example. On the other hand, physiological or pharmacological interventions with concomitant rapid changes in heart rate may be studied best with the first-pass technique. For both techniques, a steady-state heart rate is necessary, but only five or six heartbeats are required for first-pass studies compared to at least two minutes of heartbeats for the gated studies.

CLINICAL APPLICATIONS

DETECTION AND EVALUATION OF CORONARY ARTERY DISEASE. In patients with coronary artery disease who have not yet sustained an acute myocardial infarction, resting ventricular performance is usually normal because the myocardium is not ischemic. When these patients are stressed, an imbalance between oxygen supply and demand develops, resulting in ischemia. This, in turn, causes a fall in global left ventricular ejection fraction and the development of regional wall motion abnormalities. When radionuclide angiocardiography is applied during exercise in normal patients, left ventricular ejection fraction rises significantly compared to levels at rest, with no left ventricular wall motion abnormalities.[69,70] In patients with coronary artery disease and angina, left ventricular ejection fraction falls during exercise and new regional wall motion abnormalities may develop. The normal increase in ejection fraction with exercise is due primarily to a decrease in end-systolic volume, while the exercise-induced decrease in ejection fraction in patients with angina is due to an increase in end-systolic volume.[75] In patients with coronary artery disease without angina there is usually no change in ejection fraction during exercise, since there is no significant change in end-systolic volume.

The criteria for an abnormal left ventricular ejection fraction response with exercise vary considerably from laboratory to laboratory. Most groups, however, require at least a 5 or 10 per cent increase in ejection fraction to consider the result normal. In normal patients with high resting ejection fractions (>75 per cent), there may be no change in ejection fraction with exercise. In addition to the measurement of global left ventricular function, the cineangiocardiograms obtained at rest and during exercise are evaluated to detect any new wall motion abnormalities. The numerical analyses described previously can also be applied to assess regional and global ventricular performance during exercise.

At first glance, this technique would seem to be particularly accurate for the diagnosis of coronary artery disease.

Okada et al. reviewed the literature from 1978 to 1980[76] and found that the sensitivity for detection of regional wall motion abnormalities (the percentage of coronary artery disease patients with this finding) was 73 per cent, while the specificity (the percentage of normal subjects without regional asynergy) was 100 per cent. There was considerable variability in the sensitivity rates from study to study, however, with a range of less than 50 per cent to 100 per cent. It would seem that the sensitivity for detecting wall motion abnormalities should not be high with this method, since only one projection is obtained and the image has poor resolution because of the short acquisition time. The sensitivity of this method for detecting an abnormal left ventricular ejection fraction response in patients with coronary artery disease was 87 per cent with a specificity of 93 per cent.

Other factors will play a major role in determining left ventricular response with exercise. For example, inadequate stress due to peripheral vascular disease or the concurrent administration of beta-adrenergic blocking drugs may result in normal responses in spite of coronary artery disease.[77] It has also been shown that the sensitivity of the test is reduced in women and in men with atypical angina. The ejection fraction response is greater with upright exercise than with supine exercise.[78]

Most important in determining the specificity of the test is the definition of the control population. Exercise response is dependent on the patient's sex, resting ejection fraction, and change in end-diastolic volume.[79–81] Age is a particularly important factor. Most studies have involved control patients who were usually young individuals without cardiopulmonary disease. Patients over the age of 60, however, may demonstrate no increase in ejection fraction with exercise and may in fact demonstrate a decrease in ejection fraction due to aging rather than to coronary artery disease.[80]

In fact, an abnormal ejection fraction response to exercise is expected in any condition in which there is reduced left ventricular reserve, such as volume- or pressure-overload states and states of decreased left ventricular compliance. As a result, abnormal responses have been reported in patients with aortic stenosis,[82] aortic regurgitation,[83] mitral regurgitation,[84] mitral valve prolapse,[85] hypertrophic obstructive cardiomyopathy,[86] chronic obstructive pulmonary disease,[87] beta-thalassemia and chronic iron overload,[88] cystic fibrosis,[89] elderly patients, female patients, and patients receiving propranolol.[90–92]

When interpreting the exercise radionuclide angiocardiogram, it is clear that additional information should be incorporated into the decision-making process. For example, almost three-fourths of patients suspected of having coronary artery disease without a high pretest probability of the disease (i.e., no previous infarction or typical anginal symptoms) can be diagnosed with an 85 per cent certainty by combining the results of exercise radionuclide angiocardiography and clinical variables such as the presence of chest pain and ST-segment changes with exercise.[93] Thus, the radionuclide angiocardiogram is most useful in the noninvasive diagnosis of coronary artery disease when it is coupled with additional clinical information.

In the diagnostic evaluation of patients with suspected coronary artery disease, the exercise electrocardiogram may provide the necessary diagnostic information without resorting to additional noninvasive or invasive methods. If the exercise electrocardiogram is nondiagnostic, an exercise radionuclide study may be useful. At the present time, neither exercise radionuclide angiocardiography nor exercise myocardial perfusion scintigraphy (p. 370) appears clearly to be the procedure of choice. Radionuclide angiocardiography provides higher sensitivity but poorer specificity in patients with valvular heart disease, primary myocardial disease, or severe lung disease. Furthermore, particularly with supine bicycle ergometry, many patients may not achieve an adequate chronotropic response. The exercise radionuclide angiocardiogram does provide more complete information, particularly when imaging is performed at each stage of exercise, which allows cardiac performance to be assessed at various levels of submaximal exercise.

On the other hand, thallium scintigraphy can be performed in multiple projections immediately after exercise and provides a more reliable map of the pattern and location of the regional abnormality. Furthermore, it is more likely that the patient will achieve an adequate exercise response with thallium scintigraphy, since ordinarily the exercise is performed upright and on a treadmill. The choice between the two procedures may depend heavily on the experience of the nuclear cardiology personnel, however.

ACUTE MYOCARDIAL INFARCTION. Ventricular performance is a major factor affecting patient prognosis after acute myocardial infarction. Radionuclide angiocardiography provides information concerning global left ventricular function, the extent and location of regional abnormalities, and the presence and extent of right ventricular involvement. As a result, it provides prognostic information, since the left ventricular ejection fraction is a predictor of early mortality and the development of congestive failure or sudden death.[94,95] In addition, approximately half the patients with inferior infarction will have abnormalities in right ventricular performance.[96-98]

Ventricular function can also be used to assess patient recovery. Global and regional ventricular performance will improve gradually over the first two weeks after infarction but will show a significant improvement by two to four months if uninterrupted by complications such as reinfarction. Additional prognostic information may be gained from submaximal exercise testing of patients prior to discharge from the hospital, since the ventricular response to exercise appears useful in selecting patients at high risk for subsequent complications.[95,99]

VALVULAR HEART DISEASE. Radionuclide angiography provides the only readily available, noninvasive means for quantifying the degree of left-sided valvular regurgitation.[67] While echocardiography offers excellent visualization of valve motion, assesses aortic dilatation, and measures the degree of mitral stenosis, the severity of regurgitation can be estimated only qualitatively, even with Doppler methods.

In addition to its ability to detect and measure left-sided regurgitation, radionuclide angiocardiography may play a role in the management of patients with aortic valve regurgitation. In these patients, the decision to intervene surgically depends on the degree of left ventricular dysfunction (p. 1114). The dysfunction may not be apparent at rest and may show up only during exercise. It has been suggested that by the time symptoms develop in these patients, irreversible myocardial dysfunction has occurred and that functional abnormalities may appear during stress even in the asymptomatic patient.[100,101] As a result, radionuclide assessment of left ventricular function during exercise has been suggested as a means of following patients with aortic regurgitation to determine the optimal time for valve replacement. While this approach appears promising, further validation is required before it can be recommended for routine clinical use.

ASSESSMENT OF VENTRICULAR DYSFUNCTION. Radionuclide angiocardiography is most useful in patients with symptoms suggesting ventricular dysfunction because it can (1) detect ventricular aneurysm, (2) distinguish regional from global dysfunction, (3) evaluate myocardial viability, (4) evaluate right and left ventricular function, and (5) evaluate the effectiveness of therapeutic interventions. It provides a noninvasive method for accurate quantitation of ventricular hemodynamics and regional wall motion in patients too ill to undergo invasive cardiac catheterization. In addition, the technique can be performed sequentially to evaluate the natural history of heart disease and the effectiveness of medical or surgical management.

The technique is comparable in sensitivity to contrast ventriculography in detecting and assessing *aneurysm* and in determining the location and extent of dyskinetic segments and the status of the remaining ventricle. These factors are particularly important in patients with coronary artery disease in whom aneurysmectomy is being considered (p. 1374).[102] As a result, the radionuclide method can be used to screen patients to separate those with diffuse hypokinesis, who are poor candidates for surgery (Fig. 11–11) from those with localized akinesis or aneurysm (Fig.

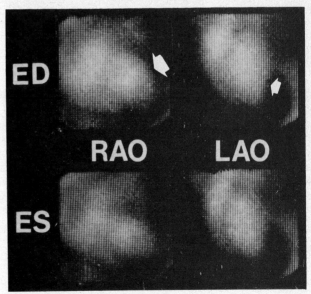

FIGURE 11–11 Equilibrium (gated) radionuclide angiocardiogram of a patient with ischemic cardiomyopathy. There is global asynergy of the markedly enlarged left ventricle (arrows). Note the small difference in size and intensity of left ventricular activity between diastole and systole. The right ventricle is normal in size and performance. ED = end-diastolic frame; ES = end-systolic frame; RAO = 30-degree right anterior oblique projection; LAO = 45-degree modified left anterior oblique projection.

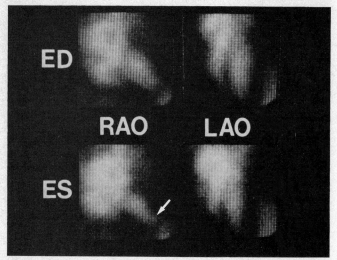

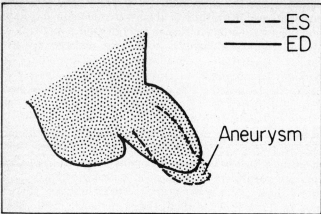

FIGURE 11–12 Equilibrium (gated) radionuclide angiocardiogram of a patient with an apical aneurysm. Note the apical dyskinesis seen best on the RAO projection (arrow). Performance is normal in the other ventricular segments. ED = end-diastolic frame; ES = end-systolic frame; RAO = 30-degree right anterior oblique projection; LAO = 45-degree modified left anterior oblique projection.

11–12), who may then undergo cardiac catheterization prior to surgery.

Regional wall motion abnormalities present at rest may be due to scar from previous myocardial infarction or to reversible ischemia of viable tissue. Since revascularization may improve regional function if the tissue is viable, it is important to *differentiate between reversible ischemia and scar*. Postextrasystolic potentiation and nitroglycerin have been used to help make this distinction, usually at the time of catheterization[103–109] (p. 1369). The exercise radionuclide angiocardiogram can be used to evaluate the change in regional wall motion after exercise.[103,109] In most patients with surgically reversible regional ventricular dysfunction (> 90 per cent), function in that region improves immediately after exercise compared to function at rest. The predictive value of this test is controversial, however, since the number of patients whose regional function does not improve after exercise but does improve after surgery varies from 16[103] to 50 per cent.[109]

Right ventricular function is seriously compromised in patients with *chronic obstructive pulmonary disease* who

have pulmonary artery hypertension or pulmonary vasoconstriction (Fig. 11–13). There is a direct relationship between right ventricular dysfunction and prognosis; right ventricular performance is also related to the magnitude of arterial hypoxemia and ventilatory impairment. Abnormal right ventricular function is a warning sign of subsequent cardiopulmonary decompensation.[110] During exercise, the majority of patients with chronic obstructive lung disease will have abnormal right ventricular reserve, as manifested by reduction in the ejection fraction.[111] This response is not necessarily due to intrinsic myocardial dysfunction but is the result of a normal response to elevated pulmonary artery (and right ventricular systolic) pressure during exercise. Left ventricular response in these patients is generally normal.[112]

Radionuclide angiocardiography provides a noninvasive method for *monitoring the acute and chronic effects of drugs* on ventricular performance. A wide variety of drugs has been studied, including inotropic agents such as digitalis and amrinone,[113,114] afterload-reducing agents such as prazosin,[115,116] bronchodilators such as aminophylline,[117] beta-adrenergic blockers such as propranolol,[118] antiarrhythmics such as disopyramide, and slow-channel calcium antagonists such as verapamil or nifedipine.[119] Individual patient response can be studied as well. Ventricular performance can be used as a guide to determine when a particular therapeutic agent has lost its effectiveness and when replacement or combinative therapy may be necessary.

Ventricular performance is an important indicator of cardiotoxicity with drugs, such as doxorubicin, that have a potentially detrimental effect on the heart[120] (p. 1690). By sequentially assessing patients who are receiving these agents, it might be possible to predict when irreversible cardiac failure might develop in an individual patient. As a result, medication can be continued as long as possible and stopped while cardiac failure is still reversible.

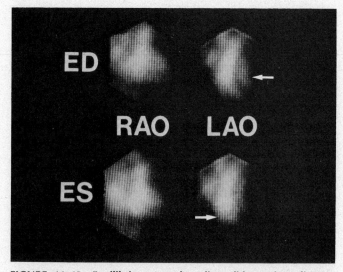

FIGURE 11–13 Equilibrium (gated) radionuclide angiocardiogram of a patient with severe chronic obstructive pulmonary disease and right sided heart failure. Note the dilated, poorly contracting right ventricle (upper arrow) and dilated right atrium. The left ventricle is normal in size and performance (lower arrow). ED = end-diastolic frame; ES = end-systolic frame; RAO = 30-degree right anterior oblique projection; and LAO = 45-degree modified left anterior oblique projection.

MYOCARDIAL PERFUSION SCINTIGRAPHY

The development of newer surgical and medical techniques for the treatment of coronary artery disease has emphasized the need for an objective measure of regional myocardial perfusion. Although the coronary arteriogram can precisely define vessel morphology (Chap. 10), the effect of a coronary artery lesion on tissue perfusion cannot be accurately determined by means of roentgenographic procedures.[121] Furthermore, objective screening procedures are needed to evaluate patients during the early stages of their disease, well before symptoms become severe enough to warrant catheterization. Radionuclide techniques that assess regional myocardial perfusion provide information useful in the detection and evaluation of coronary artery disease and in the assessment of therapies aimed at limiting the degree of ischemia and the extent of tissue necrosis.[122] It is critical to obtain *regional* information, since coronary heart disease is a regional disease with areas of normal myocardium often adjacent to severely diseased tissue. It is also critical to measure perfusion both at rest and during exercise, pacing, or some other stress, since perfusion may be normal at rest even in patients with severe coronary artery disease.

RADIOPHARMACEUTICALS FOR PERFUSION SCINTIGRAPHY

The first radioactive *potassium analogs* available for human use emitted photons that were too energetic for scintillation imaging.[123-125] Potassium-43 was the first of a number of potassium analogs with physical characteristics that were compatible with external imaging techniques.[126] Other potassium analogs have been used for myocardial scintigraphy, including cesium-129,[127] rubidium-81,[128] and thallium-201.[129] While all these radionuclides have limitations because of their long physical half-life, unsatisfactory gamma energies, or limited availability, thallium-201 has emerged clearly as the radiotracer of choice for myocardial perfusion scintigraphy.

Thallium-201 has a physical half-life of 73.1 hours and is a metallic element with properties similar to potassium.[130,131] Its physical characteristics are reasonably well suited for imaging with scintillation camera systems.[132] Characteristic x-rays are emitted in a range from 69 to 83 kev, and these photons are routinely used for external imaging. In addition, gamma emissions of 135 and 167 kev are produced during 10 per cent of the disintegrations. In routine imaging, the pulse height analyzer is centered over the lower energy characteristic x-rays. These low-energy photons result in some loss of spatial resolution because the scattered radiation cannot be separated completely from the primary photopeak. Nevertheless, this energy range does permit imaging with scintillation cameras and enables greater resolution than is obtained with potassium-43, rubidium-81, or cesium-129. Thallium-201 has a number of biological characteristics that make it particularly attractive for perfusion scintigraphy. Clearance of thallium from the blood is almost as rapid as that of potassium or rubidium, and washout from the myocardium is slower. A maximum heart-to-blood ratio is reached within 6 to 8 minutes after injection. *Distribution* of thallium and rubidium is similar throughout the left ventricle, but thallium appears to *concentrate* in myocardial tissue to a somewhat greater degree than potassium or rubidium.[129,132] Extraction of thallium by the myocardium occurs by a cell membrane transport system that can be inhibited by ouabain and is most likely due to activation of the sodium-potassium ATPase system.[133] Thallium appears to bind at two sites on the enzyme system compared to potassium, with one binding site; this may account for the prolonged clearance of thallium from the myocardium.[131]

Technetium-99m is the ideal radionuclide for Anger camera scintigraphy because of its gamma energy of 140 kev, its relatively short physical half-life (6 hours), its low radiation dose to the patient, and its general availability from a long-lived parent via a relatively inexpensive generator system. The development of a ^{99m}Tc myocardial perfusion agent would be quite attractive. A monovalent cation complex has recently been labeled with technetium-99m.[134] In most animal models, myocardial distribution of this tracer is proportional to blood flow. Further study is required to determine whether this tracer or an analog accumulates in the human heart in sufficient concentration to be clinically useful.

When cyclotron-produced positron-emitting potassium analogs and positron imaging devices are used in perfusion scintigraphy, three-dimensional reconstruction of the heart is possible. The very short half-life of these agents also permits multiple studies under various stress states as well as frequent sequential examinations to follow the course of ischemia or infarction. One of these promising tracers is *rubidium-82*, a positron emitter with a 75-second half-life.[135] Aside from the obvious advantage that results from its short half-life, this potassium analog is the daughter of strontium-82, with a 25-day half-life. Since strontium-82/rubidium-82 generator systems have been developed,[136] the parent can be stored for considerable periods of time and eluted whenever rubidium-82 is needed for injection. High-resolution scintiscans have been obtained when coincidence imaging is used with either positron cameras or positron emission–computed tomographic devices.[137] While imaging is not possible with standard Anger scintillation camera systems because of the high gamma energy (511 kev) of rubidium-82, rotating collimators have recently been developed that permit high-resolution scintigraphy after intracoronary injection of the tracer and perhaps even after intravenous injection.[138]

Another positron emitter, *nitrogen-13 ammonium*, has also been used as a marker of myocardial perfusion, and there has been a close correlation between changes in the size of the resultant perfusion defect and the clinical course of patients with acute infarction.[139] Because of the short half-life of this tracer, an on-site cyclotron is necessary for radiotracer production, markedly limiting its availability and capability.

THALLIUM-201 KINETICS

Regional alterations in myocardial perfusion can be measured when myocardial scintigraphy is performed after the intravenous injection of potassium analogs such as thallium-201. This approach is based on the indicator fractionation principle, which postulates that the uptake of these tracers by heart muscle equals the fraction of cardiac output perfusing the myocardium after the intravenous injection of the tracer.[140] Since approximately 5 per cent of the cardiac output supplies the myocardium at rest and since the myocardial extraction of thallium-201 is high, there is sufficient uptake of the tracer by the heart relative to surrounding structures to permit imaging with external detecting systems.

INITIAL DISTRIBUTION. After intravenous injection of thallium-201, the initial distribution of the tracer is equal to the product of regional myocardial blood flow times the extraction fraction, i.e., the percentage of the tracer extracted by the myocardium during a single passage through its circulation. Thus, the degree to which the distribution of thallium-201 reflects myocardial blood flow depends on an unchanging extraction fraction at different flows. However, several factors affect the extraction fraction of thallium-201 in the myocardium. At coronary flow rates while the patient is at rest, the extraction fraction is high, between 85 and 90 per cent. At high flow rates, if the increase in flow is greater than the metabolic needs of the heart, the extraction fraction is reduced, and thallium-201 uptake consequently increases at a lower rate than the increase in coronary blood flow.[141] Another factor that affects the distribution of thallium-201 is the functional integrity of the cell membrane adenosine triphosphatase, which maintains transmembrane electrochemical gradients of sodium and potassium.[142,143,143a] For example, in the presence of severe regional hypoxia with adequate perfusion, the concentration of some potassium analogs is decreased;[144] hypoxia causes a decrease in the extraction fraction of thallium-201 as well.[145] Furthermore, inhibition of either oxidative phosphorylation or glycolytic pathways reduces thallium uptake at the cellular level.[146]

Despite these limitations, regional myocardial uptake of thallium-201 correlates linearly with regional myocardial blood flow from very low flow rates to normal resting levels.[147] At flow rates above the resting level, thallium uptake increases proportionately when the increased flow levels are associated with increases in myocardial oxygen demand[148] and less than proportionately when the increases in flow exceed the metabolic needs of the heart.[141,149,150]

Exercise or other forms of stress are essential to detect coronary stenoses accurately by myocardial perfusion scintigraphy. Regions that are perfused normally at rest but exhibit reduced perfusion during exercise represent ischemic zones, while perfusion defects seen both at rest and during exercise usually represent zones of previous infarction. Abnormal perfusion during stress in patients with transient ischemia is due to a heterogeneous increase in myocardial blood flow. In normal individuals, blood flow increases uniformly throughout the left ventricle during exercise or other forms of stress-simulating interventions. In patients with coronary artery disease, the increase in blood flow to the myocardium distal to a hemodynamically significant arterial stenosis is less than normal and may in fact be absent. There is an inverse relationship between the increase in flow and the percentage of coronary artery stenosis once the lumen is narrowed by approximately 40 to 50 per cent.[151] Thus, the difference between the absolute quantity of radiotracer available for uptake by myocardial cells beyond arterial obstructions and the quantity available in beds supplied by normal coronary arteries is maximal during exercise. Since myocardial thallium clearance is high, the relative differences in regional myocardial blood flow will be reflected in disproportionate concentrations of regional myocardial radioactivity on the scintiscan.[152]

The indicator fractionation principle assumes that the tracer will remain trapped in the organ during the period of observation. This is true for microspheres injected intravenously or intra-arterially, but it is not true for thallium-201, particularly when it is injected during exercise. Redistribution of the tracer begins within 10 minutes after injection.[153] The thallium washout rate has a half-life of 4 hours after intravenous injection.[154] It is prolonged in regions of hypoperfusion[155] and is related to the rate of thallium clearance from the blood.[156]

REDISTRIBUTION. Redistribution of thallium-201 has important implications for patients with coronary artery disease, especially when imaging takes place during exercise. When myocardial perfusion scintigraphy is performed during stress, transiently ischemic myocardium can be detected.[157,158] By taking advantage of the redistribution phenomenon, one can detect exercise-induced ischemia by imaging after the exercise injection of thallium and by repeat delayed imaging when the thallium has partially cleared from the normal myocardium and partially washed into the hypoperfused areas, resulting in the disappearance of the initial perfusion defects.[159] This disappearance with time results in the accumulation of thallium in previously unperfused zones in combination with the washout of the tracers from normal myocardium.[155,160]

Perfusion defects noted on the initial postexercise thallium scintigram may be either reversible or nonreversible. In reversible defects due to transient ischemia associated with viable myocardium, thallium washout is slower in the hypoperfused region compared to normal areas, with concentrations of the tracer in the two regions eventually becoming equal. In nonreversible defects due to acute myocardial infarction or myocardial scar associated with nonviable myocardium, the initial perfusion defects persist with delayed imaging because thallium does not accumulate in the infarcted tissue and there is no washin to these nonviable zones during the redistribution phase; hence, concentrations in the infarcted and normal myocardium do not equalize with time.

The *disadvantage* of this technique is that the time during which the thallium distribution reflects myocardial blood flow is limited, lasting for only a short time after the tracer has cleared from the blood following intravenous injection. Consequently, it is essential that imaging begin very soon after injection and that imaging be performed as rapidly as possible. Furthermore, in the face of transient ischemia, the time it takes for concentrations in the ischemic and normal zones to equalize may vary considerably from patient to patient. While the use of a set time (e.g., 3 to 4 hours after injection) for redistribution imaging will differentiate transient ischemia from infarction in the majority of patients, in others redistribution will occur more slowly and further delayed imaging will be necessary to differentiate the two phenomena.

TECHNIQUE

For exercise myocardial perfusion scintigraphy, thallium-201 is injected at the time of maximal stress during a multistage treadmill test according to the Bruce protocol. The patient should not eat for at least four hours prior to the exercise test so that splanchnic uptake of the tracer is reduced to a minimum. For the detection and evaluation of coronary artery disease, drugs that protect the myocardium, such as beta-adrenergic blockers, should be discontinued for a long enough time before the study to allow the amount of drug in the blood to decrease to less than pharmacologically significant levels. (For propranolol, this would be approximately 48 hours prior to the test.) If the protective effect of the drug is being studied specifically, the dose regimen should be maintained at the levels administered prior to the test.

A 12-lead electrocardiogram is obtained prior to the test, and an intravenous line is inserted for rapid injection of the radiotracer and for emergency use if necessary. Exercise should be graded and the injection made at the time of maximal exercise, which should be maintained for at least 60 to 90 seconds following the injection to allow the tracer to be cleared from the blood. A near maximum exercise level ($\geq$ 85 per cent of predicted maximal heart rate) should be achieved to assess the extent of the disease.[161] It would appear that the heart rate response may be less critical for accurate diagnosis of coronary artery disease, although the incidence of false-negative examinations is high when the patient fails to achieve 70 per cent of the predicted maximal heart rate. Electrocardiographic monitoring should continue throughout the test and during the immediate post-test period. The exercise test should be stopped if hypotension, marked electrocardiographic evidence of ischemia, serious arrhythmias, or significant pain develops.

Imaging may begin 6 to 8 minutes after injection, allowing sufficient time for the thallium to be cleared from the blood but prior to significant redistribution. A camera and collimator with a system spatial resolution of at least 4.5 mm (full-width at half-maximum) for thallium-201 should be used for imaging. Because imaging must be performed as quickly as possible, the low-energy, all-purpose collimator is usually used, although the recently introduced high-resolution parallel square-hole collimator offers better spatial resolution with sensitivity comparable to that of the standard all-purpose collimators. With the latter collimator, care must be taken to keep the amount of the thallium-202 contaminant, with its high-energy emissions, to a minimum at the time of injection. The pulse height analyzer energy window is peaked over the low-energy (69 to 81 kev) thallium-201 photopeak. In cameras with multiple pulse height analyzer energy windows for data collection, the counts resulting from the higher energy gamma rays (135 and 165 kev) should also be collected, substantially increasing camera sensitivity and improving spatial resolution.

Projections obtained during myocardial perfusion scintigraphy include the 30- or 45-degree left anterior oblique, anterior, 70-degree left anterior oblique, and left lateral views. Since the plane of the septum can vary, patient positioning should be tailored to the individual patient and his cardiac anatomy. Care must be taken in interpreting the 70-degree LAO and the left lateral views, particularly when the patient is imaged in the supine position. Increased attenuation of the diaphragm superimposed on the inferior wall of the left ventricle may cause apparent inferior perfusion defects in patients with normal blood flow.[162] Perfusion defects seen only on these views should be confirmed with additional imaging in the 70-degree LAO or left lateral view with the patient lying left side up. At least 300,000 counts are acquired per view; when computer acquisition is used, counts on each view can be collected for a preset time, usually 6 to 10 minutes per view. With a preset time, quantitative comparisons of thallium-201 activity can be made between serial images. These projections are repeated during redistribution imaging 3 to 4 hours after injection. In addition, if perfusion defects persist and the distinction between infarction and transient ischemia is critical, repeat imaging can be performed 24 hours after injection.

Other forms of stress can be employed, including upright and supine bicycle ergometry, hand-grip exercise, and atrial pacing. Treadmill ergometry is preferable, unless patients are physically unable to run. Treadmill testing is the most likely method to force patients to adequate exercise levels and to increase coronary flow sufficiently to permit accurate interpretations of the thallium-201 images.

Pharmacological methods to increase coronary blood flow have a number of compelling advantages, however. Patients can be routinely and reproducibly stressed to a predefined endpoint, and the method can be used in patients who cannot exercise to maximum levels. Perfusion imaging can be performed after the intravenous injection of dipyridamole, a potent coronary vasodilator that produces little if any myocardial ischemia. Initial experience with this method is encouraging; accuracy in detecting coronary artery disease is comparable to that of standard exercise testing,[163–165] with an improvement in image quality. While imaging is probably safer with dipyridamole than with exercise, patients have experienced severe headaches and postural hypotension after administration of this drug. Furthermore, the relationship between increases in flow and thallium activity are probably not linear in the face of a falling extraction fraction due to increasing flow without corresponding increases in metabolic needs.

INTERPRETATION

Most commonly, image interpretation is based on analog images using Polaroid film or x-ray film for hardcopy. In our laboratory, we find Polaroid film using a triple-lens camera (each lens having a different intensity setting) the most satisfactory method for analog-image interpretation, providing a range of photographically contrast-enhanced images and protecting against the pseudodefects that may occur with computer processing (see below).

In the normal scintigram there is uniform distribution of the tracer throughout the left ventricular wall, with a decrease in concentration in the region of the apex in about half the patients (Fig. 11–14).[166] The ventricle has a horseshoe appearance, with its long axis oriented anywhere from horizontal to vertical. Activity tapers near the base of the heart. In the majority of patients, the inferior wall appears thicker than the anterolateral surface. In the central zone, a region of decreased or absent activity is noted and represents the left ventricular cavity. The right ventricular myocardium is not visualized in normal subjects at rest but may be seen as a thin wall extending from the apex

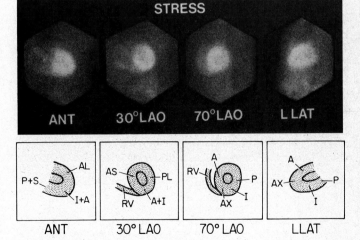

FIGURE 11–14 Normal myocardial perfusion scintigraphy with thallium-201 after stress in four different projections. Notice the uniform uptake of radiotracer throughout the left ventricular wall and the central defect due to the left ventricular cavity. ANT = anterior; 30° LAO = 30-degree left anterior oblique; 70° 70-degree left anterior oblique; LLAT = left lateral; P = posterior; S = septum; AL = anterolateral; I = inferior; A = anterior; PL = posterolateral; AX = apex; RV = right ventricle.

when the injection is made at peak stress during redistribution imaging.

Multiple oblique projections are required, since perfusion defects are seen best on a tangent. In the anterior view, the apical, inferior, and anterolateral walls are well seen. The septum and posterolateral walls are seen best on the 30- to 45-degree LAO views. The anterior free wall, inferior and posterior walls are seen best on the 70-degree LAO and left lateral views. Right ventricular activity is seen when imaging is performed after stress but is less intense than left ventricular activity.[167]

When exercise (stress) and redistribution imaging are performed, it is essential that each of the views obtained during redistribution be acquired in exactly the same position relative to the detector as the corresponding stress image. If proper technique is followed during stress and redistribution imaging, corresponding images can be evaluated for (1) reversible perfusion defects (those that appear on stress imaging but disappear after redistribution and are due to transient ischemia) (Fig. 11–15), (2) nonreversible perfusion defects (abnormalities that persist with equivalent intensity during redistribution imaging and are usually due to scar or infarction) (Fig. 11–16), and (3) normal anatomical variations (such as apical thinning and normally decreased perfusion at the base due to the aortic and mitral valves).

The greatest accuracy is achieved when perfusion defects are seen in the same segment on several views. Stenoses involving the left anterior descending coronary artery result in perfusion defects involving the anterior, septal, and lateral segments. Both the right coronary artery and the left circumflex artery perfuse the inferior and posterior segments; hence, perfusion defects in these segments may be due to stenoses involving either coronary arteries. The apex may be supplied by all three major coronary vessels.

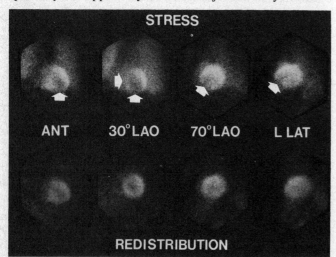

FIGURE 11–15 Myocardial perfusion scintigraphy with thallium-201 in a patient with 90 per cent stenosis of the left anterior descending artery along with less severe stenoses involving the left circumflex system. A large reversible perfusion defect involving the anteroseptal and apical segments of the left ventricle is seen best on the 30-degree LAO immediate postexercise image (arrows). The defect is not present on redistribution imaging four hours later (lower panel) because it is due to transient ischemia. Note the transiently increased lung uptake on the immediate postexercise images (upper panel). (ANT = anterior; 30° LAO = 30-degree left anterior oblique; 70° LAO = 70-degree left anterior oblique; LLAT = left lateral.)

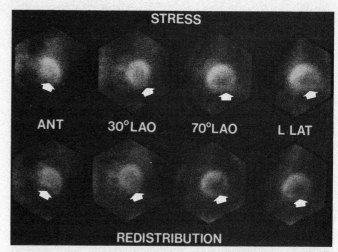

FIGURE 11–16 Myocardium perfusion scintigraphy with thallium-201 in a patient with a previous inferoposterior myocardial infarction. A large nonreversible perfusion defect involving the inferior and posterior segments of the left ventricle is seen best in the 70-degree LAO and LLAT projections. The defect is seen on the immediate poststress images (upper arrows) and involves the same area of the left ventricle on the redistribution images obtained four hours later (lower arrows). The defect is due to nonviable myocardium or to scar tissue. (ANT = anterior; 30° LAO = 30-degree left anterior oblique; 70° LAO = 70-degree left anterior oblique; LLAT = left lateral.)

In addition to interpretation of myocardial thallium-201 activity, attention should also be directed to the size of the cardiac chamber, wall thickness, and pulmonary uptake of thallium-201. An enlarged cardiac chamber may be seen at rest, indicating ventricular dilation. Cardiac chamber enlargement may be seen only during the exercise phase of the study and indicates a transient increase in end-diastolic volume, an index of diminished cardiac reserve in patients with a variety of cardiac diseases including, but not limited to, coronary artery disease. A transient increase in lung activity during exercise results from a transient increase in pulmonary blood volume and is associated with an elevated pulmonary capillary wedge pressure. The increase in pulmonary thallium-201 activity is probably due to an increase in capillary surface area and a resultant increase in tracer extraction. The ratio between lung and heart activity has been quantitated and found to be highly specific but only moderately sensitive for coronary artery disease.[168] More experience is required with this index to determine whether other cardiac or pulmonary diseases result in increased pulmonary blood volume during stress with an attendant increase in thallium activity.

QUANTIFICATION

Visual interpretation of unprocessed thallium-201 myocardial images leads to a significant degree of disagreement among observers and makes sequential assessment of regional myocardial perfusion difficult.[169] Thallium images have a relatively high level of background activity, which interferes with evaluation of the images. Computers are especially useful in thallium imaging because they allow the observer the capability for interactive image processing. It is very helpful in visualizing the subtle differences involved if one can raise the lower and upper thresholds while viewing the images. Overlaying of images is also helpful in comparing initial images with images after redistribution. In addition to simple threshold subtraction, several interpolative methods for background subtraction have been suggested. These take into account the nonuniformity of background that may result in excessive background subtraction.[170,171] Image interpretation should not depend on background-corrected images alone and must take into account the unprocessed image as well.

Quantitative computer analysis of the thallium image has been suggested as a means for standardizing the interpretation of images and eliminating the high degree of subjectivity in visual analysis.[172,173] In general, this technique evaluates the relative concentrations of thallium in the various segments of the left ventricle.[154,171,174-176] Regional activity is assessed quantitatively by breaking up the thallium myocardial image into anatomically defined left ventricular regions. Thallium-201 uptake in these left ventricular segments is considered to be pathologically reduced if count rates are less than 75 to 80 per cent of maximum left ventricular thallium-201 uptake. Thallium-201 distribution may also be analyzed quantitatively as a function of time, measuring the net rate of thallium washin or washout from the myocardium during the redistribution phase of the study.[154]

While initial experience with these quantitative techniques is promising and appears to improve the accuracy with which coronary artery disease can be detected and assessed, more experience is required before these techniques can be routinely applied. In particular, these methods depend heavily on accurate background correction, which is difficult from two-dimensional images; tomographic imaging may be required for accurate background subtraction. Furthermore, excessive contrast enhancement may result in regions of apparently reduced activity called *pseudodefects*, which are produced by a real difference in counts but are caused by statistical considerations, geometry, or inhomogeneous background activity. Accurate background correction is further complicated because thallium-201 uptake is dependent on myocardial perfusion, mass, and metabolism, and these factors determine the ratio of myocardial activity to background activity. In addition, uptake is affected by exercise, dosage and type of cardiac pharmaceuticals, equipment, and the method used for data collection, processing, and display. The accuracy of quantitative techniques is also affected by the low photon energy of thallium-201 with its high attenuation coefficient. The radiation emanating from the posterior wall of the left ventricle is markedly diminished by absorption in blood and body tissues in the anterior view. Overlying breast tissue can produce an artifactual perfusion defect as well.

TOMOGRAPHY

Many of the problems associated with conventional scintigraphy, such as superimposition of one portion of myocardium on another and the heterogeneity of background activities, are overcome by tomography. Both limited-angle and transaxial tomography can be performed using thallium-201.

Limited-angle tomography of the heart can be performed with thallium-201 and a seven-pinhole or a rotating slant-hole collimator.[177] With seven-pinhole tomography, seven two-dimensional images are obtained. The pinholes are at slightly different angles and provide seven different views of the heart. A series of two-dimensional images that focus on various depths within the chest are reconstructed from the original data. The primary advantages of this approach are that commercially available radiopharmaceuticals can be used and currently available instrumentation can be modified to obtain limited-angle tomograms. Depth resolution is poor with limited-angle tomography, and positioning of the patient is technically difficult but critical to obtaining satisfactory results. Furthermore, there does not appear to be a significant difference in accuracy between limited-angle tomography and standard two-dimensional thallium imaging.[178-180]

Transaxial computed tomography can be performed with a rotating scintillation camera system or with a multi-detector system.[181] In the rotating gamma camera system, the detector rotates 180 or 360 degrees around the patient.[182,183] The camera detector makes between 32 and 64 stops; during each of these 20- to 40-second stops, the camera acquires a two-dimensional image. The data from all 32 to 64 images or projections are summed, corrected for attenuation, and reconstructed into a transaxial image. Images of other planes, such as coronal, sagittal, or oblique sections, can be reconstructed from the data as well. Thus, imaging can be performed in planes parallel and perpendicular to the long axis of the left ventricle,[184-188] reducing interpretive errors due to reduced perfusion at the base of the heart in the region of the valve plane.

Myocardial perfusion transaxial tomography has a characteristic appearance in the normal patient (Fig. 11–17). The left ventricle appears horseshoe-shaped at the base heart, with the long axis of the horseshoe oriented between 35 and 45 degrees toward the left anterior oblique. The distribution throughout the septum and anterior and lateral walls is homogeneous. The open end of the horseshoe corresponds anatomically to the region of the aortic valve. Sections obtained at the midventricular plane appear doughnut-shaped, with uniform uptake throughout the doughnut. The central perfusion defect represents the left ventricular cavity. Slices through the apex show a round or oval region of activity with a minimal or absent central defect corresponding to a transverse section through the apical wall caudal to the cardiac chamber. Right ventricular or atrial activity is usually not detected.

In patients with myocardial infarction, regions of markedly reduced perfusion are seen in areas corresponding to the location of the infarct (Fig. 11–18). The extent of the perfusion defect is usually greater on emission tomography than on standard two-dimensional scintigraphy. Similarly, the border between the normally perfused myocardium and perfusion defect is sharper and more clearly defined on tomography, since perfused myocardium is not superimposed on the ischemic tissue as it is with conventional imaging. Tomography also improves the contrast between the myocardium and surrounding structures, such as the lung and liver. In addition to the improved accuracy over conventional two-dimensional imaging, the ability to obtain multiple transaxial slices of the area of the myocar-

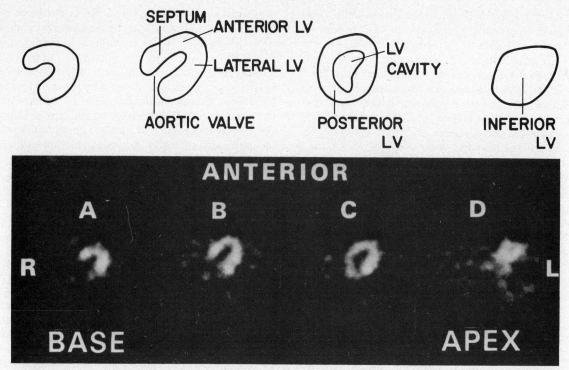

FIGURE 11–17   Normal transaxial myocardial tomograms using thallium-201 in man. The slices are oriented as though the viewer is looking from below with the anterior surface up. Slice A was taken through the base of the left ventricle. The thallium-201 uptake appears horseshoe-shaped owing to the lack of uptake in the region of the valves. Slices obtained more distally through the heart (B and C) show more of a doughnut-shape, with no radioactivity in the region of the left ventricular cavity. At the apex (D), the left ventricular wall is imaged below the cavity, and therefore uptake appears uniform. The right ventricle is not normally seen at rest. (R = right; L = left.) (From Holman, B. L., et al.: Single photon emission computed tomography of the heart in normal subjects and patients with infarction. J. Nucl. Med. *20*:736, 1979.)

dium with the perfusion defect suggests the potential for volumetric quantitation of infarction or ischemia. The ability to quantify the extent of the perfusion defect becomes increasingly important as limitation of infarct size becomes part of the therapeutic strategy in acute myocardial infarction.

CLINICAL APPLICATIONS

DIAGNOSIS OF CORONARY ARTERY DISEASE

The diagnosis of coronary artery disease is the most important application of myocardial perfusion scintigraphy with thallium-201. It is significantly more accurate for the detection of coronary artery disease than the exercise electrocardiogram[189–194] (p. 1341). In a review summarizing the results in over 1800 patients, overall sensitivity for detecting coronary artery disease using thallium-201 was 82 per cent and specificity was 91 per cent. Sensitivity for the exercise electrocardiogram was 60 per cent and specificity was 81 per cent.[76] It has been suggested that temporal and spatial quantitation and tomographic imaging may improve the accuracy of diagnosis somewhat.

Myocardial perfusion scintigraphy with thallium-201 should be used as a complement to exercise electrocardiography. The exercise ECG should be obtained first, prior to perfusion scintigraphy. Thallium-201 scintigraphy should then be carried out when the exercise ECG is nondiagnostic or is abnormal in an asymptomatic patient or when there is a moderate probability of coronary artery disease.[195]

Nondiagnostic electrocardiograms may result when the

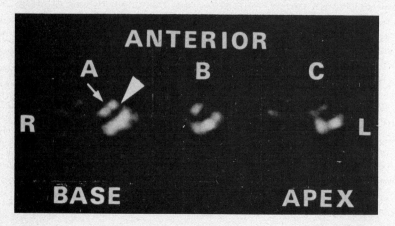

FIGURE 11–18 Transaxial myocardial tomography in a patient with anteroseptal infarct. Note some reduction in perfusion to septum (arrow) and markedly reduced perfusion to anterior wall (arrowhead). (A = slice through base of left ventricle; B = mid-ventricle; C = slice through apex; R = right; L = left.) (From Holman, B. L., et al.: Single photon emission computed tomography of the heart in normal subjects and patients with infarction. J. Nucl. Med. *20*:736, 1979.)

resting electrocardiogram is abnormal but ischemic ST-segment changes cannot be defined. This may occur in patients with left bundle branch block or in those receiving digitalis. In this group of patients, the accuracy of thallium-201 perfusion scintigraphy remains high and is therefore extremely helpful. Another cause for uninterpretable exercise electrocardiograms is failure to achieve 85 per cent of predicted maximal heart rate with no ST-segment changes (p. 1341). In this group of patients, the sensitivity and specificity of thallium-201 imaging are approximately the same as for patients who are able to achieve an adequate heart rate response.[161,196,197] These results suggest that the mechanisms underlying an abnormal stress electrocardiogram and an abnormal myocardial scintigram are different and help to explain why the sensitivities of these tests are additive. When the diagnosis of coronary artery disease is based on both an abnormal stress electrocardiogram and an abnormal thallium-201 test, the diagnostic sensitivity is substantially greater than when either test is used alone. However, it must be remembered that when the two tests are used additively, the diagnostic specificity for coronary artery disease falls substantially.

Patients with *atypical angina pectoris* are reasonable candidates for myocardial perfusion scintigraphy. The likelihood of these patients having coronary artery disease is between 30 and 50 per cent.[198] Perfusion scintigraphy is useful in this group of patients. The accuracy of the exercise electrocardiogram may be too low to affect substantially the likelihood of coronary artery disease, regardless of the outcome of the test (p. 2). The accuracy of myocardial perfusion scintigraphy is higher, so that in patients who are moderately likely to have coronary artery disease, the results of the test can be used to guide medical management. This is not true for patients with *typical angina pectoris*, in whom the likelihood of having the disease is so high prior to diagnostic testing that a normal perfusion test cannot be accepted as strong evidence that the patient does not have coronary artery disease. Similarly, in *asymptomatic* patients, the likelihood of disease is so small prior to testing that this likelihood will change little after the test.[199] Furthermore, if large numbers of asymptomatic patients are studied, a sizable number of false-positive results will occur even when the test's specificity is 90 per cent.

While the test has limited usefulness for asymptomatic patients in general, it is of value in asymptomatic patients with positive stress electrocardiograms. The prevalence of coronary artery disease in this population is approximately 30 per cent.[200] A positive thallium perfusion scintigram raises the likelihood of disease to greater than 80 per cent, while a negative test reduces it to less than 10 per cent.

DIAGNOSING THE EXTENT OF CORONARY ARTERY DISEASE. Thallium-201 perfusion scintigraphy has been most useful in providing the clinician with an objective guide to the severity of a patient's coronary artery disease and the effectiveness of medical therapy. For example, patients with coronary artery disease can be studied while taking propranolol to determine whether they are adequately protected from ischemia at the maximum exercise levels they can achieve while on the drug.

Thallium-201 perfusion scintigraphy has not been particularly useful in determining the number of stenotic coronary arteries nor in identifying which vessels are diseased. The sensitivity is approximately 60 to 80 per cent for identifying obstruction of the left anterior coronary artery, 50 to 60 per cent for the right coronary artery, and 20 to 50 per cent for the left circumflex coronary artery.[201,202] Sensitivity is affected by the severity of the stenosis,[203] with an increasing sensitivity as the degree of stenosis increases. Specific patterns of extensive coronary artery disease that involves either three vessels or the left main coronary artery are helpful when present but are seen in less than half the patients.[204]

The sensitivity for detecting the *extent* of coronary artery disease is directly related to the level of exercise attained.[162] In addition, computer processing (specifically, the measurement of thallium-201 washout at two or three points during the first 6 hours after injection of the tracer) has been suggested to improve the specificity for detecting the number and location of diseased coronary vessels;[205,206] temporal quantitation must be confirmed in other laboratories before it can be applied routinely in clinical practice.

Myocardial perfusion scintigraphy with thallium-201 may be a useful adjunct to coronary angiography for evaluating the *functional significance of coronary stenoses*. The coronary angiogram provides anatomical detail but very little information related to myocardial perfusion. While thallium-201 scintigraphy has been most useful in providing an overall estimate of the functional significance of the disease, it is less useful for defining the functional significance of a borderline coronary artery stenosis. If a perfusion defect is present in the segment supplied by the artery in question, the test result is useful, showing that the lesion is hemodynamically significant. If more severe coronary stenoses in adjacent vessels cause transient ischemia and cessation of the exercise test before the hemodynamically significant stenosis in question causes ischemia, no perfusion defect will appear in that segment.

Perfusion scintigraphy may also be useful as an adjunct to coronary angiography by *differentiating viable from nonviable myocardium*. There is a strong relationship between the degree of redistribution in a region of transient ischemia and the degree of asynergy in that myocardial segment.[207] Furthermore, the better the redistribution, the more likely the segment will contract normally after bypass surgery.[208]

Thallium-201 perfusion scintigraphy has been used to study patients after coronary bypass surgery in whom the question of *graft patency* has arisen. In patients with exercise-induced perfusion defects that become normal after operation, the likelihood of bypass graft patency is high.[209,210] If the segment was normal prior to operation, the postoperative development of transient ischemia indicates that the graft is probably occluded. If perfusion during exercise is normal after operation, the graft is probably patent. If there is no change in perfusion to the segment after surgery, graft patency cannot be predicted accurately.

OTHER CAUSES OF TRANSIENT PERFUSION DEFECTS. Many patients with transient perfusion defects on thallium-201 imaging but considered false-positives in reported studies have coronary stenoses of between 20 and 50 per cent of the vessel diameter.[211] That these patients have a higher incidence of transient ischemia than patients with less severe stenoses may indicate both the difficulty in accurately defining the degree of stenoses using coronary angiography and the possibility that what has traditionally been characterized as subcritical stenoses may result in myocardial hypoperfusion during maximal stress.

Abnormal results may also be seen in patients with *muscular myocardial bridges* without evidence of coronary atherosclerosis[212] and in patients with evidence of *diffuse cardiac disease*.[213] In patients with *aortic stenosis* and normal coronary arteries, exercise-induced subendocardial ischemia[214] or changes in left ventricular wall thickness may develop.[215] This ischemia will result in perfusion defects on thallium-201 imaging. While perfusion defects have been reported in patients with mitral valve prolapse, most studies have not substantiated this observation and have suggested the use of this test for identifying underlying coronary artery disease in patients with prolapse.[216–218]

CORONARY ARTERY SPASM. This may occur in patients without detectable coronary artery stenoses. These patients will have transient perfusion defects on thallium-201 imaging if they are injected during or immediately following spasm.[219–221] Spasm has been demonstrated during exercise in some patients with exertional chest pain and ST-wave elevation who have normal coronary arteries at angiography. Spasm may occur at rest; in this case, perfusion defects are observed even without exercise.

FIXED DEFECTS. *Nonreversible defects*, perfusion defects that are seen both during exercise and at rest, may be due to previous myocardial infarction, hypertrophic obstructive cardiomyopathy,[222] sarcoid heart disease,[223] idiopathic congestive cardiomyopathy,[224] amyloidosis, metastatic disease to the heart, and other infiltrative heart diseases.

Other causes of abnormal tests result from *technical factors*. For example, in patients with negative electrocardiographic exercise tests, the specificity of the test is quite low in women (56 per cent) compared with men (81 per cent) and is due to attenuation of myocardial activity by overlying breast resulting in an apparent perfusion defect in the myocardial segment underlying the breast.[225] As mentioned previously, perfusion defects may appear on the lateral or 70-degree LAO projection in patients studied supine because of attenuation caused by abdominal organs and the diaphragm. Because camera nonuniformity may also result in apparent defects, it is critical to pay close attention to quality control. Probably the single most common cause of apparent perfusion abnormalities is heterogeneous background lung activity, especially when lung activity is high owing to increased pulmonary blood volume. This will result in apparently decreased activity in myocardium that does not overlie the lung and is only partially corrected by interpolative background-correction programs. Emission tomography will alleviate these background problems but may introduce additional problems due to inadequate correction of attenuation.

ACUTE MYOCARDIAL INFARCTION (p. 1288). Perfusion scintigraphy at rest has been used to detect the presence of acute myocardial infarction. Wackers et al. showed defects in 165 of 200 patients (82 per cent).[226] This technique is most sensitive soon after infarction. Thus, 90 of 96 patients had abnormal scintiscans within 24 hours of infarction, while only 75 of 104 had abnormalities after 24 hours. Defects also appear to decrease in size with time, particularly when the initial study is performed within 24 hours of infarction. Since perfusion defects can be seen at rest in some patients with unstable angina and during

spasm in patients with Prinzmetal's angina, perfusion scintigraphy cannot always distinguish between these two conditions. The greatest value of this technique lies in obtaining a normal scintigram within 24 hours of suspected infarction, greatly lowering the probability that the patient has sustained acute infarction. In acute infarction the perfusion defect will decrease in size during the first week, while the defect produced by scar tissue will not change in size. Consequently, serial imaging will be necessary to distinguish old from new infarction.

Patients with unstable angina pectoris have abnormal perfusion at the time of chest pain, but they also have abnormal scintigrams after the pain has subsided.[227] Abnormal scintigrams occur more frequently in patients with a complicated course.

Perfusion scintigraphy may provide prognostic information, since it correlates well with estimates of infarct size made by serum creatine kinase curve analysis[228–230] and by pathological studies.[231–233] Initially, the thallium perfusion defect is larger than the acute infarct because of surrounding ischemia, and it may remain larger if the patient has sustained previous infarctions and has myocardial scar in addition to necrosis.

Thallium perfusion scintigraphy may be useful as a prognostic indicator if it is obtained early after the onset of symptoms.[234] Patients with large defects have an extremely high mortality rate compared to patients with smaller defects. To use this test in a predictive way, it is essential that imaging be obtained early or at a predefined time after the onset of symptoms. Since the perfusion defect will shrink with time unless the patient sustains reinfarction or extension of the infarct, it will not be possible to compare the results obtained at variable times after infarction. The predictive value of this test is enhanced when the test is combined with technetium-99m–pyrophosphate scintigraphy (see Infarct-Avid Scintigraphy), particularly with emission computed tomography.

THE RIGHT VENTRICLE. Right ventricular uptake on the resting thallium-201 images correlates with right ventricular overload (Fig. 11–19) and may be seen in either volume overload (atrial septal defect or pulmonic or tricuspid regurgitation) or pressure overload (mitral stenosis, primary pulmonary hypertension, ventricular septal defect, or Eisenmenger's syndrome). There is a direct relationship between the intensity of right ventricular uptake and the hemodynamic measurement of right ventricular work.

THROMBOLYTIC THERAPY. The intracoronary injection of thrombolytic agents such as streptokinase may reduce the extent of irreversible myocardial damage in patients with acute infarction[235,236] (p. 1324). Since a coronary artery catheter is already in place in the vessel, coronary arteriography can be performed to demonstrate the degree to which the vessel has been reopened. In addition, thallium-201 can be injected directly into the coronary artery both before and after thrombolytic therapy to determine the viability of the reperfused myocardium. Only a small amount of thallium (30 to 50 μCi) needs to be injected at each time. The advantage of this approach is that both reperfusion and integrity of the sodium-potassium pump are necessary for thallium accumulation in the cell. Further work is needed to document that the previously ischemic cells that take up thallium-201 will survive.

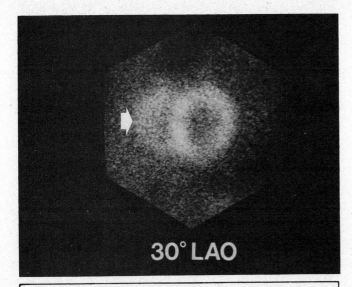

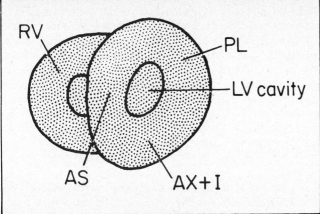

FIGURE 11–19 Myocardial perfusion scintigram in a patient with right ventricular hypertrophy. Note increased thallium-201 uptake in the right ventricle (arrow). 30° LAO = 30-degree left anterior oblique projection; RV = right ventricle; AS = anteroseptal; AX = apex; I = inferior; LV = left ventricular; and PL = posterolateral.

ASSESSMENT OF REGIONAL MYOCARDIAL PERFUSION WITH INVASIVE TECHNIQUES

A number of techniques utilizing radionuclides during or after coronary arteriography have been developed to assess fully the significance of coronary artery lesions. These "invasive" techniques suffer in that they are limited in serial evaluations of patients with coronary artery disease. Nevertheless, they do provide information complementary to that of the coronary arteriogram. Myocardial perfusion may be assessed both in the basal state and following an intervention to determine regional myocardial blood flow distal to coronary artery lesions; thus the hemodynamic significance of the latter may be assessed. It may also be possible to discover those segments of myocardium irreversibly scarred from prior infarction.

Perfusion Scintigraphy with Microparticles. Myocardial perfusion scintigraphy may be performed following intracoronary injection of either macroaggregated albumin[237,238] or radiolabeled microspheres. The primary advantages of this approach are the improved spatial resolution that results from the substantially higher target-to-background ratio and the better physical characteristics of the radiopharmaceutical when it is labeled with [99m]Tc. As already mentioned, its major limitations are the need to inject the tracer *directly* into the coronary circulation, usually at the time of coronary angiography, and the impracticality of serial studies.

Myocardial perfusion imaging yields results compatible in most cases to the anatomical lesions found at coronary arteriography[239] and left ventricular angiography. Occasionally, a region of reduced uptake is not associated with abnormal wall motion in the same location. Obstructions of major vessel branches that exceed 70 per cent of the diameter are usually associated with recognizable regional hypoperfusion on the appropriate radionuclide images. This appears to be more marked when there is a relative lack of collateral perfusion, when multiple vessels are involved, and in those cases in which extensive scarring of the myocardium has occurred.

Perfusion scintigraphy with microparticles, performed in the basal state, demonstrates abnormalities in only a portion of patients with significant coronary artery disease.[238] Presumably, in patients with normal scintigrams and coronary obstruction, the latter is not severe enough to limit the flow in the resting state nor is there any scar tissue caused by previous infarction. The finding of abnormal perfusion studies with normal coronary arteriograms may result from several factors. First, since the particles are injected directly into the coronary artery, streaming becomes a potential source of error that may result in artifactual regions of reduced perfusion. Second, other types of cardiac disease may result in increased heterogeneity of blood flow and even of regional scarring. Thus, a perfusion defect on the scintigram may not be specific for coronary artery disease. It is possible, but much less likely, that perfusion defects result from disease not detected arteriographically. Perfusion scintigraphy may also be performed after various types of intervention procedures that include the injection of contrast media.[240] Thus, it may be possible to provide information similar to that obtained with potassium analogs after exercise.

At the present time, it is questionable whether the improvement in spatial resolution obtained with microspheres compensates for the limitations presented by the need for direct injection of the tracer into the coronary arteries and for the difficulty in assessing perfusion during exercise. These problems should be kept in mind, since the difference between spatial resolution obtained with the microsphere technique and that with intravenous myocardial perfusion scintigraphy has been substantially reduced with the introduction of [201]Tl.

Intracoronary Rubidium-82. The positron emitter [82]Rb can be injected directly into the coronary arteries at the time of coronary angiography.[138] Imaging can be performed with well-shielded Anger cameras using rotating collimators. Because the half-life of the tracer is so short (75 sec), sequential imaging can be performed, with repeat injections made within 5 or 10 minutes of one another. By studying patients at rest and during atrial pacing and by injecting both the left and right coronary arteries, the effectiveness of collateral blood flow can be studied. Because the injection is arterial, catheter streaming remains a problem with this approach. Also, like the microsphere method, it does not permit quantitative measurement of flow.

Inert Gas Washout Method. The inert gas washout method provides a quantitative measure of tissue flow expressed in ml/min/100 gm. The inert gas dissolved in saline is injected directly and rapidly into the coronary artery. Once the tracer has diffused into the tissue, the organ is perfused by tracer-free blood, setting up a concentration gradient between tissue and blood. Since the tracer is not diffusion-limited, the rate at which it diffuses back into the blood depends on the flow rate through the tissue and the solubility partition coefficient between blood and tissue. The more rapid the flow rate, the more rapid the clearance, or washout, from the tissue.

Radiotracers must meet several requirements to be suitable for this technique: (1) they must be freely diffusible into the tissue in which perfusion is to be measured; (2) they cannot be diffusion-limited, since washout of the tracer would then be proportional not only to flow, but also to the time needed for the tracer to diffuse back to the capillary tissue interface; (3) they cannot be metabolized or sequestered in the tissues, since flow measurements depend on the undegraded tracer diffusing freely back into the blood; and (4) if possible, the tracers should not recirculate, since recirculation redistributes a portion of the tracer back into the organ. (If recirculation does occur, corrections must be employed.) The inert gases satisfy these conditions.

For external monitoring, the physical characteristics of the tracer become important. Xenon-133 is the tracer most frequently used. Because the energy of its photon emission is low (81 kev), scattered radiation cannot be easily eliminated from the photopeak by pulse height analysis, and this reduces the spatial resolution of the resultant data. Blood flow measurements are weighted more heavily toward superficial tissue lying closer to the external detector, since the attenuation for 81 kev photons is less than for those from deep structures. Other isotopes of xenon, such as ^{127}Xe, may reduce these problems when they become commercially available. ^{81m}Kr has also been suggested as a tracer to enable quantitation of blood flow.[241] ^{81}Rb is injected into the coronary arteries and serves as an in vivo generator, continually producing ^{81m}Kr (190 kev), which has a 13-second half-life. This technique permits quantitative measurement of transient changes in coronary blood flow following a single injection of ^{81}Rb.

There are advantages to specific flow measurements, particularly in regional perfusion studies. The geometry of the organ is not a factor when external monitoring devices are used, since flow is measured per unit weight. Furthermore, clearance rates are independent of the initial quantity of tracer reaching the tissue (the calculation depends only on the slope of the washout) and are therefore not affected by catheter streaming.

However, the inert gas washout technique has a number of inherent limitations. The relative solubility between lipid and water differs by a factor of 10 for xenon, and the blood:tissue partition coefficient (λ) is difficult to determine accurately. No method is currently available for the in vivo determination of λ. In addition, the washout curve, even the initial portion, may be influenced by cardiac fat, with its high affinity for and correspondingly slow release of xenon, thus underestimating specific flow. Errors result when there is inhomogeneous perfusion in the region in which flow is to be assessed, leading to overestimation of flow because the initial slope reflects predominantly washout of the well-perfused muscle to which the indicator is predominantly distributed. This problem has been overcome to a considerable extent by assessing regional perfusion with scintillation camera systems.

The presence of countercurrent exchange vascular systems may result in underestimation of flow values, since trapping of gas by the system causes its rate of washout to be slower than that predicted from capillary blood flow rates. It has been postulated that in subendocardial regions of heart muscle, some diffusional shunting across arterial or capillary loops may occur.[242,243] The differences in myocardial transit that result from shunting appear to be small and would therefore result in an insignificant error when the inert gas washout method is used to measure transmural flow.

Regional flow measurements present a number of additional problems. Specific flow measurement techniques assume that the perfused tissue is not diffusion-limited.[244] With xenon, the detector is more sensitive to perfusion in the myocardial wall closer to the detector, and studies in multiple projections are therefore desirable. Perfusion gradients across the ventricular wall cannot be detected with this technique. Since the ischemic myocardium will receive little indicator if ischemia occurs in only a part of the tissue included in the xenon clearance curve, the initial part of the washout curve will be determined essentially by the indicator contained in well-perfused zones.

Although the limitations of specific flow techniques must be taken into account, correlation between flow measured directly with electromagnetic flow meters and with the inert gas washout technique has been excellent,[245,246] while regional flow values obtained in the clinic have been quite reproducible and have correlated with the extent of coronary artery disease, particularly during pharmacological or physiological stress.[247]

Global myocardial blood flow has been measured using a scintillation counter as the external detector.[248] Techniques to assess regional myocardial blood flow (RMBF) have been developed recently using the inert gas washout technique with ^{133}Xe and scintillation cameras.[247,249,250] Electronic crystal-splitting techniques or multicrystal cameras allow clearance curves to be monitored from small regions of the myocardium.

Although compartmental analysis can be applied to myocardial washout curves, the initial slope method is the one usually applied. Specific flow is calculated from the equation

$$F/W = \frac{\lambda \cdot k \cdot 100}{\rho} \qquad (11)$$

where F/W is specific flow (ml/min/100 gm), λ is the blood:tissue partition coefficient, k is the slope of the washout curve, and ρ is the specific gravity of myocardium.

The inert gas washout method is most useful in assessing the effect of drugs on coronary blood flow. For example, nitroglycerin has been shown to improve flow preferentially to ischemic regions in some patients with well-developed collaterals.[251] Conversely, nitroprusside has been shown to induce a coronary steal phenomenon in some patients with coronary artery disease.[252]

MYOCARDIAL METABOLISM

Adequate cardiac function requires a sufficient supply of blood to meet the metabolic demands of the myocardium. With conventional radionuclide studies, perfusion of the myocardium and cardiac performance can be assessed. Recently, techniques have been developed to allow measurement of metabolism using the radiotracer method. Direct measurement of the uptake and utilization of fuel substrates may provide a more direct measure of the severity of myocardial ischemia, since ischemia results from a combination of inadequate blood supply and excessive demand for mechanical work. It may also be possible to understand better intrinsic disturbances in myocardial metabolism as might occur in cardiomyopathies and other diseases in which the primary etiology is alteration of biochemical pathways.

Perhaps the greatest impetus to study in this area has been the development of *positron emission tomography*. Three-dimensional reconstruction using positron emitters is based on coincidence detection. After a positron is formed through positron decay, it travels a short distance within the tissue, giving up its kinetic energy, and then interacts with an electron. Both particles are converted into annihilation photons, each with an energy of 511 kev. The photons leave the site of interaction in opposite directions, at an angle of 180 degrees. If two scintillation detectors are placed opposite one another, they will detect the annihilation photons simultaneously (coincidence detection). Scattered photons that reach only one of the detectors are rejected.

A number of approaches have been advocated for positron emission tomography.[253] In most cases, a ring of detectors is used in which each detector operates in coincidence with one or more detectors in the opposite bank. The patient is positioned within the detector ring. After imaging, the data are reconstructed into an image representing the transaxial distribution of the tracer.

Positron emission tomography has a number of advantages: (1) the field of view of the coincidence detectors is highly uniform over a large distance; (2) the coincidence counting rate remains virtually constant, regardless of the position of the radiation source within the absorber; (3) tissue attenuation is less with annihilation photons than with lower energy photon emissions of radionuclides such as technetium-99m and thallium-201; and (4) the short-lived positron-emitting radionuclides such as oxygen-15, nitrogen-13, and carbon-11 offer fundamental advantages in the study of metabolic processes. These last elements are ubiquitous in naturally occurring metabolic processes, and these nuclides are the only isotopes of these elements suitable for imaging. Thus, ^{15}O, ^{13}N, and ^{11}C can be incorporated into radiopharmaceuticals that are true metabolic substrates and consequently can be tailored to the investigation of selected metabolic pathways.[254]

MYOCARDIAL GLUCOSE UPTAKE

Regional myocardial glucose uptake can be measured using ^{18}F 2-fluoro-2-deoxyglucose (FDG).[254a] Fluorine-18 is a positron emitter with a 2-hour half-life. FDG exchanges rapidly across the capillary and cellular membranes in direct proportion to glucose transport. It competes for hexokinase and is phosphorylated to FDG-6-phosphate. Since it is not a substrate for glycolysis, it undergoes no further metabolism and therefore remains in the heart. As a result, the amount of tracer in the heart at the time of equilibrium is directly proportional to the rate of uptake of exogenous glucose.[255,256]

While the initial tissue uptake of the tracer is a function of blood flow and the concentration of tracer in the blood, at the time of equilibrium—approximately 60 to 90 minutes after injection—the tissue activity represents primarily FDG-6-phosphate.[255-258] To measure *exogenous* glucose uptake, positron emission tomography is performed 60 minutes after injection to determine the tissue concentration of the tracer. Arterial glucose and FDG plasma concentrations are also determined, and the information is fit into a three-compartment model consisting of vascular, tissue, and metabolic components.

While this technique is a satisfactory measure of exogenous glucose uptake in man, it measures the glycolytic rate only when all the extracted glucose is used for glycolysis. This occurs only when glycogen stores are depleted, as in ischemia.[259] This technique has a number of technical limitations as well, in that it requires arterial or arterialized blood sampling; a knowledge of the rate constants required for application of the three-compartment model (since these rate constants may change during disease and during ischemia); and correction for washout of the tracer from the myocardium, which occurs late after injection.

When these studies are applied to man, they have provided insights into the biochemical pathways initiated during ischemia. In patients with unstable angina, there is a regional increase in glucose uptake in the ischemic segment despite a decrease in perfusion.[260,261] Even when normal myocardium is metabolizing primarily free fatty acids and hence has low glucose uptake, regions of ischemia may show excessive glucose uptake, indicating the primary reliance on glycolysis for energy in ischemic myocardium.

FATTY ACID METABOLISM
(Also see p. 1250)

Under normal conditions, most of the energy requirements of the heart are met by oxidation of free fatty acids.[260-262] Free fatty acid metabolism has been studied in man using ^{11}C-labeled palmitic acid combined with positron emission tomography.[263,263a] The initial distribution of this tracer in the myocardium is directly proportional to myocardial blood flow.[264] Myocardial clearance depends on the oxygen demand and the availability of alternative substrates. In normal hearts, the slope of the early component of the washout curve corresponds to the rate of oxidation of ^{11}C-palmitic acid.[265-267] Abnormalities in initial clearance may be due to metabolic abnormalities in free fatty acid utilization or to alternative metabolic pathways, as may occur if free fatty acid plasma levels are low and the heart is using primarily glucose and lactic acid.[268] While this method provides a semiquantitative measure of free fatty acid utilization in the heart, accurate measurement is limited by washout of ^{11}C-palmitic acid when oxygen availability is restricted, because of reduced availability of the tracer in regions of markedly reduced flow and because other fatty acids are utilized by the heart.

Positron emission tomography using ^{11}C-palmitate has been used to identify the size and extent of myocardial infarction.[269] In normal subjects tomography shows uniform distribution of the tracer throughout the left ventricle. Tomograms from patients with previous myocardial infarction show diminished accumulation of ^{11}C-palmitate, delineating regions corresponding to the electrocardiographic focus of infarction. (Fig. 36–14, p. 1251)

Since ischemia alters the myocardial metabolism of free fatty acid by decreasing oxidation and increasing conversion to triglycerides, fatty acids labeled with positron-emitting nuclides such as ^{11}C–palmitate may be used to localize zones of transient ischemia. Because of the very short half-life of the tracer, transient changes can be documented by serial injections of the tracer. Thus, regions that are transiently ischemic will show augmented accumulation of the tracer with reperfusion, while zones of infarction will show no change in uptake on sequential studies obtained over a relatively short period of time (up to six hours). It has therefore been suggested that this method may be a useful indicator of cell viability, and since its accumulation is related to blood flow, it may be used as a marker of the severity and extent of tissue infarction.

[11]C–lactic acid and pyruvic acid may be useful markers for identifying acutely ischemic tissue.[270] Tracer clearance from the myocardium is extremely prolonged in areas of ischemia resulting in zones of increased tracer activity. This method may also prove useful in distinguishing reversible from irreversible ischemia. The underlying metabolic pathways involved in tracer retention are so far unknown.

IODINE-123 FATTY ACIDS. Positron emission tomography will be limited largely to major medical centers and applied largely to research in the foreseeable future. The technology is very expensive, requiring an on-site production facility for most of the short-lived radiopharmaceuticals; even ^{18}F-FDG must be produced nearby. As a result, this method will be used primarily to improve our understanding of the pathophysiology of cardiac disease and may eventually lead to less expensive diagnostic tools, using single photon–emitting radiotracers.

[123]I-hexadecanoic acid and ^{123}I-heptadecanoic acid have been used for measuring myocardial perfusion and fatty acid metabolism using standard single-photon imaging equipment such as Anger scintillation cameras. These tracers are extracted avidly from the blood and cleared quickly from the myocardial tissue with a half-time of approximately 25 minutes.[271] They are esterified and then undergo beta-oxidation.[272-274] The pattern of uptake and washout in the heart is similar to that for unlabeled free fatty acids.[275,276]

The major limitation of this technique is that the iodide label dissociates rather quickly from the free fatty acid. Subsequent washout of free iodide results in progressively high blood levels of the contaminant. This ^{123}I washout added to the clearance of the free fatty acid makes quantification difficult. Furthermore, the increasing background activity interferes with quantification using two-dimensional imaging or limited-angle tomography. This may explain the discordance in clearance results obtained in ischemic myocardium between ^{11}C-labeled fatty acids and ^{123}I-labeled fatty acids.[277] Corrections have been proposed for this contamination.[278]

[123]I-labeled fatty acids may also be used to measure myocardial perfusion, since their initial distribution is proportional to blood flow. The rapid washout of the ^{123}I-hexadecanoic and heptadecanoic acids makes high-quality imaging difficult and limits imaging to two-dimensional techniques and to limited-angle tomography. Other fatty acids that are more readily retained by the myocardium are more suitable for this purpose but still suffer because of the low dose of tracer that can be administered to the patient; the high cost of the pharmaceutical; and the high-energy photons associated with the tracer and with its contaminant, [124]I, which degrades spatial resolution. As a perfusion agent, the ^{123}I label offers no advantages over thallium-201 and would be clearly inferior to technetium-99m–labeled perfusion agents that localize in the human heart.

INFARCT-AVID MYOCARDIAL SCINTIGRAPHY

In infarct-avid scintigraphy, radiopharmaceuticals are sequestered by acutely infarcted myocardium, resulting in regions of increased myocardial uptake. This procedure has emerged as a useful noninvasive technique to aid in the detection, localization, and quantification of myocardial necrosis. Infarct-avid scintigraphy has potential advantages over other techniques, including serum enzyme tests, electrocardiography, and vectorcardiography, which provide indirect evidence of the presence, size, and location of an infarcted region of the myocardium. These indirect techniques are usually satisfactory for detecting infarction, particularly during its early stages, but may be less useful for measuring the extent of irreversible tissue damage.

RADIOPHARMACEUTICALS

99mTc-PYROPHOSPHATE

At the present time, 99mTc-pyrophosphate is the radiotracer of choice for imaging acute myocardial infarction in man.[279-281] Fifty per cent of the injected dose is extracted by bone and the remainder is rapidly excreted through the kidneys in normal subjects. At 90 minutes, less than 5 per cent of the injected dose remains in the blood.

99mTc-pyrophosphate uptake in acute myocardial infarction depends on a number of factors: (1) regional blood flow, (2) myocardial calcium concentration, (3) irreversible myocardial injury, and (4) time after infarction.

Blood Flow. While the uptake of 99mTc-pyrophosphate is directly related to the degree of tissue damage, the pharmaceutical must reach the damaged tissue before it can be extracted. Following acute coronary occlusion, increased concentrations of 99mTc-pyrophosphate are found in regions with only minimally reduced blood flow.[288] In animal studies, tissue concentrations have been found to be about 20 times the concentration in normal myocardium. The highest concentration ratio between damaged and normal myocardium occurs when normal local blood flow is reduced by 20 to 40 per cent. As flow is reduced further, the concentration ratios begin to fall until, in regions of minimal flow (0 to 5 per cent of normal levels), 99mTc-pyrophosphate concentrations may be normal. Furthermore, there is a greater concentration of the tracer in epicardial than in endocardial segments at the same blood flow.

There are a number of reasons for this flow-dependency.[283] The total extraction of 99mTc-pyrophosphate can be expressed as a product of the extraction fraction times flow. With marked decreases in blood flow, the amount of 99mTc-pyrophosphate that is extracted is reduced because the radiopharmaceutical does not reach the tissue. The only way extraction can keep up with marked reductions in flow is if the extraction fraction (i.e., that portion of the radiotracer removed by the tissue during a single transit through the microcirculation) increases proportionately. This does not appear to be the case for 99mTc-pyrophosphate, and as a result, the total amount of tracer extracted decreases at low flow.

A second reason for reduced tracer uptake at low flow is less direct. The calcium phosphate deposits that appear in the necrotic myocardium soon after infarction may not represent precipitation of intracellular calcium.[284-286] If the deposits are of exogenous origin, their intracellular concentrations will depend on residual blood flow to provide the calcium. Since calcium concentration within the center of the infarct is low and is probably required for binding of the radiotracer, low levels of calcium within the center of the infarct may also account for the decreased concentration of radiotracer in that region in patients with large infarcts.

Myocardial Calcium. This ion probably plays a key role in technetium-99m–pyrophosphate binding in acute infarction. Approximately 50 per cent of the radiopharmaceutical is absorbed by bone in the normal patient. The binding site in bone is probably low-density amorphous calcium phosphate. While binding is possible at both the crystalline and the amorphous calcium phosphate sites, the concentration is twice as high in amorphous calcium phosphate. Furthermore, there is a direct relationship between the number of moles of bone-seeking radiopharmaceutical and the number of moles of calcium.

Irreversibly injured myocardium contains three types of calcium phosphate: amorphous, crystalline, and hydroxyapatite-like deposits. Calcium phosphate deposits are particularly abundant in the periphery of the infarct. Regional 99mTc-pyrophosphate concentrations parallel the calcium phosphate concentrations with increased radiotracer activities in the periphery of the infarct.[284-289]

The relationship between calcium content and pyrophosphate uptake is not linear, however, probably because the avidity for radiotracer binding depends on the form of the tissue calcium deposit. Much of the calcium in necrotic myocardium is exogenous in origin and results from a complex between the calcium ions and various components of the myocardial cell.[288] Massive calcium accumulation results in precipitation of calcium phosphate deposits. Hydrolysis of amorphous calcium phosphate results in the formation of crystalline hydroxyapatite. While the hydroxyapatite is localized primarily in the mitochondria, the amorphous calcium phosphate deposits are distributed more uniformly throughout the irreversibly damaged cell. Since both the amorphous and hydroxyapatite deposits probably represent binding sites, 99mTc-pyrophosphate is found in the various cellular fractions, including the mitochondria, the microsomes, and the soluble supernatant fraction.

It has also been suggested that the lack of correlation between calcium and pyrophosphate concentrations may indicate an alternative mechanism for localization, such as binding by polynuclear complexing with denatured macromolecules. In this case, calcium may form a bridge between the denatured protein and the radiotracer.[290] Furthermore, pyrophosphate uptake may be seen in irreversibly damaged myocardium independent of the presence or absence of calcium ion in the perfusate.[291] Thus, there may be binding sites in addition to calcium phosphate deposits within the infarct.

Irreversible Tissue Damage. In man, ^{99m}Tc-pyrophosphate labels acutely necrotic myocardium. The concentration ratio between infarcted and normal myocardium may be as high as 18:1, and the distribution—even in large circumferential infarcts—may be homogeneous throughout the infarct.[292]

In the zone immediately bordering the infarct, the concentration of pyrophosphate is greater than in normal myocardium; however, the increase is less than 50 per cent higher than normal myocardium. Furthermore, this border zone of slightly increased radiotracer concentration extends only a small distance from the necrotic region.

Technetium-99m–pyrophosphate uptake may be increased in patients with unstable angina pectoris, although histopathological examination of several of these patients has indicated multifocal lesions of coagulation necrosis, myocytolysis, and replacement fibrosis.[293] Increased uptake has also been noted in patients with ventricular aneurysm and regions of ventricular dyskinesis. The increase in radiotracer uptake may persist for some time after an acute infarction. In these patients, histopathological examinations have demonstrated myocytolytic degeneration in myocardial foci that have survived initial infarction. Myocytolysis appears to result from more slowly progressive injury compared to coagulation necrosis. This chronic injury occurs in regions of previous myocardial infarction.

Time After Infarction. Uptake of the radiopharmaceutical begins to increase after four hours of permanent coronary artery occlusion.[294] In most patients with transmural myocardial infarction, faint uptake will be seen shortly after this time and will increase in intensity over the next 36 to 48 hours. Intensity will reach a peak by 48 hours and will gradually diminish over the next 5 to 7 days. The time course will vary depending on a number of factors:

1. The larger the infarct, the longer it takes for the intensity of tracer uptake to reach its peak.[295] This is because initial delivery of the radiopharmaceutical is retarded by markedly diminished perfusion, particularly in the center of the infarct. With the development of collateral vessels, more radiopharmaceutical can reach the infarct and the intensity reaches its peak.

2. The intensity will fade more slowly in large transmural infarcts because there may be continuing tissue necrosis well beyond the initial event.

3. There may be extension of the infarct or reinfarction following the initial event. Following this complication, the extent of the radiotracer uptake will increase and the intensity of uptake may also increase.

OTHER INFARCT-AVID TRACERS

The first successful attempt at infarct-avid scintigraphy in man used technetium-99m–tetracycline as the radiotracer.[296,297] Since the optimal time for imaging is 24 hours after injection and liver concentration is high, this tracer has been replaced by the bone-seeking radiotracers. Nevertheless, ^{99m}Tc-tetracycline does more accurately reflect the degree of tissue necrosis, since its myocardial uptake is inversely related to blood flow even at low flow rates.[298]

Other tracers have been suggested, including ^{99m}Tc-glucoheptonate,[299,300] ^{99m}Tc-methylene diphosphonate,[301,302] and ^{99m}Tc-imidodiphosphonate,[303] but these do not appear to have any advantage over ^{99m}Tc-pyrophosphate.

Radiolabeled Antibody Against Cardiac Myosin. Purified radiolabeled antibody against cardiac myosin has also been demonstrated in regions of acute infarction. After intravenous injection of radioiodine-labeled (FAB')$_2$ fragments of antibodies specific for cardiac myosins, concentration ratios of up to 6:1 between infarcted and normal myocardium may be found in the animal model. There is an inverse relationship between regional myocardial blood flow and uptake of the tracer even in areas of low flow.[304] After intravenous injection, well-defined areas of increased myocardial activity are found by 72 hours after permanent occlusion of a coronary artery in animals. Unfortunately, the concentration of tracer within the infarct is too low to permit external detection of the infarct within the first 24 hours after coronary occlusion unless the tracer is injected directly into the coronary artery.[305] The delay in infarct visualization is the result of prolonged clearance time of the tracer from the blood and slow entry of the tracer into the infarct.

This technique is based on the assumption that these antibodies are highly specific for myocardium and that as capillary and cellular membrane integrity is disrupted by myocardial ischemia, the antibodies attach themselves to the contractile proteins of the myocardium. Initial results demonstrate very slow blood clearance because of the relatively large size of the antibody molecules. When fragments of antimyosin antibody are used, blood clearance is significantly improved without loss of antibody specificity.

The tissue activity of the radiolabeled cardiac myosin antibody fragments is inversely related to blood flow. The radioconcentration is highest in segments of maximal flow reduction and tissue necrosis, unlike ^{99m}Tc-pyrophosphate, which concentrates most in myocardial segments with flow reductions 20 to 40 per cent of normal. Thus, the radiolabeled antibodies are similar to ^{99m}Tc-tetracycline in distribution. The high uptake in low-flow areas results from prolonged intravascular transit, which allows the radiotracer time to reach poorly perfused tissue.

Indium-111–Labeled White Blood Cells. By labeling blood cell components, physiological parameters other than tissue necrosis can be measured. Experimental acute coronary artery thrombosis and experimental infective endocarditis have been detected using indium-111–labeled platelets.[306] Although this technique is promising for evaluating coronary artery bypass graft patency and for assessing the inflammatory component of acute infarction, it is currently limited by the difficulty encountered in routine labeling of platelets.

Indium-111–labeled white blood cells provide an additional tool for visualizing acute myocardial infarctions, particularly for studying their pathophysiology.[307] Migration of polymorphous leukocytes into acutely infarcted myocardium is known to occur, and use of these labeled cells can provide useful information when one is monitoring the inflammatory response in acutely infarcted myocardium as well as the effects of therapeutic intervention.

TECHNIQUE

Patients suspected of having sustained an acute myocardial infarction are usually admitted directly to the coronary care unit. Usually they are at risk for developing either electrophysiological or hemodynamic complications; if so, imaging must be performed at the bedside using a portable scintillation camera. The camera should be a 37-photomultiplier tube, high-resolution instrument used in conjunction with a high-resolution collimator.

Patients who are clinically stable may be brought to the nuclear medicine clinical unit. In this case, the suite used for imaging should contain monitoring equipment, including an electrocardiographic monitor, defibrillator, and emergency drugs. Standard infarct imaging does not require additional equipment. Computer processing has been suggested to subtract uptake by overlying ribs in patients in whom costochondral cartilage uptake obscures the myocardial field. We have found this to be a problem in less than 1 per cent of patients. More sophisticated equipment, such as transaxial tomographic imaging systems with a rotating gamma camera or a multidetector scanning tomograph are necessary for sizing the acute infarction.

For best results, it is essential that the amount of free pertechnetate be kept to an absolute minimum. Poor labeling or rapid breakdown within the vial or syringe will lead to poor clearance of the tracer from the blood pool because of either the presence of free ^{99m}Tc-pertechnetate or excessive labeling of the patient's red blood cells with ^{99m}Tc. Poor clearance will lead to excessive blood pool activity on the scintigrams, resulting in a diffuse myocardial pattern, and may mask underlying focal uptake. Each batch of ^{99m}Tc-pyrophosphate should be tested for labeling efficiency, and free pertechnetate should be less than 1 per cent of the total activity. Once the material is labeled, breakdown will occur with time. It is critical that the radiopharmaceutical be injected shortly after it is prepared.

The specificity of infarct-avid scintigraphy with ^{99m}Tc-pyrophosphate depends on the time intervals between injection and imaging and should be performed at least three hours after the intravenous injection of 10 to 15 mCi of the tracer. When imaging is performed at 90 minutes after injection, there is a high incidence of diffuse blood pool activity, which can lead to a false-positive test for acute infarction. By delaying the imaging time from 90 minutes to three hours, the probability of acute infarction with moderately intense diffuse uptake (greater than or equal to the ribs in intensity) increases from 40 to 75 per cent.[308]

Images are obtained in the anterior, left anterior oblique, and left lateral projections, with at least 400,000 counts collected in each projection. Multiple projections permit accurate localization of the infarct uptake as distinguished from that in overlying bone.

A number of other techniques have also been suggested to improve the specificity of a diffuse pattern. Since the initial distribution of the radiotracer is intravascular, images obtained shortly after injection represent the extent of myocardial blood flow. It may be useful to subtract the initial blood pool image from the final image obtained 3 hours later. If focal myocardial uptake is present, myocardial uptake will involve a smaller area of the myocardium than on the initial blood pool image. Several techniques have been suggested for this purpose, including subjective assessment and computer subtraction.[309,310]

IMAGE INTERPRETATION

THE NORMAL IMAGE. Technetium-99m–pyrophosphate is a bone-seeking radiopharmaceutical. After injection, about half the tracer is extracted by bone and the remainder is excreted through the kidneys. In the normal image, myocardial uptake will be equal to that over the right hemithorax and there will be no identification of a discrete cardiac silhouette (Fig. 11–20). The threshold for abnormal myocardial uptake is controversial, however, and will be described in more detail in the next section. Bone uptake will usually be prominent, with activity in the sternum and anterior ribs seen on all three views. Activity from the thoracolumbar spine will be seen superimposed on the sternum in the anterior view, extending to the left of the sternum on the LAO projection, and forming the border opposite the sternum on the left lateral view. Activity in the scapula may be seen as shine-through on the anterior projection; the inferior tip of the scapula frequently shows disproportionately increased activity compared to

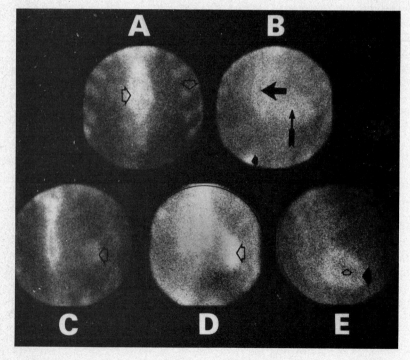

FIGURE 11–20 Scintigraphic classification of myocardial uptake of technetium-99m–pyrophosphate. *A*, Normal (horizontal arrow = sternum; vertical arrow = rib). *B*, Diffuse (upper arrow = sternum; lower arrow = kidney; vertical arrow = myocardial activity). *C*, Focal, less intense than radioactivity in sternum (arrow = focal myocardial activity). *D*, Focal, equal to or greater than radioactivity in sternum (arrow = focal myocardial activity). *E*, Massive (open arrow = central defect due to ventricular cavity; closed arrow = myocardial uptake involving entire left ventricle). (From Holman, B. L., et al.: The prognostic implications of acute myocardial infarct scintigraphy with ^{99m}Tc-pyrophosphate. Circulation *57*:320, 1978, by permission of the American Heart Association, Inc.)

the rest of the bone, and this should not be confused with uptake in the lateral wall of the myocardium.

A number of abdominal structures may be seen on the images. Activity in the renal pelvis may appear as a focal defect and could occasionally be confused with an inferior myocardial infarct, particularly if the kidney lies high in the diaphragm. Activity in the stomach indicates breakdown of the radiopharmaceutical, with free ^{99m}Tc-pertechnetate accumulating in the gastric cells of the antrum. A number of conditions that result in splenic uptake such as infarction, sarcoidosis, tuberculosis, and amyloidosis may be seen occasionally; splenic uptake is usually diffusely distributed throughout the organ and is usually too lateral and posterior to be confused with myocardial uptake. Breast uptake of the radiopharmaceutical has been reported in a wide variety of conditions and may overlie the myocardium, particularly in the anterior projection. Uptake by the breast will be anterior to the sternum and the myocardium on the left lateral projection. Burns to the skin and the underlying chest wall muscle may occur following cardioversion; while superimposition may occur on the anterior view, focal radiotracer uptake will be anterior to the sternum and to the myocardium on the left lateral view. Calcification of the costochondral junctions or the cartilaginous structures of the rib cage may result in focal uptake overlying the myocardial silhouette. While uptake in overlying rib may make interpretation difficult in a small minority of patients, only rarely will rib uptake be confused with myocardial uptake, and again, multiple images in various projections can be used to differentiate the two.

THE ABNORMAL IMAGE. A number of grading systems have been suggested for interpreting the abnormal image. Most systems are based on a grading of 0 to 4+.[281] A grade of 0 means that there is no activity in the heart and indicates a negative myocardial scintigram. A grade of 1+ represents questionable but not definite activity and is also considered to be a negative scintigraphic result. A grade of 2+ indicates definite but faint activity and an abnormal myocardial scintigram, while definite and increased activity within the myocardial image is associated with grades 3+ and 4+. In scintiscans considered to be positive (2+, 3+, and 4+), the area of increased activity (anterior, inferior, lateral, or true posterior) is also described.

Although this classification has proved useful, it suffers from several shortcomings. Grading is highly subjective and prone to interobserver error. Moreover, it does not take into account the difference in accuracy when uptake is focal or diffuse. Several alternative grading systems have been suggested to correct for these limitations.[311] In those that retain the 0 to 4+ grading, the grades are made more objective by differentiating 2+ as activity less than that in the adjacent ribs, 3+ as activity equal to that in adjacent ribs, and 4+ as activity greater than that in adjacent ribs.

A distinction must be made between *diffuse* and *focal* activity. Diffuse uptake will appear as relatively homogeneous radiotracer activity throughout the myocardium, including both ventricles and often the great vessels. Activity frequently extends to the right of the sternum; left ventricular activity does not appear as a photon-deficient area, as would be the case if the activity were primarily in the myocardial walls. In diffuse uptake, activity is most often

due to persistent radiotracer in the blood pool resulting from poor renal clearance, as may occur in impaired renal function; a particularly large left ventricular end-diastolic volume, as may occur in congestive heart failure and cardiomyopathies; and red blood cell labeling, as may occur in breakdown of the radiopharmaceutical. The specificity of the diffuse pattern for the diagnosis of acute myocardial infarction is poor.

Because the specificity of the diffuse pattern depends on the time after injection and the intensity of the pattern, we suggest the following grading system when imaging is performed 3 or more hours after injection (Fig. 11–20):

Normal (No identification of the discrete cardiac silhouette): Myocardial uptake that is equal to that over the right hemithorax.

Mild Diffuse (Low probability of acute myocardial infarction): Myocardial uptake exceeding that over the right hemithorax but less intense than that over the ribs and distributed over most or all of the myocardium.

Moderate Diffuse (Indeterminant for the diagnosis of acute infarction): Myocardial uptake equally or more intense than that over the ribs but less intense than that over the sternum.

Focal (High probability of acute infarction): Discrete myocardial uptake.

Massive (High probability of acute myocardial infarction): An increase in myocardial uptake that involves 50 per cent or more of the cardiac silhouette and is equally or more intense than uptake over the sternum. Most often there is a focal central area of decreased activity due either to the left ventricular cavity or to central necrosis.

When myocardial uptake is focal, it can be localized to one or more segments of the myocardial wall from an analysis of the scintigrams obtained in multiple projections. In patients with *anterior myocardial infarcts*, uptake involves much of the left ventricular silhouette on the anterior view; in the left lateral view, the uptake appears as a thin band directly behind the sternum, since the anterior free wall of the left ventricle is being viewed tangentially in this projection (Fig. 11–21). In patients with inferior myocardial infarction, the radiotracer appears curvilinear, usually extending from the lower portion of the sternum laterally toward the ribs on the anterior projection and from the lower portion of the sternum approximately two-thirds of the way toward the vertebrae on the left lateral view. *Inferior infarcts* are always imaged perpendicular to the collimator. The true extent of an inferior infarct can be appreciated only with the aid of single-photon transaxial tomography. *Lateral infarcts* are seen perpendicular to the collimator on the anterior view, usually lying directly under the anterior rib ends and well away from the sternum. Lateral infarcts are seen in their greatest extent on the left lateral or left anterior oblique projections. *Apical infarcts* usually result from uptake in several adjacent walls, usually the inferior and lateral or distal anterior and lateral walls. *Posterior infarction* is usually seen in conjunction with inferior wall uptake and is seen best in the left lateral projection extending superiorly and posteriorly from the inferior wall. Occasionally posterior uptake may be seen in isolation. *Right ventricular uptake* is most often seen in conjunction with inferior left ventricular activity and is appreciated best when there is also uptake in the inferior portion of the left ventricular septum. In this case, the right ventricular activity appears to the right of the septum and inferior wall. The activity may extend horizontally or at various angles from the inferior wall from a horizontal to an almost vertical orientation, depending on the ana-

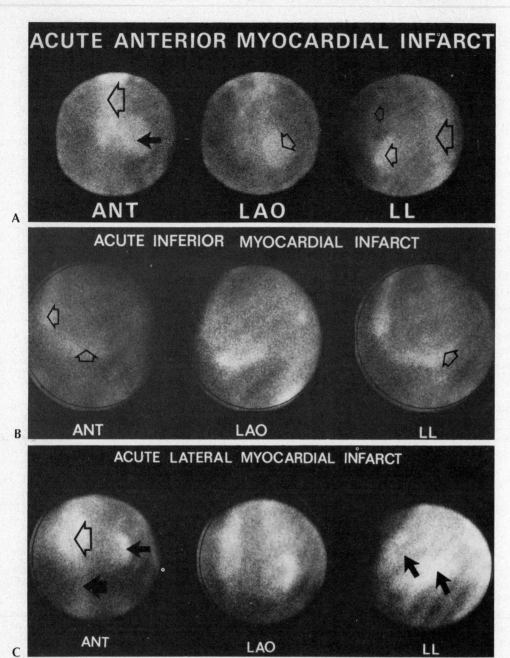

ACUTE ANTERIOR MYOCARDIAL INFARCT

A   ANT   LAO   LL

ACUTE INFERIOR MYOCARDIAL INFARCT

B   ANT   LAO   LL

ACUTE LATERAL MYOCARDIAL INFARCT

C   ANT   LAO   LL

FIGURE 11–21 *A*, Myocardial scintigraphy with ^{99m}Tc-pyrophosphate in patients with acute anterior myocardial infarct. *Anterior*: Open arrow = sternum; arrow = myocardial uptake. *Left anterior oblique*: Arrow = myocardial activity. *Left lateral*: Upper arrow = sternum; lower arrow = myocardial activity; large arrow = vertebrae. *B*, Scintigrams of a patient with acute inferior myocardial infarction. *Anterior*: Upper arrow = sternum; lower arrow = myocardial activity. *Left lateral*: Note posterior wall extension (arrow). *C*, Myocardial scintigraphy in a patient with acute lateral myocardial infarct. *Anterior*: Open arrow = sternum; lower arrow = vertebrae; upper arrow = myocardial activity. *Left lateral*: Upper arrow = ribs; lower arrow = myocardial activity.

tomical position of the right ventricle and of the right ventricular free wall (Fig. 11–22).

In patients with large anteroseptal or anterolateral or circumferential left ventricular infarcts, the pattern of uptake is massive, and in most of these patients, the scintigraphic appearance has been described as a *doughnut pattern* with intense uptake along the borders and relatively diminished intensity in the center. This pattern can be explained in two ways: First, patients presenting with this pattern have large infarcts, and animal data suggest that the central portion of the infarct takes up relatively less radiotracer than do the peripheral zones because of diminished perfusion and decreased radiotracer delivery.[288] Second, even in patients with large myocardial infarcts who present with the doughnut pattern, radiotracer uptake may be uniform throughout the area of tissue necrosis.[292] The explanation for the doughnut pattern in these patients

—and perhaps, to some extent, in all patients exhibiting this pattern—is that the intensity in any region is equal to the concentration of the tracer times the weight of the tissue within the field of view. The weight of tissue is considerable in the field of view where the left ventricular wall is being imaged tangentially and where the wall is parallel to the collimator. The weight of tissue is less where the wall is parallel to the detector. Thus, a ^{99m}Tc-pyrophosphate scan in a patient with a large left ventricular infarct has a central photopenic zone similar to the one found in a normal thallium-201 scan.

While most subendocardial and many transmural infarcts will appear normal on infarct-avid scintigraphy after the first week, many transmural infarcts will show persistent accumulation of the radiotracer for considerable periods of time after the initial episode, even when extension or reinfarction has not been documented.[312] In approxi-

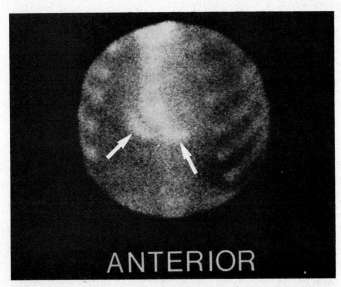

FIGURE 11–22 Infarct-avid scintigraphy with 99mTc-pyrophosphate in a patient with an acute inferior wall infarct (right arrow) with extensive right ventricular extension (left arrow).

mately 40 per cent of patients with acute myocardial infarction, activity will persist beyond the first several weeks, the intensity of uptake will gradually diminish, and the appearance and the distribution of the radiotracer will appear more diffuse than on the initial scintigrams obtained several days after infarction.

Focal uptake may also be seen in patients with valvular calcifications,[313] repeated high-energy direct-current (DC) cardioversions,[314] ventricular aneurysms,[315] myocardial contusion,[316] and metastatic carcinoma to the heart (Table 11–1). Since myocardial scintigraphy with 99mTc-pyrophosphate would be a useful technique for examining patients after resuscitation to detect acute infarction, initial case reports and animal studies that reported significant myocardial uptake after DC cardioversion in the absence of ischemic heart disease were discouraging.[314] When patients were studied systematically following cardiopulmonary resuscitation with cardioversion, however, the incidence of pyrophosphate uptake in patients without myocardial infarction was only 13 per cent.[317] With an imaging accuracy of 80 per cent, it would appear that false-positive scintiscans after electrical cardioversion occur infrequently. Similarly, valvular calcification must be extensive, and focal uptake without evidence of infarction is

TABLE 11–1 CAUSES OF 99mTC-PYROPHOSPHATE UPTAKE

FOCAL	DIFFUSE
Acute myocardial infarction	Acute myocardial infarction[†]
Recent myocardial infarction	(subendocardial)
Breast tumors	Unstable angina pectoris[†]
Left ventricular aneurysms	Cardiomyopathy[†]
Rib fractures	Left ventricular aneurysms
Skeletal muscle damage	Persistent blood pool activity
Cardioversion (secondary to skeletal muscle as well as myocardial damage)*	Myocarditis
Valvular calcification*	
Myocardial contusion	
Skin lesions*	
Calcified costal cartilage	

*Unusual.
[†]Due to blood pool activity.

unusual in such patients. Focal uptake in patients with ventricular aneurysms may represent calcification within the aneurysm, or, as in patients with recent infarction, persistent and ongoing cellular necrosis and damage. Pericarditis alone does not result in increased uptake of pyrophosphate.[318] One exception is the hypercalcemic patient with pericardial calcification.[319]

Diffuse patterns of increased uptake of 99mTc-pyrophosphate have been observed in patients with nontransmural acute myocardial infarction, idiopathic cardiomyopathy,[320] unstable angina pectoris,[321] and stable angina pectoris[320,322] and in patients with no apparent heart disease. The high incidence of diffuse uptake in nontransmural infarction and its occurrence in many other conditions suggest that the primary cause for the diffuse pattern is persistent blood pool activity. Most patients with nontransmural infarction have focal necrosis, and even in those patients with global subendocardial infarction, an area of reduced radioactivity corresponding to the left ventricular cavity is rarely seen.[318] This pattern would be observed if the uptake were primarily in the left ventricular wall,[292] but it is seen only in patients with massive transmural infarcts. Persistent blood pool activity is seen when imaging is performed too soon after injection. It occurs in patients with poor renal function, cardiac enlargement, and reduced ejection fraction. Some patients may have persistent blood pool activity without apparent explanation. In these patients, there is probably some dissociation of the 99mTc from the pyrophosphate, with subsequent binding to either a protein or a red blood cell fraction. Drugs may also cause increased retention of the label within the vascular compartment. This probably accounts for the reports of diffusely abnormal pyrophosphate scans in patients with adriamycin toxicity. Patients who receive this drug have altered tracer kinetics with increased activity outside of the intravascular component when in vivo labeling of red blood cells is performed with 99mTc-pertechnetate after pyrophosphate injection. Also, blood clearance is delayed when 99mTc-pyrophosphate is used for myocardial scintigraphy. Other interactions between drugs and radiotracers probably occur as well.

It is possible, however, that processes that affect the myocardium diffusely, resulting in tissue necrosis, may cause diffuse myocardial uptake. One such example has been demonstrated in an animal model of experimental viral myopericarditis. Extensive experience with pyrophosphate imaging in myocarditis in humans has not yet been reported.[323] Similarly, processes that result in extensive calcification within the myocardium may result in diffuse uptake of pyrophosphate. Such a pattern has been reported with amyloidosis.[324]

ASSESSMENT OF THE METHOD

The sensitivity of myocardial scintigraphy with 99mTc-pyrophosphate for the detection of acute myocardial infarction depends on a number of factors, including the criteria used for interpretation of the images and patient selection. In most large series in which patients were selected either at random or sequentially, the sensitivity of the technique was high. In 24 different series—a total of 1143 patients with documented acute myocardial infarcts—pyrophosphate scans were abnormal in 89 per cent.[308] In a similar group of 19 different series, which included a total of 1482 patients with no evidence of acute infarction, ^{99m}Tc-pyrophosphate scans were normal in 86 per cent.[308] The composite results indicate a false-negative rate of 11 per cent and a false-positive rate of 14 per cent.

These results may be deceiving, however. The low incidence of false-positive results may be attributable to the patient mix, which frequently included a spectrum of chest pain syndromes. The diagnostic problem that is usually faced, however, is in distinguishing unstable angina pectoris from acute infarction. Many patients with unstable angina have abnormal scintiscans. Among 374 patients with a clinical diagnosis of unstable angina pectoris and without clinical evidence of acute infarction, 152 (41 per cent) had positive ^{99m}Tc-pyrophosphate scans.[308]

It has generally been assumed that abnormal scintiscans obtained in patients with unstable angina pectoris represent false-positive results. However, in a small series of patients with unstable angina pectoris or symptomatic ischemic heart disease after myocardial infarction, those patients with abnormal scintigrams were found to have histopathological evidence of multifocal irreversible damage at autopsy.[325] Of those patients with clinical evidence of unstable angina pectoris studied by means of both ^{99m}Tc-pyrophosphate and sequential determination of serum MB-band creatine kinase (MB-CK) activity, total plasma CK and MB-CK activity was elevated in 22 of 36 patients with abnormal images.[326] These studies suggest that, at least in some patients with unstable angina and abnormal scintigrams, underlying tissue necrosis accounts for the uptake of pyrophosphate. Furthermore, patients with abnormal images but without clinical evidence of acute infarction have a poorer prognosis than do those with normal scintigrams (i.e., complication rates of 22 and 5 per cent, respectively).[327]

Another diagnostic problem that is overlooked when composite results are reported is the difference in sensitivity between transmural and nontransmural infarction. Infarct scintigraphy with ^{99m}Tc-pyrophosphate is most sensitive in patients with transmural infarction. However, these patients can usually be diagnosed without the aid of infarct scintigraphy. It is in patients with nontransmural infarction that the diagnosis is frequently in doubt at the time of admission. The diagnosis of nontransmural infarction may be difficult to confirm because the accompanying electrocardiographic changes may be nonspecific. Nontransmural infarction frequently occurs during surgery or in other clinical settings characterized by hemodynamic instability. Furthermore, when patients present with nonspecific ST-segment or T-wave abnormalities several days after a prolonged episode of pain, it may be impossible to establish the diagnosis of acute myocardial infarction using currently available cardiac enzyme techniques.

Although initial reports suggested that myocardial scintigraphy with ^{99m}Tc-pyrophosphate was a very sensitive method for detecting nontransmural myocardial infarction, more recent evidence suggests a substantially lower accuracy.[311] The sensitivity of the technique is high in patients with nontransmural infarction if one is willing to accept a correspondingly low specificity, since approximately 50 per cent of these patients show diffuse uptake that is indistinguishable from that seen in many patients with unstable angina pectoris but without clinical evidence of infarction. When rigid criteria are used and faint diffuse uptake is considered to be a normal finding, the sensitivity for the detection of nontransmural infarction has not been found to be as high as was initially reported. Recent studies report focal uptake in only 40 to 60 per cent of these patients.[326–328]

The incidence of diffuse uptake in patients with nontransmural infarction may be dependent on the spatial resolution of the imaging equipment. Recent studies suggest a lower incidence of diffuse uptake than has been reported previously. Massie et al. found diffuse uptake in only 19 per cent of patients with nontransmural infarction and in 10 per cent of those with stable angina pectoris,[329] whereas Jaffe et al. found focal uptake of pyrophosphate in more than 95 per cent of patients with unstable angina pectoris and elevated MB-CK activity.[326]

The failure of ^{99m}Tc-pyrophosphate scintigraphy to return to normal within one to two weeks in the majority of patients with acute infarction limits the specificity of the technique in patients with recent myocardial infarction and recurrent symptoms. In those patients with infarction and recurrent symptoms, a single study at the time when reinfarction is suspected is of value only if it is negative or intensely positive, since persistently faint or moderately intense uptake may be due to the initial infarct. Sequential scintigraphy is of value if the scintigraphic pattern follows a classic course after the recurrent symptoms. If the intensity of pyrophosphate uptake increases for the first 48 to 72 hours following the development of recurrent symptoms, with a subsequent rapid decrease in intensity, the probability of reinfarction is high. In all other cases, recurrent myocardial infarction cannot be distinguished from recent infarction without a baseline study at the time of initial infarction.

CLINICAL APPLICATIONS

Myocardial scintigraphy with ^{99m}Tc-pyrophosphate is useful in patients with *suspected acute infarction* in whom other clinical and laboratory evidence is nondiagnostic. Thus, scintigraphy is very helpful in patients who present more than 24 hours after the onset of symptoms when very sensitive serum enzyme tests such as MB-band CK may have returned to normal. The probability of acute infarction is high in patients with focal uptake, provided an infarction has not occurred within 6 to 12 months of the acute event. The size and persistence of uptake may provide predictive information as well. Usefulness of the test in the presence of moderately intense diffuse uptake is limited, however. Myocardial scintigraphy can be used to diagnose *right ventricular infarction.* Although an elevation in right ventricular filling pressure may indicate right ventricular involvement, it may also occur in the presence of cor pulmonale. Myocardial scintigraphy with ^{99m}Tc-pyrophosphate provides more direct evidence of acute infarction of the right ventricle.[330]

This technique is also of value in evaluating patients following coronary bypass surgery (Fig. 11–23). The diagnosis of myocardial infarction after cardiac surgery is complicated because chest pain, elevated enzyme levels, and

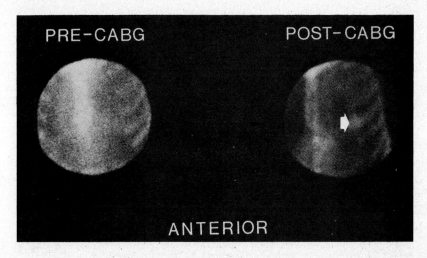

FIGURE 11–23 Infarct-avid scintigraphy with ^{99m}Tc-pyrophosphate in a patient who sustained an intraoperative infarct during coronary artery bypass graft surgery. PRE-CABG = faint diffuse myocardial uptake prior to surgery; POST-CABG = focal apical uptake of the radiotracer (arrow) in the location of the intraoperative infarct.

electrocardiographic changes may result from the operation itself.[331] Infarction occurs in about 10 per cent of these patients, however. ^{99m}Tc-pyrophosphate scintigraphy is accurate in the postoperative patient.[332,333] The importance of preoperative scintigraphy for comparison is controversial. A significant number of patients undergoing bypass surgery will have positive infarct scintigrams preoperatively.[334] In order to interpret postoperative scintigraphy in patients who suffered an infarction within one year prior to the operation, we recommend a baseline study be obtained for comparison.

Extension of an infarction or reinfarction can be determined if a baseline scintigram is available. For example, it has been observed that the abnormalities on infarct scintigraphy may become more prominent in the absence of clinically suspected infarct extension during the first 24 to 48 hours after the onset of symptoms. If serial infarct scintigrams are obtained, certain sequential abnormalities are suggestive of infarct extension. Reinfarction is likely if there is a marked increase in the size of the scintigraphic abnormality observed during the baseline examination, reappearance of an abnormality that has cleared, or appearance of a regional abnormality in an area that was previously normal.

Infarct-avid scintigraphy is useful in patients who develop symptoms suggestive of acute myocardial infarction after heavy exercise. For example, serum creatine kinase activity, including that of the MB isoenzyme fraction, is elevated in marathon runners because of skeletal muscle necrosis. Imaging with ^{99m}Tc-pyrophosphate may be useful to exclude myocardial infarction and to localize the site of tissue necrosis.[335] Similarly, scintigraphic imaging may define the extent of muscle necrosis after electrical injury.

The scintigraphic pattern of myocardial uptake provides clues to the patient's future course, both in the hospital and over the long term.[327] The complication rate, particularly during hospitalization, is directly related to the extent of uptake of pyrophosphate in patients with acute infarction (Fig. 11–24). In fact, in patients with clinical evidence of infarction and small foci of ^{99m}Tc-pyrophosphate myocardial uptake (less than 16 cm^2), complication rates are comparable to those in patients without acute infarction. On the other hand, when the extent of uptake is moderate (16 to 40 cm^2), morbidity is high (67 per cent). When the extent of uptake is considerable (greater than 40 cm^2), mortality is high (87 per cent).

A number of other observations that reflect the extent and intensity of pyrophosphate uptake also have prognostic value. In one study, 67 per cent of patients with a doughnut pattern developed left ventricular failure with infarction.[336] In another series, late complications developed in all patients with the doughnut pattern, compared with 43 per cent of the patients with focal uptake and 12 per cent of those with diffuse uptake.[337] Persistently positive

FIGURE 11–24 Complication rates versus area of technetium-99m–pyrophosphate uptake in patients with acute myocardial infarction and patterns C, D, and E. (Single bracket designates complication rate; double bracket designates mortality rate.) (From Holman, B. L., et al.: The prognostic implications of acute myocardial infarct scintigraphy with ^{99m}Tc-pyrophosphate. Circulation *57*:320, 1978, by permission of the American Heart Association, Inc.)

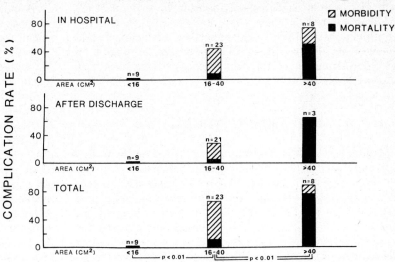

^{99m}Tc-pyrophosphate scintigrams also correlate with mortality and morbidity[295] and with elevated pulmonary artery pressure.[338]

The past decade has seen considerable interest in the concept of infarct size reduction (p. 1318). Since the incidence of pump failure is related directly to the extent of myocardial necrosis, and since at least some of the myocardium at risk may be salvageable during the early hours after infarction, a wide range of therapeutic interventions has been suggested to attempt to limit the size of an infarct. To determine the efficacy of such interventions, accurate quantification of infarct size is necessary. Myocardial scintigraphy with ^{99m}Tc-pyrophosphate allows direct visualization of the necrotic myocardium and may therefore permit accurate estimation of infarct size.

Accurate sizing of the acute infarction be measuring the extent of radiotracer uptake is limited by the geometrical constraints of standard two-dimensional imaging. Single-photon–emission computed tomography provides a three-dimensional map of radionuclide distribution and may yield more accurate assessments of infarct size. Initial studies in an animal model have demonstrated a good correlation between infarct size and measured uptake of ^{99m}Tc-pyrophosphate.[339]

Emission tomography can be performed in humans and provides a three-dimensional map of ^{99m}Tc-pyrophosphate uptake within the heart.[340] In patients with acute anterior infarction, uptake is seen within the anterior wall of the left ventricle, frequently involving the septum (Fig. 11–25). In patients with acute inferior infarction, uptake may occur in the posterior wall of the right ventricle, posterior septum, and posterolateral wall of the left ventricle as well. The advantages of tomography over other methods for in-

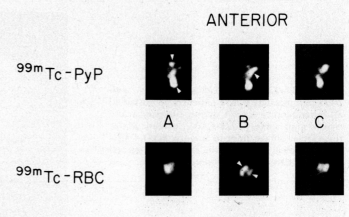

ANTERIOR

^{99m}Tc - PyP

A   B   C

^{99m}Tc - RBC

POSTERIOR

FIGURE 11–25 Transaxial tomograms obtained with technetium-99m pyrophosphate (upper panels) and technetium-99m red blood cells (lower panels) of a patient with an acute anteroseptal infarct. In upper frame A, upper arrow indicates the sternum and lower arrow indicates the spine. In upper frame B, arrow indicates ^{99m}Tc-pyrophosphate uptake in the anterior wall of the left ventricle and the septum. In lower frame B, the upper arrow indicates the right ventricular cavity and the lower arrow indicates the left ventricular cavity. A = transaxial plane corresponding to base of left ventricle; B = midventricle; C = apex.

farct sizing is that imaging need be performed only once between 1 and 10 days after infarction. Serum enzyme analysis requires frequent sampling beginning hours after the onset of symptoms. This approach appears to be promising for quantitatively estimating infarct size in humans, especially when coupled with thallium-201 to assess the volume of perfused myocardium.

PULMONARY SCINTIGRAPHY

Pulmonary scintigraphy is a safe, noninvasive method for evaluating regional myocardial perfusion and ventilation. It has been applied most widely in the diagnosis of pulmonary embolism. The radionuclide image provides a map of regional pulmonary perfusion or ventilation. Many abnormalities appear as areas of decreased isotopic uptake on the scan. The presence or absence of these areas, their size and location, and their relationship to anatomical abnormalities seen on chest x-rays provide clues to underlying pulmonary disease. Quantification of regional pulmonary function is also possible based on the relative regional distribution of the radiotracers and the change in activity levels with time.

PERFUSION SCINTIGRAPHY

Pulmonary perfusion scintigraphy is based on the principles developed by Sapirstein: regional blood flow is directly proportional to the quantity of the radiotracer in that region provided (a) that the radiotracer is completely extracted by the tissue, (b) that complete mixing of the tracer has taken place within the blood, and (c) that the radiotracer remains in the tissue and is not metabolized or released from the tissue.[341] When radioactive particles larg-

er in size than the diameter of a pulmonary capillary are injected intravenously, they are mixed in the right side of the heart and are then trapped by the capillary and precapillary vasculature. As a result, the quantity of radioactivity in any region of the lung—and hence the activity emanating from that region—is directly proportional to blood flow to that region.

A number of agents have been used to determine regional pulmonary perfusion by means of the particle-entrapment technique.[342] The first material used clinically was macroaggregated albumin (MAA) labeled with iodine-131. Subsequently, indium-labeled iron hydroxide aggregates came into use and, more recently, technetium-labeled iron hydroxide aggregates, macroaggregated albumin, and human albumin microspheres.

At the present time, either ^{99m}Tc–macroaggregated albumin or ^{99m}Tc–human albumin microspheres are in common use. ^{99m}Tc-microspheres provide a more uniform particle size than other ^{99m}Tc-labeled particles;[343] on the other hand, macroaggregated albumin has been associated with fewer instances of allergic reactions than have the microspheres.[344] The aggregated albumin particles are between 10 and 40 microns in diameter; the albumin microspheres are more uniform in size and are between 20 and 40 microns in diameter. The particles break up slowly after entrapment in the lung;

their biological half-life is approximately 7 hours in normal patients and somewhat longer in patients with pulmonary embolism or parenchymal lung disease. The fragments are then removed from the circulation by the reticuloendothelial system.

Perfusion scintigraphy is a safe procedure with a very low incidence of side effects. It has been estimated that less than 0.1 per cent of the pulmonary capillaries are occluded when 200,000 to 500,000 particles are injected. Iatrogenic impairment of lung function is unlikely, even when the organ is severely compromised by disease, because of the sparsity of occlusion and rich collateral circulation.[345,346] No change is observed in pulmonary diffusing capacity after injection of the radiopharmaceutical,[347] although fatal reactions have been reported to occur after the labeled particles were administered to patients with severe pulmonary hypertension.[348]

Images are obtained, using a standard high-resolution gamma camera, in the right and left lateral, right and left posterior oblique, and anterior and posterior positions. The posterior oblique views have been recently incorporated into the imaging regimen because they provide better delineation of the posterior and lateral basal segments of the lower lobes and eliminate much of the overlapping radioactivity seen from the opposite lung on lateral views.[349] At least 400,000 to 600,000 counts should be obtained in each view. The two lateral views should be imaged for the same time rather than for the same counts; similarly, the two oblique views should be imaged for the same time.

In the normal perfusion lung scintiscan there is uniform distribution of activity throughout the lung, with increasing radioactivity seen from the anterior to the posterior projection if the patient is injected while supine (Fig. 11-26). The margins of the lung's radioactivity are smooth and correspond to the lung outline seen on the chest radiograph. The heart and mediastinal structures produce a midline defect extending to the left, particularly on the anterior view. The heart is usually not seen on the posterior view unless it is enlarged. Occasionally, the aortic notch produces a defect in the midline, particularly when it is tortuous. Diminished perfusion may be seen in the region of an azygos lobe.[350] More subtle changes occur with changes in the position of the diaphragm, particularly if there is central eventration. In patients with diaphragmatic paralysis and those who are very obese, basilar defects in the perfusion scan may cause confusion at times.

Of the pathological conditions that can interfere with regional lung perfusion, the most important are those involving the pulmonary arterial vasculature. These include primary diseases of the pulmonary arteries, either congenital (atresia) or acquired (arteritis); extraluminal compression by interstitial fluid, tumors, lymph nodes, or other mediastinal structures; and intraluminal filling by tumor, fat, air, parasites, amniotic fluid, or blood clots.

Parenchymal diseases (inflammatory, malignant) and extrapulmonic displacement of lung tissue due to pleural effusion or cardiomegaly also compromise regional lung perfusion. Intrapulmonary shunting caused by regional hypoxia diverts blood flow and therefore radioactive particles away from that portion of the lung. Shunts from the bronchial to the pulmonary arteries in bronchiectasis and some bronchogenic carcinomas also keep the particles

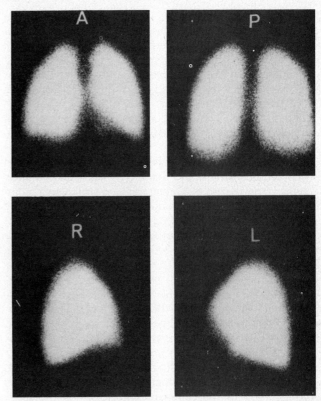

FIGURE 11-26 Normal pulmonary perfusion scintiscan. The distribution of tracer is relatively homogeneous but with a decreasing gradient toward the apex due to decreasing lung volume, an increasing gradient toward the dependent portion of the lung (posterior if injected supine) due to gravitational effects on perfusion, and no radioactivity in the mediastinum. (A = anterior view; P = posterior view; R = right lateral view; L = left lateral view.)

away from the affected areas.[351] Although clinical attention has focused primarily on the value of pulmonary scintigraphy in detecting thromboembolic disease, it is important to remember that other conditions can interfere with regional perfusion, leading to abnormal scans.

VENTILATION SCINTIGRAPHY

Ventilation scintigraphy is a helpful maneuver in distinguishing between primary perfusion abnormalities and those secondary to regional hypoxia.[352,353] Regional ventilation is usually assessed using the inert gas xenon-133. The maneuver can be performed before perfusion scintigraphy, in which case imaging is performed in the posterior projection. Alternatively, ventilation imaging can be performed after perfusion scintigraphy, in which case the physician has the flexibility to choose the projection to be used for imaging. If ventilation is assessed after perfusion scintigraphy, there is substantial scattered radiation within the xenon-133 energy window due to the higher energy technetium-99m. This interference must be overcome by using higher doses of xenon-133.

Areas of poor ventilation represent deficits in activity on the initial breathholding scintiscan, while regions of relatively increased activity indicate abnormal ventilation during the washout phase. The abnormal retention of xenon during the washout phase is due to air-trapping. The initial breathholding study alone is insufficient because patients with parenchymal disease may have normal ventilation in areas of reduced perfusion on the single-breath image but will trap xenon during the washout phase.[354] When initial breathholding imaging is used alone, without the washout phase of the study, the specificity for detection of pulmonary embolism is only 80 per cent; however, when the additional information obtained from the washout phase of the study is added, the specificity increases to over 90 per cent.

A number of other radiopharmaceuticals have been used for ventilation scintigraphy. Xenon-127 has a photon energy higher than that of technetium-99m. Ventilation scintigraphy can therefore be performed after perfusion imaging with far less interference from technetium-99m. At the present time, xenon-127 is not widely available; it is expensive and requires recycling because of its costs and long half-life.

An alternative approach uses the rubidium-81/krypton-81m generator. The patient inhales krypton-81m during normal respiration.[355,356] Because the primary photopeak of krypton-81m is 190 kev, higher spatial resolution can be obtained than with xenon-133, and imaging can be performed following the perfusion study with little scattered radiation from technetium-99m. The primary disadvantage of this radiotracer—one that will severely limit its implementation in the community hospital—is the short half-life of its parent compound, rubidium-81 (4 hours). Since the physical half-life of this radiotracer is very short (13 seconds), the continual inhalation of krypton-81m results in images that depict the balance between regional ventilation and radioactive decay of the tracer. After about 30 seconds of inhalation, a steady state is reached, and the activity represents the distribution of tidal ventilation.[356] Thus, information contained in a single krypton-81m ventilation scan is only a crude representation of regional ventilation. The short time required for imaging, its simplicity, and the low absorbed radiation dose enable serial high-resolution images of ventilatory flow to be obtained in multiple views. However, because of the short half-life, washout studies cannot be obtained.

PULMONARY EMBOLISM
(See also p. 1586)

The single most important application of pulmonary scintigraphy is in the diagnosis of pulmonary embolism. The clinical manifestations of pulmonary embolism are frequently vague and nonspecific[357] (p. 1586). The most frequent signs and symptoms are tachypnea (92 per cent), dyspnea (81 per cent), pleuritic chest pain (72 per cent), apprehension (59 per cent), cough (54 per cent), and rales (53 per cent). Signs and symptoms more specific for the diagnosis of pulmonary embolism occur much less frequently. For example, hemoptysis is seen in only 34 per cent of patients, cyanosis in 18 per cent, and thrombophlebitis in 33 per cent.

The value of pulmonary scintigraphy in detecting acute pulmonary emboli is based, in part, on its high sensitivity, since a normal lung scan virtually rules out clinically significant pulmonary emboli within the previous 48 hours.[358]

Theoretically, microemboli might produce perfusion defects beyond the resolution of present instrumentation, or clots in the central pulmonary artery that only partially occlude the lumen might not affect regional blood flow. Nevertheless, a well-documented case of acute pulmonary embolism with a technically adequate normal perfusion scan obtained within 48 hours of the onset of symptoms has yet to be recorded.

The abnormal scintigram presents more of a problem. Diagnostic information must be garnered from clues derived from the anatomical distribution of the perfusion defects, the relationship between the degree of impairment in regional perfusion and ventilation, and the stability of the perfusion defects over time. In general, acute pulmonary emboli produce sharply delineated polysegmental or lobar defects (Fig. 11–27).[359] These are unlike the anatomically less well-defined defects seen in chronic lung disease. A large proportion of patients with lobar defects have pulmonary embolism, for example.[360,361] On the other hand, subsegmental defects are the predominant perfusion abnormality in only a small fraction of patients with clinically apparent pulmonary embolism. Unilateral absence of perfusion is not pathognomonic of pulmonary embolism; it is also seen in bronchogenic carcinoma, the hyperlucent emphysematous lung, and pulmonary artery atresia.

Most patients with pulmonary emboli have multiple perfusion defects. In one series, for example, only 16 of 104 patients with abnormal lung scintigrams had single perfusion defects.[360] Of these, only three were present in patients with pulmonary embolism. Thus, 93 per cent of patients with pulmonary emboli have multiple perfusion defects. In patients with multiple perfusion defects, 52 per cent of patients with pulmonary embolism have perfusion defects in-

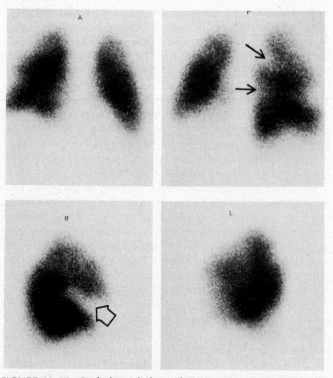

FIGURE 11–27 Perfusion scintiscan demonstrating absent perfusion to a segment of the right middle lobe (open arrow) with additional subsegmental perfusion defects (arrows).

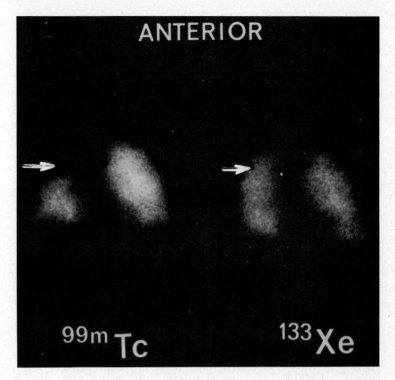

FIGURE 11–28 Perfusion scintiscan demonstrating that perfusion to the right upper lung field is absent (left, arrow). Single-breath ventilation scintiscan demonstrating normal ventilation in this region (right, arrow). Ventilation-perfusion mismatch is consistent with pulmonary embolism.

volving lobar areas. Only 8 per cent of patients without pulmonary emboli had similar findings. Segmental defects occurred with about equal frequency (22 to 33 per cent) in patients with pulmonary embolism and in patients with chronic lung disease. Patients with pulmonary emboli rarely have small subsegmental defects as their largest perfusion defects (2 to 8 per cent).[362] Nevertheless, the pattern of perfusion abnormalities is only a fair discriminator of pulmonary embolism and, if possible, should not constitute the only radiodiagnostic criterion.

Ventilation scintigraphy is a helpful maneuver in distinguishing between primary perfusion abnormalities and those secondary to regional hypoxia.[352-354] In patients with pulmonary emboli, the perfusion abnormality clearly exceeds any abnormality in ventilation (Fig. 11–28). In patients with acute bronchospasm or chronic lung disease, the compromise of regional ventilation usually matches or exceeds that of perfusion. In patients with normal or near-normal chest x-rays, this comparison between perfusion and ventilation is particularly useful in differentiating pulmonary lung disease from pulmonary emboli.

Interpretation becomes more difficult when the chest x-ray is abnormal in the region of the perfusion defect. The pulmonary density seen on the x-ray may represent parenchymal pulmonary disease or may be secondary to pulmonary infarction. Since ventilation will be affected in either case, ventilation scintigraphy is of limited value unless other perfusion defects are present. The size relationship of the perfusion defect and the density on chest x-ray may be helpful, however.[363] If the perfusion defect is small relative to the density on the x-ray, the probability of pulmonary embolism is low (7 per cent). When the perfusion defect is substantially larger than the roentgenographic abnormality, the probability of pulmonary embolism is increased (89 per cent). The perfusion defect must be substantially larger or smaller than the corresponding radiographic abnormalities for these diagnostic criteria to apply. Otherwise, a

scintigram with a perfusion defect and accompanying chest x-ray density with no other diagnostic clues is indeterminant for the diagnosis of pulmonary embolism.

Natural evolution of the appearance on perfusion scans after an acute episode is also a useful indicator of pulmonary embolism (Fig. 11–29).[364-366] In general, perfusion scintigraphy returns to normal soon after the embolic event. The rapidity of improvement seems to depend on the patient's age and cardiovascular status and the amount of lung involved. In the absence of heart failure, even major occlusions may revert to normal within weeks. Recurrent embolism is often characterized by the appearance of new regions of involvement as old ones disappear. Frag-

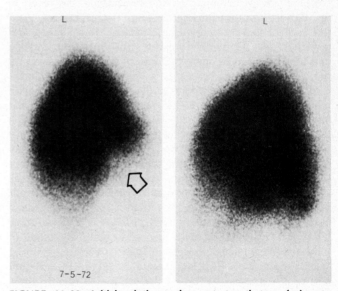

FIGURE 11–29 Initial scintiscan demonstrates that perfusion to most of left lower lobe is absent (left, arrow). Repeat scintigraphy (right) demonstrates markedly improved perfusion to this region six days later. This rapid resolution in the face of a normal chest x-ray is consistent with pulmonary embolism.

TABLE 11–2   THE ROLE OF SCINTIGRAPHY IN PULMONARY EMBOLISM (PE)

LARGEST PERFUSION DEFECT	X-RAY	VENTILATION	INTERPRETATION	STRATEGY
Normal			No pulmonary embolism within past 48 hours	No pulmonary angiography
Subsegmental		Indicated only if large subsegmental deficit; then interpretation same as segmental or lobar below	Low probability of PE ($<5\%$)	Pulmonary angiography only if clinical suspicion is high
Segmental or lobar	Normal in region of defect	Perfusion-ventilation match	Low probability of PE	Pulmonary angiography only if clinical suspicion is high
Segmental or lobar	Abnormal density in region of defect	Not indicated	Indeterminate	Pulmonary angiography recommended
Segmental or lobar	Normal in region of defect	Perfusion-ventilation mismatch	High probability of PE ($>90\%$)	Treat
Segmental or lobar	Normal in region of defect	Cannot be performed	Moderate probability of PE (25% in segmental and 80% in lobar defects)	Pulmonary angiography recommended

mentation of large central thromboemboli can produce new subsegmental defects, however. Because of this natural evolution, it is often difficult to document reembolization in patients already receiving therapy for previous pulmonary emboli.

Conditions other than acute pulmonary embolism can result in ventilation/perfusion mismatches (normal ventilation in regions of decreased or absent perfusion).[367] The ventilation/perfusion mismatch is, after all, evidence only of a vascular rather than a parenchymal etiology. In parenchymal disease, regional hypoxia results in a reflex reduction in decreased pulmonary blood flow to that region. Vascular diseases, such as previous pulmonary embolism, pulmonary artery agenesis or stenosis, vasculitis (polyarteritis nodosa), tuberculosis, pulmonary artery sarcoma, hemangioendotheliomatosis, and pulmonary venoocclusive disease would be expected to result in ventilation/perfusion mismatches. There are sporadic reports of parenchymal lung disease, including emphysema, radiation therapy, intravenous drug abuse, bronchogenic carcinoma, lymphangitic carcinomatosis, and pneumonia that result in ventilation/perfusion mismatch. Despite this extensive differential diagnosis, ventilation/perfusion mismatches and perfusion defects involving large subsegments, segments, and lobes are due to acute pulmonary embolism in over 90 per cent of the cases.

A reasonable strategy can be developed in patients with suspected pulmonary embolism based on the perfusion and ventilation studies (Table 11–2). Patients with normal perfusion scintigrams have not had clinically significant embolism within the previous 48 hours. Pulmonary angiography is not ordinarily indicated in these patients. If the perfusion scintigram contains small subsegmental defects as the predominant perfusion abnormality, the likelihood of pulmonary embolism is low (less than 5 per cent). Unless clinical suspicion of pulmonary embolism is high or other laboratory or radiographic evidence is highly suggestive of pulmonary embolism, the patient can be considered to be free of recent emboli. If a segmental or large subsegmental perfusion defect is the largest perfusion abnormality present, and the ventilation study cannot be performed because of the patient's clinical condition or because an abnormality is present in that region on the chest radiography, the probability of embolization is moderate and a pulmonary arteriogram is necessary for documentation of the disease.

While the presence of a lobar defect increases the likelihood of pulmonary embolism, pulmonary angiography is still necessary to document the disease if ventilation scintigraphy cannot be performed or if additional segmental defects do not accompany it. If a large subsegmental or lobar defect is associated with a ventilation/perfusion mismatch, and multiple perfusion defects are present, the likelihood of pulmonary embolism is very high and treatment should be begun immediately. Care must be taken in patients with severe chronic lung disease in which the changes due to pulmonary embolism may be masked by the parenchymal disease. Angiography should be performed in these patients if the perfusion scans are not normal or exhibit only small subsegmental defects.

References

CARDIAC PERFORMANCE

1. Blumgart, H. L., and Weiss, S.: Studies on the velocity of blood flow. II. The velocity of blood flow in normal resting individuals, and a critique of the method used. J. Clin. Invest. 4:15, 1927.
2. Cohn, P. F., Gorlin, R., Cohn, L. H., and Collins, J. J., Jr.: Left ventricular ejection fraction as a prognostic guide in surgical treatment of coronary and valvular heart disease. Am. J. Cardiol. 34:136, 1974.
3. Nelson, G. R., Cohn, P. F., and Gorlin, R.: Prognosis in medically treated coronary artery disease: The value of ejection fraction compared with other measurements. Circulation 52:408, 1975.
4. Feild, B. J., Russell, R. O., Jr., Dowling, J. T., and Rackley, C. E.: Regional left ventricular performance in the year following myocardial infarction. Circulation 46:679, 1972.
5. Watson, L. E., Dickhaus, D. W., and Martin, R. H.: Left ventricular aneurysm: Preoperative hemodynamics, chamber volume, and results of aneurysmectomy. Circulation 52:868, 1975.
6. Schelbert, H. R., Henning, H., Ashburn, W. L., Verba, J. W., Karliner, J. S., and O'Rourke, R. A.: Serial measurements of left ventricular ejection fraction by radionuclide angiography early and late after myocardial infarction. Am. J. Cardiol. 38:407, 1976.
7. Rigo, P., Murray, M., Strauss, H. W., Taylor, D., Kelly, D., Weisfeldt, M., and Pitt, B.: Left ventricular function in acute myocardial infarction evaluated by gated scintigraphy. Circulation 50:678, 1974.
8. Karliner, J. S., Gault, M. D., Eckberg, D., Mullins, C. B., and Ross, J., Jr.: Mean velocity of fiber shortening: A simplified measure of left ventricular myocardial contractility. Circulation 44:323, 1971.
9. Ashburn, W. L., Schelbert, H. R., and Verba, J. W.: Left ventricular ejection fraction: A review of several radionuclide angiographic approaches using the scintillation camera. Progr. Cardiovasc. Dis. 20:267, 1978.
10. Bodenheimer, M. M., Banka, V. S., and Helfant, R. H.: Nuclear cardiology. I. Radionuclide angiographic assessment of left ventricular contraction: Uses, limitations, and future directions. Am. J. Cardiol. 45:661, 1980.
11. Marshall, R. C., Berger, H. J., Costin, J. C., Freedman, G. S., Wolberg, J., Cohen, L. S., Gottschalk, A., and Zaret, B. L.: Assessment of cardiac performance with quantitative radionuclide angiocardiography. Circulation 56:820, 1977.

12. Wackers, F. J., Giles, R. W., Hoffer, P. B., Lange, R. C., Berger, H. J., and Zaret, B. L.: Gold-195m, a new generator-produced short-lived radionuclide for sequential assessment of ventricular performance by first pass radionuclide angiocardiography. Am. J. Cardiol. 50:89, 1982.

13. Holman, B. L., Neirinckx, R. D., Treves, S., and Tow, D. E.: Cardiac imaging with tantalum-178. Radiology 131:525, 1979.

14. Treves, S., Cheng, C., Samuel, A., Lambrecht, R., Babchyck, B., Zimmerman, R., and Norwood, W.: Iridium-191 angiocardiography for the detection and quantitation of left-to-right shunting. J. Nucl. Med. 21:1151, 1980.

15. Schelbert, H. R., Verba, J. W., Johnson, A. D., Brock, G. W., Alazraki, N. P., Rose, F. J., and Ashburn, W. L.: Nontraumatic determination of left ventricular ejection fraction by radionuclide angiocardiography. Circulation 51:902, 1975.

16. Jengo, J. A., Mena, I., Blaufuss, A., and Criley, J. M.: Evaluation of left ventricular function (ejection fraction and segmental wall motion) by single pass radioisotope angiography. Circulation 57:326, 1978.

17. Parker, J. A., and Treves, S.: Radionuclide detection, localization and quantitation of intracardiac shunts and shunts between the great arteries. Progr. Cardiovasc. Dis. 20:121, 1977.

18. Lane, S. D., Patton, D. D., Staab, E. V., and Baglan, R. J.: Simple technique for rapid bolus injection. J. Nucl. Med. 13:118, 1972.

19. Oldendorf, W. H.: Measurement of the mean transit time of cerebral circulation by external detection of an intravenously injected radioisotope. J. Nucl. Med. 3:382, 1962.

20. Treves, S., Maltz, D. L., and Adlestein, S. J.: Intracardiac shunts. In James, A. E., Wagner, H. N., and Cooke, R. E. (eds.): Pediatric Nuclear Medicine. Philadelphia, W. B. Saunders Co., 1974, p. 231.

21. Donato, L.: Basic concepts of radiocardiography. Semin. Nucl. Med. 3:111, 1973.

22. Ellis, J. H., and Steele, P. P.: Value of combined hemodynamic and radiocardiographic studies in acute respiratory failure. In Serafini, A. N., Gilson, A. J., and Smoak, W. M. (eds.): Nuclear Cardiology. New York, Plenum Press, 1977, p. 187.

23. Parker, H., Van Dyke, D., Weber, P., Davies, H., Steele, P., and Sullivan, R.: Evaluation of central circulatory dynamics with the radionuclide angiocardiogram. In Wagner, H. (ed.): Diagnostic Nuclear Cardiology. St. Louis, The C. V. Mosby Co., 1974.

24. Pierson, R. N., Jr., and Van Dyke, D. C.: Analysis of left ventricular function. In Pierson, R. N., Kriss, J. P., Jones, R. H., and MacIntyre, W. J. (eds.): Quantitative Nuclear Cardiology. New York, John Wiley and Sons, 1975, p. 123.

25. Hamilton, W. F., Moore, J. W., Kinsman, J. M., and Spurling, R. G.: Studies on the circulation. IV. Further analysis of the injection method and of changes in hemodynamics under physiological and pathological conditions. Am. J. Physiol. 99:534, 1931–32.

26. Razzak, M. A., Botti, R. E., MacIntyre, W. J., and Pritchard, W. H.: Consecutive determination of cardiac output and renal blood flow by external monitoring of radioactive isotopes. J. Nucl. Med. 11:190, 1970.

27. Thompson, H. K., Starmer, C. E., Whalen, R. E., and McIntosh, H. D.: Indicator transit time considered as a gamma variate. Circ. Res. 14:502, 1964.

28. Starmer, C. E., and Clark, D. O.: Computer computations of cardiac output using the gamma function. J. Appl. Physiol. 28:219, 1970.

29. Steadham, R. E., and Blackwell, L. H.: A new method for the determination of the area under a cardiac output curve. I.E.E.E. Trans. Biomed. Engin. 17: 335, 1970.

30. Kriss, J. P., Enright, L. P., Hayden, W. G., Wexler, L., and Shumway, N. E.: Radioisotope angiocardiography: Wide scope applicability in diagnosis and evaluation of therapy in diseases of the heart and great vessels. Circulation 43: 792, 1971.

31. Mann, T., Goldberg, S., Mudge, G. H., and Grossman, W.: Factors contributing to altered left ventricular diastolic properties during angina pectoris. Circulation 59:14, 1979.

32. Hirota, Y.: A clinical study of left ventricular relaxation. Circulation 62:756, 1980.

33. Ludbrook, P. A., Byrne, J. D., and McKnight, R. C.: Influence of right ventricular hemodynamics on left ventricular diastolic pressure-volume relations in man. Circulation 59:21, 1979.

34. Polak, J. F., Kemper, A. J., Bianco, J. A., Parisi, A. F., and Tow, D. E.: Resting early peak diastolic filling rate: A sensitive index of myocardial dysfunction in patients with coronary artery disease. J. Nucl. Med. 23:471, 1982.

35. Bonow, R. O., Bacharach, S. L., Green, M. V., Kent, K. M., Rosing, D. R., Lipson, L. C., Leon, M. B., and Epstein, S. E.: Left ventricular diastolic filling in patients with coronary artery disease (abstr). Circulation 62:III-77, 1980.

36. Tobinick, E., Schelbert, H. R., Henning, H., LeWinter, M., Taylor, A., Ashburn, W. L., and Karliner, J. S.: Right ventricular ejection fraction in patients with acute anterior and inferior myocardial infarction assessed by radionuclide angiography. Circulation 57:1078, 1978.

37. Berger, H. J., Matthay, R. A., Marshal, R. A., Gottschalk, A., Cohen, L. S., and Zaret, B. L.: Noninvasive radionuclide technique for right ventricular ejection fraction in man. Circulation 54(Suppl.):II-109, 1976.

38. Berger, H. J., Matthay, R. A., Loke, J., Marshall, R. C., Gottschalk, A., and Zaret, B. L.: Assessment of cardiac performance with quantitative radionuclide angiocardiography: Right ventricular ejection fraction with reference to findings in chronic obstructive pulmonary disease. Am. J. Cardiol. 51:897, 1978.

39. Sandler, H., and Dodge, H. T.: Use of single pace cineangiograms for the calculation of left ventricular volume in man. Am. Heart J. 75:325, 1968.

40. Folse, R., and Braunwald, E.: Pulmonary vascular dilution curves recorded by external detection in the diagnosis of left-to-right shunts. Br. Heart J. 24:166, 1962.

41. Carter, S. A., Bajec, D. F., Yannicelli, E., and Wood, E. H.: Estimation of left-to-right shunt from arterial dilution curves. J. Lab. Clin. Med. 55:77, 1960.

42. Alazraki, N. P., Ashburn, W. L., and Hagan, A.: Detection of left-to-right cardiac shunts with the scintillation camera pulmonary dilution curve. J. Nucl. Med. 13:142, 1972.

43. Maltz, D. L., and Treves, S.: Quantitative radionuclide angiocardiography: Determination of Q_p:Q_s in children. Circulation 47: 1040, 1973.

44. Greenfield, L. D., and Bennett, L. R.: Detection of intracardiac shunts with radionuclide imaging. Semin. Nucl. Med. 3:139, 1973.

45. Greenfield, L. D., Vincent, W. R., Graham, L. S., and Bennett, L. R.: Evaluation of intracardiac shunts. CRC Crit. Rev. Clin. Radiol. Nucl. Med. 6:217, 1975.

46. Braunwald, E., Long, R. T. L., and Morrow, A. G.: Injections of radioactive krypton (Kr^{85}) solution in the detection and localization of cardiac shunts. J. Clin. Invest. 38:990, 1959.

47. Bosnjakovic, B., Bennett, L., and Vincent, W.: Diagnosis of intracardiac shunts without cardiac catheterization. Circulation 44:II-144, 1971.

48. Polak, J. F., Podrid, P. J., Lown, B., and Holman, B. L.: Ventricular postextrasystolic potentiation in the dog: A study using list mode radionuclide ventriculography. J. Nucl. Med. (in press).

49. Rabinovitch, M. A., Stewart, J., Chan, W., Dunlap, T. E., Kalff, V., Clare, J., Thrall, J. H., and Pitt, B.: Scintigraphic demonstration of ventriculo-atrial conduction in the ventricular pacemaker syndrome. J. Nucl. Med. 23:795, 1982.

50. Bacharach, S. L., Green, M. V., Borer, J. S., Hyde, J. E., Farkas, S. P., and Johnson, G. S.: Left-ventricular peak ejection rate, filling rate, and ejection fraction—frame rate requirements at rest and exercise. J. Nucl. Med. 20:189, 1979.

51. Maddox, D. E., Holman, B. L., Wynne, J., Idoine, J., Parker, J. A., Uren, R., Neill, J. M., and Cohn, P. F.: The ejection fraction image: A noninvasive index of regional left ventricular wall motion. Am. J. Cardiol. 41:1230, 1978.

52. Parker, J. A., Secker-Walker, R. H., Hill, R. L., Siegel, B. A., and Potchen, E. J.: A new technique for the calculation of left ventricular ejection fraction. J. Nucl. Med. 13:649, 1972.

53. Secker-Walker, R. H., Resnick, L., Kunz, H., Parker, J. A., Hill, R. L., and Potchen, E. J.: Measurement of left ventricular ejection fraction. J. Nucl. Med. 14:798, 1973.

54. Slutsky, R., Karliner, J., Ricci, D., Kaiser, R., Pfisterer, M., Gordon, D., Peterson, K., and Ashburn, W.: Left ventricular volumes by gated equilibrium radionuclide angiography: A new method. Circulation 60:556, 1979.

55. Konstam, M. A., Wynne, J., Holman, B. L., Brown, E. J., Neill, J. M., and Kozlowski, J.: Use of equilibrium (gated) radionuclide ventriculography to quantitate left ventricular output in patients with and without left-sided valvular regurgitation. Circulation 64:578, 1981.

56. Maddox, D. E., Holman, B. L., Wynne, J., Idoine, J., Parker, J. A., Uren, R., Neill, J. M., and Cohn, P. F.: Ejection fraction image: A noninvasive index of regional left ventricular wall motion. Am. J. Cardiol. 41:1230, 1978.

57. Holman, B. L., Wynne, J., Idoine, J., Zielonka, J., and Neill, J.: The paradox image: A noninvasive index of regional left ventricular dyskinesis. J. Nucl. Med. 20:1237, 1979.

58. Holman, B. L., Wynne, J., Idoine, J., and Neill, J.: Disruption in the temporal sequence of regional ventricular contraction. Circulation 61:1075, 1980.

59. Botvinick, E. H., Frais, M. A., Shosa, D. W., O'Connell, J. W., Pacheco-Alvarez, J. A., Scheinman, M., Hattner, R. S., Morady, F., and Faulkner, D. B.: An accurate means of detecting and characterizing abnormal patterns of ventricular activation by phase image analysis. Am. J. Cardiol. 50:289, 1982.

60. Pavel, D., Swlryn, S., Lam, W., Byrom, E., Shelkh, A., and Rosen, K.: Ventricular phase analysis of radionuclide gated studies (abstr.). Am. J. Cardiol. 45:398, 1980.

61. Maddox, D. E., Wynne, J., Uren, R., Parker, J. A., Idoine, J., Siegel, L. C., Neill, J. M., Cohn, P. F., and Holman, B. L.: Regional ejection fraction: A quantitative radionuclide index of regional left ventricular performance. Circulation 59:1001, 1979.

62. Silber, S., Schwaiger, M., Klein, U., and Rudolph, W.: Quantitative Beurteilung der linksventrikulären Funktion mit der Radionuklid-Ventrikulographie. Herz 5:146, 1980.

63. Slutsky, R., Hooper, W., Gerber, K., Battler, A., Froelicher, V., Ashburn, W., and Karliner, J.: Assessment of right ventricular function at rest and during exercise in patients with coronary artery disease: A new approach using equilibrium radionuclide angiography. Am. J. Cardiol. 45:63, 1980.

64. Holman, B. L., Wynne, J., Zielonka, J. S., and Idoine, J.: A simplified technique for measuring right ventricular ejection fraction using the equilibrium radionuclide angiocardiogram and the slant-hole collimator. Radiology 138: 429, 1981.

65. Rigo, P., Alderson, P. O., Robertson, R. M., Becher, L. C., and Wagner, H. N., Jr.: Measurement of aortic and ventral regurgitation by gated cardiac blood pool scans. Circulation 60:306, 1979.

66. Nicod, P., Corbett, J. R., Firth, B. G., Dehmer, G. J., Izquierdo, C., Markham, R. V., Jr., Hillis, L. D., Willerson, J. T., and Lewis, S. E.: Radionuclide techniques for valvular regurgitant index: Comparison in patients with normal and depressed ventricular function. J. Nucl. Med. 23:763, 1982.

67. Alderson, P. O.: Radionuclide quantification of valvular regurgitation. J. Nucl. Med. 23:851, 1982.

68. Tu'meh, S. S., Tracy, D., Wynne, J., Konstam, M. A., Kozlowski, J. F., Neu-

mann, A. L., and Holman, B. L.: Scintigraphic diagnosis of tricuspid regurgitation. Radiology 145:463, 1982.

69. Borer, J., Bacharach, S. L., Green, M. V., Kent, K. M., Epstein, S. E., and Johnston, G. S.: Real-time radionuclide cineangiography in the noninvasive evaluation of global and regional left ventricular function at rest and during exercise in patients with coronary-artery disease. N. Engl. J. Med. 296:839, 1977.

70. Borer, J., Bacharach, S. L., and Green, M. V.: Radionuclide cineangiography in the clinical assessment of patients with coronary and valvular heart diseases. Progr. Nucl. Med. 6:151, 1980.

71. Bodenheimer, M. M., Banka, V. S., Fooshee, C. M., Gillespie, J. A., and Helfant, R. H.: Detection of coronary heart disease using radionuclide determined regional ejection fraction at rest and during handgrip exercise: Correlation with coronary arteriography. Circulation 58:640, 1980.

72. Wainwright, R. J., Brennand-Roper, D. A., Cueni, T. A., Sowton, E., Hilson, A. J. W., and Maisey, M. N.: Cold pressor test in detection of coronary heart-disease and cardiomyopathy using technetium-99m gated blood-pool imaging. Lancet 2:320, 1979.

73. Peter, C. A., and Jones, R. H.: Effects of isometric handgrip and dynamic exercise on left-ventricular function. J. Nucl. Med. 21:1131, 1980.

74. Wynne, J. W., Borwo, K. M., Holman, B. L., and Mudge, G. H., Jr.: Cold pressor radionuclide ventriculography: Clinical utility. Br. Heart J. (in press).

75. Slutsky, R., Karliner, J., Ricci, D., Schuler, G., Pfisterer, M., Peterson, K., and Ashburn, W.: Response of left ventricular volume to exercise in man assessed by radionuclide equilibrium angiography. Circulation 60:565, 1979.

76. Okada, R. D., Boucher, C. A., Strauss, H. W., and Pohost, G. M.: Exercise radionuclide imaging approaches to coronary artery disease. Am. J. Cardiol. 46:1188, 1980.

77. Marshall, R. C., Wisenberg, G., Schelbert, H. R., and Henze, E.: Effect of oral propranolol on rest, exercise and postexercise left ventricular performance in normal subjects and patients with coronary artery disease. Circulation 63:572, 1981.

78. Poliner, L. R., Dehmer, G. J., Lewis, S. E., Parkey, R. W., Blomqvist, C. G., and Willerson, J. T.: Left ventricular performance in normal subjects: A comparison of the responses to exercise in the upright and supine positions. Circulation 62:528, 1980.

79. Jones, R. H., McEwan, P., Newman, G. E., Port, S., Rerych, S. K., Scholz, P. M., Upton, M. T., Peter, C. A., Austin, E. H., Leong, K., Gibbons, R. J., Cobb, F. R., Coleman, R. E., and Sabiston, D. C.: Accuracy of diagnosis of coronary artery disease by radionuclide measurements of left ventricular function during rest and exercise. Circulation 64:586, 1981.

80. Port, S., Cobb, F. R., Coleman, R. E., and Jones, R. H.: Effect of age on the response of the left ventricular ejection fraction to exercise. N. Engl. J. Med. 303:1133, 1980.

81. Gibbons, R. H., Lee, J. L., Cobb, F. R., Coleman, R. E., and Jones, R. H.: Ejection fraction response to exercise in patients with chest pain, coronary artery disease, and normal coronary arteriograms. Circulation 66:643, 1982.

82. Borer, J. S., Bacharach, S. L., Green, M. V., Kent, K. M., Rosing, D. R., Seides, S. F., McIntosh, C. L., Conkle, D., Morrow, A. G., and Epstein, S. E.: Left ventricular function in aortic stenosis: Response to exercise and effects of operation (abstr). Am. J. Cardiol. 41:382, 1978.

83. Borer, J. S., Bacharach, S. L., Green, M. V., Kent, K. M., Henry, W. L., Rosing, D. R., Seides, S. F., Johnston, G. S., and Epstein, S. E.: Exercise-induced left ventricular dysfunction in symptomatic and asymptomatic patients with aortic regurgitation: Assessment with radionuclide cineangiography. Am. J. Cardiol. 42:351, 1978.

84. Borer, J. S., Gottdiener, J. S., Rosing, D. R., Kent, K. M., Bacharach, S. L., Green, M. V., and Epstein, S. E.: Left ventricular function in mitral regurgitation: Determination during exercise (abstr). Circulation 60(Suppl.):II-38, 1979.

85. Ahmad, M., Sullivan, T., Haibach, H., Sandock, K., Logan, K., and Holmes, R.: Exercise induced changes in left ventricular function in patients with mitral valve prolapse (abstr). Clin. Res. 27:146, 1979.

86. Borer, J. S., Bacharach, S. L., Green, M. V., Kent, K. M., Maron, B. J., Rosing, D. R., Seides, S. F., and Epstein, S. E.: Obstructive vs. nonobstructive symmetric septal hypertrophy: Differences in left ventricular function with exercise (abstr). Am. J. Cardiol. 41:379, 1978.

87. Slutsky, R., Ackerman, W., Hooper, W., Battler, A., Karliner, J., Ashburn, W., and Moser, K.: The response of left ventricular ejection fraction and volume to supine exercise in patients with severe COPD (abstr). Circulation 60 (Suppl.):II-234, 1979.

88. Leon, M. B., Borer, J. S., Bacharach, S. L., Green, M. V., Benz, E. J., Griffith, P., and Nienhuis, A. W.: Detection of early cardiac dysfunction in patients with severe beta-thalassemia and chronic iron overload. N. Engl. J. Med. 301:1143, 1979.

89. Chipps, B. E., Alderson, P. O., Roland, J. M. A., Yang, S., van Aswegen, A., Rosenstein, B. L., and Wagner, H. N.: Ventricular function at rest and during exercise in cystic fibrosis (abstr). J. Nucl. Med. 20:637, 1979.

90. Port, S., Cobb, F. R., and Jones, R. H.: Effects of propranolol on left ventricular function in normal men (abstr). J. Nucl. Med. 60 (Suppl.):II-91, 1979.

91. Wisenberg, G., Marshal, R., Schelbert, H.,and Rue, C.: The effects of oral propranolol on left ventricular function at rest and during exercise in normal patients and in patients with coronary artery disease as determined by radionuclide angiography (abstr). J. Nucl. Med. it 20:639, 1979.

92. Ehrhardt, J. C., Verani, M. S., and Marcus, M. L.: Exercise isotope ventriculogram: Use in assessing change in left ventricular function (abstr). Circulation 56 (Suppl.):II-141, 1977.

93. Gibbons, R. J., Lee, K. L., Pryor, D., Harrell, F. E., Jr., Coleman, R. E., Cobb, F. R., Rosati, R. A., and Jones, R. H.: The use of radionuclide angiography in the diagnosis of coronary artery disease: A logistic regression analysis. Circulation (in press).

94. Nesto, R. W., Cohn, L. H., Collins, J. J., Wynne, J., Holman, L., and Cohn, P. F.: Inotropic contractile reserve: A useful predictor of increased 5 year survival and improved postoperative left ventricular function in patients with coronary artery disease and reduced ejection fraction. Am. J. Cardiol. 50:39, 1982.

95. Borer, J. S., Rosing, D. R., Miller, R. H., Stark, R. M., Kent, K. M., Bacharach, S. L., Green, M. V., Lake, C. R., Cohen, H., Holmes, D., Donohue, D., Baker, W., and Epstein, S. E.: Natural history of left ventricular function during 1 year after acute myocardial infarction: Comparison with clinical, electrocardiographic and biochemical determinations. Am. J. Cardiol. 46:1, 1980.

96. Reduto, L. A., Berger, H. J., Gottschalk, A., and Zaret, B. L.: Sequential radionuclide assessment of left and right ventricular performance after acute transmural myocardial infarction. Ann. Intern. Med. 89:441, 1978.

97. Shah, P. K., Pichler, M., Berman, D. S., Singh, B. N., and Swan, H. J. C.: Left ventricular ejection fraction and first third ejection fraction determined by radionuclide ventriculography in early stages of first transmural myocardial infarction: Relation to short-term prognosis. Am. J. Cardiol. 45:542, 1980.

98. Rigo, P., Murray, M., Taylor, D. R., Weisfeldt, M. L., Kelley, D. T., Strauss, H. W., and Pitt, B.: Right ventricular dysfunction detected by gated scintigraphy in patients with acute inferior myocardial infarction. Circulation 52:268, 1975.

99. Pulido, J. I., Doss, J., Twieg, D., Blomqvist, G. C., Faulkner, D., Horn, V., DeBates, D., Tobey, M., Parkey, R. W., and Willerson, J. T.: Submaximal exercise testing after acute myocardial infarction: Myocardial scintigraphic and electrocardiographic observations. Am. J. Cardiol. 42:19, 1978.

100. Borer, J. S., Bacharach, S. L., Green, M. V., Kent, K. M., Henry, W. L., Rosing, D. R., Seides, S. F., Johnston, G. S., and Epstein, S. E.: Exercise-induced left and right ventricular dysfunction in symptomatic and asymptomatic patients with aortic regurgitation: Assessment with radionuclide cineangiography. Am. J. Cardiol. 42:351, 1978.

101. Borer, J. S., Rosing, D. R., Kent, K. M., Bacharach, S. L., Green, M. V., McIntosh, C. J., Morrow, A. G., and Epstein, S. E.: Left ventricular function at rest and during exercise after aortic valve replacement in patients with aortic regurgitation. Am. J. Cardiol. 44:1297, 1979.

102. Watson, L. E., Dickhaus, D. W., and Martin, R. H.: Left ventricular aneurysm. Preoperative hemodynamics, chamber volume, and results of aneurysmectomy. Circulation 52:868, 1975.

103. Rozanski, A., Berman, D., Gray, R., Diamond, G., Raymond, M., Prause, J., Maddahi, J., Swan, H. J. C., and Matloff, J.: Preoperative prediction of reversible myocardial asynergy by postexercise radionuclide ventriculography. N. Engl. J. Med. 307:212, 1982.

104. Bodenheimer, M. M., Banka, V. S., Hermann, G. A., Trout, R. G., Pasdar, H., and Helfant, R. H.: Reversible asynergy. Circulation 53:792, 1976.

105. Chatterjee, K., Swan, H. J. C., Parmley, W. W., Sustaita, H., Marcus, H. S., and Matloff, J.: Influence of direct myocardial revascularization on left ventricular asynergy and function in patients with coronary heart disease: With and without previous myocardial infarction. Circulation 47:276, 1973.

106. Popio, K. A., Gorlin, R., Bechtel, D., and Levine, J. A.: Postextrasystolic potentiation as a predictor of potential myocardial viability. Am. J. Cardiol. 39:944, 1977.

107. Righetti, A., Crawford, M. H., O'Rourke, R. A., Schelbert, H., Daily, P. O., and Ross, J., Jr.: Intraventricular septal motion and left ventricular function after coronary bypass surgery: Evaluation with echocardiography and radionuclide angiography. Am. J. Cardiol. 39:372, 1977.

108. Helfant, R. H., Pine, R., Meister, S. G., Feldman, M. S., Trout, R. G., and Banka, V. S.: Nitroglycerin to unmask reversible asynergy: Correlation with post coronary bypass surgery. Circulation 50:108, 1974.

109. DePuey, E. G., Mammen, G. P., Rivas, A. H., Thompson, W. L., Sonnemaker, R. E., Mathur, V., Burdine, J. A., Garcia, E., and Hall, R. J.: Post-exercise potentiation of wall motion to identify myocardial viability. Texas Heart Inst. J. 9:127, 1982.

110. Berger, H. J., Matthay, R. A., Loke, J., Marshall, R. C., Gottschalk, A., and Zaret, B. L.: Assessment of cardiac performance with quantitative radionuclide angiocardiography: Right ventricular ejection fraction with reference to findings in chronic obstructive pulmonary disease. Am. J. Cardiol. 41:897, 1978.

111. Berger, H. J., and Matthay, R. A.: Noninvasive radiographic assessment of cardiovascular function in acute and chronic respiratory failure. Am. J. Cardiol. 47:950, 1981.

112. Matthay, R. A., Berger, J. H., Davies, R. A., Loke, J., Mahler, D. A., Gottschalk, A., and Zaret, B. L.: Right and left ventricular exercise performance in chronic obstructive pulmonary disease: Radionuclide assessment. Ann. Intern. Med. 93:234, 1980.

113. Morrison, J., Coromilas, J., Robbins, M., Ong, L., Eisenberg, S., Stechel, R., Zema, M., Reiser, P., and Scherr, L.: Digitalis and myocardial infarction in man. Circulation 62:8, 1978.

114. Wynne, J., Malacoff, R. F., Benotti, J. R., Curfman, G. D., Grossman, W., Holman, B. L., Smith, T. W., and Braunwald, E.: Oral amrinone in refractory congestive heart failure. Am. J. Cardiol. 45:1245, 1980.

115. Goldman, S. A., Johnson, L. L., Escala, E., Cannon, P. J., and Weiss, M. B.: Improved exercise ejection fraction with long-term prazosin therapy in patients with heart failure. Am. J. Med. 68:36, 1980.

116. Colucci, W. S., Wynne, J., Holman, B. L., and Braunwald, E.: Long-term therapy of heart failure with prazosin: A randomized double blind trial. Am. J. Cardiol. 45:337, 1980.

117. Matthay, R. A., Berger, H. J., Loke, J., Gottschalk, A., and Zaret, B. L.: Effects of aminophylline upon right and left ventricular performance in chronic obstructive pulmonary disease: Noninvasive assessment by radionuclide angiocardiography. Am. J. Med. 65:903, 1978.

118. Bonow, R. O., Leon, M. B., Rosing, D. R., Kent, K. M., Lipson, L. C., Bacharach, S. L., Green, M. V., and Epstein, S. E.: Effect of propranolol and verapamil on left ventricular diastolic filling in patients with coronary artery disease (abstr). Circulation 62:III-85, 1980.

119. Malacoff, R. F., Lorell, B. H., Mudge, G. H., Jr., Holman, B. L., Idoine, J., Bifolck, L., and Cohn, P. F.: Beneficial effects of nifedipine on regional myocardial blood flow in patients with coronary artery disease. Circulation 65:I-32, 1982.

120. Alexander, J., Dainiak, N., Berger, H. J., Goldman, L., Johnstone, D., Reduto, L., Duffy, T., Schwartz, P., Gottschalk, A., and Zaret, B. L.: Serial assessment of doxorubicin cardiotoxicity with quantitative radionuclide angiocardiography. N. Engl. J. Med. 300:278, 1979.

MYOCARDIAL SCINTIGRAPHY

121. Abrams, H. L., and Adams, D. F.: The coronary arteriogram. Structural and functional aspects. N. Engl. J. Med. 281:1276, 1969.

122. Bodenheimer, M. M., Banka, V. S., and Helfant, R. H.: Nuclear cardiology. II. The role of myocardial perfusion imaging using thallium-201 in diagnosis of coronary heart disease. Am. J. Cardiol. 45:674, 1980.

123. Bennett, K. R., Smith, R. O., Lehan, P. H., and Hellems, H. K.: Correlation of myocardial 42K uptake with coronary arteriography. Radiology 102:117, 1972.

124. Carr, E. A., Jr., Beierwaltes, W. H., Wegst, A. V., and Bartlett, J. D., Jr.: Myocardial scanning with rubidium-86. J. Nucl. Med. 3:76, 1962.

125. Carr, E. A., Jr., Walker, B. J., and Bartlett, J., Jr.: The diagnosis of myocardial infarcts by photoscanning after administration of cesium131. J. Clin. Invest. 42:922, 1963.

126. Hurley, P. J., Cooper, M., Reba, R. C., Poggenburg, K. J., and Wagner, H. N., Jr.: 143KCl: A new radiopharmaceutical for imaging the heart. J. Nucl. Med. 12:516, 1971.

127. Romhilt, D. W., Adolph, R. J., Sodd, V. C., Levenson, N. I., August, L. S., Nishiyama, H., and Berke, R. A.: Cesium-129 myocardial scintigraphy to detect myocardial infarction. Circulation 48:1242, 1973.

128. Martin, N. D., Zaret, B. L., McGowan, R. L., Wells, H. P., Jr., and Flamm, M. D.: Rubidium-81: A new myocardial scanning agent. Radiology. 111:651, 1974.

129. Lebowitz, E., Greene, M. W., Bradley-Moore, P., Atkins, H., Ansari, A., Richards, P., and Belgrave, E.: 201Tl for medical use. J. Nucl. Med. 14:421, 1973.

130. Gehring, P. J., and Hammond, P. B.: The interrelationship between thallium and potassium in animals. J. Pharmacol. Exp. Ther. 55:187, 1967.

131. Britten, J. S., and Blank, M.: Thallium activation of the (Na^+-K^+)-activated ATPase of rabbit kidney. Biochim. Biophys. Acta 159:160, 1968.

132. Strauss, H. W., Harrison, K., Langan, J. K., Lebowitz, E., and Pitt, B.: Thallium-201 for myocardial imaging. Relation of thallium-201 to regional myocardial perfusion. Circulation 51:641, 1975.

133. Zimmer, L., McCall, D., D'Addabbo, L., and Whitney, K.: Kinetics and characteristics of thallium exchange in cultured cells (abstr). Circulation 60 (Suppl.):II-138, 1979.

134. Deutsch, E., Bushong, W., Glavan, K. A., Elder, R. C., Sodd, V. J., Scholz, K. L., Fortman, D. L., and Lukes, S. J.: Heart imaging with cationic complexes of technetium. Science 214:85, 1981.

135. Budinger, T. F., Yano, Y., and Hoop, B.: A comparison of 82Rb+ and 13NH3 for myocardial positron scintigraphy. J. Nucl. Med. 16:429, 1975.

136. Yano, Y., and Anger, H. O.: Visualization of heart and kidneys in animals with ultrashort-lived 82Rb and the positron scintillation camera. J. Nucl. Med. 9:413, 1968.

137. Vokelman, J., Van Dyke, D., and Yano, Y.: Myocardial scanning with rubidium-82. Stokely Laboratory Reports. Berkeley, CA, University of California Press, 1972, p. 775.

138. Harper, P. V., Ryan, J. W., Al-Sadir, J., Chua, K. G., Resnekov, L., Neirinckx, R., Loberg, M., and the Los Alamos Medical Radioisotope Group: Intracoronary use of rubidium-82. J. Nucl. Med. 23:P69, 1982.

139. Walsh, W. F., Fill, H. R., and Harper, P. V.: Nitrogen-13–labeled ammonia for myocardial imaging. Semin. Nucl. Med. 7:59, 1977.

140. Sapirstein, L. A.: Fractionation of the cardiac output of rats with isotopic potassium. Circ. Res. 4:689, 1956.

141. Weich, H. F., Strauss, H. W., and Pitt, B.: The extraction of Tl-201 by the myocardium. Circulation 56:188, 1977.

142. Case, R. B.: Ion alterations during myocardial ischemia. Cardiology 56:245, 1971.

143. Parker, J. O., Chiong, M. A., West, R. O., and Case, R. B.: The effect of ischemia and alterations of heart rate on myocardial potassium balance in man. Circulation 42:205, 1970.

143a. Goldhaber, S. Z., Newell, J. B., Alpert, N. M., Andrews, E., Pohost, G. M., and Ingwall, J. S.: Effects of ischemic-like insult on myocardial thallium-201 accumulation. Circulation 67:778, 1983.

144. Levenson, N. I., Adolph, R. J., Romhilt, D. W., Gabel, M., Sodd, V. C., and August, L. S.: Effect of myocardial hypoxia and ischemia on myocardial scintigraphy. Am. J. Cardiol. 35:251, 1975.

145. Adolph, R., Romhilt, D., Nishiyama, H., Sodd, V., Blue, J., and Gabel, M.: Use of positive and negative imaging agents to visualize myocardial ischemia. Circulation 54(Suppl.):II-220, 1976.

146. McCall, D., Zimmer, L., D'Addabbo, L., and Whitney, K.: Modification of 204Tl uptake in cultured myocardial cells. Circulation 60:II-220, 1976.

147. Mueller, T. M., Marcus, M. L., Ehrhardt, J. C., Kerber, R. E., Brown, D. D., and Abboud, F. M.: Limitations of thallium-201 myocardial perfusion scintigrams. Circulation 54:640, 1976.

148. Nielson, A., Morris, K. G., Murdock, R. H., Bruno, F. P., and Cobb, F. R.: Linear relationship between distribution of thallium-201 and blood flow in ischemic and nonischemic myocardium during exercise. Circulation 60 (Suppl.):II-148, 1979.

149. Strauss, H. W., and Pitt, B.: Noninvasive detection of subcritical coronary arterial narrowings with a coronary vasodilator and myocardial perfusion imaging. Am. J. Cardiol. 39:403, 1977.

150. Gould, K. L.: Noninvasive assessment of coronary stenoses by myocardial perfusion imaging during pharmacologic coronary vasodilatation. I. Physiological basis and experimental validation. Am. J. Cardiol. 41:267, 1978.

151. Holman, B. L., Cohn, P. F., Adams, D. F., See, J. R., Roberts, B. H., Idoine, J., and Gorlin, R.: Regional myocardial blood flow during hyperemia induced by contrast agent in patients with coronary artery disease. Am. J. Cardiol. 38:416, 1976.

152. Zaret, B. L., Strauss, H. W., Martin, N. D., Wells, H. P., Jr., and Flamm, M. D., Jr.: Noninvasive regional myocardial perfusion with radioactive potassium. Study of patients at rest, with exercise, and during angina pectoris. N. Engl. J. Med. 288:809, 1973.

153. Schwartz, J. S., Ponto, R., Carlyle, P., Forstrom, L., and Cohn, J. N.: Early distribution of thallium-201 after temporary ischemia. Circulation 57:332, 1978.

154. Garcia, E., Maddahi, J., Berman, D., and Waxman, A: Space/time quantitation of thallium-201 myocardial scintigraphy. J. Nucl. Med. 22:309, 1981.

155. Grunwald, A., Watson, D., Holzgrefe, H., Irving, J., and Beller, G. A.: Myocardial thallium-201 kinetics in normal and ischemic myocardium. Circulation 64:610, 1981.

156. Okada, R., Jacobs, M., Daggett, W., Leppo, J., Strauss, H. W., Newell, J. B., Moore, R., Boucher, C. A., O'Keefe, D., and Pohost, G. M.: Thallium-201 kinetics in nonischemic canine myocardium. Circulation 65:70, 1982.

157. Berger, H. J., and Zaret, B. L.: Nuclear cardiology. N. Engl. J. Med. 305:799 and 855, 1981.

158. Jengo, J. A., Freeman, R., Brizendine, M., and Mena, I.: Detection of coronary artery disease: Comparison of exercise stress radionuclide angiocardiography and thallium stress perfusion scanning. Am. J. Cardiol. 45:535, 1980.

159. Pohost, G. M., Zir, L. M., Moore, R. H., McKusick, K. A., Guiney, T. E., and Beller, G. A.: Differentiation of transiently ischemic from infarcted myocardium by serial imaging after a single dose of thallium-201. Circulation 55:294, 1977.

160. Leppo, J., Rosenkrantz, J., Rosenthal, R., Bontemps, R., and Yipintsoi, T.: Quantitative thallium-201 redistribution with a fixed coronary stenosis in dogs. Circulation 63:632, 1981.

161. McLaughlin, P. R., Martin, R. P., Doherty, P., Daspit, S., Goris, M., Haskell, W., Lewis, S., Kriss, J. P., and Harrison, D. C.: Reproducibility of thallium-201 myocardial imaging. Circulation 55:497, 1977.

162. Johnstone, D. E., Wackers, F. J., Berger, H. J., Hoffer, P. B., Kelley, M. J., Gottschalk, A., and Zaret, B. L.: Effect of patient positioning on left lateral thallium-201 myocardial images. J. Nucl. Med. 20:183, 1979.

163. Francisco, D. A., Collins, S. M., Go, R. T., Ehrhardt, J. C., Van Kirk, O. C., and Marcus, M. L.: Tomographic thallium-201 myocardial perfusion scintigrams after maximal coronary artery vasodilation with intravenous dipyridamole. Circulation 66:370, 1982.

164. Heiss, H. W.: Coronary blood flow at rest and during exercise. In Rackman, H., and Hahn, C. H. (eds.): Ventricular Function at Rest and During Exercise. Berlin, Springer-Verlag, 1976, p. 17.

165. Albro, P. C., Gould, K. L., Westcott, R. J., Hamilton, G. W., Ritchie, J. L., and Williams, D. L.: Noninvasive assessment of coronary stenoses by myocardial imaging during pharmacologic coronary vasodilatation. III. Clinical trial. Am. J. Cardiol. 41:279, 1978.

166. Strauss, H. W., and Pitt, B.: Thallium-201 as a myocardial imaging agent. Semin. Nucl. Med. 7:49, 1977.

167. Wackers, F. J., Klay, J. W., Laks, H., Schnitzer, J., Zaret, B. L., and Geha, A. S.: Pathophysiological correlates of right ventricular thallium-201 uptake in a canine model. Circulation 64:1256, 1981.

168. Boucher, C. A., Zir, L. M., Beller, G. A., Okada, R. D., McKusick, K. A., Strauss, H. W., and Pohost, G. M.: Increased lung uptake of thallium-201 during exercise myocardial imaging: Hemodynamic and angiographic implications of patients with coronary artery disease. Am. J. Cardiol. 46:189, 1980.

169. Okada, R. D., Boucher, C. A., Kirshenbaum, H. D., Kushner, F. G., Strauss, H. W., and Pohost, G. M.: Thallium stress test: Improved diagnostic accuracy for an individual observer using criteria derived from interobserver analysis of variance (abstr). Clin. Res 27:191, 1979.

170. Goris, M. L., Daspit, S. G., McLaughlin, P., and Kriss, J. P.: Interpolative background subtraction. J. Nucl. Med. 17:744, 1976.

171. Narahara, K. A., Hamilton, G. W., Williams, D. L., and Gould, K. L.: Myocardial imaging with thallium-201: An experimental model for analysis of the true myocardial and background image components. J. Nucl. Med. 18:781, 1977.

172. Cantez, S., Harper, P. V., Atkins, F., Sbarboro, J., and Karunaratne, H.: Tomography in cardiac imaging. J. Nucl. Med. *18*:642, 1977.

173. Atwood, E., Jensen, D., Froelicher, V., Witztum, K., Gerber, K., Gilpin, E., and Ashburn, W.: Agreement in human interpretation of analog thallium myocardial perfusion images. Circulation *64*:601, 1981.

174. Meade, R. C., Bamrah, V. S., Horgan, J. D., Ruetz, P. P., Kronenwetter, C., and Yeh, E.: Quantitative methods in the evaluation of thallium-201 myocardial perfusion images. J. Nucl. Med. *19*:1175, 1978.

175. Koral, K. F., Rogers, W. L., and Knoll, G. F.: Digital tomographic imaging with time-modulated pseudorandom coded aperture and Anger camera. J. Nucl. Med. *16*:402, 1975.

176. Burow, R. D., Pond, M., Schafer, A. W., and Becker, L.: "Circumferential profiles:" A new method for computer analysis of thallium-201 myocardial perfusion images. J. Nucl. Med. *20*:771, 1979.

177. Vogel, R. A., Kirsh, D. L., LeFree, M. T., Rainwater, O. J., Jensen, D. P., and Steele, P. P.: Thallium-201 myocardial perfusion scintigraphy: Results of standard and multi-pinhole tomographic techniques. Am. J. Cardiol. *43*:787, 1979.

178. Berman, D., Staniloff, H., Freeman, M., Garcia, E., Pantaleo, N., Maddahi, J., Waxman, A., Forrester, J., and Swan, H. J. C.: Thallium-201 stress myocardial scintigraphy: Comparison of multiple pinhole tomography with planar imaging in the assessment of patients undergoing coronary arteriography. Am. J. Cardiol. *45*:481, 1980.

179. Green, A., Alderson, P., Berman, D., Caldwell, J., Thrall, J., and Vogel, R.: A multicenter comparison of standard and 7 pinhole tomographic myocardial perfusion imaging: ROC analysis of qualitative visual interpretation. J. Nucl. Med. *21*:P70, 1980.

180. Berman, D., Garcia, E., Maddahi, J., and Forrester, J.: Quantitative analysis of thallium-201 distribution and washout for comparison of multiple pinhole tomography with planar imaging. Circulation *62*:III-103, 1980.

181. Holman, B. L., Hill, T. C., Wynne, J., Lovett, R. D., Zimmerman, R. E., and Smith, E. M.: Single photon transaxial emission computed tomography of the heart in normal subjects and in patients with infarction. J. Nucl. Med. *20*:736, 1979.

182. Coleman, R. E., Jaszczak, R. J., and Cobb, F. R.: Comparison of 180° and 360° data collection in thallium-201 imaging using single-photon emission computerized tomography (SPECT): Concise communication. J. Nucl. Med. *23*:655, 1982.

183. Tamaki, N., Muaki, T., Ishii, Y., Fujita, T., Yamamoto, K., Minato, K., Yonekura, Y., Tamaki, S., Kambara, H., Kawai, C., and Torizuka, K.: Comparative study of thallium emission myocardial tomography with 180° and 360° data collection. J. Nucl. Med. *23*:661, 1982.

184. Ritchie, J. L., Olson, D. O., Williams, D. L., Harp, G., Caldwell, J. H., and Hamilton, G. W.: Transaxial computed tomography with ²⁰¹Tl in patients with prior myocardial infarction (abstr). J. Nucl. Med. *22*:P11, 1981.

185. Coleman, R. E., Cobb, F. R., and Jaszczak, R. J.: Thallium studies using single photon emission computed tomography (SPECT) (abstr). J. Nucl. Med. *22*:P11, 1981.

186. Borello, J. A., Clinthorne, N. H., Rogers, W. L., Thrall, J. H., and Keyes, J. W., Jr.: Oblique-angle tomography: A restructuring algorithm for transaxial tomographic data. J. Nucl. Med. *22*:471, 1981.

187. Besozzi, M. C., Rizi, H. R., Rogers, W. L., Clinthorne, N., Pitt, B., Thrall, J. H., and Keyes, J. W., Jr.: Rotating gamma camera ECT of Tl-201 in the human heart (abstr). J. Nucl. Med. *22*:P11, 1981.

188. Rizzi, R. H., Pasyk, S., Fiedler, V. H., Mori, K. W., Lucchesi, B., Pitt, B., and Keyes, J. W., Jr.: Tl-201 transaxial ECT: In vivo quantification of myocardial ischemia in dogs. J. Nucl. Med. *22*:P11, 1981.

189. Ritchie, J. L., Zaret, B. L., Strauss, H. W., Pitt, B., Berman, D. S., Schelbert, H. R., Ashburn, W. L., Berger, H. J., and Hamilton, G. W.: Myocardial imaging with thallium-201: A multicenter study in patients with angina pectoris or acute myocardial infarction. Am. J. Cardiol. *42*:345, 1978.

190. Verani, M. S., Marcus, M. L., Razzak, M. A., and Ehrhardt, J. C.: Sensitivity and specificity of thallium-201 perfusion scintigrams under exercise in the diagnosis of coronary artery disease. J. Nucl. Med. *19*:773, 1978.

191. Blood, D. K., McCarthy, D. M., Sciacca, R. R., and Cannon, P. J.: Comparison of single-dose and double-dose thallium-201 myocardial perfusion scintigraphy for the detection of coronary artery disease and prior myocardial infarction. Circulation *58*:777, 1978.

192. Ritchie, J. L., Trobaugh, G. B., Hamilton, G. W., Gould, K. L., Narahara, K. A., Murray, J. A., and Williams, D. L.: Myocardial imaging with thallium-201 at rest and during exercise: Comparison with coronary arteriography and resting and stress electrocardiography. Circulation *56*:66, 1977.

193. Botvinick, E. H., Taradash, M. R., Shames, D. M., and Parmley, W. W.: Thallium-201 myocardial perfusion scintigraphy for the clinical clarification of normal, abnormal and equivocal electrocardiographic stress tests. Am. J. Cardiol. *41*:43, 1978.

194. Bailey, I. K., Griffith, L. S. C., Rouleau, J., Strauss, H. W., and Pitt, W.: Thallium-201 myocardial perfusion imaging at rest and during exercise. Comparative sensitivity to electrocardiography in coronary artery disease. Circulation *55*:79, 1977.

195. McCarthy, D. M., Blood, D. K., Sciacca, R. R., and Cannon, P. J.: Single dose myocardial perfusion imaging with thallium-201: Application in patients with nondiagnostic electrocardiographic stress tests. Am. J. Cardiol. *43*:899, 1979.

196. Berger, B. C., Watson, D. D., Taylor, G. T., Craddock, G. B., Martin, R. P., and Beller, G. A.: Sensitivity of quantitative thallium-201 scintigraphy following nondiagnostic exercise stress. Circulation *60*:II-72, 1979.

197. Iskandrian, A. S., and Segal, B. I.: Value of exercise thallium-201 imaging in patients with diagnostic and nondiagnostic exercise electrocardiograms. Am. J. Cardiol. *48*:233, 1981.

198. Diamond, G. A., and Forrester, J. S.: Analysis of probability as an aid in the clinical diagnosis of coronary-artery disease. N. Engl. J. Med. *300*:1350, 1979.

199. Ritchie, J. L.: Myocardial perfusion imaging. Am. J. Cardiol. *49*:1341, 1982.

200. Caralis, D. G., Bailey, I., Kennedy, H. L., and Pitt, B.: Thallium-201 myocardial imaging in evaluation of asymptomatic individuals with ischaemic ST segment depression on exercise electrocardiogram. Br. Heart J. *42*:562, 1979.

201. Rigo, P., Bailey, I. K., Griffith, L. S. C., Pitt, B., Burow, R. D., Wagner, H. N., Jr., and Becker, L. C.: Value and limitations of segmental analysis of stress thallium myocardial imaging for localization of coronary artery disease. Circulation *61*:973, 1980.

202. Lenaers, A.: Thallium-201 myocardial perfusion scintigraphy during rest and exercise. Cardiovasc. Radiol. *2*:195, 1979.

203. Massie, B. M., Botvinick, E. H., and Brundage, B. H.: Correlation of thallium-201 scintigrams with coronary anatomy: Factors affecting region-by-region sensitivity. Am. J. Cardiol. *44*:616, 1979.

204. Dash, H., Massie, B. M., Botvinick, E. H., and Brundage, B. H.: The noninvasive identification of left main and three-vessel coronary artery disease by myocardial stress perfusion scintigraphy and treadmill exercise electrocardiography. Circulation *60*:276, 1979.

205. Beller, G. A., Watson, D. D., Berger, B. C., Martin, R. D., and Taylor, G. J.: Detection of multivessel disease by exercise thallium-201 scintigraphy. Am. J. Cardiol. *45*:482, 1980.

206. Garcia, E., Maddahi, J., Berman, D. S., Waxman, A., and Swan, H. J. C.: A comprehensive model for space-time quantitation of sequential thallium-201 myocardial scintigrams. Circulation *62* (Suppl):II-75, 1980.

207. Bodenheimer, M. M., Banka, V. S., Fooshee, C., Hermann, G. A., and Helfant, R. H.: Relationship between regional myocardial perfusion and the presence, severity and reversibility of asynergy in patients with coronary heart disease. Circulation *58*:789, 1978.

208. Rozanski, A., Berman, D., Gray, R., Levy, R., Raymond, M., Maddahi, J., Pantaleo, N., Waxman, A. D., Swan, H. J. C., and Matloff, G.: Use of thallium-201 redistribution scintigraphy in the preoperative differentiation of reversible and nonreversible myocardial asynergy. Circulation *64*:936, 1981.

209. Greenberg, B. H., Hart, R., Botvinick, E. H., Werner, J. A., Brundage, D. M., Shames, D. M., Chatterjee, K., and Parmley, W. W.: Thallium-201 myocardial perfusion scintigraphy to evaluate patients after coronary bypass surgery. Am. J. Cardiol. *42*:167, 1978.

210. Rehn, T., Griffith, L., Achuff, S., Pond, M., and Becker, L.: Value and limitations of thallium-201 imaging to detect bypass graft patency. Am. J. Cardiol. *43*:434, 1979.

211. Pohost, G. M., Boucher, C. A., Zir, L. M., McKusick, K. A., Beller, G. A., and Strauss, H. W.: The thallium stress test: The quantitative approach revisited. Circulation *60*:II-149, 1979.

212. Ahmad, M., Merry, S. L., and Harbach, H.: Thallium-201 scintigraphic evidence of ischemia in patients with myocardial bridges. Am. J. Cardiol. *45*:482, 1980.

213. Losse, B., Kuhn, H., Kronert, H., Rafflenbeal, D., Fernendegen, L. E., and Loogen, F.: Exercise thallium-201 myocardial perfusion imaging in patients with normal coronary angiogram and ventriculogram. Circulation *60*:II-148, 1979.

214. Bailey, I. K., Come, P. C., Kelly, D. T., Burow, R. D., Griffith, L. S. C., Strauss, H. W., and Pitt, B.: Thallium-201 myocardial perfusion imaging in aortic valve stenosis. Am. J. Cardiol. *40*:889, 1977.

215. Keyes, J. W., Orlandea, N., Heetderks, W. J., Leonard, P. F., and Rogers, W. L.: The humongotron—a scintillation camera transaxial tomograph. J. Nucl. Med. *18*:381, 1977.

216. Gaffney, F. A., Wohl, A. J., Blomqvist, C. G., Parkey, R. W., and Willerson, J. T.: Thallium-201 myocardial perfusion studies in patients with mitral valve prolapse syndrome. Am. J. Med. *64*:21, 1978.

217. Klein, G. J., Kostuk, W. J., Boughner, D. R., and Chamberlain, M. J.: Stress myocardial imaging in mitral leaflet prolapse syndrome. Am. J. Cardiol. *42*:746, 1978.

218. Massie, B., Botvinick, E. H., Shames, D., Taradash, M., Werner, J., and Schiller, N.: Myocardial perfusion scintigraphy in patients with mitral valve prolapse. Circulation *57*:19, 1978.

219. Maseri, A., Parodi, O., Severi, S., and Pesola, A.: Transient transmural reduction of myocardial blood flow, demonstrated by thallium-201 scintigraphy, as a cause of variant angina. Circulation *54*:280, 1976.

220. Ricci, D. R., Orlick, A. E., Doherty, P. W., Cipriano, P. R., and Harrison, D. C.: Reduction of coronary blood flow during coronary artery spasm occurring spontaneously and after provocation by ergonovine maleate. Circulation *57*:392, 1978.

221. Waters, D. D., Chaitman, B. R., Dupras, G., Theroux, P., and Mizgala, M. D.: Coronary artery spasm during exercise in patients with variant angina. Circulation *59*:580, 1979.

222. Bulkley, B. H., Rouleau, J., Strauss, W., and Pitt, B.: Idiopathic hypertrophic subaortic stenosis: Detection by thallium-201 myocardial perfusion imaging. N. Engl. J. Med. *293*:1113, 1975.

223. Bulkley, B. H., Rouleau, J. R., Whitaker, J. Q., Strauss, H. W., and Pitt, B.: The use of ²⁰¹thallium for myocardial perfusion imaging in sarcoid heart disease. Chest *72*:27, 1977.

224. Bulkley, B. H., Hutchins, G. M., Bailey, I., Strauss, H. W., and Pitt, B.: Thallium-201 imaging and gated cardiac blood pool scans in patients with ischemic and idiopathic congestive cardiomyopathy: A clinical and pathologic study. Circulation *55*:753, 1977.

225. Pohost, G. M., Boucher, C. A., Zir, L. M., McKusick, K. A., Beller, G. A., and Strauss, H. W.: The thallium stress test: The qualitative approach revisited. Circulation 60(Suppl.):II-49, 1979.

226. Wackers, F. J. T., Sokole, E. B., Samson, G., van der Schoot, J. B., Lie, K. I., Liem, K. L., and Wellens, H. J. J.: Value and limitations of thallium-201 scintigraphy in the acute phase of myocardial infarction. N. Engl. J. Med. 295:1, 1976.

227. Wackers, F. J. T., Lie, K. I., Liem, K. L., Sokole, E. B., Samson, G., van der Schoot, J. B., and Durrer, D.: Thallium-201 scintigraphy in unstable angina pectoris. Circulation 57:738, 1978.

228. DiCola, V. C., Downing, S. F., Donabedian, R. K., and Zaret, B. L.: Pathophysiological correlates of thallium-201 myocardial uptake in experimental infarction. Cardiovasc. Res. 11:141, 1977.

229. Henning, H., Schelbert, H. R., Righetti, A., Ashburn, W. L., and O'Rourke, R. A.: Dual myocardial imaging with technetium-99m pyrophosphate and thallium-201 for detecting, localizing and sizing acute myocardial infarction. Am. J. Cardiol. 40:147, 1977.

230. Mueller, H. S., Fletcher, J. W., and Ayres, S. M.: 201-Thallium image and creatine kinase MB infarct size—evaluation of variable treatment responses (abstr). Circulation 60:II-163, 1979.

231. Buja, L. M., Parkey, R. W., Stokely, E. M., Bonte, F. J., and Willerson, J. T.: Pathophysiology of technetium-99m stannous pyrophosphate and thallium-201 scintigraphy of acute anterior myocardial infarct in dogs. J. Clin. Invest. 57:1508, 1976.

232. Wackers, F. J., Becker, A. E., Samson, G., Sokole, E. B., van der Schoot, J. B., Vet, A. J. T. M., Lie, K. I., Durrer, D., and Wellens, H.: Location and size of acute transmural myocardial infarction estimated from thallium-201 scintiscans: A clinicopathological study. Circulation 56:72, 1977.

233. Smitherman, T. C., Osborn, R. C., and Narahara, K. A.: Serial myocardial scintigraphy after a single dose of thallium-201 in men after acute myocardial infarction. Am. J. Cardiol. 42:177, 1978.

234. Silverman, K. J., Becker, L. C., Bulkley, B. H., Burow, R. D., Mellits, E. D., Kallman, C. H. and Weisfeldt, M. L.: Value of early thallium-201 scintigraphy for predicting mortality in patients with acute myocardial infarction. Circulation 61:996, 1980.

235. Markis, J. E., Malagold, M., Parker, J. A., Silverman, K. F., Barry, W. H., Als, A. V., Paulin, J. S., Grossman, W., and Braunwald, E.: Myocardial salvage after intracoronary thrombolysis with streptokinase in acute myocardial infarction: Assessment of intracoronary thallium-201. N. Engl. J. Med. 305:777, 1981.

236. Maddahi, J., Ganz, W., Ninomiya, K., Hashida, J., Fishbein, M. C., Mondkar, A., Buchbinder, N., Marcus, H., Geft, I., Shah, P. S., Rozanski, A., Swan, H. J. C., and Berman, D. S.: Myocardial salvage by intracoronary thrombolysis in evolving acute myocardial infarction: Evaluation using intracoronary injection of thallium-201. Am. Heart J. 102:664, 1981.

237. Ashburn, W. L., Braunwald, E., Simon, A. L., Peterson, K. L., and Gault, J. H.: Myocardial perfusion imaging with radioactive-labeled particles injected directly into the coronary circulation of patients with coronary artery disease. Circulation 44:851, 1971.

238. Jansen, C., Judkins, M. P., Grames, G. M., Gander, M., and Adams, R.: Myocardial perfusion color scintigraphy with MAA. Radiology 109:369, 1973.

239. MacIntyre, W. J., Cannon, P. J., and Ashburn, W. L.: Measurements of regional myocardial perfusion. In Pierson, R. N., Jr., Kriss, J. P., Jones, R. H., and MacIntyre, W. J. (eds.): Quantitative Nuclear Cardiography. New York, John Wiley and Sons, 1975, p. 155.

240. Ritchie, J. L., Hamilton, G. W., Gould, K. L., Allen, D., Kennedy, J. W., and Hammermeister, K. E.: Myocardial imaging with indium-113m-and technetium-99m-macroaggregated albumin: New procedure for identification of stress-induced regional ischemia. Am. J. Cardiol. 35:380, 1975.

241. Idoine, J. D., Holman, B. L., Jones, A. G., Schneider, R. J., Schroeder, K. L., and Zimmerman, R. E.: Quantification of flow in a dynamic phantom using 81Rb-81mKr and a sodium iodide detector. J. Nucl. Med. 18:570, 1977.

242. Yipintsoi, T., Knapp, T. J., and Bassingthwaighte, J. B.: Countercurrent exchange of labelled water in canine myocardium. Fed. Proc. 28:645, 1969.

243. Yipintsoi, T., and Bassingthwaighte, J. B.: Circulatory transport of iodoantipyrine and water in the isolated dog heart. Circ. Res. 27:461, 1970.

244. Ter-Pogossian, M. M., Koehler, P. R., and Potchen, E. J.: In vivo autoradiography of xenon-133 distribution in the cystic human kidney. Radiology 91:358, 1968.

245. Bassingthwaighte, J. B., Strandell, T., and Donald, D. E.: Estimation of coronary blood flow by washout of diffusible indicators. Circ. Res. 23:259, 1968.

246. Shaw, D. J., Pitt, A., and Friesinger, G. C.: Autoradiographic study of the 133xenon disappearance method for measurement of myocardial blood flow. Cardiovasc. Res. 6:268, 1972.

247. Cannon, P. J., Weiss, M. B., and Casarella, W. J.: Studies of regional myocardial blood flow: Results in patients with left anterior descending coronary artery disease. Semin. Nucl. Med. 6:279, 1976.

248. Holman, B. L., Adams, D. F., Jewitt, D., Eldh, P., Idoine, J., Cohn, P. F., Gorlin, R., and Adelstein, S. J.: Measuring regional myocardial blood flow with 133Xe and the Anger camera. Radiology 112:99, 1974.

249. Cannon, P. J., Dell, R. B., and Dwyer, E. M., Jr.: Measurement of regional myocardial perfusion in man with 133xenon and a scintillation camera. J. Clin. Invest. 51:964, 1972.

250. Cannon, P. J., Dell, R. B., and Dwyer, E. M., Jr.: Regional myocardial perfusion rates in patients with coronary artery disease. J. Clin. Invest. 51:978, 1972.

251. Cohn, P. F., Maddox, D., Holman, B. L., Markis, J. E., Adams, D. F., and

See, J. R.: Effect of sublingually administered nitroglycerin on regional myocardial blood flow in patients with coronary artery disease. Am. J. Cardiol. 39:672, 1977.

252. Mann, T., Cohn, P. F., Holman, B. L., Green, L. H., Markis, J. E., and Philips, D. A.: Effect of nitroprusside on regional myocardial blood flow in coronary artery disease. Results in 25 patients and comparison with nitroglycerin. Circulation 57:732, 1978.

253. Phelps, M. E., Hoffman, E. J., Huang, S. C., and Kuhl, D. E.: ECAT: A new computerized tomographic imaging system for positron-emitting radiopharmaceuticals. J. Nucl. Med. 19:635, 1978.

254. Ter-Pogossian, M. M., Klein, M. S., Markham, J., Roberts, R., and Sobel, B. E.: Regional assessment of myocardial metabolic integrity in vivo by positron-emission tomography with 11C-labeled palmitate. Circulation 61:242, 1980.

254a. Marshall, R. C., Tillisch, J. H., Phelps, M. E., Huang, S-C., Carson, R., Henze, E., and Schelbert, H. R.: Identification and differentiation of resting myocardial ischemia and infarction in man with positron computed tomography, 18F-labeled fluorodeoxyglucose and N-13 ammonia. Circulation 67:766, 1983.

255. Phelps, M. E., Hoffman, E. J., Selin, C., Huang, S. C., Robinson, G., MacDonald, O., Schelbert, H., and Kuhl, D. E.: Investigation of [18F]2-fluoro-2-deoxyglucose for the measure of myocardial glucose metabolism. J. Nucl. Med. 19:1311, 1978.

256. Ratib, O., Phelps, M. E., Huang, S. C., Henze, E., Selin, C., and Schelbert, H. R.: Determination of myocardial metabolic rate (MRGlc) by positron computed tomography (PCT) and fluoro-18 deoxyglucose (FDG) (abstr). J. Nucl. Med. 22:P11, 1981.

257. Huang, S. C., Phelps, M. E., Hoffman, E. J., Sideris, K., Selin, C. J., and Kuhl, D. E.: Noninvasive determination of local cerebral metabolic rate of glucose in man. Am. J. Physiol. 238:E69, 1980.

258. Phelps, M. E., Huang, S. C., Hoffman, E. J., Selin, C., Sokoloff, L., and Kuhl, D. E.: Tomographic measurement of local cerebral glucose metabolic rate in man with (F-18)2-fluoro-2-deoxy-D-glucose: Validation of method. Ann. Neurol. 6:371, 1979.

259. Opie, L. H., Owen, P., and Riemersma, R. A.: Relative rates of oxidation of glucose and free fatty acids by ischemic and nonischemic myocardium after coronary ligation in the dog. Eur. J. Clin. Invest. 3:419, 1973.

260. Neely, J. R., Rovetto, M. J., and Oram, J. F.: Myocardial utilization of carbohydrate and lipids. Progr. Cardiovasc. Dis. 15:289, 1972.

261. Neely, J. R., and Morgan, H. E.: Relationship between carbohydrates and lipid metabolism and the energy balance of heart muscle. Ann. Rev. Physiol. 36:413, 1974.

262. Schelbert, H. R.: The heart. In Ell, P. J., and Holman, B. L. (eds.): Computed Emission Tomography. Oxford, Oxford University Press, 1982, p. 91.

263. Henze, E., Perloff, J. K., and Schelbert, H. R.: Alterations of regional myocardial perfusion and metabolism in Duchenne's muscular dystrophy detection by positron computed tomography (abstr). Circulation 64:IV-279, 1981.

263a. Geltman, E. M., Smith, J. J., Beecher, D., Ludbrook, P. A., Ter-Pogossian, M. M., and Sobel, B. E.: Altered regional myocardial metabolism in congestive cardiomyopathy detected by positron tomography. Am. J. Med. 74:773, 1983.

264. Schelbert, H. R., Henze, E., Huang, S. C., and Phelps, M. E.: Relationship between myocardial blood flow and uptake and utilization of free fatty acids (abstr). J. Nucl. Med. 22:P10, 1981.

265. Schön, H., Robinson, G., Barrio, J., Phelps, M., and Schelbert, H.: Extraction and clearance of C-11 palmitate in normal myocardium. Circulation 62:III-103, 1980.

266. Schön, H. R., Robinson, G., Schelbert, H. R., and Barrio, J. R.: Kinetics of C-11-labeled palmitate in ischemic myocardium (abstr). Am. J. Cardiol. 47:414, 1981.

267. Hillis, L. D., and Braunwald, E.: Myocardial ischemia. N. Engl. J. Med. 296:971, 1034, and 1093, 1977.

268. Klein, M. S., Goldstein, R. A., Welch, M. J., and Sobel, B. E.: External assessment of myocardial metabolism with [11C]palmitate in rabbit hearts. Am. J. Physiol. 237:H51, 1979.

269. Goldstein, R. A., Klein, M. S., Welch, M. J., and Sobel, B. E.: External assessment of myocardial metabolism with C-11 palmitate in vivo. J. Nucl. Med. 21:342, 1980.

270. Goldstein, R. A., Klein, M. S., and Sobel, B. E.: Detection of myocardial ischemia before infarction, based on accumulation of labeled pyruvate. J. Nucl. Med. 21:1101, 1980.

271. Poe, N. D., Robinson, G. D., Jr., and MacDonald, N. S.: Myocardial extraction of labeled long-chain fatty acid analogs. Proc. Soc. Exp. Biol. Med. 148:215, 1975.

272. Reske, S. N., Machulla, H.-J., Biersack, H. J., Lackner, K., Knopp, R., and Winkler, C.: Nicht-invasive Erfassung des regionalen myocardialen Stoffwechsels von J-123-para-Phenylpentadecansäure durch single photon tomography. Nucklearmedizin 19:558, 1982.

273. Chanussot, F., and Debry, G.: Incorporation d'acid heptadécanoïque dans les lipides hépatiques du rat Wistar. J. Physiol. (Paris) 76:831, 1980.

274. Knust, E. J., Kupfernagel, C. H., and Stocklin, G.: Long-chain F-18 fatty acids for the study of regional metabolism in heart and liver: Odd-even effects of metabolism in mice. J. Nucl. Med. 20:1170, 1979.

275. van der Wall, E. E., Westera, G., den Hollander, W., and Visser, F. C.: External detection of regional myocardial metabolism with radioiodinated hexadecanoic acid in the dog heart. Eur. J. Nucl. Med. 6:147, 1981.

276. van der Wall, E. E., Heidendal, G. A. K., den Hollander, W., Westera, G., and Roos, J. P.: Metabolic myocardial imaging with I-123 labeled heptadecanoic acid in patients with stable angina pectoris. Eur. J. Nucl. Med. 6:391, 1981.

277. Okada, R. D., Strauss, H. W., Elmaleh, D., Yasuda, T., Werre, G., and Boucher, C. A.: Myocardial kinetics of I-123 labeled-16-hexadecanoic acid (abstr). Circulation 64:IV-235, 1981.

278. van der Wall, E. E., den Hollander, W., Heidendal, G. A. K., Westera, G., Majid, P. A., and Roos, J. P.: Dynamic myocardial scintigraphy with ^{123}I-labeled free fatty acids in patients with myocardial infarction. Eur. J. Nucl. Med. 6:383, 1981.

INFARCT-AVID MYOCARDIAL SCINTIGRAPHY

279. Holman, B. L., Tanaka, T. T., and Lesch, M.: Evaluation of radiopharmaceuticals for the detection of acute myocardial infarction in man. Radiology 121: 427, 1976.

280. Bonte, F. J., Parkey, R. W., Graham, K. D., Moore, J., and Stokely, E. M.: A new method for radionuclide imaging of myocardial infarcts. Radiology 110: 473, 1974.

281. Parkey, R. W., Bonte, F. J., Meyer, S. L., Atkins, J. M., Curry, G. L., Stokely, E. M., and Willerson, J. T.: A new method for radionuclide imaging of acute myocardial infarction in humans. Circulation 50:540, 1974.

282. Zaret, B. L., DiCola, V. C., Donabedian, R. K., Puri, S., Wolfson, S., Freedman, G. S., and Cohen, L. S.: Dual radionuclide study of myocardial infarction. Relationships between myocardial uptake of potassium-43, technetium-99m stannous pyrophosphate, regional myocardial blood flow and creatine phosphokinase depletion. Circulation 53:422, 1976.

283. Schelbert, H. R., Wisenberg, G., and Henze, E.: Imaging with infarct avid agents. CRC Crit. Rev. Diagn. Imaging 16:239, 1981.

284. Jennings, R. B., Herson, P. B., and Sommers, H. M.: Structural and functional abnormalities in mitochondria isolated from ischemic dog myocardium. Lab. Invest. 20:548, 1969.

285. Shen, A. C., and Jennings, R. B.: Myocardial calcium and magnesium in acute ischemic injury. Am. J. Pathol. 67:417, 1972.

286. Sommers, H. M., and Jennings, R. B.: Experimental acute myocardial infarction: Histologic and histochemical studies of early myocardial infarct induced by temporary or permanent occlusion of a coronary artery. Lab. Invest. 13: 1491, 1964.

287. D'Agostino, A. N., and Chiga, M.: Mitochondrial mineralization in human myocardium. Am. J. Clin. Pathol. 53:820, 1970.

288. Buja, L. M., Tofe, A. J., Mukherjee, A., Parkey, R. W., Bonte, F. J., and Willerson, J. T.: Role of elevated tissue calcium in myocardial infarct scintigraphy with technetium phosphorous radiopharmaceuticals. Circulation 54:II-219, 1976.

289. Buja, L. M., Parkey, R. W., Stokely, E. M., Bonte, F. J., and Willerson, J. T.: Pathophysiology of technetium-99m stannous pyrophosphate and thallium-201 scintigraphy of acute anterior myocardial infarcts in dogs. J. Clin. Invest. 57: 1508, 1976.

290. Dewanjee, M. K.: Localization of skeletal-imaging ^{99m}Tc chelates in dead cells in tissue culture: Concise communication. J. Nucl. Med. 17:993, 1976.

291. Schelbert, H., Ingwall, J., Sybers, H., and Ashburn, W.: Uptake of Tc-99m pyrophosphate and calcium in irreversibly damaged myocardium. J. Nucl. Med. 17:534, 1976.

292. Holman, B. L., Ehrie, M., and Lesch, M.: Correlation of acute myocardial infarct scintigraphy with postmortem studies. Am. J. Cardiol. 37:311, 1976.

293. Buja, L. M., Poliner, L. R., Parkey, R. W., Pulido, J. I., Hutcheson, D., Platt, M. R., Mills, L. J., Bonte, F. J., and Willerson, J. T.: Clinicopathologic study of persistently positive technetium-99m stannous pyrophosphate myocardial scintigrams and myocytolytic degeneration after myocardial infarction. Circulation 56:1016, 1977.

294. Holman, B. L., Lesch, M., and Alpert, J. S.: Myocardial scintigraphy with technetium-99m pyrophosphate during the early phase of acute infarction. Am. J. Cardiol. 41:39, 1978.

295. Olson, H. G., Lyons, K. P., Aronow, W. S., Brown, W. T., and Greenfield, R. S.: Follow-up technetium-99m stannous pyrophosphate myocardial scintigrams after acute myocardial infarction. Circulation 56:181, 1977.

296. Holman, B. L., Dewanjee, M. K., Idoine, J., Fliegel, C. P., Davis, M. A., Treves, S., and Eldh, P.: Detection and localization of experimental myocardial infarction with ^{99m}Tc-tetracycline. J. Nucl. Med. 14:595, 1973.

297. Holman, B. L., Lesch, M., Zweiman, F. G., Temte, J., Lown, B., and Gorlin, R.: Detection and sizing of acute myocardial infarcts with ^{99m}Tc(Sn)tetracycline. N. Engl. J. Med. 291:159, 1974.

298. Holman, B. L., and Zweiman, F. G.: Time course of ^{99m}Tc(Sn)-tetracycline uptake in experimental acute myocardial infarction. J. Nucl. Med. 16:1144, 1975.

299. Rossman, D. J., Strauss, H. W., Siegel, M. E., and Pitt, B.: Accumulation of ^{99m}Tc-glucoheptonate in acutely infarcted myocardium. J. Nucl. Med. 16:875, 1975.

300. Jacobstein, J. G., Alonso, D. R., Roberts, A. J., Cipriano, P. R., Combes, J. R., and Post, M. R.: Early diagnosis of myocardial infarction in the dog with ^{99m}Tc-glucoheptonate. J. Nucl. Med. 18:413, 1977.

301. Davis, M. A., Holman, B. L., and Carmel, A. N.: Evaluation of radiopharmaceuticals sequestered by acutely damaged myocardium. J. Nucl. Med. 17:911, 1976.

302. Kung, H. F., Ackerhalt, R., and Blau, M.: Uptake of Tc-99m monophosphate complexes in bone and myocardial necrosis in animals. J. Nucl. Med. 19:1027, 1978.

303. Pereira-Prestes, A. V., Donaldson, R. M., Ell, P. J., Brown, N. J. G., Jarritt, P. H., Al-Baghdadi, T., and Elliott, A. T.: Mobile gamma cameras and ^{99m}Tc-labeled phosphates in acute myocardial infarction. Nuklearmedizin 18:73, 1979.

304. Khaw, B. A., Gold, H. K., Leinback, R. C., Fallon, J. T., Strauss, W., Pohost, G. M., and Haber, E.: Early imaging of experimental myocardial infarction by intracoronary administration of ^{131}I-labeled anticardiac myosin (Fab')$_2$ fragments. Circulation 58:1137, 1978.

305. Khaw, B. A., Beller, G. A., and Haber, E.: Experimental myocardial infarct imaging following intravenous administration of iodine-131 labeled antibody (Fab')$_2$ fragments specific for cardiac myosin. Circulation 57:743, 1978.

306. Riba, A. L., Thakur, M. L., Gottschalk, A., and Zaret, B. L.: Imaging experimental coronary artery thrombosis with indium-111 platelets. Circulation 60: 767, 1979.

307. Riba, A. L., Thakur, M. L., Gottschalk, A., Andriole, V. T., and Zaret, B. L.: Imaging experimental infective endocarditis with indium-111–labeled blood cellular components. Circulation 59:336, 1979.

308. Holman, B. L., and Wynne, J.: Infarct avid (hot spot) myocardial scintigraphy. Radiol. Clin. North Am. 18:487, 1980.

309. Berman, D. S., Amsterdam, E. A., Hines, H. H., Denaro, G. L., Salel, A. F., Ikeda, R., Jansholt, H. A., and Mason, D. T.: Problem of diffuse cardiac uptake of technetium-99m pyrophosphate in the diagnosis of acute myocardial infarction: Enhanced scintigraphy accuracy by computerized selective blood pool subtraction. Am. J. Cardiol. 40:768, 1977.

310. Cowley, M. J., Mantle, J. A., Rogers, W. J., Russell, R. O., Jr., Rackley, C. E., and Logic, J. R.: Technetium-99m stannous pyrophosphate myocardial scintigraphy. Reliability and limitations in assessment of acute myocardial infarction. Circulation 56:192, 1977.

311. Berman, D. S., Amsterdam, E. A., Hines, H. H., Salel, A. F., Bailey, G. J., DeNardo, G. L., and Mason, D. T.: New approach to interpretation of technetium-99m pyrophosphate scintigraphy in detection of acute myocardial infarction. Am. J. Cardiol. 39:341, 1977.

312. Bloor, C. M.: Functional significance of the coronary collateral circulation: A review. Am. J. Pathol. 76:562, 1974.

313. Jengo, J. A., Mena, I., Joe, S. H., and Criley, J. M.: The significance of calcific valvular heart disease in Tc-99m pyrophosphate myocardial infarction scanning: Radiographic, scintigraphic, and pathological correlation. J. Nucl. Med. 18:776, 1977.

314. Pugh, B. R., Buja, L. M., Parkey, R. W., Poliner, L. R., Stokely, E. M., Bonte, F. J., and Willerson, J. T.: Cardioversion and "false positive" technetium-99m stannous pyrophosphate myocardial scintigrams. Circulation 54:399, 1976.

315. Ahmad, M., Dubiel, J., Verdon, T. A., and Martin, R. H.: Technetium-99m stannous pyrophosphate myocardial imaging in patients with suspected myocardial infarction. Am. J. Cardiol. 37:168a, 1975.

316. Go, R. T., Chiu, C. L., Doty, D. B., Cheng, H. F., and Christie, J. H.: Radionuclide imaging of experimental myocardial contusion. J. Nucl. Med. 15:1174, 1974.

317. Davison, R., Spies, S. M., Przybylek, J., Hai, H., and Lesch, M.: Technetium-99m stannous pyrophosphate myocardial scintigraphy after cardiopulmonary resuscitation and cardioversion. Circulation 60:292, 1979.

318. Fleg, J. L., Siegel, B. A., Williamson, J. R., and Roberts, R.: ^{99m}Tc-pyrophosphate imaging in acute pericarditis: A clinical and experimental study. Radiology 126:727, 1978.

319. Janowitz, W. R., and Serafini, A. N.: Intense myocardial uptake of ^{99m}Tc-diphosphonate in a uremic patient with secondary hyperparathyroidism and pericarditis: Case report. J. Nucl. Med. 17:896, 1976.

320. Perez, L. A., Haty, D. B., and Freeman, L. M.: Localization of myocardial disorders other than infarction with ^{99m}Tc-labeled phosphate agents. J. Nucl. Med. 17:241, 1976.

321. Walsh, W., Lessem, J., Fill, H., and Harper, P. V.: Value of ^{99m}Tc-pyrophosphate myocardial scintigraphy in patients with left myocardial infarction. Am. J. Cardiol. 37:180, 1976.

322. Prasquier, R., Taradash, M. R., Botvinick, E. H., Shames, D. M., and Parmley, W. W.: The specificity of the diffuse pattern of cardiac uptake in myocardial infarction imaging with technetium-99m stannous pyrophosphate. Circulation 55:61, 1977.

323. Kadota, K., Matsumori, A., Kambara, H., and Kawai, C.: Myocardial uptake of technetium-99m stannous pyrophosphate in experimental viral myopericarditis. J. Nucl. Med. 20:1047, 1979.

324. Braun, S. D., Lisbona, R., Novales-Diaz, J. A., and Sniderman, A.: Myocardial uptake of ^{99m}Tc-phosphate tracer in amyloidosis. Clin. Nucl. Med. 4:244, 1979.

325. Poliner, L. R., Buja, L. M., Parkey, R. W., Bonte, F. J., and Willerson, J. T.: Clinicopathologic findings in 52 patients studied by technetium-99m stannous pyrophosphate myocardial scintigraphy. Circulation 59:257, 1979.

326. Jaffe, A. S., Klein, M. S., Patel, B. R., Siegel, B. A., and Roberts, R.: Abnornmal technetium-99m pyrophosphate images in unstable angina: Ischemia versus infarction? Am. J. Cardiol. 44:1035, 1979.

327. Holman, B. L., Chisholm, R. J., and Braunwald, E.: The prognostic implications of acute myocardial infarct scintigraphy with ^{99m}Tc-pyrophosphate. Circulation 57:320, 1978.

328. Malin, F. R., Rollo, D., and Gertz, E. W.: Sequential myocardial scintigraphy with technetium-99m stannous pyrophosphate following myocardial infarction. J. Nucl. Med. 19:1111, 1978.

329. Massie, B. M., Botvinick, E. H., Werner, J. A., Chatterjee, K., and Parmley, W. W.: Myocardial scintigraphy with technetium-99m stannous pyrophos-

phate: An insensitive test for nontransmural myocardial infarction. Am. J. Cardiol. *43*:186, 1979.

330. Sharpe, D. N., Botvinick, E. H., Shames, D. M., Schiller, N. B., Massie, B. M., Chatterjee, K., and Parmley, W. W.: The noninvasive diagnosis of right ventricular infarction. Circulation *57*:483, 1978.

331. Dailey, P. O., Ashburn, W., and Ross, J., Jr.: Usefulness of preoperative and postoperative Tc-99m(Sn) pyrophosphate scans in patients with ischemic and valvular heart disease. Am. J. Cardiol. *39*:43, 1977.

332. Burdine, J. A., DePuey, E. G., Orzan, F., Mathur, V. S., and Hall, R. J.: Scintigraphic, electrocardiographic, and enzymatic diagnosis of perioperative myocardial infarction in patients undergoing myocardial revascularization. J. Nucl. Med. *20*:711, 1979.

333. Platt, M. R., Parkey, R. W., Willerson, J. T., Bonte, F. J., Shapiro, W., and Sugg, W. L.: Technetium stannous pyrophosphate myocardial scintigrams in the recognition of myocardial infarction in patients undergoing coronary artery revascularization. Ann. Thorac. Surg. *21*:311, 1976.

334. Hung, J., Kelly, D. T., McLaughlin, A. F., Uren, R. F., and Baird, D. K.: Preoperative and postoperative technetium-99m pyrophosphate myocardial scintigraphy in the assessment of operative infarction in coronary artery surgery. J. Thorac. Cardiovasc. Surg. *78*:68, 1979.

335. Siegel, A. J., Silverman, L. M., and Holman, B. L.: Elevated creatine kinase MB isoenzyme levels in marathon runners. J.A.M.A. *246*:2049, 1981.

336. Rude, R. E., Parkey, R. W., Bonte, F. J., Lewis, S. E., Twieg, D., Buja, L. M., and Willerson, J. T.: Clinical implications of the technetium-99m stannous pyrophosphate myocardial scintigraphy "doughnut" pattern in patients with acute myocardial infarcts. Circulation *59*:721, 1979.

337. Ahmad, M., Logan, K. W., and Martin, R. H.: Doughnut pattern of technetium-99m pyrophosphate myocardial uptake in patients with acute myocardial infarction: A sign of poor long-term prognosis. Am. J. Cardiol. *44*:13, 1979.

338. Aldor, E., Heeger, H., Kahn, P., and Kainz, W.: Long-time follow-up scintigraphy with ^{99m}Tc-pyrophosphate after myocardial infarction. Z. Kardiol. *68*:461, 1979.

339. Keyes, J. W., Leonard, P. F., Brody, S. L., Svetkoff, D. J., Rogers, W. L., and Lucchesi, B. R.: Myocardial infarct quantification in the dog by single photon emission computed tomography. Circulation *58*:227, 1978.

340. Holman, B. L., Goldhaber, S. Z., Kirsch, C., Polak, J. F., Friedman, B. J., English, R. J., and Wynne, J.: Measurement of infarct size using single photon emission computed tomography and technetium-99m pyrophosphate: A description of the method and comparison with patient prognosis. Am. J. Cardiol. *50*:503, 1982.

PULMONARY SCINTIGRAPHY

341. Sapirstein, L. A., and Moses, L. E.: Cerebral and cephalic blood flow in man; basic considerations of the indicator fractionation technique in dynamic clinical studies with isotopes. *In* Proceedings of Symposium held at Oak Ridge Institute of Nuclear Studies, Oct. 21–25, 1963.

342. Davis, M. A., and Holman, B. L.: Radiopharmaceuticals for perfusion scanning. *In* Holman, B. L., and Lindeman, J. F. (eds.): Progress in Nuclear Medicine, Vol. 3. Regional Pulmonary Function in Health and Disease. Basel, S. Karger, 1973, p. 10.

343. Wagner, H. N., Hosain, T., and Rhodes, B. A.: Recently developed radiopharmaceuticals: Ytterbium-169 DTPA and technetium-99m microspheres. Radiol. Clin. North Am. *7*:233, 1969.

344. Neumann, R. D., Sostman, H. D., and Gottschalk, A.: Current status of ventilation-perfusion imaging. Semin. Nucl. Med. *10*:198, 1980.

345. Taplin, G. V., Johnson, D. E., Dore, E. K., and Kaplan, H. S.: Suspensions of radioalbumin aggregates for photoscanning the liver, spleen, lung, and other organs. J. Nucl. Med. *5*:259, 1964.

346. Tow, D. E., Wagner, H. N., Jr., Lopez-Majano, V., Smith, E. M., and Migita, T.: Validity of measuring regional pulmonary arterial blood flow with macroaggregates of human serum albumin. Am. J. Roentgenol. Rad. Ther. Nucl. Med. *96*:664, 1966.

347. Rootwelt, K., and Vale, J. R.: Pulmonary gas exchange after intravenous injection of ^{99m}Tc-sulphur-colloid albumin macroaggregates for lung perfusion scintigraphy. Scand. J. Clin. Lab. Invest. *30*:14, 1972.

348. Vincent, W. R., Goldberg, S. J., and Desilets, D.: Fatality immediately following rapid infusion of macroaggregates of ^{99m}Tc-albumin (MAA) for lung scan. Radiology *91*:1181, 1968.

349. Caride, V. J., Puri, S., Slavin, J. D., Lange, R. C., and Gottschalk, A.: The usefulness of posterior oblique views in perfusion lung imaging. Radiology *121*:669, 1976.

350. Polga, J. P., and Drum, D. E.: Abnormal perfusion and ventilation scintigrams in patients with azygos fissures. J. Nucl. Med. *13*:633, 1972.

351. Potchen, E. J.: Lung scintiscanning. J.A.M.A. *204*:907, 1968.

352. DeNardo, G. L., Goodwin, D. A., Ravasini, R., and Dietrich, P. A.: The ventilatory lung scan in the diagnosis of pulmonary embolism. N. Engl. J. Med. *282*:1334, 1970.

353. Farmelant, M. H., and Trainor, J. C.: Evaluation of a ^{133}Xe technique for diagnosis of pulmonary disorders. J. Nucl. Med. *12*:586, 1971.

354. Alderson, P. O., and Line, B. R.: Scintigraphic evaluation of regional pulmonary ventilation. Semin. Nucl. Med. *10*:218, 1980.

355. Li, D. K., Treves, S., Heyman, S., Kirkpatrick, J. A., Jr., Lambrecht, R. M., Ruth, T. J., and Wolf, A. P.: Krypton-81m: A better radiopharmaceutical for assessment of regional lung function in children. Radiology *130*:741, 1979.

356. Fazio, F., and Jones, T.: Assessment of regional ventilation by continuous inhalation of radioactive krypton-81m. Br. J. Med. *1*:673, 1975.

357. The Urokinase Pulmonary Embolism Trial: A national cooperative study. Circulation *47*:II-66, 1973.

358. Cook, D. J., and Lander, H.: The diagnosis of pulmonary embolism. A review with particular reference to the use of radionuclides. Postgrad. Med. J. *47*:214, 1971.

359. Poulose, K. P., Reba, R. C., Gilday, D. L., DeLand, F. H., and Wagner, H. N., Jr.: Diagnosis of pulmonary embolism. A correlative study in patients suspect for pulmonary embolism. Br. Med. J. *3*:67, 1970.

360. McNeil, B. J.: A diagnostic strategy using ventilation-perfusion studies in patients suspect for pulmonary embolism. J. Nucl. Med. *17*:613, 1976.

361. McNeil, B. J., Holman, B. L., and Adelstein, S. J.: The scintigraphic diagnosis of pulmonary embolism. J.A.M.A. *227*:753, 1974.

362. Biello, D. R., Mattar, A. G., McKnight, R. C., and Siegel, B. A.: Ventilation-perfusion studies in suspected pulmonary embolism. Am. J. Roetgenol. *133*:1033, 1979.

363. Biello, D. R., Mattar, A. G., Osei-Wusu, A., Alderson, P. O., McNeil, B. J., and Siegel, B. A.: Interpretation of indeterminate lung scintigrams. Radiology *133*:189, 1979.

364. Tow, D. E., and Wagner, H. N., Jr.: Recovery of pulmonary arterial blood flow in patients with pulmonary embolism. N. Engl. J. Med. *276*:1053, 1967.

365. Secker-Walker, R. H., Jackson, J. A., and Goodwin, J.: Resolution of pulmonary embolism. Br. Med. J. *4*:135, 1970.

366. Grossman, W., Dexter, L., and Dalen, J.: The late prognosis of acute pulmonary embolism. N. Engl. J. Med. *289*:55, 1973.

367. Lie, D. K., Seltzer, S. E., and McNeil, B. J.: V/Q mismatches unassociated with pulmonary embolism: Case report and review of the literature. J. Nucl. Med. *19*:1331, 1978.

11 CARDIAC IMAGING

B—Nuclear Magnetic Resonance Imaging of the Heart

by Adam V. Ratner and Gerald M. Pohost, M.D.

Nuclear magnetic resonance (NMR), a method first applied by chemists to characterize molecular structure, now allows high-resolution tomographic and three-dimensional imaging as well as the acquisition of metabolic information, all without the need for ionizing radiation. Images produced by NMR methods have already shown significant clinical utility, particularly in the assessment of neurological disease.[1] For example, NMR imaging of protons can differentiate gray and white matter, detect demyelination, and define cerebral infarcts and tumors. Images can be generated with spatial resolution approaching that of x-ray computed tomography.

The spectroscopic aspect of NMR promises to provide a means for in vivo assessment of the metabolic function of internal organs. While the exact role that NMR techniques will play in the assessment of cardiac disease is currently not defined, there are many applications in which NMR may provide unique or complementary information when compared to existing diagnostic methods.

GENERAL PRINCIPLES OF NMR

Nucleons (protons and neutrons), the subunits of the atomic nucleus, have an intrinsic spin. Accordingly, certain nuclei (usually with odd numbers of nucleons) have a net nuclear spin. Since the nucleus is charged and a moving charge generates a magnetic field, spinning atomic nuclei possess magnetic fields or *moments* and simulate submicroscopic bar magnets. Such nuclear magnetic moments are required for a nucleus to exhibit NMR. Medically relevant nuclei that exhibit NMR include ^{1}H (proton), ^{13}C, ^{23}Na, and ^{31}P.

In a substance containing magnetic nuclei, the magnetic moments are usually randomly oriented. However, when placed in an external magnetic field, a number of magnetic nuclei align with the field. Most of the nuclei that align are parallel with respect to the field; however, some are antiparallel. The net effect is to generate a macroscopic magnetic moment parallel to the applied magnetic field (Fig. 11–30). The magnitude of the macroscopic magnetic moment is related to the concentration of magnetic nuclei within the sample under investigation.

To detect a magnetic moment it is necessary to displace it from its equilibrium position parallel to the external field. When a magnetic nucleus is rotated away from its original orientation, it will spin or precess about an axis parallel to the extrinsic magnetic field, like a spinning top.

In practice, radiofrequency (RF) pulses are used as the energy source for perturbing the net magnetization of the sample under investigation. The net magnetic moment will be rotated away from the direction of the extrinsic field in proportion to the duration and power of the RF pulse. When the RF pulse is turned off, these nuclei precess at the resonant or Larmor frequency, which is unique for a specific nuclear species at a given magnetic field strength and is determined by the Larmor equation:

Larmor (resonant) frequency = Gyromagnetic ratio (specific for each nucleus) × Magnetic field strength

For example, the resonant frequency of protons in a magnetic field of 0.15 tesla (tesla = unit of magnetic field strength equivalent to 10,000 gauss or 10 kilogauss) is 6.25 MHz, or 6,250,000 cycles/second. For ^{31}P (naturally abundant phosphorus) the resonant frequency would be 2.53 MHz.

The precessing nuclei will release an RF signal at the same unique (Larmor) frequency when they return to their original equilibrium positions. The RF signal released after an RF pulse is known as the free induction decay (FID) and provides the data that are analyzed in both NMR spectroscopy and NMR imaging.

The return of the nuclei to the initial, aligned state is known as relaxation; the time constant describing this process is known as the relaxation time. Actually, two terms mathematically describe the duration of this relaxation process: T1 and T2. T1, the spin-lattice (or longitudinal) relaxation time, describes the time course for the rotated or energized nuclei to return to the initial aligned position and describes

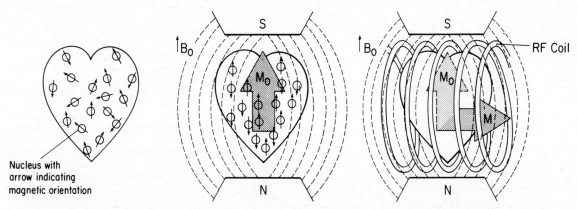

FIGURE 11–30 Nuclei with randomly oriented moments are depicted within the heart (*left*). When the heart is placed in a magnetic field (B_0), the nuclei align both parallel and antiparallel to the field (*middle*). There is, however, a net moment (M_0) that is aligned in parallel with B_0. When an RF pulse is transmitted at the Larmor frequency of the nuclei, the magnetic moment M_0 is rotated to M, in this case after a 90-degree pulse (*right*).

the process of energy transfer from the displaced nuclei to the environment. T2, the spin-spin (or transverse) relaxation time, describes the decay of the magnetic field in the transverse plane (perpendicular to the direction of the external field). During the RF pulse, nuclei precess in phase. After the RF pulse, each nucleus continues to experience not only the effects of the external static magnetic field but also the effects of the magnetic properties of neighboring nuclei. Consequently, after a time described by T2, the precession of individual nuclei drifts out of phase, and the net magnetic moment becomes smaller until the nuclei precess randomly and there is no net moment. T2 may never exceed T1 but, in certain instances, may approach it.

NMR SPECTROSCOPY

In 1946, Bloch and Purcell, motivated by theoretical considerations, independently published experimental data demonstrating the existence of NMR.[2,3] Since NMR signals are influenced by the chemical environment, NMR is capable of defining chemical composition. The frequency of a nucleus may be shifted away from the Larmor frequency by interactions of the electrons surrounding the nucleus in question, a so-called chemical shift. After an appropriate RF pulse, the resultant free induction decay signal is converted to a spectrum by using Fourier transformation. The area under each peak on the NMR spectral plot is directly related to the concentration of the chemical constituent containing that nucleus. In principle, NMR spectroscopy may be useful for the detection of many soluble body constituents and, as a result, may be useful over a wide range of medical applications. Using appropriate spectroscopic methods, investigators have studied cardiac metabolism and the effects of various interventions.

Most spectroscopic studies record the RF energy emitted by the sample after numerous bursts of radiofrequency energy. After a single burst, the resulting signal is weak and has considerable noise and by itself is inadequate for spectroscopic analysis. In order to obtain an adequate signal-to-noise ratio, many spectra are summed. Applications of proton, ^{13}C, and ^{31}P NMR spectroscopy to the study of ischemia and myocardial metabolism are summarized below.

Proton (^{1}H) Spectroscopy. Protons (^{1}H) are the most common nuclei in biology. Indeed, they compose approximately 70 per cent of the human body. Since they are so abundant and can emit stronger NMR signals than any other nuclei, protons are used for high-resolution imaging. In addition, since proton relaxation rates can be visualized by NMR imaging methods, proton spectroscopy is being used to define alterations of these proton relaxation parameters in relevant disease states.

Accordingly, Buonanno et al. have used proton spectroscopy to examine the effects of ischemia on T1 and T2 values of cerebral tissue. These investigators produced cerebral ischemia in the gerbil by ligating a carotid artery. Gerbils that were asymptomatic (demonstrated no evidence of hemiparesis) had normal relaxation times in both hemispheres, whereas symptomatic animals had significant increases in T1 and T2 in the hemisphere ipsilateral to the carotid ligation and normal values in the contralateral hemisphere.[4] With regard to myocardium, Williams et al. examined T1 in canine myocardium 30 minutes to 2 hours after coronary ligation. Significant increases in T1 were observed in ischemic myocardium compared with nonischemic myocardium[5] as early as 30 minutes after ligation.

Changes in proton relaxation parameters such as those demonstrated above suggest that, in addition to high-resolution tomography, proton NMR imaging may be useful for characterizing tissue damage during and after an ischemic insult.

[13]C Spectroscopy. Approximately 1 per cent of natural carbon atoms are stable and the NMR-sensitive ^{13}C and virtually all the rest are [12]C. NMR spectroscopy has been applied to biological systems to evaluate metabolic processes using endogenous ^{13}C or ^{13}C-labeled substrates as tracers. Using ^{13}C-labeled precursors, Alger et al. studied glucose and lipid metabolism in various organs in the rat.[6] Bailey et al. studied tricarboxylic acid cycle intermediates in isolated perfused rat hearts.[7] This method has great potential for experimental characterization of metabolic processes and may ultimately be useful for clinical assessment of myocardial metabolism.

[31]P Spectroscopy. Phosphorus-31, the naturally abundant phosphorus nucleus, is perhaps the most interesting from a biological perspective, since high-energy phosphate metabolism can be directly monitored with NMR techniques. In Figure 11–31, a schematic representation of a ^{31}P spectrum of myocardium, each peak represents a different phosphorus-containing moiety. The area under each peak is related to the relative concentration of each substance. Using ^{31}P spectroscopy in isolated working rat or rabbit hearts, it is possible to monitor the time course and reversibility of changes in high-energy phosphate concentrations with myocardial anoxia, ischemia, and infarction. In addition, the position of the inorganic phosphate peak is related to intracellular pH. Accordingly, changes in intracellular pH can be evaluated using spectroscopic monitoring of the position of the inorganic phosphorous resonance peak. Also, the concentration of magnesium (II) may be measured by examination of the position of the gamma-ATP resonance. When magnesium (II) is bound to ATP, the chemical environment surrounding the gamma phosphorus of ATP changes, altering its resonant frequency. Furthermore, enzyme kinetics and the compartmentalization of metabolites can be studied using a method that "labels" nuclei, enabling specific moieties to be followed even after chemical change. This technique is known as saturation transfer ^{31}P NMR.[8]

Phosphorus-31 spectroscopy has been used to study high-energy phosphate metabolism under normal and pathological conditions. Fossel et al. demonstrated variations in the concentrations of high-energy phosphates during different stages of the cardiac cycle.[9] They found that phosphocreatine and ATP levels were highest and inorganic phosphate levels lowest at end diastole, when aortic pressure was low. Conversely, in systole when aortic pressure was high, high-energy phosphate levels were lowest and inorganic phosphate levels were highest.

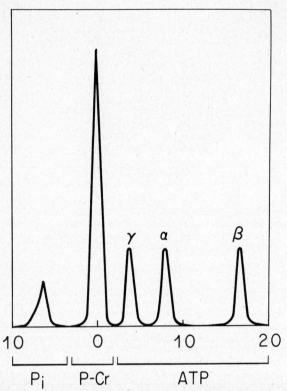

FIGURE 11–31   Schematic diagram of a ³¹P spectrum of myocardium. Each peak represents a different phosphorus-containing moiety. From left to right are inorganic phosphate (P$_i$); phosphocreatine (P-Cr); and the gamma, alpha, and beta peaks of ATP. The area under each peak is related to the concentration of each group. The distance between the inorganic phosphate and phosphocreatine peaks is related to the pH. The numbers on the abscissa denote the difference (chemical shift) in the resonant frequency of each peak from the reference peak (phosphocreatine) in parts per million.

The beneficial effects of various interventions have been evaluated using ³¹P spectroscopy. For example, Pieper et al. demonstrated that the acidosis of ischemic arrest could be significantly reduced with the addition of the beta-adrenergic blocking agent propranolol.[10] Flaherty et al. showed that potassium cardioplegia worked synergistically with hypothermia to preserve myocardial high-energy phosphates during episodes of ischemia.[11] The clinical relevance of these studies is apparent, and techniques are being developed and implemented for clinical application of NMR spectroscopy.

TOPICAL MAGNETIC RESONANCE

By application of specialized methods known as topical magnetic resonance (TMR), NMR spectroscopy can be performed in vivo in one of two ways. One method, the surface coil technique, uses radiofrequency coils placed on the surface of the subject being evaluated to delineate the region of interest. The other technique uses profiling magnetic gradients to designate a small sensitive volume from which spectra are generated. By these means, one may compare the spectra from regions of suspected disease with normal regions, serially follow the course of a disease with or without treatment, and obtain values of pH and metabolite concentrations.

In the *surface coil technique*, a small coil is placed adjacent to the physical region of interest. This technique allows signal acquisition from tissues no deeper than the radius of the coil and is most useful for studying superficial structures in vivo or excised structures. By placing a surface coil over the region of the left anterior descending coronary artery (LAD) on an excised perfused rabbit heart, Nunnally and Bottomley demonstrated that verapamil limited myocardial ischemic damage, as shown by increased high-energy phosphate concentrations after 30 minutes of LAD ligation versus the control.[12]

In the *sensitive volume technique*, a second magnetic field is established electronically that will localize the region of interest without the physical placement of a coil on the sample.[13]

Clinically, using the surface coil technique, a case of McArdle's syndrome was detected in skeletal muscle. In normal skeletal muscle, anaerobic exercise causes lactic acidosis, which shifts the inorganic phosphate resonance peak as observed in ³¹P TMR spectra. However, in McArdle's syndrome, where lactate is not produced, the inorganic phosphate resonance peak remained fixed, a finding consistent with the absence of acidosis during anaerobic exercise.[14] It should be noted that TMR is not an imaging modality but rather a technique that produces a chemical spectrum similar to that produced in a classic NMR spectrometer. The difference is that the classic spectrometer collects signals from all parts of the sample, whereas TMR allows one to localize a specific region of interest within a sample.

NMR IMAGING

NMR imaging was first performed 10 years ago by Lauterbur using a modified spectrometer.[15] As described earlier, the resonant frequency of a given nucleus is proportional to the magnetic field in which it resides. If two identical nuclei are placed in magnetic fields of different strengths, they will have different resonant frequencies. Different regions of the magnetic field will have different field strengths if a magnetic field gradient is superimposed on the static magnetic field. As a consequence, identical nuclei in different parts of the field will have different resonant frequencies. If the field strength at all parts of the imaging field is known, it is possible to determine the location of nuclei using the emitted radiofrequency.

Most current NMR imaging systems acquire data from one or more planes or from an entire volume at any given time. Volumetric acquisitions allow sampling of an entire anatomical region with selection of the planes of interest to be studied after data collection. This allows retrospective analysis of data and may be particularly useful if the precise location of the suspected disease is unknown.

Intensity in an NMR image depends primarily on several factors, including proton density, T1, T2, and motion. With different pulse sequences, one or more of the above factors may be highlighted. In initial cardiac imaging studies, the NMR imaging group at the Massachusetts General Hospital employed a pulse sequence known as steady-state free precession (SSFP). This pulse sequence generates images related to proton density as well as to both T1 and T2 and is extremely sensitive to motion. The inherent motion sensitivity of this pulse sequence has made it only of historical interest in terms of in vivo cardiac imaging. This pulse sequence is produced by rapidly transmitting pulses while not allowing enough time for either spin-lattice or spin-spin relaxation to be completed.

Saturation recovery (SR) is a pulse sequence that can produce images with both proton density and T1 components. It is produced by employing 90-degree RF pulses interspersed by some time delay, tau (τ). By selecting different tau values, one can control the degree of T1 weighting. In SR images, the longer the time between the two RF pulses, the more complete is relaxation, and there is more proton density weighting and less T1 weighting. The proton density of a given tissue tends to change substantially only late in the course of a pathological process. T1, however, appears to provide additional contrast earlier in the course of certain disease states. When further T1 contrast is desired, an inversion recovery pulse sequence may be used. This pulse sequence is characterized by an initial 180-degree or inversion pulse followed by a 90-degree "read" pulse separated from the inversion pulse by a given tau. After the "read" pulse, a period of time equivalent to at least four to five times the longest T1 present is allowed to pass before the next 180-degree pulse is transmitted, so that complete relaxation can occur. As with saturation recovery, variations in the tau value will lead to changes in tissue contrast.

A spin-echo pulse sequence is used to acquire images with T2 weighting. A spin-echo sequence commences with a 90-degree pulse followed by one or more 180-degree pulses. One such sequence is the Carr-Purcell-Meiboom-Gill (CPMG) pulse sequence, which uses several 180-degree pulses after the 90-degree pulse.

CARDIAC NMR IMAGING

Some of the early images of the heart were of poor quality because the SSFP pulse sequence used was extremely sensitive to motion. Cardiac images obtained by Smith et al. using another ungated approach produced images with substantially better definition of the myocardium.[16] Subsequently, efforts were made to synchronize the RF pulses to the cardiac cycle. This was done by gating to physiologic cardiac parameters such as the arterial pulse or the electrocardiogram. Typically, projections are acquired at the same point in successive cardiac cycles until a complete tomograph is produced (Fig. 11–32). Problems arise in patients with irregular cardiac rhythms; in such patients, image degradation can be expected owing to successive projections being acquired at different points in the cardiac cycle. The ECG tends to provide synchronization that is physiologically superior to hemodynamic parameters, since most changes in cardiac function have a greater effect on the morphology of the arterial pressure wave than on the configuration of the QRS complex. Unfortunately, ECG-gated NMR images can have a high level of noise,

since the ECG electrode acts as an antenna and transmits noise into the imaging region.

Myocardial intensity from gated saturation recovery images depends primarily on proton density with some T1 weighting. Because the RF pulses are synchronized with the cardiac cycle, T1 weighting in gated SR images of the heart depends on the heart rate. Gated inversion recovery and CPMG images have not yet been made because of the greater complexity of these pulse sequences. Gated cardiac images in man have been generated by investigators at Case–Western Reserve University Hospital.[17] These images were made using a gated saturation recovery pulse sequence, and they tend to highlight proton density.

Figure 11–33 depicts transverse section cardiac anatomy throughout the cardiac cycle. Anticipated changes in cardiac chamber size are observed during the cardiac cycle. In coronal images at end diastole (Fig. 11–34A), the signal intensity of blood in the arteries of the thorax is similar to that found in the surrounding tissue. In systole, as seen in Figure 11–34B, motion of the blood causes the signal from within the vessel to diminish. Proton NMR imaging thus differentiates moving blood from the tissue surrounding it. Kaufman, Crooks, and their associates demonstrated the feasibility of making quantitative measurements of flow and flow obstructions in models.[18,19] Thus, in addition to depicting cardiac structures with high resolution, gated proton NMR imaging may provide information concerning vascular flow.

The utility of proton NMR imaging for characterizing myocardium as ischemic or infarcted is now being explored.[19a] As stated earlier, spectroscopic studies showed that a prolonged ischemic insult may affect proton relaxation parameters in both ischemic brain and heart. Buonanno et al. showed that spectroscopically identified differences in T1 and T2 could also be seen in SSFP images of infarcted gerbil cerebral hemispheres.[4] Changes in proton signal strength in myocardium during infarction may result from the formation of edema, lipid accumulation, and fibrosis.

Studies in dogs carried out at the Massachusetts Gener-

GATED CARDIAC NMR IMAGING

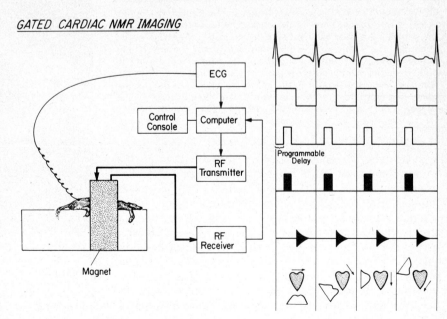

FIGURE 11–32 Schematic diagram of gating technique used in NMR tomographic imaging. A physiologic cardiac parameter such as the R wave of the ECG is converted to a digital signal in order to synchronize NMR imaging pulses with the cardiac cycle. The computer may be programmed to add some delay time to allow signal acquisition from different parts of the cardiac cycle. After the transmitter sends RF pulses into the imaging region, the returned signal (FID) is acquired by the receiver and relayed to the computer for processing of that projection. The system then waits for the next gating pulse to begin acquiring the next projection.

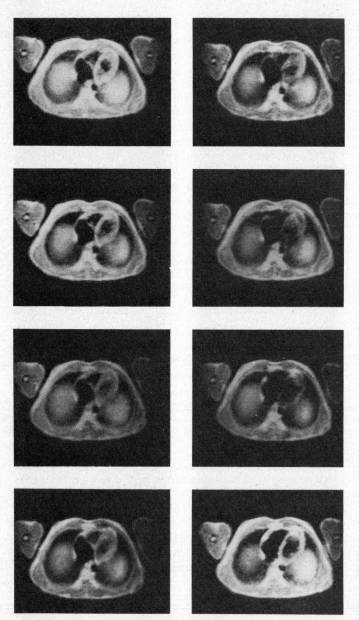

FIGURE 11–33 Gated proton NMR tomographs through the thorax acquired at different times in the cardiac cycle. Anterior is up and the patient's left is on the right side of the image. The image in the upper left was acquired in early systole and that at the lower right during end diastole. Notice the variation in chamber dimensions in both ventricles during different parts of the cardiac cycle. The descending aorta is noted just to the left of the anterior portion of the spine. Also note the presence of the tricuspid valve in some of the images. (Courtesy of Technicare Corporation, Solon, Ohio.)

al Hospital have shown that proton NMR imaging methods may be useful for assessing the response of the myocardium to an ischemic insult. In 16 dogs that underwent occlusion of the LAD for 30 minutes followed by 15 minutes of reflow, several changes were noted using gated saturation recovery proton NMR imaging. As anticipated, transient coronary occlusion was generally associated with myocardial thinning and ventricular dilatation. In addition, a region of increased signal intensity was frequently evident subjacent to the ischemic zone, suggesting anomalous blood motion in that region. During reflow, myocardial thickness, ventricular size, and the blood pool signal

tended to revert toward normal. There was no apparent change in the intensity of the myocardial signal in the ischemic zone versus the normal zone. In dogs that underwent 72 hours of occlusion of the LAD without a reflow period, myocardial thinning, ventricular dilatation, and blood stasis also appeared. There were also examples of increased myocardial signal intensity in the ischemic region, which may represent lipid accumulation or asynergy in the necrotic myocardium.[20,21] It appears that cardiac NMR imaging can depict dynamic myocardial responses secondary to ischemia and may also be useful in characterizing the degree of ischemic tissue damage (Fig. 11–35).

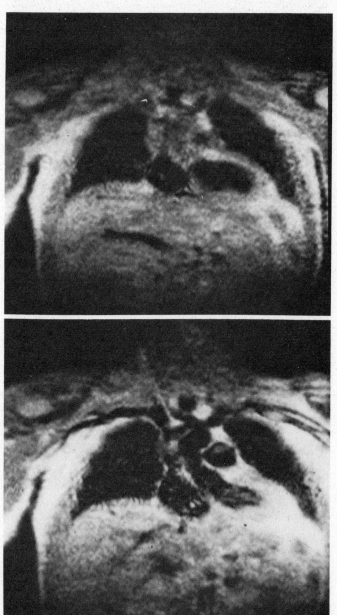

FIGURE 11–34 Gated proton NMR images of the thorax at end diastole (A) and end systole (B). Compare the chamber sizes in both images. Notice that the aortic outflow tract and its large arterial branches in the thorax, which are not well seen in A, are very well delineated in B. Motion of the blood is responsible for the heightened contrast. (Courtesy of Technicare Corporation, Solon, Ohio.)

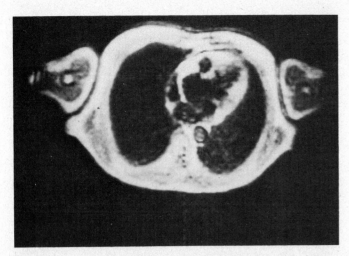

FIGURE 11–35 Gated proton NMR tomograph of a patient with a history of an old infarct. Notice the myocardial thinning and diminished signal intensity at the apex. The patient's left side is at the right side of the image. (Courtesy of Technicare Corporation, Solon, Ohio.)

CONTRAST AGENTS

Paramagnetic substances can modify the relaxation times of NMR-sensitive nuclei and as such may be useful as NMR contrast agents. In general, paramagnetic substances are those with unpaired electrons that can interact with NMR-sensitive nuclei and accelerate both spin-lattice and spin-spin relaxation, significantly shortening T1 and T2. Manganese ion (Mn^{++}) is strongly paramagnetic and has been shown in radionuclide studies to distribute in myocardium in proportion to blood flow.[22] Lauterbur et al. demonstrated spectroscopically that Mn^{++} could be used to label normal myocardium by reducing relaxation times.[23] In canine studies performed at the Massachusetts General Hospital, defects seen in Mn^{++}-enhanced NMR images corresponded closely with triphenyl tetrazolium chloride defects in both 90-minute and 24-hour coronary ligations.[24,25] Unfortunately, free Mn^{++} is a fairly toxic substance, and its clinical utility may therefore be limited.

There are several other paramagnetic substances, including molecular oxygen and stable free radicals, which may be clinically useful and not limited by toxicity. The paramagnetism of molecular oxygen may allow the in vivo assessment of blood oxygen saturation.

FUTURE IMAGING TECHNIQUES

With regard to proton imaging, an approach now being developed by Mansfield has the potential to allow acquisition of an entire tomographic image in less than 100 milliseconds.[26] Tomographic gated cardiac images, as described previously, require several minutes and the acquisition of numerous cardiac cycles. The Mansfield technique, known as "echo planar" imaging, is accomplished by using rapidly switching field gradients and can generate images in a small fraction of the cardiac cycle. Accordingly, the approach does not require gating, since each tomograph represents a single acquisition. Although images produced thus far by this technique have limited spatial resolution,

the approach may provide the basis for a future avenue of cardiac NMR imaging.

Another development with potential cardiac applicability was the demonstration by DeLayre et al. that gated ^{23}Na images could be generated from the blood pool of an isolated beating rat heart.[27]

Although ^{31}P accounts for virtually 100 per cent of natural phosphorus, the concentration of phosphorus within most biological samples is very low. This low concentration, combined with the intrinsically lower NMR sensitivity of ^{31}P, contributes to the million-fold difference in the signal strength of phosphorus NMR signals compared to proton signals. While low signal strength may preclude high-resolution imaging of this nucleus, clinically useful low-resolution images may someday be obtained. Phosphorus spectroscopy in vivo is currently possible using TMR as described earlier.

SAFETY CONSIDERATIONS

While both NMR spectroscopic and imaging techniques appear to be safe, there are a few exceptions. Patients with metallic implants (e.g., aneurysm clips) should avoid strong magnetic fields, since the magnetic forces might displace the implant and cause harm. Furthermore, persons with cardiac pacemakers should not come close to an NMR system because of the risk that pacemakers may be reprogrammed or switched into the fixed-rate mode by the magnetic field. Budinger summarizes the potential medical effects and hazards of radiofrequency and magnetic fields and concludes that no biological hazard should be anticipated with NMR imaging systems.[29]

CLINICAL UTILITY OF NMR (Table 11–3)

High-resolution gated proton NMR tomography should permit accurate evaluation of ventricular volumes, myocardial mass, and the relative positions of the cardiac chambers and great vessels. The relaxation times T1 and T2 provide the basis for characterizing myocardial disease in proton NMR imaging, but considerable investigation is still needed to establish the utility of this approach.

The contrast provided by the motion of blood within the vasculature suggests that noninvasive angiography may ultimately be feasible without the need for radiopaque contrast media. In addition, reduced blood motion can be depicted within the cardiac chambers, and consequently, NMR imaging may allow detection of conditions favorable to thrombus formation. Paramagnetic substances provide a basis for myocardial perfusion imaging.

Perhaps the most exciting potential application for cardiac NMR is in the assessment of nuclei other than the proton. Measurement of cardiac high-energy phosphate concentrations and intracellular pH using TMR or imaging approaches may have important ramifications. The ability to assess high-energy phosphates, even with limited spatial resolution, would permit evaluation and monitoring of myocardial health in ischemic or other states.

While echocardiography provides some structural information at a considerably lower cost and during real time,

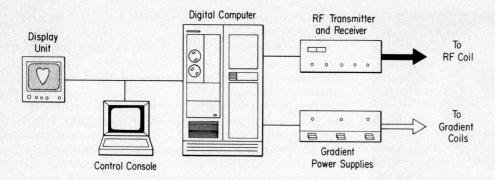

FIGURE 11-36 Schematic diagram of NMR imaging hardware.

proton NMR imaging is not impeded by bone or lung and can provide three-dimensional images as well as the potential for tissue contrast.

The ability to evaluate myocardial perfusion and viability noninvasively is limited to radionuclide approaches using thallium-201 with gamma-camera imaging[30] and positron-emission tomography using radioactive metabolic substrates. Although gamma-camera imaging can be performed at moderate cost, it requires the administration of radiopharmaceuticals with limited shelf-lives and generates reliable tomograms with difficulty. Positron methods are expensive because, for maximum flexibility, a cyclotron is needed to generate the short-lived radiopharmaceuticals. A fundamental problem with all tracer methods is that they require intravenous administration of the substance to be monitored; as a result, distribution is related not only to cell function but also to perfusion. High-energy phosphates, on the other hand, are endogenous, and their concentration directly reflects the state of myocardial health.

Although NMR imaging is at an early stage of development, its proven ability to generate high-resolution,

tomographic, and three-dimensional images without the need to employ ionizing radiation will make it a powerful diagnostic tool. In addition, the ability of NMR spectroscopy and TMR to assess metabolic function by analysis of endogenous substrates and metabolic tracers will increase our understanding of cardiac disease and its therapy.

HARDWARE CONSIDERATIONS

NMR techniques are sophisticated and represent the confluence of computer and image-processing technology with radio and magnetic phenomena.

Most NMR imaging systems, whether they utilize resistive or superconducting magnets, employ a system similar to that depicted in Figure 11-36. The central unit, the digital computer, is responsible for image data acquisition and reconstruction. Through peripheral devices such as those shown, the computer can execute the desired RF pulse sequences and make the proper gradient adjustments as well as acquire the resultant NMR signals and reconstruct them into images.

The magnet is central to an NMR system. There are two types of magnets: electromagnets and permanent magnets. Nearly all systems to date have used electromagnets, which can be either resistive

TABLE 11-3 EVALUATION OF NMR IMAGING

Advantages

High resolution (about 1 mm)
Intrinsically tomographic or three-dimensional
Ionizing radiation not employed
No interference from bone or lung
Contrast achieved between cardiovascular blood and surrounding structures without contrast media
Tissue characterization possible

Disadvantages

Relatively slow speed of image acquisition compared to x-ray and ultrasound methods
High cost of hardware and site preparation
Greater impact on cost of medical care
Potential for changing operating mode of artificial pacemaker
Potential for displacing metallic implants
Effects of long-term chronic exposure unknown

Potential Utility

Proton imaging
Noninvasive angiocardiography without contrast media
Detection of blood stasis (e.g., in left ventricle associated with myocardial infarction)
Characterization of diseased tissue using T1 and T2
Noninvasive oximetry
Rapid tomography (10 to 100 msec) using "echo-planar" technique
Tomographic myocardial perfusion imaging
Non-proton imaging using ^{13}C, ^{23}Na, and ^{31}P
  High-energy phosphate metabolism
  Intracellular pH
  ^{13}C-labeled substrate metabolism

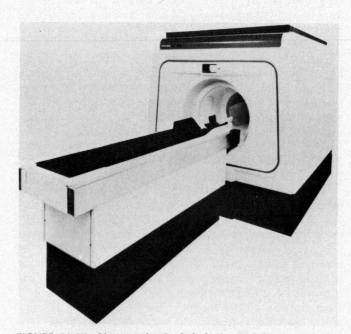

FIGURE 11-37 Photograph of whole-body NMR imaging magnet. (Courtesy of Technicare Corporation, Solon, Ohio.)

or superconducting. Superconducting magnets, although more expensive and considerably more difficult to manufacture, are necessary for work at field strengths above 2.0 to 2.5 kilogauss. Superconducting systems with fields of 3.5 to 5.0 kilogauss are being used for proton work (Fig. 11–37), and 15 kilogauss or higher field systems are used for ^{13}C and ^{31}P TMR. Resistive magnets can produce excellent images and may ultimately allow construction of computed tomography systems at a lower cost than can be produced with radiographic methods.

Resistive magnets consist of conductive copper wrapped around a central core. Such systems consume large amounts of electric current and require magnet power supplies. Superconducting systems consist of niobium alloy wire wrapped around a cylindrical core, which is surrounded by dewars of liquid helium and liquid nitrogen. This wire has an extremely high electrical resistance at room temperature but virtually no electrical resistance at the temperature of the surrounding liquid helium. The liquid nitrogen fills a dewar, which surrounds the liquid helium and serves to reduce the amount of helium boiled off. Both helium and nitrogen require periodic replenishing.

Owing largely to the dewars for the cryogens, superconducting magnets are necessarily larger than resistive magnets. Other considerations when erecting an NMR system include allocation of adequate floor space so that the magnetic field does not interfere with surrounding hospital functions and vice versa. Precautions must be taken to keep the laboratory isolated from large moving metal objects such as elevators because these objects can alter the uniformity of the magnetic field. Care must be taken to keep small ferromagnetic objects away from the NMR system, since the magnetic field can convert such objects into dangerous projectiles. Adequate space must be allocated for the requisite computer, power supplies, control console, and ancillary items crucial for patient safety.

References

1. Bydder, G. M., Steiner, R. E., Young, I. R., et al.: Clinical NMR imaging of the brain: 140 cases. Am. J. Radiol. *139*:215, 1982.
2. Bloch, F.: Nuclear induction. Physiol. Rev. *70*:460, 1946.
3. Purcell, E. M., Torrey, H. C., and Pound, R. V.: Resonance absorption by nuclear magnetic moments in a solid. Physiol. Rev. *69*:37, 1946.
4. Buonanno, F. S., Pykett, I. L., Vielma, J., et al.: Proton NMR imaging of normal and abnormal brain. Experimental and clinical observations. *In* Witcofski, R. L., Karstaedt, N., and Partain, C. L. (eds.): Proceedings of the International Symposium in NMR Imaging. Winston-Salem, N.C., Bowman Gray School of Medicine Press, 1982, pp. 147–157.
5. Williams, E. S., Kaplan, J. I., Thatcher, F., Zimmerman, G., and Knoebel, S. B.: Prolongation of proton spin-lattice relaxation times in regionally ischemic tissue from dog hearts. J. Nucl. Med. *21*:449, 1980.
6. Alger, J. R., Sillerud, L. O., Behar, K. L., Gillies, R. J., and Shulman, R. G.: In vivo carbon-13 nuclear magnetic resonance studies of mammals. Science *214*:660, 1981.
7. Bailey, I. A., Gadian, D. G., Matthews, P. M., Radda, G. K., and Seeley, P. J.: Studies of metabolism in the isolated perfused rat heart using C-13 NMR. FEBS Lett. *123*:315, 1981.
8. Ingwall, J. S.: Phosphorus nuclear magnetic resonance spectroscopy of cardiac and skeletal muscles. Am. J. Physiol. *242*:729, 1982.
9. Fossel, E. T., Morgan, H. E., and Ingwall, J. S.: Measurement of changes in high-energy phosphates in the cardiac cycle using gated P-31 NMR. Proc. Natl. Acad. Sci. *77*:3654, 1980.
10. Pieper, G. M., Todd, G. L., Wu, S. T., Salhany, J. M., Clayton, F. C., and Eliot, R. S.: Attenuation of myocardial acidosis by propranolol during ischemic

11. Flaherty, J. T., Weisfeldt, M. L., Bulkley, B. H., Gardner, T. J., Gott, V. L., and Jacobus, W. E.: Mechanisms of ischemic myocardial cell damage assessed by phosphorus-31 nuclear magnetic resonance. Circulation *65*:561, 1982.
12. Nunnally, R. L., and Bottomley, P. A.: Assessment of pharmacological treatment of myocardial infarction by phosphorus-31 NMR with surface coils. Science *211*:177, 1981.
13. Ross, B. D., Radda, G. K., Gadian, D. G., Rocker, G., Esiri, M., and Falconer-Smith, J.: Examination of a case of suspected McArdle's syndrome by P-31 NMR. N. Engl. J. Med. *304*:1338, 1981.
14. Gordon, R. E., Hanley, P. E., and Shaw, D.: Topical magnetic resonance. *In* Progress in NMR Spectroscopy, Vol. 15. New York, Pergamon Press, 1982, pp. 1–47.
15. Lauterbur, P. C.: Image formation by induced local interactions: Examples employing nuclear magnetic resonance. Nature *242*:190, 1973.
16. Smith, F. W.: Clinical application of NMR tomographic imaging. *In* Witcofski, R. L., Karstaedt, N., and Partain, C. L. (eds.): Proceedings of the International Symposium in NMR Imaging. Winston-Salem, N.C., Bowman Gray School of Medicine Press, 1982, pp. 125–32.
17. Alfidi, R. J., Haaga, J. R., El-Yousef, S. J., et al.: Preliminary experimental results in humans and animals with a superconducting, whole-body, nuclear magnetic resonance scanner. Radiology *143*:175, 1982.
18. Kaufman, L., Crooks, L. E., Sheldon, P. E., Rowan, W., and Miller, T.: Evaluation of NMR imaging for detection and quantification of obstructions in vessels. Invest. Radiol. *17*:554, 1982.
19. Crooks, L. E., Mills, C. M., Davis, P. L., et al.: Visualization of cerebral and vascular abnormalities by NMR imaging. The effects of imaging parameters on contrast. Radiology *144*:843, 1982.
19a. Ruigrok, T. J. C., van Echteld, C. J. A., Kruijff, B. de, Borst, C., and Meijler, F. L.: Protective effect of nifedipine in myocardial ischemia assessed by phosphorus nuclear magnetic resonance. J. Am. Coll. Cardiol. *1*:666, 1983.
20. Pohost, G. M., Goldman, M. R., Pykett, I. L., et al.: Gated NMR imaging in canine myocardial infarction (Abstract). Circulation *66*: 11-39, 1982.
21. Ratner, A. V., Goldman, M. R., and Pohost, G. M.: Visualization of myocardial ischemic damage using nuclear magnetic resonance imaging (Abstract). Clin. Res., *31*:213a, 1983.
22. Chauncey, D. M., Jr., Schelbert, H. R., Halpern, S. E., Delans, F., McKegney, M. L., Ashburn, W. L., and Hagan, P. L.: Tissue distribution studies with radioactive manganese: A potential agent for myocardial imaging. J. Nucl. Med. *18*:933, 1977.
23. Lauterbur, P. C., Dias, M. H. M., and Rudin, A. M.: Augmentation of tissue water proton spin-lattice relaxation rates by in vivo addition of paramagnetic ions. *In* Dutton, P. L., Leigh, J. S., and Scarpa, A. (eds.): Frontiers of Biological Energetics. New York, Academic Press, p. 752, 1981.
24. Goldman, M. R., Brady, T. J., Pykett, I. L., et al.: Quantification of experimental myocardial infarction using nuclear magnetic resonance imaging and paramagnetic ion contrast enhancement in excised canine hearts. Circulation *66*:1012, 1982.
25. Brady, T. J., Goldman, M. R., Pykett, I. L., Buonanno, F. S., Kistler, J. P., Newhouse, J. H., Burt, C. T., Hinshaw, W. S., and Pohost, G. M.: Proton nuclear magnetic resonance imaging of regionally ischemic canine hearts: Effect of paramagnetic proton signal enhancement. Radiology *144*:343, 1982.
26. Ordidge, R. J., Mansfield, P., Doyle, M., et al.: "Real-time" moving images by NMR. *In* Witcofski, R. L., Karstaedt, N., and Partain, C. L. (eds.): Proceedings of the International Symposium in NMR Imaging. Winston-Salem, N.C., Bowman Gray School of Medicine Press, 1982, pp. 89–92.
27. DeLayre, J. L., Ingwall, J. S., Malloy, C., and Fossel, E. T.: Gated sodium-23 nuclear magnetic resonance images of an isolated perfused working rat heart. Science *212*:935, 1981.
28. New, P. F. J., Rosen, B. R., Brady, T. J., et al.: Potential hazards and artifacts of ferromagnetic and nonferromagnetic surgical and dental materials and devices in NMR imaging. Radiology, *147*:139, 1983.
29. Budinger, T. F.: Thresholds for physiological effects due to RF and magnetic fields used in NMR imaging. IEEE Trans. Nucl. Sci. *NS-26*:2821, 1979.
30. Pohost G. M., and Goldhaber, S. Z.: Nuclear magnetic resonance. *In* Morganroth, J., Parisi, A., and Pohost, G. M. (eds): Noninvasive Cardiac Imaging. Chicago, Year Book Medical Publishers, Inc., 1983, pp. 423–431.

PART II

ABNORMALITIES OF CIRCULATORY FUNCTION

12 CONTRACTION OF THE NORMAL HEART

by Eugene Braunwald, M.D., Edmund H. Sonnenblick, M.D., and John Ross, Jr., M.D.

The function of the heart is to propel unoxygenated blood to the lungs and oxygenated blood to the peripheral tissues in accordance with their metabolic requirements. Heart failure may therefore be defined as the pathophysiological state in which an abnormality of cardiac function is responsible for the failure of the heart to pump blood at a rate commensurate with these requirements. To understand the disturbances in cardiac contraction that characterize heart failure, described in Chapter 13, it is necessary to comprehend the structure and function of the normal cardiac cell and of the normal contractile process, described in this chapter.

STRUCTURE OF THE MYOCARDIAL CELL

MYOCARDIAL CELLS, MYOFIBRILS, AND SARCOMERES. *Ventricular myocardial cells* (fibers) are normally 40 to 100 μ in length and 10 to 20 μ in diameter (Fig. 12–1). Numerous cross-banded strands or bundles, termed *myofibrils*, traverse the length of the fibers and, unlike the case for skeletal muscle, are incompletely separated by clefts of cytoplasm that contain mitochondria and membranous tubules (Fig. 12–1*B*).[1–4]

Myofibrils are composed of longitudinally repeating *sarcomeres* separated by two adjacent dark lines, the Z lines (Fig. 12–1*B* and *C*).[5] Sarcomeres occupy about 50 per cent of the mass of the cardiac cells and are aligned so that the ends of adjacent myofibrils are in register, giving the fiber its striated appearance.[1,2] The length of the sarcomere ranges from 1.6 to 2.2 μ, depending on muscle length. The center of the sarcomere is occupied by a dark band, the A band (the anisotropic or birefringent band that rotates polarized light); the band is composed primarily of myosin and is 1.5 μ in length. The A band is flanked by two lighter bands, termed I (isotropic) bands, which are variable in length depending on the length of the sarcomere. The bands of the sarcomere reflect the disposition of interdigitating myofilaments made up of contractile proteins (Fig. 12–1*C* and 12–3*A*). Thin filaments composed of actin are attached to each Z line and project longitudinally into the middle of the sarcomere, where they interdigitate with an array of thicker filaments composed of myosin molecules.[6] It is the interactions between the thick and thin myofilaments that generate force and shortening of the myocardium.

The *nucleus* is centrally placed within the myocardial cell. *Mitochondria*, which make up about 20 per cent of the

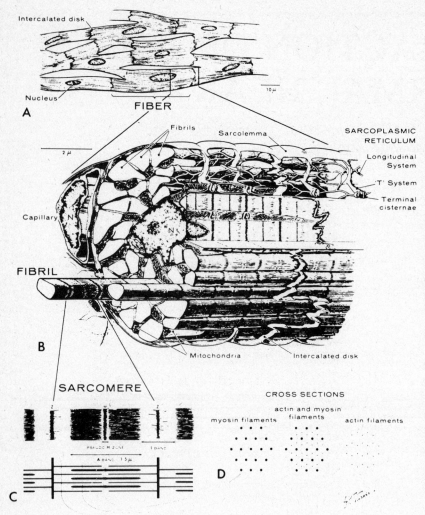

volume of the cell, are elliptically shaped, approximately 2 to 5 μ by 0.5 μ, and are situated between and in close apposition to the myofibrils as well as just beneath the sarcolemma.[7] Their platelike foldings, or cristae, which contain the enzymes of the tricarboxylic acid cycle, project inward from the surface membrane. The close proximity of the mitochondria, the organelles in which ATP is produced, to the contractile filaments may facilitate the transfer of ATP from its site of production to its site of utilization during the contractile process. *Lysosomes*, membrane-limited vesicles about 0.1 μ in diameter and located near the pole of the nucleus, contain latent hydrolytic enzymes capable of lysing cellular membranes as well as other cellular components.

Myocardial cells that initiate intrinsic activity in the heart, i.e., *pacemaker or automatic cells*, are somewhat smaller than ventricular fibers[8] (p. 605). Those which are specialized for conduction and the spread of excitation, i.e., Purkinje fibers, are very large when compared to contractile fibers; they contain fewer myofibrils and greater quantities of clear cytoplasm, fine intracellular noncontractile filaments, and glycogen in addition to having a rich external investment of capillaries and small nerves.[9]

Myocardial fibers are surrounded by a rich capillary network, and small, nonmyelinated nerves are found lying free in the extracellular space.[3] These nerves have no specific junctions with cardiac cells but do exhibit bulbous ends bearing granules that contain neurotransmitter substances. These substances are *acetylcholine*, located primarily in the atria and in automatic and conduction tissues, and *norepinephrine*, found in these tissues but also in the ventricles; both can be released to act on membrane surface receptors of adjacent cells.

SARCOLEMMA, INTERCALATED DISKS, AND SARCOPLASMIC RETICULUM. A surface membrane, the *sarcolemma*, surrounds the myocardial cells and invaginates the Z lines of the sarcomere.[1,7,7a] It is composed of a thin (7 to 9 nm), bimolecular phospholipid layer, the plasmalemma, which is the site of electrical polarization (Fig. 19–5, p. 609). Just exterior to the plasmalemma is the glycocalyx, i.e., the basement membrane, approximately 50 nm in thickness (Fig. 12–2), which in turn is composed of an inner and an outer coat. The plasmalemma is the major semipermeable membrane between the intracellular cytoplasm and the negatively charged glycocalyx to which Ca^{++} may be bound and which separates the cell from the extracellular matrix. Adjacent myocardial cells are connected end-to-end by a thickened portion of the sarcolemma, termed the *intercalated disk*,[1–3] a segment of which, i.e., the nevus or gap junction, represents a low-resistance pathway to the propagation of electrical activity between cells.[1,8] Myocardial fibers are also interconnected

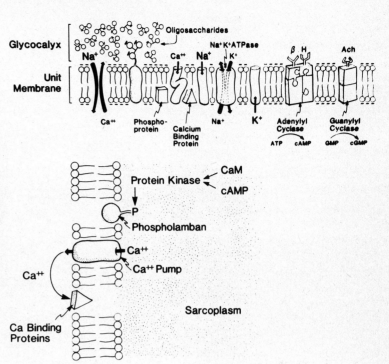

FIGURE 12–2 Schematic of the ultrastructure of the sarcolemma (*top*) and sarcoplasmic reticulum (*bottom*) of ventricular muscle cells. Both membrane systems have a lamina consisting of a sheet of lipids forming the matrix of the membrane and acting as a hydrophobic barrier. The outer surface of the sarcolemma is covered by a negatively charged glycocalyx that appears as a fuzzy layer in electron micrographs. Embedded in the sarcolemma are receptors for hormones and neurotransmitters along with the enzymes that transduce receptor binding to an alteration in intracellular concentrations of cyclic nucleotides. Major proteins in the sarcoplasmic reticulum (SR) are a calcium pump protein; calcium binding proteins that store transported calcium ions; and phospholamban, which, when phosphorylated by cAMP- or calmodulin-dependent protein kinases, alters the calcium pump and induces an increase in the rate of calcium transport into the lumen of the SR. (From Solaro, R. J.: The role of calcium in the contraction of the heart. *In* Flaim, S. F., and Zelis, R. (eds.): Calcium Blockers: Mechanisms of Action and Clinical Applications. Baltimore, Urban and Schwarzenberg, 1982, p. 25.)

by an extensive network of fine microfibrils and microthreads,[10] which play an important role in cell orientation, tissue compliance, and force transmission.

The hydrophobic phospholipid bilayer of the plasmalemma acts as an ionic barrier and maintains higher intracellular than extracellular potassium [K$^+$] concentrations and lower intracellular than extracellular sodium [Na$^+$] and calcium [Ca^{++}] concentrations. (Cytoplasmic [Ca^{++}] is of the order of 10^{-7} M; extracellular [Ca^{++}] is 10^{-3} M.) The sarcolemma possesses enzyme systems that utilize ATP for energy in order to maintain these differences in ion concentrations.[11,12] Na$^+$,K$^+$-stimulated ATPases (p. 509) are responsible for the active transport of Na$^+$ and Ca^{++} out of the cardiac cell and for the uptake of K$^+$. Near the Z lines the sarcolemma contains wide invaginations, *the T system*, which branch, both longitudinally and transversely, through the cell (Fig. 12–3). Closely coupled to but not continuous with the T system is the *sarcoplasmic reticulum* (SR), a complex network of anastomosing, membrane-limited tubular intracellular channels, approximately 300 Å in diameter, which surround each myofibril and play a critical role in excitation of the muscle.[7] Unlike the T system, the SR is not continuous with the extracellular space. Where the SR approaches the T tubules or the sarcolemma, it widens into flattened saclike enlargements (cisternae). At their junction, the SR and T tubules are separated by gaps of 10 to 12 nm. Depolarization of the sarcolemma is channeled through the T system to release Ca^{++} from the SR, which mediates myofibrillar activation (see below). Like the sarcolemma, the SR has a bilayer matrix consisting principally of phospholipids.

CONTRACTILE PROTEINS. The contractile apparatus consists of partially overlapping, rodlike myofilaments that are fixed in length, both at rest and during contraction.[1,13] The thicker filaments, composed of *myosin* molecules, are limited to the A band, are about 100 nm in diameter with tapered ends, and measure 1.5 to 1.6 μ in length.[1,14] They are created by an orderly aggregation of longitudinally stacked molecules of myosin proteins with a molecular weight of approximately 500,000 daltons and are held parallel and in register by centrally located connections at the M line. A rodlike tail, approximately 1300 nm in length, lies along the filament, and a globular bilobed head forms bridgelike outcroppings from the filament that can form a cross bridge which interacts with actin filaments[15] (Fig. 12–4). Myosin exhibits the ability to split ATP, i.e., it acts as an ATPase that is inhibited by Mg^{++} but activated by small amounts of Ca^{++}.[16] When myosin combines with actin, it forms an actomyosin complex that is enzymatically even more active in its ability to split ATP and is stimulated by both Mg^{++} and Ca^{++}. This constitutes the enzyme which is physiologically active in force development. The myosin molecule can be broken down by the proteolytic enzyme trypsin into two fragments, *light meromyosin* and *heavy meromyosin*. The latter contains bilobed globular heads (Fig. 12–4A), the site of ATPase activity.

Myosin itself can be separated into three isoenzyme components—V$_1$, V$_2$, and V$_3$—which have a different heavy-chain composition.[17,17a] Only two chemically distinct heavy-chain subunits exist, α and β.[18] V$_1$ and V$_3$ comprise $\alpha\alpha$ and $\beta\beta$ while V$_2$ is a heterodimer, $\alpha\beta$. Myosin ATPase and intrinsic muscle speed (V$_{max}$) depend on the proportions of these isoenzymes that are present, V$_1$ being fast and V$_3$ being slow.[19] As noted on page 449, hypertrophied heart muscle has a lowered V$_{max}$ and a greater amount of V$_3$.[18]

The thin filament, 1.0 μ in length in ventricular myocardium, is a double alpha-helix that consists of two strands of *actin*, has a molecular weight of 47,000 daltons and a diameter of 55 nm (Fig. 12–5).[20] Actin filaments course from the Z line through the I band and into the A band (Fig. 12–1C). The A band is the region of the sarcomere where there is overlapping of thick and thin filaments, while the I band contains only thin filaments. In atrial tissue, thin filament length is more variable.[6]

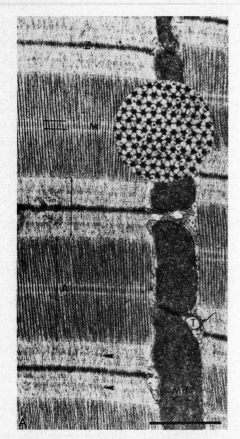

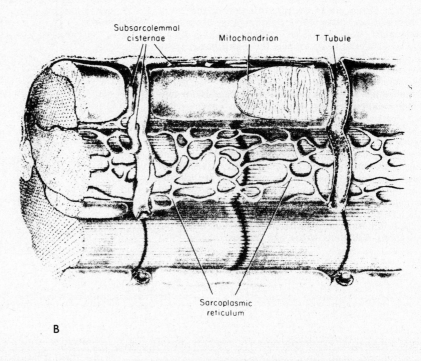

FIGURE 12–3 *A,* Longitudinal section through opossum cardiac muscle; different bands of striated muscle are clearly distinguishable. The A band (A = anisotropic) is composed of thick (myosin) filaments. Between the thick filaments, thin (actin) filaments are visible that slide between the former during contraction. Actin filaments make up the I band (I = isotropic) and are attached to the Z line (Z). Note that in the region of the M line (*inset*) some thin filaments are present equidistant from adjacent filaments. M = M line; arrows = pseudo H or L line; arrowheads = N line; curved arrow = junctional sarcoplasmic reticulum forming interior couplings with transverse tubules (T); Mit = mitochondrion. Bar = 1000 nm. (From Sommer, J. R., and Johnson, E. A.: Ultrastructure of cardiac muscle. *In* Berne, R. M. (ed.): Handbook of Physiology. Section 2, The Cardiovascular System. Vol. I, The Heart. Bethesda, American Physiological Society, 1979, pp. 113–186.)

Inset, Transverse section through region of M line. Note connections between myosin filaments and few actin filaments within the lattice. (From Robinson, T., and Winegrad, S.: Variations of thin filament lengths in heart muscle. Nature *267*:74, 1977.)

B, Schematic of T tubules and sarcoplasmic reticulum of mammalian cardiac muscle. Note how the diffuse tubular network of the sarcoplasmic reticulum forms saccular expansions, the subsarcolemmal cisternae, which are in close apposition to the sarcolemma and T tubules. (From Fawcett, D. W., and McNutt, N. S.: The ultrastructure of the cat myocardium. I. Ventricular papillary muscle. J. Cell Biol. *42*:1, 1969.)

Troponin and *tropomyosin* are regulatory proteins that constitute about 10 per cent of total myofibrillar protein and are associated with the thin filament.[21] Tropomyosin is a rodlike protein, 400 nm in length and 20 to 30 nm in width, with a molecular weight of 70,000 daltons. It comprises two helices, each of which lies slightly off the groove between the actin chains. Tropomyosin forms a continuing strand through the center of the thin filament while the troponin complex is located at intervals of 365 nm. *Troponin* can be separated into three components[22]: (1) troponin C, a "calcium-sensitizing factor" that binds Ca^{++} [23,24]; (2) troponin I, an "inhibitory factor" that inhibits the Mg^{++}-stimulated ATPase of actomyosin; and (3) troponin T, which is necessary for the entire complex to function and serves to allow attachment of the troponin complex to actin and tropomyosin.[24]

In the absence of troponin and tropomyosin, the contractile proteins actin and myosin interact and are fully activated, requiring the presence of only Mg^{++} and ATP to initiate the reaction leading to muscular contraction. When these regulatory proteins are present, however, crossbridge formation between myosin and actin is inhibited.[21] When Ca^{++} is bound to troponin C, the binding of troponin I to actin is inhibited, which in turn causes a conformational change in tropomyosin, so that the latter, instead of inhibiting, now enhances cross-bridge formation. Ca^{++} may thus be considered to be a "derepressor," since it *inactivates* an *inhibitor* of the reaction between actin and myosin. Inhibition of the interaction between actin and myosin is mediated by the ability of the Ca^{++}-troponin complex to alter the configuration of tropomyosin, which in turn changes the exposure of active sites all along the thin filaments.[21] In relaxed muscle, tropomyosin blocks the active sites of actin that react to form cross bridges with myosin.[25] With cellular depolarization, the myoplasmic $[Ca^{++}]$ rises from 10^{-7} to about 10^{-5} M. Ca^{++} is bound to troponin, and the actin rods are drawn toward the center of the sarcomere.[26] Once such a "stroke" is completed, an

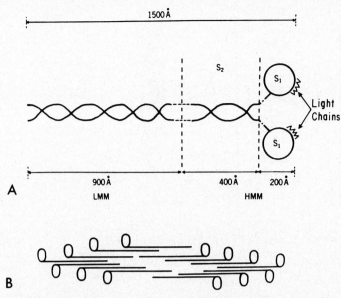

FIGURE 12–4 Structure of the myosin molecule and its aggregation into a thick filament.

A, The myosin molecule. The two-stranded portion of the molecule shows a point of cleavage between light meromyosin (LMM) and heavy meromyosin (HMM). Heavy meromyosin can be cleaved into two portions—an S_2 fragment, which is similar to the LMM portion of the molecule, and an S_1 fragment, which contains the ATPase portion of the molecule. Light chains are associated with the S_1 fragment. (From Lowey, S., et al.: Substructure of the myosin molecule. I. Subfragments of myosin by enzymatic degradation. J. Molec. Biol. *42*:1, 1969.)

B, Diagram of the aggregation of myosin filaments into a thick filament. The long portion of the molecule tends to be oriented toward the center of the filament, with the enzymatically active heads of the molecule oriented laterally. Thus, the center of this aggregation will contain no active enzyme sites.

attached myosin head ejects its ATP hydrolysis products, binds another ATP molecule, and detaches from the actin site. The myosin head then returns to its original orientation and the cycle is repeated, the head attaching to a different actin monomer farther along the thin filament[27] (Fig. 12–6). Thus, shortening of cardiac muscle involves a relative change in position of these two sets of filaments, i.e., actin filaments are displaced by the force-generating process at many cross-bridge sites. If the muscle is not permitted to shorten, i.e., during isometric contraction (in the presence of Ca^{++}), the heavy meromyosin does not undergo a conformational change, the cross bridges between ac-

tin and myosin are maintained, and ADP rather than ATP remains bound to myosin.

EXCITATION-CONTRACTION COUPLING: THE ROLE OF CALCIUM

Since the classic experiments of Ringer in 1882, it has been appreciated that cardiac contraction depends on the presence of Ca^{++}.[28] Heart muscle contains 2.5 mmol of Ca^{++} per liter of water, which is several hundred times higher than the concentration required for activation.[20] However, the higher $[Ca^{++}]$ within the relaxed cell is not directly available to initiate contraction but is bound to many structures, including the nucleus, mitochondria, sarcolemma, T system, and particularly the SR. As already indicated, Ca^{++} is required at the contractile sites to trigger the contractile process by repressing troponin, the inhibitor of the actin-myosin interaction. The key event in the initiation of contraction then is the rise in sarcoplasmic $[Ca^{++}]$.[29] The importance of this event had been suspected for many years, but there was no *direct* evidence for it in cardiac muscle until Allen and Blinks succeeded in the difficult task of using the photoprotein aequorin as an intracellular indicator of $[Ca^{++}]$ in cardiac muscle.[30,31]

The Ca^{++} flowing into the cell does not appear to activate the contractile system directly but rather is stored in the membrane sites within the cell, i.e., the T system and the SR (Fig. 12–7). The Ca^{++} that actually activates the contractile system appears to be stored in the cisternae of the SR, which have the capacity to bind Ca^{++} actively and to store it in a bound form within their lumina.[31] A minute amount of Ca^{++}, which enters the cell during the plateau of the action potential but is insufficient to stimulate the contractile apparatus, may be capable of releasing a much larger quantity of Ca^{++} from the SR, allowing activation of the contractile system. This Ca^{++}-mediated release of Ca^{++} has been termed "regenerative" or "calcium-induced" calcium release.[32,33] According to this concept, depolarization of the cell membrane causes release of Ca^{++} from a store, SR_1 (the terminal cisternae of the SR), into the cytoplasm; Ca^{++} binding by troponin molecules results in contractile activity; relaxation is brought about by the active uptake of Ca^{++} into the temporary store, SR_2 (area of the SR adjacent to the contractile proteins), and from there the Ca^{++} eventually returns to SR_1. Thus, in

FIGURE 12–5 Structure and relations of the thick (*A*) and thin (*B*) filaments. The active myosin bridges turn progressively as one moves across the filament, with a complete revolution every 429 Å. The thin filament is composed of a double-chained alpha helix of actin molecules. The troponin complex is located at every seventh actin site, while the tropomyosin molecule lies close to the ridge between the two strands of actin. Thus, each strand of seven molecules of actin is associated with one troponin complex and one long molecule of tropomyosin, which extends the length of these seven molecules of actin. (Modified from Perry, S. V.: The control of muscular contraction. Symp. Soc. Exp. Biol. *27*:531, 1973.)

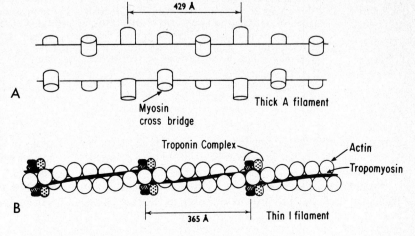

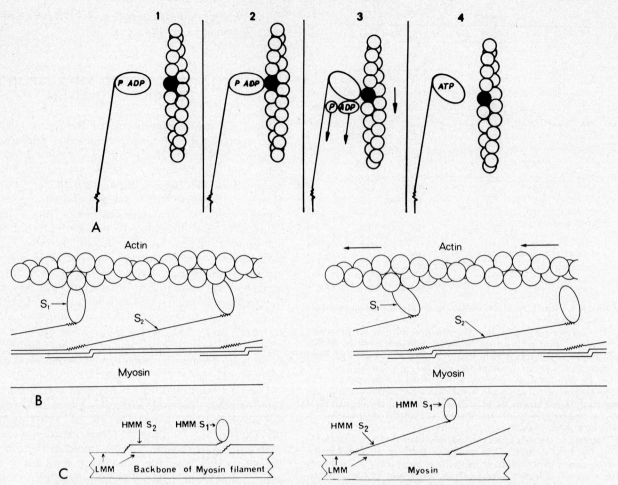

FIGURE 12–6   *A,* A possible four-stage cross-bridge cycle based on the kinetic studies of Lymn and Taylor* and the structural studies summarized by H. E. Huxley.[26] The object on the left in each section of the diagram represents the S_2 tail and S_1 head of a heavy meromyosin molecule, which is joined to the myosin filament at the base of the S_2 rod; the S_1 head (depicted here as a single head) contains ATPase. The actin filament is shown on the right. Rotation of the bridge while attached to actin moves the actin filament along. Probably ADP is released during this part of the cycle. The binding of ATP to the new empty nucleotide binding site releases the bridge and restores it to the right-angle conformation. During this process ATP is hydrolyzed; concomitantly, the affinity for actin is raised, leading to a rebinding and repetition of the cycle. (From Holmes, K. C.: The myosin cross-bridge as revealed by structure studies. *In* Riecker, G., et al. (eds.): Myocardial Failure. Berlin, Springer-Verlag, 1977, pp. 16–27.)

B, An active change in the angle of attachment of cross-bridges (S_1 subunits) to actin filaments could produce relative sliding movements between filaments maintained at constant lateral separation. Bridges can act asynchronously, since subunit and helical periodicities differ in the actin and myosin filaments. *Left,* The left-hand bridge has just attached; the right-hand bridge is already partly tilted. *Right,* The left-hand bridge has just reached the end of its working stroke; the right-hand bridge has already detached and will probably not be able to attach to this actin filament again until further sliding brings the helically arranged sites on the actin filament into a favorable orientation. (From Huxley, H. E., and Haselgrove, J. C.: The structural basis of contraction in muscle and its study by rapid x-ray diffraction methods. *In* Riecker, G., et al. (eds.): Myocardial Failure. Berlin, Springer-Verlag, 1977, pp. 4–15.)

C, In order to explain the binding of cross-bridges (S_1) to actin over a range of filament spacings, Huxley[26] envisaged the S_2 part of heavy meromyosin acting as a stiff, light rod with hinges at both ends. The S_1 is thereby allowed to be closer to either the myosin filament or the actin filament, depending on the state of the muscle. (From Holmes, K. C.: The myosin cross-bridge as revealed by structure studies. *In* Riecker, G., et al. (eds.): Myocardial Failure. Berlin, Springer-Verlag, 1977, pp. 16–27.)

---

*Lymn, R. W., and Taylor, E. W.: Mechanism of adenosine triphosphate hydrolysis by actomyosin. Biochemisty *10*:4617, 1971.

cardiac muscle, SR_l is considered to be a labile store, the Ca^{++} content of which determines the inotropic state of the muscle.[33,34]

Studies with the aequorin technique in atrial and ventricular muscle have shown that changes in the rate or pattern of stimulation, in extracellular $[Ca^{++}]$, and in catecholamines all produce a greater increase in cytoplasmic $[Ca^{++}]$.[30] Catecholamines differ from the other inotropic interventions in that they produce a smaller increase in tension production than would be expected from the increase in the cytoplasmic [Ca^{++}], presumably by reducing the sensitivity of the contractile system to Ca^{++}. This decrease in sensitivity results from an increase in the degree of phosphorylation of troponin that is brought about by the cyclic AMP–induced activation of a protein kinase.[31]

As presented in detail on pages 610 to 617, the action potential for cardiac cells is generated by the movement of ions across the cell membrane, which in turn is controlled by variations in membrane permeability and ion concentration gradient in a manner similar to that occurring in nerve cells.[35,35a] The action potential of ventricular myocardium has two components, the spike and the plateau; a large fast inward Na$^+$ current passing through "fast Na$^+$

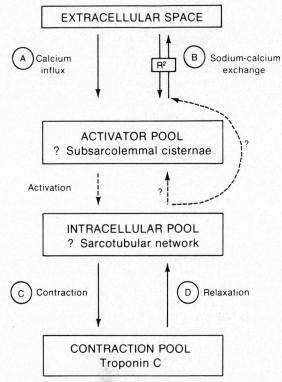

channels" is responsible for the early spike, while Ca^{++} influx into the myocardial cell occurs during the plateau phase of the action potential through a separate set of "slow channels" that are permeable primarily to Ca^{++}.[36] The latter are blocked by the organic Ca^{++}-channel blocking agents such as verapamil, nifedipine, diltiazem, and their analogs[37,,38,38a] (p. 1350) and by manganese ion, lanthanum ion, and acidosis; additional Ca^{++} channels are recruited by beta-adrenergic stimulation. Total Ca^{++} within the cell is also affected by an exchange of more than 2Na$^+$ for each Ca^{++} across the sarcolemma, the energy for which is supplied by the Na$^+$ gradient generated by the sodium pump.[39] Ca^{++} removal from the cell is enhanced when the Na$^+$ gradient is increased, and it is reduced (leading to intracellular Ca^{++} accumulation) when the gradient diminishes. The latter effect may explain the positive inotropic effect of lowering extracellular [Na$^+$] or of inhibiting the Na$^+$,K$^+$-stimulated ATPase with digitalis, which elevates intracellular [Na$^+$]; both these interventions alter the transmembrane Na$^+$ gradient and elevate intracellular [Ca^{++}] (p. 510).

As has already been pointed out, the absolute quantity of Ca^{++} that crosses the sarcolemma during the plateau (phase 2) of the action potential, i.e., during the slow inward current, is relatively small and is incapable in and of itself of bringing about full activation of the contractile apparatus. Instead, the major portion of the Ca^{++} used to activate concentration is stored within the cell, largely in the SR, in its subsarcolemmal cisternae (Fig. 12–7), or on the inner surface of the sarcolemma itself.[40] This Ca^{++} diffuses toward the myofibrils and binds to troponin, which, together with tropomyosin but in the absence of Ca^{++}, prevents the interaction between heavy meromyosin and actin. The number of contractile sites activated and therefore the resultant force generated are directly related to the quantity of Ca^{++} present in the vicinity of the myofibrils, which in turn ultimately depends on the influx of Ca^{++} that accompanied the action potential.[41] This influx, in turn, is a function of the extracellular [Ca^{++}], the duration of the action potential,[42] and the number of action potentials per unit time.[34]

Relaxation of cardiac muscle results from a cessation of the inward slow Ca^{++} current coupled with the uptake and storage of Ca^{++} by the SR, in which is embedded a 100,000-dalton membrane-bound protein, phospholamban, which spans the lipid bilayer (Fig. 12–2). This protein, a Ca^{++}-stimulated Mg-ATPase, has a very high affinity for Ca^{++} and is responsible for the active transport of Ca^{++} from the cytoplasm into the lumen of the SR. Thus, during repolarization, the SR in the presence of ATP avidly accumulates myoplasmic Ca^{++} against a concentration gradient, so that intracellular [Ca^{++}] falls to below 10^{-7} M and Ca^{++} detaches from the troponin, resulting in inhibition of the interactions between actin and myosin and hence in relaxation.[42]

INOTROPIC EFFECTS AND CALCIUM KINETICS. There is evidence that (1) the total tension developed, (2) the rate of tension development, and (3) the rate of tension decline during relaxation can be related, respectively, to (1) the quantity of Ca^{++} made available for binding to troponin, (2) the rate of Ca^{++} delivery to troponin, and (3) the rate at which Ca^{++} is removed from

FIGURE 12–7 Calcium fluxes that participate in cardiac excitation-contraction coupling represent movement of calcium between the extracellular space, an activator pool that may be related to the subsarcolemmal cisternae, an intracellular pool that is probably within the sarcoplasmic reticulum, and a contraction pool that represents calcium bound to troponin. Calcium influx (*A*) is a "downhill" flux across the sarcolemma that occurs largely as the electrogenic slow inward current. A sodium-calcium exchange (*B*) can transport calcium in either direction across the sarcolemma but is involved mainly in the "uphill" transport of calcium out of the cell in a nonelectrogenic exchange for sodium, which moves down a concentration gradient into the cell. The intracellular pool that supplies calcium to the sodium-calcium exchange has not been identified but may be related to the sarcoplasmic reticulum. A relatively small calcium flux from the activator pool may trigger the release of a larger amount of calcium from the intracellular pool ("calcium-triggered calcium release") as shown by the arrow labeled "activation." Contraction (*C*) occurs when a large amount of calcium is released from the intracellular pool, most likely when an increase in the calcium permeability of the sarcoplasmic reticulum allows this ion to become available for binding to calcium-binding sites on troponin. Relaxation (*D*) occurs when the ATP-dependent calcium pump of the sarcoplasmic reticulum pumps calcium back into the intracellular membrane system. The resulting fall in cytosolic Ca^{++} concentration causes calcium to become dissociated from its binding site on troponin. (From Katz, A. M.: Physiology of the Heart. New York, Raven Press, 1977.)

troponin.[43] Many interventions that augment or depress the contractile state of heart muscle are associated with—and indeed are caused by—alterations in Ca^{++} movement and concentrations in heart muscle.[44,45] These include the force-frequency relation,[46] i.e., the increase in contractility resulting from an increase in the frequency of contraction[47,48]; postextrasystolic potentiation (a special instance of the force-frequency relation)[49–52]; and pharmacological agents such as the cardiac glycosides (p. 510), sympathomimetic amines,[53–55] and xanthines[56]—all of which improve contractility—and agents such as beta-adrenergic blockers, some Ca^{++}-channel blockers, quinidine and other Type I antiarrhythmic agents, and barbiturates—all of which depress it. Experiments on skinned muscle cells suggest that even moderate acidosis causes a reduction in the quantity of Ca^{++} released from the SR of cardiac muscle, accounting in part for the negative inotropic effect of acidosis.[57]

One proposed mechanism of action of *sympathomimetic amines* is shown in Figure 12–8. These drugs are thought to act on beta receptors on the cardiac sarcolemma; this process leads to the activation of adenylate cyclase, a membrane-bound enzyme that catalyzes the production of cyclic AMP from ATP in the presence of Ca^{++}. Cyclic AMP, in turn, activates a class of enzymes, the cyclic AMP–dependent protein kinases, which phosphorylate a number of cellular proteins. Activation of a protein kinase by an increase in cAMP resulting from beta-adrenergic stimulation of the heart may induce phosphorylation of a protein located near the Ca^{++} channel and regulate its open state. Such Ca^{++} channels, which are recruited by beta-adrenergic agonists, are termed "receptor-operated channels." Another protein, *phospholamban*, when phosphorylated by cAMP-dependent protein kinase, stimulates the rate of Ca^{++} uptake by the SR.[53] There is also some evidence that beta-adrenergic agonists decrease the sensitivity of the contractile system to Ca^{++} as a consequence of phosphorylation of troponin by a cyclic AMP–activated protein kinase.[55,58] Katz has proposed that the reactions summarized in Figure 12–8, resulting from myocardial beta-receptor stimulation, increase the rate of Ca^{++} transport by the SR, which in turn is responsible for both enhancement of tension development and an increased rate of relaxation.

In *summary*, beta-adrenergic agonists augment Ca^{++} influx across the sarcolemma by recruiting additional (receptor-activated) slow channels. These substances do not appear to affect the *rate* at which the Ca^{++} channels open but rather they increase the *number* of open channels.[37] The increase in the rate of relaxation of tension produced by cyclic AMP appears to be caused by enhancement of Ca^{++} accumulation by the SR.[59] Theophylline and related compounds inhibit phosphodiesterase, an enzyme responsible for the breakdown of cyclic AMP, which has an effect similar to that of catecholamines.[56] In addition, xanthines may increase the sensitivity of the contractile system to a given amount of Ca^{++}.[30]

Another cyclic nucleotide, cyclic 3′,5′-guanosine monophosphate (GMP), has been identified in the myocardium.[60] The reduction of the contractile state induced by acetylcholine is accompanied by significant *increases* in cyclic GMP, which appears to mediate effects opposing those of cyclic AMP.[61]

CONTROL OF CYTOPLASMIC [Ca^{++}]. As already indicated, cytoplasmic [Ca^{++}] is critical to the contractile state of the heart. Therefore, it is useful to recapitulate the determinants of myoplasmic [Ca^{++}].[38] At least seven mechanisms have been identified, and these are shown diagrammatically in Figure 12–9.

1. The inward movement of Ca^{++} along its concentration gradient, across the sarcolemma, i.e., the slow inward current through the Ca^{++} channels (Fig. 12–9, Mechanism 1A and 1B).[62] Ca^{++}-channel blockers act at these sites.

2. Since small quantities of Ca^{++} enter the cardiac cell with each contraction, there must be some mechanism for removal of Ca^{++} from the cell so that [Ca^{++}] remains constant in a steady state. A bidirectional Na^+-Ca^{++} exchange system mediates Ca^{++} movement across the sarcolemma. Energy required by this system for moving Ca^{++} out of the cell against a concentration gradient may be provided by the downhill movement of Na^+ into the cell along its electrochemical gradient. The direction of this exchange depends upon the relative concentrations of extracellular and intracellular Na^+ and Ca^{++}. Thus, when cardiac glycosides inhibit Na^+,K^+-ATPase and thereby inhibit the pump responsible for Na^+-K^+ exchange (Fig. 12–9, Mechanism 2A), intracellular [Na^+] is elevated. Ca^{++} enters the cell as a consequence of Na^+-Ca^{++} exchange, and this brings about a positive inotropic effect.[63]

3. The sarcolemma possesses a Ca^{++}-ATPase that extrudes Ca^{++} from the cell in an energy-requiring process (Fig. 12–9, Mechanism 3).[12]

4. A Ca^{++}-stimulated Mg-ATPase in the membrane of

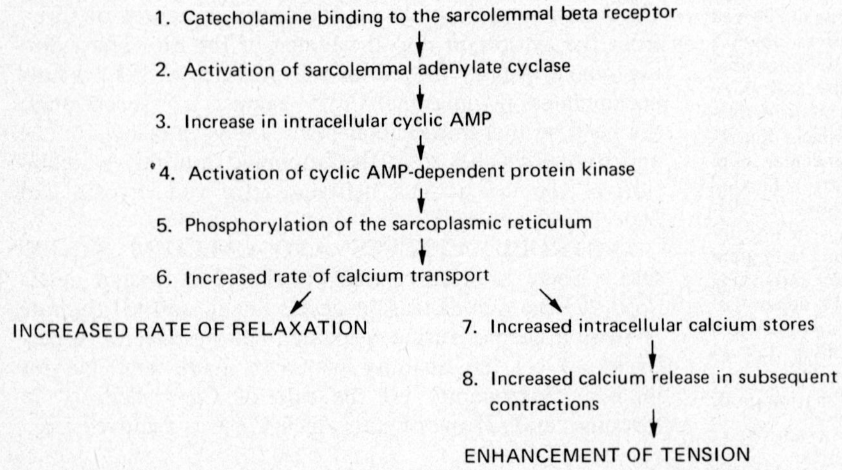

1. Catecholamine binding to the sarcolemmal beta receptor
↓
2. Activation of sarcolemmal adenylate cyclase
↓
3. Increase in intracellular cyclic AMP
↓
4. Activation of cyclic AMP-dependent protein kinase
↓
5. Phosphorylation of the sarcoplasmic reticulum
↓
6. Increased rate of calcium transport
↙ ↘
INCREASED RATE OF RELAXATION   7. Increased intracellular calcium stores
↓
8. Increased calcium release in subsequent contractions
↓
ENHANCEMENT OF TENSION

FIGURE 12–8 One mechanism by which catecholamines may modify the tension and rate of relaxation of the myocardium. This mechanism does not include the increased Ca^{++} influx into the cell resulting from catecholamine-stimulated recruitment of receptor-operated Ca^{++} channels (see text and Figure 12–9, Mechanism 1B). (From Katz, A. M., et al.: Regulation of myocardial cell function by agents that increase cyclic AMP production in the heart. *In* Fishman, A. P. (ed.): Heart Failure. Washington, D.C., Hemisphere Publishing Corp., 1978, pp. 11–28.)

CONTROL OF [Ca^{++}] IN MYOCARDIUM

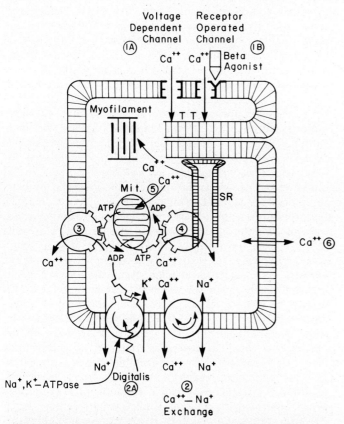

FIGURE 12–9 Determinants of [Ca^{++}] in myocardium. Numbers in circles denote the mechanisms affecting intracellular [Ca^{++}] described in the text. TT = transverse tubule; SR = sarcolemmic reticulum; Mit = mitochondrion. (From Braunwald, E.: Mechanisms of action of calcium channel blocking agents. N. Engl. J. Med. *307:* 1618, 1982.)

the SR (Fig. 12–9, Mechanism 4) transports Ca^{++} into the lumen of the SR and sequesters it there through an energy-requiring process.

5. Ca^{++} can also be taken up and released by other intracellular structures, particularly the mitochondria (Fig. 12–9, Mechanism 5) and internal aspect of the sarcolemma. When intracellular [Ca^{++}] rises, ATP, generated by the mitochondria, is involved in the uptake of Ca^{++} by these organelles; excess uptake of mitochondrial Ca^{++} in turn interferes with mitochondrial function.[64]

6. A variety of ionophores can effect the selective movement of Ca^{++} along its concentration gradient directly across the sarcolemma, i.e., not through the slow channels (Fig. 12–9, Mechanism 6).

7. The buffering of Ca^{++} by intracellular proteins such as calmodulin, troponin C, and myosin-P light chains also regulates myoplasmic [Ca^{++}].

Since cardiac contraction and relaxation are critically dependent on precisely timed modulations of myoplasmic [Ca^{++}], it is evident that abnormalities of *any* of the systems just described can affect myocardial performance.

THE CALCIUM CHANNEL

Although relatively little is known of the actual structure of ion channels in the sarcolemma, since these chan-

nels are highly specific for a given ion species, it can be assumed that the aqueous "pore" within the channel is provided with a selectivity filter that defines the type of ion that can pass through a given type of channel (Fig. 12–10). Since ion channels can be open or shut depending on the intracellular voltage, the channel also has voltage sensors, i.e., charged regions of the channel proteins that determine the state of channel "gates" as open or shut.[65]

When a propagated wave of depolarization approaches the membrane region containing the Ca^{++} channel, a reduction of membrane potential (i.e., a decrease in the electronegativity of the cell interior) causes the activation gate to open, permitting Ca^{++} to cross the membrane and pass into the cell. The gate closes when the interior of the cell has again become electronegative, i.e., when the resting level of transmembrane potential has been restored. Since the movement of Ca^{++} through these channels is controlled by electrical potentials, they have been termed voltage-dependent channels (Fig. 12–9, Mechanism 1A).

An important feature of many Ca^{++} channels is their sensitivity to control by sarcolemmal receptors. Beta$_1$-ago-

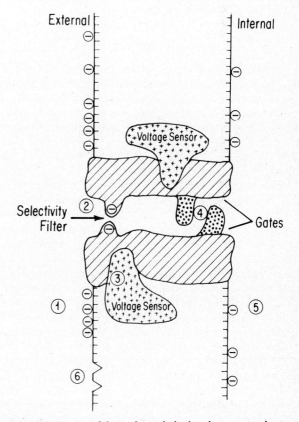

FIGURE 12–10 A calcium channel depicted as a membrane pore containing within it a negatively charged site (2) of dimensions and charge density appropriate to act as a "selectivity filter" to distinguish between different cations. Voltage sensor components (3) confer voltage-dependence on channel opening and closing and channel gates (4) determine the open or shut character of the channel. Negatively charged sites on the external (1) and internal (5) membrane surfaces serve as cation binding sites, particularly for divalent cations, by which transmembrane potential detected by voltage sensor components may be modulated. A receptor site (6) is shown adjacent to the channel. (From Triggle, D. J.: *In* Flaim, S. F., and Zelis, R. (eds.): Calcium Channel Blockers: Mechanism of Action and Clinical Applications. Baltimore, Urban and Schwarzenberg, 1982.)

nists in cardiac muscle (and alpha-adrenergic agonists in vascular smooth muscle) increase Ca^{++} influx via the slow inward current, thereby enhancing contractility, frequency and conduction velocity in the heart in the case of $beta_1$ receptors, and the degree of contraction of arterioles in the case of alpha receptors on vascular smooth muscle. Activation of adrenergic receptors does not appear to increase Ca^{++} influx by increasing the size of the Ca^{++} channels or the rates at which their gates open or close but rather appears to recruit an additional number of active channels.[66] It has been proposed that when endogenous adrenergic nervous activity is low or is blocked by an adrenergic-receptor blocker, a certain proportion of the Ca^{++} channels is unable to open in response to a depolarizing stimulus. According to this theory, physiological stimuli or drugs that activate adrenergic receptors elevate cyclic AMP levels in the myocardium, which in turn facilitates transfer of a phosphate in ATP to form a phosphoester bond with one of the proteins in an inactive Ca^{++} channel, permitting the channel to participate in Ca^{++} entry into the cell. As a consequence, adrenergic influences increase Ca^{++} influx across the sarcolemma; the channels acted upon by receptor-mediated events are termed receptor-operated channels (Fig. 12–9, Mechanism 1B).

CALCIUM-CHANNEL BLOCKERS

A number of inorganic cations such as manganese, cobalt, and lanthanum can function as general Ca^{++} antagonists and are effective in blocking a wide variety of Ca^{++}-dependent processes. This nonselectivity of action probably arises from the ability of these cations to substitute for Ca^{++} at a variety of Ca^{++} binding sites. They probably block the function of all Ca^{++} channels or actually enter the cell, where they substitute for Ca^{++} at the intracellular Ca^{++} receptors. Of far more significance to clinical medicine are the organic Ca^{++}-channel blockers. The pioneering work of Fleckenstein[67] revealed that these compounds can produce selective blockade of the slow inward current and produce electromechanical uncoupling in heart muscle.

Since organic Ca^{++}-channel blockers exert their actions at nanomolar concentrations and exhibit stereospecificity, it appears likely that they are recognized by specific structures of the Ca^{++} channel.[37,68–70] However, the diversity of molecular structures of Ca^{++}-channel blockers is consistent with differing modes and sites of action rather than with the tight binding of these drugs to a specific receptor, analogous to the receptor that binds beta-adrenergic blockers.

The action of nifedipine is consistent with the drug actually "plugging" Ca^{++} channels. In contrast, verapamil, and to a lesser extent diltiazem, are "use-dependent," i.e., their Ca^{++}-blocking activities are a function of the frequency of contraction so that they cause an inversion of the myocardium's normal force-frequency relationship, an increase in contraction frequency causing a reduction rather than an augmentation of contraction.[65] This situation is analogous to the better investigated, frequency-dependent inhibition of Na^+ channels by local anesthetics and Type I antiarrhythmic drugs and suggests that verapamil interacts preferentially with the depolarized, inactivated state of the Ca^{++} channel.

CARDIAC ADRENERGIC RECEPTORS

In 1967 Lands et al. demonstrated that beta-adrenergic receptors could be classified into two types: $beta_1$ receptors, which mediate cardiac stimulation and lipolysis, and $beta_2$ receptors, which mediate relaxation of vascular and bronchial smooth muscle.[71] The effects of catecholamines on the contractile and electrical properties of the heart are mediated predominantly by beta-adrenergic receptors, embedded in the sarcolemma (see Fig. 12–2). As determined by physiologic and radioligand-binding studies, the large majority of myocardial beta receptors are of the $beta_1$ subtype; likewise, the inotropic effects of beta-adrenergic agonists are mediated predominantly, if not exclusively, by $beta_1$ receptors.[71a] However, it has been suggested that chronotropy, i.e., sinoatrial rate, may be mediated by $beta_2$ receptors located in the sinoatrial node.[72] $Beta_1$-adrenergic receptors are located on effector cells in proximity to adrenergic synapses, while $beta_2$ receptors are located at some distance from the synapses.[73] $Beta_1$ receptors appear to respond primarily to neuronally released norepinephrine, whereas $beta_2$ receptors respond preferentially to circulating epinephrine from the adrenal medulla (and to exogenously injected agonists). Also, as in the case of alpha-adrenergic receptors (p. 914), beta-adrenergic receptors located presynaptically on the nerve fiber regulate norepinephrine release. However, as opposed to presynaptic alpha receptors, which have an inhibitory role, stimulation of presynaptic beta receptors stimulates release of norepinephrine.[74] Whereas ventricular receptors are exclusively $beta_1$,[75] approximately 25 per cent of atrial receptors are of the $beta_2$ subtype. Atrial $beta_2$ receptors, presumably located within the sinoatrial node, may mediate the chronotropic effects of catecholamines on the heart.

It appears that catecholamines exert at least some of their effects through myocardial alpha-adrenergic receptors.[75a] As with myocardial beta-adrenergic receptors, stimulation of myocardial alpha receptors augments myocardial contractility.[76,77] The subtype of myocardial alpha-adrenergic receptors is somewhat controversial, although most evidence favors the presence of only $alpha_1$ receptors.[77] A number of observations suggest that the molecular mechanism by which alpha-adrenergic receptors exert a positive inotropic effect is different from that of beta receptors. Whereas stimulation of beta-adrenergic receptors increases intracellular cyclic AMP, which is thought to mediate subsequent events, stimulation of alpha-adrenergic receptors has no effect on cyclic AMP production in myocardium. Also, alpha receptor–mediated effects on inotropy are more sensitive to the extracellular concentration of Ca^{++} or blockade of Ca^{++} influx by Ca-channel blockers than are beta-mediated effects. Based on these observations, it has been suggested that alpha-adrenergic receptors mediate an increase in inotropy almost exclusively by means of an increase in Ca^{++} influx.[78]

MECHANICS OF CARDIAC CONTRACTION

Cardiac contraction can be readily studied in vitro by mounting a mammalian papillary muscle, trabeculae carneae, or strip of atrial myocardium in an oxygenated, physiological salt solution.[79–82] The ends of the muscle are fixed, and the muscle is activated by electrical stimulation. The

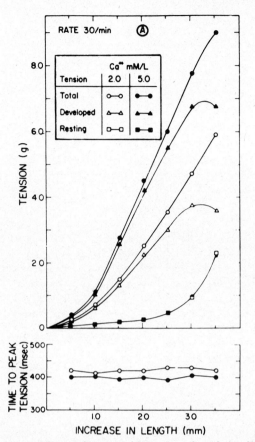

FIGURE 12–11 Effects of increased [Ca++] on the relation between muscle length and tension in an isolated cat papillary muscle. The [Ca++] in the perfusing medium has been increased from 2.0 mM to 5.0 mM. The relation between resting muscle length and tension is not altered. However, the development of tension at any given muscle length is increased at the higher [Ca++] concentration, although L_{max} is not altered. Total tension is the sum of developed and resting tension.

strength of individual isometric cardiac contractions is modified by two major influences: (1) a *change in initial muscle length*, or preload, induced by a change in the passive stretch of the muscle; and (2) a *change in contractility or inotropic state*.[80]

Development of active tension during isometric contraction by the myocardium can be altered by changing initial muscle length, and the relation between these two variables constitutes the length–active tension curve (Fig. 12–11). When a change in contractility is induced by what is termed an *inotropic intervention*, such as the addition of Ca++, digitalis, or norepinephrine to the medium, the peak force developed increases, the rate of force development rises, and the time to reach peak force shortens; these changes in contractile activity occur at a constant preload. Inotropic interventions do not generally alter the relation between the preload (the tension placed on the resting muscle) and the length of the muscle, i.e., the length–resting tension relation, an expression of the resting stiffness of the cardiac muscle.

By adjusting the initial degree of stretch placed on resting muscle, a length of the muscle can be found at which the resultant force development is maximal when the muscle is stimulated to contract isometrically; this length is termed L_{max}. The relation between developed isometric ten-

sion (i.e., the increment in tension occurring during contraction) and initial muscle length is termed the *length–active tension relation* (Fig. 12–11). By definition, the length–active tension relation at lengths below L_{max} is termed the *ascending limb* of the curve and the portion above L_{max}, the *descending limb* of the curve. When initial muscle length is altered slightly on either side of L_{max}, active tension is altered substantially; a 10 per cent reduction in muscle length below L_{max} may be responsible for a 30 per cent decrease in actively developed tension.

THE FORCE-VELOCITY RELATION. In order to analyze not only isometric contractions but also the shortening characteristics of the muscle, one end of the muscle is attached to a lever system and its degree of shortening is measured (Fig. 12–12*A*). The preload, a small weight placed on the opposite end of the lever, stretches the passive muscle; a stop is then adjusted above the tip of the lever and any weight added to the lever over and above the preload, termed the *afterload*, may be sensed by the muscle *after* the onset of contraction (Fig. 12–12*B*). The extent and maximum velocity of shortening for each contraction depend on the load (Fig. 12–12*C*), and the inverse relation between the tension (force) developed and the velocity of contraction constitutes the *force-velocity curve* (Fig. 12–12 *D*). When the load is greatest, there is no shortening, i.e., the muscle develops maximal force during isometric contraction (P_0). Conversely, when the load is smallest, the velocity of shortening is greatest. Although the velocity of shortening with zero load cannot be measured directly, since the preload provides for initial length, extrapolation of the curve back to zero load allows approximation of this maximum velocity of unloaded shortening, termed V_{max}.[79-83]

When the *initial muscle length* is altered by increasing the preload, the force-velocity curve is shifted characteristically (Fig. 12–13); the velocity of shortening at any given load is increased as is P_0. However, V_{max} is little altered by a change in initial muscle length. In contrast, when the *contractility* of the papillary muscle is augmented (Fig. 12–14), the rate of tension development is increased, as are the velocity and extent of shortening with a given load.[84] The entire force-velocity curve is shifted upward and to the right with increases in *both* P_0 and V_{max}.[81,82,85]

MUSCLE MODELS

There has been considerable interest in the development of models of muscle contraction, since they provide a method for analyzing contraction of heart muscle[86] as well as some insight into the complexities of ventricular function. Current working models include a *contractile element* (CE), which represents the actively contracting portion of the muscle, arranged in series with a passive elastic component, the *series elastic element* (SE). At rest, CE is considered to be freely extensible, so that resting tension is sustained by another elastic component arranged in parallel, the *parallel elastic component* (PE). Depending on the model chosen, PE spans both CE and SE (Maxwell model) or CE alone (Voight model).

The resting stiffness of cardiac muscle is greater than that of skeletal muscle, but the reasons for this difference are not clear.[87] Myocardial cells are smaller than skeletal muscle cells and therefore possess a relatively greater proportion of stiff sarcolemma per unit weight of tissue; intercellular collagen is also more abundant in heart muscle. The sarcomeres of cardiac muscle resist stretching beyond 2.2 μ, which may also be a factor in the stiffness of PE of heart muscle. An as yet unidentified elastic element, perhaps the protein fibrillin, may reside within the cardiac sarcomeres and be involved in maintaining rigidity.

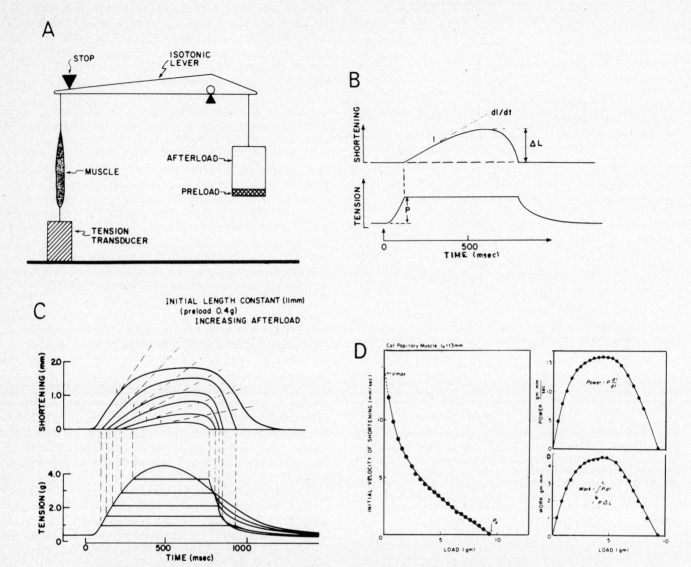

FIGURE 12–12   Use of afterloaded isotonic contractions to obtain force-velocity relations.

A, Diagrammatic representation of an isotonic lever system. A papillary muscle is placed in a bath (not shown) of Krebs-Ringer solution and stimulated by electrodes along its lateral aspect. The lower end of the muscle is attached to an extension from a tension transducer while the upper, free end is attached to the end of a lever system that is free to move. The fulcrum of the lever system is shown toward the right. Initially the stop is not above the tip of the lever, which is above the muscle. A small weight, termed a "preload," is placed on the opposite end of the lever; this preload will stretch the muscle to a length consistent with its resting length-tension relation. The stop is then fixed above the tip of the lever, so that any added weight above the preload will not be sensed by the muscle until it attempts to contract. Additional loads can be added to the preload (i.e., afterloads). Total load equals the sum of the preload and the afterload.

B, Tracings of an afterloaded isotonic contraction. The contraction is shown as a function of time, plotted along the abscissa. After stimulation at time zero, there is a short latent period followed by the generation of isometric force. When the force (P) equals the load, shortening begins, as shown in the upper half of the panel. Maximum velocity is reached shortly after shortening commences, and the tangent to this slope (dl/dt) approximates the maximum velocity of shortening with this particular load. ΔL denotes the extent of shortening. Subsequently the muscle elongates and then relaxes isometrically.

C, Effects of increasing afterloads on the course of tension development and subsequent shortening. Several superimposed contractions are displayed. The muscle develops a force equal to the afterload and thereafter shortens. As the afterload is increased, the velocity of shortening (dashed lines) and the extent of shortening decline.

D, Velocity of shortening plotted as a function of load: the force-velocity relation. As the load is increased, the velocity of shortening decreases. When the load is so high that no external shortening is recorded, velocity is zero, and the force is equivalent to the isometric contraction (P_0). When the curve is extrapolated back to zero load, V_{max} is obtained. Also shown at right are power (*top*) and work (*bottom*) curves as a function of increasing afterloads. Both power and work are zero when the load is zero or with isometric contractions, and both curves peak at an intermediate load. (From Braunwald, E., et al.: Mechanisms of Contraction of the Normal and Failing Heart. 2nd ed. Boston, Little, Brown, 1976.)

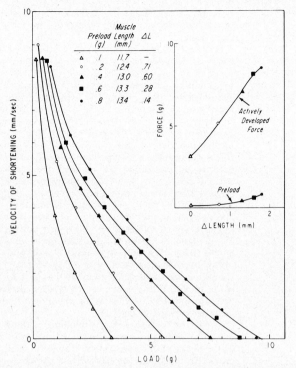

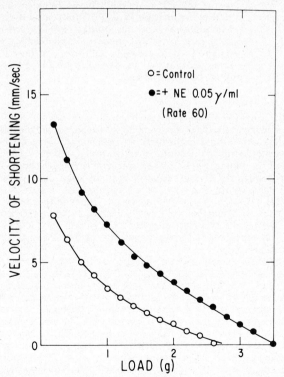

FIGURE 12–13 Relation between peak velocity of afterloaded, isotonic shortening and total load at several initial muscle lengths in a cat papillary muscle. The inset at the right shows the resting and developed active force at these various lengths. When initial muscle length is increased, the actively developed force is augmented, as is the velocity of shortening at any individual load. The maximum velocity of shortening with the preload alone is little altered. Moreover, if these curves were to be extrapolated back to zero load (V_{max}), this value would also show little or no change.

FIGURE 12–14 Effects of the addition of norepinephrine on the force-velocity relation of the cat papillary muscle. Norepinephrine induces an increase in the velocity of shortening at any load, in the maximum force of isometric contraction (P_0), and in the maximum velocity of zero load shortening (V_{max}).

The characteristics of muscular contraction are determined by the time course of activation of CE, its force-generating and shortening properties, and the stiffness of SE. The SE is a "lumped" elasticity, most of it being in elastic connections of the muscle to its points of fixation.

In the simplest model, consisting of only CE and SE, in an *isometric* contraction, with activation of the muscle, the CE shortens, stretching the springlike SE, and the force builds up at the ends of the system in a manner dependent upon the interaction of the shortening properties of the CE and compliance of the SE. On the other hand, in an *afterloaded isotonic* contraction, force is developed as shortening of the CE stretches the SE, until the force equals the load, and the load is then lifted. Muscle shortening occurs with the SE at a fixed length, and the subsequent course of shortening reflects shortening of the CE alone. Viscous elements are identified in the PE of resting heart muscle by the presence of stress relaxation, i.e., a fall in resting tension following a sustained stretch to a long length.

Contraction of muscle depends on its loading. The muscle can be permitted to shorten isotonically with just the preload, i.e., the small load that stretches the resting muscle and sets its initial length. If the ends of the muscle are fixed to prevent shortening, *isometric* force is developed. In the beating heart in vivo, contraction commences isometrically but is followed by shortening against a load, a condition mimicked in the isolated muscle by the *afterloaded isotonic contraction*, in which isometric force develops first and shortening then occurs at a constant force. In such a contraction, force is generated until it equals an imposed load, the *afterload* (Fig. 12–12*B*). The muscle then shortens, bearing the total load (afterload plus preload) until the length–active tension curve is reached. The intensity of the active state then declines; isotonic lengthening, i.e., lengthening at a constant force, occurs first and then the force itself declines. In the intact heart, the load is largely removed during relaxation owing to the closing of the aortic valve. When preload and thus the initial muscle length are increased, both developed force and the extent of afterloaded isotonic shortening are increased. When contractility is stimulated (Fig. 12–11), isometric force development and the extent of afterloaded isotonic muscle and CE shortening are increased. As already pointed out, the *force-velocity relation* obtained from afterloaded isotonic contractions helps to distinguish the two major ways in which cardiac performance is altered[80] (Figs. 12–13 and 12–14).

PROPERTIES OF THE CONTRACTILE ELEMENT

The mechanical activity of the CE reflects the summated contribution of cross bridges between myosin and actin and some form of conformational changes in the heads of the cross bridges, which then generate displacement of the actin filaments (see Fig. 12–6).[88–90] *Active state*, a term adapted from skeletal muscle physiology, has been used to describe the capacity of the CE to shorten in accordance with the force-velocity relation.[85,90,91] It is a mechanical measure of the chemical processes in the CE that generate both force and shortening.

RESTING LENGTH-TENSION RELATIONS

When relaxed heart muscle is stretched progressively, its resting tension increases slightly at first and then rises more markedly (Fig. 12–11). The stiffness of the resting muscle is represented by the slope of the curve relating the change in resting tension (ΔP) to the change in length (ΔL), which is approximately exponential. The resting length-tension relation is not generally altered by interventions that acutely alter the length–active tension curve or the force-velocity-length relation except that ischemia increases the apparent stiffness of the resting muscle (p. 1247), presumably by interfering with relaxation. Marked tachycardia also tends to increase the resting length-tension relation, because relaxation is not complete at the termination of diastole.[92] Aging also causes a significant increase in stiffness; less stress relaxation is exhibited by muscles from old compared to young adult rats, which may account, at least in part, for the age-associated changes in the resting length-tension curve.[93]

FORCE-VELOCITY-LENGTH RELATIONS

The interdependence between force, velocity, and muscle length is demonstrated as a *force-velocity-length diagram*.[94] The projection on the left of each of the panels of Figure 12–15 forms the *force-velocity*

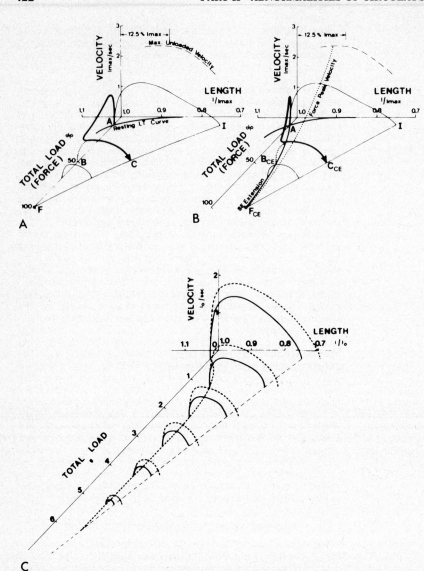

FIGURE 12–15 Three-dimensional representation of the force-velocity-length relations in the cat papillary muscle.

A, The velocity-length relations of isotonic contractions obtained at L_{max} have been replotted as a function of total load. The course of velocity of a hypothetical afterloaded isotonic contraction is superimposed (thick line). The velocity of shortening during the isometric phase of the contractions has been theoretically derived from a two-component muscle model. Velocity rises rapidly to the level appropriate for the plane of this three-dimensional composite. During isometric contraction the velocity of the contractile element falls as force rises. This velocity is not seen but is expressed in terms of the rate of force development, i.e., dP/dt. At point B, the force development equals the load, and external shortening can then proceed between points B and C. Velocity of shortening between B and C depends on the level of the force-velocity-length plane. The velocity-length relation and the maximum unloaded velocity of shortening (V_{max}) is shown on the right. Projection to the right of the plane of the force-velocity-length relation provides the force-velocity relation, while the length-tension curve is reflected on the base.

B, The force-velocity-length relations of the same muscle as shown in *A* after correction for extension of the series elastic component. The entire curve is moved to the right. The dashed line shown on the plane created by the force-velocity-length relation represents the force-velocity curve as obtained from afterloaded contractions.

C, Effect of a positive inotropic intervention (dashed line) on the force-velocity-length relation. The velocity of shortening at any given muscle length is augmented, so that the entire surface relating force-velocity and length is increased, and the extent of shortening is augmented. The projection of this surface to the right would be characterized by an increase in V_{max}. (From Brutsaert, D. L., and Sonnenblick, E. H.: Cardiac muscle mechanics in the evaluation of myocardial contractility and pump function: Problems, concepts and directions. Progr. Cardiovasc. Dis. *16*:337, 1973, by permission of Grune and Stratton.)

relation, the projection to the rear forms the *length-velocity* relation, and the base of this diagram represents the *length-tension* relation. During contraction, the muscle moves in a predictable manner across the surface, describing this relation between force, length, and velocity. With activation, the contractile elements rise onto a hypothetical force-velocity curve, with force increasing and the velocity of the contractile element decreasing until the afterload is reached, after which shortening proceeds across the surface. The force-velocity-length relation is relatively independent of time during a major portion of the shortening phase of contraction.[95] However, late in the course of contraction, shortening diverges from the velocity-length phase planes, indicating that the active state is declining.

Myocardial contractility can be described by the surface of the plane describing the force-velocity-length relation (Fig. 12–15).[94] The full activity of cardiac muscle commences rapidly after stimulation. The surface of the plane describing the force-velocity-length relation is reached rapidly, and its position may be considered to be a definition of the contractile state, since the position of this surface is essentially independent of preload and afterload. The duration of the active state is sufficient to allow shortening to occur to the same end-systolic length, regardless of the initial length if afterload and contractility remain constant.[96] This property of cardiac muscle is crucial to the use of end-systolic cardiac dimensions or volume in the assessment of cardiac contractility (p. 476).[97,98]

While force-velocity curves (Figs. 12–13 and 12–14) appear to provide valid descriptors of the contractile state in a wide variety of circumstances, an important theoretical limitation of such curves must be appreciated; the measurements to obtain each point in the curve are not made at the same time during contraction, so that the intensity of the active state might differ for each point. Thus, when the afterload is increased, velocity is measured later in time after the stimulus for contraction, and these measurements may occur at differing lengths of CE, thus distorting the enscribed curve from the "true" force-velocity curve.[94] The extrapolated V_{max} therefore could have been misleading. However, when the effects of these variables have been considered carefully, with unloading of the muscle to near zero external load once contraction has begun, the conclusions previously reached from simple afterloaded contractions have been supported.[95]

When initial muscle length is reduced by 10 per cent, actively developed tension falls about 30 per cent, but unloaded velocity does not change. In intact muscle, this dependency of force development on the length of heart muscle is related to the compliance of SE.[94] When cardiac muscle is activated and made to contract isometrically, the development of force is accompanied by an internal shortening, so that when maximal isometric force is reached, CE is actually substantially shorter and SE is longer than prior to activation. Indeed, sarcomeres actually do shorten substantially during "apparent" isometric contraction.[99-102] In contrast, isotonic contractions against very small loads do not involve the development of force, stretching of SE, and shortening of CE at the expense of SE; hence, shortening of CE is directly translated into shortening of the muscle, and velocities are measured at longer sarcomere lengths.[99] In studies in which sarcomere dynamics have been measured directly,[100] it appears that only a minor proportion of the SE is associated with the contractile machinery and cross bridges in heart muscle and that the effective SE largely reflects external elastic connections.

LENGTH-DEPENDENT ACTIVATION

In the foregoing discussion of the mechanics of muscular contraction, it has been generally assumed that inotropic interventions and changes in muscle length are independent regulators of myocardial performance. However, evidence is increasing that both inotropic interventions and changes of muscle length may act primarily through mechanisms that involve Ca^{++} activation.[31,103-108] The traditional view that length and inotropic state are independent regulators of myocardial performance was based on the observation that a decline of tension production occurs at short muscle lengths; this would be expected, because tension is lost as a consequence of the double overlap of the thin filaments in the central region of each sarcomere, resulting in interference with normal cross-bridge formation. However, tension production in cardiac muscle falls off much more steeply at muscle lengths below L_{max} than would be expected according to the sliding filament hypothesis.[105]

The inotropic effect of changes in extracellular $[Ca^{++}]$ is dependent on muscle length; the mechanical performance of cardiac muscle is more sensitive to changes in extracellular $[Ca^{++}]$ at longer than at shorter muscle lengths.[31,105,108,109] There is evidence in skeletal muscle too that the affinity of troponin for Ca^{++} is length-dependent,[110] and the same situation may well exist in cardiac muscle. It has been suggested that the same quantity of Ca^{++} released may thus be more actively bound at longer than at shorter sarcomere lengths and that an increase in muscle length (1) does not change or decreases the transsarcolemmal influx of Ca^{++}, (2) increases the release of Ca^{++} triggered by the transsarcolemmal Ca^{++} influx, and/or (3) increases the sensitivity of the myofilaments to Ca^{++}.[31]

Thus, all changes in contractile behavior may result primarily from alterations in the degree of activation of the contractile system, and therefore contractility and muscle length (preload) should not be regarded as totally independent regulators of myocardial performance. While a change in contractility relates to changes in *quantity and rate* of Ca^{++} made available to troponin C, a change in muscle length appears to alter the *sensitivity* of the sarcomere to Ca^{++}. However, the distinct differences in the effects of changes in preload and of contractility on V_{max} (Figs. 12–13 and 12–14), on the duration of the active state, and on the rate of tension development and decline all indicate that, regardless of the similarity in the fundamental molecular mechanism, consideration of preload and contractility as separate determinants of cardiac performance still remains an extremely useful working model.

THE ULTRASTRUCTURAL BASIS OF STARLING'S LAW OF THE HEART

The capacity of the intact ventricle to vary its force of contraction on a beat-to-beat basis as a function of its preload, reflected in the initial (end-diastolic) size, constitutes one of the major principles of cardiac function and is generally referred to as the *Frank-Starling phenomenon*, or *Starling's Law of the Heart*.[111,112] This fundamental property of the heart is based on the myocardial *length–active tension relation*, in which force of contraction and/or extent of shortening depends on initial muscle length,[113] which in turn is dependent on the ultrastructural disposition of thick and thin myofilaments within the sarcomeres.[114] As has already been pointed out (p. 409), the sarcomere is composed of an array of partially overlapping thick and thin filaments. A change in the length of the sarcomeres in striated muscle, whether skeletal or cardiac, creates a predictable change in the extent of overlapping between the two sets of filaments (Fig. 12–16). The critical relation between sarcomere length and isometric tension development was defined for skeletal muscle by A.F. Huxley and associates [114,115] (Fig. 12–17) who found that developed tension was constant with a sarcomere length between 2.0 and 2.2 μ but that when sarcomeres were shortened to less than 2.0 μ, the developed force fell. These changes in force development were explained by the relative position of the two sets of myofilaments within the sarcomere. The thick filaments are about 1.5 μ in length while the thin filaments

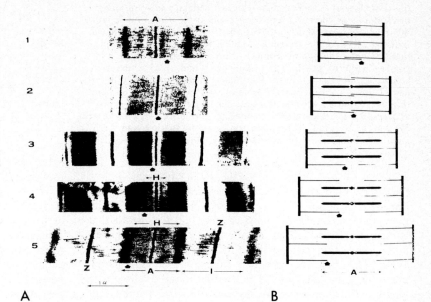

FIGURE 12–16 Relation between changes in sarcomere length and band patterns in skeletal muscle (frog sartorius). *A*, Band patterns as seen with the electron microscope. *B*, Relative disposition of the thick and thin filaments that create these patterns. The arrows in both panels denote the ends of the thin filaments that insert into the Z line to the left. In *A*, (3) represents the sarcomere at the apex of the length-active tension curve, i.e., at L_{max}. In (1) and (2), the sarcomere is shorter, whereas in (4) and (5) it is elongated. Throughout, the A band remains constant in width. The placement of filaments to provide for maximum overlap is shown in *B* (3). In (1), the sarcomere from a greatly shortened muscle is shown; the I band has disappeared, and a secondary dark band has formed at the center of the sarcomere, termed the C contraction band, and is due to the passage of thin filaments through this area. In *A* (4) and (5), an expanding H zone has appeared, owing to the withdrawal of thin filaments of constant length from the A band, as shown diagrammatically in *B* (4) and (5).

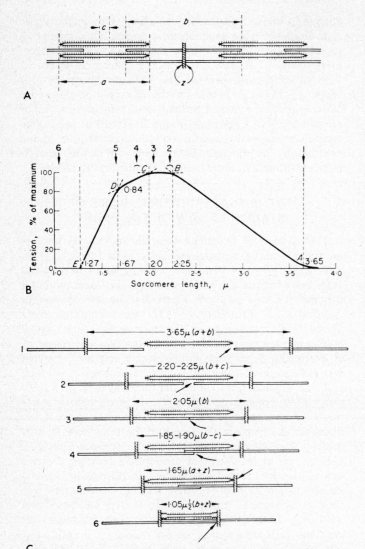

C

FIGURE 12–17 Relation between myofilament disposition and tension development in striated muscle. *A,* Diagram of myofilaments of the sarcomere drawn to scale. Thin filaments are 1.0 μ and thick filaments 1.6 μ in length. *B,* Relation between the tension development as percentage of maximum and the sarcomere length in single fibers of skeletal muscle. Numbers shown with arrows at top denote break points on the curve and correspond to the sarcomere lengths depicted diagrammatically in *C. C,* Myofilament overlap shown as a function of sarcomere length. At 3.65 μ (1) there is no overlap of myofilaments. The optimal overlap of myofilaments occurs at a sarcomere length of 2.05 to 2.25 μ (between 2 and 3). At a sarcomere length shorter than 2.0 μ (4), thin filaments pass into the opposite half of the sarcomere, and a double overlap occurs (5 and 6). Note that the central 0.2 μ of the thick filament is devoid of cross-bridges that could interact with sites on the thin filaments. (Adapted from Gordon, A. M., et al.: The variation in isometric tension with sarcomere length in vertebrate muscle fibers. J. Physiol. (Lond.) *184*:170, 1966.)

measure 1.0 μ.[13] According to the sliding filament theory, the length of both sets remains constant, both at rest and during contraction. The central region of the thick filaments contains an area approximately 0.2 μ in width that is devoid of cross bridges for the formation of force-generating cross links with actin. The optimal overlap of the 1.0 μ thin filaments with thick filaments occurs in sarcomeres between 2.0 and 2.2 μ. In this range of sarcomere lengths, the number of force-generating cross links that can be formed and the resultant developed force are maxi-

mal and constant. With sarcomeres longer than 2.2 μ, the fall in developed force may be directly related to the widening H zone and the resultant decrease in overlap between thick and thin filaments, thereby reducing the potential for cross bridge formation. At 3.65 μ, no overlap of filaments remains, and force generation ceases.[115]

When sarcomere lengths are progressively reduced below 2.0 μ, a reduction in tension development also occurs, presumably because (as pointed out earlier [p. 411]) thin filaments of 1.0 μ meet in the center of the sarcomere and bypass one another as sarcomere length is decreased further, resulting in a double overlap of filaments. As noted previously, this may interfere with the formation of cross bridges, may alter the ability of the filaments to bind Ca^{++} for activation, may reduce the sensitivity of the overlapping filaments to Ca^{++},[105] and/or may generate significant internal loads that might impair shortening of the sarcomere. Also, thin filaments may actually be repelled from the opposite half of the A band. All these factors may contribute to the fall in force development with shorter sarcomere lengths.

Although it has been suggested that thin filaments may be pulled by electrostatic forces rather than attaching physically to the thick filaments,[101,116] the concept of cross bridges between thick and thin filaments provides a useful working model that satisfactorily explains most of the observations of a variety of interventions involving cardiac contraction.

RELATION BETWEEN SARCOMERE LENGTH AND THE LENGTH-ACTIVE TENSION CURVE OF HEART MUSCLE

At L_{max}, the length of sarcomeres in mammalian ventricular myocardium averages 2.2 μ[117] (Fig. 12–18). As the resting muscle is shortened to about 85 per cent of L_{max}, sarcomere lengths decrease as a linear function of muscle length.[117,118] With further passive shortening of myocardium, however, little additional passive shortening of sarcomeres occurs, with diastolic sarcomere length remaining at 1.9 μ.

Although the structure of the sarcomere is similar in heart and skeletal muscle, important specialized differences permit cardiac muscle to function on the ascending portion of the length–active tension curve and maintain a length-dependent relation between sarcomere length and force development. First, the stiffness of the passive elastic component of cardiac muscle is such that diastolic sarcomere length is prevented from exceeding 2.3 μ, thus preventing disengagement of the myofilaments (Fig. 12–19). Second, the series elastic component is so compliant that during isometric contraction of cardiac muscle, substantial shortening of the sarcomeres occurs on the steep portion of their length–active tension curve.[119]

When cardiac muscle is stretched beyond L_{max}, resting tension rises to very high levels (Fig. 12–19), while, by definition, actively developed tension falls. However, in contrast to skeletal muscle, sarcomeres in cardiac muscle resist overstretching. With extension of the muscle to 20 per cent beyond L_{max}, sarcomeres elongate only slightly beyond 2.2 μ, but developed tension falls substantially. A decrease in overlap between thick and thin filaments, i.e., disengagement of myofilaments, cannot explain the sub-

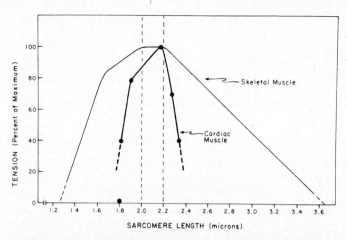

FIGURE 12–18 Relation between tension development and sarcomere length for cardiac muscle. Data were obtained by fixing cat papillary muscles with glutaraldehyde at various diastolic lengths relative to the length-tension curve and determining the average sarcomere length within the tissue using electron microscopic methods. The relation between tension development and sarcomere length obtained with skeletal fibers has been superimposed for comparison. In cardiac muscle, peak tension occurs with a diastolic sarcomere length of 2.2 μ. In skeletal muscle, there is a plateau of developed tension between sarcomere lengths of 2.2 and 2.0 μ, whereas in cardiac muscle this is not the case, and developed tension falls as sarcomere length is decreased below 2.2 μ. Furthermore, the shortest diastolic sarcomere length obtained in cardiac muscle in the absence of activation is 1.8 μ. As the papillary muscle is stretched beyond 2.2 μ, resting tension rises substantially (not shown; see Figure 12–20, p. 426) while actively developed tension falls precipitously. In contrast, in skeletal muscle, actively developed tension falls in a linear fashion between a sarcomere length of 2.2 and 3.6 μ. (From Sonnenblick, E. H., and Skelton, C. L.: Reconsideration of the ultrastructural basis of cardiac length-tension relations. Circ. Res. *35*:517, 1974, by permission of the American Heart Association, Inc.)

stantial decrements in developed force observed under these conditions; cellular damage occurs in cardiac muscle with this degree of overstretching and presumably is responsible, at least in part, for the reduction of tension development.[120]

Figure 12–19 shows the relation between average midwall sarcomere length and filling pressure for the left ventricles of the dog and cat.[121] When the left ventricle is empty, sarcomere length averages 1.9 μ, but as the left ventricle is filled, sarcomere lengths increase, so that at a filling pressure of 12 mm Hg the sarcomere length reaches 2.2 μ. With further ventricular distention, filling pressure rises markedly for small increments in ventricular volume, and only small increases in sarcomere length accompany large increases in intraventricular pressure. The same relation holds for the right ventricle but is scaled to lower filling pressures.[122] The relation between tension developed by the cat papillary muscle over a range of sarcomere lengths has been superimposed on the sarcomere resting length-tension relation in Figure 12–19. The optimal sarcomere length for maximum tension development (i.e., 2.2 μ) corresponds to the upper limits of normal ventricular filling pressure. When diastolic sarcomere length is related simultaneously to ventricular filling pressure and to active tension development, it becomes apparent that the apex of the sarcomere length–active tension curve and the normal upper limit of ventricular filling pressure coincide. Thus, the ventricle normally starts to contract when end-diastolic

sarcomere lengths are along the upper half of the ascending portion of the sarcomere length–active tension curve.

In studies of the relation between sarcomere length and ventricular performance in the intact ejecting heart, the canine left ventricle has been fixed in situ during end diastole and end systole.[123,124] Diastolic sarcomere lengths in the midwall of the left ventricle averaged 2.07 μ when filling pressure ranged from 6 to 8 mm Hg.[124] At end systole, when the ventricle had ejected about two-thirds of its end-diastolic volume, the average sarcomere length shortened to 1.8 μ (Fig. 12–20), and when contractility of the ventricle was augmented by postextrasystolic potentiation, maximum systolic emptying was increased substantially and end-systolic sarcomere lengths were 1.6 μ.

Sarcomeres tend to be longest in the midwall of the ventricle and reach a maximal length (2.25 μ) at filling pressures of 10 mm Hg, when subendocardial and subepicardial sarcomeres are shorter.[121] As filling pressure is raised further, sarcomere length increases across the entire wall; this recruitment of shorter sarcomeres from across the wall may constitute one of the principal functional reserves of the Frank-Starling mechanism.[125]

The relative degree of sarcomere shortening cannot be the same across the ventricular wall during ejection; geo-

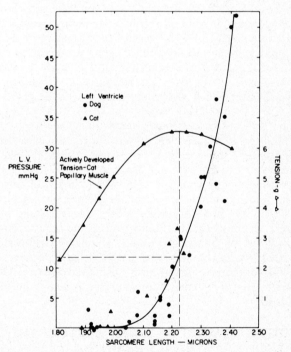

FIGURE 12–19 Relation between left ventricular pressure and average sarcomere length in the midwall of a canine left ventricle. The upper curve represents the relation between tension development and sarcomere length, as obtained from studies of cat papillary muscle. The lower curve relates left ventricular filling pressure to midwall sarcomere length for both dog and cat. At a left ventricular filling pressure of 12 mm Hg, which approximates the upper limit of normal filling pressure in the intact animal, average midwall sarcomere length is about 2.2 μ. This sarcomere length is also associated with the upper limits of the length–active tension curve, as shown by the vertical dashed line. Further increments in filling pressure yield only minor further increments in sarcomere length for very large increments in filling pressure. (From Spotnitz, J. H., et al.: Relation of ultrastructure to function in the intact heart: Sarcomere structure relative to pressure-volume curves of the intact left ventricles of dog and cat. Circ. Res. *18*:49, 1966, by permission of the American Heart Association, Inc.)

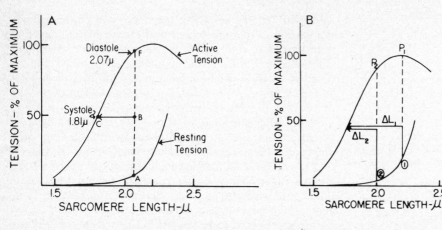

FIGURE 12–20 *A*, Relation between average diastolic sarcomere lengths as noted in the midwall of the normal diastolic and systolic left ventricle of the dog and the sarcomere length-tension curve of the isolated cat papillary muscle. In the intact dog, normal diastole is associated with a diastolic sarcomere length of 2.07 μ. During systole, sarcomeres in the intact heart shorten to an average of 1.81 μ. This provides for a 13 per cent change in sarcomere length, which would produce an ejection fraction of 55 per cent when considered in terms of a thick-walled model of the left ventricle.

B, Effects of altering initial muscle lengths on shortening of afterloaded sarcomeres. During an afterloaded isotonic contraction (1), the sarcomere begins to shorten from a diastolic length of 2.20 μ (point 1) and to become 1.81 μ (ΔL_1). The isometric force associated with this sarcomere length is noted at P_1. When diastolic sarcomere length is reduced to 2.0 μ (point 2), the sarcomere with the same afterload will shorten to the same point on the length–active tension curve (ΔL_2). This will result in a shortening from 2.00 to 1.81 μ. In this instance the associated isometric force occurs at P_2. Note that despite a minor change in peak developed isometric force, a substantial change in afterloaded isotonic shortening occurs at the same afterload. This would produce a substantial change in the stroke volume when extrapolated to the intact heart; e.g., in a 100-gram canine left ventricle, a change in diastolic sarcomere length from 2.0 to 2.2 μ in the midwall would increase stroke volume from 17 to 42 ml, with end-diastolic volume increasing from 40 to 65 ml. (From Ross, J., Jr., et al.: Architecture of the heart in systole and diastole: Technique of rapid fixation and analysis of left ventricular geometry. Circ. Res. *27*:409, 1967, by permission of the American Heart Association, Inc.)

metrical considerations dictate that epicardial fibers must shorten relatively less than endocardial fibers. Nevertheless, when sarcomere lengths obtained from the intact heart are superimposed on the initial sarcomere length-tension curve (Fig. 12–20*A*), the normal sarcomere might be considered to start to contract at point A. Were the ends of the muscle fixed, the isometric force at point F would be developed. With an afterload, force is developed to point B, after which shortening occurs between points B and C from a sarcomere length of 2.07 μ to 1.81 μ. As diastolic sarcomere length is altered along the ascending limb of the sarcomere length–active tension curve, both peak isometric force development and the extent of shortening at any given load are changed (Fig. 12–20*B*). The extent of this shortening is of great physiological importance, since it ultimately determines the quantity of blood ejected by the intact ventricle at any given diastolic fiber length. The basis for the Frank-Starling mechanism in the intact heart (discussed in the next section) is apparent in Figure 12–20*B*, in which it is clear that small changes in diastolic sarcomere length can mediate relatively large changes in the extent of sarcomere shortening at any afterload.

DETERMINANTS OF CONTRACTION OF THE INTACT HEART

Although the geometry of the intact ventricle is far more complex than that of papillary muscle, with its parallel, longitudinally disposed fibers, if certain analogies are drawn and assumptions made, it becomes apparent that the basic mechanisms that influence the contraction of isolated cardiac muscle (described above) affect the performance of the whole heart in a similar manner.[94,125–129]

CHANGES IN VENTRICULAR SIZE AND SHAPE

The dimensions of the ventricular cavities, thickness of the ventricular walls, and intrinsic mechanical properties of cardiac tissue are the determinants of passive elasticity or stiffness of the ventricle and therefore of diastolic tension. In this manner they determine the filling of the ventricles, ultimately affecting the length of the sarcomeres at the onset of systole and thereby the contractile events. The shape of the ventricles, the angles of adjacent muscle fibers, and the thickness of the ventricular walls also determine the distribution of active forces within the ventricular myocardium throughout systole and hence affect the extent and speed of muscle shortening. In addition to the changes that occur normally during the cardiac cycle and that are produced by acute physiological stresses, the shape of the ventricle often undergoes major alterations consequent to chronic cardiac disorders, such as valvular abnormalities, or local scarring due to coronary heart disease. The model often applied when one is considering the left ventricle as a thick-walled ellipsoid of revolution, which has practical utility in the calculation of left ventricular volume (p. 471).

The myocardial fibers are arranged in a spiral fashion around the central cavity of the left ventricle. The subendocardial and the subepicardial fibers run largely parallel to the long axis of the cavity, and the midwall fibers are mostly circumferential, i.e., perpendicular to the long axis. All the fibers tend to be perpendicular to the radius of the cavity. During contraction, the myocardial fibers shorten and thicken (Fig. 12–21), and as a consequence the left ventricular cavity decreases circumferentially and longitudinally and the wall thickens. The generation of intraventricular pressure and the displacement of blood from the left ventricular cavity are produced by a combination of fiber shortening and thickening.

During isovolumetric left ventricular contraction, the chordae tendineae become tense, the mitral valve closes, and the ellipsoidal left ventricle becomes more spherical, with slight apex-to-base shortening and a small increase in the minor ventricular diameter. These changes in left ventricular dimensions prior to ejection appear most marked when measured on the external surface of the heart.[130,131] The tendency toward sphericalization and wall thickening

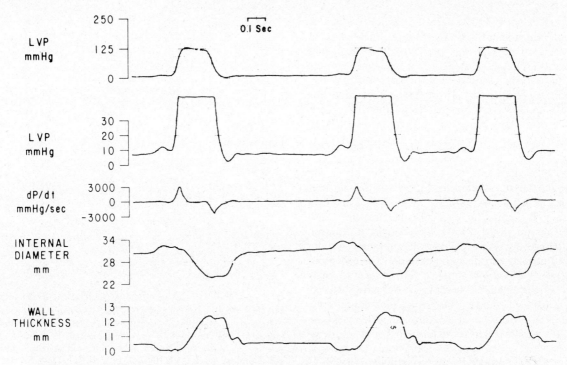

FIGURE 12–21 High-speed tracings obtained in a normal conscious, chronically instrumented dog with sinus arrhythmia. LVP = left ventricular pressure (in the top two tracings, at high and low amplification). dP/dt = the first derivative of left ventricular pressure. The internal diameter of the left ventricle was measured by means of a pair of ultrasonic crystals placed on the endocardium near the minor equator. The wall thickness of the left ventricle was measured by means of a pair of miniature ultrasonic crystals juxtaposed across the free wall near the minor equator. (From Theroux, P., Ross, J., Jr., et al.: Unpublished observations.)

during isovolumetric contraction and toward ellipticalization and wall thinning during isovolumetric relaxation is more pronounced when ventricular size is reduced, as occurs during thoracotomy (i.e., in the absence of a negative intrapleural pressure) or with occlusion of venous inflow into the heart.[132] During ejection, the minor (transverse) axis shortens by only 9 per cent.[132,133] Thus, shortening of the internal minor axis diameter accounts for approximately 85 to 90 per cent of the stroke volume. Measurements of casts of canine left ventricles arrested at end diastole and end systole have provided similar values and in addition have shown that the ratio of the major-to-minor axis changed from an average of 1.49 in diastole to 1.93 in systole.[123]

Similar changes in shape occur in the human left ventricle studied by means of angiography. As the left ventricle empties during systole, the inner surface decreases proportionately more than the external surface, as dictated by the geometry of the heart. Since muscle mass remains constant, an increase in wall thickness must occur; direct measurements of the left ventricular wall in intact animals[133,134] as well as cineangiography in patients[135] have confirmed that left ventricular wall thickness increases by 25 and 35 per cent during systole.

DIASTOLIC PROPERTIES OF THE VENTRICLES

Certain terms are commonly used to describe the mechanical properties of cardiac muscle.[136,137] Since there has been confusion about their meaning, they will be defined

explicitly here. *Stress* is the force per unit of cross-sectional area, frequently expressed as gm/cm²; *strain* is the fractional (or percentage of) change in dimension or size from the unstressed dimension that results from the application of stress; *elasticity* is the property of recovery of a deformed material after removal of the stress; *creep* is the time-dependent strain of tissue maintained at a constant level of stress after a rapid change in stress; *stress relaxation* is the time-dependent reduction of stress when tissue is maintained at a constant level of strain after a rapid change in strain. Like most biological materials, cardiac muscle exhibits a curvilinear relation between passive (diastolic) stress and strain (see Fig. 12–11); this property is responsible for the nonlinear pressure-volume curve (Fig. 12–22) and stress-strain relation of the intact ventricle. *Elastic stiffness* defines the ratio of stress to strain at any defined point of the curve relating these two variables. The *elastic stiffness constant* is the slope of the straight line relating elastic stiffness to the corresponding stress. The term elastic stiffness, sometimes called *volume stiffness* or *chamber stiffness*, has also been used to refer to the stiffness of the ventricular chamber and, by simplification, has been defined as the ratio of the change in pressure (dP) to the change in volume (dV). When the stress-strain relation is analyzed, the term *myocardial stiffness* has been employed to differentiate those effects due to changes in the stiffness properties of each unit of muscle as opposed to those due to increased muscle mass alone, which can affect *chamber stiffness*; thus, in some patients with concentric left ventricular hypertrophy, chamber stiffness is increased and myocardial stiffness is normal, whereas in others, both are elevated.[137] The terms *compliance* and *distensibility* represent the inverse of elastic stiffness, i.e., in referring to isolated muscle it is the ratio of a change in strain relative to a change in stress (d_e/d_s). In the ventricle these terms have been used to refer to the ratio dV/dP. The term *specific compliance* introduces a correction for the initial volume. Efforts to correct this value for ventricles of different sizes have also led to such expressions as $\dfrac{dV/dP}{V}$, where V in the denominator represents end-diastolic volume.

The diastolic pressure-volume relation of the normal mammalian left ventricle is curvilinear (Figs. 12–22 and 12–23).[138,139] At a low ventricular end-diastolic pressure there is a relatively gentle slope, with large changes in volume being accompanied by small changes in pressure. At the upper limits of normal end-diastolic pressure, the curve becomes steeper[140,141] and approximates an exponential relation, so that as the chamber becomes progressively filled during each diastole, instantaneous ventricular compliance (dV/dP) decreases; the inverse of compliance, i.e., elastic stiffness (dP/dV) bears a linear relation to the pressure in the normal dog left ventricle at diastolic pressures exceeding 3 mm Hg.[142] The slope of the line relating dP/dV to P represents the elastic stiffness constant of the chamber; it is relatively independent of ventricular shape and therefore may be useful for detecting changes in wall stiffness.[135,136] However, caution must be used in drawing conclusions from measuring these variables in one ventricle when the effects of changes in the volume of the other ventricle and the elastic limits of the pericardium cannot be excluded.

Although by definition, and as is apparent from Figures

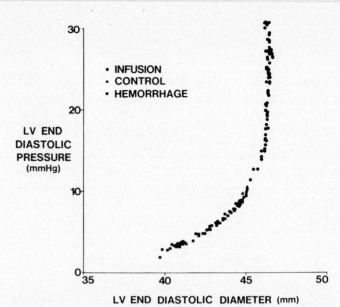

FIGURE 12–23   LVEDP-LVEDD curve constructed from an experiment in an intact dog. LVEDP and LVEDD fell with hemorrhage (squares) and returned to the same control levels (triangles) with reinfusion. With subsequent saline infusion (circles), LVEDP rose considerably, while LVEDD rose only slightly. (From Boettcher, D. H., et al.: Extent of utilization of the Frank-Starling mechanism in conscious dogs. Am. J. Physiol. *234*:H338, 1978.)

12–22 and 12–23, the compliance of the ventricle changes as it fills, an alteration of the compliance of the chamber as a whole can be identified by a change in the shape and position of the curve relating ventricular diastolic volume or dimensions to pressure.[131] As has already been pointed out (p. 421), excluding the incomplete relaxation that occurs in tachycardia and myocardial ischemia, interventions that alter myocardial contractility acutely do not cause significant shifts in the ventricle's diastolic pressure-volume relation. The small changes in the relation reported in some studies may be secondary to effects on time-dependent, inertial, and viscous properties and to the influence of filling of the opposite ventricle (p. 429). Since the diastolic pressure-volume relation is curvilinear, left ventricular diastolic compliance is determined by both the diastolic pressure-volume relation and the level of diastolic pressure at any instant, the so-called operating diastolic pressure (Fig. 12–22).[143] Therefore, ventricular compliance declines, i.e., the chamber elastic stiffness increases as it fills. Increased diastolic filling, as occurs with acute aortic regurgitation, and, conversely, reduced ventricular preload, as occurs after administration of nitroglycerin, result in increased and reduced stiffness, respectively, as the ventricle moves up or down its pressure-volume curve.[143]

Ventricular (chamber) stiffness is a function of muscle stiffness as well as of the thickness and geometry of the ventricle. If the stiffness of cardiac tissue (myocardial stiffness) is increased, as may occur with a fibrous scar or with infiltration of amyloid, but the thickness of the ventricular wall remains normal, ventricular (chamber) stiffness will be increased. An increase in chamber stiffness will also occur if the stiffness of each individual unit of myocardial tissue (myocardial stiffness) is normal but the ventricular wall becomes thicker.

In the intact heart, *stress relaxation* is of significance

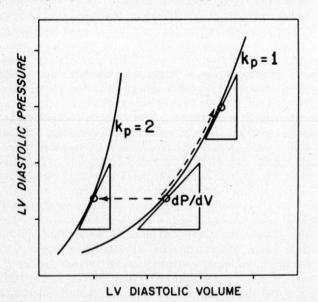

FIGURE 12–22   Diagrammatic representation of left ventricular (LV) diastolic pressure-volume relationships. *Right,* An increase in operative chamber stiffness (dP/dV) occurs in the absence of any change in the modulus of chamber stiffness (K_p). *Left,* An increase in operative chamber stiffness occurs as a result of an increase in the modulus of chamber stiffness (relative to the curve on the right). Because operative chamber stiffness depends on the modulus of stiffness and the level of operative filling pressure, this comparison is made at equivalent levels of pressure. (From Gaasch, W. H., et al.: Left ventricular compliance: Mechanisms and clinical implications. Am. J. Cardiol. *38*:645, 1976.)

only when large increases in ventricular diastolic pressure and volume occur abruptly. For example, there is a small drop in ventricular end-diastolic pressure (about 1 mm Hg) when systolic pressure is suddenly elevated by 70 to 80 per cent in the isovolumetrically contracting left ventricle, which is held at a constant volume. This suggests the presence of viscous elements, but these changes are of relatively minor significance in the intact heart.[144] *Creep*, a time-dependent shift of the left ventricular diastolic pressure-volume relation, has also been documented in the conscious dog after large increases in systolic and diastolic pressures (ventricular diastolic volume being larger at the same levels of diastolic pressure).[145]

The normal *right ventricle is more compliant than the left*, not because of any intrinsic difference in myocardial stiffness but because of its thinner wall.[122] In the isolated, nonbeating normal dog heart, when the left and right ventricles are filled simultaneously to a pressure of 10 mm Hg, the volume of the right ventricle is about 35 per cent greater than that of the left, and the upper limit of normal for right ventricular end-diastolic pressure in man is about one-half (6 mm Hg) that of the left ventricle (12 mm Hg).[140] In man, the end-diastolic volumes of the two ventricles are approximately equal,[146] and therefore the ejection fractions of the two ventricles are normally similar as well.

Ventricular Interdependence. Alterations in the filling of one ventricle can substantially alter the diastolic pressure-volume relation of the opposite chamber.[140] Therefore, when right ventricular volume changes significantly, changes in left ventricular end-diastolic pressure may not be a reliable guide even to directional changes of the diastolic volume of the left ventricle.[147,148] Studies in which the pericardium is intact have shown that not only the diastolic pressure but also the shape of the left ventricle is altered by increased right ventricular filling, which can result in encroachment of the interventricular septum on the left ventricular cavity.[149] Alterations in the right ventricular pressure-volume relation that occur after an alteration in left ventricular loading may not reflect a change in right ventricular myocardial or chamber stiffness but rather may be secondary to changes in the volume of the left ventricle within a pericardial sac that restrains changes in the volume of the entire heart.[150]

ROLE OF THE PERICARDIUM (See also p. 1471)

Experimental data indicate that the normal pericardium has an important effect on the diastolic properties of the ventricles during acute volume overload and therefore could be important during acute heart failure. During acute volume loading in the dog, intrapericardial pressure rises when overall cardiac volume (both right and left heart chambers) is increased beyond the limit of pericardial distensibility, i.e., the pericardium becomes restrictive. This factor may also play a role in the large decreases in left ventricular filling pressures that are observed during nitroprusside vasodilator therapy in human heart failure (p. 1473) when heart size decreases within the pericardial sac, which is no longer restrictive.

Figure 12–24 shows data from a conscious experimental animal instrumented for the measurement of left ventricular segment dimensions and left ventricular end-diastolic pressure; with the pericardium intact, overtransfusion pro-

duced a marked shift upward and to the left of the entire diastolic pressure-dimension curve of the left ventricle. Infusion of nitroprusside under these conditions caused a partial shift downward of the entire curve, the degree of the shift being equal to the fall of intrapericardial pressure. Thus, although a portion of the drop in cardiac filling pressure produced by nitroprusside was due to a reduction of cardiac volume, a portion of the fall resulted from the shift of the entire curve due to lowering of the elevated intrapericardial pressure. In contrast, when the pericardium was removed and the same animal was studied several days later, acute volume overloading, followed by the administration of nitroprusside, moved the left ventricle upward and downward on a single diastolic pressure-dimension curve.[151] Further research is needed to establish

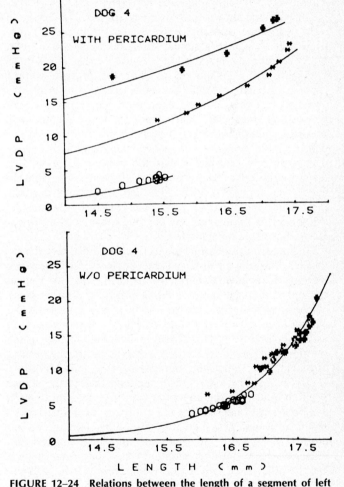

FIGURE 12–24 Relations between the length of a segment of left ventricle and left ventricular diastolic pressure (LVDP) in a conscious dog. Points were obtained during slow cardiac filling (diastasis). *Upper panel*, Relation with the *pericardium intact* before (open symbols) and after intravenous infusion of dextran to produce acute cardiac dilatation (asterisks, upper curve); the middle curve (x's) shows the effect of an intravenous infusion of nitroprusside in the presence of such acute cardiac dilatation. *Lower panel*, the same dog studied *without (W/O) the pericardium* (after its surgical removal). The same interventions, volume loading and nitroprusside, are carried out. The ventricle now appears to be operating on a single diastolic pressure–length relation. (Adapted from Shirato, K., et al.: Alteration of the left ventricular diastolic pressure–segment length relation produced by the pericardium: Effects of cardiac distention and afterload reduction in conscious dogs. Circulation *57:* 1191, 1978. By permission of the American Heart Association, Inc.)

the importance of such effects of the pericardium in human subjects.

While a reduction of left ventricular compliance occurs during angina pectoris (p. 1247), presumably as a consequence of impaired ventricular relaxation, this is not sufficient to account for the marked shifts in the left ventricular pressure-volume relations observed in pacing-induced angina signifying an apparent increase in elastic stiffness, when the pericardium is intact.[152] Furthermore, opposite shifts that suggest *increased* ventricular compliance occur with the administration of nitroglycerin and nitroprusside,[140,141] whereas shifts that suggest *decreased* compliance occur when systemic arterial pressure is raised by angiotensin II. These shifts of the pressure-volume relation may result in part from alterations of extrinsic pressures acting on the left ventricle, which is contained within a relatively stiff container, the pericardial sac. For example, it has been shown that for every 1.0 mm Hg change in right ventricular diastolic pressure, pressure in the left ventricle will change in a similar direction by about 0.5 mm Hg.[149,152] Thus, merely altering pressure on the right side of the heart can be expected to shift the pressure-volume curve of the left ventricle. As nitroprusside and nitroglycerin, through their dilating actions on the systemic vascular bed, reduce left ventricular diastolic volume and pressure, pulmonary artery pressure declines, right ventricular diastolic pressure and volume fall, and a secondary decline in left ventricular diastolic pressure occurs. This does not reflect a true change in left ventricular compliance. The opposite occurs when left ventricular diastolic (and hence pulmonary artery) pressure rises with the development of angina pectoris or upon infusion of a pressor agent such as angiotensin II.[153]

An important consequence of the shape of the left ventricular diastolic pressure-volume curve is the ventricle's inability to augment volume much above that existing at the upper limits of normal filling pressure, despite stress. Thus, in experiments carried out in intact, conscious, reclining dogs in the basal state, in which ventricular end-diastolic pressure was greatly elevated by volume expansion, by inducing global myocardial ischemia, or by augmenting afterload, left ventricular dimensions rose only slightly[154] (Fig. 12–23). This observation suggests that in the supine position, and with the animal at rest, at a basal heart rate, left ventricular muscle fibers are already near their maximal length and that operating from this baseline an increase of preload is *not* an important mechanism responsible for the augmentation of cardiac performance. On the other hand, when ventricular end-diastolic pressure and volume are lowered by hemorrhage, tachycardia, assumption of the upright posture, or opening of the chest, changes in cardiac performance can result from large alterations in ventricular dimensions as a consequence of augmenting blood volume or afterload. Therefore in the resting, reclining, conscious dog, the left ventricle operates near the bend of its pressure-volume curve, end-diastolic dimensions are nearly maximal, and cardiac performance cannot be augmented substantially through an increase in preload; rather, it requires an increase in contractility expressed as more complete systolic emptying from the same end-diastolic volume and an increase in heart rate, to augment cardiac output. Similar considerations apply to patients.[155]

The classic experiments of Starling,[112] Wiggers,[156] Sarnoff,[157] and their coworkers were carried out at unphysiological, high heart rates, with ventricular end-diastolic volumes far from maximal, allowing them to observe a distinct augmentation of ventricular diastolic dimensions with a variety of interventions. However, even in the conscious, intact organism, variations in ventricular performance as a consequence of alterations in preload are not totally unphysiological. They operate on a beat-to-beat basis in maintaining balanced outputs from the two ventricles during normal respiration[157] and allow for an increase in end-diastolic volume during exercise in the upright position, i.e., when baseline volume is not maximal.

PERFORMANCE OF THE INTACT VENTRICLE

The three determinants of performance of isolated cardiac muscle—preload, afterload, and contractility—also affect the performance of the intact ventricle. In addition, heart rate represents a fourth determinant of performance per unit time.

THE CARDIAC CYCLE. The relations between left ventricular pressure, the diameter of the minor equator at the endocardial surface of the left ventricular wall, and the wall thickness in a conscious dog are shown in Figure 12–21, and the events of the cardiac cycle are shown diagrammatically in Figure 12–25. Ventricular end diastole is followed by a brief period of isovolumetric left ventricular contraction, the maximum rate of pressure change (peak dP/dt) occurring just prior to the onset of ejection.[157a] The onset of inward motion of the ventricular wall then commences as blood is ejected into the aorta, and the rate of wall shortening becomes maximal near the middle of ejection. Wall thickness increases during shortening, becoming maximal at the end of ejection. Following isovolumetric relaxation, during which peak negative dP/dt is reached, a rapid increase in the diameter of the ventricle occurs during early diastole, followed by a slow phase of filling in mid-diastole (diastasis); a second, rapid increase in diameter takes place in late diastole, as a consequence of atrial contraction. The time course of changes in ventricular volume closely parallel those shown for ventricular internal diameter during each cardiac cycle. This relation between ventricular pressure and volume can also be plotted as a pressure-volume loop (Fig. 12–26) in a manner analogous to the sarcomere length-pressure (Fig. 12–19) and length-tension (Fig. 12–20) relations. This provides a convenient framework for understanding the responses of individual left ventricular contractions to alterations in preload, afterload, and contractility.

The pressure-volume loop of the left ventricle can be related to the performance of isolated cardiac muscle, in which the active isometric length-tension curve provides the limit of shortening for isotonic contractions. The linear relation between the end-systolic volume and the end-systolic pressure of the left ventricle is analogous to this length-tension relation and has been well defined in the isolated heart preparation[158,159] (Fig. 12–26, upper panel). It has also been studied in conscious animals by infusing a range of doses of a vasoconstrictor (that does not itself

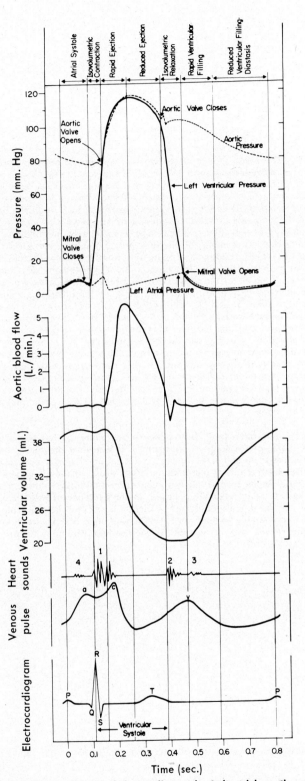

FIGURE 12–25 Events of the cardiac cycle. Left atrial, aortic, and left ventricular pressure pulses are correlated in time with aortic flow, ventricular volume, heart sounds, venous pulse, and electrocardiogram to provide a complete cardiac cycle in the dog. (From Berne, R. M., and Levy, M. N.: Cardiovascular Physiology. 3rd ed. St. Louis, The C. V. Mosby Co., 1977.)

have appreciable inotropic effects, such as the alpha-adrenergic agonist phenylephrine.[160] In man, the end-systolic ventricular volume can be determined by obtaining two or more angiocardiograms during infusion of such a vasoconstrictor, and the end-systolic values are then related to the corresponding ventricular or aortic pressure at the end of ventricular ejection; noninvasive techniques for measuring ventricular dimensions or volume (echocardiography and radionuclide methods) can also be employed. The linear end-systolic pressure-volume relation of the left ventricle has been found to shift downward and to the right in the presence of myocardial disease and to shift upward and to the left (with steepening of its slope) during acute positive inotropic interventions in experimental animals and in man (Fig. 12–26, lower panel).[161]

This relation is of particular importance because it defines the level of inotropic state under acutely changing conditions *independent* of the end-diastolic volume (preload) and the systolic aortic or ventricular pressure (as a measure of afterload). Thus, a given cardiac cycle arrives at end ejection and falls in this linear relation, regardless of the starting point for end-diastolic volume and the level of aortic pressure encountered during ejection, and the entire end-systolic pressure-volume relation is shifted acutely only by a change in inotropic state (Fig. 21–26). However, it should be recognized that under conditions in which there are *chronic* changes in the shape and size of the ventricle or in the thickness of its wall, systolic pressure is not indicative of the level of afterload; under these conditions the end-systolic pressure-volume relation does not define the level of inotropic state, and the wall force must be calculated in order to determine the linear relations between end-systolic volume and end-systolic wall force, which does identify the status of contractility.[162]

In comparing the whole heart to isolated muscle, heart volume and pressure are analogous to muscle length and tension. More complex formulations have also been developed; thus, the average circumferential wall stress (force per unit of cross-sectional area of wall) is related directly to the product of intraventricular pressure and internal radius and inversely to wall thickness. In the simplest versions of Laplace's law for a spherical ventricle, $\sigma = Pa/2h$ and, for an ellipsoidal ventricle, $\sigma = \dfrac{Pb}{h} \cdot \dfrac{1-b^2}{2c^2}$ where σ = average circumferential wall stress, P = intraventricular pressure, h = wall thickness; and b and c = the semiminor and semimajor axes at the endocardial surface.[136,158] In the ejecting ventricle, the extent and rate of wall shortening — and thus indirectly the stroke volume — are analogous to the extent and velocity of shortening of isolated muscle. The ventricular pressure during ventricular ejection is closely related to the afterload, although geometrical factors must be considered in order to calculate wall forces in the heart.

In order to clarify these concepts further, the relation between left ventricular systolic pressure and stroke volume was examined in the intact canine ventricle, while ventricular end-diastolic volume was held constant, and the force-velocity relation of the whole ventricle was calculated[163,164] (Fig. 12–27). Aortic pressure was varied independently of ventricular end-diastolic volume by rapid infusion or withdrawal of blood from the aorta during a single diastolic interval while the aortic valve was closed. The next cardiac cycle was then initiated from the same ven-

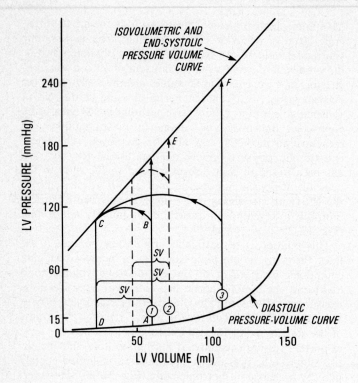

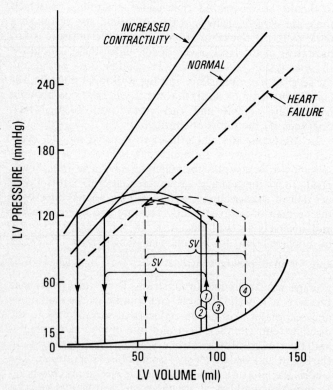

FIGURE 12–26 Effects of several interventions on pressure-volume loops of the left ventricle (LV) shown diagrammatically.

Upper panel, Effects of varying preload and afterload (with level of contractility remaining constant). Contraction 1 commences at end diastole (A) and is isovolumetric (arrow A to B) until the onset of ejection (B); the end of ejection or end-systolic volume (C) is followed by isovolumetric relaxation (C to D), and then filling of the ventricle occurs along the diastolic pressure-volume curve (from D to A). When a contraction originating from the same diastolic volume as contraction 1 is forced to contract isovolumetrically (top arrows), a point on the volume-isovolumetric systolic pressure curve is generated; if beats originating at larger end-diastolic volumes (contractions 2 and 3) are forced to contract isovolumetrically, points E and F are generated on that curve. This active pressure-volume curve provides the limit for the end-systolic volume of ejecting contractions. Ejecting contraction 3 shows that increasing end-diastolic volume causes an increase in stroke volume (SV) when aortic pressure is relatively constant. Ejecting contraction 2 (dashed lines) shows the effect of increasing systolic aortic pressure; when compared with contraction 1, SV is actually less, despite an increased end-diastolic volume, because of the higher level of aortic pressure or afterload.

Lower panel, Effects of increasing contractility (positive inotropic agent) and decreasing contractility (heart failure) on left ventricular pressure-volume loops. Contraction 1 is a normal pressure-volume loop, at a normal level of contractility. Contraction 2 shows that when contractility is increased, a larger stroke volume is generated from a similar or even slightly reduced end-diastolic volume, aortic pressure being relatively constant. In the presence of heart failure, SV may be diminished despite a slightly larger end-diastolic volume at a comparable level of aortic pressure (dashed line, contraction 3); however, SV may be restored if end-diastolic volume is further increased (contraction 4).

tricular end-diastolic volume but could be subjected to a wide range of predetermined pressures, i.e., afterloads. This experimental design mimics that of the isolated muscle contracting under variably afterloaded conditions, when a force-velocity relation is determined from a constant resting muscle length or preload (see Fig. 12–12). The ventricle became shorter auxotonically, i.e., against a *varying* afterload as ventricular wall tension declined when radius fell during ejection, rather than in a manner analogous to the usual papillary muscle preparation, which contracts isotonically, i.e., against a constant afterload.

Increases in stroke volume and peak flow rate occurred when aortic pressure was lowered, and the opposite effect was observed when the pressure was elevated. Thus, an inverse relation was observed between myocardial wall stress and the velocity of circumferential fiber shortening (V_{CF}). When aortic pressure was increased to a sufficiently high level during diastole, the ventricle could be forced to contract isovolumetrically. Peak stress (P_0) as well as shortening velocities at all levels of afterload were altered by inotropic influences when ventricular end-diastolic volume was constant. These experiments indicate that the mamma-

FIGURE 12–27 Diagram of a method of calculating force-velocity relationships in the intact ventricle. The equations assume a spherical model, the transected ventricle being shown at end diastole and during systole, when the instantaneous force-velocity relation is calculated. The wall-thickness (h) has increased from end diastole, and the instantaneous volume (V) can be computed from the aortic flow tracing (shown diagrammatically at the upper right) by subtracting the ejected volume (EV) (the cross-hatched area) from the end-diastolic volume (EDV). The instantaneous mean wall stress can then be calculated by solving the equation under heading A for the volume of the sphere to yield the inner radius (r_i). Since the ventricular wall becomes increasingly thick during systole, the velocity of the circumferential fibers (V_{CF}), calculated under heading B, employs values of both the inner radius (r_i) and the outer radius (r_o) to arrive at the midwall radius. The first equation under heading B represents differentiation of the equation for the volume of the sphere; the second equation represents the rate of shortening of the circumferential fibers (V_{CF}). Under heading C, the approach for calculating the velocity of the contractile elements (V_{CE}) is shown; the two-component model for muscle described by A. V. Hill is utilized in which the rate of stretch of the series elastic component (V_{SE}) is directly proportional to the rate of tension development (dT/dt) and is inversely proportional to the stiffness of the series elastic component (dT/dl). V_{CE} is equal to V_{SE} during isovolumetric contraction, whereas during shortening, V_{CE} equals $V_{CF} + V_{SE}$. (From Braunwald, E., et al.: Mechanisms of Contraction of the Normal and Failing Heart. 2nd ed. Boston, Little, Brown, 1976.)

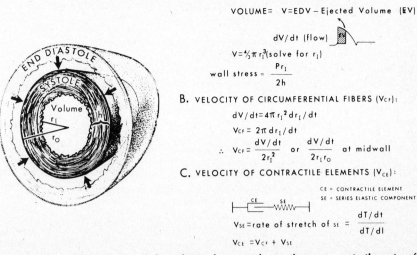

A. INSTANTANEOUS WALL STRESS:

$$\text{VOLUME} = V = EDV - \text{Ejected Volume (EV)}$$

dV/dt (flow)

$$V = \tfrac{4}{3}\pi r_i^3 \text{ (solve for } r_i)$$

$$\text{wall stress} = \frac{P r_i}{2h}$$

B. VELOCITY OF CIRCUMFERENTIAL FIBERS (V_{CF}):

$$dV/dt = 4\pi r_i^2 dr_i/dt$$

$$V_{CF} = 2\pi dr_i/dt$$

$$\therefore V_{CF} = \frac{dV/dt}{2 r_i^2} \text{ or } \frac{dV/dt}{2 r_i r_o} \text{ at midwall}$$

C. VELOCITY OF CONTRACTILE ELEMENTS (V_{CE}):

CE = CONTRACTILE ELEMENT
SE = SERIES ELASTIC COMPONENT

$$V_{SE} = \text{rate of stretch of SE} = \frac{dT/dt}{dT/dl}$$

$$V_{CE} = V_{CF} + V_{SE}$$

lian ventricle as a whole responds in a manner similar to that of isolated cardiac muscle.

Preload

Starling's Law of the Heart, which states that "the mechanical energy set free on passage from the resting to the contracted state is a function of the length of the muscle fiber, i.e., of the area of chemically active surfaces,"[112] is an expression of the length–active tension curve, reflecting the functional consequences of variations in preload. In the intact heart, ventricular end-diastolic wall stress or tension is analogous to the preload of isolated muscle and ultimately determines the resting length of the sarcomeres (see Fig. 12–19).

The influence of alterations in preload independent of alterations in frequency, afterload, and inotropic state for the isotonically contracting canine left ventricle are shown diagrammatically in Figure 12–28A. Increases in preload augment the stroke volume as well as the extent and velocity of wall shortening.[164a] As in isolated muscle, in force-velocity curves obtained in the isotonically contracting heart, the maximum velocity of wall shortening estimated at zero force (V_{max}) does not appear to be altered by changing preload.[163,164] If ejection is prevented and the ventricle contracts isovolumetrically, a direct correlation between preload, as reflected in the end-diastolic volume, and peak left ventricular systolic pressure or calculated wall stress can also be shown (analogous to the length–active tension curve of isolated muscle). These relationships constitute expressions of the Frank-Starling mechanism and provide the basis for ventricular function curves in the normally ejecting heart, which relate ventricular end-diastolic volume or pressure to stroke volume and stroke work.[157] Any of the curves discussed above can, of course, be shifted up or down by positive and negative inotropic influences, respectively (see Fig. 12–26).

ATRIAL CONTRIBUTION TO PRELOAD. Atrial

muscle behaves in accord with Starling's law, with increasing stretch resulting in a more forceful contraction.[165] When properly timed, atrial contraction augments ventricular filling and preload. Rapid ventricular filling induced by atrial contraction at the end of diastole abruptly elevates ventricular end-diastolic pressure and volume. This allows a lower mean right or left atrial pressure to exist throughout most of diastole than would be the case if atrial contraction were ineffective (as in atrial fibrillation) or ill-timed (as in nodal rhythm or atrioventricular dissociation).[166] The atrial contribution to ventricular filling is of particular importance in the presence of ventricular hypertrophy and other states of reduced ventricular compliance. In these conditions, the loss of atrial systole reduces ventricular end-diastolic pressure and volume, ultimately impairing myocardial performance.[166a]

DESCENDING LIMB OF STARLING'S CURVE. The question of whether a descending limb of cardiac function exists in the whole left ventricle has been of great interest.[167] In the isovolumetrically contracting isolated canine left ventricle, no reduction of developed wall stress or systolic pressure occurred until the ventricular end-diastolic pressure exceeded 60 mm Hg; when diastolic ventricular pressure was further elevated to 100 mm Hg, developed pressure declined by only 7.5 per cent. At these extremely high end-diastolic pressures, sarcomere lengths averaged 2.27 to 2.30 μ.[168] Based on this and earlier work showing that midwall sarcomere lengths did not exceed 2.27 μ at left ventricular end-diastolic pressures up to 40 mm Hg,[169] may be postulated that the descending limb of ventricular performance, when observed in ejecting heart, is not caused by operation of the heart on a descending limb of the sarcomere length-tension relation,[170] i.e., it is not a consequence of the disengagement of actin and myosin myofilaments. However, a descending limb of curves that relate left ventricular end-diastolic pressure to stroke work was demonstrated in dogs when volume loading was carried out to achieve end-diastolic pressures exceeding 30 mm

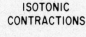

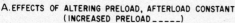

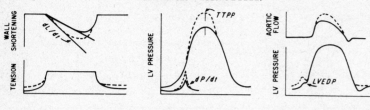

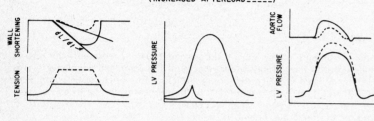

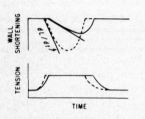

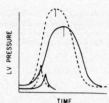

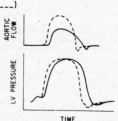

FIGURE 12–28 Effects of changing preload, afterload, and inotropic state on contractions of the whole heart. The upper row of panels (*A*) shows the effects of increasing preload when afterload and contractility are held constant, the middle row (*B*) shows the effects of increasing afterload when preload and contractility are held constant, and the bottom row (*C*) shows the effects of increasing the inotropic state when preload and afterload are held constant. Dashed lines show effects of intervention. Each of the three panels arranged vertically on the left (under the column labeled isotonic contractions) shows the extent of wall shortening, shortening velocity (dL/dt), and tension in superimposed tracings obtained in the isotonic canine left ventricular preparation. The tracings in the middle column (isovolumetric contractions) show isovolumetric left ventricular (LV) pressure tracings, the first derivatives (dP/dt), and time to peak pressure (TTPP). It should be noted that, by definition, an isovolumetric contraction is not afterloaded (since no shortening occurs) and therefore is unchanged in *B*, center panel. The tracings in the right column (normally ejecting contractions) show the effects of these three interventions on superimposed left ventricular contractions ejecting into the aorta, with left ventricular pressure and blood flow in the aortic root being shown. Left ventricular end-diastolic pressure (LVEDP) is also indicated.

Hg, after mean aortic pressure had initially been elevated.[171] Under these circumstances, slight further increases in aortic pressure occurred during the volume loading, which elevated left ventricular filling pressures above 30 mm Hg. It was concluded that the descending limb of function in the ejecting ventricle is only apparent and actually results from reduced myocardial wall shortening due to an increased afterload, when the ventricle is unable to compensate by further increases in sarcomere length. It has also been proposed that the descending limb of function induced in the failing human heart by infusion of a vasopressor agent[172] is due to such an effect of augmented afterload, when preload reserve is absent.[173] The development of mitral regurgitation consequent to ventricular dilatation can also depress forward stroke volume and result in an *apparent* depression of ventricular performance as preload is elevated to very high levels.

In summary, alterations in preload, operating through changes in end-diastolic sarcomere length, serve as an important determinant of the performance of the intact ventricle and provide the basis for the function curves of the intact ventricle. The ability to augment preload provides a functional reserve to the heart in situations of acute stress and operates on a beat-to-beat basis in maintaining balanced outputs of the two ventricles during such normal maneuvers as respiration.[157] The possibility of increasing preload provides a reserve mechanism and allows some augmentation of cardiac performance during severe stresses

such as maximum exercise performed in the upright position.[174]

CONTROL OF PRELOAD IN THE INTACT ORGANISM

In the intact organism, preload is determined largely by venous return and total blood volume and its distribution (Fig. 12–29)[175,176] as well as by the activity of the atrium.

Venous Return. In the absence of heart failure in the intact organism, most changes in cardiac output can be accounted for largely by changes in the *return* of blood to the heart, which in turn alters the preload. In the absence of heart failure, simple augmentation of myocardial contractility, as occurs with administration of a cardiac glycoside or institution of sustained postextrasystolic potentiation (paired electrical stimulation), has little effect on cardiac output.[177] In contrast, relatively large changes in output occur during maneuvers that alter venous return, such as lower body positive or negative pressure, positive-pressure respiration, a sudden change in posture, and rapid changes in blood volume.

Conditions that lower peripheral vascular resistance are among the most important of those augmenting venous return and include the opening of arteriovenous fistulas and conditions that mimic the latter, such as patent ductus arteriosus, fever, beriberi, pregnancy, and Paget's disease. (These and other chronic high-output states are discussed in Chapter 24.) A reduction in vascular resistance also occurs during *exercise*, when the arterioles supplying the ex-

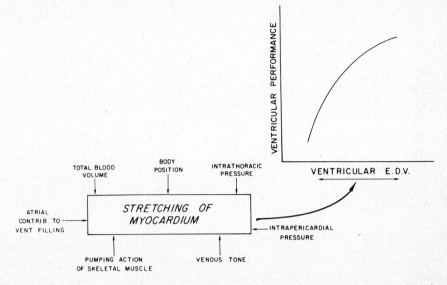

FIGURE 12–29 *Bottom left*, Major influences that determine the degree of stretching of the myocardium, i.e., the magnitude of end-diastolic volume (E.D.V.). *Top right*, Diagram of a Frank-Starling curve, relating ventricular E.D.V. to ventricular performance. (From Braunwald, E., et. al.: Mechanisms of Contraction of the Normal and Failing Heart. 2nd ed. Boston, Little, Brown, 1976.)

ercising muscle dilate; in severe *anoxia*, when generalized vascular dilation occurs; and in the presence of *anemia*, when blood viscosity and hence resistance to flow in the vascular bed are reduced.

Total Blood Volume. When blood volume is rapidly reduced, cardiac output and particularly stroke volume decline. However, in the intact organism, small (less than 15 per cent of control) or gradual reductions in blood volume can be tolerated with barely perceptible changes in cardiac output, as a consequence of a number of compensatory mechanisms resulting from activation of the adrenergic nervous system.

Distribution of Blood Volume. At any given total blood volume, the ventricular end-diastolic volume is a function of the distribution of blood between the intra- and extrathoracic compartments. The principal determinants of this distribution are as follows.

Body Position. Gravitational forces pool blood in the dependent portions of the body, and assumption of the upright posture therefore increases extrathoracic blood volume at the expense of intrathoracic and ventricular end-diastolic volumes, thereby reducing preload and cardiac output. The effects of negative pressure (suction) applied to the lower extremities and trunk with the subject supine mimic those of assumption of the upright posture, while inflation of a lower-body positive-pressure suit, immersion of the lower extremities and trunk into water, or the absence of gravitational force during space flight increases intrathoracic blood volume and preload.

Intrathoracic Pressure. The negative intrathoracic pressure normally increases thoracic blood volume, improving cardiac filling and augmenting preload and thereby cardiac performance. The intrathoracic pressure becomes most negative during inspiration and approximates atmospheric pressure during expiration. Accordingly, the gradient for venous return (and therefore right ventricular stroke volume) rises during inspiration when the intrathoracic pressure declines. Elevation of mean intrathoracic pressure, as occurs with the application of positive-pressure respiration or the development of pneumothorax, tends to impede total venous return to the heart, diminishes intrathoracic blood volume, and ultimately reduces ventricular performance.[178]

Intrapericardial Pressure. (See also Chapter 43). When pericardial pressure is elevated, as occurs in pericardial effusion, there is interference with cardiac filling, and the resultant reduction in ventricular diastolic volume (preload) reduces ventricular performance. With marked elevations of intrapericardial pressure, cardiac tamponade may occur, which is characterized by marked lowering of stroke volume and arterial pressure with circulatory collapse. Chronic constrictive pericarditis also impedes ventricular filling and thereby lowers stroke volume.[179]

Venous Tone. Smooth muscle in the walls of the veins responds to a variety of neural and humoral stimuli[180]; venoconstriction occurs during exercise, anxiety, deep respiration, or marked hypotension, tending to augment intrathoracic blood volume.[181] A variety of drugs act on venous smooth muscle. Thus, sympathomimetic agents produce venoconstriction,[180] while ganglionic blocking agents and sympatholytic and norepinephrine-depleting drugs or agents such as nitroglycerin that are direct venodilators[182,183] produce extrathoracic pooling and thereby ultimately reduce preload and cardiac output.[184] Extravascular compression of the veins by skeletal muscle plays an important role in augmenting venous return by exercising skeletal muscle.[185]

Atrial Contribution to Ventricular Filling (see p. 433). A vigorous, appropriately timed atrial contraction augments ventricular filling and end-diastolic volume.[165,166]

Afterload

When applied to the intact ventricle, afterload may be defined as the tension, force, or stress (force per unit of cross-sectional area) acting on the fibers in the ventricular wall *after* the onset of shortening, and it is a key determinant of the quantity of blood ejected by the ventricle.[187,188] In the intact heart, abrupt alterations in the impedance to left ventricular ejection cause reciprocal changes in the stroke volume of the left ventricle[159,160,187–189] (Fig. 12–26).

The influence of variations in afterload on the performance of the intact ventricle can be studied using the isotonically contracting heart preparation in which the other two determinants of ventricular performance (preload and contractility) are held constant (Fig. 12–28B). Increasing the afterload reduces both stroke volume and the extent

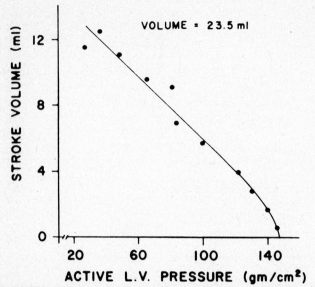

FIGURE 12–30 Relation between left ventricular systolic pressure (active L.V. pressure) and stroke volume in a series of contractions in the isotonically contracting canine left ventricle, in which left ventricular end-diastolic volume was held constant at 23.5 ml. The inverse relation between active pressure and stroke volume is apparent. (From Burns, J. W., et al.: Mechanics of isotonic left ventricular contractions. Am. J. Physiol. *224*:725, 1973.)

and velocity of wall shortening. Curves showing inverse relationships between afterload and stroke volume (Fig. 12–30), extent of wall shortening, and velocity of shortening can be constructed.[163,164,190]

The low impedance to left ventricular ejection (reduction in afterload) produced by mitral regurgitation,[191,192] patent ductus arteriosus, ventricular septal defect, or arteriovenous fistula can increase the extent of shortening and the ejection fraction. In the acutely pressure- and/or volume-overloaded ventricle, when sarcomere length is optimal and there is no preload reserve, any alteration in afterload causes a reciprocal change in stroke volume.[171] It is clear that the more severely depressed the inotropic state of the heart, the greater the influence of a change in afterload on the extent of myocardial fiber shortening. These considerations are relevant to the use of vasodilating agents to augment cardiac output in patients with left ventricular failure (Fig. 16–17, p. 537) and the use of pressor agents in the assessment of left ventricular function (p. 484).

When the ventricle is not operating along the steep portion of its diastolic pressure-volume curve, i.e., when there is still some preload reserve, an elevation of afterload often results in a compensatory elevation of ventricular end-diastolic volume, i.e., a rise in ventricular preload, which enhances myocardial contraction. However, as a consequence of the operation of Laplace's law (p. 431), this compensatory elevation of preload elevates myocardial tension development (afterload) further, and this in turn reduces myocardial fiber shortening. However, geometrical considerations dictate that the relative extent of myocardial fiber shortening required to maintain stroke volume constant is less in the larger ventricle. Hence, stroke volume may remain constant even though myocardial fiber shortening declines. If afterload rises, and if inflow into the ventricle is not restricted and preload can also rise, stroke volume can

be maintained. In accord with these considerations, the normal subject responds to a pressor agent by maintaining stroke volume and increasing stroke work while augmenting left ventricular end-diastolic pressure and volume, i.e., the increase in afterload is met by an increase in preload, whereas in the diseased heart stroke volume and stroke work tend to fall because there is little, if any, preload reserve[172] (see Fig. 14–21, p. 485). Thus, the response to increased aortic pressure is dependent in significant measure both on the level of myocardial contractility and on the preload, in that a moderate pressor stress will ordinarily produce little change in stroke volume in the normal heart but will augment stroke volume in heart failure. When there is relative hypovolemia, and preload cannot rise appropriately, an increase in afterload will reduce the stroke volume in the normal heart.

HOMEOMETRIC AUTOREGULATION, OR THE "ANREP EFFECT." A positive inotropic effect has been said to follow abrupt elevation of systolic aortic and left ventricular pressure.[157,193–197] This response was first described by Von Anrep in 1912[198] and has been termed the "Anrep effect," or homeometric autoregulation. This effect occurs during the first minutes after aortic pressure is abruptly elevated, with end-diastolic pressure and circumference then tending to fall as stroke volume and stroke work recover. Force-velocity analyses of the left ventricle in anesthetized dogs suggest that it constitutes a small net positive inotropic effect.[195]

Homeometric autoregulation is most marked in the anesthetized state, and studies in conscious animals show that the initial increases in end-diastolic pressure and dimension are minimal at slow heart rates; however, during tachycardia greater initial increases in end-diastolic pressure and dimensions observed during aortic pressure elevation were followed by a much more marked Anrep effect.[199] These observations, together with the finding that reactive hyperemia in the myocardium occurs if aortic pressure is lower early during the Anrep effect but not after the effect is complete, support the concept that the phenomenon is related to recovery from transient subendocardial ischemia.[199]

CONTROL OF AFTERLOAD IN THE INTACT ORGANISM. In the intact organism, afterload is determined largely by peripheral vascular resistance, the physical characteristics of the arterial tree, and the volume of blood that it contains at the onset of ejection. The critical role played by ventricular afterload in cardiovascular regulation is summarized in Figure 12–31. While increases in both preload and contractility increase myocardial fiber shortening, increases in afterload reduce it; the extent of myocardial fiber shortening and of left ventricular size determines stroke volume. Arterial pressure, in turn, is related to the product of cardiac output and systemic vascular resistance, while afterload is a function of left ventricular size and arterial pressure. For example, when vasoconstriction raises arterial pressure, afterload is also augmented, which, through a negative feedback mechanism, tends to depress myocardial fiber shortening, stroke volume, and cardiac output; the latter, in turn, restores arterial pressure to its previous level.

When left ventricular function is impaired, afterload becomes an increasingly important determinant of cardiac performance. Afterload may rise as a consequence of vasoconstriction resulting from the influence on the arterial bed

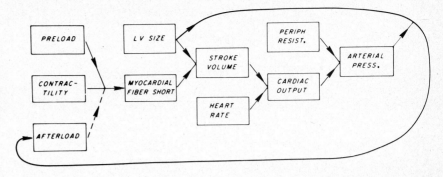

FIGURE 12–31 Schema showing interactions between various components regulating cardiac activity. Solid lines indicate an increasing effect; broken line represents a depressing effect. Note that left ventricular (L.V.) size is a determinant of both stroke volume and afterload. (Reprinted by permission from Braunwald, E.: Regulation of the circulation. N. Engl. J. Med. *290*:1124, 1974.)

of neural, humoral, and structural changes that occur in response to a fall in cardiac output. This increased afterload may reduce cardiac output further; on the other hand, pharmacological reductions of afterload may be beneficial in elevating cardiac output (p. 534).

In summary, when acute changes in arterial pressure occur, the resultant alteration in afterload has an important effect on cardiac performance (Fig. 12–30). An understanding of the effects of changes in afterload is central to an appreciation of the effects of conditions such as systemic or pulmonary arterial hypertension and obstruction to ventricular ejection by valvular disease (aortic and pulmonic stenosis), which increase afterload, and of mitral regurgitation and ventricular septal defect, which reduce it. Adaptation to a chronic increase in afterload by means of wall hypertrophy, in which a gradual increase in wall thickness occurs and tends to return wall stress and wall shortening characteristics toward normal,[200] is discussed in Chapter 13.

Contractility (Inotropic State)

The term "contractility," or "inotropic state," has a different connotation from the term "performance." For practical purposes, it is useful to regard a *change in contractility as an alteration in cardiac performance that is independent of changes resulting from variations in preload or afterload.* When loading conditions remain constant, an improvement in contractility augments cardiac performance (a positive inotropic effect) while a depression in contractility lowers cardiac performance (a negative inotropic effect).

The effects of an increase in contractility induced by a positive inotropic agent such as a catecholamine have been studied in the isotonically contracting heart preparation in which the other determinants of performance (preload, afterload, and contraction frequency) can be held constant.[164,200a] As in isolated muscle, increases in the velocity and extent of wall shortening and increased stroke volume occur while the duration of contraction is shortened (Fig. 12–28C). The force-velocity relation is shifted upward, P_0 and V_{max} both increase (Fig. 12–14), and curves relating diastolic volume to active peak isovolumetric pressure are shifted upward (Fig. 12–26). Acute administration of negative inotropic agents produce the opposite effects.[201]

THE INTERVAL-STRENGTH RELATION. In the intact ventricle, as in isolated cardiac muscle, premature depolarization results in a reduced mechanical contraction, the extent of the reduction being directly proportional to the degree of prematurity. However, the ensuing contrac-

tion is then more forceful than normal, the degree of augmentation being greater the earlier the extra depolarization is introduced.[49-51] This phenomenon, termed "postextrasystolic potentiation," is clearly *independent* of variations in preload, since it occurs in the isovolumetrically contracting heart in which preload is fixed.[202,203] In the intact organism, when the premature beat is followed by a compensatory pause, the ventricular end-diastolic volume may be augmented, and this increased preload may contribute along with the greater contractility to the enhanced performance that characterizes the postextrasystolic contraction. Postextrasystolic potentiation can be sustained and results in a striking augmentation of myocardial contractility when pairs of stimuli are delivered repetitively to the intact ventricle. In this technique, termed "paired electrical stimulation," the second stimulus is placed immediately after the electrical refractory period and results in only a small secondary contraction.[50,51] It is likely that the additional activation promotes an increased availability of Ca^{++} at the contractile sites. Despite its striking positive inotropic effect, paired electrical stimulation does not increase cardiac output in the nonfailing heart of the intact dog or of human subjects but does have this effect in the presence of experimental heart failure.[204]

Control of Contractility in the Intact Organism

The factors that modify cardiac contractility of the myocardium may be considered to operate by modifying the level of ventricular performance at any given ventricular end-diastolic volume, i.e., the relative position of the entire Frank-Starling curve (Fig. 12–32).

Sympathetic Nerve Activity. The quantity of norepinephrine (NE) released by sympathetic nerve endings in the heart is probably the most important factor regulating myocardial contractility under physiological conditions. Rapid changes in contractility in the intact organism are effected by variations in the impulse traffic in the cardiac adrenergic nerves. Beta-adrenergic receptor blocking agents and NE-depleting drugs interfere with the myocardial response to sympathetic nerve stimuli.

Circulating Catecholamines. When stimulated by nerve impulses, the adrenal medulla releases epinephrine, which is carried by the bloodstream to the myocardium, where it acts upon beta receptors to augment contractility. This mechanism is slower than the response to NE release by cardiac nerves but may be of physiological importance in conditions such as hypovolemia and a variety of chronic stresses, including congestive heart failure.

Interval-Strength Relation. As described above, myo-

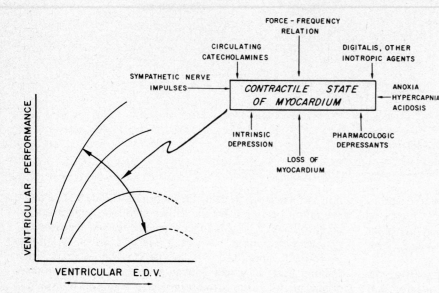

FIGURE 12–32 *Top right,* Diagram showing the major influences that elevate or depress the contractile state of the myocardium. *Bottom left,* Effect of alterations in the contractile state of the myocardium on the level of ventricular performance at any given level of ventricular end-diastolic volume. (From Braunwald, E., et al.: Mechanisms of Contraction of the Normal and Failing Heart. 2nd ed. Boston, Little, Brown, 1976.)

cardial contractility may be influenced profoundly by the rate and rhythm of cardiac contraction. For example, a ventricular extrasystole augments contractility, although to a decreasing extent, for several cardiac cycles. A simple increase in frequency in the physiological range also augments cardiac contractility, but this effect is more prominent in isolated heart muscle or in the intact heart with depressed function than it is in the normal heart of the intact organism.

Exogenous Inotropic Agents. The cardiac glycosides, sympathomimetic agents, Ca^{++}, caffeine, theophylline, amrinone, and their derivatives (see Chap. 16) all augment cardiac contractility.

Physiological and Pharmacological Depressants. These include anoxia,[205] ischemia (Chap. 36),[206] acidosis,[207] and local anesthetics (Chap. 20), barbiturates, and most general anesthetics.

Loss of Contractile Mass. When a portion of the ventricle becomes necrotic, as occurs in ischemic heart disease, the overall performance of the ventricle at any given end-diastolic volume is reduced, even though the contractility of the remaining myocardium may be normal (Chap. 37).

Intrinsic Myocardial Depression. Although, as indicated in Chapter 13, the fundamental mechanism responsible for depression of myocardial contractility in heart failure still remains to be elucidated, it is now apparent that the contractile state of each unit of myocardium is depressed in this condition.

Heart Rate

Accelerating the frequency of contraction generally does not induce a shift of the ventricular function curve, i.e., the relation between ventricular end-diastolic pressure and stroke work, in the open-chest anesthetized dog; however, it does increase stroke power (rate of performance of stroke work) at any given level of filling pressure,[157,208] a finding consistent with improvement of myocardial contractility and with observations on the effects of increases in the frequency of contraction in isolated cardiac muscle. Pacing-induced increases in contraction frequency, unac-

companied by sympathetic stimulation of the ventricle, also increase the calculated V_{max} and elevate the force-velocity relation of the ventricle in the anesthetized open-chest dog.[47]

The positive inotropic effect resulting from an increase in the frequency of contraction is more prominent in the anesthetized animal, in the depressed heart, and in isolated cardiac muscle than in the normal heart of the intact, conscious dog.[48] In the last situation, venous return to the heart is reflexly and metabolically stabilized, so that artificially varying heart rate between about 60 and 160 beats/minute has little effect on cardiac output, despite the above-mentioned modest changes in contractility that accompany changes in heart rate.[208,208a] However, if the diastolic volume of the heart is maintained, by increasing venous return as heart rate is increased, an elevation of frequency will augment cardiac output, and during exercise, tachycardia normally plays the major role in increasing cardiac output. However, since an increased heart rate augments the total fraction of each cardiac cycle occupied by systole, the corresponding reduction in the duration of diastole at very rapid rates can interfere with ventricular filling, ultimately limiting the rise in cardiac output associated with tachycardia.

Since, at a constant stroke volume, cardiac output is a linear function of heart rate, the ability to alter the latter is a critically important mechanism in the adjustment of cardiac output.[208b] The importance of heart rate in the maintenance of cardiac output is reflected in the inability of patients or experimental animals with fixed heart rates to elevate cardiac output appropriately, even when myocardial function is entirely normal. Under normal circumstances, heart rate is determined largely by the slope of phase 4 (spontaneous depolarization) of the sinoatrial node (p. 616); the intrinsic rhythmicity may be altered by a variety of influences, such as temperature and metabolism, rising with fever and thyrotoxicosis and falling with hypothermia and hypothyroidism. The two neurotransmitters released by autonomic nerves innervating the sinoatrial node play a critical role in the control of heart rate; acetylcholine slows while NE accelerates the slope of diastolic depolarization.

NEURAL CONTROL OF CARDIAC CONTRACTION

The autonomic nervous system is of critical importance in the moment-to-moment regulation of heart rate and contractility and of the capacitance and resistance of the vascular bed, thereby controlling cardiac output, blood flow distribution, and arterial pressure. Neural regulation is capable of producing considerable changes in cardiocirculatory function within seconds, before more slowly acting mechanisms, such as those mediated by the metabolic stimuli, circulating catecholamines, and the renin-angiotensin system, exert any effect.

ANATOMICAL CONSIDERATIONS. Sympathetic and parasympathetic preganglionic cells represent the final common pathways of neural impulses to the cardiovascular system. These cells receive both excitatory and inhibitory impulses from all levels of the central nervous system but most importantly from the cardiovascular center in the medulla and from spinal neurons. The medullary cardiovascular centers, operating independently of higher structures, are capable of regulating cardiac contractility and rate, arterial pressure, and even blood flow distribution, but under normal conditions their activity is regulated by influences from higher centers, notably the cerebral cortex, especially its cingulate gyrus, the hypothalamus, and the reticular substance in the pons and the mesencephalon. The impulse traffic from the vasomotor center is heightened by wakefulness, pain, mental and muscular effort, or emotional stress. Tonic activity in the medullary cardiovascular-excitatory center is constantly inhibited by impulses from the cardiovascular mechanoreceptors (both the high-pressure receptors in the carotid sinuses, aorta, and left ventricle and the low-pressure receptors in the atria, pulmonary vascular bed, and ventricles), but the medullary centers also receive input from chemoreceptors in skeletal muscle, skin, the viscera, and the special senses.

The cell bodies of the sympathetic preganglionic neurons lie in the intermediolateral horns of the spinal cord; most of their axons leave the spinal cord through the anterior roots of the thoracic and first two lumbar spinal nerves, synapse with postganglionic neurons in the chains of ganglia on each side of the spinal cord or in the peripheral sympathetic ganglia, and then traverse peripheral sympathetic nerves or spinal nerves to the heart and blood vessels. Some preganglionic sympathetic nerve fibers pass directly through the sympathetic chains, through the splanchnic nerves, and into the adrenal medulla where they synapse with secretory cells, which are analogous to postganglionic neurons. Catecholamines (predominantly epinephrine) may be released thereby from the adrenal medulla into the bloodstream at times when sympathetic efferent activity involving other organs is heightened. These two means of sympathetic stimulation (neural and humoral) supplement each other, the former acting rapidly but often briefly and the latter acting slowly but in a more sustained fashion.

While considerable overlap of autonomic innervation exists within most portions of the heart, certain regions receive their major supply from restricted sources. The sympathetic nerves originating from the right stellate ganglion are distributed primarily to the sinoatrial node and the right atrium, while the left ventrolateral cardiac nerve provides the primary supply to the posterolateral surfaces of the left atrium and ventricle; the central representation of these nerves may allow selective and rapid regulation of cardiac function. Contractility of both the epicardial and endocardial surfaces of the left ventricle can be independently altered, and it is now clear that certain nerves preferentially supply nodal tissues while others innervate contractile tissues.[209] The sympathetic nerve endings in the atria and ventricles are interposed between muscle bundles. The terminal innervation of the heart is a plexiform structure, the so-called *perimuscular* or *perimysial plexus*, which extends around the muscle cells in close apposition to, but without penetrating, the myocardial cells. The cardiac muscle cells and innervating fibers might be considered to be analogous to a neuromuscular unit in skeletal muscle. When the rate of liberation of the neurotransmitter exceeds the capacity of the enclosed units to utilize or metabolize it, it may overflow into vascular channels.[210,211]

The NE present in the heart is synthesized and then stored in the sympathetic nerve fibers rather than in the myocardial cells per se. Chemical sympathectomy with 6-hydroxydopamine, cardiac denervation, and treatment with catecholamine-depleting drugs such as reserpine all result in a striking reduction in NE content of the heart as well as in the disappearance of histochemical fluorescence. Sympathetic nerve endings contain neurosecretory granules ranging in size from 400 to 700 nm, and the depolarization of the neurons triggers the release of NE from these vesicles and thence from the adrenergic neuron.

The effects of released NE are terminated by three mechanisms (Fig. 12–33): (1) reuptake into the adrenergic neuron by means of an energy-dependent pump; once inside the neuron, much of the transmitter is again taken up into the neurosecretory granules and is available for subsequent re-release; (2) escape of NE into the circulation is metabolized by catechol-O-methyl transferase (COMT) to normetanephrine, some of which is further converted into vanillylmandelic acid (VMA) via the action of monoamine oxidase (MAO); and finally (3) conversion of NE intraneuronally to 3,4-dihydroxymandelic acid by MAO and then to VMA by COMT. The heart and other organs exhibit supersensitivity to NE after surgical denervation or the administration of cocaine. Both these interventions block the neuronal uptake of NE, thus making a larger quantity of neurotransmitter available for binding to the receptor sites.

The peripheral effects mediated by NE and epinephrine have been classified as alpha or beta. An important effect of NE is to cause vasoconstriction, an action on postsynaptic alpha$_1$ receptors on vascular smooth muscle. However, NE also acts on receptors on the neuron terminal itself. These *presynaptic* alpha receptors (termed alpha$_2$ receptors) serve as feedback inhibitors of the release of NE from the neuron terminal and reduce the release of neurotransmitter. The mechanisms by which NE acts upon cardiac beta and alpha receptors is discussed on page 418.

As we have seen, NE, the natural transmitter for sympathetic neurons, has both alpha and beta receptor–stimulating properties. When NE is given systemically, the alpha vasoconstrictor action predominates, and the elevation of arterial pressure results in reflex bradycardia and an increase in stroke volume and coronary blood flow but no change in cardiac output. *Epinephrine*, synthesized only

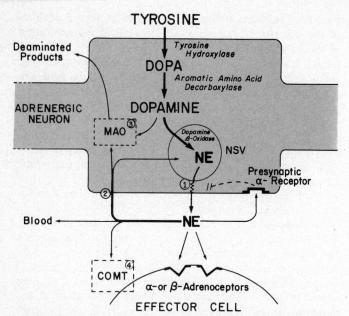

FIGURE 12–33 Synthesis, storage, secretion, and disposition of the adrenergic neurotransmitter norepinephrine (NE). A varicosity of the adrenergic neuron is depicted diagrammatically. Multiple varicosities occur at intervals along the terminal segments of peripheral adrenergic neurons and are juxtaposed to effector sites within target organs. Tyrosine is transported into the adrenergic neuron to provide substrate for the synthesis of NE. The rate-limiting enzyme is tyrosine hydroxylase, and the final enzyme, dopamine β-oxidase, is located within the neurosecretory vesicle (NSV).

1, Depolarization of the neuron leads to release of NE by a calcium-dependent process of "excitation-secretion coupling." in which the neurosecretory vesicle fuses with the neuronal membrane and by exocytosis discharges its soluble contents, including NE and dopamine β-oxidase.

2, Much of the NE released into the synaptic cleft between the neuron and the effector cell is removed from this area by a specialized membrane transport system, known as the NE pump, which transports NE back into the neuron against a concentration gradient. This transport system is relatively unspecific and is responsible for the uptake of a number of ring-substituted amines such as tyramine, ephedrine, and guanethidine. It is competitively inhibited by the tricyclic antidepressants. Released NE may act on adrenoreceptors, "spill" into the bloodstream, or be metabolized extraneuronally (see *4*).

3, The major pathway for intraneuronal bioinactivation of NE (and dopamine) is via monoamine oxidase (MAO).

4, Extraneuronally, a major pathway of NE metabolism is via catechol-O-methyl transferase (COMT), to which NE is exposed at some effector cells and in remote organs such as the liver. (From Oates, J. A., and Shand, D. G.: Clinical pharmacology of the autonomic nervous system. *In* Isselbacher, K. J., et al. (eds.): Harrison's Principles of Internal Medicine. 9th ed. New York, McGraw-Hill Book Co., 1980, p. 390.)

in the adrenal medulla, also has combined alpha and beta actions, but its beta effects are more striking than those of NE, especially in low doses; therefore, it produces tachycardia and an elevation of cardiac output. *Dopamine* (p. 542) is the third naturally occurring catecholamine that subserves a transmitter function in the central nervous system. When infused, it has both alpha and beta effects and in addition acts on what appear to be specific dopamine receptors. At low doses (1 to 5 μg/kg/min, administered intravenously), it dilates mesenteric and renal vessels, producing increased renal blood flow and sodium excretion by its action on dopamine receptors. At slightly higher doses

(5 to 10 μg/kg/min), beta stimulation increases cardiac output with relatively little tachycardia. At even higher doses (>10 μg/kg), tachycardia and alpha stimulation occur. *Isoproterenol* is a synthetic compound with pure beta-agonist activity, causing a reduction in peripheral vascular resistance with an increase in heart rate and contractility and thus an increase in cardiac output.

CARDIAC CONTROL IN THE INTACT ORGANISM (Fig. 12–34)

In the normal state, interference with one or even more of the above-mentioned mechanisms that affect cardiac performance may not influence the cardiac output. For example, a moderate reduction of blood volume or loss of the atrial contribution to ventricular contraction can ordinarily be sustained without a reduction of cardiac output in the resting state. Presumably, other factors such as an increase in adrenergic nerve impulse traffic, which augments contractility, and venoconstriction, which increases ventricular filling, can compensate for this depression.[212] Mechanisms are also available to prevent unnecessary elevation of cardiac output. For example, in normal subjects, expansion of blood volume, a simple increase in heart rate induced by atropine or pacing, or augmentation of myocardial contractility by means of cardiac glycosides does not increase cardiac output[213,214]; the latter reduces the frequency of adrenergic nerve impulses to the heart, thereby tending to oppose the direct inotropic effect.[215] More importantly, since the normal heart is capable of expelling all the blood returned to it under most physiological conditions, cardiac output is ordinarily a function of venous return, not of the level of contractility.[177] The latter does not limit the volume of blood ejected by the heart in the normal subject except perhaps under the most severe stress, and therefore stimulation of myocardial contractility alone would not be expected to elevate cardiac output in a normal subject at rest or during mild activity unless there is a simultaneous reduction in peripheral arterial resistance (as occurs with isoproterenol administration).[216] In the presence of congestive heart failure, on the other hand, cardiac output is usually limited by the contractile state of the myocardium, and a positive inotropic influence raises cardiac output.[204]

Circulatory Adjustment During Exercise

Peripheral Circulatory Responses. As important as the heart may be in mediating the body's response to exercise, alterations in the peripheral circulation are of at least equal significance. Indeed, the elevation of cardiac output achieved in the resting state through infusion of a maximal dose of isoproterenol, which greatly augments cardiac rate and contractility, does not approach the level commonly observed during exercise. Changes in the peripheral circulation act in concert to augment the capacity of the vascular bed to return blood to the heart.[217] Perhaps the most important of these is the vasodilation that takes place in the blood vessels supplying the exercising muscles. The marked reduction in systemic vascular resistance acts in a

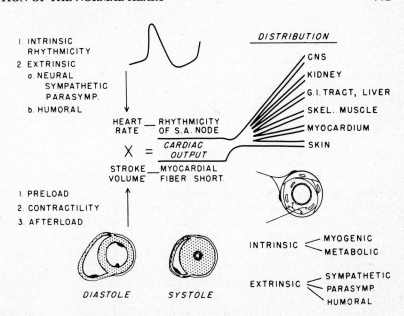

FIGURE 12–34 Schema of factors affecting systemic circulation. In the center, cardiac output is shown with its two determinants, heart rate and stroke volume; the former is a function of the automaticity of the sinoatrial (S.A.) node, while the latter is dependent on the extent of myocardial fiber shortening. The principal determinants of heart rate and stroke volume are listed at the extreme left. Distribution of cardiac output through various vascular beds is shown at the upper right (CNS = central nervous system). The two principal influences (intrinsic and extrinsic) on the lumen of the peripheral resistance vessels and their major determinants are shown at the lower right. (Reprinted by permission from Braunwald, E.: Regulation of the circulation. N. Engl. J. Med. *290*:1124, 1974.)

manner analogous to the opening of multiple arteriovenous fistulas and greatly reduces the resistance to the return of blood ejected from the left ventricle back to the right atrium. Vascular dilatation also tends to reduce afterload and thereby facilitates left ventricular emptying. However, despite profound vasodilation in the metabolizing muscles during exercise, arterial pressure tends to rise, primarily as a consequence of the elevation of cardiac output but also as a result of vasoconstriction, which occurs in many vascular beds other than in the heart and the exercising limbs.[218] Other factors that facilitate venous return during exercise include the rhythmic tensing of the skeletal muscles, not only of the exercising limbs but of the abdomen and thorax as well, which compresses the veins and displaces blood centrally.[217]

Ventricular Volumes and Dimension. The cardiac response to exercise is complex and involves the interaction of changes in heart rate, contractility, preload, and afterload. In man, the elevation of cardiac output that occurs during mild exercise in the supine position results almost exclusively from an increase in heart rate, with stroke volume showing little change.[219] In contrast, in individuals at rest in the erect position, stroke volume is less than in the supine position but increases markedly during strenuous exertion; these increases in stroke volume contribute substantially to the elevation of cardiac output. Indeed, during maximal treadmill exercise, stroke volume increases to approximately twice the levels present at rest in the upright position.[220,221]

The effects of *light* muscular exercise in the supine position on ventricular dimensions have been studied in patients by determining the distances between roentgenopaque markers sewn onto the epicardium.[222] End-diastolic dimensions in both ventricles decreased slightly[223,224] while myocardial contractility rose, as attested to by a shift of the force-velocity relation.[224] Maximal exercise in the dog[174] or strenuous exercise in semirecumbent[225] or upright[226] humans results in an increase in end-diastolic dimensions.

Heart Rate. The ability to alter heart rate is an extremely important mechanism for the adjustment of cardiac output during exercise. Indeed, changes in heart rate normally account in large measure for changes in cardiac

output. The increase in cardiac output that occurs in man during light to moderate exercise in the supine position is accompanied by a parallel augmentation of heart rate, while, as just noted, the stroke volume remains essentially unchanged. When heart rate fails to rise normally, as in patients with heart block, the maximal cardiac output that can be achieved during exercise is reduced.

The Adrenergic Nervous System. The effects of adrenergic blockade have been studied in an effort to elucidate the role of adrenergic nervous activity in the cardiovascular response to exercise. Beta blockade reduces the endurance for maximal activity, cardiac output, mean arterial pressure, left ventricular minute work, and maximal oxygen uptake and increases the arteriovenous oxygen difference and central venous pressure in normal human subjects during maximal exercise in the upright position.[220] This intervention has no significant effect on ventricular dimensions recorded at rest in the supine position, indicating that there is little tonic adrenergic support under these circumstances. However, after beta blockade, little augmentation of the contractile state was observed during exercise; despite some elevations of heart rate, ventricular end-diastolic dimensions do not decrease during exercise, as is the case in the unblocked state.[224]

The Frank-Starling Mechanism. The finding that with light exercise, performed in the supine position, ventricular end-diastolic dimensions decline has been used to support the view that the Frank-Starling mechanism is *not* involved in the cardiac response to exercise.[225,226] In the intact subject the increase in end-diastolic volume that occurs during light exercise may not be evident because of the opposing effects of the tachycardia per se and the increased sympathetic activity normally occurring during exercise, both of which contribute to the reduction of end-diastolic dimensions; indeed, in the presence of beta blockade, exercise no longer reduces end-diastolic size. This conclusion is consonant with studies on denervated dogs[227] in which exercise results in small but significant increases in ventricular end-diastolic dimensions as well as stroke volume.

There is considerable evidence that the *intensity* of exercise also conditions the cardiac response to this stimulus. Indeed, since, as already noted, stroke volume may double in normal human subjects during maximal exercise in the erect posture,[220,221] and since the ratio between stroke volume and end-diastolic volume (i.e., the ejection fraction) is normally in the range of 0.67, ventricular end-diastolic volume *must* increase during maximal exercise. The extent to which the Frank-Starling mechanism is utilized during heavy exercise in normal, healthy dogs has been investigated against this background.[174] Profound increases in heart rate (often exceeding 300 beats/min) occur while cardiac output rises four- to fivefold and stroke volume increases by 50 per cent; increases in contractility are also profound. These values probably represent *physiological maxima* in conscious dogs, since the increases in contractility exceed those resulting from maximally tolerable doses of isoproterenol or norepinephrine. Reductions in end-systolic diameter occur, and in contrast to the findings in supine human subjects carrying out mild exercise, small *increases* in end-diastolic diameter and pressure are consistently noted. Thus, a small augmentation of preload clearly remains a mechanism by which the heart can augment its performance during severe exertion. Greater increases in end-diastolic size are observed during exercise when heart rate is held constant, indicating again that the tachycardia occurring during exercise counteracts the increase in dimensions that would otherwise occur and that might be considered to mask the contribution of the Frank-Starling mechanism.

Beta-adrenergic receptor blockade imposes significant limitations on normal dogs' performance during maximal exercise. The increases in contractility are largely prevented, and the tachycardia and increases in stroke volume and cardiac output are blunted. While slightly greater increases in end-diastolic size occur during exercise after beta blockade, these are not sufficient to augment stroke volume normally.[174] Thus, in the normal dog, activation of beta receptors is responsible for approximately half the increment in heart rate during severe exercise and for an even greater fraction of the augmentation of contractility.

Integrated Responses. The concept that emerges from these observations is that simple tachycardia and adrenergic stimulation of the myocardium are complementary influences, both resulting in improvement of myocardial contractility during exercise, the latter to a greater extent than the former. Adrenergic stimulation of the heart also shortens the duration of systole, thereby providing more time for diastolic filling at any heart rate, further favoring an augmentation of cardiac output. Since the tachycardia that normally occurs during exercise is dependent only in part on sympathetic nerve stimuli and circulating catecholamines but is also due to withdrawal of vagal restraint, an elevation of cardiac output can still occur despite adrenergic blockade. However, the degree of improvement of contractility occurring during exercise is reduced during sympathetic blockade, and, as a consequence, the elevation of cardiac output that can occur under these circumstances is limited.[220,222]

Thus, the normal cardiac response to exercise involves the integrated effects on the myocardium of an increase in heart rate, adrenergic stimulation, and the operation of the Frank-Starling mechanism. During submaximal levels of exertion, cardiac output can rise when one or even two of these influences are inhibited. However, during maximal levels of muscular exercise, the ventricular myocardium requires all three influences to sustain a level of activity suf-

ficient to satisfy the greatly augmented oxygen requirements of the exercising skeletal muscles.

Other Adjustments. Several other systems aid in the augmented delivery of oxygen to the metabolizing tissues during exercise. Among these are (1) a large increase (up to threefold) in the extraction of oxygen from blood perfusing skeletal muscle; (2) the augmented activity of thoracic and abdominal respiratory muscles during exercise, which aids substantially in displacing blood from the peripheral venous system to the heart; (3) augmentation of the oxygen-carrying capacity of the arterial blood, a phenomenon particularly prominent in species such as the dog and cat, in which splenic contraction can contribute a substantial quantity of red cell mass to the circulation; (4) rightward displacement of the oxygen-hemoglobin dissociation curve, which facilitates the unloading of oxygen from red cells to the peripheral tissues; and (5) in highly trained athletes, the development of cardiac dilatation and hypertrophy with enlargement of the ventricular chambers. This last adaptation, together with a slower than normal heart rate at rest and during exertion, appears to allow a higher and more sustained level of cardiac output.

Although so-called athlete's heart was at one time considered to represent an abnormal state, it is now felt that the cardiac enlargement and hypertrophy that occur during this type of physiological hypertrophy represent a useful adaptive mechanism, undoubtedly important to the elevated maximal oxygen uptake observed in such individuals.[228] Thus, increased left ventricular dimensions and wall thickness[229] are associated with elevations of stroke volume and right ventricular end-diastolic dimensions at rest; however, the ejection fraction and normalized mean velocity of wall shortening of the left ventricle in the endurance athlete are normal.[230] Many such individuals show electrocardiographic evidence of ventricular hypertrophy as well.[230]

CLINICAL CORRELATIONS

A few examples will serve to demonstrate that the principles of circulatory regulation described above are readily applicable to a variety of clinical situations. For instance, the mechanical lesions characteristic of congenital and rheumatic valvular disease result in abnormalities of ventricular preload or afterload or both. In obstruction to left ventricular outflow, for example, the increase in afterload tends, in the absence of compensatory features, to depress stroke volume and hence cardiac output. Increased afterload imposed by the aorta, which has become stiffer with age, limits the stroke volume response to exercise.[231] The development of left ventricular hypertrophy reduces the stress on each unit of myocardium, despite an elevated intraventricular pressure. In this manner hypertrophy tends to maintain the afterload of each myocardial cell at or close to normal, although there is, of course, a limit to the compensation that can be provided by this mechanism.

Of the many congenital and valvular abnormalities that produce alterations in ventricular preload, perhaps the most straightforward to consider is atrial septal defect (pp. 958 and 1027); as a result of the interatrial communication and the greater compliance of the right ventricle than the left, the preload placed on the right ventricle is greatly augmented and the stroke volume of the right ventricle greatly exceeds that of the left. This congenital lesion is usually well tolerated unless pulmonary artery pressure rises, thereby elevating right ventricular afterload. Lesions such as ventricular septal defect, patent ductus arteriosus, and mitral regurgitation are more complex in that a measure of compensation for the increased preload that is placed on the left ventricle is provided by the lowered afterload that results from unloading of the ventricle through the regurgitant mitral valve, the septal defect, or the aorta–pulmonary artery communication.[191]

References

1. Sommer, J. R., and Waugh, R. A.: The ultrastructure of the mammalian cardiac muscle cell—with special emphasis on the tubular membrane systems. Am. J. Pathol. 82:192, 1976.
2. McNutt, N. S., and Weinstein, R. S.: Membrane ultrastructure at mammalian intracellular junctions. Progr. Biophys. 20:45, 1973.
3. Fawcett, D. W., and McNutt, N. S.: The ultrastructure of the cat myocardium. I. Ventricular papillary muscle. J. Cell Biol. 42:1, 1969.
4. Sommer, J. R., and Johnson, E. A.: Ultrastructure of cardiac muscle. In Berne, R. M. (ed.): Handbook of Physiology. Section 2, The Cardiovascular System. Vol. I, The Heart. Bethesda, American Physiological Society, 1979, pp. 113–186.
5. Page, E., Polimeni, P. I., Zak, R., Early, J., and Johnson, M.: Myofibrillar mass in rat and rabbit heart muscle. Circ. Res. 30:430, 1972.
6. Robinson, T. F., and Winegrad, S.: The measurement and dynamic implications of thin filament lengths in heart muscle. J. Physiol. (Lond.) 286:607, 1979.
7. Adams, R. J., and Schwartz, A.: Comparative mechanisms for contraction of cardiac and skeletal muscle. Chest 78:123, 1980.
7a. Langer, G. A.: The structure and function of the myocardial cell surface. In Levy, M. N., and Vassalle, M. (Eds.): Excitation and Neural Control of the Heart. Baltimore, Williams & Wilkins, 1982, pp. 79–92.
8. Navaratnam, V.: The structure of cardiac muscle. In Dickinson, C. J., and Marks, J. (eds.): Developments in Cardiovascular Medicine. Cambridge, MIT Press, 1978, pp. 119–128.
9. Thornell, L., and Erickson, A.: Filament systems in the Purkinje fibers of the heart. Am. J. Physiol. 241:H-291, 1981.
10. Robinson, T. F., and Winegrad, S.: A variety of intercellular connections in heart muscle. J. Molec. Cell Cardiol. 13:185, 1981.
11. Schwartz, A.: Active transport in mammalian myocardium. In Langer, G. A., and Brady, A. J. (eds.): The Mammalian Myocardium. New York, John Wiley and Sons, 1974, pp. 81–104.
12. Caroni, P., and Carafoli, E.: An ATP-dependent Ca^{2+}-pumping system in dog heart sarcolemma. Nature 283:765, 1980.
13. Huxley, H. E.: The double array of filament in cross-striated muscle. J. Biophys. Biochem. Cytol. 3:631, 1957.
14. Page, S.: Measurement of structural parameters in cardiac muscle. CIBA Foundation Symposium 24 (New Series), Amsterdam, Elsevier, 1974, p. 13.
15. Lowey, S., Slayter, H. S., Weeds, A. G., and Baker, H.: Substructure of the myosin molecule. I. Subfragments of myosin by enzymic degradation. J. Molec. Biol. 42:1, 1969.
16. Scheuer, J., and Bhan, A. K.: Cardiac contractile proteins. Adenosine triphosphatase activity and physiological function. Circ. Res. 45:1, 1979.
17. Hoh, J. F. Y., McGrath, P. A., and Hale, P. T.: Electrophoretic analysis of multiple forms of rat cardiac myosin: Effect of hypophysectomy and thyroxine replacement. J. Molec. Cell Cardiol. 10:1053, 1978.
17a. Samuel, J-L., Rappaport, L., Mercadier, J-J., Lompre, A-M., Sartore, S., Triban, C., Schiaffino, S., and Schwartz, K.: Distribution of myosin isozymes within single cardiac cells. An immnohistochemical study. Circ. Res. 52:200, 1983.
18. Mercadier, J. J., Lompre, A. M., Wisnewsky, C., Samuel, J. L., Bercovici, J., Swynghedauw, B., and Schwartz, K.: Myosin isoenzymic changes in several models of rat cardiac hypertrophy. Circ. Res. 49:525, 1981.
19. Schwartz, K., Lecarpentier, Y., Martin, J. L., Lompre, A. M., Mercadier, J. J., and Swynghedauw, B.: Myosin isoenzymic distribution correlates with speed of myocardial contraction. J. Molec. Cell. Cardiol. 13:1071, 1981.
20. Katz, A. M.: Contractile proteins of the heart. Physiol. Rev. 50:63, 1970.
21. Weber, A., and Murray, J. M.: Molecular control mechanisms in muscle contraction. Physiol. Rev. 53:612, 1973.
22. Ebashi, S.: Regulatory mechanism of muscle contraction with special reference to Ca-troponin-tropomyosin system. Essays Biochem. 10:1, 1974.
23. Potter, J. D., and Gergely, J.: Troponin, tropomyosin and actin interactions in the Ca++ regulation of muscle contraction. Biochemistry 13:2697, 1974.
24. Greaser, M. L., Yamaguchi, M., Brekke, C., Potter, J., and Gergely, J.: Troponin subunits and their interactions. Cold Spring Harbor Symp. Quant. Biol. 37:235, 1973.
25. Spudich, J. A., Huxley, H. E., and Finch, J. F.: Regulation of skeletal muscle contraction. II. Structural studies of the interaction of the tropomyosin-troponin complex with actin. J. Molec. Biol. 72:619, 1972.
26. Huxley, H. E.: Muscular contraction and cell motility. Nature 243:445, 1973.
27. Julian, F. J., Moss, R. L., and Sollins, M. R.: The mechanism for vertebrate striated muscle contraction. Circ. Res. 42:2, 1978.
28. Ringer, S.: A further contribution regarding the influence of the different constituents of the blood on the contraction of the heart. J. Physiol. (Lond.) 4:30, 1882.
29. Fabiato, A., and Fabiato, F.: Calcium and cardiac excitation-contraction coupling. Ann. Rev. Physiol. 41:473, 1979.
30. Allen, D. G., and Blinks, J. R.: Calcium transients in aequorin-injected frog cardiac muscle. Nature 273:509, 1978.
31. Jewell, B. R.: Activation of contraction in cardiac muscle. Mayo Clin. Proc. 57(Suppl.):6, 1982.
32. Winegrad, S.: Electromechanical coupling in heart muscle. In Berne, R. M. (ed.): Handbook of Physiology. Section 2, The Cardiovascular System. Vol. I, The Heart. Bethesda, American Physiological Society, 1979, pp. 393–428.
33. Fabiato, A.: Calcium release in skinned cardiac cells: Variations with species, tissues and development. Fed. Proc. 41:2238, 1982.
34. Allen, D. G., Jewell, B. R., and Wood, E. H.: Studies of the contractility of mammalian myocardium at low rates of stimulation. J. Physiol. 254:1, 1976.
35. Baker, P. F., Hodgkin, A. L., and Ridgeway, E. B.: Depolarization and calcium entry in squid giant axon. J. Physiol. (Lond.) 218:709, 1971.
35a. Coraboeuf, E.: Ionic basis of electrical activity in cardiac tissues. In Levy, M. N., and Vassalle, M. (Eds.): Excitation and Neural Control of the Heart. Baltimore, Williams & Wilkins, 1982, pp. 1–36.
35b. Glitsch, H. G.: Characteristics of active sodium transport in intact cardiac cells. In Levy, M. N., and Vassalle, M. (Eds.): Baltimore, Williams & Wilkins, 1982, pp. 36–58.
36. Reuter, H., and Scholz, H.: A study of the ion selectivity and the kinetic properties of the calcium dependent slow inward current in mammalian cardiac muscle. J. Physiol. (Lond.) 264:12, 1977.
37. Flaim, S. F., and Zelis, R. (eds.): Calcium Blockers. Baltimore, Urban and Schwartzenberg, 1982, 303 pp.
38. Braunwald, E.: Mechanisms of action of calcium channel blocking agents. N. Engl. J. Med. 307:1618, 1982.
38a. Keung, E. C. H., and Aronson, R. S.: Physiology of calcium current is cardiac muscle. Prog. Cardiovasc. Dis. 25:279, 1983.
39. Langer, G. A.: Sodium-calcium exchange in the heart. Ann. Rev. Physiol. 44:435, 1982.
40. Philipson, K. D., Bers, D. M., Nishimoto, A. Y., and Langer, G. A.: Binding of Ca^{2+} and Na^{2+} to sarcolemmal membranes: Relation to control of myocardial contractility. Am. J. Physiol. 238:H373, 1980.
41. McDonald, T. F., Pelzer, D., and Trautwein, W.: Does the calcium current modulate the contraction of the accompanying beat? A study of E-C coupling in mammalian ventricular muscle using cobalt ions. Circ. Res. 49:576, 1981.
42. Inesi, G.: Active transport of calcium ion in sarcoplasmic membranes. Ann. Rev. Phys. Bioeng. 1:191, 1973.
43. Maughan, D. W., Low, E. S., and Alpert, N. R.: Isometric force development, isotonic shortening, and elasticity measurements from Ca^{2+}-activated ventricular muscle of the guinea pig. J. Gen. Physiol. 71:431, 1978.
44. Langer, G. A.: Heart: Excitation-contraction coupling. Ann. Rev. Physiol. 35:55, 1973.
45. Sperelakis, N., and Schneider, J. A.: A metabolic control mechanism for calcium ion influx that may protect the ventricular myocardial cell. Am. J. Cardiol. 37:1079, 1976.
46. Johnson, E. A.: Force-interval relationship of cardiac muscle. In Berne, R. M. (ed.): Handbook of Physiology. Section 2, The Cardiovascular System. Vol. I, The Heart. Bethesda, American Physiological Society, 1979, pp. 475–496.
47. Covell, J. W., Ross, J., Jr., Taylor, R., Sonnenblick, E. H., and Braunwald, E.: Effects of increasing frequency of contraction on force-velocity relation of left ventricle. Cardiovasc. Res. 1:2, 1967.
48. Higgins, C. B., Vatner, S. F., Franklin, D., and Braunwald, E.: Extent of regulation of the heart's contractile state in the conscious dog by alteration in the frequency of contraction. J. Clin. Invest. 52:1187, 1973.
49. Hoffman, B. F., Bindler, E., and Suckling, E. E.: Postextrasystolic potentiation of contraction in cardiac muscle. Am. J. Physiol. 185:95, 1956.
50. Ross, J., Jr., Sonnenblick, E. H., Kaiser, G. A., Frommer, P. L., and Braunwald, E.: Electroaugmentation of ventricular performance and oxygen consumption by repetitive application of paired electrical stimuli. Circ. Res. 16:332, 1965.
51. Braunwald, E., Sonnenblick, E. H., Frommer, P. L., and Ross, J., Jr.: Paired electric stimulation of the heart: Physiologic observations and clinical implications. Adv. Intern. Med. 13:61, 1967.
52. Cranefield, P. F.: The force of contraction of extrasystoles and the potentiation of force of the post-extrasystolic contraction: A historical review. Bull. N. Y. Acad. Med. 41:419, 1965.
53. Katz, A. M., Bailin, G., Kirchberger, M. A., and Today, M.: Regulation of myocardial cell function by agents that increase cyclic AMP production in the heart. In Fishman, A. P. (ed.): Heart Failure. Washington, D.C., Hemisphere Publishing Corp., 1978, pp. 11–28.
54. Keely, S. L., and Corbin, J. D.: Involvement of cAMP-dependent protein kinase in the regulation of heart contractile force. Am. J. Physiol. 233:H269, 1977.
55. Hicks, M. J., Shigekawa, M., and Katz, A. M.: Mechanism by which cyclic adenosine 3':5'-monophosphate–dependent protein kinase stimulates calcium transport in cardiac sarcoplasmic reticulum. Circ. Res. 44:384, 1979.
56. Luttgau, H. C.: Caffeine, calcium and the activation of contraction. In Cuth-

bert, A. W. (ed.): Calcium and Cellular Function. New York, St. Martins Press, 1970, pp. 241–248.

57. Fabiato, A., and Fabiato, F.: Effects of pH on the myofilaments and sarcoplasmic reticulum of skinned cells from cardiac and skeletal muscles. J. Physiol. 276:233, 1978.

58. Ray, K. P., and England, P. J.: Phosphorylation of the inhibitory subunit of troponin and its effect on the calcium dependence of cardiac myofibril adenosine triphosphatase. FEBS Lett. 70:11, 1976.

59. Fabiato, A., and Fabiato, F.: Cyclic AMP-induced enhancement of calcium accumulation by the sarcoplasmic reticulum with no modification of the sensitivity of the myofilaments to calcium in skinned fibres from a fast skeletal muscle. Biochim. Biophys. Acta 539:253, 1978.

60. Goldberg, N. D.: Cyclic nucleotides and cell function. Hosp. Pract. 9:127, 1974.

61. Nawrath, H.: Does cyclic GMP mediate the negative inotropic effect of acetylcholine in the heart? Nature 267:72, 1977.

62. Carmeliet, E.: The slow inward current: Nonvoltage-clamp studies. In Zipes, D. P., Bailey, J. C., and Elharrar, V. (eds.): The Slow Inward Current and Cardiac Arrhythmias. The Hague, Martinus Nijhoff, 1980.

63. Barry, W. H., Biedert, S., Miura, D. S., and Smith, T. W.: Changes in cellular Na, K and Ca contents, monovalent cation transport rate, and contractile state during washout of cardiac glycosides from cultured chick heart cells. Circ. Res. 49:141, 1981.

64. Solaro, R. J.: The role of calcium in the contraction of the heart. In Flaim, S. F., and Zelis, R. (eds.): Calcium Blockers. Baltimore, Urban and Schwarzenberg, 1982, pp. 21–36.

65. Triggle, D. J., and Swamy, V. C.: Pharmacology of agents that affect calcium: Agonists and antagonists. Chest 78(Suppl.):174, 1980.

66. van Breemen, C., Aaronson, P., and Loutzenhiser, R.: Na-Ca interactions in mammalian smooth muscle. Pharmacol. Rev. 30:167, 1979.

67. Fleckenstein, A.: Calcium Antagonism in Heart and Smooth Muscle. New York, Jonh Wiley and Sons, 1983.

68. Braunwald, E.: Calcium-channel blockers: Pharmacologic considerations. Am. Heart J. 104:665, 1982.

69. Antman, E. M., Stone, P. H., Muller, J. E., and Braunwald, E.: Calcium channel blocking agents in the treatment of cardiovascular disorders. Part I. Basic and clinical electrophysiologic effects. Ann. Intern. Med. 93:875, 1980.

70. Stone, P. H., Antman, E. M., Muller, J. E., and Braunwald, E.: Calcium channel blocking agents in the treatment of cardiovascular disorders. Part II. Hemodynamic effects and clinical applications. Ann. Intern. Med. 93:886, 1980.

71. Lands, A. M., Arnold, A., McAuliff, J. P., Ludena, R. P., and Brown, T. G.: Differentiation of receptor systems activated by sympathomimetic amines. Nature 214:597, 1967.

71a. Watanabe, A. M.: Recent advances in knowledge about beta-adrenergic receptors: Application to clinical cardiology. J. Am. Coll. Cardiol. 1:82, 1983.

72. Carlsson, E., Dahlot, C. G., Hedberg, A., Persson, H., and Tangstrand, B.: Differentiation of cardiac chronotropic and inotropic effects of beta adrenoceptor agonists. Naunyn-Schmiedeberg's Arch. Pharmacol. 300:101, 1977.

73. Wilffart, B., Tummermans, P. B. M. W. M., and van Zwieten, P. A.: Extrasynaptic location of alpha-2 and non-innervated beta-2 adrenoceptors in the vascular system in the pithed normotensive rat. J. Pharmacol. Exp. Ther. 221:762, 1982.

74. Langer, S. Z.: Presynaptic regulation of catecholamines. Pharmacol. Rev. 32:337, 1981.

75. Hedberg, A., Minneman, K. P., and Molinoff, P. B.: Differential distribution of beta-1 and beta-2 adrenergic receptors in cat and guinea-pig heart. J. Pharmacol. Exp. Ther. 213:503, 1980.

75a. Schumann, H. J.: What role do alpha and beta adrenoceptors play in the regulation of the heart. Europ. Heart J. 4(Suppl. A):55, 1983.

76. Lee, J. C., Fripp, R. R., and Downing, S. E.: Myocardial responses to alpha-adrenoceptor stimulation with methoxamine hydrochloride in lambs. Am. J. Physiol. 242:H405, 1982.

77. Colucci, W. S., and Braunwald, E.: Adrenergic receptors: New concepts and implications for cardiovascular therapeutics. In Conti, C. R. (ed.): Cardiac Clinics. Philadelphia, F. A. Davis, 1983.

78. Wagner, J., and Shumann, H.-J.: Different mechanisms underlying the stimulation of myocardial alpha- and beta-adrenoceptors. Life Sci. 24:2045, 1979.

79. Abbott, B. C., and Mommaerts, W. F. H. M.: A study of inotropic mechanisms in the papillary muscle preparation. J. Gen. Physiol. 42:533, 1959.

80. Sonnenblick, E. H.: Force-velocity relations in mammalian heart muscle. Am. J. Physiol. 202:931, 1962.

81. Sonnenblick, E. H.: Determinants of active state in heart muscle: Force, velocity, instantaneous muscle length and time. Fed. Proc. 24:1396, 1965.

82. Brady, A. J.: Time and displacement dependence of cardiac contractility: Problems in defining the active state and force-velocity relations. Fed. Proc. 24:1410, 1965.

83. deClerck, N. M., Claes, V. A., and Brutsaert, D. L.: Force velocity relations of single cardiac muscle cells. J. Gen. Physiol. 69:221, 1977.

84. Brady, A. J.: Mechanical properties of cardiac fibers. In Berne, R. M. (ed.): Handbook of Physiology. Section 2, The Cardiovascular System. Vol. I, The Heart. Bethesda, American Physiological Society, 1979, pp. 461–474.

85. Sonnenblick, E. H.: Active state in heart muscle: its delayed onset and modification by inotropic agents. J. Gen. Physiol. 50:661, 1967.

86. Parmley, W. W., and Sonnenblick, E. H.: Series elasticity: In relation to contractile element velocity and proposed muscle models. Circ. Res. 20:112, 1967.

87. Grimm, A. F., and Whitehorn, W. V.: Characteristics of resting tension of myocardium and localization of its elements. Am. J. Physiol. 210:1362, 1966.

88. Huxley, A. F., and Simmons, R. M.: Mechanical transients and the origin of muscular force. Cold Spring Harbor Symp. Quant. Biol. 37:669, 1973.

89. Podolsky, R. J., and Nolan, A. C.: Muscle contraction transients, crossbridge kinetics and the Fenn effect. Cold Spring Harbor. Symp. Quant. Biol. 37:661, 1973.

90. Edman, K. A. P., and Nilsson, L.: Time course of the active state in relation to muscle length and movement: A comparative study on skeletal muscle and myocardium. Cardiovasc. Res. 5(Suppl. 1):3, 1971.

91. ter Keurs, H. E. D. J., Rijnsburger, W. H., van Heuningen, R., and Negelsmit, M. J.: Tension development and sarcomere length in rat cardiac trabeculae. Circ. Res. 46:703, 1980.

92. Braunwald, E., Frye, R. L., and Ross, J., Jr.: Studies on Starling's law of the heart: Determinants of the relationship between end-diastolic pressure and circumference. Circ. Res. 8:1254, 1960.

93. Weisfeldt, M. L., Loeven, W. A., and Shock, N. W.: Resting and active mechanical properties of trabeculae carneae from aged male rats. Am. J. Physiol. 220:1921, 1971.

94. Brutsaert, D. L., and Sonnenblick, E. H.: Cardiac muscle mechanics in the evaluation of myocardial contractility and pump function: Problems, concepts and directions. Progr. Cardiovasc. Dis. 16:337, 1973.

95. Henderson, A. H., Van Ocken, E., and Brutsaert, D. L.: A reappraisal of force-velocity measurements in isolated heart muscle preparation. Europ. J. Cardiol. 1:105, 1973.

96. Strobeck, J. E., Krueger, J. W., and Sonnenblick, E. H.: Lead and time considerations in the force-length relation of heart muscle. Fed. Proc. 39:175, 1980.

97. Grossman, W., Braunwald, E., Mann, T., McLaurin, L. P., and Green, L. H.: Contractile state of the left ventricle in man as evaluated from endsystolic pressure-volume relations. Circulation 56:845, 1977.

98. Suga, H., and Yamakoshi, K.: Effects of stroke volume and velocity of ejection on end-systolic pressure on canine left ventricle. Circ. Res. 40:445, 1977.

99. Krueger, J. W., and Pollack, G. H.: Myocardial sarcomere dynamics during isometric contraction. J. Physiol. 251:627, 1973.

100. Pollack, G. H., and Huntsman, L. L.: Sarcomere length-active force relations in living mammalian cardiac muscle. Am. J. Physiol. 227:383, 1974.

101. Vassale, D. V., and Pollack, G. H.: The force-velocity relation and stepwise shortening in cardiac muscle. Cir. Res. 51:37, 1982.

102. Van Henningen, R., Rijnsburger, W. H., and ter Keurs, H. E. D. J.: Sarcomere length control in striated muscle. Am. J. Physiol. 242:H411, 1982.

103. Fabiato, A., and Fabiato, F.: Dependence of the contractile activation of skinned cardiac cells on the sarcomere length. Nature 256:54, 1975.

104. Jewell, B. R.: A reexamination of the influence of muscle length on myocardial performance. Circ. Res. 40:221, 1977.

105. Fabiato, A., and Fabiato, F.: Dependence of calcium release, tension generation, and restoring forces on sarcomere length in skinned cardiac cells. Europ. J. Cardiol. 4(Suppl.):13, 1976.

106. Tarr, M., Trank, J. W., Goertz, K. K., and Leiffer, P.: Effect of initial sarcomere length on sarcomere kinetics and force development in single frog atrial cardiac cells. Circ. Res. 49:767, 1981.

107. Gordon, A. M., and Pollack, G. H.: Effects of calcium on the sarcomere length-tension relation in rat cardiac muscle. Circ. Res. 47:610, 1980.

108. Brady, A. J.: Mechanical properties of cardiac fibers. In Berne, R. M. (ed.): Handbook of Physiology. Section 2, The Cardiovascular System. Vol. I, The Heart. Bethesda, American Physiological Society; 1979, pp. 461–474.

109. Huntsman, L. L., and Stewart, D. K.: Length-dependent calcium inotropism in cat papillary muscle. Circ. Res. 40:366, 1977.

110. Endo, M.: Stretch-induced increase in activation of skinned muscle fibres by calcium. Nature (New Biol.) 237:211, 1972.

111. Frank, O.: On the dynamics of cardiac muscle. (Transl. by C. B. Chapman and E. Wasserman.) Am. Heart J. 58:282 and 467, 1959.

112. Starling, E. H.: Linacre Lecture on the Law of the Heart (1915). London, Longmans, Green and Co., Ltd., 1918.

113. Ramsey, R. W., and Street, S. F.: The isometric length-tension diagram of isolated skeletal muscle fibers of the frog. J. Cell. Comp. Physiol. 15:11, 1940.

114. Gordon, A. M., Huxley, A. F., and Julian, F. J.: The variation in isometric tension with sarcomere length in vertebrate muscle fibers. J. Physiol. (Lond.) 184:170, 1966.

115. Gordon, A. M., Huxley, A. F., and Julian, F. J.: Tension development in highly stretched vertebrate muscle fibers. J. Physiol. 184:143, 1966.

116. Noble, M. I. M., and Pollack, G. H.: Molecular mechanisms of contraction. Circ. Res. 40:333, 1977.

117. Sonnenblick, E. H., Spiro, D., and Cottrell, J. S.: Fine structural changes in heart muscle in relation to the length-tension curve. Proc. Natl. Acad. Sci. (USA) 49:193, 1963.

118. Grimm, A. F., Katele, K. V., Kubota, R., and Whitehorn, W. V.: Relation of sarcomere length and muscle length in resting myocardium. Am. J. Physiol. 218:1412, 1970.

119. Pollack, G. H., and Krueger, J. W.: Sarcomere dynamics in intact cardiac muscle. Europ. J. Cardiol. 4:53, 1976.

120. Sonnenblick, E. H., Skelton, C. L., Spotnitz, W. D., and Feldman, D.: Redefinition of the ultrastructural basis of cardiac length-tension relations. Circulation 48(Suppl. 4):65, 1973.

121. Spotnitz, H. M., Sonnenblick, E. H., and Spiro, D.: Relation of ultrastructure

to function in the intact heart: Sarcomere structure relative to pressure-volume curves of the intact left ventricles of dog and cat. Circ. Res. *18*:49, 1966.

122. Leyton, R. A., Spotnitz, H. M., and Sonnenblick, E. H.: Cardiac ultrastructure and function: Sarcomeres in the right ventricle. Am. J. Physiol. *221*:902, 1971.

123. Ross, J., Jr., Sonnenblick, E. H., Covell, J. W., Kaiser, G. A., and Spiro, D.: Architecture of the heart in systole and diastole: Technique of rapid fixation and analysis of left ventricular geometry. Circ. Res. *21*:409, 1967.

124. Sonnenblick, E. H., Ross, J., Jr., Covell, J. W., Spotnitz, H. M., and Spiro, D.: Ultrastructure of the heart in systole and diastole. Circ. Res. *21*:423, 1967.

125. Yoran, C., Covell, J. W., and Ross, J., Jr.: Structural basis for ascending limb of left ventricular function. Circ. Res. *32*:297, 1973.

126. Elzinga, G., and Westerhof, N.: "Pressure-volume" relations in isolated cat trabecula. Circ. Res. *49*:388, 1981.

127. Weber, K. T., and Janicki, J. S.: Muscle-pump function of the intact heart. *In* Fishman, A. P. (ed.): Heart Failure. Washington, D.C., Hemisphere Publishing Co., 1978, pp. 29–42.

128. Suga, H., Kitabatake, A., and Sagawa, K.: End-systolic pressure determines stoke volume in the isolated canine left ventricle under a constant contractile state. Circ. Res. *44*:238, 1979.

129. Braunwald, E., and Ross, J., Jr.: Control of cardiac performance. *In* Berne, R. M. (ed.): Handbook of Physiology. Section 2, The Cardiovascular System. Vol. I, The Heart. Bethesda, American Physiological Society, 1979, pp. 533–580.

130. Hawthorne, E. W.: Instantaneous dimensional changes of the left ventricle in dogs. Circ. Res. *9*:110, 1961.

131. Karliner, J. S., Bouchard, R. J., and Gault, J. H.: Dimensional changes of the human left ventricle prior to aortic valve opening: A cineangiographic study in patients with and without left heart disease. Circulation *44*:312, 1971.

132. Rankin, J. S., McHale, P. A., Arentzen, C. E., Ling, D., Greenfield, J. C., Jr., and Anderson, R. W.: The three dimensional dynamic geometry of the left ventricle in the conscious dog. Circ. Res. *39*:304, 1976.

133. Bove, A. A., and Lynch, P. R.: Measurement of canine left ventricular performance by cineradiography of the heart. J. Appl. Physiol. *29*:877, 1970.

134. Sasayama, S., Franklin, D., Ross, J., Jr., Kemper, W. S., and McKown, D.: Dynamic changes in left ventricular wall thickness and their use in analyzing cardiac function in the conscious dog. Am. J. Cardiol. *38*:870, 1976.

135. Sandler, H., and Alderman, E.: Determination of left ventricular size and shape. Circ. Res. *34*:1, 1974.

136. Mirsky, I.: Elastic properties of the myocardium: A quantitative approach with physiological and clinical applications. *In* Berne, R. M. (ed.): Handbook of Physiology. Section 2, The Cardiovascular System. Vol. I, The Heart. Bethesda, Md., American Physiological Society, 1979, pp. 497–532.

137. Peterson, K. L., Tsuji, J., Johnson, A., DiDonna, J., and LeWinter, M.: Diastolic left ventricular pressure-volume and stress-strain relations in patients with valvular aortic stenosis and left ventricular hypertrophy. Circulation *58*:77, 1978.

138. Mirsky, I., and Rankin, J. S.: The effects of geometry , elasticity, and external pressures on the diastolic pressure-volume and stiffness-stress relations. How important is the pericardium? Circ. Res. *44*:601, 1979.

139. Grossman, W., and McLaurin, L. P.: Diastolic properties of the left ventricle. Ann Intern. Med. *84*:316, 1976.

140. Taylor, R. R., Covell, J. W., Sonnenblick, E. H., and Ross, J., Jr.: The dependence of ventricular distensibility in the filling of the opposite ventricle. Am. J. Physiol. *213*:711, 1967.

141. Covell, J. W., and Ross, J., Jr.: Nature and significance of alterations in myocardial compliance. Am. J. Cardiol. *32*:449, 1973.

142. Diamond, G., Forrester, J. S., Hargis, J., Parmley, W. W., Danzig, R., and Swan, H. J. C.: The diastolic pressure-volume relationship of the canine left ventricle. Circ. Res. *29*:297, 1971.

143. Gaasch, W. H., Levine, H. J., Quinones, M. A., and Alexander, J. K.: Left ventricular compliance: Mechanisms and clinical implications. Am. J. Cardiol. *38*:645, 1976.

144. Pouleur, H., Karliner, J. S., LeWinter, M. M., and Covell, J. W.: Diastolic viscous properties of the intact canine left ventricle. Circ. Res. *45*:410, 1979.

145. LeWinter, M. M., Engler, R., and Pavelec, R. S.: Time-dependent shifts of the left ventricular diastolic filling relationship in conscious dogs. Circ. Res. *45*:641, 1979.

146. Gentzler, R. D., II, Briselli, M. F., and Gault, J. H.: Angiographic estimation of right ventricular volume in man. Circulation *50*:324, 1974.

147. Santamore, W. P., Lynch, P. R., Meier, G., Heckman, J., and Bove, A. A.: Myocardial interaction between the ventricles. J. Appl. Physiol. *4*:362, 1976.

148. Spann, J. F., Covell, J. W., Eckberg, D. L., Sonnenblick, E. H., Ross, J., Jr., and Braunwald, E.: Contractile performance of the hypertrophied and chronically failing cat ventricle. Am. J. Physiol. *223*:1150, 1972.

149. Bemis, C. E., Serur, J. R., Borkenhagen, D., Sonnenblick, E. H., and Urschel, C. W.: Influence of right ventricular filling pressure on left ventricular pressure and dimension. Circ. Res. *34*:498, 1974.

150. Parmley, W. W., Chuck, L., Chatterjee, K., Swan, H. J. C., Klausner, S. C., Glantz, S. A., and Ratshin, R. A.: Acute changes in the diastolic pressure-volume relationship of the left ventricle. Europ. J. Cardiol. *4*(Suppl.):105, 1976.

151. LeWinter, M. M., and Porsche, R.: Influence of the pericardium on left ventricular end-diastolic pressure-segment relations during early and late stages of experimental chronic volume overload in dogs. Circ. Res. *50*:501, 1981.

152. Mann, T., Goldberg, S., Mudge, G. H., Jr., and Grossman, W.: Factors con-

tributing to altered left ventricular diastolic properties during angina pectoris. Circulation *59*:14, 1979.

153. Shirato, K., Shabetai, R., Bhargava, V., Franklin, D., and Ross, J., Jr.: Alteration of the left ventricular diastolic pressure-segment length relation produced by the pericardium: Effects of cardiac distention and afterload reduction in conscious dogs. Circulation *57*:1191, 1978.

154. Boettcher, D. H., Vatner, S. F., Heyndrickx, G. R., and Braunwald, E.: Extent of utilization of the Frank-Starling mechanism in conscious dogs. Am. J. Physiol. *3*:338, 1978.

155. Parker, J. O., and Case, R. B.: Normal left ventricular function. Circulation *60*:4, 1979.

156. Wiggers, C. J., and Katz, L. N.: Contour of the ventricular volume curves under different conditions. Am. J. Physiol. *58*:439, 1922.

157. Sarnoff, S. J., and Mitchell, J. H.: Control of the function of the heart. *In* Hamilton, W. F., and Dow, P. (eds.): Handbook of Physiology. Section 2, Circulation. Vol. I. Bethesda, Md., American Physiological Society. 1962, pp. 489–532.

157a.Strobeck, J. E., and Sonnenblick, E. H.: Myocardial and ventricular function. Cardiovasc. Rev. Rep. *4*:568, 1983.

158. Suga, H., Sagawa, K., and Shoukas, A. A.: Load independence of the instantaneous pressure-volume ratio of the canine left ventricle and effects of epinephrine and heart rate on the ratio. Circ. Res. *32*:314, 1973.

159. Sagawa, K.: The end systolic pressure-volume relation of the ventricle: Definition, modifications and clinical use. Circulation *63*:1223, 1981.

160. Mahler, F., Covell, J. W., and Ross, J., Jr.: Systolic pressure-diameter relations in the normal conscious dog. Cardiovasc. Res. *9*:447, 1975.

161. Weber, K. T., and Janicki, K. T.: The dynamics of ventricular contraction: Force, length and shortening. Fed. Proc. *39*:188, 1980.

162. Mehmel, H. C., Stocking, B., Ruffmann, K., Olhausen, K. V., Schuler, G., and Kubler, W.: The linearity of the end-systolic pressure–volume relationship in man and its sensitivity for assessment of left ventricular function. Circulation *63*:1216, 1981.

163. Ross, J., Jr., Covell, J. W., Sonnenblick, E. H., and Braunwald, E.: Contractile state of heart characterized by force-velocity relations in variably afterloaded and isovolumic beats. Circ. Res. *18*:149, 1966.

164. Burns, J. W., Covell, J. W., and Ross, J., Jr.: Mechanics of isotonic left ventricular contractions. Am. J. Physiol. *224*:725, 1973.

164a.Ross, J., Jr.: Mechanisms of cardiac contraction. What roles for preload, afterload and inotropic state in heart failure? Eur. Heart J. *4*(Suppl. A):19, 1983.

165. Williams, J. F., Jr., Sonnenblick, E. H., and Braunwald, E.: Determinants of atrial contractile force in intact heart. Am. J. Physiol. *209*:1061, 1965.

166. Braunwald, E., and Frahm, C. J.: Studies on Starling's law of the heart. IV. Observations on hemodynamic functions of left atrium in man. Circulation *24*:633, 1961.

166a.Linderer, T., Chatterjee, K., Parmley, W. W., Sievers, R. E., Glantz, S. A., and Tyberg, J. V.: Influence of atrial systole on the Frank-Starling relation and the end-diastolic pressure-diameter relation of the left ventricle. Circulation *67*: 1045, 1983.

167. Katz, A. M.: Editorial—The descending limb of the Starling curve and the failing heart. Circulation *32*:871, 1965.

168. Monroe, R. G., Gamble, W. J., LaFarge, C. G., Kumar, A. E., and Manasek, F. J.: Left ventricular performance at high-end diastolic pressures in isolated, perfused dog hearts. Circ. Res. *26*:85, 1970.

169. Ross, J., Jr., Sonnenblick, E. H., Taylor, R. R., Spotnitz, H. M., and Covell, J. W.: Diastolic geometry and sarcomere lengths in the chronically dilated canine left ventricle. Circ. Res. *28*:49, 1971.

170. Grimm, A. F., Lin, H. L., and Grimm, B. R.: Left ventricular free wall and intraventricular pressure-sarcomere length distributions. Am. J. Physiol. *239*: H101, 1980.

171. MacGregor, D. C., Covell, J. W., Mahler, F., Dilley, R. B., and Ross, J., Jr.: Relations between afterload, stroke volume, and the descending limb of Starling's curve. Am. J. Physiol. *227*:884, 1974.

172. Ross, J., Jr., and Braunwald, E.: The study of left ventricular function in man by increasing resistance to ventricular ejection with angiotensin. Circulation *29*:739, 1964.

173. Ross, J., Jr.: Afterload mismatch and preload reserve: a conceptual framework for the analysis of ventricular function. Progr. Cardiovasc. Dis. *18*:255, 1976.

174. Vatner, S. F., Franklin, D., Higgins, C. B., Patrick, T., and Braunwald, E.: Left ventricular response to severe exertion in untethered dogs. J. Clin. Invest. *51*:3052, 1972.

175. Braunwald, E.: Regulation of the circulation. N. Engl. J. Med. *290*:1124 and 1420, 1974.

176. Parker, J. O., and Case, R. B.: Normal left ventricular function. Circulation *60*:4, 1979.

177. Braunwald, E.: Editorial—On the difference between the heart's output and its contractile state. Circulation *43*:171, 1971.

178. Braunwald, E., Binion, J. T., Morgan, W. L., Jr., and Sarnoff, S. J.: Alterations in central blood volume and cardiac output induced by positive pressure breathing and counteracted by metaraminol (Aramine). Circ. Res. *5*:670, 1957.

179. Shabetai, R., Fowler, N. O., and Guntheroth, W. G.: The hemodynamics of cardiac tamponade and constrictive pericarditis. Am. J. Cardiol. *26*:480, 1970.

180. Braunwald, E., Ross, J., Jr., Kahler, R. L., Gaffney, T. E., Goldblatt, A., and Mason, D. T.: Reflex control of the systemic venous bed: Effects on venous

tone of vasoactive drugs, and of baroreceptor and chemoreceptor stimulation. Circ. Res. *12*:539, 1963.

181. Shepherd, J. T., and Vanhoutte, P. M.: Veins and Their Control. Philadelphia, W. B. Saunders Co., 1975, 269 pp.

182. Mason, D. T., and Braunwald, E.: Effects of guanethidine, reserpine and methyldopa on reflex venous and arterial constriction in man. J. Clin. Invest. *43*:1449, 1964.

183. Mason, D. T., and Braunwald, E.: The effects of nitroglycerin and amyl nitrite on arteriolar and venous tone in the human forearm. Circulation *32*:755, 1965.

184. Williams, J. F., Jr., Glick, G., and Braunwald, E.: Studies on cardiac dimensions in intact unanesthetized man. V. Effects of nitroglycerin. Circulation *32*:767, 1965.

185. Guyton, A. C., Douglas, B. H., Langston, J. B., and Richardson, T. Q.: Instantaneous increase in mean circulatory pressure and cardiac output at onset of muscular activity. Circ. Res. *11*:431, 1962.

186. Braunwald, E.: Determinants of cardiac function. N. Engl. J. Med. *296*: 86, 1977.

187. Sonnenblick, E. H., and Downing, J. E.: Afterload as a primary determinant of ventricular performance. Am. J. Physiol. *204*:604, 1962.

188. Ford, L. E.: Effect of afterload reduction on myocardial energetics. Circ. Res. *46*:161, 1980.

189. Wilcken, D. E. L., Charlier, A. A., Hoffman, J. I. E., and Guz, A.: Effects of alterations in aortic impedance on the performance of the ventricles. Circ. Res. *14*:283, 1964.

190. Piene, H., and Covell, J. W.: A force-length-time relationship describes the mechanics of canine left ventricular wall segments during auxotonic contractions. Circ. Res. *49*:70, 1981.

191. Urschel, C. W., Covell, J. W., Sonnenblick, E. H., Ross, J., Jr., and Braunwald, E.: Myocardial mechanics in aortic and mitral valvular regurgitation: The concept of instantaneous impedance as a determinant of the performance of the intact heart. J. Clin. Invest. *47*:867, 1968.

192. Urschel, C. W., Covell, J. W., Sonnenblick, E. H., Ross, J., Jr., Gault, J. H., and Braunwald, E.: The effects of decreased aortic compliance on the performance of the left ventricle. Am. J. Physiol. *214*:298, 1968.

193. Bugge-Asperheim, B., and Kill, F.: Cardiac response to increased aortic pressure: Changes in output and left ventricular pressure pattern at various levels of inotropy. Scand. J. Clin. Lab. Invest. *24*:345, 1969.

194. Sarnoff, S. J., Mitchell, J. H., Gilmore, J. P., and Remensnyder, J. P.: Homeometric autoregulation of the heart. Circ. Res. *8*:1077, 1960.

195. Clancy, R. L., Graham, T. P., Jr., Ross, J., Jr., Sonnenblick, E. H., and Braunwald, E.: The influence of aortic pressure-induced homeometric autoregulation on myocardial performance. Am. J. Physiol. *214*:1186, 1968.

196. LaFarge, C. G., Monroe, R. G., Gamble, W. J., Rosenthal, A., and Hammond, R. P.: Left ventricular pressure and norepinephrine efflux from the innervated heart. Am. J. Physiol. *219*:519, 1970.

197. Furnival, C. M., Linden, R. J., and Snow, H. M.: Inotropic changes in the left ventricle: The effect of changes in heart rate, aortic pressure and end-diastolic pressure. J. Physiol. (Lond.) *211*:359, 1970.

198. Von Anrep, G.: On the part played by the suprarenals in the normal vascular reactions of the body. J. Physiol. (Lond.) *45*:307, 1912.

199. Vatner, S. F., Monroe, R. G., and McRitchie, R. J.: Effects of anesthesia, tachycardia, and autonomic blockade on the Anrep effect in intact dogs. Am. J. Physiol. *226*:1450, 1974.

200. Sasayama, S., Ross, J., Jr., Franklin, D., Bloor, C., Bishop, S., and Dilley, R. B.: Adaptations of the left ventricle to chronic pressure overload. Circ. Res. *38*:172, 1976.

200a. Katz, A. M.: Regulation of myocardial contractility 1958–1983. J. Am. Coll. Cardiol. *1*:126, 1983.

201. Ross, J., Jr., Covell, J. W., and Sonnenblick, E. H.: The mechanics of left ventricular contraction in acute experimental cardiac failure. J. Clin. Invest. *46*:299, 1967.

202. Sibens, A. A., Hoffman, B. F., Cranefield, P. F., and Brooks, C. M.: Regulation of contractile force during ventricular arrhythmias. Am. J. Physiol. *197*:971, 1959.

203. Lendrum, B., Feinberg, H., Boyd, E., and Katz, L. N.: Rhythm effects on contractility of beating isovolemic left ventricle. Am. J. Physiol. *199*:1115, 1960.

204. Frommer, P. L., Robinson, B. F., and Braunwald, E.: Paired electrical stimulation. A comparison of the effects on performance of the failing and nonfailing heart. Am. J. Cardiol. *18*:738, 1966.

205. Beierholm, E. A., Grantham, R. N., O'Keefe, D. D., Laver, M. B., and Daggett, W. M.: Effects of acid-base changes, hypoxia, and catecholamines on ventricular performance. Am. J. Physiol. *228*:1555, 1975.

206. Braunwald, E.: Symposium on protection of the ischemic myocardium. Circulation *53*(Suppl. 1):217, 1976.

207. Williamson, J. R., Schaffer, S. W., Ford, C., and Safen, B.: Contribution of tissue acidosis to ischemic injury in the perfused rat heart. Circulation *53* (Suppl. 1):3, 1976.

208. Mitchell, J. H., Wallace, A. G., and Skinner, N. S., Jr.: Intrinsic effects of heart rate on left ventricular performance. Am. J. Physiol. *205*:41, 1963.

208a. Narahara, K. A., and Blettel, L.: Effect of rate on left ventricular volumes and ejection fraction during chronic ventricular pacing. Circulation *67*:323, 1983.

208b. Narahara, K. A., and Blettel, M. L.: Effect of rate on left ventricular volumes and ejection fraction during chronic ventricular pacing. Circulation *67*:323, 1983.

209. Randall, W. C. (ed.): Neural Regulation of the Heart. New York, Oxford University Press, 1977, 440 pp.

210. Rolett, E. S.: Adrenergic mechanisms in mammalian myocardium. *In* Langer, G. A., and Brady, A. J. (eds.): The Mammalian Myocardium. New York, John Wiley and Sons, 1974, pp. 219–250.

211. Yamaguchie, N., de Champlain, J., and Nadeau, R.: Correlation between the response of the heart to sympathetic stimulation and the release of endogenous catecholamines into the coronary sinus of the dog. Circ. Res. *36*:662, 1975.

212. Martin, R. H., Lim, S. T., and VanCitters, R. L.: Atrial fibrillation in the intact anesthetized dog: Hemodynamic effects during rest, exercise, and beta-adrenergic blockade. J. Clin. Invest. *46*:205, 1967.

213. Frye, R. L., and Braunwald, E.: Studies on Starling's law of the heart. I. The circulatory response to acute hypervolemia and its modification by ganglionic blockade. J. Clin. Invest. *39*:1043, 1960.

214. Sonnenblick, E. H., Williams, J. F., Jr., Glick, G., Mason, D. T., and Braunwald, E.: Studies on digitalis. XV. Effects of cardiac glycosides on myocardial force-velocity relations in nonfailing human heart. Circulation *34*:532, 1966.

215. Daggett, W. M., and Weisfeldt, M. L.: Influence of sympathetic nervous system on response of normal heart to digitalis. Am. J. Cardiol. *16*:394, 1965.

216. Liedtke, A. M., Buoncristiani, J. F., Kirk, E. S., Sonnenblick, E. H., and Urschel, C. W.: Regulation of cardiac output after administration of isoproterenol and ouabain. Cardiovasc. Res. *6*:325, 1972.

217. Guyton, A. C.: The relationship of cardiac output and arterial pressure control. Circulation *64*:1079, 1981.

218. Vatner, S. F., Higgins, C. B., White, S., Patrick, T., and Franklin, D.: The peripheral vascular response to severe exercise in untethered dogs before and after complete heart block. J. Clin. Invest. *50*:1950, 1971.

219. Ross, J., Jr., Gault, J. H., Mason, D. T., Linhart, J. W., and Braunwald, E.: Left ventricular performance during muscular exercise in patients with and without cardiac dysfunction. Circulation *34*:597, 1966.

220. Epstein, S. E., Robinson, B. F., Kahler, R. L., and Braunwald, E.: Effects of beta-adrenergic blockade on the cardiac response to maximal and submaximal exercise in man. J. Clin. Invest. *44*:1745, 1965.

221. Robinson, B. F., Epstein, S. E., Kahler, R. L., and Braunwald, E.: Circulatory effects of acute expansion of blood volume: Studies during maximal exercise and at rest. Circ. Res. *19*:26, 1966.

222. Braunwald, E., Goldblatt, A., Harrison, D. C., and Mason, D. T.: Studies on cardiac dimensions in intact, unanesthetized man. III. Effects of muscular exercise. Circ. Res. *13*:460, 1963.

223. Caldwell, J. H., Stewart, D. K., Dodge, H. T., Frimer, M., and Kennedy, J. W.: Left ventricular volume during maximal supine exercise. A study using metallic epicardial markers. Circulation *58*:732, 1978.

224. Sonnenblick, E. H., Braunwald, E., Williams, J. F., Jr., and Glick, G.: Effects of exercise on myocardial force-velocity relations in intact unanesthetized man: Relative roles of changes in heart rate, sympathetic activity, and ventricular dimensions. J. Clin. Invest. *44*:2051, 1965.

225. Weiss, J. L., Weisfeldt, M. L., Mason, S. V., Garrison, J. B., Livengood, S. V., and Fortuin, N. J.: Evidence of Frank-Starling effect in man during severe semi-supine exercise. Circulation *59*:655, 1979.

226. Rerych, S. K., Scholz, P. M., Sabiston, D. C., Jr., and Jones, R. H.: Effects of exercise training on left ventricular function in normal subjects: A longitudinal study by radionuclide angiography. Am. J. Cardiol. *45*:244, 1980.

227. Bruce, T. A., Chapman, C. P., Baker, O., and Fisher, J. N.: Role of autonomic and myocardial factors in cardiac control. J. Clin. Invest. *42*:721, 1963.

228. Saltin, B., and Astrand, P. O.: Maximal oxygen uptake in the athlete. J. Appl. Physiol. *23*:353, 1967.

229. Morganroth, J., Maron, B. J., Henry, W. L., and Epstein, S. E.: Comparative left ventricular dimensions in trained athletes. Ann. Intern. Med. *82*:521, 1975.

230. Roeske, W. R., O'Rourke, R. A., Klein, A., Leopold, G., and Karliner, J. S.: Noninvasive evaluation of ventricular hypertrophy in professional athletes. Circulation *53*:286, 1976.

231. Yin, F. C. P., Weisfeldt, M. L., and Milnor, W. R.: Role of aortic input impedance in the decreased cardiovascular response to exercise with aging in dogs. J. Clin. Invest. *68*:28, 1981.

13 PATHOPHYSIOLOGY OF HEART FAILURE

by Eugene Braunwald, M.D.

Heart (or cardiac) failure, the pathophysiological state in which an abnormality of *cardiac* function is responsible for failure of the heart to pump blood at a rate commensurate with the requirements of the metabolizing tissues, is frequently, but not always, caused by a defect in myocardial contraction, i.e., by *myocardial failure*. However, in some patients with heart failure, a similar clinical syndrome is present, but there is no detectable abnormality of *myocardial* function; in such cases heart failure is brought about by conditions in which the normal heart is suddenly presented with a load that exceeds its capacity or in which ventricular filling is impaired.[1] Heart failure must be distinguished from conditions in which there is circulatory congestion consequent to abnormal salt and water retention (the so-called congested state) but in which there is no disturbance of cardiac function per se.[2] A distinction must also be made between heart failure and *circulatory failure*, in which an abnormality of some component of the circulation—the heart, the blood volume, the concentration of oxygenated hemoglobin in the arterial blood, or the vascular bed—is responsible for inadequate cardiac output.

Thus, myocardial failure, heart failure, and circulatory failure are not synonymous but refer to progressively broader entities. Myocardial failure, when sufficiently severe, always produces heart failure, but the converse is not necessarily the case, since a number of conditions in which the heart is suddenly overloaded (e.g., acute aortic regurgitation secondary to acute infective endocarditis) can produce heart failure in the presence of normal myocardial function. Also, conditions such as tricuspid stenosis and constrictive pericarditis, which interfere with cardiac filling, can produce heart failure without myocardial failure. Heart failure, in turn, always produces circulatory failure, but again the converse is not necessarily the case, since a variety of noncardiac conditions, e.g., hypovolemic shock (Chap. 18) or extremely severe anemia, beriberi, and other

high-output states (Chap. 24), can produce circulatory failure at a time when cardiac function is normal or only modestly impaired.

COMPENSATORY MECHANISMS

In the presence of a defect in myocardial contraction or an excessive hemodynamic burden placed on the ventricle or both, the heart depends upon three principal compensatory mechanisms for maintenance of its pumping function: (1) the Frank-Starling mechanism, in which an increased preload (i.e., lengthening of sarcomeres to provide optimal overlap between thick and thin myofilaments) acts to sustain cardiac performance (p. 423); (2) increased release of catecholamines by adrenergic cardiac nerves and the adrenal medulla, which augments myocardial contractility (p. 439); and (3) myocardial hypertrophy with or without cardiac chamber dilatation, in which the mass of contractile tissue is augmented. Initially, these three compensatory mechanisms may be adequate to maintain the pumping performance of the heart at a relatively normal level, although intrinsic myocardial contractility may be substantially reduced. However, each of these mechanisms has a limited potential and ultimately fails. The clinical syndrome of heart failure occurs as a consequence of the limitations and/or the ultimate failure of these compensatory mechanisms.[3]

Cardiac output is often depressed in the basal state in patients with the common forms of heart failure secondary to ischemic heart disease, hypertension, primary myocardial disease, valvular disease, and pericardial disease (so-called low-output heart failure) but tends to be elevated in patients with heart failure associated with conditions of reduced afterload and/or hypermetabolism, such as hyperthyroidism, anemia, arteriovenous fistula, beriberi, and

Paget's disease (so-called high-output heart failure, Chap. 24). The mechanisms responsible for the development of heart failure in patients whose cardiac output is initially high are complex and depend on the specific underlying disease process and its effect on the myocardium. In most of these conditions, the heart is called upon to pump an abnormally large volume of blood in order to deliver an adequate quantity of oxygen to the metabolizing tissues. This increased volume load exerts an effect on the myocardium resembling that produced by regurgitant valvular lesions or cardiac left-to-right shunts. In some patients with high-output heart failure, severe anemia or thiamine deficiency impairs myocardial function.

In the absence of the shunting of blood in the periphery, the inadequate delivery of oxygen to the metabolizing tissues characteristic of heart failure is reflected in an abnormally widened arterial–mixed venous oxygen difference. In mild cases this abnormality may not be present in the basal state and may become evident only during the stress of increased activity. In the presence of the peripheral arteriovenous shunting of blood and heart failure (as occurs, for example, in beriberi heart disease), although the arterial–mixed venous oxygen difference may be normal or even narrowed, the venous oxygen content proximal to the shunt—if it could be measured—would be reduced, reflecting an augmented extraction of oxygen by inadequately perfused tissues.

When the volume of blood delivered into the systemic vascular bed is chronically reduced, and when one or both ventricles fail to expel the normal fraction of its end-diastolic volume, a complex sequence of adjustments occurs that ultimately results in an abnormal accumulation of fluid. These adjustments are described in detail on pages 1748 to 1752. Although many of the clinical manifestations of heart failure are secondary to this excessive retention of fluid, the expansion of blood volume also constitutes an important compensatory mechanism that tends to maintain cardiac output by elevating ventricular preload, since the myocardium operates on an ascending limb of a depressed function curve[4-7] (Figure 12–32, p. 438), and the augmented ventricular end-diastolic volume must be regarded as helping to maintain cardiac output, except in the terminal stages of heart failure. Elevation of ventricular end-diastolic volume and pressure, in accordance with the Frank-Starling mechanism, raises ventricular performance but at the same time causes pulmonary or systemic venous congestion and promotes the formation of pulmonary or peripheral edema.

Redistribution of left ventricular output is one of a number of peripheral mechanisms brought into play to conserve the limited cardiac output. Vasoconstriction, mediated largely by the adrenergic nervous system, is primarily responsible for this redistribution of peripheral blood flow, which occurs when an additional burden (such as exercise, fever, or anemia) is imposed on the circulation in the presence of impaired myocardial function, preventing cardiac output from rising normally. As heart failure advances, redistribution of left ventricular output ultimately occurs even in the basal state.[8-13] This redistribution maintains the delivery of oxygen to vital organs such as the heart and brain, whereas blood flow to less critical areas such as the skin is reduced.

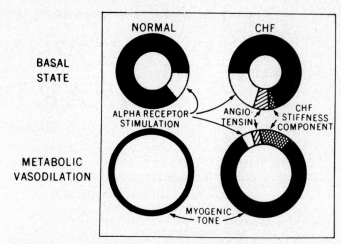

FIGURE 13–1   Determinants of vasomotor tone in the basal state and under conditions of metabolic vasodilation in normal subjects and in patients with congestive heart failure (CHF). The lumina of the blood vessels are drawn to scale from data derived from the study of blood flow in human limbs. Blood vessels in CHF are more constricted than normal vessels. The estimated relative contribution of alpha receptor stimulation, angiotensin, and the "stiffness factor" to this vasoconstriction in CHF is portrayed. (Reproduced with permission from Zelis, R., and Flaim, S. F.: Peripheral vascular mechanisms mediating vasoconstriction. *In* Braunwald, E., Mock, M. B., and Watson, J. [eds.]: Congestive Heart Failure: Current Research and Clinical Applications. New York, Grune and Stratton, 1982, p. 115.)

Alterations in autonomic control of the heart and peripheral circulation vary with the model and etiology of heart failure, as well as with the nature and severity of the inciting stimulus. Activation of the autonomic nervous system acts to maintain cardiac output by increasing myocardial contractility and raising heart rate; in severe heart failure, vasoconstriction mediated by the sympathetic nervous system and circulating angiotensin II tends to sustain arterial pressure and diverts blood flow from the cutaneous, splanchnic, and renal beds to preserve perfusion of the coronary and cerebral beds.[14] In patients with moderate heart failure, these changes occur primarily during exercise, whereas in patients with severe heart failure they are present at rest. Renal vasoconstriction and the activation of the renin-angiotensin-aldosterone system result in sodium retention (p. 1749).

Increased vascular sodium content and raised interstitial pressure resulting from sodium and water retention lead to stiffening, thickening, and compression of the blood vessel walls, which prevents a normal vasodilator response during exercise (Fig. 13–1). Inadequate perfusion of skeletal muscle, in turn, leads to earlier dependence on anaerobic metabolism, lactic acidemia, an excessive oxygen debt, weakness, and fatigue. The veins in the extremities of patients with heart failure are constricted, apparently as a consequence of compression by increased tissue pressure, by circulating venoconstrictors (norepinephrine and angiotensin II), and, to a lesser extent, by the activity of the sympathetic nervous system. Venoconstriction in the extremities results in displacement of blood to the heart and lungs and presumably to the splanchnic venous bed.

A progressive *decline in the affinity of hemoglobin for oxygen* due to an increase in 2,3-diphosphoglycerate (DPG) also occurs in heart failure.[15] This rightward shift in the oxygen-hemoglobin dissociation curve represents a significant compensatory mechanism to facilitate oxygen transport; increased DPG, tissue acidosis, and the slow circulation time characteristic of heart failure act synergistically to maintain the delivery of oxygen to the metabolizing tissues in the face of a reduced cardiac output.

CONTRACTILITY OF HYPERTROPHIED AND FAILING MYOCARDIUM

When an excessive pressure or volume load is imposed on a ventricle, myocardial hypertrophy develops, providing a fundamental compensatory mechanism that permits the ventricle to sustain this burden.[16] A ventricle subjected to an abnormally elevated load for a prolonged period, however, may fail to maintain compensation despite the presence of ventricular hypertrophy, and pump failure may occur.

STUDIES ON ISOLATED MUSCLE. There has been substantial interest in the analysis of the behavior of isolated muscle removed from animals in which the heart was subjected to a controlled major stress. A convenient experimental model of ventricular pressure overload is the cat with pulmonary artery constriction. Papillary muscles are removed from the right ventricles in which either hypertrophy or overt failure has developed, and the excised muscle is then studied in vitro.[17,18] Right ventricular hypertrophy and failure both reduce the maximum velocity of unloaded shortening (V_{max}) below the values observed in muscles obtained from normal cats; the changes are more marked in muscles obtained from animals in which heart failure was present than in those with hypertrophy alone (Figs. 13–2 and 13–3). Heart failure depresses the maximal isometric tension, but hypertrophy without failure produces only borderline depression of this variable.

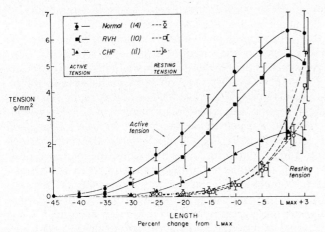

FIGURE 13–2 Relation between muscle length and tension of papillary muscles from normal (circles), hypertrophied (squares), and failing (triangles) right ventricles. Open symbols = resting tension; filled symbols = actively developed tension. Each value is the average of the group; vertical lines with cross bars = ± 1 SEM. Tension is corrected for cross-sectional area (g/mm²). Numbers in parentheses = number of animals. (From Spann, J. F., Jr., Buccino, R. A., Sonnenblick, E. H., and Braunwald, E.: Contractile state of cardiac muscle obtained from cats with experimentally produced ventricular hypertrophy and heart failure. Circ. Res. *21*:341, 1967, by permission of the American Heart Association, Inc.)

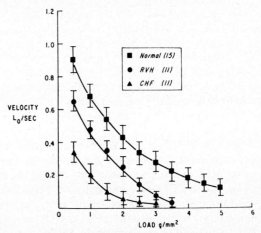

FIGURE 13–3 Force-velocity relations of the three groups of cat papillary muscles. Average values ± SEM are given for each point. Velocity has been corrected to muscle lengths per second (L₀/sec). Numbers in parentheses = number of animals. (From Spann, J. F., Jr., Buccino, R. A., Sonnenblick, E. H., and Braunwald, E.: Contractile state of cardiac muscle obtained from cats with experimentally produced ventricular hypertrophy and heart failure. Circ. Res. *21*: 341, 1967, by permission of the American Heart Association, Inc.)

The findings summarized above are, in general, consonant with those of a number of other investigations on cardiac muscle isolated from animals with experimentally produced pressure overload. For example, the trabecular muscles removed from the left ventricles of the rat in which left ventricular hypertrophy has been created by aortic constriction also exhibit a depression in the velocity of isotonic shortening, although no reduction in the development of isometric tension was demonstrated;[19] similar findings were made in papillary muscles of rats with renovascular hypertension.[20] The force and rate of force development are also depressed in muscles obtained from hearts with totally different forms of heart failure, i.e., from Syrian hamsters with hereditary cardiomyopathy,[21] as well as in papillary muscles removed from the left ventricles of patients with heart failure due to chronic valvular disease.[22] Papillary muscles obtained from rats rendered diabetic with streptozotocin exhibited normal force development but reduced velocity of shortening.[23]

In contrast to the depressed performance of cardiac muscle removed from cardiomyopathic or pressure-overloaded hearts, contractility is normal in papillary muscles removed from cats with a volume overload resulting from an experimentally produced atrial septal defect.[24] It should also be noted that although the length–active tension curve, the maximal rate of isometric force development, and force-velocity relations are all significantly depressed in cat papillary muscles removed 6 weeks after pulmonary artery banding, in some,[25] but not all,[18] studies these variables returned to normal when the elevated pressure was maintained for prolonged periods. These observations emphasize the important temporal relationships between the imposition of a load, its nature (volume or pressure), severity, time, and the resultant depression of the contractile state.

Electron microscopic studies of myocardium removed from overloaded, dilated hearts fixed at the elevated filling pressures that existed during life have revealed sarcomere lengths averaging 2.2 μm—no longer than those at the apex of the length–active tension curve of normal cardiac muscle[26]—indicating that the depressed contractility of failing heart muscle is *not* due to an enlarging H zone, i.e., the disengagement of actin and myosin filaments. Thus, the depression of contractility in failing heart muscle appears to be related to an *intrinsic defect of the muscle* rather than to its operation on the descending limb of the Frank-Starling curve.[5]

STUDIES ON INTACT HEARTS.   In general, changes in performance of the intact heart are similar to those observed in isolated cardiac tissue obtained from hearts subjected to abnormal hemodynamic loads. Thus, the contractile performance of the intact right ventricles of cats with pulmonary artery constriction reveals a marked depression paralleling that observed in the isolated papillary muscles removed from these ventricles.[27] When compared with normal values, the active tension developed by the right ventricle at equivalent end-diastolic fiber lengths is markedly reduced in cats with heart failure (Fig. 13–4). Studies involving manipulations of end-diastolic volume revealed that these failing hearts ordinarily function on the *ascending* limb of a *depressed* length–active tension curve rather than on the descending limb of a normal curve. Thus, as the ventricle fails, it moves to the right along a depressed length–active tension curve, so that it requires an abnormally elevated end-diastolic volume (and often an elevation of end-diastolic pressure as well) to generate a level of tension equal to that achieved by the normal heart at a normal end-diastolic volume. The similar level of active tension at spontaneously occurring end-diastolic volumes in normal and failing cat hearts is evidence of the

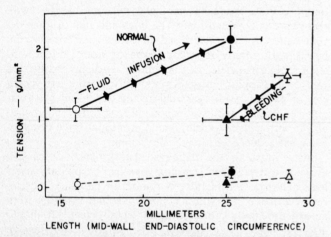

FIGURE 13–4 Length-tension relationships in the intact ventricle. Acute manipulation of end-diastolic volume to obtain ventricular Frank-Starling curves. Lines represent segments of active and resting length-tension curves (Frank-Starling relationship) of five normal (circles) and five failing (triangles) ventricles. Solid lines represent active tension, whereas dashed lines refer to resting or diastolic tension. Open symbols refer to values obtained at spontaneously occurring end-diastolic volume, whereas solid symbols refer to values obtained after volume infusion in normal cats and bleeding of cats with heart failure. Average values ± SEM are shown. Active and resting tensions are expressed on the ordinate, and normalized end-diastolic circumference, or muscle length, on the abscissa. (From Spann, J. F., Jr., Covell, J. W., Eckberg, D. L., Sonnenblick, E. H., Ross, J., Jr., and Braunwald, E.: Contractile performance of the hypertrophied and chronically failing cat ventricle. Am. J. Physiol. *223*: 1150, 1972.)

compensation afforded the depressed myocardium by cardiac dilatation. Contractile tension is thus preserved, but at the expense of an increased end-diastolic pressure and volume. However, the velocity of myocardial fiber shortening and the velocity of contraction at any given load are depressed despite the normal levels of tension development.

Although cardiac output and left ventricular end-diastolic pressure are normal at rest in spontaneously hypertensive rats with chronic pressure overload,[28] the left ventricular ejection fraction is depressed.[29,30] When such rats are stressed with infusions of fluid, the stroke volume and cardiac output rise subnormally. Left ventricular performance, reflected in the ejection fraction as well as in maximal cardiac output and pressure development, is also depressed in rats with myocardial infarction produced by coronary artery ligation.[31] Chronic left ventricular volume overload, produced by creating a large arteriovenous fistula, causes depression of a variety of indices of contractility.[32] Thus, there is substantial evidence that both chronic pressure and volume overload depress contractility of the intact heart. In addition, left ventricular function has also been found to be depressed in isolated but intact hearts removed from rats with experimentally induced diabetes mellitus.[33]

MANIFESTATIONS OF DEPRESSED CONTRACTILITY.   When all of the studies on isolated muscle and intact hearts are taken together, it may be concluded that the depression of the cardiac contractile state observed in the hypertrophied and failing ventricle, however caused, represents an *intrinsic* property of the muscle. This depression is evident in vitro, when the muscle's physical and chemical milieu is controlled, and it is therefore not dependent on any altered humoral or other environmental factors existing in vivo. Although contractility is depressed in the intact ventricle and in isolated muscles with many preparations subjected to pressure overload, the cardiac index and stroke volume in the basal state are often maintained despite markedly depressed levels of contractility.

It appears, then, that when the ventricle is stressed, by either a pressure or a volume overload, the initial response is an increase in the length of sarcomeres, so that the overlap between myofilaments is optimal, i.e., approximately 2.2 μm (p. 423). This is followed by an increase in the total muscle mass. If the overload is not extreme, this adaptation at first can allow maintenance of a high systolic pressure or augmented cardiac output without a depression of contractility. If the intrinsic contractile state of each unit of myocardium becomes depressed, the increased muscle mass, operating in conjunction with increased sympathetic stimulation, maintains overall circulatory compensation. If the overload persists, Meerson has proposed that some of the hypertrophied cells become necrotic,[34] which places an additional load on the surviving cells and may thereby result in a vicious cycle, ultimately causing heart failure.

In its mildest form, the depression of contractility is manifest by a reduction in the maximal velocity of shortening of unloaded myocardium (V_{max}) but by little, if any, decrease in the development of maximal isometric force (P_0). As the intrinsic contractile state of each unit of myocardium becomes further depressed, a more extensive reduction in V_{max} occurs, and this is now accompanied by a decline in P_0. At this point, circulatory compensation is still provided by an increase in muscle mass and cardiac dilatation, which tend to maintain wall stress at normal levels. Cardiac output and stroke volume are maintained in the basal state, but ejection fraction is depressed, as are the maximal levels of cardiac output and left ventricular systolic pressure that can be attained during stress. As contractility declines further, overt congestive heart failure, as manifested by a depression of cardiac output and work and/or an elevation of ventricular end-diastolic volume and pressure, becomes manifest. In addition, although an improvement in function can occur in failing muscle in response to positive inotropic stimuli such as digitalis, the *degree* of augmentation falls, and at a late stage, the contractility of even the stimulated heart is subnormal.

Reversibility of Cardiac Depression. The depression of myocardial contractility in papillary muscles removed from cats with pressure overload–induced hypertrophy is reversible when the hypertrophy is reversed by unbanding the pulmonary artery.[35] Sustained treatment of hypertension also reverses the impairment of contractility.[20,29,30]

CAUSES OF HYPERTROPHY. The character of the stress (increased preload, increased afterload, or primary depression of contractility) responsible for inciting the hypertrophy also appears to play a critical role in determining whether or not it is detrimental to myocardial contractility. When volume overload is produced by the creation of an aortocaval fistula, sarcomere length initially rises to the optimal level of 2.2 μm. Then progressive left ventricular dilatation and moderate left ventricular hypertrophy occur without clinical evidence of heart failure, and the length–active tension relations of the dilated, hypertrophied ventricle remain essentially normal.[36] Within 1 week of the creation of such a fistula, left ventricular end-diastolic pressure rises and then remains constant, whereas the left ventricular end-diastolic diameter continues to increase progressively. Following chronic adjustment to the shunt, the end-diastolic volume increases at any given end-diastolic pressure (Fig. 13–5); myocardial function, as reflected in the velocity of circumferential fiber shortening, may be normal or depressed. The performance of the chronically volume-overloaded ventricle is characterized by normal or nearly normal performance of each unit of myocardium, allowing delivery of a stroke volume greater than normal.[37] The chronic ventricular dilatation is associated with diastolic sarcomere lengths that are optimal (2.2 μm).

Thus, despite the augmented volumes and filling pressures, there is *no* disengagement of thick and thin myofilaments.

Following the initial increase in stroke volume, mediated by increased sarcomere length during the acute phase of volume overloading, progressive cardiac dilatation subsequently occurs, whereas end-diastolic sarcomere lengths remain relatively constant. Cardiac dilatation presumably results from an increase in the size of myocardial cells, from a greater number of sarcomeres developing in series during the process of hypertrophy, and perhaps from slippage between adjacent fibers and fibrils[38]—changes that may be irreversible[32] and may further impair contractile performance. Thus, in summary, the ventricle ordinarily compensates for a volume overload with both a change in ventricular geometry and an increase in the number of sarcomeres, resulting in an augmented stroke volume. In the compensated state of chronic volume overloading, the combination of ventricular dilatation and hypertrophy allows enhancement of overall cardiac performance, with normal function of each unit of an enlarged ventricle operating at an optimal sarcomere length.[38] However, in the presence of a very large volume overload and clinical evidence of congestive heart failure, myocardial contractility does become seriously depressed.[32]

Effects of Depressed Contractility. The effects of depression of myocardial contractility on the myocardial force-velocity relations are shown schematically in Figure 13–6.[38] Mild depression of contractility permits normal extent and velocity of shortening of cardiac muscle through operation of the Frank-Starling mechanism, and the stress of any augmentation of afterload can be met only with further augmentation of preload. With marked depression of contractility, no preload reserve is available, and any augmentation of afterload results in a marked reduction in the extent and velocity of shortening. Under these circumstances, a reduction of preload will depress ventricular performance (but may be helpful clinically by reducing ventricular filling pressure and thereby reducing the symptoms of pulmonary congestion, Figure 16–12, p. 531), but a reduction of afterload will improve ventricular performance.

Cardiac Response in Various Forms of Volume and Pressure Overloading

Since alterations in afterload are important determinants of the dynamics of cardiac contraction (Figure 12–30, p.

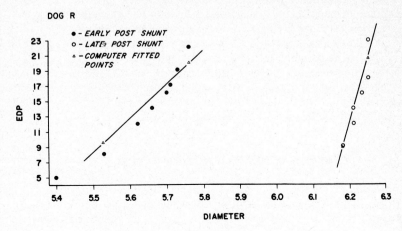

FIGURE 13–5 Relations between left ventricular end-diastolic pressure (EDP, mm Hg) and left ventricular diameter at end diastole (cm) in one dog studied early and late during the course of chronic volume overloading by means of an arteriovenous fistula. Each curve relating end-diastolic pressure to end-diastolic diameter was obtained by acute transfusion and bleeding. The shift to the right and increase in the slope of the pressure-diameter relation between the early postshunt study (closed circles) and the study many weeks after the occurrence of chronic cardiac dilatation (closed triangles) are apparent; the slope change reflects a reduction in diastolic compliance. (From McCullagh, W. H., et al.: Left ventricular dilatation and diastolic compliance changes during chronic volume overloading. Circulation 45:943, 1972, by permission of the American Heart Association, Inc.)

CHRONIC MYOCARDIAL FAILURE

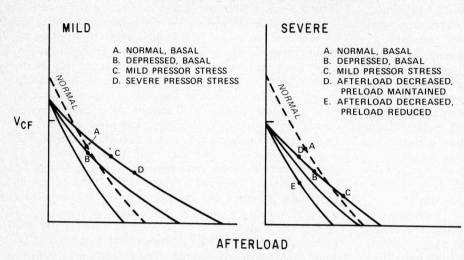

FIGURE 13–6 Alterations of force-velocity relations during afterload changes in the presence of left ventricular failure. *Left panel*, A normal force-velocity curve is indicated by the dashed line, and the normal basal state by point A. With mild depression of the inotropic activity in the basal state, through some encroachment on the Frank-Starling reserve, V_{CF} can be maintained near normal (point B). Some preload reserve may remain, and a mild pressor stress produced by infusion of a peripheral vasoconstrictor may cause little reduction in V_{CF} (point C). However, a more marked increase in afterload will result in a substantial drop in V_{CF} and stroke volume (point D). *Right panel*, With severe depression of the myocardial inotropic activity under basal conditions, V_{CF} is depressed to below the normal range (point B). Since the preload reserve has been fully utilized in the basal state, any afterload increase of even moderate degree will result in a marked drop in V_{CF} and stroke volume (point C). A reduction in afterload with preload maintained constant results in restoration of V_{CF} or stroke volume to near normal (point D), but if preload is allowed to fall substantially, such an afterload reduction may result in no change or even a fall in V_{CF} and stroke volume (point E). (From Ross, J., Jr.: Afterload mismatch and preload reserve: A conceptual framework for the analysis of ventricular function. Prog. Cardiovasc. Dis. *18*:255, 1976, by permission of Grune and Stratton.)

436), it is not surprising that cardiac performance differs in various lesions depending on the precise alterations in pressure and volume overloading. For example, with equivalent total and effective stroke volumes, left ventricular function is more severely stressed, with greater end-diastolic pressure and volume, in aortic than in mitral regurgitation.[39-41] In the latter, the regurgitant volume is delivered into the low-pressure left atrium, whereas in aortic regurgitation the regurgitant volume must be ejected into the high-pressure aorta. For similar reasons, left ventricular function appears to be less impaired in ventricular septal defect than in patent ductus arteriosus with similar degrees of left-to-right shunt.[42] Ventricular septal defect resembles mitral regurgitation in that the shunted flow is ejected directly into the low-pressure right ventricle, and there is a rapid fall in tension during systole as the result of a greater reduction in instantaneous impedance to left ventricular emptying, whereas patent ductus arteriosus is similar to aortic regurgitation in that the entire left ventricular stroke volume, including the shunted blood, is ejected into the high-pressure aorta. Therefore, at identical levels of pulmonary blood flow, left ventricular end-diastolic pressure and volume, systolic tension, work, and duration of ejection are all greater, whereas the ventricular ejection rate and fraction are lower in experimentally produced patent ductus arteriosus than in ventricular septal defect. Furthermore, conditions in which the impedance offered to ejection is considerably reduced, such as mitral regurgitation and ventricular septal defect, impose a smaller increase in myocardial oxygen requirements than do patent ductus and aortic regurgitation.[43]

Patterns of Ventricular Hypertrophy

The development of ventricular hypertrophy constitutes one of the principal mechanisms by which the heart compensates for an increased load. Grossman et al. examined systolic and diastolic wall stresses in normal subjects and in well-compensated patients with chronically pressure-overloaded and volume-overloaded left ventricles.[44] Left ventricular systolic stress, end-diastolic pressure, and mass were increased approximately equally in both the pressure-

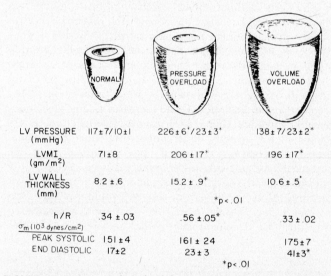

	NORMAL	PRESSURE OVERLOAD	VOLUME OVERLOAD
LV PRESSURE (mmHg)	117±7/10±1	226±6*/23±3*	138±7/23±2*
LVMI (gm/m²)	71±8	206±17*	196±17*
LV WALL THICKNESS (mm)	8.2±.6	15.2±.9*	10.6±.5*
		*p<.01	
h/R	.34±.03	.56±.05*	33±.02
σ_m (10³ dynes/cm²)			
PEAK SYSTOLIC	151±4	161±24	175±7
END DIASTOLIC	17±2	23±3	41±3*
		*p<.01	

FIGURE 13–7 Mean values for left ventricular (LV) pressure, mass index (LVMI), left ventricular wall thickness, the ratio of wall thickness to radius (h/R), and peak systolic and end-diastolic meridional wall stress in patients with normal (6 subjects), pressure-overloaded (6 subjects), and volume-overloaded (18 subjects) ventricles. Although mass is increased similarly in both pressure- and volume-overloaded groups, the increase is accomplished primarily by wall thickening in the pressure-overloaded group. The h/R ratio is normal in volume-overload hypertrophy, indicating a "magnification" type of growth. In pressure overload, concentric hypertrophy is quantified by the increase in h/R. Patients were compensated with respect to heart failure, and peak systolic tension (σ_m) was not statistically different from normal. However, end-diastolic stress was consistently elevated in the volume-overloaded group. See text for details. (From Grossman, W., et al.: Wall stress and patterns of hypertrophy in the human left ventricle. J. Clin. Invest. *56*:56, 1975.)

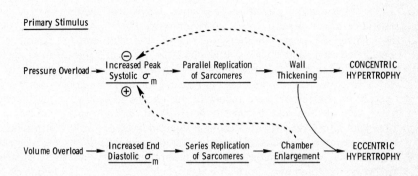

FIGURE 13–8 Hypothesis relating wall stress and patterns of hypertrophy. (From Grossman, W., et al.: Wall stress and patterns of hypertrophy in the human left ventricle. J. Clin. Invest. *56*:56, 1975.)

and the volume-overload groups. There was a substantial increase in wall thickness in the pressure-overloaded ventricles, but only a mild increase in wall thickness in the volume-overloaded ventricles (Fig. 13–7). The latter was just sufficient to counterbalance the increased radius, so that the ratio of wall thickness (h) to radius (R) remained normal for the patients with volume-overload hypertrophy, although it was substantially increased in patients with pressure-overload hypertrophy, in which there was disproportionate thickening of the ventricular wall.

These observations are in concert with those of other investigators who have indicated that myocardial hypertrophy develops in a manner that maintains systolic stress within normal limits.[45–48] When the primary stimulus to hypertrophy is pressure overload, the resultant acute increase in systolic wall stress leads to parallel replication of sarcomeres, wall thickening, and concentric hypertrophy (Fig. 13–8). The wall thickening is just sufficient to return systolic stress to normal. On the other hand, when the primary stimulus is ventricular volume overload, increased diastolic wall stress leads to replication of sarcomeres in series, fiber elongation, and chamber enlargement. This, in turn, results in an increased systolic stress (by the Laplace relationship), which then causes wall thickening of sufficient magnitude to return systolic stress to normal. Thus, in compensated subjects, both volume and pressure overload alter ventricular geometry and wall thickness, so that systolic stress is not changed greatly.

An inverse correlation between circumferential wall stress and both ejection fraction and velocity of fiber shortening has been described in patients with aortic stenosis, with relationships between stress and shortening indistinguishable from those of normal subjects, suggesting that intrinsic myocardial function is normal in most patients with pressure-overload hypertrophy due to aortic stenosis and with depressed ejection fractions and velocity of fiber shortening. Such impairment of ventricular emptying and shortening occurred only when wall thickening (as reflected in the ratio h/R) was not appropriately elevated (Fig. 13–9).[49] These observations suggest that left ventricular wall thickness is a critical determinant of ventricular performance in patients with pressure-overload hypertrophy due to aortic stenosis. Poor cardiac performance in such patients is not necessarily caused by an intrinsic depression of myocardial contractility, but rather it could be secondary to inadequate hypertrophy leading to increased wall stress (afterload), which is responsible for in-

adequate muscle shortening. Obviously, it is possible that myocardial ischemia and intrinsic depression of contractility can also contribute to the depression of cardiac performance. Indeed, such depression in intrinsic contractility

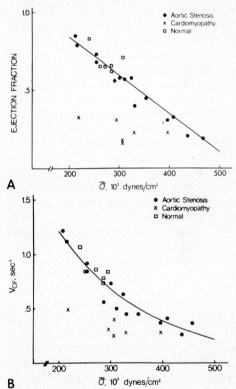

FIGURE 13–9 Relationship between wall stress and muscle fiber shortening characteristics. *A,* Ejection fraction. The line represents the best curve derived from linear regression analysis of the data for patients with aortic stenosis. In these patients, normal values for ejection fraction are associated with normal levels of wall stress, whereas decreasing values for ejection fraction are associated with increasing levels of wall stress. Values for normal controls fall on or near the regression line for the aortic stenosis group. Patients with cardiomyopathy, however, have depressed ejection fractions, regardless of the level of stress. *B,* Mean midwall velocity of circumferential fiber shortening (V_{CF}). Values for patients with aortic stenosis are well approximated as an exponential function of wall stress. Normal patients, again, exhibit a relationship similar to those with aortic stenosis. Patients with cardiomyopathy show depressed values for V_{CF} for any corresponding wall stress. $\bar{\sigma}$ = Mean midwall circumferential stress. (From Gunther, S., and Grossman, W.: Determinants of ventricular function in pressure overload hypertrophy in man. Circulation *59*:679, 1979, by permission of the American Heart Association, Inc.)

has been documented in some patients with aortic stenosis and heart failure.[50]

The experimental studies of Sasayama, Ross, and their associates are in accord with this hypothesis. They found that when the aorta in conscious dogs was suddenly constricted, left ventricular systolic pressure rose and the left ventricular wall became thinned; this was associated with a large increase in wall stress, whereas the extent and velocity of shortening were reduced. During the next few weeks the left ventricle became hypertrophied, and therefore wall stress decreased, although systolic pressure remained elevated and shortening returned to normal levels. Interestingly, when the constriction was suddenly released, wall stress declined and shortening increased.[51]

DIASTOLIC PROPERTIES OF THE LEFT VENTRICLE (See also p. 427)

The diastolic properties of the ventricle are defined by its curvilinear pressure-volume relation (Figure 12–22, p. 428). The slope of a tangent (dP/dv) to this curvilinear relation defines the *chamber stiffness* at any level of filling pressure. An increase in chamber stiffness may occur (1) secondary to a rise in filling pressure,[52] i.e., by moving up on the pressure-volume curve; (2) by a shift to a steeper pressure-volume curve at the same ventricular end-diastolic pressure; or (3) through a combination of these two mechanisms. The second of these mechanisms, i.e., an alteration of ventricular (chamber) stiffness, in turn, can result from (1) an increase in intrinsic myocardial stiffness, as might occur with amyloid infiltration, fibrosis, or hypertrophy alone, without a change in ventricular mass; (2) a change in ventricular mass and wall thickness but without any alteration in intrinsic myocardial stiffness; or (3) a combination of these two mechanisms.

Since ventricular volume is also a determinant of chamber stiffness, disease states that modify ventricular size will alter chamber stiffness as a consequence of simple changes of ventricular volume in the absence of a change in myocardial stiffness. Thus, in acute volume overload, as might occur in acute aortic or mitral regurgitation or in acute left ventricular failure due to myocarditis, the left ventricle appears to move up to the steep portion of its pressure-volume curve and the end-diastolic pressure can rise sharply.

CHRONIC CHANGES IN VENTRICULAR DIASTOLIC PRESSURE-VOLUME RELATIONS. In contrast to the relative constancy of the passive pressure-volume relation of the left ventricle during acute interventions, prominent changes in this relation frequently occur with chronic heart disease, thus making the ventricular end-diastolic pressure an unreliable guide to end-diastolic volume.[53] Changes in compliance and substantial shifts in the diastolic pressure-volume curve of the left ventricle can be demonstrated experimentally during sustained volume overloading. Dogs with a chronic arteriovenous fistula demonstrate a progressive increase in left ventricular end-diastolic volume, without further elevation of the left ventricular end-diastolic pressure beyond that observed during the early, acute phase of the volume overloading. A rightward displacement (along the volume axis) of the entire diastolic pressure-dimension relationship occurs, and the slope of this curve is steeper, indicating increased chamber stiffness (Fig.

13–5).[36] Some patients with severe overloading due to chronic aortic regurgitation demonstrate similar shifts of the left ventricular diastolic pressure-circumference relation.

An increase in intrinsic myocardial (as opposed to chamber) stiffness has been described in the ventricular myocardium of dogs subjected to pulmonary artery constriction.[54] When spontaneously hypertensive rats exhibit a depression of ventricular contractility, they also evidence an increase of myocardial stiffness, even without an increase of left ventricular (chamber) stiffness.[55] An increase in myocardial stiffness that may be reversed following surgical treatment has also been reported in patients with aortic stenosis.[48] Thus, it has been postulated that in aortic stenosis, the development of concentric hypertrophy mitigates the increased systolic tension that would otherwise be required to eject blood across the narrowed orifice. An elevation of diastolic ventricular pressure is required to fill the hypertrophied ventricle. However, some patients have not only increased chamber stiffness but increased muscle stiffness as well, and in them the rise in left ventricular diastolic pressure is particularly striking.[48]

The dilated left ventricles of patients with chronic volume overload or with congestive (dilated) cardiomyopathy may be associated with little elevation of left ventricular end-diastolic pressure, indicating a shift of the pressure-volume curve to the right, i.e., along the volume axis (Fig. 13–5).[56] In contrast, concentric left ventricular hypertrophy, as occurs in aortic stenosis, hypertension, and hypertrophic cardiomyopathy, frequently changes the shape and position of the normal pressure-volume relation, so that at any diastolic volume, ventricular diastolic pressure is abnormally elevated, representing a shift to the left along the volume axis. Myocardial stiffness may or may not be altered in the presence of myocardial hypertrophy secondary to pressure overload.[57] However, the speed of ventricular relaxation is impaired in patients with marked left ventricular hypertrophy, regardless of whether it is due to pressure (aortic stenosis) or volume (aortic regurgitation) overload.[58]

ISCHEMIC HEART DISEASE. Marked changes can occur in the diastolic properties of the left ventricle in ischemic heart disease. First of all, ventricular relaxation may be slowed in the presence of acute, reversible myocardial ischemia.[59] Myocardial infarction causes complex changes in ventricular pressure-volume relations,[60] the results depending on (1) whether the infarcted tissue or the entire ventricle is studied, (2) the size of the infarct, and (3) the time following infarction that the study is carried out. In experimental infarction, the infarcted muscle initially exhibits *increased* stiffness,[61] perhaps related to the stress placed on the noncontracting tissue by the neighboring normal muscle.[62] Edema and the fibrocellular infiltration can contribute to further late stiffening of the necrotic tissue.[63] In a rat model of well-healed infarction, the diastolic pressure-volume relationship is shifted so that at low distending pressures, volume is increased—i.e., the chamber displays decreased stiffness—whereas at higher pressures the slope of the pressure-volume curve is normal. The left ventricular diastolic volume is increased at any diastolic pressure, the extent of displacement of the pressure-volume curve being a function of infarct size.[31]

CLINICAL IMPLICATIONS. Changes in the diastolic properties of the ventricular chambers are of clinical as well as theoretical importance. Thus, impairment of cardiac relaxation and leftward displacement of the ventricular diastolic pressure-volume curve can interfere with ventricular filling; this situation constitutes a major hemodynamic abnormality in hypertrophic cardiomyopathy as well as other conditions characterized by concentric ventricular hypertrophy and by reversible myocardial ischemia. At any given diastolic volume, ventricular end-diastolic pressure and pulmonary venous pressures rise. Tachycardia, by reducing the duration of diastole, intensifies this abnormality, whereas bradycardia reduces it. When the pressure-volume curve is shifted by ischemia, the treatment of the ischemia (with a beta-adrenergic blocker or calcium channel blocker[64]) improves diastolic relaxation and lowers ventricular diastolic (and pulmonary venous) pressure.

The contribution of atrial contraction to ventricular filling is particularly important in conditions in which ventricular stiffness is increased. Thus, loss of a properly synchronized, powerful atrial contraction in patients with impaired cardiac relaxation or leftward displacement of the ventricular pressure-volume curve (higher pressure at any volume) or both, as occurs in atrial fibrillation or atrioventricular dissociation, raises atrial pressure or lowers cardiac output or both. Pericardial tamponade and constrictive pericarditis also change the apparent diastolic properties of the heart (Figure 43–17, p. 1490). Early filling is unimpaired in constrictive pericarditis because the myocardium is normal. However, filling is abruptly halted in mid-diastole by the constricted pericardium, which imposes its properties on those of the ventricle.

The fact that the normal left ventricle operates just below the bend of the pressure-volume curve (Figure 12–22, p. 428) explains why an acute volume overload or impairment of contractility will result in a marked rise in left ventricular diastolic pressure, which can lead to pulmonary edema as the ventricle moves up to the steep portion of its pressure-volume curve. The rightward displacement of the curve—i.e., an increase in volume at any level of pressure—as occurs with chronic volume overload or cardiomyopathy, is a helpful change, since it lowers the pressure necessary to provide the high preload required by the diseased left ventricle.

MECHANISM OF DEPRESSED CONTRACTILITY

Considerable effort has been directed toward elucidating the fundamental mechanism responsible for the relative decrease in the useful external work of the myocardium in the common forms of low-output heart failure. The available evidence for the mechanism of myocardial failure analyzed in terms of energy supply, production, storage, and utilization, as well as the structure and function of the contractile proteins, is conflicting. Although a number of metabolic alterations have been identified in the failing, hemodynamically overloaded heart, it is not clear which is the *primary* defect responsible for heart failure and which are *secondary* compensatory mechanisms that aid these hearts in coping with the overload. Therefore, although a single unifying biochemical defect responsible for heart

failure has not been identified, a number of possible abnormalities have been excluded, and there is increasing evidence for several possible defects that might be responsible. Some of the confusion in this field results undoubtedly from the various models of heart failure employed, from species differences, from variations in the nature of the inciting stimulus, and from the rate and severity of its applications.[65,66]

Myocardial Energy Production

In early studies, measurements of coronary blood flow utilizing coronary sinus catheterization, both in humans and in dogs with low-output heart failure, showed that the coronary blood flow per gram of myocardium does not differ significantly from normal.[67] However, other observations on the relation between left ventricular performance and myocardial oxygen consumption have shown that when contractility becomes acutely depressed, myocardial oxygen consumption also declines.[68] Patients with chronic impairment of left ventricular performance and reduction of the velocity of myocardial fiber shortening also exhibit reduction of coronary blood flow and myocardial oxygen consumption per unit of muscle.[69] Papillary muscles removed from cats with pressure overload–induced right ventricular hypertrophy exhibit a depression of both contractility and oxygen consumption per unit of tension development.[18] Thus, although ischemia clearly can impair cardiac contraction, heart failure can certainly occur in the presence of both adequate myocardial perfusion and oxygen availability. In several preparations, failing heart muscle appears to require less oxygen than does normal muscle.

MITOCHONDRIAL FUNCTION

Considerable dispute has centered on the question of whether or not mitochondrial oxidative phosphorylation, i.e., energy production, is abnormal in heart failure. Some investigators have shown that experimentally produced heart failure is characterized by a defect in mitochondrial energy production.[70] The respiratory control index, i.e., the ratio of active phosphorylating respiration to baseline respiration, and the rate of oxygen consumption during active phosphorylation have been reported to be markedly reduced in mitochondria obtained from hearts with experimentally produced failure. Similarly, mitochondria isolated from the hearts of hamsters with hereditary cardiomyopathy[71] and the cardiomyopathy produced by potassium depletion[72] exhibit depression of respiratory activity. Homogenates prepared from hamster hearts with hereditary cardiomyopathy exhibit severe depression of the ability to oxidize fatty acids and acetate.[73] Mitochondria obtained from failing *human* cardiac muscle have also shown reduced oxygen consumption during active phosphorylation and reduced rates of NADH-linked respiratory activity.[70] In contrast to these observations, other data indicate that electron transport and the tightness of respiratory control are normal in mitochondria obtained from failing human hearts[74] and cat hearts with experimental heart failure produced by pressure overload.[75]

Mitochondria obtained from hypertrophied, nonfailing rabbit hearts have shown significantly *increased* respiratory activity compared with those of normal hearts, without a change in the ADP/O ratio, i.e., in the rate of energy production to oxygen consumption, or in the tightness of respiratory control, permitting an *increase* in the capacity for synthesizing ATP; in contrast, mitochondria obtained from rabbit hearts with congestive heart failure have shown respiratory rates near or below normal, a decreased respiratory control index, and some lowering of the ADP/O ratio.[76]

Sordahl has suggested that in the phase of compensatory hypertrophy the ability of mitochondria to generate ATP is increased, but that in the late phase of hypertrophy there is a reduction in the quantity of mitochondria as well as in the capacity of individual mitochondria to generate ATP. According to this concept, a primary cause of contractile failure of the hypertrophic heart might be an inability of the energy-producing system, i.e., the mitochondria, to keep pace with the needs of the contractile apparatus.[77]

Failing muscles removed from cats subjected to an acute pressure overload exhibit decreased efficiency, i.e., increased O_2 uptake for any level of tension development. The mitochondria from these papillary muscles exhibit an increase in the rate of O_2 consumption in state 4—i.e., basal (so-called nonphosphorylating)—respiration.[77,78] Ruthenium red, a compound that blocks the mitochondrial uptake of Ca^{++}, reduces the rate of state 4 respiration to normal in these mitochondria, suggesting that nonphosphorylating mitochondrial respiration, linked to Ca^{++} transport and perhaps due to increased cycling of Ca^{++} across the mitochondrial membranes, is responsible for the abnormal myocardial O_2 consumption and the reduced external efficiency that characterizes hypertrophy induced by the acute imposition of a pressure load. Following unbanding of the pulmonary artery, myocardial hypertrophy, the accompanying depression of contractility, elevation of O_2 consumption, and the abnormality of state 4 mitochondrial respiration all return to normal.[35] In addition, no abnormality of mitochondrial function (or, as already noted, of contractility) has been noted in hypertrophy produced by moderately severe volume overload.[24]

The explanation for the conflicting data concerning mitochondrial respiration in experimental heart failure, summarized above, is not clear. It may be related to differences in species or in the nature, severity, and rate of application of the inciting stimulus. However, since, in some studies, oxidative phosphorylation appears to be sustained until very late in the course of heart failure, it is unlikely that the observed changes in mitochondrial function are causally related to the development of heart failure. However, they may well be important in *perpetuating* chronic heart failure.

Myocardial Energy Supplies

In order to determine whether energy supplies are adequate in cardiac hypertrophy and failure, the contents of high-energy phosphate were compared in the papillary muscles of normal cats, cats with hypertrophy without failure, and cats with overt right ventricular failure induced by pulmonary artery constriction. Both the ATP and the creatine phosphate (CP) concentrations were normal in the papillary muscles removed from failing hearts and from nonfailing, hypertrophied hearts which were studied in vitro.[79] Since, as already pointed out (Figs. 13–2 and 13–3), the mechanical performance of these isolated muscles was impaired, *their depression of contractility could not be attributed to a reduction of total myocardial high-energy stores.*[79,80] In addition, there appear to be no reductions of ATP and CP concentrations in papillary muscles removed from failing human hearts.[74] Thus, it would appear that, just as is the case for abnormalities of mitochondrial function, defects in energy production and the total reserve of high-energy phosphate compounds are not *primarily* responsible for the reduced contractility of the hypertrophied or failing heart. However, the possibility that the reduction of a small compartment of ATP vital for ionic movement and muscular contraction plays a key role in the depression of contractility characteristic of heart failure has not been excluded.

One form of heart failure *primarily* related to a reduction of myocardial energy stores is that due to phosphate deficiency. Chronic hypophosphatemia induced by dietary means is associated with reversible depression of myocardial performance in isolated muscle as well as in the intact heart of animals and humans, presumably as a consequence of reduced ATP stores.[81]

Myocardial Energy Utilization

External efficiency, i.e., the ratio of work performed to oxygen utilized, is usually decreased in chronic myocardial failure, probably as a consequence of an abnormality in the conversion of metabolic energy to contractile work. Other possibilities, however, such as abnormalities of cellular alignment with ineffective coordination of contraction, must also be considered.

Insofar as the *quantity* of the contractile apparatus is concerned, in a model of stable pressure-induced hypertrophy, the fraction of cell volume composed of myofibrils has been reported to increase.[82] Patients having aortic stenosis without heart failure exhibited a normal fraction of myofibrils per cell, whereas those with left ventricular failure showed a significant reduction in cell volume occupied by myofibrils, suggesting that this decrease in the quantity of the contractile machinery may be responsible for the cardiac decompensation.[83]

DEPRESSION OF MYOSIN ATPase. There is considerable evidence implicating abnormalities of contractile proteins in heart failure. First of all, the finding that the reduced velocity of contraction of the hypertrophied myocardium occurs in chemically skinned ventricular fiber suggests that this change reflects intrinsic alterations in the contractile apparatus. The activity of myofibrillar ATPase has been found to be reduced in the hearts of patients who died of heart failure[84,85] and in dogs with naturally occurring heart failure.[86] Furthermore, reductions in the activities of myofibrillar ATPase, actomyosin ATPase, or myosin ATPase occur in heart failure induced in cats by pulmonary artery constriction,[87] in guinea pigs with constriction of the ascending aorta,[88] and in dogs with marked constriction of the pulmonary artery or aorta.[89] These depressions of enzymatic activity could occur if an altered low molecular weight subunit of the myosin molecule, i.e., the portion of the molecule responsible for the ATPase activity, were produced in the overloaded heart and if it reduced contractility by lowering the rate of interaction between actin and myosin filaments.

It has been shown that cardiac myosin, like skeletal muscle, is composed of several polymorphic forms, termed isozymes.[90–92] Thus adaptation of cardiac performance appears to be mediated by a change in myosin. Thyroxin administration,[93] exercise,[94] and mild pressure overload[95] increase the work of the heart and produce a shift in isomyosin synthesis toward a myosin with increased ATPase activity.[90] However, a marked increase in cardiac work produced by volume or pressure overload or both, acting presumably by stretching the muscle fiber, induces the preferential synthesis of a cardiac myosin isoenzyme having specific immunological and electrophoretic properties and a depressed ATPase activity.[96,97] Since there are no differences between the light chains of myosin from normal and from hypertrophied human hearts,[98] it is likely that the molecular basis for the variations in the properties of the myosin is confined to the heavy chains.

The synthesis of a myosin with abnormally low intrinsic ATPase activity could explain many of the functional changes in failing heart muscle, such as depression of the force-velocity curve (Fig. 13–3), but it has also been proposed that such a biochemical abnormality might actually be beneficial in heart failure, since it would be expected to *increase* the quantity of mechanical energy derived from each mole of ATP utilized, albeit at the expense of a slowing of the maximum rate at which blood is ejected;[80] this suggestion is compatible with the finding of reduced O_2 consumption per unit of tension development of papillary muscles obtained from cats with gradually increasing pressure overload.[18] Further support for a change in the contractile proteins as a cause of some forms of heart failure comes from the finding that doxorubicin (Adriamycin)–induced cardiomyopathy (p. 1691) is associated with the synthesis of abnormally stimulated myosin ATPase.[99]

Excitation-Contraction Coupling

The critical role played by Ca^{++} in the initiation of contraction and as a determinant of the contractile state is discussed on pages 413 to 418. Studies of a number of in vitro

systems indicate that the delivery of Ca^{++} for activation of the contractile process is impaired in heart failure.[99a] A variety of cellular structures, including the sarcolemma, the sarcoplasmic reticulum (SR), and the mitochondria, affect the myoplasmic ionic calcium concentration $[Ca^{++}]$ (Figure 12–9, p. 417). It has been proposed that structural damage to these organelles or changes in the intracellular concentrations of other cations, adenonucleotides, or free fatty acids may interfere with mechanisms regulating myoplasmic $[Ca^{++}]$ and thereby participate in the production of heart failure.

The uptake of Ca^{++} by SR is dependent on a Ca^{++}-activated ATPase. Depressed activity of this enzyme, leading to defects in Ca^{++} accumulation by the SR, could play a role in the development of myocardial failure, in that a reduction in Ca^{++} pumping could be responsible for a reduction of Ca^{++} bound to the SR and eventually for less Ca^{++} available for "regenerative release" (p. 415) for the contractile process (Fig. 13–10).

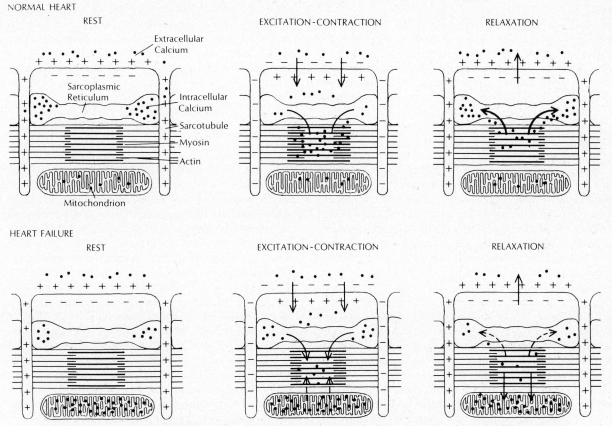

FIGURE 13–10 Hypothetical abnormality in excitation-contraction in heart failure. In the *normal heart* at rest, extracellular calcium is concentrated in the region of the sarcolemmal membrane and its invaginations (sarcotubular system); intracellular calcium sequestered chiefly in the sarcoplasmic reticulum is awaiting delivery to the contractile apparatus. With excitation of the cell membrane and depolarization, there is rapid entry of extracellular calcium; spread of electrical activity via the sarcotubules causes release of intracellular calcium and activation of contraction. For muscle to relax, intracellular calcium must be recaptured by the sarcoplasmic reticulum; efflux of calcium across the cell membrane probably also occurs. In contrast, according to the sequence of events postulated to occur in *heart failure*, ineffective calcium pumping by the sarcoplasmic reticulum may alter the normal relaxation process, rendering the mitochondria the dominant calcium uptake mechanism and a source of activator calcium for contraction. If so, in resting muscle, relatively little calcium would be available for release from the sarcoplasmic reticulum to activate contraction. Although the mitochondria may contain an ample amount, it is likely to be released slowly; thus, with depolarization, a diminished amount of calcium might be supplied to the contractile proteins. Whether the depressed myocardial contractility characteristic of heart failure develops on this basis remains to be determined. (From Chidsey, C. A.: Calcium metabolism in the normal and failing heart. *In* Braunwald, E. [ed.]: The Myocardium: Failure and Infarction. New York, HP Publishing Co., 1974, p. 37.)

The aforementioned reduction in contractility of papillary muscle obtained from cats with constriction of the pulmonary artery (Figs. 13–2 and 13–3) is accompanied by reduction in the muscle's resting membrane potential, maximum rate of rise, and overshoot, as well as in the duration of the action potential.[100] Although the precise mechanism responsible for these changes in electrical properties is unknown, they may be related to alterations in cellular concentrations of Na^+ and K^+ and thereby affect the entry of Ca^{++} into the myocardium. Although the contractility of muscle obtained from failing hearts is markedly reduced in a medium containing a normal amount of Ca^{++} (i.e., 2.5 mM), in a medium containing 11 mM Ca^{++}, the contractility of both hypertrophied, failing muscles and normal muscles becomes augmented to similar levels.[101] The ATPase isolated from the SR obtained from the right ventricles of dogs with heart failure has been found to be depressed,[102] and in failing calf hearts the rate of Ca^{++} uptake by the SR and the activity of microsomal Ca^{++}-activated ATPase obtained are reduced to about 50 per cent of normal.[103]

A disturbance in the uptake of Ca^{++} by the SR could also interfere with cardiac performance in another manner, i.e., inadequate reduction of the intracellular $[Ca^{++}]$ at the end of systole could result in delayed or incomplete relaxation. It has been demonstrated in studies employing murexide, a dye that rapidly binds Ca^{++} in solution,[104] that the rate of Ca^{++} uptake by the SR obtained from failing heart muscle in humans,[105] rabbits,[106] and hamsters[107] is slowed and the total binding of Ca^{++} is reduced.

Experimental heart failure in the rabbit produced by aortic regurgitation appears to be associated with a significant alteration in the intracellular distribution of Ca^{++}. Although total intracellular $[Ca^{++}]$ is normal, mitochondrial $[Ca^{++}]$ is greatly increased.[108] The rate and binding of Ca^{++} to the SR are reduced (Fig. 13–10), and it is possible that if the SR can no longer maintain the myoplasmic $[Ca^{++}]$ low enough to initiate muscle relaxation, the mitochondria might become an important storage site as a source of activator Ca^{++} for muscle contraction.[109] Thus, although the total *quantity* of Ca^{++} available to the myocardial cell may not necessarily be diminished in heart failure, *distribution* of this cation might well become altered. With greater quantities of Ca^{++} accumulated in the mitochondria, contractility might then be reduced by limiting the amount of Ca^{++} available to activate the myofilaments; moreover, if enough Ca^{++} enters the mitochondria, their function may become impaired, i.e., uncoupling of oxidative phosphorylation can occur. Interestingly, the uptake of Ca^{++} by the SR is significantly reduced in rabbits with aortic regurgitation which were sacrificed *before* the objective signs of heart failure had developed. This finding, very early in the course of failure, suggests that this reduction of Ca^{++} uptake is responsible for, rather than a consequence of, impaired contractility.[110]

The hamster with hereditary cardiomyopathy offers the opportunity for study of the function of the SR in a naturally occurring form of myocardial failure. There is a depression of the rate of Ca^{++} binding by the SR, and this depression becomes more severe as heart failure progresses;[111] the Ca^{++} content bound to the sarcolemma is reduced.[112] Abnormalities of phospholipid and cholesterol composition of the SR, which have been described in the cardiomyopathic hamster,[113] might explain these changes. In addition, both the rate and the extent of energy-linked Ca^{++} binding by mitochondria have been reported to be greatly reduced in these failing hearts.[111]

Abnormalities in the accumulation of Ca^{++} by the SR have been demonstrated in other forms of heart failure as well, including round heart disease, a naturally occurring model of congestive cardiomyopathy in turkeys,[114] spontaneously failing dog heart-lung preparation,[115] failing ischemic heart muscle,[116] the substrate-depleted failing rat heart, and the heart with isoproterenol-induced necrosis,[117] as well as the heart in which hypertrophy and failure are caused by bacterial infection. In the depressed contractile state characteristic of chronic K^+ deficiency, Ca^{++} uptake of SR isolated from K^+-deficient hearts is reduced, whereas mitochondrial Ca^{++} binding is increased.[118] Cardiac muscle removed from patients with severe heart failure who were recipients of cardiac transplants has yielded SR with slower rates of Ca^{++} accumulation and reduced release of Ca^{++} compared with normal animal heart preparations.[105,119] Thus, although disturbances of Ca^{++} transport frequently accompany and may be causally related to heart failure, the nature of the abnormality of Ca^{++} transport appears to vary in different types of heart failure.[110, 120–122]

ALTERATIONS IN THE FUNCTION OF THE ADRENERGIC NERVOUS SYSTEM

In view of the well-established importance of the adrenergic nervous system in normal regulation of cardiac performance (p. 439), considerable attention has been directed to the activity of this system in patients with heart failure. Measurements of the concentration of norepinephrine (NE) in arterial blood provide an index of the activity of this system at rest and during exercise. Either no change or small increases occur during exercise in normal subjects or patients without heart failure, whereas much greater elevations occur in patients with heart failure, presumably reflecting greater activity of the adrenergic nervous system during exercise in these patients[123–125,125a] (Fig. 13–11A). Measurements of 24-hour urinary NE excretion revealed marked elevations in patients with heart failure,[126] indicating that the activity of the adrenergic nervous system (and presumably secretion of catecholamines by the adrenal medulla) was also augmented at rest (Fig. 13–11B).

The elevation of plasma NE concentration that occurs in patients with heart failure correlates directly with the degree of left ventricular dysfunction,[127] as reflected in the height of the pulmonary capillary wedge pressure, in the duration of the preejection period, and in the ratio of the preejection to the left ventricular ejection period, and correlates inversely with cardiac index and left ventricular ejection time.[128–130] The finding that plasma lymphocytes from patients with severe heart failure fail to generate normal amounts of cyclic adenosine monophosphate (AMP) after beta-adrenergic receptor stimulation with isoproterenol suggests that beta-adrenergic receptors may be desensitized in patients with heart failure and raises the possibility that this desensitization contributes to the observed alterations in myocardial contractility.[127] The obser-

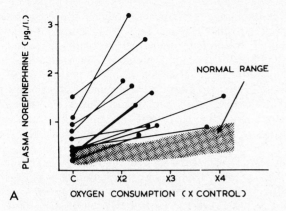

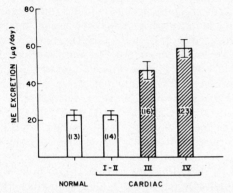

FIGURE 13–11 Measurements of concentration of norepinephrine (NE) in patients with congestive heart failure and in normal control subjects. *A*, Changes in plasma norepinephrine during exercise in congestive heart failure. Oxygen consumption during the exercise period is expressed in multiples of the resting oxygen consumption. C = control or resting values. The normal range is represented by the stippled area. *B*, Urinary NE excretion in normal control subjects, in cardiac patients without failure (Classes I and II, New York Heart Association Classification), and in patients with failure (Classes III and IV). Average values ± SEM are shown. (From Braunwald, E., Ross, J., Jr., and Sonnenblick, E. H.: Mechanisms of Contraction of the Normal and Failing Heart. 2nd ed. Boston, Little, Brown and Co., 1976.)

vation of reduced beta-adrenergic receptor density in circulating lymphocytes of patients with heart failure[131] is consistent with "down regulation" of receptors as a consequence of the elevation of circulating NE.

Further abnormality of adrenergic nervous activity is reflected in the very low concentrations of NE in atrial tissue[126] removed at operation from patients with heart failure (Fig. 13–12*A*). In some patients with heart failure, extremely low values were found, with NE concentrations less than 10 per cent of normal. NE concentrations were also markedly depressed in papillary muscles removed from the left ventricles of patients undergoing mitral valve replacement and who had been in severe left ventricular failure.[22]

In dogs with right ventricular failure produced by the creation of pulmonary stenosis and tricuspid regurgitation,[132] the reduction of cardiac NE concentrations was shown *not* to be the result of a simple dilution of sympathetic nerve endings in a hypertrophied muscle mass, since the total ventricular content of NE was lower both in the hypertrophied right ventricle and in the nonhypertrophied left ventricle (Fig. 13–12*B*). In NE-depleted failing hearts, fluorescence is absent in the terminal varicosities of sympathetic fibers in close association with cardiac muscle cells. Following relief from pulmonary constriction, many indices of contractile function of the hypertrophied or failing cat right ventricle returned to normal, but NE depletion persisted.[133]

In addition to NE depletion, ventricles obtained from patients with heart failure demonstrated a marked reduction of beta receptor density, isoproterenol-mediated adenylate cyclase stimulation, and muscle contraction[134] (Fig. 13–13). Local NE stores do *not* play any role in the intrinsic contractile state of cardiac muscle. Thus, no differences in contractility were found in papillary muscles removed from normal cats and from cats with NE depletion produced by chronic cardiac denervation or reserpine pretreatment;[135] length-tension curves, force-velocity relations, and the augmentation of isometric tension achieved by postextrasystolic potentiation and by increasing the frequency

FIGURE 13–12 Effects of heart failure on cardiac stores of norepinephrine (NE). *A*, Concentration of NE in biopsy specimens of the atrial appendage taken during cardiac operations from 34 patients without heart failure (Classes I and II) and 49 patients with heart failure (Classes III and IV). Average values ± SEM are included. *B*, Total ventricular NE content in normal dogs and in dogs with pulmonary stenosis, tricuspid regurgitation, and congestive heart failure (CHF). Average values ± SEM are given. RV = right ventricle; LV = left ventricle. (From Braunwald, E., Ross, J., Jr., and Sonnenblick, E. H.: Mechanisms of Contraction of the Normal and Failing Heart. 2nd ed. Boston, Little, Brown and Co., 1976.)

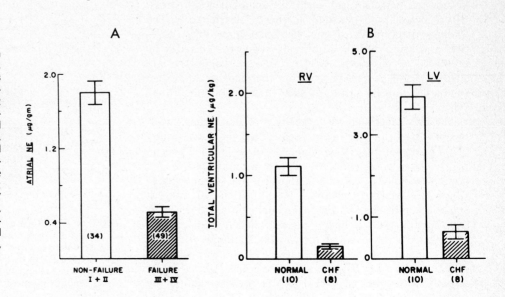

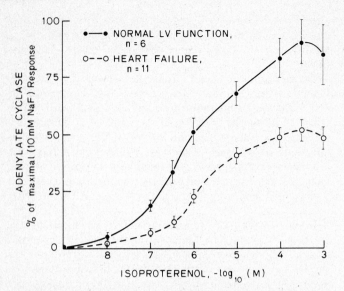

FIGURE 13–13 l-Isoproterenol–stimulated adenylate cyclase activity in human left ventricles in normal human hearts (solid circles) and failing human hearts (open circles), expressed as a percentage of the response to 10 mM sodium fluoride (NaF) stimulation (mean ± SEM). (Reproduced with permission from Bristow, M. R., Ginsburg, R., Minobe, W., et al.: Decreased catecholamine sensitivity and beta-adrenergic receptor density in failing human hearts. N. Engl. J. Med. *307*:205, 1982.)

of contraction were not altered from the normal state in NE-depleted muscles.

MECHANISM OF CARDIAC NOREPINEPHRINE DEPLETION IN HEART FAILURE. After the production of heart failure in the guinea pig and in the dog, the ventricular NE concentration falls markedly, and the infusion of NE raises cardiac NE stores substantially less than in normal animals.[136] This reduced capacity to retain administered NE might be due either to a reduction in the total number of neurons in the heart or to a diminution of the number of intraneuronal binding sites. However, there is no evidence for any *qualitative* abnormality in the distribution of the reduced quantities of NE taken up by the failing heart. Compared with the control values, the cardiac turnover of NE is greatly augmented in the cardiomyopathic Syrian hamster and approaches the values observed in normal hamsters subjected to immobilization stress, which produces a massive adrenergic discharge.[137] The findings that prolonged immobilization leads to a reduction in cardiac NE in both strains and that this can be prevented by ganglionic blockage suggest that in the late stage of hamster cardiomyopathy, the increase in cardiac sympathetic tone is responsible for the reduction in cardiac NE.[138]

The biosynthesis of NE normally proceeds through a series of steps from tyrosine to dopa to dopamine, the immediate precursor of NE (Figure 12–33, p. 440). Tyrosine hydroxylase, which catalyzes the first reaction (tyrosine to dopa), normally is the rate-limiting enzyme in the synthesis of NE. Marked reductions in the activity of this enzyme accompanied cardiac NE depletion of dogs with experimental heart failure,[139] whereas no alterations in enzyme activity occurred in the hearts of animals in which NE depletion had been experimentally produced with reserpine, suggesting that this reduction in enzyme activity is responsible for cardiac NE depletion in heart failure. In

the cardiomyopathic hamster, however, there is no reduction of tyrosine hydroxylase activity during the development of heart failure,[140] although with the decline of cardiac NE, there is an accumulation of cardiac dopamine. The acute increase in cardiac sympathetic tone induced by immobilization stress in normal hamsters mimics this alteration in cardiac catecholamine distribution (increase of dopamine and reduction of NE) in heart failure and can be restored to normal in these animals by ganglionic blockade. These findings suggest that the increase in cardiac sympathetic tone leads to a shift in the rate-limiting step for NE synthesis from the hydroxylation of tyrosine to the hydroxylation of dopamine. Thus, although there is clear evidence for a defect in cardiac NE synthesis in heart failure, the specific step that is responsible is still in dispute.

A marked decline in cardiac NE stores has been reported to occur in both normal and necrotic regions of the heart following experimental myocardial infarction.[141,142] However, cardiac NE content begins to increase in these areas 2 weeks after infarction, until normal levels are reached at 6 weeks. These studies support the concept that the depletion of NE stores may be reversible, but, as already noted, this is not a universal finding.[133]

CONSEQUENCES OF CARDIAC NE DEPLETION. In view of the strongly positive inotropic effect exerted by the NE released from its nerves, the adrenergic nervous system may be considered to provide important potential support to the failing myocardium. However, with supramaximal stimulation of the cardiac sympathetic nerves, the increments in heart rate and contractile force that occur in animals with heart failure and cardiac NE depletion are abolished or are much smaller than those in normal dogs[143] (Fig. 13–14). Thus, it is likely that when heart failure is accompanied by depletion of cardiac NE stores, the

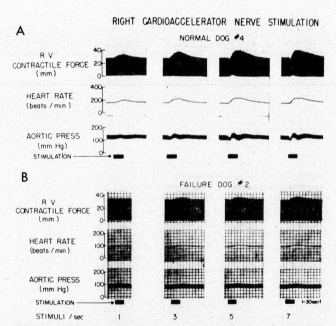

FIGURE 13–14 Records showing the effect of right cardioaccelerator stimulation in a normal dog (*A*) and in a dog with congestive heart failure (*B*). (From Covell, J. W., Chidsey, C. A., and Braunwald, E.: Reduction of the cardiac response to postganglionic sympathetic nerve stimulation in experimental heart failure. Circ. Res. *19*:51, 1966, by permission of the American Heart Association, Inc.)

quantity of NE released by the sympathetic nerve endings in the heart is deficient in relation to the impulse traffic along these nerves. Furthermore, the reduction in beta receptor density in failing heart muscle[134] further limits the response. Therefore, although cardiac stores of NE are not fundamental to maintenance of the *intrinsic* contractile state of the myocardium, diminished release of the neurotransmitter and of beta receptor density in heart failure may be responsible for loss of the much-needed adrenergic support of the failing heart and in this manner could intensify the severity of the congestive heart failure state.

ADRENERGIC SUPPORT OF THE FAILING HEART. The importance of the adrenergic nervous system in maintaining ventricular contractility when myocardial function is depressed in congestive heart failure is shown by the effects of adrenergic blockade. Pharmacological blockade of the sympathetic nervous system may cause sodium and water retention as well as intensification of heart failure.[144,145] Therefore, caution must be exercised in using adrenergic blocking agents in the treatment of patients with limited cardiac reserve. Additional important evidence indicating that the NE-depleted failing heart is supported by circulating catecholamines comes from experiments on calves with experimentally produced heart failure and cardiac NE depletion in which beta-adrenergic blockade intensifies heart failure, presumably by blocking the inotropic action of circulating epinephrine.[146] Thus, the failing heart appears to be increasingly dependent on this extracardiac adrenergic support supplied by circulating catecholamines for the maintenance of cardiac function. However, this generalized adrenergic stimulation resulting from circulating catecholamines may also exert undesirable side effects, because it elevates vascular resistance and may therefore present the heart with an excessive afterload.

The possibility of defective adrenergic control of heart rate in patients with heart failure has been studied by observing the reflex chronotropic responses to upright tilt and to nitroglycerin-induced hypotension.[147] An attenuation of the normal increase in heart rate in patients with heart failure both before and after administration of atropine confirmed that a defect exists in the adrenergic component of baroreceptor-mediated control of heart rate in patients with cardiac dysfunction; the severity of this defect was, in general, proportional to the impairment of cardiac reserve. Similar observations have been made in dogs

with experimental heart failure during carotid occlusion.[148,149] A reduction in responsiveness of the beta receptors could be excluded as a cause of impaired sympathetic influence, because there was a normal response to isoproterenol,[147] indicating that the sympathetically mediated heart rate response results from NE depletion. In addition, the heart rate during maximal exercise was reduced in patients with cardiac dysfunction,[147] suggesting that the ability of the sympathetic nervous system to speed the heart is impaired in these subjects. Thus, cardiac dysfunction appears to be associated with a marked impairment of autonomically mediated changes in heart rate.

An inappropriately depressed increase in heart rate in humans[150] and in dogs[149] with heart failure was also observed when arterial pressure was reduced through administration of vasodilators (nitroprusside, hydralazine, prazosin, and teprotide); whereas the changes in mean arterial pressure observed in response to the vasodilators were similar in patients with heart failure and control subjects, the changes in heart rate after vasodilators correlated significantly with the changes in concentration of circulating NE and with the sum of circulating NE and epinephrine. In normal individuals, both heart rate and catecholamine concentrations rose, whereas in patients with heart failure, in whom resting catecholamine levels were increased, cardiac acceleration was blunted, and catecholamine concentration failed to rise further.[150]

ADRENERGIC NERVOUS FUNCTIONS IN THE PERIPHERAL CIRCULATION. Substantial changes also occur in the function of the adrenergic nerves that innervate peripheral blood vessels in heart failure. Thus, whereas adrenergically mediated vasoconstriction normally occurs in the vessels supplying the splanchnic viscera and kidneys during exercise, neurogenic vasoconstriction is even more important when augmentation of cardiac output is seriously limited, as happens in heart failure. Figure 13–15 contrasts values in a normal dog with those in a dog with heart failure produced experimentally by inducing tricuspid regurgitation and constriction of the pulmonary artery. In the latter, exercise induced a much more marked reduction in mesenteric blood flow and elevation of mesenteric vascular resistance than it did in the normal dog.[8] Similar changes during exercise were observed in other major visceral vascular beds, such as the renal bed. Evidence that this intense vasoconstriction during exercise is mediat-

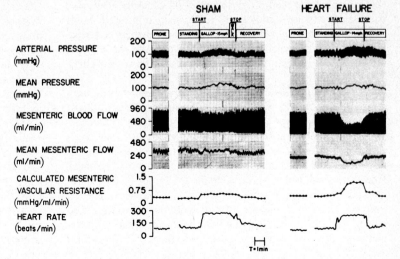

FIGURE 13–15 Tracings comparing the effects of similar levels of severe exercise in a sham-operated dog (*left*) and in a dog with heart failure (*right*). In contrast to the normal response observed in the sham-operated animal, mean arterial pressure rose only slightly, mesenteric blood flow decreased, and mesenteric resistance rose profoundly in the dog with heart failure. (From Higgins, C. B., et al.: Alterations in regional hemodynamics in experimental heart failure in conscious dogs. Trans. Assoc. Am. Physicians 85:267, 1972.)

HEART FAILURE

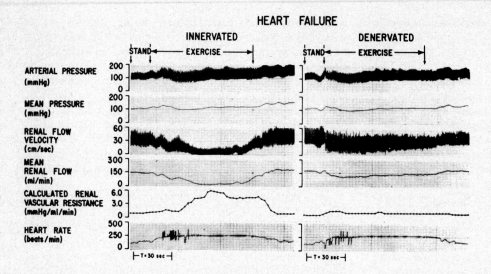

FIGURE 13–16 Tracings comparing the alterations in renal hemodynamics during exercise in the innervated kidney and contralateral denervated kidney in a dog with experimental heart failure. (From Higgins, C. B., et al.: Alterations in regional hemodynamics in experimental heart failure in conscious dogs. Trans. Assoc. Am. Physicians 85:267, 1972.)

ed by the adrenergic nervous system is provided by observations on dogs with experimentally produced heart failure in which one kidney was denervated. Blood flow through the normal kidney declined precipitously during exercise, and calculated renal vascular resistance increased markedly. In contrast, little change in renal blood flow and calculated renal vascular resistance occurred in the denervated kidney[8] (Fig. 13–16). In addition to the abnormally intense peripheral vasoconstriction occurring in heart failure, other defects in adrenergic control of the peripheral vascular bed in heart failure have been identified. These include a diminution of reflex elevation of vascular resistance with carotid hypotension[148] as well as a blunting of the vasoconstrictor response to adrenergic nerve stimulation[151] in experimental heart failure.

PARASYMPATHETIC FUNCTION IN HEART FAILURE

Cardiac enlargement, with or without heart failure, is associated with marked disturbances of parasympathetic as well as sympathetic function.[152,153] The parasympathetic restraint on sinoatrial node automaticity is markedly reduced in patients with heart disease who also exhibit less heart rate slowing for any given elevation of systemic arterial pressure than do normal subjects. The sensitivity of the baroreceptor reflex to increase in pressure has also been shown to be significantly reduced in dogs with heart failure.[148] Cardiomyopathic hamster hearts display a reduction in the activity of choline acetyltransferase, an enzyme that provides an estimate of the density of parasympathetic innervation.[153,154]

Although the mechanism responsible for the demonstrated impairment of parasympathetic function in heart failure is not clear,[155] this disturbance may be of considerable functional importance, since the ability to alter heart rate constitutes an extremely important mechanism for the adjustment of cardiac output; indeed, in normal subjects alterations in heart rate account in large measure for changes in cardiac output. In patients with heart failure, exercise does not elevate stroke volume normally, and when this limitation of stroke volume is combined with defective control of heart rate as a consequence of abnormal-

ities of both the sympathetic and the parasympathetic limbs of the autonomic nervous system, this inability to raise cardiac output appropriately is readily appreciated.

ABNORMALITIES IN AFFERENT IMPULSES. Heart failure also interferes with the afferent limbs of cardiovascular reflexes. According to the schema proposed by Gauer and Henry,[156] under normal circumstances, elevated left atrial pressure increases left atrial stretch and stimulates left atrial stretch receptors.[157] The increased activity of both myelinated and nonmyelinated (C-fiber) afferents[158] normally inhibits the release of ADH, thereby increasing water excretion, which in turn reduces plasma volume, and left atrial pressure returns to normal. In addition, enhanced left atrial stretch receptor activity depresses renal efferent sympathetic nerve activity and increases renal blood flow and glomerular filtration rate, thereby enhancing the ability of the kidney to reduce plasma volume. Indeed, in patients with myocardial infarction and acute heart failure, urine flow and glomerular filtration rate (and sometimes even sodium excretion) are increased despite the decline in arterial pressure. Presumably, activation of atrial or ventricular receptors from a rise in left atrial pressure or bulging left ventricle is responsible.[159] However, in chronic heart failure, in spite of the augmented stretch of left atrial receptors in heart failure, ADH titers remain high and renal blood flow remains low.[160-162] Zucker et al.[163] observed that the decreased sensitivity of left atrial stretch receptors in dogs with heart failure is the result of cardiac dilatation and alterations in atrial compliance and is reversible following reversal of heart failure.[164] This resetting of atrial receptors may be responsible for the inappropriately high plasma ADH levels[165] and may contribute to the peripheral edema, ascites, and hyponatremia often seen in patients with chronic heart failure (Chap. 52). Although ADH is a pressor substance, the concentrations in patients with heart failure, while elevated, are probably insufficient to contribute to the observed elevation of systemic vascular resistance.

This resetting of the sensitivity of cardiac receptors may have even broader significance in heart failure. Thus the initial response in acute heart failure consists of an increase in renin activity, as well as in circulating angiotensin II and aldosterone concentrations. As a result, there is sodium and water retention, and with expansion of the blood volume the signal for activation of the renin-angiotensin-aldosterone axis is turned off, presumably as a result of stimulation of cardiac receptors. With chronic heart failure and its attendant cardiac distention and decreased sensitivity of these receptors, the reflex inhibition of renin release and sympathetic activity disappears, and the activity of both of these systems (i.e., the renin-angiotensin-aldosterone axis and the adrenergic drive to the heart, to the peripheral vascular bed, and to the adrenal medulla) is enhanced, resulting in the sodium retention, tachycardia, and vasoconstricted state characteristic of heart failure.[159]

THE RENIN-ANGIOTENSIN SYSTEM. Sympathetic stimulation of $beta_1$ adrenergic receptors in the juxtaglomerular apparatus is probably the principal mechanism responsible for activation of the renin-angiotensin-aldosterone axis in acute heart failure (Figure 26–21, p. 868; Figure 52–3, p. 1750). However, in patients with severe chronic heart failure, especially following salt restriction and diuretic treatment, reduction of the sodium presented to the macula densa also contributes to the release of renin. Elevated plasma renin activity is a common finding in patients with heart failure.[129,130,130a] Angiotensin II is a potent vasoconstrictor and contributes, along with increased adrenergic activity, to the excessive elevation of systemic vascular resistance in these patients. Aldosterone, in turn, has potent sodium-retaining properties. Therefore, it is not surprising that interruption of the renin-angiotensin-aldosterone axis by means of an angiotensin conversion inhibitor reduces systemic vascular resistance, diminishes afterload, and thereby elevates cardiac output in heart failure (p. 539). In addition, converting enzyme inhibition often acts as a diuretic, presumably by lowering angiotensin II–stimulated production of aldosterone.

CONCLUSIONS

It may be useful to consider normal and impaired myocardial function, whatever the etiology and pathogenesis, within the framework of the familiar Frank-Starling mechanism.[166] The normal relation between ventricular end-diastolic volume and performance is shown in Figure 13–17, curve 1. Normally, assumption of the upright posture reduces venous return; as a consequence, at any particular level of exercise, cardiac output tends to be lower in the upright than in the recumbent position. On the other hand, the hyperventilation of exercise, the pumping action of the exercising muscles, and the venoconstriction that occur all tend to augment ventricular filling. Simultaneously, the increase in sympathetic nerve impulses to the myocardium and in the concentration of circulating catecholamines and the tachycardia that occur during exercise all augment the myocardial contractility and the stroke volume, with either no change or even a reduction in end-diastolic pressure and volume. This state is represented by a shift from point A to point B in Figure 13–17. Vasodilation occurs in the exercising muscles, reducing peripheral vascular resistance and aortic impedance. This ultimately allows achievement of a greatly elevated cardiac output during exercise at an arterial pressure only slightly greater than that in the resting state. During intense exercise, cardiac output can rise to a maximal level if use is made of

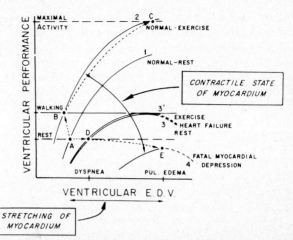

FIGURE 13–17 Diagram showing the interrelationship of influences on ventricular end-diastolic volume (EDV) through stretching of the myocardium and the contractile state of the myocardium. Levels of ventricular EDV associated with filling pressures that result in dyspnea and pulmonary edema are shown on the abscissa. Levels of ventricular performance required during rest, walking, and maximal activity are designated on the ordinate. The dotted lines are the descending limbs of the ventricular performance curves, which are rarely seen during life but which show what the level of ventricular performance would be if end-diastolic volume could be elevated to very high levels. (From Braunwald, E., Ross, J., Jr., and Sonnenblick, E. H.: Mechanisms of Contraction of the Normal and Failing Heart. Boston, Little, Brown and Co., 1968.)

the Frank-Starling mechanism, as reflected in increases in the left ventricular end-diastolic volume and pressure (Figure 13–17, point C).

In heart failure, the fundamental abnormality resides in depressions of the myocardial force-velocity relation and of the length–active tension curve, reflecting reductions in the myocardial contractile state. In many cases, such as those represented by Figure 13–17, curve 3, cardiac output and external ventricular performance at rest are within normal limits, but are maintained at these levels only because the end-diastolic fiber length and the ventricular end-diastolic volume are above normal, i.e., through the operation of the Frank-Starling mechanism. The elevations of left ventricular end-diastolic volume and pressure are associated with greater than normal levels of the pulmonary capillary pressure, contributing to the dyspnea experienced by patients with heart failure (Fig. 13–17, point D).

Since heart failure is frequently accompanied by reductions in (1) cardiac NE stores, (2) myocardial beta-receptor density, (3) catecholamine sensitivity, and (4) inotropic response to impulses in the cardiac adrenergic nerves, ventricular performance curves cannot be elevated to normal levels by the adrenergic nervous system, and the normal improvement of contractility that takes place during exercise is attenuated or even prevented (Fig. 13–17, curves 3 and 3'). The factors that tend to augment ventricular filling during exercise in the normal subject push the failing myocardium even farther along its flattened length–active tension curve, and although left ventricular performance may be improved slightly, this occurs only as a consequence of an inordinate elevation of ventricular end-diastolic volume and pressure and therefore of pulmonary capillary pressure. The elevation of the latter intensifies dyspnea and therefore plays an important role in limiting the intensity of exercise that the patient can perform. According to this concept, left ventricular failure becomes fatal when the myocardial length–active tension curve becomes depressed (Fig. 13–17, curve 4) to the point at which either cardiac performance fails to satisfy the requirements of the peripheral tissues even at rest or the left ventricular end-diastolic and pulmonary capillary pressures are elevated to levels that result in pulmonary edema, or both (Fig. 13–17, point E).

References

1. Braunwald, E., Mock, M. B., and Watson, J. (eds.): Congestive Heart Failure: Current Research and Clinical Applications. New York, Grune and Stratton, 1982, 384 pp.
2. Eichna, L. S.: Circulatory congestion and heart failure. Circulation 22:864, 1960.
3. Braunwald, E.: The Myocardium: Failure and Infarction. New York, H. P. Publishing Co., 1974, 409 pp.
4. Guyton, A. C.: The relationship of cardiac output and arterial pressure control. Circulation 64:1079, 1981.
5. Katz, A. M.: The descending limb of the Starling curve and the failing heart (Editorial). Circulation 32:871, 1965.
6. Ross, J., Jr., and Braunwald, E.: Studies on Starling's law of the heart. IX. The effects of impeding venous return on performance of the normal and failing human left ventricle. Circulation 30:719, 1964.
7. Braunwald, E., Ross, J., Jr., and Sonnenblick, E. H.: Mechanisms of Contraction of the Normal and Failing Heart. 2nd ed. Boston, Little, Brown and Co., 1976, 417 pp.
8. Vanhoutte, P. M.: Adjustments in the peripheral circulation in chronic heart failure. Eur. Heart J. 4(Suppl. A):67, 1983.
9. Higgins, C. B., Vatner, S. F., Franklin, D., and Braunwald, E.: Effects of experimentally produced heart failure on the peripheral vascular response to severe exercise in conscious dogs. Circ. Res. 31:186, 1972.
10. Wade, O. L., and Bishop, J. M.: Cardiac Output and Regional Blood Flow. London, Blackwell Scientific Publications, 1962, 134 pp.
11. Zelis, R. J., Longhurst, J., Capone, R. J., and Lee, G.: Peripheral circulatory control mechanisms in congestive heart failure. Am. J. Cardiol. 32:481, 1973.
12. Zelis, R. D., Mason, D. T., and Braunwald, E.: A comparison of the effects of vasodilator stimuli on peripheral resistance vessels in normal subjects and in patients with congestive heart failure. J. Clin. Invest. 47:960, 1968.
13. Zelis, R. G., Mason, D. T., and Braunwald, E.: Partition of blood flow to the cutaneous and muscular beds of the forearm at rest and during leg exercise in normal subjects and in patients with heart failure. Circ. Res. 24:799, 1969.
14. Zelis, R., and Flaim, S. F.: Peripheral vascular mechanisms mediating vasoconstriction. In Braunwald, E., Mock, M. B., and Watson, J. (eds.): Congestive Heart Failure: Current Research and Clinical Applications. New York, Grune and Stratton, 1982, p. 115.
15. Woodson, R. D., Torrance, J. D., Shappell, S. D., and Lenfant, C.: The effect of cardiac disease on hemoglobin-oxygen binding. J. Clin. Invest. 49:1349, 1970.
16. Krayenbuehl, H. P., Hess, O. M., Schneider, J., and Turina, M.: Physiologic or pathologic hypertrophy. Eur. Heart J. 4(Suppl. A):29, 1983.
17. Spann, J. F., Jr., Buccino, R. A., Sonnenblick, E. H., and Braunwald, E.: Contractile state of cardiac muscle obtained from cats with experimentally produced ventricular hypertrophy and heart failure. Circ. Res. 21:341, 1967.
18. Cooper, G., IV, Tomanek, R. J., Ehrhardt, J. C., and Marcus, M. L.: Chronic progressive pressure overload of the cat right ventricle. Circ. Res. 48:488, 1981.
19. Bing, O. H. L., Matsushita, S., Fanburg, B. L., and Levine, H. J.: Mechanical properties of rat cardiac muscle during experimental hypertrophy. Circ. Res. 28:234, 1971.
20. Capasso, J. M., Strobeck, J. E., Malhotra, A., Scheuer, J., and Sonnenblick, E. H.: Contractile behavior of rat myocardium after reversal of hypertensive hypertrophy. Am. J. Physiol. 242:H882, 1982.
21. Forman, R., Parmley, W. W., and Sonnenblick, E. H.: Myocardial contractility in relation to hypertrophy and failure in myopathic Syrian hamsters. J. Mol. Cell. Cardiol. 4:203, 1972.
22. Chidsey, C. A., Sonnenblick, E. H., Morrow, A. G., and Braunwald, E.: Norepinephrine stores and contractile force of papillary muscle from the failing human heart. Circulation 33:43, 1966.
23. Fein, F. S., Kornstein, L. B., Strobeck, J. E., Capasso, J. M., and Sonnenblick, E. H.: Altered myocardial mechanics in diabetic rats. Circ. Res. 47:922, 1980.
24. Cooper, G., IV, Puga, F., Zujko, K. J., Harrison, C. E., and Coleman, H. N.: Normal myocardial function and energetics in volume-overload hypertrophy in the cat. Circ. Res. 32:140, 1973.
25. Williams, J. F., Jr., and Potter, R. D.: Normal contractile state of hypertrophied myocardium after pulmonary artery constriction in the cat. J. Clin. Invest. 54:1266, 1974.
26. Ross, J., Jr., Sonnenblick, E. H., Taylor, R. R., and Covell, J. W.: Diastolic geometry and sarcomere length in the chronically dilated canine left ventricle. Circ. Res. 28:49, 1971.
27. Spann, J. F., Jr., Covell, J. W., Eckberg, D. L., Sonnenblick, E. H., Ross, J., Jr., and Braunwald, E.: Contractile performance of the hypertrophied and chronically failing cat ventricle. Am. J. Physiol. 223:1150, 1972.
28. Pfeffer, M. A., Pfeffer, J. M., and Frohlich, E. M.: Pumping ability of the hypertrophying left ventricle in the spontaneously hypertensive rat. Circ. Res. 38:423, 1976.
29. Pfeffer, J. M., Pfeffer, M. A., Mirsky, E., and Brauwald, E.: Regression of left ventricular hypertrophy and prevention of left ventricular dysfunction by captopril in the spontaneously hypertensive rat. Proc. Natl. Acad. Sci. 79:3310, 1982.
30. Pfeffer, J. M., Pfeffer, M. A., Fletcher, P., Fishbein, M. C., and Braunwald, E.: Favorable effects of therapy on cardiac performance in spontaneously hypertensive rats. Am. J. Physiol. 242:H776, 1982.
31. Fletcher, P. J., Pfeffer, J. M., Pfeffer, M. A., and Braunwald, E.: Left ventricular diastolic pressure-volume relations in rats with healed myocardial infarction. Effects on systolic function. Circ. Res. 49:618, 1981.
32. Pinsky, W. W., Lewis, R. M., Hartley, C. J., and Entman, M. L.: Permanent changes of ventricular contractility and compliance in chronic volume overload. Am. J. Physiol. 237:H575, 1979.
33. Penpargkul, S., Schaible, T., Yipintsoi, T., and Scheuer, J.: The effect of diabetes on performance and metabolism of rat hearts. Circ. Res. 47:911, 1980.
34. Meerson, F. Z.: The myocardium in hyperfunction, hypertrophy, and heart failure. Circ. Res. 25(Suppl. 2):1, 1969.
35. Cooper, G., IV, Satava, R. M., Harrison, C. E., and Coleman, H. N.: Normal myocardial function and energetics after reversing pressure-overload hypertrophy. Am. J. Physiol. 226:1158, 1974.
36. McCullagh, W. H., Covell, J. W., and Ross, J., Jr.: Left ventricular dilatation and diastolic compliance changes during chronic volume overloading. Circulation 45:943, 1972.
37. Ross, J., Jr.: Adaptations of the left ventricle to chronic volume overload. Circ. Res. 35(Suppl. 2):64, 1974.
38. Ross, J., Jr.: Afterload mismatch and preload reserve: A conceptual framework for the analysis of ventricular function. Prog. Cardiovasc. Dis. 18:255, 1976.
39. Braunwald, E., Welch, G. H., Jr., and Sarnoff, S. J.: Hemodynamic effects of quantitatively varied experimental mitral regurgitation. Circ. Res. 5:539, 1957.
40. Welch, G. H., Jr., Braunwald, E., and Sarnoff, S. J.: Hemodynamic effects of quantitatively varied experimental aortic regurgitation. Circ. Res. 5:546, 1957.
41. Urschel, C. W., Covell, J. W., Sonnenblick, E. H., Ross, J., Jr., and Braunwald, E.: Myocardial mechanics in aortic and mitral valvular regurgitation: The concept of instantaneous impedance as a determinant of the performance of the intact heart. J. Clin. Invest. 47:867, 1968.
42. Mason, D. T.: Regulation of cardiac performance in clinical heart disease: Interactions between contractile state, mechanical abnormalities and ventricular compensatory mechanisms. Am. J. Cardiol. 32:437, 1973.
43. Urschel, C. W., Covell, J. W., Graham, T. P., Clancy, R. L., Ross, J., Jr., Sonnenblick, E. H., and Braunwald, E.: Effects of acute valvular regurgitation on the oxygen consumption of the canine heart. Circ. Res. 23:33, 1968.
44. Grossman, W., Jones, D., and McLaurin, L. P.: Wall stress and patterns of hypertrophy in the human left ventricle. J. Clin. Invest. 56:56, 1975.
45. Sandler, H., and Dodge, H. T.: Left ventricular tension and stress in man. Circ. Res. 13:91, 1963.
46. Hood, W. P., Jr., Rackley, C. E., and Rolett, E. L.: Wall stress in the normal and hypertrophied human left ventricle. Am. J. Cardiol. 22:550, 1968.
47. Donner, R., Carabello, B. A., Black, I., and Spann, J. F.: Left ventricular wall stress in compensated aortic stenosis in children. Am. J. Cardiol. 51:946, 1983.
48. Peterson, K. L., Tsuji, J., Johnson, A., DiDonna, J., and LeWinter, M.: Diastolic left ventricular pressure-volume and stress-strain relations in patients with valvular aortic stenosis and left ventricular hypertrophy. Circulation 58:77, 1978.
49. Gunther, S., and Grossman, W.: Determinants of ventricular function in pressure overload hypertrophy in man. Circulation 59:679, 1979.
50. Spann, J. F., Bove, A. A., Natarajan, G., and Kreulen, T.: Ventricular performance, pump function and compensatory mechanisms in patients with aortic stenosis. Circulation 62:576, 1980.
51. Sasayama, S., Ross, J., Jr., Franklin, D., Bloor, C. M., Bishop, S., and Dilley, R. B.: Adaptations of the left ventricle to chronic pressure overload. Circ. Res. 38:172, 1976.
52. Gaasch, W. H., Levine, H. J., Quinones, M. A., and Alexander, J. K.: Left ventricular compliance: Mechanisms and clinical implications. Am. J. Cardiol. 38:645, 1976.
53. Braunwald, E., and Ross, J., Jr.: The ventricular end-diastolic pressure: Appraisal of its value in the recognition of ventricular failure in man (Editorial). Am. J. Med. 34:147, 1963.
54. Mirsky, I., and Laks, M. M.: Time course of changes in the mechanical properties of the canine right and left ventricles during hypertrophy caused by pressure overload. Circulation 46:530, 1980.
55. Mirsky, I., Pfeffer, J. M., Pfeffer, M. A., and Braunwald, E.: The contractile state as a major determinant in the evolution of left ventricular dysfunction in the spontaneously hypertensive rat. Circ. Res. (In press.)
56. Lewis, B. S., and Gotsman, M. S.: Current concepts of left ventricular relaxation and compliance. Am. Heart J. 99:101, 1980.
57. Williams, J. F., Jr., Potter, R. D., Hern, D. L., Matthew, B., and Deiss, W. P., Jr.: Hydroxyproline and passive stiffness of pressure-induced hypertrophied kitten myocardium. J. Clin. Invest. 69:309, 1982.

58. Eichhorn, P., Grimm, J., Koch, R., Hess, O., Carroll, J., and Krayenbuehl, H. P.: Left ventricular relaxation in patients with left ventricular hypertrophy secondary to aortic valve disease. Circulation 65:1395, 1982.

59. Serizawa, T., Carabello, B. A., and Grossman, W.: Effect of pacing-induced ischemia on left ventricular diastolic pressure—volume relations in dogs with coronary stenosis. Circ. Res. 46:430, 1980.

60. Forrester, J., Diamond, G., Parmley, W. W., and Swan, H. J. C.: Early increase in left ventricular compliance following myocardial infarction. J. Clin. Invest. 51:598, 1972.

61. Pirzada, F. A., Ekong, E. A., Vokonas, P. S., Apstein, C. S., and Hood, W. B., Jr.: Experimental myocardial infarction. XIII. Sequential changes in left ventricular pressure-length relations in the acute phase. Circulation 53:970, 1976.

62. Swan, H. J. C., Forrester, J. S., Diamond, G., Chatterjee, K., and Parmley, W. W.: Hemodynamic spectrum of myocardial infarction and cardiogenic shock. Circulation 40:1097, 1972.

63. Diamond, G., and Forrester, J. S.: Effect of coronary artery disease and acute myocardial infarction on left ventricular compliance in man. Circulation 45:11, 1972.

64. Lorell, B. M., Turi, Z., and Grossman, W.: Modification of left ventricular response to pacing tachycardia by nifedipine in patients with coronary artery disease. Am. J. Med. 71:667, 1981.

65. Entman, M. L., VanWinkle, W. B., Tate, C. A., and McMillin-Wood, J.B.: Pitfalls in biochemical studies of hypertrophied and failing myocardium. In Braunwald, E., Mock, M. B., and Watson, J. (eds.): Congestive Heart Failure: Current Research and Clinical Applications. New York, Grune and Stratton, 1982, p. 51.

66. Maughan, D., Low, E., Litten, R., Brayden, J., and Alpert, N. R.: Calcium-activated muscle from hypertrophied rabbit heart. Circ. Res. 44:279, 1979.

67. Bing, R. J.: Metabolic activity of intact heart. Am. J. Med. 30:679, 1961.

68. Graham, T. P., Jr., Ross, J., Jr., and Covell, J. W.: Myocardial oxygen consumption in acute experimental cardiac depression. Circ. Res. 21:123, 1967.

69. Henry, P. D., Eckberg, D., Gault, J. H., and Ross, J., Jr.: Depressed inotropic state and reduced myocardial oxygen consumption in the human heart. Am. J. Cardiol. 31:300, 1973.

70. Schwartz, A., Sordahl, L. A., Entman, M. L., Allen, J. C., Reddy, Y. S., Goldstein, M. A., Luchi, R. J., and Wyborny, L. E.: Abnormal biochemistry in myocardial failure. Am. J. Cardiol. 32:407, 1973.

71. Schwartz, A., Lindenmayer, G. E., and Harigaya, S.: Respiratory control and calcium transport in heart mitochondria from the cardiomyopathic Syrian hamster. Trans. N.Y. Acad. Sci. 30(Suppl. II):951, 1968.

72. Harrison, C. E., Jr., Cooper, G., IV, Zujko, K. J., and Coleman, H. N., III: Myocardial and mitochondrial function in potassium depletion cardiomyopathy. J. Mol. Cell. Cardiol. 4:633, 1972.

73. Kako, K. J., Thornton, M. J., and Hegtveit, H. A.: Depressed fatty acid and acetate oxidation and other metabolic defects in homogenates from hearts of hamsters with hereditary cardiomyopathy. Circ. Res. 34:570, 1974.

74. Chidsey, C. A., Weinbach, E. C., Pool, P. E., and Morrow, A. G.: Biochemical studies of energy production in the failing human heart. J. Clin. Invest. 45: 40, 1966.

75. Sobel, B. E., Spann, J. F., Jr., Pool, P. E., Sonnenblick, E. H., and Braunwald, E.: Normal oxidative phosphorylation in mitochondria from the failing heart. Circ. Res. 21:355, 1967.

76. Sordahl, L. A., Wood, W. G., and Lazarus, M.: Alterations in heart mitochondria during hypertrophy and progressive failure: Increases and decreases in function and structure. Circ. Res. 42(Suppl. 2):51, 1970.

77. Sordahl, L. A.: Some biochemical lesions in myocardial disease. Tex. Rep. Biol. Med. 38:121, 1979.

78. Cooper, G., IV, Satava, R. M., Harrison, C. E., and Coleman, H. N.: Mechanisms for the abnormal energetics of pressure-induced hypertrophy of cat myocardium. Circ. Res. 33:213, 1973.

79. Pool, P. E., Spann, J. F., Jr., Buccino, R. A., Sonnenblick, E. J., and Braunwald, E.: Myocardial high energy phosphate stores in cardiac hypertrophy and heart failure. Circ. Res. 21:365, 1967.

80. Katz, A. M.: Biochemical "defect" in the hypertrophied and failing heart. Circulation 47:1076, 1973.

81. Capasso, J. M., Aronson, R. S., Strobeck, J. E., and Sonnenblick, E. H.: Effects of experimental phosphate deficiency on action potential characteristics and contractile performance of rat myocardium. Cardiovasc. Res. 16:71, 1982.

82. Page, E., and McCallister, L. P.: Quantitative electron microscopic description of heart muscle cells. Application to normal, hypertrophied and thyroxin-stimulated hearts. Am. J. Cardiol. 31:172, 1973.

83. Schwarz, F., Schaper, J., Kittstein, D., Flameng, W., Walter, P., and Schaper, W.: Reduced volume fraction of myofibrils in myocardium of patients with decompensated pressure overload. Circulation 63:1299, 1981.

84. Alpert, N. R., and Gordon, M. S.: Myofibrillar adenosine triphosphate activity in congestive failure. Am. J. Physiol. 202:940, 1962.

85. Gordon, M. S., and Brown, A. L.: Myofibrillar adenosine triphosphate activity of human heart tissue and congestive failure: Effects of ouabain and calcium. Circ. Res. 19:534, 1966.

86. Luchi, R. J., Dritcher, E. M., and Thyrum, P. T.: Reduced cardiac myosin adenosine triphosphate activity in dogs with spontaneously occurring heart failure. Circ. Res. 24:513, 1969.

87. Chandler, B. M., Sonnenblick, E. H., Spann, J. R., Jr., and Pool, P. E.: Association of depressed myofibrillar adenosine triphosphatase and reduced contractility in experimental heart failure. Circ. Res. 21:717, 1967.

88. Draper, M., Taylor, N., and Alpert, N. R.: Alteration in contractile protein in hypertrophied guinea pig hearts. In Alpert, N. (ed.): Cardiac Hypertrophy. New York, Academic Press, 1971, pp. 315–331.

89. Wikman-Coffelt, J., Kamiyama, T., Salel, A. F., and Mason, D. T.: Differential responses of canine myosin ATPase activity and tissue gases in the pressure-overloaded ventricle dependent upon degree of obstruction—mild versus severe pulmonic and aortic stenosis. In Kobayashi, T., Yoshio, I., and Rona, G. (eds.): Recent Advances in Studies on Cardiac Structure and Metabolism. Vol. 12. Cardiac Adaption. Baltimore, University Park Press, 1978, pp. 367–372.

90. Wikman-Coffelt, J., Parmley, W. W., and Mason, D. T.: Relation of myosin isozymes to the heart as a pump. Am. Heart J. 103:934, 1982.

91. Houser, S. R., Freeman, A. R., Jaeger, J. M., Breisch, E. A., Coulson, R. L., Carey, R., and Spann, J. F.: Resting potential changes associated with Na-K pump in failing heart muscle. Am. J. Physiol. 240:H168, 1981.

92. Gorza, L., Pauletto, P., Pessina, A. C., Sartore, S., and Schiaffino, S.: Isomyosin distribution in normal and pressure-overloaded rat ventricular myocardium. An immunohistochemical study. Circ. Res. 49:1003, 1981.

93. Flink, I. L., Rader, J. H., and Morkin, E.: Thyroid hormone stimulates synthesis of cardiac myosin isozymes. J. Biol. Chem. 254:3105, 1979.

94. Scheuer, J., and Bhan, A.: Cardiac contractile proteins, adenosine triphosphate activity and physiological function. Circ. Res. 45:1, 1979.

95. Wikman-Coffelt, J., Fenner, C., Walsh, R., Salel, A., Kamiyama, T., and Mason, D. T.: Comparison of mild vs. severe pressure overload on the enzymatic activity of myosin in the canine ventricles. Biochem. Med. 14:139, 1975.

96. Lompre, A.-M., Schwartz, K., d'Albis, A., Lacombe, G., Van Thiem, N., and Swynghedauw, B.: Myosin isoenzyme redistribution in chronic heart overload. Nature 282:105, 1979.

97. Wikman-Coffelt, J., Parmley, W. W., and Mason, D. T.: The cardiac hypertrophy process. Analyses of factors determining pathological vs physiological development. Circ. Res. 45:697, 1979.

98. Klotz, C., Leger, J. J., and Elzinga, M.: Comparative sequence of myosin light chains from normal and hypertrophied human hearts. Circ. Res. 50:201, 1982.

99. Lewis, W., Kleinerman, J., and Puszkin, S.: Interaction of adriamycin in vitro with cardiac myofibrillar proteins. Circ. Res. 50:547, 1982.

99a. Fleckenstein, A.: Calcium Antagonism in Heart and Smooth Muscle. New York, John Wiley and Sons, 1983.

100. Gelband, H., and Bassett, A. L.: Depressed transmembrane potentials during experimentally induced ventricular failure in cats. Circ. Res. 32:625, 1973.

101. Kaufmann, R. L., Hamburger, H., and Wirth, H.: Disorder in excitation-contraction coupling of cardiac muscle from cats with experimentally produced right ventricular hypertrophy. Circ. Res. 28:346, 1971.

102. Mead, R. J., Peterson, M. B., and Welty, J. D.: Sarcolemmal and sarcoplasmic reticular ATPase activities in the failing canine heart. Circ. Res. 29:14, 1971.

103. Suko, J., Vogel, J. H. K., and Chidsey, C. A.: Intracellular calcium and myocardial contractility. III. Reduced calcium uptake and ATPase of the sarcoplasmic reticular fraction prepared from chronically failing calf hearts. Circ. Res. 27:235, 1970.

104. Ohnishi, T., and Ebashi, S.: Spectrophotometric measurement of instantaneous calcium binding to the relaxing factor of muscle. J. Biochem. 54:506, 1963.

105. Harigaya, S., and Schwartz, A.: Rate of calcium binding and uptake in normal animal and failing human cardiac muscle. Circ. Res. 25:781, 1969.

106. Sordahl, L. A., Wood, W. G., and Schwartz, A.: Production of cardiac hypertrophy and failure in rabbits with ameroid clips. J. Mol. Cell. Cardiol. 1:341, 1970.

107. McCollum, W. B., Crow, C., Harigaya, S., Bajusz, E., and Schwartz, A.: Calcium binding by cardiac relaxing system isolated from myopathic Syrian hamsters. J. Mol. Cell. Cardiol. 1:445, 1970.

108. Ito, Y., and Chidsey, C. A.: Intracellular calcium and myocardial contractility. IV. Distribution of calcium in the failing heart. J. Mol. Cell. Cardiol. 4:507, 1972.

109. Sordahl, L. A., McCollum, W. B., Wood, W. G., and Schwartz, A.: Mitochondria and sarcoplasmic reticulum function in cardiac hypertrophy and failure. Am. J. Physiol. 224:497, 1973.

110. Ito, Y., Suko, J., and Chidsey, C. A.: Intracellular calcium and myocardial contractility. V. Calcium uptake of sarcoplasmic reticulum fractions in hypertrophied and failing rabbit hearts. J. Mol. Cell. Cardiol. 6:237, 1974.

111. Sulakhe, P. V., and Dhalla, N. S.: Excitation-contraction coupling in heart. VII. Calcium accumulation in subcellular particles in congestive heart failure. J. Clin. Invest. 50:1019, 1971.

112. Ma, T. S., and Bailey, L. E.: Excitation-contraction coupling in normal and myopathic hamster hearts II: Changes in contractility and Ca pools associated with development of the cardiomyopathy. Cardiovasc. Res. 13:499, 1979.

113. Owens, K., Ruth, R. C., Weglicki, W. B., Stam, A. C., and Sonnenblick, E. H.: Fragmented sarcoplasmic reticulum of the cardiomyopathic Syrian hamster: Lipid composition, Ca^{++} transport, and Ca^{++}-stimulated ATPase. In Dhalla, N. S. (ed.): Myocardial Biology: Recent Advances in Studies on Cardiac Structure and Metabolism. Baltimore, University Park Press, 1974, pp. 541–550.

114. Staley, N. A., Noren, G. R., and Einzig, S.: Early alterations in the function of sarcoplasmic reticulum in a naturally occurring model of congestive cardiomyopathy. Cardiovasc. Res. 15:276, 1981.

115. Gertz, E. W., Hess, M. L., Lain, R. F., and Briggs, F. N.: Activity of the vesicular calcium pump in the spontaneously failing heart-lung preparation. Circ. Res. 20:477, 1967.

116. Lee, K. S., Ladinsky, H., and Stuckey, J. H.: Decreased Ca^{2+} uptake by sar-

coplasmic reticulum after coronary artery occlusion for 60 and 90 minutes. Circ. Res. *20*:439, 1967.

117. Varley, K. G., and Dhalla, N. S.: Excitation-contraction coupling in heart: XII. Subcellular calcium transport in isoproterenol-induced myocardial necrosis. Exp. Mol. Pathol. *19*:94, 1973.

118. Kim, N. D., and Harrison, C. E.: $^{45}Ca^{2+}$ accumulation by mitochondria and sarcoplasmic reticulum in chronic potassium depletion cardiomyopathy. *In* Dhalla, N. S., and Rona, G. (eds.): Myocardial Biology. Vol. 4. Baltimore, University Park Press, 1972, pp. 551–562.

119. Lindenmayer, G. E., Sordahl, L. A., Harigaya, S., Allen, J. C., Besch, H. R., Jr., and Schwartz, A.: Some biochemical studies on subcellular systems isolated from fresh recipient human cardiac tissue obtained during transplantation. Am. J. Cardiol. *27*:277, 1971.

120. Khatter, J. C., and Prasad, K.: Myocardial sarcolemmal ATPase in dogs with induced mitral insufficiency. Cardiovasc. Res. *10*:637, 1976.

121. Prasad, K., Khatter, J. C., and Bharadwaj, B.: Intra- and extracellular electrolytes and sarcolemmal ATPase in the failing heart due to pressure overload in dogs. Cardiovasc. Res. *13*:95, 1979.

122. Braunwald, E., and Ross, J., Jr.: Control of Cardiac Performance. *In* Berne, R. M. (ed.): Handbook of Physiology. Section 2, The Cardiovascular System, Vol. 1, The Heart. Bethesda, American Physiological Society, 1979, pp. 533–580.

123. Chidsey, C. A., Harrison, D. C., and Braunwald, E.: Augmentation of plasma norepinephrine response to exercise in patients with congestive heart failure. N. Engl. J. Med. *267*:650, 1962.

124. Goldstein, D. S.: Plasma norepinephrine as an indicator of sympathetic neural activity in clinical cardiology. Am. J. Cardiol. *48*:1147, 1981.

125. Maurer, W., Ablasser, A., Tschada, R., Hausen, M., Saggau, W., and Kubler, W.: Myocardial catecholamine metabolism in patients with chronic aortic regurgitation. Circulation *66*(Suppl. 1):139, 1982.

125a. Malliani, A., and Pagani, M.: The role of the sympathetic nervous system in congestive heart failure. Eur. Heart J. *4*(Suppl. A):49, 1983.

126. Chidsey, C. A., Braunwald, E., and Morrow, A. G.: Catecholamine excretion and cardiac stores of norepinephrine in congestive heart failure. Am. J. Med. *39*:442, 1965.

127. Thomas, J. A., and Marks, B. H.: Plasma norepinephrine in congestive heart failure. Am. J. Cardiol. *41*:233, 1978.

128. Cody, R. J., Franklin, K. W., Kluger, J., and Laragh, J. H.: Sympathetic responsiveness and plasma norepinephrine during therapy of chronic congestive heart failure with captopril. Am. J. Med. *72*:791, 1982.

129. Levine, T. B., Francis, G. S., Goldsmith, S. R., Siomon, A. B., and Cohn, J. N.: Activity of the sympathetic nervous system and renin-angiotensin system assessed by plasma hormone levels and their relation to hemodynamic abnormalities in congestive heart failure. Am. J. Cardiol. *49*:1659, 1982.

130. Kluger, J., Cody, R. J., and Laragh, J. H.: The contributions of sympathetic tone and the renin-angiotensin system to severe chronic congestive heart failure: Response to specific inhibitors (prazosin and captopril). Am. J. Cardiol. *49*:1667, 1982.

130a. Turini, G. A., Waeber, B., and Brunner, H. R.: The renin-angiotensin system in refractory heart failure: Clinical, hemodynamic and hormonal effects of captopril and enalapril. Eur. Heart J. *4*(Suppl. A):189, 1983.

131. Colucci, W. S., Alexander, R. W., Williams, G. H., Rude, R. E., Holman, B. L., Konstam, M. A., Wynne, J., Mudge, G. H., Jr., and Braunwald, E.: Decreased lymphocyte beta-adrenergic-receptor density in patients with heart failure and tolerance to the beta-adrenergic agonist pirbuterol. N. Engl. J. Med. *305*:185, 1981.

132. Chidsey, C. A., Kaiser, G. A., Sonnenblick, E. H., Spann, J. F., Jr., and Braunwald, E.: Cardiac norepinephrine stores in experimental heart failure in dogs. J. Clin. Invest. *43*:2386, 1964.

133. Coulson, R. L., Yazdanfar, S., Rubio, E., Bove, A. A., Lemole, G. M., and Spann, J. F.: Recuperative potential of cardiac muscle following relief of pressure overload hypertrophy and right ventricular failure in the cat. Circ. Res. *40*:41, 1977.

134. Bristow, M. R., Ginsburg, R., Minobe, W., Cubicciotti, R. S., Sageman, W. S., Lurie, K., Billingham, M. E., Harrison, D. C., and Stinson, E. B.: Decreased catecholamine sensitivity and beta-adrenergic-receptor density in failing human hearts. N. Engl. J. Med. *307*:205, 1982.

135. Spann, J. F., Jr., Sonnenblick, E. H., Cooper, T., Chidsey, C. A., Willman, V. L., and Braunwald, E.: Cardiac norepinephrine stores and the contractile state of heart muscle. Circ. Res. *19*:317, 1966.

136. Spann, J. F., Jr., Chidsey, C. A., Pool, P. E., and Braunwald, E.: Mechanism of norepinephrine depletion in experimental heart failure produced by aortic constriction in guinea pig. Circ. Res. *17*:312, 1965.

137. Sole, M. J., Lo, C., Laird, O., Sonnenblick, E. H., and Wurtman, R. J.: Norepinephrine turnover in the heart and spleen of the cardiomyopathic Syrian hamster. Circ. Res. *37*:855, 1975.

138. Sole, M. J.: Alterations in sympathetic and parasympathetic neurotransmitter activity. *In* Braunwald, E., Mock, M. B., and Watson, J. (eds.): Congestive Heart Failure: Current Research and Clinical Applications. New York, Grune and Stratton, 1982, p. 101.

139. Pool, P. E., Covell, J. W., Levitt, M., Gibb, J., and Braunwald, E.: Reduction of cardiac tyrosine hydroxylase activity in experimental congestive heart failure. Its role in depletion of cardiac norepinephrine stores. Circ. Res. *20*:349, 1967.

140. Sole, M. J., Kamble, A. B., and Hussain, M. N.: A possible change in the rate-limiting step for cardiac norepinephrine synthesis in the cardiomyopathic Syrian hamster. Circ. Res. *41*:814, 1977.

141. Rutenberg, H. L., and Spann, J. F., Jr.: Alterations in cardiac sympathetic neurotransmitter activity in congestive heart failure. Am. J. Cardiol. *32*:472, 1973.

142. Mathes, P., Cowan, C., and Gudbjarnarson, S.: Storage and metabolism of norepinephrine after experimental myocardial infarction. Am. J. Physiol. *220*:27, 1971.

143. Covell, J. W., Chidsey, C. A., and Braunwald, E.: Reduction of the cardiac response to postganglionic sympathetic nerve stimulation in experimental heart failure. Circ. Res. *19*:51, 1966.

144. Gaffney, T. E., and Braunwald, E.: Importance of the adrenergic nervous system in the support of circulatory function in patients with congestive heart failure. Am. J. Med. *34*:320, 1963.

145. Epstein, S. E., and Braunwald, E.: The effect of beta-adrenergic blockade on patterns of urinary sodium excretion: Studies in normal subjects and in patients with heart disease. Ann. Intern. Med. *75*:20, 1966.

146. Vogel, J. H. K., and Chidsey, C. A.: Cardiac adrenergic activity in experimental heart failure assessed with beta-receptor blockade. Am. J. Cardiol. *24*:198, 1969.

147. Goldstein, R. E., Beiser, G. D., Stampfer, M., and Epstein, S. E.: Impairment of autonomically mediated heart rate control in patients with cardiac dysfunction. Circ. Res. *36*:571, 1975.

148. Higgins, C. B., Vatner, S. F., Eckberg, D. L., and Braunwald, E.: Alterations in the baroreceptor reflex in conscious dogs with heart failure. J. Clin. Invest. *51*:715, 1972.

149. White, C. W.: Reversibility of abnormal arterial baroreflex control of heart rate in heart failure. Am. J. Physiol. *241*(Heart Circ. Physiol. 10):H778, 1981.

150. Cohn, J. N., Taylor, N., Vrobel, T., and Moskowitz, R.: Contrasting effect of vasodilators on heart rate and plasma catecholamines in patients with hypertension and heart failure. Clin. Res. *26*(Abstr.):547A, 1978.

151. Mark, A. L., Mayer, H. E., Schmid, P. G., Heistad, D. D., and Abboud, F. M.: Adrenergic control of the peripheral circulation in cardiomyopathic hamsters with heart failure. Circ. Res. *33*:74, 1973.

152. Eckberg, D. L., Drabinsky, M., and Braunwald, E.: Defective cardiac parasympathetic control in patients with heart disease. N. Engl. J. Med. *285*:877, 1971.

153. Roskoski, R., Jr., Schmid, P. G., Mayer, H. E., and Abboud, F. M.: In vitro acetylcholine biosynthesis in normal and failing guinea pig hearts. Circ. Res. *36*:547, 1975.

154. Schmid, P. G., Lund, D. D., and Roskoski, R., Jr.: Efferent autonomic dysfunction in heart failure. *In* Abboud, F. M., Fozzard, H. A., Gilmore, J. P., and Reis, D. J. (eds.): Disturbances in Neurogenic Control of the Circulation. Bethesda, Md., American Physiological Society, 1981, p. 138.

155. Amorim, D. S., Heer, K., Jenner, D., Richardson, P., Dargie, H. J., Brown, M., Olsen, E. G. J., and Goodwin, J. F.: Is there autonomic impairment in congestive (dilated) cardiomyopathy? Lancet *1*:525, 1981.

156. Gauer, O. H., and Henry, J. P.: Neurohumoral control of plasma volume. *In* Guyton, A. C., and Cowley, A. W. (eds.): International Review of Physiology. Cardiovascular Physiology II. Baltimore, University Park Press, 1976, pp. 145–190.

157. Nonidez, J. F.: Identification of the receptor areas in the venae cavae and pulmonary veins which initiate reflex cardiac acceleration (Bainbridge's reflex). Am. J. Anat. *61*:203, 1937.

158. Thoren, P., and Ricksten, S.-E.: Cardiac C-fiber endings in cardiovascular control under normal and pathophysiological conditions. *In* Abboud, F. M., Fozzard, H. A., Gilmore, J. P., and Reis, D. J. (eds.): Disturbances in Neurogenic Control of the Circulation. Bethesda, Md., American Physiological Society, 1981, p. 17.

159. Abboud, F. M., Thames, M. C., and Mark, A. L.: Role of cardiac afferent nerves in regulation of circulation during coronary occlusion and heart failure. *In* Abboud, F. M., Fozzard, H. A., Gilmore, J. P., and Reis, D. J. (eds.): Disturbances in Neurogenic Control of the Circulation. Bethesda, Md., American Physiological Society, 1981, p. 65.

160. Belleau, L., Mion, H., Simard, S., Granger, P., Bertranou, E., Nowacynski, W., Boucher, R., and Genest, J.: Studies on the mechanism of experimental congestive heart failure in dogs. Can. J. Physiol. Pharmacol. *48*:450, 1970.

161. Zehr, J. E., Hawe, A., Tsakiris, A. G., Rastelli, G. C., McGoon, D. C., and Segar, W. E.: ADH levels following nonhypotensive hemorrhage in dogs with chronic mitral stenosis. Am. J. Physiol. *221*:312, 1971.

162. Greenberg, T. T., Richmond, W. H., Stocking, R. A., Gupta, P. D., Meehan, J. P., and Henry, J. P.: Impaired atrial receptor responses in dogs with heart failure due to tricuspid insufficiency and pulmonary artery stenosis. Circ. Res. *32*:424, 1973.

163. Zucker, I. H., Earle, A. M., and Gilmore, J. P.: The mechanism of adaptation of left atrial stretch receptors in dogs with chronic congestive heart failure. J. Clin. Invest. *60*:323, 1977.

164. Zucker, I. H., Earle, A. M., and Gilmore, J. P.: Changes in the sensitivity of left atrial receptors following reversal of heart failure. Am. J. Physiol. *237*:H555, 1979.

165. Riegger, G. A. J., Liebau, G., and Kocksiek, K.: Antidiuretic hormone in congestive heart failure. Am. J. Med. *72*:49, 1982.

166. Weber, K. T., and Janicki, J. S.: The heart as a muscle-pump system and the concept of heart failure. Am. Heart J. *98*:371, 1979.

14

ASSESSMENT OF CARDIAC FUNCTION

by Eugene Braunwald, M.D.

THEORETICAL CONSIDERATIONS

Assessment of cardiac function is a challenging and critically important task in the evaluation of patients with real or suspected heart disease. Since the heart's prime function is to deliver sufficient oxygenated blood to meet the metabolic requirements of the tissues, it is understandable that measurement of cardiac output has become a time-honored method for assessing cardiac performance and that therapeutic interventions in patients with heart disease are frequently evaluated in terms of their effects on cardiac output. Determination of cardiac output does indeed provide a useful measure of the pumping ability of the heart; however, we have seen from the discussion in Chapter 12 that cardiac output is dependent on two other influences in addition to contractility—preload and afterload.* Therefore, measurement of cardiac output alone is of limited value in the characterization of cardiac function.[1]

At any level of contractility, the extent of myocardial fiber shortening, and therefore the stroke volume, varies directly with the preload and inversely with the afterload.[2] When the latter is progressively raised, an increasing proportion of the muscle's contractile energy is expended in the generation of tension and a correspondingly smaller fraction in myocardial fiber shortening (Fig. 12–12, p. 420). For example, when aortic impedance† is progressively

---

*Heart rate, the fourth determinant of cardiac performance (p. 438), is so easily measurable that it will not be considered further, although it is recognized that changes in heart rate per se affect myocardial contractility.

†Aortic impedance is defined as the sum of the external factors that oppose ventricular ejection. It is the ratio of pressure to flow in the aorta and is determined by the physical properties of blood and the vascular wall; it includes the viscosity and density of blood, the diameter of the aorta and the viscoelasticity of the aortic wall, and the reflected pressure and flow waves generated in distal parts of the arterial tree; aortic impedance is generally expressed as the sum of a series of sinusoidal functions of pressure and flow waves ("harmonics") superimposed on the mean pressure and flow.[3]

raised while ventricular end-diastolic volume is held constant, stroke volume declines until a level of impedance is reached at which the maximum force-generating capacity of the myocardium is exceeded, and ventricular ejection ceases, i.e., the contraction becomes isovolumetric. Conversely, when the aortic impedance falls (afterload is reduced), stroke volume rises. From these considerations, it is clear that when changes in afterload occur, reciprocal changes in cardiac output take place that need not reflect changes in myocardial contractility (Fig. 12–30, p. 436). For example, an increase in cardiac output in a patient with heart failure following relief of severe aortic stenosis or the successful treatment of hypertension may be due to reduction in afterload or an improvement in contractility or both. Similarly, the elevated cardiac output associated with severe anemia (low blood viscosity), fever (arteriolar dilatation), or patent ductus arteriosus (arteriovenous fistula) may be explained in part or entirely by a reduction in aortic impedance, which reduces afterload (Fig. 12–26, p. 432, and Fig. 24–1, p. 808); again, an augmentation of contractility such as occurs with stimulation of cardiac sympathetic nerves need not necessarily be invoked.

The effects of simple alterations of preload on cardiac output are even more widely appreciated. Thus, the depression of cardiac output that occurs with hypovolemia (e.g., hemorrhagic shock), displacement of blood from the thorax (e.g., positive-pressure ventilation), or cardiac compression (e.g., pericardial tamponade) may be explained solely by a reduction of preload (Fig. 12–28, p. 434, and Fig. 12–29, p. 435), and the elevation of cardiac output that occurs in some patients with polycythemia vera or acute glomerulonephritis does not reflect an augmentation of contractility but rather a higher preload resulting from the hypervolemia (p. 820).

When myocardial contractility is normal, cardiac output is dependent more upon peripheral factors and their influence on ventricular preload and afterload than on the exact level of myocardial contractility. For example, both digitalis glycosides and paired electrical stimulation exert powerful inotropic influences yet do not raise cardiac output in normal human subjects or experimental animals. By contrast, in the presence of myocardial failure these stimuli significantly elevate cardiac output.[4]

The relation between a chain and its links may be a useful, though obviously oversimplified, analogy for explaining the relation between cardiac output and myocardial contractility; the total weight that the chain can support will increase only if its weakest link is strengthened. Thus, in a patient with heart failure and a depressed myocardium, stimulation of contractility, which may be thought of as strengthening the weakest link in the chain of factors controlling cardiac output, will elevate cardiac output. On the other hand, when one or both of the other links of the chain (i.e., preload and/or afterload) are limiting, it is not surprising that strengthening a link that is not weakest (i.e., improving myocardial contractility) does not improve cardiac output.

From the foregoing discussion, and as is evident from Figure 12–31 (p. 437), cardiac output can be lowered by reduction of contractility and preload, and by elevation of afterload—operating singly or in combination—and it is not possible to deduce from the measurement of a reduced cardiac output that contractility is depressed. Conversely, cardiac output may be normal when depression of contractility is accompanied by an augmented preload or a reduced afterload or both. Therefore, assessment of cardiac performance should include—but must not be limited to—measurement of cardiac output, i.e., it should also provide an analysis both of contractility and of the heart's loading conditions.

It is often desirable in the clinical care of patients with heart disease to ascertain the basal level of myocardial contractility and in other instances to determine the effects of therapeutic interventions, such as a drug or an operation, on contractility. In isolated cardiac muscle or in the isolated heart, the individual influence of each of the three major determinants of cardiac performance (preload, afterload, and contractility) can be analyzed by maintaining two of these three variables constant and determining the effects of changing the third on muscle or cardiac performance. However, it is far more difficult to make analogous measurements in patients with heart disease in whom preload or afterload, or both, may be abnormal and cannot be controlled or held constant. For example, it is often desirable to ascertain in a patient with valvular heart disease, ventricular hypertrophy, and symptoms of heart failure whether it is the abnormality in loading produced by the valvular lesion or a depression of myocardial contractility (or a combination of these two factors) that is responsible for the clinical manifestations. Similarly, it is frequently necessary to study the effects on myocardial contractility of a pharmacological agent that may also act on the arterial and venous beds and therefore may change preload and afterload. Such considerations have led to the search for methods of evaluating ventricular function that go beyond simple analysis of the pumping function of the ventricle and that are directed toward quantification of contractility. Although a number of indices of contractility have been proposed and investigated empirically, conclusions drawn about them have involved an element of circular reasoning,

since, unfortunately, there is no *absolute* hemodynamic or mechanical measure of this property of the myocardium with which these indices can be compared.

The Frank-Starling Mechanism

The earliest efforts to separate loading conditions from contractility in assessing ventricular performance utilized the Frank-Starling relation, i.e., the relation between ventricular filling pressure or end-diastolic volume, on the one hand, and ventricular mechanical activity, as expressed in the pressure generated, the volume output, or the product of these two variables (i.e., stroke work), on the other. It was shown in the heart-lung preparation that the stroke volume is a function both of diastolic fiber length (i.e., of preload) and of contractility. The failing heart was found to deliver a smaller than normal stroke volume from a normal or elevated end-diastolic volume.[5] Later, Sarnoff and his collaborators examined ventricular stroke work over a range of mean atrial or ventricular end-diastolic pressures and termed the resulting relation "the ventricular function curve."[6] A family of such curves reflects a spectrum of contractile states, and the position of a given curve provides a description of ventricular contractility (Fig. 12–32, p. 438). Movement along a single curve (Fig. 12–29, p. 435) represents the operation of the "Frank-Starling principle," where stroke work or volume varies directly with changes in preload. By contrast, upward or

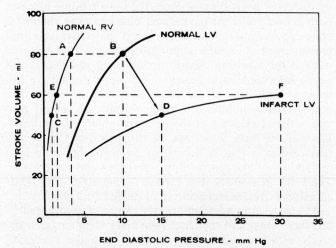

FIGURE 14–1 Schematic right ventricular (RV) and left ventricular (LV) function curves before and after left ventricular infarction. The normal RV function curve is to the left of the normal LV function curve, since, at any stroke volume, RV end-diastolic pressure is less than LV end-diastolic pressure. However, since the two ventricles have the same average stroke volume in a steady state, they operate on the same horizontal line. Under normal circumstances, the right ventricle would be at point A and the left ventricle at point B, both with a stroke volume of 80 ml. Following infarction, which predominantly affects the left ventricle, the LV curve is shifted down and to the right (point D), although the RV curve may not be initially affected. Stroke volume decreases to 50 ml, and the function of the right ventricle moves to point C. A volume load at this point might increase stroke volume to 60 ml, and the function of the right ventricle would move to point E, whereas that of the left ventricle would move to point F. At this high filling pressure, the patient might well go into pulmonary edema. (From Parmley, W. W.: Hemodynamic monitoring in acute ischemic disease. *In* Fishman, A. P. [ed.]: Heart Failure. New York, McGraw-Hill Book Co., 1978, p. 113.)

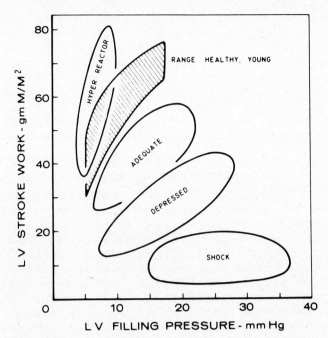

FIGURE 14-2 Hemodynamic consequences of myocardial infarction expressed as varying levels of left ventricular function. The cross-hatched area represents the range of left ventricular (LV) function in healthy, young individuals. Following acute myocardial infarction, there is wide variability in the hemodynamic response. Some patients with small infarcts and increased sympathetic tone may be in the normal or supernormal range. As the size of the infarct increases, however, function is progressively shifted down and to the right, so that all patients with cardiogenic shock fall in the lower right-hand group. (From Parmley, W. W.: Hemodynamic monitoring in acute ischemic disease. *In* Fishman, A. P. [ed.]: Heart Failure. New York, McGraw-Hill Book Co., 1978, p. 114.)

downward displacement of the *entire* curve (Fig. 12–32, p. 438) represents a positive or negative inotropic effect, i.e., an augmentation or depression of contractility, respectively (Figs. 14–1 and 14–2). In experimental animal preparations, ventricular function curves are usually recorded at a constant mean arterial pressure,[4] since the level of stroke work is pressure-dependent, just as the work of isolated muscle is afterload-dependent (Fig. 12–12, p. 420). Thus, at any level of contractility, stroke work is influenced also by the afterload, being low when outflow pressure is very low, increasing to a maximal level as pressure is raised, and again declining to zero when the afterload is so high as to prevent ventricular ejection (i.e., when ventricular contraction is isovolumetric and stroke volume is zero).[7] It should be recognized that even when outflow pressure is held constant, the standard ventricular function curve (Fig. 12–29, p. 435) represents a complex interaction of preload and afterload, since as preload is augmented and heart size increases, according to Laplace's law (p. 431), afterload rises at a constant aortic pressure.

ASSESSING CARDIAC PERFORMANCE BASED ON PRESSURES, FLOWS, VOLUMES, AND DIMENSIONS

Despite the theoretical limitations alluded to above, the simplest, most straightforward approaches for assessing resting levels of contractility and their changes are still based on measurements of intravascular and intracardiac pressures, stroke volume (or cardiac output), and ventricular volume and/or dimensions.

CARDIAC INDEX. The normal range for the cardiac index in the basal (resting) state and the supine position is wide—between 2.5 and 4.2 liters/min/square meter—making this variable a very *insensitive* assessment of cardiac function; it can be within normal limits, decline by almost 40 per cent as a consequence of myocardial failure, and still remain within these limits. Therefore, when the cardiac index falls below normal, it usually represents a gross disturbance in *circulatory*, though not necessarily *cardiac*, performance (p. 447), and such a degree of impairment is usually readily detectable clinically. Despite these limitations, measurement of cardiac index in the basal state is of value, since it provides an assessment of the heart's most critical function, i.e., the delivery of blood to the metabolizing tissues.

A measurement that detects milder degrees of cardiac impairment with greater sensitivity than does the measurement of cardiac output in the basal state is the level of cardiac output in response to the stress of exercise. Most commonly, the effect of exercise on cardiac output is determined in the cardiac catheterization laboratory as the patient pedals a stationary bicycle in the supine position, and both oxygen consumption and cardiac output are measured at rest and during exercise (p. 294). The increase in cardiac output is a function not only of the heart's pumping capacity but also of the severity of exercise, which can be expressed by the patient's total oxygen consumption. The increase in cardiac output normally exceeds 6 ml/min for each ml increase in oxygen consumption per minute.

INTRACARDIAC PRESSURES. The accuracy of the assessment of cardiac performance can be increased by adding a measurement of ventricular filling pressure* to that of cardiac (or stroke) index. In the basal state, when the ventricular end-diastolic pressure is abnormally elevated *and* cardiac performance (expressed as cardiac [or stroke] index or work) is depressed, myocardial contractility is *probably* impaired. However, elevation of ventricular filling pressure does not necessarily indicate an elevation of end-diastolic volume, since ventricular compliance may be reduced (Fig. 12–22, p. 428). Such a reduction of compliance may be caused, for example, by pericardial disease, by restrictive endocardial or myocardial disease, by cardiac hypertrophy, or by myocardial ischemia; it can elevate the ventricular filling pressure while end-diastolic volume remains normal.

Despite the problems mentioned above, the combination of ventricular end-diastolic pressure and cardiac output or work is often helpful (Figs. 14–1 and 14–2). For example,

---

*Ventricular filling pressure refers to ventricular end-diastolic pressure, or an index thereof; in the absence of disease of the atrioventricular valve, this is reflected in the mean atrial or, preferably, the mean diastolic atrial pressure or the atrial pressure at the *z* point, i.e., at the time of onset of ventricular contraction. In the case of the left ventricle, the mean pulmonary capillary wedge pressure or, in the case of the right ventricle, the central venous pressure provides a reasonably accurate approximation of ventricular end-diastolic pressure, except when there is a tall *a* wave in the ventricular pressure pulse, in which case the end-diastolic ventricular pressure exceeds the mean atrial pressure, or when there is a tall *v* wave, in which case the mean atrial pressure exceeds the end-diastolic ventricular pressure.

the finding of the combination of a normal cardiac index (>2.5 $1/min/m^2$) and ventricular filling pressure (<12 mm Hg) is a more accurate indicator of normal contractility than is either measurement alone. However, a further obvious limitation of this combination of measurements emerges when cardiac output (or work) is depressed while filling pressure is within the normal range (6 to 12 mm Hg) or low (<6 mm Hg); such findings could reflect a depression of contractility and/or a reduction of preload in the presence of normal contractility.

One approach to overcome the problems described above is to measure cardiac performance (cardiac or stroke index or work) both in the basal state and after preload has been raised by increasing intravascular volume. Normally, an elevation of preload is accompanied by a clear-cut increase in cardiac output. In addition, the effects of an intervention on the slope of the relation between filling pressure and cardiac work can be evaluated. For example, as shown in Figure 14–3, in a patient recovering from myocardial infarction, cessation of the infusion of glucose-insulin-potassium depressed the ventricular function curve.[8]

From the foregoing consideration of the importance of ventricular compliance, measurement of ventricular end-diastolic volume obviously is superior to that of filling pressure in the assessment of left ventricular preload (end-diastolic fiber stretch). Angiographic techniques, described below, provide the most widely accepted means for measuring ventricular cavity volumes as well as wall thickness and thereby allow calculation of the extent and velocity of

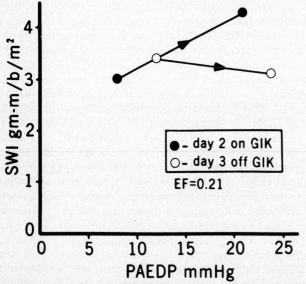

FIGURE 14–3 The hemodynamic effect of glucose-insulin-potassium (GIK) solution on left ventricular (LV) function is illustrated by the slope of the ventricular function curve in a patient with acute myocardial infarction. After the patient had been on the GIK solution for 2 days, the slope of the function curve was steeper than on day 3, 24 hours after the GIK solution had been discontinued. These changes indicate the positive inotropic effect of the metabolic solution on the viable and/or marginally ischemic myocardium surrounding the infarction site. Ventricular function is expressed as the relation between pulmonary artery end-diastolic pressure (PAEDP), reflecting left ventricular filling pressure and left ventricular stroke work index (SWI). (Reproduced with permission from Rackley, C. E., Russell, R. O., Jr., Rogers, W. J., et al.: Clinical experience with glucose-insulin-potassium therapy in acute myocardial infarction. Am. Heart J. *102*:1038, 1981.)

wall shortening and of regional abnormalities of wall motion and, when combined with pressure measurements, estimation of ventricular compliance and the forces acting within the wall that oppose shortening. Such calculations permit left ventricular performance to be analyzed in terms used for describing isolated heart muscle (Chap. 12); when the results are expressed in units corrected for muscle length or circumferences of the ventricle, comparisons can be made between individuals with widely differing heart sizes.

Quantitative Angiocardiography

TECHNIQUES. Measurements of the volumes of cardiac chambers can be made utilizing either large, cut films or cineangiograms (single plane or biplane).[9] Cineangiography, which is emerging as the method of choice, provides a larger number of sequential observations per unit of time (30 to 60 frames per second), whereas the large, cut films, which are exposed less frequently (6 to 12 per second), produce sharper margins of the opacified chambers. Although contrast material can be injected into the pulmonary artery and left atrium, the left ventricle is outlined more clearly by means of direct injection into its cavity; therefore, this latter mode is used in most patients, except in those with severe aortic regurgitation, in whom the contrast material may be injected into the aorta, with the resultant reflux outlining the left ventricular cavity. Digital subtraction augiography utilizing peripheral vein injections may also be employed.[9a,9b]

Unless the effects of premature contractions and of the resultant postextrasystolic potentiation are to be examined specifically,[10] ventricular irritability should be avoided during injection by assuring that the tip of the catheter is not in contact with the myocardium and that a multiholed catheter is used to diminish the impact of the jet of contrast agent striking the endocardium. If premature contractions are induced, the results are subject to serious misinterpretation, since the premature contraction itself and the first and second postpremature beats may result in marked changes in cardiac function. However, since the contrast material is usually injected within 2 to 3 seconds and filming is carried out within 5 to 8 seconds, one to two cycles are usually available for analysis even if a single premature contraction occurs at the beginning of the injection. Injection of the contrast agent does not begin to produce hemodynamic changes (except for premature beats) until approximately the sixth beat post injection.[11] Moreover, the hyperosmolarity produced by the contrast agent increases the blood volume, which begins to raise preload and heart rate within 30 seconds of the injection, an effect which may persist for as long as 2 hours. Accordingly, when multiple observations in a comparable state are desired, it is essential to monitor hemodynamics to assure that they have returned to control levels before the angiogram is repeated. Ordinarily, the exposure of each pair of angiographic films or cineangiographic frames is recorded on a multichannel recorder and related to a simultaneously recorded electrocardiogram and to intracardiac pressure.

In calculating ventricular volume or, for that matter, ventricular dimension, from radiographs, it is essential to take into account and apply appropriate correction factors for magnification as well as for distortion resulting from nonparallel x-ray beams.[12–14] In order to apply these correction factors, care must be exercised to determine the tube-to-patient and tube-to-film distances with great accuracy. With cine technique, correction is best accomplished by filming a calibrated grid at the position of the ventricle.[15]

NONINVASIVE METHODS FOR ASSESSING CARDIAC PERFORMANCE

Cardiac catheterization and quantitative angiography are the standard tools for evaluating the function and contractility of the heart, but these invasive procedures are not free of risk or discomfort, and they are not suitable for multiple application in the same patient. Therefore, as has already been pointed out, there has been a continuing search for reliable noninvasive methods of assessing cardiac performance. Such methods are particularly needed in detecting serial changes in cardiac function with time and in evaluating both acute and chronic effects of drug therapy and cardiac operations. Discussed elsewhere are the three principal noninvasive methods for assessing cardiac performance: systolic time intervals (p. 55), M-mode and cross-sectional echocardiography[15a] (p. 102), and radionuclide angiography (p. 357). The last two techniques are alternatives to contrast angiography for measurement of ventricular volume and/or dimensions, and both allow the noninvasive estimation of ejection phase indices. Afterload can be estimated from systemic arterial pressure and ventricular wall thickness in patients other than those with aortic stenosis; wall thickness can be determined by echocardiography.

Mean velocity of circumferential fiber shortening (V_{CF}) can be simply determined from echocardiographic measurements of end-diastolic and end-systolic dimensions. Since the ventricle is approximately circular at its minor axis, the circumference is equal to $\pi \cdot D$. Mean V_{CF} is therefore the difference between end-diastolic and end-systolic circumference (in centimeters) divided by the product of the duration of ejection (in seconds) and the end-diastolic circumference (in centimeters). Values of V_{CF} obtained by echocardiography compare closely with those determined from cineangiograms.[16]

Prolongation of the preejection period (PEP) and shortening of the left ventricular ejection time (LVET) reflect reduced left ventricular dP/dt and stroke volume, respectively, and there is an empirical inverse correlation between the ratio PEP/LVET (which is elevated in left ventricular dysfunction) and ejection fraction (EF).[17]

LEFT VENTRICULAR VOLUME. The area-length method developed by Dodge is still the most useful for calculating left ventricular volume[12,18] (Fig. 14–4). The longest length of the ventricular chamber, i.e., from the apex to the root of the aortic valve, is measured directly, and the diameter of the ventricle is calculated from the formula $D = 4A/\pi L$, where D = calculated diameter in centimeters; L = length in centimeters; and A = area of left ventricular cavity in square centimeters determined by planimetry. Ordinarily this calculation is made for films exposed in both anteroposterior (AP) and lateral projections. The shape of the left ventricle usually resembles a prolate ellipsoid, with one major and two minor diameters.[12,19,20] With this assumption, left ventricular volume is calculated from the formula

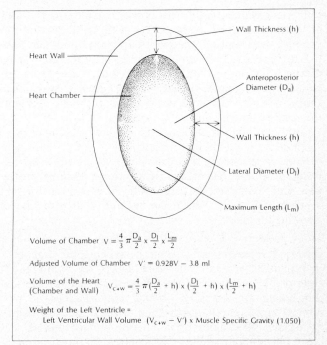

Volume of Chamber $V = \frac{4}{3}\pi \frac{D_a}{2} \times \frac{D_l}{2} \times \frac{L_m}{2}$

Adjusted Volume of Chamber $V' = 0.928V - 3.8$ ml

Volume of the Heart (Chamber and Wall) $V_{c+w} = \frac{4}{3}\pi\left(\frac{D_a}{2} + h\right) \times \left(\frac{D_l}{2} + h\right) \times \left(\frac{L_m}{2} + h\right)$

Weight of the Left Ventricle = Left Ventricular Wall Volume $(V_{c+w} - V') \times$ Muscle Specific Gravity (1.050)

FIGURE 14–4 Diagram illustrating the approach used to calculate left ventricular volume by means of quantitative angiocardiography. Margins of the projected image of the left ventricular chamber are traced, and maximum length is measured in the anteroposterior and lateral views. Minor axes are derived from the planimetered areas of the chamber in both views; all dimensions are corrected to allow for distortion due to nonparallel x-rays. Left ventricular volumes are calculated using the formula for the volume of an ellipsoid, since (with regression-equation adjustment) this has given results that tally closely with directly measured ventricular volume. To determine left ventricular mass, volume of the ventricular chamber is subtracted from volume of chamber plus wall; multiplying wall volume by the specific gravity of cardiac muscle converts volume to heart weight or mass. (From Dodge, H. T.: Hemodynamic aspects of cardiac failure. *In* Braunwald, E. [ed.]: The Myocardium: Failure and Infarction. New York, HP Publishing Co., 1974, p. 70.)

$$V = 4/3\pi \, (L/2) \cdot (D_{AP}/2) \cdot (D_{lat}/2)$$

where V = volume in milliliters; L = longest length in centimeters in the AP or lateral projection; and D_{AP} and D_{lat} = the diameters (minor axes) in centimeters calculated from the AP and lateral projection angiocardiograms, respectively. These diameters, in turn, are calculated from the formula for the area of an ellipse (A) as follows:

$$D = \frac{4A}{\pi L}$$

A, the area of the opacified ventricle, can be conveniently determined by a hand or electronic planimeter and an X-Y platter.[15] *Actual* ventricular volume is determined from the calculated volume using the aforementioned correction factors and a regression formula that takes into account the volume occupied by the papillary muscles and chordae tendineae within the ventricular chamber (see adjusted volume, Fig. 14–4). Studies based on human autopsy specimens as well as on models and casts thereof have proved the accuracy of this approach.[9]

Left ventricular stroke volume is calculated as the difference between end-systolic and end-diastolic volumes. An important validation of the angiographic method for measuring ventricular volume has been provided by the observation that the stroke volume, calculated by angiocardiography, correlates closely with that determined by the Fick or indicator dilution method.[21] When the ventricular stroke volume (determined by angiocardiography) and the effective forward stroke volume (determined by the Fick or indicator dilution method) are not equal, such as occurs with aortic or mitral valvular regurgitation or with intracardiac shunts, the difference between the two represents the regurgitant (or shunt) flow.

Although biplane angiographic methods are superior to single-plane methods for the calculation of left ventricular volume, a reasonable approximation can be obtained utilizing either the AP or the right anterior oblique projection and assuming that the two diameters of the left ventricle are equal. Ventricular volume is then calculated from the formula

$$V = L \cdot D^2 \cdot CF^3 \cdot \pi/6$$

where CF represents a one-dimensional correction factor.[9]

In patients with ischemic heart disease, the right and left anterior oblique views of the left ventricle are the optimal projections for assessing regional abnormalities of wall motion. However, standardization of the degree of obliquity, usually 30 degrees right anterior oblique and 60 degrees left anterior oblique, is required for application of any particular correction factor in the calculation of ventricular volume. A close correlation has been found between left ventricular volume determined in the right anterior oblique view and true cardiac volume; however, the overestimation of true volume is greater than that using the biplane oblique volume method, and appropriate corrections must be made.[22]

Just as the prolate ellipsoid provides a frame of reference for the shape of the left ventricle, the right ventricle is shaped like a pyramid with a triangular base, and the formula for deriving the volume of this geometrical figure should be employed in the calculation of right ventricular volume.[23] The atria resemble ellipsoids, and their volumes can be determined using the area-length method.[24]

LEFT VENTRICULAR MASS. This value can also be determined by angiocardiography. Wall thickness, as visualized and measured along the free lateral wall of the left ventricle just below the equator during diastole (best measured on the AP or RAO angiogram), is added to the major and minor semiaxes to compute the volume of the chamber plus wall. This volume minus the chamber volume equals wall volume. The product of wall volume and the specific gravity of heart muscle (1.050) equals left ventricular mass.[25] Thus, left ventricular mass (M) in grams can be calculated from the formula

$$M = ([4/3 \cdot \pi \frac{(L + 2h)}{2} \cdot \frac{(D_{AP} + 2h)}{2} \cdot \frac{(D_{lat} + 2h)}{2}]$$
$$- V) \cdot (1.050)$$

where h = left ventricular wall thickness in centimeters; 1.050 = specific gravity of heart muscle; D_{AP} and D_{lat} are the ventricular diameters in centimeters in the AP and lateral views, respectively; and V = left ventricular volume in cubic centimeters. A major assumption made with this method and one that undoubtedly introduces some inaccuracy is that left ventricular wall thickness is uniform around the entire left ventricular cavity. However, this method has been validated by postmortem studies comparing actual and calculated left ventricular weights.[15]

LEFT VENTRICULAR FORCES. The *forces* acting within the ventricular wall can be calculated from knowledge of the dimensions of the left ventricular cavity, wall thickness, and pressure.[26] *Tension* (force/cm), which, according to Laplace's law, is a product of the intraventricular pressure and radius (p. 431), may be defined as the force acting on a hypothetical slit in the ventricular wall that would tend to pull its edges apart. *Wall stress* is the force or tension (in dynes) per unit of cross-sectional area of the ventricular wall (in square centimeters). From a clinical viewpoint, the most useful calculation is *circumferential wall stress*, which is the largest force generated and supported within the ventricular wall at the equator

$$CWS = \frac{(P \cdot b)}{h} (1 - b^2/2a^2 - h/2b + h^2/8a^2)$$

where CWS = circumferential wall stress in dynes/square centimeters $\times$ 10^3; P = left ventricular pressure in dynes/square centimeters; and a and b are the major and minor semiaxes (i.e., half the longest lengths), respectively, in centimeters and h = left ventricular wall thickness in centimeters.[27]

Simultaneous recording of a biplane angiogram and intraventricular pressure pulse (recorded preferably with a high-fidelity micromanometer to avoid the artifacts inherent in the usual catheter–external manometer systems) allows calculation of *left ventricular tension* and *stress* throughout the cardiac cycle. Another method of analyzing the instantaneous force-velocity-length relations of the left ventricle consists of recording left ventricular pressure simultaneously with left ventricular diameter across the minor axis of the left ventricle recorded by means of an M-mode echocardiogram[27a]* (Fig. 5–16, p. 98). This combination of measurements provides all the data necessary to calculate ventricular circumferential fiber shortening, at either the endocardium or the midwall, and midwall circumferential stress, using minor modifications of the equations presented above.[28]

Ventricular *preload* may be expressed as end-diastolic wall stress and *afterload* as peak or mean systolic wall stress. During ejection, as the left ventricular cavity decreases in size and wall thickness increases, systolic wall stress (and tension) declines rapidly even though pressure is maintained (Fig. 14–5). *Left ventricular power* can be calculated as the product of intracavitary pressure and the rate of change of ventricular volume. Simultaneously recorded ventricular volumes and pressures during diastole allow the calculation of *left ventricular chamber and muscle compliance*[29] (Fig. 12–22, p. 428).

VENTRICULAR WALL MOTION. Quantitative angiography also permits study of ventricular wall motion. The most gross focal abnormalities of the extent of contraction can be appreciated by visual inspection of cineventriculograms. Segments of abnormal ventricular contraction can be localized by superimposing end-diastolic and

---

*However, use of M-mode echocardiography is based on the assumption of uniform wall motion; this assumption can be made with reasonable assurance in conditions that affect left ventricular function uniformly, such as dilated cardiomyopathy, or aortic regurgitation, but is not warranted in conditions that produce localized or regional dysfunction, such as coronary artery disease.

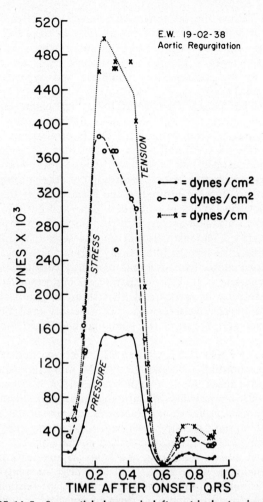

E.W. 19-02-38
Aortic Regurgitation

— = dynes/cm²
o—o = dynes/cm²
x····x = dynes/cm

DYNES × 10³

STRESS

TENSION

PRESSURE

0.2 0.4 0.6 0.8 1.0
TIME AFTER ONSET QRS

FIGURE 14–5 Sequential changes in left ventricular tension, stress, and pressure are illustrated throughout the cardiac cycle in a patient with aortic regurgitation. Note that tension, but particularly stress, declines during ejection (i.e., while the left ventricular volume decreases), although left ventricular pressure is maintained. (From Rackley, C. E.: Quantitative evaluation of left ventricular function by radiographic techniques. Circulation *54*:862, 1976, by permission of the American Heart Association, Inc.)

end-systolic outlines of the left ventricular cavity and tracing both the central x-ray beam and the cavity silhouette on paper or by using a computer (Fig. 10–48, p. 339).[30] *Akinesis* is present when a portion of each of the two silhouettes shares a common line; *dyskinesis* is present when the end-systolic silhouette extends outside the end-diastolic silhouette. The abnormally contracting segments (both akinetic and dyskinetic) are expressed as percentages of the total end-diastolic circumference (Fig. 14–6). *Hypokinesis* (focal decreases in the extent of contraction) as well as *asynchrony* (abnormalities of timing of contraction) are less severe disturbances of contraction. High filming rates, with analysis of wall motion from multiple cine frames, and the use of computer techniques to assist in data reduction and analysis are necessary for the detection of these more subtle abnormalities.[31] By use of such techniques, it is apparent that focal hypokinesis that cannot readily be detected by visual inspection of cineangiograms is a common disturbance and that abnormalities of timing of segmental wall motion are nearly as common as abnormalities of the extent of contraction. Focal hypokinesis is often associated with hyperkinesis of other wall regions, presumably as a compensatory mechanism.[25,31] Two-dimensional echocardiography[32,33] (p. 102) and radionuclide angiography (p. 357) have provided useful approaches for assessing wall motion noninvasively.

Applications

VENTRICULAR VOLUME. The normal left ventricular end-diastolic volume averages 70 ± 20 (SD) ml/square meter.[15,25] When ventricular end-diastolic volume is clearly elevated (i.e., >108 ml/square meter, or >2 SD's above the normal average) and *total* stroke volume and/or cardiac index and work are either reduced or within normal limits, while heart rate and afterload are normal, cardiac contractility is depressed.

EJECTION FRACTION. The ratio of stroke volume to end-diastolic volume, the ejection fraction (EF), is a

FIGURE 14–6 Systolic (dashed) and diastolic (solid) lateral and anteroposterior (AP) angiocardiograms are superimposed with a central lead marker as a reference point. The abnormally contracting segments are enclosed by brackets on the diastolic silhouette. (From Rackley, C. E.: Quantitative evaluation of left ventricular function by radiographic techniques. Circulation *54*:862, 1976, by permission of the American Heart Association, Inc.)

LATERAL VIEW

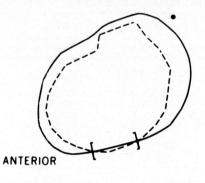

ANTERIOR

AP VIEW

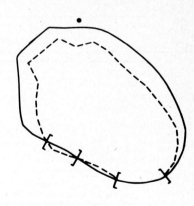

Abnormally Contracting Segments (ACS) =

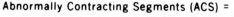

akinetic or dyskinetic length of end-diastolic circumference
―――――――――――――――――――――――――――――――――――――― × 100
total end-diastolic circumference

global index of the extent of ventricular fiber shortening and has been considered, on the basis of a number of empirical studies, to provide one of the most useful measures of left ventricular pump function. EF averages 0.67 ± 0.08 (SD) in normal subjects[15,25] and ranges from 0.45 to 0.70 in experimental animals, depending on the heart rate, the method used to measure cardiac volume, and whether the animal is anesthetized or awake.[34] EF is closely related to and can be predicted accurately from the percentage of shortening during systole of left ventricular minor axis dimension, and this provides the basis for assessing ejection fraction by echocardiography (p. 103).[35,36] Most commonly, the diameter perpendicular to the midpoint of the long axis is used, and its fractional shortening (FS) is calculated as follows

$$FS = \frac{\text{(Left ventricular) end-diastolic dimension} - \text{End-systolic dimension}}{\text{End-diastolic dimension}}$$

and is expressed as a percentage.

In addition to myocardial contractility, both preload and afterload affect EF, FS, and the mean velocity of circumferential fiber shortening (V_{CF}). The last-named, expressed in circumferences per second, is calculated as the quotient of circumferential fiber shortening during ejection (in circumferences) and ejection time (in seconds). The lower limit of normal for mean V_{CF} is 1.1 circumferences per second.[37] Studies in conscious or lightly sedated baboons[38] and conscious human subjects[39] have shown that moderate changes in preload have little effect on mean or maximum velocity of fiber shortening. However, when end-diastolic volume (preload) is acutely reduced or aortic pressure (afterload) is acutely elevated or both, the so-called *ejection phase indices of ventricular performance* (i.e., EF, FS, and mean and peak V_{CF}) all decline (Fig. 12–28, p. 434). Conversely, the ejection phase indices may be normal in conditions in which afterload is reduced, such as mitral regurgitation, even when contractility is depressed (p. 1079). These findings suggest that *changes* in EF, FS, and V_{CF}, like changes in stroke volume, do not simply reflect variations in contractility. However, as will be pointed out below, the ejection phase indices are often useful for determining the level of contractility in the basal state in the presence of chronic heart disease, in which the influence of changes in preload and afterload tends to be corrected for by compensatory dilatation and hypertrophy[40] (Table 14–1).

VENTRICULAR DIMENSIONS. The extent and velocity of ventricular wall shortening during ejection have been employed to determine the effects of a variety of interventions on contractility using implanted ultrasonic dimension gauges in conscious dogs and primates[35] and by cineradiographic recording of the motion of radiopaque markers sutured to the epicardium at the time of cardiac operations in patients.[41] Mean and peak V_{CF} can be used to evaluate acute inotropic interventions provided that afterload remains constant or almost so.[42] V_{CF} probably shows little change fortuitously during acute elevations in preload alone had afterload remained constant.[35,36,43,44] The mean and peak V_{CF} incorporate the important element of the velocity of myocardial fiber shortening and appear to be more sensitive measures of contractility than EF and FS, which simply reflect the pumping function of the ventricle.

LEFT VENTRICULAR MASS. Left ventricular wall thickness normally averages 10.9 ± 2.0 mm (SD)[15] and left ventricular mass 92 ± 16 gm/square meter body surface area.[9,24] Chronic cardiac dilatation secondary to valvular or primary myocardial disease increases left ventricular mass, as does chronic pressure overload. Characteristically, hypertrophy due to pressure overload is characterized by an increased muscle mass resulting from an augmentation of wall thickness with, at first, little change in ventricular chamber volume (concentric hypertrophy); in contrast, hypertrophy due to volume overload of myocardial disease is characterized by an increased muscle mass resulting from ventricular dilatation, with a slight increase in wall thickness (eccentric hypertrophy [Fig. 13–7, p. 452). There is often a correlation between stroke work of the left ventricle and left ventricular mass in chronic valvular heart disease, but no such relation exists in primary myocardial disease[24] (Table 14–1).

TABLE 14–1   LEFT VENTRICULAR VOLUME DATA IN PATIENTS

Group	Number of Patients	End-Diastolic Volume (ml/m²)	Stroke Volume (ml/m²)	Mass (gm/m²)	Ejection Fraction
Normal*	–	70 ± 20.0	45 ± 13.0	92 ± 16.0	0.67 ± 0.08
AS	14	84 ± 22.9	44 ± 10.1	172 ± 32.7	0.56 ± 0.17
AR	22	193 ± 55.4	92 ± 30.9	223 ± 73.0	0.56 ± 0.13
AS and AR	13	138 ± 36.5	75 ± 19.1	231 ± 56.9	0.53 ± 0.10
MS	37	83 ± 21.2	43 ± 11.9	98 ± 24.1	0.57 ± 0.14
MR	29	160 ± 53.1	87 ± 21.3	166 ± 49.9	0.47 ± 0.10
MS and MR	29	106 ± 34.4	58 ± 14.7	119 ± 27.8	0.57 ± 0.12
A and M combined	45	130 ± 55.8	69 ± 25.5	156 ± 55.9	0.55 ± 0.12
Myocardial disease	15	199 ± 75.7	44 ± 14.5	145 ± 27.6	0.25 ± 0.09

*Normal values from Kennedy, J. W., et al.: Quantitative angiocardiography. The normal left ventricle in man. Circulation *34*:272, 1966.
AS = aortic valve stenosis with peak systolic pressure gradient > 30 mm Hg.
AR = aortic valve insufficiency with regurgitant flow > 30 ml per beat.
MS = mitral valve area < 1.5 sq cm.
MR = mitral valve regurgitant flow > 20 ml per beat.
A and M combined = combined aortic and mitral valve disease.
Myocardial disease = primary cardiomyopathy or myocardial disease secondary to coronary atherosclerosis.
From Dodge, H. T., and Baxley, W. A.: Left ventricular volume and mass and their significance in heart disease. Am. J. Cardiol. *23*:528, 1969.

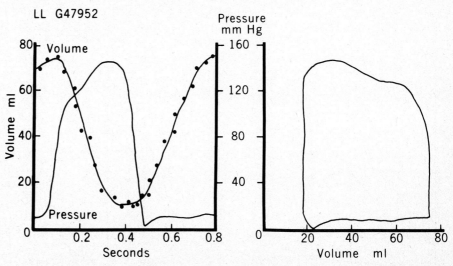

LL G47952

FIGURE 14–7 Volume and pressure changes obtained from a patient with a normal left ventricle are displayed on the left, timed with respect to onset of the QRS complex in the electrocardiogram. On the right, pressure and volume are related to construct a pressure-volume loop. (From Grossman, W. [ed.]: Cardiac Catheterization and Angiography. 2nd ed. Philadelphia, Lea and Febiger, 1980.)

THE PRESSURE-VOLUME LOOP. When ventricular pressure and volume are related to each other over an entire cardiac cycle, a pressure-volume loop can be constructed (Fig. 14–7). The timing of valve opening and closing can be indicated on such a loop; the height and width of the loop are determined by the systolic pressure and stroke volume, respectively.[25] The area subtended by the systolic portion of the curve provides a measure of stroke work performed by the left ventricle during systole, whereas the area subtended by the diastolic limb provides a measure of diastolic work performed *on* the left ventricle in distending it during diastole. Net work is the difference between the two. Diastolic work may be thought of as the energy supplied to the ventricle required for "priming the pump." In the absence of valvular regurgitation, diastolic work is largely generated by the left atrium and right ventricle, and its elevation is the physiological basis, at least in part, for the right ventricular failure observed in patients with left ventricular failure and secondary pulmonary hypertension.[25] With left ventricular failure and a rise in left ventricular diastolic pressure, there is an increase in diastolic work relative to systolic work and thus a decrease in net work. Charac-

teristic changes in the left ventricular pressure-volume loops occur in various disease states (Fig. 14–8 and Table 14–1).

VENTRICULAR END-SYSTOLIC PRESSURE-VOLUME RELATIONS. The extent of myocardial fiber shortening reflects the interaction of preload, afterload, and contractility. As afterload increases, the extent of systolic fiber shortening declines (Fig. 12–30, p. 436, and Fig. 24–3, p. 808) resulting in progressively greater end-systolic fiber lengths[45–48] (Fig. 12–26, p. 432). Thus, end-systolic fiber length is a direct function of afterload (Fig. 14–9). Myocardial contractility can be evaluated by making use of this fundamental property of heart muscle and focusing attention on the relation of the residual volume, i.e., the volume of blood remaining in the ventricle at the end of systole, and the ventricular pressure at that instant. At any level of contractility the end-systolic volume to which a ventricle contracts is a linearly increasing function of end-systolic ventricular pressure. End-systolic volume varies inversely and end-systolic pressures vary directly with contractility (Fig. 14–9). There is little difference between the end-systolic pressure-volume relation in isovolumetric and ejecting contractions. Indeed, the virtual identity of isometric and

FIGURE 14–8 Left ventricular pressure-volume curves from patients with different varieties of heart disease. The height of each curve is determined by systolic pressure and the width by stroke volume. The two smallest curves—one from a patient with mitral stenosis, the other from a patient with primary cardiomyopathy—indicate similar stroke volumes; however, in the latter, the dilated left ventricle is functioning at an inappropriately large volume, and the ejection fraction is low. The curve in mitral insufficiency demonstrates volume overload by the large excursion along the volume axis and the absence of an isovolumetric contraction period. The shape of the curve in aortic stenosis shows the effect of pressure overload. In aortic stenosis and insufficiency the curve demonstrates the influence of pressure and volume overload, with the large

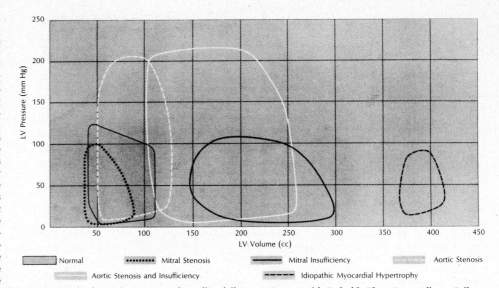

area subtended by the curve. (From Dodge, H. T.: Hemodynamic aspects of cardiac failure. *In* Braunwald, E. [ed.]: The Myocardium: Failure and Infarction. New York, HP Publishing Co., 1974, p. 70.)

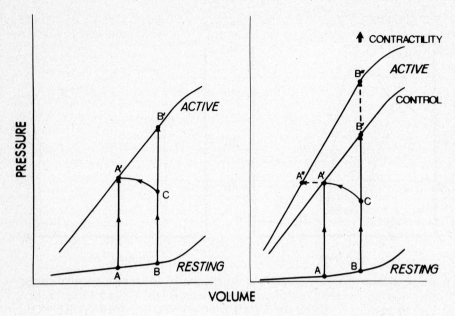

FIGURE 14–9 Schematic representation of the theoretical relationship of ventricular preload, afterload, and contractility for isovolumetric and ejecting beats. *Left,* Isovolumetric (A → A', B → B') and ejecting (B → C → A') pathways illustrate the identity of isovolumetric and ejecting end-systolic pressure-volume relations. *Right,* The effect of increased myocardial contractility is to produce a higher pressure in isovolumetric beats (B' → B") and a smaller end-systolic volume in ejecting beats (B → C → A' → A"). Note that end-systolic volume at the higher contractile state (A") is independent of end-diastolic volume or preload, in that it is the final volume for ejecting beats originating from both the higher (B → C → A' → A") and lower (A → A' → A") preloads. (From Grossman, W., Braunwald, E., Mann, T., McLaurin, L. P., and Green, L. H.: Contractile state of the left ventricle in man as evaluated from end-systolic pressure-volume relations. Circulation *56*:845, 1977, by permission of the American Heart Association, Inc.)

isotonic length-tension curves has been demonstrated in isolated cat papillary muscle[49,50] (Fig. 14–10) and in the intact heart[51-55] (Fig. 14–11). Figure 14–11*B* shows the pressure-volume diagrams from a left ventricle connected to a pump system, which allowed the ventricle to eject the fluid at any desired afterload.[54] The large dots, which represent the peak pressures that this ventricle reached in isovolumetric contractions, lie very close to the solid lines, which connect the end-systolic pressure-volume relations of ejecting beats. Figure 14–11*C* shows pressure-volume

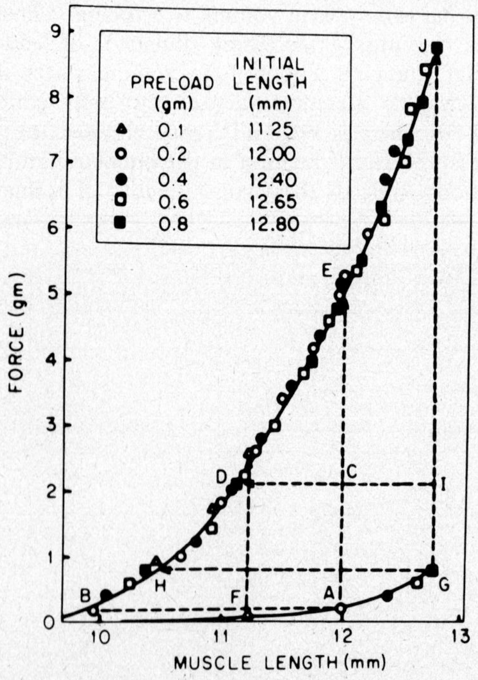

FIGURE 14–10 Force-length relation in cat papillary muscle. No distinct end-systolic length-tension relation resulted from different modes of contraction, such as isometric (F to D), isotonic (A to B), and afterloaded isotonic contractions (G to I to D). (From Downing, S. E., and Sonnenblick, E. H.: Cardiac muscle mechanics and ventricular performance. Force and time parameters. Am. J. Physiol. *207*: 705, 1964.)

loops from a left ventricle that ejected blood from different end-diastolic volumes but at identical systolic pressures. The end-systolic pressure-volume relations are identical. When the ventricle contracted at different afterloads,[51,52] the left ventricular end-systolic pressure-volume relations again formed a straight line. Figure 14–11*D* shows the effects of decreasing venous return; there was a progressive reduction in end-diastolic and end-systolic diameters as well as left ventricular wall stress. However, the stress-diameter relation remained constant.[56]

The end-systolic pressure-volume relationship for both isovolumetric and ejecting contractions can be expressed as

$$P_{es} = E_{es}(V_{es} - V_d)$$

where P_{es} and V_{es} are end-systolic pressure and end-systolic volume, respectively; E_{es} is the slope of the line relating these two variables (the solid lines in Figure 14–11); and V_d is the intercept of this line on the volume axis (Fig. 14–11*C*). Thus, E_{es} is a numerical expression of myocardial contractility; a higher value indicates a steeper slope and a smaller end-systolic volume, i.e., more complete systolic emptying at any given end-systolic pressure.

There appear to be a number of theoretical advantages to the use of end-systolic pressure–volume relations as an approach to the assessment of myocardial contractility.[56a] First, since afterload is already incorporated into the calculation of E_{es}, the observed changes assess contractility directly rather than the mixture of changes in contractility and afterload that affect the ejection phase indices;[57] and second, since E_{es} is independent of preload,[51,55] difficulties with the ejection phase indices that are affected by end-diastolic volume[58] are obviated.[56] E_{es} can be measured by rearranging the equation as follows:

$$E_{es} = P_{es}/(V_{es} - V_d)$$

P_{es} and V_{es} can be measured relatively easily in patients; the determination of V_d requires measurement of P_{es} and V_{es} from contractions at a constant contractility but at different afterloads. P_{es} and V_{es} can be measured at two pressures by either raising resistance with phenylephrine or lowering

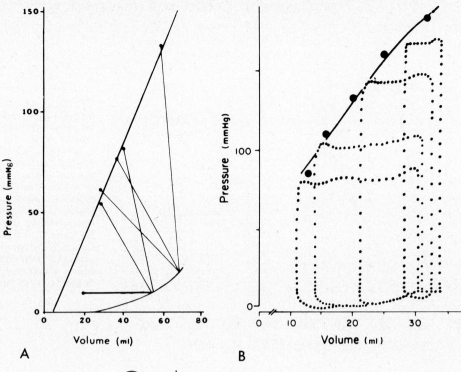

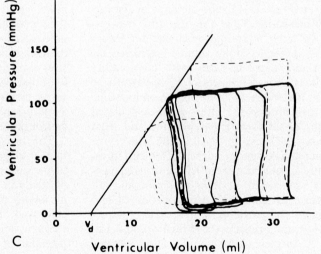

FIGURE 14–11 Pressure-volume (P-V) diagrams in canine ventricles. *A*, P-V diagram obtained in an isolated left ventricle that was filled with air and connected to an air chamber. The ventricle compressed air during systole. (From Monroe, R. G., and French, G. N.: Left ventricular pressure-volume relationships and myocardial oxygen consumption in the isolated heart. Circ. Res. *9*:362, 1961, by permission of the American Heart Association, Inc.). *B*, P-V diagram obtained in an isolated left ventricle that ejected liquid against a hydraulic servo-controlled loading system. The large dots near the solid line represent the peak isovolumetric pressures at various volumes.) (From Weber, K. T., et al.: Left ventricular force-length relations of isovolumic and ejecting beats. Am. J. Physiol. *231*:337, 1976.) *C*, P-V diagram obtained in a left ventricle ejecting blood. Volume was measured by a cardiometer while venting the right ventricles. (From Sagawa, K.: The ventricular pressure-volume diagram revisited. Circ. Res. *43*:677, 1978, by permission of the American Heart Association, Inc.) *D*, Beat-to-beat changes in left ventricular stress-diameter loop during a decrease in venous return in an open-chest dog. The dotted line corresponds to the end-systolic–stress endsystolic diameter line. The stress-diameter relations are linear during most of the ejection. The slope of this linear phase is much less affected by the maneuver than is the end-systolic diameter. (Reproduced with permission from Pouleur, H., Rousseau, M. F., van Eyll, C., van Mechelen, H., Brasseur, L. A., and Charlier, A. A.: Assessment of left ventricular contractility from late systolic stress-volume relations. Circulation *65*:1204, 1982, by permission of the American Heart Association, Inc.)

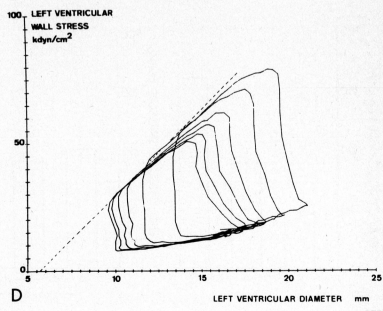

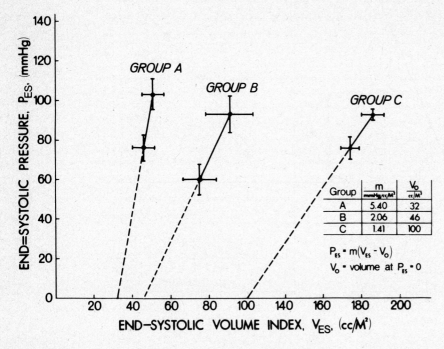

FIGURE 14–12 Average values for left ventricular end-systolic volume and pressure at two levels of systolic load are plotted for subjects with normal contractile function (group A, ejection fraction $\geq$ 0.60), intermediate function (group B, ejection fraction = 0.41 to 0.59), and poor contractile function (group C, ejection fraction $\leq$ 0.40). Points represent average values, and brackets indicate standard errors of the means. Volumes are index for body surface area in square meters. (From Grossman, W., Braunwald, E., Mann, T., McLaurin, L. P., and Green, L. H.: Contractile state of the left ventricle in man as evaluated from end-systolic pressure-volume relations. Circulation *56*:845, 1977, by permission of the American Heart Association, Inc.)

it with nitroglycerin (Fig. 14–12). The method can be further simplified by measuring V_{es} at the operating end-systolic pressure, if the latter is normal or almost so. Under these circumstances the end-systolic volume (corrected for body surface area) correlates inversely with contractility (Fig. 14–13). Although measurements of P_{es} appear to be useful clinically,[59,60] it is more accurate to use end-systolic wall *stress* rather than pressure;[60–63] stress can be calculated from considerations of intraventricular pressure and from cavity diameter and thickness (p. 472).[61] The use of M-mode or two-dimensional echocardiography,[61,63] cuff pressure (in the absence of obstruction to left ventricular outflow) to estimate ventricular systolic pressure, and an indirect carotid pulse to aid in the determination of end systole are all helpful in providing a noninvasive assessment of the end-systolic pressure (or stress)–volume (dimension) index. A further useful simplification of this index can be derived by determining the ratio of peak systolic pressure/end-systolic volume, the former parameter determined by sphygmomanometry and the latter by radionuclide ventriculography.[64–66,66a,66b] Normally, this ratio rises markedly during exercise but fails to do so in patients with left ventricular dysfunction. The end-systolic pressure/volume ratio at rest and during exercise appears to be a more sensitive index than the ejection fraction (at rest and during exercise) in identifying ventricular dysfunction.

The left ventricular end-systolic pressure–volume relation is of particular value in assessing contractility in patients with mitral regurgitation, in whom this is otherwise particularly difficult.[60] Since isovolumetric systole is absent in mitral regurgitation, isovolumetric indices cannot be employed. The reduced afterload and augmented preload characteristic of mitral regurgitation complicate the interpretation of the ejection phase indices as well. The relation

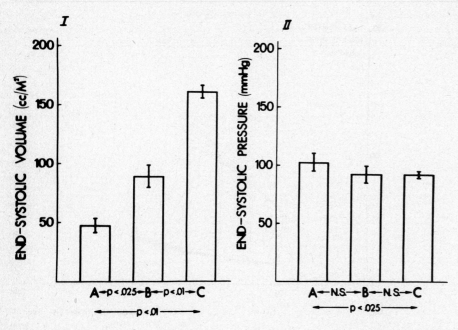

FIGURE 14–13 Values for end-systolic volume and pressure in groups A, B, and C (defined in legend to Figure 14–12). Resting end-systolic volume closely reflects overall left ventricular contractile performance, as indicated by the clear separation of groups A, B, and C. Bars represent mean values, and brackets indicate standard errors of the means. (From Grossman, W., Braunwald, E., Mann, T., McLaurin, L. P., and Green, L. H.: Contractile state of the left ventricle in man as evaluated from end-systolic pressure-volume relations. Circulation *56*:845, 1977, by permission of the American Heart Association, Inc.)

between arterial pressure and wall stress, determined by echocardiography, has been used to classify patients with hypertension into those with normal or impaired left ventricular function.[65] The left ventricular stress-dimension relation, determined noninvasively, has also been found helpful in identifying positive inotropic interventions.[63]

WALL MOTION ABNORMALITIES. The mildest disturbance of ventricular performance in ischemic heart disease consists of focal abnormality of contraction in the presence only of a reduction in diastolic distensibility but with a normal end-diastolic volume and EF.[67] A slightly more severe disturbance consists of a normal EF at rest, but a failure to rise during exercise. This is followed by a reduced EF and an elevated filling pressure in the presence of a normal end-diastolic volume at rest. The elevated filling pressure reflects reduced compliance of the scarred ventricle rather than systolic failure. Similar abnormalities may occur with acute ischemia and may be induced by stress through atrial pacing or by exercise. When abnormal wall motion involves more than approximately one-sixth of the endocardial surface, the ventricular end-diastolic volume at rest rises. Cardiac output declines with abnormal contraction involving more than approximately one-fourth of the endocardial surface.[67]

VENTRICULAR dP/dt. Since *changes* in the maximum rate of rise of ventricular pressure (peak dP/dt) are known to be highly sensitive to acute *changes* in contractility[68,69] (Fig. 14–14), measurement of ventricular dP/dt may be employed along with ventricular end-diastolic volume and filling pressure in the assessment of *directional changes* in contractility with an intervention. Peak dP/dt cannot be reliably measured with the catheter-manometer systems ordinarily used during cardiac catheterization, unless special precautions are taken to prevent artifacts and the frequency response of the system is carefully determined.[70] High-fidelity catheter-tip micromanometers should be employed, but even with these, artifacts due to flicking catheter motion during the cardiac cycle must be assiduously avoided.

Peak dP/dt is largely independent of changes in

afterload, provided it occurs *before* aortic valve opening.[44,71] Studies carried out in both dogs[72] and human patients[44] have shown that peak dP/dt is little altered by steady-state alterations in aortic pressure, and although it appears to be much more markedly affected by changes in contractility than by alterations in preload, the latter influence cannot be disregarded; therefore, even when contractility is constant, a large change in preload can cause a modest alteration in dP/dt in the same direction. Another difficulty with peak dP/dt is that it cannot be corrected for changes in muscle mass produced by ventricular hypertrophy. Although peak dP/dt, in general, correlates with the basal level of contractility, it is not as useful for assessing this property of cardiac function as are the ejection phase indices (see below).

ASSESSING CARDIAC PERFORMANCE BASED ON FORCE-VELOCITY-LENGTH CONCEPTS

In the final analysis, irrespective of theoretical considerations, any index that is proposed for assessing ventricular function must be reproducible in the same individual under constant conditions and must be capable of differentiating patients with normal cardiac function from those with reduced cardiac function.[73] The principles of myocardial muscle mechanics, outlined in Chapter 12, have provided a framework for analysis for two classes of indices: one group based on events during isovolumetric contraction and a second group based on events during ejection. These indices are employed for two purposes: (1) determining absolute levels of contractility, i.e., whether the basal level of contractility is normal or not; and (2) determining directional changes of contractility, i.e., whether any given intervention exerts a positive or negative inotropic effect.

Isovolumetric Phase Indices. V_{max}, the maximum velocity of shortening of the unloaded contractile elements (CE), theoretically provides a measure of myocardial contractility independent of preload or afterload. Controversy continues to surround calculation of CE V_{max}, both in isolated muscle and, even more so, in the intact heart, in which case the calculation must be based on many assumptions.[74] Despite these difficulties, however, observations in the intact left ventricle (p. 435) indicate that its V_{max}, determined by extrapolation of the force-velocity relation derived from multiple variably afterloaded beats, is, like the V_{max} of isolated cardiac muscle, not significantly al-

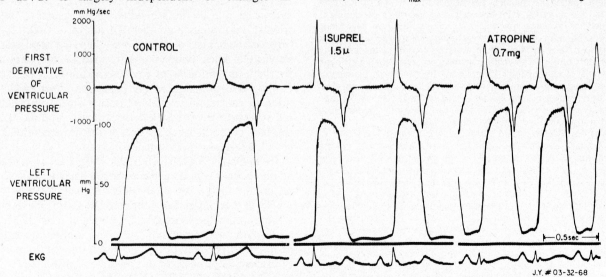

FIGURE 14–14 Serial recordings of left ventricular pressure and of the first derivative of left ventricular pressure (dP/dt) in a 12-year-old girl with mild pulmonic valvular stenosis. The first record (control) is in the basal state, the middle record after the administration of 1.5 μg isoproterenol, and the final record after 0.7 mg atropine. (From Gleason, W. L., and Braunwald, E.: Studies on the first derivative of the ventricular pressure pulse in man. J. Clin. Invest. *41*:80, 1962.)

tered by alterations of preload within the physiological range but is markedly sensitive to inotropic stimuli.[75]

CE velocity in the intact heart has been estimated assuming a muscle model in which CE and SE (series elastic element) are in series (p. 419). At any instant the velocity of SE extension (V_{SE}), and hence of V_{CE}, is directly proportional to the rate of force development (dF/dt) and is inversely related to the stiffness of SE.[76] When ejection of the canine ventricle is prevented experimentally and the calculated V_{CE} is plotted against the corresponding wall stress, an inverse relation between V_{CE} and stress is described.[77] V_{max} has been estimated from isovolumetric contractions by extrapolation of the V_{CE} stress relation to zero stress; maximum isovolumetric wall stress (P_o) can also be calculated. Such force-velocity curves obtained from the intact dog ventricle during inotropic interventions[77] exhibit changes resembling those calculated in a similar manner, albeit with fewer assumptions, from isometric twitches as well as from variably afterloaded contractions in isolated cardiac muscle.

It is obviously impractical in patients to determine V_{max} either in variably afterloaded or completely isovolumetric beats. However, a mathematical derivation of CE V_{max} can be obtained in the normally ejecting heart, using only the isovolumetric phase of contraction and employing one of the so-called isovolumetric phase indices described below. In one approach that has been applied clinically,[78] V_{CE} is calculated as dP/dt/KP (where K is an assumed stiffness constant for the series elastic element) and is plotted against instantaneous wall stress (calculated from intraventricular pressure, volume, and wall thickness) during the isovolumetric phase of left ventricular systole, and the curve is then extrapolated to zero stress to obtain V_{max}. However, if it is further assumed that contraction of the myocardium during isovolumetric contraction is truly isometric, then pressure and wall stress are linearly related to one another, and no calculation of wall stress is required to determine V_{max};[79] calculated V_{CE} is simply plotted against the instantaneous intraventricular pressure and extrapolated to zero pressure. This index of V_{max} is relatively independent of acute changes in preload at low left ventricular end-diastolic pressures[80] but declines at end-diastolic pressures exceeding 10 mm Hg.[81]

Determination of V_{max} in the intact heart, as described above, requires a number of assumptions concerning the characteristics of the SE and PE (parallel elastic elements) and the type of muscle model that exists in the intact heart,[73] little information is available about how chronic heart disease alters these characteristics.[74] Furthermore, the validity of the assumption that isovolumetric contraction is truly isometric has been questioned.[82] Since this estimate of V_{max} declines as left ventricular end-diastolic pressure rises,[37] it will underestimate contractility when ventricular compliance is reduced, as occurs in ventricular hypertrophy. In addition, this index of V_{max} may be maintained in the presence of acute ischemia despite depression of pump performance, presumably because it reflects the behavior of normal muscle in series with nonfunctioning segments of myocardium. In addition to these theoretical objections, errors in calculating V_{max} can arise from artifacts in measuring dP/dt from inadequate catheter-manometer systems; from whipping motion of the catheter; and from the presence of mitral regurgitation, which prevents even brief periods of isovolumetric contraction. Despite these limitations, when data derived from analysis of the isovolumetric phase are considered to be only *empirical indices of the inotropic state* rather than *true measures of behavior of CE*, they can be useful for detecting *changes* in myocardial contractility with an intervention.

Some of the difficulties cited above involving the calculation of V_{max} can be partially avoided by the selection of certain points on the curve relating dP/dt/DP, where DP is the developed left ventricular pressure (i.e., left ventricular pressure minus end-diastolic pressure) to the corresponding DP. These measures tend to be relatively independent of changes in afterload, since they are usually computed at a DP of 40 mm Hg, a level of pressure generation which in most clinical circumstances occurs before the opening of the aortic valve.[83] The ratio dP/dt/DP at a DP of 40 mm Hg, although somewhat less sensitive to acute changes in contractility than simple peak dP/dt, is nonetheless useful for assessing *directional* changes in contractility,[42,44,83,84] since it is unaffected by changes in afterload and is relatively insensitive to changes in preload. The peak level of dP/dt/TP, termed "V_{pm}" (where TP refers to total pressure development), is also relatively independent of both preload and afterload but sensitive to changes in the inotropic state,[85,86] and it has been advocated as an index of the contractility in the basal state, as discussed further below.

Ejection Phase Indices. The most commonly used ejection phase indices include ejection fraction (EF), peak and mean fractional shortening (FS) of ventricular myocardium, and peak and mean velocity of circumferential fiber shortening.[73] Contractility can be evaluated using high-fidelity catheter-tip manometers and cineangiography[87] or a catheter-tip velocity flow meter in the ascending aorta[88] to determine the instantaneous relation between wall stress or tension and midwall or endocardial shortening velocity throughout ejection. Ejection phase indices can also be obtained noninvasively by echocardiography.[61,64] V_{CF} at peak wall stress has been chosen for many calculations, since at that instant the rate of change in wall force (and therefore the rate of change in the length of SE) is zero, and V_{CF} equals V_{CE}.

DETERMINATION OF DIRECTIONAL CHANGES IN CONTRACTILITY

At constant levels of ventricular filling pressure, end-diastolic volume or dimensions (as evidence of constant ventricular preload); aortic or left ventricular systolic pressure (as evidence of constant afterload); and a variety of measures of left ventricular performance, such as the ejection phase indices (EF, peak and mean FS, and V_{CF}) as well as stroke volume, stroke work, stroke power, and peak left ventricular dP/dt (see below), all vary as functions of myocardial contractility. Thus, acute enhancement or depression of contractility may be assumed to occur if any of these indices of mechanical performance increases while filling pressure or end-diastolic volume and aortic pressure remain unchanged or vary in a manner that affects performance in a direction *opposite* to the change in contractility.[58,89] For example, at a similar aortic pressure, the finding of a reduction of stroke volume or dP/dt while ventricular filling pressure or end-diastolic volume remains constant or rises reflects a depression of contractility.

Although the absolute levels of ventricular filling pressure do not correlate with end-diastolic volume in chronic heart disease[25,90] (Fig. 14–8), acute *changes* in ventricular filling pressure are *directionally* similar to changes in end-diastolic volume (except in the presence of myocardial ischemia or marked tachycardia [p. 428]). Therefore, a *change* in ventricular filling pressure can be related to a *change* in one of the hemodynamic measures of left ventricular performance enumerated above in order to assess *directional* changes of contractility.[58,89] This approach is not applicable when preload or afterload or both are altered by the intervention so as to cause a change in performance in the same direction as the presumed effect of the alteration in contractility, such as occurs when ventricular filling pressure rises or left ventricular systolic pressure declines or both occur as one of the aforementioned indices of ventricular performance increases.

ISOVOLUMETRIC PHASE INDICES. In assessing acute *changes* in contractility, there does not seem to be an advantage in the use of derived measures such as "V_{max}," which is calculated from the isovolumetric phase pressure tracings, over the more directly obtained peak $dP/dt/DP_{40}$, since both these isovolumetric phase indices are highly responsive to changes in the inotropic state and are relatively insensitive to changes in preload and afterload.[42]

EJECTION PHASE INDICES. Changes in the relation between the velocity or extent of myocardial wall shortening (measured from cineangiographic frames,[91] echocardiograms, or a catheter-tip velocity meter[88]) and the simultaneous ventricular wall stress at any given length

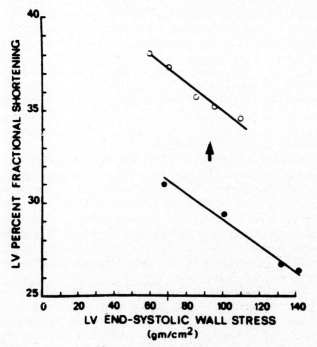

FIGURE 14–15 Comparison of the LV end-systolic wall stress-shortening lines joining points at different afterloads for control (closed circles) and increased (open circles) contractile states produced by dobutamine in a representative subject. With the dobutamine infusion, the percentage of ΔD is higher for any level of end-systolic wall stress. (Reproduced with permission from Borow, K. M., Green, L. H., Grossman, W., and Braunwald, E.: Left ventricular end-systolic stress-shortening and stress-length relations in humans. Am. J. Cardiol. *50*:1301, 1982.)

reflect acute changes in contractility. For instance, an augmentation of instantaneous velocity of minor axis shortening (V_{CF}) at any given ventricular length and wall stress signifies an improvement of contractility. The relation between end-systolic meridional wall stress and of left ventricular fractional shortening provides a sensitive index by which an inotropic intervention can be assessed[63] (Fig. 14–15).

DETERMINATION OF CONTRACTILITY IN THE BASAL STATE

ISOVOLUMETRIC PHASE INDICES. As already stated, these isovolumetric phase indices—$dP/dt/DP_{40}$, peak dP/dt, V_{pm}, and V_{max}—are usually of little value in assessing *basal levels* of contractility and in *comparing* contractility in different patients or in any given patient at different times.[73] Empirically, it has been observed that of these several indices, V_{pm}—i.e., the physiological maximum observed velocity of myocardial shortening, calculated as the maximum $dP/dt/P$—is superior to the others in separating *groups* of patients with normal and depressed contractility, but even this index is unreliable in classifying individual patients.[92] Although the average values of normal subjects and of patients with left ventricular dysfunction differ significantly, there is sufficient overlap so that any given patient cannot be reliably assessed by V_{pm} or any other isovolumetric phase index.

EJECTION PHASE INDICES. In contrast to the above-mentioned limitations of the isovolumetric phase indices, the ejection phase indices—EF, FS, and mean and

peak V_{CF} as well as the rate of left ventricular wall thickening during systole[93]—and the closely related mean systolic ejection rate can be employed to define basal contractility (Fig. 14–16) despite their sensitivity to variations in loading. Acute elevations of afterload cause an inverse change in ejection phase indices; however, these indices are less sensitive to changes in preload. In experimental animals, both FS and V_{CF} remain normal when measured at various time intervals following a chronic volume overload despite progressive cardiac dilatation, unless acute cardiac failure occurs.[95] Therefore compensation of the heart by chronic dilatation and hypertrophy for a chronic volume overload does *not* preclude the usefulness of ejection phase indices for assessing the basal level of contractility. Ejection phase indices may also be useful in assessing basal levels of contractility in the chronically pressure-overloaded heart that

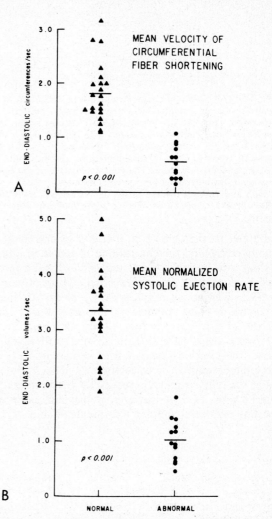

FIGURE 14–16 *A*, Mean velocity of circumferential fiber shortening (mean V_{CF}) plotted in circumferences per second (corrected for end-diastolic circumference). *B*, Mean systolic ejection rate (corrected for end-diastolic volume). Triangles represent patients with normal ventricular function; circles represent patients with clearly abnormal ventricular function as determined from other criteria. In addition to significant separation between the two groups, there is little overlap among individual patients. The superiority of these two ejection phase indices in separating these two groups of patients compared with the isovolumetric phase indices is evident. (From Peterson, K. L., et al.: Comparison of isovolumic and ejection phase indices of myocardial performance in man. Circulation *49*:1088, 1974, by permission of the American Heart Association, Inc.)

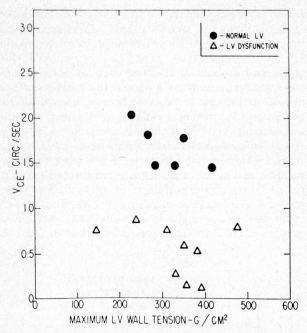

FIGURE 14–17   Velocity of circumferential fiber shortening at maximal wall tension (V_{CE}, contractile element velocity) plotted against corresponding values of maximum tension in subjects with normal left ventricles (solid circles) and patients with left ventricular disease (open triangles) are plotted against corresponding levels of left ventricular wall tension. Circ = circumferences. (From Gault, J. H., Ross, J., Jr., and Braunwald, E.: The contractile state of the left ventricle in man: Instantaneous tension-velocity-length relations in patients with and without disease of the left ventricular myocardium. Circ. Res. **22**:451, 1968, by permission of the American Heart Association, Inc.)

has adapted to the change in afterload by means of concentric hypertrophy, thereby tending to maintain afterload or restore it to normal. As left ventricular hypertrophy develops, in dogs with chronic experimental aortic constriction, FS as well as mean and peak V_{CF} at first decline but then return to and stabilize at normal levels.[96] Indeed, when the obstruction develops slowly and compensatory hypertrophy keeps pace with it, so that wall stress does not rise, the ejection phase indices remain normal.[97] The lower limit of normal of calculated V_{CE} (i.e., V_{CF} at peak stress at the minor equator) exceeds 1.4 circumferences per second[87,98] (Fig. 14–17). However, it may not be essential to use this relatively complex measurement, since V_{CE} (i.e.,

V_{CF} at the time of maximal wall stress) correlates well with mean V_{CF}, calculated from changes in dimensions and ejection time.[94] The aforementioned relation between left ventricular end-systolic stress and per cent fractional shortening, determined noninvasively,[63] provides a useful, practical framework for assessing left ventricular contractility (Fig. 14–18). It is particularly useful in patients with reduced ejection phase indexes to distinguish reduced myocardial shortening due to excessive afterload from depressed myocardial contractility.

FORCE - VELOCITY - LENGTH RELATIONS. The usefulness of force-velocity concepts for assessing left ventricular contractility has been demonstrated in patients before and after aortic valve replacement for free *aortic regurgitation*.[98] Although all patients studied demonstrated an improved forward cardiac index, increased aortic diastolic pressure, and decreased left ventricular end-diastolic pressure postoperatively, the majority manifested no improvement in the depressed V_{CF}.

Under conditions of chronic pressure overload, such as occurs in *aortic stenosis*, the ventricle compensates by means of hypertrophy, adding more contractile units in parallel in an attempt to maintain afterload relatively constant. It has been pointed out that if hypertrophy is inadequate or fails to keep pace with an increasingly severe pressure overload, wall stress rises, and in keeping with the inverse force-velocity relation of cardiac muscle, there are reciprocal obligatory declines in the various ejection phase indices.[26,97] Therefore, for these indices to provide an index of contractility, they must be related to wall stress. In some patients with pressure overload, wall stress is elevated, and contractility, as reflected in the fiber shortening–wall stress relation, is normal despite absolute depressions of the ejection phase indices. A true depression of contractility is present when these indices of shortening are lowered even when the existing level of afterload is taken into account (Fig. 13–9, p. 453). These observations illustrate the usefulness of characterizing myocardial function by utilizing force-velocity concepts.[99]

Studies in experimental animals have demonstrated that acute *mitral regurgitation* is associated with a marked reduction in intramyocardial wall tension (i.e., afterload) but enhanced ventricular emptying and increased EF, FS, and V_{CF}.[100,101] In patients with severe mitral regurgitation in the clinically compensated state, these ejection phase indices

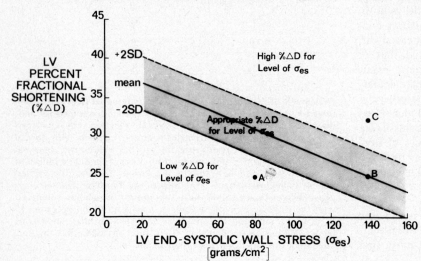

FIGURE 14–18   Diagram of the LV end-systolic wall stress (σ_{es}-shortening percentage of ΔD) relation. This relation may be useful in distinguishing depressed myocardial shortening due to excessive afterload (point B) from an intrinsic contractile abnormality (point A). Hypercontractile states would be characterized by a higher than predicted percentage of ΔD for any σ_{es} (point C versus point B). (Reproduced with permission from Borow, K. M., Green, L. H., Grossman, W., and Braunwald, E.: Left ventricular end-systolic stress-shortening and stress-length relations in humans. Am. J. Cardiol. **50**:1301, 1982.)

are also elevated. Although left ventricular fiber shortening and ejection phase indices may be normal[102] in patients with chronic mitral regurgitation in heart failure, it is impaired in patients with left ventricular failure due to cardiomyopathy, aortic stenosis, and chronic aortic regurgitation. A likely explanation for this difference between mitral regurgitation and these other causes of left heart failure is that in mitral regurgitation there is a low-impedance systolic leak into the left atrium, which reduces left ventricular afterload, increases myocardial fiber shortening, and reduces end-systolic volume.[100,102,103]

Thus, in chronic severe mitral regurgitation, myocardial contraction is affected by two opposing influences: the tendency of a low-impedance leak to increase myocardial shortening and of impaired myocardial function secondary to prolonged volume overload to reduce it. The important implication of this observation is that values for ejection phase indices in the normal range in patients with severe mitral regurgitation often represent impaired myocardial function and moderately reduced values are usually indicative of much more severe myocardial impairment than are similar values recorded in patients with cardiomyopathy, aortic stenosis, or chronic aortic regurgitation. Many patients with chronic mitral regurgitation, marked left ventricular dilatation, low-normal ejection fraction, and eccentric cardiac hypertrophy manifest progressive worsening of myocardial shortening and lack of regression of hypertrophy after mitral valve replacement presumably as a consequence of the increase in left ventricular afterload with abolition of the regurgitant leak.[104]

Patients with *cardiomyopathy* without clearly abnormal hemodynamic function, i.e., without volume or pressure overload, can be distinguished from normal subjects by the presence of depressed ejection phase indices and lower levels of V_{CE}.[91,92]

In conclusion, the ejection phase indices are more useful than the isovolumetric phase indices for the evaluation of basal levels of contractility. However, unlike the isovolumetric phase indices, the ejection phase indices are exquisitely sensitive to afterload.[44,105]

When a ventricle is stressed by a hemodynamic overload, at first it utilizes all its compensatory mechanisms to maintain normal mechanical performance, and the ejection phase indices are maintained within normal limits. However, when the Frank-Starling mechanism, the development of hypertrophy, and endogenous adrenergic stimulation are all maximally utilized and contractility becomes impaired, an abnormally elevated afterload results in reduced myocardial performance, as reflected in depressed ejection phase indices, a mechanical expression of depressions of contractility, which may occur despite maintenance of a normal cardiac output at rest.[105] With further depressions of contractility, these indices decline more, ultimately resulting in a reduction in stroke volume, a rise in ventricular filling pressure, and the clinical manifestations of heart failure (described in Chap. 15).

ASSESSMENT OF THE VENTRICULAR RESPONSE TO STRESS

A number of approaches have been used to detect mild to moderate left ventricular dysfunction, when the basal

values for left ventricular performance—including the filling pressure, cardiac index, and ventricular stroke and minute work—ejection fraction, and other ejection indices are all within the normal range. In many such patients the cardiovascular response to stress is nonetheless subnormal. The stresses most commonly employed are isotonic exercise, isometric exercise, pacing, and increased afterload.

As pointed out earlier (p. 294), during *dynamic exercise* in the supine posture, the cardiac output normally rises by more than 6 ml/min for each milliliter of increase in oxygen consumption/min;[106] stroke volume and ejection fraction usually rise, and left ventricular end-diastolic pressure at rest is less than 12 mm Hg and rises slightly, remains unchanged, or decreases slightly. With impairment of left ventricular function, however, the left ventricular end-diastolic pressure rises by more than 3 mm Hg, usually to exceed 12 mm Hg, and stroke volume and ejection fraction either remain constant or decline.[107-109] There are various intermediate degrees of impairment between the normal response and that of the failing left ventricle to the stress of isotonic exercise[108,109a] (Figs. 14–19 and 14–20A). When dynamic exercise is carried out in the erect position, end-diastolic volume may rise in normal subjects,[110] and both end-diastolic and end-systolic volumes rise markedly in patients with impaired left ventricular function (Fig. 14–20B). It is important to recognize that the response to exercise is altered by age and physical training. In elderly normal subjects (> 65 years) during upright exercise, ejection fraction declines rather than increases,[111] as it does in normal young subjects. It is possible that stiffening of the arterial system with age results in a greater afterload during exercise and thereby reduces the ejection fraction.[112] Although both untrained and trained healthy young subjects experienced increased ejection fraction during supine exercise, untrained subjects tended to have an increase in end-dia-

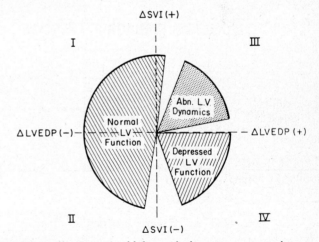

FIGURE 14–19 Patterns of left ventricular response to supine muscular exercise. Normal LV function (quadrants I and II, crosshatched area) includes a variable change in stroke volume, usually an increase, and a fall or no change in LVEDP. Abnormal left ventricular dynamics (quadrant III, stippled area) is associated with an increase in stroke volume index (SVI) and an increase in LVEDP. Depressed LV function (quadrant IV, cross-hatched area) is characterized by no change or a fall in SVI and an increase in LVEDP. The areas between the shaded sectors include responses that cannot be definitively classified. (From Ross, J., Jr., and Braunwald, E.: Left ventricular performance during muscular exercise in patients with and without cardiac dysfunction. Circulation *34*:597, 1966, by permission of the American Heart Association, Inc.)

stolic volume, whereas trained subjects showed decreased end-systolic volume.[113] Obviously, these variations must be kept in mind in interpreting the results of patients with suspected heart disease.

Isometric exercise, usually sustained handgrip,[114] has the advantage over isotonic exercise in that it requires minimal movement of the patient and therefore allows simultaneous measurements, such as phonocardiograms and echocardiograms.[115] It is a simple, convenient test of left ventricular function.[116] The centrally mediated increase in heart rate, arterial pressure, and cardiac output appears to be designed to maintain flow in the compressed vascular bed of skeletal muscle.[117] The normal left ventricle responds to the stress of isometric exercise with little change or a decline in filling pressure and end-diastolic volume, but with an increase in stroke work. In contrast, the ventricle whose function is impaired displays an increase in filling pressure and end-diastolic volume, but little change or an actual fall in stroke work[118,119] (Fig. 14–20B).

The response of stroke volume, stroke work, and ventricular end-diastolic pressure before and during an *increase in left ventricular afterload* induced by the infusion of a pressor agent such as angiotensin is another useful method of evaluating the left ventricle under stress.[120] Whereas the normal left ventricle responds to this stress with little change or even an increase in stroke volume, an increase in stroke work, and a small rise in filling pressure and end-diastolic volume, when left ventricular contractility is impaired, filling pressure rises markedly, but stroke volume falls, whereas stroke work either remains constant or declines (Fig. 14–21).

With *atrial pacing* in normal subjects, cardiac output and arterial pressure remain constant and stroke volume varies inversely with heart rate;[121] both end-diastolic and end-systolic volumes decline, whereas ejection fraction shows little change. In patients with ischemic heart disease, atrial pacing may cause ischemia with an elevation of left ventricular end-diastolic pressure if the tachycardia produces ischemia (Fig. 14–20D).[108]

The left ventricular responses to these various forms of stress are useful not only in detecting the impairment of myocardial functional reserve but also in expressing the se-

RESPONSE OF THE LEFT VENTRICLE TO SUPINE EXERCISE

	ΔEF	ΔEDV	ΔESV	ΔSV
NORMAL CONTROLS	↑	→	↓	↑
CORONARY PATIENTS WITHOUT ANGINA	→	→	→↑	↑→
CORONARY PATIENTS WITH ANGINA	↓	↑→	↑	↓→

A

RESPONSE OF THE LEFT VENTRICLE TO ERECT EXERCISE

	ΔEF	ΔEDV	ΔESV	ΔSV
NORMAL CONTROLS	↑	→↑	↓	→↑
CORONARY PATIENTS WITHOUT ANGINA	→	↑	→↑	→↑
CORONARY PATIENTS WITH ANGINA	↓	↑↑	↑↑	↑→↓

B

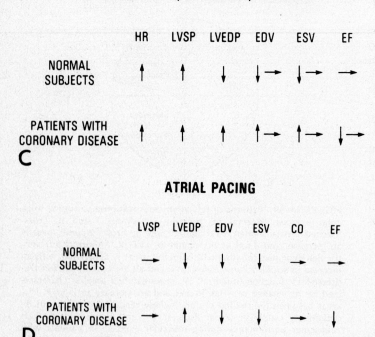

ISOMETRIC (HANDGRIP) EXERCISE

	HR	LVSP	LVEDP	EDV	ESV	EF
NORMAL SUBJECTS	↑	↑	↓	↓→	↓→	→
PATIENTS WITH CORONARY DISEASE	↑	↑	↑	↑→	↑→	↓→

C

ATRIAL PACING

	LVSP	LVEDP	EDV	ESV	CO	EF
NORMAL SUBJECTS	→	↓	↓	↓	→	→
PATIENTS WITH CORONARY DISEASE	→	↑	↓	↓	→	↓

D

FIGURE 14–20 *A*, Response of ejection fraction (EF), end-diastolic volume (EDV), end-systolic volume (ESV), and stroke volume (SV) to supine exercise. ↑ = an increase; → = little change; ↓ = a decrease. *B*, Hemodynamic responses to erect bicycle exercise. Abbreviations and symbols as in *A*. *C*, Hemodynamic responses to handgrip exercise. HR = heart rate; LVEDP = left ventricular end-diastolic pressure; LVSP = left ventricular systolic pressure; other abbreviations and symbols as in *A*. *D*, Hemodynamic response to atrial pacing. CO = cardiac output; other abbreviations and symbols as in *A*. (Reproduced with permission from Slutsky, R.: Response of the left ventricle to stress. Am. J. Cardiol. *47*:357, 1981.)

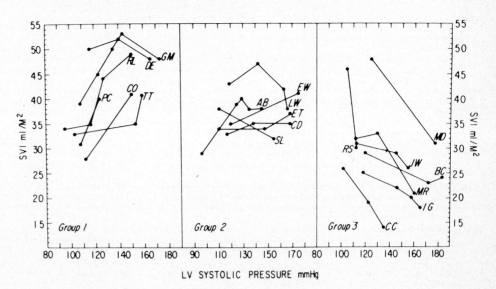

FIGURE 14–21 Relations between elevations of left ventricular (LV) systolic pressure and the stroke volume index (SVI) induced by angiotensin infusion in a group of patients with normal left ventricular function (Group 1), minor left ventricular dysfunction (Group 2), and cardiac dilatation and severe left ventricular dysfunction (Group 3). In each group, substantial and comparable increases in left ventricular end-diastolic pressure also occurred. (From Ross, J., Jr., and Braunwald, E.: A study of left ventricular function in humans by increasing resistance to ventricular ejection with angiotensin. Circulation 29:739, 1964, by permission of the American Heart Association, Inc.)

verity of this impairment quantitatively and for studying the effects of interventions such as drugs on the diseased heart faced with an increased load. Considerable effort is now under way to apply such stresses in a standardized manner by employing noninvasive techniques to evaluate the effects on ventricular performance.

CONCLUSIONS

The isovolumetric phase indices are most useful for measuring *acute directional changes* in contractility. Left ventricular $dP/dt/DP_{40}$ is relatively simple to obtain and has the advantage over maximum dP/dt in that it is relatively independent of the time and level of arterial pressure at the instant of aortic valve opening; it is insensitive to changes in afterload but increases slightly with large changes in preload. Although V_{max}, calculated using developed pressure, is not preload- or afterload-dependent, its determination is beset by many serious theoretical problems, and it appears to have little advantage over V_{pm}, i.e., the maximum $dP/dt/P$ or $dP/dt/DP_{40}$.

Stroke volume and stroke work are useful for detecting acute changes in contractility if they can be related to directional changes in ventricular end-diastolic volume or filling pressure or if they can be determined at various levels of ventricular filling pressure. The ejection phase indices (ejection fraction, fractional shortening of the ventricular circumference or a ventricular dimension, and the mean and peak velocities of circumferential fiber shortening) are responsive to acute changes in contractility and are relatively insensitive to acute changes in preload, but they are markedly influenced by acute alterations in afterload, so that they cannot be used to assess variations in contractility when acute changes in aortic pressure occur. However, the end-systolic pressure-volume (or stress-dimension) relation can be used to assess changes in contractility even when afterload varies, and this relation is preload-independent as well.

A number of invasive and noninvasive approaches appear useful for separating *groups of patients* with normal left ventricular function from those with abnormal function. Of the isovolumetric phase indices, V_{pm} and V_{max} based on total pressure appear to be the most reliable, although considerable overlap exists between individuals in normal and abnormal groups.

Ejection phase indices are capable of detecting depressed contractility in the basal state in individual patients and are clearly preferable to the isovolumetric phase indices for this purpose. End-systolic pressure-volume, stress-dimension, and stress-shortening relations provide a particularly useful approach to assessing basal levels of contractility in individual patients.

Determination of the effect of an acute stress, such as isotonic or isometric exercise, or of pressure overloading by pharmacological means on stroke volume, stroke work, filling pressure, or ejection phase indices may be useful in detecting reductions of myocardial reserve when no abnormality is apparent in the basal state. Noninvasive techniques may be used for assessing left ventricular ejection phase indices and are particularly useful in serial assessments of cardiac performance in individual patients.

References

1. Braunwald, E.: On the difference between the heart's output and its contractile state (Editorial). Circulation 43:171, 1971.
2. Ross, J., Jr.: Cardiac function and myocardial contractility: A perspective. J. Am. Coll. Cardiol. 1:52, 1983.
3. Nichols, W. W., Conti, C. R., Walker, W. E., and Milnor, W. R.: Input impedance of the systemic circulation in man. Circ. Res. 40:451, 1977.
4. Frommer, P. L., Robinson, B. F., and Braunwald, E.: Paired electrical stimulation. A comparison of the effects on performance of the failing and nonfailing heart. Am. J. Cardiol. 18:738, 1966.
5. Starling, E. H.: Linacre Lecture on the Law of the Heart (1915). London, Longmans, 1918.
6. Sarnoff, S. J., and Mitchell, J. H.: Control of function of heart. In Hamilton, W. F., and Dow, P. (eds.): Handbook of Physiology. Section 2. Circulation, Vol. 1. Washington, D.C., American Physiological Society, 1962, pp. 489–532.
7. Suga, H., Sagawa, K., and Demer, L.: Determinants of instantaneous pressure in canine left ventricle: Time and volume specification. Circ. Res. 46:256, 1980.
8. Rackley, C. E., Russell, R. O., Rogers, W. J., Mantle, J. A., McDaniel, H. G., and Papapietro, S. E.: Clinical experience with glucose-insulin-potassium therapy in acute myocardial infarction. Am. Heart J. 102:1038, 1981.
9. Rackley, C. E.: Quantitative evaluation of left ventricular function by radiographic techniques. Circulation 54:862, 1976.
9a. Tobis, J., Nalcioglu, O., Johnston, W. D., Seibert, A., Iseri, L. T., Roeck, W., and Henry, W. L.: Digital aniography in assessment of ventricular function and wall motion during pacing in patients with coronary artery disease. Am. J. Cardiol. 51:668, 1983.
9b. Kronenberg, M. W., Price, R. R., Smith, C. W., Robertson, R. M., Perry, J. M., Pickens, D. R., Domanski, M. J., Partain, C. L., and Friesinger, G. C.: Evaluation of left ventricular performance using digital subtraction angiography. Am. J. Cardiol. 51:837, 1983.
10. Popio, K. A., Gorlin, R., Bechtel, D., and Levine, J. A.: Postextrasystolic po-

tentiation as a predictor of potential myocardial viability: Preoperative analyses compared with studies after coronary bypass surgery. Am. J. Cardiol. 39:944, 1977.

11. Vine, D. L., Hegg, T. D., Dodge, H. T., Stewart, D. K., and Frimer, M.: Immediate effect of contrast medium injection on left ventricular volumes and ejection fraction. Circulation 56:379, 1977.

12. Dodge, H. T., Sheehan, F. H.: Quantitative contrast angiography for assessment of ventricular performance in heart disease. J. Am. Coll. Cardiol. 1:73, 1983.

13. Dodge, H. T., Sandler, H., Baxley, W. A., and Hawley, R. R.: Usefulness and limitations of radiographic methods for determining left ventricular volume. Am. J. Cardiol. 18:10, 1966.

14. Rackley, C. E., and Hood, W. P., Jr.: Quantitative angiographic evaluation and pathophysiological mechanisms in valvular heart disease. Prog. Cardiovasc. Dis. 15:427, 1973.

15. Rackley, C. F., Hood, W. P., and Grossman, W.: Measurements of ventricular volume, mass and ejection fraction. In Grossman, W. (ed.): Cardiac Catheterization and Angiography. 2nd Ed. Philadelphia, Lea and Febiger, 1980, pp. 232–244.

15a. Tortoledo, F. A., Quinones, M. A., Fernandez, G. C., Waggoner, A. D., and Winters, W. L., Jr.: Quantification of left ventricular volumes by two-dimensional echocardiography: A simplified and accurate approach. Circulation 67: 579, 1983.

16. Fortuin, N. J., and Pawsey, C. G. K.: The evaluation of left ventricular function by echocardiography. Am. J. Med. 63:1, 1977.

17. Garrard, G. L., Jr., Weissler, A. M., and Dodge, H. T.: The relationship of alterations in systolic time intervals to ejection fraction in patients with cardiac disease. Circulation 42:455, 1970.

18. Rackley, C. E., Hood, W. P., Jr., Wilcox, B. P., and Peters, R. M.: Quantitation of myocardial function in valvular heart disease. In Brewer, L. A. (ed.): Prosthetic Heart Valves. Springfield, Ill., Charles C Thomas, 1969, p. 342.

19. Davila, J. C., and Sanmarco, M. E.: An analysis of the fit of mathematical models applicable to the measurement of left ventricular volume. Am. J. Cardiol. 18:31, 1966.

20. Herman, H. J., and Bartle, S. H.: Left ventricular volumes by angiocardiography: Comparison of methods and simplification of techniques. Cardiovasc. Res. 4:404, 1968.

21. Dodge, H. T., Hay, R. E., and Sandler, H.: An angiocardiographic method for directly determining left ventricular stroke volume in man. Circ. Res. 11:739, 1962.

22. Wynne, J., Green, L. H., Mann, T., Levin, D., and Grossman, W.: Estimation of left ventricular volumes in man from biplane cineangiograms filmed in oblique projections. Am. J. Cardiol. 41:726, 1978.

23. Sandler, H., and Dodge, H. T.: Angiographic methods for determination of left ventricular geometry and volume. In Mirsky, I., Ghista, D. N., and Sandler, H. (eds.): Cardiac Mechanics: Physiological, Clinical and Mathematical Considerations. New York, John Wiley and Sons, 1974.

24. Graham, T. P., Jr., Atwood, G. F., Faulkner, S. L., and Nelson, J. H.: Right atrial volume measurements from biplane cineangiocardiography. Circulation 49:709, 1974.

25. Dodge, H. T.: Hemodynamic aspects of cardiac failure. In Braunwald, E. (ed.): The Myocardium: Failure and Infarction. New York, H. P. Publishing Co., 1974, pp. 70–79.

26. Sandler, H., and Dodge, H. T.: Left ventricular tension and stress in man. Circ. Res. 13:91, 1963.

27. Mirsky, I.: Elastic properties of the myocardium: A quantitative approach with physiological and clinical applications. In Berne, R. M. (ed.): Handbook of Physiology. Section 2, The Cardiovascular System. Vol. 1, Heart. Bethesda, Md. American Physiological Society, 1979, p. 501.

27a. Lehmann, K. G., Johnson, A. D., and Goldberger, A. L.: Mitral valve E point-septal separation as an index of left ventricular function with valvular heart disease. Chest 83:102, 1983.

28. Peterson, K. L.: Instantaneous force-velocity-length relations of the left ventricle: Methods, limitations and applications in humans. In Fishman, A. P. (ed.): Heart Failure. Washington, D.C., Hemisphere Publishing Co., 1978, pp. 121–132.

29. Smith, M., Russell, R. O., Jr., Feild, B. J., and Rackley, C. E.: Left ventricular compliance and abnormally contracting segments in post–myocardial infarction patients. Chest 65:368, 1974.

30. Herman, M. V., Heinle, R. A., Klein, M. D., and Gorlin, R.: Localized disorders in myocardial contraction: Asynergy and its role in congestive heart failure. N. Engl. J. Med. 277:222, 1967.

31. Dodge, H. T., Stewart, D. K., and Frimer, M.: Implications of shape, stress and wall dynamics in clinical heart disease. In Fishman, A. P. (ed.): Heart Failure. Washington, D.C., Hemisphere Publishing Co., 1978, p. 43.

32. Glover, M. U., Hagan, A. D., Cohen, A., Mazzoleni, A., Schvartzman, M., Warren, S. E., and Vieweg, W. V. R.: Two-dimensional echocardiography in predicting left ventricular wall motion abnormalities and left ventricular function. South. Med. J. 75:313, 1982.

33. Rein, A. J. J. T., Lewis, N., Sapoznikov, D., Gotsman, M. S., and Lewis, B. S.: Quantitation of regional ventricular asynergy using real-time two-dimensional echocardiography. Isr. J. Med. Sci. 18:457, 1982.

34. Tsakiris, A. G., Donald, D. E., Sturm, R. E., and Wood, E. H.: Volume, ejection fraction, and internal dimensions of left ventricle determined by biplane videometry. Fed. Proc. 28:1358, 1969.

35. Stamm, R. B., Carabello, B. A., Mayers, D. L., and Martin, R. P.: Two-dimensional echocardiographic measurement of left ventricular ejection fraction: Prospective analysis of what constitutes an adequate determination. Am. Heart J. 104:136, 1982.

36. Quinones, M. A., Waggoner, A. D., Reduto, L. A., Nelson, J. G., Young, J. B., Winters, W. L., Jr., Ribeiro, L. G., and Miller, R. R.: A new simplified and accurate method for determining ejection fraction with two-dimensional echocardiography. Circulation 64:744, 1981.

37. Peterson, K. L., Sklovan, D., Ludbrook, P., Uther, J. B., and Ross, J., Jr.: Comparison of isovolumic and ejection phase indices of myocardial performance in man. Circulation 49:1088, 1974.

38. Zimpfer, M., and Vatner, S. F.: Effects of acute increases in left ventricular preload on indices of myocardial function in conscious, unrestrained and intact, tranquilized baboons. J. Clin. Invest. 67:430, 1981.

39. Nixon, J. V., Murray, R. G., Leonard, P. D., Mitchell, J. H., and Blomqvist, C. G.: Effect of large variations in preload on left ventricular performance characteristic in normal subjects. Circulation 65:698, 1982.

40. Dodge, H. T., and Baxley, W. A.: Left ventricular volume and mass and their significance in heart disease. Am. J. Cardiol. 23:528, 1969.

41. Braunwald, E., Goldblatt, A., Harrison, D. C., and Mason, D. T.: Studies on cardiac dimensions in intact unanesthetized man. III. Effects of muscular exercise. Circ. Res. 13:460, 1963.

42. Mahler, F., Covell, J. W., O'Rourke, R. A., and Ross, J., Jr.: Effects of acute changes in loading and inotropic state on left ventricular performance and contractility measures in the conscious dog. Am. J. Cardiol. 35:626, 1975.

43. Burns, J. W., Covell, J. W., and Ross, J., Jr.: Mechanics of isotonic left ventricular contractions. Am. J. Physiol. 224:725, 1973.

44. Quinones, M. A., Gaasch, W. H., and Alexander, J. K.: Influence of acute changes in preload, afterload, contractile state and heart rate on ejection and isovolumic indices of myocardial contractility in man. Circulation 53:293, 1976.

45. Grossman, W., Braunwald, E., Mann, T., McLaurin, L. P., and Green, L. H.: Contractile state of the left ventricle in man as evaluated from end-systolic pressure-volume relations. Circulation 56:845, 1977.

46. Frank, O.: Zur Dynamik des Herzmuskels. Zeitschr. Biologie 32:370, 1895.

47. Imperial, E. S., Levy, M. N., and Zieske, H., Jr.: Outflow resistance as an independent determinant of cardiac performance. Circ. Res. 9:1148, 1961.

48. Tsakiris, A. G., Donald, D. E., Sturm, R. E., and Wood, E. H.: Volume, ejection fraction and internal dimensions of the left ventricle determined by biplane videometry. Fed. Proc. 28:1358, 1969.

49. Downing, S. E., and Sonnenblick, E. H.: Cardiac muscle mechanics and ventricular performance. Force and time parameters. Am. J. Physiol. 207:705, 1964.

50. Noble, M. I. M.: Problems concerning the application of concepts of muscle mechanics to the determination of contractile state of the heart. Circulation 45: 252, 1972.

51. Sagawa, K.: The ventricular pressure-volume diagram revisited. Circ. Res. 43: 677, 1978.

52. Taylor, R. R., Covell, J. W., and Ross, J., Jr.: Volume-tension diagrams of ejecting and isovolumic contractions in left ventricle. Am. J. Physiol. 216: 1097, 1969.

53. Suga, H., Katabatake, A., and Sagawa, K.: End-systolic pressure determines stroke volume from fixed end-diastolic volume in the isolated canine left ventricle under a constant contractile state. Circ. Res. 44:238, 1979.

54. Weber, K. T., and Janicki, J. S.: Muscle-pump function of the intact heart. In Fishman, A. P. (ed.): Heart Failure. Washington, D.C., Hemisphere Publishing Co., 1978, pp. 29–42.

55. Mahler, F., Covell, J. W., and Ross, J., Jr.: Systolic pressure-diameter relations in the normal conscious dog. Cardiovasc. Res. 9:447, 1975.

56. Pouleur, H., Rousseau, M. F., van Eyll, C., van Mechelen, H., Brasseur, L. A., and Charlier, A. A.: Assessment of left ventricular contractility from late systolic stress-volume relations. Circulation 65:1204, 1982.

56a. Sunagawa, K., Maughan, W. L., and Sagawa, K.: Effect of regional ischemia on the left ventricular end-systolic pressure-volume relationship of isolated canine hearts. Circ. Res. 52:170, 1983.

57. Ross, J., Jr., and Peterson, K.: On assessment of the cardiac inotropic state. Circulation 47:435, 1973.

58. Mitchell, J. H., Wildenthal, K., and Mullins, C. B.: Geometrical studies of the left ventricle utilizing biplane cinefluorography. Fed. Proc. 28:1334, 1969.

59. Mehmel, H. C., Stockins, B., Ruffmann, K., Olshausen, K. V., Schuler, G., and Kobler, W.: The linearity of the end-systolic pressure-volume relationship in man and its sensitivity for assessment of left ventricular function. Circulation 63:1216, 1981.

60. Carabello, B. A., Nolan, S. P., and McGuire, L. B.: Assessment of preoperative left ventricular function in patients with mitral regurgitation: Value of the end-systolic wall stress–end-systolic volume ratio. Circulation 64:1212, 1981.

61. Reichek, N., Wilson, J., Sutton, M. St.J., Plappert, T. A., Goldberg, S., and Hirshfeld, J. W.: Noninvasive determination of left ventricular end-systolic stress: Validation of the method and initial application. Circulation 65:99, 1982.

62. Sagawa, K.: The end-systolic pressure-volume relation of the ventricle: Definition, modifications and clinical use (Editorial). Circulation 63:1223, 1981.

63. Borow, K. M., Green, L. H., Grossman, W., and Braunwald, E.: Left ventricular end-systolic stress-shortening and stress-length relations in humans. Am. J. Cardiol. 50:1301, 1982.

64. Slutsky, R., Karliner, J., Gerber, K., Battler, A., Froelicher, V., Gregoratos, G., Peterson, K., and Ashburn, W.: Peak systolic blood pressure/end-systolic volume ratio: Assessment at rest and during exercise in normal subjects and patients with coronary heart disease. Am. J. Cardiol. 46:813, 1980.

65. Takahashi, M., Sasayama, S., Kawai, C., and Kotoura, H.: Contractile performance of the hypertrophied ventricle in patients with systemic hypertension. Circulation 62:116, 1980.

66. Watkins, J., Slutsky, R., Tubau, J., and Karliner, J.: Scintigraphic study of relation between left ventricular peak systolic pressure and end-systolic volume in patients with coronary artery disease and normal subjects. Br. Heart J. *48*: 39, 1982.

66a. Iskandrian, A. S., Hakki, A-H., Bemmis, C. E., Kane, S. A., Boston, B., and Amenta, A.: Left ventricular end-systolic pressure-volume relation. A combined radionuclide and hemodynamic study. Am. J. Cardiol. *51*:1057, 1983.

66b. Magorien, D. J., Shaffer, P., Bush, C. A., Magorien, R. D., Kolibash, A. J., Leier, C. V., and Bashore, T. M.: Assessment of left ventricular pressure-volume relations using gated radionuclide angiography, echocardiography, and micromanometer pressure recordings. A new method for serial measurements of systolic and diastolic function in man. Circulation *67*:844, 1983.

67. Rackley, C. E., Russell, R. O., Jr., Mantle, J. A., and Rogers, W. J.: Modern approach to the patient with acute myocardial infarction. Curr. Prob. Cardiol. Vol. 1, No. 10, 1977, 49 pp.

68. Gleason, W. L., and Braunwald, E.: Studies on the first derivative of the ventricular pressure pulse in man. J. Clin. Invest. *41*:80, 1962.

69. Mason, D. T.: Usefulness and limitations of the rate of rise of intraventricular pressure (dp/dt) in the evaluation of myocardial contractility in man. Am. J. Cardiol. *23*:516, 1969.

70. Fry, D. L., Noble, F. W., and Mallos, A. J.: An evaluation of modern pressure recording systems. Circ. Res. *5*:40, 1957.

71. Wallace, A. G., Skinner, N. S., Jr., and Mitchell, J. H.: Hemodynamic determinants of the maximal rate of left ventricular pressure. Am. J. Physiol. *205*: 30, 1963.

72. Furnival, C. M., Linden, R. J., and Snow, H. M.: Inotropic changes in the left ventricle: The effect of changes in heart rate, aortic pressure and end-diastolic pressure. J. Physiol. (Lond.) *211*:359, 1970.

73. Karliner, J. S., Peterson, K. L., and Ross, J., Jr.: Left ventricular myocardial mechanics: Systolic and diastolic function. *In* Grossman, W. (ed.): Cardiac Catheterization and Angiography. 2nd Ed. Philadelphia, Lea and Febiger, 1980, pp. 245–267.

74. Ross, J., Jr., and Sobel, B. E.: Regulation of cardiac contraction. Ann. Rev. Physiol. *34*:47, 1972.

75. Burns, J. W., Covell, J. W., and Ross, J., Jr.: Mechanics of isotonic left ventricular contractions. Am. J. Physiol. *224*:725, 1973.

76. Yeatman, L. A., Jr., Parmley, W. W., Urschel, C. W., and Sonnenblick, E. H.: Dynamics of contractile elements in isometric contractions of cardiac muscle. Am. J. Physiol. *220*:534, 1971.

77. Ross, J., Jr., Covell, J. W., Sonnenblick, E. H., and Braunwald, E.: Contractile state of heart characterized by force-velocity relations in variably afterloaded and isovolumic beats. Circ. Res. *18*:149, 1966.

78. Hugenholtz, P. G., Ellison, R. C., Urschel, C. W., Mirsky, I., and Sonnenblick, E. H.: Myocardial force-velocity relationships in clinical heart disease. Circulation *41*:191, 1970.

79. Mirsky, I., and Parmley, W. W.: Force-velocity studies in isolated and intact heart muscle. *In* Mirsky, I., Ghista, D. N., and Sandler, H. (eds.): Cardiac Mechanics: Physiological, Clinical and Mathematical Considerations. New York, John Wiley and Sons, 1974, pp. 87–112.

80. Wolk, M. J., Keefe, J. F., Bing, O. H. L., Finkelstein, L. J., and Levine, H. J.: Estimation of V_{max} in auxotonic systoles from the rate of relative increase of isovolumic pressures: (dP/dt)dP. J. Clin. Invest. *50*:1276, 1971.

81. Grossman, W., Haynes, F., Paraskos, J. A., Saltz, S., Dalen, J. E., and Dexter, L.: Alterations in preload and myocardial mechanics in the dog and in man. Circ. Res. *31*:83, 1972.

82. Van Den Box, G. C., Elzinga, G., Westerhof, N., and Noble, M. I. M.: Problems in the use of indices of myocardial contractility. Cardiovasc. Res. *7*:834, 1973.

83. Mason, D. T., Braunwald, E., Covell, J. W., Sonnenblick, E. H., and Ross, J., Jr.: Assessment of cardiac contractility: The relation between the rate of pressure rise and ventricular pressure during isovolumic systole. Circulation *44*:47, 1971.

84. Davidson, D. M., Covell, J. W., Malloch, C. I., and Ross, J., Jr.: Factors influencing indices of left ventricular contractility in the conscious dog. Cardiovasc. Res. *8*:299, 1974.

85. Mehmel, H., Krayenbuehl, H. P., and Rutishauser, W.: Peak measured velocity of shortening in the canine left ventricle. J. Appl. Physiol. *29*:637, 1970.

86. Nejad, N. S., Klein, M. D., Mirsky, I., and Lown, B.: Assessment of myocardial contractility from ventricular pressure recordings. Cardiovasc. Res. *5*:15, 1971.

87. Gault, J. H., Ross, J., Jr., and Braunwald, E.: The contractile state of the left ventricle in man: Instantaneous tension-velocity-length relations in patients with and without disease of the left ventricular myocardium. Circ. Res. *22*: 451, 1968.

88. Peterson, K. L., Uther, J. B., Shabetai, R., and Braunwald, E.: Assessment of left ventricular performance in man: Instantaneous tension-velocity-length relations obtained with the aid of an electromagnetic velocity catheter in the ascending aorta. Circulation *47*:924, 1973.

89. Ross, J., Jr.: The assessment of myocardial performance in man by hemodynamic and cineangiographic techniques. Am. J. Cardiol. *23*:511, 1969.

90. Braunwald, E., and Ross, J., Jr.: The ventricular end-diastolic pressure. An appraisal of its value in the recognition of ventricular failure in man (Editorial). Am. J. Med. *34*:147, 1963.

91. Glick, G., Sonnenblick, E. H., and Braunwald, E.: Myocardial force-velocity relations studied in intact unanesthetized man. J. Clin. Invest. *44*:978, 1965.

92. Peterson, K. L., Sklovan, D., Ludbrook, P., Uther, J. B., and Ross, J., Jr.: Comparison of isovolumic and ejection phase indices of myocardial performance in man. Circulation *49*:1088, 1974.

93. Gould, K. L.: Analysis of wall dynamics and directional components of left ventricular contraction in man. Am. J. Cardiol. *38*:322, 1976.

94. Karliner, J. S., Gault, J. H., Eckberg, D. L., Mullins, C. B., and Ross, J., Jr.: Mean velocity of fiber shortening: A simplified measure of left ventricular myocardial contractility. Circulation *44*:323, 1971.

95. Ross, J., Jr., and McCullagh, W. H.: The nature of enhanced performance of the dilated left ventricle during chronic volume overloading. Circ. Res. *30*:549, 1972.

96. Sasayama, S., Theroux, P., Romero, M., Bishop, S., Bloor, C., Franklin, D., and Ross, J., Jr.: Adaptations of the left ventricle to chronic pressure overload. Am. J. Cardiol. *35*:167, 1975.

97. Carabello, B. A., Mee, R., Collins, J. J., Jr., Kloner, R. A., Levin, D., and Grossman, W.: Experimental model for chronic gradually developing subcoronary aortic stenosis in the dog: Evidence for normal contractile function in hypertrophied hearts. (To be published.)

98. Gault, J. H., Covell, J. W., Braunwald, E., and Ross, J., Jr.: Left ventricular performance following correction of the free aortic regurgitation. Circulation *42*:773, 1970.

99. Carabello, B. A., Green, L. H., Grossman, W., Cohn, L. H., Koster, J. K., and Collins, J. J., Jr.: Hemodynamic determinants of prognosis of aortic valve replacement in critical aortic stenosis and advanced congestive heart failure. Circulation *62*:42, 1980.

100. Urschel, C. W., Covell, J. W., Sonnenblick, E. H., Ross, J., Jr., and Braunwald, E.: Myocardial mechanics in aortic and mitral valvular regurgitation: The concept of instantaneous impedance as a determinant of the performance of the intact heart. J. Clin. Invest. *47*:867, 1968.

101. Ross, J., Jr.: Left ventricular function and the timing of surgical treatment in valvular heart disease. Ann. Intern. Med. *94*:498, 1981.

102. McDonald, I. G.: Echocardiographic assessment of left ventricular function in mitral valve disease. Circulation *53*:865, 1976.

103. Vokonas, P. S., Gorlin, R., Cohn, P. F., Herman, M. V., and Sonnenblick, E. H.: Dynamic geometry of the left ventricle in mitral regurgitation. Circulation *48*:786, 1973.

104. Schuler, G., Peterson, K. L., Johnson, A., Francis, G., Dennosh, G., Utley, J., Daily, P., Ashburn, W., and Ross, J., Jr.: Temporal response of left ventricular performance to mitral valve surgery. Circulation *59*:1218, 1979.

105. Ross, J., Jr.: Afterload mismatch and preload reserve: A conceptual framework for the analysis of ventricular function. Prog. Cardiovasc. Dis. *18*:255, 1976.

106. Grossman, W., and McLaurin, L. P.: Dynamic and isometric exercise during cardiac catheterization. *In* Grossman, W. (ed.): Cardiac Catheterization and Angiography. 2nd Ed. Philadelphia, Lea and Febiger, 1980, pp. 215–222.

107. Ross, J., Jr., Gault, J. H., Mason, D. T., Linhart, J. W., and Braunwald, E.: Left ventricular performance during muscular exercise in patients with and without cardiac dysfunction. Circulation *34*:597, 1966.

108. Slutsky, R.: Response of the left ventricle to stress: Effects of exercise, atrial pacing, afterload stress and drugs. Am. J. Cardiol. *47*:357, 1981.

109. Gelberg, H. J., Rubin, S. A., Ports, T. A., Brundage, B. H., Parmley, W. W., and Chatterjee, K.: Detection of left ventricular functional reserve by supine exercise hemodynamics in patients with severe, chronic heart failure. Am. J. Cardiol. *44*:1062, 1979.

109a. Boucher, C. A., Wilson, R. A., Kanarek, D. J., Hutter, A. M., Jr., Okada, R. D., Libethson, R. R., Strauss, H. W., and Pohost, G. M.: Exercise testing in asymptomatic or minimally symptomatic aortic regurgitation: Relationship of left ventricular ejection fraction to left ventricular filling pressure during exercise. Circulation *67*:1091, 1983.

110. Upton, M. T., Rerych, S. K., Roeback, J. R., Jr., Newman, G. E., Douglas, J. M., Jr., Wallace, A. G., and Jones, R. H.: Effect of brief and prolonged exercise on left ventricular function. Am. J. Cardiol. *45*:1154, 1980.

111. Port, S., Cobb, F. R., Coleman, R. E., and Jones, R. H.: Effect of age on the response of the left ventricular ejection fraction to exercise. N. Engl. J. Med. *303*:1133, 1980.

112. Yin, F. C. P., Weisfeldt, M. L., and Milnor, W. R.: Role of aortic input impedance in the decreased cardiovascular response to exercise with aging in dogs. J. Clin. Invest. *68*:28, 1981.

113. Bar-Shlomo, B.-Z., Druck, M. N., Morch, J. E., Jablonsky, G., Hilton, J. D., Feiglin, D. H. I., and McLaughlin, P. R.: Left ventricular function in trained and untrained healthy subjects. Circulation *65*:484, 1982.

114. Donald, K. W., Lind, A., McNicol, G. W., Humphreys, P. W., Taylor, S. H., and Staunton, H. P.: Cardiovascular responses to sustained (static) contractions. Circ. Res. *21* (Suppl. 1):15, 1967.

115. Corya, B. C., and Rasmussen, S.: Assessing left ventricular function with intervention echocardiography. J. Cardiovasc. Med. *6*:574, 1981.

116. Amende, I., Krayenbuehl, H. P., Rutishauser, W., and Wirz, D.: Left ventricular dynamics during handgrip. Br. Heart J. *34*:688, 1972.

117. Awan, N., Vismara, L. N., Miller, R. R., DeMaria, A. N., and Mason, D. T.: Effects of isometric exercise and increased arterial impedance on left ventricular function in severe aortic valvular stenosis. Br. Heart J. *39*:651, 1977.

118. Helfant, R. H., deVilla, M., and Meister, S. G.: Effect of sustained isometric handgrip exercise on left ventricular performance. Circulation *44*:982, 1971.

119. Kivowitz, C., Parmley, W. W., Donoso, R., Marcus, H., Ganz, W., and Swan, H. J. C.: Effects of isometric exercise on left cardiac performance: The grip test. Circulation *44*:994, 1971.

120. Ross, J., Jr., and Braunwald, E.: A study of left ventricular function in man by increasing resistance to ventricular ejection with angiotensin. Circulation *29*: 739, 1964.

121. Parker, J. D.: Atrial pacing: Pacing ventricular function curves. *In* Grossman, W. (ed.): Cardiac Catheterization and Angiography, 2nd Ed. Philadelphia, Lea and Febiger, 1980, pp. 223–231.

15
CLINICAL MANIFESTATIONS OF HEART FAILURE

by Eugene Braunwald, M.D.

It is impossible thoughtfully to survey, in the light of early experience, the field of medical work covering diseases of the heart without realizing the central problem to be failure of the heart to accomplish its work in lesser or greater degree. . . . The very essence of cardiovascular practice is recognition of early heart failure and discrimination between different grades of failure. . . . When a patient seeks advice and heart disease is suspected, or is known to be present, two questions are of chief importance. Firstly, has the heart the capacity to do the work demanded of it when the body is at rest? Secondly, what is the condition of the heart's reserve? These questions can be correctly answered in almost all cases by simple interrogations and by bedside signs.

In this, the opening paragraph of his classic text *Diseases of the Heart*, published in 1933, Sir Thomas Lewis identified the diagnosis and assessment of heart failure as the cardinal problem in clinical cardiology.[1] Now, a half century later, the situation has changed little, in that a principal complication of virtually all forms of heart disease is heart failure, defined as the pathophysiological state in which an abnormality of cardiac function is responsible for the failure of the heart to pump blood at a rate commensurate with the requirements of the metabolizing tissues (p. 447). Included in this definition is a wide spectrum of clinical-physiological states, ranging from the rapid impairment of pumping function, occurring when a massive myocardial infarction or tachy- or bradyarrhythmia develops suddenly, to the gradual impairment of myocardial function, observed only during stress and occurring in a patient whose heart sustains a pressure or volume overload for a prolonged period.[2]

The clinical manifestations of heart failure vary enormously and depend on a variety of factors, including the age of the patient, the extent and rate of development of the impairment of cardiac performance, the etiology of the heart disease, the precipitating causes of heart failure, and the specific chambers involved in the disease process.[3]

FORMS OF HEART FAILURE
Forward vs. Backward Heart Failure

The clinical manifestations of heart failure arise as a consequence of inadequate cardiac output and/or damming up of blood behind one or both ventricles. These two principal mechanisms are the basis of the so-called forward and backward pressure theories of heart failure. The *backward failure hypothesis*, first proposed in 1832 by James Hope, indicates that when the ventricle fails to discharge its contents, blood accumulates and pressure rises in the atrium and the venous system emptying into it.[4] There is substantial physiological evidence in favor of this theory. As discussed on page 475, the inability of cardiac muscle to shorten against a load alters the relationship between ventricular end-systolic pressure and volume, so that residual volume rises. The following sequence of adaptations then occurs that at first tends to maintain normal cardiac output: (1) Ventricular end-diastolic volume and pressure increase; (2) the volume and pressure rise in the atrium behind the failing ventricle; (3) the atrium contracts more vigorously (a manifestation of Starling's Law of the Atrium);[5] (4) the pressure rises in the venous bed behind (upstream to) the failing ventricle; (5) the capillary pressure upstream to the failing ventricle rises; (6) transudation of fluid from the capillary bed into the interstitial space (pulmonary or systemic) rises; and (7) extracellular fluid volume increases. Many of the symptoms characteristic of heart failure result from this sequence of events and the subsequent increase in fluid in the interstitial spaces of the lungs, liver, subcutaneous tissues, and serous cavities.

Cardiac output in the basal state is a relatively *insensitive* index of cardiac function. (p. 469). In many patients a portion of or, indeed, the entire sequence of events outlined above may be well established while cardiac output *at rest* is still within normal limits. Indeed, the backward pressure theory of heart failure reflects one of the principal compensatory mechanisms in heart failure, i.e., the operation of Starling's Law of the Heart,[6] in which distention of the ventricle helps to maintain cardiac output. The failing ventricle operates on an ascending, albeit depressed and flattened, function curve[7] (Figure 13–17, p. 463), and the augmented ventricular end-diastolic volume and pressure characteristic of heart failure must be regarded as aiding in the maintenance of cardiac output. When this compensatory mechanism is interfered with (e.g., by means of dietary sodium restriction and treatment with diuretics), there may be clinical improvement due to loss of extracellular fluid volume, with its accompanying reduction in tissue congestion, but at the same time cardiac output may decline,[8] and the symptoms secondary to a reduction of cardiac output may actually intensify. Thus, although many of the clinical manifestations of heart failure are secondary to excessive retention of fluid, the elevation of preload constitutes an important compensatory mechanism.

Hope's backward pressure theory of cardiac failure incorporates the concept that the cardiac chambers may fail independently and that an imbalance in performance of the ventricles may result. If one considers, for simplicity, the development of left ventricular failure consequent to aortic stenosis or of right ventricular failure secondary to pulmonic stenosis, the initial clinical manifestations of each relate primarily to the damming up of blood behind the affected ventricle. An important extension of the backward failure theory is the sequential development of right ventricular failure as a consequence of left ventricular failure (Fig. 15–1). According to this concept, the elevation of left ventricular diastolic, left atrial, and pulmonary venous pressures results in backward transmission of pressure and leads to pulmonary hypertension, which ultimately causes right ventricular failure. Often, pulmonary vasoconstriction plays a part in this form of pulmonary hypertension as well (p. 828).

Eighty years after publication of Hope's work, Mackenzie proposed the *forward failure hypothesis*, which relates clinical manifestations of heart failure to inadequate delivery of blood into the arterial system.[9] According to this hypothesis, the principal clinical manifestations of heart failure are due to reduced cardiac output, which results in diminished perfusion of vital organs, including the brain, leading to mental confusion; skeletal muscles, leading to weakness; and kidneys, leading to sodium and water retention through a series of complex mechanisms (Chap. 52). This renal effect, in turn, augments extracellular fluid volume and ultimately leads to symptoms due to congestion of organs and tissues. The heart then fails "as a whole," since there can be no imbalance between the output of the two ventricles in the steady state.

Although these two seemingly opposing views concerning the pathogenesis of heart failure led to lively controversy during the first half of this century, it no longer seems fruitful to make a rigid distinction between backward and forward heart failure, since both mechanisms operate in the majority of patients with *chronic* heart failure. Exceptions may occur, however, and some patients, particularly those with *acute* decompensation, develop relatively pure forms of forward or backward failure. An example of relatively pure forward failure occurs in the patient with acute right ventricular failure secondary to massive pulmonary embolism in whom shock—perhaps even death—due to inadequate cardiac output may ensue within minutes or hours. Although right ventricular diastolic pressure and volume and right atrial and systemic venous pressure all rise markedly, the patient may succumb before sufficient extracellular fluid has accumulated to produce symptoms of systemic venous congestion. This presentation may be contrasted with that of the patient who develops chronic cor pulmonale as a result of multiple pulmonary emboli and gradually rising pressures in the pulmonary artery, right side of the heart, and systemic venous bed. Cardiac

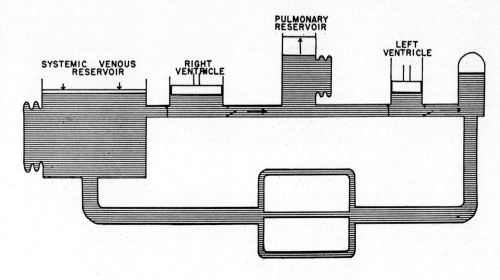

FIGURE 15–1 Diagram of the circulation explaining the etiology of pulmonary congestion. Since the capacity of the systemic venous reservoir is much larger than that of the pulmonary venous reservoir, transfer of small quantities of blood from the systemic circulation would produce a relatively large increase in pulmonary vascular volume and pressure. A slight imbalance in output between the right and left ventricles could produce significant pulmonary congestion. A sustained increase in left ventricular filling pressure could produce chronic pulmonary congestion without appreciable increase in total blood volume. (From Rushmer, R. F.: Cardiac compensation, hypertrophy and myopathy and congestive heart failure. *In* Rushmer, R. F. [ed.]: Cardiovascular Dynamics. Philadelphia, W. B. Saunders Co., 1976, p. 532.)

output and perfusion of the renal bed may be normal, at least in the resting state, but abnormal retention of extracellular fluid volume, with congestive hepatomegaly, ankle edema, and ascites, may occur. Such a patient manifests relatively pure backward failure.

Similar considerations apply to disorders affecting the left ventricle. For instance, a massive myocardial infarction may result in either (1) forward failure with a marked reduction of left ventricular output and cardiogenic shock (p. 591) and clinical manifestations secondary to impaired perfusion (hypotension, mental confusion, oliguria, and so on) or (2) backward failure with a transient inequality of output between the two ventricles, resulting in acute pulmonary edema. More commonly, patients with large myocardial infarctions develop a combination of forward and backward failure, with symptoms resulting from both inadequate cardiac output and pulmonary congestion. Early in the course of acute myocardial infarction, patients might succumb to these forms of heart failure long before renal retention of salt and water can occur. However, if the patient survives the acute insult, expansion of the extracellular fluid volume and manifestations resulting therefrom usually occur.

The relative importance of forward and backward failure in the genesis of clinical manifestations of heart failure also depends on the specific anatomical abnormality. For instance, in conditions involving interference with filling of the right side of the heart, i.e., tricuspid stenosis or constrictive pericarditis, systemic venous pressure is markedly elevated; one can readily appreciate how this leads to systemic venous congestion, capillary transudation, hepatomegaly, edema, and ascites, i.e., to backward heart failure. Patients with chronic left ventricular failure secondary to coronary artery disease or hypertension may exhibit marked accumulation of sodium and water in the systemic venous bed with no or only minimal elevation of systemic venous pressure. In these patients, accumulation of fluid is largely due to impairment of renal perfusion, i.e., forward heart failure accompanied by excessive renal tubular sodium reabsorption.

There is general agreement that fluid retention in heart failure (Figure 52-3, p. 175) is due in part to reduction in glomerular filtration rate and in part to activation of the renin-angiotensin-aldosterone system.[10] Reduced cardiac output is associated with a lowered glomerular filtration rate and an increased elaboration of renin, which, through the activation of angiotensin, results in the release of aldosterone. The combination of impaired hepatic function due to hepatic venous congestion and reduced hepatic blood flow interferes with the metabolism of aldosterone,[11,12] further raising its plasma concentration and augmenting the retention of sodium and water.

Right-sided vs. Left-sided Heart Failure

Implicit in the backward failure theory is the idea that fluid localizes behind the specific cardiac chamber that is initially affected. Thus, symptoms secondary to pulmonary congestion initially predominate in patients with left ventricular infarction, hypertension, and aortic and mitral valve disease, i.e., they manifest *left heart failure*. With time, however, fluid accumulation becomes generalized, and ankle edema, congestive hepatomegaly, ascites, and

pleural effusion occur, i.e., the patients later exhibit *right heart failure* as well. Less commonly, prolonged right ventricular failure with massive accumulation of extracellular fluid may be associated with dyspnea, particularly when the patient is in the supine position and when large pleural effusions are present.

Although a disturbance of contractile function initially takes place in the ventricle subjected to the abnormal burden, with the passage of time the other ventricle undergoes changes as well. For example, the depletion of norepinephrine that occurs in experimental animals subjected to ventricular pressure overload is not confined to the stressed ventricle, but also involves the opposite ventricle[13,14] (Figure 13-12, p. 459). Similarly, alterations in the activity of actomyosin ATPase have been observed in both ventricles of animals in which the hemodynamic burden was placed on only one.[15] These findings are not suprising when one considers that both ventricles share a common wall—the interventricular septum—and that the muscle bundles constituting the ventricles are continuous. Thus, specific lesions that place an abnormal load on only one ventricle may eventually be responsible for failure of the heart as a whole.

Acute vs. Chronic Heart Failure

As has already been pointed out, the clinical manifestations of heart failure depend importantly on how rapidly the syndrome develops and specifically on whether sufficient time has elapsed for compensatory mechanisms to become operative and for fluid to accumulate in the interstitial space. For example, when a previously normal person suddenly develops a serious anatomical or functional abnormality of the heart (such as massive myocardial infarction, heart block with a very slow ventricular rate [<40/min], a tachyarrhythmia with a very rapid rate [>180/min], rupture of a valve secondary to infective endocarditis, or occlusion of a large segment of the pulmonary vascular bed by a pulmonary embolus), either a marked, sudden reduction in cardiac output with symptoms due to inadequate organ perfusion and/or acute congestion of the venous bed behind the affected ventricle will occur. If the same anatomical abnormality develops gradually, a host of compensatory mechanisms, especially cardiac hypertrophy, will allow the patient to adjust to and tolerate not only the anatomical abnormality but also a reduction in cardiac output, with less difficulty. Frequently, the clinical manifestations of chronic heart failure are suppressed by treatment. Under these circumstances, an acute event such as an infection, an arrhythmia, or discontinuation of therapy may precipitate manifestations of acute heart failure.

Low-output vs. High-output Heart Failure

Low cardiac output characterizes heart failure occurring in most forms of heart disease, i.e., congenital, valvular, rheumatic, hypertensive, coronary, and cardiomyopathic. A variety of high-output states, including thyrotoxicosis, arteriovenous fistula, beriberi, Paget's disease of bone, anemia, and pregnancy (described in detail in Chap. 24), lead to heart failure as well. Low-output heart failure is characterized by clinical evidence of impairment of the peripheral circulation, with peripheral vasoconstriction and cold, pale, and sometimes cyanotic extremities; in late stages, as the stroke volume declines, the pulse pressure narrows. In contrast, in high-output heart failure the extremities are usually warm and flushed, and the pulse pressure is widened or at least normal. The ability of the heart to deliver the quantity of oxygen required by the metabolizing tissues is reflected in the arterial–mixed venous oxygen difference, which is abnormally widened (i.e., > 5.0 ml/dl in the basal state) in patients with low-output heart failure but is normal or even reduced in high-output states, owing to elevation of the mixed venous oxygen saturation by the admixture of blood that has been shunted away from metabolizing tissues. However, the arterial–mixed venous oxygen difference still exceeds the level that existed *prior* to the development of heart failure, and cardiac output, though frequently elevated in absolute terms, is lower than it had been before the development of heart failure.

Heart Failure in the Neonate and Infant

Heart failure in the neonate or infant has a different clinical expression from that in the older child or adult[16] (Table 29–4, p. 948). Feeding difficulties, failure to gain weight and grow, tachypnea, and excessive diaphoresis are manifestations of heart failure occurring in the first year of life. Obstruction of the airways due to enlargement of the left atrium and main pulmonary artery may result in either emphysematous expansion of the left lung or, in more severe cases, atelectasis. Excessive sweating and repeated pulmonary infections are common features of heart failure in infants. Tachypnea accompanies a reduction in tidal volume, which is secondary to the presence of interstitial pulmonary edema. Respiratory distress is manifested by flaring of the alae nasi, grunting, and retraction of the ribs, features rarely seen in adults. Peripheral perfusion is poor, with cool limbs and delayed capillary filling. Hepatomegaly is a common manifestation of both left and right heart failure in infants, as is a paradoxical pulse secondary to wide variations in ventricular filling as a consequence of marked swings in intrapulmonary pressure. Peripheral edema, ascites, and pulsus alternans occur far less frequently in infants than in older children or adults with heart failure. On the other hand, facial edema, an uncommon finding in adults, is more common than peripheral edema in infants.

Because of the short neck of infants, distention of the jugular veins is difficult to detect. However, prominence of the veins on the back of the hand is a valuable sign of systemic venous congestion. Although most neonates and infants with cardiac failure have heart disease that is obvious on clinical examination, it is sometimes difficult to distinguish respiratory distress arising from cardiac disease from that associated with primary pulmonary disorders. Specifically, heart failure may be confused with bronchiolitis, asthma, or pneumonia. The presence of cyanosis and heart murmurs on physical examination and of cardiomegaly and pulmonary congestion on radiological examination are helpful though not decisive signs in the differential diagnosis.

CAUSES OF HEART FAILURE

It is useful to divide the causes of heart failure into three separate categories: (1) *underlying causes*, comprising the structural abnormalities—congenital or acquired—that affect the peripheral and coronary vessels, pericardium, myocardium, or cardiac valves and lead to the increased hemodynamic burden or myocardial or coronary insufficiency responsible for heart failure; (2) *fundamental causes*, comprising the biochemical and physiological mechanisms through which either an increased hemodynamic burden or a reduction in oxygen delivery to the myocardium results in impairment of myocardial contraction (Chap. 13); and (3) *precipitating causes*, comprising the specific causes or incidents that precipitate heart failure in approximately 50 per cent of episodes of clinical heart failure.[17]

It is helpful to recognize both the underlying and the precipitating causes of heart failure. Appropriate management of the underlying heart disease (e.g., surgical correction of a congenital heart defect or of an acquired valvular abnormality or pharmacological management of hypertension) may prevent the development or recurrence of heart failure. Similarly, treatment of the precipitating cause will usually rapidly terminate an episode of heart failure and may be life-saving.

Overt heart failure may, of course, also be precipitated if there is progression of the underlying heart disease. A previously stable, compensated patient may develop heart failure that is apparent clinically for the first time when the intrinsic process has advanced to a critical point, such as with progressive obliteration of the pulmonary vascular bed in a patient with cor pulmonale or further narrowing of a stenotic aortic valve. Alternatively, decompensation may occur as a result of failure or exhaustion of the compensatory mechanisms but without any change in the volume load on the heart.

Precipitating Causes of Heart Failure

Inappropriate Reduction of Therapy. Perhaps the most common cause of decompensation in a previously compensated patient with heart failure is inappropriate relaxation in the intensity of treatment—be it dietary sodium restriction, reduced physical activity, a drug regimen, or, most commonly, a combination of these measures. Many patients with serious underlying heart disease, regardless of whether they previously experienced heart failure, may be relatively asymptomatic for as long as they carefully adhere to their treatment regimen. However, without proper instruction, the patient who has become asymptomatic may incorrectly assume that his underlying condition has been cured and may voluntarily diminish the intensity of therapy, precipitating a bout of congestive heart failure. Perhaps the most serious example of this situation is the patient who adjusts his digitalis dosage on the basis of symptoms, discontinuing the drug when there are no symptoms of heart failure but taking three, four, or even more times the maintenance dose when symptoms of heart failure are present. Obviously, this practice can lead to wide variations in digitalis levels, exacerbation of heart failure, and digitalis intoxication.

Dietary excesses of sodium, incurred particularly on vacations or holidays or during an illness of the spouse responsible for preparing the patient's meals, are related frequent causes of sudden cardiac decompensation.

Arrhythmias (see also Chap. 21). Cardiac arrhythmias are far more common in patients with underlying structural heart disease than in normal subjects and commonly precipitate or intensify heart failure. Arrhythmias impair cardiac function through several mechanisms. (1) *Tachyarrhythmias* reduce the time available for ventricular filling, When there is already an impairment of ventricular filling, as in mitral stenosis or ventricular hypertrophy, tachycardia will raise left atrial pressure and reduce cardiac output further. In addition, tachyarrhythmias increase myocardial oxygen demands and, in a patient with obstructive coronary artery disease, may induce or intensify myocardial ischemia, which, in turn, impairs both cardiac relaxation and systolic function, thereby raising left atrial pressure further and causing symptoms secondary to pulmonary congestion. (2) *Marked bradycardia* in a patient with underlying heart disease usually depresses cardiac output, since stroke volume may already be maximal and cannot rise further to maintain cardiac output. (3) *Dissociation between atrial and ventricular contraction*, which occurs in many arrhythmias, results in loss of the atrial booster pump mechanism, which impairs ventricular filling, lowers cardiac output, and raises atrial pressure.[18] This loss is particularly deleterious in patients with impaired ventricular filling due to concentric cardiac hypertrophy, e.g., in systemic hypertension, aortic stenosis, and hypertrophic obstructive cardiomyopathy. (4) *Abnormal intraventricular conduction*, which occurs in many arrhythmias such as ventricular tachycardia, impairs myocardial performance because of loss of the normal synchronicity of ventricular contraction.

Systemic Infection. Although patients with congestive heart failure are particularly susceptible to pulmonary infections, *any* infection may precipitate cardiac failure. The mechanisms include increased total metabolism as a consequence of fever, discomfort, and cough, which increase the hemodynamic burden on the heart; the accompanying sinus tachycardia, secondary to fever and discomfort, plays an additional adverse role.

Pulmonary Embolism. Patients with congestive heart failure, particularly when confined to bed, are at high risk of developing pulmonary emboli, which may increase the hemodynamic burden on the right ventricle by elevating right ventricular systolic pressure further and may cause fever, tachypnea, and tachycardia, the deleterious effects of which have already been discussed.

Physical, Environmental, and Emotional Excesses. Intense, prolonged exertion or severe fatigue, such as may result from prolonged travel or emotional crises, and a severe climatic change, such as to a hot, humid environment, are relatively common precipitants of cardiac decompensation.

Cardiac Infection and Inflammation. Myocarditis due to a recurrence of acute rheumatic fever (p. 1646) or to infective endocarditis (p. 1152) or as a consequence of a variety of allergic inflammatory or infectious processes (including viral myocarditis) (p. 1432) may impair myocardial function directly and exacerbate existing heart disease. The anemia and tachycardia that accompany these processes are also deleterious. In patients with infective endocarditis, additional valvular damage may also precipitate cardiac decompensation.

High-Output States. As indicated in Chapter 24, anemia, thyrotoxicosis, or pregnancy and other high-output states by themselves rarely, if ever, produce heart failure; however, the development of these conditions in the presence of underlying heart disease often precipitates heart failure. In these states the requirements of the peripheral tissues for oxygen can be satisfied only by an increase in cardiac output. Although the normal heart is capable of augmenting its output, this may not be true of the diseased heart. Thus, acute heart failure may be precipitated in patients with underlying heart disease who develop one of the hyperkinetic circulatory states.

Development of an Unrelated Illness. Heart failure may be precipitated in patients with compensated heart disease when an unrelated illness develops. For example, renal failure may further impair the ability of patients with heart failure to excrete sodium and thus may intensify the accumulation of fluid. Similarly, blood transfusion or the administration of sodium-containing fluid in the postoperative state may result in sudden heart failure in patients with underlying heart disease. Prostatic obstruction in the elderly male, parenchymal liver disease, and administration of corticosteroids or estrogens with sodium-retaining properties may also precipitate heart failure in patients with underlying heart disease.

Administration of a Cardiac Depressant or Salt-Retaining Drug. A variety of drugs depress cardiac function; these include alcohol, beta-adrenergic blocking agents, disopyramide (p. 659), and antineoplastic drugs such as adriamycin and cyclophosphamide (p. 1690). Others, such as estrogens, androgens, glucocorticoids, and nonsteroidal antiinflammatory agents, may cause salt and water retention. Any of these drugs, when administered to a patient with heart disease, can precipitate or aggravate heart failure.

Development of a Second Form of Heart Disease. Patients with one form of heart disease often remain compensated until they develop a second form of heart disease. For example, a patient with chronic hypertension and left ventricular hypertrophy but without left ventricular failure may be asymptomatic until a myocardial infarction develops (which may be silent) and precipitates sudden heart failure.

It is essential to make a careful and systematic search for one or more of these precipitating causes in all patients with congestive heart failure, since lack of recognition or treatment or both may be responsible for otherwise refractory heart failure. In most instances these precipitating causes can be treated effectively, after which appropriate measures should be instituted to avoid any recurrence. When a precipitating cause of heart failure can be identified, it generally signifies a better prognosis than when a similar degree of heart failure is due simply to progression of the underlying cardiac disease.

SYMPTOMS OF HEART FAILURE

Respiratory Distress

Breathlessness, a cardinal manifestation of left ventricular failure, may present with progressively increasing severity as (1) exertional dyspnea, (2) orthopnea, (3) paroxysmal nocturnal dyspnea, (4) dyspnea at rest, and (5) acute pulmonary edema.

Dyspnea (see also p. 1789). The principal difference between exertional dyspnea in normal subjects and in cardiac patients is the degree of activity necessary to induce the symptom. Indeed, at first, exertional dyspnea may simply represent an aggravation of the breathlessness that occurs in normal subjects during activity. Patients usually report that a specific task which they were able to carry out without difficulty for many years, e.g., climbing three flights of stairs, evokes more breathlessness than previously or requires them to stop briefly midway or both. As left ventricular failure advances, the intensity of exercise resulting in breathlessness declines progressively. Engorged pulmonary vessels and interstitial pulmonary edema reduce the compliance of the lungs and increase airway resistance, which increases the work of the respiratory muscles required for ventilation. However, there is no close correlation between subjective exercise capacity and objective left ventricular performance at rest in patients with heart failure.[19]

Orthopnea. This symptom may be defined as dyspnea that develops in the recumbent position and is relieved by sitting or standing. In the recumbent position there is reduced pooling of fluid in the lower extremities and abdomen; movement of fluid from the dependent parts into the circulation causes displacement of blood from the extrathoracic to the thoracic compartment.[20] The failing left ventricle, operating on the flat portion of its depressed Starling curve (see Figure 13–17, p. 463), cannot accept and pump out the extra volume of blood delivered to it by the competent right ventricle, and pulmonary venous and capillary pressures rise further.

The patient with orthopnea generally elevates his head on several pillows to prevent nocturnal breathlessness and the development of paroxysmal nocturnal dyspnea (see below); in fact, the severity of orthopnea is conveniently estimated from the number of pillows required. Patients frequently awaken short of breath if the head has slipped off the pillows and they then often seek and find relief by sitting in front of an open window. In advanced left ventricular failure, orthopnea may be so severe that the patient cannot lie down at all and must spend the entire night in the sitting position. Often such patients are observed sitting at the side of the bed, slumped over a night table or bedside stand.

A nonproductive *cough* in patients with heart failure is often a "dyspnea equivalent." It may be caused by pulmonary congestion, occurs under the same circumstances as dyspnea (i.e., during exertion or recumbency), and is relieved by treatment of heart failure.

Paroxysmal Nocturnal Dyspnea. These attacks may be considered exaggerations of orthopnea. They usually occur at night, and the patient awakens with a feeling of extreme suffocation, sits bolt upright, and gasps for breath. Bronchospasm, which may be caused by congestion of the bronchial mucosa and which increases ventilatory difficulty and the work of breathing, is a common complicating factor of paroxysmal nocturnal dyspnea. The commonly associated wheezing is responsible for the alternate name of this condition, *cardiac asthma.* In contrast to orthopnea, which may be relieved by sitting upright at the side of the bed with the legs dependent, attacks of paroxysmal nocturnal dyspnea generally persist even in this position. The reason for the common occurrence of these episodes at night is not clear, but it seems likely that the combination of (1) reduced adrenergic drive to the left ventricle during sleep, (2) elevation of thoracic blood volume during recumbency, and (3) normal nocturnal depression of the respiratory center, plays a major role. Attacks of paroxysmal dyspnea rarely occur during the daytime and are provoked by effort or excitement.

Pulmonary Edema. The most severe form of breathlessness, pulmonary edema, is associated with a number of unique pathophysiological and clinical features and is described in Chapter 17.

MECHANISMS OF DYSPNEA. Increased awareness of respiration or difficulty in breathing is associated with pulmonary capillary hypertension and results from an elevation of left atrial or left ventricular filling pressure. Patients with left ventricular failure typically exhibit a restrictive ventilatory defect, characterized by a reduction of vital capacity as a consequence of the replacement of the air in the lungs with blood or interstitial fluid or both. Consequently, the lungs become stiffer, air trapping occurs because of earlier than normal closure of dependent airways,[21] and the work of breathing is increased because higher intrapleural pressures are required to distend the stiff lungs.[22] Tidal volume is reduced, and respiratory frequency rises in a compensatory fashion (Fig. 15–2). En-

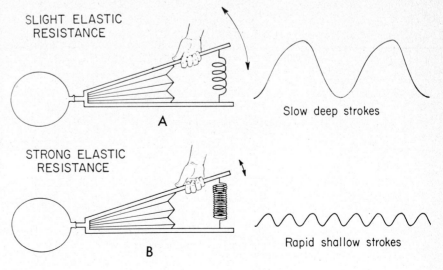

FIGURE 15–2 Mechanism for tachypnea in heart failure. To pump equal volumes of air per unit time against strong elastic resistance, a spring-loaded bellows should be operated with short rapid strokes to achieve greatest efficiency and reduce the total work. Congested lungs tend to resist normal inspiratory distention, so that rapid shallow breathing tends to reduce the work of breathing, particularly when respiratory minute volume must be increased, as during exertion. This suggests that the breathing pattern observed in patients with congestive heart failure may actually minimize the excess work of breathing imposed by the rigidity of the lungs. (From Rushmer, R. F.: Cardiac compensation, hypertrophy and myopathy and congestive heart failure. *In* Rushmer, R. F. [ed.]: Cardiovascular Dynamics. Philadelphia, W. B. Saunders Co., 1976, p. 532.)

SLIGHT ELASTIC RESISTANCE

A

Slow deep strokes

STRONG ELASTIC RESISTANCE

B

Rapid shallow strokes

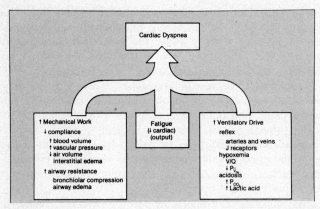

FIGURE 15–3 Factors that induce an increase in mechanical work of ventilation and ventilatory drive in states of pulmonary venous hypertension resulting from increased left heart filling pressure. The simultaneous occurrence of these factors and muscular fatigue converge to produce the sensation of dyspnea. (Reproduced with permission from Turino, G. M.: Origins of cardiac dyspnea. Primary Cardiol. 7:76, 1981.)

gorgement of blood vessels may reduce the caliber of the peripheral airways, increasing the airway resistance. In addition, there are alterations in the distribution of ventilation and perfusion (p. 1783), resulting in widened alveolar-arterial differences for oxygen, hypoxemia, and an increased ratio of dead space to tidal volume. Whatever abnormalities in mechanics and gas exchange function of the lung exist at rest are aggravated during exercise when pulmonary venous and capillary pressures rise further. Transudation of fluid from the intravascular to the extravascular space results in greater stiffening of the lungs, an augmentation in the work of breathing, and increased resistance to air flow.[23] There is an increased ventilatory drive, as a consequence of the stimulation of stretch receptors in the pulmonary vessels and interstitium, as well as a result of hypoxemia and metabolic acidosis. The increased work of breathing, combined with a low cardiac output and resulting impaired perfusion of the respiratory mus-

cles, causes fatigue[24] and ultimately the sensation of dyspnea[25] (Fig. 15–3).

Thus, dyspnea (during exertion or at rest) and orthopnea are clinical expressions of pulmonary venous and capillary congestion. Paroxysmal nocturnal dyspnea reflects the presence of *interstitial* edema, whereas pulmonary edema, in which there is transudation and expectoration of blood-tinged fluid (Chap. 17), is a manifestation of *alveolar* edema. The precise mechanism (or mechanisms) responsible for the respiratory distress of heart failure have not been definitively elucidated,[26] but a number of factors may be in operation (Figs. 15–3 and 15–4). It is well known that dyspnea occurs whenever the work of respiration is excessive. Increased force generation is required for the respiratory muscles to move a given volume of air if the compliance of the lungs is reduced or the resistance to air flow is increased; both these changes occur in left heart failure. Although patients are more likely to become dyspneic when the work of respiration is augmented, this increased work does not account for the perceptual difference between a deep breath with a normal mechanical load and a normal-sized breath with an increased mechanical load. The amount of work may be the same with both breaths, but the normal breath with the increased load will be associated with discomfort. A more appealing theory of the mechanism of dyspnea involves the inappropriateness of length to tension in the respiratory muscles. It has been proposed that discomfort arises when there is misalignment of the nerve spindles, which sense tension, in relation to muscle length. This misalignment could lead to the sensation of getting an insufficient breath for the tension generated by the respiratory muscles.[27]

DIFFERENTIATION BETWEEN CARDIAC AND PULMONARY DYSPNEA (see also Chap. 54).   In most patients with dyspnea, there is obvious clinical evidence of disease of either the heart or the lungs, but in some the differentiation between cardiac and pulmonary dyspnea may be difficult. The dyspnea of chronic obstructive lung disease tends to develop more gradually than that of heart disease; exceptions, of course, occur in patients with *ob-*

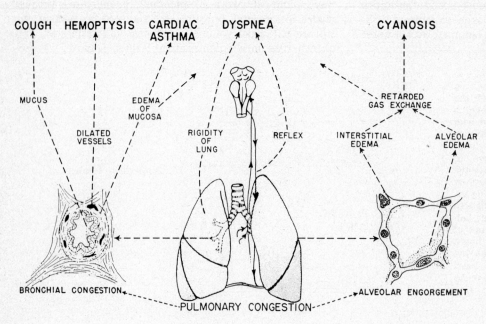

FIGURE 15–4 Etiology of respiratory symptoms from pulmonary congestion. Since most bronchial capillaries drain by way of the pulmonary veins, congestion develops simultaneously in alveolar and bronchial vascular networks. Bronchial congestion tends to stimulate production of mucus, leading to a productive cough. The distended bronchial capillaries may rupture, causing the patient to cough up blood-tinged sputum (hemoptysis). Edema of the bronchial mucosa increases resistance to air flow, producing respiratory distress similar to asthma. Dyspnea results primarily from reflexes initiated by vascular distention but may be supplemented by increased rigidity of the lungs and by impaired gas exchange resulting from interstitial edema and the accumulation of fluid in alveolar sacs. (From Rushmer, R. F.: Cardiac compensation, hypertrophy and myopathy and congestive heart failure. In Rushmer, R. F. [ed.]: Cardiovascular Dynamics. Philadelphia, W. B. Saunders Co., 1976, p. 532).

structive lung disease who experience an episode of infectious bronchitis, pneumonia or pneumothorax or an exacerbation of asthma. Like patients with cardiac dyspnea, patients with chronic obstructive lung disease may also waken at night with dyspnea, but this is usually associated with sputum production; the dyspnea is relieved after the patient rids himself of secretions by coughing rather than specifically by sitting up.

Acute cardiac asthma (paroxysmal nocturnal dyspnea with prominent wheezing) usually occurs in patients who have obvious clinical evidence of heart disease and may be further differentiated from acute bronchial asthma by the presence of diaphoresis, more bubbly airway sounds, and the more common occurrence of cyanosis. The difficulty in distinguishing between cardiac and pulmonary dyspnea may be compounded by the coexistence of diseases involving both organ systems. Thus, patients with a history of chronic bronchitis or asthma who develop left ventricular failure tend to develop particularly severe bronchoconstriction and wheezing in association with bouts of paroxysmal nocturnal dyspnea and pulmonary edema.

Pulmonary function testing should be carried out in patients in whom the etiology of dyspnea is unclear despite detailed clinical evaluation. The results may be helpful in determining whether dyspnea is produced by heart disease, lung disease, a combination of the two, or anxiety. In addition to the usual clinical means of assessing patients for heart disease (Chaps. 1 and 2), the arm-to-tongue circulation time may be useful, since in patients with cardiac dyspnea, this value usually exceeds the upper limit of normal (16 seconds) by 4 seconds or more (unless high-output heart failure is present).

The major alterations in pulmonary function tests in congestive heart failure are reductions of vital capacity, total lung capacity, pulmonary diffusion capacity at rest and particularly during exercise, and pulmonary compliance; resistance to air flow is moderately increased. Often there is hyperventilation at rest and during exercise, an increase in dead space, and some abnormalities of ventilation-perfusion relations with slight reductions in arterial pCO_2 and pO_2.

Rarely, it may be difficult to differentiate between cardiac dyspnea, dyspnea based on *malingering,* and dyspnea due to an *anxiety neurosis.* Careful observation for the appearance of effortless or irregular respiration during exercise testing often helps to identify the patient in whom dyspnea is related to these two noncardiac causes. Patients whose anxiety neurosis focuses on the heart may fear the presence of (nonexistent) heart disease and may exhibit sighing respiration and difficulty in taking a deep breath as well as dyspnea at rest. Their breathing pattern is not rapid and shallow, as in cardiac dyspnea. In some patients, a "therapeutic test" is helpful, and amelioration of dyspnea accompanied by a weight loss exceeding 2 kg induced by administration of a diuretic supports a cardiac origin for the dyspnea. Conversely, failure of these measures to achieve weight reduction in excess of 2 kg and to diminish dyspnea weighs heavily against a cardiac origin.

Other Symptoms

Fatigue and Weakness. Although these symptoms, often accompanied by a feeling of heaviness in the limbs, are generally related to poor perfusion of the skeletal muscles in patients with a lowered cardiac output, they may also be caused by sodium depletion, hypovolemia or both, as a consequence of excessive treatment with diuretics and restriction of dietary sodium.

Urinary Symptoms. *Nocturia* occurs relatively early in the course of heart failure. Urine formation is suppressed during the day when the patient is upright and active; this is due, at least in part, to a redistribution of blood flow away from the kidneys during activity[28] (see Figure 13–16, p. 462). When the patient rests in the recumbent position at night, the deficit in cardiac output in relation to oxygen demands is reduced, renal vasoconstriction diminishes, and urine formation increases. This diurnal pattern of urine flow characteristic of heart failure contrasts sharply with that existing in renal failure, in which urine formation occurs at a reasonably constant rate, both day and night. *Oliguria* is a sign of late cardiac failure and is related to the suppression of urine formation as a consequence of severely reduced cardiac output.

Cerebral Symptoms. Confusion, impairment of memory, anxiety, headache, insomnia, bad dreams or nightmares, and rarely psychosis with disorientation, delirium, and even hallucinations may occur in elderly patients with advanced heart failure, particularly in those with accompanying cerebral arteriosclerosis.

Symptoms of Predominant Right Heart Failure. Breathlessness, the cardinal manifestation of left ventricular failure, is uncommon in isolated right ventricular failure because pulmonary congestion is usually absent. Indeed, when a patient with mitral stenosis or left ventricular failure develops right ventricular failure, the more severe forms of dyspnea (i.e., paroxysmal nocturnal dyspnea and episodic pulmonary edema) tend to diminish in frequency and intensity, because the inability of the right ventricle to augment its output prevents the temporary imbalance between blood flow into and out of the pulmonary vascular bed. On the other hand, when cardiac output becomes markedly reduced in patients with terminal right heart failure, as may occur in the terminal phases of primary pulmonary hypertension and of pulmonary thromboembolic disease, severe dyspnea (air hunger) may occur, presumably as a consequence of the reduced cardiac output, poor perfusion of respiratory muscle, hypoxemia, and metabolic acidosis. In addition, dyspnea may be a prominent symptom in some patients with right ventricular failure and anasarca, hydrothorax, and ascites as a consequence of lung compression; these patients may even have orthopnea.

As in patients with predominant left ventricular failure, fatigue, a sense of heaviness of the limbs, and anorexia may be troubling symptoms in patients with predominant right heart failure. In patients with severe obstruction of right ventricular outflow of any cause and right ventricular failure, right ventricular stroke volume cannot be augmented, and dizziness and syncope may occur on exertion, just as in patients with aortic stenosis.

Congestive hepatomegaly may produce pain in the right upper quadrant or epigastrium, generally described as a dull ache or heaviness. This discomfort, which is caused by stretching of the hepatic capsule, may be severe when the liver enlarges rapidly, as in acute right heart failure. In contrast, chronic hepatic enlargement is generally painless. Other gastrointestinal symptoms, including anorexia, nausea, a sense of fullness after meals, and constipation, occur owing to congestion of the liver and gastrointestinal tract. In severe, preterminal heart failure, inadequate bowel perfusion can cause abdominal pain, distention, and bloody stools. Nausea, anorexia, and emesis may also be due to cardiac drugs, particularly digitalis (p. 525) and quinidine (p. 656).

FUNCTIONAL CLASSIFICATION. A classification of patients with heart disease based on the relation between symptoms and the amount of effort required to provoke them has been developed by the New York Heart Association.[29] Although there are obvious limitations to assigning numerical values to subjective findings, this classification is extremely useful in comparing groups of patients as well as the same patient at different times.

Class I—*No limitation:* Ordinary physical activity does not cause undue fatigue, dyspnea, or palpitation.
Class II—*Slight limitation of physical activity:* Such patients are comfortable at rest. Ordinary physical activity results in fatigue, palpitation, dyspnea, or angina.
Class III—*Marked limitation of physical activity:* Although patients are comfortable at rest, less than ordinary activity will lead to symptoms.
Class IV—*Inability to carry on any physical activity without discomfort:* Symptoms of congestive failure are present even at rest. With any physical activity, increased discomfort is experienced. As discussed on page 13, the accuracy and reproducibility of this classification are limited. To overcome these limitations, Goldman et al. have developed a useful classification based on the estimated metabolic cost of various activities (Table 1–2, p. 13).[30]

PHYSICAL FINDINGS

General Appearance. Patients with mild or moderate heart failure appear to be in no distress after a few minutes of rest. However, they may be obviously dyspneic during and immediately after activity, such as coming to the physician's office or undressing. Patients with left ventricular failure may become uncomfortable if asked to lie flat for more than a few minutes. Those with severe heart failure appear anxious and may exhibit signs of air hunger. Patients with heart failure of recent onset appear acutely ill but are usually well nourished, whereas those with chronic cardiac failure often appear malnourished and wasted. Chronic, marked elevation of systemic venous pressure may produce exophthalmos and severe tricuspid regurgitation and may lead to visible systolic pulsation of the eyes.[31]

Reduced Stroke Volume. In mild or moderately severe heart failure, stroke volume is normal at rest; in severe heart failure, it is reduced, and this reduction is reflected in a diminished pulse pressure and dusky discoloration of the skin. With very severe failure, particularly if cardiac output drops acutely, systolic arterial pressure may be reduced. The pulse may be rapid, weak, and thready.

Adrenergic Activity. Increased activity of the adrenergic nervous system is a principal compensatory mechanism for support of the circulation in the presence of reduced cardiac output (p. 458). It is responsible for a number of physical signs, including peripheral vasoconstriction, which is manifested as pallor and coldness of the extremities and cyanosis of the digits. There may be diaphoresis with tachycardia, loss of normal sinus arrhythmia, and obvious distention of the peripheral veins secondary to venoconstriction. Diastolic arterial pressure may even be slightly elevated.

Pulmonary Rales. Moist rales that result from the transudation of fluid into the alveoli are heard over the lung bases and are often accompanied by some dullness to percussion. They are characteristic of congestive heart failure of at least moderate severity. (In acute pulmonary edema, coarse, bubbling rales and wheezes are heard over both lung fields and are accompanied by the expectoration of frothy, blood-tinged sputum [p. 570].) With congestion of the bronchial mucosa, excessive bronchial secretions or bronchospasm or both may give rise to rhonchi and wheezes. Rales are usually bilateral, but if unilateral they usually occur on the right side. When rales are audible *only* over the left lung in a patient with heart failure, they may signify the presence of pulmonary embolism to that lung.

Systemic Venous Hypertension (see also pp. 20 to 21). This can be detected more readily by inspection of the jugular veins, which provides a useful index of right atrial pressure. The upper limit of normal of the jugular venous pressure is approximately 4 cm above the sternal angle. When tricuspid regurgitation is present, the *v* wave and *y* descent are most prominent; however, with impedance to right ventricular filling (tricuspid stenosis) or right ventricular emptying (pulmonary hypertension, pulmonic stenosis), the *a* wave is most prominent. Normally, the jugular venous pressure declines on exertion, but in patients with heart failure it rises. Rarely, venous pressure may be so high that the peripheral veins on the dorsum of the hands or in the temporal region are dilated.

Congestive Hepatomegaly. The liver often enlarges *before* overt edema develops, and it may remain so even after other symptoms of right-sided heart failure have disappeared. Inspection of the abdomen may reveal epigastric fullness and, on percussion, dullness in the right upper quadrant. If hepatomegaly has occurred rapidly and relatively recently, the liver is usually tender owing to stretching of its capsule. In long-standing heart failure this tenderness disappears, even though the liver remains enlarged.

In patients with tricuspid regurgitation, the prominent right atrial *v* wave may be transmitted to the liver, which pulsates during systole (Fig. 15–5). A prominent presystolic pulsation in the liver due to an enlarged right atrial *a* wave can occur in tricuspid stenosis, constrictive pericarditis, restrictive cardiomyopathy, pulmonary hypertension, and pulmonic stenosis. In patients with mild right heart failure, the jugular venous pressure may be normal at rest but rises to abnormal levels with compression of the abdomen, a sign known as the *abdominojugular reflux*. In order to elicit this sign, the periumbilical region should be compressed firmly, gradually, and continuously for 1 minute while the veins of the neck are observed. The patient should be advised to avoid straining or holding his breath. A positive test, i.e., expansion of the jugular veins during and immediately after compression, usually reflects the combination of a congested abdomen (particularly the liver) and inability of the right side of the heart to accept or

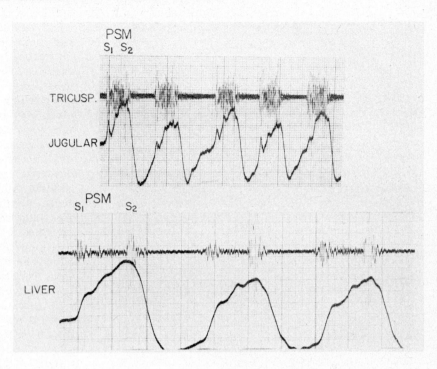

FIGURE 15–5 Jugular venous and hepatic pulse tracings and phonocardiogram from a 42-year-old woman with mitral stenosis and marked tricuspid regurgitation. A pansystolic murmur (PSM) was heard in the tricuspid area. Atrial fibrillation was present. The phonocardiogram shows the pansystolic murmur in the tricuspid region. Graphs of the jugular vein and liver show "ventricularization" of the systolic pulse wave. The rise of the regurgitant venous and liver pulses is synchronous with the first sound. Paper speed at the top tracing is 25 mm/sec, in the bottom tracing 75 mm/sec. (From Dressler, W.: Pulsations of the cervical veins and liver. *In* Dressler, W. [ed.]: Clinical Aids in Cardiac Diagnosis. New York, Grune and Stratton, 1970, p. 190, by permission of Grune and Stratton.)

eject this transiently increased venous return. Thus, a positive abdominojugular reflux is helpful in differentiating hepatic enlargement due to heart failure from that due to other conditions.

Edema. Although a cardinal manifestation of congestive heart failure, edema does not correlate well with the level of systemic venous pressure. As already noted, in patients with chronic left ventricular failure and a low cardiac output, extracellular fluid volume may be sufficiently expanded to produce edema in the presence of normal or only minimal elevations of systemic venous pressure. A substantial gain of extracellular fluid volume, a minimum of 5 liters in adults, must usually take place before peripheral edema is manifested. Therefore, edema may develop over a number of days and may not be present initially in patients with acute heart failure and marked systemic venous hypertension.

Edema is usually symmetrical and generally occurs first in the dependent portions of the body, where the systemic venous pressure rises to its highest levels. Accordingly, cardiac edema in ambulatory patients is usually first noted in the feet or ankles at the end of the day and generally resolves after a night's rest. In bedridden patients it is most commonly found over the sacrum. Facial edema seldom appears in adults but, as mentioned earlier, may occur in infants and young children. Late in the course of heart failure, edema may become massive and generalized (anasarca); it can involve the upper extremities, the thoracic and abdominal walls, and particularly the genital area. Rarely, when edema is severe and develops suddenly, it may cause rupture of the skin and extravasation of fluid. Long-standing edema results in pigmentation, reddening, and induration of the skin of the lower extremities, usually the dorsum of the feet and the pretibial areas. In patients with hemiplegia, edema is usually more marked on the paralyzed side.

Hydrothorax. Since the pleural veins drain into both the systemic and the pulmonary venous beds, hydrothorax is observed most commonly in patients with hypertension involving both venous systems, but it may also occur when there is marked elevation of pressure in either venous bed. An increase in capillary permeability probably also plays a role in the pathogenesis of cardiac hydrothorax, since the protein content of the pleural fluid is usually significantly greater (2 to 3 gm/dl) than that found in edema fluid (0.5 gm/dl). Hydrothorax is usually bilateral, but when unilateral it is usually confined to the right side of the chest and is caused most commonly by severe systemic venous hypertension, as occurs in tricuspid stenosis or constrictive pericarditis. Conversely, if the hydrothorax is limited to the left side, it is most commonly secondary to pulmonary venous hypertension (e.g., mitral stenosis). When hydrothorax develops, dyspnea usually becomes intensified owing to a further reduction in vital capacity. Although the excess fluid in hydrothorax is usually resorbed as the condition of the heart improves, interlobar effusions sometimes persist.

Ascites. This complication occurs in patients with increased pressure in the hepatic veins and in the veins draining the peritoneum (Fig. 15–6). Ascites usually reflects long-standing systemic venous hypertension, and in patients with organic tricuspid valve disease and chronic constrictive pericarditis, it may be more prominent than subcutaneous edema. As in the case of hydrothorax, there is increased capillary permeability because the protein content is similar to that of hepatic lymph, i.e., four to six times that of edema fluid. Protein-losing enteropathy may occur in patients with visceral congestion,[32] and the resultant reduced plasma oncotic pressure may lower the threshold for the development of ascites.

CARDIAC FINDINGS

Cardiomegaly. This finding is nonspecific and occurs in the majority of patients with chronic heart failure. Notable exceptions are heart failure due to chronic constrictive pericarditis, restrictive cardiomyopathy, and a variety

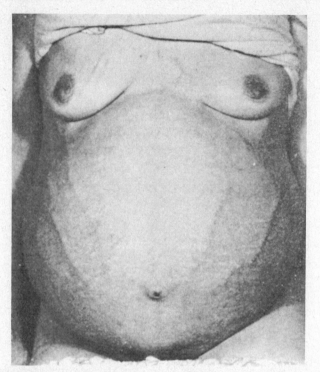

FIGURE 15–6 Gross ascites due to congestive heart failure. The everted umbilicus, distended abdominal veins, and striae are typical. (From Oram, S.: Heart failure. *In* Oram, S. [ed.]: Clinical Heart Disease. 2nd ed. London, William Heinemann Medical Books, Ltd., 1981, p. 666.)

of acute insults such as acute myocardial infarction, the sudden development of arrhythmias, or rupture of a valve or chordae tendineae; in such circumstances heart failure may occur before the heart has had a chance to enlarge.

Gallop Sounds. Protodiastolic sounds, generally emanating from the left ventricle (but occasionally from the right) and occurring 0.13 to 0.16 second after the second heart sound, are common findings in healthy children and young adults. Such physiological sounds are rarely audible in healthy persons after the age of 40 years but occur in patients of all ages with heart failure and are referred to as protodiastolic, or S_3, gallops. Thus, in older adults, they generally signify the presence of heart failure (p. 50). Protodiastolic gallops are caused by the sharp deceleration of ventricular inflow that occurs immediately after the early filling phase, perhaps accompanied by simultaneous closure of the atrioventricular valve; a reduction in ventricular distensibility, i.e., the ventricle operating on the steep portion of its diastolic pressure-volume curve (see Figure 12–23, p. 428), may contribute to their genesis. In patients with mitral or tricuspid regurgitation or left-to-right shunts, torrential flow into the ventricle in early diastole contributes to the generation of an S_3 (p. 50), but under these conditions this sound is not to be interpreted as signifying the presence of heart failure. In heart failure the atrioventricular pressure gradient during early filling may be high as a consequence of elevated atrial pressure, and the distensibility of the ventricle may be altered, resulting in a protodiastolic gallop. Thus, a protodiastolic gallop sound is an excellent sign of heart failure when other causes, such as a physiological S_3 occurring in a healthy child or young adult, constrictive pericarditis, mitral and tricuspid regurgitation, or a left-to-right shunt, can be excluded.

Left ventricular gallop sounds are best heard at the apex with the patient in the left lateral recumbent position and are frequently palpable, whereas right ventricular gallop sounds are best heard at the left sternal edge in the fourth or fifth interspace with the patient supine. Protodiastolic gallop sounds originating from the left ventricle tend to be louder *after* inspiration, whereas those originating from the right ventricle are best heard *during* inspiration. Gallop sounds are more readily audible in the presence of a rapid heart rate and may sometimes be elicited by a brief bout of exercise.

Pulsus Alternans (see also p. 25). This condition is characterized by a regular rhythm with alternation of strong and weak contractions (Fig. 15–7). It should be distinguished from the alternation of strong and weak beats that occurs in pulsus bigeminus, in which the weak beat follows the strong beat by a shorter time interval than the strong beat follows the weak, whereas in pulsus alternans they are equally spaced or the weak beat is slightly closer to the succeeding than to the preceding beat. Severe pulsus alternans may be detected either by palpation of the peripheral pulses (the femoral more readily than the brachial, radial, or carotid) or by sphygmomanometry. As the cuff is slowly deflated, only alternate beats are audible for a variable number of millimeters of Hg below the systolic level, depending on the severity of the alternans, and then all beats are heard. Occasionally, the weak beat is so small that the aortic valve is not opened, and this results in an apparent halving of the pulse rate, a condition referred to as *total alternans*. Pulsus alternans may be accompanied by alternation in the intensity of the heart sounds and of existing heart murmurs. With total alternans there is a first heart sound for each contraction, but the second heart sound may be absent, with the weak contractions owing to failure of the semilunar valves to open.

Pulsus alternans occurs most commonly in heart failure secondary to increased resistance to left ventricular ejection, as occurs in systemic hypertension and aortic stenosis, as well as in coronary atherosclerosis and cardiomyopathy. It is frequently associated with a ventricular protodiastolic gallop sound (S_3), usually signifies advanced myocardial disease, and often disappears with treatment of heart failure. Rarely, it may also occur in normal persons during tachycardia or following a single premature beat. In patients with heart failure, pulsus alternans can often be elicited by reduction in systemic venous return, as occurs with assumption of the erect posture or application of venous tourniquets, and it is reduced by an increase in venous return, as in recumbency or with exercise. In patients with heart disease, it tends to be present during tachycardia and is often initiated by a premature beat (Fig. 15–7).

Pulsus alternans is attributed to an alternation in the stroke volume ejected by the left ventricle[33] and ultimately to a deletion in the number of contracting cells in every other cycle due to incomplete recovery. Alternans is almost always concordant in the two sides of the circulation, i.e., the strong and weak beats occur simultaneously in the two ventricles. Rarely, pulsus alternans is accompanied by electrical alternans; however, the latter condition is usually not due to mechanical alternans but rather to alternating position of the heart within the fluid-filled pericardial sac (Figure 5–75, p. 132).

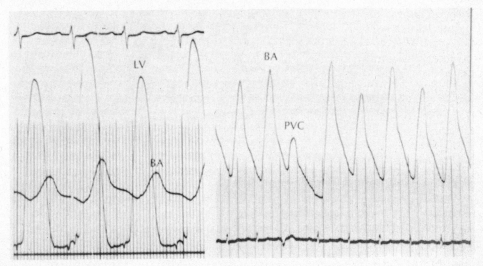

FIGURE 15–7 Pulsus alternans: *Left,* A classic strong-weak-strong-weak pattern in both brachial and left ventricular pulse pressures in tracings from a patient with aortic stenosis. *Right,* Premature ventricular contraction precipitates pulsus alternans, facilitating detection of this sign of left ventricular failure. (From Perloff, J. K.: The clinical manifestations of cardiac failure in adults. Hosp. Pract. *5:*43, 1970; and Braunwald, E. [ed.]: The Myocardium: Failure and Infarction. New York, HP Publishing Co., 1974, p. 93.)

Accentuation of P_2. With the development of left ventricular failure, pulmonary artery pressure rises, and P_2 becomes accentuated—often louder than A_2—and more widely transmitted. As the patient improves, P_2 becomes softer.

Systolic murmurs are common in heart failure owing to the relative mitral or tricuspid regurgitation that may occur secondary to ventricular dilatation. Often these murmurs diminish or disappear when compensation is restored.

Fever. A low-grade temperature ($<38°C$), which results from cutaneous vasoconstriction and therefore impairment of heat loss, may occur in severe heart failure; fever usually subsides when compensation is restored. Greater elevations of temperature often signify the presence of an infection, pulmonary infarction, or infective endocarditis.

Cardiac Cachexia. Long-standing, severe congestive heart failure, particularly of the right ventricle, may lead to anorexia, owing to hepatic and intestinal congestion and sometimes to digitalis intoxication. Occasionally, there is impaired intestinal absorption of fat[34] and rarely protein-losing enteropathy.[32] Patients with heart failure may also exhibit an increase in total metabolism, secondary to (1) an augmentation of myocardial oxygen consumption, as occurs in patients with aortic stenosis and hypertension; (2) excessive work of breathing; and (3) low-grade fever. The combination of a reduced caloric intake and increased caloric expenditure may lead to marked weight loss and, in severe cases, to cardiac cachexia.[35] In some patients the cachexia may be severe enough to suggest the presence of disseminated malignant disease.

Cheyne-Stokes Respiration. This condition, also known as periodic or cyclic respiration, is characterized by the combination of depression in the sensitivity of the respiratory center to carbon dioxide and left ventricular failure.[36,37] During the apneic phase, arterial pO_2 falls and pCO_2 rises; this combination excites the depressed respiratory center, resulting in hyperventilation and subsequently hypocapnia, followed by another period of apnea. The principal cause of Cheyne-Stokes respiration is a cerebral lesion such as cerebral arteriosclerosis, stroke, or head injury. These causes are often exaggerated by sleep, barbiturates, and narcotics, all of which further depress the sensitivity

of the respiratory center. Left ventricular failure, which prolongs the circulation time from the lung to the brain, results in a sluggish response of the system and is responsible for the oscillations between apnea and hyperpnea and prevents return to a steady state of ventilation and blood gases. Occasionally, the patient with heart failure awakens at night with dyspnea precipitated by periodic (Cheyne-Stokes) respiration; this form of nocturnal dyspnea is not considered as ominous as classic paroxysmal nocturnal dyspnea.[38]

PATHOLOGICAL FINDINGS

Lungs. The lungs are enlarged, firm, dark, and filled with bloody fluid. When pulmonary congestion has been long-standing, they are brown with deposition of hemosiderin and usually do not seep edema fluid. On microscopic examination, the capillaries are engorged and there is thickening of the alveolar septa as well as extravasation of large mononuclear cells containing red blood cells or hemosiderin granules or both.[39] Often the pulmonary vessels show medial hypertrophy and intimal hyperplasia (p. 831).

Liver. In acute right heart failure, the liver is enlarged, firm, and filled with fluid. On microscopic examination, the central hepatic veins and sinusoids are dilated. With long-standing right heart failure, the liver returns to normal size, subsequently atrophies, and becomes "nutmeg" in appearance as a consequence of the dark red areas of central venous congestion and the lighter, fatty area in the periphery of the lobule. Cardiac cirrhosis is characterized by central lobular necrosis and atrophy as well as extensive fibrous retraction;[40] sometimes there is sclerosis of the hepatic veins. Since cardiac cirrhosis develops as a function of the level of hepatic venous pressure and the duration of its elevation, it is not surprising that it occurs most commonly in patients with chronic constrictive pericarditis and organic tricuspid valve disease who often have prolonged elevation of systemic venous pressure. In patients with left ventricular failure, central hepatic necrosis without evidence of passive congestion may be present.[41] Liver biopsies in patients with acute heart failure exhibiting fulminant hepatic failure showed replacement of hepatocytes by red blood cells.[42] Presumably, the hypoxia caused by hypoperfusion produces hepatocyte necrosis;[43] erythrocytes may then enter the space of Disse between damaged endothelial cells. These changes resulting from acute heart failure may be transient if there is hemodynamic recovery.

Other Viscera. Patients with chronic hepatic venous hypertension develop portal hypertension that results in congestive splenomegaly. On microscopic examination, the spleen reveals dilatation of the sinusoids and fibrosis, and there is chronic passive congestion of the pancreas and of the veins and capillaries of the gastrointestinal tract. Rarely, intense mesenteric vasoconstriction without thrombotic or embolic occlusion of a mesenteric artery may lead to a hemorrhagic, nonbacterial enterocolitis,[44] with hemorrhagic necrosis.

Chronic venous congestion also occurs in the kidney and brain, with dilatation and engorgement of the capillaries. Small infarcts are frequently observed in the spleen and kidneys of patients with long-standing atrial fibrillation.

LABORATORY FINDINGS

Proteinuria and a high urine specific gravity are common findings in heart failure. Blood urea nitrogen and creatinine levels are often moderately elevated secondary to reductions in renal blood flow and glomerular filtration rate[10] (p. 1750). The erythrocyte sedimentation rate is usually quite low secondary to impaired fibrinogen synthesis and resultant decreased fibrinogen concentrations.

SERUM ELECTROLYTES. Serum electrolyte values are generally normal in patients with heart failure prior to treatment. However, in severe heart failure, prolonged, rigid sodium restriction, coupled with intensive diuretic therapy as well as the inability to excrete water, may lead to hyponatremia (p. 1750). The hyponatremia is dilutional and occurs despite an expansion of extracellular fluid volume and an increase in total body sodium. It may be accompanied by, and presumably is caused in part by, elevated concentrations of circulating vasopressin.[45] Serum potassium levels are usually normal, although the prolonged administration of kaliuretic diuretics, such as the thiazides or loop diuretics, may result in hypokalemia (p. 531). Hyperkalemia may occur in patients with very severe heart failure who show marked reductions in glomerular filtration rate and inadequate delivery of sodium to the distal tubular sodium-potassium exchange sites, particularly if these patients are also receiving potassium-retaining diuretics (p. 1752).

Congestive hepatomegaly and cardiac cirrhosis are often associated with impaired hepatic function, characterized by abnormal values of serum glutamic oxaloacetic transaminase (SGOT) and other liver enzymes.[46,47] Hyperbilirubinemia, secondary to an increase in both the directly and the indirectly reacting bilirubins, is common, and in severe cases of acute (right or left) ventricular failure, frank jaundice may occur. Acute hepatic venous congestion can result in severe jaundice with a bilirubin level as high as 15 to 20 mg/dl, elevation of SGOT to more than 10 times the upper limit of normal, and elevation of the serum alkaline phosphatase level, as well as prolongation of the prothrombin time. Both the clinical and the laboratory pictures may resemble viral hepatitis, but the impairment of hepatic function is rapidly ameliorated by successful treat-

ment of heart failure. In patients with long-standing cardiac cirrhosis, albumin synthesis may be impaired, with resultant hypoalbuminemia, intensifying the accumulation of fluid. Hepatic hypoglycemia, fulminant hepatic failure, and hepatic coma are rare, late, and sometimes terminal complications of cardiac cirrhosis.[48–51]

Venous pressure can be conveniently measured with a spinal fluid manometer while the patient is in the recumbent position and the arm is abducted from the thorax. The baseline for the measurement should be 5 cm below the sternal angle, i.e., the estimated position of the right atrium. The venous pressure is often elevated (i.e., > 12 cm H_2O) at rest, but in mild or borderline cases it may be normal at rest but rises with hepatic compression or during exercise.

Circulation time can be measured by rapid intravenous injection of 3 to 5 ml of 20 per cent dehydrocholic acid (Decholin), with a bitter taste designating the endpoint. The normal range in adults is 9 to 16 seconds. Circulation time varies directly with the volume of blood in which the indicator is diluted and inversely with the velocity of blood flow. Therefore, pulmonary and/or systemic venous congestion, as well as reduced cardiac output, causes prolongation. Because of the high velocity of blood flow, circulation time tends to be normal or even shortened in patients with high-output heart failure. Although circulation time is not a particularly sensitive test for heart failure, it may be useful in differentiating between pulmonary or cardiac dyspnea and between low- and high-output cardiac failure.

THE VALSALVA MANEUVER. This maneuver—forced expiration against a closed glottis—is helpful in the diagnosis of heart failure.[52] The standard test consists of asking the patient to blow against an aneroid manometer and to maintain a pressure of 40 mm Hg for 30 seconds. The Valsalva maneuver raises intrathoracic pressure, venous return to the heart diminishes, stroke volume falls, and venous pressure rises. Arterial pressure tracings normally show four distinct phases (Fig. 15–8): (1) an initial rise in arterial pressure, which represents transmission to the periphery of the increased intrathoracic pressure; (2) with continuation of the strain and the accompanying reduction of venous return, reductions in systolic, diastolic, and pulse pressures accompanied by a reflex increase in heart rate; (3) on release of the strain, a sudden drop of arterial pressure equivalent to the fall in intrathoracic pressure; and (4) an overshoot of arterial pressure to above control levels, with a wide pulse pressure and bradycardia due to the combination of the inrush into the heart of blood that had been dammed up in the venous bed and reflex vasoconstriction and tachycardia secondary to the low perfusion pressure of the carotid and baroreceptors during phase 3.

In heart failure[52] (Fig. 15–9), phases 1 and 3 are normal, i.e., there is normal transmission of the elevated intrathoracic pressure into the arterial tree during phase 1 and sudden loss of this with the release of the strain during phase 3. However, since the heart operates on the flat portion of its Starling curve (see Figure 13–17, p. 463), the impedance of venous return during phase 2 does not affect stroke volume. Therefore the baroreceptor reflex is not activated, and there is no overshoot upon release of the

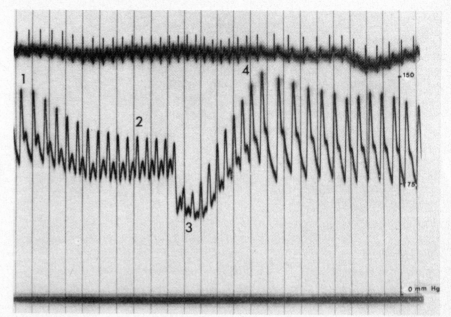

FIGURE 15–8 Normal response to Valsalva maneuver. Intraarterial pressure tracing. The four phases (see text) are denoted. (From Oram, S.: Further bedside examination. *In* Oram, S. [ed.]: Clinical Heart Disease. 2nd ed. London, William Heinemann Medical Books, Ltd., 1981, p. 668.)

strain. This results in a "square-wave" appearance of the tracing. Although the Valsalva maneuver can be recorded most accurately through an indwelling needle, careful palpation of the pulse in normal individuals allows detection of phases 2 and 4 and their absence, in particular, slowing of the pulse in phase 4 in heart failure.[53]

The Chest Roentgenogram
(See also Chap. 6)

Two principal features of the chest roentgenogram are useful in the patient with congestive heart failure.

The *size and shape of the cardiac silhouette* provide important information concerning the precise nature of the underlying heart disease. Both the cardiothoracic ratio (see Figure 6–16, p. 158) and the heart volume determined on the plain film (see Figure 6–17, p. 159) are relatively spe-

cific but insensitive indicators of increased left ventricular end-diastolic volume and reduced ejection fraction.

In the presence of normal pulmonary capillary and venous pressure in the erect position, the lung bases are better perfused than the apices, and the vessels supplying the lower lobes are significantly larger than are those supplying the upper lobes. With elevation of left atrial, pulmonary venous, and capillary pressures, interstitial and perivascular edema develops and is most prominent at the lung bases because hydrostatic pressure is greater there.[54] The resultant compression of pulmonary vessels in the lower lobes causes equalization in size of the vessels to the apices and bases when pulmonary capillary pressure is slightly elevated, i.e., approximately 13 to 17 mm Hg.[55,56] With greater pressure elevation (approximately 18 to 23 mm Hg), actual pulmonary vascular redistribution occurs, i.e., further constriction of vessels leading to the lower lobes and dilatation of vessels leading to the upper lobes.

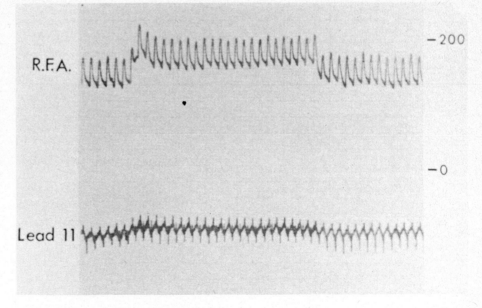

FIGURE 15–9 Valsalva maneuver in congestive heart failure showing the "square-wave" response. (From Oram, S.: Further bedside examination. *In* Oram, S. [ed.]: Clinical Heart Disease. 2nd ed. London, William Heinemann Medical Books, Ltd., 1981, p. 668.)

When pulmonary capillary pressures exceed approximately 20 to 25 mm Hg, interstitial pulmonary edema occurs. This may be of several varieties: (1) *septal*, producing Kerley's lines (i.e., sharp, linear densities of interlobular interstitial edema); (2) *perivascular*, producing loss of sharpness of the central and peripheral vessels; and (3) *subpleural*, producing spindle-shaped accumulations of fluid between the lung and adjacent pleural surface. When pulmonary capillary pressure exceeds 25 mm Hg, alveolar edema, with a cloudlike appearance and concentration of the fluid around the hili in a "butterfly pattern," and large pleural effusions may occur.[56] With elevation of systemic venous pressure, the azygos vein and superior vena cava may enlarge.[57]

References

1. Lewis, T.: Diseases of the Heart. New York, The Macmillan Co., 1933, p. 1.
2. Braunwald, E., Mock, M. B., and Watson, J. (eds.): Congestive Heart Failure. Current Research and Clinical Applications, New York, Grune and Stratton, 1982, 384 pp.
3. O'Brien, C. P.: Approaches to heart failure. *In* Brandenburg, R. O. (ed.): Office cardiology. Cardiovasc. Clin. *10*:33, 1980.
4. Hope, J. A.: Treatise on the Diseases of the Heart and Great Vessels. London, Williams-Kidd, 1832.
5. Williams, J. F., Jr., Sonnenblick, E. H., and Braunwald, E.: Determinants of atrial contractile force in intact heart. Am. J. Physiol. *209*:1061, 1965.
6. Starling, E. H.: Linacre Lecture on the Law of the Heart (1915). London, Longmans, 1918.
7. Ross, J., Jr., and Braunwald, E.: Studies on Starling's law of the heart. IX. The effects of impeding venous return on performance of the normal and failing human left ventricle. Circulation *30*:719, 1964.
8. Stampfer, M., Epstein, S. E., Beiser, G. D., and Braunwald, E.: Hemodynamic effects of diuresis at rest and during intense upright exercise in patients with impaired cardiac function. Circulation *37*:900, 1968.
9. Mackenzie, J.: Disease of the Heart. 3rd ed. London, Oxford University Press, 1913.
10. Hricik, D. E., and Kassirer, J. P.: Azotemia in cardiac failure. J. Cardiovasc. Med. (In press.)
11. Davis, J. O.: The mechanism of salt and water retention in cardiac failure. In Braunwald, E. (ed.): The Myocardium: Failure and Infarction. New York, HP Publishing Co., 1974, pp. 80–92.
12. Tan, S. Y., and Mulrow, P. J.: Aldosterone in hypertension and edema. *In* Bondy, P. K., and Rosenberg, L. E. (eds.): Metabolic Control and Disease. 8th ed. Philadelphia, W. B. Saunders Co., 1980, p. 1516.
13. Spann, J. F., Chidsey, C. A., Pool, P. E., and Braunwald, E.: Mechanism of norepinephrine depletion in experimental heart failure produced by aortic constriction in the guinea pig. Circ. Res. *17*:312, 1965.
14. Chidsey, C. A., Kaiser, G. A., Sonnenblick, E. H., Spann, J. F., and Braunwald, E.: Cardiac norepinephrine stores in experimental heart failure in the dog. J. Clin. Invest. *43*:2386, 1964.
15. Chandler, B. M., Sonnenblick, E. H., Spann, J. F., and Pool, P. E.: Association of depressed myofibrillar adenosinetriphosphate and reduced contractility in experimental heart failure. Circ. Res. *21*:717, 1967.
16. Artman, M., and Graham, T. P., Jr.: Congestive heart failure in infancy: Recognition and management. Am. Heart J. *103*:1040, 1982.
17. Sodeman, W. A., and Burch, G. E.: The precipitating causes of congestive heart failure. Am. Heart J. *15*:22, 1938.
18. Braunwald, E., and Frahm, C. J.: Studies on Starling's law of the heart. IV. Observations on the hemodynamic functions of the left atrium in man. Circulation *24*:633, 1961.
19. Franciosa, J. A., Park, M., and Levine, T. B.: Lack of correlation between exercise capacity and indexes of resting left ventricular performance in heart failure. Am. J. Cardiol. *47*:33, 1981.
20. Perera, G. A., and Berliner, R. W.: The relation of postural hemodilution to paroxysmal dyspnea. J. Clin. Invest. *22*:25, 1943.
21. Collins, J. V., Clark, T. J. H., and Brown, D. J.: Airway function in healthy subjects and in patients with left heart disease. Clin. Sci. Molec. Med. *49*:217, 1975.
22. Marshall, R., McIroy, M. B., and Christie, R. V.: The work of breathing in mitral stenosis. Clin. Sci. *17*:667, 1958.
23. Fishman, A. P. (ed.): Pulmonary Diseases and Disorders. New York, McGraw-Hill Book Co., 1980, pp. 44–67.
24. Macklem, P. T.: Respiratory muscles: The vital pump. Chest *78*:753, 1980.

25. Turino, G. M.: Origins of cardiac dyspnea. Primary Cardiol. *7*:76, 1981.
26. Fishman, A. P., and Ledlie, J. F.: Dyspnea. Bull. Eur. Physiopathol. Resp. *15*: 789, 1979.
27. Campbell, E. J. M., Agostoni, E., and Newsom Davis, J.: The Respiratory Muscles: Mechanisms and Neural Control. 2nd ed. Philadelphia, W. B. Saunders Co., 1970.
28. Higgins, C. B., Vatner, S. F., Franklin, D., and Braunwald, E.: Effects of experimentally produced heart failure on the peripheral vascular response to severe exercise in conscious dogs. Circ. Res. *31*:186, 1972.
29. Criteria Committee, New York Heart Association, Inc.: Diseases of the Heart and Blood Vessels. Nomenclature and Criteria for Diagnosis. 6th ed. Boston, Little, Brown and Co., 1964, p. 114.
30. Goldman, L., Hashimoto, B., Cook, E. F., and Loscalzo, A.: Comparative reproducibility and validity of symptoms for assessing cardiovascular functional class. Advantages of a new specific activity scale. Circulation *64*:1227, 1981.
31. Earnest, D. L., and Hurst, J. W.: Exophthalmos, stare and increase in intraocular pressure and systolic propulsion of the eyeballs due to congestive heart failure. Am. J. Cardiol. *26*:351, 1970.
32. Strober, W., Cohen, L. S., Waldmann, T. A., and Braunwald, E.: Tricuspid regurgitation: A newly recognized cause of protein-losing enteropathy, lymphocytopenia and immunologic deficiency. Am. J. Med. *44*:842, 1968.
33. Gleason, W. L., and Braunwald, E.: Studies on Starling's law of the heart. VI. Relationships between left ventricular end-diastolic volume and stroke volume in man with observations on the mechanism of pulsus alternans. Circulation *25*: 841, 1962.
34. Berkowitz, D., Croll, M. N., and Likoff, W.: Malabsorption as a complication of congestive heart failure. Am. J. Cardiol. *11*:43, 1963.
35. Pittman, J. G., and Cohen, P.: The pathogenesis of cardiac cachexia. N. Engl. J. Med. *27*:403, 1964.
36. Brown, H. W., and Plum, F.: The neurological basis of Cheyne-Stokes respiration. Am. J. Med. *30*:849, 1940.
37. Lange, R. L., and Hecht, H. H.: The mechanism of Cheyne-Stokes respiration. J. Clin. Invest. *41*:42, 1962.
38. Rees, P. J., and Clark, T. J. H.: Paroxysmal nocturnal dyspnoea and periodic respiration. Lancet *2*:1315, 1979.
39. Friedman-Mor, Z., Chalon, J., Turndorf, H., and Orkin, L. R.: Cardiac index and incidence of heart failure cells. Arch. Pathol. Lab. Med. *102*:418, 1978.
40. Moschcowitz, E.: The morphology and pathogenesis of cardiac fibrosis of the liver. Ann. Intern. Med. *36*:933, 1952.
41. Cohen, J. A., and Kaplan, M. M.: Left-sided heart failure presenting as hepatitis. Gastroenterology *74*:583, 1978.
42. Kanel, G. C., Ucci, A. A., Kaplan, M. M., and Wolfe, H. J.: A distinctive perivenular hepatic lesion associated with heart failure. Am. J. Clin. Pathol. *73*: 235, 1980.
43. Nouel, O., Henrion, J., Bernuau, J., DeGott, C., Rueff, B., and Benhamou, J.-P.: Fulminant hepatic failure due to transient circulatory failure in patients with chronic heart disease. Dig. Dis. Sci. *25*:49, 1980.
44. Wilson, R., and Qualheim, R. E.: A form of acute hemorrhagic enterocolitis afflicting chronically ill individuals. Gastroenterology *27*:431, 1954.
45. Szatalowicz, V. L., Arnold, P. E., Chaimovitz, C., Bichet, D., Beri, T., and Schrier, R. W.: Radioimmunoassay of plasma arginine vasopressin in hyponatremic patients with congestive heart failure. N. Engl. J. Med. *305*:263, 1981.
46. West, M., Pilz, C. G., and Zimmerman, H. J.: Serum enzymes in disease: III. Significance of abnormal serum enzyme levels in cardiac failure. Am. J. Med. Sci. *241*:350, 1960.
47. Kaplan, M. M.: Liver dysfunction secondary to congestive heart failure. Practical Cardiol. *6*:39, 1980.
48. Kaymakcalan, H., Dourdourekas, D., Szanto, P. B., and Steigmann, F.: Congestive heart failure as cause of fulminant hepatic failure. Am. J. Med. *65*:384, 1978.
49. Dunn, G. D., Hayes, P., Breen, K. J., and Schenker, S.: The liver in congestive heart failure. A review. Am. J. Med. Sci. *265*:174, 1973.
50. Benzing, G., III, Schubert, W., Hug, G., and Kaplan, S.: Simultaneous hypoglycemia and acute congestive heart failure. Circulation *40*:209, 1969.
51. Kisloff, B., and Schaffer, G.: Fulminant hepatic failure secondary to congestive heart failure. Am. J. Dig. Dis. *21*:895, 1976.
52. Gorlin, R., Knowles, J. H., and Storey, C. F.: The Valsalva maneuver as a test of cardiac function. Pathologic physiology and clinical significance. Am. J. Med. *22*:197, 1957.
53. Elisberg, E. I.: Heart rate response to the Valsalva maneuver as a test of circulatory integrity. J.A.M.A. *186*:200, 1963.
54. Jefferson, K., and Rees, S.: Pulmonary venous hypertension. *In* Jefferson, K., and Rees, S. (eds.): Clinical Cardiac Radiology. London, Butterworth and Co., 1973, pp. 84–94.
55. Levin, D. C., Hessel, S. J., Mann, T., Swensson, R. G., Grossman, W., Baumstark, A., and Abrams, H. L.: Estimation of pulmonary capillary wedge pressure from chest radiographs. Radiology (in press).
56. Spindola-Franco, H.: Plain film diagnosis of congestive heart failure. J. Med. Soc. N.J. *75*:783, 1978.
57. Daves, M. L.: Cardiac Roentgenology. Chicago, Year Book Medical Publishers, 1981, pp. 78–86.

16 THE MANAGEMENT OF HEART FAILURE

by Thomas W. Smith, M.D., and Eugene Braunwald, M.D.

INTRODUCTION

Three general approaches are employed in the treatment of heart failure:

1. *Removal of the Underlying Cause.* This—the most desirable approach—involves surgical correction of structural abnormalities responsible for heart failure, such as congenital malformations and acquired valvular lesions, or medical treatment of conditions such as infective endocarditis or hypertension.

2. *Removal of the Precipitating Cause.* The recognition, prompt treatment, and, whenever possible, prevention of the specific causes or incidents that produce or exacerbate heart failure, such as infections, arrhythmias, and pulmonary emboli (p. 491), are critical to successful management of heart failure.

3. *Control of the Congestive Heart Failure State.* This approach, the subject of this chapter, may be divided into three categories (Table 16–1):

a. *Improvement of the heart's pumping performance,* which consists of efforts to restore the contractility of the failing heart toward normal.

b. *Reduction of the heart's workload,* which involves reduction of the demands placed on the heart to generate pressure and/or to pump blood.

c. *Control of excessive salt and water retention,* i.e., control of the expansion of extracellular fluid volume, which is the principal cause of many manifestations of heart failure, such as dyspnea and edema.

In each of these last three categories, a number of therapeutic measures are available. As outlined in Table 16–2, numbers 2 (digitalis) and 6 (other inotropic agents) contribute to the direct improvement of the heart's pumping performance; numbers 1 (restriction of physical activity) and 5 (vasodilators) involve reducing the heart's workload; while numbers 3 (restriction of sodium intake), 4 (diuretics), and 7 (physical removal of excess fluid) involve control of excessive salt and water retention.

TABLE 16–1 CONTROL OF CONGESTIVE HEART FAILURE

1. *Improvement of Pumping Performance*
  (A) Digitalis glycoside
  (B) Sympathomimetic agents
  (C) Other positive inotropic agents
  (D) Pacemaker
2. *Reduction of Workload*
  (A) Physical and emotional rest
  (B) Treatment of obesity
  (C) Vasodilator therapy
  (D) Assisted circulation
3. *Control of Excessive Salt and Water Retention*
  (A) Low-sodium diet
  (B) Diuretics
  (C) Mechanical removal of fluid
    (1) Thoracentesis
    (2) Paracentesis
    (3) Dialysis
    (4) Phlebotomy

TABLE 16–2   OUTLINE OF TREATMENT OF CHRONIC CONGESTIVE HEART FAILURE*

1. *Restriction of Physical Activity*
   (A) Discontinue exhausting sports and heavy labor
   (B) Discontinue full-time work or equivalent activity, introduce rest periods during the day
   (C) Confine to house
   (D) Confine to bed-chair
2. *Digitalis Glycoside*
   (A) Usual maintenance dose
   (B) Maximally tolerable dose
3. *Restriction of Sodium Intake*
   (A) Eliminate saltshaker at table (Na = 1.6 to 2.8 gm)
   (B) Eliminate salt in cooking and at table (Na = 1.2 to 1.8 gm)
   (C) Institute A and B above plus low-sodium diet (Na = 0.2 to 1.0 gm)
4. *Diuretics*
   (A) Moderate diuretics (thiazide†)
   (B) "Loop" diuretic (ethacrynic acid or furosemide)
   (C) "Loop" diuretic plus distal tubular (potassium-sparing) diuretic
   (D) "Loop" diuretic plus thiazide and distal tubular diuretic
5. *Vasodilators*
   (A) Hydralazine plus isosorbide dinitrate combination or prazosin
   (B) Captopril
   (C) Intravenous nitroprusside
6. *Other Inotropic Agents* (dopamine, dobutamine)
7. *Special Measures* (thoracentesis, paracentesis, dialysis, assisted circulation, cardiac transplantation)

*Numbers and letters correspond to Figure 16–1.
†Thiazide or a diuretic of approximately equal potency, such as metolazone.

THERAPEUTIC STRATEGY IN THE TREATMENT OF HEART FAILURE

CHRONIC HEART FAILURE. A condition as variable as congestive heart failure cannot be treated according to a simple formula. Intelligent management depends on an appreciation of the nature of the underlying condition and the rapidity of its progression; the presence of associated illnesses; the patient's age, occupation, personality, life style, family setting, and ability and motivation to cooperate with treatment; and, importantly, the response to therapeutic measures.[1] With the recognition that wide differences exist among individual patients, Figure 16–1 is presented as a general guide to the therapy of adult patients with chronic congestive heart failure in whom the underlying disease is not amenable to further treatment and in whom precipitating causes have been eliminated to the maximum extent possible. The course of heart failure is rarely smoothly progressive; rather, it is usually punctuated by a series of abrupt downward steps due to acute decompensation, generally as a consequence of one of the precipitating causes of heart failure described on p. 492. When the precipitating cause has been removed and treatment has been intensified, the patient's previous condition is often restored. In other patients there are long periods—many months or even years—when the course is stable without any discernible deterioration.

Ordinarily, treatment of heart failure is not begun until the first symptoms of diminished cardiac reserve occur, i.e., until the patient enters New York Heart Association Class II. The general strategy is to utilize, first, relatively simple means, such as administration of digitalis glycosides or diuretics, mild restriction of physical activity, and reduction of sodium dietary intake. If symptoms and signs of heart failure persist despite these measures, progressively stricter and more aggressive measures must be employed. As has been pointed out elsewhere (p. 493), the earliest symptoms of heart failure usually appear during heavy exertion. When symptoms of dyspnea on exertion or orthopnea are due to ischemia-induced impairment of ventricular diastolic relaxation rather than to diminished systolic contraction, specific measures to reduce myocardial ischemia are in order (see Chapter 40). When it has become clear that these symptoms are indeed related to impaired cardiovascular reserve, two forms of treatment are begun simultaneously: discontinuation of intense physical exertion, i.e., heavy labor and competitive or exhausting sports (1A*); and improvement of the pumping performance of the heart with a usual maintenance dose of a digitalis glycoside (2A*). Obese patients should be encouraged to lose weight, and systemic hypertension, if present, must be treated vigorously. Most patients initially respond to these relatively simple measures, but if symptoms secondary to extracellular fluid accumulation again appear, dietary sodium intake should be restricted. This may consist merely of eliminating the saltshaker at the table (3A*). If heart failure persists or advances despite these measures, an oral diuretic such as a thiazide or an agent of similar potency should be administered (4A*).

When, despite the measures outlined above, a patient is symptomatic upon ordinary exertion such as nondemanding work, shopping, cleaning the home, i.e., when de-

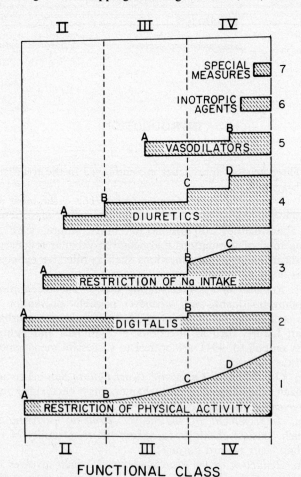

FIGURE 16–1   Strategy of treatment of chronic congestive heart failure in the adult. Various modes of therapy and the intensity of their application at various stages of the patient's course are plotted. For further explanation, see Table 16–2.

terioration into functional Class III (p. 496) has occurred, certain of the measures already taken should be intensified. Full-time work or its equivalent is reduced, the patient is advised to take one or two rest periods during the day (1B*), and a more powerful diuretic—furosemide or ethacrynic acid—is substituted for the thiazide (4B*). When a patient becomes a "late Class III" and is increasingly symptomatic upon ordinary activity, vasodilators may be given (5A*). In some clinical circumstances (e.g., mitral regurgitation), vasodilators may be of particular value and should be considered earlier in the clinical course.

In patients who are symptomatic at rest or with minimal activity, i.e., functional Class IV, confinement to the home is necessary (1C*), and the dose of the cardiac glycoside is cautiously raised to achieve the maximum level consistent with an adequate margin of safety (2B*). All salt is eliminated at the table and in cooking (3B*), and a potassium-sparing diuretic that acts on the distal tubule, such as spironolactone or triamterene, is added to the "loop" diuretic (4C*). If further deterioration occurs, hospitalization is usually required. Other inotropic agents such as a sympathomimetic amine (6*) are administered, physical activity is drastically curtailed (1D*), a low-sodium (200 mg) diet is instituted (3C*), the number and/or dose of diuretics is increased (4D*), intravenous vasodilators may be administered (5B*), and the application of special measures (7*) such as the physical removal of fluid (thoracentesis, paracentesis, or dialysis) or, under special circumstances, the application of assisted circulation or cardiac transplantation may be considered.

To reemphasize the importance of individualizing the treatment of heart failure, a few explanations of this therapeutic strategy are in order.

1. It appears more logical to commence therapy by improving cardiac contractility with a cardiac glycoside and to reduce or eliminate those activities that usually precipitate symptoms of cardiac failure (i.e., to diminish the discrepancy between the heart's ability to pump blood and the requirements of the metabolizing tissues [Fig. 16–2]) as opposed to commencing therapy with diuretics, which treat a complication of heart failure (i.e., the abnormal retention of sodium and water). Nevertheless, certain subsets of patients, such as those with mild symptoms and signs of failure whose physical activity is limited by age or other infirmity, may be treated initially with thiazide diuretics with a more favorable risk-benefit ratio. Also, certain patients with an unusual propensity to develop overt digitalis toxicity may be more appropriately treated initially with a diuretic.

2. Restriction of physical activity is carried out in a manner so as to disturb the patient's life style as little as possible (p. 506).

3. Similarly, restriction of sodium intake need be only mild initially and consist of eliminating the saltshaker at the table, unless heart failure is severe. The availability of potent diuretics allows the patient to eat a nutritious and palatable diet for the major portion of the course of the disease.

4. There is considerable debate about when in the course of heart failure vasodilator treatment should be initiated. It has been proposed that the treatment of heart failure can begin with these drugs rather than with digitalis or diuretics. While the efficacy of this mode of therapy is unquestioned, many patients do not derive long-term benefit (or cannot tolerate side effects) from the chronic oral use of vasodilators (p. 541). Furthermore, in the absence of pulmonary congestion, vasodilators produce little if any rise in cardiac output and may cause a dangerous fall in arterial pressure. Accordingly, it is recommended that vasodilator therapy be begun when the patient has become symptomatic upon mild activity despite optimal use of digitalis and loop diuretics. It is appropriate to use these agents *before* rigid dietary sodium restriction, multiple diuretics, or intravenous inotropic agents are employed.

Since there are many exceptions to this general thera-

*These number and letter designations refer to both Figure 16–1 and Table 16–2.

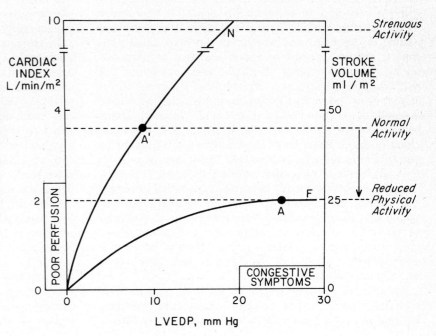

FIGURE 16–2 Diagram demonstrating the relationship between left ventricular end-diastolic pressure (LVEDP) and cardiac index (left ordinate) or stroke volume (right ordinate) in a normal (N) and a failing (F) heart. The upper limit of normal of LVEDP (12 mm Hg) and lower limit of normal of CI (2.2 liters/min/m²) are shown, as are the values associated with congestive symptoms (LVEDP > 20 mm Hg) and with impaired perfusion (< 2.2 liters/min/m²). A and A′ represent the operating points at rest of a hypothetical patient with heart failure and of a normal person, respectively. Reduction of physical activity allows the failing heart to meet the demands of the metabolizing tissues. A positive inotropic agent displaces the curve from F toward N.

peutic strategy, a few examples are provided to demonstrate how it may be modified in specific circumstances:

1. If a patient's livelihood is dependent on physical labor and transfer to a more sedentary occupation cannot be readily accomplished, moderate restriction of sodium intake and diuretics can be begun along with digitalis, and marked restriction of physical activity can be deferred, often for a number of years. Also, the administration of digitalis (with or without ancillary use of verapamil or a beta-adrenergic blocking agent), by controlling ventricular rate in a patient with atrial fibrillation and limitation of functional activity, may restore the patient to near-normal cardiac reserve, and restriction of physical activity can be avoided.

2. Occasional patients with left ventricular failure exhibit symptoms of paroxysmal nocturnal dyspnea that are particularly troublesome, yet they are able to engage in almost normal physical activity during the day. In such patients the paroxysmal nocturnal dyspnea can often be prevented by the administration in the evening of a long-acting venodilator such as nitroglycerin ointment or other transdermal preparation, or by the intensification of diuretic therapy, and they can be maintained in functional Class II.

3. Some patients cannot tolerate vasodilators. They become severely hypotensive, develop an adverse reaction to one of the drugs after prolonged use (e.g., the lupus-like syndrome due to hydralazine), or are unwilling (or unable) to take multiple medications several times a day. Such patients may fare better with more rigid restriction of dietary sodium at an early stage of the disease, and the vasodilator can be held in reserve until later.

4. Occasional patients are particularly prone to accumulate fluid in serous cavities, in which case thoracentesis and/or paracentesis may rapidly relieve dyspnea and need not be reserved until a more advanced phase of the illness.

ACUTE HEART FAILURE (see also p. 571). Treatment of patients with acute congestive cardiac failure usually involves a choice among diuretics, vasodilators, and inotropic agents. In selecting from these three modes of therapy it is well to ascertain by clinical or laboratory means whether cardiac output and arterial pressure are normal or depressed and whether or not myocardial ischemia is present. It must be appreciated that although *diuretics* diminish filling pressure and symptoms of pulmonary congestion, they do not usually increase cardiac output or relieve hypoperfusion; indeed, they may have precisely the opposite effect (Fig. 16–12). *Inotropic agents* increase cardiac output but differ widely in their effects on blood pressure. Selection of the specific agent(s) should be influenced by the effect on vascular resistance that is desired. By virtue of increasing myocardial oxygen demands, inotropic agents potentially aggravate myocardial ischemia. In the presence of ischemia, therefore, afterload-reducing agents that increase cardiac output without this potential adverse effect of inotropic agents may be desirable. However, *vasodilators* may lower arterial pressure, which can interfere with perfusion of the coronary bed, thereby potentially intensifying ischemia.

An effective therapeutic strategy for most patients with acute heart failure can be developed when these principles are kept in mind. Thus, congestion without hypoperfusion should be treated with diuretics. If blood pressure is elevated or normal, vasodilators are indicated if heart failure is severe. The combination of congestion and hypoperfusion should be treated with a vasodilator and diuretic as long as arterial pressure is not depressed, and with positive inotropic agents when blood pressure is depressed.

In transient acute heart failure (e.g., that following acute cardiopulmonary bypass), the most effective therapy may consist of a short period of additional inotropic support with infusion of a sympathomimetic agent, or of reduction of the cardiac workload by applying intraaortic balloon counterpulsation.

General Measures

REST. Reduced physical activity is critical in the care of patients with heart failure throughout their entire course (Fig. 16–1). The intensity of the restriction should depend, of course, on the severity of the heart failure. Until relatively recently it was common practice to reduce markedly the physical activity of patients with enlarged hearts in functional Class II; as a consequence, these patients led unnecessarily restricted lives for many years. Now, the usual recommendation is to tailor the degree of physical activity depending on the symptoms in patients with impaired cardiac reserve. For example, if dyspnea occurs only while a patient is loading cartons into a truck or climbing four flights of stairs, he or she should be advised to make every effort to discontinue these particular activities. If it is essential for them to be continued, they should be carried out more slowly and should be interrupted by rest periods. Competitive or exhausting sports should be discontinued. As is the case in patients with angina pectoris (p. 1346), regular physical activity to a level which does not regularly produce symptoms is desirable in patients with congestive heart failure. Often relatively minor adjustments in activity will allow a patient with mild heart failure to remain gainfully employed or a homemaker to continue routine tasks. Insofar as recreation is concerned, again, minor adjustments, such as the use of a golf cart, may allow the patient many hours of pleasurable activity.

In patients with more severe heart failure, i.e., those in functional Class III, the problem of continued employment becomes more difficult. Such patients are usually unable, and should not be encouraged, to work full-time, even at a relatively sedentary job. This should not mean, however, that total unemployment is necessary or even desirable. Often an adjustment of the work schedule is feasible, e.g., a reduction of the working day from 8 to 5 or 6 hours, with two mandatory one-hour rest periods, or a four-day work week, with a day in the middle of the week during which the patient remains at home to rest. Evening activities should be curtailed but need not be discontinued. Even some patients who are in functional Class IV and are confined to the home are able to lead more satisfying and productive lives by working for two or three hours a day at a desk.

In contrast to the situation in chronic heart failure, in which the patient is urged to remain active short of becoming symptomatic, *physical activity should be rigidly restricted in the presence of acute cardiac decompensation.*

Under these circumstances it is almost always desirable to hospitalize the patient, since this will facilitate work-up and the search for a precipitating cause and will allow adjustment of medication and institution of additional therapeutic measures while the patient is under observation. Hospitalization also facilitates more rigid restriction of sodium intake than is usually possible at home and allows more rigorous control of the restriction of physical activity. Although physical rest plays a crucial role in the treatment of heart failure, complete physical rest does not mean complete rest in bed. Indeed, patients are usually more comfortable and the venous return (and therefore the cardiac preload) is lower when the patient is sitting rather than supine. Also, patients should not be forced to use the bedpan, and trips to the bathroom can usually be allowed. On the other hand, too much relaxation of the rules restricting physical activity can obviate the value of physical rest. For examples, frequent walks to another room on the hospital floor to visit with family or friends, watch television, eat, or use the telephone may nullify the potential benefit of rest.

The hazards of phlebothrombosis and pulmonary embolization should be recognized, and deep-breathing exercises, leg exercises, and elastic stockings are advisable. The use of anticoagulants (minidose heparin, p. 1588) should be considered in patients with heart failure with or without a previous history of thromboembolic disease.

Emotional and mental rest are as important as physical rest. Hospitalization is often beneficial because it removes the patient from a situation that is anxiety-provoking. Since emotional stress can retard convalescence from an episode of acute congestive heart failure, visitors and incoming telephone calls should be limited. The physician should serve as a thoughtful, sympathetic listener with whom the patient can discuss a variety of problems. In particular, the patient must be given a realistic appraisal of the prognosis, and it must be emphasized that if a precipitating cause of heart failure can be identified, acute cardiac decompensation does not signify a hopeless outlook. It is important that the patient sleep well each night, and the use of flurazepam, 15 to 30 mg, as a hypnotic may be advisable. Diazepam, 2 to 5 mg twice a day, may be helpful as well in patients with marked anxiety.

There is no formula for deciding on the duration of rigid restriction of physical activity for patients with acute cardiac decompensation. It should depend principally on the patient's response to the overall treatment program. As a general rule, it is advisable to maintain the patient at rest as long as *more* than a trace of ankle edema or a few moist rales at the lung bases persist. At this point the patient can usually be discharged to continue convalescence at home or in a nursing home. Although the restriction of physical activity can be relaxed at this point, it should continue in a modified form for two to four weeks, depending on the rigidity of the patient's convalescence.

DIET. Before effective oral diuretics were available, diet played a more important role in the control of salt and water retention than it does today. It is now possible to recommend only modest restriction of sodium intake in most patients with heart failure, with intensification of the diuretic regimen to prevent accumulation of extracellular fluid. Nonetheless, restriction of sodium intake remains one of the cornerstones of the treatment of congestive heart failure. The normal daily sodium content of the unrestricted American diet ranges from 3.0 to 6.0 gm; simple elimination of the saltshaker at the table and a few common foods such as pretzels, popcorn, salted nuts, potato chips, candy bars, smoked and salt-cured meats (including ham, bacon, and sausage), delicatessen meats, herring, and condiments such as olives and pickles will reduce this to approximately half (1.5 to 3.0 gm). Potassium chloride (salt substitute) may be used in place of ordinary table salt. There is no need to eliminate the salt in cooking and to make the diet unpalatable unless fluid retention occurs despite intensive use of diuretics. Indeed, the monotony and unpalatability of a low-sodium diet has caused unnecessary hardship to patients and their families and has often interfered with adequate nutrition.

Reduction of sodium intake to between 1.2 and 1.5 gm/day can be achieved by simply eliminating all salt from cooking and from the table. If it is necessary to reduce the sodium intake to 0.2 gm daily in patients with Class IV congestive heart failure, many common foods must be eliminated. Spices and herbs should be used to flavor the food in place of sodium chloride, and as wide a variety of foods as possible should be employed to diminish the monotony. A variety of books and pamphlets are available to aid in the preparation of salt-poor diets. It must be recognized that while the elimination of dietary salt may be necessary in patients with severe heart failure, this can result in a marked reduction of caloric intake, leading to malnutrition and even cardiac cachexia (p. 499).

Opinion concerning *water intake* in heart failure has varied widely in the past. At one time rigid restriction of water intake was advised; then it became clear that the total extracellular fluid volume was primarily dependent on the body sodium content. For some years it was thought that excessive water intake (exceeding 3 liters/day) would increase the elimination of salt, i.e., it would "flush out" sodium. There is no evidence in favor of this concept, and therefore it is advisable simply to leave the water intake to the patient's own desire. However, in far-advanced congestive heart failure the ability to excrete a free-water load may be impaired, with resulting dilutional hyponatremia (p. 1750). Only under these circumstances is it desirable to restrict water intake so that the serum sodium concentration does not fall below approximately 130 mEq/liter. Modest reductions of serum sodium (i.e., to 130 to 142 mEq/liter) do not usually require specific therapy.

OXYGEN. The use of oxygen in patients with pulmonary edema and with acute myocardial infarction is discussed elsewhere (pp. 571 and 1303). Oxygen inhalation, most conveniently by means of nasal prongs at 4 to 6 liters/min, should be employed in patients with other forms of congestive heart failure if the arterial oxygen saturation falls below 90 per cent. Oxygen therapy is particularly useful in patients with heart failure precipitated by pulmonary infection or pulmonary infarction. Many patients consider the inhalation of oxygen a sign of terminal illness, and it is important to explain to them that in most instances its use is temporary.

PHYSICAL REMOVAL OF FLUID. Ordinarily, mechanical removal of fluid from the pleural and abdominal cavities is unnecessary in patients with congestive heart failure, because these collections are generally easily mobilized and eliminated with effective diuresis. Occasionally, patients with advanced congestive heart failure who are resistant to diuretic therapy may regain their sensitivity following mechanical removal of fluid. In some patients with acute respiratory distress in whom the lungs are compressed by large pleural effusion(s) and/or by diaphragms elevated by ascites, mechanical removal of the effusions can bring rapid relief of dyspnea. Mechanical removal of fluid may be associated with a risk, albeit a small one in experienced hands, of pneumothorax or infection. Drainage of ascitic fluid should be carried out slowly, i.e., not more than 1600 ml/hr, and the total quantity of pleural fluid re-

moved on a single occasion should not usually exceed 1500 ml; otherwise, fluid may move rapidly from the circulation into the abdominal or pleural cavity, and cardiovascular collapse may occur.

Removal of excess fluid by *peritoneal dialysis* or, preferably, *hemodialysis with ultrafiltration* has been employed successfully in patients with congestive heart failure resistant to diuretic therapy.

Severe constipation and consequent straining at stool should be avoided in patients with heart failure. Dioctyl sodium sulfosuccinate, 50 to 200 mg daily, is useful as a stool softener. In addition, a mild laxative may be necessary in patients whose physical activity has been restricted.

DIGITALIS GLYCOSIDES

For 200 years, digitalis glycosides have occupied a prominent place in the management of congestive heart failure and certain arrhythmias. Withering recognized in 1785 that optimal use of digitalis requires considerable knowledge and skill on the part of the physician because of the unusually narrow therapeutic:toxic dose ratio of this group of drugs.[2] A sound understanding of the actions and pharmacokinetics of these drugs is essential to minimize the ever-present risk of toxicity and to provide maximum benefit to the patient.

In the discussion that follows, the term *digitalis* is used to refer to any of the steroid or steroid glycoside compounds that exert typical positive inotropic and electrophysiological effects on the heart. Although there are important differences in pharmacokinetics among the more than 300 known compounds with these properties, their pharmacological actions are fundamentally similar, and detailed consideration will therefore be limited to those agents that are in common clinical use.

SOURCES.   The majority of digitalis drugs in routine clinical use today are steroid glycosides derived from the leaves of the common flowering plant known as foxglove, or *Digitalis purpurea* (digitoxin, gitalin, digitalis leaf), or from the leaves of *D. lanata* (digoxin, lanatoside C, deslanoside). Ouabain, an exception, is obtained from seeds of *Strophanthus gratus.*

STRUCTURE.   The steroid nucleus common to all cardiac glycosides contains an α, β-unsaturated lactone

ring attached at the C-17 position. Without attached sugars, the steroid and unsaturated lactone part of the molecule is called the *genin* or *aglycone*. Although possessing characteristic digitalis-like pharmacological properties, genins are usually less potent and have more transient actions than do the parent glycosides. Figure 16–3 shows the structure of digoxin; digitoxin differs from digoxin only in the absence of the hydroxyl group at C-12. It is apparent from structure-activity comparisons that considerable variation in the steroid nucleus as well as sugar substituents attached at the C-3 position occurs among the cardioactive glycosides. Potent cardioactivity does, however, require the unsaturated lactone ring, the C-14 β-hydroxyl group, and *cis* fusion of the C and D rings.[2a,3]

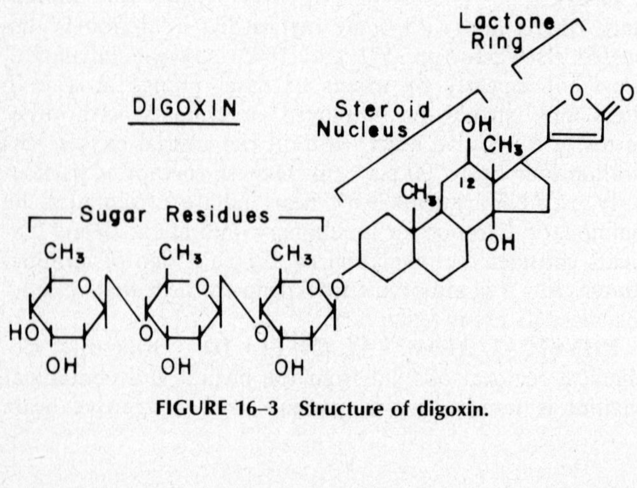

MECHANISMS OF CARDIAC GLYCOSIDE ACTION

INOTROPY.   The entire spectrum of myocardial cellular activity has been studied in search of the cellular or molecular mechanism underlying the positive inotropic action of digitalis.[4-7] While controversy persists regarding the basic mechanism of digitalis-induced inotropy, it is apparent that cardiac glycosides increase the force and velocity of contraction of the normal as well as the failing heart.

Any comprehensive model of cardiac glycoside–induced inotropy must take into account several fundamental observations, including the following: digitalis glycosides exert a positive inotropic effect on cardiac muscle but not on skeletal muscle[8]; the extent of the positive inotropic response is dependent on contraction frequency, declining on either side of an optimum value[9]; and the magnitude and rate of onset of positive inotropy are dependent on the concentration of a number of ions, including potassium, sodium, calcium, and magnesium.[10] There is not a close correlation between cardiac catecholamine content and the response to cardiac glycosides.[11] Furthermore, marked positive inotropic effects persist in the presence of full β-adrenergic blocking doses of drugs such as propranolol.[12] Therefore the major inotropic effects of cardiac glycosides are not mediated by catecholamine release or increased sensitivity to catecholamines. Adenylate cyclase activity, although thought to participate in the mediation of posi-

FIGURE 16–3   Structure of digoxin.

tive inotropic effects of β-adrenergic agonists and glucagon, does not appear to be influenced by digitalis glycosides.[13]

Actin, myosin, and the troponin-tropomyosin regulatory system have all been postulated as possible sites of cardiac glycoside action, but convincing evidence is lacking for a primary interaction between these proteins and digitalis glycosides at relevant concentrations.[14] Also, there is no evidence that digitalis has a direct effect on intermediary metabolism or on myocardial energetics, although cardiac glycosides share with other positive inotropic agents the tendency to increase myocardial oxygen consumption. In the failing heart, digitalis may actually reduce myocardial oxygen consumption by decreasing heart size and hence wall tension through the Laplace relation.[15]

CALCIUM AND CARDIAC GLYCOSIDES. Central to the problem of elucidating the mechanism by which digitalis exerts its positive inotropic effect is the still incomplete understanding of myocardial excitation-contraction coupling. As discussed on pages 417 and 613, the slow inward current that occurs during the plateau phase of the myocardial action potential has been well documented to be carried, in large part, by Ca^{++}; this influx of Ca^{++} appears to be related to excitation-contraction coupling. An increase in the magnitude of slow inward current in cardiac Purkinje and myocardial fibers exposed to cardiotonic steroids has been reported and may be related, at least in part, to inhibition of the Na pump, as discussed below.[16–18] In any case, the absence of definable primary changes in other cellular functions has led most investigators to conclude that cardiac glycosides, by some mechanism, increase the availability of Ca^{++} to the contractile element at the time of excitation-contraction coupling. In principle, this could be brought about by an increase in the steady-state contractile Ca^{++} pool as a result of increased influx or decreased efflux of Ca^{++}, or by increased influx of Ca^{++} during the action potential, with enhanced excitation-contraction coupling, balanced by increased efflux with no increase in net steady-state myocardial Ca^{++}. This effect appears to require an intact sarcolemma, since inotropic effects of digitalis are absent in mechanically skinned myocardial fibers[19] despite intact sarcoplasmic reticulum and contractile element structures. The complexity of myocardial Ca^{++} compartmentalization precludes any simple experimental approach to these problems, but cardiac glycoside–induced increases in a rapidly exchangeable Ca^{++} pool that appear to be linked to the contractile state of the cell have been reported.[20–22] Direct evidence for an increase in the intracellular Ca^{++} transient following exposure to digitalis is now available from the studies of Blinks and colleagues with the photoactive calcium-sensitive protein aequorin.[22a] Digitalis seems to exert no consistent effect on Ca^{++} transport by the sarcoplasmic reticulum.[4]

Na^+,K^+-ATPase AND CARDIAC GLYCOSIDES. The noteworthy lack of well-defined effects of digitalis on other cellular functions has led to continuing investigative interest in the uniquely specific ability of cardioactive steroids to inhibit transmembrane movement of Na^+ and K^+ by inhibition of the Mg^{++}- and ATP-dependent, Na^+- and K^+-activated transport enzyme complex known as Na^+,K^+-ATPase. Following the observation that cardiac glycosides inhibit monovalent cation transport in the red cell,[23]

Na^+,K^+-ATPase was identified as a membrane-bound transport enzyme system[24] and was postulated to be the pharmacological receptor for digitalis glycosides.[25] Labeled cardiac glycosides bind to Na^+,K^+-ATPase in a saturable manner, and the rate of this interaction is increased by Na^+ and decreased by K^+.[26]

Circumstantial evidence implicating Na^+,K^+-ATPase as a receptor for the inotropic action of cardiac glycosides includes the following observations:

1. Na^+,K^+-ATPase is inhibited by cardioactive but not by inactive digitalis analogs, and a reasonably close relation exists between potency of Na^+,K^+-ATPase inhibition and cardiac activity.[6,24,27]

2. Species cardiac sensitivity to digitalis glycosides is directly correlated with the ability of glycosides to inhibit myocardial Na^+,K^+-ATPase from that species.[25] In the rat, for example, which is notably resistant to the cardiac effects of digitalis, myocardial Na^+,K^+-ATPase is about 100 times less sensitive to cardiac glycosides than is enzyme derived from sensitive species.[28]

3. The time course of Na^+,K^+-ATPase inhibition closely parallels that of the inotropic effect in the hearts of several species, in terms of both onset and offset of effects.[22,29,30]

4. The positive inotropic effects of cardiac glycosides are enhanced under conditions that increase intracellular Na^+ concentration, such as paired stimulation or the presence of grayanotoxins, which increase Na^+ influx.[31] Conversely, digitalis-induced inotropy is delayed under conditions that decrease intracellular Na^+ concentration such as a low [Na^+] in the extracellular milieu[31] or the presence of tetrodotoxin.[32]

5. A number of interventions, such as lowering temperature, raising extracellular [K^+], or lowering pH, all have a parallel tendency to reduce both the inotropic effect on isolated heart muscle and the inhibitory effect of cardiac glycosides on Na^+,K^+-ATPase.[7]

6. Another intervention that inhibits the activity of Na^+,K^+-ATPase, reduction of extracellular [K^+], exerts similar positive inotropic effects, a similar degree of Na^+,K^+-ATPase inhibition, and similar enhancement of intracellular [Na^+].[33,34]

7. Doses of cardiac glycosides producing a positive inotropic effect in the intact dog have been shown to inhibit Na^+,K^+-ATPase activity in myocardial enzyme preparations from the heart of the same animal.[35] Studies employing myocardial biopsies in dogs have demonstrated that sustained subtoxic plasma and myocardial cardiac glycoside levels sufficient to produce a positive inotropic effect result in appreciable inhibition of myocardial monovalent cation transport capacity.[36,37]

8. Elevated extracellular [K^+] has been shown to slow the uptake of cardiac glycosides by myocardial tissue,[38] to slow the onset of inotropic effect,[38] and to slow the rate of binding of cardiac glycosides to myocardial Na^+,K^+-ATPase.[26] The ability of potassium to suppress clinical digitalis toxicity adds further substance to this line of reasoning.

9. At least one group of compounds, the erythrophleum alkaloids, differs chemically from the cardiac glycosides yet shares both the positive inotropic effect and the ability specifically to inhibit Na^+,K^+-ATPase.[39]

10. Inhibitors of Na^+,K^+-ATPase such as N-ethylmaleimide and p-chloromercuribenzoate have been shown to produce positive inotropic effects, and these effects are accompanied by inhibition of the Na^+ pump.[40] Furthermore, monovalent cations such as Rb^+ and Tl^+ that are capable of inhibiting Na^+,K^+-ATPase in the presence of Na^+ and K^+ produce sustained positive inotropic effects in isolated heart preparations[40]; concentrations of Tl^+ and digitalis that are equieffective in inhibiting the activity of the Na^+ pump produce similar increases in myocardial contractility.

The interaction between cardiac glycosides and Na^+,K^+-ATPase has been studied in considerable detail,[5] and these studies have been aided by advances in the purification and characterization of the transport enzyme itself. As isolated from kidney,[41] shark rectal gland,[42] or avian salt gland,[43] the Na^+,K^+-ATPase complex includes a large polypeptide chain of about 100,000 daltons that undergoes transphosphorylation from the γ phosphate of ATP; a smaller sialoglycoprotein of about 50,000 daltons; and a somewhat variable phospholipid content, without which the enzyme is inactive. A 12,000-dalton proteolipid component has been described in Na^+,K^+-ATPase from pig kidney[44]; further studies are required to determine whether this component is also present in highly purified enzyme from other organs and species.

One cardiac glycoside binding site appears to be present per large polypeptide chain.[45] Na+,K+-ATPase purified from cardiac muscle has characteristics similar to those of the highly purified enzyme from the above-noted sources.[46] The sarcolemma is assumed to be the principal site of this enzyme complex in heart muscle. Optimal binding of cardiac glycosides to Na+,K+-ATPase under physiological circumstances requires the presence of Na++, Mg++, and ATP.[5]

Monovalent Cation Transport Inhibition and Inotropy

Although a highly specific interaction between cardiac glycosides and Na+,K+-ATPase has been defined, the relationship between this interaction and the well-known effects of digitalis on the intact heart has been elusive. As early as 1931, Calhoun and Harrison observed a decrease in myocardial [K+] after toxic doses of cardiac glycosides.[47] Many subsequent studies have documented decreases in intracellular [K+] and, in many cases, increases in intracellular [Na+] in response to large toxic doses of cardiac glycosides, while results with smaller subtoxic but still inotropic doses have often been more equivocal.[4]

Studies with isotopic uptake and washout techniques have provided evidence that positive inotropic responses are accompanied by a net loss of K+ and a net uptake of Na+, accompanied by a net uptake of cellular Ca++.[21] The appearance of toxic manifestations, such as ectopic beats and contracture, was accompanied by further changes of still greater magnitude. Positive inotropic responses were not observed without evidence of some degree of inhibition of Na+ transport. Direct evidence supporting cardiac glycoside–induced increases in intracellular [Na+] comes from impalement of cardiac cells with Na+-sensitive microelectrodes.[48-50]

From these and other experiments it has been argued that inhibition of active cellular Na+ transport may result in enhancement of Ca++ uptake, which in turn produces a positive inotropic response analogous to that which follows an increase in contraction frequency in the "treppe" or Bowditch staircase phenomenon.[51] The mechanism of this effect might be enhanced exchange of intracellular Na+ for extracellular Ca++ such as has been observed in the squid giant axon[52] as well as mammalian myocardium.[53] This proposed sequence is shown in schematic form in Figure 16–4. Such a mechanism would be consistent with the known dependence of cardiac glycoside–induced inotropy on both the number and the rate of contractions following exposure to the drug.[9] The transmembrane Na+ influx occurring with each action potential, together with diminished outward Na+ pumping, would lead to the increased intracellular Na+ concentration proposed to promote transmembrane exchange of Na+ and Ca++. At rapid heart rates, Na+ influx might be of sufficient magnitude to provide the maximum utilizable intracellular Na+, thus perhaps explaining the diminished effects of cardiac glycosides at these high frequencies.[9]

Akera and Brody and their colleagues have advanced a hypothesis that takes into account most of the observations noted above.[4,40,54] This hypothesis is based on binding to and inhibition of Na+,K+-ATPase by cardiac glycosides. This in turn reduces the activity of the

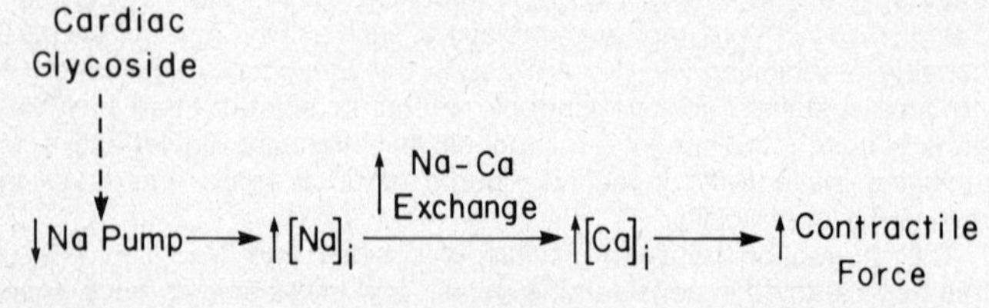

Na+ pump, resulting in an enhanced transient increase in intracellular Na+ close to the sarcolemma that occurs only during the early portion of each cardiac cycle. The transient increase in Na+ is postulated to result in enhanced Ca++ influx, presumably through the Na+-Ca++ exchange carrier mechanism, and hence in enhanced activation of contractile elements. This hypothesis differs from that advanced by other authors in that the increase in intracellular Na+ is presumed to be cyclic and not cumulative.

Studies with spontaneously contracting cultured chick embryo ventricular cells have demonstrated direct correlations between ouabain-induced enhancement of the contractile state and inhibition of monovalent cation active transport as well as increased cell content of both Na+ and Ca++.[22] These data support the hypothesis that inhibition of the Na+ pump by cardiac glycosides is causally related to the development of positive inotropy and are consistent with modulation of Ca++ content by Na+ via the Na+-Ca++ exchange carrier mechanism. Further support is provided by studies showing that another intervention, decreasing extracellular [K+], produces equivalent positive inotropic effects together with similar Na+ and K+ transport inhibition, similar increases in intracellular [Na+], and similar enhancement of Na+-Ca++ exchange compared with cardiac glycosides.[33]

Alternatively, it may be that the positive inotropic response in the mammalian heart, although dependent upon a specific interaction between cardiac glycosides and Na+,K+-ATPase, does not depend upon inhibition of the Na+ and K+ pumping function of the enzyme per se. The present state of knowledge does not preclude the possibility of more direct interactions between this enzyme system and the release of Ca++ during excitation-contraction coupling that could be modified by cardiac glycosides.[55,56] Other studies have provided evidence in support of the hypothesis that the interaction of cardiac glycosides with Na+,K+-ATPase inhibits outward pumping of both Na+ and Ca++ from the myocardial cell, resulting in an increase in the Ca++ pool available for excitation-contraction coupling.[57]

Despite this weight of evidence implicating Na+,K+-ATPase as a receptor for the inotropic effects of digitalis, findings from some laboratories do not support the concept that positive inotropy results from inhibition of this enzyme system.[58] Further detailed discussions of the vast experimental literature on mechanisms of cardiac glycoside action are found in several reviews.[5,6,40,51,56,59-62]

Myocardial Uptake and Subcellular Localization

Availability of radioactively labeled cardiac glycosides has allowed detailed studies of uptake by intact heart muscle and of subcellular localization. A general conclusion that can be drawn is that more polar glycosides, such as ouabain, principally undergo specific binding to membrane receptor sites that have many of the properties of Na+, K+-ATPase.[4,5] Less polar glycosides are bound nonspecifically to lipid membrane sites, and there is a high degree of nonspecific binding of nonpolar glycosides such as digitoxin. Digoxin is intermediate both in polarity and in specificity of binding.

The degree of specific binding to myocardial cell membrane components is dependent upon Na+ and K+ concentrations, with low extracellular K+ and high Na+ promoting binding.[5,6] Therefore, it is not surprising that electrolyte disturbances may exert clinically important effects on the myocardial uptake and hence actions of cardiac glycosides. Goldman et al. showed that hyperkalemia inhibited the positive inotropic effect of digoxin in addition to diminishing digoxin binding by the intact canine heart.[63] Mg++ depletion with resultant hypomagnesemia may predispose to digitalis toxicity.[64]

Cardiac glycosides can inhibit monovalent cation transport only when present at the outer cell surface in the red blood cell[65,66] and in the squid giant axon.[67] The myocardial receptor is also likely to be accessible only at the outer cell surface, although studies with ouabain and digoxin covalently coupled to macromolecular carrier molecules such as albumin, which are too large to enter intact cells, have not provided conclusive proof of this hypothesis.[68] Cell fractionation procedures have shown that binding of cardiac glycosides to myocardium of sensitive species is mainly in the "microsomal" membrane fraction. No high-affinity binding site with requisite properties for a cardiac glycoside receptor has yet been identified in myocardium that could be separated from Na+,K+-ATPase.[69]

Cardiac
Glycoside

FIGURE 16–4 Schematic representation of the mechanism of inotropic action of cardiac glycosides. Binding of digitalis to NaK-ATPase inhibits this enzyme and hence the active outward transport of Na+ across the myocardial cell membrane. Na+ pump inhibition thus leads to increased intracellular Na+ ([Na]i) content and activity, which in turn enhances Na-Ca exchange with consequent increase in Ca influx, decrease of Ca efflux, or both. The resulting increase in intracellular Ca ([Ca]i) is presumed to mediate the observed increase in myocardial contractile force.

Electrophysiological Effects (See also p. 238)

Major electrophysiological effects of digitalis on the heart are summarized in Table 16–3. The 80- to 90-mV transmembrane resting potential of cardiac cells (see Figure 19–6, p. 611) is maintained by Na^+ and K^+ gradients (particularly the latter), which in turn are dependent upon the integrity of the active Na^+-K^+ pump mechanism discussed above. It is therefore not surprising that agents such as cardiac glycosides that inhibit the pump mechanism have profound effects on the electrophysiology of the intact heart as well as on isolated muscle preparations. Unlike the controversial subject of the mechanism of inotropic cardiac glycoside effects, there is general agreement that inhibition of Na^+,K^+-ATPase underlies direct toxic effects on cardiac rhythm. Cells in various parts of the heart show differing sensitivities to digitalis (Table 16–3), and both direct and neurally mediated effects must be dissected before conclusions can be drawn about the mechanisms involved.[70]

Although usually absent or clinically inapparent at conventional doses, glycoside-induced depression of intraatrial conduction, manifested by increases in P-A interval and atrial effective and functional refractory periods, has been documented.[71] The relative importance of direct and autonomically mediated effects of digoxin has been assessed in man by studying patients undergoing cardiac transplantation.[72,73] Evaluation of sinus node function showed no change in sinus cycle length after administration of digoxin to patients with hearts denervated by transplantation. Sinoatrial conduction time was unchanged by digoxin in the majority of patients, while first-degree sinoatrial node exit block occurred in one patient and 2:1 sinoatrial node exit block developed in a second.[72] Digoxin did not produce significant changes in atrial effective or functional refractory periods nor in atrioventricular nodal effective or functional refractory periods in denervated patients.[73] These findings, as well as experimental observations in the dog,[74] underscore the importance of the autonomic nervous system in the modulation of automaticity and conduction by digitalis.

In studies on the cellular electrophysiological effects of digitalis on human atrial fibers obtained at operation, ouabain initially induced increases in maximum diastolic potential, action-potential amplitude, and upstroke velocity of phase 0 depolarization and decreases in duration and automaticity of the action potential.[75] These effects were identical to those produced by acetylcholine and were blocked by atropine. After more prolonged ouabain exposure, opposite responses emerged, and delayed afterdepolarizations and tachyarrhythmias occurred. Thus, the acetylcholine-like effects of digitalis decreased automaticity and increased maximum diastolic potential, while direct effects decreased maximum diastolic potential, increased automaticity, and induced tachyarrhythmias in isolated human atrial fibers.[75]

Most of the antiarrhythmic effects of digitalis are the result of its action on the atria and atrioventricular junction.[70] Within the specialized conduction tissues of the heart the refractory period is increased by digitalis, and conduction velocity is diminished, tending to slow the ventricular response to atrial fibrillation and atrial flutter or to prolong the P-R interval in the presence of normal sinus rhythm. In atrial and ventricular myocardium, the refractory period tends to be shortened, and the more rapid recovery time is reflected in a shortening of the Q-T interval. Effects of digitalis on AV conduction occur predominantly at the level of the AV node, rather than more distally in the His-Purkinje system.[76]

Detailed in vitro studies of the effects of digitalis glycosides on cardiac transmembrane action potentials have been carried out for the most part in the mammalian ventricular Purkinje fiber, and the effects observed are generally assumed to be relevant to electrophysiological changes occurring in other cardiac cells. At low concentrations, the resting potential, action potential amplitude, and time course of depolarization and repolarization remain unchanged at a time when inotropic effects are first apparent. At higher concentrations of cardiac glycosides and particularly at more rapid rates of stimulation, there is progressive loss of resting potential, and changes occur in the time course of depolarization and repolarization, including decreased slope of the upstroke of the action potential, shortening of the plateau phase, and increased rate of spontaneous diastolic depolarization. The sensitivity of canine Purkinje fibers to ouabain increases with age,[77] consistent with the clinical observation that younger patients tend to require (and to tolerate) greater cardiac glycoside doses on the basis of dosage per unit of body weight or per square meter of body surface area.[78]

Further details concerning the electrophysiological effects of cardiac glycosides may be found in the discussions of Smith et al.,[61] Hoffman and Bigger,[3] and Weingart.[79]

TABLE 16–3 SOME MAJOR EFFECTS OF DIGITALIS ON THE ELECTROPHYSIOLOGICAL PROPERTIES OF THE HEART

PROPERTY	EFFECT
Pacemaker Automaticity	
SA node	→ ↓ (↑ after atropine or toxic doses)
Purkinje fibers	↑
Excitability	
Atrium	→*
Ventricle	Variable*
Purkinje fibers	↑*
Membrane Responsiveness	
Atrium	Variable* (↓ after atropine)
Ventricle	↓ (toxic doses)
Purkinje fibers	↓ (toxic doses)
Conduction Velocity	
Atrium, ventricle	↑ (slight)*
AV node	↓
Purkinje fibers	↓
Effective Refractory Period	
Atrium	↓ (↑ after atropine)
Ventricle	↓
AV node	↑
Purkinje fibers	↑*

Key: The arrows indicate the direction, not the magnitude, of the changes indicated: ↑ = increased; ↓ = decreased; → = no significant change.

*Decreased with high toxic doses of digitalis.

From Moe, G. K., and Farah, A. E.: Digitalis and allied cardiac glycosides. *In* Goodman, L. S., and Gilman, A. (eds.): The Pharmacological Basis of Therapeutics. 5th ed. New York, The Macmillan Co., 1975, p. 661.

Neurally Mediated Effects

Substantial progress has been made in recent years in the delineation of neurally mediated effects of cardiac glycosides.[61,79a] Direct nerve recordings have shown that cardiac glycosides can influence preganglionic cardiac sympathetic nerve activity in anesthetized cats.[80,81] In the toxic range, sympathetic nerve activity was substantially augmented, and high-intensity bursting was temporally correlated with ventricular tachyarrhythmias, including fatal ventricular fibrillation. Spinal-cord section at the C1 level prevented these effects and resulted in an increase in the dose of ouabain required to produce ventricular arrhythmias.[81–83] Propranolol administration reduced ouabain-induced neural hyperactivity and usually converted ventricular arrhythmias to normal sinus rhythm. These studies support the concept that neural activation by cardiac glycosides may play an important part in the development of cardiac rhythm disturbances.

Studies in a cat experimental model indicate that an important locus of neural augmentation of digitalis-induced arrhythmias lies within an area of the medulla 2 mm above to 2 mm below the obex.[82] Taken together with observations of the effects of highly polar glycosides derivatives that do not appear to cross the normal blood-brain barrier,[84] these findings implicate the area postrema as a likely site of digitalis-induced neural activation. Neurally mediated effects of cardiac glycosides are discussed in greater detail in a recent review.[61]

HEMODYNAMIC EFFECTS

MYOCARDIAL CONTRACTILITY. For many decades after the introduction of digitalis into clinical use, clinicians overlooked what is now considered to be one of its major actions; augmentation of the force of myocardial contraction. The drug was not recommended for the treatment of heart failure with normal rhythm but was instead reserved for patients with rapid heart rates. Early in the twentieth century, a series of clinical observations led to recognition that the beneficial effects of digitalis in congestive heart failure were not solely dependent on cardiac rate but were mediated through a positive inotropic effect on the myocardium.[85]

Improved techniques of pharmacological investigation allowed documentation of the positive inotropic actions of digitalis. Wiggers and Stimson showed that digitalis increases the rate of rise in intraventricular pressure during isovolumetric systole when heart rate and aortic pressure are kept constant.[86] The experiments of Cattell and Gold in 1938 showed directly that ouabain increased the force of contraction in isolated, electrically driven cat papillary muscles.[87] The inotropic action of digitalis is manifest in normal as well as in failing heart muscle.[88,89]

The effect of digitalis on the intact heart is reflected in the ventricular function curve (Fig. 16–2), in which glycoside administration causes the curve to shift upward and to the left, so that at any given ventricular filling pressure more stroke work is generated in the presence of digitalis than in control circumstances. Figure 16–5 shows an experimental approach in which the velocity of contraction is examined at varying loads. It is apparent that maximum tension development is greater after strophanthidin administration. In addition, the time needed to reach a given tension is less at each successive load studied. These effects on the force-velocity relation are similar to those resulting from the action of catecholamines but are independent of cardiac norepinephrine stores, since similar results have been observed in reserpine-treated or chronically denervated hearts[11] or after beta-adrenergic blockade.[12] The *absolute* increase in tension development induced by digitalis is at

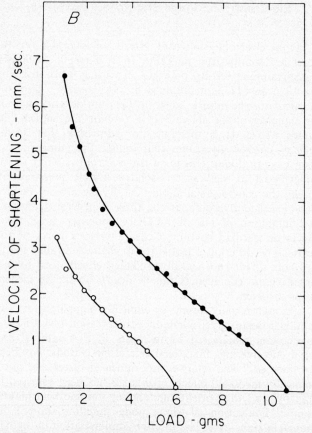

FIGURE 16–5 Force-velocity curves for normal cat papillary muscle before and after (●——●) addition of strophanthidin to the bath. The drug increases the maximum velocity of shortening as well as maximum isometric force developed. (From Sonnenblick, E. H., Williams, J. F., Jr., Glick, G., Mason, D. T., and Braunwald, E.: Studies on digitalis. XV. Effects of cardiac glycosides on myocardial force-velocity relations in the nonfailing human heart. Circulation *34*:532, 1966, by permission of the American Heart Association, Inc.)

least as great in the normal as in the failing myocardium. However, since the failing myocardium has a lower peak tension, the *relative* augmentation of tension is greater.[90]

Administration of cardiac glycosides results in no change or a slight decline in cardiac output in normal subjects.[91,92] This is not surprising, since cardiac output is determined not only by contractile state but also by preload, afterload, and heart rate (p. 441). It is now clear that digitalis augments the contractile state of the nonfailing myocardium in the intact human heart, but adjustments in other determinants of cardiac output prevent an appreciable increase in cardiac output.[88,93]

The effects of digitalis on cardiac function of patients in normal sinus rhythm have undergone considerable study recently, prompted in part by several publications questioning the value of cardiac glycosides in this setting.[94] Studies using both noninvasive and invasive techniques have now documented sustained improvement in cardiac performance of patients with chronic congestive heart failure.[94] The clinical response, however, is critically dependent on patient selection and on the nature and extent of ventricular dysfunction. Arnold and colleagues documented favorable hemodynamic effects of digoxin in a series of patients with functional class III or IV heart failure.[95] Lee et al., using a double-blind placebo-controlled trial design, reported clinical improvement in 14 of 25 patients during outpatient digoxin administration. If one excludes patients with normal left ventricular ejection fractions and those with steady-state serum digoxin concentrations of 0.5 ng/ml or less from the group reported by Lee et al., then 14 of the 16 patients (all of whom had depressed left ventricular ejection fractions and an audible S_3 gallop) who might have been expected to respond favorably showed objective improvement on digoxin.[96] Murray and colleagues likewise found that both intravenous ouabain and maintenance oral digoxin exerted a modest positive inotropic effect in patients with cardiac failure in sinus rhythm, but hemodynamic benefit was significant only during exertion in this group of 10 patients.[97] However, a group of 30 patients, most of whom were elderly and had ischemic heart disease, studied with a placebo-controlled trial design by Fleg et al., showed no detectable deterioration during the period of digoxin withdrawal.[98] These authors concluded that long-term digoxin therapy has only a minor effect on cardiac performance that is without apparent clinical importance in a "representative" population of ambulatory patients, a little over half of whom were in functional class II; only one subject in this series had an S_3 gallop. These studies emphasize the importance of patient selection in predicting clinical responses to cardiac glycosides of patients with normal sinus rhythm.

DIGITALIS IN HEART FAILURE. The foregoing observations provide a basis for understanding the mechanisms whereby digitalis ameliorates the signs and symptoms of congestive heart failure. As various pathological processes (such as ischemia, volume or pressure loading, or intrinsic cardiac muscle defects) decrease contractility, compensatory reserve mechanisms are brought into play. Elevations in end-diastolic pressure and volume result in increased contractile force through the Frank-Starling mechanism, increased sympathetic tone tends to increase the contractile state, and ventricular hypertrophy may provide more contractile elements. However, each of these three compensatory mechanisms has a price: pulmonary or peripheral edema occurs when end-diastolic ventricular pressures rise excessively; tachycardia may be an undesirable effect of excess sympathetic tone; and increased myocardial oxygen consumption results with all three compensatory mechanisms. If cardiac disease progresses and contractility continues to diminish, the consequences of one of these compensatory mechanisms will become dominant (e.g., pulmonary edema) or the compensatory mechanisms will become insufficient to maintain cardiac output.

Under these circumstances, administration of cardiac glycosides will improve the depressed contractile state, decreasing encroachment on compensatory mechanisms and improving cardiac reserve. The ventricular function curve is shifted upward (Fig. 16–2), so that for any given ventricular end-diastolic pressure, cardiac output is greater. The clinical consequence is a reduction in end-diastolic pressure (and hence diminished pulmonary and systemic venous pressure) and increased cardiac output.

Of major clinical importance is the selection of appropriate endpoints or therapeutic goals in the use of digitalis. Although experimental studies have indicated that the positive inotropic action of cardiac glycosides increases progressively until toxic arrhythmias appear,[99,100] the limited clinical evidence available suggests that little if any further benefit is to be expected by increasing digoxin doses to levels resulting in serum concentrations in excess of about 1.5 to 2.0 ng/ml in patients with congestive heart failure and normal sinus rhythm.[94] Nevertheless, digitalization is not an all-or-none state and the degree of positive inotropic action of the drug increases in a graded manner with increasing dose, at least to the point where steady-state serum digoxin levels are in the range usually considered to be therapeutic. The clinician's task is to determine the appropriate dose consistent with an adequate margin of safety.

DIGITALIS AND THE NONFAILING HEART. Although general agreement exists regarding the beneficial effect of digitalis glycosides in the treatment of the failing heart, considerably less evidence is available to support their usefulness in the absence of overt heart failure. Digitalis is often administered to patients with mitral stenosis regardless of the type of rhythm. It is clearly beneficial in slowing the ventricular response to atrial fibrillation, and thereby allowing more complete diastolic filling of the left ventricle. In the presence of right ventricular failure, benefit results from increased contractility and reduced end-diastolic pressure. However, in patients with mitral stenosis and normal sinus rhythm who were studied during maximal exercise, ouabain produced no significant change in heart rate and had no beneficial effect on cardiac output, oxygen consumption, or severity of pulmonary hypertension.[101]

The therapeutic value of digitalis in the hypertrophied or dilated nonfailing heart remains unclear. With the development of hypertrophy, and before the onset of overt failure, the work capacity of the myocardium at any given left ventricular end-diastolic pressure tends to be decreased, and digitalis exerts a positive inotropic action,[102] augments the capacity for performance of cardiac work, and reduces end-systolic volume and end-diastolic pressure.[102] If cardiac output has not been reduced, it does not increase as a result of digitalis administration, but the same stroke work and cardiac output can be delivered from a lower ventricular filling pressure. Thus, digitalis should provide a greater inotropic reserve. However, there is little objective evidence that these considerations can be translated directly into clinical practice. The therapeutic value of digitalis in patients without heart failure (either in altering their prognosis or in retarding the progress of hypertrophy or dilatation) has not been determined in long-term studies. Nevertheless, in the early stages of heart failure, cardiac output may be impaired only on exertion, with a normal output at rest. The clinical diagnosis of this intermediate state between compensation and frank failure is often difficult to make. It is likely that digitalis would improve exercise performance of such patients by increasing cardiac output during exercise and by preventing an undue rise in end-diastolic pressure.

Extracardiac Hemodynamic Effects. Whereas the direct cardiac effects of digitalis are of primary importance to an understanding of the hemodynamic effects of the drug, it is clear that extracardiac effects are also involved. Digitalis glycosides constrict isolated arterial and venous segments,[103,104] and arteriolar and venous constriction has been demonstrated in intact laboratory animals. Elevation of total systemic arteriolar resistance has been demonstrated in normal human subjects.[105] These effects appear to be mediated both by the local action of digitalis on vascular smooth muscle and indirectly through the sympathetic nervous system.[106] The latter effect appears to be the predominant mechanism whereby the drug increases the vascular resistance of skeletal muscle. Cross-circulation experiments have shown that the central nervous system may mediate a substantial portion of the vasoconstrictor effect of digoxin.[107] Neurogenic coronary vasoconstrictor effects of digoxin and acetylstrophanthidin have also been documented in a canine model of acute global myocardial ischemia.[108] These effects could be blocked with phenoxybenzamine and hence appear to be mediated by a digitalis-evoked increase in sympathetically mediated vasoconstriction.[108]

Peripheral vasoconstrictor effects of ouabain have also been documented clinically,[109] including observations in patients with cardiogenic shock[110] in whom the vasoconstrictor effect preceded the positive inotropic effect. In some cases this effect was associated with increased left ventricular end-diastolic pressures. These observations indicate the need for caution when digitalis glycosides are administered acutely, particularly in situations in which transient increases in peripheral resistance would be deleterious. There is also evidence that increased mesenteric vascular resistance can compromise splanchnic blood flow, possibly subjecting the patient with marginal perfusion to increased risk of ischemic bowel necrosis.[111]

In clinical circumstances in which the intravenous use of digitalis is required, gradual administration of glycosides over several minutes is preferred to a rapid bolus injection. This preference has recently been confirmed in a clinically relevant study of the effects of ouabain on coronary and systemic vascular resistance and myocardial oxygen consumption in patients undergoing cardiac catheterization.[112] Ten-second and 2-minute intravenous infusions of ouabain produced increases in mean arterial pressure and systemic vascular resistance, while a 15-minute infusion of the same dose produced no significant change in either variable. Coronary vascular resistance increased after the 10-second infusion but did not change after the 15-minute infusion. The 10-second infusion was also associated with transient deterioration of myocardial lactate metabolism. These findings demonstrate that rapid intravenous infusion of a cardiac glycoside produces systemic and coronary arteriolar constriction that may lead to clinical deterioration. These effects can and should be avoided with slower administration of the drug.

Digitalis produces generalized venoconstriction in the normal dog. This action is particularly marked in the hepatic veins and leads to pooling of blood in the portal venous system and consequently diminished venous return. Effects are probably less striking in man.

In congestive heart failure, sympathetic augmentation of contractility is important in maintaining cardiac output, as discussed in Chapter 13. This increase in sympathetic nervous activity, producing systemic arteriolar and venous constriction, may serve to maintain blood pressure in the face of diminished cardiac output and to redistribute this reduced output among various regional circulations.[113] In most cases, when digitalis is given to patients with heart failure, generalized vasodilation occurs instead of the vasoconstriction observed in normal persons[105]—an effect presumably related to increased cardiac output mediated by the positive inotropic action of the drug and resulting in reflex withdrawal of sympathetic vasoconstriction. This withdrawal may account for the observation that venous pressure is often lowered before diuresis occurs after the administration of digitalis.[105]

Diuresis is a characteristic and important manifestation of digitalis action in edematous patients with congestive heart failure. Digitalis has been shown to inhibit tubular reabsorption of sodium.[114] Direct infusion of ouabain into the renal artery produces substantial inhibition of renal Na^+,K^+-ATPase and impairment of both concentrating and diluting ability.[115] However, relatively large doses are needed to demonstrate these effects, and it is unlikely that any direct renal action of digitalis plays an important part in the diuresis that occurs in the treatment of congestive heart failure. Rather, it is through an improvement of cardiac output and therefore in renal hemodynamics that glycosides induce diuresis.

Finally, a major hemodynamic effect of digitalis in enhancing cardiac performance lies in its ability to slow the ventricular response to supraventricular tachyarrhythmias, particularly in conditions such as mitral stenosis. Slowing of sinus tachycardia in patients with congestive heart failure is often pronounced, through withdrawal of enhanced sympathetic tone, when the failure state is ameliorated by virtue of increased cardiac contractility and output. In usual doses,

digitalis has no pronounced direct effect on sinoatrial pacemaker automaticity.

PHARMACOKINETICS AND BIOAVAILABILITY

Many important aspects of pharmacokinetic patterns of commonly used cardiac glycosides were outlined as a result of the studies of Gold and Modell and their coworkers in the 1940's.[116–118] More recent contributions to the current understanding of digitalis pharmacokinetics have been reviewed recently.[61] Table 16–4 summarizes data related to absorption, onset of action, and excretion times and patterns for cardiac glycosides commonly used in the United States. It is important to recognize that the values cited are averages and that substantial individual variation is to be expected. Extensive discussions of the pharmacokinetics of cardiac glycosides are available in the volume edited by Greeff.[119]

DIGOXIN. This glycoside has become the digitalis preparation predominantly used in hospitalized patients and to only a slightly lesser extent in outpatients, principally because of the flexibility in its route of administration and its intermediate duration of action. Digoxin is excreted exponentially, with a half-life of about 36 to 48 hours in subjects with normal renal function, resulting in the loss of about one-third of body stores daily.[120] Although the drug is excreted for the most part in unchanged form, some patients excrete appreciable quantities of the relatively inactive metabolite dihydrodigoxin, which appears to arise through bacterial biotransformation in the gut lumen.[61,121,122,122a] Renal excretion of digoxin is proportional to glomerular filtration rate (and hence to creatinine clearance) and is largely independent of rate of urine flow in patients with reasonably intact renal function.[61] In patients with prerenal azotemia, digoxin clearance was reported to correlate more closely with urea clearance than with creatinine clearance, suggesting that digoxin may undergo some degree of tubular reabsorption under these circumstances.[123] This point remains unsettled, however, and evidence for secretion of digoxin at the tubular level in man has also been reported[61] and appears to be more pronounced prior to puberty.[124] With daily maintenance therapy, a steady state is reached when daily losses are matched by daily intake. For patients not previously given digitalis, institution of daily maintenance therapy without a loading dose results in development of steady-state plateau concentrations after four to five half-lives, or about seven days, in subjects with normal renal function.[125] If the half-life of the drug is prolonged, the length of time before a steady state is reached on a daily maintenance dose is prolonged accordingly. Because of the high degree of tissue binding of digoxin, the drug is not effectively removed from the body by dialysis.[126] Similarly, it has been shown that cardiopulmonary bypass[127] and exchange transfusion[128] remove only minor amounts of digoxin from the body. Serum digoxin levels and pharmacokinetics are essentially the same before and after the loss of large amounts of adipose tissue in massively obese subjects,[129] suggesting that lean body mass should be used when dosage is being calculated. Acute vasodilator therapy with nitroprusside or hydralazine tends to increase renal digoxin clearance without changing glomerular filtration rate, and

TABLE 16–4 CARDIAC GLYCOSIDE PREPARATIONS

AGENT	GASTRO-INTESTINAL ABSORPTION	ONSET OF ACTION* (MIN)	PEAK EFFECT (HR)	AVERAGE HALF-LIFE**	PRINCIPAL METABOLIC ROUTE (EXCRETORY PATHWAY)	AVERAGE DIGITALIZING DOSE		USUAL DAILY ORAL MAINTE-NANCE DOSE§††
						Oral†	Intra-Venous†	
Ouabain	Unreliable	5 to 10	½ to 2	21 hours	Renal; some gastro-intestinal excretion	——	0.30 to 0.50 mg	——
Deslano-side	Unreliable	10 to 30	1 to 2	33 hours	Renal	——	0.80 mg	——
Digoxin	55 to 75%¶ 90 to 100%#	15 to 30	1½ to 5	36 to 48 hours	Renal; some gastro-intestinal excretion	1.25 to 1.50 mg#	0.75 to 1.00 mg#	0.25 to 0.50 mg
Digitoxin	90 to 100%	25 to 120	4 to 12	4 to 6 days	Hepatic‖; renal excretion of metabo-lites	0.70 to 1.20 mg	1.00 mg	0.10 mg
Digitalis leaf	About 40%	——	——	4 to 6 days	Similar to digitoxin	0.08 to 1.20 g	——	0.10 g

*For intravenous dose.
**For normal subjects (prolonged by renal impairment with digoxin, ouabain, and deslanoside and probably by severe hepatic disease with digitoxin and digitalis leaf).
†Divided doses over 12 to 24 hours at intervals of 6 to 8 hours.
††Given in increments for initial subcomplete digitalization, to be supplemented by further small increments as necessary.
§Average for adult patients without renal or hepatic impairment; varies widely among individual patients and requires close medical supervision.
¶For tablet form of administration (may be less in malabsorption syndromes and in formulations with poor bioavailability).
‖ Enterohepatic cycle exists.
#Ninety to 100 per cent gastrointestinal absorption has been reported for the new encapsulated gel formulation Lanoxicaps®, available in capsules containing 0.05, 0.10, and 0.20 mg. When this product is used, the average digitalizing dose should be lowered about 20 per cent.
Modified from Smith, T. W.: Drug therapy: Digitalis glycosides. N. Engl. J. Med. 288:719, 1973.

may necessitate adjustment of maintenance digoxin dosage.[130]

Infants and children absorb and excrete digoxin in much the same way as adults do,[131] although recent evidence suggests that secretion at the renal tubular level may be quantitatively more important in prepubertal subjects.[124] Digoxin doses in neonates and infants are substantially larger than those in adults when calculated on the basis of milligrams per kilogram of body weight or per square meter of body surface area.[78,132] These higher doses result in relatively higher serum digoxin concentrations, which are generally well tolerated.[78,132] Fetal umbilical-cord venous blood digoxin concentrations at term have been found to be similar to those in the venous blood of the mother maintained on digoxin, documenting transplacental passage of the drug.[78]

An important interaction between digoxin and quinidine has been described that leads to an approximately two-fold increase in serum digoxin concentration when conventional quinidine doses are added to a standard maintenance digoxin regimen (p. 519).[133] This increase is associated in some instances with the development of digoxin-toxic rhythm disturbances.[61] A decrease in digoxin dosage, in addition to frequent assessment of serum digoxin concentration and clinical status, is advisable when quinidine is given concurrently. Interactions of digoxin with quinidine, verapamil, tiapamil, nifedipine, and amiodarone are discussed on p. 519.

DIGITOXIN. This glycoside is the least polar and most slowly excreted of the cardiac glycosides in common use. Since it constitutes the principal active agent in digitalis leaf, the two preparations will be considered together.

Gastrointestinal absorption of digitoxin is a passive process and is thought to be essentially complete, although patients with malabsorption syndromes or other gastrointestinal diseases have not been studied extensively.

Digitoxin binds avidly to human serum albumin, and about 97 per cent of the serum or plasma content of the drug is bound to albumin at clinically relevant concentrations.[134] It therefore differs considerably in this respect from digoxin, which is only about 23 per cent bound to plasma proteins.[134] Renal clearance of the native compound is relatively minor compared with digoxin,[135,136] and extensive metabolism of digitoxin occurs, presumably in the liver. An enterohepatic cycle exists for digitoxin and can be interrupted by resins, such as cholestyramine, which bind digitoxin in the gut lumen.[137] A modest acceleration of the excretion of digitoxin has been documented in human subjects given cholestyramine,[138] but the clinical efficacy of this approach in patients with digitoxin intoxication remains to be proved. Digoxin is not ordinarily a quantitatively important metabolic product of digitoxin in man. It is of interest that drugs known to increase the activity of hepatic microsomal enzyme systems, such as phenobarbital and phenylbutazone, can accelerate the metabolism of digitoxin in some patients. Although digitoxin can be displaced from its serum albumin binding sites by high concentrations of other drugs, including phenylbutazone, warfarin, tolbutamide, sulfadimethoxine, and clofibrate, these effects are probably not of consequence at the plasma concentrations encountered in clinical use.[139]

Half-times of digitoxin in plasma appear to vary relatively little from patient to patient, usually remaining in the range of 4 to 6 days irrespective of renal function. Administration of daily maintenance doses of digitoxin without a loading dose will result in gradual digitalization, with the 4- to 6-day half-life of the drug resulting in establishment of the final steady-state plateau after 3 to 4 weeks.

DESLANOSIDE (CEDILANID-D). This agent is structurally identical to digoxin except for the presence of an additional terminal glucose residue. This alteration results in poor gastrointestinal absorption, and thus the drug is recommended only for parenteral use. Its half-life is essentially identical to that of digoxin. Although its onset of action is somewhat more rapid, it probably enjoys no substantial advantages over parenteral use of digoxin unless rapidity of effect is an overriding consideration; however, if this is the case, ouabain may be preferable.

OUABAIN AND ACETYLSTROPHANTHIDIN. *Ouabain* is the most polar and rapidly acting of the cardiac glycosides currently available for routine clinical use. Like the other cardiac glycosides, its excretion from the body follows first-order pharmacokinetics, with a fixed proportion of the residual drug in the body being excreted each day. For ouabain, the plasma half-life in normal subjects is about 21 hours—similar to the half-life of positive inotropic effect and of ventricular rate slowing in patients with atrial fibrillation.[140] The quantity of ouabain in the body, and also the risk of toxicity, in a patient placed on a regular maintenance dosage schedule without a loading dose will continue to rise for four to five half-lives (4 to 5 days) until a plateau is reached. Impairment of renal function will prolong the half-life of ouabain and also the period during which accumulation will continue.

Although ouabain is predominantly excreted unchanged via the renal route, its gastrointestinal excretion is substantial after intravenous administration in both dog and man.[141] The drug appears to enter the gastrointestinal tract by pathways other than the biliary tract. In normal human subjects, urinary excretion accounted for an average of only 47 per cent of the intravenous dose. Ouabain is poorly absorbed from the gastrointestinal tract and is not available for oral use.

Acetylstrophanthidin, a rapidly acting synthetic C-3 acetyl ester of the aglycone strophanthidin, has been used in both experimental and clinical investigations but is available for clinical use only on an investigative basis. In human subjects, the principal exponential decline of plasma acetylstrophanthidin commences 10 to 30 minutes after intravenous infusion, and the mean half-life in plasma is 2.3 hours, in keeping with the known short duration of clinical effect. Urinary excretion averages only 22 per cent of the intravenous dose.[142]

Detailed reviews of cardiac glycoside pharmacokinetics and metabolism are available.[61,143]

BIOAVAILABILITY

Three decades ago, Gold and his colleagues evaluated the relative efficacy of cardiac glycosides given by oral and parenteral routes. The ventricular rate of patients in atrial fibrillation was used as a quantitative indicator of digitalis effect.[116] Oral digoxin was found to be about two thirds as effective in slowing the ventricular rate as an equivalent intravenous dose,[118] whereas digitoxin was almost equally effective when given by either route.[116] Thus, the bioavailability of digoxin as determined by this clinical bioassay was about 67 per cent, whereas that of digitoxin was nearly 100 per cent.

A number of subsequent studies have documented incomplete absorption of digoxin from the gastrointestinal tract.[144,145] Individual patient variation, circumstances of drug administration, and characteristics of the pharmaceutical preparation ingested are all known to affect digoxin bioavailability.[146] Patients with malabsorption syndromes may absorb digoxin poorly and erratically.[147] However, patients with maldigestion due to pancreatic insufficiency, despite comparable degrees of steatorrhea, appear to absorb the drug more normally. Administration of digoxin after meals is likely to decrease peak serum levels achieved, but total absorption is not affected to any noteworthy degree. Absorption of digoxin tends to be enhanced by drugs that decrease gastrointestinal motility and to be reduced by drugs that increase motility, particularly if the preparations have limited bioavailability. In addition, nonabsorbed substances, such as cholestyramine, colestipol, kaolin and pectin (Kaopectate), and nonabsorbable antacids, when taken concurrently can interfere with gastrointestinal absorption of digoxin; neomycin has also been shown to interfere with digoxin absorption. Because of previously documented variations in the bioavailability of commercially available digoxin preparations, bioavailability specifications provided by the FDA and USP are currently in effect.[148–150]

Biological availability uniformly approaching 100 per cent probably cannot be achieved with any oral digoxin preparation, but a recently marketed encapsulated gel preparation is reported to have 90 to 100 per cent bioavailability. After intravenous administration of digoxin, 6-day urinary recovery by radioimmunoassay averaged 76 per cent of the administered dose. Intramuscular digoxin caused severe pain at the injection site, and bioavailability was only 83 per cent that of intravenous digoxin. Digoxin elixir was significantly more bioavailable (65 per cent of intravenous) than the tablet form studied (55 per cent of intravenous).[149]

Since the studies of Gold et al., oral absorption of digitoxin has generally been considered to be virtually 100 per cent, and no recent studies have cast doubt on that estimate. As with digoxin, binding to nonabsorbable substances such as cholestyramine can interfere with initial absorption.[138] Patients receiving such anion-exchange resins in addition to a cardiac glycoside should be instructed to ingest the cardiac glycoside two hours before the resin to minimize this effect.

CLINICAL USE OF DIGITALIS

A sound working knowledge of the pharmacokinetics of the commonly used cardiac glycosides is essential to the optimal use of these drugs. Computer programs and nomograms[151,152] can provide initial approximations of optimal dose, but further dosage adjustments based on close clinical observation of the patient are often required. In many cases the variability in serum digoxin concentrations among different patients remains unexplained even after adjustments for dose, body size, and renal function have been made and measurement of digoxin concentrations and their use for feedback dosage adjustments have been suggested.[153]

The clinical use of cardiac glycosides is complicated by the absence of a readily measurable therapeutic objective (except in certain atrial arrhythmias), the lack of reliable means to predict individual cardiac responses, and the difficulty in defining proximity to toxicity. The acetylstrophanthidin tolerance test has been used investigatively[154,155] but carries potential risk and is not generally available for clinical use. Other experimental approaches employ electrical pulses to assess the degree of digitalization, on the basis of the observation that cardioversion may elicit rhythm disturbances in digitalized patients.[156]

CONGESTIVE HEART FAILURE. Cardiac glycosides are of potential value in most patients with symptoms and signs of *congestive heart failure* due to ischemic, valvular, hypertensive, or congenital heart disease, dilated cardiomyopathies, and cor pulmonale. Improvement of depressed myocardial contractility increases cardiac output, promotes diuresis, and reduces the filling pressure of the failing ventricle(s), with consequent reduction of pulmonary vascular congestion and central venous pressure.

As previously noted, digitalis is of no demonstrable benefit in isolated *mitral stenosis* with normal sinus rhythm unless right ventricular failure has supervened. Similarly, little benefit may result in patients with *pericardial tamponade* or *constrictive pericarditis* except when there is invasion of the myocardium in the latter. Hypertrophic obstructive cardiomyopathy represents another process in which digitalis is often of little value and may actually be deleterious because it can increase left ventricular outflow obstruction by augmenting the contractility of the hypertrophic outflow-tract segment. It is our impression that patients with left ventricular hypertrophy and well-preserved left ventricular ejection fractions, even in the presence of symptoms related to elevated filling pressures, benefit little from digitalis. In the later stages of hypertrophic cardiomyopathy, in which ventricular dilation and congestive problems may predominate over obstructive ones, cardiac glycosides may be beneficial. Patients who develop congestive heart failure in response to a specific precipitating stress (p. 491) may benefit from temporary use of digitalis but will not necessarily require long-term maintenance digitalization. The risk:benefit ratio must be reassessed with any change in clinical status and will often be found to favor discontinuation of digitalis when an acute stress such as infection, anemia, or thyrotoxicosis is no longer present.[62]

Digitalis glycosides may improve symptoms of angina pectoris when it coexists with cardiomegaly and congestive heart failure. As discussed subsequently, however, an increase in angina may occur unless the tendency toward increased oxygen consumption is offset by decreased ventricular size and wall tension.

Prophylactic digitalization of the patient with diminished cardiac reserve about to undergo a major stress such as surgery remains controversial (p. 1821). In the absence of obvious cardiomegaly or other evidence of overt congestive heart failure, most clinicians prefer to withhold digitalis until a specific indication arises. Prophylactic digitalization has been recommended for patients undergoing aortocoronary bypass surgery on the basis of a significant reduction in

supraventricular arrhythmias.[157] Evidence of a difference in ultimate outcome between digitalized and nondigitalized patients was not documented, however, and another study of 140 consecutive patients undergoing myocardial revascularization showed a *higher* incidence of supraventricular tachyarrhythmias in patients receiving prophylactic digitalis.[158]

The availability of reliable pervenous catheter endocardial pacing techniques has helped to resolve the problem of digitalis use in patients with marginal atrioventricular conduction or established atrioventricular block. One can now carry out pacemaker implantation at minimal risk even in severely ill patients and then give digitalis without fear of aggravating conduction problems.

Arrhythmias (See also Chapter 22).   Digitalis is of potential use in the management of four types of supraventricular tachyarrhythmias.

1. *Paroxysmal superventricular tachycardia* (p. 702), whether of atrial or atrioventricular junctional origin, usually responds to digitalization when simpler measures such as carotid sinus pressure alone have failed. Many clinicians now prefer to use verapamil as the drug of first choice in this clinical setting (p. 665). When digitalis is used, carotid sinus pressure should be repeated during the course of digitalization, since the combination of partial digitalization and carotid sinus pressure will often succeed when neither measure alone suffices. Maintenance digitalization usually abolishes or reduces the frequency of recurrent attacks. Use of digitalis in the setting of paroxysmal supraventricular tachycardia demands that digitalis intoxication be excluded as a cause of the arrhythmia.

2. *Atrial fibrillation* with a rapid ventricular response is one of the most common indications for the use of digitalis. Both vagal and direct mechanisms result in increased blockade of impulses arriving at the atrioventricular junction, with slowing of the ventricular rate. Conversion to normal sinus rhythm may occur in the course of digitalization. Addition of beta-adrenergic blocking agents or verapamil[159] may be useful in circumstances in which the ventricular rate is difficult to control without the emergence of toxic symptoms (e.g., untreated thyrotoxicosis) and congestive heart failure is absent or minimal.

3. *Atrial flutter*, usually accompanied by 2:1 atrioventricular block in untreated cases, can often be managed with digitalis in doses sufficient to produce a degree of atrioventricular blockade that results in a ventricular rate in the range of 70 to 100/min. This effect may require doses considerably in excess of the usual range. As in atrial fibrillation, when the arrhythmia is poorly tolerated by the patient, it is often advisable to attempt direct-current cardioversion before administration of doses of digitalis that would render the procedure hazardous.

4. *Wolff-Parkinson-White syndrome* tachyarrhythmias (p. 712) may be terminated or prevented by digitalis in cases in which preferential effects on conduction or refractoriness in the normal or anomalous conduction pathways result in interruption of the reentrant circus movement. Other antiarrhythmic drugs may be more effective in other cases. Sellers et al. concluded on the basis of detailed electrophysiological studies of responses to digoxin in 21 patients that no a priori prediction about the effect of digitalis on the antegrade conduction of accessory pathways can be made, suggesting that formal electrophysiological studies are indicated in many of these patients to predict their response to maintenance digoxin therapy.[160] Potential hazards of digitalis use in patients with the Wolff-Parkinson-White syndrome and episodes of atrial fibrillation are discussed on page 718.

DOSAGE SCHEDULES

Specific recommendations for digoxin dosage have been developed on the basis of the pharmacokinetic principles previously discussed. Usually there is no reason to use a loading dose far in excess of what the steady-state body content will be with the usual maintenance dose. A patient with entirely normal renal function who excretes 37 per cent of the digoxin in his body each day will, on a maintenance dose of 0.25 or 0.50 mg/day, have a steady-state total body content of about 0.67 or 1.35 mg, respectively. If a reasonable estimate of 75 per cent absorption of the tablet form of digoxin is made, estimates for the loading dose become 0.5 and 1.0 mg, respectively, for maintenance doses of 0.25 and 0.50 mg/day. This amount can be given over a period of a day or so in several increments, or the same level of digitalization can be achieved over a period of about a week in a patient with normal renal function by administration of the daily maintenance dose without any loading dose. The latter procedure is often preferable in outpatient practice. It must be remembered, however, that severe renal impairment will prolong the half-life of digoxin to a maximum of about 4.4 days and hence extend the period required to reach a steady-state plateau to a maximum of about 3 weeks. Lean body mass should be considered in selection of both loading and maintenance digoxin doses. In adult patients with cardiac disease, initial intravenous loading doses of about 0.50 to 0.75 mg/45 kg (100 lb) of body weight, given in increments, are unlikely to cause toxicity and can be supplemented by further increments if indicated by the clinical course.

The maintenance digoxin dose required to replace daily losses will vary from about 37 per cent of the total body content in patients with normal renal function to nonrenal losses averaging about 14 per cent in patients who are essentially anephric. Between the extremes of normal renal function and no renal function, digoxin excretion is linearly related to glomerular filtration rate or creatinine clearance (C_{Cr}). A reasonable approximation of daily percentage of loss of digoxin is as follows[161]:

$$14 + \frac{C_{Cr} \text{ in ml/min}}{5}$$

Since accurate creatinine clearance values will often not be immediately available, one can use the following estimate based on a stable serum creatinine in mg/100 ml, abbreviated as c:

$$C_{Cr} \text{ (men)} = \frac{100}{c} - 12$$

and

$$C_{Cr} \text{ (women)} = \frac{80}{c} - 7$$

These expressions can be combined so that

$$\% \text{ daily loss (men)} = 11.6 + \frac{20}{c}$$

and

$$\% \text{ daily loss (women)} = 12.6 + \frac{16}{c}$$

The daily maintenance digoxin dose is intended to replace daily losses after an appropriate loading dose, so that the above value for daily percentage of loss multiplied by the loading dose that produced a satisfactory therapeutic response gives a reasonable initial approximation of the proper daily maintenance dose. Jelliffe and Brooker have developed a useful nomogram for digoxin therapy that takes into account body weight and renal function and provides guidelines for determining both loading and maintenance doses.[152]

The recommended oral loading dose of digoxin, based on *lean body weight* and administered in the form of digoxin elixir, is 25 to 35 μg/kg for full-term infants; 35 to 60 μg/kg for infants from 1 to 24 months; 30 to 40 μg/kg for ages 2 to 5 years; 20 to 35 μg/kg for 5 to 10 years; and 10 to 15 μg/kg for children over 10 years. For premature infants a loading dose of 20 to 30 μg/kg is recommended. Daily maintenance doses *for patients with normal renal function* are estimated as 20 to 30 per cent of the oral loading dose for premature infants and as 25 to 35 per cent of the oral loading dose for full-term infants through children 10 years of age and older. Parenteral (intravenous) loading and maintenance dose recommendations are approximately 75 per cent of the oral dosages.[162]

For digitoxin, half-lives usually range within 20 per cent of a mean value of 4.8 days, and relatively little variation in the body pool would be expected among individual patients receiving a given maintenance dose of the drug. The average steady-state digitoxin pool in a patient receiving 0.1 mg/day is about 0.8 mg, and as with digoxin, there is usually no reason to give a loading dose substantially in excess of the expected steady-state body pool achieved with usual maintenance doses. A loading dose of about 0.010 to 0.012 mg/kg allows compensation for variations in body size. Gradual digitalization without a loading dose is feasible with digitoxin, but because four to five half-lives are required to reach the steady-state plateau, this will take 3 to 4 weeks.

Estimates of loading and maintenance doses based on the above considerations are average values intended only as initial approximations and in no way diminish the need for further adjustments based on frequent and careful observation of the patient.

THERAPEUTIC ENDPOINTS

In addressing the difficult problem of defining the elusive state of optimal digitalization, one might begin by stating that it is not necessarily the largest dose that can be tolerated without emergence of overt toxicity. The toxic:therapeutic ratio for cardiac glycosides is small at best, and the availability of other measures of treating heart failure, particularly potent oral diuretics and vasodilators, usually obviates balancing therapy at the edge of toxicity. Electrocardiographic ST-segment and T-wave changes of "digitalis effect" are, unfortunately, limited indicators of the state of digitalization. The perils of depending on slowing of sinus tachycardia to gauge the adequacy of digitalis dosage are well known.

In patients with atrial flutter or fibrillation, control of the ventricular response provides a relatively straightforward endpoint. Failure of atropine or exercise to increase the ventricular response has been used as an additional indicator of "full digitalization" in such patients, but overly vigorous pursuit of this goal may result in unduly slow resting heart rates or other evidence of impending or overt toxicity.

When congestive heart failure is the indication for use of digitalis, it is helpful to remember that positive inotropy is a graded response that is appreciable at doses well short of "maximally tolerated doses." As already stated, available data suggest that further inotropic benefit may not occur clinically beyond serum digoxin levels in the 1.0 to 2.0

TABLE 16–5 FACTORS INFLUENCING INDIVIDUAL SENSITIVITY TO DIGITALIS

Type and severity of underlying cardiac disease
Serum electrolyte derangements
    Hypokalemia or hyperkalemia
    Hypomagnesemia
    Hypercalcemia
    Hyponatremia
Acid-base imbalance
Concomitant drug administration
    Anesthetics
    Catecholamines and sympathomimetics
    Antiarrhythmic agents
Thyroid status
Renal function
Autonomic nervous system tone
Respiratory disease

ng/ml range.[62] Carotid sinus massage can provide useful bedside clues to impending digitalis excess. Rhythm disorders such as second-degree atrioventricular block, accelerated atrioventricular junctional rhythm, and ventricular premature beats or bigeminy may emerge in response to carotid sinus stimulation before they occur spontaneously.[163]

INDIVIDUAL SENSITIVITY TO DIGITALIS. It is considerably easier to calculate theoretical body pools of cardiac glycosides than to decide, at the bedside, when optimal digitalization has been achieved in an individual patient. A number of factors influencing individual sensitivity to cardiac glycosides are listed in Table 16–5. Changes in absorption or bioavailability increase the probability of suboptimal digitalization because of fluctuations that can occur on a supposedly fixed dosage regimen. Such changes are reflected by changes in serum glycoside concentrations, however, and do not represent an actual change in sensitivity to the drug's effects. Quite distinct from the clinical problem of variable bioavailability is the enhanced sensitivity to lower serum concentrations of cardiac glycosides noted in up to 10 to 15 per cent of patients.

ELECTROLYTE AND ACID-BASE DISTURBANCES. Disturbances of potassium homeostasis clearly influence the action of digitalis.[61,164] Myocardial concentrations of digoxin tend to decrease with increasing serum potassium concentration. Furthermore, hypokalemia has a primary arrhythmogenic effect, both decreasing the effective refractory period of Purkinje cells and shortening the coupling interval for ventricular premature beats.[165] Depression of atrioventricular nodal conduction can occur with both digitalis excess and either very low or extremely high levels of serum K^+.[166,167] Diuretic therapy, insulin administration or carbohydrate loading, renal disease, and acid-base disturbances must all be borne in mind as potential causes of clinically significant alterations in potassium homeostasis, which can, in turn, affect importantly the response to cardiac glycoside.

Disturbances in serum levels of other electrolytes may also influence myocardial sensitivity to digitalis, although less profoundly than K^+ concentration. Administration of Mg^{++} salts suppresses digitalis-induced arrhythmias and hypomagnesemia appears to predispose to digitalis toxicity.[168] There is some evidence that the digitalis-induced K^+ efflux from the myocardium is reduced by Mg^{++} salts.[169] Magnesium depletion may become clinically important with the chronic administration of diuretic agents[170] and

with gastrointestinal disease, diabetes mellitus, or poor nutritional states. Moreover, in patients with congestive heart failure, significant depletion of total body Mg^{++} stores may occur owing to prolonged secondary aldosteronism. The frequency and clinical importance of Mg^{++} depletion in digitalis therapy remain unresolved.[171,172]

Elevated serum Ca^{++} levels increase ventricular automaticity, and this effect is at least additive to and perhaps synergistic with the effects of digitalis. In one early study, ventricular ectopic activity occurred at lower doses of ouabain in hypercalcemic patients.[173] Furthermore, patients with digitalis intoxication have been reported to respond successfully to calcium-chelating agents.[174] The clinician should be alert for the possibility of enhanced digitalis sensitivity when treating hypercalcemic patients or when administering calcium parenterally to digitalized patients.

The interactions of digitalis with acid-base disturbances are complex. Perturbations in potassium homeostasis that follow shifts in hydrogen ion concentration obviously will affect myocardial binding of cardiac glycosides and the development of digitalis-related arrhythmias, as will primary changes in serum K^+ concentration. Similarly, acid-base status will influence the serum levels of ionized Ca^{++}, with attendant effects on automaticity. Whether alkalosis itself, independent of these changes, increases sensitivity to digitalis is controversial.[175,176] Acidosis independent of changes in $[K^+]$ does not appear to enhance sensitivity to the arrhythmogenic effects of digitalis[177] and may even render the myocardium more resistant to digitalis intoxication.[178]

DRUG INTERACTIONS. Concomitant drug administration may interact with the effects of digitalis through several mechanisms. As noted above, certain drugs such as cholestyramine and neomycin may decrease oral absorption of digoxin, thereby altering the serum and myocardial levels ultimately achieved. In addition, nonabsorbable antacids and Kaopectate may have a similar effect in some patients.

Drugs that affect metabolism or excretion of various digitalis preparations will influence toxicity through variations in the levels of serum and myocardial digitalis achieved rather than through altered sensitivity to the action of the glycosides themselves. Quinidine reduces both the renal and nonrenal elimination of digoxin and also appears to decrease the apparent volume of distribution of this glycoside.[179] The net result is an increase in serum digoxin concentration that averages two-fold in patients in whom conventional doses of quinidine are added to a maintenance digoxin regimen[179]; unfortunately, individual responses to quinidine may vary substantially and close surveillance of clinical status (and, if possible, serum digoxin concentration) is needed to reduce the risk of precipitating overt digoxin toxicity. Preliminary studies of a possible interaction between digitoxin and quinidine have yielded conflicting results, and this issue remains unsettled.[61] Procainamide and disopyramide do not appear to alter serum digoxin levels, but verapamil does increase serum digoxin concentration by decreasing volume of distribution and clearance of digoxin.[180,181] Other calcium channel blocking agents, including nifedipine and tiapamil, can also increase serum digoxin levels,[182,183] and both short- and long-term amiodarone administration has been found to increase steady-state serum digoxin concentration.[184,185] Other newly introduced drugs will require close surveillance for interactions with cardiac glycosides.

Diuretic agents potentially enhance the occurrence of digitalis toxicity both by decreasing glomerular filtration rate and through a variety of electrolyte disturbances, including hypokalemia, hypomagnesemia, and (for thiazide diuretics) hypercalcemia. By counteracting the cardiac toxic manifestations of digitalis excess, concurrent administration of some antiarrhythmic agents may create the impression of a relative resistance to digitalis toxicity.

Several anesthetic agents are arrhythmogenic, and experimental studies suggest that this effect may be synergistic with digitalis enhancement of ventricular automaticity in the case of cyclopropane[186] and succinylcholine.[187] The profound systemic effects of general anesthesia introduce many variables that could affect digitalis sensitivity, thus greatly complicating the detailed assessment of individual anesthetic agents. The interrelationships between catecholamines and sympathomimetic drugs and cardiac glycosides are intriguing but incompletely characterized. Several experimental studies have demonstrated that catecholamine-induced increases in ventricular automaticity add to the arrhythmogenic effects of digitalis[188]; however, detailed clinical correlation has not been forthcoming. It is reasonable for the clinician to assume that sympathomimetic agents increase the likelihood of enhanced automaticity of ectopic pacemakers in patients receiving digitalis.

TYPE AND SEVERITY OF UNDERLYING HEART DISEASE

The effects of digitalis on the heart are modified by the type and severity of the underlying heart disease.[189] This is dramatically demonstrated in otherwise healthy subjects who ingest massive doses of digitalis. Toxicity in such situations is frequently manifested by progressively diminished atrioventricular conduction or by sinoatrial exit block, rather than by enhanced automaticity and ventricular ectopic activity as seen in patients with underlying heart disease.[190,191] In many patients with ischemic, myocardial, or valvular heart disease the effects of digitalis are superimposed on an electrophysiologically unstable condition with preexisting abnormalities of impulse formation and conduction. The more severe and advanced the heart disease, the more likely the occurrence of focal ischemia, myocardial fibrosis, and ventricular dilatation with stretching of Purkinje fibers and resultant tendency toward increased automaticity. The clinical observation that digitalis toxicity is particularly common in patients with amyloidosis involving the heart may be accounted for, at least in part, by digoxin binding by amyloid fibrils.[192]

DIGITALIS AND ISCHEMIC HEART DISEASE. The use of digitalis in patients with ischemic heart disease deserves special attention. In experiments employing an isolated canine cardiac preparation, it was shown that acetylstrophanthidin administration increased myocardial oxygen consumption in the normal heart, whereas consumption was decreased in the failing heart.[193] The increase in oxygen consumption in the normal heart can be explained by the increased velocity of contraction and increased wall tension. In the failing heart, decreased oxygen consumption can be explained by a decrease in left ventricular end-diastolic pressure, resulting in a reduction in end-diastolic volume and consequently, on the basis of the Laplace relation, a decline in intramyocardial tension.

Changes in oxygen consumption are always the net result of two opposing effects of digitalis: a potential reduction in wall tension and an increase in contractility. Thus, in the failing heart the net result depends on the balance of these effects, and either a diminution of oxygen consumption or no change may be observed. In the nonfailing heart, oxygen consumption increases with digitalis administration.[194] These considerations are of clinical importance when a decision must be made about whether to use digitalis in patients with coronary disease. Angina pectoris has been observed to improve after digitalization in patients with heart failure but occasionally to worsen in those who are well compensated. An objective study of the effect of ouabain on the response of the left ventricle in patients with angina pectoris showed that the depressed myocardial performance noted on exercise was improved by digitalization in the majority of patients studied.[195] Despite these beneficial effects on left ventricular performance, however, there was no consistent alteration in exercise tolerance or the pressure-rate product at which angina occurred. Other studies have demonstrated an increased cardiac output on exercise after digitalization, suggesting that the reduction in myocardial oxygen consumption that followed digitalis-induced improvement in left ventricular function probably masked any increase caused by its positive inotropic action.[196] No deterioration of myocardial metabolism with acute ouabain administration was found in patients with chronic coronary artery disease either at rest[197] or with pacing-induced myocardial ischemia.[198] Improved myocardial perfusion judged by means of thallium-201 scans was found in response to maintenance doses of digoxin in patients with coronary artery disease and left ventricular dysfunction.[199] The combination of propranolol and digoxin in patients with angina pectoris appears to be advantageous in the subgroup with angina pectoris and abnormal ventricular function or large hearts.[200]

There are still many unanswered questions concerning the role of digitalis therapy after acute myocardial infarction. There is little to be gained from administration of the drug to patients who have uncomplicated infarction without cardiomegaly (p. 1315).[201] There is limited clinical documentation of its value in cardiogenic shock, a syndrome in which no pharmacological agent has been demonstrated to be highly effective. Indeed, rapid digitalization may occasionally be harmful, owing to the vasoconstrictor properties of the drug.[202] Small increases in cardiac index and stroke work as well as a reduction in left ventricular end-diastolic pressure have been observed after digitalization in patients with left ventricular failure following myocardial infarction.[203] Although ouabain did not alter cardiac output in another series of patients with acute myocardial infarction,[204] it caused significant improvement in other indices of left ventricular performance, such as end-diastolic pressure and stroke work. Similar benefits were noted in patients convalescing from myocardial infarction.[205]

The issue of increased susceptibility to the toxic effects of digitalis in recent or acute myocardial infarction remains controversial. In animal models, the dose of digitalis required to reach a toxic endpoint clearly is reduced after experimentally induced myocardial infarction.[206,207] However, in a study of patients with acute myocardial infarction, 89 per cent tolerated a full dose of acetylstrophanthidin, suggesting no significant enhancement of sensitivity to the drug.[155] In patients with acute myocardial infarction treated with intravenous digoxin using a double-blind randomized protocol, no difference in incidence of rhythm disturbances was found between digoxin-treated and control patients.[208] There appears to be no convincing evidence for an increased incidence of arrhythmias complicating digitalization in patients with acute infarction when serum levels do not exceed the conventional therapeutic range.[209]

The clearest indication for digitalis after acute myocardial infarction is in the treatment of atrial fibrillation with a rapid ventricular rate. Electrical cardioversion may be preferred in the treatment of other supraventricular tachyarrhythmias.[210]

Evidence based on a retrospective analysis by Moss et al.[211] suggests that mortality within the first 4 months after myocardial infarction may be increased in a high-risk subset of patients with congestive heart failure and ventricular arrhythmias, but this finding has not yet been confirmed by prospective studies, and, indeed, has been contested.[211a]

In summary, current evidence indicates that digitalis has no well-defined role in the management of acute myocardial infarction without congestive heart failure or supraventricular tachyarrhythmias. Judicious patient selection and management of drug doses will minimize the potentially deleterious effects of digitalis in acute myocardial infarction.

ADVANCED AGE. Advanced age per se has been considered by some to be a risk factor in the development of digitalis toxicity because of an enhanced sensitivity to the drug.[212,213] However, diminished glomerular filtration rate with age will alone lead to prolonged half-life of digoxin and thus to increased serum levels and an increased probability of toxicity on a given dosage regimen. Advanced age is frequently associated with other factors that increase the likelihood of digitalis intoxication, including more severe heart disease; impairment of pulmonary, renal, and neurological function; and an increased number of concurrent medications.

RENAL FAILURE (See also page 1759). Renal failure, particularly in patients requiring hemodialysis, is a disease state in which factors influencing digitalis absorption and elimination and rapid shifts of electrolytes profoundly affect the response to digitalis. The marked diminution of glomerular filtration rate with renal failure prolongs the half-life of digoxin and thus increases serum digoxin levels. Toxicity from this predictable response can be avoided by careful and frequent adjustments of dosage to correlate with the level of renal function present. Less predictably, dialysis can cause at least a transient decrease in serum potassium that will increase the tendency toward digitalis-induced arrhythmias. Depending on the magnesium content of the dialysate and the use of magnesium-containing antacids by the patient, there may be significant aberrations of serum magnesium levels in patients on dialysis.[172] Some evidence suggests that increased serum levels of digoxin may reflect a decreased volume of distribution, so that relatively higher levels may be needed to achieve a

certain effect.[214] The clinician is well advised to use the minimum drug dosage that produces the desired clinical effect in this condition noted for its extreme fluctuations in fluid and electrolyte balance.

THYROID DISEASE. It is well known that thyroid disease alters digitalis pharmacokinetics. In hypothyroid patients the serum digoxin half-life is consistently prolonged, while in those with hyperthyroidism serum digoxin levels tend to be decreased.[215] Since some studies have not documented significant changes in metabolism or serum half-life of digoxin in hyperthyroid patients,[216] it has been suggested that an increased distribution space for digoxin may exist. This hypothesis is of interest in light of experimental findings indicating higher levels of Na^+,K^+-ATPase activity in the myocardium[217] and other tissues of hyperthyroid animals.[218] In any event the apparent resistance or sensitivity to digitalis in thyroid disease is dependent, at least in part, on changes in the pharmacokinetics of digoxin. Changes in the response of the heart to a given serum level of drug probably also occur (for example, the difficulty in controlling the ventricular response in patients with thyrotoxicosis and atrial fibrillation), but these changes have not been well defined either in the experimental laboratory or in the clinical setting. As discussed previously, autonomic neural influences on the effect of digitalis on the heart have long been appreciated. Such changes in autonomic tone may to some extent explain the apparent resistance to digitalis effect seen in thyrotoxicosis.

PULMONARY DISEASE. There has been considerable interest in the use of digitalis in patients with pulmonary disease.[219] A number of authors have noted that ventricular ectopic activity consistent with digitalis toxicity frequently occurs in patients with respiratory disease who are receiving digitalis.[220-222] Such reports are difficult to interpret, however, because respiratory failure and hypoxemia frequently provoke arrhythmias indistinguishable from those associated with digitalis excess.[223,224] A population of 931 patients admitted consecutively to a medical service and studied prospectively demonstrated an increased incidence of rhythm disturbances consistent with digitalis toxicity among patients with acute or chronic lung disease.[225]

When excessive sensitivity to digitalis in patients with pulmonary disease was investigated utilizing acetylstrophanthidin tolerance testing, it was observed that of 18 patients with chronic lung disease who did not receive digitalis previously, six demonstrated increased sensitivity, all of whom had cor pulmonale and hypercapnia and five of whom were hypoxemic.[226] These findings are corroborated by the relatively frequent discordance between serum digoxin levels and tolerance to acetylstrophanthidin in patients with pulmonary disease.[227] In a group of patients with severe respiratory failure, 18 had rhythm disturbances consistent with digitalis toxicity at a time when serum digoxin levels were within a range not usually associated with toxicity.[228] Only the presence of more severe hypoxemia distinguished these patients from those with pulmonary disease who appeared toxic only at higher serum concentrations.

Therefore the evidence is highly suggestive that pulmonary disease predisposes to the development of digitalis intoxication at relatively low serum concentrations. It would appear that hypoxemia is an important factor associated with this enhanced sensitivity to digitalis. However, the degree of hypoxemia may be merely an index of the severity of the respiratory failure and its associated physiological derangements rather than a factor that by itself is causally related to digitalis sensitivity. Although not adequately subdivided into acute or chronic respiratory illnesses, the available epidemiological data suggest that patients with stable chronic lung disease are at increased risk of developing digitalis intoxication. Particularly as a result of diuretic therapy, these patients are subject to derangements in potassium homeostasis and the development of metabolic alkalosis—both predisposing to digitalis toxicity. What role exogenous catecholamines and the sympathomimetic agents commonly used in the therapy of chronic airway disease may have in the development of digitalis-related arrhythmias is not known. No published studies have shown convincing enhancement of ventricular ectopic activity in patients receiving catecholamines by inhalation in either the presence or the absence of digitalis.

From the data available, then, it is reasonable for the clinician to assume that patients with a variety of pulmonary diseases may be sensitive to the arrhythmogenic effects of digitalis at relatively low serum concentrations.

SERUM OR PLASMA CONCENTRATIONS OF DIGITALIS GLYCOSIDES

It has long been apparent clinically that alterations in cardiac rhythm as well as extracardiac manifestations of digitalis action, such as gastrointestinal and central nervous system symptoms, are dose-related.[229] It has now been demonstrated convincingly in a number of studies that plasma digitalis concentrations are also correlated with the amount of drug administered.[189] One would therefore expect that a correlation would exist between plasma digitalis concentration and the symptoms and signs of toxicity. In both animal and human studies, after attainment of equilibrium, a relatively constant ratio of plasma to myocardial digoxin concentration has been observed,[230,231] although not all the digoxin present in myocardium is bound to specific receptors relevant to the pharmacological action of the drug. As discussed earlier, the available evidence that digitalis glycosides act on receptors similar or identical to Na^+,K^+-ATPase and hence in close proximity to the cell surface suggests that digitalis concentration at these receptor sites would be influenced readily by the concentration in plasma. Animal experiments have confirmed the expected relation between plasma digoxin concentrations and electrophysiological effects on the heart.[232]

The availability of methods for measuring serum or plasma digitalis concentrations* in the clinical laboratory has led to extensive studies concerning the relation between serum levels and manifestations of toxicity in man.[61] Methods practically applicable to evaluation of patient serum samples are based on physicochemical separation, inhibition of Na^+,K^+-ATPase or its transmembrane cation transport function, or competitive protein binding employing either a specific antibody or a preparation containing Na^+,K^+-ATPase. Available methods are discussed in detail elsewhere.[233]

RADIOIMMUNOASSAY. Most published clinical studies have employed specific antibody as the binding protein in a competitive binding assay. This procedure is readily adaptable to the clinical laboratory. Small volumes of serum or plasma may be used directly, without prior extraction, necessitating a minimal number of manipulations. Appropriately selected antisera have exceptionally high degrees of affinity and specificity for the cardiac glycoside of interest, allowing the measurement of subnanogram amounts.[234] However, as with other radioimmunoassays, these are subject to certain pitfalls that may cause erroneous results if careful attention is not paid to selection of antisera, assurance of purity of standards and tracers, and appropriate counting techniques.[235]

Further details of available techniques for measurement of circulating cardiac glycoside concentrations are provided in reviews of this subject.[61,233,234] With the proliferation of commercial kits for measuring cardiac glycoside concentrations, it is particularly important for the clinician and clinical investigator to be certain that the values reported by the laboratory are accurate. Moreover, uncertainty can be introduced if sufficient time has not elapsed since the last previous dose to allow full equilibration of the drug between intravascular and peripheral compartments. In practice, a safe time for sampling of serum or plasma is 6 hours or more after the last dose of the cardiac glycoside.

CLINICAL CORRELATIONS. Although several techniques have been used to measure the concentrations of digoxin and digitoxin, there is substantial agreement regarding these values in patients receiving usual maintenance doses of these drugs.[61] Mean serum or plasma digoxin concentrations in groups of patients without evidence of toxicity average about 1.4 ng/ml. As would be expected, increasing digoxin doses or decreasing renal function is correlated with higher mean serum levels. Mean serum digoxin concentrations tend to be two to three times higher in patients with clinical evidence of digoxin toxicity, and the difference in mean levels is statistically significant in the vast majority of studies.[61] It must be emphasized that overlap of levels between groups with and without evidence of toxicity has been observed in most series and tends to be more pronounced in prospective, blind studies than in retrospective studies.[225] Despite this overlap, use of serum digoxin concentration measurements to guide therapy has been associated with a reduction in the incidence of digitalis toxicity.[236]

Analogous data correlating serum digitoxin concentrations with clinical state[61] indicate that although levels average about 10-fold higher than those of digoxin because of digitoxin binding to serum proteins, patients with clinical evidence of toxicity again have mean levels about two times higher than those without evidence of a toxic response. As in the case of digoxin, substantial overlap in levels occurs among groups of patients with and without evidence of toxicity despite the statistically significant differences in mean serum concentrations.

Although cardiac digitalis toxicity is accompanied by relatively well-defined relations between rhythm disturbance and serum glycoside concentration, it is more difficult to correlate therapeutic effects with serum levels in

---

*Serum and plasma digoxin, digitoxin, and ouabain concentrations are equivalent and will hereafter be referred to as serum concentrations.

man. A correlation has been reported between plasma digoxin levels and slowing of previously rapid ventricular rates in patients with atrial fibrillation.[237] Another measure of the degree of digitalization is the cumulative dose of acetylstrophanthidin required to reach a toxic endpoint.[227] Substantial variation in acetylstrophanthidin sensitivity was demonstrated among individual patients at any given serum digoxin level, indicating a continuing need to correlate serum digoxin concentration with other, independent methods of assessing myocardial sensitivity to cardiac glycosides.

The multifactorial determinants of digitalis intoxication and the overlap in serum digitalis concentrations between toxic and nontoxic states preclude the use of these levels as a sole guide to digitalis dosage. A Bayesian approach (page 273) to the use of serum digoxin levels in clinical decision making is logical and theoretically attractive.[238] Serum levels considered within a particular clinical context together with other available information can be a valuable aid to therapeutic decision-making. Suspected manifestations of digitalis intoxication in the absence of an adequate history, fluctuating renal function, presence of overt or suspected malabsorption, and use of preparations of uncertain bioavailability are among the circumstances in which knowledge of the serum level is most helpful. More generally, it is our opinion that measurement of serum cardiac glycoside concentrations is indicated whenever an unanticipated response to these drugs (either suspected toxicity or absence of an expected therapeutic effect) is encountered.

DIGITALIS TOXICITY

Toxic manifestations of digitalis persist as one of the most prevalent adverse drug reactions encountered in clinical practice.[61,239,240] The true incidence is difficult to determine accurately but at present is probably in the range of 5 to 15 per cent in hospitalized patients receiving these drugs. The variability in available estimates relates to differing definitions of digitalis intoxication, the retrospective nature of many studies, and differences in the groups under study. In a prospective investigation, 931 consecutive admissions to a single medical facility were studied. Of these, 15 per cent of patients had taken digitoxin, digoxin, or digitalis leaf up to 48 hours or less before admission. Digitalis intoxication was diagnosed electrocardiographically by the presence of typical disturbances of impulse formation and conduction that disappeared when the drug was withheld. Of the digitalized patients, 23 per cent fulfilled criteria for definite digitalis toxicity and another 6 per cent were judged to be possibly toxic. Other prospective studies have reported a comparable incidence of toxicity.[61] There is some evidence that increased understanding of pharmacokinetics and the use of serum level data to guide therapy have reduced this alarming incidence,[236] but constant vigilance on the part of the physician is required.

Mechanisms of Digitalis Intoxication (See also p. 238)

The major manifestations of digitalis intoxication include gastrointestinal and central nervous system symptoms and disturbances of cardiac rhythm. Anorexia, nausea, and vomiting are probably mediated by chemoreceptors located in the area postrema of the medulla rather than by a direct irritant effect of the drug on the gastrointestinal tract.[241] The precise mechanism underlying this and other central nervous system effects remains unclear, but several studies have demonstrated the presence of digoxin in the cerebrospinal fluid of patients treated with this drug.[242,243] Therefore, the drug clearly penetrates the blood-brain barrier in appreciable amounts and may, in addition, exert effects in regions that lack a normal blood-brain barrier, such as the area postrema of the medulla.[82,244]

The genesis of cardiac arrhythmias depends, at least in part, on the effect of the drug on the electrical activity of cardiac cells. Digitalis-induced disturbances of impulse formation and conduction are conventionally explained in terms of alterations in refractory period, impulse transmission, and automaticity of cardiac tissues, although alterations in sympathetic activity and changes in vagal tone may also be of considerable importance in some situations, as discussed previously. Interesting data have been obtained from experiments in which isolated canine Purkinje fibers were perfused with the blood of intact donor dogs and ouabain-induced changes in the donor dog's electrocardiogram were correlated with changes in the Purkinje fiber transmembrane potential[245,246] (Fig. 16–6). At the time of onset of early ouabain toxicity in the donor dog, defined as junctional or ventricular premature contractions or junctional tachycardia, Purkinje fiber recordings showed decreases in action-potential amplitude, resting membrane potential, maximum velocity of the upstroke of the action potential, action-potential duration, and plateau phase. Slowing of conduction was also apparent, often varying in extent from cycle to cycle. With further progression of toxicity to ventricular tachycardia in the donor dog, changes in transmembrane potential became still more marked, as shown in Figure 16–6.

In additional experiments, increased automaticity was found to occur at the time of early toxicity at plasma potassium concentrations below 4 mEq/liter. Increased automaticity was more frequent when Purkinje fibers had been stretched and in the presence of hypokalemia, which correlates well with clinical observations of increased frequency of digitalis toxicity in the dilated failing heart as well as in the presence of hypokalemia. Additional evidence bearing on the particular sensitivity of Purkinje fibers to the toxic electrophysiologic effects of digitalis comes from studies showing greater effects of acute and chronic digoxin administration on monovalent cation transport in Purkinje fibers compared with adjacent working myocardium.[37]

Regarding the cellular mechanism of digitalis toxicity, until recently most investigators favored a sequence in which digitalis-induced inhibition of Na^+ and K^+ transport caused increased intracellular $[Na^+]$, decreased intracellular $[K^+]$, and gradual depolarization. This in turn

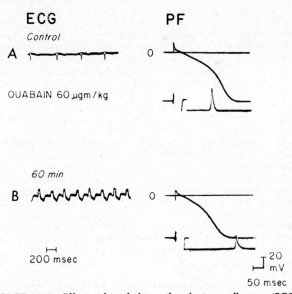

FIGURE 16–6 Effects of ouabain on the electrocardiogram (ECG) of an intact donor dog and on the Purkinje fiber (PF) action potential of an isolated preparation perfused with blood from the donor dog. Sinus rhythm (panel A) is succeeded by ventricular tachycardia (panel B) 60 minutes after administration of a toxic dose of ouabain. At the onset of ventricular tachycardia, the Purkinje fiber action potential shows significant loss of amplitude, duration, and maximum velocity of the phase 0 upstroke. The lower trace in each PF panel shows the first derivative of voltage with respect to time during phase 0. (From Rosen, M. R., et al.: Correlation between effects of ouabain on the canine electrocardiogram and transmembrane potentials of isolated Purkinje fibers. Circulation 47:65, 1973, by permission of the American Heart Association, Inc.)

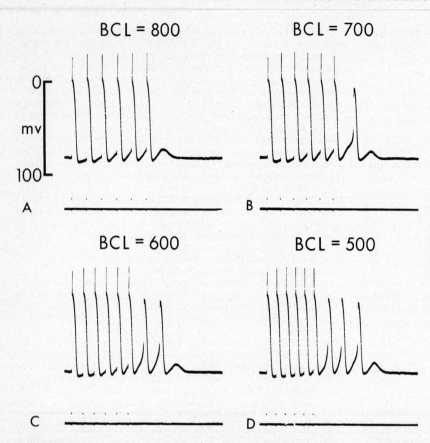

FIGURE 16–7 Sequential development (*A* to *D*) of a train of spontaneous beats due to transient depolarizations (also called oscillatory afterpotentials) in a canine Purkinje fiber exposed to acetylstrophanthidin and then driven at varying basic cycle lengths (BCL), indicated in milliseconds at the top of each panel. (From Ferrier, G. R., et al.: A cellular mechanism for the generation of ventricular arrhythmias by acetylstrophanthidin. Circ. Res. *32*:600, 1973, by permission of the American Heart Association, Inc.)

led to increased automaticity, conduction disturbances, and finally inexcitability. Recent experimental evidence suggests that cardiac glycosides promote a hitherto unrecognized mechanism of spontaneous activity in specialized cardiac conducting tissue. The underlying cellular event is a depolarizing afterpotential that has been variously called "enhanced diastolic depolarization,"[247] "low-amplitude potential,"[248] "transient depolarization,"[249] or "oscillatory afterpotentials" (p. 620), shown in Figure 16–7. In panel A, a transient depolarization follows a train of six action potentials. It falls short of threshold in this instance but can influence conduction of subsequent impulses.[250] With increased driving frequency, as shown in panel B, the transient depolarization reaches threshold, and excitation occurs. The counterpart of this event in the intact heart would be a ventricular premature beat. Panels C and D show multiple repetitive responses to further increases in driving frequency, which may be analogous to the beat dependence of digitalis-induced ectopic activity in intact hearts of experimental animals.[251,252]

The cellular mechanism underlying the transient depolarization phenomenon has been studied in calf Purkinje fibers using voltage-clamp techniques.[253] A transient inward current closely related to transient depolarizations was observed in response to the cardiotonic steroid strophanthidin and was temporally coincident with phasic increases in tension ("aftercontraction").[254] Further evidence suggests that elevated levels of free intracellular calcium may be a crucial factor,[254,255] just as has been discussed earlier with respect to the mechanism of positive inotropic action of digitalis. The mechanism involved in the generation of digitalis-induced transient depolarizations clearly differs both from that underlying normal phase 4 spontaneous depolarization and from the slow inward current.[256]

Potential or overt toxic effects of digitalis on cardiac electrophysiology will now be briefly summarized:

SINUS NODE AND ATRIUM

Digitalis-induced slowing of the sinus rate in patients without congestive heart failure is usually minor in degree and is largely mediated by vagal effects on the sinoatrial node. Patients with transplanted, denervated hearts do not respond to conventional doses of digoxin with any change in sinus rate.[257] As far as direct effects of digitalis are concerned, the atrium seems more sensitive than the sinus node.

Experimentally, at higher doses, there is a depression in sinus node automaticity.[258,259] A combination of vagal and direct effects on the sinus node probably contributes to sinus bradycardia as well as to occasional cases of sinoatrial arrest or exit block seen in digitalis intoxication. This bradycardia predisposes to the emergence of junctional ventricular escape rhythms.

Digitalis, even in therapeutic doses, can impair sinoatrial conduction. Although usually well tolerated in patients with sick sinus syndrome, occasionally sinus node dysfunction is precipitated by digoxin, even in doses not usually associated with toxicity. Digitalis shortens the refractory period of the atrial myocardium in experimental studies, but has relatively minor and variable effects in the human heart.[61]

ATRIOVENTRICULAR NODE

The effective refractory period of the atrioventricular node is prolonged by digitalis. As with the sinus node, this longer period is in part related to increased vagal activity and in part to direct action on nodal fibers, although the vagal effect appears to predominate in subjects without intrinsic diseases of the cardiac conduction system.[190] Decreased amplitude and upstroke velocity of the action potential from the node itself and from nodal-His fibers have been recorded by means of microelectrode studies of isolated tissues in response to cardiac glycosides.[260]

The therapeutic effect of digitalis in slowing ventricular response in atrial flutter or fibrillation depends in part on the entry of concealed atrial impulses into the atrioventricular node, with failure to reach the His-Purkinje system by virtue of decremental conduction within the node (p. 624). When atrioventricular block of second or third degree occurs as a result of digitalis intoxication, however, the principal mechanism is failure of propagation within the atrioventricular node.[260]

HIS-PURKINJE SYSTEM

Digitalis-induced increases in the automaticity of the His-Purkinje system may come about because of enhanced spontaneous diastolic (phase 4) depolarization or the more recently described transient depolarization mechanism discussed above and elsewhere.[61] The appearance of new pacemakers is manifest clinically by premature junctional or ventricular beats or by accelerated junctional or ventricular rhythms. The nonuniform effect of digitalis on ventricular and Purkinje fibers and simultaneous enhancement of automaticity, depression of conduction velocity, and local block may also predispose to arrhythmias based on reentry mechanisms that may progress to ventricular tachycardia and fibrillation.[61]

Clinical Manifestations

Gastrointestinal Symptoms. Anorexia is often an early manifestation of digitalis intoxication.[225] Nausea and vomiting follow as clear consequences of digitalis overdose and result from central nervous system mechanisms.[241] It may be difficult, in clinical situations, to attribute these symptoms to digitalis, since they may also be caused by cardiac failure or by associated illnesses.

Neurological Symptoms. These include headache, fatigue, malaise, neuralgic pain, disorientation, confusion, delirium, and seizures. Visual symptoms are not infrequent and include scotomas, flickering, halos, and changes in color perception.[261] As with gastrointestinal symptoms, it is often difficult to determine whether neurological symptoms are a consequence of digitalis excess, associated fluid and electrolyte disturbances, or associated illnesses.

Cardiac Toxicity (see also pages 238 to 242). Cardiac toxicity manifested by arrhythmias can take the form of essentially every known rhythm disturbance.[61] Common arrhythmias include atrioventricular junctional escape rhythms, ventricular bigeminy or trigeminy, nonparoxysmal atrioventricular junctional tachycardia, unifocal or multifocal ectopic ventricular beats, and ventricular tachycardia. Atrioventricular junctional exit block, paroxysmal atrial tachycardia with atrioventricular block, sinus arrest, and Mobitz type I (Wenckebach) second-degree atrioventricular block also occur. This list should not be considered exhaustive. There are no unequivocal electrocardiographic features that distinguish digitalis-toxic rhythm disturbances from rhythms due to intrinsic cardiac disease, although rhythms combining features of increased automaticity of ectopic pacemakers with impaired conduction, such as paroxysmal atrial tachycardia with atrioventricular dissociation and an accelerated atrioventricular junctional pacemaker, strongly suggest digitalis toxicity. However, even rhythms such as atrial tachycardia with AV block, considered typical of digitalis toxicity, are frequently due to underlying heart disease rather than to digitalis excess.[262] The difficulty in determining whether or not ventricular ectopic activity is due to digitalis excess is exemplified by a study in which 142 patients with this rhythm disturbance, most of whom were on maintenance digoxin doses, were given incremental doses of the rapidly acting agent acetylstrophanthidin to determine their response.[263] Frequency of ventricular premature beats decreased in 46 per cent of patients, remained unchanged in 26 per cent, and increased in 28 per cent in response to the additional doses of digitalis. The cause of an arrhythmia may at times be clarified (but not defined with complete certainty) by demonstration of a reversion to normal rhythm when the drug is withheld. Clinical and electrocardiographic findings associated with digitalis toxicity have been reviewed extensively.[61,264–266]

Other Manifestations. Allergic skin lesions are rare but have been reported.[267] Gynecomastia is occasionally induced in men,[268] and sexual dysfunction has been reported.[269]

Massive Cardiac Glycoside Overdose

Digitalis overdose, either suicidal or accidental, is occasionally encountered as a life-threatening problem.[190,191,270] Patients without underlying heart disease tend to tolerate large doses, with serum digoxin concentrations ranging as high as 10 to 15 ng/ml.[190]

The principal manifestations in patients without intrinsic heart disease are most often sinus bradycardia; atrioventricular block of first, second, or third degree; or sinoatrial exit block. Atropine alone is often successful in reversing these manifestations but is not invariably effective.[61,190] Ventricular pacing with a pervenous endocardial catheter electrode is usually successful, although ventricular standstill unresponsive to pacing has been reported.[190]

Patients with preexisting heart disease tend to be more difficult to manage, in that ectopic ventricular arrhythmias are frequently the initial manifestation of digitalis intoxication.[190] Phenytoin, lidocaine, procainamide, and potassium have been used in treatment.[61] Direct-current cardioversion may also be required for refractory, life-threatening supraventricular or ventricular tachycardia or for ventricular fibrillation, despite the known hazards of this therapeutic modality in patients with digitalis toxicity. Not infrequently, the ventricular arrhythmias in this group lead to a fatal outcome despite the most vigorous therapeutic efforts.

Refractory hyperkalemia can occur at extremely high digoxin doses and serum concentrations.[190,191,271] Greater elevations of serum K^+ concentration were associated with worsening prognosis in a large series of patients after massive doses, usually of digitoxin.[272] It is likely that elevation of serum potassium is a consequence of inhibition of Na^+,K^+-ATPase throughout the body, with consequent impairment of monovalent cation transport across cell membranes.

The half-time for digoxin clearance from plasma is shortened when levels are very high.[190,273] This effect may be related to an altered ratio between plasma and tissue concentrations, allowing a relatively large quantity of the drug to be presented to the kidney for excretion.

Treatment of Digitalis Intoxication

The key to successful treatment is early recognition that an arrhythmia is related to digitalis intoxication. The more common manifestations—including occasional ectopic beats, marked first-degree atrioventricular block, or atrial fibrillation with a slow ventricular response—require only temporary withdrawal of the drug, electrocardiographic monitoring (if indicated) until the arrhythmia has disappeared, and subsequent adjustment of the dosage schedule to prevent recurrence. Rhythm disturbances that impair cardiac output because of too rapid or too slow ventricular rates, or those that portend ventricular fibrillation, require more active intervention. Ventricular tachycardia due to digitalis intoxication demands immediate vigorous treatment. Sinus bradycardia, sinoatrial arrest, and atrioventricular block of second or third degree are sometimes treated effectively with atropine, as previously indicated. Occasionally, electrical pacing will be required. It has been recommended that nonparoxysmal atrioventricular junctional rhythms with rates greater than 90 or with exit block be treated actively.[274] Atrioventricular junctional escape rhythms may simply be monitored if the rate is satisfactory.

Phenytoin and Lidocaine (see also pages 653 and 661). Phenytoin and lidocaine are useful drugs in the treatment of ectopic arrhythmias due to digitalis toxicity.[61] They have little adverse effect on sinoatrial rate, atrial conduction, atrioventricular conduction, or conduction in the

His-Purkinje system.[275-277] Indeed, phenytoin may improve sinoatrial block and atrioventricular conduction under some circumstances.[277,278] A recommended regimen for phenytoin is 100 mg administered by slow intravenous infusion every 5 minutes until onset of toxicity or control of the arrhythmia, followed by an oral maintenance dose of 400 to 600 mg/day if control of the arrhythmia is achieved. Lidocaine is given intravenously in 100-mg bolus doses every 3 to 5 minutes, followed by the continuous infusion of 15 to 50 μg/kg of body weight/min as required to maintain control of the rhythm disturbances.

Potassium. Therapy with potassium is recommended for ectopic tachyarrhythmias when hypokalemia is present but must be used with caution in other circumstances because of the risks associated with hyperkalemia.[61] Particular care is necessary when conduction disturbances are present, since elevations of plasma potassium concentration may impair atrioventricular conduction.[279]

Propranolol. Propranolol has been useful in the treatment of some digitalis-toxic arrhythmias. Because of its antiadrenergic effects, it causes a decrease in automaticity, whereas by virtue of its direct myocardial effects, it shortens the refractory period of atrial muscle, ventricular muscle, and Purkinje fibers; slows the rate of depolarization; and slows conduction velocity.[280] Potential undesirable effects include depression of atrioventricular conduction and of sinoatrial and atrioventricular junctional pacemakers, with asystole or marked bradycardia, and depression of myocardial contractility with hemodynamic deterioration.

Quinidine and Procainamide (see also pages 656 and 657). Quinidine and procainamide carry a risk of cardiac toxicity, such as depression of the sinoatrial node and of atrioventricular and His-Purkinje conduction, as well as the potential for eliciting ventricular arrhythmias. They are also capable of depressing myocardial contractility. Quinidine may actually intensify digitalis intoxication by raising serum level, as discussed on p. 519. Other agents are usually preferable for use in digitalis intoxication.[274]

Direct-Current Countershock (see also page 669). Whereas countershock is generally inadvisable in the presence of digitalis intoxication because of the severe arrhythmias that may ensue, it must occasionally be used when all other methods have failed in the face of a life-threatening rhythm disturbance. The risk is decreased when lower energy levels are employed.[61,281] In contrast to the increased risk reported in the presence of overt digitalis toxicity, cardioversion appears to be a benign procedure in patients without digitalis-induced rhythm disturbances.[282]

Steroid-Binding Resins. As previously noted (p. 514), digitoxin undergoes some enterohepatic circulation, and agents that bind the drug within the gastrointestinal lumen should shorten its half-life. Cholestyramine induced a reduction in serum half-life of chloroform-extractable activity from 6.0 to 4.5 days after tritiated digitoxin administration in man,[138] and colestipol appears to have a similar effect.[283] These effects may provide a means of reducing the duration of digitoxin toxicity but are probably not of sufficient magnitude or rapidity to be of great importance in the management of severe, life-threatening toxicity. Although digoxin has only a minimal enterohepatic circulation,[144] cholestyramine tends to interfere with its initial absorption from the gastrointestinal tract.[284]

Reversal of Toxicity by Specific Antibody. The use of cardiac glycoside–specific antibodies and their Fab fragments for treatment of advanced digitalis intoxication has been studied in considerable detail.[285-287] A possible mechanism for the reversal of both inotropic and arrhythmogenic effects of cardiac glycosides was suggested in experiments demonstrating that high-affinity cardiac glycoside–specific antibodies are able to reverse established glycoside-induced inhibition of myocardial Na$^+$,K$^+$-ATPase[288] and monovalent cation active transport.[289]

Fab fragments provide advantages over purified intact antibodies as potential therapeutic agents. Each intact IgG antibody molecule of molecular weight 150,000 is cleaved by the proteolytic enzyme papain into an Fc fragment and two Fab fragments, each of which contains a specific binding site and has a molecular weight of 50,000. This smaller molecular species has a greater rate and volume of distribution after intravenous infusion and reverses experimentally induced digoxin-toxic arrhythmias more rapidly than does intact antibody.[287] The smaller size of the Fab molecule also allows it to pass through the mammalian glomerulus, unlike intact IgG. Fab fragments are excreted to an appreciable extent in the urine, but intact IgG is not.[290] Whereas injection of intact antibody markedly prolongs the plasma half-life of digoxin (although it is largely antibody-bound), digoxin bound to Fab fragments is excreted much more rapidly.[291] Rapid reversal of otherwise lethal experimentally induced digitoxin toxicity with specific antibodies and Fab fragments has been demonstrated,[292] together with substantial acceleration by Fab of the renal excretion of digitoxin. This rapid renal excretion of Fab fragments may be of importance in reducing the immunogenicity of the foreign protein.[293]

A series of 26 patients with life-threatening digoxin or digitoxin toxicity has been treated with purified digoxin-specific Fab fragments.[191] All these patients had advanced cardiac rhythm disturbances and in 9 cases hyperkalemia was present as well, owing, in the majority, to ingestion of very large digitalis doses accidentally or with suicidal intent. All patients treated had an initial favorable response to intravenously administered Fab. Four patients eventually died as a result of cerebral or myocardial damage from prolonged low output states prior to Fab administration; available Fab supplies were insufficient to provide adequate treatment in a fifth case. In the remaining 21 patients, cardiac arrhythmias and hyperkalemia were reversed rapidly with full recovery.[191] Efforts are underway to make this therapeutic modality more widely available.

DIURETICS

A diuretic is a drug that increases urinary excretion of salt and water. Certain agents *indirectly* increase urine production by enhancing renal blood flow and the rate of glomerular filtration. Examples of such agents are digitalis, which effects a diuresis indirectly by enhancing cardiac output, and dopamine, which not only increases cardiac output but also acts directly on the renal vasculature; the diuretic action of albumin and dextran is through expansion of plasma volume. Most diuretics, however, act *directly* on the kidney to inhibit solute and water absorption, thereby increasing urine volume. While it is generally assumed that diuretics exert their favorable clinical effects by promoting excretion of excess salt and water and reducing abnormally elevated preload, there is evidence that furosemide administration can produce a diuresis accompanied by improved performance of the failing left ventricle and reduced afterload without alteration of the left ventricular diastolic dimension as an index of preload.[294]

Nonreabsorbable solutes such as mannitol are freely filtered at the glomerulus. Since their osmotic effects inhibit water reabsorption, thereby causing a diuresis, such substances are termed osmotic diuretics.[295] Many pharmacological agents interfere with active ion transport, resulting in increased urine flow secondary to the enhanced excretion of ions and the water they osmotically obligate (Fig. 16–8). The precise cellular sites of action of most diuretics are not known. They may interfere with any of the three steps in the sequence of sodium reabsorption: (1) the entry of the solute into the cell, (2) the generation and utilization of energy for sodium transport, and (3) the transfer of sodium from the cell to peritubular blood through the antiluminal membrane.[296,297] *Water diuresis* may be induced by agents such as demeclocycline or lithium that block the cellular action of vasopressin, which normally allows the reabsorption of water along the distal nephron and collecting system.

SITES AND MECHANISMS OF ACTION OF DIURETIC AGENTS (See Figures 16–9 and 16–10 and Table 16–6)

PROXIMAL TUBULE

Since 50 to 75 per cent of filtered sodium and water is reabsorbed by the proximal tubule, substances that inhibit transport in this segment of the nephron would be expected to be potent diuretic agents.[298] Although no available diuretic completely prevents proximal tubular sodium reabsorption, the carbonic anhydrase inhibitors such as acetazolamide act primarily by inhibiting proximal reabsorption. It has been shown under experimental conditions that thiazide diuretics,[299,300] metolazone, and furosemide[301] possess mild carbonic anhydrase inhibitory activity, but this action does not appear to be clinically important. Acetazolamide is actively absorbed and concentrated within cells of the proximal tubule and causes diuresis by inhibiting the formation of hydrogen ions needed to reabsorb filtered sodium bicarbonate. The demands of electroneutrality require that sodium and, to a lesser extent, potassium be retained in the tubular lumen to offset the accumulating negative charge from unreabsorbed bicarbonate anion, causing a sodium, potassium, and bicarbonate diuresis. The effectiveness of carbonic anhydrase inhibitors is proportional to the filtered load of bicarbonate. It follows that their efficacy is impaired by metabolic acidosis and enhanced by metabolic alkalosis.[302] Moreover, because these agents induce loss of $NaHCO_3$, they induce metabolic acidosis, which progressively limits their effectiveness.

A significant fraction of proximal sodium and chloride reabsorption is passive, being dependent on the generation of a favorable chloride gradient between tubular fluid and plasma. The active reabsorption of

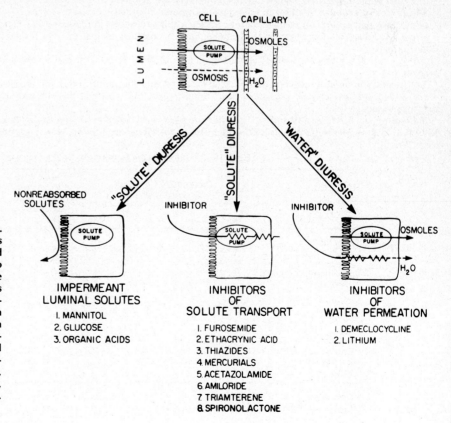

FIGURE 16–8 General mechanisms of diuresis. Glomerular filtrate is absorbed in renal tubules by the active transport of solute (osmoles) and the passive transport of water (osmosis). Two types of diuresis can occur due to interference with tubular absorption: (1) "Solute" diuresis follows the glomerular filtration of nonreabsorbable solute or in consequence of the inhibition of solute pumps. (2) "Water" diuresis is seen when the osmotic permeability to water is decreased selectively. (From Grantham, J. J., and Chonko, A. M.: The physiological basis and clinical use of diuretics. *In* Brenner, B. M., and Stein, J. H. (eds.): Sodium and Water Homeostasis. Vol. I. New York, Churchill Livingstone, 1978, p. 179.)

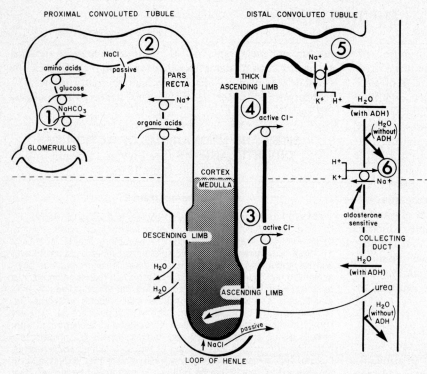

FIGURE 16–9 Transport functions of the various anatomical segments of the mammalian nephron. Fluid reabsorption across the proximal tubule is isosmotic and accounts for approximately two-thirds of the reabsorption of filtered Na^+ and H_2O. $NaHCO_3$ is reabsorbed by a nonelectrogenic mechanism, most likely via H^+ secretion. The active transport of these solutes results in transepithelial concentration and effective osmotic pressure gradients promoting H_2O flow across the proximal tubule into the peritubular capillaries. The rise in tubular fluid Cl^- concentration is a consequence of the decreased luminal HCO_3^- concentration and becomes an important force for the outward passive transport of Cl^- down its concentration gradient. The pars recta of the proximal tubule is capable of active electrogenic transport of Na^+. Normally, approximately one-third of the glomerular filtrate enters the descending limb of Henle's loop. Because the thin descending limb is incapable of active outward NaCl transport and is characterized by low permeability to Na^+ but high H_2O permeability, H_2O is extracted passively as the fluid approaches the end of Henle's loop. Hypertonic fluid with a greater NaCl concentration but lower urea concentration than the surrounding medullary interstitium thus enters the thin ascending limb of Henle. This segment differs from the descending limb in that it is largely impermeable to H_2O and urea but highly permeable to NaCl. These characteristics allow for passive diffusion of NaCl out of the ascending limb. Active electrogenic transport of Cl^- across the water-impermeable thick ascending limb of Henle, with Na^+ following passively, allows for separation of solute and water. Tubular fluid therefore becomes dilute, and the medullary interstitium becomes hypertonic. Irrespective of the final osmolality of the urine, the fluid that enters the distal convoluted tubule is always hypo-osmotic. This segment exhibits active Na^+ reabsorption. All but the terminal portion of the distal convoluted tubule is impermeable to H_2O, even in the presence of ADH. Aldosterone exerts its effect in this segment by enhancing Na^+ reabsorption, which is variably coupled to K^+ and H^+ secretion. The cortical and papillary portions of the collecting duct are sites where ADH exerts its principal effect. The permeability of these segments to H_2O in the absence of ADH is very low but can be greatly enhanced in the presence of ADH. These segments are also characterized by active Na^+ reabsorption, which appears to depend on the presence of mineralocorticoids. In the absence of ADH, the collecting tubule is impermeable to H_2O, so that hypotonic tubule fluid courses through it. However, in the presence of ADH, water is avidly absorbed here, resulting in hypertonic final urine.

The sites of diuretic action, shown as circled numbers, are as follows:

Site 1: Proximal tubule. Sensitive to inhibitors of carbonic anhydrase.

Site 2: Proximal tubule. An osmotic diuretic acting at this site results in *increased* free-water production and *increased* potassium loss.

Site 3: Medullary diluting segment of ascending limb. A diuretic acting at this site results in *decreased* free-water production and *increased* potassium loss.

Site 4: Cortical diluting segment of ascending limb. A diuretic acting at this site results in *decreased* free-water production and *increased* potassium loss.

Site 5: Aldosterone-insensitive portion of distal tubule. A diuretic acting at this site produces *decreased* potassium loss.

Site 6: Aldosterone-sensitive portion of distal tubule. A diuretic acting at this site produces *decreased* potassium loss but acts only in the presence of aldosterone.

(From Brenner, B. M., and Hostetter, T.: Disturbances of renal function. *In* Petersdorf, R. G., Adams, R. D., Braunwald, E., Isselbacher, K. J., Wilson, J. D., and Martin, J. M. (eds.): Principles of Internal Medicine. 10th ed. New York, McGraw-Hill Book Co., 1983, p. 1602.)

TABLE 16–6   EFFECTS OF DIURETICS ON ELECTROLYTE EXCRETION

AGENT	CHANGES IN URINARY ELECTROLYTES				MAXIMAL FRACTIONAL EXCRETION OF SODIUM (%)	INHIBITORY FACTORS		SITE(S) OF ACTION (SEE FIGURE 16–19 FOR SITE NUMBERS)
	Na^+	K^+	Cl^-	HCO_3^-		*Acidosis*	*Alkalosis*	
Weak Diuretics								
Acetazolamide	↑	↑	↓	↑	~4	+		1
Spironolactone	↑	↓	↑	↑	~2			6
Triamterene	↑	↓	↑	- ↑	~2			5
Amiloride	↑	↓	↑	↑	~2			5
Moderately Effective Diuretics								
Thiazide compounds	↑	↑	↑	↑	~8			4
Potent Diuretics								
Organomercurials	↑	↑	↑		~20		+	3,4
Furosemide	↑	↑	↑		~23			3,4
Ethacrynic acid	↑	↑	↑		~23			3,4?,5,6

From Brater, D. C., and Thier, S. O.: Renal disorders. *In* Melmon, K. L., and Morrelli, H. F. (eds.): Clinical Pharmacology. New York, The Macmillan Co., 1978, p. 349.

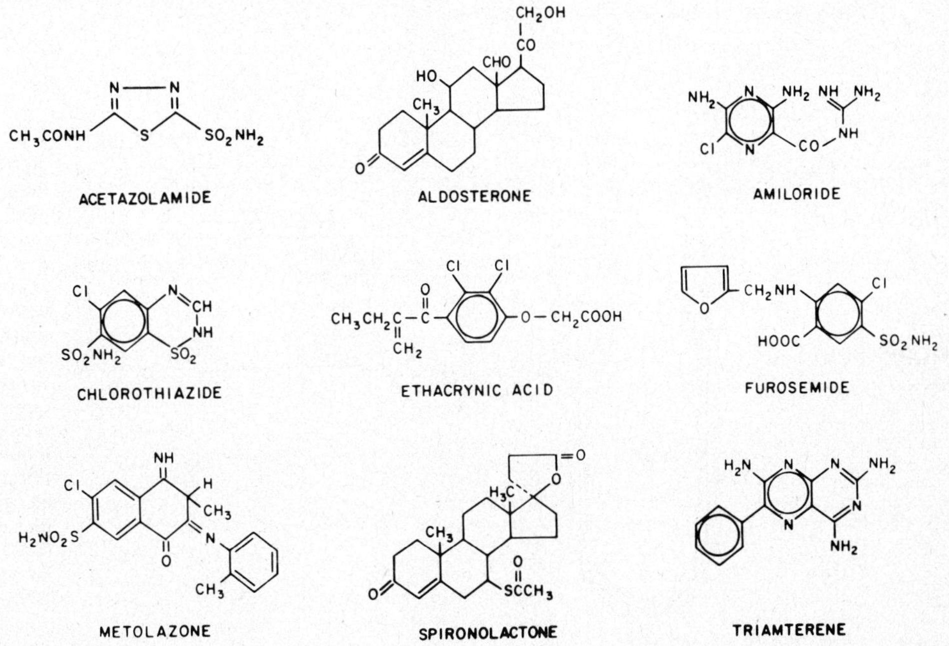

FIGURE 16–10 Structures of diuretics.

sodium bicarbonate and water increases this luminal concentration of chloride, thereby creating a favorable chemical gradient for the passive movement of chloride into the peritubular blood. The positive luminal charge engendered by loss of chloride enables sodium to move passively down its electrochemical gradient into the blood. Water passively follows NaCl along its osmotic gradient.[303] Reduction of proximal tubular bicarbonate reabsorption by inhibition of carbonic anhydrase will therefore appreciably decrease sodium and chloride transport. However, the increased delivery of sodium chloride to the distal tubule merely results in enhanced reabsorption there, and as a consequence, carbonic anhydrase inhibition may produce little diuresis. However, when distal reabsorption is interfered with by another diuretic, such as ethacrynic acid or chlorothiazide, acetazolamide's inhibition of proximal reabsorption is unmasked.[302] In some patients who develop normokalemic hypochloremic alkalosis as a consequence of treatment with furosemide and spironolactone, inhibitors of proximal tubular reabsorption may be effective.[304]

LOOP OF HENLE

The thin and thick portions of the ascending limb of Henle's loop are impermeable to water but permeable to solute (Fig. 16–9). Sodium chloride *passively* exits from the thin segment, whereas *active* chloride transport, accompanied passively by sodium, accounts for loss of solute from the thick ascending segment.[305,306] Loss of luminal solute but retention of water renders luminal fluid dilute and interstitial tissue concentrated. In the distal tubule and early cortical collecting duct, water moves out of the lumen, down its osmotic gradient, but the relative impermeability of these segments to urea causes the luminal urea concentration to increase. In the late medullary collecting duct, urea moves passively into the interstitium where it accumulates and exerts a major osmotic effect on the water-permeable but sodium chloride–impermeable descending limb. Water leaves this segment—in response to a high concentration of urea in the interstitium—causing the remaining sodium chloride concentration to increase progressively. The luminal solute concentration is increased above that of the interstitium, allowing sodium chloride to exit *passively* from the thin ascending limb.

Diuretics such as *furosemide, ethacrynic acid*, and the *organic mercurials*, which act, in part, by inhibiting chloride transport in the ascending limb, enhance the excretion not only of that solute but also of water, by removing the gradient for passive water movement from the descending limb of Henle's loop and the medullary collecting duct

into the renal interstitium. The mechanism by which these diuretics inhibit chloride reabsorption in the ascending limb has not been elucidated, although considerable evidence supports the view that they block the entry of chloride into the cell at the luminal membrane (Fig. 16–11). It has also been proposed that chloride transport in the ascending limb is in some way dependent on Na^+,K^+ATPase activity and that this inhibition of ATPase activity[307] plays a role in the diuretic effects of furosemide, ethacrynic acid, and the mercurials. Indeed, furosemide has been shown to inhibit selectively Na^+,K^+-ATPase in the loop of Henle,[308] but the relationship between this inhibition and its diuretic effects is still debated.[296,297] Some studies have suggested that the diuretic effect of ethacrynic acid may, at least in part, be related to its inhibition of prostaglandin degradation.[309] Both furosemide and ethacrynic acid inhibit adenylate cyclase[310] and prostaglandin dehydrogenase[311] and increase the urinary excretion of prostaglandin E_2.[309] Since indomethacin, aspirin, and presumably other prostaglandin synthetase inhibitors can blunt the natriuretic effect of furosemide,[312,313] the possibility that local prostaglandins may be involved in mediating the action of furosemide in the tubule must be considered. This change in sodium excretion may be caused by inhibition of the increased renal blood flow usually associated with furosemide administration. Another possibility is that indomethacin reduces the renal clearance of furosemide.

There is agreement that the loop diuretics, furosemide and ethacrynic acid, exert their effects on the luminal membrane and therefore must be secreted from peritubular capillaries into the proximal tubular fluid.[314–319] At least in the case of furosemide, the efficiency of this transport system is one determinant of the magnitude of the diuresis; the time-course of furosemide excretion is another. Progressive reabsorption of diuretic-free glomerular filtrate causes relatively high concentrations of the drug to be presented to the ascending limb of Henle's loop, where furosemide, ethacrynic acid, and mercurials exert their direct tubular effects. The observation that probenecid (an inhibi-

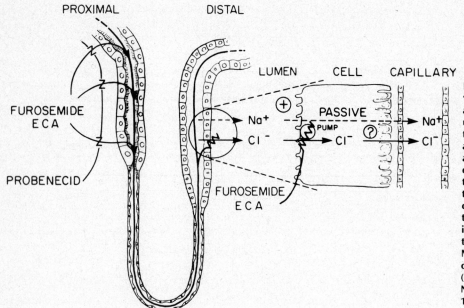

FIGURE 16–11 The mechanism of action of "loop" diuretics. Furosemide and ethacrynic acid (ECA) are actively secreted into the urine in the proximal tubule by a process that is inhibited by probenecid. Ethacrynic acid is modified to the cysteine adduct, the active form of the drug in the urine. These diuretics interfere with chloride transport at the luminal membrane of the ascending limb to decrease net solute absorption. Consequently, the drugs interfere with the formation of dilute urine and the concentration of interstitial solutes by a single inhibitory action. (From Grantham, J. J., and Chonko, A. M.: The physiological basis and clinical use of diuretics. *In* Brenner, B. M., and Stein, J. H. (eds.): Sodium and Water Homeostasis. Vol 1. New York, Churchill Livingstone, 1978, p. 178.)

tor of aryl acid transport) in the proximal tubule blocks the diuresis caused by furosemide supports this sequence of events.[320]

THE DISTAL NEPHRON

Thiazides act in the distal convoluted tubule,[300] perhaps by reducing the permeability of the luminal membrane to both sodium and chloride. However, they also enhance the excretion of potassium both by increasing its delivery to the distal tubule and by enhancing its secretion along this segment.[321] The molecular basis of the diuretic effect of the thiazides is still unknown.

Sodium chloride absorption and sodium-potassium exchange in the distal convoluted tubule, cortical collecting tubules, and perhaps the papillary collecting ducts are modulated by aldosterone. *Spironolactone* inhibits sodium reabsorption and potassium secretion indirectly by binding both to cytosolic and to nuclear protein receptors of aldosterone, displacing the hormone, and thereby preventing its effect.[322] Thus, it is a true competitive inhibitor of aldosterone, and its diuretic and antikaliuretic effects are dependent upon the presence of this hormone. Two other diuretics, *triamterene* and *amiloride*, also inhibit both the distal reabsorption of sodium and the secretion of potassium. However, these agents differ from spironolactone in that they are effective even in the absence of aldosterone. It has been proposed that they reduce the sodium permeability of the luminal surface of the tubular cell membrane, thus lowering the sodium available for transport across the antiluminal membrane[323]; this effect, in turn, is thought to interfere with potassium secretion.[324] In addition to their effects on distal sodium and potassium transport (perhaps secondary to potassium retention[325]), triamterene,[323] amiloride,[323] and spironolactone[326] are all capable of inhibiting urinary hydrogen ion secretion. There is evidence that furosemide and ethacrynic acid, in addition to their primary effect on the thick segment of the ascending limb of the loop of Henle, also act on the *collecting tubules* by inhibiting the action of vasopressin.[327,328]

PRINCIPLES OF DIURETIC ACTION

Diuretics stimulate regulatory processes that tend to counter their renal effects. Diuresis-induced plasma volume contraction, acting through a series of complex physical and hormonal signals, enhances tubular avidity for sodium, thereby tending to neutralize the diuretic effect. As a consequence, the efficacy of any diuretic in an intact system is much less than would be predicted from its action in an isolated preparation. Also, when a diuretic is given repeatedly, its activity diminishes as a result of progressively increased fractional reabsorption of sodium in the portion of the nephron unaffected by the diuretic. In this manner, salt balance is reestablished, albeit at a lower total body sodium than before diuretic administration. Hypovolemia may enhance sodium reabsorption by suppression of the postulated natriuretic hormone[329] and by activation of the renin-angiotensin system, which stimulates release of aldosterone. Other mediators, such as catecholamines and prostaglandins, may also affect the "tubuloglomerular feedback" system, which accounts for increased proximal tubular reabsorption of sodium in response to hypovolemia.

Since renal blood flow usually falls to a greater extent than does glomerular filtration during hypovolemia, a greater fraction of blood delivered to the kidney is filtered. Removal of a greater amount of protein-free fluid at the glomerulus causes the albumin concentration of postglomerular and peritubular blood to increase, and this increased oncotic pressure enhances the proximal reabsorption of sodium. Diuretics acting on the more distal nephron become progressively less effective as the glomerular filtration rate falls and increased reabsorption of sodium occurs in the proximal tubule. Therefore, drugs that act at different sites, such as furosemide and acetazolamide, tend to have additive diuretic effects. The combination of furosemide and metolazone has been reported to be effective in some patients with refractory edema,[330] and Wollam et al. have reported a successful diuretic response to combined hydrochlorothiazide and furosemide therapy in patients with renal insufficiency (serum creatinine range 1.3 to 4.9 mg/dl) who had a poor response to either drug alone.[331] We have found this combination to be effective in patients with refractory congestive heart failure without intrinsic renal disease. Also, intermittent courses of acetazolamide may induce diuresis in patients with refractory heart failure who have developed normokalemic hypochloremic alkalosis as a result of treatment with furosemide and spironolactone.[304] In addition, diuretics that act at the same site via different mechanisms, such as spironolactone and triamterene, may be additive. The action of one diuretic may counteract an undesirable effect of a second agent. Thus, spironolactone may reduce the potassium loss caused by thiazides without interfering with their diuretic action. It should be recognized that some degree of salt restriction is essential if negative sodium balance is to be achieved with potent but short-acting diuretics such as furosemide, because sodium lost after diuretic administration will otherwise be regained by renal conservation throughout the remainder of the day.[332]

RENAL BLOOD FLOW AND GLOMERULAR FILTRATION RATE.

The acute administration of either furosemide or ethacrynic acid causes a significant increase in renal blood flow and reduction of renal vascular resistance.[333] Since both these agents also cause an increase in renal renin release, and since the renin-angiotensin system mediates vasoconstriction, some other prominent vasodilatory influence (perhaps enhanced synthesis of prostaglandin E[309,311]) must override this effect. In contrast, thiazides and acetazolamide diminish renal blood flow.[309,334] If as a consequence of diuretic administration plasma volume decreases and the left ventricular function curve moves to the left, (Figure 16–12), cardiac output, renal blood flow, and glomerular filtration rate will all decline, reducing the effectiveness of additional diuretic administration.

Some diuretics reduce the glomerular filtration rate, related in part to lowered extracellular fluid volume and consequent lowering of cardiac output. In the case of furosemide, there is an initial rise in glomerular filtration rate, and, as extracellular fluid volume is reduced, renal blood flow and glomerular filtration rate fall. In contrast, ethacrynic acid may cause a fall in filtration rate despite concurrent replacement of fluid losses.[335] Since these diuretics increase peripheral venous compliance and reduce venous return[336-338]—actions independent of their renal effects—it is possible that renal blood flow and filtration rate may fall despite maintenance of extracellular fluid volume. The thiazides, mercurials, and carbonic anhydrase inhibitors also cause a decrease in glomerular filtration rate when diuretic losses are replaced. There is evidence that these effects may be secondary to an intrarenal feedback mechanism that couples distal salt delivery with filtration rate in individual nephrons.[339-341]

POTASSIUM EXCRETION. Urinary potassium excretion is dependent, in part, on the rate of volume flow past the distal convoluted and cortical collecting tubules. Therefore, acetazolamide, furosemide, ethacrynic acid, the thiazides, and osmotic diuretics such as mannitol tend to enhance urinary potassium loss.[342] In addition, activation of the renin-angiotensin-aldosterone system, which occurs in heart failure and also as a result of the contraction of the extracellular fluid volume induced by diuresis, further increases potassium secretion in the distal nephron. The aldosterone component of potassium-wasting becomes blunted, since hypokalemia decreases the adrenal secretion of aldosterone.[343] Also, contraction of the extracellular fluid compartment enhances the proximal reabsorption of glomerular filtrate, thereby reducing flow into the distal nephron and thus inhibiting further excretion of potassium. Thus, enhanced potassium excretion is usually not sustained if the extracellular fluid volume has been markedly contracted.[344] Indeed, urinary potassium loss and resultant potassium depletion are most pronounced in patients receiving diuretics with large sodium chloride and water intake.[345] Metabolic alkalosis is also a potent stimulus to distal potassium secretion and further loss of potassium into the urine.[346] Under these circumstances, supplemental intake of potassium chloride and administration of spironolactone or triamterene may be necessary.

COMPLICATIONS OF DIURETIC THERAPY
(See Table 16–7)

The increased distal delivery of sodium and water during diuretic therapy enhances secretion of potassium and hydrogen ions. *Potassium depletion*, in turn, further enhances hydrogen ion secretion and increases ammonia production through stimulation of renal glutaminase activity. The consequent reduction of hydrogen ion concentration produces a *metabolic alkalosis*. With contraction of the extracellular fluid volume and loss of sodium chloride ("contraction alkalosis"), there is increased reabsorption of sodium bicarbonate, maintaining the *metabolic alkalosis*.[347,348] Contraction alkalosis will usually respond to reduction of the dose of diuretic and reexpansion of the extracellular fluid volume[347] as well as to potassium

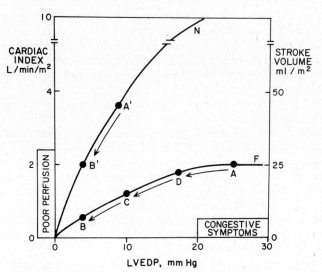

FIGURE 16–12 Effect of venodilator or diuretic therapy in a normal (N) subject (A′ → B′) and in patients with heart failure (F) and markedly elevated left ventricular filling pressure (A → D), moderately elevated filling pressure (D → C), and normal filling pressure (C → B). In all instances venodilators or diuretic therapy results in a decline in filling pressure; except in the patient with marked elevation of filling pressure, cardiac output declines.

TABLE 16–7   COMPLICATIONS OF DIURETIC TREATMENT

DIURETIC	HYPER-URICEMIA	HYPO-KALEMIA	HYPER-KALEMIA	ACIDOSIS	ALKALOSIS	OTHER
Osmotic	−	+	−	−	+ (Contraction)	Hyper- or hypoosmolality
Acid-forming salts	−	+	−	+	−	
Organomercurials	−	+	+ (Rare, acute)	−	+	Tubular necrosis, hyper-sensitivity reactions
Acetazolamide	?	+	−	+	−	Urinary tract calculi, hepatic coma
Thiazides	+	+	−	−	+	Cutaneous vasculitis, agranulocytosis, thrombocytopenia, anemia, pancreatitis, glucose intolerance, hepatic coma
Ethacrynic acid	+	+	−	−	+	Hyper- and hypoglycemia, gastrointestinal bleeding, deafness, hepatic coma
Furosemide	+	+	−	−	+	Glucose intolerance, deafness, hepatic coma
Spironolactone	−	−	+	−	−	Gynecomastia
Triamterene	−	−	+	+	−	Azotemia, muscle cramps
Amiloride	−	−	+	+	−	Azotemia

From Brater, D. C., and Thier, S. O.: Renal disorders. *In* Melmon, K. L., and Morrelli, H. F. (eds.): Clinical Pharmacology. New York, The Macmillan Co., 1978, p. 349.

supplementation.[348] Diuretic-induced potassium depletion clearly predisposes some patients without overt cardiac disease to high-grade ventricular arrhythmias,[349] and this tendency is an even greater potential problem in patients with known cardiac disease. It must also be remembered, however, that *hyperkalemia* is also a serious risk in patients receiving potassium-sparing diuretics, especially in the elderly, in those with impaired renal function, and in those with diabetes mellitus.[350] Beta-adrenergic blocking agents will tend to accentuate any tendency to hyperkalemia in all of these states. These agents act, in part, by reducing renin release as well as by diminishing the extrarenal capacity for potassium uptake.[351]

Metabolic acidosis may occur as a complication of treatment with acetazolamide, which causes a sodium bicarbonate diuresis by reducing its proximal reabsorption. Spironolactone, by antagonizing aldosterone, may also limit the ability to excrete hydrogen ions, resulting in a hyperchloremic metabolic acidosis.[326]

Hyponatremia, an important complication of diuretic therapy, results from an imbalance between water ingestion and renal diluting capacity. Furosemide, ethacrynic acid, and thiazides inhibit free water generation and cause excretion of relatively concentrated urine. When water intake is increased, hyponatremia may occur.[352] In addition, stimuli for the secretion of antidiuretic hormone (ADH), including volume contraction,[353] morphine, pain, and mechanical ventilation, may be present in these patients. Since total body sodium is usually normal or increased in patients with heart failure receiving diuretics, restriction of water intake below external and insensible loss (usually ≤ 1000 ml/day) will increase the serum sodium concentration. Temporary interruption of diuretic therapy and, if possible, improvement of cardiac function with inotropic agents or treatment of a precipitating cause of heart failure are useful measures.

Hyperuricemia is a common complication of chronic diuretic therapy with thiazides, furosemide, and ethacrynic acid. Furosemide and ethacrynic acid compete with uric acid for secretion by the proximal organic acid transport system. This competition plus enhanced proximal and distal reabsorption of uric acid (caused by diuretic-induced contraction of the extracellular fluid volume) combine to elevate sodium uric acid. Most patients tolerate hyperuricemia well and require no specific treatment.[354] Sustained plasma urate concentrations up to 10 mg/100 ml appear to have no deleterious effect on renal function. Occasionally clinical gout develops, particularly in patients with a previous history of gout or hyperuricemia. Levels higher than 10 mg/100 ml may warrant the use of allopurinol.[355] It appears unlikely that moderate hyperuricemia (men < 13 mg/dl; women < 10 mg/dl) exerts a deleterious effect on renal function.[356] At higher levels or in patients with a history of gout, allopurinol can be used with diuretics.[355] There seem to be few indications for uricosuric agents in asymptomatic hyperuricemic patients.[357] Indeed, before they are used uric acid excretion should be measured, because if hyperuricemia is caused by overproduction of uric acid, a uricosuric agent can lead to urate nephropathy or stones.

Carbohydrate intolerance, especially in the presence of latent diabetes mellitus, occurs in patients treated with thiazides[358] and less commonly in those receiving furosemide and ethacrynic acid. This complication may simply lead to loss of control of blood sugar concentration. Ketoacidosis rarely if ever develops. However, hyperosmolar nonketotic coma may develop in patients with Type II diabetes who become severely volume depleted.[354] Thiazide diuretics also exert an adverse effect, albeit a small one, on serum lipoproteins, lowering HDL cholesterol and raising LDL cholesterol as well as triglycerides.[359,360]

Ototoxicity caused by furosemide and ethacrynic acid is usually dose-related and occurs most commonly in patients with renal insufficiency. Hearing loss is usually, but not always, reversible.[298] Thiazides diminish the renal excretion of calcium, and *hypercalcemia* is an occasional complication of their use. It occurs, in particular, in patients with hyperparathyroidism.

Endocrine disorders, particularly gynecomastia, impotence, diminished libido, and irregular menses, may result from chronic administration of spironolactone, which appears to antagonize androgen activity.[361]

INDIVIDUAL DIURETICS (See Table 16-8 and Figure 16-10)

THIAZIDES. The thiazides can induce a maximal increase in sodium excretion to 3 to 6 per cent of the filtered load, placing them in the "moderately potent" category. Their major natriuretic activity occurs as a result of their ability to block sodium reabsorption at the cortical diluting site in the late ascending limb of the loop of Henle and the early distal convoluted tubule (see Fig. 16-9). Thiazides cause the excretion of equivalent quantities of sodium and chloride. Although the diuretic response to thiazides is not affected by alkalosis or acidosis, their administration may lead to metabolic alkalosis. These agents have achieved preeminence in the treatment of mild to moderate congestive heart failure because of their relative safety and their record of side effects that are usually managed easily.

The thiazides are relatively ineffective in patients with glomerular filtration rates below 30 ml/min,[362] which may account for their lack of effectiveness in the therapy of severe congestive heart failure, in which renal blood flow is markedly reduced. The dosages and durations of action of various thiazides are shown in Table 16-8.

METOLAZONE. This is a quinethazone derivative, the site of action and the potency of which are similar to those of chlorothiazide.[363,364] However, unlike the thiazides,[365] metolazone in usual doses does not generally reduce renal blood flow or glomerular filtration rate[363,366]—a fact of importance in patients whose renal hemodynamics are already compromised. Thus, unlike the thiazides, metolazone may be effective in patients with markedly reduced renal function.[366] Metolazone has a duration of action of 24 to 48 hours,[363] much longer than that of most of the thiazides. Both the thiazides and metolazone are weak carbonic anhydrase inhibitors and therefore exert a mild inhibitory effect on proximal tubular sodium reabsorption.[363,364,367]

ETHACRYNIC ACID AND FUROSEMIDE. Although ethacrynic acid and furosemide are quite dissimilar structurally, they are similar in their functional characteristics (Figs. 16-10 and 16-11). Both drugs are powerful diuretics capable of increasing the fractional sodium excretion to more than 20 per cent of the filtered load for short periods.

The maximal single oral or intravenous dose of furosemide or ethacrynic acid ranges from 200 to 250 mg. Higher doses are given to patients with acute or chronic renal failure and occasionally effect an increased urine volume. In some patients with heart failure large doses of either of these loop diuretics given orally may yield a poor response, while a much smaller intravenous dose may be effective. Both drugs have a rapid onset and short duration of action and inhibit active chloride reabsorption in the ascending limb of the loop of Henle. Their diuretic effect may also be due to some extent to reversal of the shunting of blood from cortical to juxtamedullary nephrons, which is common in heart failure. These agents can cause hypovolemia, potassium depletion, and alkalosis secondary to loss of potassium and hydrogen ions. Like the thiazides, their activity is not affected by alkalosis or acidosis. Furosemide also exerts a weak effect on the proximal tubule as a carbonic anhydrase inhibitor. These drugs are equipotent, and there is little reason to choose between them except for patients who are allergic to sulfa drugs, in which case ethacrynic acid should be employed. Gastrointestinal distress and ototoxicity occur more commonly with ethacrynic acid than with furosemide.

SPIRONOLACTONE, TRIAMTERENE, AND AMILORIDE. These three diuretics are relatively weak and rarely are used as the sole diuretic agent. Rather, they are usually added to thiazides or "loop" diuretics, where they exert an additive diuretic effect and, in addition, antagonize the kaliuretic actions of the most potent diuretics. Since triamterene and amiloride act directly on distal tubular cells to diminish potassium secretion, they are capable of antikaliuretic effects independent of the presence or absence of aldosterone.[368] Triamterene and amiloride act more

TABLE 16-8 CHARACTERISTICS OF DIURETICS

GENERIC NAME	BRAND NAME	HOW SUPPLIED	USUAL DOSAGE	ONSET OF EFFECT	PEAK EFFECT	DURATION
Acetazolamide	Diamox	250-mg tablet	250 to 375 mg/day	1 hr	2 to 4 hr	8 hr
Chlorothiazide	Diuril	500-mg tablet	500 to 1000 mg/day	1 hr	4 hr	6 to 12 hr
Hydrochlorothiazide	HydroDiuril	50-mg tablet	50 to 100 mg/day	2 hr	4 hr	12 hr or more
Trichlormethiazide	Metahydrin, Naqua	4-mg tablet	4 to 8 mg/day	2 hr	6 hr	24 hr
Chlorthalidone	Hygroton (generic)	100-mg tablet	100 mg/day	2 hr	6 hr	24 hr or more
Meralluride	Mercuhydrin	10-ml vial	0.50 to 2.00 ml IM 3 times/week	2 hr	6 to 9 hr	12 to 24 hr
Mercaptomerin	Thiomerin	10-ml vial	0.25 to 2.00 ml IM 3 times/week	2 hr	6 to 9 hr	12 to 24 hr
Metolazone	Zaroxolyn	2.5-, 5-, and 10-mg tablets	5 to 10 mg/day	1 hr	2 to 4 hr	24 to 48 hr
Triamterene	Dyrenium	100-mg capsule	100 to 300 mg/day	2 hr	6 to 8 hr	12 to 16 hr
Spironolactone	Aldactone	25-mg tablet	25 mg 4 times/day	Gradual onset	1 to 2 days after initiation of therapy	2 to 3 days after cessation of therapy
Furosemide	Lasix	40-mg tablet	40 to 120 mg/day	Oral, 1 hr; IV, 5 min	Oral, 1 to 2 hr; IV, 30 min	Oral, 6 hr; IV, 2 hr
Ethacrynic acid	Edecrin	50-mg tablet	50 to 100 mg/day	Oral, 30 min; IV, 15 min	Oral 2 hr; IV, 45 min	Oral, 6 to 8 hr; IV, 3 hr

Adapted from Frazier, H. S., and Yager, H.: The clinical use of diuretics; renal regulation of salt and water balance. N. Engl. J. Med. *288*:248, 1973.

rapidly than does spironolactone—within hours versus two to three days—but unlike the aldosterone antagonists, they may produce azotemia. It must be recognized that all three drugs inhibit the exchange of potassium not only for sodium but also for hydrogen and may induce metabolic acidosis as well as hyperkalemia. Amiloride may cause anorexia, nausea, and vomiting.[367] Unlike triamterene it does not cause renal calculi; unlike spironolactone, it does not cause gynecomastia. Potassium-sparing diuretics should be used with caution in patients with renal failure, diabetes, or advanced age.

Mercurial Diuretics.   While quite effective when administered par-

enterally, these agents are ineffective when given orally. They are rarely used because more effective, less toxic drugs, such as furosemide and ethacrynic acid, are available and can be given orally. Mercurials inhibit the reabsorption of sodium in the thick portion of the ascending limb of the loop of Henle and in the distal convoluted tubule. Potassium secretion tends to be reduced, so that urinary losses of this electrolyte are less prominent than after doses of thiazides, ethacrynic acid, or furosemide, which produce comparable losses of sodium. Metabolic alkalosis, however, is a frequent sequela of diuresis with mercurials. Sudden death, presumably from cardiac arrhythmia, is a rare complication of intravenous administration. Renal failure, nephrotic syndrome, and hemorrhagic colitis may occur with chronic therapy, particularly in patients with renal insufficiency, and probably represent a form of heavy-metal poisoning.[369]

VASODILATORS

GENERAL CONSIDERATIONS

Cardiac function can be profoundly affected by alterations in the resistance and capacitance of the peripheral vascular bed. Thus, it has been appreciated for many years that both in animals with experimentally induced mitral regurgitation[370,371] and in patients with this valvular lesion[372] the volume of regurgitant flow varies directly, and the forward stroke volume varies inversely, with afterload. The response of the left ventricle to an augmentation of afterload induced by the infusion of a pressor agent is a direct function of myocardial contractility (see Figure 14–21, p. 485); when contractility is normal, elevating afterload leads to a marked increase in stroke work, with little elevation of ventricular end-diastolic volume of pressure and little decline in stroke volume. In patients with impaired contractility, however, as afterload is increased, stroke volume falls, and left ventricular end-diastolic pressure and volume rise, often sharply.[373] Arterial counterpulsation, a mechanical technique that reduces left ventricular afterload (p. 593), appears to have been the first deliberate clinical use of afterload reduction in the treatment of left ventricular failure,[374] although effective treatment of hypertension has undoubtedly achieved this goal in many instances since the introduction of antihypertensive drugs.

Majid et al. took an important step forward when they infused the alpha-adrenergic blocking agent phentolamine into normotensive patients with persistent left ventricular dysfunction after myocardial infarction and demonstrated that the induced fall in systemic vascular resistance was accompanied by considerable elevation of cardiac output and reduction of pulmonary artery pressure.[375] Since that report, vasodilators have appropriately achieved wide use in the treatment of heart failure.[376–379]

With few exceptions, vasodilators do not exert a direct effect on the heart, but their ability to relax vascular smooth muscle, directly or indirectly, can result in profound improvement in both the clinical and hemodynamic state of the patient. By dilating arterioles and/or veins, these agents have the capacity to alter profoundly the loading conditions on the heart and thereby to modify cardiac performance. *Arteriolar dilatation* results in a reduction in afterload and may augment cardiac output, while venodilatation produces a reduction in preload, lowers

ventricular filling pressure, and thereby may diminish symptoms of pulmonary congestion. However, like all other drugs useful in the management of congestive heart failure, vasodilator agents must be used with caution and a thorough understanding of their mechanism of action, since their inappropriate administration can result in deterioration rather than improvement of the patient's circulatory status.

Venodilators result in a redistribution of the blood volume. Since the capacity of the venous bed (also referred to as the "capacitance bed") is large, a relatively small reduction in venous tone can result in the pooling of substantial quantities of blood in this bed and its redistribution from the pulmonary to the systemic circuit.[380] Patients with heart failure often exhibit intense and inappropriate venoconstriction,[381] thus augmenting pulmonary blood volume and contributing to pulmonary congestion. The hemodynamic effects of a pure venodilator resemble those of a diuretic (Fig. 16–12) and result in a shift to the left on the left ventricular function curve. In a normal subject this reduction in preload can result in an undesirable decline of cardiac output (A' → B'). However, it is not sufficiently appreciated that in a patient with heart failure but normal filling pressure, venodilatation (or further diuresis) may also result in a decline in cardiac performance (C → B). Only in the patient with heart failure and an elevated filling pressure can venodilatation (or diuresis) reduce filling pressure and thereby produce relief of symptoms of pulmonary congestion without depressing cardiac output (A → D). Many patients with heart failure present with a moderate elevation of filling pressure (D); in them the cardiac output response will be intermediate between that observed in patients with marked elevation (A) and those without elevation (C) of filling pressure; i.e., they will experience some clinical improvement resulting from reduction of the moderately elevated pulmonary capillary pressure but at the expense of some reduction in cardiac output (D → C). Fundamental aspects of the effects of afterload reduction on myocardial energetics have been reviewed by Ford,[382] and Packer and LeJemtel have reviewed the conceptual framework for vasodilator therapy in heart failure.[383]

CHOICE OF VASODILATOR.   From a theoretical point of view, therefore, one would expect the administration of a pure venodilator to be (1) *desirable* in patients whose principal clinical manifestation of heart failure is

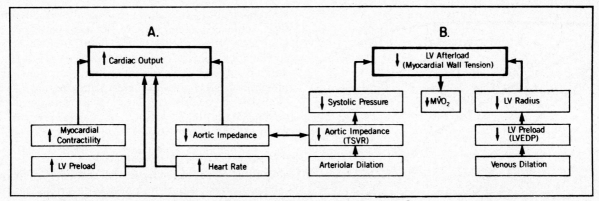

FIGURE 16–13   *A,* Representation of four principal determinants of cardiac output (CO). *B,* Representation of two major determinants of left ventricular (LV) afterload. TSVR indicates total systemic vascular resistance. LVEDP = left ventricular end-diastolic pressure; MVO_2 = myocardial oxygen requirements. Arteriolar dilation raises CO (reduces fatigue), decreases LV afterload, and diminishes MVO_2 (antianginal effect). Venous dilation decreases LVEDP (reduces dyspnea), decreases LV afterload, and diminishes MVO_2 (anti-ischemic effect). Combined arteriolar and venous dilation raises CO, decreases LVEDP, diminishes LV afterload, and reduces MVO_2. (Reproduced with permission from Mason, D. T., Awan, N. A., Joye, J. A., Lee, G., DeMaria, A. N., and Amsterdam, E. A.: Treatment of acute and chronic congestive heart failure by vasodilator-afterload reduction. Arch. Intern. Med. *140*:1577, 1980.)

pulmonary congestion secondary to elevated left ventricular filling pressure rather than to a lowered cardiac output and resultant poor perfusion, (2) *contraindicated* in patients in whom the preload or filling pressure has already been restored to normal by means of diuretic therapy and/or dietary sodium restriction, and (3) *useful in combination with arteriolar dilators* in patients whose clinical manifestations of failure are related to both reduction of perfusion and pulmonary congestion.[384]

Arteriolar dilators act as *afterload reducing agents.* As shown in Figures 16–13 and 16–14, as well as in Figures 12–28 (p. 434) and 12–30 (p. 436), at any level of preload and myocardial contractility, the extent of myocardial fiber shortening (and therefore stroke volume) is inversely related to the afterload. As discussed elsewhere (p. 435), afterload is related to the instantaneous wall stress in the muscle fibers of the ventricle. Therefore, it is also closely related to the aortic impedance, i.e., the instantaneous relationship between pressure and flow in the aorta during ejection. Impedance, in turn, is closely related to systemic vascular resistance, i.e., the average relationship between pressure and flow. Just as the effects of venodilatation and the resultant reduction of ventricular preload are dependent on the filling pressure (Fig. 16–12), so are the effects of afterload dependent on myocardial contractility. Figures 16–14 and 16–15 display the effects of afterload reduction on ventricular fiber shortening in normal and failing hearts. In the normal heart (Fig. 16–14) a reduction of afterload (from B to C) results in only a minor augmentation of myocardial fiber shortening (B → F to C → G). In contrast, an identical reduction in afterload results in a substantial augmentation of myocardial fiber shortening in the failing heart (B → D to C → E). In the intact heart, as outlined in Figure 16–15, the consequences of increased afterload thus are substantially greater in the presence of heart failure than when normal contractile function is present.

In patients with congestive heart failure the arterial vascular bed (just like the venous bed) is often inappropriately constricted. (Fig. 16–16).[381] The vasoconstriction is related to that observed in other conditions such as hypovolemic shock, in which there is a reduction of cardiac output, and it represents a fundamental response of the organism, the survival value of which is to maintain the perfusion pressure of vital organs, such as the brain and the heart, at the expense of less immediately essential vascular beds, such as the skin, gut, and kidney. While this maintenance of perfusion pressure may be a desirable evolutionary development insofar as hypovolemic shock is concerned, it plays a deleterious role in patients with congestive heart failure. (Presumably there is little evolutionary selective advantage to the survival of individuals with heart failure.) At least four mechanisms appear to be involved in the inappropriate elevation of systemic vascular

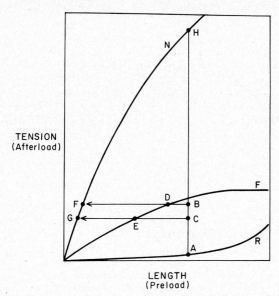

FIGURE 16–14   Length-tension relations in normal (N) and failing (F) heart muscle. R = length–resting tension curve for both normal and failing heart muscle. The effects of reducing afterloads from B to C on shortening are contrasted. In the normal muscle, shortening increases only slightly (from B → F to C → G). In failing muscle, there is substantial enhancement of shortening (B → D to C → E). H represents isometric tension development by normal muscle.

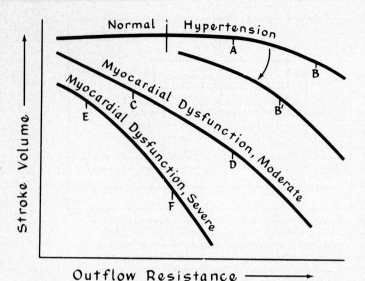

FIGURE 16–15 Relation of left ventricular stroke volume to systemic outflow resistance in normal and diseased hearts. A family of curves may be described, depending on the severity of the myocardial disease. If cardiac function is normal, a rise in resistance results in hypertension, since cardiac output remains fairly constant. Heart failure in a hypertensive patient could be shown by a move to either point B, a high resistance with normal function, or point B', which represents a shift to a slightly depressed ventricular function curve. When myocardial dysfunction is more severe, as shown by the lower two curves, blood pressure is no longer directly determined by resistance, since stroke volume and resistance are inversely related. Consequently, arterial pressure may be similar at points E and F despite marked differences in cardiac output and resistance. It is also apparent that a reduction in outflow resistance will not affect significantly the stroke volume of the normal ventricle. However, it can produce a marked increase in the stroke volume of the failing ventricle (F → E). (Reproduced with permission from Cohn, J. N., and Franciosa, J. A.: Vasodilator therapy of cardiac failure. N. Engl. J. Med. *297*:27, 1977.)

resistance, arterial pressure, and therefore ventricular afterload in patients with congestive heart failure: (1) increased sympathetic vasoconstrictor tone; (2) elevated concentrations of circulating catecholamines; (3) elaboration of renin, with resultant increase in the potent vasoconstrictor angiotensin II; and (4) increased thickness of arteriolar walls, presumably related to extracellular fluid accumulation in the blood vessels themselves.[385,386]

Arteriolar dilators (afterload-reducing agents) are capable of augmenting stroke volume (and cardiac output) in patients with heart failure (Fig. 16–17, A → H) and in this manner reduce symptoms caused by poor perfusion. The reduction in vascular resistance induced by the vasodilator will be offset by the large increase in cardiac output, and arterial pressure may decline only slightly or not at all. In normal subjects the reduction of systemic vascular resistance induced by afterload-reducing agents is associated with no or only small increases in cardiac output (A' → H'), and their administration may result in a marked reduction of arterial pressure accompanied by a reflex tachycardia. In patients with depressed contractility and normal preload, arterial dilatation may produce a small augmentation of cardiac output (C → H''), but in contrast to the situation existing in patients with an elevated preload, arterial pressure may decline to dangerously low levels.

A number of vasodilators act on both the arterial and

the venous beds (so-called "balanced" vasodilators), and their actions are intermediate between those of pure venous and pure arterial dilators and resemble those of a combination of arterial and venodilators (Fig. 16–17). In normal subjects, vasodilators cause reductions in filling pressure, arterial pressure, and cardiac output (A' → P'). Similarly, in patients with heart failure without an elevated preload, both filling pressure and arterial pressure decline, while cardiac output remains constant or falls slightly (C → P''). Patients with heart failure and pulmonary congestion display decisively favorable effects (A → P), with augmentation of cardiac output and reduction of pulmonary capillary pressure but little decline in arterial pressure or elevation of heart rate.

From these considerations, it is apparent that patients with depressed myocardial contractility *and* an elevated preload are likely to benefit significantly from vasodilator therapy, with an increase in cardiac output resulting chiefly from arterial dilators, a reduction in pulmonary congestion resulting from venodilators, and a combination of effects resulting from "balanced" dilators. Patients with heart disease but with normal or almost normal hemodynamics (cardiac output and filling pressure) are unlikely to benefit from the use of vasodilators; indeed, they are likely to experience a reduction of cardiac output and/or arterial pressure. In patients with heart disease, impaired myocardial contractility, and normal preload (often achieved by means of vigorous diuretic therapy), the effects of vasodilator therapy are more difficult to predict; venodilators usually decrease left ventricular performance; arteriolar dilators or balanced dilators may achieve a modest increase in cardiac output, but often at the expense of perfusion pressure. It therefore becomes evident that (in the absence of mitral regurgitation) vasodilator therapy is not desirable in the earliest stages of heart failure but is more appropriate when the use of other measures is inadequate to maintain cardiac output and filling pressure at or near normal.

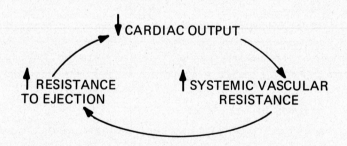

IS THE SYSTEMIC VASCULAR RESISTANCE HIGHER THAN NECESSARY FOR OPTIMAL CARDIOVASCULAR FUNCTION?

FIGURE 16–16 Potential vicious circle of chronic heart failure. With the onset of heart failure, cardiac output decreases. As a compensatory mechanism to maintain arterial blood pressure, systemic vascular resistance increases. This further increases the resistance or impedance to ejection of the left ventricle, which will result in a further reduction in cardiac output. The patient will spiral down this cycle until a new steady-state relation is reached in which cardiac output may be lower and systemic vascular resistance higher than is really optimal for the benefit of the patient. (From Parmley, W. W., and Chatterjee, K.: Vasodilator therapy. Curr. Probl. Cardiol. Vol. 2, No. 12, 1978, p. 15.)

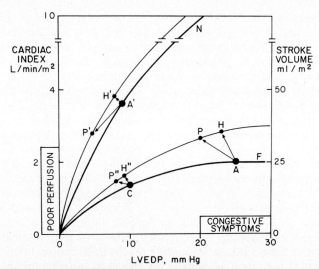

FIGURE 16–17 Effects of various vasodilators on the relationship between left ventricular end-diastolic pressure (LVEDP) and cardiac index or stroke volume in normal (N) and failing (F) hearts. H represents hydralazine or any other pure arterial dilator. It produces only a minimal increase in cardiac index in the normal subject (A′ → H′) or in the patient with heart failure with normal LVEDP (C → H″). In contrast, it elevates output in the patient with heart failure and elevated LVEDP (A → H). P represents a balanced vasodilator, such as sodium nitroprusside or prazosin. It reduces filling pressure in all patients, elevates cardiac output in patients with heart failure and elevated LVEDP (A → P), lowers cardiac output in normal subjects (A′ → P′), and has little effect on cardiac output in heart failure patients with normal filling pressures (C → P″).

Although the classification of vasodilators as predominant arterial or venodilators or as "balanced" vasodilators has proved to be useful in understanding their action and in the rational selection of a particular agent for a specific patient, the intimate interactions between cardiac preload and afterload that exist in the intact circulation must be considered. Since afterload, i.e., myocardial systolic wall tension, is a function not only of intraventricular pressure but also of ventricular volume, it may be readily appreciated that a venodilator that reduces preload will also lower afterload by reducing ventricular volume without altering systemic vascular resistance. Conversely, an arterial dilator that diminishes arterial pressure and thereby enhances stroke volume and ventricular emptying, i.e., reduces ventricular volume in both systole and diastole, will also reduce preload. The lower filling pressure will result in greater reduction of systolic wall tension (afterload) than of arterial pressure.

Since wall tension is a principal determinant of myocardial oxygen consumption ($M\dot{V}O_2$) and since both arteriolar and venodilators reduce wall tension in patients with heart failure, vasodilators reduce $M\dot{V}O_2$ while increasing cardiac output. These actions of vasodilators compare favorably with those of (1) positive inotropic agents, which (like vasodilators) augment cardiac output but either increase $M\dot{V}O_2$ or maintain it at a constant level; or (2) beta-adrenergic blocking agents, which (like vasodilators) reduce $M\dot{V}O_2$ but depress cardiac performance.

MONITORING. The use of vasodilators in the treatment of acute myocardial infarction is discussed in detail elsewhere (p. 1314). When these agents are used in patients with coronary artery disease, it is important to bear in mind that reductions in coronary perfusion pressure in the face of critical coronary obstruction can further impair blood flow through narrowed, though not occluded, coronary arteries, or through collaterals. Therefore, vasodilator therapy must be employed cautiously in patients with coronary artery disease, particularly those with acute myocardial infarction or other acute ischemia syndromes, to avoid the intensification of ischemia. Arterial pressure should be monitored carefully during vasodilator therapy in patients with known or suspected coronary artery disease. In view of the importance of ventricular filling pressure as a determinant of the response to vasodilators (Figs. 16–12 and 16–17), the monitoring of pulmonary artery or pulmonary capillary wedge pressure by means of a Swan-Ganz catheter is extremely helpful in regulating the dose of vasodilators during intravenous therapy. Since, in addition to the reduction in pulmonary wedge pressure, the elevation of cardiac output is an important endpoint, it is desirable to make serial measurements of cardiac output in acutely ill patients receiving intravenous vasodilators. In patients without ischemic heart disease, monitoring of intraarterial pressure during *intravenous* vasodilator therapy may be desirable but is not essential as long as pressure is measured indirectly at frequent intervals. Invasive monitoring is obviously not practical or necessary for patients treated for prolonged periods with agents administered orally, sublingually, or in ointment form. However, it is highly desirable to make frequent measurements of arterial pressure in the supine and upright positions when therapy is initiated or the dosage is being adjusted.

VASODILATOR AGENTS

SODIUM NITROPRUSSIDE. Probably the most widely used vasodilator in the treatment of *acute* congestive heart failure, sodium nitroprusside is ultrashort-acting and must be given intravenously. It acts directly to relax vascular smooth muscle in both arterioles and veins. For many years sodium nitroprusside has been employed successfully to treat hypertensive crisis (p. 923) but was introduced for the treatment of congestive heart failure only as recently as 1972.[387–390] Since sodium nitroprusside is a balanced (arteriolar and venous) dilator, its hemodynamic action in the presence of severe impairment of left ventricular function is both to increase cardiac output and to diminish pulmonary congestion (Fig. 16–17). The initial infusion rate in adults is usually about 10 μg/min and is increased by increments of 5 to 10 μg/min every 5 minutes until the desired effect is achieved or hypotension or other side effects limit further dose increments. The maximum dose in adults is 500 μg/min.

The most important hazardous effect is hypotension, which is actually an extension of its therapeutic action and is reversed within 10 minutes after discontinuation of the drug. If this waiting period would pose a danger, hypotension can be treated more rapidly by infusion of a vasoconstrictor such as phenylephrine or norepinephrine, a combination vasoconstrictor–positive inotropic agent. Nitroprusside releases hydrocyanic acid, which theoretically could lead to cyanide poisoning.[391] However, this is an extremely uncommon complication, since hydrocyanic acid is converted to thiocyanate in the presence of thiosulfate. Thiocyanate is excreted by the kidney, and in the presence of renal insufficiency the infusion of large doses of nitro-prusside for prolonged periods may lead to thiocyanate toxicity, which is characterized by convulsions, psychosis, abdominal pain, hypothyroidism, muscle twitching, and dizziness. Therefore, when patients receive nitroprusside for more than a few days, serum levels of thiocyanate should be measured and not allowed to exceed 6 mg/100 ml. Methemoglobinemia and vitamin B_{12} deficiency are two other rare complications of nitroprusside therapy.[376]

PHENTOLAMINE. This agent was the first vasodila-tor used to increase cardiac output in patients with heart failure.[375] Phentolamine is a complex drug, having at least three actions: (1) it is an alpha-1 (post-synaptic) and al-pha-2 (pre-synaptic) -adrenergic receptor blocker of both arterioles and veins, but predominantly of the former[392]; (2) it is a direct relaxant of vascular smooth muscle[393]; and (3) it releases cardiac norepinephrine stores and thereby exerts transient positive chronotropic and inotropic effects. Like nitroprusside, phentolamine has a short duration of action when used intravenously, and excessive hypotension is its major adverse effect. The initial dose in adult pa-tients is 0.1 mg/min, and it may be increased in steps of 0.1 mg/min every 5 minutes to a maximum of 2.0 mg/min. It has been reported to be effective in the treat-ment of low-output chronic heart failure[394] and pulmonary edema.[395] In addition to gastrointestinal symptoms of nau-sea, vomiting, and abdominal pain, the aforementioned tachycardia and the high cost of the drug make phentol-amine less desirable than nitroprusside in the treatment of acute heart failure.

TRIMETHAPHAN. This is a short-acting ganglionic blocking agent which, like sodium nitroprusside, has been used for a number of years in the treatment of hyperten-sive crisis and aortic dissection. It is effective when admin-istered intravenously and acts on both the arteriolar and the venous beds. The principal disadvantages of trimetha-phan are that it may cause serious orthostatic hypotension and may produce respiratory arrest.[378] Thus it does not ap-pear to be as useful as sodium nitroprusside.

NITRATES. Nitroglycerin and the closely related long-acting nitrates, such as isosorbide dinitrate and penta-erythritol tetranitrate, are vasodilators that act on vascular smooth muscle, principally on the venous and to a lesser extent on the arteriolar bed. These drugs are available in a variety of formulations[396] and can be administered by vari-ous routes (pp. 1346 to 1349), making them useful in a number of situations. In normal individuals and in patients with heart failure but without elevated filling pressure, the prominent venodilator action results in reduction of cardi-ac output and often postural hypotension as well (see Fig-ure 16–12). This hypotensive response, which had been observed many years ago in some patients with acute myo-cardial infarction without heart failure, was responsible for the proscription of the use of nitroglycerin in this condi-tion. However, in patients with heart failure and elevated pulmonary capillary pressure, even when secondary to myocardial infarction, nitroglycerin reduces ventricular fill-ing pressure and relieves congestive symptoms. The slight arteriolar dilating effects of the drug are sufficient to cause a modest increase in cardiac output as well if ventricular filling pressures are maintained in an adequate range.

Sublingual nitroglycerin is usually administered in a dose of 0.4 mg; the effect usually begins within 2 minutes, be-

comes maximal in 8 minutes, and persists for 15 to 30 minutes. When left ventricular filling pressure is elevated to 20 mm Hg, it usually declines to approximately 10 mm Hg within 5 to 10 minutes.[397] Although the slight reduc-tion of arterial pressure may be accompanied by a mild ac-celeration of heart rate, $M\dot{V}O_2$ declines, and this is the major mechanism for the antianginal effect of the drug (p. 1346). Since the absorption of sublingual nitroglycerin may be erratic, continuous *intravenous infusion of nitroglycerin* has been employed to produce a sustained, controllable ef-fect in patients with acute heart failure and pulmonary congestion in whom predominant venodilation is desired.[398] The initial dose is about 10 μg/min and may be increased by increments of 10 μg/min every 5 minutes to a maximal dose of 100 μg/min. For prolonged duration of action, *topical nitroglycerin* may be used; effects of the ointment last at least 3 hours. Depending on the dose desired, a 0.5- to 4.0-inch strip is applied to the skin, usually on the chest. Although topical administration does not make ni-troglycerin ointment convenient for ambulatory patients, an advantage of this formulation is that it can be readily removed in case of adverse effects. It can be conveniently applied before retiring and is useful to combat attacks of paroxysmal nocturnal dyspnea. A transdermal administra-tion system provides a steady rate of absorption and stable venous plasma level for 24 hrs. It is more convenient than the ointment for ambulatory patients and allows shower-ing. The dosage is proportional to the size of the adhesive bandage, which ranges from 5 to 20 cm².

Isosorbide dinitrate is available in sublingual and oral formulations. The sublingual dose is 2.5 to 10 mg every 2 hours, and the oral dose is 20 to 60 mg every 4 hours. In addition, other long-acting nitrates such as oral pentae-rythritol tetranitrate (10 to 40 mg four times a day) or oral controlled-released nitroglycerin preparation (one 6.5-mg capsule every 4 hours) have been employed to achieve a prolonged nitrate effect and have been found useful in the treatment of chronic heart failure.[399,399a] The side effects of all nitrates include headache and postural hypotension, but these symptoms are more prominent in patients with mild than with severe heart failure and can be controlled by decreasing the dose. Methemoglobinemia, an extremely rare complication, may occur with long-term use of large doses.

HYDRALAZINE. This orally effective vasodilator acts directly on arteriolar smooth muscle. The usual dose ranges from 25 to 100 mg three to four times daily, and its effects commence within 30 minutes and persist for about 6 hours. Hydralazine's predominant action on the arterial bed results in an increase in cardiac output with relatively minor reductions in ventricular filling pressure and arterial pressure or increases in heart rate in patients with heart failure.[376,400,401]

The degree of left ventricular enlargement,[402] as well as the level of peripheral vascular resistance, appears to be an important determinant of the response to hydralazine in patients with chronic heart failure, patients with marked cardiomegaly and markedly elevated systemic vascular re-sistance exhibiting the most salutary responses. Side effects include vascular headaches, flushing, nausea, and vomiting, which often disappear with continued therapy. Drug fever and skin rash are seen occasionally; fluid retention and in-creased edema occur commonly when this drug, as well as other vasodilators, is administered over the long term. However, this latter complication usually responds readily to an increase in the dosage of diuretics. In addition to fluid retention, tolerance to the favorable hemodynamic effects of hydralazine develops in a minority of patients, apparently due to an altered responsiveness of vascular smooth muscle to the drug.[403] A more serious adverse effect, a systemic lupus erythematosus–like syndrome, is seen in approximately 15 per cent of patients receiving 400 mg of hydralazine daily; an even higher proportion of patients develops circulating antinuclear antibodies. Although this lupus-like syndrome is not usually observed in patients who receive less than 200 mg of the drug daily, the average dose required for effective afterload reduction is about 75 mg four times a day, making this troublesome complication a real threat to patients receiving hydralazine. Hydralazine is metabolized principally by acetylation, and patients in whom this process is slow are more likely to develop both the lupus-like syndrome and a peripheral neuropathy due to pyridoxine deficiency. Fortunately, the lupus-like syndrome subsides when hydralazine is discontinued. The latter complication can be treated or prevented by pyridoxine administration.

The ultimate role of hydralazine in the management of chronic congestive heart failure remains somewhat controversial. While some studies have yielded generally favorable results in longer-term follow-up, especially when hydralazine is used in combination with nitrates,[404] a recent trial at two centers did not demonstrate a difference between hydralazine and placebo in long-term treatment of chronic heart failure.[405] Patient selection is undoubtedly a critical variable in comparing results of different studies.

Minoxidil is a potent vasodilator that has hemodynamic effects similar to those of hydralazine; it may be a useful alternative drug because of its different spectrum of side effects.[406]

PRAZOSIN. This antihypertensive drug, a quinazoline derivative, is a potent alpha-adrenergic receptor blocking agent, the action of which is limited to the vascular adrenergic (alpha$_1$) receptors with little effect on presynaptic (alpha$_2$) receptors (Fig. 27–9, p. 914).[407] As a consequence, neuronally released norepinephrine is available to act on the alpha$_2$ receptors, inhibiting its own release and preventing the development of reflex tachycardia. In this manner prazosin differs from phentolamine and phenoxybenzamine, which block both presynaptic (alpha$_2$) and postsynaptic (alpha$_1$) receptors. In addition, prazosin exerts direct relaxing effects on vascular smooth muscle,[408] but this mechanism is probably not important at clinically relevant serum or tissue levels of the drug.[407]

Prazosin is an orally effective, balanced vasodilator, equieffective on arterioles and veins. Thus the circulatory effects of prazosin resemble those of intravenous nitroprusside.[409,410] An oral dose shows maximum effectiveness in 45 minutes and persists for 6 hours. Tolerance to the drug has been reported,[411] but recent studies indicate that if the dose is raised and the frequent tendency toward salt and water retention is countered by appropriate increases in diuretic dose, prazosin remains effective for at least several months.[412,413,413a] The vascular headaches, flushing, and lupus-like syndrome that occur with the use of hydralazine are not observed with prazosin. However, polyarthralgias, transient headache, mild nausea, urinary incontinence,

rashes, mental depression, and dry mouth have been reported in addition to fluid retention.[414] An important problem with the use of the drug, although quite uncommon in patients with congestive heart failure, is the so-called "first dose phenomenon," in which transient faintness, dizziness, palpitation, and, rarely, syncope occur after the initial dose of prazosin, owing to postural hypotension. The initial oral dose is therefore quite low, 1 mg, and this may be adjusted upward during the first few days of administration to avoid hypotension but should not exceed 10 mg three times a day.

ANGIOTENSIN-CONVERTING ENZYME INHIBITION. The renin-angiotensin system is activated in many patients with congestive heart failure, and levels of circulating angiotensin II are often elevated.[415] This has led to clinical use of captopril[416–419] and more recently, enalapril[419a], an orally active drug that blocks the enzymatic conversion of angiotensin I to angiotensin II, in the management of heart failure.[416–419] Inhibition of converting enzyme would be expected to act as a particularly potent dilator of those arterioles that are highly sensitive to angiotensin II, such as the renal arterial bed.[420,421] Also, by interfering with the breakdown of bradykinin, converting enzyme inhibition increases the level of this vasodilator; this action, as well as possible increases in circulating prostaglandins, may play a role in the vasodilator action of these drugs.[422,423] Captopril is a balanced vasodilator with actions on both the arteriolar and venous beds,[424] and it causes marked reductions in systemic vascular resistance and in left and right ventricular filling pressures. Cardiac output rises, but there is usually no change in heart rate.[425–427] Thus, captopril has been reported to improve hemodynamics in patients with congestive heart failure that is poorly controlled by digitalis and diuretics,[416–418,428,429,429a,429b] to restore responsiveness to diuretics, to lower serum creatinine, and to restore serum sodium levels in azotemic hyponatremic patients with heart failure.[419]

Converting enzyme inhibitors may also induce a favorable redistribution of blood flow, with less vasodilatation in vascular beds in the limb than in other systemic beds.[430] The lack of arterial unsaturation, regularly observed with the use of other vasodilators,[431] suggests that, in contrast to other vasodilators, converting enzyme inhibitors do not produce significant pulmonary arteriovenous shunting. This class of drugs offers a promising approach to vasodilation, both acutely and chronically, not only by reducing arteriolar tone but perhaps also by effecting a more favorable redistribution of cardiac output. Adverse side effects include impairment of renal function[432] and occasionally the development of nephrotic syndrome with biopsy evidence of membranous glomerulonephritis.[433]

CLINICAL APPLICATIONS

The use of vasodilators in two specific situations, acute pulmonary edema and acute myocardial infarction, is discussed elsewhere (p. 1314).

LEFT VENTRICULAR FAILURE. Vasodilator therapy has proved to be most effective in patients with *acute* left ventricular decompensation. The intravenous infusion of sodium nitroprusside is generally associated with sub-

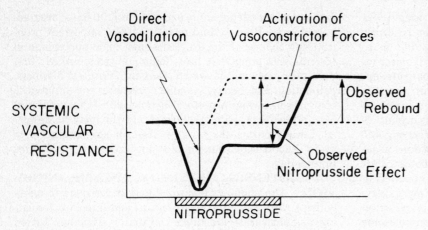

FIGURE 16–18 Schematic representation of events proposed to occur during nitroprusside infusion and withdrawal. Net effects observed are due to immediate direct vasodilator actions of the drug combined with secondary delayed but sustained activation of reflex vasoconstrictor forces. Unopposed effects of this reflex vasoconstrictor tone are presumed to mediate the rebound events observed upon abrupt vasodilator withdrawal. (Reproduced with permission from Packer, M., and LeJemtel, T. H.: Physiologic and pharmacologic determinants of vasodilator response: A conceptual framework for rational drug therapy for chronic heart failure. Prog. Cardiovasc. Dis. *24*:279, 1982, by permission of Grune and Stratton.)

stantial clinical improvement, rapid clearing of rales, elevation of cardiac output, improvement of peripheral perfusion, and augmented responsiveness to diuretics. When left ventricular filling pressure has declined to approximately 15 mm Hg and cardiac output has risen to above 2.1 liters/min/m², an attempt should be made to wean the patient from the intravenous vasodilator and to convert to one of the oral (or transdermal) medications. Although the infusion can usually be discontinued after 48 to 72 hours, it may be necessary to continue it for as long as 7 to 10 days in patients with severe heart failure. The major problem with sodium nitroprusside infusion is hypotension, and if, in a previously normotensive patient, systolic arterial pressure falls to below 90 mm Hg or decreases by more than 30 mm Hg from the control level, the drug should be discontinued or the dosage reduced. In patients who become hypotensive but require vasodilator therapy to improve perfusion, a combination of nitroprusside and an inotropic agent (dopamine or dobutamine) should be considered (p. 542). Particular care must be taken to avoid hypotension (and therefore hypoperfusion of myocardium in the distribution of stenotic coronary vessels) in patients with known or suspected coronary artery disease.

Transient myocardial depression during the perioperative period in patients undergoing cardiac surgery may be associated with an elevated systemic vascular resistance, and in such cases sodium nitroprusside may be useful. In patients with perioperative depression of cardiac function and hypotension, a sympathomimetic agent and/or intraaortic balloon counterpulsation is usually used in combination with the vasodilator.[376]

Infusion of sodium nitroprusside for several days may also be effective in *chronic heart failure* that has become refractory to digitalis and diuretic therapy.[383,434] Patients with borderline hypotension (systolic pressure 95 to 110 mm Hg) and borderline elevations of left ventricular filling pressure (12 to 15 mm Hg) derive little benefit from nitroprusside, because the venodilator action results in further reduction of filling pressure with little change in cardiac output. When filling pressure has been reduced to normal levels by nitroprusside and the principal hemodynamic abnormality is low cardiac output, cautious expansion of blood volume with dextran and the simultaneous administration of nitroprusside can result in a striking elevation in cardiac output.[400] Rebound increases in systemic vascular resistance above baseline, with consequent reduction in cardiac output, have been reported immediately after withdrawal of nitroprusside and are most pronounced in patients who developed tachycardia during infusion of the drug.[383] As shown schematically in Figure 16–18, this phenomenon is presumably due to vasoconstrictor influences,

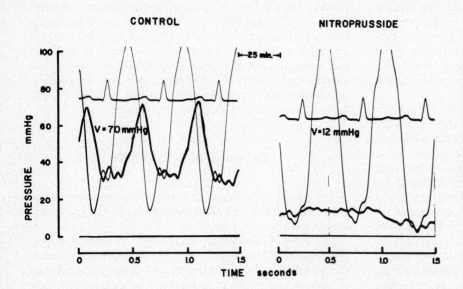

FIGURE 16–19 In a patient with acute, severe mitral regurgitation, the effects of nitroprusside on pulmonary capillary wedge (heavier pressure tracing) and left ventricular (LV) pressures are shown. In the control tracing, note the large regurgitant *v* waves in the wedge tracing peaking to 70 mm Hg with LV end-diastolic pressure of approximately 32 mm Hg. During administration of sodium nitroprusside (25 minutes later), the pulmonary capillary wedge pressure was markedly reduced and the *v* waves were only 12 mm Hg. Similarly, LV end-diastolic pressure was markedly reduced, despite an increase in peak LV systolic pressure. (From Chatterjee, K., et al.: Beneficial effects of vasodilator agents in severe mitral regurgitation due to dysfunction of subvalvar apparatus. Circulation *48*:684, 1973, by permission of the American Heart Association, Inc.)

the magnitude of which will vary substantially among patients. When encountered, the problem can be handled by gradual tapering of nitroprusside dosage.

MECHANICAL LESIONS. In patients with mitral regurgitation or ventricular septal defect,[435] the abnormal flow (regurgitant or shunt) is a direct function of the systemic vascular resistance; reduction of the latter augments systemic output and diminishes the load on the left ventricle by reducing the abnormal flow. Ordinarily when these lesions are severe enough to cause heart failure, they should be treated surgically, but when they occur in the course of acute myocardial infarction, it may be best to defer operation, if the patient's condition is stable, for several weeks after the infarct for technical reasons (p. 1318). Treatment with vasodilators, at first with sodium nitroprusside and then sustained with long-acting drugs administered orally, can often stabilize the patient's condition during the interval[376,436] (Fig. 16–19).

Increased systemic vascular resistance also augments the regurgitant volume in patients with aortic regurgitation, and vasodilator therapy will reduce the regurgitation and increase the forward stroke volume and cardiac output[437,437a] (Fig. 16–20). However, caution must be exercised in the treatment of aortic regurgitation with vasodilators, since these drugs may lower further the already depressed aortic diastolic pressure and interfere with coronary filling.

Vasodilator therapy is of comparatively little benefit to patients with obstructive valvular lesions, i.e., mitral and aortic stenosis,[378] unless they are associated with severe left ventricular dysfunction. Although systemic vasodilators often have relatively little effect on the pulmonary vascular bed, oral hydralazine has been reported to have favorable hemodynamic effects in some patients with cor pulmonale,[438] and prazosin can improve right ventricular function by lowering left ventricular diastolic pressure and, secondarily, pulmonary artery and right ventricular systolic pressure in patients with severe congestive heart failure.[439] When high concentrations of inhaled oxygen are used to counteract the pulmonary vasoconstrictor actions of hypoxia, oxygen may be considered to be a right ventricular afterload reducing agent.

Long-Term Therapy

Bearing in mind that vasodilators improve cardiac performance at rest and at submaximal workloads[413,440,440a] but often fail to improve maximal exercise capacity,[441] two groups of patients are good candidates for chronic vasodilator therapy: (1) patients whose conditions have been stabilized by means of an intravenously administered vasodilator but who continue to display abnormal hemodynamics, and (2) patients who have not received intravenous vasodilators previously but who are symptomatic despite optimal treatment with cardiac glycosides and diuretics.

Balanced vasodilator regimens available for chronic use in patients expected to benefit from reduction in both preload and afterload include the following:

1. *Oral hydralazine combined with sublingual or oral isosorbide dinitrate* or with a transdermal nitroglycerin dosage form. Although this combination is effective in many patients, and its actions resemble those of intravenous sodium nitroprusside,[442] postural hypotension is often a limiting factor in chronic use.[443] The side effects associated with chronic administration (particularly the lupus-like syndrome) in some patients may make it difficult or impossible to sustain this therapy for indefinite periods.

2. *Oral prazosin* provides balanced arterial and venous actions. In view of its effectiveness over several months[412,444,445] and the relative freedom from major side effects that cannot be adequately treated,[407] oral prazosin is a useful agent for chronic vasodilator treatment, provided that the need for dose adjustment upward and augmentation of diuretic dosage is recognized in view of decreased responsiveness with continued therapy.[412]

3. *Oral captopril* also provides a balanced vasodilator effect on both arterial and venous beds and has been shown to exert sustained favorable effects on the circulation in patients with refractory congestive heart failure who have not responded well to other vasodilator regimens.[446] Doses ranging from 75 to 450 mg per day in divided doses have been found to be effective.

Despite the most careful patient selection and clinical management, some patients with refractory congestive heart failure either do not respond favorably to vasodilator therapy or discontinue it because of side effects. Thus, in a series of 34 patients with refractory heart failure reported by Walsh and Greenberg, only about one fourth of patients in whom vasodilator therapy was initiated experienced sustained clinical benefit.[447] Important reasons for this lack of sustained clinical benefit include the development of drug-specific tolerance that can be counteracted by switching to another vasodilator[403] as well as the activa-

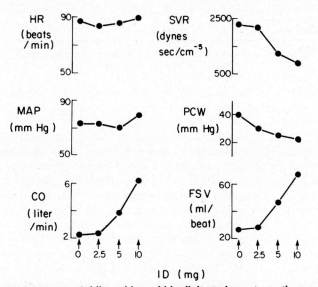

FIGURE 16–20 **Sublingual isosorbide dinitrate in acute aortic regurgitation.** The hemodynamic response to sublingual isosorbide dinitrate (ID) is illustrated in a 67-year-old woman with acute bacterial endocarditis and severe congestive heart failure secondary to acute, severe aortic regurgitation. Note the marked increase in forward cardiac output (CO), which accompanied the reduction in systemic vascular resistance (SVR), following sublingual doses up to 10 mg. Pulmonary capillary wedge (PCW) pressure fell, and there was no change in heart rate (HR) or mean arterial pressure (MAP). The patient's heart failure improved considerably over the two-week period before corrective operation. FSV = forward stroke volume. (From Chatterjee, K., and Parmley, W. W.: The role of vasodilator therapy in heart failure. Progr. Cardiovasc. Dis. *19*:301, 1977, by permission of Grune and Stratton.)

tion by vasodilator drugs of neurohumoral forces that promote peripheral vasoconstriction and tachycardia[448] and sodium retention.[449] Franciosa has reviewed the clinical status of long-term vasodilator therapy in the chronic heart failure setting.[434]

The contribution of vasodilator therapy to the support of the circulation may be difficult to assess in patients with severe heart failure who are already receiving oral vasodilator therapy. If clinical circumstances dictate, hospitalization may be advisable, and the effects of raising the dose of vasodilator may be assessed. Occasionally it is desirable to substitute or add a course of therapy with intravenous sodium nitroprusside and/or a sympathomimetic amine (p. 546).

SYMPATHOMIMETIC AMINES

Catecholamines and other sympathomimetic amines (Fig. 16–21) exert potent inotropic effects by interacting with myocardial (beta$_1$) adrenergic receptors. For many years attempts were made to utilize these properties in the treatment of heart failure, but these efforts were largely unsuccessful because of the other effects of these agents (Tables 16–9 and 16–10). Thus, isoproterenol, and to a lesser extent epinephrine, causes tachycardia and hypotension by stimulating beta$_1$-adrenergic receptors in the sinoatrial node and beta$_2$ receptors in the systemic vascular bed. Norepinephrine, on the other hand, by stimulating alpha-adrenergic receptors, causes vasoconstriction and hypertension. Two agents introduced relatively recently, dopamine and dobutamine, produce less tachycardia and fewer peripheral vascular effects and are used frequently in the treatment of acute heart failure.

DOPAMINE

This endogenous catecholamine, the immediate precursor of norepinephrine (Fig. 12–33, p. 440), stimulates myocardial contractility by acting directly on beta$_1$-adrenergic

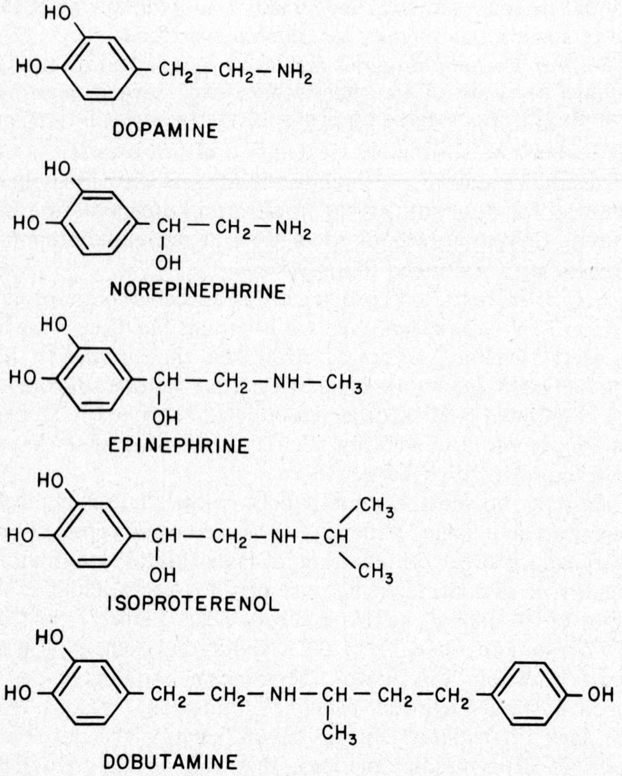

TABLE 16–9   SOME RECEPTOR ACTIONS OF CATECHOLAMINES

ADRENERGIC RECEPTOR	SITE	ACTION
Beta$_1$	Myocardium	Increase atrial and ventricular contractility
	Sinoatrial node	Increase heart rate
	Atrioventricular conduction system	Enhance atrioventricular conduction
Beta$_2$	Arterioles	Vasodilation
	Lungs	Bronchodilation
Alpha	Peripheral arterioles	Vasoconstriction

TABLE 16–10   ADRENERGIC RECEPTOR ACTIVITY OF SYMPATHOMIMETIC AMINES

	ALPHA PERIPHERAL	BETA$_1$ CARDIAC	BETA$_2$ PERIPHERAL
Norepinephrine	++++	++++	0
Epinephrine	++++	++++	++
Dopamine*	++++	++++	++
Isoproterenol	0	++++	++++
Dobutamine	+	++++	++
Methoxamine	++++	0	0

*Causes renal and mesenteric dilatation by stimulating dopaminergic receptors.
Both tables from Sonnenblick, E. H., et al.: Dobutamine: A new synthetic cardioactive sympathetic amine. N. Engl. J. Med. *300*:18, 1979.

receptors in the myocardium and indirectly by releasing norepinephrine from sympathetic nerve terminals, which in turn also stimulates beta$_1$ receptors[450] (Tables 16–9 and 16–10). All *cardiac* effects of dopamine are antagonized by beta-adrenergic blockers.[450] However, there is considerable evidence that the vasodilation mediated by dopamine is secondary to activation of specific dopaminergic receptors.[451,452] Dopamine-induced vasodilation, which is not blocked by propranolol and therefore is not related to activation of beta$_2$ receptors, occurs in the renal, mesenteric, coronary, and cerebral vascular beds.[450] This vasodilation is not due to release of acetylcholine,[450,453] histamine,[450] or prostaglandins.[454] However, dopaminergic vasodilation is antagonized by phenothiazines, such as chlorpromazine, and butyrophenone compounds, such as haloperidol.[455] Dopamine also causes vasodilation of dog hind limb vasculature that can be prevented by section of the nerves innervating these vessels,[456] and it has been suggested that this response is due to a ganglionic blocking action of this amine[457] or to inhibition of transmission in the postganglionic sympathetic nerve.[458] Dopamine-induced diuresis is common in patients with heart failure and is secondary to a combination of inotropic and renal vasodilator effects[450]; studies in both dog[459] and man[460] have demonstrated that dopamine preferentially dilates vessels in the renal cortex.

FIGURE 16–21   Chemical structures of sympathomimetic amines.

When larger doses of dopamine are administered, the dilation is reversed, and dopamine causes constriction of arteries and veins in all vascular beds.[450] Although the vasoconstriction has been attributed to action of the drug on alpha-adrenergic receptors,[450,461] the doses of the alpha-receptor blockers phentolamine and phenoxybenzamine required to prevent the dopamine-induced vasoconstriction are higher than those required to antagonize the vasoconstriction caused by other alpha-adrenergic agonists. Dopamine-induced contractions of isolated canine vessels can be attenuated by concentrations of the serotonin-blocking agent cyproheptadine that do not antagonize the actions of norepinephrine. These findings suggest that dopamine may cause contraction of vascular smooth muscle, in part, by action on serotonin- or tryptamine-sensitive receptors.[456]

Because dopamine in small and large doses acts on receptors that mediate opposing effects in animal experiments, it is not surprising that the effects of this drug on vascular resistance and arterial pressure are dose-dependent in patients as well. With infusion rates of 2 to 5 μg/kg/min, cardiac contractility, cardiac output, and renal blood flow increase, with little change in heart rate and either a reduction or no change in total peripheral resistance.[462] With higher infusion rates (5 to 10 μg/kg/min), arterial pressure, peripheral resistance, and heart rate increase[463] and renal blood flow may decline.

Like other sympathomimetic amines that increase cardiac contractility, dopamine increases coronary blood flow[450,464] secondary to the increase in myocardial oxygen consumption that results from increased cardiac work.[465] Direct coronary vasodilation through action on dopaminergic receptors is a secondary mechanism involved in the increase in coronary flow.[466] However, as is the case in other vascular beds, large doses of dopamine may increase coronary artery resistance by direct action on receptors mediating constriction.[450] Ultimately, the effects of dopamine, like those of other catecholamines, depend on myocardial oxygen utilization and coronary blood flow, which in turn are affected by the sum total of its several actions. Augmented heart rate, contractility, and arterial pressure will increase oxygen utilization, whereas reduced peripheral resistance and heart size will decrease oxygen utilization. Stimulation of dopaminergic receptors increases coronary blood flow, while stimulation of alpha-adrenergic receptors decreases it.

In early investigations, Goldberg et al. found that in patients with heart failure, dopamine increased sodium excretion and cardiac output[467,468]; infusion rates of 2.1 to 5.8 μg/kg/min increased cardiac index ($+26$ per cent) without significant change in heart rate or total body oxygen consumption. Peripheral resistance was reduced, and pulmonary resistance, when elevated, also fell. Left ventricular dP/dt increased by 58 per cent, glomerular filtration rate by 38 per cent, renal plasma flow by 79 per cent, and sodium excretion by an average of 48 per cent.[468] Thus, in patients with congestive heart failure, dopamine exerts important beneficial hemodynamic and renal effects. However, care must be taken to adjust the infusion rate carefully to prevent excessive positive inotropic effect, tachycardia, and increased peripheral resistance.

In normotensive patients with otherwise refractory heart failure, infusions are begun at low rates (0.5 to 1.0 μg/kg/min) and are gradually increased until urine flow is augmented or until increments in diastolic pressure and heart rate are observed. The infusion rate should then be decreased or the infusion discontinued. In patients with cardiogenic shock, both the vasoconstrictor and the more intense inotropic effects of higher doses may be desirable (pp. 595 and 1317).

USE IN CARDIAC SURGERY

Dopamine has become widely used for the treatment of acute heart failure during and after cardiac surgery. In a comparison of the effects of three catecholamines in 22 patients with low cardiac output states following surgery, dopamine increased cardiac index by 1.10 liters/min/m², mean arterial blood pressure by 7 mm Hg, heart rate by 19 beats/min, and urine flow by 75 ml/hr. In contrast, norepinephrine increased cardiac index by much less (only 0.20 liter/min/m²) and mean arterial pressure by much more (23 mm Hg), while heart rate rose by 9 beats/min and urine flow *decreased* by 8 ml/hr. Isoproterenol resembled dopamine by increasing cardiac index by 0.95 liter/min/m² but caused a more severe tachycardia, increasing heart rate by 28 beats/min. Urine flow increased by 28 ml/hr, while mean arterial pressure decreased by 7 mm Hg. These observations demonstrate the superiority of dopamine over previously used sympathomimetic agents in this clinical setting.[469] Sometimes the use of sympathomimetic amines permits the discontinuation of cardiopulmonary bypass in patients who cannot be weaned from the pump. Here also dopamine appears to be superior to isoproterenol.[451] Combined use of intraaortic balloon counterpulsation with dopamine and nitroprusside has been reported to be effective in patients with low cardiac output and elevated systemic vascular resistance following cardiopulmonary bypass.[470]

DOBUTAMINE

Dobutamine is a synthetic cardioactive sympathomimetic amine that stimulates beta₁-, beta₂-, and alpha-adrenergic receptors.[471-474] Radioligand binding studies suggest that beta₁ activity predominates over beta₂, and that alpha₁ predominates over alpha₂ activity of this drug.[475] Under some circumstances, dobutamine has been shown to exert alpha-adrenergic antagonist activity in vascular tissue.[476] At equivalent cardiac contractile force responses, dobutamine exerts a much weaker beta₂-adrenergic action than does isoproterenol and a much weaker alpha-adrenergic action than does either norepinephrine or dopamine. Injections of dobutamine into the femoral vascular bed cause slight vasoconstriction at low doses and a biphasic vasoconstrictor-vasodilator response at higher doses; phenoxybenzamine blocks the vasoconstrictor component and propranolol blocks the vasodilator component.[451]

In contrast to dopamine, which increases renal blood flow in all dose ranges, dobutamine does not alter renal blood flow but does cause a redistribution of cardiac output in favor of the coronary and skeletal muscle beds over the mesenteric and renal vascular beds.[477,477a] Gillespie and colleagues administered dobutamine to patients with acute myocardial infarction and found that the drug improved hemodynamic parameters without provoking undesirable effects and without increasing the extent of myocardial injury.[478] Favorable hemodynamic effects sustained for weeks to a few months in patients with congestive cardiomyopathy treated for two or three days with intravenous dobutamine have been reported.[479,479a] Improvement in cardiac index (mean increase 54 per cent) and stroke work index (mean increase 65 per cent) has also been reported in response to dobutamine infusion in patients with chronic heart failure associated with ischemic heart disease, with infrequent precipitation of overt myocardial ischemia.[480]

Adverse Effects of Dopamine and Dobutamine. Cardiac arrhythmias constitute the most serious adverse effect of sympathomimetic amines. The electrophysiological properties of dopamine and dobutamine resemble those of other sympathomimetic amines[450,481,482] and consist of an acceleration of the spontaneous depolarization of sino-atrial cells, thereby increasing heart rate, accelerating diastolic depolarization and facilitating activation of latent pacemaker cells, shortening the refractory period of atrial and ventricular muscle, and speeding atrioventricular conduction. Ventricular arrhythmias have been observed with the use of both drugs.[450,483-485] Since ventricular arrhythmias are more prone to develop with increased peripheral resistance during halothane anesthesia, dobutamine is less likely to cause such arrhythmias than are vasoconstricting doses of dopamine.[486] In patients with coronary artery disease, both dobutamine and dopamine may precipitate angina pectoris.[450,483,487]

In patients with preexisting vascular disease, dopamine may cause gangrene of the digits.[488,489] Tissue necrosis similar to that produced by norepinephrine can also occur if an infusion of dopamine extravasates into tissue; this can be prevented by infiltrating the area promptly with 5 to 10 mg of phentolamine diluted in saline. Dopamine differs from the other catecholamines in that it causes nausea and vomiting in some patients, an effect more commonly observed with high doses.[450,460] Since the cardiovascular effects of dopamine (in contrast to dobutamine) are potentiated by prior therapy with monoamine oxidase inhibitors,[450] the dose of dopamine in such patients should be reduced to approximately 10 per cent of the usual dose.

Comparisons Between Dopamine and Dobutamine.[489a,489b] There has been considerable interest in comparing the effects of dobutamine and dopamine in patients with severe congestive heart failure. In one study dobutamine raised cardiac index while lowering left ventricular end-diastolic pressure and leaving mean aortic pressure unchanged.[490] Dopamine also improved cardiac index but at the expense of a greater increase in heart rate than occurred with dobutamine. Dopamine was ineffective in lowering left ventricular end-diastolic pressure but increased mean aortic pressure. Because dobutamine has little effect on two major determinants of myocardial oxygen consumption, i.e., heart rate and aortic pressure, and reduces a third, i.e., ventricular filling pressure—a determinant of ventricular size, it may be superior to dopamine in patients with low-output syndrome associated with ischemic heart disease. In these patients, heart rate and arterial pressure rise and end-diastolic pressure remains constant.[490]

In another study comparing the acute hemodynamic effects of dobutamine and dopamine in patients with chronic low-output cardiac failure, it was observed that at dosages adjusted to achieve similar increments in cardiac output, dobutamine reduced left ventricular filling pressure from an average of 25 to 17 mm Hg, while dopamine increased it to 30 mm Hg.[491] This response to dopamine was probably the result of its vasoconstrictor actions and illustrates the potential advantages of using a more cardioselective agent such as dobutamine when the desired goal of therapy is to improve ventricular function by direct inotropic stimulation.

In a comparison between the two sympathomimetic amines in patients with severe heart failure, dobutamine in doses up to 10 μg/kg/min progressively increased cardiac output while decreasing systemic and pulmonary vascular resistance and filling pressure, without a significant effect on heart rate and ventricular irritability. In contrast, dopamine at doses above 4 μg/kg/min increased not only cardiac output but also filling pressure and ventricular ectopic activity; at doses greater than 6 μg/kg/min, dopamine increased heart rate and systemic and pulmonary resistance. Infusion rates above 4 μg/kg/min had little additional effect on cardiac output, presumably because of the increase in systemic vascular resistance.[492]

The heart rate–systolic blood pressure product, an index related to myocardial oxygen demands, increases with both agents but more so with dopamine than with dobutamine. Furthermore, at any increase in the heart rate–systolic pressure product, the increase in cardiac output with dobutamine is nearly twice as great as with dopamine. With prolonged infusions of optimal doses of both agents (dopamine 3.7 to 4.0 μg/kg/min and dobutamine 7.3 to 7.7 μg/kg/min), only dobutamine *maintained* the elevations in stroke volume, cardiac output, urinary sodium excretion, urine flow rate, and creatinine clearance.[492]

Thus, the hemodynamic effects are adverse in *normotensive* patients with advanced heart failure, i.e., left ventricular filling pressures rise, with agents such as norepinephrine or dopamine in large doses, which cause vasoconstriction, but often respond well to vasodilator therapy, to dobutamine, or to a combination of a vasodilator and dopamine or dobutamine. Since the inotropic effects of dopamine are in part mediated by release of endogenous cardiac catecholamines, which may be depleted in patients with chronic heart failure (p. 459), low doses of this drug may be insufficient to achieve the desired inotropic effect of an increase in cardiac output, while larger doses may produce unwanted vasoconstriction.

Although dopamine can improve renal and mesenteric perfusion by selective nonbeta-adrenergic vasodilation (and this unique property of dopamine is not shared by dobutamine[472]), this beneficial effect on regional perfusion is often reversed when dopamine is given in the large doses sometimes required to achieve a sufficient inotropic effect. It is possible, however, to use dopamine in low doses (1.2 to 2.5 μg/kg/min) to provide selective vasodilation in mesenteric and renal vascular beds and combine it with dobutamine, or with a vasodilator, to achieve optimal hemodynamic improvement (p. 547). In patients

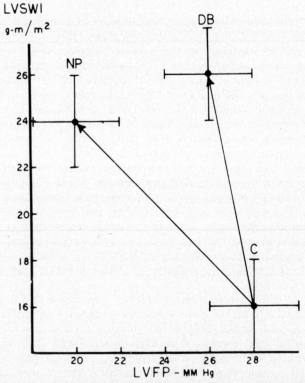

FIGURE 16–22 Left ventricular stroke work index (LVSWI) is plotted on the vertical axis, and left ventricular filling pressure (LVFP) is plotted on the horizontal axis. C = control; NP = nitroprusside; DB = dobutamine. The plots move upward and to the left during infusion of both agents, suggesting improved ventricular performance. Data are from 19 patients in chronic low-output (Class III or IV) congestive heart failure despite use of digitalis and diuretics. (From Berkowitz, C., et al.: Comparative responses to dobutamine and nitroprusside in patients with chronic low output cardiac failure. Circulation *56*:918, 1977, by permission of the American Heart Association, Inc.)

with frank hypotension, dopamine, with its greater vasoconstrictor properties, may be superior to dobutamine.

In a comparison between sodium nitroprusside and dobutamine, it was found that both drugs reduced systemic vascular resistance.[493] The reduction produced by dobutamine results primarily from withdrawal of compensatory vasoconstriction, as a consequence of elevation of cardiac output,[494] the direct peripheral vasodilator effect of dobutamine playing only a minor role.[495,496] On the other hand, sodium nitroprusside infusion reduces systemic vascular resistance more than does dobutamine, suggesting that dobutamine might be preferable to nitroprusside for augmenting cardiac output in borderline hypotensive patients or in patients with preexisting vascular disease, particularly those with coronary artery disease, in whom blood flow to vital organs may be largely dependent upon arterial pressure. Nitroprusside, however, is more effective than dobutamine in lowering elevated filling pressure (Fig. 16–22). Dobutamine consistently increases heart rate, albeit only moderately, in patients with heart failure,[482,483,491,497,498] whereas sodium nitroprusside, which lacks direct chronotrophic activity, has a variable effect on heart rate in patients with heart failure.[499] When increases in heart rate do occur during nitroprusside infusion, they probably result from compensatory reflexes[500] secondary to excessive hypotension.[501,502] Therefore, nitroprusside is preferable to dobutamine for emergency treatment of patients who require rapid reduction of pulmonary venous pressure.

ORALLY ACTIVE SYMPATHOMIMETIC AMINES

Several orally active beta-adrenergic agonists have undergone clinical study recently, although none of these newer agents is available for routine clinical use in the United States at this time.

Pirbuterol has been found to have favorable hemodynamic effects in patients with refractory congestive heart failure that may derive from both vasodilator and positive inotropic actions.[446] Awan and colleagues have documented improved cardiac output with lowered ventricular filling pressures in patients with chronic severe congestive heart failure[503] and found responses to an oral dose of pirbuterol similar to those observed with intravenous dopamine.[504] Dawson et al. also observed improved pump performance of the heart in patients with chronic heart failure in response to oral pirbuterol,[505] and Rude and colleagues observed substantial acute hemodynamic improvement in patients with chronic congestive heart failure, with no evident increased requirement for coronary blood flow or myocardial oxygen delivery.[506] No provocation of myocardial ischemia was noted in six patients with coronary artery disease and chronic congestive heart failure refractory to digitalis and diuretics. Of concern, however, is the finding of Colucci et al. that tolerance to the favorable hemodynamic effects of pirbuterol developed over a one-month period of chronic administration of the drug. This was accompanied by decreased numbers of beta-adrenergic receptors on lymphocytes of these patients, suggesting a possible mechanism for reduced responsiveness after long-term therapy with pirbuterol.[507]

Prenalterol is an orally active beta$_1$ selective adrenergic agonist with positive inotropic effects that has undergone recent clinical testing. At appropriate doses, positive inotropic effects have been observed with little increase in heart rate,[508–512,512a] but increased ventricular ectopic activity has also been observed in some patients.[509]

Other beta-adrenergic agonists originally introduced as bronchodilators, including *terbutaline*[513] and *salbutamol*,[514] have also been found to exert favorable hemodynamic effects owing to vasodilator and/or positive inotropic properties.

AMRINONE

Appreciable clinical experience has accumulated with amrinone, an orally active drug still in investigational status at this writing with both vasodilator and positive inotropic properties initially thought to act through a mechanism separate from those of the cardiac glycosides or sympathomimetic amines.[515] Recent evidence suggests, however, that amrinone acts as a phosphodiesterase inhibitor, thus increasing intracellular cyclic AMP levels.[516,517,517a] Since the initial report of Benotti et al.,[518] several studies have documented substantial increases in cardiac output and left ventricular ejection fraction together with lowered ventricular filling pressures in patients with severe congestive heart failure.[519–521]

Favorable hemodynamic effects were not associated with adverse effects on myocardial oxygen consumption or coronary blood flow requirements in patients with congestive heart failure due to coronary artery disease.[522] Improved exercise capacity has also been documented in selected patients with heart failure in response to amrinone given acutely[523,524] and chronically.[523,525] A combination of amrinone and hydralazine produced greater hemodynamic benefit than either agent alone.[526] Side effects, including dose-related thrombocytopenia, have been relatively frequent in clinical testing and require further study. Recently, milrinone, a congener of amrinone, has been found to have about 15 times the potency of the parent compound and far fewer side effects.[526a,526b] Although it appears to be an effective drug in the treatment of refractory heart failure, its ultimate clinical role remains to be determined.

REFRACTORY AND INTRACTABLE HEART FAILURE

Heart failure is considered to be *refractory* when it persists or the patient's condition deteriorates despite intensive therapy. It is defined as *intractable* when it is resistant to all known therapeutic measures. The first step in treating a patient in refractory failure is to exclude any underlying disease that might be reversible. Thus, both the nature and hemodynamic consequences of the underlying illness should be reassessed, and surgical treatment should be considered or reconsidered; often cardiac catheterization and angiography should be carried out or repeated at this time. For example, resection of a large ventricular aneurysm might have been deferred as long as the patient responded to medical treatment for heart failure because of the potentially high surgical risk, but reconsideration might be in order when such a response wanes. Similar considerations may apply to patients with known multivessel coronary artery disease or advanced valvular heart disease and poor left ventricular function. Other forms of heart disease that may lead to refractory heart failure and that are treatable surgically but are not readily recognized on clinical examination include cardiac tumors (Chap. 42), endomyocardial fibrosis (p. 1427), and constrictive pericarditis without calcification. Such conditions should at least be considered and, if possible, excluded assuming that the heart failure state is refractory.

In the absence of any correctable underlying heart disease, one must next consider whether some precipitating cause has not been properly identified and treated. A number of possibilities should come to mind:

1. Could the patient be "cheating" on the restricted sodium diet?

2. Is the patient not complying with the medication schedule prescribed, despite protestations to the contrary?

3. Has excessive diuresis occurred, and are lethargy and weakness due not to refractory heart failure but rather to a low cardiac output state secondary to an inadequate preload?

4. Could digitalis intoxication be present? Digitalis toxicity can occur despite a serum glycoside level in the usual therapeutic range and can cause fatigue, lethargy, and anorexia that may mimic refractory heart failure.

5. Has the patient been receiving optimal doses of cardiac glycosides? A glycoside level in the usual therapeutic range does not necessarily mean that the patient has been receiving the optimal dose of the glycoside. A greater inotropic effect may sometimes be provided by the addition of a very small dose of digitalis (0.125 mg digoxin daily or every other day) above the maintenance dose without precipitating signs or symptoms of toxicity.

6. Has an electrolyte imbalance, such as hypokalemic alkalosis or hyponatremia, developed as a consequence of excessive diuresis and severe restriction of sodium intake?

7. Could the patient be suffering from unrecognized pulmonary embolism (p. 1578)? This condition is often silent and manifests itself only by slight tachycardia, anxiety, tachypnea, and intensification of heart failure. Densities on the chest roentgenogram may make it difficult or impossible to interpret lung scans, and a pulmonary angiogram may be required to establish the diagnosis. Although this procedure is not without risk, a positive result may lead to treatment such as anticoagulants and/or vena caval interruption that could prevent further emboli and prove to be life-saving.

8. Could pulmonary infection be present? Pneumonitis may be difficult to recognize in patients with chronic congestive heart failure who often have a chronic low-grade fever as well as increased interstitial markings on chest roentgenogram and pulmonary rales on clinical examination. Is the suspicion of pulmonary infection high enough to warrant sputum culture and consideration of a course of antibiotics?

9. Could hyperthyroidism or infective endocarditis be present? Thyrotoxicosis (often apathetic in the elderly) and infective endocarditis in the presence of heart failure may not present with typical clinical manifestations, but their presence can lead to refractory heart failure. Should tests including an assessment of thyroid function and multiple blood cultures be obtained?

10. Could the diagnosis of refractory heart failure be incorrect, and could the patient with established heart disease be suffering from an unrelated illness, such as an occult neoplasm, viral hepatitis, or hepatic cirrhosis?

11. Could alcohol be playing a role? Alcohol is a potent myocardial depressant. In addition to producing cardiomyopathy (p. 1406), it can contribute to the heart failure state when it is not the primary cause of heart failure but is superimposed on some other form of heart disease.

12. Does the patient have inappropriate bradycardia due to sinus node dysfunction or atrioventricular block that could be corrected by means of a pacemaker?

13. Is the patient receiving any medications with salt-retaining (e.g., corticosteroids, estrogens, non-steroidal antiinflammatory drugs) or negative inotropic (e.g., disopyramide,[527] beta-adrenergic blocking agents, verapamil[528]) effects?

14. Is vasodilator therapy causing an increased tendency to salt and fluid retention?

15. Can *any* aspect of therapy be intensified without producing untoward effects?

These and related questions can usually be answered only if the patient is hospitalized; if *every* aspect of the diagnosis, including underlying and precipitating causes of heart failure, is carefully assessed; and if *every* aspect of therapy is meticulously reconsidered. If the patient has been placed at rest and has received optimal doses of cardiac glycosides and diuretics, and if electrolyte imbalance has been corrected and large volumes of fluid in the serous cavities not mobilized by diuretics have been removed mechanically, then the patient should receive a course of intravenous therapy with a vasodilator, a sympathomimetic agent, or both for 4 to 7 days. Individual use of vasodilators or of sympathomimetic amines has been discussed previously (pp. 534 and 542). In addition, combinations of nitroprusside or nitroglycerin[502] and dobutamine or dopamine have been remarkably effective. The *combined administration* of a sympathomimetic amine and vasodilator may be of benefit in patients with severe heart failure in whom the use of one of these agents alone is insufficient. Thus, in one series of patients with severe chronic congestive heart failure, nitroprusside alone reduced left ventricular end-diastolic pressure from 25 to 14 mm Hg and increased cardiac index from 2.4 to 3.0 liters/min/m². Dopamine alone caused a greater elevation of cardiac index, to 3.4 liters/min/m², but did not reduce end-diastolic pressure. Simultaneous infusion of the two agents resulted in favorable alterations in *both* hemodynamic variables: left ventricular end-diastolic pressure declined to 16 mm Hg and cardiac index rose to 3.5 liters/min/m².[529]

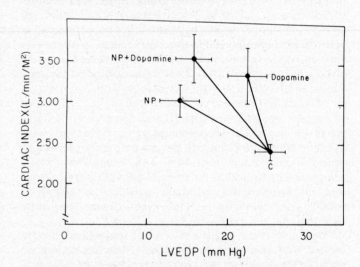

FIGURE 16–23 Effect of nitroprusside (NP), dopamine, and the combination of NP and dopamine on left ventricular end-diastolic pressure and cardiac index. Data are from 9 patients with chronic congestive heart failure (Class III) despite use of digitalis and diuretics; digitalis was discontinued 72 hours before this study. (From Miller, R. R., et al.: Combined dopamine and nitroprusside therapy in congestive heart failure. Circulation 55:881, 1977, by permission of the American Heart Association, Inc.)

Thus, the combination of dopamine and nitroprusside provides the principal beneficial actions of both drugs in patients with heart failure. The combination raises cardiac output considerably while markedly reducing elevated filling pressure (Fig. 16–23). Combined use of digoxin with nitroprusside has also been shown to be more effective than nitroprusside alone in heart failure complicating acute myocardial infarction.[530] Such treatment can, of course, be carried out only in the hospital, with careful monitoring of filling pressure, cardiac output, and arterial pressure. If it is successful and the patient can be weaned from the intravenous therapy, larger doses of oral vasodilators and experimental drugs such as oral sympathomimetics or amrinone (or its congener, milrinone, p. 545) may provide sustained benefit.

Heart failure can properly be termed intractable if it persists despite the application of all the measures cited above. Then, the possibilities of cardiac transplantation and assisted circulation may be considered in selected instances.

OTHER MEASURES
Cardiac Transplantation

This procedure was first performed in humans in 1967.[531,532] Despite its technical feasibility, the high mortality rates resulting from graft rejection led to its abandonment in most institutions. As of May 1, 1983, a total of 263 transplants had been carried out at Stanford University Medical Center, where experience with cardiac transplantation has been most extensive. One hundred and seven of these patients are current survivors, and the longest living recipient underwent transplantation 13.3 years ago. Currently the one-year survival rate after cardiac transplantation at Stanford is 82 per cent, which is comparable to the results obtained with cadaver kidney programs.[533,534] Recent improved results reflect the potency and effectiveness of the immunosuppressive agent, Cyclosporin A.[534a]

Potential recipients of cardiac transplants must have advanced heart disease, should be in Class IV with intractable heart failure (as defined above, on p. 545), and should have a poor prognosis for one-year survival. Candidates should be stable psychologically and should have a history of compliance with medical therapy. Since younger patients have better survival rates, 50 years is the usual upper age limit for potential recipients. Contraindications to cardiac transplantation include severe pulmonary hypertension, parenchymal pulmonary disease, recent pulmonary infarction, donor-specific cytotoxic antibodies, active infection, diabetes mellitus requiring insulin, and other diseases considered likely to limit survival or rehabilitation. Over half the recipients at Stanford Medical Center have had coronary artery disease, while the remainder have had idiopathic, viral, or rheumatic cardiomyopathies. Thus, the ideal recipient has been a young person who is dying of end-stage cardiac disease and who is otherwise vigorous, emotionally stable, and willing to risk a complex procedure and course for the chance of functional improvement. Combined transplantation of the heart and lungs has been employed successfully in the treatment of irreversible, severe pulmonary hypertension.[535]

The majority of heart donors have sustained irreversible cerebral damage due to trauma or intracranial hemorrhage. However, donor supply remains critical, and the experience at Stanford has been that an appreciable number (approximately one third) of recipients awaiting transplant die before a suitable donor heart becomes available. The success of using hearts removed from donors and transported under conditions of hypothermic ischemia for up to 3 hours has broadened the sources of donor supply.[536] It is likely that continuous hypothermic perfusion with an oxygenated hyperosmolar solution will extend the duration of possible storage to 24 hours.[537] Other than choosing a heart from a donor less than 35 years of age of appropriate weight, ABO type, and absence of a positive lymphocyte cross match, no prospective histocompatibility typing has been used for cardiac transplantation. The results of HLA typing have been disappointing in predicting long-term survival.

After placing the recipient on cardiopulmonary bypass, the heart is removed, leaving the posterior walls of the atria with their venous connections in place.[532] The donor atria are sutured to the corresponding structures of the in situ residual atria of the recipient, and the great vessels are anastomosed last. Alternatively, in *heterotopic heart transplantation*, the recipient's heart is left in situ, and the donor heart is placed in parallel, with anastomoses between the two right atria, pulmonary arteries, left atria, and aortae. The stated advantage of this technique is that should acute donor heart failure occur, chances for the patient's survival are improved by his own heart; retransplantation is possible if the donor heart becomes nonfunctional because of rejection or any other reason.[538] Immunosuppression has been accomplished with high-dose prednisone and azathioprine and antithymocyte globulin, the dosage being adjusted according to the patient's course. More recently, the combination of cyclosporin-A, a fungal metabolite which is a cyclic oligopeptide, and low-dose prednisone has proved to be a promising immunosuppressive regimen.[539]

In the absence of rejection, the transplanted heart, which of course is denervated and lacks autonomic neural control, has the capacity to maintain a normal resting cardiac output. During exercise, stroke volume rises first, after which increased levels of circulating catecholamines cause tachycardia. As a consequence of this near-normal circulatory response, the transplanted heart has allowed functional rehabilitation in 90 per cent of the long-term survivors in the Stanford program.[540,541]

Transplant recipients are monitored in order to detect a fall in electrocardiographic QRS voltage (reflecting myocardial edema), atrial arrhythmias, and an S_3 gallop as early manifestations of the rejection process. These changes can be confirmed by histopathological examination of tissue obtained by percutaneous transvenous (internal jugular) biopsy of the right ventricular endomyocardium (p. 297).[542] Acute rejection can be treated successfully in more than 90 per cent of patients by high-dose boluses of methylprednisolone and antithymocyte globulin. Infections complicating intense immunosuppression are still the major hazard to survival. Continued medical surveillance is required at 2- to 4-week intervals. In the late postoperative course the threat of rejection continues, but its likelihood is considerably less than it is earlier in the course. However, accelerated coronary atherosclerosis, presumably due to rejection-induced injury to the coronary arterial intima, develops in the transplanted heart of a small number of patients. As in kidney transplant programs involving chronic immunosuppression, malignant neoplasms, usually of the lymphoreticular type, have been observed in a few recipients.

Patients who survive for three months have a better than 75 per cent two-year survival rate. Patients younger than 40 years and those who have had previous cardiac surgery associated with blood transfusions exhibit even better survival. Subsequent attrition is approximately 5 per cent per year and reflects the continuing hazards threatening immunosuppressed patients.[543] Despite advances in distant heart procurement procedures,[536] it is likely that the supply of donor hearts will continue to be a limiting factor in the number of cardiac transplants performed.

MECHANICAL CIRCULATORY SUPPORT

INTRAAORTIC BALLOON COUNTERPULSATION. This method of partial circulatory support is described on page 1317 and is illustrated in Figure 18–10 (p. 593). The phased inflation during diastole of a balloon inserted into the descending aorta through the femoral artery generally increases cardiac output by 10 to 20 per cent and elevates arterial diastolic pressure while reducing arterial systolic pressure.[544-548] A major application of this technique has been in patients with acute left ventricular failure secondary to acute myocardial infarction (cardiogenic shock), but it has also been utilized to support the circulation in patients with acute ischemic syndromes who are undergoing cardiac catheterization, angiocardiography, and coronary arteriography.[549] Of increasing importance is the use of intraaortic balloon counterpulsation during the perioperative period in patients undergoing cardiac surgery and developing acute heart failure. Usually this method of therapy is applied for 24 to 48 hours, after which an attempt is made to wean the patient from the support provided by the balloon. In some instances, counterpulsation has been continued for as long as two weeks.

The principal advantage of the technique is its relative simplicity and low risk. Ease of insertion of the device has been improved by the introduction of percutaneous methods not requiring surgical cutdown (p. 298). The major disadvantage is that it offers only modest circulatory support (elevation of cardiac index up to 0.8 liter/min/m²) and cannot sustain life in extremely severe heart failure or in the presence of chaotic cardiac rhythms.

TEMPORARY LEFT VENTRICULAR ASSISTANCE. For patients who cannot be resuscitated or sustained by pharmacologic therapy and intraaortic balloon assistance, a more effective means of circulatory support is required. In patients in whom recovery of left ventricular function is anticipated and where removal of the pump is expected, several groups have developed left ventricular assist devices consisting of a pump with afferent and efferent conduits attached to the left ventricular apex and ascending thoracic aorta, respectively[550-552,552a,552b] (Fig. 16–24). The inflow and outflow conduits each contain a xenograft (porcine) valve to provide unidirectional flow. The pneumatic power source and control circuit are extracorporeal, and the pump itself rests on the anterior chest wall. Pumping is accomplished by the introduction of carbon dioxide under pressure into the space between the flexible bladder and rigid housing. Stroke volumes of 85 ml and rates of 100 beats/min can be achieved.

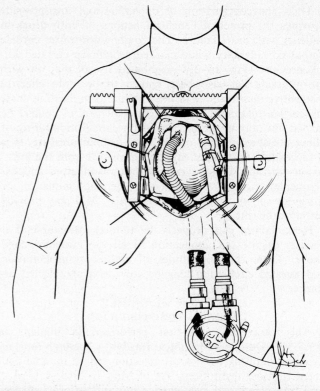

FIGURE 16–24 Pneumatically powered ventricular-assist pump as employed after cardiac operation but before chest closure. Blood is removed from the left atrium and pumped into the ascending aorta. (Reproduced with permission from Pierce, W. S., et al.: Ventricular-assist pumping in patients with cardiogenic shock after cardiac operations. N. Engl. J. Med. *305*:1606, 1981.)

Clinical trials are currently underway in patients who have had corrective cardiac surgery and in whom (1) pump oxygenator dependence develops in spite of intensive treatment with conventional measures, including intraaortic balloon counterpulsation, and (2) refractory cardiogenic shock occurs within 72 hours of the operation. In addition, it is being tested in patients with terminal heart failure secondary to acute (presumably viral) myocarditis and in patients with acute myocardial infarction and refractory cardiogenic shock.

When the left ventricular assist device is first applied to the patient, it handles almost the total left-heart output, while the patient's left ventricle performs little work. If, as a result of this "rest" period for 48 to 72 hours, the myocardium recovers, the left ventricle may be allowed to resume pumping a gradually increasing fraction of systemic blood flow, and attempts to wean the patient from the assist device are undertaken. Temporary reductions in the output of the mechanical device are made, and if adequate cardiac output and arterial pressures are maintained without a marked increase in left atrial pressure, withdrawal of mechanical support can be planned. Severe right-heart failure leads to inadequate left-heart filling, and the low preload precludes adequate inflow into the left ventricular assist device. Inotropic support of the right heart with catecholamines is therefore frequently necessary.

Norman, Cooley, and colleagues have developed an intracorporeal (abdominal) left ventricular assist device that is undergoing clinical testing,[553] and Rose et al. have reported clinical experiences in 16 patients with perioperative myocardial infarction and shock who could not be weaned from cardiopulmonary bypass despite use of inotropic agents and the intraaortic balloon pump and were treated with partial left heart (left atrium–aorta) bypass; eight patients survived.[554]

There is increasing evidence that approximately 25 per cent of patients whose hearts cannot sustain life despite pharmacologic therapy and intraaortic balloon counterpulsation can be maintained alive, survive discontinuation of left ventricular assistance, and leave the hospital. Obviously, long-term survival from this temporary period of support can be attained only if the cardiac insult is reversible.

PERMANENT LEFT VENTRICULAR ASSISTANCE. Patients whose left ventricles have sustained permanent damage and in whom recovery of function sufficient to support the circulation is not anticipated would be candidates for permanent left ventricular assistance. Potential candidates are patients with end-stage left ventricular disease, resulting from ischemic or other cardiomyopathies, patients with left ventricular infarction and shock, and postoperative patients with intractable left ventricular failure who are dependent on and cannot be weaned from temporary left ventricular assistance. These permanent devices, currently undergoing refinement and chronic testing in animals, are similar to those described above for temporary left ventricular assistance, except that the pump which fills from the left atrium or left ventricle and ejects blood into the aorta is implanted into the thorax or abdominal cavity. The energy source for these pumps is external and either an air tube or a wire passes through the skin. The native heart remains in situ, and survival requires continued function of the right ventricle. Such devices have functioned in calves for several months,[555,556] but at the time of this writing they have not been employed successfully for prolonged periods in human patients.

THE TOTAL ARTIFICIAL HEART. Also known as the biventricular replacement device, the *total* artificial heart involves the use of two mechanical pumps that replace the natural ventricles and support both the systemic and pulmonary circulations. With such a device the natural heart is excised. The contemplated use of the total arti-

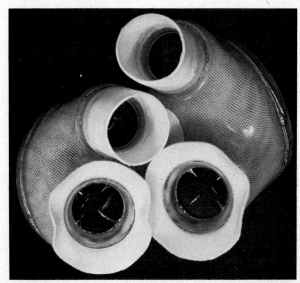

FIGURE 16–26 Utah total artificial heart. (Reproduced with permission from DeVries, W. C.: The total artificial heart. In Sabiston, D. C., Jr., and Spencer, F. C. (Eds.): Surgery of the Chest, 4th Ed. Philadelphia, W. B. Saunders Company, 1983.)

ficial heart is in patients who could not otherwise survive and in whom the natural heart is permanently useless or even a threat to life, such as patients with large left ventricular infarctions and with rupture of the left ventricle or an irreparable ventricular septal defect or patients in whom catastrophic injury to the heart occurs during operation.

Since the first report describing the implantation of an artificial heart in an experimental animal in 1958, progress has been made, albeit gradually, toward the goal of developing a practical, totally implanted device that will support the circulation and allow a comfortable existence.[557] When successful clinical cardiac transplantation was first accomplished, the concept that a mechanical heart would become a useful therapeutic device was in doubt. However,

JARVIK ELLIPTICAL ARTIFICIAL HEART VENTRICLE

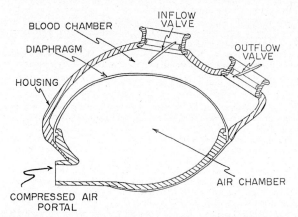

FIGURE 16–25 Cutaway of pneumatic ventricle. (Reproduced with permission from DeVries, W. C.: The total artificial heart. In Sabiston, D. C., Jr., and Spencer, F. C. (Eds.): Surgery of the Chest, 4th Ed. Philadelphia, W. B. Saunders Company, 1983.)

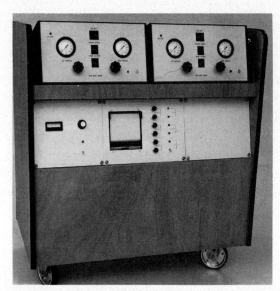

FIGURE 16–27 Utah heart drive system. (Reproduced with permission from DeVries, W. C.: The total artificial heart. In Sabiston, D. C., Jr., and Spencer, F. C. (Eds.): Surgery of the Chest, 4th Ed. Philadelphia, W. B. Saunders Company, 1983.)

the serious problems faced in obtaining donor hearts and in coordinating donor heart availability and recipient need have forced a reevaluation of transplantation as the ultimate solution to intractable heart failure.

A variety of devices is now being tested in experimental animals. A promising artificial heart recently developed[557a] consists of an electronic control system and two smooth-surfaced, sac-type pumps made of segmental polyurethane (Fig. 16–25 and 16–26). Two pneumatic power units (Fig. 16–27) pulse air intermittently to move the diaphragm, thereby moving blood into and out of the blood chamber (Fig. 16–25). Four pyrolitic carbon disc valves assure the unidirectional blood flow. A similar device[556,558] totally assumed the function of the heart for as long as six months in calves, which ate well and gained weight, and for more than three months in one patient, Dr. Barney Clark. The control system has the capability of balancing the output automatically during exercise. Bulky, electrically driven air-powered units (Fig. 16–27) positioned alongside the recipient power the artificial ventricles through air tubes. Current research centers on the development of pumps powered by implanted compact electrical motors.[556,558,559] At this time it appears that the problems inherent in the development of a totally implanted heart capable of permanent support of the circulation, although they have not been solved, are not insurmountable.

References

Digitalis Glycosides

1. Opie, L. H.: Principles of therapy for congestive heart failure. Europ. Heart J. 4(Suppl. A):199, 1983.
2. Withering, W.: An account of the foxglove and some of its medical uses, with practical remarks on dropsy, and other diseases. In Willis, F. A., and Keys, T. E. (eds.): Classics of Cardiology. New York, Henry Schuman, Inc., 1941, p. 231.
2a. Marshall, P. G.: Steroids: Cardiotonic glycosides and aglycons: Toad poisons. In Coffey, S. (ed.): Rodd's Chemistry of Carbon Compounds. 2nd ed. Vol. 2D, Steroids. Amsterdam, Elsevier Publishing Co., 1970, p. 360.
3. Hoffman, B. F., and Bigger, J. T., Jr.: Digitalis and allied cardiac glycosides. In Gilman, A. G., Goodman, L. S., and Gilman, A. (eds.): The Pharmacological Basis of Therapeutics. 2nd ed. New York, Macmillan Publishing Company, Inc., 1980.
4. Lee, K. S., and Klaus, W.: The subcellular basis for the mechanism of inotropic action of cardiac glycosides. Pharmacol. Rev. 23:193, 1971.
5. Schwartz, A., Lindenmayer, G. E., and Allen, J. C.: The sodium-potassium adenosine triphosphatase: Pharmacological, physiological and biochemical aspects. Pharmacol. Rev. 27:1, 1975.
6. Akera, T., and Brody, T. M.: The role of Na^+,K^+-ATPase in the inotropic action of digitalis. Pharmacol. Rev. 29:187, 1977.
7. Smith, T. W., and Barry, W. H.: Monovalent cation transport and mechanisms of digitalis-induced inotropy. Yale Symposium, 1982, in press.
8. Moran, N. C.: The effects of cardiac glycosides on mechanical properties of heart muscle. In Marks, B. H., and Weissler, A. M. (eds.): Basic and Clinical Pharmacology of Digitalis. Springfield, Ill., Charles C Thomas, 1972, p. 94.
9. Koch-Weser, J., and Blinks, J. R.: Analysis of the relation of the positive inotropic action of cardiac glycosides to the frequency of contraction of heart muscle. J. Pharmacol. Exp. Ther. 136:305, 1962.
10. Farah, A. E.: The effects of the ionic milieu on the response of cardiac muscle to cardiac glycosides. In Fisch, C., and Surawicz, B. (eds.): Digitalis. New York, Grune and Stratton, 1969, p. 55.
11. Spann, J. F., Jr., Sonnenblick, E. H., Cooper, T., Chidsey, C. A., Willman, V. L., and Braunwald, E.: Studies on digitalis. XIV. Influence of cardiac norepinephrine stores on the response of isolated heart muscle to digitalis. Circ. Res. 19:326, 1966.
12. Koch-Weser, J.: Beta-receptor blockade and myocardial effects of cardiac glycosides. Circ. Res. 28:109, 1971.
13. Entman, M. L., Cook, J. W., Jr., and Bressler, R.: The influence of ouabain and alpha angelica lactone on calcium metabolism of dog cardiac microsomes. J. Clin. Invest. 48:229, 1969.
14. Katz, A. M.: Contractile proteins of the heart. Physiol. Rev. 50:63, 1970.
15. Coleman, H. N.: Role of acetylstrophanthidin in augmenting myocardial oxygen consumption. Circ. Res. 21:487, 1967.
16. Weingart, R., Kass, R. S., and Tsien, R. W.: Is digitalis inotropy associated with enhanced slow inward calcium current? Nature 273:389, 1978.

17. Lederer, W. J., and Eisner, D. A.: The effects of sodium pump activity on the slow inward current in sheep cardiac Purkinje fibers. Proc. Roy. Soc., Series B.
18. Marban, E., and Tsien, R. W.: Enhancement of cardiac calcium current during digitalis inotropy: Positive feedback regulation by intracellular calcium? J. Physiol. (London) 329:589, 1982.
19. Fabiato, A., and Fabiato, F.: Activation of skinned cardiac cells. Subcellular effects of cardioactive drugs. Eur. J. Cardiol. 1:145–155, 1973.
20. Bailey, L. E., and Harvey, S. C.: Effect of ouabain on cardiac ^{45}Ca kinetics measured by indicator dilution. Am. J. Physiol. 216:123, 1969.
21. Langer, G. A., and Serena, S. D.: Effects of strophanthidin upon contraction and ionic exchange in rabbit ventricular myocardium: Relation to control of active state. J. Molec. Cell. Cardiol. 1:65, 1970.
22. Biedert, S., Barry, W. H., and Smith, T. W.: Inotropic effects and changes in sodium and calcium contents associated with inhibition of monovalent cation active transport by ouabain in cultured myocardial cells. J. Gen. Physiol. 74:479, 1979.
22a. Morgan, J. P., and Blinks, J. R.: Intracellular Ca^{++} transients in the cat papillary muscle. Can. J. Physiol. Pharmacol. 60:524, 1982.
23. Schatzmann, H. J.: Herzglykoside als Hemmstoffe für den activen Kalium- and Natriumtransport durch die Erythrocytenmembran. Helv. Physiol. Pharmacol. Acta 11:346, 1953.
24. Skou, J. C.: Enzymatic basis for active transport of Na^+ and K^+ across cell membrane. Physiol. Rev. 43:596, 1965.
25. Repke, K., Est, M., and Portius, H. F.: Über die Ursache der Speciesunterschiede in der Digitalisempfindlichkeit. Biochem. Pharmacol. 14:1785, 1965.
26. Schwartz, A., Matsui, H., and Laughter, A. H.: Tritiated digoxin binding to Na^+, K^+-activated adenosine-triphosphatase: Possible allosteric site. Science 160:323, 1968.
27. Flasch, H., and Heinz, N.: Correlation between inhibition of NaK-membrane-ATPase and positive inotropic activity of cardenolides in isolated papillary muscles of guinea pig. Naunyn Schmiedebergs Arch. Pharmakol. 304:37–44, 1978.
28. Allen, J. C., and Schwartz, A.: A possible biochemical explanation for the sensitivity of the rat to cardiac glycosides. J. Pharmacol. Exp. Ther. 168:42, 1969.
29. Akera, T., Baskin, S. I., Tobin, T., and Brody, T. M.: Ouabain: Temporal relationship between the inotropic effect and the in vitro binding to, and dissociation from, (Na^+,K^+)-activated ATPase. Naunyn Schmiedebergs Arch. Pharmakol. 277:151, 1973.
30. Ku, D., Akera, T., Pew, C. L., and Brody, T. M.: Cardiac glycosides: Correlation among Na^+,K^+-ATPase, sodium pump and contractility in the guinea pig heart. Naunyn Schmiedebergs Arch. Pharmakol. 285:185, 1974.
31. Akera, T., Olgaard, M. K., Temma, K., and Brody, T. M.: Development of the positive inotropic action of ouabain: Effects of transmembrane sodium movement. J. Pharmacol. Exp. Ther. 203:675, 1977.
32. Wasserman, O., and Holland, W. C.: Effects of tetrodotoxin and ouabain on atrial contractions. Pharmacol. Res. Commun. 1:236, 1969.
33. Barry, W. H., Liechty, L., Beaudoin, D., and Smith, T. W.: Comparison of effects of a low extracellular potassium concentration and cardiac glycoside on contractility, monovalent cation transport and Na-Ca exchange in cultured ventricular cells. Trans. Assoc. Amer. Phys. 95:12, 1982.
34. Eisner, D. A., and Lederer, W. J.: The role of the sodium pump in the effects of potassium-depleted solutions on mammalian cardiac muscle. J. Physiol. (London) 294:279–301, 1979.
35. Akera, T., Larsen, F. S., and Brody, T. M.: Correlation of cardiac sodium- and potassium-activated adenosine triphosphatase activity with ouabain-induced inotropic stimulation. J. Pharmacol. Exp. Ther. 173:145, 1970.
36. Hougen, T. J., and Smith, T. W.: Inhibition of myocardial monovalent cation active transport by subtoxic doses of ouabain in the dog. Circ. Res. 42:856, 1978.
37. Somberg, J. C., Barry, W. H., and Smith, T. W.: Differing sensitivities of Purkinje fibers and myocardium to inhibition of monovalent cation transport by digitalis. J. Clin. Invest. 67:116–123, 1981.
38. Prindle, K. H., Jr., Skelton, C. L., Epstein, S. E., and Marcus, F. I.: Influence of extracellular potassium concentration on myocardial uptake and inotropic effect of tritiated digoxin. Circ. Res. 28:337, 1971.
39. Bonting, S. L., Hawkins, N. M., and Canady, M. R.: Studies of sodium-potassium activated adenosine triphosphatase. VII. Inhibition by erythrophleum alkaloids. Biochem. Pharmacol. 13:13, 1964.
40. Akera, T.: Membrane adenosine triphosphatase: A digitalis receptor? Science 198:569, 1977.
41. Kyte, J.: Purification of the sodium- and potassium-dependent adenosine triphosphatase from canine renal medulla. J. Biol. Chem. 246:4157, 1971.
42. Hokin, L. E., Dahl, J. L., Deupree, J. D., Dixon, J. F., Hackney, J. F., and Perdue, J. F.: Studies on the characterization of the sodium-potassium transport adenosine triphosphatase. X. Purification of the enzyme from the rectal gland of a Squalus acanthias. J. Biol. Chem. 248:2593, 1973.
43. Hopkins, B. E., Wagner, H., Jr., and Smith, T. W.: Sodium- and potassium-activated adenosine triphosphatase of the nasal salt gland of the duck (Anas platyrhynchos): Purification, characterization, and NH_2-terminal amino acid sequence of the phosphorylating polypeptide. J. Biol. Chem. 251:4365, 1976.
44. Forbush, B., III, Kaplan, J. H., and Hoffman, J. F.: Characterization of a new photoaffinity derivative of ouabain: Labelling of the large polypeptide and of a proteolipid component of the Na,K-ATPase. Biochemistry 17:3667, 1978.
45. Kyte, J.: The titration of the cardiac glycoside binding site of the $(Na^+ + K^+)$-adenosine triphosphatase. J. Biol. Chem. 247:7634, 1972.

46. Pitts, B. J. R., and Schwartz, A.: Improved purification and partial characterization of (Na+,K+)-ATPase from cardiac muscle. Biochim. Biophys. Acta 401:184, 1975.

47. Calhoun, J. A., and Harrison, T. R.: Studies in congestive heart failure. IX. The effect of digitalis on the potassium content of the cardiac muscle of dogs. J. Clin. Invest. 10:139, 1931.

48. Ellis, D.: The effects of external cations and ouabain on the intracellular sodium activity of sheep heart Purkinje fibers. J. Physiol. (London) 273:211, 1977.

49. Lee, C. O., Kang, D. H., Sokol, J. H., and Lee, K. S.: Relation between intracellular Na ion activity and tension of sheep cardiac Purkinje fibers exposed to dihydro-ouabain. Biophys. J. 29:315, 1980.

50. Cohen, C. J., Fozzard, H. A., and Shen, S-S.:Increase in intracellular sodium ion activity during stimulation in mammalian cardiac muscle. Circ. Res. 50:651, 1982.

51. Langer, G. A.: Relationship between myocardial contractility and the effects of digitalis on ionic exchange. Fed. Proc. 36:2231, 1977.

52. Baker, P. F., Blaustein, M. P., Hodgkin, A. L., and Steinhardt, R. A.: The influence of calcium on sodium efflux in squid axons. J. Physiol. (London) 200:431, 1969.

53. Glitsch, H. G., Reuter, H., and Scholz, H.: The effect of the internal sodium concentration on calcium fluxes in isolated guinea pig auricles. J. Physiol. (London) 209:25–43, 1970.

54. Akera, T., Bennett, R. T., Olgaard, M. K., and Brody, T. M.: Cardiac (Na+ + K+)-adenosine triphosphatase inhibition by ouabain and myocardial sodium: A computer simulation. J. Pharmacol. Exp. Ther. 199:287, 1976.

55. Gervais, A., Lane, L. K., Anner, B. M., Lindenmayer, G. E., and Schwartz, A.: A possible molecular mechanism of the action of digitalis: Ouabain action on calcium binding to sites associated with a purified sodium-potassium-activated adenosine triphosphatase. Circ. Res. 40:8, 1977.

56. Lüllman, H., and Peters, T.: Action of cardiac glycosides on the excitation-contraction coupling in heart muscle. Progr. Pharmacol. 2:1, 1979.

57. Schon, R., Schonfeld, W., Menke, K.-H., and Repke, K. R. H.: Mechanism and role of Na+/Ca++ competition in (NaK)-ATPase. Acta Biol. Med. Germ. 29:643, 1972.

58. Okita, G. T.: Dissociation of Na+,K+-ATPase inhibition from digitalis inotropy. Fed. Proc. 36:2275, 1977.

59. Schwartz, A.: Brief reviews: Is the cell membrane Na+,K+-ATPase enzyme system the pharmacological receptor of digitalis? Circ. Res. 39:2, 1976.

60. Noble, D.: Mechanism of action of therapeutic levels of cardiac glycosides. Cardiovasc. Res. 14:495–514, 1980.

61. Smith, T. W., Antman, E. M., Friedman, P. L., Blatt, C. M., and Marsh, J. D.: Digitalis glycosides: Mechanisms and manifestations of toxicity. Progr. Cardiovasc. Dis. In Press.

62. Smith, T. W., and Barry, W. H.: The role of NaK-ATPase as a cardiac glycoside receptor. In Haft, J., and Karliner, J. (eds.): Textbook on Cardiac Receptors. In Press.

63. Goldman, R. H., Deutscher, R. N., Schweizer, E., and Harrison, D. C.: Effect of a pharmacologic dose of digoxin on inotropy in hyper- and normokalemic dogs. Am. J. Physiol. 223:1438, 1972.

64. Seller, R. H.: The role of magnesium in digitalis toxicity. Am. Heart J. 82:511, 1971.

65. Hoffman, J. F.: The red cell membrane and the transport of sodium and potassium. Am. J. Med. 41:666, 1966.

66. Perrone, J. R., and Blostein, R.: Asymmetric interaction of inside-out and right-side-out erythrocyte membrane vesicles with ouabain. Biochim. Biophys. Acta 291:680, 1973.

67. Caldwell, P. C., and Keynes, R. D.: The effect of ouabain on the efflux of sodium from a squid axon. J. Physiol. (London) 148:8P, 1959.

68. Smith, T. W., Wagner, H., Jr., Markis, J. E., and Young, M.: Studies on the localization of the cardiac receptor. J. Clin. Invest. 51:1777, 1972.

69. Smith, T. W., Wagner, H., Jr., and Young, M.: Cardiac glycoside interaction with solubilized myocardial sodium- and potassium-dependent adenosine triphosphatase. Molec. Pharmacol. 10:626, 1974.

70. Rosen, M. R., Wit, A. L., and Hoffman, B. F.: Electrophysiology and pharmacology of cardiac arrhythmias. IV. Cardiac antiarrhythmic and toxic effects of digitalis. Am. Heart J. 89:391, 1975.

71. Dhingra, R. C., Amat-Y-Leon, F., Wyndham, C., Wu, D., Denes, P., and Rosen, K. M.: The electrophysiological effects of ouabain on sinus node and atrium in man. J. Clin. Invest. 56:555, 1975.

72. Goodman, D. J., Rossen, R. M., Ingham, R., Rider, A. K., and Harrison, D. C.: Sinus node function in the denervated human heart: Effects of digitalis. Br. Heart J. 37:612, 1975.

73. Goodman, D. J., Rossen, R. M., Cannom, D. S., Rider, A. K., and Harrison, D. C.: Effect of digoxin on atrioventricular conduction: Studies in patients with and without cardiac autonomic innervation. Circulation 51:251, 1975.

74. Kim, Y. I., Noble, R. J., and Zipes, D. P.: Dissociation of the inotropic effect of digitalis from its effect on atrioventricular conduction. Am. J. Cardiol. 36:459, 1975.

75. Hordof, A. J., Spotnitz, A., Mary-Rabine, L., Edie, R., and Rosen, M. R.: The cellular electrophysiologic effects of digitalis on human atrial fibers. Circulation 54:223, 1978.

76. Przybyla, A. C., Paulay, K. L., Stein, E., and Damato, A. N.: Effects of digoxin on atrioventricular conduction patterns in man. Am. J. Cardiol. 33:344, 1974.

77. Rosen, M. R., Hordof, A. J., Hodess, A. B., Verosky, M., and Vulliemoz, Y.: Ouabain-induced changes in electrophysiologic properties of neonatal, young

and adult canine cardiac Purkinje fibers. J. Pharmacol. Exp. Ther. 194:255, 1975.

78. Rogers, M. C., Willerson, J. T., Goldblatt, A., and Smith, T. W.: Serum digoxin concentrations in the human fetus, neonate, and infant. N. Engl. J. Med. 287:1010, 1972.

79. Weingart, R.: Influence of cardiac glycosides on electrophysiologic processes. In Greeff, K. (ed.): Cardiac Glycosides. Vol. 56, Part I, Handbook of Experimental Pharmacology. Berlin, Springer-Verlag, 1981.

79a.Gillis, R. A., and Quest, J. A.: The role of the nervous system in the cardiovascular effects of digitalis. Pharmacol. Rev. 31:19–97, 1979.

80. Pace, C. B., and Gillis, R. A.: Neuroexcitatory effects of digoxin in the cat. J. Pharmacol. Exp. Ther. 199:583, 1976.

81. Gillis, R. A., Raines, A., Sohn, Y. J., Levitt, B., and Standaert, F. G.: Neuroexcitatory effects of digitalis and their role in the development of cardiac arrhythmias. J. Pharmacol. Exp. Ther. 183:154, 1972.

81a.Levitt, B., Cagin, N. A., Somberg, J., Bounous, H., Mittag, T., and Raines, A.: Alteration of the effects and distribution of ouabain by spinal cord transection in the cat. J. Pharmacol. Exp. Ther. 185:24, 1973.

82. Somberg, J. C., and Smith, T. W.: Localization of the neurally mediated arrhythmogenic properties of digitalis. Science 204:321, 1979.

83. Somberg, J. C., Risler, T., and Smith, T. W.: Neural factors in digitalis toxicity: Protective effect of C-1 spinal cord transection. Am. J. Physiol. 235:H531–536, 1978.

84. Mudge, G. H., Jr., Lloyd, B. L., Greenblatt, D. J., and Smith, T. W.: Inotropic and toxic effects of a polar cardiac glycoside derivative in the dog. Circ. Res. 43:847, 1978.

85. Smith, T. W.: The future of inotropic drugs in clinical practice. Eur. Heart J. 3:149, 1982.

86. Wiggers, C. J., and Stimson, B.: Studies on cardiodynamic action of drugs. III. The mechanism of cardiac stimulation by digitalis and g-strophanthin. J. Pharmacol. Exp. Ther. 30:251, 1927.

87. Cattell, M., and Gold, H.: The influence of digitalis glycosides on the force of contraction of mammalian cardiac muscle. J. Pharmacol. Exp. Ther. 62:116, 1938.

88. Braunwald, E., Bloodwell, R. D., Goldberg, L. I., and Morrow, A. G.: Studies on digitalis. IV. Observations in man on the effects of digitalis preparations on the contractility of the non-failing heart and on total vascular resistance. J. Clin. Invest. 40:52, 1961.

89. Cotten, M. deV., and Stopp, P. E.: Action of digitalis on the nonfailing heart of the dog. Am. J. Physiol. 192:114, 1958.

90. Spann, J. F., Jr., Buccino, R. A., Sonnenblick, E. H., and Braunwald, E.: Contractile state of cardiac muscle obtained from cats with experimentally produced ventricular hypertrophy and heart failure. Circ. Res. 21:341, 1967.

91. Burwell, C. S., Neighbors, DeW., and Regen, E. M.: The effect of digitalis upon the output of the heart in normal man. J. Clin. Invest. 5:125, 1927.

92. Harvey, R. M., Ferrer, M. I., Cathcart, R. T., and Alexander, J. K.: Some effects of digoxin on the heart and circulation in man: Digoxin in enlarged hearts not in clinical congestive failure. Circulation 4:366, 1951.

93. Sonnenblick, E. H., Williams, J. F., Jr., Glick, G., Mason, D. T., and Braunwald, E.: Studies on digitalis. XV. Effects of cardiac glycosides on myocardial force-velocity relations in the nonfailing human heart. Circulation 34:532, 1966.

94. Smith, T. W.: Medical treatment of advanced congestive heart failure: Digitalis and diuretics. In Braunwald, E., Moch, M. B., and Watson, J. T. (eds.): Congestive Heart Failure. New York, Grune and Stratton, Inc., 1982, pp. 261–278.

95. Arnold, S. B., Byrd, R. C., Meister, W., Melmon, K., Cheitlin, M. D., Bristow, J. D., Parmley, W. W., and Chatterjee, K.: Long-term digitalis therapy improves left ventricular function in heart failure. N. Engl. J. Med. 303:1443–1448, 1980.

96. Lee, D. C.-S., Johnson, R. A., Bingham, J. B., Leahy, M., Dinsmore, R. E., Goroll, A. H., Newell, J. B., Strauss, H. W., and Haber, E.: Heart failure in outpatients. A randomized trial of digoxin versus placebo. N. Engl. J. Med. 306:699–705, 1982.

97. Murray, R. G., Tweddel, A. C., Martin, W., Pearson, D., Hutton, I., and Lawrie, T. D. V.: Evaluation of digitalis in cardiac failure. Br. Med. J. 284:1526–1528, 1982.

98. Fleg, J. L., Gottlieb, S. H., and Lakatta, E. G.: Is digoxin really important in treatment of compensated heart failure? Am. J. Med. 73:244–250, 1982.

99. Williams, F. J., Jr., Klocke, F. J., and Braunwald, E.: Studies on digitalis. XIII. A comparison of the effects of potassium on the inotropic and arrhythmia-producing actions of ouabain. J. Clin. Invest. 45:346, 1965.

100. Klein, M., Nejad, N. S., Lown, B., Hagemeijer, F., and Barr, I.: Correlation of the electrical and mechanical changes in the dog heart during progressive digitalization. Circ. Res. 29:635, 1971.

101. Beiser, G. D., Epstein, S. E., Stampfer, M., Robinson, B., and Braunwald, E.: Studies on digitalis. XVII. Effects of ouabain on the hemodynamic response to exercise in patients with mitral stenosis in normal sinus rhythm. N. Engl. J. Med. 278:131, 1968.

102. Mason, D. T., Zelis, R., and Amsterdam, E. A.: Unified concept of the mechanism of action of digitalis: Influence of ventricular function and cardiac disease on hemodynamic response to fundamental contractile effect. In Marks, B. H., and Weissler, A. M. (eds.): Basic and Clinical Pharmacology of Digitalis. Springfield, Ill., Charles C Thomas, 1972, p. 206.

103. Ross, J., Jr., Waldhausen, J. A., and Braunwald, E.: Studies on digitalis. I. Direct effects on peripheral vascular resistance. J. Clin. Invest. 39:930, 1960.

104. Goldman, M. R., Wold, S. W., Rulten, D. L., and Powell, W. J., Jr.: Effect of

ouabain on total vascular capacity in the dog. J. Clin. Invest. 69:175–184, 1982.

105. Mason, D. T., and Braunwald, E.: Studies on digitalis. X. Effects of ouabain on forearm vascular resistance and venous tone in normal subjects and in patients in heart failure. J. Clin. Invest. 43:532, 1964.

106. Stark, J. J., Sanders, C. A., and Powell, W. J., Jr.: Neurally mediated and direct effects of acetylstrophanthidin on canine skeletal muscle vascular resistance. Circ. Res. 30:274, 1972.

107. Garan, H., Smith, T. W., and Powell, W. J., Jr.: The central nervous system as a site of action for the coronary vasoconstrictor effect of digoxin. J. Clin. Invest. 54:1365, 1974.

108. Sagar, K. B., Hanson, E. C., and Powell, W. J.: Neurogenic coronary vasoconstrictor effects of digitalis during acute global ischemia in dogs. J. Clin. Invest. 60:1248, 1977.

109. Kumar, R., Yankopoulos, N. A., and Abelmann, W. H.: Ouabain-induced hypertension in a patient with decompensated hypertensive heart disease. Chest 63:105, 1973.

110. Cohn, J. N., Tristani, F. E., and Khatri, I. M.: Cardiac and peripheral vascular effects of digitalis in clinical shock. Am. Heart J. 78:318, 1969.

111. Shanbour, L. L., and Jacobson, E. D.: Digitalis and the mesenteric circulation. Am. J. Dig. Dis. 17:826, 1972.

112. DeMots, H., Rahimtoola, S. H., McAnulty, J. H., and Porter, G. A.: Effects of ouabain on coronary and systemic vascular resistance and myocardial oxygen consumption in patients without heart failure. Am. J. Cardiol. 41:88, 1978.

113. Zelis, R., and Mason, D. T.: Compensatory mechanisms in congestive heart failure: The role of the peripheral resistance vessels. N. Engl. J. Med. 282:962, 1970.

114. Strickler, J. C., and Kessler, R. H.: Direct renal action of some digitalis steroids. J. Clin. Invest. 40:311, 1961.

115. Torretti, J., Hendler, E., and Weinstein, E.: Functional significance of Na-K-ATPase in the kidney: Effects of ouabain inhibition. Am. J. Physiol. 222:1398, 1972.

116. Gold, H., Cattell, M., Modell, W., Kwit, N. T., Kramer, M. L., and Zahm, W.: Clinical studies on digitoxin (Digitaline Nativelle): With further observations on its use in the single average full dose method of digitalization. J. Pharmacol. Exp. Ther. 82:187, 1944.

117. Gold, H., Modell, W., Kwit, N. T., Shane, S. J., Dayrit, C., Kramer, M. L., Zahm, W., and Otto, H. L.: Comparison of ouabain with strophanthidin-3-acetate by intravenous injection in man. J. Pharmacol. Exp. Ther. 94:39, 1948.

118. Gold, H., Cattell, M., Greiner, T., Hanlon, L. W., Kwit, N. T., Modell, W., Cotlove, E., Benton, J., and Otto, H. L.: Clinical pharmacology of digoxin. J. Pharmacol. Exp. Ther. 109:45, 1953.

119. Cardiac Glycosides. Part II: Pharmacokinetics and Clinical Pharmacology. In Greeff, K. (ed.): Handbook of Experimental Pharmacology, Vol. 56. Berlin, Springer-Verlag, 1981.

120. Smith, T. W.: Drug therapy: Digitalis glycosides. N. Engl. J. Med. 288:719, 1973.

121. Peters, V., Falk, L. C., and Kalman, S. M.: Digoxin metabolism in patients. Arch. Intern. Med. 138:1074–1076, 1978.

122. Lindenbaum, J., Tse-Eng, D., Butler, V. P., Jr., and Rund, D. G.: Urinary excretion of reduced metabolites of digoxin. Am. J. Med. 71:67–74, 1981.

122a. Lindenbaum, J., Rund, D. G., and Butler, V. P., Jr.: Inactivation of digoxin by the gut flora: reversal by antibiotic therapy. N. Engl. J. Med. 305:789, 1981.

123. Halkin, H., Sheiner, L. B., Peck, C. C., and Melmon, K. L.: Determinants of the renal clearance of digoxin. Clin. Pharmacol. Ther. 385:394, 1975.

124. Linday, L. A., Engle, M. A., and Reidenberg, M. M.: Maturation and renal digoxin clearance. Clin. Pharmacol. Ther. 30:735–738, 1981.

125. Marcus, F. L., Burkhalter, L., Cuccia, C., Pavlovich, J., and Kapadia, G. G.: Administration of tritiated digoxin with and without a loading dose: A metabolic study. Circulation 34:865, 1966.

126. Ackerman, G. L., Doherty, J. E., and Flanigan, W. J.: Peritoneal dialysis and hemodialysis of tritiated digoxin. Ann. Intern. Med. 67:718, 1967.

127. Coltart, D. J., Chamberlain, D. A., Howard, M. R., Kettlewell, M. G., Mercer, J. L., and Smith, T. W.: The effect of cardiopulmonary bypass on plasma digoxin concentrations. Br. Heart J. 33:334, 1971.

128. Coltart, D. J., Watson, D., and Howard, M. R.: Effect of exchange transfusions on plasma digoxin levels. Arch. Dis. Child. 47:814, 1972.

129. Ewy, G. A., Groves, B. M., Ball, M. F., Nimmol, L., Jackson, B., and Marcus, F.: Digoxin-metabolism in obesity. Circulation 44:810, 1971.

130. Cogan, J. J., Humphreys, M. H., Carlson, C. J., Benowitz, N. L., and Rapaport, E.: Acute vasodilator therapy increases renal clearance of digoxin in patients with congestive heart failure. Circulation 64:973, 1981.

131. Dungan, W. T., Doherty, J. E., Harvey, C., Char, F., and Dalrymple, G. V.: Tritiated digoxin. XVIII. Studies in infants and children. Circulation 46:983, 1972.

132. O'Malley, K., Coleman, E. N., Doig, W. B., and Stevenson, I. H.: Plasma digoxin levels in infants. Arch. Dis. Child. 48:55, 1973.

133. Leahey, E. B., Jr., Reiffel, J. A., Drusin, R. E., Heissenbuttel, R. H., Lovejoy, W. P., and Bigger, J. T., Jr.: Interaction between quinidine and digoxin. J.A.M.A. 240:533, 1978.

134. Lukas, D. S., and DeMartino, A. G.: Binding of digitoxin and some related cardenolides to human plasma proteins. J. Clin. Invest. 48:1041, 1969.

135. Storstein, L.: Studies on digitalis. I. Renal excretion of digitoxin and its cardioactive metabolites. Clin. Pharmacol. Ther. 16:14, 1974.

136. Storstein, L.: Studies on digitalis. II. The influence of impaired renal function on the renal excretion of digitoxin and its cardioactive metabolites. Clin. Pharmacol. Ther. 16:25, 1974.

137. Okita, G. T.: Distribution, disposition and excretion of digitalis glycosides. In Fisch, C., and Surawicz, B. (eds.): Digitalis. New York, Grune and Stratton, 1969, p. 13.

138. Caldwell, J. H., Bush, C. A., and Greenberger, N. J.: Interruption of the enterohepatic circulation of digitoxin by cholestyramine. II. Effect on metabolic disposition of tritium-labeled digitoxin and cardiac systolic intervals in man. J. Clin. Invest. 52:2638, 1971.

139. Solomon, H. M., and Abrams, W. B.: Interactions between digitoxin and other drugs in man. Am. Heart J. 83:277, 1972.

140. Selden, R., and Smith, T. W.: Ouabain pharmacokinetics in dog and man: Determination by radioimmunoassay. Circulation 45:1176, 1972.

141. Selden, R., Margolies, M. N., and Smith, T. W.: Renal and gastrointestinal excretion of ouabain in dog and man. J. Pharmacol. Exp. Ther. 188:615, 1974.

142. Selden, R., Klein, M. D., and Smith, T. W.: Plasma concentration and urinary excretion kinetics of acetylstrophanthidin. Circulation 47:744, 1973.

143. Cardiac Glycosides. Part II: Pharmacokinetics and Clinical Pharmacology. In Greeff, K. (ed.): Handbook of Experimental Pharmacology, Volume 56. Berlin, Springer-Verlag, 1981.

144. Doherty, J. E., Flanigan, W. J., Murphy, M. L., Bulloch, R. T., Dalrymple, G. V., Beard, O. W., and Perkins, W. H.: Tritiated digoxin. XIV. Enterohepatic circulation, absorption and excretion studies in human volunteers. Circulation 42:867, 1970.

145. Beermann, B., Hellstrom, K., and Rosen, A.: The absorption of orally administered (12α-³H) digoxin in man. Clin. Sci. 43:507, 1972.

146. Greenblatt, D. J., Smith, T. W., and Koch-Weser, J.: Bioavailability of drugs: The digoxin dilemma. Clin. Pharmacokinet. 1:36–51, 1976.

147. Heizer, W. D., Smith, T. W., and Goldfinger, S. E.: Absorption of digoxin in patients with malabsorption syndromes. N. Engl. J. Med. 285:257, 1971.

148. Lindenbaum, J., Mellow, M. H., Blackstone, M. O., and Butler, V. P.: Variation in biologic availability of digoxin from four preparations. N. Engl. J. Med. 285:1344, 1971.

149. Greenblatt, D. J., Smith, T. W., and Koch-Weser, J.: Bioavailability of drugs: The digoxin dilemma. Clin. Pharmacokinet. 1:36, 1976.

150. Harter, J. G., Skelly, J. P., and Steers, A. W.: Digoxin—The regulatory viewpoint. Circulation 49:395, 1974.

151. Jelliffe, R. W., Buell, J., and Kalaba, R.: Reduction of digitalis toxicity by computer-assisted glycoside dosage regimens. Ann. Intern. Med. 77:891, 1972.

152. Jelliffe, R. W., and Brooker, G.: A nomogram for digoxin therapy. Am. J. Med. 57:63, 1974.

153. Peck, C. C., Sheiner, L. B., Martin, C. M., Combs, D. L., and Melmon, K. L.: Computer-assisted digoxin therapy. N. Engl. J. Med. 289:441, 1973.

154. Lown, B., Hagemeijer, F., Barr, I., and Klein, M.: Digitalis intoxication: Clinical and experimental assessment of the degree of digitalization. In Marks, B. H., and Weissler, A. M. (eds.): Basic and Clinical Pharmacology of Digitalis. Springfield, Ill., Charles C Thomas, 1972, p. 299.

155. Lown, B., Klein, M. D., Barr, I., Hagemeijer, F., Kosowsky, B. D., and Garrison, H.: Sensitivity to digitalis drugs in acute myocardial infarction. Am. J. Cardiol. 30:388, 1972.

156. Kleiger, R., and Lown, B.: Cardioversion and digitalis. II. Clinical studies. Circulation 33:878, 1966.

157. Johnson, L. W., Dickstein, R. A., Freuhan, C. T., Kane, P., Potts, J. L., Smulyan, H., Webb, W. R., and Eich, R. H.: Prophylactic digitalization for coronary artery bypass surgery. Circulation 53:819, 1976.

158. Tyras, D. H., Stothert, J. C., Jr., Kaiser, G. C., Barner, H. B., Codd, J. E., and Willman, V. L.: Supraventricular tachyarrhythmias after myocardial revascularization: A randomized trial of prophylactic digitalization. J. Thorac. Cardiovasc. Surg. 77:310, 1979.

159. Schwartz, J. B., Keefe, D., Kates, R. E., Kirsten, E., and Harrison, D. C.: Acute and chronic pharmacodynamic interaction of verapamil and digoxin in atrial fibrillation. Circulation 65:1162–1170, 1982.

160. Sellers, T. D., Bashore, T. M., and Gallagher, J. J.: Digitalis in pre-excitation syndrome—Analysis during atrial fibrillation. Circulation 56:260, 1977.

161. Jelliffe, R. W.: Factors to consider in planning digoxin therapy. J. Chron. Dis. 24:407, 1971.

162. Package Insert—Lanoxin Brand of Digoxin. Burroughs Wellcome Company, March, 1981.

163. Lown, B., and Levine, S. A.: The carotid sinus: Clinical value of its stimulation. Circulation 23:766, 1961.

164. Sampson, J. J., Albertson, E. C., and Kondo, B.: The effect on man of potassium administration in relation to digitalis glycosides with special reference to blood serum potassium, the electrocardiogram and ectopic beats. Am. Heart J. 26:164, 1943.

165. Fisch, C.: Relation of electrolyte disturbances to cardiac arrhythmias. Circulation 47:408, 1973.

166. Davidson, S., and Surawicz, B.: Ectopic beats and atrioventricular conduction disturbances. Arch. Intern. Med. 120:280, 1967.

167. Fisch, C., Martz, B. C., and Priebe, F. H.: Enhancement of potassium-induced atrioventricular block by toxic doses of digitalis drugs. J. Clin. Invest. 39:1885, 1960.

168. Ghani, M. F., and Smith, J. R.: The effectiveness of magnesium chloride in the treatment of ventricular tachyarrhythmias due to digitalis intoxication. Am. Heart J. 88:621, 1974.

169. Neff, M. S., Mendelssohn, S., Kim, K. E., Banach, S., Swartz, C., and Seller, R. H.: Magnesium sulfate in digitalis toxicity. Am. J. Cardiol. 29:377, 1972.

170. Editorial: Calcium, magnesium, and diuretics. Br. Med. J. 1:170, 1975.

171. Holt, D. W., and Goulding, R.: Magnesium depletion and digoxin toxicity. Br. Med. J. 1:627, 1975.

172. Beller, G. A., Hood, W. B., Jr., Smith, T. W., Abelmann, W. H., and Wacker, W. E. C.: Correlation of serum magnesium levels and cardiac digitalis intoxication. Am. J. Cardiol. 33:225, 1974.

173. Gold, H., and Edwards, D. J.: The effects of ouabain on the heart in the presence of hypercalcemia. Am. Heart J. 3:45, 1927.

174. Surawicz, B.: Use of the chelating agent, EDTA, in digitalis intoxication and cardiac arrhythmias. Progr. Cardiovasc. Dis. 2:432, 1959.

175. Warren, M. C., Gianelly, R. E., Cutler, S. L., and Harrison, D. C.: Digitalis toxicity. II. The effect of metabolic alkalosis. Am. Heart J. 75:358, 1968.

176. Galmarini, D., Campdonico, J. F., and Wenk, R. D.: Effect of alkalosis on ouabain toxicity in the dog. J. Pharmacol. Exp. Ther. 186:199, 1973.

177. Williams, J. F., Jr., Boyd, D. C., and Border, J. F.: Effects of acute hypoxia and hypercapnic acidosis on the development of acetylstrophanthidin induced arrhythmias. J. Clin. Invest. 47:1885, 1968.

178. Tisi, G. M., and Moser, K. M.: Effect of acute changes in pO_2, pCO_2, and pH on digitalis toxicity. Circulation 36:11, 1967.

179. Bigger, J. T.: The quinidine-digoxin interaction. Int. J. Cardiol. 1:109–116, 1981.

180. Pedersen, K. E., Dorph-Pedersen, A., Hvidt, S., Klitgaard, N. A., and Nielsen-Kudsk, F.: Digoxin-verapamil interaction. Clin. Pharmacol. Ther. 30:311–316, 1981.

181. Klein, H. O., Lang, R., Weiss, E., Segni, E. D., Libhaber, C., Guerrero, J., and Kaplinsky, E.: The influence of verapamil on serum digoxin concentration. Circulation 65:998–1003, 1982.

182. Belz, G. G., Aust, P. E., and Munkes, R.: Digoxin plasma concentrations and nifedipine. Lancet 1:844–845, 1981.

183. Lessem, J., and Bellinetto, A.: Interaction between digoxin and calcium antagonists. Am. J. Cardiol. 49:1025, 1982.

184. Moysey, J. O., Jaggarao, N. S. V., Grundy, E. N., and Chamberlain, D. A.: Amiodarone increases plasma digoxin concentrations. Br. Med. J. 282:272–273, 1981.

185. Nademanee, K., Kannan, R., Hendrickson, J., Burnam, M., Kay, I., and Singh, B.: Amiodarone-digoxin interaction during treatment of resistant cardiac arrhythmias. Am. J. Cardiol. 49:1026, 1982.

186. Morrow, D. H., and Townley, N. T.: Anesthesia and digitalis toxicity: An experimental study. Anesth. Analg. 43:510, 1964.

187. Dowdy, E. G., and Fabian, L. W.: Ventricular arrhythmias induced by succinylcholine in digitalized patients. Anesth. Analg. 42:501, 1963.

188. Becker, D. J., Nankin, P. M., Bennett, L. D., Kimball, S. G., Sternberg, M. S., and Wasserman, F.: Effect of isoproterenol in digitalis cardiotoxicity. Am. J. Cardiol. 10:242, 1962.

189. Smith, T. W.: Contribution of quantitative assay technics to the understanding of the clinical pharmacology of digitalis. Circulation 46:188, 1972.

190. Smith, T. W., and Willerson, J. T.: Suicidal and accidental digoxin ingestion: Report of five cases with serum digoxin level correlations. Circulation 44:29, 1971.

191. Smith, T. W., Butler, V. P., Jr., Haber, E., Fozzard, H., Marcus, F. I., Bremner, W. F., Schulman, I. C., and Phillips, A.: Treatment of life-threatening digitalis intoxication with digoxin-specific Fab fragments: Experience in 26 cases. N. Engl. J. Med. 307:1357, 1982.

192. Rubinow, A., Skinner, M., and Cohen, A. S.: Digoxin sensitivity in amyloid cardiomyopathy. Circulation 63:1285–1288, 1981.

193. Covell, J. W., Braunwald, E., Ross, J., Jr., and Sonnenblick, E. H.: Studies on digitalis. XVI. Effects on myocardial oxygen consumption. J. Clin. Invest. 45:1535, 1966.

194. Sonnenblick, E. H., Ross, J., Jr., and Braunwald, E.: Oxygen consumption of the heart: Newer concepts of its multifactorial determination. Am. J. Cardiol. 22:328, 1968.

195. Glancy, D. L., Higgs, L. M., O'Brien, K. P., and Epstein, S. E.: Effects of ouabain on the left ventricular response to exercise in patients with angina pectoris. Circulation 43:45, 1971.

196. Sharma, B., Majid, P. A., Meeran, M. K., Whitaker, W., and Taylor, S. H.: Clinical, electrocardiographic and haemodynamic effects of digitalis (ouabain) in angina pectoris. Br. Heart J. 34:631, 1972.

197. DeMots, H., Rahimtoola, S. H., Kremkau, E. L., Bennett, W., and Mahler, D.: Effects of ouabain on myocardial oxygen supply and demand in patients with chronic coronary artery disease: A hemodynamic, volumetric, and metabolic study in patients without heart failure. J. Clin. Invest. 58:312, 1976.

198. Loeb, H. S., Streitmatter, N., Braunstein, D., Jacobs, W. R., Croke, R. P., and Gunnar, R. M.: Lack of ouabain effect on pacing-induced myocardial ischemia in patients with coronary artery disease. Am. J. Cardiol. 43:995, 1979.

199. Vogel, R., Kirch, D., LeFree, M., Frischknecht, J., and Steele, P.: Effects of digitalis on resting and isometric exercise myocardial perfusion in patients with coronary artery disease and left ventricular dysfunction. Circulation 56:355, 1977.

200. Crawford, M. H., LeWinter, M. M., O'Rourke, R. A., Karliner, J. S., and Ross, J.: Combined propranolol and digoxin therapy in angina pectoris. Ann. Intern. Med. 83:449, 1975.

201. Karliner, J. S., and Braunwald, E.: Present status of digitalis treatment of acute myocardial infarction. Circulation 45:891, 1972.

202. Cohn, J. N., Tristani, F. E., and Khatri, I. M.: Cardiac and peripheral vascular effects of digitalis in clinical cardiogenic shock. Am. Heart J. 78:318, 1969.

203. Ratshin, R. A., Rackley, C. E., and Russell, R. O., Jr.: Hemodynamic evaluation of left ventricular function in shock complicating myocardial infarction. Circulation 45:127, 1972.

204. Rahimtoola, S. H., Sinno, M. Z., Chuquimia, R., Loeb, H. S., Rosen, K. M., and Gunnar, R. M.: Effects of ouabain on impaired left ventricular function in acute myocardial infarction. N. Engl. J. Med. 287:527, 1972.

205. Rahimtoola, S. H., DiGilio, M. M., Sinno, M. Z., Loeb, H. S., Rosen, K. M., and Gunnar, R. M.: Effects of ouabain on impaired left ventricular function during convalescence after acute myocardial infarction. Circulation 44:866, 1971.

206. Morris, J. J., Jr., Taft, C. V., Whalen, R. E., and McIntosh, H. D.: Digitalis and experimental myocardial infarction. Am. Heart J. 77:342, 1969.

207. Kumar, R., Hood, W. B., Jr., Joison, J., Gilmour, D. P., Norman, J. C., and Abelmann, W. H.: Experimental myocardial infarction. VI. Efficacy and toxicity of digitalis in acute and healing phase in intact conscious dogs. J. Clin. Invest. 49:358, 1970.

208. Reičansky, I., Conradson, T. B., Holmberg, S., Rydén, L., Waldenström, A., and Wennerblom, B.: The effect of intravenous digoxin on the occurrence of ventricular tachyarrhythmias in acute myocardial infarction in man. Am. Heart J. 91:705, 1976.

209. Rahimtoola, S. H., and Gunnar, R. M.: Digitalis in acute myocardial infarction: Help or hazard? Ann. Intern. Med. 82:234, 1975.

210. Selzer, A.: The use of digitalis in acute myocardial infarction. Progr. Cardiovasc. Dis. 10:518, 1968.

211. Moss, A. J., Davis, H. T., Conard, D. L., DeCamilla, J. J., and Odoroff, C. L.: Digitalis-associated cardiac mortality after myocardial infarction. Circulation 64:1150, 1981.

211a. Ryan, T. J., Bailey, K. R., McCabe, C. H., Luk, S., Fisher, L. D., Mock, M. B., and Killip, T.: The effects of digitalis on survival in high-risk patients with coronary artery disease. The coronary artery surgery study (CASS). Circulation 67:735, 1983.

212. Dall, J. L.: Digitalis intoxication in the elderly. Lancet 1:194, 1965.

213. Hermann, G. R.: Digitoxicity in the aged. Geriatrics 21:109, 1966.

214. Szefler, S. J., and Jusko, W. J.: Decreased volume of distribution of digoxin in a patient with renal failure. Res. Commun. Chem. Pathol. Pharmacol. 6:1095, 1973.

215. Croxson, M. S., and Ibbertson, H. K.: Serum digoxin in patients with thyroid disease. Br. Med. J. 3:566, 1975.

216. Doherty, J. E., and Perkins, W. H.: Digoxin metabolism in hypo- and hyperthyroidism: Studies with tritiated digoxin in thyroid disease. Ann. Intern. Med. 64:489, 1966.

217. Curfman, G. D., Crowley, T. J., and Smith, T. W.: Thyroid-induced alterations in myocardial sodium- and potassium-activated adenosine triphosphatase, monovalent cation active transport, and cardiac glycoside binding. J. Clin. Invest. 59:586, 1977.

218. Ismail-Beigi, F., and Edelman, I. S.: The mechanism of the calorigenic action of thyroid hormone: Stimulation of $Na^+ + K^+$-activated adenosine-triphosphatase. J. Gen. Physiol. 57:710, 1971.

219. Green, L. H., and Smith, T. W.: The use of digitalis in patients with pulmonary disease. Ann. Intern. Med. 87:459, 1977.

220. Hargreave, F. D.: Digitalis and cor pulmonale. Br. Med. J. 2:943, 1965.

221. Carazza, L. J., and Pastor, B. H.: Cardiac arrhythmias in chronic cor pulmonale. N. Engl. J. Med. 259:862, 1958.

222. Rodensky, P. L., and Wasserman, F.: Observations on digitalis intoxication. Arch. Intern. Med. 108:171, 1961.

223. Hudson, L. D., Kurt, T. L., Petty, T. L., and Genton, E.: Arrhythmias associated with acute respiratory failure in patients with chronic airway obstruction. Chest 63:661, 1973.

224. Thomas, A. J., and Valabhji, P.: Arrhythmia and tachycardia in pulmonary heart disease. Br. Heart J. 31:491, 1969.

225. Beller, G. A., Smith, T. W., Abelmann, W. H., Haber, E., and Hood, W. B., Jr.: Digitalis intoxication: Prospective clinical study with serum level correlations. N. Engl. J. Med. 284:989, 1971.

226. Baum, G. L., Dick, M. M., Schotz, S., and Gumpel, R. C.: Digitalis toxicity in chronic cor pulmonale. South. Med. J. 49:1037, 1956.

227. Klein, M. D., Lown, B., Barr, I., Hagemeijer, F., Garrison, H., and Axelrod, P.: Comparison of serum digoxin level measurement with acetyl strophanthidin tolerance testing. Circulation 49:1053, 1974.

228. Harrison, D. C., Robinson, M. D., and Kleiger, R. E.: Role of hypoxia in digitalis toxicity. Am. J. Med. Sci. 256:352, 1968.

229. Lely, A. H., and van Enter, C. H. J.: Non-cardiac symptoms of digitalis intoxication. Am. Heart J. 83:149, 1972.

230. Doherty, J. E., and Perkins, W. H.: Tissue concentration and turnover of tritiated digoxin in dogs. Am. J. Cardiol. 17:47, 1966.

231. Doherty, J. E., Perkins, W. H., and Flanigan, W. J.: The distribution and concentration of tritiated digoxin in human tissues. Ann. Intern. Med. 66:116, 1967.

232. Barr, I., Smith, T. W., Klein, M. D., Hagemeijer, F., and Lown, B.: Correlation of the electrophysiologic action of digoxin with serum digoxin concentration. J. Pharmacol. Exp. Ther. 180:710, 1972.

233. Smith, T. W., and Curfman, G. D.: Radioimmunoassay of cardiac glycosides. In Strauss, W., and Pitt, B. (eds.): Cardiovascular Nuclear Medicine. 2nd ed. St. Louis, C. V. Mosby Co., 1979, p. 394.

234. Smith, T. W., and Haber, E.: The current status of cardiac glycoside assay techniques. *In* Yu, P. N., and Goodwin, J. F. (eds.): Progress in Cardiology. Philadelphia, Lea and Febiger, 1973, p. 49.

235. Smith, T. W., and Haber, E.: Clinical value of the radioimmunoassay of the digitalis glycosides. Pharmacol. Rev. 25:219, 1973.

236. Duhme, D. W., Greenblatt, D. J., and Koch-Weser, J.: Reduction of digoxin toxicity associated with measurement of serum levels. Ann. Intern. Med. 80:516, 1974.

237. Chamberlain, D. A., White, R. J., Howard, M. R., and Smith, T. W.: Plasma digoxin concentrations in patients with atrial fibrillation. Br. Med. J. 3:429, 1970.

238. Eraker, S. A., and Sasse, L.: The serum digoxin test and digoxin toxicity: A Bayesian approach to decision-making. Circulation 64:409–420, 1981.

239. Hurwitz, N., and Wade, O. L.: Intensive hospital monitoring of adverse reactions to drugs. Br. Med. J. 1:531, 1969.

240. Ogilvie, R. I., and Ruedy, J.: Adverse drug reactions during hospitalization. Canad. Med. Assoc. J. 97:1450, 1967.

241. Borison, H. L., and Wang, S. C.: Physiology and pharmacology of vomiting. Pharmacol. Rev. 5:193, 1953.

242. Gayes, J. M., Greenblatt, D. J., Lloyd, B. L., Harmatz, J. S., and Smith, T. W.: Cerebrospinal fluid digoxin concentrations in humans. J. Clin. Pharmacol. 18:16, 1978.

243. Allonen, H., Andersson, K.-E., Iisalo, E., Kanto, J., Strömblad, L. G., and Wettrell, G.: Passage of digoxin into cerebrospinal fluid in man. Acta Pharmacol. Toxicol. 41:193, 1977.

244. Somberg, J. C., Kuhlman, J. E., and Smith, T. W.: Localization of the neurally mediated coronary vasoconstrictor properties of digitalis in the cat. Circ. Res. 49:226–233, 1981.

245. Rosen, M. R., Gelband, H., and Hoffman, B. F.: Correlation between effects of ouabain on the canine electrocardiogram and transmembrane potentials of isolated Purkinje fibers. Circulation 47:65, 1973.

246. Rosen, M. R., and Gelband, H.: Effect of ouabain on canine Purkinje fibers in situ or perfused with blood. J. Pharmacol. Exp. Ther. 186:366, 1973.

247. Davis, L. D.: Effect of changes in cycle length on diastolic depolarization produced by ouabain in canine Purkinje fibers. Circ. Res. 32:206, 1973.

248. Rosen, M. R., Gelband, H., Merker, C., and Hoffman, B. F.: Mechanisms of digitalis toxicity. Effects of ouabain on phase 4 of canine Purkinje fiber transmembrane potentials. Circulation 47:681, 1973.

249. Ferrier, G. R., Saunders, J. H., and Mendez, C.: A cellular mechanism of the generation of ventricular arrhythmias by acetylstrophanthidin. Circ. Res. 32:600, 1973.

250. Saunders, J. H., Ferrier, G. R., and Moe, G. K.: Conduction block associated with transient depolarizations induced by acetylstrophanthidin in isolated canine Purkinje fibers. Circ. Res. 32:610, 1973.

251. Zipes, D. P., Arbel, E., Knope, R. F., and Moe, G. K.: Accelerated cardiac escape rhythms caused by ouabain intoxication. Am. J. Cardiol. 33:248, 1973.

252. Ferrier, J. R.: Digitalis arrhythmias: Role of oscillatory afterpotentials. Progr. Cardiovasc. Dis. 19:459, 1977.

253. Lederer, W. J., and Tsien, R. W.: Transient inward current underlying arrhythmogenic effects of cardiotonic steroids in Purkinje fibers. J. Physiol. (London) 263:73, 1976.

254. Kass, R. S., Lederer, W. J., Tsien, R. W., and Weingart, R.: Role of calcium ions in transient inward currents and aftercontractions induced by strophanthidin in cardiac Purkinje fibers. J. Physiol. (London) 281:187, 1978.

255. Tsien, R. W., Weingart, R., Lederer, W. J., and Kass, R. S.: On the inotropic and arrhythmogenic effects of digitalis. *In* Riecker, G., Weber, A., and Goodwin, J. (eds.): Myocardial Failure. New York, Springer-Verlag, 1977, p. 331.

256. Kass, R. S., Tsien, R. W., and Weingart, R.: Ionic basis of transient inward current induced by strophanthidin in cardiac Purkinje fibers. J. Physiol. (London) 281:209, 1978.

257. Goodman, D. J., Rossen, R. M., Ingham, R., Rider, A. K., and Harrison, D. C.: Sinus node function in the denervated human heart. Effect of digitalis. Br. Heart J. 37:612–618, 1975.

258. Hoffman, B. F., and Singer, D. H.: Effects of digitalis on electrical activity of cardiac fibers. Progr. Cardiovasc. Dis. 7:226, 1964.

259. James, T. N., and Nadeau, R. A.: The chronotropic effect of digitalis studied by direct perfusion of the sinus node. J. Pharmacol. 139:42, 1960.

260. Watanabe, Y., and Dreifus, L. S.: Interactions of lanatoside C and potassium on atrioventricular conduction in rabbits. Circ. Res. 27:931, 1970.

261. Lely, A., and van Enter, C.: Large-scale digitoxin intoxication. Br. Med. J. 3:737, 1970.

262. Storstein, O., and Rasmussen, K.: Digitalis and atrial tachycardia with block. Br. Heart J. 36:171, 1974.

263. Lown, B., Graboys, T. B., Podrid, P. J., Cohen, B. H., Stockman, M. B., and Gaughan, C. E.: Effect of a digitalis drug on ventricular premature beats. N. Engl. J. Med. 296:301, 1977.

264. Chung, E. K.: Principles of Cardiac Arrhythmias. Baltimore, Williams and Wilkins, 1971.

265. Fisch, C., Zipes, D. P., and Noble, R. J.: Digitalis toxicity: Mechanism and recognition. *In* Yu, P. N., and Goodwin, J. F. (eds.): Progress in Cardiology. Vol. 4. Philadelphia, Lea and Febiger, 1975, p. 35.

266. Wellens, H. J. J.: The electrocardiogram in digitalis intoxication. *In* Yu, P. N., and Goodwin, J. F. (eds.): Progress in Cardiology. Vol. 5. Philadelphia, Lea and Febiger, 1976, p. 271.

267. Brauner, G. J., and Greene, M. H.: Digitalis allergy: Digoxin-induced vasculitis. Cutis 10:441, 1972.

268. LeWinn, E. B.: Gynecomastia during digitalis therapy: Report of eight additional cases with liver-function studies. N. Engl. J. Med. 248:316, 1953.

269. Neri, A., Aygen, M., Zuckerman, A., and Bahary, C.: Subject of assessment of sexual dysfunction of patients on long-term administration of digoxin. Arch. Sexual Behav. 9:343–347, 1980.

270. Bismuth, C., Motte, G., Conso, F., Chauvin, M., and Gaultier, M.: Acute digitoxin intoxication treated by intracardiac pacemaker: Experience in sixty-eight patients. Clin. Toxicol. 10:443, 1977.

271. Citrin, D., Stevenson, I. H., and O'Malley, K.: Massive digoxin overdose: Observations on hyperkalaemia and plasma digoxin levels. Scott. Med. J. 17:275, 1972.

272. Gaultier, M., Fournier, E., Efthymiou, M. L., Frejaville, J. P., Jouannot, P., and Dentan, M.: Intoxication digitalique aiguë (70 observations). Bull. Soc. Med. Hop. Paris 119:247, 1968.

273. Hobson, J. D., and Zettner, A.: Digoxin serum half-life following suicidal digoxin poisoning. J.A.M.A. 223:147, 1973.

274. Bigger, J. T., Jr., and Strauss, H. C.: Digitalis toxicity: Drug interactions promoting toxicity and the management of toxicity. Semin. Drug Treat. 2:147, 1972.

275. Bigger, J. T., Jr., and Mandel, W. J.: Effect of lidocaine on the electrophysiological properties of ventricular muscle and Purkinje fibers. J. Clin. Invest. 49:63, 1970.

276. Bigger, J. T., Jr., Bassett, A. L., and Hoffman, B. F.: Electrophysiological effects of diphenylhydantoin on canine Purkinje fibers. Circ. Res. 22:221, 1968.

277. Strauss, H. C., Bigger, J. T., Jr., Bassett, A. L., and Hoffman, B. F.: Actions of diphenylhydantoin on the electrical properties of isolated rabbit and canine atria. Circ. Res. 23:463, 1968.

278. Helfant, R. H., Scherlag, B. J., and Damato, A. N.: The electrophysiological properties of diphenylhydantoin sodium as compared to procaine amide in the normal and digitalis-intoxicated heart. Circulation 36:108, 1967.

279. Fisch, C., Knoebel, S. B., Feigenbaum, H., and Greenspan, K.: Potassium and the monophasic action potential, electrocardiogram, conduction and arrhythmias. Progr. Cardiovasc. Dis. 8:387, 1966.

280. Davis, L. D., and Temte, J. V.: Effects of propranolol on the transmembrane potentials of ventricular muscle and Purkinje fibers of the dog. Circ. Res. 22:661, 1968.

281. Lown, B., Kleiger, R., and Williams, J.: Cardioversion and digitalis drugs: Changed threshold to electric shock in digitalized animals. Circ. Res. 17:519, 1965.

282. Ditchey, R. V., and Karliner, J. S.: Safety of electrical cardioversion in patients without digitalis toxicity. Ann. Intern. Med. 95:676–679, 1981.

283. Bazzano, G., and Bazzano, G. S.: Digitalis intoxication: Treatment with a new steroid-binding resin. J.A.M.A. 220:828, 1972.

284. Goldfinger, S. E., Heizer, W. D., and Smith, T. W.: Absorption of digoxin in patients with malabsorption syndrome. *In* Storstein, O. (ed.): International Symposium on Digitalis. Oslo, Gyldendal Norsk Forlag, 1973, p. 224.

285. Smith, T. W., Butler, V. P., Jr., and Haber, E.: Cardiac glycoside-specific antibodies in the treatment of digitalis intoxication. *In* Haber, E., and Krause, R. M. (eds.): Antibodies in Human Diagnosis and Therapy. New York, Raven Press, 1977.

286. Butler, V. P., Jr., Smith, T. W., Schmidt, D. H., and Haber, E.: Immunological reversal of the effects of digoxin. Fed. Proc. 36:2235, 1977.

287. Lloyd, B. L., and Smith, T. W.: Contrasting rates of reversal of digoxin toxicity by digoxin-specific IgG and Fab fragments. Circulation 58:280, 1978.

288. Smith, T. W.: Ouabain-specific antibodies: Immunochemical properties and reversal of Na+, K+-activated adenosine triphosphatase inhibition. J. Clin. Invest. 51:1583, 1972.

289. Hougen, T. J., Lloyd, B. L., and Smith, T. W.: Effects of inotropic and arrhythmogenic digoxin doses and of digoxin-specific antibody on myocardial monovalent cation transport in the dog. Circ. Res. 44:23, 1979.

290. Waldmann, T. A., and Strober, W.: Metabolism of immunoglobulins. Progr. Allergy 13:1, 1969.

291. Butler, V. P., Jr., Schmidt, D. H., Smith, T. W., Haber, E., Raynor, B. D., and McMartini, P.: Effects of sheep digoxin-specific antibodies and their Fab fragments on digoxin pharmacokinetics in dogs. J. Clin. Invest. 59:345, 1977.

292. Ochs, H. R., and Smith, T. W.: Reversal of advanced digitoxin toxicity and modification of pharmacokinetics by specific antibodies and Fab fragments. J. Clin. Invest. 60:1303, 1977.

293. Smith, T. W., Lloyd, B. L., Spicer, N., and Haber, E.: Immunogenicity and kinetics of distribution and elimination of sheep digoxin-specific IgG and Fab fragments in the rabbit and baboon. Clin. Exp. Immunol. 36:384, 1979.

Diuretics

294. Wilson, J. R., Reichek, N., Dunkman, W. B., and Goldberg, S.: Effect of diuresis on the performance of the failing left ventricle in man. Am. J. Med. 70:234, 1981.

295. Gennari, F. J., and Kassirer, J. P.: Osmotic diuresis. N. Engl. J. Med. 291:714, 1974.

296. Grantham, J. J., and Chonko, A. M.: The physiologic basis and clinical use of diuretics. *In* Brenner, B. M., and Stein, J. H. (eds.): Contemporary Issues in Nephrology: Sodium and Water Homeostasis. Vol. 1. New York, Churchill Livingstone, 1978, p. 178.

297. Warnock, D. G., and Eveloff, J.: NaCl entry mechanism in the luminal membrane of the renal tubule. Am. J. Physiol. 242:F561–F574, 1982.

298. Reineck, H. J., and Stein, J. H.: Mechanisms of action and clinical uses of diuretics. In Brenner, B. M., and Rector, F. C. (eds.): The Kidney. 2nd ed. Philadelphia, W. B. Saunders Co., 1981.

299. Beyer, K., and Baer, J.: Physiologic basis for the action of newer diuretic agents. Pharmacol. Rev. 13:517, 1961.

300. Kunau, R. T., Weller, D. R., and Webb, H. L.: Clarification of the site of action of chlorothiazide in the rat nephron. J. Clin. Invest. 56:401, 1975.

301. Stein, J. H., Wilson, C. B., and Kirkendall, W. M.: Differences in the acute effects of furosemide and ethacrynic acid in man. J. Lab. Clin. Med. 71:654, 1968.

302. Chou, S., Porush, J. G., Slater, P. A., Flombaum, C. D., Shafi, T., and Fein, P. A.: Effects of acetazolamide on proximal tubule Cl, Na, HCO₃ transport in normal and acidotic dogs during distal blockade. J. Clin. Invest. 60:162, 1977.

303. Rector, F. C., Martinez-Maldonado, M., Brunner, F. P., and Seldin, D. W.: Evidence of passive reabsorption of sodium chloride in the proximal tubule of rat kidney. J. Clin. Invest. 45:1060, 1966.

304. Khan, M. I.: Treatment of refractory congestive heart failure and normokalemic hypochloremic alkalosis with acetazolamide and spironolactone. Can. Med. Assoc. J. 123:883, 1980.

305. Burg, M. B., and Green, N.: Function of the thick ascending limb of Henle's loop. Am. J. Physiol. 224:659, 1973.

306. Rocha, A. S., and Kokko, J. P.: Sodium chloride and water transport in the medullary thick ascending limb of Henle: Evidence for active chloride transport. J. Clin. Invest. 52:612, 1973.

307. Burg, M., and Stoner, L.: Renal tubular chloride transport and mode of action of some diuretics. Ann. Rev. Physiol. 38:37, 1976.

308. Schmidt, U., and Dubach, U. C.: The behavior of Na-K activated adenosine triphosphate in various structures in the rat nephron after furosemide application. Nephron 7:447, 1970.

309. Patak, R., Rosenblatt, S., Fadem, S., Lifschitz, M. D., and Stein, J. H.: Diuretic induced changes in renal blood flow and prostaglandin E excretion in the dog. Am. J. Physiol. 236:F494, 1979.

310. Ebel, H.: Effects of diuretics on renal Na-K ATPase and adenyl cyclase. Naunyn Schmiedebergs Arch. Pharmakol. 281:301, 1974.

311. Abe, K., Yasuima, M., Cheiba, L., Irokawa, N., Ipo, P., and Yoshinaga, K.: Effect of furosemide on urinary excretion prostaglandin E in normal volunteers and patients with essential hypertension. Prostaglandins 14:513, 1977.

312. Patak, R. V., Mookerjee, B. K., Bentzel, C. J., Hysert, P. E., Babej, M., and Lee, J. B.: Antagonism of the effects of furosemide by indomethacin in normal and hypertensive man. Prostaglandins 10:649, 1975.

313. Bailie, M. D., Barbour, J. A., and Hook, J. B.: Effects of indomethacin on furosemide-induced changes in renal blood flow. Proc. Soc. Exp. Biol. Med. 148:1173, 1975.

314. Bowman, R. H.: Renal secretion of [³⁵S] furosemide and its depression by albumin binding. Am. J. Physiol. 229:93, 1975.

315. Burg, M. B.: The mechanism of action of diuretics in renal tubules. In Wesson, L. G., and Fanelli, G. M. (eds.): Recent Advances in Renal Physiology and Pharmacology. Baltimore, University Park Press, 1974, pp. 99–109.

316. Charnock, J. S., and Almeida, A. F.: Ethacrynic acid accumulation by renal tissue. Biochem. Pharmacol. 21:647, 1972.

317. Mitch, W. E., and Wilcox, C. S.: Disorders of body fluids, sodium and potassium in chronic renal failure. Am. J. Med. 72:536, 1982.

318. Essig, A.: Competitive inhibition of renal transport of p-aminohippurate by analogues of chlorothiazide. Am. J. Physiol. 201:303, 1961.

319. Hirsch, G. H., Pakuts, A. P., and Bayne, A. J.: Furosemide accumulation by renal tissue. Biochem. Pharmacol. 24:1943, 1975.

320. Hook, J. B., and Williamson, H. E.: Influence of probenecid and alterations in acid base balance on the saluretic activity of furosemide. J. Pharmacol. Exp. Ther. 149:404, 1965.

321. Costanzo, L. S., and Windhager, E. E.: Calcium and sodium transport by the distal convoluted tubule of the rat. Am. J. Physiol. 4:F492, 1978.

322. Edelman, I., and Fimognari, G.: On the biochemical mechanisms of action of aldosterone. Recent Prog. Hormone Res. 24:1, 1968.

323. Crabbe, J.: A hypothesis concerning the mode of action of amiloride and triamterene. Arch. Int. Pharmacodyn. Ther. 173:474, 1968.

324. Stoner, L. C., Burg, M. B., and Orloff, J.: Ion transport in cortical collecting tubule; effect of amiloride. Am. J. Physiol. 227:453, 1974.

325. Tannen, R. L.: Relationship of renal ammonia production and potassium homeostasis. Kidney Int. 11:453, 1977.

326. Manuel, M. A., Beirne, G. J., Wagnild, J. P., and Weiner, M. W.: An effect of spironolactone on urinary acidification in normal man. Arch. Intern. Med. 134:472, 1974.

327. Abramow, M.: Effects of ethacrynic acid on the isolated collecting tubule. J. Clin. Invest. 53:796, 1974.

328. Hantman, D., Rossier, B., Zohlman, R., and Schrier, R.: Rapid correction of hyponatremia in the syndrome of inappropriate secretion of antidiuretic hormone: An alternative treatment to hypertonic saline. Ann. Intern. Med. 78:870, 1973.

329. deWardener, H. E.: Natriuretic hormone. Clin. Sci. Molec. Med. 53:1, 1977.

330. Epstein, M., Lepp, B. A., Hoffman, D. S., and Levinson, R.: Potentiation of furosemide by metolazone in refractory edema. Current Therap. Res. 21:656, 1977.

331. Wollam, G. L., Tarazi, R. C., Bravo, E. L., and Dristan, H. P.: Diuretic potency of combined hydrochlorothiazide and furosemide therapy in patients with azotemia. Am. J. Med. 72:929, 1982.

332. Wilcox, C. S., Mitch, W. E., Kelly, R. A., Skorecki, K., Meyer, T., Friedman, P., and Souney, P.: Effect of salt intake on sodium homeostasis during furosemide administration. Kidney Int. 21:160, 1982.

333. Stein, J. H., Lameire, N. H., and Earley, L. E.: Renal hemodynamic factors in the regulation of sodium excretion. In Andriole, T. E., Hoffman, J. F., and Fanestil, D. D. (eds.): Physiology of Membrane Disorders. New York, Plenum Press, 1978, p. 739.

334. Mathisen, O., Raeder, M., Sejersted, O. M., and Kiil, F.: Effect of acetazolamide on glomerulo-tubular balance and renal metabolic rate. Scand. J. Clin. Lab. Invest. 36:617, 1976.

335. Clapp, J. R., Nottebohm, G. A., and Robinson, R. R.: Proximal site of action of ethacrynic acid. Importance of filtration rate. Am. J. Physiol. 220:1355, 1971.

336. Ogilvie, R. I., and Ruedy, J.: Hemodynamic effects of ethacrynic acid in anephric dogs. J. Pharmacol. Exp. Ther. 176:389, 1971.

337. Ogilvie, R. I., and Schlieper, E.: Comparative effects of ethacrynic acid, furosemide and diazoxide in the perfused dog hindlimb. Canad. J. Physiol. Pharmacol. 49:1038, 1971.

338. Dikshit, K., Vyden, J. D., Forrester, J. S., and Swan, H. J. C.: Renal and extrarenal hemodynamic effects of furosemide in congestive heart failure after acute myocardial infarction. N. Engl. J. Med. 288:1087, 1973.

339. Wright, F. S.: Intrarenal regulation of glomerular filtration rate. N. Engl. J. Med. 291:135, 1974.

340. Wright, F. S., and Schnermann, J.: Interference with feedback control of glomerular filtration rate by furosemide, triflocin and cyanide. J. Clin. Invest. 53:1695, 1974.

341. Seely, J. F., and Dirks, J. H.: Editorial: Site of action of diuretic drugs. Kidney Int. 11:1, 1977.

342. Giebisch, G.: Effects of diuretics on renal transport of potassium. In Martinez-Maldonado, M. (ed.): Methods in Pharmacology. Vol. 4A. Renal Pharmacology. New York, Plenum Press, 1976, pp. 121–164.

343. Sealey, J. E., and Laragh, J. H.: A proposed cybernetic system for sodium and potassium homeostasis: Coordination of aldosterone and intrarenal physical factors. Kidney Int. 6:281, 1974.

344. Davidson, C., McLachlan, M. S. F., Burkinshaw, L., and Morgan, D. B.: Effect of long-term diuretic treatment on body potassium in heart disease. Lancet 2:1044, 1976.

345. Venkata, C., Ram, S., Garrett, B. N., and Kaplan, M.: Moderate sodium restriction and various diuretics in the treatment of hypertension. Arch. Intern. Med. 141:1015, 1981.

346. Seldin, D. W., and Rector, F. C., Jr.: The generation and maintenance of metabolic alkalosis. Kidney Int. 1:306, 1972.

347. Editorial: Hypokalemia and diuretics—Analysis of publications. Br. Med. J. 1:905, 1980.

348. Garella, S., Chazan, J. A., and Cohen, J. J.: Saline-resistant metabolic alkalosis or "chloride-wasting nephropathy." Ann. Intern. Med. 73:31, 1970.

349. Holland, O. B., Nixon, J. V., and Kuknert, L.: Diuretic-induced ventricular ectopic activity. Am. J. Med. 70:762, 1981.

350. Kelly, R. A., Wilcox, C. S., and Mitch, W. E.: Diuretics: An update. J. Cardiovasc. Med. 7:1153, 1982.

351. Rosa, R. M., Silva, P., Young, J. B., Landsberg, L., Brown, R. S., Rowe, J. W., and Epstein, F. N.: Adrenergic modulation of extrarenal potassium disposal. N. Engl. J. Med. 302:431, 1980.

352. Kennedy, R. M., and Earley, L. E.: Profound hyponatremia resulting from thiazide induced decrease in urinary diluting capacity in a patient with primary polydipsia. N. Engl. J. Med. 282:1185, 1970.

353. Verney, E. V.: Croonian Lecture: The anti-diuretic hormone and the factors which determine its release. Proc. Roy. Soc. Lond. (Series B) 135:25, 1947.

354. Davies, D. L., and Wilson, G. M.: Diuretics: Mechanism of action and clinical application. Drugs 9:178, 1975.

355. Berger, L., and Yü, T.: Renal function in gout. IV. An analysis of 524 gouty subjects including long-term follow-up studies. Am. J. Med. 59:605, 1975.

356. Fessel, W. J.: Renal outcomes of gout and hyperuricemia. Am. J. Med. 67:74, 1979.

357. Johnson, M. W., and Mitch, W. E.: The risks of asymptomatic hyperuricaemia and the use of uricosuric diuretics. Drugs 21:220, 1981.

358. Glodner, M. G., Zarowitz, H., and Akgun, F.: Hyperglycemia and glucosuria due to thiazide derivatives administered in diabetes mellitus. N. Engl. J. Med. 262:403, 1960.

359. Helgsland, A., Huermann, I., Holme, I., and Leren, P.: Serum triglycerides and serum uric acid in untreated and thiazide-treated patients with mild hypertension. Am. J. Med. 64:34, 1978.

360. Bauer, J. H., Brooks, C. S., Weinstein, I., Wilcox, H. H., Heimberg, M., Burch, R. N., and Barkley, R.: Effects of diuretic and propranolol on plasma lipoprotein lipids. Clin. Pharmacol. Therap. 30:35, 1981.

361. Loreaux, L., Menard, R., Taylor, A., Patpita, J. C., and Santen, R.: Spironolactone and endocrine dysfunction. Ann. Intern. Med. 85:630, 1976.

362. Reubi, F. C.: The action and use of diuretics in renal disease. In Friedberg, C. K. (ed.): Heart, Kidney and Electrolytes. New York, Grune and Stratton, 1962, p. 169.

363. Steinmuller, S. R., and Puschett, J. B.: Effects of metolazone in man: Comparison with chlorothiazide. Kidney Int. 1:169, 1972.

364. Fernandez, P. C., and Puschett, J. B.: Proximal tubular actions of metolazone and chlorothiazide. Am. J. Physiol. 225:954, 1973.

365. Heinemann, H. O., Demartini, E. E., and Laragh, J. H.: The mode of action and use of chlorothiazide on renal excretion of electrolytes and free water. Am. J. Med. *26*:853, 1959.

366. Craswell, P. W., Ezzat, E., Kopstein, J., Varghese, Z., and Moorhead, J. F.: Use of metolazone, a new diuretic, in patients with renal disease. Nephron *12*:63, 1973.

367. Multicenter Diuretic Cooperative Study Group. Arch. Intern. Med. *141*:482, 1982.

368. Crosley, A. P., Jr., Ronquillo, L. M., Strickland, W. H., and Alexander, F.: Triamterene, a new natriuretic agent: Preliminary observations in man. Ann. Intern. Med. *56*:241, 1962.

369. Frazier, H. S., and Yager, H.: The clinical use of diuretics. N. Engl. J. Med. *288*:246 and 455, 1973.

Vasodilators

370. Wiggers, C. J., and Feely, H.: The cardiodynamics of mitral insufficiency. Heart *9*:141, 1921–22.

371. Braunwald, E., Welch, G. H., Jr., and Sarnoff, S. J.: Hemodynamic effects of quantitatively varied experimental mitral regurgitation. Circ. Res. *5*:539, 1957.

372. Braunwald, E., Welch, G. H., Jr., and Morrow, A. G.: The effects of acutely increased systemic resistance on the left atrial pressure pulse: A method for the clinical detection of mitral insufficiency. J. Clin. Invest. *37*:35, 1958.

373. Ross, J., Jr., and Braunwald, E.: The study of left ventricular function in man by increasing resistance to ventricular ejection with angiotensin. Circulation *29*:739, 1964.

374. Clauss, R. H., Birtwell, W. C., Albertel, G. A., Lunzer, S., Taylor, W. J., Fosberg, A. M., and Harkin, D. E.: Assisted circulation. I. The arterial counterpulsator. J. Thorac. Cardiovasc. Surg. *41*:447, 1961.

375. Majid, P. A., Sharma, B., and Taylor, S. H.: Phentolamine for vasodilator treatment of severe heart failure. Lancet *2*:719, 1971.

376. Massie, B. M., Chatterjee, K., and Parmley, W. W.: Vasodilator therapy for acute and chronic heart failure. *In* Yu, P. N., and Goodwin, J. F. (eds.): Progress in Cardiology. Vol. 8. Philadelphia, Lea and Febiger, 1979.

377. Mason, D. T. (ed.): Symposium on vasodilator and inotropic therapy of heart failure. Am. J. Med. *65*:101, 1978.

378. Cohn, J. N., and Franciosa, J. A.: Vasodilator therapy of cardiac failure. N. Engl. J. Med. *297*:27 and 254, 1977.

379. Cohn, J. N.: Vasodilators: Rationale, application, and future prospects. *In* Braunwald, E., Mock, M. B., and Watson, J. (eds.): Congestive Heart Failure: Current Research and Clinical Applications. New York, Grune and Stratton, 1982, p. 279.

380. Braunwald, E., Ross, J., Jr., Kahler, R. L., Gaffney, T. E., Goldblatt, A., and Mason, D. T.: Reflex control of the systemic venous bed: Effects on venous tone of vasoactive drugs and of baroreceptor and chemoreceptor stimulation. Circ. Res. *12*:539, 1963.

381. Zelis, R., and Flaim, S. F.: Alterations in vasomotor tone in congestive heart failure. Prog. Cardiovasc. Dis. *24*:437–459, 1982.

382. Ford, L. E.: Effect of afterload reduction on myocardial energetics. Circ. Res. *46*:161–166, 1980.

383. Packer, M., and LeJemtel, T. H.: Physiologic and pharmacologic determinants of vasodilator response: A conceptual framework for rational drug therapy for chronic heart failure. Prog. Cardiovasc. Dis. *24*:275–292, 1982.

384. Miller, R. M., Fennell, W. H., Young, J. B., Palomo, A. R., and Quinones, M. A.: Differential systemic arterial and venous actions and consequent cardiac effects of vasodilator drugs. Prog. Cardiovasc. Dis. *24*:353–374, 1982.

385. Zelis, R., Mason, D. T., and Braunwald, E.: A comparison of the effects of vasodilator stimuli on peripheral resistance vessels in normal subjects and in patients with congestive heart failure. J. Clin. Invest. *47*:960, 1968.

386. Zelis, R., Lee, G., and Mason, D. T.: Influence of experimental edema on metabolically determined blood flow. Circ. Res. *34*:482, 1974.

387. Franciosa, J. A., Guiha, N. M., Limas, C. J., Rodriguera, E., and Cohn, J. N.: Improved left ventricular function during nitroprusside infusion in acute myocardial infarction. Lancet *1*:650, 1972.

388. Pepine, C. J., Nichols, W. W., Curry, R. C., Jr., and Conti, C. R.: Aortic input impedance during nitroprusside infusion. A reconsideration of afterload reduction and beneficial action. J. Clin. Invest. *64*:643, 1979.

389. Pouleur, H., Covell, J. W., and Ross, J., Jr.: Effects of nitroprusside on venous return and central blood volume in the absence and presence of acute heart failure. Circulation *61*:328, 1980.

390. Cogan, J. J., Humphreys, M. H., Carlson, C. J., and Rapaport, E.: Renal effects of nitroprusside and hydralazine in patients with congestive heart failure. Circulation *61*:316, 1980.

391. Davies, D. W., Kadar, D., Steward, D. J., and Munro, I. R.: A sudden death associated with the use of sodium nitroprusside for induction of hypotension during anesthesia. Canad. Anaesth. Soc. J. *22*:547, 1975.

392. Miller, R. R., Vismara, L. A., Williams, D. O., Amsterdam, E. A., and Mason, D. T.: Pharmacological mechanisms for left ventricular unloading in clinical congestive heart failure: Differential effects of nitroprusside, phentolamine, and nitroglycerin on cardiac function and peripheral circulation. Circ. Res. *39*:127, 1976.

393. Taylor, S. H., Sutherland, G. R., MacKenzie, M. B., Staunton, H. P., and Donald, K. W.: The circulatory effects of intravenous phentolamine in man. Circulation *31*:741, 1955.

394. Stern, M. A., Gohlke, H. K., Loeb, H. S., Croke, R. P., and Gunnar, R. M.: Hemodynamic effects of intravenous phentolamine in low output cardiac failure. Dose-response relationships. Circulation *58*:157, 1978.

395. Henning, R. J., Shubin, H., and Weil, M. H.: Afterload reduction with phentolamine in patients with acute pulmonary edema. Am. J. Med. *63*:568, 1977.

396. Warren, S. E., and Francis, G. S.: Nitroglycerin and nitrate esters. Am. J. Med. *65*:53, 1978.

397. Williams, D. O., Amsterdam, E. A., and Mason, D. T.: Hemodynamic effects of nitroglycerin in acute myocardial infarction. Decrease in ventricular preload at the expense of cardiac output. Circulation *51*:421, 1975.

398. Flaherty, J. T., Reid, P. R., Kelly, D. T., Taylor, D. R., Weisfeldt, M. L., and Pitt, B.: Intravenous nitroglycerin in acute myocardial infarction. Circulation *51*:132, 1975.

399. Franciosa, J. A., and Cohn, J. N.: Sustained hemodynamic effects without tolerance during long-term isosorbide dinitrate treatment of chronic left ventricular failure. Am. J. Cardiol. *45*:648, 1980.

399a. Leier, C. V., Huss, P., Magorien, R. D., and Unverferth, D. V.: Improved exercise capacity and differing arterial and venous tolerance during chronic isosorbide dinitrate therapy for congestive heart failure. Circulation *67*:817, 1983.

400. Pierpont, G. L., Brown, D. C., Franciosa, J. A., and Cohn, J. N.: Effect of hydralazine on renal failure in patients with congestive heart failure. Circulation *61*:323, 1980.

401. Packer, M., Meller, J., Medina, N., Gorlin, R., and Herman, M. V.: Dose requirements of hydralazine in patients with severe chronic congestive heart failure. Am. J. Cardiol. *45*:655, 1980.

402. Packer, M., Meller, J., Medina, N., Gorlin, R., and Herman, M. V.: Importance of left ventricular chamber size in determining the response to hydralazine in severe chronic heart failure. N. Engl. J. Med. *303*:250–255, 1980.

403. Packer, M., Meller, J., Medina, N., Yushak, M., and Gorlin, R.: Hemodynamic characterization of tolerance to long-term hydralazine therapy in severe chronic heart failure. N. Engl. J. Med. *306*:57–62, 1982.

404. Massie, B., Ports, T., Chatterjee, K., Parmley, W., Ostland, J., O'Young, J., and Haughom, F.: Long-term vasodilator therapy for heart failure: Clinical response and its relationship to hemodynamic measurements. Circulation *63*: 269–278, 1981.

405. Franciosa, J. A., Weber, K. T., Levine, T. B., Kinasewitz, G. T., Janicki, J. S., West, J., Henis, M. M., and Cohn, J. N.: Hydralazine in the long-term treatment of chronic heart failure: Lack of difference from placebo. Am. Heart J. *104*:587–594, 1982.

406. Franciosa, J. A., and Cohn, J. N.: Effects of minoxidil on hemodynamics in patients with congestive heart failure. Circulation *63*:652–657, 1981.

407. Colucci, W. S.: Alpha-adrenergic receptor blockade with prazosin: Consideration of hypertension, heart failure, and potential new applications. Ann. Intern. Med. *97*:67–77, 1982.

408. Lowenstein, J., and Steele, J., Jr.: Prazosin. Am. Heart J. *95*:262, 1978.

409. Awan, N. A., Miller, R. R., and Mason, D. T.: Comparison of effects of nitroprusside and prazosin on left ventricular function and the peripheral circulation in chronic refractory congestive heart failure. Circulation *57*:152, 1978.

410. Mehta, J., Iacona, M., Feldman, R. L., Pepine, C. J., and Conti, C. R.: Comparative hemodynamic effects of intravenous nitroprusside and oral prazosin in refractory heart failure. Am. J. Cardiol. *41*:925, 1978.

411. Packer, M., Meller, J., Gorlin, R., and Herman, H. V.: Hemodynamic and clinical tachyphylaxis to prazosin-mediated afterload reduction in severe congestive heart failure. Circulation *59*:531, 1979.

412. Colucci, W. S., Wynne, J., Holman, B. L., and Braunwald, E.: Chronic therapy of heart failure with prazosin: A randomized double-blind trial. Am. J. Cardiol. *45*:337–344, 1980.

413. Goldman, S. A., Johnson, L. L., Escala, E., Cannon, P. J., and Weiss, M. D.: Improved exercise ejection fraction with long-term prazosin therapy in patients with heart failure. Am. J. Med. *68*:36–42, 1980.

413a. Rutishauser, W.: A review of the long-term effects of prazosin and hydralazine in chronic congestive heart failure. Europ. Heart J. *4*(Suppl. A):149, 1983.

414. Awan, N. A., Miller, R. R., Miller, M. P., Specht, K., Vera, Z., and Mason, D. T.: Clinical pharmacology and therapeutic application of prazosin in acute and chronic refractory congestive heart failure. Balanced systemic venous and arterial dilation improving pulmonary congestion and cardiac output. Am. J. Med. *65*:146, 1978.

415. Dzau, V. J., Colucci, W. S., Hollenberg, N. K., and Williams, G. H.: Relation of the renin-angiotensin-aldosterone system to clinical state in congestive heart failure. Circulation *63*:645–651, 1981.

416. Levine, T., Franciosa, J. A., and Cohn, J. N.: Acute and long-term response to an oral converting enzyme inhibitor, captopril, in congestive heart failure. Circulation *62*:35–41, 1980.

417. Dzau, V. J., Colucci, W. S., Williams, G. H., Curfman, G., Meggs, L., and Hollenberg, N. K.: Sustained effectiveness of converting-enzyme inhibition in patients with severe congestive heart failure. N. Engl. J. Med. *302*:1373–1379, 1980.

418. Ader, R., Chatterjee, K., Ports, T., Brundage, B., Hiramatsu, B., and Parmley, W.: Immediate and sustained hemodynamic and clinical improvement in chronic heart failure by an oral angiotensin-converting enzyme inhibitor. Circulation *61*:931–937, 1980.

419. Dzau, V. J.: Angiotensin-converting enzyme inhibition in the treatment of hypertension and congestive heart failure. *In* Isselbacher. K. J., et al. (eds.):

Updates of Internal Medicine, IV. New York, McGraw-Hill, 1982, pp. 137–146.

419a. Cody, R. J., Covit, A. B., Schaer, G. L., and Laragh, J. H.: Evaluation of a long-acting converting enzyme inhibitor (Enalapril) for the treatment of chronic congestive heart failure. J. Am. Coll. Cardiol. *1*:1154, 1983.

420. Fouad, F. M., Ceimo, J. M. K., Tarazi, R. C., and Bravo, E. L.: Contrasts and similarities of acute hemodynamic responses to specific antagonism of angiotensin II ([Sar¹, Thr⁸] A II) and to inhibition of converting enzyme (Captopril). Circulation *61*:163, 1980.

421. Vrobel, T., and Cohn, J. N.: Comparative hemodynamic effects of converting enzyme inhibitor and sodium nitroprusside in severe heart failure. Am. J. Cardiol. *45*:331, 1980.

422. Swartz, S. L., Williams, G. H., Hollenberg, N. K., Crantz, F. R., Moore, T. J., Levine, L., Sasahara, A. A., and Dluhy, R. G.: Endocrine profile in the long-term phase of converting-enzyme inhibition. Clin. Pharmacol. Ther. *28*:499, 1980.

423. Lijnen, P., Fagard, R., Staessen, J., VerSchueren, L. J., and Amery, A.: Role of various vasodepressor systems in the acute hypotensive effect of captopril in man. Eur. J. Clin. Pharmacol. *20*:1, 1981.

424. Levine, T. B., Franciosa, J. A., and Cohn, J. N.: Acute and long-term responses to an oral converting-enzyme inhibitor, captopril, in congestive heart failure. Circulation *62*:35, 1980.

425. Gavras, H., Faxon, D. P., Berkoben, J., Brunner, H. R., and Ryan, T. J.: Angiotensin converting enzyme inhibition in patients with congestive heart failure. Circulation *58*:770, 1978.

426. Curtiss, C., Cohn, J. N., Vrobel, T., and Franciosa, J. A.: Role of the renin-angiotensin system in the systemic vasoconstriction of chronic congestive heart failure. Circulation *58*:763, 1978.

427. Creager, M. A., Halperin, J. L., Bernard, D. B., Faxon, D. P., Melidossian, C. D., Gavras, H., and Ryan, T. J.: Acute regional circulatory and renal hemodynamic effects of converting-enzyme inhibition in patients with congestive heart failure. Circulation *64*:483, 1981.

428. Maslowski, A. H., Ikram, H., Nicholls, M. G., and Espiner, E. A.: Haemodynamic, hormonal and electrolyte responses to captopril in resistant heart failure. Lancet *1*:71, 1981.

429. Davis, R., Ribner, H. S., Keung, E., LeJemtel, T. H., and Sonnenblick, E. H.: Treatment of chronic congestive heart failure with captopril, an oral inhibitor of angiotensin-converting enzyme. N. Engl. J. Med. *301*:177, 1979.

429a. Kramer, B. L., Massie, B. M., and Topic, N.: Controlled trial of captopril in chronic heart failure: A rest and exercise hemodynamic study. Circulation *67*:807, 1983.

429b. Awan, N. A., Amsterdam, E. A., Hermanovich, J., Bommer, W. J., Needham, K. E., and Mason, D. T.: Long-term hemodynamic and clinical efficacy of captopril therapy in ambulatory management of severe chronic congestive heart failure. Am. Heart J. *103*:474, 1982.

430. Faxon, D. P., Creager, M. A., Halperin, J. L., Gavras, H., Coffman, J. D., and Ryan, T. J.: Central and peripheral hemodynamic effects of angiotensin inhibition in patients with refractory congestive heart failure. Circulation *61*:925, 1980.

431. Pierpont, G. L., Hale, K. A., Franciosa, J. A., and Cohn, J. N.: Relationship between pulmonary vascular and hypoxemic effects of vasodilators in left ventricular failure. Circulation *56*(Suppl. III):III–163, 1977 (abstract).

432. Collste, P., Haglund, K., Lundgren, G., Magnusson, G., and Ostman, J.: Reversible renal failure during treatment with captopril. Br. Med. J. *2*:612–613, 1979.

433. Case, D. B., Atlas, S. A., Mouradian, J. A., Fishman, R. A., Sherman, R. L., and Laragh, J. H.: Proteinuria during long-term captopril therapy. J.A.M.A. *244*:346–349, 1980.

434. Franciosa, J. A.: Effectiveness of long-term vasodilator administration in the treatment of chronic left ventricular failure. Prog. Cardiovasc. Dis. *24*:319–330, 1982.

435. DiSegni, E., Kaplinsky, E., Klein, H. O., and Levy, M.: Treatment of ruptured interventricular septum with afterload reduction. Arch. Intern. Med. *138*:1427, 1978.

436. Greenberg, B. H., Massie, B. M., Brundage, B. H., Botvinick, E. H., Parmley, W. W., and Chatterjee, K.: Beneficial effects of hydralazine in severe mitral regurgitation. Circulation *58*:273, 1978.

437. Greenberg, B. H., DeMots, H., Murphy, E., and Rahimtoola, S.: Beneficial effects of hydralazine on rest and exercise hemodynamics in patients with chronic severe aortic insufficiency. Circulation *62*:49–55, 1980.

437a. Fioretti, P., Benussi, B., Scardi, S., Klugmann, S., Brower, R. W., and Camerini, F.: Afterload reduction with nifedipine in aortic insufficiency. Am. J. Cardiol. *49*:1728–1732, 1982.

438. Rubin, L. J., and Peter, R. H.: Hemodynamics at rest and during exercise after oral hydralazine in patients with cor pulmonale. Am. J. Cardiol. *47*:116–122, 1981.

439. Colucci, W. S., Holman, L., Wynne, J., Carabello, B., Malacoff, R., Grossman, W., and Braunwald, E.: Improved right ventricular function and reduced pulmonary vascular resistance during prazosin therapy of congestive heart failure. Am. J. Med. *71*:75–80, 1981.

440. Weber, K. T., Kinasewitz, G. T., West, J. S., Janicki, J. S., Reichek, N., and Fishman, A. P.: Long-term vasodilator therapy with trimazosin in chronic cardiac failure. N. Engl. J. Med. *303*:242, 1980.

440a. Lemke, R., Trompler, A., Kaltenbach, M., and Bussmann, W. D.: Wirkung von Prazosin bei der therapierefraktären chronischen Herzinsuffizienz. Dtsch. Med. Wschr. *104*:1769, 1979.

441. Franciosa, J. A., and Cohn, J. N.: Immediate effects of hydralazine isosorbide dinitrate combination on exercise capacity and exercise hemodynamics in patients with left ventricular failure. Circulation *59*:1085, 1979.

442. Pierpont, G. L., Cohn, J. N., and Franciosa, J. A.: Combined oral hydralazine-nitrate therapy in left ventricular failure. Hemodynamic equivalency to sodium nitroprusside. Chest *73*:8, 1978.

443. Massie, B., Kramer, B., and Haughom, F.: Postural hypotension and tachycardia during hydralazine-isosorbide dinitrate therapy for chronic heart failure. Circulation *63*:658–644, 1981.

444. Aronow, W. S., Lurie, M., Turbow, M., Whittaker, K., VanCamp, S., and Hughes, D.: Effects of prazosin vs. placebo on chronic left ventricular heart failure. Circulation *59*:344, 1979.

445. Aronow, W. S., and Danahy, D. T.: Efficacy of trimazosin and prazosin therapy on cardiac and exercise performance in outpatients with chronic congestive heart failure. Am. J. Med. *65*:155, 1978.

446. Sharma, B., Hoback, J., Francis, G. S., Hodges, M., Asinger, R. W., Cohn, J. N., and Taylor, C. R.: Pirbuterol: A new oral sympathomimetic amine for the treatment of congestive heart failure. Am. Heart J. *102*(Part 2):533–541, 1981.

447. Walsh, W. F., and Greenberg, B. H.: Results of long-term vasodilator therapy in patients with refractory congestive heart failure. Circulation *64*:499–505, 1981.

448. Packer, M., Meller, J., Medina, N., Yushak, M., and Gorlin, R.: Determinants of drug response in severe chronic heart failure. I. Activation of vasoconstrictor forces during vasodilator therapy. Circulation *64*:505–514, 1981.

449. Colucci, W. S., Williams, G. H., Alexander, R. W., and Braunwald, E.: Mechanisms and implications of vasodilator tolerance in the treatment of congestive heart failure. Am. J. Med. *71*:89–99, 1981.

Sympathomimetic Amines

450. Goldberg, L. I.: Cardiovascular and renal actions of dopamine: Potential clinical applications. Pharmacol. Rev *24*:1, 1972.

451. Goldberg, L. I., Hsieh, Y.-Y., and Resnekov, L.: Newer catecholamines for treatment of heart failure and shock: An update on dopamine and a first look at dobutamine. Progr. Cardiovasc. Dis. *19*:327, 1977.

452. Goldberg, L. I.: The dopamine vascular receptor: New areas for biochemical pharmacologists. Biochem. Pharmacol. *24*:651, 1975.

453. Toda, N., Hojo, M., Sakae, K., and Usui, H.: Comparison of the relaxing effect of dopamine with that of adenosine, isoproterenol and acetylcholine in isolated canine coronary arteries. Blood Vessels *12*:290, 1975.

454. Dressler, W. E., Rossi, G. V., and Orzechowski, R. F.: Evidence that renal vasodilation by dopamine in dogs does not involve release of prostaglandin. J. Pharm. Pharmacol. *27*:203, 1975.

455. Yeh, B. K., McNay, J. L., and Goldberg, L. I.: Attenuation of dopamine renal and mesenteric vasodilation by haloperidol: Evidence for a specific receptor. J. Pharmacol. Exp. Ther. *168*:303, 1969.

456. Gilbert, J. C., and Goldberg, L. I.: Characterization by cyproheptadine of the dopamine-induced contraction in canine isolated arteries. J. Pharmacol. Exp. Ther. *193*:435, 1975.

457. Willems, L. J., and Bogaert, M. G.: Dopamine-induced neurogenic vasodilation in isolated perfused muscle preparation of the dog. Naunyn Schmiedebergs Arch. Pharmakol. *286*:413, 1975.

458. Enero, M. A., and Langer, S. Z.: Inhibition of dopamine of ³H-noradrenaline release elicited by nerve stimulation of the isolated cat's nictitating membrane. Naunyn Schmiedebergs Arch. Pharmakol. *289*:179, 1975.

459. Hardaker, W. T., Jr., and Wechsler, A. S.: Redistribution of renal intracortical blood flow during dopamine infusion in dogs. Circ. Res. *33*:437, 1973.

460. Hollenberg, N. K., Adams, D. F., Mendell, P., Abrams, H. L., and Merrill, J. P.: Renal vascular responses to dopamine. Haemodynamics and angiographic observations in normal man. Clin. Sci. Molec. Med. *45*:733, 1973.

461. Goldberg, L. I., and Toda, N.: Dopamine-induced relaxation of isolated canine renal, mesenteric and femoral arteries contracted with prostaglandin-F₂α. Circ. Res. *36*(Suppl. I):I-97, 1975.

462. Goldberg, L. I.: Dopamine: Clinical uses of an endogenous catecholamine. N. Engl. J. Med. *291*:707, 1974.

463. Allwood, M. J., and Ginsburg, J.: Peripheral vascular and other effects of dopamine infusion in man. Clin. Sci. *27*:271, 1964.

464. Vincenti, F., and Goldberg, L. I.: Combined use of dopamine and prostaglandin A₁ in patients with acute renal failure and hepatorenal syndrome. Prostaglandins *15*:463, 1978.

465. Brooks, H. L., Stein, P. D., Matson, J. L., and Hyland, J. W.: Dopamine-induced alterations in coronary hemodynamics in dogs. Circ. Res. *24*:699, 1969.

466. Toda, N., and Goldberg, L. I.: Effects of dopamine on isolated canine coronary arteries. Cardiovasc. Res. *9*:384, 1975.

467. Goldberg, L. I., McDonald, R. H., Jr., and Zimmerman, A. M.: Sodium diuresis produced by dopamine in patients with congestive heart failure. N. Engl. J. Med. *269*:1060, 1963.

468. Rosenblum, R., Tai, A. R., and Lawson, D.: Dopamine in man: Cardiorenal hemodynamics in normotensive patients with heart disease. J. Pharmacol. Exp. Ther. *183*:256, 1972.

469. Marino, R. J., Romagnoli, A., and Keats, A. S.: Selective venoconstriction by

dopamine in comparison with isoproterenol and phenylephrine. Anesthesiology *43*:570, 1975.

470. Sturm, J. T., Guhrman, T. M., Sterling, R., Turner, S. A., Igo, S. R., and Norman, J. C.: Combined use of dopamine and nitroprusside therapy in conjunction with intra-aortic balloon pumping for the treatment of post-cardiotomy low-output syndrome. J. Thorac. Cardiovasc. Surg. *82*:13–17, 1981.

471. Tuttle, R. R., and Mills, J.: Dopamine development of a new catecholamine to selectively increase cardiac contractility. Circ. Res. *36*:185, 1975.

472. Vatner, S. F., Higgins, C. B., and Braunwald, E.: Effects of norepinephrine on coronary circulation and left ventricular dynamics in the conscious dog. Circ. Res. *34*:812, 1974.

473. Sonnenblick, E. H., Frishman, W. H., and LeJemtel, T. H.: Dobutamine: A new synthetic cardioactive sympathetic amine. N. Engl. J. Med. *300*:17, 1979.

474. Fuchs, R. M., Rutlen, D. L., and Powell, W. J., Jr.: Effect of dobutamine on systemic capacity in the dog. Circ. Res. *46*:133, 1980.

475. Williams, R. S., and Bishop, T.: Selectivity of dobutamine for adrenergic receptor subtypes: *In vitro* analysis by radioligand binding. J. Clin. Invest. *67*:1703–1711, 1981.

476. Fleisch, J. H., and Spaethe, S. M.: Vasodilation and aging evaluated in the isolated perfused rat mesenteric vascular bed: Preliminary observations on the vascular pharmacology of dobutamine. J. Cardiovasc. Pharmacol. *3*:187, 1981.

477. Robie, N. W., and Goldberg, L. I.: Comparative systemic and regional hemodynamic effects of dopamine and dobutamine. Am. Heart J. *90*:340, 1975.

477a.Magorien, R. D., Unverferth, D. V., Brown, G. P., and Leier, C. V.: Dobutamine and hydralazine: Comparative influences of positive inotropy and vasodilation on coronary blood flow and myocardial energetics in non-ischemic congestive heart failure. J. Am. Coll. Cardiol. *1*:499, 1983.

478. Gillespie, J. A., Ambos, H. D., Sobel, B. E., and Roberts, R.: Effects of dobutamine in patients with acute myocardial infarction. Am. J. Cardiol. *39*:588, 1977.

479. Unverferth, D. V., Magorien, R. D., Lewis, R. P., and Laier, C. V.: Long-term benefit of dobutamine in patients with congestive cardiomyopathy. Am. Heart J. *100*:622–630, 1980.

479a.Applefeld, M. M., Newman, K. A., Grove, W. R., Stutton, F. J., Roffman, D. S., Reed, W. P., and Linberg, S.: Intermittent, continuous outpatient dobutamine infusion in the management of congestive heart failure. Am. J. Cardiol. *51*:455, 1983.

480. Bendersky, R., Chatterjee, K., Parmley, W. W., Brundage, B. H., and Ports, T. A.: Dobutamine in chronic ischemic heart failure: Alterations in left ventricular function and coronary hemodynamics. Am. J. Cardiol. *48*:554, 1981.

481. Aronson, R. S., and Gelles, J. M.: Electrophysiologic effects of dopamine on sheep cardiac Purkinje fibers. J. Pharmacol. Exp. Ther. *188*:596, 1974.

482. Loeb, H. S., Sinno, M. Z., Saudye, A., Towne, W. D., and Gunnar, R. M.: Electrophysiologic properties of dobutamine. Circ. Shock *1*:217, 1974.

483. Loeb, H. S., Khan, M., Klodnycky, M. L., Sinno, M. Z., Towne, W. D., and Gunnar, R. M.: Haemodynamic effects of dobutamine in man. Circ. Shock *2*:29, 1975.

484. Tinker, J. H., Tarhan, S., White, R. D., Pluth, J. R., and Barnhorst, D. A.: Dobutamine for inotropic support during emergence from cardiopulmonary bypass. Anesthesiology *44*:281, 1976.

485. Lipp, H., Falicov, R. E., Resnekov, L., and King, S.: The effects of dopamine on depressed myocardial function following coronary embolization in the closed-chest dog. Am. Heart J. *84*:208, 1972.

486. Holloway, G. A., Jr., and Frederickson, E. L.: Dobutamine, a new beta agonist. Anesth. Analg. *53*:616, 1974.

487. Pozen, R. G., DiBianco, R., Katz, R. J., Bortz, R., Myerburg, R. J., and Fletcher, R. D.: Myocardial metabolic and hemodynamic effects of dobutamine in heart failure complicating coronary artery disease. Circulation *63*:1279–1285, 1981.

488. Alexander, C. S., Sako, Y., and Mikulic, E.: Pedal gangrene associated with the use of dopamine. N. Engl. J. Med. *293*:591, 1975.

489. Greene, S. I., and Smith, J. W.: Dopamine gangrene. N. Engl. J. Med. *294*:114, 1976.

490. Stoner, J. D., Bolen, J. L., and Harrison, D. C.: Comparison of dobutamine and dopamine in treatment of severe heart failure. Br. Heart J. *39*:536, 1977.

491. Loeb, H. S., Bredakis, J., and Gunnar, R. M.: Superiority of dobutamine over dopamine for augmentation of cardiac output in patients with chronic low output cardiac failure. Circulation *55*:375, 1977.

492. Leier, C. V., Heban, P. T., Huss, P., Bush, C. A., and Lewis, R. P.: Comparative systemic and regional hemodynamic effects of dopamine and dobutamine in patients with cardiomyopathic heart failure. Circulation *58*:466, 1978.

493. Berkowitz, C., McKeever, L., Croke, R. P., Jacobs, W. R., Loeb, H. S., and Gunnar, R. M.: Comparative responses to dobutamine and nitroprusside in patients with chronic low output cardiac failure. Circulation *56*:918, 1977.

494. Mason, D. T., and Braunwald, E.: Studies on digitalis. X. Effects of ouabain on forearm vascular resistance and venous tone in normal subjects and in patients in heart failure. J. Clin. Invest. *43*:532, 1964.

495. Robie, N. W., Nutter, D. O., Moody, C., and McNay, J. L.: In vivo analysis of adrenergic receptor activity of dobutamine. Circ. Res. (Abstract) *34*:663, 1974.

496. Vatner, S. F., McRitchie, R. J., and Braunwald, E.: Effects of dobutamine on left ventricular performance, coronary dynamics, and distribution of cardiac output in conscious dogs. J. Clin. Invest. *53*:1265, 1974.

497. Akhtar, N., Mikulic, E., Cohn, J. N., and Chaudhry, M. H.: Hemodynamic effect of dobutamine in patients with severe heart failure. Am. J. Cardiol. *36*:202, 1975.

498. Loeb, H. S., Khan, M., Saudye, A., and Gunnar, R. M.: Acute hemodynamic effects of dobutamine and isoproterenol in patients with low output cardiac failure. Circ. Shock *3*:55, 1976.

499. Guiha, N. H., Cohn, J. N., Mikulic, E., Franciosa, J. A., and Limas, C. J.: Treatment of refractory heart failure with infusion of nitroprusside. N. Engl. J. Med. *291*:587, 1974.

500. Palmer, R. F., and Lasseter, K. C.: Drug therapy: Sodium nitroprusside. N. Engl. J. Med. *292*:294, 1975.

501. Faxon, D. P., Gross, S., Flessas, A. P., Tilney, C., and Ryan, T. J.: The significance of heart rate response to nitroglycerin. Am. J. Cardiol. (Abstract) *39*:298, 1977.

502. Gagnon, R. M., Fortin, L., Boucher, R., Gilbert, S., Morrisette, M., Present, S., Lemire, J., and David, A.: Combined hemodynamic effects of dobutamine and IV nitroglycerin in congestive heart failure. Chest *78*:694, 1980.

Refractory and Intractable Heart Failure

503. Awan, N. A., Evenson, M. K., Needham, K. E., Evans, T. O., Hermanovich, J., Taylor, C. R., Amsterdam, E., and Mason, D. T.: Hemodynamic effects of oral pirbuterol in chronic severe congestive heart failure. Circulation *63*:96–101, 1981.

504. Awan, N. A., Needham, K. E., Evenson, M. K., and Mason, D. T.: Comparison of hemodynamic actions of pirbuterol and dobutamine on cardiac function in severe congestive heart failure. Am. J. Cardiol. *47*:665–669, 1981.

505. Dawson, J. R., Canepa-Anson, R., Kuan, P., Whitaker, N. H. G., Carnie, J., Warnes, C., Ruben, S. R., Poole-Wilson, P. A., and Sutton, G. C.: Treatment of chronic heart failure with pirbuterol: Acute haemodynamic responses. Br. Med. J. *282*:1423–1426, 1981.

506. Rude, R. E., Turi, Z., Brown, E. J., Lorell, B. H., Colucci, W. S., Mudge, G. H., Jr., Taylor, C. R., and Grossman, W.: Acute effects of oral pirbuterol on myocardial oxygen metabolism and systemic hemodynamics in chronic congestive heart failure. Circulation *64*:139–145, 1981.

507. Colucci, W. S., Alexander, R. W., Williams, G. H., Rude, R. E., Holman, B. L., Konstam, M. A., Wynne, J., Mudge, G. H., Jr., and Braunwald, E.: Decreased lymphocyte beta-adrenergic-receptor density in patients with heart failure and tolerance to the beta-adrenergic agonist pirbuterol. N. Engl. J. Med. *305*:185–190, 1981.

508. Hutton, I., Murray, R. G., Boyes, R. N., Rae, A. P., and Hillis, W. S.: Haemodynamic effects of prenalterol in patients with coronary heart disease. Br. Heart J. *43*:134–137, 1980.

509. Kirlin, P. C., and Pitt, B.: Hemodynamic effects of intravenous prenalterol in severe heart failure. Am. J. Cardiol. *47*:670–675, 1981.

510. Awan, N. A., Needham, K. E., Evenson, M. K., Wyn, A., and Mason, D. T.: Hemodynamic actions of prenalterol in severe congestive heart failure due to chronic coronary disease. Am. Heart J. *101*:158–161, 1981.

511. Tweddel, A. C., Murray, R. G., Pearson, D., Martin, W., and Hutton, I.: Cardiovascular effects of prenalterol on rest and exercise haemodynamics in patients with chronic congestive heart failure. Br. Heart J. *47*:375–380, 1982.

512. Drexler, H. J., Lollgen, H., and Just, H.: Short- and long-term effects of hydralazine and combined hydralazine-prenalterol therapy in severe chronic congestive heart failure. Klin. Wochenschr. *59*:647, 1981.

512a.Fitzpatrick, D., Ikram, H., Nicholls, G., and Espiner, E. A.: Hemodynamic, hormonal and electrolyte responses to prenalterol infusion in heart failure. Circulation *67*:613, 1983.

513. Slutsky, R.: Hemodynamic effects of inhaled terbutaline in congestive heart failure patients without lung disease: Beneficial cardiotonic and vasodilator beta-agonist properties evaluated by ventricular catheterization and radionuclide angiography. Am. Heart J. *101*:556–560, 1981.

514. Sharma, B., and Goodwin, J. F.: Beneficial effects of salbutamol on cardiac function in severe congestive cardiomyopathy: Effect on systolic and diastolic function of the left ventricle. Circulation *58*:449, 1978.

515. Alousi, A. A., Farah, A. E., Lesher, G. Y., and Opalka, C. J., Jr.: Cardiotonic activity of amrinone. Circ. Res. *45*:666–677, 1979.

516. Endoh, M., Yamashita, S., and Taira, N.: Positive inotropic effect of amrinone in relation to cyclic nucleotide metabolism in the canine ventricular muscle. J. Pharmacol. Exp. Ther. *221*:775–783, 1982.

517. Honerjäger, P., Schäfer-Korting, M., and Reiter, M.: Involvement of cyclic AMP in the direct inotropic action of amrinone: Biochemical and functional evidence. Naunyn Schmiedebergs Arch. Pharmacol. *318*:112–120, 1981.

517a.Scholz, H.: Pharmacological actions of various inotropic agents. Europ. Heart J. *4*(Suppl. A):161, 1983.

518. Benotti, J. R., Grossman, W., Braunwald, E., Davolos, D. D., and Alousi, A. A.: Hemodynamic assessment of amrinone: A new inotropic agent. N. Engl. J. Med. *299*:1373–1377, 1978.

519. LeJemtel, T. H., Keung, E., Sonnenblick, E. H., et al.: Amrinone: A new nonglycosidic, non-adrenergic cardiotonic agent effective in the treatment of intractible myocardial failure in man. Circulation *59*:1098–1104, 1979.

520. LeJemtel, T. H., Keung, E., Ribner, H. S., Davis, R., Wexler, J., Blaufox, M. D., and Sonnenblick, E. H.: Sustained beneficial effects of oral amrinone on cardiac and renal function in patients with severe congestive heart failure. Am. J. Cardiol. *45*:123–129, 1980.

521. Wynne, J., Malacoff, R. F., Benotti, J. R., Curfman, G. C., Grossman, W., Holman, B. L., Smith, T. W., and Braunwald, E.: Oral amrinone in refractory congestive heart failure. Am. J. Cardiol. *45*:1245–1249, 1980.

522. Benotti, J. R., Grossman, W., Braunwald, E., and Carabello, B. A.: Effects of amrinone on myocardial energy metabolism and hemodynamics in patients

with severe congestive heart failure due to coronary artery disease. Circulation 62:28–34, 1980.

523. Weber, K. T., Andrews, V., Janicki, J. S., Wilson, J. R., and Fishman, A. P.: Amrinone and exercise performance in patients with chronic heart failure. Am. J. Cardiol. 48:164–169, 1981.

524. Siskind, S. J., Sonnenblick, E. H., Forman, R., Scheuer, J., and LeJemtel, T. H.: Acute substantial benefit of inotropic therapy with amrinone on exercise hemodynamics and metabolism in severe congestive heart failure. Circulation 64:966–973, 1981.

525. Maskin, C. S., Forman, R., Klein, N. A., Sonnenblick, E. H., and LeJemtel, T. H.: Long-term amrinone therapy in patients with severe heart failure. Am. J. Med. 72:113–118, 1982.

526. Siegel, L. A., Keung, E., Siskind, S. J., Forman, R., Feinberg, H., Strom, J., Efstathakis, D., Sonnenblick, E. H., and LeJemtel, T. H.: Beneficial effects of amrinone-hydralazine combination on resting hemodynamics and exercise capacity in patients with severe congestive heart failure. Circulation 63:838–844, 1981.

526a. McDowell, A., Baim, D., Cherniles, J., Bekele, T., Braunwald, E., and Grossman, W.: Hemodynamic effects of a new inotropic agent (WIN 47203) in patients with refractory heart failure. J. Am. Coll. Cardiol. 1:675, 1983.

526b. Maskin, C. S., Sinoway, L., Chadwick, B., Sonnenblick, E. H., and LeJemtel, T. H.: Sustained hemodynamic and clinical effects of a new cardiotonic agent, WIN 47203, in patients with severe congestive heart failure. Circulation 67: 1065, 1983.

527. Podrid, P. J., Schoenberger, A., and Lown, B.: Congestive heart failure caused by oral disopyramide. N. Engl. J. Med. 302:614–617, 1980.

528. Chew, C. Y. C., Hecht, H. S., Collett, J. T., McAllister, R. G., and Singh, B. N.: Influence of severity of ventricular dysfunction on hemodynamic responses to intravenously administered verapamil in ischemic heart disease. Am. J. Cardiol. 47:917–922, 1981.

529. Miller, R. R., Awan, N. A., Joye, J. A., Maxwell, K. S., DeMaria, A. N., Amsterdam, E. A., and Mason, D. T.: Combined dopamine and nitroprusside therapy in congestive heart failure. Circulation 55:881, 1977.

530. Raabe, D. S., Jr.: Combined therapy with digoxin and nitroprusside in heart failure complicating acute myocardial infarction. Am. J. Cardiol. 43:990, 1979.

Other Measures

531. Barnard, C. N.: The operation. S. Afr. Med. J. 41:1271, 1967.

532. Stinson, E. B., Dong, E., Jr., Iben, A. R., and Shumway, N. E.: Cardiac transplantation in man. III. Surgical aspects. Am. J. Surg. 118:182, 1969.

533. Schroeder, J. S.: Current status of cardiac transplantation—1978. J.A.M.A. 241:2069, 1979.

534. Watson, D. C., Reitz, B. A., Baumgartner, W. A., Raney, A. A., Oyer, P. E., Stinson, E. B., and Shumway, N. E.: Distant heart procurement for transplantation. Surgery 86:56, 1979.

534a. Hess, M. L. Hastillo, A., Thompson, M., Copeland, J., and Stinson, E. B.: Status of cardiac transplantation 1981–1982. The national registry report. J. Am. Coll. Cardiol. 1:721, 1983.

535. Reitz, B. A., Wallmork, J. L., Hunt, S. A., Pennock, J. L., Billingham, M. E., Oyer, P. E., Stinson, E. B., and Shumway, N. E.: Heart-lung transplantation. N. Engl. J. Med. 306:557, 1982.

536. Billingham, M. E., Baumgartner, W. A., Watson, D. C., Reitz, B. A., Masek, M. A., Raney, A. A., Oyer, P. E., Stinson, E. B., and Shumway, N. E.: Distant heart procurement for human transplantation. Circulation 62(Suppl. I): 11–19, 1980.

537. Wiscomb, W., Cooper, D. K. C., Hassoulas, J., Rose, A. G., and Barnard, C. N.: Orthotopic transplantation of the baboon heart after 20 to 24 hours' preservation by continuous hypothermic perfusion with an oxygenated hyperosmolar solution. J. Thorac. Cardiovasc. Surg. 83:133, 1982.

538. Losiman, J. G., and Barnard, C. N.: Heterotopic heart transplantation: A valid alternative to orthotopic transplantation: Results, advantages and disadvantages. J. Surg. Res. 32:297, 1982.

539. Oyer, P. E., Jamieson, S. W., and Stinson, E. B.: Cardiac transplantation for end-stage congestive heart failure. In Braunwald, E., Mock, M. B., and Watson, J. (eds.): Congestive Heart Failure. New York, Grune and Stratton, 1982, pp. 317–328.

540. Hunt, S. A., Rider, A. K., Stinson, E. B., Griepp, R. B., Schroeder, J. S., Harrison, D. C., and Shumway, N. E.: Does cardiac transplantation prolong life and improve its quality? An updated report. Circulation 54(Suppl. III):III–56, 1976.

541. Christopherson, L. K., Griepp, R. B., and Stinson, E. B.: Rehabilitation after cardiac transplantation. J.A.M.A. 236:2082, 1976.

542. Caves, P. K., Stinson, E. B., Billingham, M. E., and Shumway, N. E.: Serial transvenous biopsy of the transplanted human heart: Improved management of acute rejection episodes. Lancet 1:821, 1974.

543. Mason, J. W., Stinson, E. B., Hunt, S. A., Schroeder, J. S., and Rider, A. K.: Infections after cardiac transplantation: Relation to rejection therapy. Ann. Intern. Med. 85:69, 1976.

544. Miller, M. G., Weintraub, R. M., Hedley-Whyte, J., and Restall, D. S.: Surgery for cardiogenic shock. Lancet 2:1342, 1974.

545. Weber, K. T., and Janicki, J. S.: Intraaortic balloon counterpulsation: A review of physiological principles, clinical results, and device safety. Ann. Thorac. Surg. 17:602, 1974.

546. Weil, M. H., and Shubin, H.: Shock following acute myocardial infarction: Current understanding of hemodynamic mechanisms. Progr. Cardiovasc. Dis. 11:1, 1968.

547. Moulopoulos, S. D., Topaz, S., and Kolff, W. J.: Diastolic balloon pumping (with carbon dioxide) in the aorta—a mechanical assistance to the failing circulation. Am. Heart J. 63:669, 1962.

548. Bregman, D.: Assessment of intra-aortic balloon counterpulsation in cardiogenic shock. Crit. Care Med. 3:90, 1975.

549. Leinbach, R. C., Dinsmore, R. E., Mundth, E. D., Buckley, M. J., Dunkman, W. B., Austen, W. G., and Sanders, C. A.: Selective coronary and left ventricular cineangiography during intraaortic balloon pumping for cardiogenic shock. Circulation 45:845, 1972.

550. Bernhard, W. F., Berger, R. L., Stetz, J., Carr, J., Colo, N., McCormick, J., and Fishbein, M.: Temporary left ventricular bypass: Factors affecting patient survival. Circulation 60(Suppl. II):131, 1979.

551. Pierce, W. S., Parr, G. V. S., Myers, J. L., Pae, W. E., Jr., Bull, A. P., and Waldhausen, J. A.: Ventricular-assist pumping in patients with cardiogenic shock after cardiac operations. N. Engl. J. Med. 305:1606, 1981

552. Berger, R. L., Merin, G., Carr, J., Sossman, H. A., and Bernhard, W. F.: Successful use of a left ventricular assist device in cardiogenic shock from massive post-operative myocardial infarction. J. Thorac. Cardiovasc. Surg., 78:626, 1980.

552a. Golding, L. R., Jacobs, G., Groves, L. K., Gill, C. C., Nose, Y., and Loop, F. D.: Clinical results of mechanical support of the failing left ventricle. J. Thorac. Cardiovasc. Surg. 83:597, 1982.

552b. Turina, M.: Surgical and mechanical support of the failing heart. Europ. Heart J. 4(Suppl. A):211, 1983.

553. Norman, J. C., Duncan, J. M., Frazier, O. H., Hallman, G. L., Ott, D. A., Ruel, G. J., and Cooley, D. A.: Intracorporeal (abdominal) left ventricular assist devices or partial artificial hearts. Arch. Surg. 116:1441–1445, 1981.

554. Rose, D. M., Culvin, S. B., Culliford, A. T., Cunningham, J. N., Adams, P. X., Glassman, E., Isom, O. W., and Spencer, F. C.: Long-term survival with partial left heart bypass following perioperative myocardial infarction and shock. J. Thorac. Cardiovasc. Surg. 83:483–492, 1982.

555. Oyer, P. E., Stinson, E. B., Portner, P. M., Ream, A. K., and Shumway, N. E.: Development of a totally implantable, electrically actuated left ventricular assist system. Am. J. Surg. 140:17, 1980.

556. Pierce, W. S.: The use of mechanical circulatory support in advanced congestive heart failure. In Braunwald, E., Mock, M. B., and Watson, J. (eds.): Congestive Heart Failure. New York, Grune and Stratton, 1982, pp. 329–340.

557. Lawson, J. H., Fukumasu, H., Olsen, D. B., Jarvik, K., Kessler, T. R., Coleman, D., Blaylock, R., and Kolff, W. J.: Six-month survival of a calf with an artificial heart. J. Thorac. Cardiovasc. Surg. 78:150, 1979.

557a. Büchert, E. S., Affeld, K., Baer, P., et al.: Total artificial heart replacement. Int. J. Artif. Organs 2:141, 1979.

558. Pierce, W. S., Myers, J. L., Donachy, J. H., Rosenberg, G., Landis, D. L., Prophet, A., and Snyder, A. J.: Approaches to the artificial heart. Surgery 137:137, 1981.

558a. DeVries, W. C.: The total artificial heart. In Sabiston, D. C., Jr., and Spencer, F. C. (Eds.): Surgery of the Chest, 4th Ed. Philadelphia, W. B. Saunders Co., 1983.

559. Jarvik, R. K.: The total artificial heart. Sci. Am. 244:74, 1981.

17

PULMONARY EDEMA: CARDIOGENIC AND NONCARDIOGENIC

by Roland H. Ingram, Jr., M.D., and Eugene Braunwald, M.D.

HISTORY

As an easily diagnosable clinical and pathological entity, pulmonary edema was clearly defined in 1819 by Laennec as "an infiltration of serum into the pulmonary tissue, carried to a degree such that it significantly diminishes [the lungs'] permeability to air."[1] From the standpoint of the clinician, this definition prevailed until 1956, when Visscher and colleagues restated the same basic idea more prosaically by defining pulmonary edema as a pathological state in which there is abnormal extravascular water storage in the lung.[2] This later definition thus allowed the identification of pulmonary edema at an earlier stage, in that diminished "permeability to air" was not a criterion. This review contained a clear, concise, and detailed summary of experimental studies up to that time, including the classic treatise by C. K. Drinker.[3] Although the principles of transcapillary liquid exchange were well established, the first experimentally quantitative assessment of the edema process in the lung was made in 1959 by Guyton and Lindsey.[4] Over the ensuing years, significant strides have been made in terms of not only more precise quantitation but also a deeper understanding of the structural and functional relationships of this process, which in turn has improved our understanding of edema in the lung.

THE ALVEOLAR-CAPILLARY MEMBRANE AND PULMONARY EDEMA

Structure of the Alveolar-capillary Membrane. The barrier between pulmonary capillaries and alveolar gas consists of a series of three anatomical layers with distinct structural characteristics (Fig. 17–1). The cytoplasmic projections of the capillary endothelial cells join by abutment or interdigitation or overlap to form a continuous cytoplasmic tube. At the overlapping junctions of these cytoplasmic projections are clefts of varying sizes, averaging approximately 40 μm in width, which provide communication between pulmonary capillaries and the interstitial space. Because these clefts can be widened with relatively small increases in vascular pressure, they are referred to as "loose" junctions. Although thin cytoplasmic projections result in maximal area for gas exchange with minimal tissue mass, these tenuous projections and junctions may be unusually vulnerable to disruption.[7]

The interstitial space varies in thickness and may contain connective tissue fibrils, fibroblasts, and macrophages between the capillary endothelium and the alveolar epithelium. There are no lymphatics in the alveolar-capillary interstitium.[5] This interstitial space of the alveolar-capillary septum is continuous with the wider and more compliant space surrounding terminal bronchioles, small arteries, and veins, and it is in this latter portion of the interstitial space that lymphatic channels first appear.[5] The lymphatics serve to remove solutes, colloids, and liquid derived from the blood vessels. Because of the increased compliance of the nonalveolar interstitial space, liquid is more apt to increase

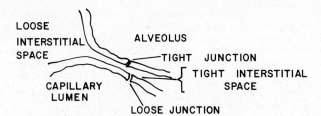

FIGURE 17–1 Schematic representation of the ultrastructure of the alveolar-capillary membrane. (Labeling corresponds to the discussion in the text.)

here once the pumping capacity of the lymphatic channels is exceeded.

The lining of the alveolar wall, which is continuous with the bronchial epithelium, is composed predominantly of large squamous cells (Type I) with thin cytoplasmic projections. Many fewer granular pneumocytes (Type II) join with the Type I cells to form the alveolar epithelium. Similar to the junctions of capillary endothelium, the projections of the alveolar cells abut and overlap. In contrast to the endothelial junctions, which allow for variable continuity between blood vessels and interstitial space, the alveolar epithelial clefts are obliterated by complete fusion of the membranes of the adjacent cells. Because the alveolar intercellular unions require much greater distending forces for their disruption than do the capillary endothelial connections, the former are referred to as "tight" junctions. The *tightness* of these junctions helps to forestall alveolar flooding, which represents the third and final stage of pulmonary edema. Although its principal function is to maintain alveolar stability, surfactant, the hydrophobic lipoprotein that lines the alveoli, may represent an additional mechanism for maintaining a dry alveolus.

Principles Governing Capillary-interstitial Liquid Exchange in the Lung. As in other tissues, there is normally a continuous exchange of liquid, colloid, and solutes between the vascular bed and interstitium.[8] A pathological state exists only when there is an increase in the net flux of liquids, colloids, and solutes from the vasculature into the interstitial space. Over the years experimental studies have confirmed that the basic principles outlined in the classic Starling equation apply to the lung as well as to the systemic circulation. The equation describes the net flux of liquid between capillaries and interstitium in terms of a permeability coefficient (K_f) and the balance of the total forces tending to move liquid out of the capillary into the interstitial space and those that act to move liquid into the capillary from the interstitial space. Liquid accumulation in the lung is determined by the net flux between the vascular and interstitial spaces (which is in turn determined by the algebraic sum of vascular and interstitial hydrostatic and colloid osmotic pressures) and the rate of lymphatic drainage. That is to say, there will be an undetectable net accumulation of liquid in the lung with time if the rate of transudation of liquid from the blood vessels to the interstitial space is equal to the rate of removal of liquid from the interstitial space by way of the lymphatics ($\dot{Q}_{lymph}$). The rate of transudation from blood vessels can be expressed either as the balance of those forces acting to move liquid out of and those acting to move liquid into the vessels (Eq. 1) or as the balance of hydrostatic and colloid osmotic forces (Eq. 2):

$$\dot{Q}_{(iv-int)} \propto K_f[(P_{iv} + \Pi_{int}) - (P_{int} + \Pi_{iv})] \tag{1}$$
$$\underset{\text{Outward}}{\phantom{K_f[(P_{iv} + \Pi_{int})}} \underset{\text{Inward}}{\phantom{- (P_{int} + \Pi_{iv})]}}$$
force   force

$$\dot{Q}_{(iv-int)} = K_f[(P_{iv} - P_{int}) - \sigma_f(\Pi_{iv} - \Pi_{int})] \tag{2}$$
Hydrostatic   Colloid osmotic
force   force

where $\dot{Q}$ = net rate of transudation (flow) of fluid from blood vessels to interstitial space

P_{int} = interstitial hydrostatic pressures
P_{iv} = intravascular hydrostatic pressures
Π_{int} = interstitial colloid osmotic pressure
Π_{iv} = intravascular colloid osmotic pressure
σ_f = reflection coefficient for proteins
K_f = apparent liquid filtration coefficient

Although the traditional Starling relationship has in the past been considered to apply to the transfer of liquid between pulmonary vasculature and alveolar space, it is clear from both the structural and the functional standpoints outlined above that this relationship applies mainly to the transfer between blood vessels and interstitial space. Although the equations are straightforward and set the stage for designating cardiogenic versus noncardiogenic pulmonary edema, there are many specific points to be made with regard to quantitative assessments.

What can be measured? An estimate of pulmonary capillary pressure (P_{iv}) can be obtained from capillary wedge or left atrial pressure measurements. Also, plasma colloid osmotic pressure (Π_{iv}) can be determined by means of an osmometer. However, accurate measurements of interstitial fluid colloid osmotic pressures (Π_{int}) and interstitial hydrostatic pressures (P_{int}) continue to be elusive. With regard to Π_{int}, it has been frequently assumed in experimental studies that values obtained for lymph or for the free space of implanted capsules are representative of interstitial fluid. However, Staub has pointed out that such assumptions are ill-founded, since interstitial liquid is not homogeneous, and lymph from the lung collected experimentally may be contaminated with lymph from other tissues. Interstitial hydrostatic pressure is equally elusive, but the assumption is often made that pleural pressures or hydrostatic pressures in implanted capsules are closely related to interstitial pressure.[5] Recent direct measurements using micropipettes inserted into the perivascular interstitium of hilar vessels of dog lungs indicate, indeed, that P_{int} is more negative than pleural pressure and that the difference increases at higher lung volumes.[9] However, the difference is small, and pleural pressure is probably sufficiently close to interstitial hydrostatic pressure to be useful as a clinical index. Recently it has been suggested that the mean negative intrapleural pressures seen in asthma may promote the formation and accumulation of interstitial liquid.[10]

It is worthwhile to note that the reflection coefficient (σ_f in Equation 2 above) is often considered to be 1.0 in experimental studies, i.e., the capillary membrane does not allow colloids to pass. In fact, as can be anticipated from the existence of the clefts described above and possibly through pinocytotic vesicles in the capillary endothelial projections, macromolecules can and do pass into the interstitial space. This is reflected by the fact that the mean lymph to plasma protein ratio is 0.75. The larger the molecule, the higher the reflection coefficient and the smaller the lymph to plasma ratio.[11] Hence the lymphatic proteins are predominantly of the smaller variety. Any disruption of the endothelial barrier produced either by increasing P_{iv} or by direct toxins will result in greater passage of macromolecules into the interstitium, which in turn increases Π_{int} and results in the passage of greater quantities of liquid.

As stated above, the lymphatics play a key role in removing liquid from the interstitial space, and unless the pumping capacity of the lymphatic channels is exceeded, edema will occur.

$$\dot{Q}_{(iv-int)} - \dot{Q}_{lymph} = \text{Rate of accumulation} \tag{3}$$

where Q = flow, iv = intravascular, and int = interstitial.

Although there is no direct way to measure lymph flow in humans, on the basis of extrapolation from animal data, Staub has estimated that an average 70-kg person at rest has a $\dot{Q}_{lymph}$ of approximately 20 ml per hour.[12] Experimentally, lymph flow rates of up to 10 times control values have been reported. Thus, it is possible that lymphatic pumping capacity can be as much as 200 ml per hour in an average-sized adult. It is probable that there would be some measurable accumulation of liquid in the lung before this capacity were reached, but it should be clear that there is an enormous lymphatic reserve. Given the capacity of lymphatic pumping, it can readily be comprehended that complete interruption of lymph flow, as with experiments on isolated lungs or in animals that have had surgical excision and reimplantation of the lung,[13] would result in much more rapid accumulation of interstitial liquid at any given rate of transudation from vessels.

Studies in the dog by Sampson and colleagues have shown that with chronic elevations of left atrial pressure, the pulmonary lymphatic system hypertrophies and is able to transport greater quantities of capillary filtrate during acute edematogenic incidents, thus prolonging survival.[14] On the basis of these experimental findings it is tempting to speculate that chronic increases in left atrial pressure in human disease might result in the same adaptive changes in the lymphatics that protect the lungs from edema during acute insults.

Since the lymphatic channels are so important in determining the net accumulation of interstitial liquid in the lung, it is worthwhile to consider how liquids and colloids get into these channels and the manner by which they are then transferred to the systemic circulation.[15] Normally, filtered liquid does not accumulate in the less compliant interstitial space of the alveolar-capillary septum but moves into the more compliant interstitial space that surrounds the bronchioles, venules, and arterioles. As noted earlier, it is in this latter interstitial space that the lymphatic channels are found.

How do liquids and colloids move from the tight interstitium of the alveolar-capillary septum to the more compliant interstitial space? It has been suggested that the forces resulting from the geometrical configuration of adjacent alveoli serve as a means of collecting liquid.[16] Figure 17-2 shows this configuration schematically. Through the Laplace relationship, the smaller radius of curvature at the corners results in greater local recoil pressures (hence more negative interstitial pressures) than occur at portions with greater radii of curvature. The resulting hydrostatic gradient would result in transfer of liquid to those junctions with smaller radii of curvature.[5] Indeed, after subpleural injections of dye-containing saline into cat lung, rapid accumulation of dye at such corners has been demonstrated. Within several minutes, the dye appears in the loose connective tissue spaces where the lymph capillaries are located.[5] Thus, there is a relatively direct pathway from the alveolar-capillary septum to the site of lymphatic channels. How liquids and colloids get into the lymphatic channels is not known. Increased permeability of the lymphatic walls with passive movement according to hydrostatic pressure gradients has been suggested,[17] yet with no experimental support. It has also been suggested that the pinocytotic vesicles within the lymphatic capillary endothelium serve to transfer liquid and protein into these channels; however, two studies have failed to demonstrate active transport.[18,19] Some structural data have supported the proposition that the fine fibrillar attachments of connective tissue to the edges of the cytoplasmic projections at points of juncture serve as one-way valve mechanisms.[20] These fibrils are thought to expand the lymph-capillary lumen and open junctions during tissue swelling, thus opening the drainage pathway when tissue pressure rises. Conversely, as lymph pressure rises, the junctions close.

Once inside the lymphatic channels, liquids and colloids are driven to major channels and ultimately to the systemic venous circulation. It had long been thought that only extrinsic forces were responsible for the propulsion of lymph through these valved channels, i.e., respiratory movements and vascular pulsations were thought to massage the

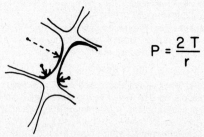

FIGURE 17-2 Schematic representation of the junction of several alveoli. The radii of curvature of a single alveolus vary considerably. The portion of the alveolar wall at which the radius of curvature is small (solid arrows) will tend toward greater local recoil pressures according to the Laplace relationship (P = 2T/r, where P = transmural pressure, T = surface tension, and r = the local radius of curvature). Since pressure in communicating alveoli is the same relative to atmospheric pressure, differences in transmural pressure result in different local interstitial pressures. It is in that portion of the interstitial space beneath smaller radii that liquid would first accumulate under conditions of increased transduction. These portions of the wall with greater radii of curvature (dashed arrow) would have smaller transmural pressures and hence would accumulate less liquid.

lymphatics and result in unidirectional movement due to the valves in the lymphatic capillaries. Although there is no doubt that extrinsic forces influence the rate of lymph movement, it is now well established that lymphatic capillaries are actively contractile.[21] Factors that control or regulate contraction of lymphatic capillaries and any change in their contractile properties under conditions of increased liquid and colloid filtration remain to be elucidated.

Quantitation of Pulmonary Edema

Direct Measures. Constant weighing of an isolated perfused lung has often been used as an index of edema based simply upon weight gain. However, as pointed out above, an isolated lung has no active lymphatic pump; hence the findings in this preparation do not take into account the important role that lymphatics play in vivo. The most commonly used and still standard quantitative assessment of pulmonary edema in experimental studies is the ratio of wet-to-dry lung weight. All the blood possible is drained from the vessels, and the lung is weighed, desiccated, and weighed again. This technique invariably includes the effects of a variable amount of retained blood and clearly measures the end result of a prolonged experiment rather than giving insights into the rate of change in response to a perturbation across the alveolar-capillary membrane.[22]

Indirect Measures. Recently, attempts have been made to gain quantitative information concerning the rate of change in lung water both during experimental interventions in animals and for assessment of disease and effects of treatment in human beings. These include the measurement of transthoracic electrical impedance, emission or absorption of radiation, and simultaneous indicator-dilution curves. The potential advantage of these less invasive measures lies in the fact that multiple determinations can be made for rapid assessment of changes in response to interventions.

Transthoracic electrical impedance measurements were initially thought to hold great promise for the quantitation of pulmonary edema in its early stage[23] (Stage 2). However, despite its noninvasiveness and rapidity, this method can be considered neither quantitative nor sensitive.

Methods employing *detection of radiation* assess either the appearance or the disappearance of radioactive substances introduced through the airways or blood vessels (emission) or the changes in absorption of roentgen rays or gamma irradiation across the chest from external sources (absorption). Emission techniques, although not completely tested, do not show great promise for clinical use. In contrast, quantitation of roentgen ray transmission using a filtered, monochromatic roentgen source and a photomultiplier detector offers some promise,[24] as does computerized axial tomography. The latter has been combined with radionuclide emission to quantitate edema in an experimental setting.[25] Intravascular marker (^{14}CO) signals were subtracted from those of a marker contained in both intra- and extravascular spaces ($C^{15}O_2$) to give extravascular lung water. Although interesting and possibly sensitive, the application of this technique requires expensive and rarely available equipment, including a cyclotron for generation of short-lived isotopes and a positron camera. Thus, to date, methods involving the use of radiation or radioisotopes have not been systematically applied to the study of pulmonary edema, either experimentally or clinically.

Simultaneous indicator-dilution curves derived from measurements of a detectable tracer substance that remains in the vasculature and one that quickly diffuses into the interstitial space offer the advantages of safety, theoretical soundness, and a numerical value.[26,26a] Theoretically, the tracer for water must equilibrate with tissue water during a single-transit interval. However, this condition is rarely met, since, in human lungs, only about half the interstitial lung water is measured by this technique.[5] Thus, although the double indicator-dilution method is simple, safe, and rapid, it is relatively insensitive and therefore does not serve a useful function in detecting the interstitial phase of acute pulmonary edema. Certainly, with the alveolar flooding in Stage 3, more water is in contact with the microvasculature than at any other stage, so that, as would be expected, the technique shows quite high values at a time when both the clinical and the routine radiographic methods of diagnosis probably suffice.

To sum up, attempts to quantitate pulmonary edema in its various stages of development are not yet sufficiently successful in terms of accuracy, sensitivity, and reproducibility to be clinically applicable.

Sequence of Liquid Accumulation in the Lung During Pulmonary Edema.
Whether initiated by an imbalance of Starling forces or by primary damage to the

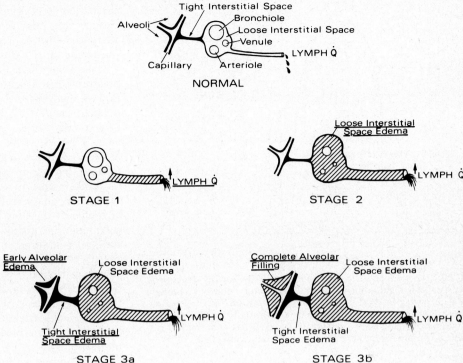

FIGURE 17–3 Schematic representation of alveolar-capillary membrane, loose interstitial space, and lymphatic system at the several stages of pulmonary edema—from the normal situation to fully developed alveolar edema, the new feature at each stage being underlined. (Drawn from Staub, N.C., et al.: Pulmonary edema in dogs, especially the sequence of fluid accumulation in lungs. J. Appl. Physiol. *22*: 227, 1967.)

various components of the alveolar-capillary membranes, the sequence of liquid exchange and accumulation in the lungs is the same and can be represented as three separate stages, the last of which has two substages that occur closely in time.[27,28] These three stages are shown schematically in Figure 17–3. As discussed above, the top portion demonstrates that normally there is continuous movement of liquid and colloid from the vessels to the interstitial space and that lymphatic channels constantly pump this liquid and colloid into the systemic venous system to maintain a constant interstitial volume.

In *Stage 1*, there is an increase in mass transfer of liquid and colloid from blood capillaries through the interstitium. The pulmonary capillary endothelial junctions may have been widened by an increase in filtrative forces or by toxic damage. Despite the increased filtration, there is no measurable increase in interstitial volume because there is an equal increase in lymphatic outflow. The stimulus or mechanism for increased lymph flow is not clear, yet it is possible that small increases in interstitial volume that defy detection by present techniques stimulate stretch receptors, resulting in tachypnea and, in turn, extrinsically augmenting lymphatic pumping.[7] Furthermore, it is possible that the same stimulus somehow augments the intrinsic lymphatic pumping capacity.

When the filtered load from the pulmonary capillaries is sufficiently large, the pumping capacity of the lymphatics is approached or exceeded, and liquid and colloid then begin to accumulate in the more compliant interstitial compartment surrounding bronchioles, arterioles, and venules. This is designated *Stage 2*.

With further increments in filtered load, the volume limits of the loose interstitial spaces are exceeded, causing distention of the less compliant interstitial space of the alveolar-capillary septum. Pressures sufficient to disrupt the tight junctions of the alveolar membranes ensue, and

alveolar edema results. In early alveolar edema (*Stage 3a*), liquid accumulates at the corners of alveolar-capillary membranes where the radii of curvature are the smallest. Alveolar flooding (*Stage 3b*) occurs when alveoli reach a critical configuration at which inflation pressures can no longer maintain the existing configuration, and the alveolar gas volume rapidly decreases, being replaced by liquid and macromolecules. At this final stage of alveolar flooding, disruption of all components of the alveolar-capillary membrane occurs, irrespective of the initiating events.

Gravity-dependent Distribution of Pulmonary Edema and Redistribution of Pulmonary Blood Flow. The foregoing discussion dealt with the forces across the alveolar-capillary membranes as if they were homogeneously distributed throughout the lung. However, it is well known that neither lung tissue forces nor intravascular pressures are homogeneous and that major interregional nonhomogeneities exist owing to the differential effects of gravity on blood, gas-containing lung tissue, and air. Since blood is more dense (i.e., heavier) than gas-containing lung, the effects of gravity are much greater on the distribution of blood flow than on the distribution of tissue forces in the lung. From apex to base, the effective perfusion pressure of the pulmonary circulation (P_{pa}) increases by approximately 1.00 cm H_2O/cm vertical distance, whereas pleural pressures (P_{pl}) increase by only 0.25 cm H_2O/cm vertical distance.[29] Pulmonary capillaries (or alveolar vessels) are exposed to alveolar pressure (P_{alv}), which does not vary from apex to base. In contrast, pulmonary arteries, arterioles, veins, and venules (extraalveolar vessels) are exposed to pleural pressure, which does vary from apex to base. The consequences of these differences in forces on ventilation-perfusion relationships have been well described.[30] As shown in Figure 17–4, in Zone 1, arterial pressure is less than alveolar pressure; thus there is no flow. Indeed, rapid-freezing techniques in animals have

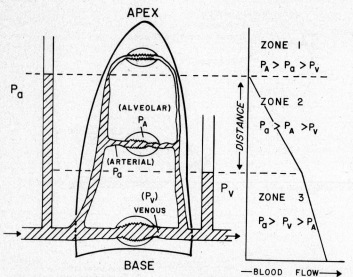

FIGURE 17–4 Schematic representation of the gravity-dependent, apex-to-base distribution of pulmonary blood flow in an upright lung according to West.[30] Pulmonary artery pressure (P_a) and pulmonary venous pressure (P_v) increase on a hydrostatic basis as the base is approached. Alveolar pressure (P_A) is constant with vertical distance. (The three zones are described at length in the text.)

confirmed that apical capillaries are bloodless.[31] On the other hand, gamma-emitting isotope studies in normal humans indicate that, although blood flow is strikingly diminished at the apex, no *true* Zone 1 (with total absence of flow) exists.[32]

In Zone 2, arterial pressure exceeds alveolar pressure, which in turn exceeds venous pressure. Here, each vessel is similar to a collapsible tube in a pressure chamber, and an analogy has been drawn between these vessels and a Starling resistor. An interesting property of the Starling resistor is as follows: When chamber pressure (analogous to alveolar pressure) exceeds the downstream pressure (analogous to venous pressure), the pressure drop for flow is not equal to the difference between upstream (arterial) and downstream (venous) pressures but rather to the difference between upstream (arterial) and chamber (alveolar) pressures. It is in this zone that large increases in flow occur per unit of distance of descent down the lung. These are due to large increases in perfusing pressures with no change in alveolar pressures.

In Zone 3, venous pressure exceeds alveolar pressure, resulting in distention of collapsible capillaries. Mean intravascular pressures are greatest in this zone; hence, with elevations of venus pressure or with disruption of alveolar-capillary membranes, edema formation is both more rapid and greatest here. It is only in this zone that the usual calculation of pulmonary vascular resistance holds true, and it is the only zone in which a valid pulmonary capillary wedge pressure measurement can be obtained. Increases in blood flow with increasing distance from the apex are more gradual in this zone because increases in pulmonary arterial pressures are offset by identical increases in venous pressures. The basis for the increase in flow with distance is the greater mean distending intravascular pressure with greater distention of the vessels as the base is approached.

Thus, in normal, erect humans, perfusion is greater in the basilar lung regions than in the more apical ones. Deviation from this gravity-dependent pattern has been called *vascular redistribution.* There are several ways to view the phenomenon of redistribution. Any encroachment of Zone 1 upon Zone 2 secondary to increased pulmonary venous pressure is, in a sense, redistribution, since regional blood flow is distributed differently after such a change. In like manner, greater relative perfusion of Zone 2 with increases in pulmonary artery pressure distributes more blood to the apex. However, true redistribution is generally considered to be a relative reduction in perfusion of the bases with a relative increase in apical perfusion. This phenomenon is most likely due to compression of the lumina of basilar vessels secondary to the greater and more rapid formation of edema at the lung bases and the tendency for extravascular liquid formed elsewhere to gravitate toward the bases.[5] In addition, pulmonary arteriolar constriction secondary to alveolar hypoxia, which may also contribute to this redistribution, is more prominent at the lung bases.[33] Several experimental studies either imply[34] or demonstrate[35] that vascular redistribution occurs only *after* the acute onset of alveolar edema. If this were the case in human disease, as it seems likely to be, redistribution should be no more subtle a finding than auscultatory abnormalities.

The situation with *chronic* elevations of left atrial pressure, as in mitral stenosis or chronic congestive heart failure, should be contrasted with that of acute pulmonary edema. Clinical experience with such chronic conditions suggests that redistribution of flow does occur with minimal or no evidence of interstitial edema and in the absence of alveolar edema. Because of the pathological changes found in such lungs at postmortem examination,[36] i.e., interstitial fibrosis of basilar lung regions and narrowing of basilar arteries and arterioles by lesions that often occur with pulmonary hypertension, it is more likely that redistribution is secondary to such changes.

CLASSIFICATION OF PULMONARY EDEMA

The two most common forms of pulmonary edema are those initiated by an imbalance of Starling forces and those initiated by disruption of one or more components of the alveolar-capillary membrane (Table 17–1).[37,37a] Less often, lymphatic insufficiency can be involved as a predisposing, if not initiating, factor in the genesis of edema. Although the initiating or primary mechanism may be clearly identifiable, multiple factors come into play during the development of edema, and irrespective of the initiating event, the stage of alveolar flooding is characterized most often by disruption of the alveolar-capillary membrane.

IMBALANCE OF STARLING FORCES. *Increased pulmonary capillary pressure* is a straightforward initiating event, whether due to mitral stenosis, left ventricular failure, or pulmonary venoocclusive disease.[38] Although pulmonary capillary wedge pressures must be abnormally high to increase the flow of interstitial liquid, at a time when edema is clearly present, these pressures may not correlate with the severity of pulmonary edema.[39] In fact, pulmonary capillary wedge pressures may have returned to normal at a time when there is still considerable pulmonary edema, since the rate of removal of both interstitial and alveolar edema appears to be relatively slow.[38] Other

TABLE 17-1 CLASSIFICATION OF PULMONARY EDEMA BASED UPON INITIATING MECHANISM

I. Imbalance of Starling Forces
  A. Increased pulmonary capillary pressure
    1. Increased pulmonary venous pressure without left ventricular failure (e.g., mitral stenosis)
    2. Increased pulmonary venous pressure secondary to left ventricular failure
    3. Increased pulmonary capillary pressure secondary to increased pulmonary arterial pressure (so-called overperfusion pulmonary edema)*
  B. Decreased plasma oncotic pressure
    1. Hypoalbuminemia secondary to renal, hepatic, protein-losing enteropathic, or dermatological disease or nutritional causes**
  C. Increased negativity of interstitial pressure
    1. Rapid removal of pneumothorax with large applied negative pressures (unilateral)
    2. Large negative pleural pressures due to acute airway obstruction along with increased end-expiratory volumes (asthma)*
  D. Increased interstitial oncotic pressure
    1. No known clinical or experimental example
II. Altered Alveolar-capillary Membrane Permeability (Adult Respiratory Distress Syndrome)
  A. Infectious pneumonia—bacterial, viral, parasitic
  B. Inhaled toxins (e.g., phosgene, ozone, chlorine, Teflon fumes, nitrogen dioxide, smoke)
  C. Circulating foreign substances (e.g., snake venom, bacterial endotoxins, alloxan†, alpha-naphthyl thiourea†)
  D. Aspiration of acidic gastric contents
  E. Acute radiation pneumonitis
  F. Endogenous vasoactive substances (e.g., histamine, kinins*)
  G. Disseminated intravascular coagulation
  H. Immunological—hypersensitivity pneumonitis, drugs (nitrofurantoin), leukoagglutinins
  I. Shock lung in association with nonthoracic trauma
  J. Acute hemorrhagic pancreatitis
III. Lymphatic Insufficiency
  A. Post lung transplant
  B. Lymphangitic carcinomatosis
  C. Fibrosing lymphangitis (e.g., silicosis)
IV. Unknown or Incompletely Understood
  A. High-altitude pulmonary edema
  B. Neurogenic pulmonary edema
  C. Narcotic overdose
  D. Pulmonary embolism
  E. Eclampsia
  F. Post cardioversion
  G. Post anesthesia
  H. Post cardiopulmonary bypass

*Not certain to exist as a clinical entity.
**Not certain that this, as a single factor, leads to clinical pulmonary edema.
†Predominantly an experimental technique.

factors obscure the relationship between the severity of edema and measured pulmonary capillary pressures in addition to slower rates of removal after edema has collected. The rate of increase in lung liquid at any given elevation of capillary pressure is related to the functional capacity of lymphatics,[40,41] which may vary from patient to patient, and to variations in interstitial oncotic and hydrostatic pressures.[38]

The question of increased capillary pressures secondary to increased pulmonary artery pressure due to overperfusion is difficult to place in a clinical context.[41a] Indeed, experimental resection of well over half the pulmonary capillary bed has been shown to produce pulmonary edema.[42] The most relevant clinical observation has been the description of pulmonary edema in one lung or lobe following the creation of an end-to-end shunt from a systemic artery to a single pulmonary artery for the treatment of cyanotic congenital heart disease.[43] The question might be raised of why pulmonary edema does not occur with severe pulmonary hypertension (e.g., primary pulmonary hypertension). The obvious answer is that the arteriolar bed is severely narrowed in the latter instance, and thus capillaries are not exposed to the increased pressure, whereas in the former instance, the arteriolar bed is not narrowed, and increased pressures are found in the pulmonary capillaries.

Hypoalbuminemia is well known to produce dependent systemic edema without elevations of systemic venous pressures. In contrast, pulmonary edema does *not* develop with hypoalbuminemia alone. Hypoalbuminemia may alter the fluid conductivity of the interstitial gel so that liquid moves more easily between capillaries and lymphatics to add to the lymphatic safety factor.[44] Thus, there must be, in addition to hypoalbuminemia, some elevations of pulmonary capillary pressure, albeit only small increases are necessary before pulmonary edema ensues. Indeed, in such patients, only moderate fluid overload can precipitate overt pulmonary edema in the absence of left ventricular failure.

Increased negativity of interstitial pressure due to rapid removal of pleural air for relief of a relatively complete pneumothorax may be associated with pulmonary edema. Usually, the pneumothorax has been present for several hours to days, allowing time for alterations in surfactant, so that large negative pressures are necessary to open collapsed alveoli.[45,46] In this instance the edema is unilateral and is most often only a radiographic finding with few clinical findings.

Large negative pleural pressures thought to approximate interstitial pressures have been shown experimentally to increase the rate of edema formation in dogs.[47] Stalcup and Mellins have shown that the degree of negativity of the mean intrapleural pressure in asthma correlates with the severity of an attack and have speculated that there might be associated pulmonary edema, although it is radiographically inapparent owing to the hyperinflation of the lung in this condition.[10] This interesting hypothesis should be tested, since asthma is a common condition that is often treated with large volumes of intravenous fluids. Animal experiments involving inspiratory loading and increased lung volume as a means of increasing pleural pressure swings have demonstrated increases in left atrial transmural pressures along with diminution in left ventricular end-diastolic dimensions and decreases in cardiac output.[48–50] Thus, it is possible that diminution of left ventricular diastolic filling and an elevation of left atrial pressures accompany such large negative intrapleural pressures.

There is no known clinical or experimental example of pulmonary edema initiated by *increased interstitial oncotic pressure.* However, after the appearance of increased concentrations of macromolecules in the liquid of the interstitium or in alveoli, extravascular oncotic forces undoubtedly serve to intensify and perpetuate the process of edema formation.

PRIMARY ALVEOLAR-CAPILLARY MEMBRANE DAMAGE. Many diverse medical and surgical conditions are associated with pulmonary edema that appears to be due not to primary alteration in Starling forces but rather to damage of the alveolar-capillary membrane. These conditions include acute pulmonary infections and pulmonary effects of gram-negative septicemia and non-thoracic trauma as well as any condition associated with disseminated intravascular coagulation.[51–53] Despite the diversity of underlying causes, once diffuse alveolar-capillary injury has occurred, the pathophysiological and clinical sequence of events is quite similar in most patients. Because of the resemblance of the clinical picture to that seen with respiratory distress of the neonate, these conditions have been referred to as the *adult respiratory distress syndrome* (ARDS).[54] This similarity includes the superimposition of secondary factors, either occurring spontaneously or induced by therapeutic interventions, that serve to perpetuate or worsen the clinical course. An example of a spontaneously occurring secondary factor is the appearance of left ventricular failure with elevation of pulmonary capillary pressure during the course of the illness; a frequent consequence of therapeutic intervention is fluid over-load of the patient due to the administration of excessive volumes of intravenous fluids.

Direct evidence for increased capillary permeability has come mainly from experimental studies in which pulmonary edema has been produced by endotoxin infusion;[55] hemorrhagic shock;[56,57] infusion of oleic acid;[58] and inhalation of high concentrations of oxygen[59] or toxic gases, such as phosgene,[60] ozone,[61] and nitrogen dioxide.[62] Reliable clinical data are far more difficult to obtain, since (1) macromolecules in alveolar liquid may be diluted by tracheobronchial secretion, resulting in an underestimation of the extent of the alveolar-capillary leak, and (2) such macromolecules, secondary to previously elevated capillary pressures, can be present at a time when intravascular pressures have returned to normal levels, hence leading to the erroneous conclusion that alveolar-capillary membrane damage was the primary event. Nonetheless, clinical studies of ARDS with normal pulmonary capillary wedge pressures have been reported and have shown either an elevation of protein in the liquid aspirated from the tracheobronchial tree[63,64] or appearance in this liquid of foreign macromolecules injected intravenously.[65] Thus, it is probable, though not yet proved, that increased permeability of the alveolar-capillary membrane is an initiating event in most of the cases designated as ARDS.

There are many similarities between ARDS from diverse etiologies and the respiratory distress syndrome seen in infants, which is due only to immaturity of the surfactant system. Although surfactant deficiency cannot be assigned a *primary* role in the pathogenesis of ARDS, there are many data to support the idea that changes in the properties of surfactant are added to the initial impairment and serve to perpetuate pulmonary dysfunction. Impairment of surfactant has been shown to occur with cardiogenic pulmonary edema,[66] exposure to various plasma constituents,[67] and high concentrations of oxygen[68] and in association with systemic hypotension.[69] Closely related to the pulmonary edema in the ARDS is that which is commonly associated with all forms of shock—the so-called "shock lung." The theories of pathogenesis of shock lung are shown in Table 17–2. (For further discussion of ARDS and shock lung, see p. 583.)

TABLE 17–2   THEORIES OF PATHOGENESIS OF SHOCK LUNG

I   Hemodynamic
    A. Backward theory—pulmonary venular constriction (?centrally mediated; ?cerebral hypoxia)
    B. Forward theory—pulmonary hypertension. See IV, Microemboli (below)
II   Circulating humoral agent(s)
    A. Soluble factor(s) released from extrapulmonary cells injures vascular endothelium
III   Cellular agent(s)
    A. Locally released in lung injures vascular endothelium
IV   Microemboli—altered permeability arises from diffuse microembolization of lung
    A. Subtheories: why emboli form
        1. Exogenous from transfusions
        2. Increased rate of formation (platelet, leukocyte, or erythrocyte aggregates)
        3. Decreased breakdown (altered fibrinolysis)
        4. Decreased removal by reticuloendothelial system (liver)
            a. Humoral—deficient opsonin
            b. Decreased hepatic phagocytosis
    B. Mechanism of injury
        1. Hemodynamic (forward theory—severe, unevenly distributed pulmonary arterial hypertension transmitted to pulmonary capillaries, leading to shear stress and mechanical injury)
        2. Chemical (endothelium is injured by clot products: platelet, leukocyte, or erythrocyte aggregates)

From Robin, E. D.: Permeability pulmonary edema, *In* Fishman, A. P., and Renkin, E. M. (eds.): Pulmonary Edema. Bethesda, American Physiological Society, 1979, p. 217.

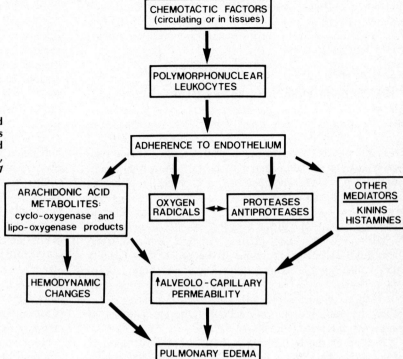

FIGURE 17–5 Flow chart showing the proposed mechanisms for chemotaxin and leukocyte interactions to produce alveolar-capillary membrane damage and pulmonary edema. (After Repine, J. E., Bowman, C. M., and Tate, R. M.: Neutrophils and lung edema. Chest *81* (Suppl.): 5, 1982.)

Recent experimental data strongly imply either a causal or a major and necessary role for interaction of polymorphonuclear leukocytes in the blood and circulating or cellular chemotactic macromolecules for the initiation, perpetuation, or amplification of lung injury leading to ARDS. The precise sequence of events is not truly settled but comprises some combination of items II, III, IVA, and B in Table 17–2. Figure 17–5 gives the elements of the potential role of leukocytes and chemotactic agents.[70] Chemotaxins in the circulating blood (e.g., the fifth component of complement, C5a) or from alveolar macrophages can recruit polymorphonuclear leukocytes, cause them to adhere to the pulmonary capillary endothelium, and activate them to produce several toxic substances that alter alveolar-capillary membrane permeability or cause circulatory changes or both. Because of the location of the polymorphonuclear leukocytes, their peripheral depletion and pulmonary vascular sequestration in many forms of acute lung injury, and their ability, when activated, to produce arachidonic acid metabolites (by both cyclo- and lipo-oxygenase pathways), oxygen radicals, proteases, and other mediators that alter permeability and influence vasomotoricity, the hypothesis is an appealing one.

Since these chemotaxins can arrive from distal sources in the body to inflict injury or can be derived from the alveolar macrophages of the alveolar side, systemic events such as gram-negative septicemia, distal events such as pancreatitis, and local pulmonary events such as inhalational injury can all be accommodated by this hypothesis.[71,72] Moreover, since the leukocyte aggregates often include platelets, the thrombocytopenic and consumptive coagulopathic states often accompanying ARDS can be explained. Recent clinical studies appear to support this hypothesis.[71] Bronchoalveolar lavage liquid from patients with ARDS has shown a predominance of neutrophils, leukocytic elastase, and partially inactivated alpha$_1$ antitrypsin.[73,74] Further, there is a strong correlation between neutrophil-aggregating activity in the plasma and the subsequent development of ARDS in clinical conditions that are often associated with this syndrome.[75] To date, no observations are available to refute this hypothesis, yet the many potential and complex interactions await elucidation before preventive or therapeutic measures can be devised and translated into clinical practice for the avoidance or arrest of lung injury.

LYMPHATIC DYSFUNCTION. Abnormalities in pulmonary lymphatics can produce abnormalities of liquid transport in the lung. However, the question remains whether such alterations alone ever account for pulmonary edema. Experimental studies have been in direct conflict on this point.[40,76] From the clinical standpoint, however, there are clear examples to suggest the importance of pulmonary lymphatics. In silicosis, with the invariably associated obliterative lymphangitis, only moderate elevations of left atrial pressures result in impressive pulmonary edema.[41] Similar observations have been made following lung transplantation with complete disruption of lymphatics[13] and in association with obstruction of lymphatics due to lymphangitic carcinomatosis.[77]

There are experimental studies showing that lymphatic dysfunction can be present *without structural abnormalities.* For example, Hall and colleagues have shown that the normal rhythmic contractions of pulmonary lymphatic vessels in sheep disappear when the animals are anesthetized.[78] Cessation of lymphatic pumping would be expected to result in a net gain of interstitial liquid, and this may leave a clinical counterpart of pulmonary edema following anesthesia or sedative drug overdose. Impairment of lymphatic flow with a net gain of lung liquid content has also been shown to occur in sheep given continuous positive airway pressure.[79] The clinical occurrence or importance of this finding has yet to be established, but the question is a significant one, since both continuous positive airway pressure and positive end-expiratory pressure with mechanical ventilation are often used to improve gas exchange in patients with pulmonary edema.

FORMS OF UNKNOWN PATHOGENESIS

High-altitude Pulmonary Edema (HAPE). Victims of this disorder are those persons usually in their teens or early twenties who have quickly ascended to altitudes in excess of 2700 meters and who have often engaged in strenuous physical exercise at that altitude.[80,81] At one time this syndrome was considered to be rare; however, recent estimates place the incidence at 6.4 clinically apparent cases per 100 exposures to high altitude in persons less than 21 years of age and 0.4 case per 100 exposures in those older than 21 years.[82] Gradual ascent, allowing time for acclimatization, and limiting physical exertion upon more rapid ascent are thought to be preventive. Usually within one day of ascent, affected patients complain of cough, dyspnea, and, in some cases, chest pain in association with tachycardia, bilateral rales, and cyanosis accompanied by radiographic evidence of discrete patches of pulmonary infiltrate (Fig. 17–6).

Reversal of this syndrome is both rapid (less than 48 hours) and certain either by returning the patient to a lower altitude or by administering a high inspiratory concentration of oxygen. Sleeping below 8000 ft, gradual acclimatization, and avoidance of heavy exertion for the first 2 or 3 days at high altitude appear to be preventive. Although formerly thought to occur only in persons from low altitudes who ascend quickly for mountaineering or skiing,[83,84] it has recently been documented to occur among natives of high-altitude regions upon their return from altitudes below 2200 meters.[85] No single mechanism satisfactorily explains the pathogenesis of HAPE, yet several possible mechanisms have been proposed. Although most

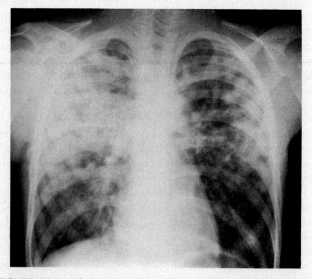

FIGURE 17–6   Chest x-ray of a 10-year-old boy in whom pulmonary edema developed on his return to his home at an elevation of 3100 meters after a visit to low altitude. Note patchy infiltrates scattered throughout both lung fields. Normal heart size indicates absence of left heart failure. (From Grover, R. F., et al.: High-altitude pulmonary edema. *In* Fishman, A. P., and Renkin, E. M. (eds.): Pulmonary Edema. Bethesda, American Physiological Society, 1979, p. 229.)

have shown pulmonary arterial hypertension, the pulmonary capillary wedge pressures have been near normal,[86] a finding which has led to the suggestion that direct disruption of the walls of small arteries proximal to the hypoxically constructed arterioles in patients with hyperresponsive pulmonary vessels may be responsible.[87] Clearly, none of the catheterization data have been obtained during the development of, nor at the peak of, pulmonary edema, so that transitory elevations of pulmonary capillary pressures could have been present and could have returned to normal at the time of measurement. However, in view of the existing data showing normal pulmonary capillary wedge pressures, other mechanisms have been proposed. The direct effect of alveolar hypoxia on increasing alveolar-capillary membrane permeability was initially considered,[88] yet more recent studies do not support that idea.[89] Transient intravascular coagulation secondary to hypoxic sequestration of platelets in the pulmonary circulation has also been implicated;[90] however, it is possible that the intravascular coagulation is secondary to alveolar-capillary membrane disruption rather than a cause. At this point, it is fair to state that the pathogenesis is unknown,[91] but the response to simple treatment is dramatic.

Neurogenic Pulmonary Edema.   Central nervous system disorders ranging from head trauma to grand mal seizures can be associated with acute pulmonary edema (without detectable left ventricular disease). An early experimental model for this syndrome, consisting of fibrin injections into the fourth ventricle of dogs,[92] has been used to show that sympathectomy completely prevented the accumulation of lung liquid.[93] Indeed, observation that a variety of sympatholytic drugs serve to prevent neurogenic pulmonary edema makes it likely that the sympathetic nervous system plays a key role. Although not completely supported by direct measurements, the current idea is that sympathetic overactivity produces shifts of blood volume from the systemic to the pulmonary circulation, with secondary elevations of left atrial and pulmonary capillary pressures.[94] Thus, it would appear that an imbalance of Starling forces is the basis for this form of pulmonary edema, although capillary pressure quickly returns to normal after the acute and transitory sympathetic discharge. An unusually timely set of observations made on a patient with a pulmonary arterial catheter who experienced a grand mal seizure lent support to this idea. Wray and Nicotra observed transitory and severe elevations of pulmonary capillary wedge pressure in this patient during and immediately following the seizure.[95] Pulmonary edema diagnosed by both radiographic and clinical criteria was clearly present after wedge pressures had returned to normal levels. It should be emphasized that although sympatholytics prevent neurogenic pulmonary edema, they appear to have no place in the *treatment* of this syndrome, since pulmonary capillary pressures have returned to near normal when the syndrome is diagnosed.

The idea of a transitory sympathetic neural discharge of sufficient magnitude to account for high-pressure pulmonary edema as the basis for the neurogenic variety has not gone without challenge. Hakim et al. have presented data showing modest increases in pulmonary endothelial permeability without elevation of pressures produced by stellate ganglion stimulation in dogs,[96] and Simon and coworkers have demonstrated neurally mediated elevations in permeability during status epilepticus in anesthetized and paralyzed sheep, also without elevations of pulmonary capillary pressures.[97] Both of these observations, though demonstrating only a modest effect, suggest that neural mechanisms can alter membrane permeability. However, whether these changes are of sufficient magnitude to produce pulmonary edema is open to question. Nonetheless, in viewing the available data, we think the hemodynamic hypothesis to be the most appealing.

Narcotic Overdose Pulmonary Edema. Acute pulmonary edema is a well-recognized sequence of heroin overdose.[98] Because of the illicit traffic in this drug given by the intravenous route, the syndrome was initially thought to be due to injected impurities rather than to the heroin itself. However, since oral methadone or dextropropoxyphene can also be associated with pulmonary edema,[99,100] the syndrome cannot be attributed to injected impurities.

The well-known respiratory depressant effects of opiates lead to severe hypoxemia and hypercapnia with respiratory acidosis, which may account for the cerebral edema seen in many of these patients.[101] Cerebral edema, along with opiate-induced hypothalamic dysfunction,[102] raises the possibility of a neurogenic mechanism. Transient impairment of lymphatic pumping capacity may be a contributory factor.[78] The fact that edema fluid contains protein concentrations nearly identical to those found in plasma[103] and that pulmonary capillary wedge pressures, when measured, are normal[104] would appear to argue for an alveolar-capillary membrane leak as the initiating cause. In animal experiments, histamine has been shown to be released in the lung after both heroin and morphine administration.[105] Thus, it is possible that the well-known effects of histamine on vascular permeability might play a role in this syndrome. However, there is not sufficient experimental or clinical evidence in support of such a role. As with several other pulmonary edema syndromes of uncertain etiology that develop quickly, the possibility must be considered that transitory pulmonary capillary pressure elevations account for the edema and that the reported normal measurements were made during the phase of resolution.

Pulmonary Embolism. Acute pulmonary edema in association with either a massive embolus or multiple smaller emboli has been well described and most often attributed to concomitant left ventricular dysfunction due to a combination of hypoxemia and encroachment of the interventricular septum on the left ventricular cavity. Although this sequence is quite likely to be applicable in the case of massive embolism, whether it applies equally well to instances of multiple small emboli or microemboli is open to question. There are data to suggest, in the latter instance,

that an increase in permeability of the alveolar-capillary membrane occurs.[52] Figure 17–7 outlines a hypothesis that implicates both clotting factors and formed elements in the pathogenesis of a pulmonary capillary leak due to microembolism.[106] Thrombin generated by the clotting process and in association with the embolus causes aggregation of platelets, complement activation, and leukostasis. It is proposed that the sequence then follows that outlined in Figure 17–5. Experimental support for this notion comes from the blunting of the capillary leak process following defibrinogenation[107] or leukocyte depletion.[108]

Eclampsia. Acute pulmonary edema frequently complicates eclampsia.[109] Multiple factors such as cerebral dysfunction with massive sympathetic discharge, left ventricular dysfunction secondary to acute systemic hypertension, hypervolemia, hypoalbuminemia (secondary to renal losses), and disseminated intravascular coagulation probably play a role in the pathogenesis.

Post Cardioversion. Although pulmonary edema has been documented to occur following cardioversion,[110] the mechanism is poorly understood. Ineffective left atrial function immediately following cardioversion has been suggested as a contributing factor, yet left ventricular dysfunction and neurogenic mechanisms are also possible.

Post Anesthesia. In previously healthy subjects, pulmonary edema has been found in the early postanesthesia period without a clear relationship to fluid overload or any subsequent evidence of left ventricular disease.[111] The basis for this disorder is unknown, but it is tempting to invoke some role for temporary lymphatic dysfunction under anesthesia, as previously shown in sheep.[78]

Post Cardiopulmonary Bypass. Although all patients who undergo cardiopulmonary bypass obviously have significant heart disease, the development of edema has been associated with normal left atrial pressures.[112,113] Alterations of surfactant due to prolonged collapse of the lung during the procedure, with subsequent need to apply high negative intrapleural pressures for reexpansion, and release of toxic substances have been suggested as mechanisms. The matter is not settled, but the syndrome is fortunately rare.

CARDIOGENIC PULMONARY EDEMA

CLINICAL MANIFESTATIONS. It would be satisfying to relate signs, symptoms, radiographic changes, and measurable dysfunction to all three stages of pulmonary edema. Unfortunately, in its earliest stage—i.e., increased lymph flow without net gain of interstitial liquid—there is currently no reliable way to detect pulmonary edema clinically or to quantitate it. If the process is initiated by an in-

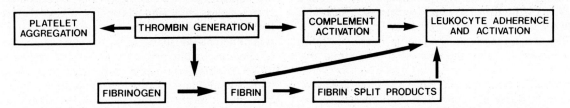

FIGURE 17–7 Flow chart showing the proposed mechanism for microembolic generation of increased permeability through the route shown in Figure 17–5. (After Malik, A. B., Tahamont, M. V., Minnear, F. L., Johnson, A., and Kaplan, J. E.: Lung fluid and protein exchange after pulmonary vascular thrombosis. Chest *81*:5, 1982.)

crease in left atrial or pulmonary venous pressures, prominent pulmonary veins with secondary prominence of pulmonary arteries would be an expected radiographic finding. Although earlier studies were able to relate vascular dimensions to intravascular pressures, those measurements were made only under conditions of *chronic* pressure elevations;[114] therefore, the findings might not apply to acute changes. Nonetheless, it is likely, given the pressure-diameter characteristics of both pulmonary veins and pulmonary arteries, that acute changes could be easily detectable radiographically, especially if serial films were available. Concerning measurable dysfunction, Hogg and coworkers were able to demonstrate in animal studies an increase in resistance of peripheral airways during pulmonary venous hypertension and to show that this finding could be attributed to competition for space between vessels and airways within the bronchovascular sheaths, with consequent compression of small airways.[115] There is some indirect evidence that the same phenomenon may be seen in human disease in which there is increased pulmonary blood volume.[116] Compromise of the lumina of small airways, predominantly in the more dependent portions of the lung, would be expected to increase both the alveolar-to-arterial difference for oxygen and the wasted ventilation ratio and to lead to a measurable increase in closing volume (Chap. 54). Since such mild changes in other settings rarely lead to symptoms, it is doubtful that any symptoms, except for exertional dyspnea, would accompany these abnormalities in Stage 1 edema. In like manner, physical findings in the lungs would be scarce except for mild inspiratory rales due to opening of closed airways.

Interstitial (or Stage 2) edema presents similar problems, in that correlative studies are scarce or nonexistent. Radiographic changes have been attributed to the increase in liquid in the loose interstitial space contiguous with the perivascular tissue of larger vessels and containing venules and arterioles. These changes (p. 173) are a loss of the normally sharp radiographic definition of pulmonary vascular markings, haziness and loss of demarcation of hilar shadows, and thickening of interlobular septa (Kerley B lines). Competition for space between vessels, airways, and increased liquid within the loose interstitial space produces greater compromise of small airway lumina than does Stage 1 edema. Thus, greater hypoxemia, more wasted ventilation, and more impressive elevations of closing volume occur. Indeed, in the setting of acute myocardial infarction, the degree of hypoxemia correlates with the degree of elevation of the pulmonary capillary wedge pressure.[117] *Tachypnea* is a frequent finding with interstitial edema and has been attributed to stimulation by the edema of interstitial J-type receptors or to stretch receptors in the interstitium rather than to hypoxemia, which is rarely of sufficient magnitude to stimulate breathing.[7] Although the tachypnea itself is a sign of dysfunction, it serves to augment the pumping action of lymphatic vessels and may serve to minimize or delay the increase in interstitial liquid.

With the onset of alveolar flooding, or Stage 3 edema, gas exchange is extremely abnormal, with severe hypoxemia and hypocapnia. Alveolar flooding can proceed to such a degree that many large airways are filled with blood-tinged foam that can be expectorated. Although hy-

pocapnia is the rule, it has been well documented that hypercapnia with acute respiratory acidemia can occur in more severe cases.[118] It is in such instances that morphine, with its well-known respiratory depressant effects, should be used with caution.

As indicated above, pulmonary edema developing during acute myocardial infarction most often is thought to be due to pulmonary capillary hypertension, yet recent experimental data in dogs with acute ligation of coronary arteries indicate another possible contributory mechanism. Richeson et al. showed that edema developing after coronary artery ligation occurred when pulmonary capillary pressures were normal and that the increases in lung water were blocked when animals were pretreated with indomethacin.[119] This finding suggests that inhibition of cyclooxygenase or cyclic nucleotide phosphodiesterase reduced pulmonary edema secondary to increased permeability of the alveolar-capillary membrane. Whether and to what extent these findings will apply to the human illness must await further study. Occasionally, patients with acute myocardial infarction and pulmonary edema present with normal pulmonary capillary wedge pressures.[120] It is possible that delay in radiographing clearance after a fall in pulmonary venous pressure is responsible, but it is also possible that in some patients an increase in permeability of the alveolar-capillary membrane secondary to low cardiac output, i.e., a form of "cardiogenic shock" lung, causes the pulmonary edema.

DIAGNOSIS. Acute cardiogenic pulmonary edema is the most dramatic symptom of left heart failure. Impaired left ventricular function, mitral stenosis, or whatever cause of elevated left atrial and pulmonary capillary pressures leading to cardiogenic pulmonary edema interferes with oxygen transfer in the lungs and, in turn, depresses arterial oxygen tension. At the same time the sensation of suffocation intensifies the patient's fright, elevates heart rate, and further restricts ventricular filling. The increased discomfort and work of breathing place an additional load on the heart, and cardiac function becomes further depressed by the hypoxia. If this vicious cycle is not interrupted, it may rapidly lead to death.

Acute cardiogenic pulmonary edema differs from orthopnea and paroxysmal nocturnal dyspnea in the more rapid development of extreme pulmonary capillary hypertension. Acute pulmonary edema is a terrifying experience for both patient and bystander; usually extreme breathlessness develops suddenly, and the patient becomes extremely anxious, coughs, and expectorates pink, frothy liquid, causing him to feel as if he is literally drowning. The patient usually sits bolt upright, exhibits air hunger, and may thrash about. The respiratory rate is elevated, the alae nasi are dilated, and there is inspiratory retraction of the intercostal spaces and supraclavicular fossae that reflects the large negative intrapleural pressures required for inspiration. The patient often grasps the sides of the bed in order to allow use of the accessory muscles of respiration. Respiration is noisy, with loud inspiratory and expiratory gurgling sounds that are often easily audible across the room. Sweating is profuse, and the skin is usually cold, ashen, and cyanotic, reflecting low cardiac output and increased sympathetic drive.

On auscultation the lungs are noisy, with rhonchi,

wheezes, and moist and fine crepitant rales that appear at first over the lung bases but then extend upward to the apices as the condition worsens. Cardiac auscultation may be difficult because of the respiratory sounds, but a third heart sound and an accentuated pulmonic component of the second heart sound are frequently present.

The patient may suffer from intense precordial pain if the pulmonary edema is secondary to acute myocardial infarction. Unless cardiogenic shock is present, arterial pressure is usually elevated above the patient's normal level as a result of excitement and sympathetic vasoconstriction. Because of the presence of systemic hypertension, it may be inappropriately suspected that the pulmonary edema is due to hypertensive heart disease. However, it should be noted that this condition is now quite rare, and if arterial pressure is elevated, examination of the fundi will usually indicate whether or not hypertensive heart disease is actually present (p. 17). Obviously, if the attack is not terminated, arterial pressure declines preterminally.

It may be difficult to differentiate severe bronchial asthma from acute pulmonary edema, since both conditions may be associated with extreme dyspnea, pulsus paradoxicus, demands for an upright posture, and diffuse wheezes that interfere with cardiac auscultation. In bronchial asthma, there is most often a history of previous similar episodes, and the patient is frequently aware of the diagnosis. During the acute attack, the asthmatic patient does not usually sweat profusely, and arterial hypoxemia, though present, is not usually of sufficient magnitude to produce cyanosis. In addition, the chest is hyperexpanded and hyperresonant, and use of accessory muscles is prominent. The wheezes are more high-pitched and musical than in pulmonary edema, and other adventitious sounds such as rhonchi and rales are less prominent in asthma. The patient with acute pulmonary edema most often perspires profusely and is frequently cyanotic owing to desaturation of arterial blood *and* decreased cutaneous blood flow. The chest is often dull to percussion, there is no hyperexpansion, accessory muscle use is less prominent than in asthma, and moist, bubbly rales and rhonchi are heard in addition to wheezes. The radiological changes in pulmonary edema are discussed on page 174 and illustrated in Figures 6–38 through 6–42, pages 173 to 175.

Measurement of pulmonary artery wedge pressure by means of a Swan-Ganz catheter may be critical to the differentiation between pulmonary edema secondary to an imbalance of Starling forces, i.e., cardiogenic pulmonary edema, and that secondary to alterations of the alveolar-capillary membrane. Specifically, a pulmonary capillary wedge or pulmonary artery diastolic pressure exceeding 25 mm Hg in a patient without previous pulmonary capillary pressure elevation (or exceeding 30 mm Hg in a patient with chronic pulmonary capillary pressure elevation) and with the clinical features of pulmonary edema strongly suggests that the edema is cardiogenic in origin.

Following effective treatment of the pulmonary edema, the patient is often rapidly restored to the condition that existed before the attack, although he usually feels exhausted; between attacks of pulmonary edema there may be few symptoms or signs of heart failure.

TREATMENT. In the treatment of acute pulmonary edema, a physician cannot usually work alone, since multiple simultaneous maneuvers are required. Therefore, if logistics and time permit, the patient should be transferred to an intensive care unit, and cardiac rhythm should be monitored. However, it is important to emphasize that transfer of the patient and institution of monitoring *must not delay initial therapy*, which must often be begun in the house or ambulance. While initial treatment is under way, it is frequently advisable to place an arterial catheter to record intraarterial pressure and obtain frequent samples for arterial blood gas measurements. If possible, a Swan-Ganz catheter should be inserted, so that pulmonary arterial diastolic and capillary wedge pressures can be measured and monitored.

The strategy of treatment of cardiogenic pulmonary edema is threefold: (1) a series of nonspecific measures are applied; (2) the precipitating factor is identified, if possible, and treated; and (3) attention is directed to the underlying condition, which is then corrected, if possible.

Nonspecific Measures

1. *Inhalation of oxygen-enriched inspired gas*, often with the aid of mechanical ventilation, is useful, as discussed below (p. 574).

2. The patient should be placed in the *sitting position*. Often this is not necessary, because the patient recognizes that distress is increased when he lies down and that he is more comfortable sitting up. However, it is often helpful to seat the patient at the side of the bed or in a chair in order to lower the feet and thereby further diminish venous return.

3. *Morphine sulfate* remains an extremely valuable drug in the treatment of cardiogenic pulmonary edema. By its narcotic action it diminishes the patient's distress, reduces the work of breathing, and, perhaps most importantly, diminishes the sympathetically induced venous and arteriolar constriction. Thus, even though morphine is not a direct vasodilator, in the setting of acute pulmonary edema it results in arteriolar and especially in venous dilation.[121]

Three to 5 mg of morphine sulfate may be injected intravenously over a 3-minute period, while the patient is observed for both its beneficial action (i.e., relief of pulmonary edema) and its principal adverse effect (i.e., respiratory depression). This dose may usually be repeated two or three times at 15-minute intervals, if necessary. When the situation is somewhat less urgent, 8 to 15 mg of morphine sulfate may be injected subcutaneously or intramuscularly, and this dose can be repeated every 3 to 4 hours. Morphine antagonists should be readily available whenever morphine is administered. Morphine should be avoided if acute pulmonary edema is associated with intracranial bleeding; disturbed consciousness; bronchial asthma; chronic pulmonary disease; or reduced ventilation, as reflected in an elevated arterial P_{CO_2}.

4. *Reduction of preload* can be accomplished by applying rotating tourniquets of wide, soft rubber tubing or blood pressure cuffs to the extremities. These should be placed several inches below the groin and shoulders, and the cuffs should be inflated to approximately 10 mm Hg below diastolic pressure, thus permitting arterial inflow to the limbs but restricting venous outflow. Only three of the four extremities should be compressed at one time, and every 15 to 20 minutes one of the tourniquets should be released and rotated to the free extremity.

5. *Furosemide* or *ethacrynic acid*, 40 to 60 mg injected intravenously over a 2-minute period, is another mainstay of therapy. With furosemide, diuresis commences within 5 minutes, reaches a peak effect at approximately 30 minutes, and lasts for approximately 2 hours.[122,123] However, pulmonary edema is relieved even before diuresis has occurred, suggesting that the initial effect of furosemide is not on the kidney but on venodilation.[124] In addition, there is evidence that furosemide reduces afterload and may act in part to relieve pulmonary edema by improving left ventricular emptying (p. 527).[125]

6. Since acute cardiogenic pulmonary edema, even in patients without hypertensive heart disease, is frequently associated with elevation of arterial and left ventricular end-diastolic pressures, cardiac output is depressed and systemic vascular resistance is elevated. Diuretic therapy, although of considerable value in reducing pulmonary capillary pressure, often does little to elevate cardiac output. *Vasodilators* promptly reduce systemic and pulmonary vascular pressures and relieve symptoms of acute pulmonary edema. A most appropriate vasodilator is *nitroprusside*, which has a dual action: (1) it lowers systemic vascular resistance (afterload), thereby elevating cardiac output; and (2) it produces venodilatation (preload), thereby reducing pulmonary capillary pressure. A useful regimen is as follows: An initial dose of 20 µg/min can be employed with the dose increased by increments of 5 µg/min every 5 minutes until pulmonary edema is relieved or until systemic arterial systolic pressure falls below approximately 100 mm Hg. If possible, arterial pressure should be recorded directly by means of an indwelling cannula during administration of this agent.

Nitroglycerin, 0.3 to 0.6 mg sublingually, also reduces ventricular preload by inducing venous dilation. The difficulty with this drug is that buccal absorption may be erratic. In addition, some patients develop marked reductions in arterial pressure. The hypotensive effect may be beneficial in patients with acute cardiogenic pulmonary edema secondary to hypertension. However, it may be hazardous in patients with pulmonary edema secondary to acute myocardial infarction in whom arterial pressure is normal or reduced. Arterial pressure usually declines little in patients with hypervolemia and systemic edema.

7. The combination of morphine, rotating tourniquets, a diuretic, and sublingual nitroglycerin generally diminishes preload sufficiently to obviate *phlebotomy*. Although the removal of approximately 500 ml of blood certainly diminishes preload, it is a time-consuming and often cumbersome procedure for an acutely ill patient, and it is therefore rarely, if ever, necessary to employ this technique.

8. In a patient known not to be receiving *digitalis*, a rapidly acting cardiac glycoside given intravenously may be helpful, depending on the etiology of the pulmonary edema. It is most useful in patients in whom pulmonary edema is secondary to severe mitral stenosis, in whom atrial fibrillation or other supraventricular tachycardias and an excessive ventricular rate have developed, and in whom the abbreviated diastolic filling period has caused increased left atrial pressure (Chap. 32). The slowing of ventricular rate accomplished by the glycoside, either by conversion of the arrhythmia to sinus rhythm or by increasing the effective refractory period of the atrioventricular conduction system, can exert a rapid and salutary effect. Specific glycosides and dosages are discussed in Chapter 16.

The problem is much more difficult in patients with acute pulmonary edema with sinus rhythm who have been taking an unknown dose of digitalis. Time usually does not allow one to wait for a serum glycoside level, and one must decide whether the pulmonary edema has been precipitated by digitalis intoxication or whether the patient requires more drug on the basis of clinical examination and the electrocardiogram (Chap. 16). A history of previous digitalis intoxication and/or nausea, vomiting, paroxysmal atrial tachycardia with atrioventricular block, nonparoxysmal atrioventricular junctional tachycardia, frequent ventricular premature contractions, ventricular tachycardia, and hypokalemia all imply digitalis intoxication (p. 523). If these signs are absent, it is well to remember that when a patient on a maintenance dose of a cardiac glycoside suddenly develops atrial fibrillation or other supraventricular tachycardia, the ventricular rate may be almost as rapid as if he had not been receiving the glycoside previously, and almost full doses may be required to slow the ventricular rate.

9. *Aminophylline* (theophylline ethylenediamine) is particularly useful when bronchospasm complicates pulmonary edema or in the occasional patient in whom it is not clear whether the attack of breathlessness is due to bronchial or cardiac asthma. Aminophylline is useful because it exerts a direct myocardial stimulating effect, analogous to that of caffeine. The reduction of ventricular filling pressure induced by aminophylline is caused not only by its positive inotropic effect but by mild venodilatation as well. In addition, it is a central nervous system stimulant, although less so than caffeine, and it exerts a mild diuretic effect.

The usual dose is 5 mg/kg intravenously in 10 minutes, followed by a constant infusion of 0.9 mg/kg/hr. This dose should be decreased in older persons and in those with hepatic or renal dysfunction.[126] Optimal blood levels range from 10 to 20 mg/liter. Measurements of blood levels are important in the clinical use of this drug, since there are surprisingly wide individual variations in the kinetics of aminophylline degradation and since symptoms of nausea and vomiting are frequently due to other drugs used in the treatment of pulmonary edema rather than to aminophylline. Other side effects include headache, flushing, palpitations, precordial pain, hypotension, and, rarely, convulsions. The more serious side effects are sudden death from ventricular arrhythmias and hypotension due to vasodilation. Arterial unsaturation may occur owing to pulmonary vasodilatation and perfusion of poorly ventilated alveoli in patients with pulmonary edema.[127]

Identification and Treatment of Precipitating Factors. In most patients with pulmonary edema, it is possible to identify one or more precipitating factors, similar to those that exacerbate congestive heart failure (p. 491). Most frequently, pulmonary edema is brought on by acute myocardial ischemia or infarction, the development of a tachyarrhythmia, fluid overloading, an infection in a patient with established underlying heart disease, pulmonary embolism (Chap. 46), thyrotoxicosis (Chaps. 24 and 51), or severe anemia (Chaps. 24 and 49).

In addition to applying the nonspecific measures for the treatment of pulmonary edema outlined above, additional attention must be directed to identifying and treating the precipitating factors (e.g., lowering body temperature in a patient with a high fever or treating thyroid storm or severe anemia). If acute pulmonary edema has been precipitated by a *tachyarrhythmia* that does not respond to appropriate medical therapy (Chap. 21) and does not appear to be secondary to digitalis intoxication, it may be necessary to institute cardioversion with direct-current countershock (p. 669). On the other hand, if acute pulmonary edema occurs in a patient with a *bradyarrhythmia* that does not respond to appropriate medical therapy, a temporary pacemaker should be inserted and the heart rate restored to normal (Chap. 22).

If acute pulmonary edema is precipitated or aggravated by a *hypertensive crisis*, treatment of the pulmonary edema clearly requires a rapid-acting hypotensive drug such as sodium nitroprusside (as discussed above). Alternatively, diazoxide, 300 mg as an intravenous bolus, may be employed (Chap. 27).

Recognition and Treatment of the Underlying Condition. After emergency therapeutic measures have been instituted, an attempt must be made rapidly to establish the diagnosis of the underlying cardiac disorder responsible for the pulmonary edema, when this is not already clear. Obviously, the history, physical examination, chest x-ray, and electrocardiogram are of great value. The echocardiogram may be helpful in the diagnosis of mitral valve disease, particularly silent mitral stenosis, as well as in the recognition of left atrial myxoma, which may be responsible for acute pulmonary edema (Chap. 42). The diagnosis of congestive cardiomyopathy and idiopathic hypertrophic subaortic stenosis, both of which may be responsible for pulmonary edema, can also be strongly suggested by the echocardiogram. Although the echocardiogram may be enormously helpful in establishing an anatomical diagnosis, it must be recognized that the *quality* of echocardiographic tracings may be poor in patients who are acutely ill.

Catheterization of the right side of the heart and pulmonary artery with a Swan-Ganz catheter is useful not only in the diagnosis of pulmonary edema, as indicated above, but also in aiding in the recognition of underlying cardiac disorders such as ventricular septal defect and mitral regurgitation, which may be responsible for pulmonary edema in patients with acute myocardial infarction. In addition, blood cultures for infective bacterial endocarditis and emergency creatine kinase (CK) determinations for the diagnosis of acute myocardial infarction are critical tests in a patient in whom the cause of the pulmonary edema is obscure. Radioisotope angiography (Chap. 11) may be helpful in revealing the status of left ventricular function.

Rarely, *surgical treatment* is necessary to relieve pulmonary edema in patients with acute infective endocarditis (Chap. 33), prosthetic valve dysfunction (Chap. 32), prolapsing atrial myxoma (Chap. 42), end-stage critically severe aortic or mitral stenosis, ventricular septal defect, or mitral regurgitation complicating acute myocardial infarction (Chap. 38). Whenever possible, the patient's condition should first be stabilized, so that operation is not carried out on an emergent basis. Occasionally, however, when pulmonary edema persists despite optimal application of the nonspecific measures and removal of the precipitating factors, preoperative stabilization is not possible, and emergency surgery must be employed as a life-saving maneuver.

Long-term Management. The initial management of pulmonary edema, outlined above, blends in with the long-term management of heart failure described in Chapter 16. If the patient's underlying heart disease is known, it is necessary to assess its severity, attempt to ascertain the precipitating cause of the pulmonary edema, and develop a therapeutic strategy to prevent its recurrence. In many instances this consists merely of instructing the patient to remain on a salt-poor diet and of continuing cardiac glycoside and diuretic administration. In other instances, the development of pulmonary edema in a patient with chronic heart disease signals a process of such severity that, following recovery from the acute decompensation, it may be advisable to assess the patient's hemodynamic status and consider or reconsider surgical treatment. If the patient is seen for the first time during an acute episode of pulmonary edema, and the nature of the underlying heart disease is not clear, a detailed cardiac work-up should be undertaken soon after recovery in order to elucidate the nature and severity of the underlying disorder with a view to its possible operative correction.

PULMONARY EDEMA SECONDARY TO ALTERATIONS OF THE ALVEOLAR-CAPILLARY MEMBRANE

CLINICAL MANIFESTATIONS. Since the sequence of liquid accumulation is similar whether primary membrane damage or alteration of Starling forces is responsible, both radiographic and clinical signs described above also apply in patients with pulmonary edema due to primary alterations of the alveolar-capillary membrane.[128] At the time of initial injury and for several hours thereafter, the patient may be free of respiratory symptoms or signs. The earliest sign is an increase in respiratory frequency followed shortly by dyspnea. Arterial blood gas measurement in the earlier period will disclose a depressed Po_2 despite a decreased Pco_2, so that the alveolar-to-arterial difference for oxygen is increased. At this point, oxygen given by mask or nasal prongs results in a significant increase in the arterial Po_2. Physical examination may be unremarkable, although a few fine inspiratory rales may be audible. With progression, the patient becomes cyanotic and increasingly dyspneic and tachypneic. Rales are more prominent and easily heard throughout both lung fields along with regions of tubular breath sounds. At this stage, hypoxemia cannot be corrected by the simple administration of oxygen, and mechanical ventilatory assistance or control must be initiated in order to provide adequate oxygenation of arterial blood. Should this more aggressive therapy be delayed, the combination of increasing tachypnea and smaller tidal volumes results in a rising Pco_2 and further fall in Po_2 to near fatal levels.

THERAPY. Whatever the underlying cause of pulmonary edema, analysis of arterial blood to assess the type and degree of gas exchange abnormality is necessary, followed by institution of appropriate inhalation therapeutic measures. When there is hypoxemia (PaO_2 < 60 mm

Hg) without hypercapnia, oxygen enrichment of the inspired gas may suffice and can be given by nasal prongs, Venturi masks, or reservoir bag masks, depending upon the degree of oxygen enrichment required to elevate the PaO_2 sufficiently. If arterial oxygen tensions cannot be maintained at or near 60 mm Hg despite 100 per cent oxygen at 20 liters per minute, or if there is progressive hypercapnia, intubation and institution of mechanical ventilation are usually necessary.

In the instance of progressive hypoxemia without hypercapnia, the role of mechanical ventilation is not to increase alveolar ventilation but to increase mean lung volume during the respiratory cycle, which in turn opens more alveoli for gas exchange. If hypoxemia is not corrected by mechanical ventilation or if toxic doses of oxygen are necessary for prolonged periods, further improvements in arterial oxygenation at the same inspired oxygen concentration or equivalent levels of arterial oxygenation at lower concentrations of oxygen can be achieved by increasing end-expiratory lung volumes by the addition of positive end-expiratory pressure (PEEP).[129] Since maintenance of oxygenation is absolutely necessary for survival, reports that mechanical ventilation with positive end-expiratory pressure actually increases the liquid content of the lung[79] may unsettle the physician who must utilize these techniques but will make him or her aware that this form of treatment should be discontinued as soon as possible.

Two complications of mechanical ventilation with positive end-expiratory pressure deserve special mention. The first is that high intrathoracic pressures and increasing lung volumes serve to impede venous return and increase the afterload to the right ventricle, with attendant decreases in cardiac output.[48] In the case of cardiogenic pulmonary edema, the impedance of venous return may provide some benefit with decreases in central pressures but no decline in cardiac output. However, in other forms of pulmonary edema, a fall in cardiac output may be detrimental to the oxygen transport system. A fall in blood pressure or urine output or both may be the only indication that a severe diminution in cardiac output has occurred unless cardiac output is monitored during this form of therapy. The predominant basis for the decrease in cardiac output is increased intrathoracic pressure, which directly impedes venous return.[48,49] An additional contribution may come from greater pulmonary vascular resistance due to increased lung volume.[48] The result of increased right ventricular afterload is a displacement of the interventricular septum, which impedes left ventricular diastolic filling.[50,130,131,132] It is also likely that direct compression of the left ventricle by the inflated lung also restricts diastolic filling.[133,134] The second complication of mechanical ventilation, barotrauma (pneumomediastinum, pneumothorax, and subcutaneous emphysema), requires appropriate decompressive therapy.[135]

When it is not possible to maintain oxygenation utilizing the above techniques, extracorporeal membrane oxygenators have been tried with the hope that life could be maintained during critical periods while reparative processes in the heart or lung or both are taking place. However, a National Heart, Lung, and Blood Institute trial designed to evaluate this heroic and costly form of life support has not been shown to improve the clinical outcome.

When hypercapnia with respiratory acidosis is present, mechanical ventilatory support may be necessary for improving alveolar ventilation in addition to improving oxygenation. If hypercapnia has resulted from excessively vigorous use of morphine, antagonist drugs might avert the need for mechanical ventilation.

In any situation in which cardiac output is diminished and arterial oxygenation is impaired, there may be insufficient oxygen delivered for aerobic metabolic demands; hence anaerobic metabolism with excessive production of lactic acid results in metabolic acidemia. Clearly, the primary aim is to improve both cardiac output and arterial oxygenation; however, sodium bicarbonate may be given intravenously as a temporary measure while more basic

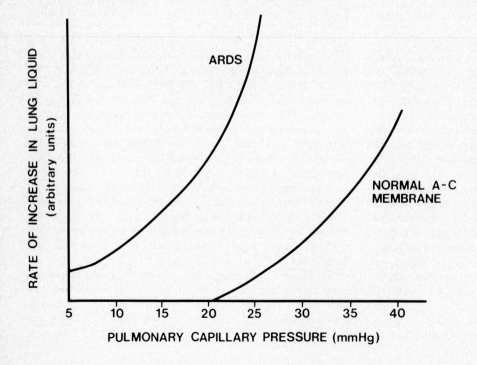

FIGURE 17–8 Schematic representation of the deleterious effects of acceptably normal capillary pressures in combination with pulmonary capillary leak. (Based upon the data of Prewitt, R. M., McCarthy, J., and Wood, L. D. H.: Treatment of acute low pressure pulmonary edema in dogs: Relative effects of hydrostatic and oncotic pressure, nitroprusside, and positive end-expiratory pressure. J. Clin. Invest. *67*:409, 1981.)

therapeutic measures are undertaken. Occasionally, when large quantities of sodium bicarbonate are required, there is a danger of sodium overload.

Measures aimed against increased capillary permeability in ARDS are frustratingly nonspecific and have not been shown to alter the time course or outcome of the illness. A possible exception is the use of specific antibiotic therapy directed against a causative or complicating bacterial infection. Adrenal glucocorticosteroid therapy leads the list of nonspecific measures that have yet to be of proven benefit.[38] In cases of pulmonary edema related to or complicated by disseminated intravascular coagulation, low molecular weight dextran and heparin have been used without any clear evidence of an effect on the severity of the lung lesion.[38]

An obvious and not often emphasized principle is to maintain pulmonary capillary pressures at the lowest possible levels (i.e., compatible with maintaining cardiac and urinary outputs and blood pressure) when there is increased permeability. Prewitt et al. have shown, using a dog model of oleic acid–induced pulmonary edema, that the rate of formation of pulmonary edema is cut to less than half when pulmonary capillary wedge pressures are decreased from 12 to 6 mm Hg.[136] The principle is schematized in Figure 17–8.

Since both increases in pulmonary capillary pressure and primary alveolar-capillary damage result in interstitial edema and alveolar flooding with liquid-containing erythrocytes and macromolecules, indicating severe membrane disruption, it is difficult to evolve a rationale for the use of intravenous colloids such as albumin or high molecular weight dextrans. In fact, large molecular weight compounds administered intravenously have been shown to appear rapidly in alveolar liquid.[65] Furthermore, there is experimental evidence that the administration of colloid to dogs with experimental lung injury actually *slows* the resolution of ultrastructural changes in the interstitium.[137] Since there is no firm clinical evidence that treatment with protein-containing solutions results in more rapid recovery from acute pulmonary edema,[135] and since there are strong intuitive reasons and some experimental data to suggest detrimental results, the use of albumin and other colloids should generally be avoided. There are, however, two situations in which albumin can be reasonably considered. First, if there is hypoalbuminemia, administration of albumin in addition to interventions designed to lower pulmonary capillary pressures seems rational. Second, the suggestion has been made that albumin might hasten the rate of resolution of pulmonary edema once alveolar-capillary membrane integrity has been reestablished.[138]

References

1. Laennec, R. T. H.: Traité de l'Auscultation Médiate. Vol. 2. Paris, Brosson and Chaude, 1819, p. 9.
2. Visscher, M. B., Haddy, F. J., and Stephens, G.: The physiology and pharmacology of lung edema. Pharmacol. Rev. 8:389, 1956.
3. Drinker, C. K.: Pulmonary Edema and Inflammation. Cambridge, Harvard University Press, 1945.
4. Guyton, A. C., and Lindsey, A. W.: Effect of elevated left atrial pressure and decreased plasma protein concentration on the development of pulmonary edema. Circ. Res. 7:649, 1959.
5. Staub, N. C.: Pulmonary edema. Physiol. Rev. 54:678, 1974.
6. Yu, P. N.: Pulmonary edema. Circulation 63:724, 1981.
7. Szidon, J. P., Pietra, G. G., and Fishman, A. P.: The alveolar-capillary membrane and pulmonary edema. N. Engl. J. Med. 286:1200, 1972.
8. Guyton, A. C., Parker, J. C., Taylor, A. E., Jackson, T. E., and Moffatt, D. S.: Forces governing water movement in the lung. In Fishman, A. P., and Renkin, E. M. (eds.): Pulmonary Edema. Bethesda, American Physiological Society, 1979, p. 70.
9. Lai-Fook, S. J.: Perivascular interstitial fluid pressure measured by micropipettes in isolated dog lung. J. Appl. Physiol. 52:9, 1982.
10. Stalcup, S. A., and Mellins, R. B.: Mechanical forces producing pulmonary edema in acute asthma. N. Engl. J. Med. 297:592, 1977.
11. Parker, J. C., Parker, R. E., Granger, D. N., and Taylor, A. E.: Vascular permeability and transvascular fluid and protein transport in the dog lung. Circ. Res. 48:549, 1981.
12. Staub, N. C.: Pulmonary edema due to increased microvascular permeability to fluid and protein. Circ. Res. 43:143, 1978.
13. Ersalan, S., Turner, M. D., and Hardy, J. D.: Lymphatic regeneration following lung reimplantation in dogs. Surgery 56:970, 1964.
14. Sampson, J. J., Leeds, S. E., Uhley, H. N., and Friedman, M.: The lymphatic system and pulmonary disease. In Mayerson, H. S. (ed.): Lymph and the Lymphatic System. Springfield, Ill., Charles C Thomas, 1968, p. 200.
15. Carlson, R. W., Schaeffer, R. C., Jr., Michaels, S. G., and Weil, M. H.: Pulmonary edema fluid. Circulation 60:1161, 1979.
16. Bruderman, I., Somers, K., Hamilton, W. K., Tooley, W. H., and Butler, J.: Effect of surface tension on circulation in the excised lungs of dogs. J. Appl. Physiol. 19:707, 1964.
17. Yoffey, J. M., and Courtice, F. C.: Lymphatics, Lymph and the Lymphomeyloid Complex. London, Academic Press, 1970.
18. Rusznyak, J., Földi, M., and Szabo, G.: Lymphatics and Lymph Circulation: Physiology and Pathology. 2nd ed. Oxford, Pergamon Press, 1967.
19. Hammersen, F.: Ultrastructure and functions of capillaries and lymphatics. Arch. Physiol. 336 (Suppl.):S43, 1972.
20. Casley-Smith, J. R.: The role of the endothelial intercellular junctions in the functioning of the initial lymphatics. Angiologica 9:106, 1972.
21. Hall, J. G., Morris, B., and Wooley, G.: Intrinsic rhythmic propulsion of lymph in the unanesthetized sheep. J. Physiol. 180:336, 1965.
22. Lambert, R. K., and Gremels, H.: On the factors concerned in the production of pulmonary edema. J. Physiol. (London) 61:98, 1926.
23. Rush, S., Abildskov, J. A., and McFee, R.: Resistivity of body tissues at low frequencies. Circ. Res. 12:40, 1963.
24. Vanselow, K., and Heuck, F.: Theoretische Untersuchungen über eine Messmethode zur quantitativen Bestimmung des Wasser-Luft-Verhältnisses des Lungengewebes. Fortschr. Röntgenstr. 100:441, 1964.
25. Ahluwalia, B. D., Brownell, G. L., Hales, C. A., and Kazemi, H.: An index of pulmonary edema measured with emission computed tomography. J. Comput. Assist. Tomogr. 5:690, 1981.
26. Chinard, F. P.: Estimation of extravascular lung water by indicator-dilution techniques. Circ. Res. 37:137, 1975.
26a. Sibbald, W. J., Warshawski, F. J., Short, A. K., Harris, J., Lefcoe, M. S., and Holliday, R. L.: Clinical studies of measuring extravascular lung water by the thermal dye technique in critically ill patients. Chest 83:725, 1983.
27. Fishman, A. P.: Pulmonary edema. In Fishman, A. P. (ed.): Pulmonary Diseases and Disorders. New York, McGraw-Hill Book Co., 1980, p. 733.
28. Staub, N. C., Nagano, H., and Pearce, M. L.: Pulmonary edema in dogs, especially the sequence of fluid accumulation in lungs. J. Appl. Physiol. 22:227, 1967.
29. Agostoni, E.: Mechanics of the pleural space. Physiol. Rev. 52:57, 1972.
30. West, J. B.: Ventilation Blood Flow and Gas Exchange. Oxford, Blackwell Scientific Publications, 1970.
31. Glazier, J. B., Hughes, J. M. B., Maloney, J. E., and West, J. B.: Measurements of capillary dimensions and blood volume in rapidly frozen lung. J. Appl. Physiol. 26:65, 1969.
32. Dollery, C. T., Heimberg, P., and Hugh-Jones, P.: Relationships between blood flow and clearance rate of radioactive carbon dioxide and oxygen in normal and oedematous lungs. J. Physiol. (London) 162:93, 1962.
33. Dawson, A.: Regional pulmonary blood flow in sitting and supine man during and after acute hypoxia. J. Clin. Invest. 48:301, 1969.
34. Ritchie, B. C., Schauberger, G., and Staub, N. C.: Inadequacy of perivascular edema hypothesis to account for distribution of pulmonary blood flow in lung edema. Circ. Res. 24:807, 1969.
35. Muir, A. L., Hogg, J. C., Naimark, A., Hall, D. L., and Chernecki, W.: Effect of alveolar liquid on distribution of blood flow in dog lungs. J. Appl. Physiol. 39:885, 1975.
36. Parker, F., Jr., and Weiss, S.: The nature and significance of the structural changes in the lungs in mitral stenosis. Am. J. Pathol. 12:573, 1936.
37. Ayres, S. M.: Mechanisms and consequences of pulmonary edema: Cardiac lung, shock lung, and principles of ventilatory therapy in adult respiratory distress syndrome. Am. Heart J. 103:97, 1982.
37a. Sprung, C. L., Rackow, E. C., Fein, I. A., Jacob, A. I., and Isikoff, S. K.: The spectrum of pulmonary edema: Differentiation of cardiogenic, intermediate, and noncardiogenic forms of pulmonary edema. Ann. Rev. Respir. Dis. 124:718, 1981.
38. Robin, E. D., Cross, C. E., and Zelis, R.: Pulmonary edema. N. Engl. J. Med. 288:239 and 292, 1973.
39. Pietra, G. G., Szidon, J. P., Leventhal, M. M., and Fishman, A. P.: Hemoglobin as a tracer in hemodynamic pulmonary edema. Science 166:1643, 1969.

40. Földi, M.: Diseases of Lymphatics and Lymph Circulation. Springfield, Ill., Charles C Thomas, 1969.

41. Cross, C. E., Shaver, J. A., Wilson, R. J., and Robin, E. D.: Mitral stenosis and pulmonary fibrosis: Special reference to pulmonary edema and lung lymphatic function. Arch. Intern. Med. 125:248, 1970.

41a. Landolt, C. C., Matthay, M. A., Albertine, K. H., Roos, P. J., Wiener-Kronish, J. P., and Staub, N. C.: Overperfusion, hypoxia, and increased pressure cause only hydrostatic pulmonary edema in anesthetized sheep. Circ. Res. 52:335, 1983.

42. Hultgren, H. N., and Grover, R. F.: Circulatory adaptation to high altitude. Annu. Rev. Med. 19:119, 1968.

43. Albers, W. H., and Nadas, A. S.: Unilateral chronic pulmonary edema and pleural effusion after systemic-pulmonary arterial shunts for cyanotic congenital heart disease. Am. J. Cardiol. 19:861, 1967.

44. Kramer, G. C., Harms, B.A., Gunther, R. A., Renkin, E. M., and Demling, R. H.: The effects of hypoproteinemia on blood-to-lymph fluid transport in sheep lung. Circ. Res. 49:1173, 1981.

45. Ziskind, M. M., Weil, H., and George, R. A.: Acute pulmonary edema following the treatment of spontaneous pneumothorax with excessive negative intrapleural pressure. Am. Rev. Respir. Dis. 92:632, 1965.

46. Trapnell, D. H., and Thurston, J. G. B.: Unilateral pulmonary oedema after pleural aspiraton. Lancet 1:1367, 1970.

47. Mellins, R. B., Levine, O. R., Skalak, R., and Fishman, A. P.: Interstitial pressure in the lungs. Circ. Res. 24:197, 1969.

48. Scharf, S. M., Caldini P., and Ingram, R. H., Jr.: Cardiovascular effects of increasing airway pressure. Am. J. Physiol. 1:35, 1977.

49. Scharf, S. M., Brown, R., Saunders, N. A., Green, L. H., and Ingram, R. H., Jr.: Changes in left ventricular size and configuration with positive end-expiratory pressure. Circ. Res. 44:672, 1979.

50. Scharf, S. M., and Brown, R.: Influence of the right ventricle on canine left ventricular function with PEEP. J. Aopl. Physiol. 52:254, 1982.

51. Malik, A. B., and Staub, N. C. (eds.): Mechanisms of Lung Microvascular Injury. New York, New York Academy of Sciences, 1982.

52. Staub, N. C.: Pulmonary edema due to increased microvascular permeability. Ann. Rev. Med. 32:291, 1981.

53. Carlson, R. W., Schaeffer, R. C., Jr., Puri, V. K., Brennan, A. P., and Weil, M. H.: Hypovolemia and permeability pulmonary edema associated with anaphylaxis. Crit. Care Med. 9:883, 1981.

54. Ashbaugh, D. G., Bigelow, D. B., Petty, T. L., and Levine, B. E.: Acute respiratory distress in adults. Lancet 2:319, 1967.

55. Snell, J. D., Jr., and Ramsey, L. H.: Pulmonary edema as a result of endotoxemia. Am. J. Physiol. 217:170, 1969.

56. Ratliff, N. B., Wilson, J. W., Horckel, D. B., and Martin, A. M., Jr.: The lung in hemorrhagic shock. II. Observations on alveolar and vascular ultrastructure. Am. J. Pathol. 58:353, 1970.

57. Moss, G. S., Das Gupta, T. K., Newson, B., and Nyhus, L. M.: Morphologic changes in the primate lung after hemorrhagic shock. Surg. Gynecol. Obstet. 134:3, 1972.

58. Parker, F. B., Jr., Wax, S. D., Kusajima, K., and Webb, W. R.: Hemodynamic and pathological findings in experimental fat embolism. Arch. Surg. 108:70, 1974.

59. Kapanci, Y., Weibel, E. R., Kaplan, H. P., and Robinson, P. V. M.: Pathogenesis and reversibility of the pulmonary lesions of oxygen toxicity in monkey. II. Ultrastructural and morphometric studies. Lab. Invest. 20:101, 1969.

60. Cameron, G. R., and Courtice, F. C.: The production and removal of oedema fluid in the lungs after exposure to carbonyl chloride (phosgene). J. Physiol. (London) 105:175, 1946.

61. Bils, R. F.: Ultrastructural alterations of alveolar tissue of mice. III. Ozone. Arch. Environ. Health 20:468, 1970.

62. Sherwin, R. P., and Richters, V.: Lung capillary permeability: nitrogen dioxide exposure and leakage of tritiated serum. Arch. Intern. Med. 128:61, 1971.

63. Gelb, A, F., and Klein, E.: Hemodynamic and alveolar protein studies in noncardiac pulmonary edema. Am. Rev. Respir. Dis. 114:831, 1976.

64. Sprung, C. L., Rackow, E. C., Fein, I. A., Jacob, A. I., and Isikoff, S. K.: The spectrum of pulmonary edema: differentiation of cardiogenic, intermediate, and noncardiogenic forms of pulmonary edema. Am. Rev. Respir. Dis. 124:718, 1981.

65. Robin, E. D., Carey, L. C., Grenvik, A., Glauser, F., and Gaudio, R.: Capillary leak syndrome with pulmonary edema. Arch. Intern. Med. 130:66, 1972.

66. Pattle, R. E.: Properties, function, and origin of the alveolar lining layer. Nature (London) 175:1125, 1955.

67. Said, S. I., Avery, M. E., Davis, R. K., Banjaree, C. M., and El-Gohar, M.: Pulmonary surface activity in induced pulmonary edema. J. Clin. Invest. 44:458, 1965.

68. Miller, W. W., Waldhausen, J. A., and Rashkind, W. J.: Comparison of oxygen poisoning of the lung in cyanotic and acyanotic dogs. N. Engl. J. Med. 282:943, 1970.

69. Henry, J. N.: The effect of shock on pulmonary alveolar surfactant. Its role in refractory respiratory insufficiency of the critically ill or severely injured patient. J. Trauma 8:756, 1968.

70. Repine, J. E., Bowman, C. M., and Tate, R. M.: Neutrophils and lung edema. Chest 81(Suppl.):5, 1982.

71. Rinaldo, J. E., and Rogers, R. M.: Adult respiratory-distress syndrome: Changing concepts of lung injury and repair. N. Engl. J. Med. 306:900, 1982.

72. Brigham, K. L., Loyd, J. E., Newman, J. H., Snapper, J. R., Ogletree, M. L.,

and English, D. K.: Granulocytes in acute lung vascular injury in unanesthetized sheep. Chest 81 (Suppl.):5, 1982.

73. Lee, C. T., Fein, A. M., Lippman, M., Holtzman, H., Kimbel, P., and Weinbaum, G.: Elastolytic activity in pulmonary lavage fluid from patients with adult respiratory distress syndrome. N. Engl. J. Med. 304:192, 1981.

74. Cohen, A. B., and Cochrane, C. G.: Studies on the pathogenesis of the adult respiratory distress syndrome. J. Clin. Invest. 69:543, 1982.

75. Hammerschmidt, D. E., Weaver, L. J., Hudson, L. D., Craddock, P. R., and Jacob, H. S.: Association of complement activation and elevated plasma-C5a with adult respiratory distress syndrome: Pathophysiological relevance and possible prognostic value. Lancet 1:947, 1980.

76. Magno, M., and Szidon, J. P.: Hemodynamic pulmonary edema in dogs with acute and chronic lymphatic ligation. Am. J. Physiol. 231:1777, 1976.

77. Trapnell, D. H.: Radiological appearances of lymphangitis carcinomatosa of the lung. Thorax 19:251, 1964.

78. Hall, J. G., Morris, B., and Wooley, G.: Intrinsic rhythmic propulsion of lymph in the unanesthetized sheep. J. Physiol. (London) 180:336, 1965.

79. Permutt, S.: Mechanical influences on water accumulation in the lungs. In Fishman, A. P., and Renkin, E. M. (eds.): Pulmonary Edema. Bethesda, American Physiological Society, 1979, p. 175.

80. Sutton, J. R., and Lassen, N.: Pathophysiology of acute mountain sickness and high altitude pulmonary oedema. An hypothesis. Bull. Eur. Physiopathol. Respir. 15:1045, 1979.

81. Lockhart, A., and Saiag, B.: Altitude and the human pulmonary circulation. Clin. Sci. 60:599, 1981.

82. Hultgren, H. N.: High altitude pulmonary edema. Adv. Cardiol. 5:24, 1970.

83. Hultgren, H. N., Spickard, W. B., Hellriegel, K., and Houston, C. S.: High altitude pulmonary edema. Medicine (Baltimore) 40:289, 1961.

84. Fred, H. L., Schmidt, A. M., Bates, T., and Hecht, H. H.: Acute pulmonary edema of altitude: Clinical and physiologic observations. Circulation 25:929, 1962.

85. Scoggin, C. H., Myers, T. M., Reeves, J. T., and Grover, R. F.: High altitude pulmonary edema in the children and young adults of Leadville, Colorado. N. Engl. J. Med. 297:1269, 1977.

86. Hultgren, H. N., Lopez, C. E., Lundberg, E., and Miller, H.: Physiologic studies of pulmonary edema at high altitude. Circulation 29:393, 1964.

87. Whayne, T. F., Jr., and Severinghaus, J. W.: Experimental hypoxic pulmonary edema in the rat. J. Appl. Physiol. 25:279, 1968.

88. Warren, M. F., and Drinker, C. K.: The flow of lymph from the lungs of the dog. Am. J. Physiol. 136:207, 1942.

89. Goodale, R. L., Goetzman, B., and Visscher, M. B.: Hypoxia and iodoacetic acid and alveolo-capillary membrane permeability to albumin. Am. J. Physiol. 219:1226, 1970.

90. Gray, G. W., Bryan, A. C., Freedman, M. H., Houston, C. S., Lewis, W. F., McFadden, D. M., and Newell, G.: Effect of altitude exposure on platelets. J. Appl. Physiol. 39:648, 1975.

91. Grover, R. F., Hyers, R. M., McCurty, I. F., and Reeves, J. T.: High-altitude pulmonary edema. In Fishman, A. P., and Renkin, E. M. (eds.): Pulmonary Edema. Bethesda, American Physiological Society, 1979, p. 229.

92. Cameron, G. R., and De, S. N.: Experimental pulmonary oedema of nervous origin. J. Pathol. Bacteriol. 61:375, 1949.

93. Sarnoff, S. J., and Sarnoff, L. C.: Neurohemodynamics of pulmonary edema. II. The role of sympathetic pathways in the elevation of pulmonary and systemic vascular pressures following the intracisternal injection of fibrin. Circulation 6:51, 1952.

94. Theodore, J., and Robin, E. D.: Speculations on neurogenic pulmonary edema (NPE). Am. Rev. Respir. Dis. 113:405, 1976.

95. Wray, N. P., and Nicotra, M. B.: Pathogenesis of neurogenic pulmonary edema. Am. Rev. Respir. Dis. 118:783, 1978.

96. Hakim, T. S., van der Zee, H., and Malik, A. B.: Effects of sympathetic nerve stimulation on lung fluid and protein exchange. J. Appl. Physiol. 47:1025, 1979.

97. Simon, R. P., Bayne, L. L., Tranbaugh, R. F., and Lewis, F. R.: Elevated pulmonary lymph flow and protein content during status epilepticus in sheep. J. Appl. Physiol. 52:91, 1982.

98. Steinberg, A. D., and Karliner, J. S.: The clinical spectrum of heroin pulmonary edema. Arch. Intern. Med. 122:122, 1968.

99. Fraser, D. W.: Methadone overdose: Illicit use of pharmaceutically prepared narcotics. J.A.M.A. 217:1387, 1971.

100. Bogartz, L. J., and Miller, W. C.: Pulmonary edema associated with propoxyphene intoxication. J.A.M.A. 215:259, 1971.

101. Richter, R. W., Baden, M. N., and Pearson, J.: Cerebral edema seen in many "sudden death" heroin victims. J.A.M.A. 212:967, 1970.

102. Jaffe, J. H.: Narcotic analgesics. In Goodman, L. S., and Gilman, A. (eds.): The Pharmacological Basis of Therapeutics. 4th ed. New York, Macmillan, 1970, p. 237.

103. Katz, S., Aberman, A., Frand, U. I., Stein, I. M., and Fulop, M.: Heroin pulmonary edema: Evidence for increased pulmonary capillary permeability. Am. Rev. Respir. Dis. 106:472, 1972.

104. Gopinathan, K., Saroja, D., Spears, J. R., Gelb, A., and Emmanuel, G. E.: Hemodynamic studies in heroin induced acute pulmonary edema. Circulation 42 (Suppl. 3):44, 1970.

105. Brashear, R. E., Kelly, M. T., and White, A. C.: Elevated plasma histamine after heroin and morphine. J. Lab. Clin. Med. 83:451, 1974.

106. Malik, A. B., Tahamont, M. V., Minnear, F. L., Johnson, A., and Kaplan, J.

E.: Lung fluid and protein exchange after pulmonary vascular thrombosis. Chest 81:5, 1982.

107. Johnson, A., and Malik, A. B.: Effect of defibrinogenation on lung water accumulation after pulmonary microembolism in dogs. J. Appl. Physiol. 49:841, 1980.

108. Flick, M. R., Perel, A., and Staub, N. C.: Leukocytes are required for increased lung microvascular permeability after microembolization in sheep. Circ. Res. 48:344, 1981.

109. Rovinsky, J. J., and Guttmacher, A. F.: Medical, Surgical, and Gynecologic Complications of Pregnancy. 2nd ed. Baltimore, Williams and Wilkins Co., 1965.

110. Resnekow, L., and McDonald, L.: Complications in 220 patients with cardiac dysrhythmias treated by phased direct current shock and indications for electroconversion. Br. Heart J. 29:926, 1967.

111. Cooperman, L. H., and Price, H. L.: Pulmonary edema in the operative and postoperative period: A review of 40 cases. Ann. Surg. 172:883, 1970.

112. Rittenhouse, E. A., and Merendino, K. A.: Acute pulmonary edema in the absence of left ventricular failure. Circulation 40:823, 1969.

113. Culliford, A. T., Thomas, S., and Spencer, F. C.: Fulminating noncardiogenic pulmonary edema: A newly recognized hazard during cardiac operations. J. Thorac. Cardiovasc. Surg. 80:868, 1980.

114. Teichmann, V., Jezek, V., and Herles, F.: Relevance of width of right descending branch of pulmonary artery as a radiological sign of pulmonary hypertension. Thorax 25:91, 1970.

115. Hogg, J. C., Agarawal, J. B., Gardiner, A. J. S., Palmer, W. H., and Macklem, P. T.: Distribution of airway resistance with developing pulmonary edema in dogs. J. Appl. Physiol. 32:20, 1972.

116. DeTroyer, A., Yernault, J., and Englert, M.: Mechanics of breathing in patients with atrial septal defect. Am. Rev. Respir. Dis. 115:413, 1977.

117. Fillmore, S. J., Giumaraes, A. C., Scheidt, S. S., and Killip, T.: Blood gas changes and pulmonary hemodynamics following acute myocardial infarction. Circulation 45:583, 1972.

118. Aberman, A., and Fulop, M.: The metabolic and respiratory acidosis of acute pulmonary edema. Ann. Intern. Med. 76:173, 1972.

119. Richeson, J. F., Paulshock, C., and Yu, P. N.: Non-hydrostatic pulmonary edema after coronary artery ligation in dogs. Circ. Res. 50:301, 1982.

120. Timmis, A. D., Fowler, M. B., Burwood, R. J., Gishen, P., Vincent, R., and Chamberlain, D. A.: Pulmonary oedema without critical increase in left atrial pressure in acute myocardial infarction. Br. Med. J. 283:636, 1981.

121. Vismara, L. A., Leaman, D. M., and Zelis, R.: The effects of morphine on venous tone in patients with acute pulmonary edema. Circulation 54:335, 1976.

122. Iff, H. W., and Flenley, D. C.: Blood-gas exchange after furosemide in acute pulmonary edema. Lancet 1:616, 1971.

123. Scheinman, M., Brown, M., and Rapaport, E.: Hemodynamic effects of ethacrynic acid in patients with refractory acute left ventricular failure. Am. J. Med. 50:291, 1971.

124. Dikshit, K., Vyden, J. K., Forrester, J. S., Chatterjee, K., Prakash, R., and Swan, H. J. C.: Renal and extrarenal hemodynamic effects of furosemide in congestive heart failure after acute myocardial infarction. N. Engl. J. Med. 288: 1087, 1973.

125. Wilson, J. R., Reichek, N., Dunkman, W. B., and Goldberg, S.: Effect of diuresis on the performance of the failing left ventricle in man. Am. J. Med. 70: 234, 1981.

126. Mitenko, P. A., and Ogilvie, R. I.: Rational intravenous doses of theophylline. N. Engl. J. Med. 289:600, 1973.

127. Tai, E., and Read, J.: Response of blood gas tensions to aminophylline and isoprenaline in patients with asthma. Thorax 22:543, 1967.

128. Hildner, F. J.: Pulmonary edema associated with low left ventricular filling pressures. Am. J. Cardiol. 44:1410, 1979.

129. Rizk, N. W., and Murray, J. F.: PEEP and pulmonary edema. Am. J. Med. 72:381, 1982.

130. Cassidy, S. S., and Mitchell, J. H.: Effects of positive pressure breathing on right and left ventricular preload and afterload. Fed. Proc. 40:2178, 1981.

131. Jardin, F., Farcot, J.-C., Boisante, L., Curien, N., Margairaz, A., and Bourdarias, J.-P.: Influence of positive end-expiratory pressure on left ventricular performance. N. Engl. J. Med. 304:387, 1981.

132. Lorell, B. H., Palacios, I., Daggett, W. M., Jacobs, M. L., Fowler, B. N., and Newell, J. B.: Right ventricular distension and left ventricular compliance. Am. J. Physiol. 240:H87, 1981.

133. Wead, W. B., and Norton, J. F.: Effects of intrapleural pressure changes on canine left ventricular function. J. Appl. Physiol. 50:1027, 1981.

134. Fewell, J. E., Abendschein, D. R., Carlson, C. J., Rapaport, E., and Murray, J. F.: Continuous positive-pressure ventilation does not alter ventricular pressure-volume relationship. Am. J. Physiol. 240:H821, 1981.

135. Pontoppidan, H., Wilson, R. S., Rie, M. A., and Schneider, R. C.: Respiratory intensive care. Anesthesiology 47:96, 1977.

136. Prewitt, R. M., McCarthy, J., and Wood, L. D. H.: Treatment of acute low pressure pulmonary edema in dogs: Relative effects of hydrostatic and oncotic pressure, nitroprusside, and positive end-expiratory pressure. J. Clin. Invest. 67: 409, 1981.

137. Lowe, R. J., and Moss, G. S.: Pulmonary failure after trauma. Surg. Annu. 8: 63, 1976.

138. Tullis, J. L.: Albumin. I. Background and use. J.A.M.A. 237:355 and 460, 1977.

18 CARDIAC AND NONCARDIAC FORMS OF ACUTE CIRCULATORY FAILURE (SHOCK)

by Burton E. Sobel, M.D.

Viewed quite simply, the systemic circulation comprises a pump (the left ventricle) in series with a compliant system of conduits (the arteries) that direct blood to the resistance vessels (the arterioles), which in turn lead to a network of vessels in which exchange of gas and metabolites occurs (the capillary bed) and then to a capacitance system (the venous bed) that returns the blood to the right atrium. *Circulatory failure* occurs when transport of blood through this circuit is not sufficient to provide oxygen and nutrients to vital organs or to remove accumulating metabolites at rates commensurate with metabolic requirements. *Transient* circulatory failure, occurring, for example, as a consequence of brief asystole, is frequently manifested by syncope, discussed in Chapter 28. Circulatory failure that results from depression of cardiac function and gives rise to maldistribution of the vascular volume with accumulation of blood in the systemic and/or pulmonary venous beds is termed *congestive heart failure* and is discussed in Chapters 13 and 15. Acute severe circulatory failure, regardless of etiology, has been termed *shock*. Cardiac function may be normal, at least initially, in many forms of circulatory failure, such as those that occur when the vascular volume is inadequate or when vascular tone is impaired.

The common denominator of shock, regardless of its etiology, is *reduction of blood flow to vital organs* due to reduction of total cardiac output or maldistribution of flow or both. Although specific entities give rise to shock with disparate clinical and hemodynamic characteristics, shock is often associated with profound arterial hypotension, restlessness and impaired cerebration, diminished urine output, and tachypnea. Depression of the central nervous system with somnolence is typically observed, and in late stages, coma ensues.

Laboratory findings may differ depending on the specific etiology, and the stage at which the patient is being studied, but profound derangements are generally evident. Hemodilution occurs in hemorrhagic shock when sufficient time has elapsed to permit the transfer of interstitial fluid into the vascular space, but hemoconcentration is characteristic of shock due to dehydration or loss of vascular volume accompanying conditions such as burns or acute pancreatitis. Hyperglycemia resulting from diminished pancreatic perfusion and from the effects of epinephrine on glycogenolysis is common. Accumulation of H^+ and lactate in hypoperfused organs and consequently in the blood contributes to systemic acidosis along with accumulation of other anions because of impaired renal excretion. Tests of renal and liver function are abnormal, arteriovenous oxygen differences are typically elevated when cardiac output is reduced, and pH and the chest roentgenogram may exhibit infiltration and edema associated with "shock lung." When the shock state is associated with infection with gram-negative organisms, there may be increased cardiac output early in the course and a reduced arteriovenous oxygen difference due to arteriovenous shunting. Respiratory alkalosis with a depressed pCO_2 is frequently superimposed on the metabolic acidosis, since the respiratory system is driven by acidemia and by reflex responses to altered fluid in the lung. Disseminated intravascular coagulation with severe thrombocytopenia sometimes occurs. Increased blood viscosity and aggregation of erythrocytes may aggravate hypoperfusion of the microcirculation.[1-7]

ETIOLOGY AND PROGNOSIS

Although the clinical syndrome of shock results from multiple pathophysiological mechanisms, it is convenient to characterize shock in terms of the primary etiology (Table 18–1). Even such a simple classification, which divides the etiology of shock into four categories—cardiogenic, obstructive, oligemic, and distributive—emphasizes the diversity of etiologies leading to shock, and within a single category of shock, the dominant physiological derange-

ments change as a function of time and therapy. Thus, we are faced with a complex array of syndromes with varying hemodynamic characteristics. In addition, elements of more than one etiology are frequently present simultaneously in an individual patient. However, as already stated, *the common denominator of all forms and etiologies of shock is impaired perfusion of and oxygen delivery to vital organs.*

Although prolonged shock from any cause is incompatible with survival, prompt and appropriate intervention can reverse most forms of shock rapidly. A wide variety of responses to treatment can be expected. At one end of the spectrum is the young, otherwise healthy person who experiences acute, massive hemorrhage and for whom adequate blood replacement is provided promptly. If bleeding can be controlled quickly and the complications of transfusion can be avoided, survival, restitution of normal hemodynamics, and no permanent sequelae can be anticipated. At the other end of the spectrum is the elderly patient with multisystem disease and cardiogenic shock due to acute myocardial infarction; this condition is associated with an extremely high mortality (75 to 90 per cent) despite therapy.[6-8] Survival in conditions such as endotoxin shock ranges from 40 to 80 per cent[9-11] and appears to be dependent upon factors such as the age and sex of the patient, the duration of shock prior to specific therapy, the specific infecting organisms, appropriate selection of antibiotic therapy, hepatic function, and the status of the immune system. In all forms of shock, survival is inversely related to the duration of hypoperfusion and is improved by therapy aimed at correcting both the cause, such as myocardi-

---

TABLE 18–1   ETIOLOGIES OF SHOCK

Cardiogenic
1. Secondary to arrhythmias
   a. Bradyarrhythmias
   b. Tachyarrhythmias
2. Secondary to cardiac mechanical factors
   a. Regurgitant lesions
      (1) Acute mitral or aortic regurgitation
      (2) Rupture of interventricular septum
      (3) Massive left ventricular aneurysm
   b. Obstructive lesions
      (1) Left ventricular outflow tract obstruction, e.g., congenital or acquired valvular aortic stenosis and hypertrophic obstructive cardiomyopathy
      (2) Left ventricular inflow tract obstruction, e.g., mitral stenosis, left atrial myxoma, atrial thrombus
3. Myopathic
   a. Impairment of left ventricular contractility, as in acute myocardial infarction or congestive cardiomyopathy
   b. Impairment of right ventricular contractility due to right ventricular infarction
   c. Impairment of left ventricular relaxation or compliance as in restrictive or hypertrophic cardiomyopathy

Obstructive (due to factors extrinsic to cardiac values and myocardium)
1. Pericardial tamponade
2. Coarctation of aorta
3. Pulmonary embolism
4. Primary pulmonary hypertension

Oligemic
1. Hemorrhage
2. Fluid depletion or sequestration due to vomiting, diarrhea, dehydration, diabetes mellitus, diabetes insipidus, adrenal

cortical failure, peritonitis, pancreatitis, burns, ascites, villous adenoma, or pheochromocytoma

Distributive
1. Septicemic
   a. Endotoxic
   b. Secondary to specific infection, such as dengue fever
2. Metabolic or toxic
   a. Renal failure
   b. Hepatic failure
   c. Severe acidosis or alkalosis
   d. Drug overdose
   e. Heavy metal intoxication
   f. Toxic shock syndrome (possibly due to a staphylococcal exotoxin)
   g. Malignant hyperthermia
3. Endocrinologic
   a. Uncontrolled diabetes mellitus with ketoacidosis or hyperosmolar coma
   b. Adrenal cortical failure
   c. Hypothyroidism
   d. Hyper- or hypoparathyroidism
   e. Diabetes insipidus
   f. Hypoglycemia secondary to excess exogenous insulin or a beta-cell tumor
4. Microcirculatory impairment due to altered blood viscosity
   a. Polycythemia vera
   b. Hyperviscosity syndromes, including multiple myeloma, macroglobulinemia, and cryoglobulinemia
   c. Sickle cell anemia
   d. Fat emboli
5. Neurogenic
   a. Cerebral
   b. Spinal
   c. Dysautonomic
6. Anaphylactic

al failure or septicemia, and the manifestations, such as hypoxemia and acidemia.

STAGES OF SHOCK

Oligemic shock has been divided into reversible and irreversible stages. This type of shock reflects decreased tissue perfusion due to diminished effective blood volume and is manifested by systemic hypotension and tachycardia. It is almost always reversible early in its course. Thus, patients suffering from simple hemorrhage and exhibiting profound hypotension when first seen respond dramatically to prompt replacement of blood and may show no sequelae of the insult after several days. Early in the evolution of such a process, compensatory mechanisms are called into play in part as a response to declining systemic arterial and right-sided filling pressures and to acidosis. Compensation usually fails if blood volume depletion exceeds 20 per cent, at which time systemic manifestations of shock, including hypotension and tachycardia, appear and are accompanied by progressive manifestations of injury to vital organs.[12] Although integrated reflex and neurohumoral control of the peripheral circulation may protect the patient during the early stages of shock, it may also mask the underlying disorder unless there is reason for a high index of suspicion. Accordingly, the nature of such compensation merits special consideration.

When systemic arterial pressure falls, decreased afferent activity emanates from baroreceptors in the carotid and aortic arteries.[13] Under physiological conditions, increased afferent activity in the baroreceptors inhibits sympathoadrenal efferent activity and vasoconstrictor tone and augments parasympathetic efferent activity to the heart via the vagi. In hypotension, this inhibition of the sympathoadrenal system is withdrawn, and vagal efferent activity is enhanced. Reflex vasoconstriction, tachycardia, and augmented cardiac output result, reflecting the increases in rate and contractility.[14]

Reflex responses are also modulated by afferent impulses originating in the atrial and ventricular myocardium.[15,16] Vagal afferent fibers from the heart and coronary vascular bed may be stimulated by metabolites accumulating locally or by changes in stretch or pressure.[17-20] Chemical, pharmacological, or electrical stimulation of selected afferents in the left ventricle elicits bradycardia as well as arterial and venous dilation,[17] possibly contributing to the syncope and exacerbation of hypotension associated with some forms of cardiogenic shock. Stimulation of other ventricular afferents gives rise to reflex tachycardia, increased contractility, and sympathetic vasoconstrictor impulses to the kidneys.

Stretch receptors in the atria and in the cavae (involved in the Bainbridge reflex) influence the flow of sympathetic impulses to the heart and kidneys as well as the secretion of antidiuretic hormone (ADH) (p. 462). Thus, shock in which left atrial pressure is elevated, i.e., cardiogenic shock, may be accompanied by renal vasodilatation, decreased circulating ADH, and a relative preservation of normal urine output, in contrast to shock in which left atrial pressure is low, which may be accompanied by pro-

found renal vasoconstriction, high ADH levels, and therefore oliguria out of proportion to the reduction of renal perfusion. Secretion of both ADH and aldosterone is influenced by reflexes involving stretch receptors in the right atrium (p. 462). Thus, decreased stretch augments efferent renal sympathetic activity, increases renin secretion and consequently angiotensin II concentration, and ultimately increases aldosterone secretion, which tends to limit excretion of sodium and water and thereby maintains blood volume.

In concert, the reflex response to hypotension resulting from oligemia is compensatory, since the decline in perfusion pressure of vital organs is limited by vasoconstriction, tachycardia, and augmented cardiac contractility. However, redistribution of blood flow occurs as well. In many forms of shock, cutaneous, skeletal muscle, renal, and splanchnic perfusion decrease primarily because of vasoconstriction mediated by the rich alpha-adrenergic innervation of the arterioles supplying these organs.[21]

Reflex responses to oligemia also result in characteristic humoral changes. Plasma renin activity increases as a consequence of sympathetic stimulation of the juxtaglomerular apparatus as well as the direct response of the kidney to reduced glomerular filtration. Elevated circulating angiotensin II contributes to maintenance of systemic vascular resistance along with the markedly increased circulating catecholamines released from the adrenal medulla and nerve endings. Elaboration of aldosterone released in response to angiotensin II, and of ADH released in response to reflex stimulation mediated by a reduction of atrial pressure, potentiates maintenance of vascular volume and systemic arterial pressure. Vasoactive prostaglandins, catabolized by the lung under physiological conditions, may accumulate. Together, these substances affect hemodynamics not only by influencing vascular volume and tone but also by modulating central and peripheral adrenergic activity.[22-27]

When oligemia is so severe that compensatory mechanisms cannot maintain adequate pressure for perfusion of vital organs, or when the metabolic derangements overpower compensatory mechanisms, decompensation occurs, manifested by a marked decline in systemic arterial pressure, diminished cardiac output, and the biochemical changes of ischemia and hypoxia in vital organs (Fig. 18–1). Anaerobic glycolysis compensates for diminished oxygen delivery and leads to the production of lactate and its elaboration from skeletal muscle, liver, and other organs into the circulation, resulting in progressive lactic acidosis. Diminished hepatic metabolism of circulating lactate, coupled with decreased renal excretion, potentiates the acidosis. Impaired pulmonary function causes hypoxemia, and the ensuing ventilatory response, mediated reflexly by chemoreceptor stimulation, leads to hypocapnia. Hyperglycemia in response to catecholamine stimulation of glycogenolysis, coupled with inhibition of insulin release, is a typical finding until glycogen stores are depleted, at which point hypoglycemia may supervene. Despite the lipolytic actions of catecholamines, the concentration of circulating free fatty acids may fall, possibly because of limited perfusion of adipose tissue. In endotoxic shock, hypertriglyceridemia may be prominent, possibly because of depressed lipoprotein lipase activity in adipose tissue and the myocardium.[28]

FIGURE 18–1 Diagram depicting the vicious circle typically manifested in shock associated with a low cardiac output. Regardless of etiology, impairment of vasomotor tone mediated by manifestations of tissue hypoxia including local acidosis contributes to reduced venous return and consequent further diminution of cardiac output with progressive reduction of effective vascular volume and perfusion of vital organs, including the heart itself. An analogous picture evolves even when the shock state is initially associated with a high cardiac output, such as in cases of distributive shock due to sepsis. Under these conditions, reduction of effective vascular volume ultimately compromises cardiac output progressively. (From Messmer, K.: Pathophysiological aspects and problems of shock. Triangle, *13*:85, 1974.)

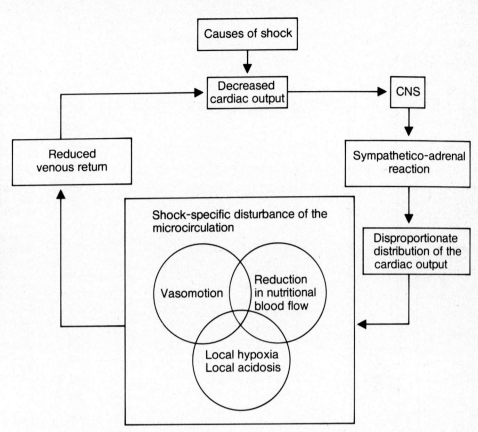

Circulating levels of lysosomal hydrolases increase not only because of liberation of these enzymes from damaged ischemic cells, primarily in splanchnic organs, but also because of impaired function of the reticuloendothelial system—an important site of enzyme removal under physiological conditions.[29–32]

COMPENSATED AND DECOMPENSATED SHOCK

In animals subjected to hemorrhage, a phenomenon referred to as "taking up" can be demonstrated. When blood pressure is reduced profoundly by bleeding, but this blood is reinfused within one to two hours, restoration of circulatory integrity can be anticipated. However, if the interval of hypotension is prolonged, reinfusion of blood is not associated with a corresponding augmentation of arterial pressure. Thus, vasodilatation within some elements of the vascular bed leads to pooling of blood, and augmentation of blood volume fails to increase the "effective" vascular volume, i.e., the blood that actually perfuses metabolizing tissues.[33]

It has been difficult to delineate the mechanisms involved in the *irreversibility* of shock in humans because of generalizations derived from experimental animal models, in which the responsible factors may be quite different. For example, in dogs subjected to hemorrhage, irreversibility appears to be related to associated endotoxemia and its sequelae. Loss of the intestinal epithelium's barrier function to bacteria and bacterial products is the putative factor.[34] However, irreversible shock occurs in germ-free

animals,[35] and evidence to corroborate an endotoxic mechanism in oligemic shock in man has been lacking.

Irreversibility of shock has also been attributed to the effects of numerous humoral agents, many of which seem to be released from cells subjected to ischemia (Fig. 18–2), including histamine,[36] serotonin, kinins, lactate, hydrogen ions, proteases, catecholamines, prostaglandins, angiotensin II, and lysosomal enzymes.[22–27,37–39] A decline in plasma histaminase activity may account, in part, for the increased concentrations of circulating histamine.[39] Physiological decompensation may be mediated in part by late inhibition of adrenergic vascular control due to inhibitory actions of prostaglandins on the peripheral adrenergic nervous system.[40] Thus, inhibitors of prostaglandin synthesis help to maintain vascular tone in animal preparations subjected to shock.

Marked and sustained increases in the blood levels of vasopressin and angiotensin II accompany hemorrhagic shock.[23,41–43] Both of these hormones are powerful constrictors of the mesenteric vascular bed and may contribute to ischemia of the gut and liver, potentially contributing to irreversibility. Administration of a nonapeptide that blocks conversion of angiotensin I to angiotensin II (the physiologically active moiety) precluded the development of intense vasoconstriction and increased the survival of dogs subjected to hemorrhage. In addition, administration of the angiotensin-converting inhibitor to dogs with experimentally induced diabetes insipidus maintained peripheral vascular conductance and cardiac output in the face of hemorrhage. Accordingly, prevention of intense mesenteric vasoconstriction mediated by angiotensin II and ADH ap-

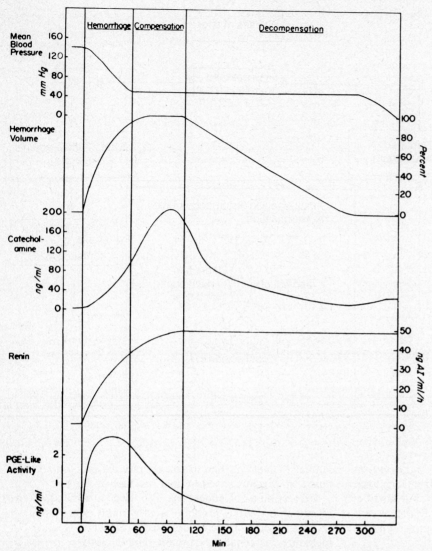

FIGURE 18–2 Diagrammatic representation of the characteristic temporal profile of plasma catecholamines, renin, and prostaglandin E (PGE)–like activity in dogs subjected to hemorrhage sufficient to induce a decline of mean arterial blood pressure to approximately 50 mm Hg. Decompensation (manifested by the need for progressive infusion of blood to maintain the same mean arterial pressure) was characterized by an associated decline in levels of plasma catecholamines and PGE-like activity but a persistent elevation of plasma renin activity. (From Jakschik, B. A., et al.: Profile of circulating vasoactive substances in hemorrhagic shock and their pharmacologic manipulation. J. Clin. Invest. *54*:842, 1974.)

pears to be protective in the canine model of hemorrhagic shock.

Several observations also suggest that shock is mediated in part by endorphins released from the pituitary gland,[44] since opiate antagonists such as naloxone maintain hemodynamics and prolong survival in experimental animals subjected to hemorrhagic shock.[45,46] Thromboxanes have also been implicated because of the elevated levels which occur, the prevalence of disseminated intravascular coagulation, and the protective effects of thromboxane synthetase inhibitors in endotoxic shock in animals.[47,48] Prostacyclin (PGI$_2$), a physiological antagonist of thromboxane A$_2$, may reverse lethal endotoxemia under some circumstances,[49] and both PGI$_2$ and PGI$_2$-analogs are undergoing clinical trials for evaluation of treatment of shock.

Ischemia due to hypoperfusion is responsible for profound organ damage in shock. Mucosal lesions in the small intestine occur in patients as well as in experimental animals in shock.[50] Ultrastructural alterations in pancreatic tissue from patients in shock are more likely due to the direct effects of ischemia than to injury mediated by activation of lysosomal enzymes.[51] Damage to the renal tubules with back-diffusion of glomerular filtrate as well as redistribution of renal blood flow contributes to oliguria.[52,53] The resting transmembrane potential of skeletal muscle de-

clines in hemorrhagic shock, a finding indicative of impaired membrane transport function secondary to ischemia.[54]

Disseminated intravascular coagulation, induced by thromboplastic substances released into the circulation,[4] may also play an important role in potentiating regional ischemia by impairing flow through the microcirculation. This may be accentuated by arteriolar and venular constriction, even though perfusion pressure is maintained.

It appears likely that irreversible shock results from destruction of cells in vital organs due to the combined effects of ischemia and of noxious circulating and local metabolites. The onset of irreversible shock in animals correlates with accumulated oxygen debt exceeding 120 ml/kg of body weight.[55]

ROLE OF THE HEART IN IRREVERSIBLE SHOCK. Prolonged shock, regardless of its etiology, leads to impairment of cardiac function (Fig. 18–3). Adequate ventricular function is dependent on aerobic metabolism of the myocardium, which like any other organ, is dependent on an adequate oxygen supply. In experimental animals in which the oxygen delivered to the heart can be manipulated by changes in the hemoglobin content of the blood, impaired ventricular performance in association with hemorrhagic shock has been directly related to oxy-

FIGURE 18–3 The interaction of factors that compromise cardiac output in noncardiac shock syndromes. The inadequate preload, consequent to hypovolemia, capillary damage, or failure of vascular autoregulation, initiates a series of responses that further compromises cardiac output and tissue perfusion, ultimately leading to microcirculatory failure. (Reproduced with permission from Shine, K. I.: Aspects of the management of shock. Ann. Intern. Med. *93*:723, 1980.)

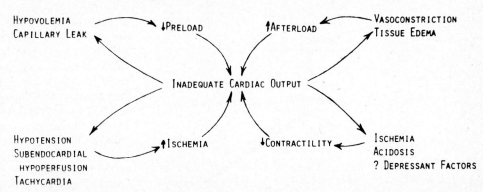

gen availability.[56-58] Depletion of cellular ATP may lead to irreversible myocardial injury through several mechanisms, including failure to maintain cation transport, with consequent cell swelling, or activation of lytic enzymes capable of degrading cell membranes.

Although contributing factors such as metabolic acidosis, loss of sympathetic stimulation to the heart,[59] circulating myocardial depressant factors,[60] and limited substrate availability[61] may all play a role in the impairment of myocardial contractility in shock, irreversibility of shock from any cause may depend in part on deterioration of cardiac function.[62,63] Preservation of myocardial function may be afforded by calcium antagonists such as verapamil, which exert favorable hemodynamic and metabolic effects and prolong survival in dogs subjected to hemorrhagic shock.[64] Since the coronary vascular bed can be constricted by alpha-adrenergic stimulation[65] (p. 1242), with resultant diminution of myocardial oxygen availability, the massive adrenergic stimulation that accompanies shock may contribute to the limitation of myocardial oxygen availability, which impairs cardiac performance and leads in turn to irreversibility.

EFFECTS OF SHOCK ON TARGET ORGANS

It is convenient to consider the pathophysiology of shock in terms of the initiating cause(s), the effects of the shock state on target organs, and the vicious circles that contribute to perpetuation and progression of the syndrome. Before considering specific categories of shock classified according to initiating cause (Table 18–1), the effects on target organs are discussed.

THE LUNG (See also page 566)

Pulmonary failure is one of the most important potentially lethal complications of shock. (Prior to the use of dialysis, renal failure predominated in this regard.) Indeed, among patients with noncardiogenic shock, pulmonary failure is the most common cause of death, affecting an estimated 150,000 patients annually with a case fatality rate exceeding 50 per cent.[66] Atelectasis and infection are contributing but probably not primary factors. The syndrome, now frequently referred to as the adult respiratory distress syndrome (ARDS), shock lung, post-transfusion lung, or stiff lung, cannot be explained in simple terms. Distressingly often, ARDS follows shock, regardless of its etiology, within 24 to 72 hours,[67] although most frequently it follows massive hemorrhage or trauma. Interstitial and alveolar pulmonary edema are the hallmarks of ARDS. Pathogenetic factors include (1) increased permeability of the alveolar-capillary membrane; (2) increased capillary hydrostatic pressure; (3) decreased plasma oncotic pressure; (4) interference with function of the pulmonary lymphatics, especially by depressant drugs or anesthetics; (5) deficient production of surfactant (Fig. 18–4);[68] (6) loss of alveolar type I cells, and their replacement with type II cells; (7) capillary obliteration; and, as a late event, (8) extensive fibrosis.[66] In addition to shock, exposure of the lung to high concentrations of inspired oxygen or other toxins causes similar injury to the alveolar-capillary membrane.[69]

The initial phase of ARDS may occur when cardiac output is still depressed or has already been restored after having been depressed. Interstitial edema accompanied by hypocapnia is an important initial finding. Factors responsible for this early accumulation of fluid in the lungs include (1) an increase in the permeability of the pulmonary capillaries to plasma proteins secondary to the effects of ischemia on the lung, with platelet aggregation, oxygen toxicity, and deleterious humoral stimuli playing contributory roles;[70] (2) a lowering of plasma oncotic pressure, sometimes potentiated by the administration of excessive volumes of crystalloid solutions; and (3) an elevated pulmonary capillary pressure. In addition, complement-mediated aggregation of neutrophils, associated with release of proteases and potentially responsive to administration of corticosteroids, contributes to pulmonary capillary stasis and endothelial injury.[66,71] Once protein has extravasated into the pulmonary interstitial or alveolar space, its oncotic pressure may enhance further accumulation of fluid.

ARDS is characterized by tachypnea and diffuse, bilateral inspiratory rales in association with severe hypoxemia and radiographic opacification of both lung fields.[72-77] Pulmonary compliance and functional residual capacity are both reduced, and ventilation-perfusion ratios are altered markedly, causing venous admixture and, as the process becomes more advanced, intrapulmonary right-to-left shunting, a condition in which the depressed arterial pO_2 is not responsive to ventilation with 100 per cent O_2. Although ischemia of the alveolar-capillary membrane alone does not appear to give rise to ARDS, the pathophysiology does appear to reflect increased membrane permeability

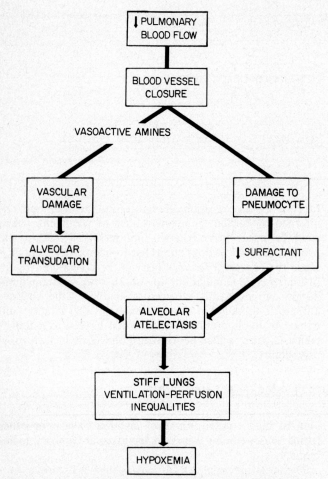

FIGURE 18-4   Pathways involved in the genesis of adult respiratory distress syndrome (ARDS) accompanying shock. (From Kones, R. J.: Cardiogenic Shock. New York, Futura Publishing Co., 1974.)

as well as augmented filtration due to altered pulmonary hemodynamics.[78] Exposure of the lung to bacterial insults occurring concomitantly with shock of another etiology potentiates pulmonary failure,[79] as does excessive administration of intravenous crystalloid solutions.[80,81] Impaired function of the reticuloendothelial system, reflecting, in part, deficiency of fibronectin, a serum opsonin, results in reduced clearance not only of bacterial components in septic shock but also of fibrin and fibrinogen degradation products and injured platelets—all of which contribute to formation of pulmonary edema.[82] This phenomenon has given rise to trials of the administration of fibronectin to patients with shock of diverse etiologies, including the toxic shock syndrome.[83-85] The possible role of neural stimulation in causing damage to the alveolar-capillary membrane has been suggested by studies in which unilateral pulmonary denervation conferred protection on the denervated lung in experimental animals subjected to hemorrhagic shock.[86-88] Impaired integrity of the alveolar-capillary membrane may be a consequence of the same circulating metabolites as those potentially contributing to irreversible injury in other organs.

Since solutions containing albumin or other colloids can extravasate into the lung when the integrity of the alveolar-capillary membrane has been compromised,[89] excessive administration of such fluids to patients with ARDS may

actually exacerbate the syndrome. On the other hand, diminution of intravascular colloid osmotic pressure correlates with increased mortality in patients with shock (Fig. 18-5), perhaps because it is a critical factor in the development of pulmonary edema.[90,91] The mechanisms underlying this decrease have not been totally elucidated, but in some instances inappropriate administration of colloid-free fluid can be implicated. Other factors underlying the progression of ARDS include perivenular leakage, potentiated by histamine and bradykinin[92] with increased filtration and pulmonary lymphatic flow early in shock; inadequate delivery of oxygen to fulfill the high oxygen requirements of Type II alveolar cells, which are responsible for synthesis of surfactant; sequestration of platelets and polymorphonuclear leukocytes[93] with liberation of proteases; immunological factors; pulmonary vasoconstrictor effects of acidosis;[94] and consequences of decreased ventilation-perfusion ratios induced by atelectasis and edema. The suggestion that impaired production of pulmonary surfactant may underlie or contribute to ARDS is based on analysis of bronchoalveolar lavage fluid,[95] and the potential importance of pulmonary venoconstriction in the genesis of the syndrome has been demonstrated in experiments on sheep. Altered pulmonary vasoreactivity contributing to edema formation may be mediated by increased synthesis of vasodilatory prostaglandins in arteries and of thromboxane-like vasoconstrictor compounds in veins; these vasoactive substances may act directly on pulmonary vascular tissue or may alter vascular responsiveness to neurohumoral agents such as norepinephrine and serotonin.[96]

TREATMENT OF ARDS (see also p. 573). Since ARDS potentiates the severity of shock and may be lethal even if circulatory failure is corrected, aggressive therapy is required. Tracheal intubation is often necessary to prevent or treat hypoxemia and permit control of pulmonary secretions. The concentration of inhaled oxygen (FIO_2) should not be elevated above the level needed to maintain arterial pO_2 within the range of 60 to 90 mm Hg and should not

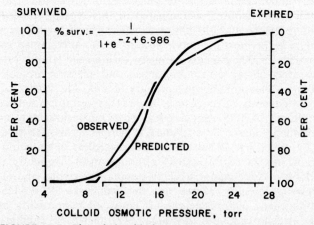

FIGURE 18-5   The relationship between survival and plasma colloid osmotic pressure among 99 patients with shock due to diverse etiologies. The mean survival time for patients who expired was 5.4 days. Based on the lowest value for colloid osmotic pressure obtained in serial determination, correct classification (survival versus mortality) was obtained with the use of the equation shown in the inset in 79 per cent of cases. (From Morissette, M., et al.: Reduction in colloid osmotic pressure associated with fatal progression of cardiopulmonary failure. Crit. Care Med. *3*:115, 1975.)

exceed 0.60. Positive end-expiratory pressure (PEEP) or continuous positive airway pressure (CPAP) may diminish intrapulmonary right-to-left shunting by recruiting previous closed alveolar units and should be employed when an FIO$_2$ of 0.60 fails to maintain an arterial pO$_2$ of 60 mm Hg.[97] The use of PEEP or CPAP in patients with ARDS may not decrease cardiac output, particularly when left ventricular end-diastolic pressure exceeds 15 mm Hg. A paradoxical increase in cardiac output may, in fact, occur because of the salutary effects of improved oxygenation of the blood on a failing left ventricle.

Maintenance of normal levels of vascular volume is desirable; colloid should not be administered in excess, and crystalloids should be administered only in volumes that replace losses. In fact, augmentation of pulmonary blood flow per se, by expansion of blood volume or administration of dopamine or isoproterenol, may accentuate venous admixture due to further mismatch of ventilation and perfusion.[98] Intravascular colloid osmotic pressure can be stabilized by the judicious intravenous administration of loop diuretics, furosemide or ethacrynic acid; the use of albumin is fraught with difficulty because of the rapidity with which it leaves the circulation and enters the pulmonary interstitium and alveoli.

Vigorous treatment of sepsis is necessary, and supportive measures designed to stabilize cardiac rhythm and function are helpful. Glucocorticoids may modify the course of the syndrome favorably, particularly when they are administered soon after the onset of the insult.[100-103] Potential benefit may also accrue from inhibition of complement-mediated neutrophil aggregation and proteolysis and

an increase in lung vascular permeability.[66] Although cyclooxygenase inhibitors, anticoagulants, and fibronectin have not yet been proven helpful, they and agents that elevate serum antiprotease acitivity, such as Danazol, are being evaluated intensively.[104] When shock is treated successfully and the underlying initiating cause is removed, abnormalities of pulmonary function or sequelae of ARDS sometimes persist.[105] The value of antifibrotic agents such as penicillamine or analogs of proline has not yet been established but is under investigation.

THE HEART

CARDIAC METABOLISM IN SHOCK. Under physiological conditions, the heart derives its energy almost exclusively from oxidative processes in mitochondria (Chap. 36). Oxidation of fatty acids and pyruvate predominates, but when the supply of these preferred substrates or of oxygen is limited, aerobic glycolysis is unable to meet the heart's metabolic needs. Net glycogenolysis does not occur in well-oxygenated myocardium, even in the face of maximal adrenergic stimulation.[106] However, myocardial anoxia or ischemia leads to rapid depletion of glycogen stores mediated by the phosphorylase reaction (Fig. 18–6). Under anaerobic conditions, myocardial viability appears to depend, in part, on glycolysis, since supplementation of perfusates with glucose improves ventricular performance[107] and maintains the biochemical integrity of anoxic tissue.[108] Nevertheless, the ability of anaerobic metabolism alone to maintain high-energy phosphate stores is limited, and myo-

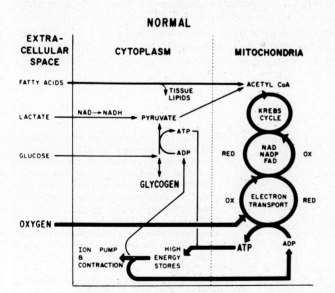

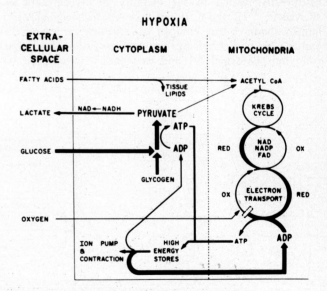

FIGURE 18–6 Diagrammatic representations of the major energy-producing pathways of intermediary metabolism in normal (left) and hypoxic (right) myocardium. Under physiological conditions, energy production depends on oxidation of fatty acids and carbohydrates, with a final common pathway being oxidation of acetyl-CoA via the tricarboxylic acid cycle (the Krebs cycle) with associated electron transport through intermediates such as reduced (RED) and sequentially oxidized (OX) pyridine nucleotides (NAD and NADP) and flavoprotein (FAD) intermediates and a final electron-acceptor role for oxygen, which is converted to water. The concomitant production of ATP permits the cell to maintain vital functions and provide chemical energy in a form suitable for mediating contraction of myofibrillar proteins. Under conditions of tissue hypoxia, such as those accompanying shock, oxidation of acetyl-CoA is inhibited because of the lack of a terminal electron acceptor (oxygen). Thus, formation of ATP depends virtually exclusively on anaerobic glycolysis, which cannot proceed beyond formation of lactate and which gives rise to a much smaller amount of ATP per mole of glucose metabolized than is the case when oxidative metabolism is present. (From Kones, R. J.: Cardiogenic Shock. New York, Futura Publishing Co., 1974.)

cardial viability is compromised in the presence of anoxia, despite maximal anaerobic glycolysis.[109] In ischemic myocardium glycolytic flux is limited not only by the intrinsic activity of enzymes that participate in the pathway but also because of inhibition of rate-limiting reactions by intracellular acidosis.[110] Under these conditions, fatty acids are preferentially incorporated into triglycerides rather than oxidized,[111] with consequent intracellular accumulation of neutral fat. The accentuation of glycolysis leads to myocardial lactate production,[112,113] along with the liberation of inorganic phosphate, reflecting a net degradation of high-energy phosphates. Increased efflux of potassium accompanies these changes, probably as a consequence of impaired cation transport, and it is often associated with cell swelling.[114]

End products of degradation of purine nucleotides, such as inosine and hypoxanthine, appear in the coronary venous blood of ischemic myocardium because nucleotide synthesis in the myocardium is not maintained effectively by salvage pathways utilizing purine bases.[115,116] Severe or persistent ischemia leads to liberation of enzymes from the heart,[117–121] in proportion to the quantity of myocardium which manifests irreversible injury, and reflects loss of integrity of cell membranes. An increased proportion of free as opposed to latent lysosomal enzyme activity in extracts of ischemic myocardium and liberation of lysosomal enzymes into the blood stream after ischemic injury to the heart have also been described.[122]

The most common etiology of cardiogenic shock is myocardial ischemia secondary to coronary artery disease (Chap. 36), and impairment of cardiac function appears to be directly related to the quantity of myocardium destroyed.[123,124] However, it must be appreciated that prolonged shock of any etiology can elicit some myocardial damage by compromising coronary perfusion, as judged from morphological[124,125] and enzymatic[126] criteria. In pa-

tients who die as a consequence of cardiogenic shock secondary to myocardial infarction, the myocardium usually exhibits a central area of necrosis, with less severe injury in peripheral regions, suggesting that the myocardial damage is progressive and occurs over time (Fig. 37–7, p. 1271). Continued late release of enzymes, such as the "myocardial" isoenzyme of creatine kinase, into the peripheral blood in patients with cardiogenic shock is compatible with this interpretation. The metabolic derangements responsible for the sudden cessation of contractility in segments of ischemic myocardium have not been identified with certainty. However, rapid declines in intracellular pH may play a role.[127] Some of the early biochemical changes may be reversible if myocardial ischemia is rapidly corrected, in which case depressed cardiac function may be prolonged but will ultimately return to normal.[128] However, even in noncardiogenic shock, the heart may sustain irreversible injury as a result of severe systemic hypotension from any cause.

Typically, in patients with cardiogenic shock, the pulmonary artery occlusive pressure or left ventricular filling pressure is elevated much more than the right ventricular filling pressure (or central venous pressure), unless shock is a consequence of right ventricular infarction, in which case right ventricular diastolic and central venous pressures are elevated. Under these circumstances pulmonary arterial occlusive pressure is normal if there is little or no involvement of the left ventricle, or, as occurs much more commonly, if there is also left ventricular infarction, the pulmonary artery occlusive pressure is elevated.

CARDIAC FUNCTION IN NONCARDIOGENIC SHOCK. Irreversible shock, even when it is noncardiogenic in origin and, indeed, even in the absence of intrinsic heart disease, is frequently accompanied by severe left ventricular dysfunction and sometimes by irreversible damage to the myocardium. Because the myocardium extracts rela-

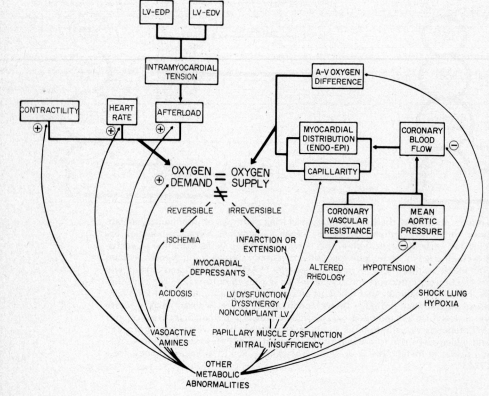

FIGURE 18–7 Changes in left ventricular end-diastolic pressure (LV-EDP) and end-diastolic volume (LV-EDV) are represented as important contributors to intramyocardial wall tension, which is of course also influenced by ventricular afterload. Parameters influencing myocardial oxygen supply are depicted on the right side of the diagram and those affecting myocardial oxygen demand are on the left side. Positive feedback loops (depicted by plus signs) exacerbate the imbalance between myocardial oxygen supply and demand and are potentiated by factors delineated in the diagram with arrows. Factors diminishing myocardial perfusion also exacerbate the disparity between myocardial oxygen supply and demand via negative feedback loops (depicted by minus signs) and are potentiated by manifestations of impaired ventricular function, as indicated by the arrows. ENDO and EPI refer to endocardial and epicardial perfusion, respectively. (From Kones, R. J.: Cardiogenic Shock. New York, Futura Publishing Co., 1974.)

tively large quantities of oxygen under physiological conditions, even modest reductions of coronary perfusion may impair cardiac performance seriously, particularly when some degree of coronary artery obstruction is present (Fig. 18–7).[129] Once myocardial viability has been compromised, correction of an independent underlying cause of shock, such as repletion of blood volume, will not restore ventricular function. This chain of events is particularly hazardous because progressive impairment of cardiac function with decreased ventricular compliance and elevation of left ventricular diastolic pressure further compromises coronary perfusion, particularly to the subendocardium, and thereby intensifies the cardiac insult. Efflux of potassium,[130] acidosis,[127] and the effects of circulating catecholamines and cardiac sympathetic efferent activity may elicit coronary constriction. Reflex sympathetic stimulation of the heart augments myocardial oxygen requirements under conditions in which oxygen delivery is severely limited. Peripheral vasoconstriction augments impedance to left ventricular outflow, further increasing the metabolic requirements of the heart. Consequently, cardiac performance may be impaired further, exacerbating the shock state and leading to a vicious circle of myocardial injury.

Prolonged noncardiogenic shock also impairs ventricular function by causing maldistribution of coronary perfusion. There is a progressive increase in coronary resistance, a decline in the ratio of subendocardial to subepicardial perfusion, and a reduction in the percentage of coronary flow occurring during diastole. Hypertonic mannitol reduces the early alterations in coronary perfusion and limits the increase in myocardial water content, suggesting that the early subendocardial ischemia may be related, in part, to cell swelling or interstitial edema induced by shock. Also, the finding that alpha-adrenergic blockade decreases the maldistribution and overall reduction of flow[131] suggest a neural component.

Arrhythmia is a common consequence of impaired myocardial perfusion in shock of any etiology. The frequent tachyarrhythmias and the less common bradyarrhythmias are likely to intensify shock because they further impair cardiac output. In addition, because of the increase in myocardial oxygen requirements accompanying tachycardia, myocardial viability may be compromised further.

When shock is present, regardless of its etiology, the sensitivity of the myocardium to the toxic effects of pharmacological agents may increase. For example, accumulation of radiolabeled digoxin in the myocardium is substantially greater in experimental animals subjected to hemorrhagic shock than in the hearts of normal animals. Diminished peripheral perfusion, with relative preservation of myocardial blood flow and transiently elevated plasma digoxin, may be one factor accounting for increased digitalis toxicity in patients with grossly impaired circulatory function.[132]

The Kidney

Renal responses may perpetuate shock because of this organ's elaboration of vasoactive substances such as renin, its failure to excrete potentially noxious metabolites such as lactate and other organic acids, and the derangements of electrolytes and acid-base balance accompanying acute renal failure. Under physiological conditions, renal blood flow is regulated, in part, by efferent activity from the thora-columbar sympathetic system. Renal vascular tone is influenced by reflex responses activated by carotid, aortic, and cardiopulmonary receptors and is mediated by altered sympathetic outflow to the heart and vasculature.[133,134] Alpha-adrenergic stimulation diminishes renal perfusion, and alpha-adrenergic antagonists inhibit renal arterial constriction in hemorrhagic shock.[135]

The renal manifestations of shock are similar to those of acute renal failure secondary to ischemia of any cause. Brief insults may elicit promptly reversible derangements, but more prolonged hypotension (lasting for one hour or more) may give rise to acute tubular necrosis, with variably persistent impairment of renal function despite restoration of renal blood flow. Based on observations in animal models and fragmentary and somewhat indirect data from clinical studies, several processes affecting the renal tubules have been implicated as factors contributing to the persistent impairment of renal function in response to an ischemic insult. These include (1) acute tubular necrosis with back-diffusion of filtrate; (2) tubular obstruction with casts and proteinaceous debris;[136,137] and (3) leakage of filtrate across damaged tubular epithelium, with interstitial edema and tubular collapse. Renal damage may also be exacerbated by agents used in the treatment of shock, such as vasopressors and low molecular weight dextran, which persist for prolonged intervals in the circulation. Plasma exchange may be helpful in removing the offending agent and potentiating recovery of renal function.[138] Severe constriction of the afferent arterioles, mediated by catecholamines, angiotensin, or renal sympathetic nerve activity, reduces glomerular filtration pressure directly, induces swelling of glomerular endothelium, and impairs the permeability of glomerular capillary endothelium. All of these processes may reduce glomerular filtration rate and interfere with renal function, even after renal blood flow has been restored.

The morphological changes in the kidney in shock are variable, ranging from no abnormalities to varying degrees of tubular necrosis with disrupted, necrotic, or regenerating tubular epithelium, intratubular casts, interstitial edema, and cellular infiltration. However, the renal histopathological changes often do not correlate closely with and are far less impressive than the functional changes.

The *oliguria of shock* may be a manifestation not only of an overall reduction of renal blood flow, but also of a diminished ratio of cortical to medullary perfusion.[139,140] This redistribution of intrarenal flow may depend, in part, on several vasoactive substances, including prostaglandins and angiotensin II. It is possible that specific prostaglandins modulate the vascular responses to adrenergic stimulation in the kidney both by inhibiting release of the neurotransmitter and by antagonizing its effect on the target tissue.[141]

In shock of any etiology glomerular filtration may be diminished disproportionately to cardiac output and to the reduction of renal blood flow.[142] Thus, in dogs subjected to hemorrhagic shock, renal blood flow may not be reduced in proportion to the decline in mean arterial pressure because of selective vasodilation of the efferent arterioles, which results in partial maintenance of renal blood flow due to decreased renal vascular resistance, but a diminution in the effective glomerular filtration pressure occurs.[143] The overall reduction of renal blood flow is less than the reduction in cardiac output in cardiogenic shock as well,[144] apparently, in part, because of renal vasodilatory reflexes initiated by stimulation of cardiac afferent nerve endings.

Other factors contributing to the oliguria of shock include profound stimulation of sodium and free water reabsorption mediated by the high circulating levels of aldosterone and ADH as well as enhanced back-diffusion through the tubules, whose function has been compromised by the direct effects of ischemia. After as little as 60 minutes of hypotension, edema within renal tubular cells leads to occlusion of tubular lumina, associated with mitochondrial damage that is detectable on electron microscopy.[145] Despite the potent effects of mineralocorticoids and ADH on the kidneys, urine osmolarity may decline relatively early during the evolution of shock. Decreased renal perfusion impairs the delivery of sodium and urea to the renal medulla, impairing maintenance of the hypertonic interstitial milieu responsible for removal of free water from urine in the collecting ducts and giving rise to an often reversible concentrating defect.[146]

In patients who recover from shock, hypertension and renal tubular insufficiency may supervene within 36 to 72 hours. This "post-resuscitative" syndrome has been thought to reflect acute hypervolemia due to mobilization of previously sequestered salt and water in the presence of impaired renal function.[147] When shock has been treated successfully, the development of acute renal failure may require dialysis. However, recovery of renal function is ultimately usually complete.

The Liver and Gastrointestinal Tract

Liver. Abnormalities of hepatic cell function and their clinical and laboratory manifestations accompany shock of prolonged duration. The histopathological picture can range from isolated zones of centrilobular necrosis to massive hepatic necrosis. Concomitant with these morphological manifestations, marked derangements of liver function are evident, manifested in part by markedly elevated plasma transaminase activity (SGOT and SGPT). Hypoxia appears to be the primary initiating factor. In addition to release of cytoplasmic and lysosomal enzymes in response to a prolonged period of impaired perfusion, inhibition of function of the reticuloendothelial (RE) cells is prominent. Impaired RE cell function appears to depend, in part, on a decline in circulating opsonin, an alpha$_2$-glycoprotein[84,148-151] that may contribute to the development of irreversible shock.[152]

Bowel. Hemorrhagic necrosis is the end result of ischemia of the gut, regardless of the underlying etiology of the shock. Ultrastructural alterations occur within 10 to 30 minutes after occlusion of the superior mesenteric artery in the dog and are first evident in the endoplasmic reticulum. Injury to the bowel may aggravate shock by several mechanisms, including sequestration of fluid in the gut lumen, and absorption of bacteria and a variety of toxins. When extensive submucosal hemorrhage occurs, remarkably large quantities of blood may be sequestered within the bowel itself, intensifying shock. Severe ischemia causes hyperperistalsis, followed by distention, impaired mobility, and, rarely, transmural infarction with perforation. Although recovery of intestinal function is usually prompt and complete in patients who survive an episode of shock, residual abnormalities of absorption may persist for several months after a severe episode of bowel ischemia, and strictures of the large bowel may develop after ischemic colitis. Among patients in whom shock is treated successfully, ultimate survival is usually not jeopardized by persistent or recurrent sequelae affecting the gastrointestinal tract.[153]

The Gastrointestinal Tract and Irreversibility The possibility that metabolites released from the ischemic gastrointestinal tract contribute to the evolution of irreversible shock has been suggested as a result of several lines of investigation. In addition to endotoxin (implicated in septic shock) and vasoactive substances such as histamine, lysosomal hydrolases and peptides capable of depressing the function of myocardium (myocardial depressant factor [MDF]) or the reticuloendothelial system in vitro (reticuloendothelial depressant substance [RDS]) have been implicated. MDF is alleged to be a small peptide that originates in ischemic pancreatic tissue by activation of lysosomal hydrolases in response to ischemia, is transported via lymphatics into the systemic circulation, and is capable of depressing contractility of papillary muscle preparations.[38] Blood-borne MDF activity appears to increase in parallel with impairment of cardiac performance in experimental models of cardiogenic as well as hemorrhagic shock.[154,155]

The Blood

Changes in Viscosity. Certain forms of shock, particularly those induced by thermal injury or sepsis, are associated with intravascular aggregation of erythrocytes, leukocytes, and platelets and with increased viscosity. These changes may contribute to the elevation of vascular resistance.[156,157] Increased blood viscosity has also been implicated in the late hepatic failure following burn or septic shock. Several strategies have been invoked to diminish the deleterious influence of aggregation and increased viscosity on microcirculatory hemodynamics, including administration of sufficient low molecular weight dextran or hydroxyethyl starch to produce modest hemodilution, avoidance of the use of large quantities of bank blood which becomes progressively prone to microaggregation with storage, and use of effective blood micropore filters.

Hemoglobin-O_2 Dissociation. Changes in blood-oxygen affinity do not play a major role in the pathogenesis of oligemic shock. Although the hemoglobin-oxygen dissociation curve is shifted slightly to the right[158] (providing delivery of more oxygen to the tissues at any given arterial oxygen tension), neither the shape of the curve nor the erythrocyte 2,3-DPG content changes markedly. Patients with cardiogenic shock exhibit elevations of P_{50} (the partial pressure of oxygen at 50 per cent saturation), indicating decreased affinity of hemoglobin for oxygen (Fig. 18–8).[159] Similar directional changes have been detected in patients with acute myocardial infarction without shock.[160] Although such shifts in the oxygen dissociation curve may be protective by enhancing delivery of oxygen to tissues, high values of P_{50} alone cannot enhance oxygen delivery when *arterial* hypoxemia is severe.

The Brain

Cerebral vascular resistance is controlled primarily by blood CO_2 tension, with increases causing vascular dilatation.[161] In addition, dim-

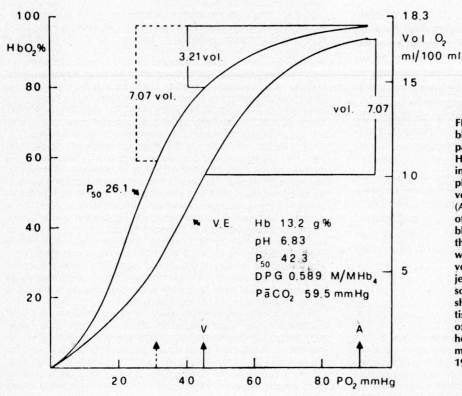

FIGURE 18–8 An oxygen dissociation curve of blood from a normal subject (left) and from a patient (V.E.) with cardiogenic shock (right). Hematological and metabolic parameters are indicated in the inset. DPG refers to diphosphoglycerate content of the red cells. The solid vertical arrows indicate the values of arterial (A) and venous (V) pO_2 required for extraction of 7.07 ml O_2/100 ml blood in the patient's blood. The dotted vertical arrow indicates the theoretical value of venous oxygen tension that would be required for extraction of the same volume of oxygen from blood of a normal subject. The change in position of the oxygen dissociation curve associated with cardiogenic shock may facilitate delivery of oxygen to the tissue. (From Agostoni, A., et al.: Hemoglobin oxygen affinity in patients with low-output heart failure and cardiogenic shock after acute myocardial infarction. Eur. J. Cardiol. *3*:53, 1975.)

inution of the arterial pO_2, common in many forms of shock, also causes cerebral dilation, thereby facilitating oxygenation of the brain. However, this is opposed by the constrictor influences resulting from the hypocapnia associated with hyperventilation.

Cerebral blood flow exhibits autoregulation (Fig. 26–38, p. 893), with flow varying only slightly with marked changes in systemic arterial pressure. However, when mean systemic pressure declines below approximately 60 mm Hg, a marked reduction in cerebral perfusion occurs.[162] As a consequence, cerebral perfusion is protected to a considerable extent when mean systemic arterial pressure remains above 60 mm Hg in the absence of intrinsic cerebrovascular disease. Although cerebral perfusion and therefore brain oxygen tension do not decline appreciably until mean arterial pressure is diminished profoundly, even modest reductions of cerebral perfusion are reflected by a shift toward reduction of cytochrome *c* oxidase, a sensitive reflection of perturbed intracellular metabolism.[163] The mechanisms accounting for cerebral autoregulation are incompletely understood. One factor appears to be the Bayliss effect, namely, contraction of vessels in response to increased pressure and relaxation in response to decreased pressure on the basis of intrinsic properties of vessel walls. Additional mechanisms include responses to regional alterations in CO_2 tension. Humoral factors may participate as well.[164] Clinically, it is clear that the central nervous system is remarkably well protected in shock; if recovery occurs, survival is rarely accompanied by neurologic defects unless an intercurrent cerebrovascular accident has occurred.

A SUMMARY OF MECHANISMS OF SHOCK

Compensatory mechanisms in response to volume depletion of 20 to 40 per cent and the consequent decline of systolic arterial pressure to approximately 70 mm Hg involve carotid and aortic baroreceptors, cardiopulmonary mechanoreceptors, afferent renal arterioles, the macula densa, and the target organs themselves, resulting in an integrated neurohumoral response. Massive sympathetic nerve stimulation to the vasculature and peripheral organs and augmentation of circulating levels of ACTH, glucocorticoids, renin, angiotensin II, ADH, aldosterone, prosta-

glandins, histamine, and catecholamines result. Vasoconstriction maintains systemic arterial pressure at the expense of diminution of blood flow and its normal distribution. A shift to anaerobic metabolism and intracellular acidosis occurs as ATP stores decline in the absence of adequate oxygenation. Acidosis further compromises energy supply in vital organs by inhibiting glycolysis and it may also contribute to irreversible cellular injury by activation of lysosomal enzymes. Systemic acidosis is exacerbated by renal functional impairment. The breakdown of permeability barriers in the gastrointestinal tract and lung leads to fluid sequestration, further reduction of effective vascular volume, interference with the function of these organs, and the release of vasodilator substances such as histamine and prostaglandins, which cannot be adequately metabolized or removed because of compromised hepatic parenchymal and reticuloendothelial cell function.

Release of thromboplastic substances into the circulation, coupled with the high concentration of circulating catecholamines, potentiates microaggregation of blood elements within the systemic and pulmonary circulations, and contributes to pulmonary venous and arterial vasoconstriction and impaired alveolar ventilation, diminished lung compliance, and increased work of breathing, thereby intensifying systemic hypoxia. Coronary perfusion is limited by the decreased perfusion pressure, alpha-adrenergic stimulation, and massive increases in circulating angiotensin II. Derangements in acid-base, electrolyte, metabolic, and neurohumoral factors may precipitate arrhythmias, further compromising cardiac function. When myocardial oxygen requirements cannot be met, ventricular compliance and contractility decrease, cardiac output declines further, and coronary perfusion is diminished because of decreased cardiac output and increased cardiac interstitial pressure due to myocardial cell swelling and edema.

TREATMENT OF SHOCK

GENERAL PRINCIPLES

The therapy of shock can be divided into three categories: *primary therapy*, which is directed toward the presumed initiating cause of the syndrome (such as hemorrhage, myocardial infarction, septicemia) (Table 18–1); *secondary therapy*, which consists of the restoration of impaired hemodynamics and perfusion; and *tertiary therapy*, which consists of the prevention and treatment of complications of shock, such as ARDS (p. 573) and acute renal failure (p. 587).

Selection of *primary therapy* is usually straightforward. For example, primary therapy of cardiogenic shock utilizes approaches designed to protect ischemic myocardium and improve myocardial perfusion in an effort to restore the compromised functional capacity of the heart (Chap. 38). Primary therapy of shock due to obstruction of flow, such as pericardial tamponade, is directed toward relieving the compressive force of the pericardial effusion or constricting tissue (Chap. 43). Oligemic shock requires repletion of vascular volume with fluid selected to conform to the nature of the fluid lost. Septicemic shock requires aggressive treatment of infection. Shock initiated by metabolic factors or

drugs requires correction of the insult or removal of the agent.

Secondary therapy requires prompt characterization of the hemodynamic pattern. Intraarterial pressure should be measured directly, since marked vasoconstriction can result in spuriously low estimates of arterial pressure based on indirect measurements obtained using a blood pressure cuff. Although detailed objective characterization of hemodynamic, respiratory, and metabolic parameters is useful and readily attainable by monitoring the patient as therapy is being implemented, initial selection of secondary therapy depends on prompt clinical assessment of salient features of the circulation, including (1) vascular volume, which must include a consideration of both total blood volume and plasma volume; (2) right ventricular filling pressure, generally reflected by central (systemic) venous pressure; (3) left ventricular filling pressure; and (4) total peripheral resistance.

Vascular Volume. When vascular volume is depleted, postural hypotension and sinus tachycardia usually occur. Tachycardia may be absent in some older individuals or patients with heart disease. Filling pressures of the left and right ventricles are generally low, as is systemic venous

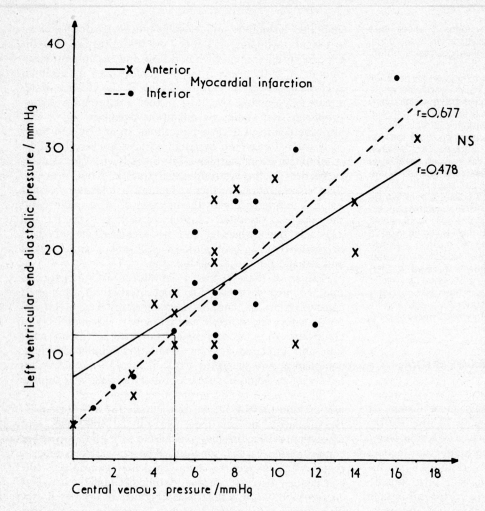

FIGURE 18–9 Comparisons of left ventricular end-diastolic pressure and central venous pressure in patients with anterior and inferior transmural myocardial infarction. The inset indicates the upper limit of normal of values for each of these parameters. The relationship between the two values is not close, and the correlation coefficients (least-squares linear regression) are low. Although there is no statistically significant difference (NS) between the regression lines obtained from patients with inferior compared to anterior myocardial infarction, the elevation of central venous pressure tended to be somewhat higher than the elevation of left ventricular end-diastolic pressure in patients with inferior compared to anterior infarction, probably because of more extensive involvement of the right ventricle. (From Bleifeld, W., et al.: Acute myocardial infarction. V. Left and right ventricular haemodynamics in cardiogenic shock. Br. Heart J. *36*:822, 1974.)

pressure. Cardiomegaly is uncommon, and pulmonary rales and edema are absent. Unfortunately, *central venous pressure is not a good index of blood volume.* Central venous pressure may not decline despite severe oligemia because of widespread venoconstriction, impaired right ventricular function, or transmission of increased intrathoracic pressure associated with mechanical ventilatory support.[165] In patients with heart disease, central venous pressure provides relatively little insight into the adequacy of left ventricular filling and is not a generally reliable criterion when adjustments in intravenous fluid or pharmacological therapy are to be made (Fig. 18–9). With depletion of vascular volume, the pulmonary artery occlusive pressure—an index of mean left atrial pressure, which, in the absence of mitral valve disease, reflects left ventricular diastolic pressure—is generally low. If the cause of shock is blood loss, hemodilution becomes evident after several hours, although initially the hematocrit is normal. If hypovolemia results primarily from loss of plasma (e.g., in pancreatitis, burn, or uncontrolled diabetes mellitus with protracted osmotic diuresis and ketoacidosis), hemoconcentration will be evident.

Right Ventricular Filling Pressure. Elevation of right ventricular filling pressure is characteristic of shock due to cor pulmonale or acute pulmonary embolism (Chap. 46), right ventricular infarction (Chap. 37), or cardiac tamponade (Chap. 43).

Left Ventricular Filling Pressure. Markedly augmented left ventricular filling pressure is characteristic of cardi-

ogenic shock and is associated with cardiomegaly and signs and symptoms of pulmonary edema. When cardiogenic shock is initially suspected but features of elevated left ventricular filling pressure are absent, relative or absolute hypovolemia may be responsible.

Peripheral Resistance. Elevation of total peripheral resistance is accompanied by signs of excessive sympathetic activity such as cold, pale, clammy skin, diaphoresis, tachycardia, and oliguria. Although this constellation of signs is typical of shock of many etiologies, it must be emphasized that septicemic, neuropathic, and metabolic forms of shock are often associated with vasodilatation and decreased total peripheral resistance ("warm shock").

Management of the patient in shock requires objective monitoring of intraarterial pressure; right atrial, pulmonary artery, and pulmonary arterial occlusive pressures; and cardiac output. Many of these measurements are facilitated by the use of a Swan-Ganz thermodilution catheter. Other important measurements include arterial pH; hematocrit, platelets, and other coagulation parameters; serum sodium, potassium, bicarbonate, chloride, albumin, calcium, creatinine, urea nitrogen, glucose, lactate, and pyruvate; urine output, osmolality and sodium, potassium, creatinine, and urea concentrations.[166–168] Continuous electrocardiographic monitoring is required for the detection of arrhythmias. Since mechanical ventilatory assistance or support is so often essential, monitoring should include assessment of the arterial pO_2, alveolar-arterial O_2 gradient, mixed venous oxygen tension (a useful adjunct for prevention of oxygen toxicity resulting from unnecessarily high fractions of oxygen in the inspired air), the adequacy of ventilation based on arterial pCO_2, and ventilatory efficiency from analysis of the ratio of dead-space volume to tidal volume, readily calculated from the alveolar gas equation.

Because the lung is so often involved in shock (p. 583) and because vigorous, early treatment of ARDS is essential, several principles must be kept in mind. These include (1) provision of sufficient colloid to maintain vascular volume but avoidance of excessive crystalloid or colloid infusions in order to minimize extravasation into the lung, with fluid management guided by monitoring pulmonary artery wedge pressure and, if possible, colloid osmotic pressure; (2) prevention of atelectasis by appropriate use of mechanical ventilatory support, with intermittent hyperinflation of the lungs and meticulous attention to removal of secretions; (3) maintenance of oxygenation with an inspired oxygen concentration sufficiently high to maintain arterial pO_2 in the range of 60 to 70 mm Hg but in any case less than 60 per cent, since maintained higher concentrations may produce oxygen toxicity; and (4) use of positive end-expiratory pressure to improve oxygenation.

SPECIFIC SHOCK SYNDROMES

CARDIOGENIC SHOCK

Cardiogenic shock may be defined as severe circulatory failure due to a primary defect in the pumping function of the heart (Table 18–1). Cardiogenic shock includes shock that (1) accompanies acute myocardial infarction, the most common form; (2) is secondary to acute impairment of myocardial function as a consequence of a chronic, progressive cardiomyopathy, such as end-stage congestive or ischemic cardiomyopathy or myocarditis; and (3) is due to mechanical factors in which the initiating cause may be sudden obstruction to flow or regurgitation. Examples of this category include cardiac tamponade (p. 1480) and rupture of the interventricular septum, or papillary muscle, in which case the contractile function of the uninvolved myocardium may be preserved initially, but the pumping ability of the heart is greatly compromised, and in which early surgical intervention may be lifesaving.[169] Other rare mechanical factors include intracardiac obstruction to blood flow by an atrial thrombus or myxoma.

Most commonly, cardiogenic shock results from impaired left ventricular function due to myocardial infarction secondary to underlying coronary artery disease. A closely related syndrome of acute pump failure occurs after cardiopulmonary bypass, particularly when extensive coronary artery disease is present. However, under these conditions, the impaired ventricular function is often transitory, presumably because it is not necessarily associated with extensive necrosis. Patients with post–cardiac surgery cardiogenic shock often respond well to temporary circulatory support with intraaortic balloon counterpulsation and positive inotropic agents. Alternatively, shock may result from profound right ventricular dysfunction secondary to right ventricular infarction.[170-175] Recognition of this entity is essential because it is often amenable to successful treatment, incorporating expansion of vascular volume and pharmacological stimulation of cardiac contractility. Right ventricular infarction can be distinguished from acute cor pulmonale accompanying massive pulmonary embolism by the low pulmonary artery pressure with right ventricular infarction, and from pericardial tamponade by the disproportionate elevation of right-sided diastolic pressures with right ventricular infarction in contrast to the four-chamber diastolic pressure elevation typical of tamponade (p. 1480).

Brady- or tachyarrhythmias are rarely of sufficient severity to compromise cardiac performance so as to cause cardiogenic shock in a patient with an otherwise normal heart. However, when concomitant diffuse coronary atherosclerosis, cardiomyopathy, or valvular lesions interfere with ventricular filling or outflow, ventricular performance may be profoundly compromised by almost any arrhythmia. Supraventricular or ventricular tachycardias may impair ventricular filling because of the limited time available for flow across the atrioventricular valves. Tachycardias augment myocardial oxygen requirements and, under conditions in which oxygen supply is limited, may cause myocardial ischemia and thereby interfere with cardiac function. Ventricular arrhythmias may impair ventricular function by inducing asynchronous contraction. Since stroke volume cannot increase in many forms of heart disease, cardiac output may decline precipitously in the presence of bradycardia. Any arrhythmia that interferes with the normal sequence of atrial and ventricular contraction may significantly diminish cardiac output in patients with compromised cardiac function, since ventricular performance is dependent on appropriate atrial transport of blood into the ventricle at the end of diastole and the consequent augmentation of preload (p. 433). Therefore, in patients with massive myocardial infarction who are in borderline compensation, it is not uncommon to observe a precipitous decline in cardiac output and the development of cardiogenic shock, even though the ventricular rate remains almost constant when the mechanism changes transiently from sinus to accelerated idioventricular rhythm. (p. 1286).

Cardiogenic shock associated with coronary artery disease generally reflects primarily impairment of left ventricular function. On the other hand, the responsible lesion may be a right ventricular infarct, in which case the hemodynamic picture is dominated by manifestations of right ventricular dysfunction.

Cardiogenic shock accompanying a large acute infarction of the left ventricle is the prototype of this form of shock. Indeed, when the term "cardiogenic shock" is used without qualification, it generally refers to shock of this type. Most patients with cardiogenic shock accompanying myocardial infarction exhibit three-vessel coronary disease with extensive involvement of the left anterior descending coronary artery,[176] and the underlying infarction usually involves large portions of the left ventricle.[123,124] In fact, the magnitude of hemodynamic impairment appears to be directly related to the amount of myocardium involved, with shock likely when the cumulative volume of infarcted tissue constitutes 40 per cent or more of the left ventricle. It is not yet clear whether the specific location of involved ventricular myocardium (i.e., anterior wall, diaphragmatic wall, apex, septum, etc.) is a significant determinant of the presence or absence of shock, unless specialized regions such as the conduction system or valvular supporting apparatus are involved.[204]

CLINICAL FEATURES. Cardiogenic shock accompanies myocardial infarction in 10 to 15 per cent of patients who survive sufficiently long to reach the hospital.[8,167,176,177] The primary defect is severe impairment of left ventricular contractile function with resultant circulatory failure. The patient is generally restless and confused but may be stuporous, with cool, moist skin reflecting reflex sympathetic reduction of cutaneous perfusion and stimulation of diaphoresis. Core temperature may be reduced, peripheral pulses are generally rapid and thready, arterial pressure is reduced, and pulse pressure is narrow. Early in the course, pressure may not be reduced despite profound impairment of perfusion of vital organs. Diminished urine output is characteristic, and persistent or recurrent chest pain is common.

Disturbances of cardiac rhythm of almost any type, including sinus tachycardia, ventricular tachyarrhythmias and premature complexes, sinus bradycardia, atrioventricular block, and supraventricular tachycardias, are common. In the absence of hypovolemia, the clinical features of acute pulmonary edema may be present (chap. 17) with bronchospasm, suffocating dyspnea, copious pulmonary secretions, and profound cyanosis. Rapid shallow respirations are typical, but Cheyne-Stokes respiration may supervene, especially when patients are treated aggressively with narcotics or when there is concomitant cerebrovascular disease. If right ventricular failure occurs, either consequent to pulmonary hypertension, secondary to left ventricular failure or primarily as a result of right ventricular infarction, systemic venous distention may be evident rather than the virtual absence of visible peripheral veins due to venoconstriction.

Cardiac signs include diminished intensity of heart sounds, reflecting greatly reduced contractility, the other auscultatory manifestations of acute myocardial infarction, pericarditis, papillary muscle dysfunction, or left or right ventricular failure. Cardiomegaly is common, but if there is concomitant hypovolemia, as may result from excessive prolonged diaphoresis, vomiting, or prior treatment with diuretics, the heart may not be enlarged. Laboratory findings include those associated with myocardial infarction, congestive heart failure, and shock. Thus, metabolic (often lactic) acidosis, hypocapnia and hypoxemia, hypo- or hyperkalemia and azotemia, markedly elevated activity of plasma enzymes, leukocytosis, and numerous nonspecific laboratory manifestations of massive neurohumoral stimulation and progressive organ injury are prevalent.

HEMODYNAMICS. Because impaired myocardial contractility secondary to loss of contractile mass is the primary defect responsible for the syndrome of cardiogenic shock secondary to acute myocardial infarction, cardiac output is invariably low, even when ventricular filling pressure is increased by intravenous administration of colloid. The elevation of left ventricular filling pressure[167,168] is usually in excess of that expected from the only modest increase in left ventricular end-diastolic volume because of reduction in left ventricular compliance.[179,180] In the presence of associated hypovolemia, left ventricular preload may not be adequate despite normal or even modestly elevated left ventricular end-diastolic pressure because of diminished ventricular compliance, and it may be necessary to augment ventricular filling pressure substantially above normal with the use of intravenous infusion of colloid to improve cardiac output, by taking maximum advantage of the Frank-Starling mechanism.[167,180,181]

The presence of reduced cardiac output, associated with systemic hypotension, in the face of an elevated left ventricular filling pressure, is the hallmark of cardiogenic shock. Since left ventricular filling pressure is often estimated from pulmonary artery occlusive pressure (an index of left atrial pressure), mitral regurgitation or impairment of left ventricular filling by mitral stenosis, thrombus, or tumor must be excluded to establish that the left ventricular diastolic pressure is truly elevated. The low cardiac output is associated with depressions of stroke volume, left ventricular work and isovolumetric and ejection phase indices of contractility. The elevation of pulmonary artery resistance and pressure, augmented by hypoxemia and acidosis, contribute to the development of right ventricular failure.[182]

On the other hand, right ventricular failure may also result from right ventricular infarction in the absence of marked elevation of pulmonary artery pressure. Regardless of its cause, right ventricular failure is accompanied by elevation of right atrial and central venous pressures; right ventricular failure may be complicated by tricuspid regurgitation, due either to dilatation of the tricuspid annulus or to ischemia or infarction of right ventricular papillary muscles. In the absence of right ventricular failure and despite profound cardiogenic shock, central venous pressure may be normal or only slightly elevated, and accordingly, monitoring of this parameter may be a misleading guide to therapy (Fig. 18–8).

The neurohumoral response to severe left ventricular failure usually includes an elevated systemic vascular resistance, although not all patients with cardiogenic shock exhibit peripheral vasoconstriction.[183–185] Thus, the typical hemodynamic picture of cardiogenic shock includes systolic arterial pressure less than 80 mm Hg, diastolic pressure less than 50 mm Hg, mean arterial pressure less than 60 mm Hg, mean central venous pressure greater than 9 mm Hg; pulmonary artery occlusive pressure greater than 18 mm Hg; heart rate greater than 95 beats/min; cardiac index less than 1.8 l/min/m²; and total peripheral resistance greater than 2000 dyne-sec-cm⁻⁵.

Pulmonary complications of cardiogenic shock are common because the same factors that affect the lung in shock of any etiology exist in this condition (p. 583) but are intensified by the pulmonary venous hypertension characteristic of cardiogenic shock. Impairment of pulmonary function exaggerates arterial hypoxemia, thereby exacerbating the functional deterioration of the heart (p. 438). The increased work of breathing in cardiogenic shock diverts an inappropriate fraction of the cardiac output to the respiratory muscles, further impairing perfusion of other beds (Fig. 54–10, p. 1789).

A variety of pharmacological agents commonly used in the treatment of patients with acute myocardial infarction exert negative inotropic effects, particularly antiarrhythmic, beta-adrenergic blocking, and central nervous system depressant agents, and the use of these drugs may contribute to the impairment of cardiac output. Tolerance of ischemic myocardium to cardiac glycosides is decreased,[186] and the vasoconstrictor actions of these compounds may influence the coronary bed itself.[187] Occult hypovolemia or unrecognized vasovagal reactions superimposed on the underlying cardiogenic process may intensify the shock and limit the efficacy of therapy directed against the primary disorder.

MANAGEMENT
(See also Chapter 38, pp. 1316 to 1318)

Primary Therapy. When cardiogenic shock is due to a mechanical defect, such as rupture of the interventricular septum, acute mitral regurgitation due to papillary muscle rupture or dysfunction, or ventricular aneurysm, primary therapy consists of surgical correction of the lesion. Unfortunately, emergency surgery is plagued by technical difficulties related to repair of tissue undergoing active necrosis, and results have been somewhat disappointing. If systemic hemodynamics can be stabilized by means of medical management or appropriate use of intraaortic balloon counterpulsation (IABP) for one week or longer, surgical results are generally more favorable.[169,188,189] In present practice, the balloon is inserted percutaneously or via an arterial cutdown into the thoracic aorta via the femoral artery. Phased pulsations synchronized with the electrocar-

diogram are utilized to commence inflation at the time of closure of the aortic valve and to initiate deflation just prior to the onset of systole. The augmented coronary perfusion pressure during diastole facilitates coronary blood flow, since coronary vascular resistance is minimal during this portion of the cardiac cycle (Fig. 18–10). Since the balloon is deflated throughout systole, the left ventricle ejects against a lower impedance. Hemodynamic changes generally include a 10 to 20 per cent increase in cardiac output, a reduction in systolic and increase in diastolic arterial pressure with little change in mean pressure, a diminution of heart rate, and an increase in urine output.[190–196]

Serious complications of IABP are infrequent but include damage to or perforation of the aortic wall, ischemia distal to the site of insertion of the balloon in the femoral artery, thrombocytopenia hemolysis, renal emboli, and mechanical failures such as rupture of the balloon.[197] Although left ventricular rupture has been observed in as many as 7 per cent of patients,[196] this phenomenon appears to be a manifestation of the underlying extensive transmural infarction rather than a complication of IABP itself. Use of echocardiography to evaluate the dimensions of the aorta and location and function of the balloon may help to minimize some of these complications.[198] Contraindications to IABP include aortic regurgitation and aortic aneurysm; tachyarrhythmias or irregular rhythms are relative contraindications and must be controlled for effective functioning of the device.

Unfortunately, IABP often fails to stabilize the hemodynamic status of patients with cardiogenic shock secondary to mechanical lesions, such as ventricular septal defect or mitral regurgitation, long enough to defer surgical intervention for even a few days.[190] Under these circumstances, surgery should not be deferred. In cases of emergency surgery for mechanical causes of cardiogenic shock, patient

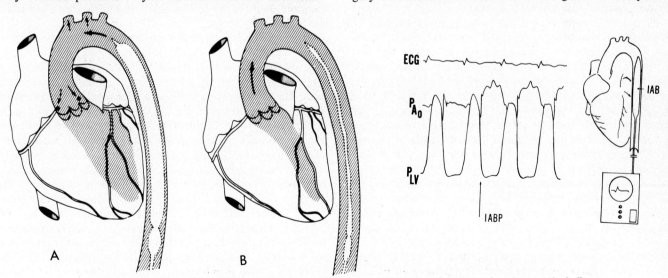

FIGURE 18–10 The relationship between the cardiac cycle and balloon inflation when intraaortic balloon counterpulsation is being utilized. During diastole (panel A) the balloon is inflated, augmenting the prevailing pressure in the proximal aorta and hence coronary arterial perfusion pressure. During systole (panel B) the left ventricular chamber dimension decreases with antegrade ejection of blood into the proximal aorta. During this portion of the cardiac cycle the balloon is deflated, facilitating ejection of blood into the periphery where systemic arterial resistance vessels are dilated maximally because of the preceding inhibition of perfusion by the inflated balloon during diastole. As shown in the inset on the right, utilization of intraaortic balloon counterpulsation (IABP) results in augmentation of diastolic arterial blood pressure (P_{Ao}) with a modest reduction in systolic left ventricular pressure (P_{LV}). (From Bolooki, H.: Clinical Application of Intra-aortic Balloon Pump. New York, Futura Publishing Co., 1977.)

survival may exceed 40 per cent,[191-193] far better than the almost uniformly dismal outlook for such patients without surgical intervention.[190,194] Even in patients whose hemodynamic status is stabilized by IABP, surgical treatment should be undertaken promptly to avoid the development of complications such as renal failure, ARDS, or infection. IABP, while useful as a "holding maneuver," does not constitute adequate therapy. In patients with cardiogenic shock and mechanical lesions, surgery may be deferred in the rare instance when weaning from IABP is possible within 12 to 24 hours and if hemodynamic stability is then maintained without the mechanical support. IABP also permits additional diagnostic studies, such as coronary angiography and ventriculography, to be performed with considerable safety in patients with cardiogenic shock.[195-200] Although survival is better in patients operated upon relatively late, i.e., more than two weeks after the development of the mechanical lesion, this may be related to patient selection; patients who are more gravely ill simply do not survive that long.

Results in patients with cardiogenic shock without mechanical lesions demonstrate conclusively that hemodynamic improvement can be achieved with IABP. Unfortunately, the large majority of such patients soon become balloon-dependent. However, IABP does permit support of the circulation, so that patients can be studied intensively in relative safety, and in some cases it makes possible detection and then surgical correction of mechanical lesions that would otherwise have been impossible.[200,201] Another mechanical approach employed recently to support the circulation in patients with cardiogenic shock is ventricular-assist pumping. This modality is particularly promising for patients undergoing open heart surgical procedures who develop post–cardiac surgery cardiogenic shock and who cannot otherwise be weaned successfully from cardiopulmonary bypass[202] (Fig. 16–24, p. 548).

From a theoretical point of view, primary therapy of cardiogenic shock due to impaired contractility of the left ventricle should include improvement of oxygen delivery to the heart; reduction of myocardial oxygen requirements; facilitation of removal of metabolites accumulating in the myocardium; protection of ischemic, reversibly injured myocardium; and support of the circulation during an interval sufficiently long to permit development of coronary collaterals to sustain jeopardized but still viable myocardium. Despite some promising results in studies in experimental animals, it is not yet clear whether any pharmacological or metabolic regimen implemented after the onset of shock in patients will accomplish these goals. However, very early (less than 4 hours) reperfusion, either surgically or by direct infusion of a thrombolytic agent into the occluded coronary artery, may result in survival of a number of patients with cardiogenic shock. However, the appropriate comparisons have not yet been made with appropriate control groups. Other than the above-mentioned anecdotal reports, the mortality associated with cardiogenic shock approaches 100 per cent when criteria for the diagnosis are rigorous.[6,8,203,204]

Secondary Therapy. Despite the lack of proof that pharmacological protection of ischemic myocardium, untilizing approaches considered in detail in Chapter 38, will reduce mortality associated with cardiogenic shock, it is sensible to predicate therapy in part on approaches designed to preserve jeopardized myocardium. General support for the patient with cardiogenic shock is vital. Relief of pain with adequate doses of morphine may reduce unrecognized vasovagal contributions to circulatory impairment, diminish profuse diaphoresis and the associated fluid loss that can complicate management, and reduce adrenergic stimulation of the heart, thereby diminishing tachyarrhythmias and potentially harmful excess metabolic requirements.

Rarely, cardiogenic shock may be complicated by a significant component of excess vagal tone, usually manifested by sinus bradycardia and other bradyarrhythmias accompanying the profound hypotension and common during the earliest phases of myocardial infarction. Atropine may be particularly helpful in reversing hemodynamic abnormalities under these circumstances.[205] Other general measures are helpful, including reduction of fever, treatment of nausea and vomiting, administration of oxygen and ventilatory assistance if hypoxemia persists, prompt treatment of arrhythmias, treatment of bronchospasm with aminophylline, and correction of electrolyte and acid-base abnormalities.

The principles underlying the medical management of cardiogenic shock include (1) maximization of ventricular performance by adjustment of left ventricular filling pressure to provide an optimal preload; (2) modification of peripheral vascular resistance to optimize impedance to left ventricular ejection; (3) stimulation of contractility, qualified by the proviso that augmentation of oxygen requirements in jeopardized ischemic tissue may be deleterious; (4) vigorous treatment of brady- and tachyarrhythmias; (5) maintenance of the physiological sequential relationship between atrial and ventricular contraction to facilitate atrial transport and the maintenance of ventricular filling pressure; and (6) control of heart rate to facilitate ventricular filling.

Since preload is an important determinant of ventricular performance (p. 433), blood volume should be adjusted so as to optimize cardiac output without causing pulmonary edema. Because of the diminished compliance of the left ventricle in myocardial ischemia, the ideal filling pressure is generally higher than the upper limit of normal and is in the range of 18 to 22 mm Hg. The use of a fluid challenge by means of graded administration of low molecular weight dextran in 50-ml increments with serial assessment of pulmonary artery occlusive pressure and cardiac output is helpful,[180] especially when hypovolemia is suspected.[167] In some patients whose left ventricular filling pressures are near the upper limits of normal (12 mm Hg), expansion of blood volume to achieve an increase in occlusive pressure to approximately 20 mm Hg will be sufficient to raise cardiac output and arterial pressure and thereby abolish shock. On the other hand, when left ventricular filling pressure exceeds 20 mm Hg and/or when pulmonary edema is present, diuresis with intravenous furosemide or ethacrynic acid should be carried out. Furosemide may reduce pulmonary capillary pressure well before it induces diuresis because of its effects on reducing venous capacitance[243] and ventricular afterload[206] (p. 527). Not only will this maneuver diminish pulmonary edema, but since it reduces ventricular dimensions, it also lowers left ventricular wall tension, a principal determinant of myocardial oxygen consumption.

If systolic arterial blood pressure remains depressed, signs of poor peripheral perfusion do not resolve, and total peripheral resistance and left ventricular filling pressure remain markedly elevated, increasing cardiac output by stimulating myocardial contractility with agents such as dopamine or dobutamine may be helpful. *Dopamine* (p. 542) may improve cardiac output by increasing contractility.[206a] At low doses (less than 2 to 5 μg/kg/min), its vasodilatory effect on the renal and other vascular beds may modestly augment renal perfusion and decrease total peripheral resistance. At doses of 5 to 8 μg/kg/min, its positive inotropic effects on beta-1 receptors in the myocardium becomes dominant and at doses in excess of 8 μg/kg/min, it exerts a vasoconstrictor effect by stimulating alpha-adrenergic receptors. Despite its relatively modest positive chronotropic effect, infusion of dopamine must be titrated carefully to avoid precipitating ventricular arrhythmias or severe peripheral vasoconstriction, which occurs at high doses (greater than 20 μg/kg/min). Cardiac output and renal blood flow may be enhanced by the combined use of an alpha-adrenergic blocking agent such as phentolamine to counteract the vasoconstriction induced by dopamine alone.[207] Despite the absence of definitive effects on long-term survival, dopamine, alone or in combination with prazosin (an alpha-adrenergic receptor antagonist) or salbutamol (a beta₂-agonist, currently investigational in the United States), has improved hemodynamics and short-term survival.[209–212]

Dobutamine, another catecholamine congener, acts on beta₁-, beta₂-, and alpha-adrenergic receptors, although its beta₂-agonist and alpha- actions are markedly less than those of isoproterenol or norepinephrine, respectively. Its potential advantage compared to dopamine is its consistent *reduction* of systemic vascular resistance.[213] Isoproterenol has also been used to treat cardiogenic shock because of its positive inotropic effects. However, tachycardia, arrhythmia, increased myocardial oxygen requirements, excessive peripheral vasodilatation, and precipitous declines in systemic arterial pressure are major disadvantages. Its use should probably be discontinued or, at most, reserved for rare circumstances in which peripheral vasoconstriction is extreme and accompanied by bradycardia.

It is tempting, on theoretical grounds and on the basis of studies in patients without shock,[214] to utilize vasodilator agents to diminish impedance to left ventricular ejection and to reduce myocardial oxygen requirements. However, therapy with vasodilators alone or even in combination with other agents such as salbutamol[215] or modalities such as intraaortic balloon counterpulsation in patients with cardiogenic shock is potentially hazardous and has not yet proven to be helpful. Peripheral perfusion may increase in some organ beds, and under some circumstances so may cardiac output, but the decline of peripheral resistance in a setting of profound systemic hypotension may decrease systemic diastolic perfusion pressure and hence coronary perfusion pressure. Since left ventricular filling pressure usually must be maintained in the range of 20 mm Hg to optimize cardiac output, any further decline in systemic arterial diastolic pressure produced by a vasodilator will not be offset by a decrease in diastolic tension

within the ventricular wall, and hence the net driving pressure supporting coronary perfusion diminishes, potentially exacerbating myocardial ischemia.

For many years alpha-adrenergic agonists provided the sole pharmacological approach to the treatment of cardiogenic shock. Use of these drugs was predicated on the concept (now recognized to be overly simplistic) that peripheral vascular resistance and arterial pressure should be augmented. Such a view neglects the primacy of the need for enhancement of *perfusion* rather than of arterial *pressure*. Agonists with both alpha- and beta-receptor actions, such as norepinephrine, then became the mainstay of treatment, because their combined effects on the heart and peripheral vascular resistance may raise arterial pressure when the circulatory system is responsive to no other drug. Metaraminol, by virtue of its direct alpha-agonistic and indirect beta-agonistic properties, mediated by local catecholamine release, has also been utilized widely. However, it has now become clear that these agents not only fail to improve overall mortality associated with cardiogenic shock but may actually exert substantial deleterious effects on the heart.[177] Although some increase in cardiac output and systemic arterial pressure can be achieved with agents such as norepinephrine, the lowest effective doses necessary should be used to avoid additional damage to the heart secondary to greater ischemia and afterload.[220]

In addition to beta-adrenergic agonists, other agents with positive inotropic effects—particularly digitalis glycosides—have been utilized. Although the beneficial effects of digitalis on ventricular performance in congestive heart failure are unequivocal (p. 513), and the net effects of digitalis on ischemic myocardium are protective in the presence of heart failure,[217] the relative inefficacy of digitalis in the setting of cardiogenic shock may be explained on both theoretical and empirical grounds. Tolerance to the drug under these circumstances is diminished, and its propensity to produce arrhythmia is accentuated.[186,218] The peripheral and coronary vasoconstrictor actions of intravenous glycosides may be deleterious in that they elevate arterial pressure (afterload) and reduce coronary blood flow. Alterations in pH and electrolyte status reduce the toxic/therapeutic ratio. Perhaps most important, the primary defect in cardiogenic shock is impaired cardiac contractility due to limited coronary perfusion and therefore impaired delivery of oxygen and substrate, so that the efficacy of glycosides for improving cardiac function may be severely limited. Uncontrolled or recurrent supraventricular tachyarrhythmias unresponsive to vagotonic maneuvers are the principal indication for use of parenteral digitalis glycosides in patients with cardiogenic shock. Digitalis may exert some beneficial effect on ventricular performance in cardiogenic shock even when these specific indications are absent, but a favorable effect on the overall course of the syndrome is unproven. Accordingly, doses should be modest to avoid inducing serious toxic effects when major benefits cannot be anticipated.

SHOCK DUE TO LEFT VENTRICULAR OUTFLOW TRACT OBSTRUCTION

Profound reduction of left ventricular output causing cardiogenic shock may be due to anatomical obstruction of the aortic outflow tract at the supra-, infra-, or aortic valvular levels. Lesions include supravalvular aortic stenosis (Chaps. 29 and 30), congenital or acquired valvular aortic stenosis (Chap. 32), or hypertrophic obstructive cardiomyopathy (Chap. 41). Any of these lesions, when sufficiently severe, may produce chronic heart failure, but if this is not treated surgically, cardiac output may continue to decline to levels that ultimately result in cardiogenic shock. At this juncture, surgical correction, while long overdue, may still be the only life-saving therapy. It is important to be aware that left ventricular outflow obstruction due to hypertrophic obstructive cardiomyopathy may be exacerbated by agents with positive inotropic effects, particularly beta-adrenergic agonists. Thus, these drugs may exaggerate the hemodynamic disturbance and should be avoided (p. 1418). Similarly, agents such as nitrates, which cause venous pooling of blood and hence diminished ventricular volume, may intensify the obstruction associated with hypertrophic cardiomyopathy and contribute to hemodynamic deterioration. Administration of calcium antagonists such as verapamil in doses of 80 to 120 mg orally at 6-hour intervals may improve ventricular performance by diminishing systolic dynamic obstruction, increasing diastolic compliance, or both[229] (p. 1420). Vasodilator agents are contraindicated in patients with shock due to obstruction to left ventricular outflow.[264]

OTHER TYPES OF OBSTRUCTIVE SHOCK. A variety of other conditions can impair outflow from the heart and cause systemic hypoperfusion and hypotension. One category comprises lesions affecting left ventricular inflow, including critical, far-advanced mitral stenosis (p. 1064); "ball-valve" thrombus that occludes flow through the mitral valve; and left atrial myxoma, which can produce the same hemodynamic abnormalities. Although ball-valve thrombi and myxomas generally give rise to intermittent circulatory insufficiency with syncope, transitory pulmonary venous hypertension, and/or postural hypotension, propagation of the thrombus with persistent occlusion of the atrioventricular orifice or persistent occlusion due to myxoma can also lead to shock (Chap. 42).

Pericardial tamponade is a prime example of obstructive shock and is discussed on page 1480.

HEMORRHAGIC SHOCK

PRIMARY THERAPY. Rapid loss of 30 per cent or more of the blood volume generally produces oligemic shock. Although this form of shock is accompanied by hemodilution, reexpansion of the plasma volume evolves slowly, with effects on the hematocrit often not evident for 3 to 6 hours. Additional blood loss must be halted as soon as hemodynamics have been stabilized by rapid repletion of vascular volume, preferably with type-specific whole blood or washed red blood cells and frozen plasma, but if necessary with colloid and crystalloid solutions. If volume repletion is initiated after more than a short interval following the onset of shock, administration of blood substantially in excess of the amount lost may be required.[12] When more than 2 liters is required, fresh blood is desirable to avoid thrombocytopenia and dilution of clotting factors. Although crystalloids such as normal saline or Ringer's lactate solution can be utilized initially, adequate amounts of colloid to maintain vascular volume should be included. Despite its availability, plasma is not necessarily the colloid of choice because of the risk of hepatitis. Albumin is useful, but the half-life of intravenously administered purified albumin is short. Dextran may interfere with coagulation or with blood-typing because of nonspecific agglutination of red cells and may induce a hypersensitivity reaction. Plasma expanders such as hydroxyethyl starch may not have these disadvantages.[221]

SECONDARY THERAPY. The hemodynamic picture that accompanies hemorrhagic shock is dominated by the direct consequences of a diminished blood volume (decreased cardiac output and systemic arterial pressure) and the sympathoadrenal response manifested by tachycardia, cutaneous vasoconstriction, venoconstriction, and redistribution of organ blood flow in relation to regional sympathetic tone. Capillary filtration may be enhanced because of the increased venous tone, and accordingly alpha-adrenergic blockade may be useful in association with expansion of vascular volume.[222] However, adequate and prompt repletion of vascular volume is usually sufficient without this adjunct.

If the hemodynamic derangements induced by hemorrhagic shock are not corrected promptly, impaired cardiac function may result and may subsequently contribute to the reduced cardiac output apparently on the basis of damage sustained as a consequence of myocardial ischemia[58,223] (Fig. 18–3). Although administration of large quantities of bank blood might depress cardiac contractility by chelating free calcium in the plasma with citrate, other manifestations of hypocalcemia, such as tetany, are usually evident first. Nevertheless, in rare circumstances, administration of intravenous calcium may be helpful when hypocalcemia is suggested by prolongation of the Q-T interval on the electrocardiogram or is documented by measurement of plasma ionized calcium.[224]

The use of glucocorticoids has been advocated for the treatment of shock of virtually all etiologies, including hemorrhagic shock.[225-228] Their use has been recommended because of their (1) potential direct stimulation of cardiac function;[229] (2) inhibition of vasoconstrictor actions of catecholamines and vasopressin; (3) restoration of phagocytic function of the reticuloendothelial system;[227] (4) diminution of platelet aggregation; (5) reduction of postganglionic sympathetic nerve transmission;[230] (6) stabilization of lysosomal membranes;[231] (7) blockade of alpha-adrenergic receptors or direct vasodilation;[232,233] (8) protection of the lung and prevention of ARDS;[234] and (9) favorable effects on the oxygen affinity of hemoglobin with enhanced oxygen delivery to the tissues.[235] However, their clinical efficacy in shock, with the exception of shock due to adrenocortical failure and possibly septic shock, has not been established.

When arterial pressure cannot be restored promptly by restitution of intravascular volume, it may be necessary to support the circulation with the use of vasoactive drugs. The previous reliance on norepinephrine, indirectly acting sympathomimetics such as metaraminol, and alpha-adrenergic agonists has been modified by favorable experience with other agents such as dopamine (2 to 5 μg/kg/min), a drug with positive inotropic effects and dopaminergic vasodilatory effects on mesenteric, renal, and cerebral vessels. As already noted, at higher doses dopamine may produce vasoconstriction. Its combined actions of increasing cardiac output and maintaining perfusion of vital organs have made it a valuable agent in the treatment of oligemic shock.[236-238]

Pure alpha- or beta-adrenergic agonists should not be used routinely for the treatment of oligemic shock, since nutritive flow may not be enhanced even though arterial pressure or cardiac output may be increased. Similar limitations apply to alpha-adrenergic receptor blocking agents to reduce vasoconstriction, since the potential advantages of vasodilatation are frequently outweighed by a decline in systemic pressure from already low levels, with consequent further compromise of perfusion of the heart and other vital organs.

Nonhemorrhagic Oligemic Shock

Reduction of effective vascular volume may result from sequestration of fluid in a "third space" in disorders such as hemorrhagic pancreatitis, burns, surgical wounds, or trauma to skeletal muscle; in the abdominal cavity with ascites; or in the intestinal lumen with obstructive or adynamic ileus. Excessive filtration of plasma sometimes accompanies pheochromocytoma with manifestations of postural hypotension and occasionally shock due to the combined effects of diminished plasma volume and rarely myocarditis, apparently induced by catecholamines (p. 1734).[239,240] The more commonly manifested vasoconstrictor effects of the circulating catecholamines released by the tumor may be masked by the profound diminution of blood volume with or without accompanying cardiac dysfunction.

Oligemic shock may also occur in association with: (1) salt-wasting nephritis; (2) protracted fluid loss from the gastrointestinal tract due to vomiting or diarrhea, cholera, or gastroenteritis in infancy;[241-243] (3) uncontrolled diabetes mellitus; (4) diabetes insipidus; (5) sodium depletion accompanying adrenocortical failure; (6) excessive diuresis induced pharmacologically; (7) or any other condition in which components of the vascular volume are sequestered or lost. The hemodynamic hallmark is hypotension, generally accompanied by arteriolar vasoconstriction and tachycardia. Systemic venous pressure is reduced, and oliguria is usually prominent. Because of the loss of plasma volume and retention of red cells, hemoconcentration is a prominent feature.

Primary therapy of nonhemorrhagic, oligemic shock consists of rapid replacement of lost fluid. Shock accompanying pheochromocytoma necessitates infusion of plasma, albumin, or another plasma expander and crystalloid solution. In the absence of unrecognized complicating factors (such as marked sodium loss and impaired vascular tone in the case of an Addisonian crisis, or impaired cardiac function accompanying profound myxedema), early oligemic shock responds promptly to adequate repletion of plasma volume, as long as additional fluid losses are controlled and the initiating cause is corrected.

Acute renal failure often accompanies intravascular hemolysis, particularly when the latter is associated with severe or persistent hypotension, despite the lack of demonstrable nephrotoxic effects of pure hemoglobin. Its etiology appears to depend in part upon deleterious effects of other, not yet delineated constituents of the red cell stroma. Administration of mannitol may be helpful in preventing or minimizing irreversible renal damage.[244] When a diuretic phase follows early renal failure associated with rhabdomyolysis, hypercalcemia may occur, presumably from remobilization of calcium previously deposited in damaged muscle,[245] as well as transient secondary hyperparathyroidism. Unrecognized or inadequately treated electrolyte abnormalities, including alterations in plasma ionized calcium, may be responsible for the occurrence of severe arrhythmias and even sudden death.

DISTRIBUTIVE SHOCK

Shock due to sepsis, neurological disturbances, anaphylaxis, and metabolic, toxic, or endocrine depression of vasomotor tone share the common features of inappropriate vasodilatation, causing maldistribution of vascular volume, reduction of systemic arterial pressure, and impaired perfusion of vital organs.[246] Calculated total peripheral vascular resistance is generally markedly decreased and arterial pressure is reduced, but cardiac output may be normal, increased, or reduced. Cutaneous vasodilatation is often present, and the patient exhibits so-called warm shock.

SEPTIC SHOCK (Table 18–2)

In septic shock severe infection leads to circulatory collapse.[246-249] The clinical picture frequently includes chills, rigors, and fever as high as 106°F (41°C). Cerebral function is frequently impaired, venous pressure is markedly reduced, and oliguria is prominent. When the cutaneous bed is dilated, the patient is often alert, the skin is warm and dry, and cardiac output is frequently increased, even though perfusion of many tissues is reduced. While vasodilatation often predominates early in the pyrogenic phase, later in the course profound vasoconstriction occurs, peripheral resistance rises, and cardiac output declines; at this stage the prognosis is ominous.[250]

The most common offending agents are gram-negative enteric bacilli, although other bacterial organisms, including gram-positive cocci, gram-negative diplococci, and clostridia, as well as nonbacterial organisms, including viruses, rickettsia, and fungi, may be responsible.[251] Compromise of a host by immunosuppressive drugs, antimetabolite therapy, or prolonged administration of glucocorticoids may predispose to the condition. "Warm shock" is particularly prominent when the initiating bacteremia is due to gram-negative enteric bacteria, presumably because of the effects of endotoxin. A substantial fraction of the blood volume pools in the venous bed, with consequent reduction of effective circulating volume. Metabolic acidosis, elevation of plasma lactate, low arteriovenous oxygen content, differences due to arteriovenous shunting, fever, and leukopenia followed by leukocytosis are typical.

Endotoxins, i.e., large macromolecular lipopolysaccharide complexes derived from the cell walls of a variety of gram-negative bacilli, produce shock when injected intravenously into experimental animals, resulting in pathophysiological disturbances that resemble septic shock in man (Fig. 18–11). Hepatic and splanchnic venoconstriction limits venous return to the heart, contributing to the decline in cardiac output and to systemic arterial hypotension. Endothelial damage, aggregation of cellular blood elements leading to thrombocytopenia and leukopenia, and stasis and microthrombi in the microcirculation contribute to impaired perfusion of vital organs.

Because endotoxin can activate the coagulation, fibrinolytic, complement, and kallikrein systems, both hyper- and hypocoagulability may occur. Activation of complement and the production of kinins appear to contribute to enhanced vascular permeability; bradykinin may contribute to the decline in systemic arterial resistance and to bradycardia. Prostaglandins are also involved, since inhibition of prostaglandin synthesis favorably modifies the hemodynamic response to the insult.[252]

Since endotoxin can activate hepatic glycogenolysis, the initial hyperglycemia—characteristic of all forms of shock because of the effect of glucocorticoids and catecholamines—may be accentuated. A secondary hypoglycemia is common when carbohydrate reserves have been depleted.[253] The disturbances of carbohydrate metabolism

TABLE 18–2 PATHOPHYSIOLOGIC SEQUELAE OF ENDOTOXEMIA

Activation of Hageman factor
Hypotension (kinin system)
Disseminated intravascular coagulation
Changes in peripheral blood levels (granulocytes and lymphocytes)
Activation of fibrinolytic pathways
Activation of classic and alternative pathways of complement
Release of vasoactive and coagulation-promoting substances from
   platelets
Endothelial damage
Release of effector substances from neutrophils and mononuclear cells

Reproduced with permission from Shine, K. I., Kuhn, M., Young, L. S., and Tillisch, J. H.: Aspects of the management of shock. Ann. Intern. Med. *93*:723, 1980.

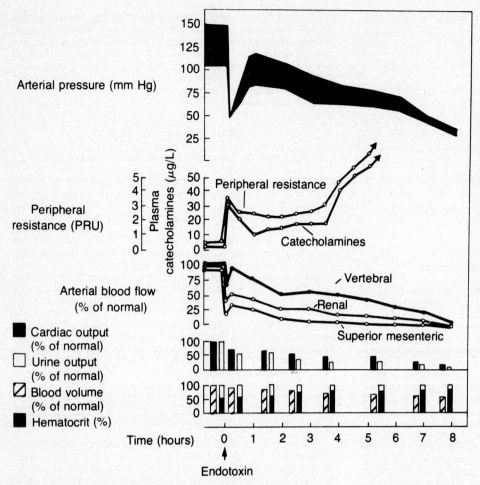

FIGURE 18-11 Characteristic hemodynamic changes induced experimentally in dogs subjected to endotoxic shock. Early in the evolution of shock, peripheral vascular resistance is inappropriately low with respect to arterial blood pressure despite the elevation of plasma catecholamines. Late in the evolution of the condition, peripheral vascular resistance increases markedly but systemic arterial blood pressure continues to decline. Progressive hemoconcentration accompanies the diminution of vascular volume. Both reflect effusion of plasma into the interstitial fluid space, further compromising cardiac output, systemic arterial pressure, and urine output. (From Niazi, Z., et al.: Use of monitoring to improve survival in shock. Geriatrics *30*:93, 1975.)

include hypoinsulinemia, mediated in part by alpha-adrenergic inhibition of insulin secretion.[253,254]

Primary Therapy. Primary therapy of septic shock includes administration of antibiotics once specimens of blood, urine, sputum, cerebrospinal fluid, and, when present, wound exudates have been obtained for culture and sensitivity tests. Initial selection of antibiotic therapy must frequently be made on an empirical basis, depending on the probable source of infection and organism involved. An aminoglycoside should be administered for suspected enteric organisms, with carbenicillin when *Pseudomonas* is suspected; penicillinase-resistant penicillins or cephalosporins are often the agents of choice when the probability of infection with a gram-positive organism is higher. Suspected *Bacteroides fragilis* infection should be treated with clindamycin.

Secondary Therapy. Large volumes of fluid and plasma expanders are needed to sustain effective vascular volume and maintain normal plasma oncotic pressure. The hemodynamic response to intermittent fluid challenges, analogous to that utilized in patients with cardiogenic shock (p. 1317), can be employed to assess the adequacy of vascular volume. If systemic hypotension persists, agents such as dopamine may be useful. Alpha-adrenergic agonists should not be utilized, since they may further compromise perfusion of vital organs in the face of vasoconstriction.

The possible benefit of corticosteroids in the treatment of septic shock remains controversial. Doses utilized have been as much as 50- to 100-fold greater than those required for replacement therapy in patients with adrenocortical failure. Dexamethasone (40 mg intravenously followed by 20 mg at 4-hour intervals) has been employed to increase cardiac output and decrease peripheral arterial resistance, improve oxygenation, and decrease metabolic acidosis.[255] Gastrointestinal bleeding may be a relative contraindication to treatment with these agents.

The efficacy of other suggested measures, such as glucose-insulin-potassium,[256] antihistamines to antagonize vasodilatation mediated by histamine release,[257] and inhibitors of prostaglandin synthesis,[258] has not yet been established. When disseminated intravascular coagulation has been documented, heparin should be administered,[259] al-

though controlled studies have not demonstrated improved survival. When there is widespread fibrinolysis, the use of agents such as epsilon-aminocaproic acid may be justified.[259]

NEUROGENIC SHOCK

Central nervous system disease, including cerebrovascular disorders, marked or rapid elevations of cerebrospinal fluid pressure from any cause, hypertensive encephalopathy, hemorrhage into the basal ganglia or into the cerebellum; vascular or traumatic injury to the spinal cord; deep general or spinal anethesia; or toxic depression of the nervous system by heat stroke, dehydration, drug overdose, or other metabolic insults may result in shock mediated in part by profound disturbance of autonomic nervous system function. Often vasodilatation, vagotonia, and suppression of sympathetic support of vascular tone with shock accompanied by bradycardia are prominent. Primary therapy consists of treatment of the underlying disturbance. Supportive therapy, primarily vigorous administration of colloid and crystalloid solutions, is similar to that utilized in the *distributive shock* of other etiologies, such as sepsis.[246,260-262] Infusion of agents with positive inotropic effects, such as dopamine, or alpha-adrenergic agonists such as methoxamine and phenylephrine may be useful, but only as a temporizing measure, until expansion of blood volume can be achieved. With the exception of neurogenic shock related to visceral pain, which may respond dramatically to analgesics, the outcome of neuropathic shock is generally grave.

SHOCK DUE TO METABOLIC, TOXIC, OR ENDOCRINE FACTORS

Drug abuse or suicide attempts with agents such as barbiturates, phenothiazines, glutethemide, diazepam, and other central nervous system depressants may give rise to shock, as may hepatic and renal failure, uncontrolled diabetes mellitus, anoxia, hypercarbia, and respiratory and metabolic acidosis (including lactic ketoacidosis), hyperosmolality,[263] alkalosis,[264] dehydration, and hypoglycemia.[263] Excessive transfusions with banked blood and chelation of calcium without adequate replacement, or injudicious administration of vasodilators or diuretics, may cause shock in patients whose circulation is already compromised. Heavy metal intoxication, often complicated by vomiting and diarrhea, intoxication with carbon monoxide, ingestion of ethylene glycol with resultant metabolic acidosis, and toxicity from venoms may all impair maintenance of vascular tone, with consequent development of shock.

Addisonian crisis, whether due to (1) disease intrinsic to the adrenal cortex (sometimes manifest only with surgical or traumatic stress); (2) hemorrhagic infarction of the adrenal glands precipitated by meningococcal infection; or (3) hemorrhage into the adrenals associated with excessive anticoagulation, may cause shock not only because of failure of sodium retention secondary to mineralocorticoid deficiency, but also because of diminished cardiac contractility and impaired vascular tone.[265-267] Pressor reactivity to catecholamines is reduced by adrenalectomy in experimental animals and can be restored by the administration of adrenocorticoid hormones.[265] Shock due to adrenocortical failure responds initially to the administration of large volumes of saline, and the accompanying hypoglycemia responds to hypertonic glucose. However, the administration of mineralocorticoids and glucocorticoids is necessary as well.

Circulatory collapse with mortality exceeding 50 per cent may accompany other serious endocrine disturbances, including myxedema (p. 1729) and hyperparathyroidism.[263] Myxedema leads to depressed myocardial contractility, myocardial injury, and hypovolemia (p. 1730). It should be suspected when shock is accompanied by hypothermia, an inappropriately slow heart rate, low voltage on the electrocardiogram, soft heart sounds, an inactive precordium, ascites or other serous effusions, and the stigmata of myxedema, such as thickened, dry skin. Circulatory collapse is an end-stage manifestation of profound thyroid deficiency and may be due in part to the loss of the permissive role of thyroid hormone in the maintenance of receptors to adrenergic agonists.[268,269]

The success of therapy of these forms of shock is dependent on the recognition of the etiology, on the prompt implementation of primary treatment directed against the specific impairment, and on appropriate attention to accompanying alterations in blood volume and electrolyte balance.

ANAPHYLACTIC SHOCK

Anaphylactic shock is a disorder that generally occurs precipitously in response either to exposure to an antigen in the natural environment or as a result of drug administration. In sensitized individuals, the antigen interacts with an IgE-specific antibody on mast cells and other cell surfaces. Mediators liberated from sensitized mast cells (Fig. 18–12) include histamine and leukotrienes. Other substances that are involved include prostaglandins, thromboxane A$_2$, kinins, chemotactic factors, and catecholamines. Tissue mast cells and basophils in the peripheral blood are important sources of these mediators.[270-272]

Life-threatening anaphylaxis occurs within minutes after exposure to the antigen and is manifested by marked respiratory distress and bronchospasm, plasma volume depletion with hemoconcentration, circulatory collapse, decreased cardiac output, increased peripheral resistance, and frequently urticaria. Supraventricular and ventricular tachyarrhythmias are common. Milder forms of anaphylactic shock present with partial airway obstruction, hives, tachycardia, and mild hyper- or hypotension.

The diagnosis of anaphylactic shock is usually based on the history and knowledge of the setting in which the episode occurs, as well as recognition of the unique combination of bronchospasm and cardiovascular collapse often accompanied by cutaneous manifestations. However, in some cases, the diagnosis is confounded when vascular collapse occurs without antecedent respiratory compromise.[274]

Primary Therapy. Primary therapy includes immediate vigorous efforts to eliminate or reduce exposure to antigen, e.g., by placing a tourniquet above an injection site when the episode occurs after administration of heterologous protein or a pharmacological agent; by using epinephrine (0.1 mg intravenously and 0.4 mg subcutaneously)

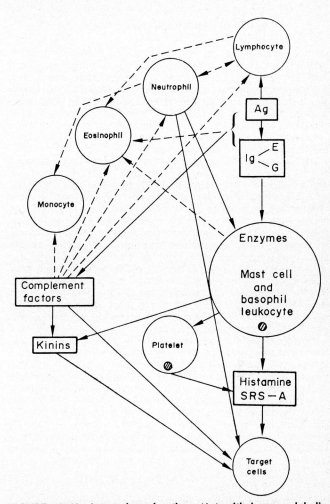

FIGURE 18–12 Interaction of antigen (Ag) with immunoglobulins (Ig), particularly of the E and G classes, influences a variety of cells, including mast cells and lymphocytes, to release mediators that either directly affect target cells in the lung and other organs or induce liberation of other mediators from platelets and other cells that, in turn, impinge on target cells. (From Austen, K. F., and Becker, E. L. (eds.): Biochemistry of the Acute Allergic Reactions—Second International Symposium. London, Blackwell Scientific Publications, 1971.)

both to support the circulation and to enhance intracellular cyclic AMP levels, thereby inhibiting release of mediators; or by further augmenting intracellular cyclic AMP levels with the use of a phosphodiesterase inhibitor such as aminophylline (500 mg intravenously over 10 to 20 minutes). Administration of antihistamines such as diphenhydramine hydrochloride (50 to 100 mg intravenously over an interval of several minutes) may be helpful but is rarely definitive. Glucocorticoids may reduce the likelihood of protracted anaphylaxis but are of little help in treating the acute episode. Epinephrine remains the mainstay of primary therapy. Intramuscular injections are advantageous when cutaneous vasoconstriction is prominent.

Secondary Therapy. Systemic arterial pressure should be maintained with infusion of large volumes of crystalloid solutions and oxygenation by mechanical support of respiration.[272,274] Since loss of plasma volume is a major consequence of anaphylactic shock, the efficacy of vasoconstrictor agents such as norepinephrine is questionable. Ventilation must be supported immediately with oxygen delivered through an endotracheal tube, since laryngeal edema may occur rapidly. Because of the possibility of recurrent anaphylaxis, it is essential to observe the patient for at least several hours after the circulatory and respiratory status have been restored to normal. The patient must be instructed to avoid subsequent exposure to the offending antigen and provided with such ancillary devices as bracelets describing his or her susceptibility to an allergic reaction.

PULMONARY EMBOLISM (See also Chapter 46)

Antecedent shock is common when massive pulmonary embolism causes death. On the other hand, except for transitory increases of pulmonary arterial pressure, marked derangements of circulatory function are uncommon in the vast majority of patients with pulmonary emboli. Even when the hemodynamic concomitants of the immediate insult of massive pulmonary embolism are marked, persistent circulatory insufficiency is rare. The improvement in hemodynamics reflects primarily two mechanisms—fibrinolysis and distal migration of emboli within the pulmonary vasculature.[275]

The primary hemodynamic manifestations of massive pulmonary emboli include pulmonary arterial hypertension; right ventricular failure with elevation of right ventricular end-diastolic and right atrial pressure, sometimes associated with tricuspid regurgitation; increased systemic venous pressure; and diminished cardiac output. Left ventricular filling pressure is generally normal or reduced, and total peripheral vascular resistance is increased. Supraventricular arrhythmias are common, but if the magnitude of the insult is so severe that systemic perfusion is impaired, arrhythmias of all types may occur. Despite massive pulmonary embolism, death is uncommon when anticoagulation is implemented promptly to prevent further embolization. Partial resolution of obstruction due to emboli within the pulmonary vasculature can be detected with angiographic and isotopic techniques within days[276] and may be complete as early as two weeks after the onset of the episode.[275]

Primary therapy of shock associated with massive pulmonary embolism includes prevention of further embolization with anticoagulation or an umbrella inserted into the inferior vena cava, relief of dynamic factors adding to the obstruction such as hypoxemia and the associated pulmonary arterial vasoconstrictor response, and the use of systemic fibrinolytic therapy (urokinase or streptokinase).[276] Secondary therapy is directed toward supporting the circulation with cardiac glycosides and vigorously treating the arrhythmias that are commonly associated. Pulmonary embolectomy is indicated only if the patient is in extremis despite the above-mentioned measures, combined with the use of isotropic agents such as dopamine.

SHOCK DUE TO MISCELLANEOUS CAUSES

Shock may occur in relatively unusual conditions such as *malignant hyperthermia*, a hereditary disorder in which profound hyperpyrexia, marked elevations of plasma creatine kinase activity, and circulatory collapse occur in response to anesthesia or other stresses.[277–279] In this disorder, refractory shock may follow triggering events unless the diagnosis is suspected and appropriate precautions are taken to avoid use of agents likely to precipitate the syndrome. The shock appears to be due to profound augmentations in anaerobic metabolism resulting from compensatory responses to an intrinsic defect in calcium binding by the sarcoplasmic reticulum.[278,280] Dantrolene sodium in doses of 1 to 10 mg/kg intravenously appears to be effective in blunting the abnormal metabolic activity and aborting the syndrome.[280] Once circulatory failure has occurred, the outlook is poor despite supportive therapy.

Cyclic episodes of shock have been observed in syndromes such a *periodic edema, angioneurotic edema* associated with hereditary deficiency of an inhibitor of the complement system, *periodic fever,* and *hyperglobulinemias.*[281,282] Effective management of these disorders is directed toward the primary derangement and prevention of shock.

References

1. Shine, K. I., Kuhn, M., Young, L. S., and Tillisch, J. H.; Aspects of the management of shock. Ann. Intern. Med. 93:723, 1980.
2. Eldridge, F. L.: Relationship between lactate turnover rate and blood concentration in hemorrhagic shock. J. Appl. Physiol. 37:321, 1974.
3. Messmer, K., and Sunder-Plassmann, L.: Microcirculatory and rheologic changes in shock. In Shoemaker, W. C., and Taveres, B. L. (eds.): Current Topics in Critical Care Medicine. Basel, S. Karger, 1976, p. 16.
4. Hardaway, R. M., Dixon, R. S., Foster, E. F., Karabin, B. L., Schifres, F. D., and Meyers, T.: The effect of hemorrhagic shock on disseminated intravascular coagulation. Ann. Surg. 184:43, 1976.
5. Kantrowitz, A., Krakauer, J. S., Butner, A. M., Freed, P. S., Jaron, D., Rosenbaum, A., and Goodman, P. M.: Phase-shift balloon pumping in cardiogenic shock. Progr. Cardiovasc. Dis. 12:293, 1969.
6. Scheidt, S., Ascheim, R., and Killip, T., III: Shock after acute myocardial infarction. Am. J. Cardiol. 26:556, 1970.
7. Gunnar R. M., Cruz, A., Boswell, J., Co, B. S., Pietras, R. J., and Tobin, J. R., Jr.: Myocardial infarction with shock: Hemodynamic studies and results of therapy. Circulation 33:753, 1966.
8. Cohn, J. N., and Franciosa, J. A.: Pathophysiology of shock in acute myocardial infarction. In Yu, P. N., and Goodwin, J. F. (eds.): Progress in Cardiology. Philadelphia, Lea and Febiger, 1973, p. 207.
9. Lees, N. W.: The diagnosis and treatment of endotoxin shock. Anaesthesia 31:897, 1976.
10. Hassen, A.: Gram-negative bacteremic shock. Med. Clin. North Am. 57:1403, 1973.
11. McArdle, C. S., MacDonald, J. A. E., and Ledingham, I. M.: A three year retrospective analysis of septic shock in a general hospital. Scott. Med. J. 20:79, 1975.
12. Pardy, B. J., and Dudley, H. A. F.: Sequential patterns of haemodynamic and metabolic changes in experimental hypovolaemic shock. I. Responses to acute haemorrhage. Br. J. Surg. 66:84, 1979.
13. Bronk, D. W., and Stella, G.: Afferent impulses in the carotid sinus nerve: I. The relation of the discharge from single end organs to arterial blood pressure. J. Cell. Physiol. 1:113, 1932.
14. Abboud, F. M., Heistad, D. D., Mark, A. L., and Schmid, P. D.: Reflex control of the peripheral circulation. Progr. Cardiovasc. Dis. 17:371, 1976.
15. Paintal, A. S.: Cardiovascular receptors. In Neil, E. (ed.): Enteroceptors. Berlin, Springer-Verlag, 1972, p. 1.
16. Oberg, B., and Thoren, P.: Increased activity in left ventricular receptors during hemorrhage or occlusion of caval veins in the cat—A possible cause of the vaso-vagal reaction. Acta Physiol. Scand. 85:164, 1972.
17. Mark, A. L., Abboud, F. M., Schmid, P. G., and Heistad, D. D.: Reflex vascular responses to left ventricular outflow obstruction and activation of ventricular baroreceptors in dogs. J. Clin. Invest. 52:1147, 1973.
18. Jarisch, A., and Zotterman, Y.: Depressor reflexes from the heart. Acta Physiol. Scand. 16:31, 1948.
19. Davies, G. S., and Comroe, J. H.: Chemoreflexes from the heart and lungs. Physiol. Rev. 34:167, 1954.
20. Linden, R. J.: Function of cardiac receptors. Circulation 48:463, 1973.
21. Green, H. D., and Kepchar, J. H.: Control of peripheral resistance in major systemic vascular beds. Physiol. Rev. 39:617, 1959.
22. Jakschik, B. A., Marshall, G. R., Kourik, J. L., and Needleman, P.: Profile of circulating vasoactive substances in hemorrhagic shock and their pharmacologic manipulation. J. Clin. Invest. 54:842, 1974.
23. Hall, R. C., and Hodge, R. L.: Changes in catecholamine and angiotensin levels in the cat and dog during hemorrhage. Am. J. Physiol. 221:1305, 1971.
24. Scornik, O. A., and Paladini, A. C.: Angiotensin blood levels in hemorrhagic hypotension and other related conditions. Am. J. Physiol. 206:553, 1964.
25. Hollenberg, N. K., Waters, J. R., Toews, M. R., Davies, R. O., and Nickerson, M.: Nature of cardiovascular decompensation during hemorrhagic hypotension. Am. J. Physiol. 219:1476, 1970.
26. Starke, K., Werner, U., Hellerforth, R., and Schumann, H. J.: Influence of peptides on the output of noradrenaline in isolated rabbit hearts. Eur. J. Pharmacol. 9:136, 1970.
27. Collier, J. G., Herman, A. G., and Vane, J. R.: Appearance of prostaglandins in the renal venous blood of dogs in response to acute systemic hypotension produced by bleeding or endotoxin. J. Physiol. 230:19, 1973.
28. Bagby, G. J., and Spitzer, J. A.: Lipoprotein lipase activity in rat heart and adipose tissue during endotoxin shock. Am. J. Physiol. 238:H325, 1980.
29. Tung, S. H., Bettice, J., Wang, B. C., and Brown, E. G., Jr.: Intracellular and extracellular acid-base changes in hemorrhagic shock. Respir. Physiol. 26:229, 1976.
30. Daniel, A. M., Pierce, C. H., MacLean, L. E., and Shizgal, H. M.: Lactate metabolism in the dog during shock from hemorrhage, cardiac tamponade or endotoxin. Surg. Gynec. Obstet. 143:581, 1976.
31. Arfman, R. C., Loegering, D. J., and Smith, J. J.: Changes in plasma levels of lysosomal and nonlysosomal enzymes during hemorrhagic hypotension. Proc. Soc. Exp. Biol. Med. 149:1029, 1975.
32. Roberts, R., and Sobel, B. E.: The inactivation and clearance of enzymes. In Hearse, D. J., and DeLeiris, J. (eds.): Enzymes in Cardiology: Diagnosis and Research. Chichester, England, John Wiley and Sons, Ltd., 1979.
33. Wiggers, C. J.: The present status of the shock problem. Physiol. Rev. 22:74, 1942.
34. Fine, J.: Septic shock. J.A.M.A. 188:127, 1964.
35. McNulty, W. P., Jr., and Linares, R.: Hemorrhagic shock of germfree rats. Am. J. Physiol. 198:141, 1960.
36. Krause, S. M., and Hess, M. L.: Diphenhydramine protection of the failing myocardium during gram-negative endotoxemia. Circ. Shock 6:75, 1979.
37. Rocha e Silva, M., Jr.: Participation of the kinin-system in different kinds of shock. In Bertelli, A., and Back, N. (eds.): Shock: Biochemical, Pharmacological, and Clinical Aspects. New York, Plenum Press, 1970, p. 135.
38. Lefer, A. M.: Blood-borne humoral factors in the pathophysiology of circulatory shock. Circ. Res. 32:129, 1973.
39. Rai, V., Pandey, S. K., Singh, R. H., and Udupa, K. N.: Systemic histamine and histaminase changes during haemorrhagic shock. Indian J. Exp. Biol. 14:187, 1976.

40. Bond, R. F., Bond, C. H., Peissner, L. C., and Manning, E. S.: Prostaglandin modulation of adrenergic vascular control during hemorrhagic shock. Am. J. Physiol. 241:H85, 1981.

41. Errington, M. L., and Rocha e Silva, M., Jr.: Vasopressin clearance and secretion during haemorrhage in normal dogs and in dogs with experimental diabetes insipidus. J. Physiol. 227:395, 1972.

42. Regoli, D., and Vane, J. R.: The continuous estimation of angiotensin formed in the circulation of the dog. J. Physiol. 183:513, 1966.

43. Errington, M. L., and Rocha e Silva, M., Jr.: On the role of vasopressin and angiotensin in the development of irreversible haemorrhagic shock. J. Physiol. 242:119, 1974.

44. Holaday, J. W., O'Hara, M., and Faden, A. I.: Hypophysectomy alters cardiorespiratory variables: Central effects of pituitary endorphins in shock. Am. J. Physiol. 241:H479, 1981.

45. Curtis, M. T., and Lefer, A. M.: Protective actions of naloxone in hemorrhagic shock. Am. J. Physiol. 239:H416, 1980.

46. Holaday, J. W., and Faden, A. I.: Naloxone reversal of endotoxin hypotension suggests role of endorphins in shock. Nature 275:450, 1978.

47. Cook, J. A., Wise, W. C., and Halushka, P. V.: Elevated thromboxane levels in the rat during endotoxic shock. J. Clin. Invest. 65:227, 1980.

48. Wise, W. C., Cook, J. A., Halushka, P. V., and Knapp, D. R.: Protective effects of thromboxane synthetase inhibitors in rats in endotoxic shock. Circ. Res. 46:854, 1980.

49. Krausz, M. M., Utsunomiya, T., Feuertein, G., Wolfe, J. H. N., Shepro, D., and Hechtman, H. B.: Prostacyclin reversal of lethal endotoxemia in dogs. J. Clin. Invest. 67:1118, 1981.

50. Haglund, U., Hulten, L., Ahren, C., and Lundgren, O.: Mucosal lesions in the human small intestine in shock. Gut 16:979, 1975.

51. Jones, R. T., Garcia, J. H., Mergner, W. J., Pendergrass, R. E., Valigorsky, J. M., and Trump, B. F.: Effects of shock on the pancreatic acinar cell. Arch. Pathol. 99:634, 1975.

52. Passmore, J. C., Leffler, C. W., and Neiberger, R. E.: A critical analysis of renal blood flow distribution during hemorrhage in dogs. Circ. Shock 5:327, 1978.

53. Dunnill, M. D., and Jerrome, D. W.: Renal tubular necrosis due to shock: Light-and-electron-microscope observation. J. Pathol. 118:109, 1976.

54. Arango, A., Illner, H., and Shires, G. T.: Role of ischemia in the induction of changes in cell membrane during hemorrhagic shock. J. Surg. Res. 20:473, 1976.

55. Guyton, A. C.: Circulatory Physiology. Philadelphia, W. B. Saunders Co., 1973.

56. Wiggers, C. H., and Werle, J. M.: Cardiac and peripheral resistance factors as determinants of circulatory failure in hemorrhagic shock. Am. J. Physiol. 136:421, 1942.

57. Jones, C. E., Smith, E. E., DuPont, E., and Williams, R. D.: Demonstration of nonperfused myocardium in late hemorrhagic shock. Circ. Shock 5:97, 1978.

58. Lee, J. C., and Downing, S. E.: Myocardial oxygen availability and cardiac failure in hemorrhagic shock. Am. Heart J. 92:201, 1976.

59. Siegel, H. W., and Downing, W. E.: Reduction of left ventricular contractility during acute hemorrhagic shock. Am. J. Physiol. 218:772, 1980.

60. Lefer, A. M.: Myocardial depressant factor and circulatory shock. Klin. Wochenschr. 52:358, 1974.

61. Kashyap, M. L., Tay, J. S. L., Sothy, S. P., and Morrison, J. A.: Role of adipose tissue in free fatty acid metabolism in hemorrhagic hypotension and shock. Metabolism 24:855, 1975.

62. Guntheroth, W. G., Jacky, J. P., Kawabori, I., Stevenson, J. G., and Moreno, A. H.: Left ventricular performance in endotoxin shock in dogs. Am. J. Physiol. 242:H172, 1982.

63. Parker, J. L., and Adams, H. R.: Contractile dysfunction of atrial myocardium from endotoxin-shocked guinea pigs. Am. J. Physiol. 240:H954, 1981.

64. Hackel, D. B., Mikat, E. M., Reimer, K., and Whalen, G.: Effects of verapamil on heart and circulation in hemorrhagic shock in dogs. Am. J. Physiol. 241:H12, 1981.

65. Feigl, E. O.: Control of myocardial oxygen tension by sympathetic coronary vasoconstriction in the dog. Circ. Res. 37:88, 1975.

66. Rinaldo, J. E., and Rogers, R. M.: Adult respiratory-distress syndrome: Changing concepts of lung injury and repair. N. Engl. J. Med. 306:900, 1982.

67. Weil, M. H., Carlson, R., Schaeffer, R., Jr., and Shubin, H.: Acute respiratory failure associated with shock. Antibiot. Chemother. 21:106, 1976.

68. Hopewell, P. H., and Murray, J. F.: The adult respiratory distress syndrome. In Creger, W. P., Coggins, C. H., and Hancock, E. W. (eds.): Annual Review of Medicine: Selected Topics in Clinic Sciences. Vol. 27. Palo Alto, Calif., Annual Reviews, Inc., 1976, p. 343.

69. Katzenstein, A., Bloor, C. M., and Leibow, A. S.: Diffuse alevolar damage—the role of oxygen, shock, and related factors. Am. J. Pathol. 85:210, 1976.

70. Gump, F. E., Mashima, R., Jorgensen, S., and Kinney, J. M.: Simultaneous use of three indicators to evaluate pulmonary capillary damage in man. Surgery 70:262, 1971.

71. Hammerschmidt, D. E., White, J. G., and Craddock, P. R.: Corticosteroids inhibit complement-induced granulocyte aggregation: A possible mechanism for their efficacy in shock states. J. Clin. Invest. 63:798, 1979.

72. Robin, E. D., Carey, L. C., Grenvik, A., Glauser, F., and Gaudio, R.: Capillary leak syndrome with pulmonary edema. Arch. Intern. Med. 130:66, 1972.

73. Ratliff, N. B., Young, W. G., Jr., Hackel, D. B., Mikat, E., and Wilson, J. W.: Pulmonary injury secondary to extracorporeal circulation. J. Thorac. Cardiovasc. Surg. 65:425, 1973.

74. Petty, T. L., and Ashbaugh, D. G.: The adult respiratory distress syndrome: Clinical features, factors influencing prognosis and principles of management. Chest 60:233, 1971.

75. Joffe, N., and Simon, M.: Pulmonary oxygen toxicity in the adult. Radiology 92:460, 1969.

76. Burford, T. H., and Burback, B.: Traumatic wet lung: Observations on certain physiologic fundamentals of thoracic trauma. J. Thorac. Surg. 14:415, 1945.

77. Senior, R. M., Wessler, S., and Avioli, L. V.: Pulmonary oxygen toxicity. J.A.M.A. 127:1373, 1971.

78. Tiefenbrun, J., Dikman, S., and Shoemaker, W. C.: The correlation of sequential changes in the distribution of pulmonary blood flow in hemorrhagic shock with the histopathologic anatomy. Surgery 78:618, 1975.

79. Esrig, B. C., and Fulton, R. L.: Sepsis, resuscitated hemorrhagic shock and "shock lung": An experimental correlation. Ann. Surg. 182:218, 1975.

80. Gaisford, W. D., Pandley, N., and Jensen, C. G.: Pulmonary changes in treated hemorrhagic shock: II. Ringer's lactate solution versus colloid infusion. Am. J. Surg. 124:738, 1972.

81. Jenkins, M. T., Jones, R. F., Wilson, B., and Moyer, C. A.: Congestive atelectasis—a complication of the intravenous infusion of fluids. Ann. Surg. 132:327, 1950.

82. Dillon, B. C., and Saba, T. M.: Fibronectin deficiency and intestinal transvascular fluid balance during bacteremia. Am. J. Physiol. 242:H557, 1982.

83. McKenna, U. G., Meadows, J. A., III, Brewer, N. S., Wilson, W. R., and Perrault, J.: Toxic shock syndrome, a newly recognized disease entity: Report of 11 cases. Mayo Clin. Proc. 55:663, 1980.

84. Blumenstock, F. A., Saba, T. M., Weber, P., and Lafin, R.: Biochemical and immunological characterization of human opsonic a_2SB glycoprotein: Its identity with cold-insoluble globulin. J. Biol. Chem. 253:4287, 1978.

85. Saba, T. M., and Jaffe, E.: Plasma fibronectin (opsonic glycoprotein): Its synthesis by vascular endothelial cells and role in cardiopulmonary integrity after trauma as related to reticuloendothelial function. Am. J. Med. 68:577, 1980.

86. Moss, G., and Stein, A. A.: The centrineurogenic etiology of the respiratory distress syndrome: Protection by unilateral chronic pulmonary denervation in hemorrhagic shock. J. Trauma 16:361, 1976.

87. Lopes, O. U., Pontieri, V., Rocha e Silva, M., Jr., and Velasco, I. T.: Hyperosmotic NaCl and severe hemorrhagic shock: Role of the innervated lung. Am. J. Physiol. 241:H883, 1981.

88. Valesco, I. T., Pontieri, V., Rocha e Silva, M., Jr., and Lopes, O. U.: Hyperosmotic NaCl and severe hemorrhagic shock. Am. J. Physiol. 239:H664, 1980.

89. Holcroft, J. W., and Trunkey, D. D.: Pulmonary extravasation of albumin during and after hemorrhagic shock in baboons. J. Surg. Res. 18:91, 1975.

90. Moss, G., and Stein, A. A.: The respiratory distress syndrome: Hypoalbuminemia as a predisposing factor. Crit. Care Med. 4(Abstract):95, 1976.

91. Morissette, M., Weil, M. H., and Shubin, H.: Reduction in colloid osmotic pressure associated with fatal progression of cardiopulmonary failure. Crit. Care Med. 3:115, 1975.

92. Attar, S. M. A., Tingey, H. B., McLaughlin, J. S., and Cowley, R. A.: Bradykinin in human shock. Surg. Forum 18:46, 1967.

93. Hallett, J. W., Jr., Sneiderman, C. A., and Wilson, J. W.: Pulmonary effects of arterial infusion of filtered blood in experimental hemorrhagic shock. Surg. Gynecol. Obstet. 138:517, 1974.

94. Shubrooks, S. J., Jr., Schneider, B., Dubin, H., and Turino, G. M.: Acidosis and pulmonary hemodynamic in hemorrhagic shock. Am. J. Physiol. 225:225, 1973.

95. Petty, T. L., Reiss, O. K., Paul, G. W., Silvers, G. W., and Elkins, N. D.: Characteristics of pulmonary surfactant in adult respiratory distress syndrome associated with trauma and shock. Am. Rev. Respir. Dis. 115:531, 1977.

96. Greenberg, S., McGowan, C., and Glenn, T. M.: Pulmonary vascular smooth muscle function in porcine splanchnic arterial occlusion shock. Am. J. Physiol. 241:H34, 1981.

97. Demling, R. H., Selinger, S. L., Bland, R. D., and Staub, N. C.: Effect of acute hemorrhagic shock on pulmonary microvascular fluid filtration and protein permeability in sheep. Surgery 77:512, 1975.

98. Jardin, F., Eveleigh, M. C., Gurdjian, F., Delille, F., and Margairaz, A.: Venous admixture in human septic shock: Comparative effects of blood volume expansion, dopamine infusion and isoproterenol infusion on mismatching of ventilation and pulmonary blood flow in peritonitis. Circulation 60:155, 1979.

99. Woolverton, W. C., Brigham, K. L., and Staub, N. C.: Effect of continuous positive airway pressure breathing on pulmonary fluid filtration and content in sheep. Physiologist 16:490, 1973.

100. James, P. M., Jr.: Treatment of shock lungs. Am. Surg. 41:451, 1975.

101. Harken, A. H., Brennan, M. F., Smith, B., and Barsamian, E. M.: The hemodynamic response to positive end-expiratory ventilation in hypovolemic patients. Surgery 76:786, 1974.

102. Chinard, F. P., Enns, T., and Nolan, M. D.: Permeability characteristics of alveolar-capillary barrier. Trans. Assoc. Am. Phys. 75:253, 1962.

103. Staub, N. C.: Pathogenesis of pulmonary edema. Am. Rev. Respir. Dis. 109:358, 1974.

104. Gadek, J. E., Fulmer, J. D., Gelfand, J. A., Frank, M. M., Petty, T. L., and Crystal, R. G.: Danazol-induced augmentation of serum α_1-antitrypsin levels in individuals with marked deficiency of this antiprotease. J. Clin. Invest. 66:82, 1980.

105. Simpson, D. L., Goodman, M., Spector, S. L., and Petty, T. L.: Long-term follow-up and bronchial reactivity testing in survivors of the adult respiratory distress syndrome. Am. Rev. Respir. Dis. 117:449, 1978.

106. Sobel, B. E., and Mayer, S. E.: Cyclic adenosine monophosphate and cardiac contractility. Circ. Res. 32:407, 1973.

107. Weissler, A. M., Kruger, F. A., Baba, N., Scarpelli, D. G., Leighton, R. F., and Gallimore, J. K.: Role of anaerobic metabolism in the preservation of functional capacity and structure of anoxic myocardium. J. Clin. Invest. 47:403, 1968.

108. Henry, P. D., Sobel, B. E., and Braunwald, E.: Protection of hypoxic guinea pig hearts with glucose and insulin. Am. J. Physiol. 226:309, 1974.

109. Clark, A. J., Gaddie, R., and Stewart, C. P.: The anaerobic activity of the isolated frog's heart. J. Physiol. 75:321, 1932.

110. Kubler, W., and Spieckermann, P. G.: Regulation of glycolysis in the ischemic and the anoxic myocardium. J. Mol. Cell. Cardiol. 1:351, 1970.

111. Brachfeld, N., Ohtaka, Y., Klein, I., and Kawade, M.: Substrate perference and metabolic activity of the aerobic and the hypoxic turtle heart. Circ. Res. 31:453, 1972.

112. Huckabee, W. E.: Relationships of pyruvate and lactate during anaerobic metabolism. I. Effects of infusion of pyruvate or glucose and of hyperventilation. J. Clin. Invest. 37:244, 1958.

113. Mueller, H., Ayres, S. M., Gregory, J. J., Giannelli, S., Jr., and Grace, W. J.: Hemodynamics, coronary blood flow, and myocardial metabolism in coronary shock; response to l-norepinephrine and isoproterenol. J. Clin. Invest. 49:1885, 1970.

114. Whalen, D. A., Jr., Hamilton, D. C., Ganote, C. E., and Jennings, R. B.: Effect of a transient period of ischemia on myocardial cells. I. Effects on cell volume regulation. Am. J. Pathol. 74:381, 1974.

115. Remme, W. J., de Jong, J. W., and Verdouw, P. D.: Effects of pacing-induced myocardial ischemia on hypoxanthine efflux from the human heart. Am. J. Cardiol. 40:55, 1977.

116. de Jong, J. W., and Goldstein, S.: Changes in coronary venous inosine concentration and myocardial wall thickening during regional ischemia in the pig. Circ. Res. 35:111, 1974.

117. Sobel, B. W.: Salient biochemical features in ischemic myocardium. Circ. Res. 35(Suppl.):III-173, 1974.

118. Agress, C. M., Jacobs, H. I., Glasner, H. F., Lederer, M. A., Clark, W. G., Wroblewski, F., Karmen, A., and LaDue, J. S.: Serum transaminase levels in experimental myocardial infarction. Circulation 11:711, 1955.

119. Nachlas, M. D., Friedman, M. D., and Cohen, S. P.: A method for the quantitation of myocardial infarcts and the relation of serum enzyme levels to infarct size. Surgery 55:700, 1964.

120. Kjekshus, J. K., and Sobel, B. E.: Depressed myocardial creatine phosphokinase activity following experimental myocardial infarction in rabbit. Circ. Res. 27:403, 1970.

121. Shell, W. E., Kjekshus, J. K., and Sobel, B. E.: Quantitative assessment of the extent of myocardial infarction in the conscious dog by means of analysis of serial changes in serum creatine phosphokinase activity. J. Clin. Invest. 50:2614, 1971.

122. Weissmann, G., Hoffstein, S., Gennaro, D., and Fox, A. C.: Lysosomes in ischemic myocardium with observations on the effects of methylprednisolone. In Lefer, A. M., Kelliher, G. J., and Rovetto, M. J. (eds.): Pathophysiology and Therapeutics of Myocardial Ischemia. New York, Spectrum Publications, Inc., 1977, p. 367.

123. Harnarayan, C., Bennett, M. A., Pentecost, B. L., and Brewer, D. B.: Quantitative study of infarcted myocardium in cardiogenic shock. Br. Heart J. 32:728, 1970.

124. Page, D. L., Caulfield, J. B., Kastor, J. A., DeSanctis, R. W., and Sanders, C. A.: Myocardial changes associated with cardiogenic shock. N. Engl. J. Med. 285:133, 1971.

125. Tennant, R., and Wiggers, C. J.: The effect of coronary occlusion on myocardial contraction. Am. J. Physiol. 112:351, 1935.

126. Gutovitz, A. L., Sobel, B. E., and Roberts, R.: Progressive nature of myocardial injury in selected patients with cardiogenic shock. Am. J. Cardiol. 41:469, 1978.

127. Steenberger, C., Deleeuw, G., Rich, T., and Williamson, J. R.: Effects of acidosis and ischemia on contractility and intracellular pH of rat heart. Circ. Res. 41:469, 1978.

128. Braunwald, E., and Kloner, R. A.: The stunned myocardium: Prolonged, postischemic ventricular dysfunction. Circulation 66:1146, 1982.

129. da Luz, P. L., Weil, M. H., and Shubin, H.: Current concepts on mechanisms and treatment of cardiogenic shock. Am. Heart J. 92:103, 1976.

130. Borda, L., Schuchleib, R., and Henry, P. D.: Effects of potassium on isolated canine coronary arteries: Modulation of adrenergic responsiveness and release of norepinephrine. Circ. Res. 41:778, 1977.

131. Carlson, E. L., Selinger, S. L., Utley, J., and Hoffman, J. I. E.: Intramyocardial distribution of blood flow in hemorrhagic shock in anesthetized dogs. Am. J. Physiol. 230:41, 1976.

132. Lloyd, B. L., and Taylor, R. R.: Augmentation of myocardial digoxin concentration in hemorrhagic shock. Circulation 51:718, 1975.

133. Peterson, D. F., and Brown, A. M.: Pressor reflexes produced by stimulation of afferent fibers in the cardiac sympathetic nerves of the cat. Circ. Res. 28:605, 1971.

134. Malliani, A., Peterson, D. F., Bishop, V. S., and Brown, A. M.: Spinal sympathetic cardiocardiac reflexes. Circ. Res. 30:158, 1972.

135. Bradfonbrener, M., and Geller, H. M.: Effect of dibenamine on renal blood flow in hemorrhagic shock. Am. J. Physiol. 171:482, 1952.

136. Stein, J. H., Lifschitz, M. D., and Barnes, L. D.: Current concepts on the pathophysiology of acute renal failure. Am. J. Physiol. 234:F171, 1978.

137. Levinsky, N. G.: Pathophysiology of acute renal failure. N. Engl. J. Med. 296:1453, 1977.

138. Van Den Berg, C. J., and Pineda, A. A.: Plasma exchange in the treatment of acute renal failure due to low molecular-weight dextran. Mayo Clin. Proc. 55:387, 1980.

139. Hollenberg, N. K., Adams, D. F., Oken, D. E., Abrams, H. L., and Merrill, J. P.: Acute renal failure due to nephrotoxins: Renal hemodynamic and angiographic studies in man. N. Engl. J. Med. 282:1329, 1970.

140. Vatner, S. F.: Effects of hemorrhage on regional blood flow distribution in dogs and primates. J. Clin. Invest. 54:225, 1974.

141. Fink, G. D., Chapnick, B. M., Goldberg, M. R., Paustian, P. W., and Kadowitz, P. J.: Influence of prostaglandin E_2, indomethacin, and reserpine on renal vascular responses to nerve stimulation, pressor and depressor hormones. Circ. Res. 41:172, 1977.

142. Reubi, F. C., and Vorburger, C.: Renal hemodynamics and physiopathology of acute renal failure and shock in man. In Giovannetti, S., Bonomini, V., and D'Amico, G. (eds.): Advances in Nephrology: Physiology, Hypertension, Renal Diseases, Renal Failure, Dialysis and Transplantation. Sixth International Congress of Nephrology. Basel, S. Karger, 1975, p. 554.

143. Lucas, C. E., Rector, F. E., Werner, M., and Rosenberg, I. K.: Altered renal homeostasis with acute sepsis: Clinical significance. Arch. Surg. 106:444, 1973.

144. Gorfinkel, H. J., Szidon, J. P., Hirsch, L. H., and Fishman, A. P.: Renal performance in experimental cardiogenic shock. Am. J. Physiol. 222:1260, 1972.

145. Kreisberg, J. I., Bulger, R. E., Trump, B. F., and Nagle, R. B.: Effects of transient hypotension on the structure and function of rat kidney. Virchows Arch. (Cell. Pathol.) 22:121, 1976.

146. Levinsky, N. G., Davidson, D. G., and Berliner, R. W.: Effects of reduced glomerular filtration on urine concentration in the presence of antidiuretic hormone. J. Clin. Invest. 38:730, 1959.

147. Shier, M. R., Bradley, V. E., Ledgerwood, A. M., Rosenberg, I. K., and Lucas, C. E.: Renal function and the postresuscitative hypertension syndrome. Surg. Forum 26:56, 1975.

148. Carlson, R. P., and Lefer, A. M.: Hepatic cell integrity in hypodynamic states. Am. J. Physiol. 231:1408, 1976.

149. Loegering, D. J.: Humoral factor depletion and reticuloendothelial depression during hemorrhagic shock. Am. J. Physiol. 232:H283, 1977.

150. Kaplan, J. E., and Saba, T. M.: Humoral deficiency and reticuloendothelial depression after traumatic shock. Am. J. Physiol. 230:7, 1976.

151. Loegering, D. J., and Saba, T. M.: Hepatic Kupffer cell dysfunction during hemorrhagic shock. Circ. Shock 3:107, 1975.

152. Saba, T. M.: Reticuloendothelial systemic host defense after surgery and traumatic shock. Circ. Shock 2:91, 1975.

153. Williams, L. F., Jr.: Vascular insufficiency of the intestines. Gastroenterology 61:757, 1971.

154. Okuda, M., and Fukui, T.: Myocardial depressant factor — A peptide: Its significance in cardiogenic shock. Jap. Circ. J. 38:497, 1974.

155. Lundgren, O., Haglund, U., Isaksson, O., and Abe, T.: Effects on myocardial contractility of blood-borne material released from the feline small intestine in simulated shock. Circ. Res. 38:307, 1976.

156. Meagher, D. M., Piermattei, D. L., and Swan, H.: Platelet aggregation during progressive hemorrhagic shock in pigs: Possible effects on reperfusion syndrome. J. Thorac. Cardiovasc. Surg. 62:822, 1971.

157. Bridenbaugh, G. A., and Lefer, A. M.: Influence of humoral shock factors in in vitro aggregation of dog platelets. Thromb. Res. 8:599, 1976.

158. Lecompte, F., II, Aberkane, H., Azoulay, E., Muffat-Joly, M., and Pocidalo, J. J.: Blood affinity for oxygen in experimental hemorrhagic shock with metabolic acidosis. Pfluegers Arch. 359:147, 1975.

159. Agostoni, A., Lotto, A., Stabilini, R., Bernasconi, C., Gerli, G., Gattinoni, L., Iapickino, G., and Salvade, P.: Hemoglobin oxygen affinity in patients with low-output heart failure and cardiogenic shock after acute myocardial infarction. Eur. J. Cardiol. 3:53, 1975.

160. Kostuk, W. J., Suwa, K., Bernstein, E. F., and Sobel, B. E.: Altered hemoglobin oxygen affinity in patients with acute myocardial infarction. Am. J. Cardiol. 31:295, 1973.

161. Lambertson, C. J., Semple, S. J. G., Smyth, M. G., and Gelfand, R.: H^+ and pCO_2 as chemical factors in respiratory and cerebral circulatory control. J. Appl. Physiol. 16:473, 1961.

162. Harper, A. M.: Autoregulation of cerebral blood flow: Influence of the arterial blood pressure on the blood flow through the cerebral cortex. J. Neurol. Neurosurg. Psychiatry 29:398, 1966.

163. Kariman, K., Hempel, F. G., Jobsis, F. F., Burnes, S. R., and Saltzman, H. A.: In vivo comparison of cerebral tissue PO_2 and cytochrome aa_3 reduction-oxidation state in cats during hemorrhagic shock. J. Clin. Invest. 68:21, 1981.

164. Siesjo, B. J., and Zwetnow, N. N.: The effect of hypovolemic hypotension on extra- and intracellular acid-base parameters and energy metabolites in the rat brain. Physiol. Scand. 79:114, 1970.

165. Baek, S.-M., Makabali, G. G., Bryan-Brown, C. W., Kusek, J. M., and Shoemaker, W. C.: Inadequacy of high central venous pressure as a guide to volume therapy. Surg. Forum 24:14, 1973.

166. Niazi, A., Beckman, C., Shatney, C., and Lillehei, R. C.: Use of monitoring to improve survival in shock. Geriatrics 30:93, 1975.

167. Rackley, C. E., Russell, R. O., Jr., Mantle, J. A., and Moraski, R. E.: Cardiogenic shock: Recognition and management. Cardiovasc. Clin. 7:251, 1975.

168. Forrester, J. S., Diamond, G., Chatterjee, K., and Swan, H. J. C.: Medical therapy of acute myocardial infarction by application of hemodynamic subsets (Parts I and II). N. Engl. J. Med. 295:1356, 1976.

169. Loisance, D. Y., Cachera, J. P., Poulain, H., Aubry, P. H., Juvin, A. M., and Galey, J. J.: Ventricular septal defect after acute myocardial infarction: Early repair. J. Thorac. Cardiovasc. Surg. 80:61, 1980.

170. Cohn, J. N., Guiha, N. H., Broder, M. I., and Limas, C. J.: Right ventricular infarction. Am. J. Cardiol. 33:209, 1974.

171. Strauss, H. D., Sobel, B. E., and Roberts, R.: The influence of occult right ventricular infarction on enzymatically estimated infarct size, hemodynamics and prognosis. Circulation 62:503, 1980.

172. Gewirtz, H., Gold, H. K., Fallon, J. T., Pasternak, R. C., and Leinbach, R. C.: Role of right ventricular infarction in cardiogenic shock associated with inferior myocardial infarction. Br. Heart J. 42:719, 1979.

173. Lorell, B., Leinbach, R. C., Pohost, G. M., Gold, H. K., Dinsmore, R. E., Hutter, A. M., Jr., Pastore, J. O., and DeSanctis, R. W.: Right ventricular infarction: Clinical diagnosis and differentiation from cardiac tamponade and pericardial constriction. Am. J. Cardiol. 43:465, 1979.

174. Iqbal, M. A., and Liebson, P. R.: Counterpulsation and dobutamine: Their use in treatment of cardiogenic shock due to right ventricular infarct. Arch. Intern. Med. 141:247, 1981.

175. Rackley, C. E., Russel, R. O., Mantle, J. A., Rogers, W. J., Papapietro, S. A., and Schwartz, K. M.: Right ventricular infarction and function. Am. Heart J. 101:215, 1981.

176. Wackers, F. J., Lie, K. I., Becker, A. E., Durrer, D., and Wellens, H. J. J.: Coronary artery disease in patients dying from cardiogenic shock or congestive heart failure in the setting of acute myocardial infarction. Br. Heart J. 38:906, 1976.

177. Amsterdam, E. A., DeMaria, A. N., Hughes, J. L., Hurley, E. J., Lurie, A. J., Williams, D. O., Miller, R. R., and Mason, D. T.: Myocardial infarction shock: Mechanisms and management. In Mason, D. T. (ed.): Congestive Heart Failure: Mechanisms, Evaluations and Treatment. New York, Dun-Donnelly, 1976, p. 365.

178. Bleifeld, W., Hanrather, P., Mathey, D., and Merx, W.: Acute myocardial infarction. V. Left and right ventricular haemodynamics in cardiogenic shock. Br. Heart J. 36:822, 1974.

179. Diamond, G., and Forrest, J. S.: Effect of coronary artery disease and acute myocardial infarction on left ventricular compliance in man. Circulation 45:11, 1972.

180. Russell, R. O., Jr., Rackley, C. E., Pombo, J., Hunt, D., Potanin, C., and Dodge, H. T.: Effects of increasing left ventricular filling pressure in patients with acute myocardial infarction. J. Clin. Invest. 49:1539, 1970.

181. Cohn, J. N., Luria, M. H., Daddario, R. C., and Tristani, F. E.: Studies in clinical shock and hypotension. V. Hemodynamic effects of dextran. Circulation 35:316, 1967.

182. Ferrer, M. I.: Disturbances in the circulation in patients with cor pulmonale. Bull. NY Acad. Med. 41:942, 1965.

183. Kezdi, P., Misra, S. N., Kordenat, R. D., Spickler, J. W., and Stanley, E. L.: The role of vagal afferents in acute myocardial infarction. Am. J. Cardiol. 26:642, 1970.

184. Costanin, L.: Extracardiac factors contributing to hypotension during coronary occlusion. Am. J. Cardiol. 11:205, 1963.

185. Brown, A. M.: Excitation of afferent cardiac sympathetic nerve fibres during myocardial ischaemia. J. Physiol. 190:35, 1967.

186. Kumar, R., Hood, W. B., Jr., Joison, J., Gilmour, D. P., Norman, J. C., and Abelmann, W. H.: Experimental myocardial infarction. VI. Efficacy and toxicity of digitalis in acute and healing phase in intact conscious dogs. J. Clin. Invest. 49:358, 1980.

187. Sagar, K. B., Hanson, E. C., and Powell, W. J., Jr.: Neurogenic coronary vasoconstrictor effects of digitalis during acute global ischemia in dogs. J. Clin. Invest. 60:1248, 1977.

188. Buckley, M. J., Mundth, E. D., Daggett, W. M., DeSanctis, R. M., Sanders, C. A., and Austen, W. G.: Surgical therapy for early complications of myocardial infarction. Surgery 70:814, 1971.

189. Guiliani, E. R., Danielson, G. K., Pluth, J. R., Odyniec, N. A., and Wallace, R. B.: Postinfarction ventricular septal rupture: Surgical considerations and results. Circulation 49:455, 1974.

190. Bardet, J., Masquet, C., Kahn, C., Gourgon, R., Bourdarias, J., Mathivat, A., and Bouvrian, Y.: Clinical and hemodynamic results of intraaortic balloon counterpulsation and surgery for cardiogenic shock. Am. Heart J. 93:280, 1977.

191. Miller, M. G., Weintraub, R. M., Hedley-Whyte, J., and Restall, D. S.: Surgery for cardiogenic shock. Lancet 2:1342, 1974.

192. Kantrowitz, A., Krakauer, J. S., Rosenbaum, A., Butner, A. M., Freed, P. S., and Jaron, D.: Phase-shift balloon pumping in medically refractory cardiogenic shock: Results in 27 patients. Arch. Surg. 99:739, 1969.

193. Snow, N., Lucas, A. E., and Richardson, J. D.: Intra-aortic balloon counterpulsation for cardiogenic shock from cardiac contusion. J. Trauma 22:426, 1982.

194. Mundth, E. D., Buckley, M. J., Daggatt, W. M., McEnany, M. T., Leinbach, R. C., Gold, H. K., and Austen, W. B.: Intra-aortic balloon pump assistance and early surgery in cardiogenic shock. Adv. Cardiol. 15:159, 1975.

195. Leinbach, R. C., Dinsmore, R. E., Mundth, E. D., Buckley, M. J., Dunkman, W. B., Austen, W. B., and Sanders, C. A.: Selective coronary and left ventricu-

lar cineangiography during intraaortic balloon pumping for cardiogenic shock. Circulation 45:845, 1972.

196. Scheidt, S., Wilner, G., Mueller, H., Summers, D., Lesch, M., Wolff, G., Krakauer, J., Rubenfire, M., Felming, P., Noon, G., Oldham, N., Killip, T., and Kantrowitz, A.: Intra-aortic balloon counterpulsation in cardiogenic shock: Report of a co-operative clinical trial. N. Engl. J. Med. 288:979, 1973.

197. Isner, J. M., Cohen, S. J., Viruari, R., Lawrikson, W., and Roberts, W. C.: Complications of the intra-aortic balloon counterpulsation device: Clinical and morphologic observations in 45 necropsy patients. Am. J. Cardiol. 45:250, 1980.

198. Weir, J., Yacoub, M., and Pridies, R. B.: Echocardiography of the intraaortic balloon. Br. Heart J. 37:1045, 1975.

199. Bergmann, S. R., Lerch, R. A., Fox, K. A. A., Ludbrook, P. A., Welch, M. J., Ter-Pogossian, M. M., and Sobel, B. E.: The temporal dependence of beneficial effects of coronary thrombolysis characterized by positron tomography. Am. J. Med., 73:573, 1982.

200. DeWood, M. A., Notske, R. N., Hensley, G. R., Shields, J. P., O'Grady, W. P., Spores, J., Goldman, M., and Ganji, J. H.: Intraaortic balloon counterpulsation with and without reperfusion for myocardial infarction shock. Circulation 61:1105, 1980.

201. Lamberi, J. J., Jr., Cohn, L. H., Lesch, M., and Collins, J. J., Jr.: Intraaortic balloon counterpulsation: Indications and long-term results in postoperative left ventricular power failure. Arch. Surg. 109:766, 1974.

202. Pierce, W. S., Parr, G. V. S., Myers, J. L., Pae, W. D., Jr., Bull, A. P., and Waldhausen, J. A.: Ventricular-assist pumping in patients with cardiogenic shock after cardiac operations. N. Engl. J. Med. 305:1606, 1981.

203. Swan, H. J. C., Forrester, J. S., Danzig, R., and Allen, H. N.: Power failure in acute myocardial infarction. Progr. Cardiovasc. Dis. 12:568, 1970.

204. Mundth, E. D., Buckley, M. J., Leinbach, R. C., Gold, H. K., Daggett, W. M., and Austen, W. G.: Surgical intervention for the complication of acute myocardial ischemia. Ann. Surg. 178:379, 1973.

205. Warren, J. V., and Lewis, R. P.: Beneficial effects of atropine in the prehospital phase of coronary care. Am. J. Cardiol. 37:68, 1976.

206. Dikshit, K., Vden, J. K., Forrester, J. S., Chatterjee, K., Prakash, R., and Swan, H. J. C.: Renal and extrarenal hemodynamic effects of furosemide in congestive heart failure after acute myocardial infarction. N. Engl. J. Med. 288:1087, 1973.

206a. Richard, C., Ricome, J. L., Rimailho, A., Bottineau, G., and Auzepy, P.: Combined hemodynamic effects of dopamine and dobutamine in cardiogenic shock. Circulation 67:620, 1983.

207. MacCannell, K. L., McNay, J. L., Meyer, M. B., and Goldberg, L. I.: Dopamine in the treatment of hypotension and shock. N. Engl. J. Med. 275:1389, 1966.

208. Goldberg, L. I., Hsieh, Y., and Resnekov, L.: Newer catecholamines for treatment of heart failure and shock: An update on dopamine and a first look at dobutamine. Prog. Cardiovasc. Dis. 19:327, 1977.

209. Holzer, J., Karline, J. S., O'Rourke, R. A., Pitt, W., and Ross, J., Jr.: Effectiveness of dopamine in patients with cardiogenic shock. Am. J. Cardiol. 32:79, 1973.

210. Goldberg, L. I., Talley, R. C., and McNay, J. L.: The potential role of dopamine in the treatment of shock. Progr. Cardiovasc. Dis. 12:40, 1969.

211. Oliver, L. E., Horowitz, J. D., Dynon, M. K., Jarrott, B., Brennan, J. B., Gobel, A. M., and Louis, W. J.: Use of dopamine and prazosin combined in the treatment of cardiogenic shock. Med. J. Aust. (Special Supplement, July) 26:42, 1980.

212. Timmis, A. D., Fowler, M. B., and Chamberlain, D. A.: Comparison of haemodynamic responses to dopamine and salbutamol in severe cardiogenic shock complicating acute myocardial infarction. Br. Med. J. 282:7, 1981.

213. Tuttle, R. R., and Mills, J.: Development of a new catecholamine to selectively increase cardiac contractility. Circ. Res. 36:185, 1975.

214. Shell, W. E., and Sobel, B. E.: Protection of jeopardized ischemic myocardium by reduction of ventricular afterload. N. Engl. J. Med. 291:481, 1974.

215. Fowler, M. B., Timmis, A. D., and Chamberlain, D. A.: Synergistic effects of a combined salbutamol-nitroprusside regimen in acute myocardial infarction and severe left ventricular failure. Br. Med. J. 16:435, 1980.

216. Diamond, G., Forrester, J., Danzig, R., Parmley, W. W., and Swan, H. J. C.: Haemodynamic effects of glucagon during acute myocardial infarction with left ventricular failure in man. Br. Heart J. 33:290, 1971.

217. Watanabe, T., Covell, J. W., Maroko, P. R., Braunwald, E., and Ross, J., Jr.: The effects of increased arterial pressure and positive inotropic agents on the severity of myocardial ischemia in the acutely depressed heart. Am. J. Cardiol. 30:371, 1972.

218. Williams, J. R., Jr., Boyd, D. L., and Border, J. F.: Effect of acute hypoxia and hypercapnia acidosis on the development of acetylstrophanthidin-induced arrhythmias. J. Clin. Invest. 47:1885, 1968.

219. Rosing, D. R., Kent, K. M., Maron, B. J., and Epstein, S. E.: Verapamil therapy: A new approach to the pharmacologic treatment of hypertrophic cardiomyopathy. II. Effects on exercise capacity and symptomatic status. Circulation 60:1208, 1979.

220. Johnson, A. M.: Aortic stenosis, sudden death, and the left ventricular baroceptors. Br. Heart J. 33:1, 1971.

221. Smith, J. A. R., Norman, J. N., Smith, A., and Smith, G.: Comparison of dextran 70 and hydroxyethyl starch in volume replacement. Br. J. Surg. 62:666, 1975.

222. Nickerson, M.: Sympathetic blockade in therapy of shock. Am. J. Cardiol. *12*: 619, 1963.
223. MacDonald, J. A. E., Milligan, G. F., Mellon, A., and Ledingham, I. M.: Ventricular function in experimental hemorrhagic shock. Surg. Gynecol. Obstet. *140*:572, 1975.
224. Drop, L. J., and Laver, M. B.: Low plasma ionized calcium and response to calcium therapy in critically ill man. Anesthesiology *43*:300, 1975.
225. Vargish, T., Turner, C. S., Bagwell, C. E., and James, P. M., Jr.: Dose-response relationships in steroid therapy for hemorrhagic shock. Rev. Surg. *33*: 363, 1976.
226. Weil, M. H., and Whigham, H.: Corticosteroids for reversal of hemorrhagic shock in rats. Am. J. Physiol. *209*:815, 1965.
227. Altura, B. M., and Altura, B. T.: Peripheral vascular actions of glucocorticoids and their relationship to protection in circulatory shock. J. Pharmacol. Exp. Ther. *190*:300, 1974.
228. Schumer, W., and Nyhus, L. M.: Corticocosteroid effect on biochemical parameters of human oligemic shock. Arch. Surg. *100*:405, 1970.
229. Vargish, T., Shircliff, A., and James, P. M.: Effect of steroids on cardiac function. Am. Surg. *40*:688, 1974.
230. Motsay, G. J., Romero, L. H., and Lillehei, R. C.: Use of corticosteroids in the treatment of shock. Int. Surg. *59*:593, 1974.
231. Tanaka, K., and Iizuka, Y.: Suppression of enzyme release from isolated rat liver lysosomes by non-steroidal anti-inflammatory drug. Biochem. Pharmacol. *17*:2023, 1968.
232. Lillehei, R. C., and MacLean, L. D.: Physiological approach to successful treatment of endotoxin shock in the experimental animal. Arch. Surg. *78*:116, 1959.
233. Dietzman, R. H., and Lillehei, R. C.: The treatment of cardiogenic shock. V. The use of corticosteroids in the treatment of cardiogenic shock. Am. Heart J. *75*:274, 1968.
234. Sladen, A.: Methylprednisolone: Pharmacologic doses in shock lung syndrome. J. Thorac. Cardiovasc. Surg. *71*:800, 1976.
235. Bryan-Brown, C. W.: Tissue blood flow and oxygen transport in critically ill patients. Crit. Care Med. *3*:103, 1975.
236. Reid, P. R., and Thompson, W. L.: The clinical use of dopamine in the treatment of shock. Johns Hopkins Med. J. *137*:276, 1975.
237. Dopamine for treatment of shock. The Medical Letter, Vol. 17, 1975.
238. Nagakawa, B., Goldberg, L., McCartney, J., and Matsumoto, T.: The effect of dopamine on renal microcirculation in hemorrhagic shock in dogs. Surg. Gynecol. Obstet. *142*:871, 1976.
239. Engelman, K., Watts, R. W. E., Klinenberg, J. R., Sjoerdsma, A., and Seegmiller, J. E.: Clinical, physiological and biochemical studies of a patient with xanthinuria and pheochromocytoma. Am. J. Med. *38*:839, 1964.
240. Sjoerdsma, A., Engelman, K., Waldman, T. A., Cooperman, L. H., and Hammond, W. G.: Pheochromocytoma: Current concepts of diagnosis and treatment. Ann. Intern. Med. *65*:1302, 1966.
241. Arthurson, G.: Burn shock. Triangle *13*:105, 1974.
242. Facey, F. L., Weil, M. H., and Rosoff, L.: Mechanism and treatment of shock associated with acute pancreatitis. Am. J. Surg. *111*:374, 1966.
243. Weil, M. H., and Shubin, H.: Critical Care Medicine: Current Principles and Practices. Hagerstown, MD, Harper & Row, 1976.
244. Rowland, L. P., and Penn, A. S.: Myoglobinuria. Med. Clin. North Am. *56*: 1233, 1972.
245. de Torrente, A., Berl, T., Cohn, P. D., Kawamoto, E., Hertz, P., and Schrier, R. W.: Hypercalcemia of acute renal failure: Clinical significance and pathogenesis. Am. J. Med. *61*:119, 1976.
246. Weil, M. H., and Shubin, H.: Proposed reclassification of shock states with special reference to distributive defects. *In* Hinshaw, L. B., and Cox, B. G. (eds.): The Fundamental Mechanisms of Shock. New York, Plenum Press, 1972, p. 13.
247. Wright, C. J., McLean, A. P. H., and MacLean, L. D.: Regional capillary blood flow and oxygen uptake in severe sepsis. Surg. Gynecol. Obstet. *132*: 637, 1971.
248. Hinshaw, L. B.: Role of the heart in the pathogenesis of endotoxin shock: A review of the clinical findings and observations on animal species. J. Surg. Res. *17*:134, 1974.
249. Lansing, A. M.: Septic shock. J. Canad. Med. Assoc. *89*:583, 1963.
250. Metabolic and cardiac alterations in shock and trauma. Circ. Shock *1* (Suppl.):1, 1979.
251. Weil, M. H., Shubin, H., and Nishijima, H.: Gram-negative shock: Definition, diagnosis and mechanisms. Antibiot. Chemother. *21*:178, 1976.
252. Fletcher, J. R., Ramwell, P. W., and Herman, C. M.: Postaglandins and the hemodynamic course of endotoxin shock. J. Surg. Res. *20*:589, 1976.

253. McClure, J. J.: Endotoxic shock. Vet. Clin. North Am. *6*:193, 1976.
254. Cryer, P. E., Herman, C. M., and Sode, J.: Carbohydrate metabolism in the baboon subjected to gram-negative (*Escherichia coli*) septicemia. II. Depressed insulin secretion with glucose intolerance and sensitivity to exogenous insulin. Curr. Top. Surg. Res. *3*:117, 1971.
255. Shatney, C. H., Dietzman, R. H., and Lillehei, R. C.: The effects of corticosteroids on systemic oxygenation and pulmonary shunting in septic shock: *In* Shoemaker, W. C., and Tavares, B. M. (eds.): Current Topics in Critical Care Medicine. Basel, S. Karger, 1974, p. 92.
256. Weisul, J. P., O'Donnell, T. F., Jr., Stone, M. A., and Clowes, G. H. A., Jr.: Myocardial performance in clinical septic shock: Effects of isoproterenol and glucose potassium insulin. J. Surg. Res. *18*:357, 1975.
257. Lowry, P., Blanco, T., and Santiago-Delpin, E. A.: Histamine and sympathetic blockage in septic shock. Am. J. Surg. *43*:12, 1977.
258. Fletcher, J. R., Herman, C. M., and Ramwell, P. W.: Improved survival in endotoxemia with aspirin and indomethacin pretreatment. Surg. Forum *27*:11, 1976.
259. Bergentz, S. E.: Septic shock and disturbances in coagulation. Triangle *13*:129, 1974.
260. Shubin, H., and Weil, M. H.: Shock associated with barbiturate intoxication. J.A.M.A. *215*:263, 1971.
261. Schwartzman, R. J.: Cerebrovascular disorders causing coma or shock: CVAs and hypertensive crisis. *In* Findeiss, J. C. (ed.): Emergency Management of the Critical Patient. New York, Stratton Intercontinental Publ. Co., 1975, p. 175.
262. Fauci, A. S., Wolff, S. M., and Johnson, J. S.: Effect of cyclophosphamide upon the immune response in Wegener's granulomatosis. New Engl. J. Med. *285*:1493, 1971.
263. Taylor, A. L.: Metabolic disorders causing coma and shock. *In* Findeiss, J. C. (ed.): Emergency Management of the Critical Patient. New York, Stratton Intercontinental Publ. Co., 1975, p. 175.
264. Griggs, D. M., Jr.: Cardiac output and peripheral resistance influenced by acidosis and alkalosis. *In* Oaks, W. W., and Moyer, J. H. (eds.): Pre- and Postoperative Management of the Cardiopulmonary Patient. New York, Grune and Stratton, 1970, p. 227.
265. Nahas, G. G., Brunson, J. G., King, W. M., and Cavert, H. M.: Functional and morphologic changes in heart-lung preparations following administration of adrenal hormones. Am. J. Pathol. *34*:717, 1958.
266. Grollman, A. P., and Gamble, J. L., Jr.: Metabolic alkalosis, a specific effect of adrenocortical hormones. Am. J. Physiol. *196*:135, 1959.
267. Sambhi, M. P., Weil, M. H., and Udhoji, V. N.: Pressor responses to norepinephrine in humans before and after corticosteroids. Am. J. Physiol. *203*:961, 1962.
268. Lefkowitz, R. J., Limbird, L. E., Mukherjee, C., and Caron, M. G.: The β-adrenergic receptor and adenylate cyclase. Biochem. Biophys. Acta *457*:1, 1976.
269. Fregly, M. H., Resch, G. E., Nelson, E. L., Jr., Field, F. P., and Tyler, P. E.: Effect of hypothyroidism on responsiveness to β-adrenergic stimulation. Can. J. Physiol. Pharmacol. *54*:200, 1976.
270. Piper, P. J.: Anaphylaxis and the release of active substances in the lung. Pharmacol. Ther. [B]*3*:75, 1977.
271. Wasserman, S. I., and Austen, K. F.: Arylsulfatase B of human lung: Isolation, characterization, and interaction with slow-reacting substance of anaphylaxis. J. Clin. Invest. *57*:738, 1976.
272. Lockey, R. F., and Bukantz, S. C.: Allergic emergencies. Med. Clin. North Am. *58*:147, 1974.
273. Ellis, E. F., and Henney, C. S.: Adverse reactions following administration of human gamma globulin. J. Allergy Clin. Immunol. *43*:45, 1969.
274. Austen, K. F.: Systemic anaphylaxis in the human being. N. Engl. J. Med. *291*: 661, 1974.
275. Dalen, J. E., and Alpert, J. S.: Natural history of pulmonary embolism. Progr. Cardiovasc. Dis. *17*:259, 1975.
276. The Urokinase Pulmonary Embolism Trial. Circulation *47*(Suppl. II):1, 1973.
277. Britt, B. A.: Malignant hyperthermia: A pharmacogenetic disease of skeletal and cardiac muscle. N. Engl. J. Med. *290*:1140, 1974.
278. Denborough, M. A., Forster, J. F. A., Hudson, M. C., Carter, N. G., and Zapf, P.: Biochemical changes in malignant hyperpyrexia. Lancet *1*:1137, 1970.
279. Harriman, D. G. F., Sumner, D. W., and Ellis, F. R.: Malignant hyperpyrexia myopathy. Q. J. Med. *42*:639, 1973.
280. Dantrolene for malignant hyperthermia during anesthesia. Med. Lett. Drugs Ther. *22*:61, 1980.
281. Moulds, R. F. W., and Denborough, M. A.: Biochemical basis of malignant hyperpyrexia. Br. Med. J. *2*:241, 1974.
282. Larcan, A., Laprevote, M. C., and Lambert, H.: Cyclical shock with hyperglobulinemia. Bibl. Anat. *13*:343, 1975.

19
GENESIS OF CARDIAC ARRHYTHMIAS: ELECTROPHYSIOLOGICAL CONSIDERATIONS

by Douglas P. Zipes, M.D.

ANATOMY OF THE CARDIAC CONDUCTION SYSTEM

Sinus Node. In man, the sinus node[1] is a spindle-shaped structure composed of a fibrous tissue matrix with closely packed cells. It is 10 to 20 mm long, 2 to 3 mm wide, and thick, tending to narrow caudally toward the inferior vena cava. It lies less than 1 mm from the epicardial surface, laterally in the right atrial sulcus terminalis, at the junction of the superior vena cava and right atrium[2,3] (Fig. 19–1). Supplying the sinus node is a prominent artery branching from the right (55 to 60 per cent of the time) or the left circumflex (40 to 45 per cent) coronary artery.[4] The artery may approach the node from a clockwise or counterclockwise direction around the superior vena caval–right atrial junction.[3] The relationship of the artery to the node is thought to be constant, provoking concepts of a physiological interrelation between pulsation, arterial diameter, and sinus discharge rate in a feedback control system.[5] However, more recent evidence suggests an inconsistent relationship between the artery and node and has thrown the postulated servomechanism[5] into question.[3]

Cellular Structure. Cell types in the sinus node include nodal cells, transitional cells, and atrial muscle cells. *Nodal cells* are small (5 to 10 µm), ovoid, primitive-appearing cells with cytoplasm that contains relatively few organelles and myofibrils. Although nuclei are of normal size, nodal cells contain fewer mitochondria compared to contractile cells. The mitochondria are distributed randomly and are variable in size and shape.[6] No transverse tubular system exists. Nodal cells stain poorly, have a pale appearance on light and electron microscopy, and are grouped in elongated clusters located centrally in the sinus node.[6] Although contact between nodal cells was thought to occur mainly by opposing cell membranes—a factor possibly related to the slow conduction within the sinus node—more recent studies suggest the presence of nexus connections.[7] Nodal cells are thought to be the source of normal impulse formation in the sinus node.[7-9]

Transitional cells, or T cells, are elongated cells intermediate in size and complexity between nodal cells and atrial muscle cells. These plentiful cells have large numbers of myofibrils and are heterogeneous in structure, with some T cells more organized and complex than others. T cells near nodal cells have simple intercellular connections, while more fully developed intercalated discs exist between T cells and atrial myocardium. Since nodal cells make contact only with each other or T cells, the latter may provide the only functional pathway for distribution of the sinus impulse formed in the nodal cells to

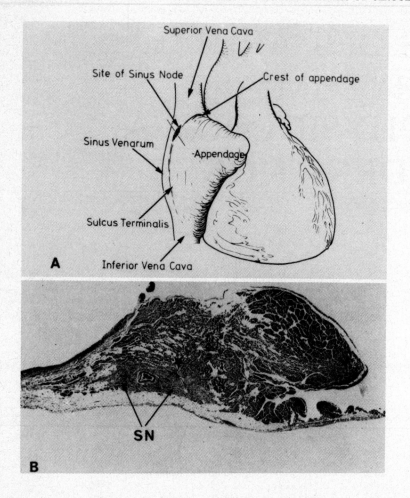

FIGURE 19-1 The human sinus node. *A*, Drawing showing location of the sinus node. *B*, Histological section taken perpendicular to the long axis of the sinus node (thin line in *A*). The sinus node (sn) rests on atrial myocardium of the crista terminalis. The star indicates a portion of nodal tissue blending with the crista terminalis. A layer of adipose tissue covers the epicardial margin of the sinus node (lower portion of the figure). (Masson's trichrome strain [X 6]. (From Becker, A. E., et al.: Functional anatomy of the cardiac conduction system. *In* Harrison, D. C. (ed.): Cardiac Arrhythmias: A Decade of Progress. Boston, G. K. Hall, 1981.)

the rest of the atrial myocardium.[2] T cells constitute a spectrum of morphologies ranging from "typical" nodal cells on the one hand and "typical" working atrial myocardium on the other.

The third cell type present in the sinus node is the working *atrial myocardial cell.* These cells extend as peninsulas into the nodal boundaries, with overlapping zones of sinus and atrial cells most prominent on the nodal surface that abuts the crista terminalis.[3]

Some investigators have described large, *clear cells* that are "Purkinje-like" anatomically and are numerous at the margins of the sinus node.[2] The nature, and even presence, of these cells is unsettled.[10]

Innervation. The sinus node is richly innervated with postganglionic adrenergic and preganglionic cholinergic nerve terminals. Biochemical evidence indicates that the concentration of norepinephrine is two to four times higher in atrial than in ventricular tissue in canine and guinea pig hearts. Although the sinus nodal region contains amounts of norepinephrine equivalent to those in other parts of the right atrium,[11] acetylcholine, acetylcholinesterase, and choline acetyltransferase (the enzyme necessary for the synthesis of acetylcholine) have all been found in greatest concentration in the sinus node, with the next highest concentration in the right and then the left atrium. The concentration of acetylcholine in the ventricles is only 20 to 50 per cent of that in the atria.[11]

In general, autonomic neural input to the heart exhibits "sidedness," with the right sympathetic and vagal nerves affecting the sinus node more than the atrioventricular (AV) node and the left sympathetic and vagal nerves affecting the AV node more than the sinus node. The distribution of neural input is somewhat more complex because of overlapping innervation and because specific branches can be shown to innervate certain regions preferentially.[12] Stimulation of the right stellate ganglion produces a sinus tachycardia, while stimulation of the left stellate ganglion generally produces a shift in the sinus pacemaker to an ectopic site and consistently shortens AV nodal conduction time and refractoriness but inconsistently speeds the sinus nodal discharge rate.[11,12] Sympathetic stimulation shortens the atrial refractory period. Stimulation of the right cervical vagus nerve

primarily slows the sinus nodal discharge rate, while stimulation of the left vagus primarily prolongs AV nodal conduction time and refractoriness.[11,12] Vagal stimulation markedly shortens atrial muscle refractoriness. In the dog, right vagal stimulation shortens the atrial muscle refractory period more in the right than in the left atrium and more in the sinus nodal area than in the rest of the right atrium.[13] Vagal stimulation also shortens atrial refractoriness in humans.[14] Vagal inhibitory effects on sinus nodal discharge rate and AV nodal conduction predominate over sympathetic excitatory effects (accentuated antagonism),[11] probably owing in part to cholinergically mediated presynaptic and postsynaptic modulation of adrenergic effects.[15]

Internodal Conduction. Whether impulses travel from the sinus to the AV node over preferentially conducting pathways—and if they do, over what kind of pathways—is still a debated issue.[10] Two lines of evidence, anatomical and functional, will be considered. As noted by James,[16] the *anterior internodal pathway* begins at the anterior margin of the sinus node and curves anteriorly around the superior vena cava to enter the anterior interatrial band, called *Bachmann's bundle.* Near the anterior margin of the interatrial septum, the fibers divide, with Bachmann's bundle continuing to the left atrium and the anterior internodal pathway diving inferiorly behind the aorta within the interatrial septum to enter the superior margin of the AV node. The *middle internodal tract* begins at the superior and posterior margins of the sinus node and travels behind the superior vena cava to the crest of the interatrial septum where the bulk of the fibers descends in the interatrial septum to the superior margin of the AV node. Prior to their plunge into the interatrial septum, a few of these fibers continue to the left atrium. The *posterior internodal tract* starts at the posterior margin of the sinus node and travels posteriorly around the superior vena cava and along the crista terminalis to the Eustachian ridge and then into the interatrial septum above the coronary sinus, joining the posterior portion of the AV node. The anterior and posterior tracts appear to be most constant. Some fibers from all three tracts bypass the crest of the AV node and enter its more distal segment.[2] Anderson and Becker contend that the internodal tissue is best referred to as the internodal atrial myocardium, not tract, because these investigators—along with other past and contemporary[10] anatomists—have been unable to demonstrate histologically discrete specialized tracts, only plain atrial myocardium. Although they question the alleged presence of Purkinje-like cells, they add that the absence of histological specialization does not preclude the existence of preferential functional conduction or cell types with different action potential contours.[3]

The functional basis for specialized tracts stems from several sources. First, cell types that differ electrophysiologically and anatomically do exist. Microelectrode studies have revealed the presence of atrial plateau fibers[17] that exhibit several electrophysiological characteristics differing from normal atrial myocardium. Conduction through these cells may be more rapid than through working atrial myocardium. On the basis of electron microscopic studies,[18] six different kinds of cells in the anterior and posterior internodal pathways have been distinguished. While it is quite clear that conduction velocity varies greatly in different areas of the atrial septum, and that the direction of the wavefront may alter the conduction velocity,[19] it is not clear that the atrial plateau fibers or any other cells are the basis for the more rapid conduction velocity. Rather, the latter may be related to orientation of muscle fibers, with more rapid propagation occurring longitudinally than transversely.[20]

Differential sensitivity of atrial fibers to potassium, giving rise to an apparent sinoventricular rhythm (i.e., impulse propagation from the sinus node to the ventricle without activating atrial myocardium),[21] and activation changes following localized surgical lesions designed to interrupt discrete pathways[22] provide further functional data to support the presence of specialized tracts. Studies involving apparent sinoventricular rhythm may be questioned on two accounts: (1) some of the examples of apparent sinoventricular conduction may actually have showed AV dissociation (i.e., the sinus impulse did not propagate to the ventricle but fortuitously had a similar rate and rhythm); and (2) loss of the P wave on the surface ECG does not rule out slow conduction through nonspecialized atrial muscle fibers. In some of the surgical studies, cuts may have been extensive enough to alter conduction through normal atrial myocardium.[20] Using multiple extracellular measurements, Spach et al.[23] concluded that the entire atrial septum conducted impulses from the sinus to the AV node and that no functional evidence existed for narrow, specialized internodal tracts of fixed location. A similar conclusion was reached by Janse and Anderson.[24] Thus, the issue is not entirely settled,[25] but the *weight of evidence does not support the presence of specialized internodal tracts resembling the bundle branches, i.e., discrete histologically identifiable tracts of tissue.*[10] However, preferential internodal conduction, i.e., more rapid conduction velocity between the nodes in some parts of the atrium compared to other parts probably does exist and may be due to fiber orientation, size, geometry, or other factors rather than to specialized tracts located between the nodes.

Interatrial Conduction. *Bachmann's bundle,* a large muscle bundle beginning along the anterior internodal pathway and traveling posteriorly around the aorta to the left atrium, appears to conduct the cardiac impulse preferentially from right to left atrium.[26] Supernormal conduction (see p. 249) has been demonstrated in Bachmann's bundle of the canine heart.[27] The middle and posterior internodal tracts may also extend fibers to the left atrium, but little is known about their anatomical or functional importance.[2]

The Atrioventricular Junctional Area (Fig. 19–2). The normal AV junctional area can be divided into distinct regions: transitional cell zone,[28] also called nodal approaches[29]; compact portion, or the AV node itself, corresponding to the "Knotenpunkten" described by Tawara[28]; and the penetrating part of the AV bundle (His bundle), which continues as nonbranching portion. Some investigators consider the branching portion of the AV bundle (i.e., the bundle branches) to be part of the AV junctional area anatomically,[28] while others,[29] relying more on electrophysiological function, separate the branching from the nonbranching portion.

Transitional Cell Zone, or Nodal Approaches. In the rabbit AV node, these are located in posterior, superficial and deep groups of cells. They differ histologically from atrial myocardium and connect the latter with the compact portion of the AV node. James[30] described some fibers passing from the posterior internodal tract to the distal portion of the AV node or His bundle that may provide the anatomical substrate for a bypass tract. However, the anatomical[28] and functional[24,31] importance of this structure is unclear (see p. 628).

The AV Node. The compact portion of the AV node is a superficial structure, lying just beneath the right atrial endocardium, anterior to the ostium of the coronary sinus, and directly above the insertion of the septal leaflet of the tricuspid valve. It is at the apex of a triangle formed by the tricuspid annulus and the tendon of Todaro, which originates in the central fibrous body, and passes posteriorly through the atrial septum to continue with the Eustachian valve (Fig. 19–2). The compact portion of the AV node is divided from and becomes the penetrating portion of the His bundle at the point where it enters the central fibrous body. In 85 to 90 per cent of human hearts, the arterial supply to the AV node is a branch from the right coronary artery that originates at the posterior intersection of the AV and interventricular grooves (crux). A branch of the circumflex coronary artery provides the AV nodal artery in the remaining hearts.[4]

The Bundle of His, or Penetrating Portion of the AV Bundle. This connects with the distal part of the compact AV node and perforates the central fibrous body, continuing through the annulus fibrosis, where it is called the nonbranching portion as its penetrates the membranous septum. Proximal cells of the penetrating portion are heterogeneous, resembling those of the compact AV node, while distal cells are similar to cells in the proximal bundle branches. Connective tissue of the central fibrous body and membranous septum encloses the penetrating portion of the AV bundle, which may send out extensions into the central fibrous body. However, large well-formed fasciculo-ventricular connections between the penetrating portion of the AV bundle and the ventricular septal crest are rarely found in adult hearts.[28] Branches from the anterior and posterior descending coronary arteries supply the upper muscular interventricular septum with blood, making the conduction system at this site more impervious to ischemic damage unless the damage is extensive.[2]

The Bundle Branches, or Branching Portion of the AV Bundle. These structures begin at the superior margin of the muscular interventricular septum, immediately beneath the membranous septum, with the cells of the left bundle branch cascading downward as a continuous sheet onto the septum beneath the noncoronary aortic cusp (Fig. 19–2). The AV bundle then may give off other left bundle

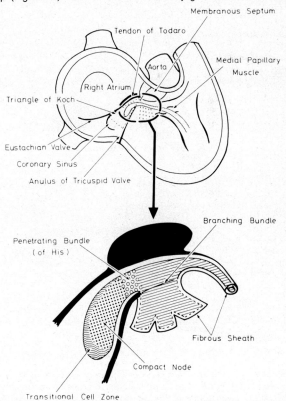

FIGURE 19–2 Schematic display of the atrioventricular junctional area. The area bounded by the dark circle in the top panel has been enlarged in the bottom panel, in which the central fibrous body (dark cap) overlies the AV node–His bundle. (See text for explanation.) (From Becker, A. E., et al.: Functional anatomy of the cardiac conduction system. *In* Harrison, D. C. (ed.): Cardiac Arrhythmias: A Decade of Progress. Boston, G. K. Hall, 1981.)

branches, sometimes constituting a true bifascicular system with an anterosuperior branch, in other hearts giving rise to a group of central fibers, and in still others appearing more as a network without a clear division into a fascicular system.[32] The right bundle branch continues intramyocardially as an unbranched extension of the AV bundle down the right side of the interventricular septum. In some hearts, the right bundle branch forms an obtuse angle with the His bundle.[33] It generally remains unbranched to the apex of the right ventricle and base of the anterior papillary muscle. In some human hearts, the His bundle traverses the right interventricular crest, giving rise to a right-sided narrow stem origin of the left bundle branch.[33] Clearly the anatomy of the left bundle branch system may be variable and may not conform to a constant bifascicular division represented as anterosuperior (thin) and posteroinferior (broad) fascicles. However, in spite of these anatomical variabilities, the concept of a trifascicular system remains useful[34] to both the electrocardiographer and the clinician.

Terminal Purkinje Fibers. These fibers connect with the ends of the bundle branches to form interweaving networks on the endocardial surface of both ventricles that transmit the cardiac impulse almost simultaneously to the entire right and left ventricular endocardial surfaces. Purkinje fibers tend to be less concentrated at the base of the ventricle and at the papillary muscle tips. They penetrate the myocardium for varying distances depending on the animal species; in man, they apparently penetrate only the inner third of the endocardium, while in the pig they almost reach the epicardium. Such variations could influence changes produced by myocardial ischemia, for example, since Purkinje fibers appear more resistant to ischemia than are ordinary myocardial fibers.[35]

Cellular Composition of the AV Junctional Area. Transitional cells are elongated, smaller than atrial cells, stain more palely, and

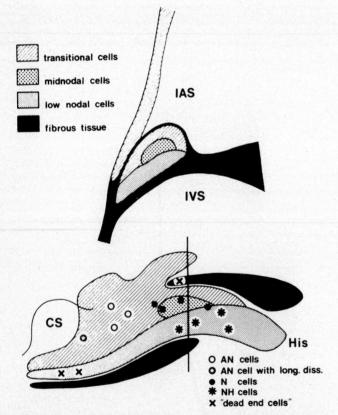

FIGURE 19–3 Diagram showing distribution of morphologically different cell types in AV node. *Upper panel,* Transverse section showing trilaminar appearance of the interior part of the node. The level of sectioning is indicated by the vertical dark line in the lower panel. *Lower panel,* Diagram of the AV node indicating the different sites identified histologically after recording typical action potentials. (From Janse, M. J., et al.: Electrophysiology and structure of the atrioventricular node of the isolated rabbit heart. *In* Wellens, J. H. H., et al. (eds.): The Conduction System of the Heart. Philadelphia, Lea and Febiger, 1976, p. 296.)

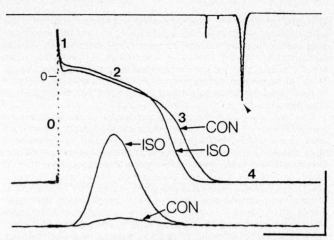

FIGURE 19–4 Recordings of canine Purkinje fiber action potential and developed tension before and during isoproterenol administration. Tracings from above downward show upstroke velocity of phase 0 (Vmax, arrowhead), action potential configuration of Purkinje fiber, and developed tension in the Purkinje fiber bundle during control (CON) and after exposure to isoproterenol (ISO, 0.1 ml/ 10^{-5} M, added directly to the tissue bath). The five phases of the action potential are indicated by the large numerals. The short horizontal line to the left with a zero near the peak of the action potential indicates the zero voltage potential. Vertical calibration: 400 V/sec for Vmax/sec, 50 mV for action potential amplitude, and 400 mg for the developed tension, respectively. Horizontal calibration: 4 msec for the upper record and 100 msec for the middle and lower records. (V = volts; mV = millivolts; msec = milliseconds.) Isoproterenol increased plateau height of the action potential and developed tension and decreased action potential duration during the terminal phase of repolarization, without significantly affecting resting membrane potential or phase 0. (From Gilmour, R. F., Jr., and Zipes, D. P.: Basic electrophysiology of the slow inward current. *In* Antman, E., and Stone, P. (eds.): Calcium Blocking Agents in the Treatment of Cardiovascular Disorders. Mt. Kisco, N.Y., Futura Publ. Co. Inc., in press.)

are separated by numerous strands of connective tissue.[36] These cells merge at the entrance of the compact portion of the AV node, which in the rabbit is surrounded by a fibrous collar that is a posterior extension of the central fibrous body. Tightly packed midnodal cells in the compact portion of the AV node are small and spherical, are not separated by muscle or connective tissue, and have very few nexuses. They interweave in interconnecting whorls of fasciculi. A group of lower nodal cells underlies the midnodal grouping and is continuous with the His bundle.[36] As will be discussed later in greater detail, the AV node is divided, based on electrophysiological characteristics, into AN, N, and NH regions[37] (Fig. 19–3). In the rabbit, the AN region corresponds to the transitional cell groups of the posterior portion of the node, the NH region to the anterior portion of the bundle of lower nodal cells, and the N region to the small enclosed node where transitional cells merge with midnodal cells. Cellular morphology alone clearly does not determine the functional characteristics of these cells, which are influenced by the overall nodal architecture as well as by the nature and direction of the excitatory wavefront. Dead-end pathways—groups of cells that form an apparent electrophysiological cul-de-sac that does not contribute to overall conduction in the node—are also found at several sites.[38] Cells in the penetrating bundle remain similar to compact AV nodal cells.

Purkinje cells are found in the His bundle and bundle branches and cover much of the endocardium of both ventricles. In the His bundle and bundle branches, Purkinje cells align to form multicellular bundles in longitudinal strands separated by collagen. They are large, clear cells (10 to 30 μm in diameter, 20 to 50 μm long) with loosely arrayed mitochondria distributed between few linearly aligned myofibrils that have few myofilaments. Round nuclei occupy the center of the cell. Although conduction of the cardiac impulse appears to be their major function, it is quite clear that free-running Purkinje fibers, sometimes called false tendons, which are composed of many Purkinje cells in a series, are capable of contraction (Fig. 19–4). While also exhibiting side-to-side connections, the major intercellular connection of Purkinje fibers is end-to-end through well-developed intercalated discs[2] (see p. 610) that may facilitate rapid longitudinal conduction.[39]

Innervation. The AV node and His bundle region are innervated by a rich supply of cholinergic and adrenergic fibers with a density exceeding that found in the ventricular myocardium.[11] Ganglia, nerve fibers, and nerve nets lie close to the AV node. Parasympathetic ganglia appear to be concentrated at the posterior margin of the AV node, between it and the anterior wall of the coronary sinus.[40] Nerves in direct contact with AV nodal fibers have been noted,[41] along with agranular and granular vesicular processes, presumably representing cholinergic and adrenergic processes.[41] Neural innervation of the AV node significantly influences conduction and refractoriness. Vagal stimulation prolongs while sympathetic stimulation shortens AV nodal conduction time and refractoriness. However, both sympathetic[42] and vagal stimulation[13] exert minimal effects on the His-Purkinje conduction time or refractoriness.

Most efferent sympathetic impulses reach the canine ventricles over the ansae subclaviae, which are branches from the stellate ganglia. Sympathetic impulses then synapse primarily in the caudal cervical ganglia and form individual cardiac nerves that are distributed to innervate relatively localized parts of the ventricles. On the right side, the major route is the recurrent cardiac nerve and, on the left, the ventrolateral cardiac nerve. The right sympathetic chain affects refractoriness primarily of the anterior portion of the ventricles while the left affects primarily the posterior surface of the ventricles,[43] although overlapping areas of distribution occur. Randall,[44] measuring contractile responses, and Kralios et al.,[45] measuring refractory period responses, have mapped the distribution of efferent cardiac sympathetic nerves to fairly localized parts of the ventricles.

The intraventricular route of sympathetic nerves generally follows coronary arteries in a base-to-apex direction. Functional data suggest that these nerves travel in the superficial layers of the epicardium and dive to innervate the endocardium.[46] According to recent evidence sympathetic afferent fibers may also be located in the epicardium of the left ventricle.[47]

Sympathetic innervation significantly influences ventricular electrophysiological properties. Stimulation of sympathetic ganglia shortens the refractory period equally in the epicardium and underlying endocardium of the left ventricular free wall,[48] although dispersion of recovery properties occurs, i.e., different degrees of shortening of refractoriness occurs when measured over an 8-mm area in the epicardium.[49] Nonuniform distribution of norepinephrine may, in part, contribute to some of the nonuniform electrophysiological effects following sympathetic neural stimulation, since the ventricular content of norepinephrine, for example, is greater at the base than at the apex of the heart,[50] with greater distribution to muscle than to Purkinje fibers.[51]

The long-disputed question of whether the vagus exerted any measurable effect on ventricular tissue is no longer in doubt. Acetylcholinesterase,[52] choline acetyltransferase (the enzyme that catalyzes the production of acetylcholine in parasympathetic nerves),[53] acetylcholine,[54] and cholinergic receptors[55] have been demonstrated in the ventricular myocardium of various species. Cholinergic effects on contractile[56] and electrophysiological[46,48,57] properties have been conclusively established. However, it is still not certain whether the vagus exerts a direct[58] or an indirect[46,48] effect on ventricular myocardium by modulating sympathetic influences. Vagal stimulation in the dog prolongs the refractory period equally in the epicardium and underlying endocardium.[48] In contrast to sympathetic fibers, efferent vagal nerves do not appear to travel in the superficial epicardium of the left ventricle[46] and conceivably could travel in the endocardium,[52] branching upward to innervate the epicardium.[59] Vagal afferents, preferentially located in the distribution supplied by the left circumflex coronary artery,[60] also do not appear to travel in the superficial epicardium.[47]

BASIC ELECTROPHYSIOLOGICAL PRINCIPLES

CELL MEMBRANE (SARCOLEMMA). The cell membrane constitutes a bilayer boundary of phospholipid molecules (Fig. 19–5). The tail end of the phospholipid molecules is nonpolar and hydrophobic, pointing toward the center of the membrane, while the head end is polar and hydrophilic, pointing toward the outer and inner layers of the membrane, in contact with the aqueous extracellular and intracellular environment. The sarcolemma, particularly the hydrophobic core, provides a high-resistance, insulated wrapping around the cell that exhibits selective permeability to ions—a property responsible for creating an electrical potential across the cell membrane.[61] Ions are positively (cations) or negatively (anions) charged atoms such as Na, K, Ca, or Cl and other molecules whose movement inside the cell or across the cell membrane constitutes a flow of current. It is the flow of current that generates signals in excitable membranes. At rest, the resistance to ion flow is greater across the cell membrane than in the cytoplasm of the cell interior. The cell membrane has openings called channels that serve as conduits through which ions move.[62] The different protein or phospholipoprotein channels are selective, favoring passage

Figure 19–5 Membrane model showing proteins embedded in the phospholipid bilayer. Proteins that span the entire bilayer can serve as ion channels by providing a hydrophilic environment through which the ions can traverse the hydrophilic phospholipid bilayer. (From Singer, S. J.: Architecture and topography of biologic membranes. *In* Weissman, G., and Clairborne, R. (eds.): Cell Membranes, Biochemistry, Cell Biology, and Pathology. New York, HP Publishing Co., 1975, pp. 35–44.)

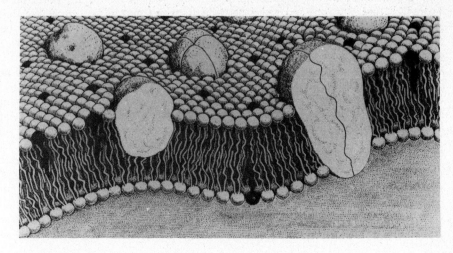

TABLE 19–1 INTRACELLULAR AND EXTRACELLULAR ION CONCENTRATIONS IN CARDIAC MUSCLE

Ion	Extracellular Concentration	Intracellular Concentration	Ratio of Extracellular to Intracellular Concentration	E_i
Na	145 mM	15 mM	9.7	+60 mV
K	4 mM	150 mM	0.027	−94 mV
Cl	120 mM	5 mM	24	−83 mV
Ca	2 mM	10^{-7} M	2×10^4	+129 mV

E_i = equilibrium potential for a particular ion.

Although intracellular Ca content is about 2 mmol/kg, most of this is bound or sequestered in intracellular organelles (mitochondria and sarcoplasmic reticulum. For the same reason, the actual free Na concentration may be less. Intracellular Cl concentration depends on the average membrane potential, if Cl is passively distributed, and therefore on heart rate.

From Sperelakis, N.: Origin of the cardiac resting potential. *In* Berne, R. M., et al. (eds.): Handbook of Physiology, The Cardiovascular System, Bethesda, Maryland, American Physiological Society, 1979, p.190.

of one ion over another. In contrast to the membrane lipids, which act primarily as inert barriers, membrane proteins appear to be responsible for most of the known biological activities of membranes.[61] Gates, influenced by the electric field and by time, control ion movement through the channels and, when opened or closed, permit or prevent ion travel, respectively.

In addition to the channels, other protein complexes serve as a major supplementary transport system through the cell membrane and provide for neutral exchange of some ions and small organic molecules along their concentration gradients (passive ion transport) and for transporting ions against their electrochemical energy gradients (active ion transport).[63,64] Some protein complexes penetrate only the outer cell membrane and may serve as receptor sites for neurotransmitters and hormones, while others, such as the adenylate cyclase system, protrude through the inner cell membrane and may be involved in various enzymatic activities. Protein molecules protruding through the entire cell membrane, such as the Na-K pump, may help regulate the ionic fluxes that determine the electrical status of the resting and excited membrane.[61,65] The Na-K pump requires adenosine triphosphate (ATP) to extrude intracellular Na against its concentration and electrical gradients and to move K intracellularly, against its concentration gradient, resulting in high concentrations of K inside and of Na outside the cell (Table 19–1). Membrane proteins are considered to be "floating," moving from one area of the membrane to another.

The cell membranes of some types of adjacent cells form close margins called *intercalated discs* (p. 410). Three types of specialized junctions make up each intercalated disc. The macula adherens or desmosome and fascia adherens form the areas of strong adhesions between cells and may provide a linkage for the transfer of mechanical energy from one cell to the next. The *nexus*, also called tight or gap junction, is a region in the intercalated disc where cells are in functional contact with each other. Membranes at these junctions are separated by only about 20 Å and are connected by a series of hexagonally packed subunit bridges. Nexuses probably provide low-resistance electrical coupling between adjacent cells[39,66,67] at their longitudinal ends. Nexuses also occur along the sides of cells, connecting lateral surfaces. The nexuses may form water-filled channels complexed with protein units that allow movement of ions and perhaps of small molecules between cells.[64] They link interiors of adjacent cells and are stable in their open state, closing when intracellular calcium rises.[61] When intracellular calcium rises, as in infarction, the nexus

may close to help "seal off" the effects of injured from noninjured cells.

In ventricular muscle cells, but apparently not in atrial or His-Purkinje cells, the cell membrane invaginates to form a transverse tubular system that introduces the cell membrane and extracellular space deep into the cells (Fig. 12–3, p. 412). Because of reduced diffusion in that space, ions, metabolites, or other constituents may be present in greater or lower concentrations than are found intra- or extracellularly. Such surface scalloping can greatly increase the surface area of the ventricular cell.

ELECTRICAL BASIS OF THE CARDIAC ACTION POTENTIAL.[65,68] The cardiac transmembrane potential consists of five phases: phase 0—the upstroke or rapid depolarization; phase 1—early rapid repolarization; phase 2—plateau; phase 3—final rapid repolarization; phase 4—resting membrane potential and diastolic depolarization (Fig. 19–4). These phases are the result of ion fluxes that are passive: ions move down electrochemical gradients established by active ion pumps and exchange mechanisms. Each ion moves primarily through its own ion-specific channel.[61] The following discussion will be clinically oriented, explaining the electrogenesis of each of these phases. For an in-depth discussion, the reader is referred to other reference sources.[69]

PHASES OF THE CARDIAC ACTION POTENTIAL

The Resting Membrane Potential. Intracellular electrical activity can be recorded by inserting a glass microelectrode with a tip diameter less than 0.5 μm into a single cell. The electrode produces minimal damage, its entry point apparently being sealed by the cell. The transmembrane potential is recorded using this electrode in reference to an extracellular ground electrode placed in the tissue bath near the cell membrane and represents the potential difference between intracellular and extracellular voltages (Fig. 19–6).

Intracellular potential during electrical quiescence in diastole is −50 to −95 mV, depending on the cell type (Table 19–2). This means that the inside of the cell is 50 to 95 mV negative relative to the outside of the cell owing to the distribution of ions such as K, Na, Cl, and Ca across the cell membrane.[64,65,70]

K is the major ion determining the resting potential. During diastole the cell membrane is quite permeable to K and relatively impermeable to Na. Because of the Na-K pump, which pumps Na out of the cell against its electrochemical gradient and simultaneously pumps K into the cell against its chemical gradient, intracellular K concen-

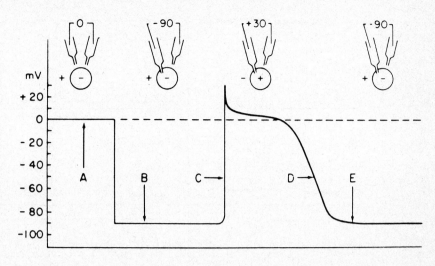

FIGURE 19–6 Demonstration of action potentials recorded during impalement of a cardiac cell. The upper row of diagrams shows a cell (circle), two microelectrodes, and stages during impalement of the cell and its activation and recovery. *A,* Both microelectrodes are extracellular, and no difference in potential exists between them (0 potential). The environment inside the cell is negative and the outside is positive, since the cell is polarized. *B,* One microelectrode has pierced the cell membrane to record the intracellular resting membrane potential, which is −90 mV with respect to the outside of the cell. *C,* The cell has depolarized and the upstroke of the action potential is recorded. At its peak voltage, the inside of the cell is about +30 mV with respect to the outside of the cell. *D,* Phase of repolarization, returning the membrane to its former resting potential (*E*). (From Cranefield, P. F.: The Conduction of the Cardiac Impulse. Mt. Kisco, N.Y., Futura Publ. Co. Inc., 1975.)

tration remains high and intracellular Na concentration remains low. This pump, fueled by an Na,K-ATPase enzyme that hydrolyzes ATP for energy, is bound to the membrane. It requires both Na and K to function and can transport three Na ions outward for two K ions inward. Therefore, the pump can be electrogenic, generating a net outward movement of positive charges.[71] The rate of Na-K pumping to maintain the same ionic gradients must increase as heart rate increases, since the cell gains a slight amount of Na and loses a slight amount of K with each depolarization. Heart rate becomes important when we consider the electrophysiological basis of some types of digitalis-induced cardiac arrhythmias, because cardiac glycosides block this pump.

Little Na, in spite of its concentration gradient, can diffuse into the cell, owing to the relative impermeability of the polarized cell membrane to Na. However, K can diffuse freely out of the cell down its concentration gradient, and does so, removing with it a positive charge and leaving the inside of the cell more negative. Negative intracellular charges, presumably due to large polyvalent ions such as proteins, do not cross the membrane and help maintain intracellular negativity. K continues to leave the cell until the forces driving it down its concentration gradient are balanced by the negative intracellular electrical charges that attract K back into the cell. The transmembrane voltage at which the electrical gradient is equal and opposite to the concentration gradient, so that the algebraic sum of these two passive forces equals zero, is the K electrochemical equilibrium potential, E_k, and is described by the Nernst equation

$$E_k = \frac{RT}{F} \ln \frac{[K]_o}{[K]_i} \tag{1}$$

where R is the gas constant, T is the absolute temperature, F is the Faraday number, ln is the logarithm to the base E, $[K]_o$ is the extracellular K concentration and $[K]_i$ the intracellular K concentration.[72]

Solving this equation predicts a transmembrane voltage of about −96 mV in cardiac muscle, which is very near the observed voltages. However, certain factors make the equation an approximation. Because the $[K]_o/[K]_i$ ratio primarily determines transmembrane voltage, the cell membrane is said to behave as a K electrode during diastole, and more closely follows the values predicted by the Nernst equation at $[K]_o$ greater than 10 mM. When $[K]_o$ is reduced, membrane permeability to K also decreases, the small inward movement of Na, negligible at high $[K]_o$, becomes more important, and the actual resting membrane voltage becomes less than that predicted by the Nernst equation for a K electrode.[73] The difference between predicted and observed voltages increases as $[K]_o$ is reduced further. The contribution of the minimal inward movement of Na to the resting membrane potential can be incorporated into an equation called the Goldman constant-field equation[74] and is a slight modification of the Nernst equation. If one assumes that the membrane is permeable to only Na and K, the resting membrane potential (V_r) would be

$$V_r = \frac{RT}{F} \ln \frac{[K]_o + P_{Na}/P_K [Na]_o}{[K]_i + P_{Na}/P_K [Na]_i} \tag{2}$$

where P_{Na}/P_K is the ratio of the sodium to the potassium permeability coefficient of the cell membrane, $[Na]_o$ is the extracellular sodium concentration, and $[Na]_i$ is the intracellular sodium concentration. The equation can be modified further to include the minimal contributions of other ions.

Calcium contributes little to the resting membrane potential, although changes in Ca concentration can affect the permeability of the cell membrane to other ions. An increase in $[Ca]_i$ increases potassium conductance. Ca is handled by several mechanisms, including uptake by the sarcoplasmic reticulum. Also, there appears to be a passive transarcolemmal Ca-Na exchange reaction.[75,76] This ex-

TABLE 19–2   PROPERTIES OF TRANSMEMBRANE POTENTIALS IN MAMMALIAN HEARTS

	SINUS NODAL CELL	ATRIAL MUSCLE CELL	AV NODAL CELL	PURKINJE FIBER	VENTRICULAR MUSCLE CELL
Resting potential (mV)	−50 to −60	−80 to −90	−60 to −70	−90 to −95	−80 to −90
Action potential					
Amplitude (mV)	60 to 70	110 to 120	70 to 80	120	110 to 120
Overshoot (mV)	0 to 10	30	5 to 15	30	30
Duration (msec)	100 to 300	100 to 300	100 to 300	300 to 500	200 to 300
Vmax (V/S)	1 to 10	100 to 200	5 to 15	500 to 700	100 to 200
Propagation velocity (M/sec)	<0.05	0.3 to 0.4	0.1	2 to 3	0.3 to 0.4
Fiber diameter (μm)	5 to 10	10 to 15	5 to 10	100	10 to 16

Modified from Sperelakis, N.: Origin of the cardiac resting potential. *In* Berne, R. M., Sperelakis, N., and Geiger, S. R. (eds.): Handbook of Physiology, The Cardiovascular System. Bethesda, Maryland, American Physiological Society, 1979, p. 190.

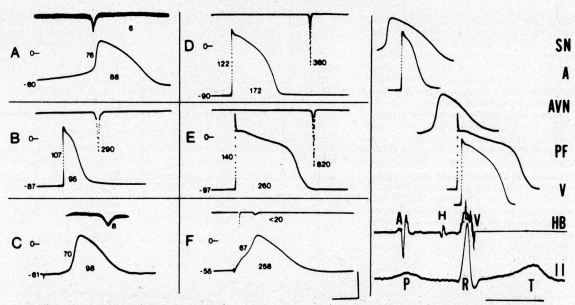

FIGURE 19–7 Action potentials recorded from different tissues in the heart (*left*), remounted along with a His bundle recording and scalar ECG from a patient (*right*) to illustrate the timing during a single cardiac cycle. In panels *A* to *F*, the top tracing is dV/dt of phase 0 and the second tracing is the action potential. For each panel, the numbers (from left to right) indicate maximum diastolic potential (mV), action potential amplitude (mV), action potential duration at 90 per cent of repolarization (msec), and Vmax of phase 0 (V/sec). Zero potential is indicated by the short horizontal line next to the zero on the upper left of each action potential. *A*, Rabbit sinoatrial node; *B*, canine atrial muscle; *C*, rabbit atrioventricular node; *D*, canine ventricular muscle; *E*, canine Purkinje fiber; *F*, diseased human ventricle. Note that the action potentials recorded in *A*, *C*, and *F* have reduced resting membrane potentials, amplitudes and Vmax compared to the other action potentials. In the right panel, SN = sinus nodal potential; A = atrial muscle potential; AVN = atrioventricular nodal potential; PF = Purkinje fiber potential; V = ventricular muscle potential; HB = His bundle recording; II = lead II. Horizontal calibration on the left: 50 msec for *A* and *C*, 100 msec for *B*, *D*, *E*, and *F*; 200 msec on the right. Vertical calibration on the left: 50 mV. Horizontal calibration on the right: 200 msec. (Modified from Gilmour, R. F., Jr., and Zipes, D. P.: Basic electrophysiology of the slow inward current. *In* Antman, E., and Stone, P. H. (eds.): Calcium Blocking Agents in the Treatment of Cardiovascular Disorders. Mt. Kisco, N.Y., Futura Publ. Co. Inc. [in press].)

change depends in part on maintenance of the Na concentration gradient by the Na-K pump (Fig. 12–2, p. 411). Under normal conditions, one internal Ca ion is probably exchanged for two or three external Na ions. Under some pathological conditions or drug actions when [Na]$_i$ is abnormally high, external Ca may be exchanged for internal Na. Cells that gain Na, in general, gain Ca—a reaction important to the genesis of some digitalis-induced arrhythmias. Further discussion about the role of calcium will be considered under the slow inward current in Chapter 21.

Phase 0—Upstroke or Rapid Depolarization. A stimulus delivered to excitable tissue evokes an action potential characterized by a sudden voltage change due to transient depolarization followed by repolarization. The action potential is conducted throughout the heart and is responsible for initiating each "heart beat." Electrical changes of the action potential follow a relatively fixed time and voltage relationship that differs according to specific cell types (Fig. 19–7). In nerve, the entire process takes several milliseconds, while action potentials in cardiac fibers last several hundred milliseconds. Normally, the action potential is independent of the size of the depolarizing stimulus, if the latter exceeds a certain threshold potential. Small subthreshold depolarizing stimuli depolarize the membrane proportional to the strength of the stimulus. However, once the stimulus is sufficiently intense to reduce membrane potential to a threshold value in the range of −70 to −65 mV for normal Purkinje fibers, more intense stimuli do not produce larger action potential responses, and an "all-or-none" response results (Fig. 19–8).

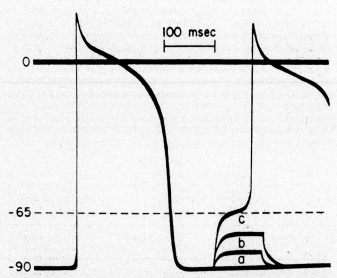

FIGURE 19–8 Excitation of a cardiac cell. The cell on the left is depolarized from −90 mV to −65 mV when the fiber is excited by any excitatory impulse that is able to reduce the resting potential to the threshold. In the panel on the right, the effects of two subthreshold stimuli, a and b, are illustrated. These do not reduce the resting membrane potential to threshold (−65 mV), and an action potential is not elicited. Stimulus c reduces the membrane potential to threshold, resulting in a regenerative action potential. (From Hoffman, B. F., and Cranefield, P. F.: Electrophysiology of the Heart. New York, McGraw-Hill Book Co., 1960.)

In contrast, hyperpolarizing pulses, i.e., stimuli that render the membrane potential more negative, elicit a response proportional to the strength of the stimulus.

The upstroke of the cardiac action potential in atrial and ventricular muscle and His-Purkinje fibers is due to a sudden increase in membrane conductance to Na. An externally applied stimulus, or a spontaneously generated local membrane circuit current in advance of a propagating action potential, depolarizes a sufficiently large area of membrane at a sufficiently rapid rate to open the Na channels and depolarize the membrane further. When the membrane voltage reaches threshold, Na rushes through ion-specific channels into the cell, down its electrochemical gradient—i.e., Na is "drawn" into the cell by the low [Na]$_i$ and the negatively charged intracellular environment. The excited membrane no longer behaves like a K electrode, i.e., exclusively permeable to K, but more closely approximates an Na electrode, and the membrane moves toward the Na equilibrium potential. The rate at which depolarization occurs during phase 0, i.e., the maximum rate of change of voltage over time, is indicated by the expression dV/dt max or $\dot{V}$max (Table 19–2), which is a measure of the rate and magnitude of Na entry into the cell and a determinant of conduction velocity for the propagated action potential.[77] The transient increase in sodium conductance lasts 1 to 2 msec. The action potential, or more properly the Na current, is said to be regenerative; that is, intracellular movement of a little Na depolarizes the membrane more, which increases conductance to Na more, which allows more Na to enter, and so on. As this is occurring, however, [Na]$_i$ and positive intracellular charges increase and reduce the driving force for Na. When the equilibrium potential (E_{Na}) for Na is reached, Na no longer enters the cell, i.e., when the driving force acting on the ion is

zero, no current will flow. In addition, Na conductance is time-dependent so that when the membrane spends some time at voltages less negative than the resting potential, Na conductance decreases. Therefore, an intervention that reduces membrane potential for a period of time—but not to threshold—partially inactivates Na channels, so that if threshold is now achieved, the magnitude and rate of Na influx are reduced.

At this point, several concepts need to be expanded. Ohm's law states that voltage equals current times resistance. The term conductance (g) is the inverse or reciprocal of resistance and is related to the ease with which ions can cross the cell membrane when driven by a potential difference across the membrane. As resistance of the membrane to passage of an ion increases, conductance decreases. Membrane permeability or conductance of the Na channel during phase 0 is regulated by two types of gates, the "m" gate and the "h" gate, which modulate Na ion passage through the channel (Fig. 19–9). This model of a gated system[78] stems from voltage clamp studies on the squid giant axon during which the voltage across a cell membrane is held constant ("clamped") at a fixed value, e.g., −50 mV, by injecting current into the fiber via a negative feedback amplifier system. The current required by the feedback system to maintain a given voltage should be equal and opposite to the currents flowing across the cell membrane in response to the voltage step. Ions carrying the current can be identified by several means, such as by varying the ionic composition of the superfusing fluid, by using compounds that block a particular channel, and by altering the stimulating sequence of the preparation.

THE GATED SYSTEM MODEL. In this model, three m (activation) gates and one h (inactivation) gate can be considered to be lined up in series in the membrane Na channel (Fig. 19–9), with

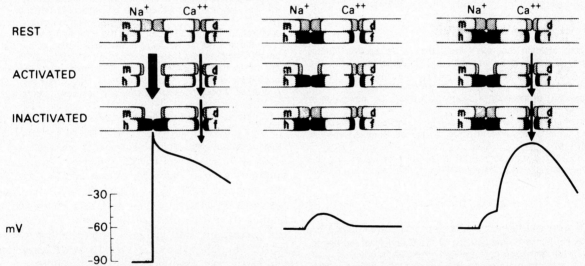

FIGURE 19–9 Schematic representation of membrane channels for rapid and slow inward currents at resting membrane potential (*top row*), during the activated state (*middle row*), and during the inactivated state (*bottom row*). Vertically separated panels depict fibers with a normal resting potential of −90 mV (*left*), with resting membrane potential reduced to less than −60 mV (*middle*), and after stimulation of the cell with catecholamine (*right*). The activation (m) and inactivation (h) gates of the fast channel and the activation (d) and inactivation (f) gates of the slow channel are depicted.

During the resting state (*left panel*), the activation gates of both channels are closed while the inactivation gates are open. When the cell is stimulated, the m gates of the fast channel open, and for a brief period of time, the open m gates and h gates allow inward sodium current to flow, depolarize the cell, and produce its upstroke. The action potential is depicted below. The h gates then close the channel and inactivate sodium conductance. When the upstroke of the action potential exceeds the threshold for activation of the slow inward current, the d gates open, allowing ingress of the slow inward current that contributes to the plateau phase of the action potential. The f gates of the slow channel close more slowly than the h gates. Although the slow inward channel remains open longer than does the fast channel, less total current flows.

When the resting membrane potential is reduced below −60 mV by increasing [K]$_o$ from 4.0 to 14.0 mm (*middle panel*), the cell depolarizes to −60 mV and the fast channel becomes inactivated because the h gates remain closed. Even though the m gate may open during activation, the amount of sodium current is too small to elicit an action potential. The inactivation gates of the slow channel (f gates) are only partially closed, and when the cell is excited after addition of catecholamine (*right panel*), the d gates open and permit flow of a slow inward current that causes a slow-response action potential. This action potential resembles those in panels *A, C,* and *F* of Figure 19–7. (From Wit, A. L., and Bigger, J. T., Jr.: Possible electrophysiological mechanisms for lethal arrhythmias accompanying myocardial ischemia and infarction. Circulation *52*(Suppl. III):96, 1975. By permission of the American Heart Association, Inc.)

the m gate on the extracellular side and the h gate on the intracellular side of the membrane. When the membrane is in a resting polarized state, the m gates are almost completely closed, the h gate is open, and no Na can cross the membrane. Although depolarization of the membrane opens the m gates and closes the h gate, the m gates open faster then the h gate closes, i.e., activation of the channel proceeds faster than inactivation can occur, and Na flows through the Na channel for about 1 msec while both gates are open simultaneously. When the membrane repolarizes to fairly high negative values, i.e., membrane potential becomes more negative than about −60 mV, the m gates shut rapidly, the h gate opens more slowly (reactivation or recovery from inactivation), and the membrane is once again capable of depolarization. Until that time, the cell is absolutely refractory, i.e., no stimulus, regardless of intensity, can activate the cell. If the membrane is activated a second time before reaching a large negative value, all the h gates have not yet reopened, so that the maximum number of Na channels that can open is reduced.[77] The resulting action potential will have reduced $\dot{V}$max, amplitude, duration, and conduction velocity (Fig. 19–10). The state of the gates at any time depends on the membrane potential and the length of time the potential has been maintained.

Using the model described above, the amount of current (I) generated by a specific ion (I_i) equals the membrane conductance for the ion (g_i) multiplied by the driving force for that ion. The driving force is the difference between the actual membrane voltage (V_m) and the equilibrium potential for that ion (E_i). Thus,

$$I_i = g_i(V_m - E_i) \qquad (3)$$

Conductance can be determined by rearranging the equation:

$$g_i = \frac{I_i}{(V_m - E_i)} \qquad (4)$$

The equations indicate that the current flow is voltage-dependent, i.e., as the voltage of the membrane (V_m) changes relative to the equilibrium potential (E_i), the electrical driving force for an ion ($V_m - E_i$) changes and so does the current. The relationship between membrane voltage, V_m, at the time of depolarization, and I_{Na}, measured in terms of $\dot{V}$max (maximum rate of rise of phase 0), is indicated by the so-called membrane responsiveness curve. Depolarization results in decreased I_{Na} and $\dot{V}$max when it occurs at reduced membrane potentials (Fig. 19–10).

Membrane voltage may also regulate current flow by altering the status of the channel gates, thereby altering conductance. For the Na channel,

$$g_{i_{Na}} = \bar{g}_{Na} M^3 h \qquad (5)$$

where $g_{i_{Na}}$ is the conductance of the Na channel at a given voltage, $\bar{g}_{Na}$ is the maximum possible conductance of the channel, m^3 represents the status of the activation gate (m = 1, the gate is open; m = 0, the gate is closed) and h represents the status of the inactivation gate (h = 1, gate open; h = 0, gate closed). Since the opening and closing of the gates is voltage- and time-dependent, the conductance of the channel (g) will be some fraction of the maximum possible conductance ($\bar{g}_{Na}$), depending on membrane voltage and the period of time during which the membrane has been at that voltage.

ACTION POTENTIALS. In normal atrial and ventricular muscle and in the fibers in the His-Purkinje system action potentials

have very rapid upstrokes with a large $\dot{V}$max and are called "fast responses." Action potentials in the normal sinus and atrioventricular (AV) nodes have very slow upstrokes with a reduced $\dot{V}$max and are called "slow responses" (Fig. 19–7). Upstrokes of "slow responses" are mediated by a slow inward, predominantly Ca current rather than the fast inward Na current.[79,80] These potentials received the name "slow response" because the time required for activation (10 to 20 msec) and inactivation (50 to 500 msec) of the slow inward current (I_{si}) is considerably longer than that for the fast inward Na current (I_{Na}). Recovery from inactivation also takes longer. Thus, the slow channel opens (activation gates "d") and closes (inactivation gates "f") more slowly than the fast channel, remains open for a longer period of time, and requires more time following a stimulus to be reactivated (Fig. 19–9). In fact, recovery of excitability outlasts full restoration of maximum diastolic potential. This means that even though the membrane potential has returned to normal, the cell has not recovered excitability completely because the latter depends on elapse of a certain amount of time (i.e., is time-dependent) and not just on recovery of a particular membrane potential. Often called the slow Ca current, I_{si} may be carried by Na under appropriate circumstances in certain fibers. Although slow channels may be 70 to 100 times more permeable to Ca than to Na, the much greater $[Na]_o$ compared to $[Ca]_o$ may permit Na to carry as much as one-third of the I_{si}.[81,82] Other divalent cations such as barium and strontium may also carry I_{si}.

The threshold for activation of I_{si}, i.e., the voltage the cell must reach to "turn on" the slow inward current, is about −30 to −40 mV. In fast-response type fibers, I_{si} is normally activated during phase 0 by the regenerative depolarization caused by the fast sodium current. Current flows through both fast and slow channels during the latter part of the action potential upstroke.[83] However, I_{si} is much smaller than the peak Na current and therefore contributes little to the action potential until the fast Na current is inactivated, after completion of phase 0.[79,84–86] Thus, I_{si} affects mainly the plateau of action potentials recorded in atrial and ventricular muscle and His-Purkinje fibers. When the fast Na current inactivates rapidly, such as in frog ventricle, I_{si} may contribute noticeably to the peak of phase 0.[87] In addition, I_{si} can be activated and may play a prominent role in partially depolarized cells in which the fast Na channels have been inactivated, if conditions are appropriate for slow-channel activation.

Other significant differences exist between the fast and slow channels (Table 19–3). The following features are of some clinical relevance. Drugs that elevate cyclic AMP levels such as beta-adrenergic agonists, phosphodiesterase inhibitors such as theophylline and the lipid-soluble derivative of cyclic AMP, dibutyryl cyclic AMP, increase I_{si}.[88] It has been proposed[88–91] that the beta-adrenergic agonist, binding to specific sarcolemmal receptors, activates adenylate cyclase and thus increases intracellular levels of cyclic AMP. The latter activates a cyclic AMP–dependent protein kinase that phosphorylates specific membrane proteins controlling the permeability of the slow channel. This increases the conductance of I_{si}, presumably by increasing the number of slow channels available for activation. No change in the time constants of activation and inactivation of I_{si} occurs. Acetylcholine reduces I_{si} in a variety of preparations, although the mechanism(s) by which this occurs

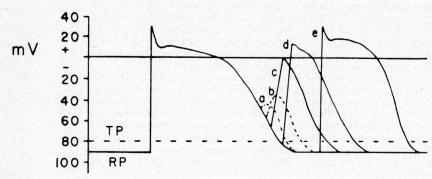

FIGURE 19–10 Schematic example of action potentials elicited during different intervals of repolarization. Late responses (e) occur after complete repolarization and produce a normal Vmax and normal conduction velocity. Earlier action potentials arise from less negative membrane potentials and result in action potentials with reduced Vmax and conduction velocity. Action potentials a and b arise from such low levels of membrane potential; they result only in a local response and do not propagate. TP= threshold potential; RP= resting potential. (From Singer, D. H., and Ten Eick, R. E.: Pharmacology of cardiac arrhythmias. Progr. Cardiovasc. Dis. *11*:488, 1969. By permission of Grune and Stratton, Inc.)

TABLE 19–3   CHARACTERISTICS OF FAST AND SLOW INWARD CURRENTS IN CARDIAC TISSUE

	FAST	SLOW
Primary charge carrier	Na	Ca (Na)
Activation threshold	−70 to −55 mV	−55 to −30 mV
Magnitude	1 to 30 μA	0.1 to 3.0 μA
Time constant of		
Activation	<1 msec	10 to 20 msec
Inactivation	<1 msec	50 to 500 msec
Inhibitors	Tetrodotoxin, local anesthetics, sustained depolarization at < −40 mV	Verapamil, D-600, nifedipine, diltiazem, Mn, Co, Ni, La
Resting membrane potential	−80 to −95 mV	−40 to −70 mV
Conduction velocity	0.3 to 3.0 M/sec	0.01 to 0.10 M/sec
Rate of rise (Vmax) of action potential upstroke	200 to 1000 V/sec	1 to 10 V/sec
Action potential amplitude	100 to 130 mV	35 to 75 mV
Response to stimulus	All-or-none	Affected by characteristics of stimulus
Recovery of excitability	Prompt, ends with repolarization	Delayed, outlasts full repolarization
Safety factor for conduction	High	Low
Major current of action potential upstroke in the following:		
SA node	−	+
Atrial myocardium	+	−
AV node (N region)	−	+
His-Purkinje system	+	−
Ventricular myocardium	+	−
Neurotransmitter influence		
Beta-adrenergic	−	↑↑
Alpha-adrenergic	−	↑(?)
Muscarinic cholinergic	−	↓ in atrium ↓ (?) in ventricle

may vary. Possibilities include a direct effect on I_{si} conductance,[92] an effect on outward K currents, and an antisympathetic effect.[86]

Fast and slow channels can be differentiated on the basis of their pharmacological sensitivity. Drugs that block the slow channel with a *fair* degree of specificity (p. 654) include verapamil, nifedipine, diltiazem, D-600 (a methoxy derivative of verapamil), and compounds like manganese, lanthanum, nickel, and cobalt. Antiarrhythmic agents such as lidocaine, quinidine, procainamide, and disopyramide (see Chap. 20) affect the fast channel and not the slow channel. The puffer fish poison, tetrodotoxin (TTX), which is too toxic to be used clinically, blocks the fast channel with considerable specificity.

While fast-response action potentials are characteristic of atrial and ventricular muscle and His-Purkinje tissue, slow-response type action potentials are found in the normal sinus and AV nodes and many kinds of diseased tissue. Normal action potentials recorded from the sinus node and the N region of the AV node have a reduced resting membrane potential, action potential amplitude, overshoot, upstroke, and conduction velocity compared to action potentials in muscle or Purkinje fibers (Fig. 19–7). Slow-channel blockers, but not TTX, suppress sinus and AV nodal action potentials.[79,93,94] The prolonged time for reactivation of the I_{si} probably accounts for the fact that these cells remain refractory longer than the time it takes

for full voltage repolarization to occur. Thus, premature stimulation immediately after the membrane potential reaches full repolarization leads to action potentials with reduced amplitudes and upstroke velocities.[95] Therefore, slow conduction and prolonged refractoriness are characteristic features of nodal cells. These cells also have a reduced "safety factor for conduction," which means that the stimulating efficacy of the propagating impulse is low and conduction block easily occurs.

These and many other observations support the conclusion that, in the *normal* heart, the I_{si} mediates not only the plateau but also the upstroke of the action potential in the sinus and AV nodes.[96,97] A small fast component, enhanced by hyperpolarization, may contribute to the slow-response upstroke of sinus nodal potentials.[94] However, the slow diastolic depolarization preceding the upstroke of sinus action potentials probably largely inactivates this fast-current component at the usual thresholds.

A variety of manipulations, including those that block or inactivate the fast inward current (such as administration of TTX or depolarization of the cell membrane with K), those that increase the slow current (such as administration of Ca or catecholamines), or those that decrease the outward potassium currents (such as barium), can transform a fast channel–dependent fiber (e.g., a Purkinje fiber) to a slow channel–dependent fiber. Whether these artificial in vitro alterations have clinical relevance is not known, but it is possible that myocardial ischemia or infarction, for example, can produce this transformation[79] (Fig. 19–7F). Current data suggest that the electrophysiological changes accompanying *acute* myocardial ischemia represent a depressed form of a fast response rather than a slow response.[98] However, probable slow-response activity has been shown in myocardium resected from patients undergoing surgery for recurrent ventricular tachyarrhythmias[99–101] (Fig. 19–11). Whether these responses play a role in the genesis of ventricular arrhythmias in these patients has not been established.

Phase 1—Early Rapid Repolarization. Following phase 0, the membrane repolarizes rapidly and transiently to near 0 mV, partly owing to inactivation of I_{Na} or activation of a transient outward current carried mostly by K ions[102] and also possibly related to Cl moving intracellularly through a Cl channel. Cl distributes itself passively according to the membrane potential. Therefore, [Cl]$_i$ is low when the membrane is polarized because of the intracellular negative environment. However, the Cl channel may open upon depolarization and permit Cl to enter the cell down its concentration gradient.[64,65,68] The increase in intracellular negative ions reduces the positive membrane voltage, and the membrane potential returns to near 0 mV, from which the plateau, or phase 2, arises. Sometimes a slight transient depolarization follows phase 1 repolarization. Phase 1 is well defined and separated from phase 2 in Purkinje fibers and some muscle fibers.

Phase 2—Plateau. During the plateau phase, which may last several hundred milliseconds, membrane conductance to all ions falls to rather low values. Potassium conductance (g_K) falls almost immediately upon depolarization, in spite of the large electrochemical gradient for K, owing to "inward-going rectification" (sometimes called "anomalous rectification," since it is opposite to that observed in the squid giant axon). This ponderous term sim-

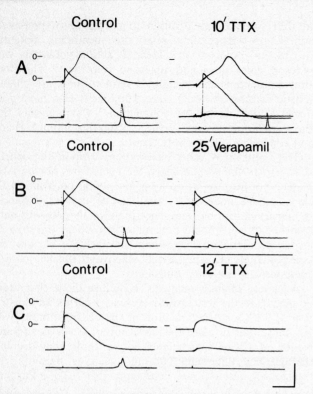

FIGURE 19–11 Effects of tetrodotoxin (TTX) and verapamil on action potentials in diseased human ventricle, removed from a patient at the time of endocardial resection for recurrent ventricular tachycardia. *A,* Action potentials and upstroke velocity recordings from an abnormal cell (upper action potential recording) and a relatively normal cell (lower action potential recording) before (*left*) and after (*right*) exposure to TTX for 10 minutes. $\dot{V}$max for the lower cell is shown in the bottom tracing. TTX produced activation delay and intermittent conduction block in the normal cell but had little effect on the action potential of the abnormal cell (right panel). Two consecutive cycles are superimposed in the right panel. *B,* After washout of TTX, the same two cells were exposed to verapamil for 25 minutes. Verapamil reduced both the action potential and the amplitude of the abnormal cell without affecting its resting membrane potential and slightly reduced both the action potential amplitude and $\dot{V}$max in the normal cell (right panel). *C,* Effects of TTX on a different specimen of myocardium from the same patient. Control recordings are shown on the left. In these cells, TTX markedly reduced action potential amplitude and $\dot{V}$max (right panel) while verapamil only slightly reduced action potential amplitude (not shown). (From Gilmour, R. F., Jr., et al.: Cellular electrophysiological abnormalities of diseased human ventricular myocardium. Am. J. Cardiol. [in press].)

ply means that the membrane passes inward current more easily than it passes outward current, or, in this instance, K can enter the cell more easily than it can exit, and therefore, in spite of at least three important outward K currents and a large electrochemical gradient, g_K is low and few K ions leave the cell. Sodium conductance (g_{Na}) is low because of inactivation of Na channels. Minor contributions to repolarization include a small inward Cl flux and electrogenic Na-K exchange, pumping out 3 Na ions in exchange for 2 K ions. The Na-K exchange does not turn on and off with each single action potential but restores the ionic gradient over a cumulative period of time. The slow inward current, active during the plateau, supplies a small inward current (compared to the Na or fast current) and balances these outward currents, and membrane voltage remains near zero for more than 100

msec.[103] A recently studied inward Na current, blocked by tetrodotoxin, also contributes to the plateau.[104]

Phase 3—Final Rapid Repolarization. In this portion of the action potential, repolarization proceeds rapidly, owing at least in part to two currents: time-dependent inactivation of the slow inward current, so that intracellular movement of positive charges decreases, and activation of an outward K current (reversal of "inward-going rectification"), so that extracellular movement of positive charges increases. The outward K current is called I_{x_1} (or I_K). The net membrane current becomes more outward, and the membrane potential shifts in a negative direction. As repolarization continues, g_K increases, and these repolarization changes self-perpetuate in a regenerative manner.

Phase 4—Resting Membrane Potential and Diastolic Depolarization. Under normal conditions, the membrane potential of atrial and ventricular muscle cells remains steady throughout diastole. Factors responsible for this resting membrane potential were described earlier. In other fibers found in certain parts of the atria, in the muscle of the mitral and tricuspid valves, in His-Purkinje fibers, and in the sinus node and distal portion of the AV node, the resting membrane potential does not remain constant in diastole but gradually depolarizes (Fig. 19–7A). If a propagating impulse does not depolarize the cell—or more likely, a group of cells—it may reach threshold by itself and produce a spontaneous action potential. The property possessed by spontaneously discharging cells is called phase 4 diastolic depolarization; when it leads to initiation of action potentials, automaticity results. The discharge rate of the sinus node normally exceeds the discharge rate of other potentially automatic pacemaker sites and thus maintains dominance of the cardiac rhythm. Normal or abnormal automaticity at other sites may discharge at rates faster than the sinus nodal discharge rate and may usurp control of the cardiac rhythm for one cycle or many. This will be discussed subsequently.

NORMAL AUTOMATICITY. The ionic basis of normal automaticity naturally must be a net gain in intracellular positive charges during diastole. This may be achieved in cardiac Purkinje fibers by a decrease in an outward K current (called the I_{K_2} or pacemaker current) while a relatively constant background current carried by Na moves intracellularly, and then a slow inward Na current depolarizes the cell to threshold.[73] The gates controlling the outward K (I_{K_2}) current open rapidly when the membrane voltage becomes more positive than −60 mV and are fully open when the membrane voltage is about 0 mV. However, because of inward-going rectification little K leaves the cell down its concentration gradient at more positive membrane potentials. As the cell repolarizes, the outward I_{K_2} current increases. After full repolarization, the I_{K_2} gates close with time (deactivate), so that when the membrane voltage is −80 to −90 mV, K cannot move extracellularly and positive ions accumulate inside the cell to produce slow diastolic depolarization. The I_{K_2} gate is not open again until the membrane potential becomes less than −60 mV, usually at the time of the next action potential. This K current does not play an important role in repolarization of the cell membrane and appears to be different from the K current (I_{K_1})—a time-independent (voltage-dependent) background current—involved in maintaining the resting potential of quiescent fibers. In summary, in Purkinje fibers there are at least three K currents: (I_{K_1}), involved in maintaining resting potential; I_{K_2}, the pacemaker current; and I_{x_1}, repolarization current.

Recently, the ionic basis of Purkinje fiber automaticity noted above has been challenged. It has been proposed that phase 4 diastolic depolarization in Purkinje fibers results primarily from activation of an inward Na current, a special pacemaker current, rather than inactivation of the outward I_{K_2} current.[105] This TTX-sensitive pacemaker current, I_F, is blocked by lidocaine and quinidine but not by procainamide.[106]

Sinus nodal cells technically do not have a "resting" membrane potential because the membrane potential continuously changes in diastole. Their maximum diastolic potential, defined as the most negative membrane potential following repolarization, is less negative than that found in atrial or ventricular muscle (Table 19–2). Since the intracellular [K] of sinus nodal cells appears similar to other cells,[107] the reduced membrane potential may be due to a higher ratio of the Na to K permeability ratio, $P_{Na/K}$. AV nodal cells also have a reduced maximum diastolic potential, possibly owing to a similar mechanism.

Diastolic depolarization in the SA node appears to result from varying degrees of inactivation of a time-dependent K current (I_{x_1} or I_k), activation of a pacemaker current (I_F), and progressive activation of the slow inward current (I_{si}). The decrease in outward K current, increase in Na influx via the pacemaker current, and Ca influx via the slow inward current gradually depolarize the cell to membrane potentials at which the slow inward current is fully activated, giving rise to the action potential upstroke.[108] Inhibitors of the slow inward current such as verapamil, D-600, and Mn^{++} suppress diastolic depolarization of the sinus node in vitro[109] and reduce the sinus nodal discharge rate in vivo.[110] TTX has little effect on diastolic depolarization of the SA node but prevents attainment of threshold in Purkinje fibers.

Whether AV nodal cells possess the property of automaticity has not been resolved. However, studies purporting to show automaticity in canine AV nodal cells have been published[111] and more recent evidence from studies of rabbit AV nodal cells suggests that they, too, exhibit automaticity.[112]

Sinus nodal discharge rate maintains dominance over latent pacemaker sites because it depolarizes more rapidly, and because of the mechanism called *overdrive suppression*.[113] This phenomenon, known since the late 19th century,[113a] refers to the observation that the escape rate of a normal pacemaker is prolonged, within certain limits, in proportion to the duration and rate of stimulation by a more rapidly discharging pacemaker[113,114] (Fig. 19–12). The mechanisms may relate to active Na extrusion that maintains diastolic depolarization of latent pacemakers to a level more negative than the threshold potential[113] and to the influence of vagal stimulation on sinus nodal discharge.

The rate of sinus nodal discharge can be varied by several mechanisms in response to autonomic or other influences. The pacemaker locus can shift within or outside[115] the sinus node to cells discharging faster or more slowly than the present rhythm. If the pacemaker site remains the same, alterations in the slope of diastolic depolarization, maximum diastolic potential, or threshold potential can speed or slow the discharge rate (Fig. 19–13). For example, if the slope of diastolic depolarization steepens and if the resting membrane potential becomes less negative or the threshold potential more negative (within limits), discharge rate increases. Opposite charges slow the discharge rate.

Passive Membrane Electrical Properties. We have just discussed many of the features of active membrane properties. In addition, it is important to be aware of some features of the passive membrane properties, such as membrane resistance, capacitance, and cable properties. The important difference between the active and passive states is that the active system responds out of propor-

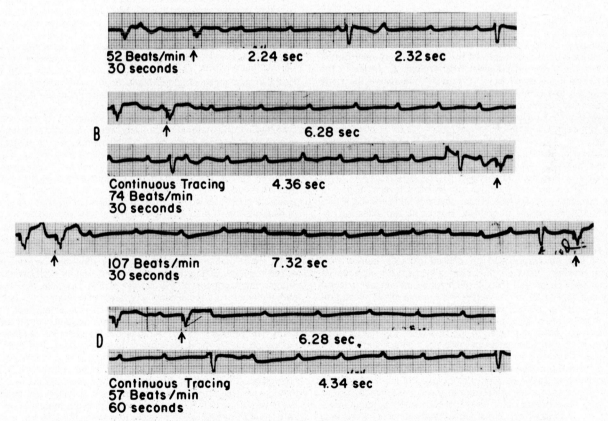

FIGURE 19–12 Overdrive suppression induced by ventricular pacing in a patient with complete AV block. The right ventricle was paced for 30 seconds at a rate of 52 bpm (A), 74 bpm (B), 107 bpm (C), and for 60 seconds at a rate of 57 bpm (D). The last two paced beats preceding termination of pacing are shown. Pacing was abruptly discontinued in each panel (first arrow) but was restarted in B and C (second arrows) because of presyncope. The interval from the last paced beat to the first idioventricular escape beat and between the first and second idioventricular escape beats is recorded in seconds below each tracing. Thus, the period of ventricular overdrive suppression occurring at termination of pacing is directly proportional—within limits—to the rate and duration of pacing. Sinus rate increases as the period of asystole progresses and, in the absence of retrograde conduction to the atria from the paced ventricular beats, it is not suppressed. (From Zipes, D. P., et al.: Artificial atrial and ventricular pacemakers in the treatment of arrhythmias. Ann. Intern. Med. *70*:885, 1969.)

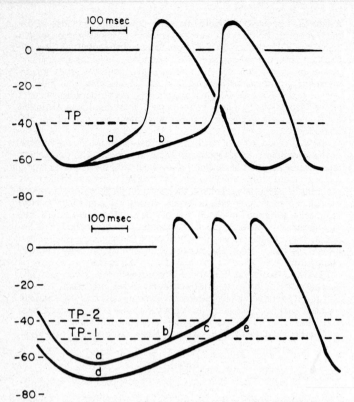

FIGURE 19–13 Significant mechanisms responsible for changes in discharge frequency of a pacemaker cell. *Top,* A decrease in the slope of phase 4 diastolic depolarization (from a to b) decreases the rate by increasing the time required for the transmembrane potential to reach the threshold potential (TP). *Bottom,* A change in the level of threshold potential from TP-1 to TP-2 increases the cycle length from a-b to a-c, and an increase in resting potential from a to d slows the discharge rate from a-c to d-e. (From Hoffman, B. F., and Cranefield, P. F.: Electrophysiology of the Heart. New York, McGraw-Hill Book Co., 1960.)

tion to the applied stimulus and thereby adds energy to the electrical system; the passive system responds proportionately to the size of the stimulus and does not add energy.[64]

Although the cardiac cell membrane is resistant to current flow, it also has capacitive properties, which means it behaves like a battery and can store charges of opposite sign on its two sides: an excess of negative charges inside the membrane balanced by equivalent positive charges outside the membrane. These resistive and capacitive charges cause the membrane to take a certain amount of time to respond to an applied stimulus, rather than responding instantly, because the charges across the capacitive membrane must be altered first. A subthreshold rectangular-shaped current pulse applied to the membrane produces a slowly rising and decaying membrane-voltage change rather than a rectangular voltage change. A value called the time constant of the membrane reflects this property and is the time taken by the membrane voltage to reach 63 per cent of its final value after application of a steady current.

When aligned end-to-end, cardiac cells, particularly the His-Purkinje system, behave like a long cable in which current flows more easily inside the cell and to the adjacent cell across the intercalated disc than it does across the cell membrane to the outside. When current is injected at a point, most of it flows along the cell but some leaks out. Because of this loss of current, the voltage change of a cell at a site distant from the point of applied current is less than the membrane-voltage change where the stimulus was given. A measure of this property of a cable is called the space or length constant (λ); it is the distance along the cable from the point of stimulation that the voltage at steady state is 1/e (37 per cent) of its value at the point of introduction. This distance is normally about 2 mm for Purkinje fibers and 0.8 mm for ventricular muscle fibers. As an example, if e is about 2.7 and a hyperpolarizing current pulse in a Purkinje fiber produces a membrane-voltage change of 15 mV at the site of current injection,

the membrane potential change one space constant (2 mm) away would be 15/2.7 = 5.5 mV.

Since the current loop in any circuit must be closed, current must flow back to its point of origin. Local circuit currents pass across nexuses between cells and exit across the sarcolemmal membrane to close the loop and complete the circuit. The outside local circuit current is the current recorded in an electrocardiogram. Through these local circuit currents the transmembrane potential of each cell influences the transmembrane potential of its neighbor because of the passive flow of current from one segment of the fiber to another across the low-resistance intercellular junctions. A cell hyperpolarized compared to its neighbor depolarizes slightly while the neighboring cell hyperpolarizes slightly. Conversely, a depolarized cell adjacent to a polarized cell polarizes slightly while the neighbor depolarizes slightly. This "electrotonic" influence of neighboring cells on each other is determined chiefly by the length constant of the fiber and is due to the passive spread of current.

As discussed earlier, the speed of conduction depends on active membrane properties such as the magnitude of the Na current, a measure of which is $\dot{V}$max. Passive membrane properties also contribute to conduction velocity and include excitability threshold,[116] which influences the capability of cells adjacent to the one that has been discharged to reach threshold; the intracellular resistance of the cell, which is determined by the free ions in the cytoplasm, the resistance of the gap junction, and the cross-sectional area of the cell.

LOSS OF MEMBRANE POTENTIAL. Most acquired abnormalities of cardiac muscle or specialized fibers that result in arrhythmias produce a loss of membrane potential, i.e., maximum diastolic potential becomes less negative.[117,118] This change should be viewed as a symptom of an underlying abnormality, like fever or jaundice, rather than a diagnostic category in and of itself, because both the ionic changes resulting in cellular depolarization and the more fundamental biochemical or metabolic abnormalities responsible for the ionic alterations are probably multicausal. Cellular depolarization can result from elevated $[K]_o$ or decreased $[K]_i$, an increase in membrane permeability to Na (P_{Na} increases), or a decrease in membrane permeability to K (P_K decreases). Reference to Equation 2 (p. 611) illustrates that these changes alone or in combination make V_r less negative. Normal cells perfused by an abnormal milieu (e.g., hyperkalemia), abnormal cells with probable membrane changes perfused by a normal milieu (e.g., healed myocardial infarction), or abnormal cells perfused by an abnormal milieu (e.g., acute myocardial ischemia and infarction) may exist alone or in combination to reduce resting membrane voltage. Each of these changes can have one or more biochemical or metabolic causes. For example, acute myocardial ischemia results in decreased $[K]_i$ and increased $[K]_o$[119,120] possibly due to reduced Na-K exchange pump activity caused by a fall in available ATP[121] as well as release of substances such as lysophosphatidylcholine.[122] Also, $[Ca]_i$ may accumulate and further reduce V_r. In the future, knowledge of the autonomic, biochemical, metabolic, or cellular changes associated with the genesis of cardiac arrhythmias may provide insight into therapy that actually reverses basic defects and restores membrane potential or other abnormalities to normal.

The reduced resting membrane potential alters depolarization and repolarization phases of the cardiac action potential. For example, partial membrane depolarization prevents attainment of the large negative potentials necessary to completely remove inactivation (h gate) of the rapid Na channel that remains from excitation in the previous cycle. The reduced number of available Na channels decreases the magnitude of the rapid Na current during phase 0. The subsequent reduction in $\dot{V}$max and action potential amplitude prolongs conduction time of the propagated impulse, at times to the point of block. Action potentials with upstrokes dependent on the rapid Na current flowing through partially inactivated Na channels are called *depressed fast responses* (Fig. 19–11*C*).[123] Their contours often resemble, and may be difficult to distinguish from, slow responses,[79,80] in which upstrokes are due to I_{si} (Fig. 19–7*F*). Membrane depolarization to levels of −60 to −70 mV may inactivate half the Na channels, while depolarization to −50 mV or less may inactivate all the Na channels. At membrane potentials positive to −50 mV, I_{si} can be activated to generate phase 0[79,80,88] if conditions are appropriate. These action potential changes are likely to be heterogeneous because of the different cardiac fibers and their different responses to a variety of interventions[35] and the heterogeneous nature of most cardiac lesions. Therefore, the degree of Na inactivation may be unequal, creating areas that conduct with minimally reduced velocity, more severely depressed zones, and areas of complete block. These uneven changes are propitious for the development of arrhythmias (Figs. 19–14 and 19–15).

Reduced membrane potential may affect action potential duration and refractory period. For example, recovery from inactivation is prolonged, because of either the depressed fast response or generation of the slow response, so that refractoriness may outlast voltage recovery of the action potential, i.e., the cell may still be refractory or partially refractory after the resting membrane potential returns to its most negative value. Further, if block of the cardiac impulse occurs in a fairly localized area without significant slowing of conduction proximal to the site of block, cells in this proximal zone exhibit short action potentials and refractory periods[124] because unexcited cells distal to the block (still in a polarized state) electrotonically speed recovery in cells proximal to the site of block. If conduction slows gradually proximal to the site of block, the duration of these action potentials and their refractory periods may be prolonged.[125]

Alterations in $[K]_o$ or $[Ca]_o$ affect the duration of action potential and refractory period as may varying levels of autonomic tone. Myocardial infarction, presumably by affecting cells directly,[126,127] or indirectly by producing metabolites[119–122] or altering autonomic tone,[128] can prolong or shorten action potential duration and refractoriness depending on the nature of the change.[129] Some cells may exhibit abnormal electrophysiological properties even though they have a relatively normal resting membrane potential. The reason for this is unclear.[100,101]

MECHANISMS OF ARRHYTHMOGENESIS. The genesis of cardiac arrhythmias is generally divided into categories of disorders of impulse formation, disorders of impulse conduction, or combinations of both.[72,130,131] Although somewhat superficial, this modified classification is still useful and will be employed in this chapter. It is important to realize, however, that our present diagnostic tools do not permit unequivocal determination of the electrophysiological mechanisms responsible for most clinically occurring arrhythmias and certainly do not allow convincing differentiation of the ionic mechanisms responsible for a particular arrhythmia. No electrocardiographic or electrophysiological criteria exist that unquestionably separate reentry from automaticity clinically nor are there tools, such as pacemakers, drugs, cardioverters, or surgery, that

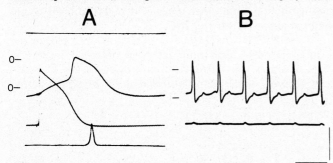

FIGURE 19–14 Unidirectional conduction in human myocardium. Action potential and upstroke velocity recordings from a cell in an abnormal area of myocardium (upper recordings) are shown during pacing in the normal myocardium at a cycle length of 1200 msec. Conduction from the normal site propagates into the abnormal site. *B* shows recordings of the same two cells in the absence of pacing, at a much slower recording speed. A spontaneously active site in the abnormal area discharges the cell being recorded in the abnormal area but fails to produce an active response in the surrounding, more normal myocardium. Only subthreshold responses are recorded. Therefore, block exists from the abnormal cell to the more normal cell (*B*) but not from the more normal cell to the abnormal cell (*A*). Vertical calibration: 50 mV and 200 V/sec. Horizontal calibration: 100 msec in *A* and 4 sec in *B*. Zero potential (short horizontal bars near peak of action potentials) is shown for both cells. (From Gilmour, R. F., Jr., et al.: Cellular electrophysiologic abnormalities of diseased human ventricular myocardium. Am. J. Cardiol. *51*:137, 1983.)

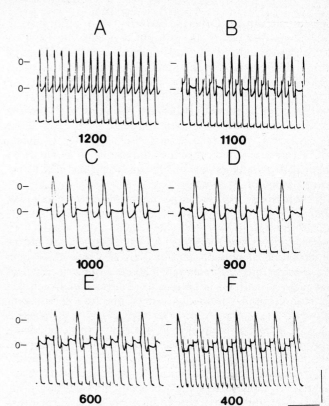

FIGURE 19–15 Rate-dependent conduction from the normal zone into the abnormal zone. Same preparation as in Figure 19–14. When the pacing cycle length in the normal zone was shortened from 1200 to 400 msec (panels A to F), increasing degrees of entrance block into the abnormal area occurred, progressing from 1:1 conduction at a cycle length of 1200 msec, to 4:3 conduction at 1100 msec, 3:2 conduction at 1000 msec, 2:1 conduction at 900 msec, 3:1 conduction at 600 msec, and 4:1 conduction at 400 msec. Vertical calibration: 50 mV. Horizontal calibration: 4 sec in *A* and *B* and 2 sec in *C* to *F*. (From Gilmour, R. F., Jr., et al.: Cellular electrophysiologic abnormalities of diseased human ventricular myocardium. Am. J. Cardiol. *51*:137, 1983.)

exert an effect specific enough to separate the two possibilities. At best, one can postulate only that a particular arrhythmia is "most consistent with" or "best explained by" one or the other electrophysiological mechanism. In the final analysis, *all* current clinical criteria established to support reentry can be mimicked by pacemaker activity and vice versa. Extracellular recordings of automatic activity (see p. 636) may allow accurate differentiation in the future. Some tachyarrhythmias may be started by one mechanism and perpetuated by another. For example, premature ventricular depolarization due to abnormal automaticity may precipitate a ventricular tachycardia sustained by reentry. Given these comments, mechanisms demonstrated to cause electrical activity in a variety of myocardial preparations will be considered and, when possible, related to clinical situations.

DISORDERS OF IMPULSE FORMATION. The category is defined as inappropriate discharge rate of the normal pacemaker, the sinus node (e.g., sinus rates too fast or too slow for the physiologic needs of the patient), or discharge from an ectopic pacemaker that controls the atrial or ventricular rhythm for one complex or more. Pacemaker discharge from ectopic sites, often called latent or subsidiary pacemakers, can occur in fibers located in several parts of the atria, the coronary sinus, atrioventricular valves, portions of the AV junction, and the His-Purkinje system. Ordinarily kept from reaching the level of threshold potential by the more rapidly firing sinus node, ectopic pacemaker activity at one of these latent sites can become manifest when sinus nodal discharge rate slows or block occurs at some level between the sinus node and the ectopic pacemaker site, permitting *escape* of the latent pacemaker at the latter's normal discharge rate. A clinical ECG correlate would be sinus bradycardia to a rate of 45 bpm that permits an AV junctional escape complex to occur at a rate of 50 bpm.

Alternatively, the discharge rate of the latent pacemaker can speed up inappropriately and usurp control of the cardiac rhythm from the sinus node that had been discharging at a normal rate. A clinical example would be interruption of normal sinus rhythm at a rate of 70 bpm by a premature ventricular complex or a burst of ventricular tachycardia. It is important to remember that such disorders of impulse formation can be due to a speeding or slowing of a *normal* pacemaker mechanism (e.g., phase 4 diastolic depolarization that is ionically normal for the sinus node or for an ectopic site such as a Purkinje fiber but occurs inappropriately fast or slow) or due to an ionically *abnormal* pacemaker mechanism. The patient with persistent sinus tachycardia at rest or sinus bradycardia during exertion exhibits inappropriate sinus nodal discharge rates, but the ionic mechanisms responsible for sinus nodal discharge may still be normal. Conversely, when a patient experiences ventricular tachycardia during an acute myocardial infarction, abnormal ionic mechanisms are probably operative to generate this tachycardia. Although pacemaker activity is generally not found in ordinary working myocardium, myocardial ischemia can conceivably bestow abnormal pacemaker properties on cells such as ventricular muscle fibers, permitting them to depolarize automatically. Based on the rate response to catecholamine administration of isolated fibers exhibiting normal phase 4 diastolic depolarization and on in vivo studies during stellate ganglion stimulation, it is likely that rates much in excess of 200 bpm are not due to enhanced normal automaticity.[12,79,131]

Mechanisms responsible for *normal* automaticity were described earlier (p. 616). *Abnormal* automaticity may arise from cells that have reduced maximum diastolic potentials, often in the range of -50 to -60 mV. This type of abnormal automaticity has been found in Purkinje fibers removed from dogs subjected to myocardial infarction,[126] in rat myocardium damaged by epinephrine (Fig. 19–16),[132] in human atrial samples,[133,134] and in ventricular myocardial specimens from patients undergoing aneurysmectomy and endocardial resection for recurrent ventricular tachyarrhythmias.[99,100] It can be produced in normal muscle[135] or Purkinje fibers[136] by appropriate interventions such as current passage that reduces diastolic potential (Fig. 19–17). Automatic discharge rate speeds up with progressive depolarization, while hyperpolarizing pulses slow the spontaneous firing. Other interventions, such as barium administration,[137] produce automaticity during which action potentials are similar to those produced by current passage. It is possible that partial depolarization and failure to reach normal maximal diastolic potential can induce automatic discharge in most if not all cardiac fibers.[131] The responsible ionic mechanisms (which are probably not the same in all the examples) are not clear, but in some preparations they may relate to reduction in an outward K current or impaired Na-K active transport.[113] In other instances, this type of abnormal automatic activity may be due to I_{si} because slow and not fast channel blockers suppress it.[99,101,135,136] Although this type of spontaneous automatic activity has been found in human atrial[133] and ventricular[99-101] fibers, its relation to the genesis of clinical arrhythmias has not been established.

Oscillatory activity may develop in cells both before and after full repolarization (Fig. 19–16). Oscillations with a variety of contours have been observed[100] and may represent another cause of automatic activity; however, their relation to clinical arrhythmias as well as their ionic causes and distinction from other types of depolarizations (see below) remain to be worked out.

TRIGGERED ACTIVITY. This newly recognized form of impulse formation has been observed in several types of fibers. Its demonstration requires a more precise consideration of the term "automaticity." Triggered activi

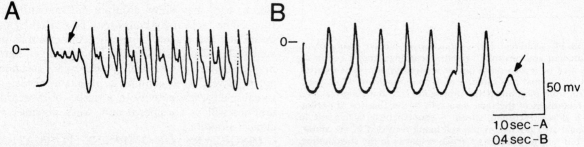

FIGURE 19–16   Triggered sustained rhythmic activity (see Fig. 19–18) recorded in rat myocardium damaged by epinephrine given 24 hours previously. *A*, Triggered activity arises from early afterdepolarizations (arrow) that occur during the plateau of the cardiac action potential. These oscillations arise from relatively low membrane potentials (< -60 mV). *B*, Spontaneous activity in the terminal phase of a triggered burst of activity is demonstrated and exhibits delayed afterdepolarizations. The delayed afterdepolarizations occur after complete repolarization, and subsequent action potentials triggered by this mechanism arise from membrane potentials of -60 to -80 mV. When a delayed afterdepolarization fails to reach threshold (end of recording, arrow), spontaneous activity ceases. (Modified from Gilmour, R. F., Jr., and Zipes, D. P.: Electrophysiological characteristics of rodent myocardium damaged by adrenaline. Cardiovasc. Res. *14*:582, 1980.)

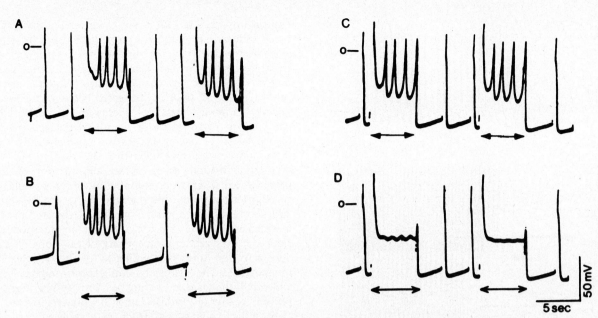

FIGURE 19–17 Abnormal automaticity during depolarization in canine Purkinje fiber. Depolarizing current pulses were delivered (across a single sucrose gap) at various times, as indicated by the intervals between arrowheads. Depolarization reduced membrane potential from −85 to −50 mV and initiated more rapid automaticity. While the fiber was at the more negative resting potential it also spontaneously discharged. Lidocaine (3 mg/L) and verapamil (3 × 10⁻⁶ M) exerted differential effects on automaticity initiated at high and low levels of transmembrane potential. *A*, Control. *B*, During superfusion with lidocaine. Lidocaine slowed the spontaneous discharge rate and reduced the amplitude of action potentials arising from the high (more negative) levels of membrane potential but did not alter action potentials or spontaneous rate at the low (less negative) level of membrane potential. *C*, Return to control after 30 minutes of washout. *D*, During superfusion with verapamil. Verapamil suppressed automaticity at the low (less negative) level of membrane potential without altering the spontaneous discharge rate at the high level of membrane potential. (From Elharrar, V., and Zipes, D. P.: Voltage modulation of automaticity in cardiac Purkinje fibers. *In* Zipes, D. P., et al. (eds.): The Slow Inward Current and Cardiac Arrhythmias. The Hague, Martinus Nijhoff, 1980, p. 357.)

ty is pacemaker activity that results *consequent to* a preceding impulse or series of impulses, without which electrical quiescence occurs (Fig. 19–18). Technically, that is not an automatic self-generating mechanism. *Automaticity* is the property of a fiber to initiate an impulse *spontaneously*, without need for prior stimulation, so that electrical quiescence does not occur. *Triggered activity* is initiated by impulses variously called low-amplitude potentials, transient depolarizations, or oscillatory afterpotentials.[138] These depolarizations may occur before or after full repolarization of the fiber (Figs. 19–16 and 19–18) and are best termed *early or late afterdepolarizations*, respectively.[139] They may arise from cells exhibiting high or low diastolic membrane potentials. Afterdepolarizations that reach threshold potential may trigger another afterdepolarization and thus self-perpetuate. Early afterdepolarizations may be precipitated by abrupt reduction in $[K]_o$, by high concentrations of catecholamines, and by some antiarrhythmic drugs[131] and may also be found in myocardium damaged by catecholamines[132] or in myocardium removed from patients who have ventricular arrhythmias.[100,101]

Delayed afterdepolarizations and triggered activity have been demonstrated in Purkinje fibers,[138,140] specialized atrial fibers[141] and ventricular muscle fibers[138] exposed to digitalis preparations and in normal Purkinje fibers exposed to Na-free superfusates.[142] When fibers in the rabbit,[143] canine,[144] simian,[145] and human[146] mitral valves and in the canine tricuspid valve[147] and coronary sinus[148] are superfused with norepinephrine, they exhibit the capacity for sustained trig-

gered rhythmic activity. In general, the fibers exhibit delayed afterhyperpolarizations (i.e., membrane potential following depolarization transiently becomes more negative than the resting potential), followed by delayed afterdepolarizations capable of reaching threshold and triggering sustained rhythmic activity. Action potentials of the mitral valve possess less negative resting membrane potentials and slower upstrokes than do action potentials in the coronary sinus and more clearly resemble slow-response action potentials. Verapamil suppresses the triggered activity in these preparations and it is possible that the slow inward current plays a role in their genesis. The membrane potential of the fibers, however—particularly those in the coronary sinus—is not sufficiently depressed to inactivate the fast response completely or to activate the slow response. Similar triggered activity not requiring norepinephrine for initiation has been recorded in the rabbit atrial pectinate muscle.[149] Triggered activity due to delayed afterdepolarizations has also been noted in diseased human atrial[150] and ventricular[100,101] fibers studied in vitro. In vivo, atrial and ventricular arrhythmias apparently due to triggered activity have been reported in the dog[151] and possibly in humans.[152–154] However, as indicated earlier, it is very difficult to be certain that a particular mechanism is operative in vivo, given our present state of knowledge. It is tempting to ascribe certain clinical arrhythmias to triggered activity, such as some atrial tachycardias that might originate in the coronary sinus, those arrhythmias in patients who have mitral valve prolapse, or those arrhyth-

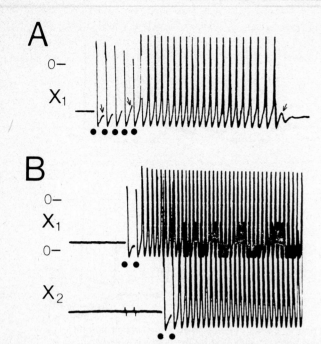

FIGURE 19–18 Triggered sustained rhythmic activity in diseased human ventricle. *A,* Spontaneous activity triggered by a series of driven action potentials (indicated by the dots) at a recording site X1. Note the gradual increase in the size of the afterdepolarizations (arrows) until the afterdepolarization reaches threshold and maintains sustained rhythmic activity after cessation of pacing. The sustained rhythmic activity finally terminates when the last afterdepolarization fails to reach threshold (arrow). *B,* Initiation of triggered activity by intracellular current injection (indicated by dots beneath the respective action potential recordings) at sites X1 and X2, which lie along the same trabeculum. Although sites X1 and X2 were only about 4 mm apart, triggered sustained rhythmic activity from one site did not propagate to the other site, indicating complete dissociation between these two sites. For current pulses, cycle length = 2000 msec; pulse duration = 10 msec; pulse intensity = 200 na. Vertical calibration: 50 mV. Horizontal calibration: 10 sec. (From Gilmour, R. F., Jr., et al.: Cellular electrophysiological abnormalities of diseased human ventricular myocardium. Am. J. Cardiol. *51*:137, 1983.)

mias precipitated by digitalis, but this approach is purely speculative at present.[155]

The ionic mechanism(s) responsible for delayed afterdepolarizations is not clear and may be varied. Because catecholamines and increases in $[Ca]_o$ enhance while verapamil suppresses activity of delayed afterdepolarizations, I_{si} is assumed to play a role. However, the negative level of resting membrane potential at which delayed depolarizations occur as well as the fact that tetrodotoxin[156,157] and antiarrhythmic agents at concentrations that affect only the fast current[158] depress or eliminate delayed afterdepolarizations caused by digitalis suggests that an inward Na current may play a role. Voltage clamp studies indicate that Na carries the inward current,[159,160] leading to the explanation that digitalis, by impairing the Na,K-ATPase exchange system, causes an increase in $[Na]_i$ which, in exchange for $[Ca]_o$, increases $[Ca]_i$. The latter in turn alters membrane conductance to a Na current that generates the afterdepolarization. Recent evidence indicates that electrogenic Na extrusion significantly influences the termination of triggered activity in the canine coronary sinus.[161]

Several features of triggered activity may have important

clinical implications. First, since triggered activity appears to be induced so easily in a variety of fibers in vitro, and since suggestive evidence supports its occurrence in vivo, triggered activity may cause some clinically occurring tachyarrhythmias yet to be defined. Second, pacing at rates more rapid than the triggered activity rate (overdrive pacing) in many instances increases the amplitude and shortens the cycle length of the afterdepolarization following cessation of pacing (overdrive acceleration)[138,162] rather than suppressing and delaying the escape rate of the afterdepolarization, as in normal automatic mechanisms[113] (Fig. 19–12). Premature stimulation exerts a similar effect; the shorter the premature interval, the larger the amplitude and shorter the escape interval of the triggered event. The mechanisms responsible for overdrive acceleration are not clear but may relate to steepening of the slope of diastolic depolarization and the influence of Na/K electrogenic pumping.[161] The clinical implication might be that tachyarrhythmias due to triggered activity may not be suppressed easily or, indeed, may be precipitated by rapid rates, either spontaneous (such as a sinus tachycardia) or pacing-induced. Finally, because a single premature stimulus can both initiate and terminate triggered activity, differentiation from reentry (see below) becomes quite difficult.[152,155]

Rhythms due to automaticity may be slow atrial, junctional and ventricular escape rhythms, certain types of atrial tachycardias (such as those produced by digitalis), accelerated junctional (nonparoxysmal junctional tachycardia), and idioventricular rhythms and parasystole (see Ch. 21).

PARASYSTOLE. Electrophysiological concepts about *parasystole* have been drastically revised in the last several years.[163-165] Classically, parasystole has been considered similar to a fixed-rate, asynchronously discharging pacemaker: its timing is not altered by the dominant rhythm, it produces depolarization when the myocardium is excitable, and the intervals between discharges are multiples of a basic interval. Complete *entrance block*, constant or intermittent,[166] insulates and protects the parasystolic focus from surrounding electrical events and accounts for such activity. Occasionally, the focus may exhibit *exit block*, during which it may fail to depolarize excitable myocardium.[167] Data from recent experiments indicate that, in fact, the dominant cardiac rhythm may modulate parasystolic discharge to speed up or slow down its rate. Experimental simulations of parasystole (using a sucrose gap technique, in which a segment of block is created in a fiber by superfusing it with a solution that prevents active impulse propagation in a localized area) demonstrate that the discharge rate of an isolated, "protected" focus can be modulated by electrotonic interactions with the dominant rhythm across an area of depressed excitability. Brief subthreshold depolarizations induced during the first half of the cardiac cycle of a spontaneously discharging pacemaker will delay the subsequent discharge, while similar depolarizations induced in the second half of the cardiac cycle will accelerate it (Figs. 19–19 and 19–20).[168] Complex interactions of complete silence, concealed or manifest bigeminy, trigeminy, quadrigeminy, and periods of more complex group beating may occur owing to the entraining effects of the dominant rhythm on the ectopic focus. Similar exam-

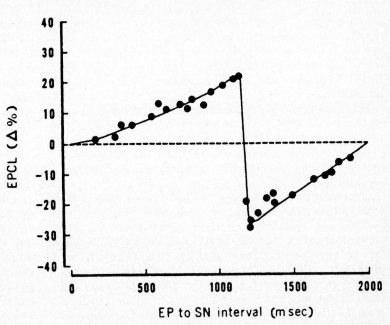

EP to SN interval (msec)

FIGURE 19–19 Phase response curve of a Purkinje fiber pacemaker mounted in a sucrose gap preparation. The x axis (EP to SN interval) represents the time after a spontaneous discharge of the pacemaker (EP) at which stimulated responses (SN) were evoked in the segment of fiber beyond the gap. The y axis (EPCL) represents the prolongation (first half) or abbreviation (second half) of the pacemaker cycle as a function of that time. EPCL = ectopic pacemaker cycle length; EP to SN interval = time after ectopic pacemaker discharge (EP) at which an evoked response (SN) was generated to simulate a ventricular response of sinus nodal (SN) origin. Intrinsic cycle length of EP, in the absence of electrotonic influence, was about 2000 msec. Abrupt phase reversal occurred at about 58 per cent of the intrinsic cycle length. These data indicate that stimulation early in the spontaneous cycle of a "parasystolic" pacemaker (EP) by a beat of sinus origin (SN) (left portion of curve) *delays* the next spontaneous discharge of EP, while stimulation late in the spontaneous cycle (right portion of the cycle) shortens the time to the next response of EP (see Figure 19–20). (From Jalife, M. J., and Moe, G. K.: A biologic model of parasystole. Am. J. Cardiol. *43*:761, 1979.)

ples have been noted in human ventricular tissue (Fig. 19–20).[101] Exactly how these observations will alter the "rules" established to diagnose parasystole electrocardiographically is still being established. However, there appear to be clinical examples[169] to support these experimental observations.

DISORDERS OF IMPULSE CONDUCTION.

Conduction delay and block can result in bradyarrhythmias or tachyarrhythmias, the former when the propagating impulse blocks and is followed by asystole or a slow escape rhythm, and the latter when the delay and block produce reentrant excitation (see below). Various factors, involving both active and passive membrane properties,[78,79,170] determine the conduction velocity of an impulse and whether or not conduction is successful. Among these factors are the stimulating efficacy of the propagating impulse, which is

related to the amplitude and rate of rise of phase 0,[171] and the excitability of the tissue into which the impulse conducts.[116,172] Over a range of take-off potentials (i.e., membrane potential at the time of excitation) that are more positive than −70 mV, action potential amplitude and rate of rise of phase 0 play prominent roles,[171] while at take-off potentials between −70 and −110 mV, conduction velocity appears to vary more directly with the level of excitability.[116,172] The explanation for this difference is as follows: At take-off potentials close to but more negative than −70 mV, the take-off potential, being closer to threshold, requires less current than a more polarized cell to reduce membrane potential to threshold potential and produce a regenerative response—i.e., the excitability threshold is reduced. Conduction improves even if action potential amplitude and V̇max are lowered. At take-off potentials less

FIGURE 19–20 Modulation of pacemaker activity by subthreshold current pulses in diseased human ventricle. *A,* Two recording sites along the same trabeculum in a spontaneously active preparation. Current pulses (indicated by the dots) of 30 msec duration were injected through the lower microelectrode at various times. The interval between the spontaneous action potentials is given in milliseconds above each cycle. Injection of a subthreshold current pulse through the lower microelectrode relatively early in the spontaneous cycle (about 680 msec after initiation of the rapid portion of the preceding action potential upstroke) produced a subthreshold depolarization in the upper recording and delayed the next spontaneous discharge by 400 msec to 1900 msec. This response would fall in the first half of the curve indicated in Figure 19–19. A current pulse of the same intensity and duration delivered later in the spontaneous cycle (950 msec after the preceding upstroke) accelerated the next discharge by 210 msec to 1390 msec, relative to the previous two action potentials. The response to this current injection falls in the second half of the graph depicted in Figure 19–19.

B, A stimulus at a precise interval in the cardiac cycle (called the singular point [in this example, 930 msec after the preceding action potential upstroke]) abolished pacemaker activity.

C, A single subthreshold pulse (dot) can also alter the contour of the subsequent spontaneous action potentials and convert biphasic action potentials to action potentials with a single active component followed by delayed afterdepolarizations (arrows). Vertical calibration: 50 mV. Horizontal calibration: 2 sec in *A* and *B* and 4 sec in *C*. (From Gilmour, R. F., Jr., et al.: Cellular electrophysiological abnormalities of diseased human ventricular myocardium. Am. J. Cardiol. *51*:137, 1983.)

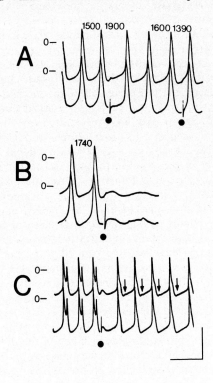

negative than −70 mV, threshold potential may become more positive (moves "away" from resting membrane potential). This factor plus Na inactivation that occurs at reduced membrane potential (see p. 613) makes action potential amplitude and $\dot{V}max$ important determinants of conduction.

Other features such as alterations in refractoriness,[173-175] electrotonic effects,[176,177] the role of intercellular connections,[178] uniformity of the propagating wavefront,[179] the role of the autonomic nervous system,[59] and the geometry of the tissue[180] may all influence conduction, to accelerate it or cause block.[174,181]

Decremental Conduction. This term is used commonly in the clinical literature but is often misapplied to describe any Wenckebach-like conduction block, i.e., responses similar to block in the AV node during which progressive conduction delay precedes the nonconducted impulse (see Ch. 21). Correctly used, decremental conduction refers to the situation in which the properties of the fiber change along its length so that the action potential loses its efficacy as a stimulus to excite the fiber ahead of it.[37,72,182,183] Thus, the stimulating efficacy of the propagating action potential diminishes progressively, possibly as a result of its decreasing amplitude and $\dot{V}max$. Whether or not decremental conduction, as defined above, accounts for Wenckebach AV block is not yet resolved.

Electrical activity during each normal cardiac cycle begins in the sinus node and continues until the entire heart has been activated. Each cell, interconnected electrically, becomes activated in turn and the cardiac impulse dies out when all fibers have been discharged and are completely refractory. During this absolute refractory period, the cardiac impulse has "no place to go" and must be extinguished. If, however, a group of fibers not activated because of unidirectional block during the initial wave of depolarization recovers excitability in time to be discharged before the impulse dies out, they may serve as a link to reexcite areas that were just discharged and have now recovered from the initial depolarization. Such a process is given various names, all meaning approximately the same thing: reentry, reentrant excitation, circus movement, reciprocal or echo beat, or reciprocating tachycardia.

McWilliam,[184] Mayer,[185] Mines,[186,187] and Garrey,[188] experimenting on the pulsating bell of the medusa, the jellyfish, turtle, and mammalian hearts, worked out the basic concepts of reentry over a 20-year period early in this century. Mines noted that to prove reentry, three features had to be established: (1) an area of unidirectional block, (2) recirculation of the impulse to its point of origin, and (3) elimination of the arrhythmia by cutting the pathway. He warned against mistaking for reentry an automatic beat that originated at one point in the circuit and traveled around the circuit in one direction because of block near its site of origin. Many investigators have continued to study these concepts over the past 70 years, but the models they have used have become more complex, making it more difficult to prove the presence of reentry. Often, the diagnosis that an arrhythmia is due to reentry is made far too liberally, based on scanty evidence and certainly not adhering to the basic criteria established by Mines.

The primary prerequisite for reentry is the development of unidirectional block due to the presence of tissue with disparate electrophysiological properties. Such asymmetrical depression of conduction occurs commonly in experimental preparations, even those having the simple, relatively uniform geometry of an isolated Purkinje fiber.[177,189] Fibers participating in the reentrant pathway may be contiguous, such as adjacent AV nodal cells or Purkinje fibers, or they may be anatomically separated, such as the AV node and an accessory pathway (see p. 714). Because the two (or more) pathways have different properties— e.g., a refractory period longer in one pathway than the other, decreased excitability in one pathway, ineffectiveness of the wavefront to activate all fibers, or other reasons— the impulse (1) blocks in one pathway (site *x* in Fig. 19–21*A*; site A in Fig. 19–21*B*) and (2) propagates slowly in the adjacent pathway (arrow from *x* to *y* in Fig. 19–21*A*; serpentine arrow, D to C, Fig. 19–21*B*). If conduction in this alternative route is sufficiently depressed, the slowly propagating impulse excites tissue beyond the blocked pathway (hatched and stippled areas in Fig. 19–21*A* and *B*) and returns in a reversed direction along the pathway initially blocked (*y* to *x* in Fig. 19–21*A*; B to A in Fig. 19–21*B*) to (3) reexcite tissue proximal to the site of block (*x* to 1 in Fig. 19–21*A*; A to D in Fig. 19–21*B*). For reentry of this type to occur, the time for conduction within the depressed but unblocked area and for excitation of the distal segments must exceed the refractory period of the initially blocked pathway (*x* in Fig. 19–21*A*; A in Fig. 19–21*B*) and the tissue proximal to the site of block (A in Fig. 19–21*A*; D in Fig. 19–21*B*). Stated another way, continuous reentry requires that the anatomical length of the circuit traveled equal or exceed the reentrant wavelength. The latter is equal to mean conduction velocity of the impulse multiplied by the longest refractory period of the elements in the circuit. Conditions that depress conduction velocity or abbreviate the refractory period will promote the development of reentry, while prolonging refractoriness and speeding conduction velocity will hinder its development. For example, if conduction velocity (0.30 M/sec) and refractoriness (350 msec) for ventricular muscle were normal, a pathway of 105 mm (0.30 M/sec ×0.35 sec) would be necessary for reentry to occur. However, under certain conditions, conduction velocity in ventricular muscle and Purkinje fibers can be very slow (0.03 M/sec),[190] and if refractoriness is not greatly prolonged (600 msec), a pathway of only 18 mm (0.03 M/sec × 0.60 sec) may be necessary. Such reasoning may have clinical implications. For example, it has been reported recently that some antiarrhythmic agents converted nonsustained ventricular tachycardia to sustained ventricular arrhythmias, possibly because the drugs greatly slowed conduction velocity with little effect on ventricular refractoriness.[191] Prior to drug therapy in these patients, when nonsustained ventricular tachycardia occurred, the reentrant impulse may have traveled too fast for the anatomical and physiological length of the circuit and may have encroached on refractory tissue, consequently causing the tachycardia to terminate.[192] Drugs that prolong conduction with little effect on refractoriness may allow sufficient time for full repolarization of the elements in the reentrant pathway and perpetuation of the ventricular tachycardia.

Reflection.[79,193,194] This can be considered as a special subclass of reentry. As in reentry, an area of conduction delay is required and the total time for the impulse to leave and return to its site of origin must exceed the refactory period of the proximal segment. Reflection differs from reentry in that the impulse does not require a circuit, as diagrammed in Figure 19–21A and B, but appears to travel along the *same* pathway in both directions. The impulse travels in one direction and meets an area of impaired conduction where active transmission pauses (Fig. 19–21C). Electrotonically (see p. 618), the impulse spans the zone of impairment, activates the distal segment, and returns electrotonically across the zone of impaired conduction to reexcite the proximal segment. A single reflection could cause a coupled premature complex, while continued reflection back and forth across an inexcitable zone could cause a tachycardia. Recent data[193] suggest that reflection and parasystole (or reentry) are part of a continuous spectrum, without a critical boundary to separate them.

Reentry is probably the cause of many tachyarrhythmias, including various kinds of supraventricular and ventricular tachycardias, flutter, and fibrillation. It is important to remember, however, that circa 1900, investigators were able to demonstrate reentry by using simple preparations. In more complex preparations, such as large pieces of tissue in vitro or the intact heart, it becomes much more difficult to prove that reentry exists. It is very hard technically to record from sufficient sites to meet Mines' criteria. Initiation or termination of tachycardia by pacing stimuli, the demonstration of electrical activity bridging diastole, fixed coupling, and a variety of other clinically used techniques,

FIGURE 19–21 Diagrams of reentry published by Schmitt and Erlanger in 1928.

A, Reentry is depicted as occurring in contiguous pathways, based on observations that these pathways can undergo functional longitudinal dissociation. Initial propagation begins at site 1 but is able to reach site 5 only in pathway B (lower arrow). Pathway A exhibits unidirectional block (from left to right) at site *x* in the cross-hatched area. The impulse can then reenter pathway A from pathway B and travel from *y* to *x*, reexciting tissue proximal to the site of block. Such concepts of reentry can be applied to any site in the heart.

B, A Purkinje fiber (D) divides into two pathways (B and C), both of which join ventricular muscle (stippled area). It is assumed that the original impulse travels down D, blocks in its anterograde direction at site A (arrow followed by double bar), but continues slowly down C (serpentine arrow) to excite ventricular muscle. The impulse then reenters the Purkinje twig at B and retrogradely excites A and D. If the impulse continues to propagate through D to the ventricular myocardium and elicits ventricular depolarization, a reentrant ventricular extrasystole results. Continued reentry of this type would produce ventricular tachycardia.

C, Reflection. Top panel, schematic representation of electrotonic transmission across an area of inexcitability in a Purkinje fiber. The central compartment (gap) of the tissue bath contains a solution that prevents active conduction in the central segment (inexcitable cable) of the Purkinje fiber. Action potentials from various locations along the Purkinje fiber are presented in panel A when transmission across the inexcitable area is unsuccessful and in panel B when transmission is successful. In panel A, the regenerative impulse encountering the region of block decays along the length of the blocked segment. In panel B, the slowly rising elec-

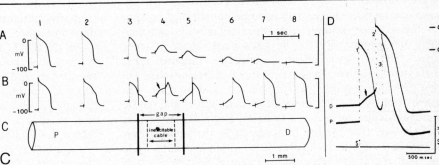

trotonic potential (arrow) resulting from the activity in the proximal tissue brings the distal segment to threshold and thus restores, after a delay, active propagation via electrotonic transmission. The amplitude of the electrotonic potential emerging from the distal end of the inexcitable cable must be sufficiently large to bring that membrane to the threshold if transmission is to succeed.

When the delay in transmission across the gap is sufficiently long, electrotonic transmission in the reverse direction over the same blocked segment can reexcite the proximal segment and generate a repetitive response, which, under these experimental conditions, is termed *reflection.* This is illustrated in panel D. The two traces were recorded from the two active segments on the proximal (P) and distal (D) sides of the inexcitable gap. The bottom trace is the stimulus marker (S). Stimulation of the proximal segment (1) was transmitted to the distal segment (2) following a slowly developing electrotonic depolarization (arrow) that reached the threshold of the tissue beyond the inexcitable gap after the delay of 300 msec. Electrotonic transmission in the reverse direction induced a closely coupled (404 msec), reflected response (3) in the proximal segment after expiration, of its refractory period. Thus, to-and-fro electrotonic transmission across an inexcitable segment of tissue occurs over the *same pathway* and must be differentiated conceptually from a micro-reentrant circuit that uses *different pathways* in each direction. (From Antzelevitch, C., and Moe, G. K.: Electrotonically-mediated delayed conduction and reentry in relation to "slow responses" in mammalian ventricular conducting tissue. Circ. Res. *49*:1129, 1981. By permission of the American Heart Association, Inc.)

while consistent with reentry, do not constitute proof of its existence.

ATRIAL FLUTTER (p. 697).   Lewis[195] considered that atrial flutter was due to a circus movement, but his evidence was not very convincing. Subsequent experiments by Rosenblueth and Garcia Ramos[196] provided more substantial evidence by showing that a well-placed cut interrupted atrial flutter initiated by rapid stimulation in dogs in which intercaval blockade had been produced. These data plus mapping studies[197,198] in animals and mapping and stimulation studies in man[199,200] provide some evidence to suggest that many forms of atrial flutter are due to reentry. Patients may also have dissimilar atrial rhythms in which all or part of one atrium exhibits atrial flutter while all or part of the other atrium has fibrillation.[201]

FIBRILLATION.   Much indirect evidence supports reentry as a cause of fibrillation,[202,203] but this is difficult to prove beyond question. Several studies have established that a critical mass of myocardium is required to maintain fibrillation,[204,205] lending support to Moe's hypothesis that multiple wavelets of reentry, influenced by the mass of the tissue, refractory periods, and conduction velocity, maintain fibrillation.[206] Lewis felt that a single wave circulating around the vena cava sent out smaller wavelets at rapid rates to activate surrounding tissue.[207] Garrey's decisive experiments,[188] in which he cut myocardium into smaller pieces that continued to fibrillate until they reached a critically small size, provided evidence against Lewis' concept and also against proponents of the hypothesis that single or multiple firing foci caused fibrillation. In the canine ventricle, the left ventricular free wall and septum appear to be required as a critical mass to maintain fibrillation, since, if they are depolarized by injecting a small amount of potassium into the left anterior descending coronary and circumflex arteries, the right ventricle stops fibrillating spontaneously.[205]

SINUS AND ATRIAL REENTRY.   Reentry in parts of the atrium has been reported to occur in several experimental models as well as in humans. The sinus node shares with the AV node electrophysiological features such as the potential for *dissociation of conduction*, i.e., an impulse can be made to conduct in some nodal fibers but not in others.[208] For example, premature stimulation can produce slow propagation in the sinus node, block in some areas, and the development of repetitive responses most likely due to reentry. Evidence from a number of studies in man[209,210] and animals[208,211] support the concept that sustained reentry in the sinus node can occur and cause supraventricular tachycardia (p. 694). Recently, Allessie et al.[211] showed that the reentrant circuit in the isolated rabbit preparation was located entirely within the sinus node and that the atrium was not an essential link. While it is possible that the sinus node responds to premature stimulation with an increase in its discharge rate, under some circumstances as a form of triggered sustained rhythmic activity or overdrive acceleration, and that supraventricular tachycardias thought to be caused by sinus nodal reentry are actually due to triggered activity, experimental evidence does not support these conclusions. The sinus node ordinarily manifests overdrive suppression after a period of rapid pacing,[212] a characteristic that may separate it from automaticity due to other slow-response models. An increase in sinus nodal discharge rate may occur transiently at times following rapid pacing, possibly owing to adrenergic stimulation or vagal withdrawal in response to the pacing-induced rate increase. Premature stimulation of the sinus node may shorten or lengthen the return cycle, depending on the coupling interval of the premature beat, which determines whether the sinus node is reset or is influenced electrotonically[213-215] or if a pacemaker shift occurs. Often, the atrial event does not reflect the true response to premature stimulation of the sinus nodal pacemaker cells. However, triggered sustained rhythmic activity in the sinus node as a cause of persistent supraventricular tachycardia does not seem likely, and the weight of evidence suggests that reentry in the sinus node is responsible for this rhythm disturbance.

Reentry within the atrium, unrelated to the sinus node, has been shown experimentally to occur in the rabbit[216,217] and dog atrium,[218] with or without an anatomical obstacle, and may be a cause of supraventricular tachycardia in man. Examples of supraventricular tachycardia purported to be due to atrial reentry have been cited,[209,220,221] but their relative infrequency in the published literature suggests that this is not a commonly recognized cause of supraventricular tachycardia in man. Distinguishing atrial tachycardia due to automaticity from atrial tachycardia sustained by reentry over very small areas, i.e., micro-reentry, is very difficult, and therefore conclusions regarding clinical electrophysiological mechanisms of this supraventricular tachycardia based on currently available information must be accepted cautiously.

Allessie et al.[216] have shown in isolated rabbit atrium that premature stimulation elicited a reentrant circuit (6 to 8 mm) with radial propagation to the periphery. The reentrant circuit propagated around a functionally inactive core and followed a course along fibers that had a shorter refractory period, blocking in one direction in fibers with a longer refractory period. An anatomical obstacle was not necessary. The refractory period and conduction velocity in the reentrant pathway determined its length. This type of reentry, called the "leading circuit concept,"[217] has a small reentrant circuit, making it difficult to distinguish from an automatic focus unless minute mapping techniques are used.

AV NODAL REENTRY.   It has been known for 75 years that stimulation of the ventricle could propagate to the atrium and then back to the ventricles,[222] sometimes being sustained to cause a reciprocating rhythm.[186,187] Although the bundle of fibers described by Kent was considered to play a role in this circus movement[186,187,223] even before the Wolff-Parkinson-White syndrome was described in man, Scherf and Shookhoff[224] ascribed the mechanism to "longitudinal functional dissociation" in the AV junction. They produced (and first used the term) "return ventricular extrasystoles" in dogs by giving quinine to delay AV nodal conduction and suggested that some fibers of the AV conduction system had shorter refractory periods and were able to conduct in one direction while conduction in other fibers with longer refractory periods was blocked. The impulse was then able to reexcite the previously refractory fibers. For a return ventricular extrasystole to occur, the R-P interval (i.e., between the onset of the QRS and the retrograde P wave) must lengthen to a critical ex-

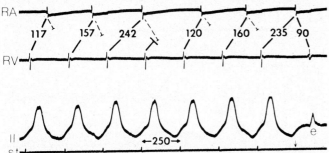

FIGURE 19–22 Return ventricular extrasystoles associated with retrograde Wenckebach conduction. A stable 4:3 retrograde Wenckebach conduction was established in a dog by rapid right ventricular pacing (left half of the figure, first four stimuli). When the eighth ventricular stimulus in the series was omitted (right half of the figure at arrow), the retrograde atrial impulse returned to the ventricle to produce a ventricular echo. Such an event can be explained by the effects of concealed reentry (see p. 247). Solid lines indicate manifest conduction and interrupted lines indicate concealed conduction. Numbers in milliseconds represent ventriculoatrial conduction time. Electrograms recorded from the epicardial surface of the right atrium (RA), right ventricle (RV), and standard lead II. St = stimulus; e = ventricular echo. (From Zipes, D. P., et al.: Some examples of Wenckebach periodicity in cardiac tissues, with an appraisal of mechanisms. *In* Rosenbaum, M. B. (ed.): Cardiac Arrhythmias. The Hague, Martinus Nijhoff [in press].)

tent, and conduction cannot block in the AV junction before the impulse reaches the site of reentry[225] (Fig. 19–22).

In canine and some human studies, the R-P interval is inversely proportional to the P-R interval,[225] i.e., the longer it takes the ventricular impulse to reach the atrium, the less time it takes the return impulse to reach the ventricle. This reciprocal relationship may result if some part of the pathway is common to both anterograde and retrograde conduction. Therefore, a longer ventriculoatrial conduction time permits a longer recovery period for the common pathway and a faster conduction time anterogradely. A short ventriculoatrial conduction time may be followed by a long atrioventricular conduction time. The final common pathway is most likely the mid and distal regions of the AV node.[125] Return extrasystoles, or echoes, can be elicited in the opposite direction as well, in contrast to the conclusions of Rosenblueth.[226] These atrial echoes have characteristics similar to ventricular echoes.[227,228]

In many patients, the ventriculoatrial conduction time may remain relatively fixed in spite of changes in the premature interval (p. 703). Longitudinal dissociation in the AV node, where reentry most likely occurs, remains a plausible mechanism. In fact, Mendez et al.[229] demonstrated that an impulse traveling from ventricle to atrium, if timed properly, did not prevent another impulse traveling simultaneously from atrium to ventricle from reaching the His bundle. For this to occur, the impulses traveling in opposite directions must be conducting in different AV nodal pathways.

Microelectrode studies on isolated rabbit AV nodal preparations provide further evidence to support these concepts of longitudinal AV nodal dissociation and reentry.[179] Cells in the upper portion of the AV node can be dissociated during propagation of premature stimuli, so that one group of cells, called alpha, can discharge in response to a premature stimulus at a time when another group of cells, called beta, fails to discharge.[125,230] The impulse can then propagate to the mid and lower portions of the AV node and turn around (without needing to activate the His bundle) to reexcite the beta group of cells and produce an atrial echo (Fig. 19–23). Experiments by Janse et al.[231] using multiple simultaneous microelectrode recordings, and by Wit et al.,[232] who created episodes of sustained AV nodal tachycardia in isolated rabbit atria, largely confirmed these observations. Although these studies provide the most conclusive animal experimental evidence supporting the presence of AV nodal reentry, they do not prove it unequivocally. In such a complex preparation, all the "rules" established by Mines cannot be met, and the evidence does not exclude, for example, the possibility of a triggered impulse responsible for the returning wavefront.

Mines postulated that reentry within AV nodal connections might be responsible for some clinically occurring arrhythmias, while several other investigators suggested similar concepts based on electrocardiograms recorded in patients.[233–236] The argument by Lewis[237] that rapid atrial conduction time should produce supraventricular tachycardia rates faster than those observed was countered by Barker, who suggested that a circus movement involving the sinus or AV nodes could explain the slower rates. Kistin, using esophageal leads,[238] offered the possibility that two or more AV nodal pathways accounted for reciprocal rhythms.

One of the first studies employing premature electrical stimulation to initiate and terminate a paroxysmal supraventricular tachycardia in situ was performed in a dog.[239] Subsequent investigations in man support the concept[240,241] that reentry, initiated by a critical degree of AV nodal conduction delay,[242,243] can be localized to the AV node, possibly occurring over functionally distinct dual AV nodal pathways.[244] The premature atrial response can block anterogradely in one AV nodal pathway that conducts more rapidly (fast pathway, or beta pathway in Figure 19–23) but has a longer refractory period than a second pathway (slow pathway, or alpha pathway in Figure 19–23). The premature atrial response travels to the ventricle over the slow (alpha) pathway and back to the atrium over the fast (beta) pathway.[198,245] Less commonly, the premature atrial response can block in the slow pathway and travel in the fast pathway anterogradely, using the slow pathway retrogradely.[246] Conceivably, some patients may have three or more pathways.[245]

In patients who have dual AV nodal physiology, both pathways exhibit electrophysiological responses in the anterograde direction characteristic of AV nodal fibers. However, in some patients, the electrophysiological features of the retrogradely conducting pathway differ greatly from those of the anterogradely conducting pathway, in response not only to atrial or ventricular pacing but also to various drugs.[221,245,247–249] Thus, it is not clear whether the retrogradely conducting pathway is extranodal, is intranodal but insulated from the rest of the AV node, or includes only a small amount of AV nodal tissue.

It is also not settled whether the retrogradely conducting pathway is distinct from the fast and slow anterogradely conducting pathways, which appear to be composed of AV nodal fibers. The geometry and direction of conduction,[250] effects of summation,[251] autonomic tone,[252] as well as the electrophysiological characteristics of the fi-

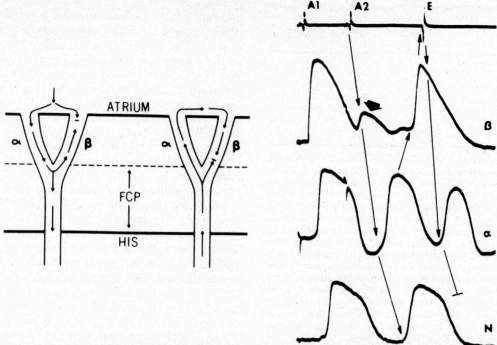

FIGURE19-23 Atrial echoes. *Left,* Schematic representation of intranodal dissociation responsible for an atrial echo. A premature atrial response fails to penetrate the beta pathway, which exhibits unidirectional block but propagates anterogradely through the alpha pathway. Once the final common pathway (FCP) is engaged, the impulse may return to the atrium via the now recovered beta pathway to produce an atrial echo. The neighboring diagram illustrates the pattern of propagation during generation of a ventricular echo. A premature response in the His bundle traverses the final common pathway, encounters a refractory beta pathway (unidirectional block), reaches the atrium over the alpha pathway, and returns through a now recovered beta pathway to produce a ventricular echo. Such events can explain the findings in Figure 19–22.

Right, Actual recordings from the atrium (top tracing), cells impaled in the beta region (second tracing), alpha region (third tracing), and N portion of the AV node (bottom tracing) in an isolated rabbit preparation. The basic response to A_1 activated both alpha and beta pathways and the N cell (first tier of action potentials). The premature atrial response, A_2, caused only a local response in the beta cell (heavy arrow), was delayed in transmission to the alpha cell, and was further delayed in propagation to the N cell. Following the alpha response, a retrograde spontaneous response occurred in the beta cell and propagated to the atrium (E). This atrial response represents an atrial echo. The echo returned to stimulate the alpha cell but was not propagated to the N cell. (From Mendez, C., and Moe, G. K.: Demonstrations of a dual AV nodal conduction system in the isolated rabbit heart. Circ. Res. *19*:378, 1966. By permission of the American Heart Association, Inc.)

bers, all may influence conduction and the response to drugs. A drug such as procainamide may effect retrograde but not anterograde AV nodal conduction in patients with presumably normal AV nodes.[253] It is likely that the anatomical as well as the electrophysiological features of AV nodal pathways may not be the same in all patients who have AV nodal reentrant supraventricular tachycardia. Recent evidence suggests that, in some patients who appear to have AV nodal reentrant supraventricular tachycardia, the retrogradely conducting pathway may exhibit electrophysiological properties consistent with AV nodal tissue but is located in an extranodal site, since it gives rise to an abnormal sequence of retrograde atrial activation.[254] The anatomical basis for such observations may be an eccentric AV node or an accessory pathway with AV nodal characteristics.

The necessary role of atrial participation in the reentrant circuit is still debated. Mendez et al.[229] demonstrated the need for the atrium in generating ventricular echoes caused by AV nodal reentrant activity in dogs, and such a circuit is implicit in their diagram in Figure 19–23. Studies in animals[227] and patients[174,255-257] have challenged the interpretations of Mendez et al. and have suggested that ventricular echoes due to AV nodal reentry can occur *without* activa-

tion of the atrium. Figure 19–24 is an example of apparent dissociation of the atrium with uninterrupted continuation of the supraventricular tachycardia, leading to the conclusion that the atrium may *not* be a necessary part of the reentrant circuit in humans (see Chap. 21). However, since rhythms in the atria may become dissimilar,[201] a portion of the atrium may control, or participate in, the cardiac rhythm without recognition of this fact from observation of a scalar ECG or, indeed, from recordings within the right atrium or coronary sinus.[258] Therefore, data refuting the role of the atrium as a necessary link in the reentrant pathway must be obtained from studies in which both atria are carefully mapped for the presence of localized atrial activity, particularly near the upper AV node.[231,232,259]

PREEXCITATION SYNDROME (See also p. 712). The accumulated anatomical and electrophysiological data support a reentrant mechanism to explain tachycardias related to an accessory pathway more than they support that mechanism for any other kind of tachycardia.[260-263] In fact, Mines[187] and deBoer[223] both attempted to explain the mechanism of paroxysmal tachycardia by reentry over the bundle described by Kent[264,265] even before the preexcitation syndrome was ever described in man.

Electrophysiological studies have demonstrated that, in

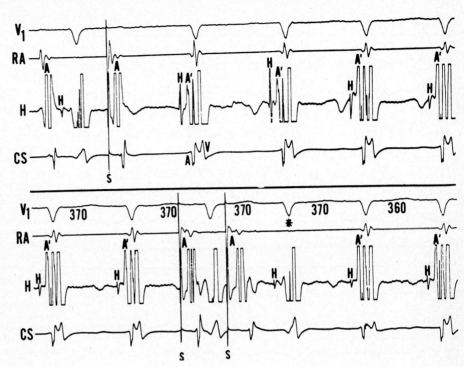

FIGURE 19–24 Dissociation of atria from ventricles without interrupting AV nodal reentrant supraventricular tachycardia. During sinus rhythm, a single premature atrial complex (S, *top panel*) was conducted with AV nodal delay (prolonged A-H interval) and initiated an AV nodal reentrant supraventricular tachycardia. Note that retrograde atrial activation (A′) occurred prior to onset of the QRS complex. Two premature atrial stimuli (S-S, *bottom panel*) captured the atria on both occasions without altering the regular cycle length of the AV nodal reentrant supraventricular tachycardia. Note that the QRS complex marked by an asterisk has no accompanying atrial complex, suggesting that atrial participation in the reentrant circuit was not required. V_1 = scalar lead; RA = right atrial electrogram; H = His bundle electrogram; CS = coronary sinus electrogram.

most patients who have reciprocating tachycardia associated with the Wolff-Parkinson-White syndrome, the accessory pathway conducts more rapidly than does the normal AV node but takes a longer time to recover excitability, i.e., the anterograde refractory period of the accessory pathway exceeds that of the AV node.[261,266] Consequently, a premature atrial complex that occurs sufficiently early blocks anterogradely in the accessory pathway and continues to the ventricle over the normal AV node and His bundle. After the ventricles have been excited, the impulse is able to enter the accessory pathway retrogradely and return to the atrium. A continuous conduction loop of this kind establishes the circuit for the tachycardia. Although exceptions occur, the usual activation wave during such a reciprocating tachycardia in a patient with an accessory pathway occurs in this fashion: anterogradely over the normal AV node–His-Purkinje system and retrogradely over the accessory pathway, resulting in a normal QRS complex (Fig. 19–25). Because the circuit requires both atria and ventricles, the term "supraventricular tachycardia" may not be precisely correct. The term "reciprocating tachycardia" or "circus movement tachycardia" has been substituted. Use of the latter terms assumes that the mechanism of the tachycardia is one of reentry. In some patients, the accessory pathway may be capable only of retrograde conduction,[262,267,268] but the circuit and mechanism of tachycardia remain the same. Less commonly, the accessory pathway may conduct only anterogradely.[262,269]

In addition to the response of the reciprocating tachycardia to premature stimulation, one of the strongest lines of evidence supporting a reentrant mechanism is that interruption of the presumed reentrant loop at widely separated points (i.e., by surgically cutting the normal AV node–His bundle pathway *or* the accessory pathway) eliminates the ability to develop supraventricular tachycardia.

Other pathways may constitute the circuit for reciprocating tachycardias in patients who have some form of the Wolff-Parkinson-White syndrome. Conduction may proceed anterogradely over the accessory pathway and retrogradely over the AV node–His bundle, so-called "antidromic tachycardia." Two accessory pathways may form the circuit. In the Lown-Ganong-Levine syndrome (short P-R interval and normal QRS complex),[270] conduction over a James fiber[271] that connects atrium to the distal portion of the AV node and His bundle may play a role, although the presence of this entity as a distinct syndrome is unsettled[31] (see p. 713).

For some patients, electrophysiological findings may be consistent with communications between the AV node and the ventricle (nodoventricular) or the His-bundle–bundle branches and the ventricle (fasciculoventricular).[272] Tachycardia in patients with nodoventricular fibers may be due to reentry using these fibers as the anterograde pathway and the His-Purkinje fibers and a portion of the AV node retrogradely. No direct relationship may exist between fasciculoventricular fibers and tachycardia. Thus, the accessory pathway concept suggested by Holzmann and Scherf[273] and Wolferth and Wood[274] can be expanded to encompass a variety of syndromes.

VENTRICULAR REENTRY (See also pp. 721 to 728). Reentry in the ventricle as a cause of sustained ventricular arrhythmias was suggested by the work of Mines.[186,187] Later, Schmitt and Erlanger[183] produced probable functional longitudinal dissociation with undirectional block in strips of turtle ventricle exposed unequally to different depressant agents. This resulted in repetitive excitation, likely due to reentry, reflection, or both, and they suggested that the event could occur in a peripheral Purkinje fiber bundle. Their diagram (Fig. 19–21A and B) has been reproduced many times. Wenckebach and Winterberg[275] raised similar possibilities. A strong objection to this explanation[276] was that the impulse conducted too quickly in cardiac tissue for a pathway to be of reasonable length to support reentry. Studies by Cranefield[189,277] and Wit[190,278] dispelled these doubts by demonstrating that high [K] could depress conduction velocity in peripheral Purkinje

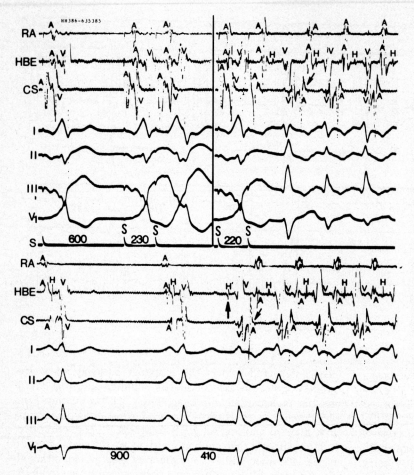

FIGURE 19–25 Spontaneous and induced initiation of paroxysmal reciprocating tachycardia in a patient with the Wolff-Parkinson-White syndrome. *Top left,* Premature left atrial stimulation (S-S) at a cycle length of 230 msec was followed by conduction over the accessory pathway to the ventricle. *Top right,* Shortening the premature interval (S-S) to 220 msec was followed by conduction to the ventricle over the normal pathway and initiation of reciprocating tachycardia, during which the earliest retrograde atrial activation was recorded in the left atrium (CS lead, arrow) followed by activity in the low right atrial (HBE) and high right atrial (RA) leads. This finding is consistent with a left-sided accessory pathway. *Bottom recording,* Premature depolarization in or near the His bundle (H', upright arrow) initiated the same tachycardia spontaneously. The QRS complex following the H' is totally normal because the impulse originates distal to the atrial insertion of the accessory pathway and therefore conducts over the normal AV node–His bundle pathway to the ventricle. Retrograde atrial activation (arrow) occurs over the left-sided accessory pathway as in the top right panel.

twigs to 0.01 to 0.10 M/sec and permit reentry, probably due to the slow response, to occur in loops of Purkinje fibers (Fig. 19–26). Spontaneous activity in unbranched fibers could also be elicited in these studies and in others using a sucrose gap technique (Fig. 19–21C). The latter studies clearly showed reflection as a cause of repetitive excitation.

Sasyniuk and Mendez[279] demonstrated repetitive firing in papillary muscle–false tendon preparations in which a premature stimulus delivered to a Purkinje fiber blocked at some Purkinje-muscle junctions, conducted through others, and propagated back to its site of origin. Reentry was facilitated in this preparation because the duration of the action potential and refractoriness shortened in the fibers proximal to the site of initial block, allowing early recovery and reexcitation. Related events may occur in damaged fibers.[280] Whether such reentry takes place in the heart in situ is not known; however, reentry has been demonstrated to occur over the bundle branches in the in situ dog heart[281–283] (Fig. 19–27) and probably in man as well.[262,284] The occurrence of bundle branch reentry explains several interesting electrocardiographic phenomena, to be discussed later (p. 727). Bundle branch reentry does not appear to be a common cause of sustained ventricular tachycardia in the dog or in man.[152,285,286,286a] More likely, reentry in ventricular muscle, with or without contribution from specialized tissue, is responsible for many ventricular tachycardias.

Reentry in ventricular muscle is difficult to prove by Mines' criteria because the large muscle mass makes complete mapping of the reentrant loop and interruption of the pathway difficult. Fontaine et al.[287] have shown that an appropriately placed ventriculotomy incision could interrupt sustained ventricular tachycardia in man. In general, experimental studies provide only supportive evidence of reentry.[288] Ischemia, both acute and chronic, has been a favorite model to investigate because it generates fragmented, delayed activation that may be conducive to the generation of reentrant excitation.[289,290] However, even the demonstration of continuous electrical activity spanning diastole that is linked temporally and perhaps causally to the generation of sustained ventricular arrhythmia[286,291,292] constitutes only circumstantial proof. For example, such continuous electrical activity could be produced by oscillatory pacemaker activity (Figs. 19–16 and 19–17) conducting with delay to the surrounding myocardium and could be unrelated to reentry. We have already indicated that initiation and termination of a sustained tachycardia is not proof of reentry, since triggered activity can respond in a similar fashion. Several recent animal studies using an extensive array of extracellular electrodes[293–296] have provided important information concerning the sequence of activation during ventricular tachyarrhythmias, strongly suggesting in some of the studies that reentry is the responsible mechanism. Even though more data meeting Mines' postulates are required to exclude completely other mechanisms responsible for ventricular tachycardia, current information suggests that a great many ventricular tachycardias occurring in man are due to reentrant excitation.

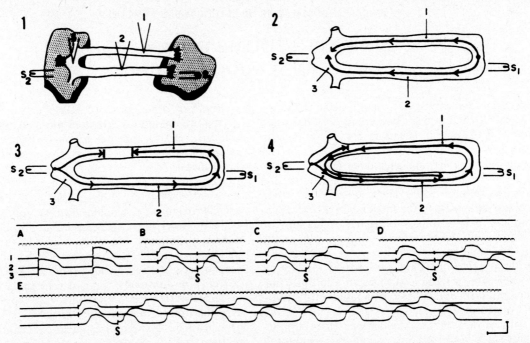

FIGURE 19–26 Sustained circus-movement "ventricular tachycardia" in an isolated preparation from a calf heart. Format of top half of figure: *Panel 1*, Schematic of preparation; stimulating electrodes at S_1 and S_2, recording microelectrodes at 1, 2, and 3; muscle = shaded area; Purkinje fibers = clear strips. *Panel 2*, Conduction of S_1 corresponding to panel B below. *Panel 3*, Conduction of S_2 corresponding to panel C below. *Panel 4*, Conduction of S_2 corresponding to panel D and E below. *Panel A*, Recordings obtained in normal Tyrode's solution. *Panels B to E*, Recordings obtained after exposure to high $[K]_o$ and epinephrine. S = premature stimulus at site 2. In panels B to E the basic drive (S_1) was applied at site 1, followed by a premature stimulus (S_2) applied at site 3. During the basic drive (S_1), activation appears almost simultaneously at sites 1 and 2 but with delay at site 3 (panel 2, above). Application of premature stimulus at S_2 in panel B causes excitation to travel from site 3 to site 2, but it does not reach site 1. Premature stimulus in panel C causes excitation to travel from site 3 to 2 and then to 1 (panel 3, above). In panel D, S_2 results in a sequence similar to that in panel C, which then continues back to site 3 and site 2 (panel 4, above). In panel E, premature stimulation results in several full circuits of this reentrant loop. Calibrations: Vertical = 100 mV; time marks are at 100-msec intervals. (From Wit, A. L., et al.: Slow conduction and reentry in the ventricular conducting system. II. Single and sustained circus movement in networks of canine and bovine Purkinje fibers. *Circ. Res.* 30:11, 1972. By permission of the American Heart Association, Inc.)

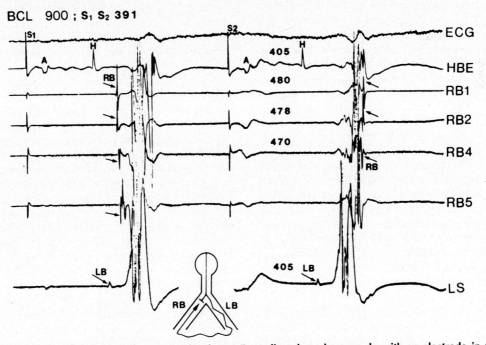

FIGURE 19–27 Reentry in the bundle branches of the dog heart. Recordings have been made with an electrode in the His bundle area (HBE), a multipolar plaque electrode sewn on the right bundle branch portraying activation from base to apex direction in electrograms RB_1 to RB_5 and from the left bundle branch (LB) in the left septal lead (LS). During the last basic cycle, S_1 applied to the atrium causes conduction to proceed from the His bundle through the left and right bundle branches to the ventricle. Note orderly progression of conduction from RB_1 to RB_5. At a premature right atrial interval of 391 msec, conduction is blocked distal to His, travels to the ventricle over the left bundle branch without any delay between left bundle branch deflections, and then activates the right bundle branch retrogradely from RB_4 to RB_2 to RB_1. Retrograde right bundle branch deflection in RB_5 cannot be seen. *Insert* shows activation sequence in bundle branches following S_2. (From Glassman, R. D., and Zipes, D. P.: Site of anterograde and retrograde functional right bundle branch block in the intact canine heart. *Circulation* 64:1277, 1981. By permission of the American Heart Association, Inc.)

APPROACH TO THE DIAGNOSIS
OF CARDIAC ARRHYTHMIAS

It is important to remember that the physician evaluates a *patient* who has a rhythm disturbance and does not evaluate a rhythm disturbance in isolation. Some rhythm disturbances are hazardous to the patient regardless of the clinical setting, while others are hazardous *because* of the clinical setting. Evaluation of the patient should usually progress from the simplest to the most complex test, from the least invasive and safest to the most invasive and risky, and from the least expensive out-of-hospital evaluations to those that require hospitalization and sophisticated, costly procedures. Occasionally, depending on the clinical circumstances, the physician may wish to proceed directly to a high-risk, expensive procedure, such as an electrophysiological study, prior to obtaining a 24-hour electrocardiographic (ECG) recording.

Patients with cardiac rhythm disturbances may present with a variety of complaints, but commonly symptoms such as palpitations, syncope, presyncope, or congestive heart failure cause them to seek a physician. Their awareness of regular or irregular cardiac rhythm varies greatly. Some patients may perceive slight variations in their heart rhythm with uncommon accuracy, while others are oblivious even to sustained episodes of ventricular tachycardia; still others complain of palpitations when they actually have regular sinus rhythm. The following tests can be used to evaluate patients who have cardiac arrhythmias.

TRANSTELEPHONIC ELECTROCARDIOGRAPHIC TRANSMISSION. Transmitters that send an electrocardiographic signal transtelephonically to a receiver unit may be used to transmit electrocardiographic information.[297] Such an instrument converts the patient's electrocardiogram to an audiotone, which, when transmitted to a recorder-receiver, is converted back to an electrocardiographic signal for interpretation. This device may be indicated when the rhythm disturbance is sufficiently infrequent that continuous ECG recording is impractical. Some recorders can store the ECG signal for later transmission. The arrhythmia must be of sufficient duration (several minutes) to permit the recording for the actual transmission or for later transmission and must not be associated with syncope or other symptoms that prevent the patient from transmitting or recording. A disadvantage to this approach is that it relies on the patient's perception of a cardiac rhythm disturbance, and many patients may be unaware of significant or serious bradyarrhythmias and tachyarrhythmias. In addition, the technique requires access to a receiver and some sort of receiving mechanism available 24 hours a day.

EXERCISE TESTING (See also pp. 257 to 278). About one-third of normal subjects develop ventricular ectopy in response to exercise testing. Ectopy is more likely to occur at faster heart rates, usually in the form of occasional, premature ventricular complexes (PVCs) of constant morphology,[298-304] or even pairs of PVCs, and is not reproducible from one stress test to the next.[298,300-302] Although multiform PVCs and ventricular tachycardia usually do not develop in normal patients, they can occur and therefore their presence does not establish the existence of ischemic or other forms of heart disease. Supraventricular premature complexes are often more common during exercise than at rest and increase in frequency with age; their occurrence does not suggest the presence of structural heart disease.[298]

Approximately 50 to 60 per cent[301-305] of patients who have coronary artery disease develop PVCs in response to exercise testing. Ventricular ectopy appears in these patients at lower heart rates (less than 130 bpm) than in the normal population and often occurs in the early recovery period as well.[306,307] The ectopy is more reproducible[301-304] during each stress test, and frequent PVCs (greater than 10/min), multiform PVCs, and ventricular tachycardia are more likely to occur in patients with coronary artery disease than in normal patients. Since exercise may suppress or exacerbate the frequency of PVCs occurring at rest, alteration in PVC frequency does not appear to be a helpful prognostic indicator.[305] The frequency of sudden cardiac death is increased in patients with coronary artery disease who develop ventricular ectopy at heart rates less than 130 bpm with exercise[301,302] and in whom the ectopy is associated with ST-segment changes, presumably as a manifestation of the relationship between ventricular ectopy and ischemia.[308]

Patients who have symptoms consistent with an arrhythmia induced by exercise (syncope, sustained palpitation, and the like) should be considered for stress testing. Stress testing may be indicated to uncover more complex grades of ectopy, to determine the relationship of the arrhythmia to activity, and to aid in choosing antiarrhythmic therapy. However, the test must be interpreted with caution because of the variability in results obtained in consecutive tests.[300,301] When two tests are performed 45 minutes apart, less ectopy is consistently recorded on the second test.[309] Hence, a decrease in the frequency of PVCs on the post-therapy test cannot be taken as absolute evidence of drug efficacy. However, the inability to reproduce sustained ventricular tachycardia on a second test, after it was produced at the first, or the absence of a deleterious effect on a second test might be helpful in assessing antiarrhythmic therapy. Stress testing appears to be more sensitive than a standard 12-lead resting ECG to detect ventricular ectopy.[300,304] However, prolonged ambulatory recording is more sensitive than exercise testing in establishing ventricular ectopy.[310] Since either technique may uncover serious arrhythmias which the other technique misses,[311] both examinations may be indicated for patients who have ischemic heart disease in whom frequent or complex ventricular ectopy is suspected.

LONG-TERM ELECTROCARDIOGRAPHIC RECORDING. Prolonged ECG recording (Holter monitoring, ambulatory monitoring) in patients engaged in normal daily activity permits quantitation of arrhythmia frequency and complexity, correlation with patient's symptoms, and evaluation of the effect of antiarrhythmic therapy on the arrhythmia.[310,312-316] In addition, such recording can document alterations in QRS, ST, and T contours, depending on the recorder used.[317] It is useful in detecting arrhythmias in symptomatic patients, correlating the ECG with symptoms, detecting pacemaker malfunction, and assessing the response to drug therapy.[317a]

Significant rhythm disturbances are fairly uncommon in healthy young persons. However, sinus bradycardia with heart rates of 35 to 40 bpm, sinus arrhythmia with pauses of even 2 seconds, Wenckebach second-degree AV block (often during sleep), a wandering atrial pacemaker, junctional escape complexes, and infrequent premature atrial complexes (PACs) and PVCs are not necessarily abnormal.[318,319,319a] Frequent ectopic complexes and complex atrial and ventricular rhythm disturbances are rarely recorded, however, and type II second-degree AV conduction disturbances are not recorded in normal patients. Elderly patients may have a greater prevalence of arrhythmias,[320] some of which may be responsible for neurological symptoms.[321,322]

A majority of patients who have ischemic heart disease, particularly those recovering from acute infarction, exhibit PVCs when monitored for periods of 6 to 24 hours. Although the presence of simple PVCs in some[323,324] but not all[325] studies appears to be of little therapeutic or prognostic significance, the following characteristics of ventricular ectopy have been reported to be associated with a worse prognosis in patients with ischemic heart disease: (1) frequent PVCs,[326–329] (2) multiform PVCs,[328–330] (3) early coupling intervals (R-on-T phenomenon),[323–330] (4) pairs of PVCs,[330] (5) bigeminy,[327,330] and (6) ventricular tachycardia.[331,332] Complexity may be related to the frequency of PVCs, and long-term recordings beyond 24 hours increases their detection.[316] There is no universal agreement as to the significance of each of these characteristics, but it is generally conceded that more complex forms of ventricular ectopy imply an increased risk of sudden cardiac death.[333–335b] Whether the ventricular ectopy is related causally to the subsequent sudden death or is only a marker identifying the patient at increased risk is unknown, but it is thought to be an independent risk factor. The frequency and complexity of ventricular rhythm disturbances recorded late in the hospital course or after hospitalization may bear no relation to those recorded during the acute phase.[336] In fact, the frequency of PVCs progressively increases over the first several weeks and months after hospitalization.[337] Serious ventricular ectopy correlates closely with the degree of impaired left ventricular function[336,338] and persistent ST-segment elevation[329] and with the extent of obstructive coronary vascular disease.[336]

Long-term ECG recording has often exposed potentially serious supraventricular tachyarrhythmias or frequent and complex ventricular ectopy in patients with hypertrophic cardiomyopathy[339,340] (p. 1415) and mitral valve prolapse[341–344] (p. 1091). Ventricular tachycardia or fibrillation does not necessarily result in patients who have complex ventricular rhythm disturbances, and sudden cardiac death has occurred in patients who have no documented arrhythmia on prolonged recordings.[345]

In patients who have otherwise unexplained syncope (Fig. 19–28) or transient vague cerebrovascular symptoms, potentially treatable rhythm disturbances are sometimes found on long-term ECG recordings to be the cause.[321,322,346,347] Such recordings may permit one to correlate symptoms with arrhythmias in several situations, including sinus node dysfunction,[348,349] the bradycardia-tachycardia syndrome,[350] and the Wolff-Parkinson-White syndrome.[351] For symptomatic patients with conduction disturbances, such as right bundle branch block and left axis deviation, invasive electrophysiological (His bundle) studies may be useful (p. 634). However, if these studies are nonrevealing particularly in patients with normal resting electrocardiograms, the diagnosis can be obtained by long-term ECG recording (Fig. 19–29). Long-term ECG recording may also be useful for documenting pacemaker malfunction[352] (p. 764).

In normal subjects and in patients with serious rhythm disturbances, the cardiac rhythm may vary markedly from one recording period to the next. To prove the efficacy of antiarrhythmic therapy, it is essential to demonstrate that the frequency of the abnormal rhythm disturbance is reduced more by the agent than by chance alone. Spontaneous reductions in the frequency of PVCs of up to 90 per cent have been demonstrated to occur between two recording periods.[314,353] Therefore, an antiarrhythmic agent must reduce the frequency of premature ventricular complexes by about 75 to 85 per cent, and the frequency of complex ventricular complexes 70 per cent, from one 24-hour recording period to another in order to be considered effective.[354]

Interpretative accuracy of long-term tape recordings varies with the system used. When technicians interpret the tape without semiautomated computer systems, an excellent qualitative analysis may be provided, i.e., detection of PVCs, ventricular tachycardia, asystolic intervals, and so forth, but not a quantitative account of the actual number of each event. With semiautomated interpreting systems, the error rate is 5 to 10 per cent of ectopic complexes. Recently developed fully automated computers reportedly miscount or misinterpret less than 3 per cent of ectopic complexes.[355,356] The clinical utility of such accuracy is questionable, since it is not clear that it really matters

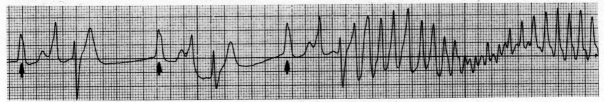

FIGURE 19–28 Onset of ventricular tachycardia–ventricular fibrillation during long-term ECG recording. This 41-year-old female presented with several episodes of presyncope. Bundle branch block and premature ventricular complexes were seen on 12-lead ECG. An electrophysiological study was totally normal (except for the presence of bundle branch block), and neither AV heart block nor ventricular tachyarrhythmias were initiated. After six weeks of *continuous* ECG recording, the patient had another syncopal spell, during which the ECG shown here was obtained. Arrows indicate sinus-initiated beats conducting with a left bundle branch block pattern. The patient could not be resuscitated.

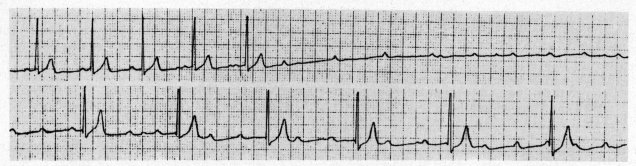

FIGURE 19–29 Paroxysmal complete atrioventricular block in a 25-year-old man with recurrent syncope for seven years. All studies, including an electrophysiological study, were totally normal. Long-term ECG recordings demonstrated intermittent complete AV block of unknown etiology. (From Zipes, D. P., and Noble, R. J.: Assessment of electrical abnormalities. *In* Hurst, J. W. (ed.): The Heart. 5th ed. New York, McGraw-Hill Book Co., 1982, pp. 333–357.)

whether a patient demonstrates 97 or 100 PVCs over a 24-hour period. All systems can potentially record more information than the physician knows how to assimilate. So long as the system detects ectopy, ventricular tachycardia, or asystolic intervals and semiquantitates those abnormalities, the physician probably receives all the clinical information that is needed. Though some physicians and regulatory agencies request information on the actual number of PVCs, until it is clearly demonstrated that reducing the number of PVCs improves prognosis, the necessity for such PVC quantitation is uncertain.

A variety of other recording devices exist that automatically record samples of the cardiac rhythm through the day or that are triggered to record a specific ECG event that occurs at a rate exceeding preset limits. Some record other physiologic signals such as respiratory rate, electroencephalogram, or blood pressure.

Invasive Electrophysiological Studies. An invasive electrophysiological procedure involves introducing multipolar catheter electrodes into the venous and/or arterial system, positioning the electrodes at various intracardiac sites to record electrical activity from portions of the atria or ventricles or from the region of the His bundle, and stimulating the atria or ventricles electrically. Such studies are performed diagnostically to provide information on the type of rhythm disturbance and insight into its electrophysiological mechanism. The procedure is used therapeutically to terminate a tachycardia by electrical stimulation as well as to evaluate effects of therapy by determining whether a particular intervention prevents electrical induction of a tachycardia.[357] Finally, these tests have been used prognostically to identify patients at risk for sudden cardiac death.[358,359] The study may be helpful in patients who have AV block, intraventricular conduction disturbance, sinus node dysfunction, tachycardia, and unexplained syncope or palpitations. It is important to remember that a negative test result—that is, not finding a particular abnormality—does not necessarily mean the patient may not experience the problem at another time. Thus, false-negative results are common with certain rhythm disturbances. A false-positive result, i.e., induction of a nonclinical arrhythmia, may be less common, depending on the stimulation protocol used, although accurate figures must be established for certain arrhythmias, like ventricular tachycardia. Several factors may explain the disparity between test results and spontaneous clinical occurrences, including altered autonomic tone in a supine patient undergoing study, therapeutic lidocaine serum concentrations resulting

from local infiltration to introduce the catheters,[360] changing anatomy after the study, and the fact that the test employs an artificial "trigger" (electrical stimulation) to induce the arrhythmia.[152]

AV BLOCK (See also pp. 730, 733, and 735). In patients with AV block, the site of block usually dictates the clinical course of the patient and whether or not a pacemaker is needed.[361,362] Generally, the site of AV block can be determined from an analysis of the scalar ECG. When the site of block cannot be determined from such an analysis, and when knowing the site of block is imperative for patient management, an invasive electrophysiological study is indicated. Candidates include patients who have second-degree AV block and bundle branch block, fixed 2:1 AV block, and syncope and AV block. Patients with block in the His-Purkinje system more commonly become symptomatic because of periods of bradycardia or asystole and require pacemaker implantation than do patients who have AV nodal block.[363–366] The mechanism responsible for the block, such as concealed His extrasystoles[367,368b] (Fig. 19–30), can sometimes be determined from such a study and can also influence the therapeutic course (p. 710).

INTRAVENTRICULAR CONDUCTION DISTURBANCE. For patients with an intraventricular conduction disturbance, an electrophysiological study provides information on the duration of the H-V interval, which can be prolonged with a normal P-R interval or normal with a prolonged P-R interval. A prolonged H-V interval is associated with a greater likelihood of developing trifascicular block, having organic disease, and higher mortality.[369] Some data suggest that finding very long H-V intervals (> 80 to 90 msec) identifies patients at significant risk of developing AV block. During the study, atrial pacing is used to uncover abnormal His-Purkinje conduction.[365,370] In addition to stressing the His-Purkinje system by pacing the atria at fast rates and short premature intervals, drug infusion, such as with procainamide or ajmaline, sometimes exposes abnormal His-Purkinje conduction.[371,372] Ajmaline may cause arrhythmias and should be used cautiously.[373]

An electrophysiological study is indicated only if the patient has symptoms that appear to be related to a bradyarrhythmia (syncope or presyncope) and when no other cause for syncope is found. For many of these patients, ventricular *tachyarrhythmias* rather than AV block may be the cause of their symptoms.[369] In patients who develop bundle branch block associated with acute anteroseptal myocardial infarction, finding a prolonged H-V in-

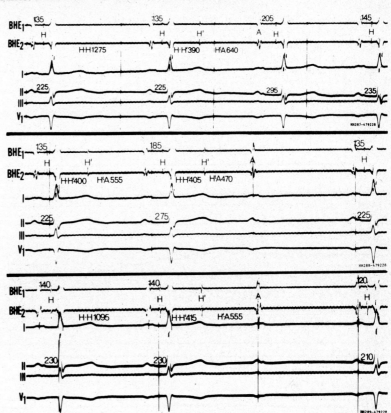

FIGURE 19-30 Concealed discharge from the bundle of His mimicking first-degree (top), type I (middle), and type II (bottom) second-degree AV block. Numbers are in milliseconds. Time lines are one second. (Magnification differs in the three panels.) Numbers in the bipolar His electrogram (BHE₁) indicate A-H intervals; the H-V interval is constant. Numbers in lead II indicate the P-R interval. H-H = interval between His responses in normal conducted cycles. H-H′ = interval between the last normal His discharge and the premature His discharge. H′-A = interval between the premature His depolarization and the next normal sinus-initiated atrial discharge. H′ invaded the AV node and lengthened the A-H interval or produced AV nodal block of the next atrial depolarization. (From Bonner, A. J., and Zipes, D. P.: Lidocaine and His bundle extrasystoles. His bundle discharge conducted normally, conducted with functional right or left bundle branch block or blocked entirely (concealed). Arch. Intern. Med. 136:700, 1976.)

terval may help identify those who are at greater risk of developing complete AV block or ventricular tachyarrhythmias and of dying.[374,375] Patients who develop bifascicular block and transient high-grade AV block during acute myocardial infarction may not require electrophysiological study, since pacemaker therapy is often recommended on the basis of their clinical course alone[375-377] (see pp. 744 and 756).

SINUS NODAL DYSFUNCTION. The demonstration of slow sinus rates, sinus exit block, or sinus pauses temporally related to symptoms strongly suggests a causal relationship and may obviate further diagnostic studies. Carotid sinus pressure that results in complete cardiac asystole with associated symptoms may expose the patient with a hypersensitive carotid sinus reflex[378] (p. 692). Carotid sinus massage must be done cautiously.[379] Neurohumoral agents or stress testing[380] may be employed to evaluate effects of autonomic tone on sinus nodal function. Atropine,[381,382] isoproterenol,[383] propranolol,[384] and combined atropine and propranolol to produce pharmacological denervation[381,385,386] have been used to identify the patient with sinus node dysfunction due to abnormal autonomic tone. Invasive electrophysiological studies to evaluate sinus node function include assessment of sinus node automaticity and sinoatrial conduction time. Electrophysiological studies should be considered in patients who have symptoms attributable to bradycardia or asystole, such as presyncope or syncope, and for whom noninvasive approaches have provided no explanation for the symptoms.

Overdrive suppression appears to be one of the more useful and sensitive tests to evaluate sinus node function.[212,387-389] The interval between the last paced high right atrial response and the first spontaneous (sinus) high right atrial response after termination of pacing is measured to determine the *sinus node recovery time.* Since spontaneous sinus cycle length influences sinus node recovery time, the *cor-*

rected sinus node recovery time may be used, calculated by subtracting the spontaneous sinus node cycle length (prior to pacing) from the sinus recovery time (Fig. 19–31). Normal values are generally less than 525 msec.[388,389] Prolonged sinus node recovery time has been found in 35 to 93 per cent of patients suspected of having sinus node dysfunction.[198,349,390] The wide range in these values probably depends on whether the patient population includes many who have ECG evidence only of sinus bradycardia.[198,349,391] Such patients often have normal corrected sinus node recovery times. After cessation of pacing, the first return sinus cycle may be normal and may be followed by secondary pauses (Fig. 19–31). Secondary pauses appear to be more common in patients whose sinus node dysfunction is caused by sinoatrial exit block. It is important to evaluate AV nodal and His-Purkinje function in patients with sinus node dysfunction, since many also exhibit impaired AV conduction.[392]

Sinoatrial conduction time can be estimated, based on the assumptions that (1) conduction times into and out of the sinus node are equal, (2) no depression of sinus node automaticity occurs, and (3) the pacemaker site does not shift following premature stimulation. Since these assumptions cannot be applied to all patients, determining sinus node conduction time is less useful than determining corrected sinus node recovery time when sinus node function in human beings is evaluated.[392a]

Marked sinus arrhythmia invalidates the calculation of sinoatrial conduction time; to eliminate its effects, brief periods of atrial pacing at rates just faster than the sinus rate have been used instead of testing during sinus rhythm.[393] The accuracy of this test is comparable to that achieved when testing during sinus rhythm.[393] Generally, measurement of sinoatrial conduction time is an insensitive indicator of sinus node dysfunction, since the time is prolonged in less than half the patients with clinical findings of sinus

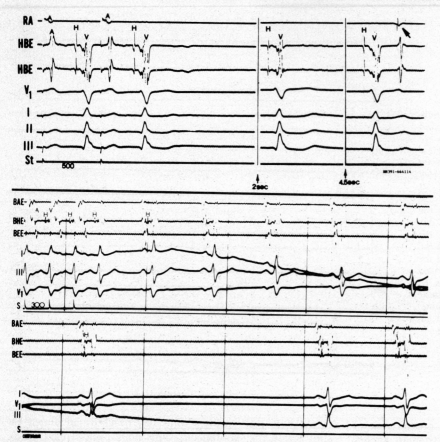

FIGURE 19–31 Abnormal response of sinus node to overdrive pacing. *Top,* After 30 sec of right atrial pacing at a cycle length of 500 msec, sinus nodal discharge (arrow) is suppressed for more than 8 sec. (Sections of 2 sec and 4.5 sec removed for mounting.) *Bottom,* Right atrial pacing at a cycle length of 300 msec was followed by initial P waves occurring at an appropriate rate. The rate then slowed progressively, with P-P prolongation reaching 3 seconds and reproducing the patient's symptoms. Continuous recording; time lines = 1 sec. RA and BAE = bipolar right atrial electrogram; HBE and BHE = bipolar His electrogram; BEE = bipolar esophageal electrogram; I, II, III, and V = scalar leads; St and S = stimulus. (Modified from Zipes, D. P., and Noble, R. J.: Assessment of electrical abnormalities. *In* Hurst, J. W. (ed.): The Heart. 5th ed. New York, McGraw-Hill Book Co., 1982, pp. 333–357.)

node dysfunction. It is least likely to be abnormal in patients with asymptomatic sinus bradycardia and is more frequently abnormal in patients with sinus node exit block or the bradycardia-tachycardia syndrome.

In contrast to these indirect measures of sinus node function, a technique has been developed recently to record sinus nodal activity with extracellular electrodes.[394] This approach may permit more accurate characterization of sinus nodal automaticity and sinoatrial conduction in humans and more reliable identification of patients who have sinus node dysfunction.

TACHYCARDIA. Electrophysiological study provides useful information in patients with tachycardias. First, it can be used to differentiate aberrant supraventricular conduction from ventricular tachyarrhythmias (p. 702). Since all the electrocardiographic manifestations of ventricular tachycardia may be mimicked, under certain circumstances, by aberrantly conducted supraventricular tachycardia, exceptions exist to the criteria that help to differentiate supraventricular tachyarrhythmias with abnormal QRS complexes from ventricular tachyarrhythmias.[395] A *supraventricular tachycardia* is recognized electrophysiologically by the presence of an H-V interval equaling or exceeding that recorded during normal sinus rhythm (Fig. 19–32). In contrast, during *ventricular tachycardia,* the H-V interval is shorter than normal or, more commonly, cannot be recorded clearly. Only two situations exist when a consistently short H-V interval occurs: during retrograde activation of the His bundle when activation originated in the ventricle or during conduction over an accessory pathway (preexcitation syndrome). A short H-V interval may occur randomly during AV dissociation when atrial activation that discharges the His bundle is superimposed on independent ventricular activation.

Atrial pacing at rates exceeding the rate of the tachycardia can be used to demonstrate ventricular origin of the wide QRS tachycardia by producing fusion and capture beats and normalization of the H-V interval (Fig. 19–33).[152] A tachycardia conducting with functional aberrancy would not be expected to respond in such a fashion. In some patients, atropine administration to improve AV nodal conduction may facilitate ventricular capture by the atria. During aberrantly conducted supraventricular tachycardia, premature ventricular stimulation sometimes can be used to eliminate the functional bundle branch block and restore normal ventricular conduction (Fig. 19–34).[396]

Initiation and termination with programmed electrical stimulation of supraventricular or ventricular tachycardia to test the potential efficacy of pharmacological, pacemaker, or surgical therapy represents a second important application of electrophysiological studies in patients with tachycardia.[397-399] One can compare the ability to initiate tachycardia after acute and after chronic administration of a drug or combination of drugs. Results from long-term ECG recordings may be insufficient, in some instances, to predict a patient's therapeutic response. For example, electrophysiological testing still provokes ventricular tachycardia in 75 to 80 per cent of patients with a history of ventricular tachycardia, at a time when the ventricular tachycardia appears to be suppressed successfully by drugs, based on results of a 24-hour ECG recording.[400] A drug that prevents electrical induction of a tachycardia induced during the control state has a high probability of achieving long-term successful suppression of spontaneous episodes.[399] A drug that fails to prevent electrical induction may still prevent spontaneous clinical episodes, depending on the drug, possibly the type of heart disease, and the mechanism of initiation and maintenance of the tachycar-

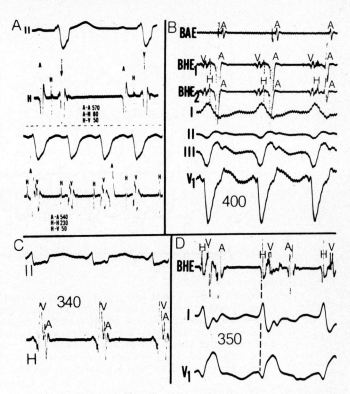

FIGURE 19–32 His bundle recording in four different patients with tachycardias. *A*, The top portion of the tracing shows His bundle recording during sinus rhythm. The H-V interval is 50 msec. The bottom portion shows His bundle recording during tachycardia. Since the QRS complex and H-V interval are the same as those recorded during sinus rhythm, this is a supraventricular tachycardia. Of note is the fact that the atria discharged at a rate that was different from (not a multiple of) the ventricular rate. Thus, AV dissociation is present during this supraventricular tachycardia. *B*, His bundle activity occurred after the onset of the QRS complex, during ventricular septal depolarization, which confirmed the diagnosis of ventricular tachycardia. (WPW had been excluded.) The R-P interval remained constant, and the atria were captured retrogradely from the ventricles. Thus, AV dissociation is not present during this ventricular tachycardia. *C*, His bundle activity was not recorded despite careful exploration of the His bundle area with the catheter electrode tip. This most likely represents ventricular tachycardia with 1:1 retrograde atrial capture, but the diagnosis cannot be as clear as in panels *B* and *D*, His bundle activity preceded the onset of ventricular septal depolarization (interrupted line) but followed the onset of the QRS complex. Thus, this must be ventricular tachycardia. Retrograde (VA) Wenckebach conduction (not shown in its entirety) was also present. (From Zipes, D. P., et al.: Clinical electrophysiology and electrocardiography. *In* Willerson, J. T., and Sanders, C. A. (eds.): The Science and Practice of Clinical Medicine. Clinical Cardiology. New York, Grune and Stratton, 1977, pp. 235–248.)

dia. Finally, the patient's hemodynamic response to the tachycardia can be assessed. Often, drugs slow the rate of a tachycardia, even though they fail to prevent its induction, and the patient has a better hemodynamic response to the tachycardia. This is not always true, and some patients experience greater hemodynamic decompensation during a ventricular tachycardia at a slower rate while receiving a drug compared to when the tachycardia was induced in a drug-free state. This difference in response can be assessed during the study.

The site of origin and/or the pathways involved in maintenance of some tachycardias can be localized by endocardial mapping. This technique has proved efficacious in patients with the Wolff-Parkinson-White syndrome or its variants[401] and in selected patients with ventricular tachycardia[287,402,403] (p. 721).

Finally, an electrophysiological study may provide some insight into possible electrophysiological mechanisms responsible for the tachycardia.[286] Conduction and refractoriness of various cardiac tissues involved in the tachycardia can be assessed. Although it is difficult in most instances to differentiate reentry from automaticity reliably (see p. 619),[152] evidence in favor of one or the other mechanism may be obtained. For example, initiation of a tachycardia by premature stimulation, especially when a critical degree of conduction delay is required, is consistent with reentry. Similarly, termination by premature stimulation that produces block in a critical site suggests reentry. However, as stated earlier (p. 620), premature stimulation can start and stop tachycardias due to triggered activity in much the same fashion. Pacing stimuli that simply reset the discharge cycle length or produce transient overdrive suppression (see Fig. 19–12) or fail to start the tachycardia when it is not present fit the concepts of automaticity. Overdrive acceleration might be more consistent with triggered activity. In selected patients, differentiation between reentry and automaticity may influence the selection of therapy, particularly as new antiarrhythmic agents, pacing, or sur-

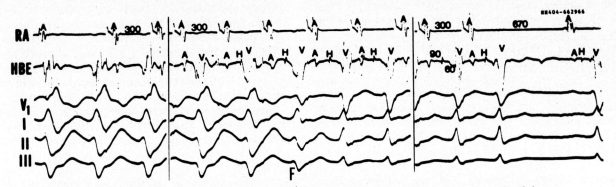

FIGURE 19–33 Termination of ventricular tachycardia by rapid atrial pacing. Ventricular tachycardia (*left panel*) with AV dissociation became captured by rapid atrial pacing (200 bpm) (*middle panel*) and was terminated after cessation of atrial pacing (*right panel*). Note fusion beat (F) in the midportion of panel 2 and normalization of the H-V interval. (From Foster, P. R., and Zipes, D. P.: Pacing and cardiac arrhythmias. *In* Mandel, W. J. (ed.): Cardiac Arrhythmias. Their Mechanisms, Diagnosis and Management. Philadelphia, J. B. Lippincott, 1980, pp. 605–624.)

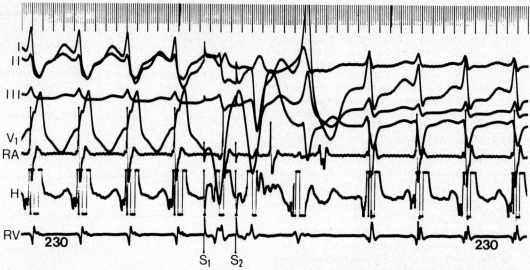

FIGURE 19–34   A wide QRS tachycardia was initiated in this patient. Despite numerous changes in catheters and in catheter positions, an adequate His bundle electrogram could not be recorded, and the diagnosis of ventricular tachycardia could not be excluded. Premature ventricular stimulation (S_1-S_2) normalized the QRS complex at an identical cycle length as the wide QRS tachycardia. Premature right ventricular stimulation thus eliminated the functional right bundle branch block and established the diagnosis of supraventricular tachycardia with aberrancy. (From Zipes, D. P., and Noble, R. J.: Assessment of electrical abnormalities. *In* Hurst, J. W. (ed.): The Heart, 5th ed. New York, McGraw-Hill Book Co., 1982, pp. 333–357.)

gical approaches are developed that may preferentially affect one or the other mechanism.

An electrophysiological study should be considered in patients who have symptomatic, recurrent, or drug-resistant tachyarrhythmias or tachyarrhythmias occurring too infrequently to permit adequate diagnostic or therapeutic assessment. Such inclusion criteria apply to patients who have supraventricular tachyarrhythmias (e.g., reciprocating tachycardia, atrial flutter, or fibrillation with a very rapid ventricular response [often, though not always associated with the Wolff-Parkinson-White syndrome]) and to patients who have symptomatic ventricular tachyarrhythmias. The studies appear useful to guide diagnosis and therapy in patients resuscitated from out-of-hospital sudden death associated with ventricular tachyarrhythmias.[404]

Electrophysiological testing may help identify patients at risk for the subsequent development of ventricular tachycardia or sudden death, not by eliciting a spontaneous premature ventricular complex, called a repetitive ventricular response following a single premature ventricular stimulus delivered during sinus rhythm or atrial pacing[359,405-409] as was originally suggested,[358] but by inducing ventricular tachycardia in susceptible patients.[410,410a]

PATIENTS WITH UNEXPLAINED PALPITATIONS OR SYNCOPE.   The three common arrhythmic causes of syncope or palpitations include sinus node dysfunction, tachyarrhythmias, and AV block. Of the three, tachyarrhythmias are probably most reliably initiated in the electrophysiology laboratory, followed by sinus node abnormalities and then His-Purkinje block. The electrophysiological study may fail to explain the patient's symptoms if the arrhythmia cannot be induced or if an abnormal rhythm is induced and the patient remains asymptomatic. However, induction of an arrhythmia that replicates the patient's symptoms may explain the cause of the palpitations or syncope. Patients considered for a study are those whose recurrent syncopal spells remain undiagnosed despite complete general and neurological

evaluation, repeated 24-hour ECG recordings, stress testing, and other noninvasive cardiac tests. The presence of palpitations alone is *not* an indication for an electrophysiological study. However, an electrophysiological study may be useful if the patient complains of symptoms such as angina, shortness of breath, or lightheadedness during the palpitations; if there is evidence that the palpitations may represent a significant rhythm disturbance, and if noninvasive studies fail to reveal a cause of the palpitations.

Sensitivity and Specificity.   Some understanding of the sensitivity and specificity of the results obtained from electrophysiological testing is required to decide which patients might benefit from such a study. Invasive electrophysiological studies provide important information when a particular abnormality can be demonstrated. Electrophysiological testing initiates paroxysmal supraventricular tachycardia due to Wolff-Parkinson-White syndrome or AV node reentry in over 90 per cent of patients who have spontaneously occurring tachycardias. The ability to precipitate ventricular tachycardia in patients who have spontaneous episodes varies with the etiology of the heart disease and nature of the ventricular tachycardia. During right ventricular pacing, ventricular tachycardia can be induced most often in patients who have ischemic heart disease and sustained ventricular tachycardia and least often in those with heart disease unrelated to ischemia and nonsustained ventricular tachycardia[411] (Fig. 19–28).

More aggressive pacing techniques (e.g., using three premature stimuli), administration of drugs (e.g., isoproterenol), or left ventricular pacing[412] may increase the success rate of ventricular tachycardia induction. The increased sensitivity of the test is paralleled by a decreased specificity because of the induction of nonclinical ventricular tachyarrhythmias. Initiation of sustained supraventricular[219] or ventricular[402,413] tachyarrhythmia during an electrophysiological study provides important information that the induced tachyarrhythmia *may* be clinically significant and responsible for the patient's symptoms. Induction of *sustained* supraventricular or ventricular tachycardia (not pleomorphic ventricular tachycardia progressing to ventricular fibrillation) during an electrophysiological study in patients who are not subject to the spontaneous development of the tachycardia appears to be uncommon, although *appropriate control groups, particularly for ventricular tachycardia, have not yet been reported.* The frequency of induction of ventricular tachycardia in patients who have no history of ventricular tachycardia but have heart disease comparable to those that do have a history of ventricular tachycardia is *not known* and needs to be established using the same stimulation protocols employed to induce ventricular tachyarrhythmias in patients with a history of ventricular tachycardia.[117] Generally, abnormalities such as sustained tachycardia, prolonged pauses following overdrive right atrial pacing, or type II AV block cannot be induced in patients who do not or may not experience these abnormalities spontaneously. In these examples, electrophysiological studies may have a high level of specificity.

Failure to initiate an arrhythmia does not exclude it as a possible cause of the patient's symptoms because of false-negative responses, as mentioned earlier. This caveat is particularly applicable to patients with sinus node dysfunction. Initiation of an abnormally long pause following overdrive pacing, for example, is uncommon in patients without abnormal sinus node function. However, as many as 50 per cent of patients with sinus bradycardia and 20 per cent of those with sinus pauses or sinus exit block may respond normally to overdrive pacing.[198,349,391] His-Purkinje block of a spontaneous or electrically-induced premature atrial complex may occur in normal patients, particularly when the basic cycle length is long and AV nodal propagation is fairly rapid (Fig. 19–35). However, development of block in the His-Purkinje system during sinus rhythm, at atrial-paced rates less than 130 to 150 bpm,[365] at premature intervals (H_1-H_2) longer than about 450 msec,[370] indicates abnormal refractoriness and/or conduction in the His-Purkinje system. However, this is often difficult to produce.

The yield from electrophysiological studies in patients who have syncope appears to vary with the population studied. In one report, such testing revealed a possible cause of the syncope in 68 per cent of 25 patients, most of whom had abnormal ECGs and forms of organic heart disease.[414] In a second study,[415] electrophysiological testing was useful in only 12 per cent of 34 patients who had a normal ECG and no evidence of organic heart disease. Thus, patient selection may influence the usefulness of such testing in patients with unexplained syncope. In these latter situations the sensitivity of the test is low.

Cognizance of the sensitivity and specificity of electrophysiological study for each rhythm disturbance is important, since the risks of these studies, although small (about 2 per cent), far exceed the risks associated with noninvasive tests used to assess electrical abnormalities.[416] Morbidity is the same as that for any cardiac catheterization procedure (p. 296) and includes any vascular complications such as bleeding, thrombosis, thrombophlebitis, pulmonary embolus, inadvertent puncture of the femoral artery, development of arteriovenous fistula, and cardiac perforation. If the left ventricle is mapped or stimulated, morbidity increases, with possible problems associated

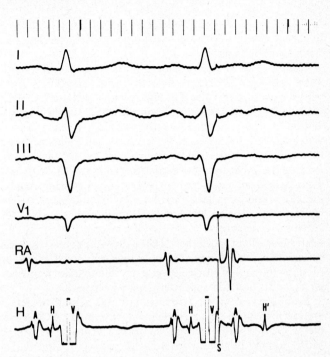

FIGURE 19–35 Premature atrial complex blocking distal to the His bundle recording site. The first two beats are of sinus origin at a cycle length of 670 msec. A premature right atrial stimulus prolongs the A-H interval from 80 msec during sinus rhythm to 150 msec. The premature His response (H′) occurs at an H-H′ interval of 370 msec, and the impulse blocks distal to the His bundle recording site. I, II, III, and V_1 = scalar leads; RA = right atrial lead; H = His bundle lead; A = atrial deflection; H′ = His bundle deflection; V = ventricular depolarization; S = premature right atrial stimulus. (Dark time lines = 50 msec.)

with an arterial puncture and left heart catheterization. If the subclavian approach is used, pneumothorax or arterial puncture may occur. Since precipitation of AV block or a tachyarrhythmia is often a desirable goal of the study, symptoms from such rhythm disturbances may result, compounding the morbidity. Mortality from the study should be near zero, although this depends on how ill the patient may be. In patients with significant myocardial dysfunction, it may be possible to precipitate a ventricular tachyarrhythmia that cannot be terminated by direct-current cardioversion or that results in cerebral, renal, or cardiac ischemia or infarction before termination.

Finally, the procedures are time-consuming[417] and expensive and require sophisticated equipment and personnel trained in catheterization techniques, cardiopulmonary resuscitation, and clinical cardiac electrophysiology. The cost of a three-day hospitalization plus electrophysiological study may exceed the cost of 20 to 25 long-term (24-hour) ECG recordings.

ESOPHAGEAL ELECTROCARDIOGRAPHY. Esophageal electrocardiography is a useful noninvasive technique to diagnose arrhythmias.[200,418,419] The esophagus is adjacent to the posterior atria, and an electrode inserted into the esophagus can record atrial potentials. Bipolar recording appears superior to unipolar recording.[200,420,421] In addition, atrial and occasionally ventricular pacing can be performed via a catheter electrode inserted into the esophagus, and initiation and termination of tachycardias can be accomplished.[422] In adults, optimum atrial recordings are obtained when the distal electrode on the esophageal lead is positioned approximately 40 cm from the patient's na-res.[419] Recently, a capsule electrode that is easily swallowed has been used to record continuous atrial electrograms from the esophagus.[418]

The esophageal atrial electrogram is useful for differentiating supraventricular tachycardia with aberrancy from ventricular tachycardia. During a wide QRS tachycardia when the ventricular rate exceeds the atrial rate, AV dissociation is often present, and the most likely diagnosis is ventricular tachycardia. If each ventricular depolarization is coupled to an atrial depolarization, either supraventricular tachycardia or ventricular tachycardia with 1:1 ventriculoatrial conduction may be present. Uncommonly, junctional tachycardia with aberrancy may mimic ventricular tachycardia, and His bundle recordings are needed for a definitive diagnosis. When the same number of atrial and ventricular depolarizations occur, the autonomic nervous system may be manipulated to evoke AV nodal block or to slow the supraventricular rate to differentiate ventricular tachycardia from supraventricular tachycardia.

Esophageal atrial electrograms are also helpful to define the mechanism of supraventricular tachycardias. For example, a narrow QRS tachycardia with a ventricular rate of 150 bpm may be due to atrial flutter with a 2:1 ventricular response, confirmed by finding an atrial rate of 300 bpm. If atrial and ventricular depolarization occur simultaneously during paroxysmal supraventricular tachycardia, reentry utilizing an accessory AV pathway (Wolff-Parkinson-White) can be excluded, and AV nodal reentry is the most likely mechanism for the tachycardia (p. 707).

BODY SURFACE MAPPING. Isopotential body surface maps are used to provide a complete picture of the effects of the currents from the heart on the body surface.[423] The potential distributions are represented by contour lines of equal potential, and each distribution is displayed instant-by-instant throughout activation or recovery, or both.

Body surface maps have been used for preliminary clinical application in the following areas:[423] localizing and sizing myocardial infarction,[424–426] detecting areas of ischemia (especially those apparent only with exercise), localizing ectopic foci[427] or accessory pathways,[428] and differentiating aberrant supraventricular conduction from ventricular origin.

DIRECT CARDIAC MAPPING: RECORDING POTENTIALS DIRECTLY FROM THE HEART. Cardiac mapping is a method whereby potentials recorded directly from the heart are spatially depicted as a function of time in an integrated manner. The location of recording electrodes (epicardial, intramural, or endocardial) and the recording mode used (unipolar versus bipolar) as well as the method of display (isopotential versus isochrone maps) depend upon the problem under consideration.

Direct cardiac mapping via catheter electrodes or at the time of cardiac surgery can be used to localize accessory pathways associated with the Wolff-Parkinson-White syndrome,[429,430] to delineate the anatomical course of the His bundle during open-heart surgery to avoid injury during procedures to correct congenital heart defects.[431] and to identify the site of rhythm disturbances in patients with supraventricular and ventricular tachyarrhythmias refractory to medical therapy; it has also fostered surgical approaches for extirpation of the latter[287,401,403,432] (p. 672). Areas of myocardial ischemia or infarction can be identified to revascularize or to define margins for surgical resection in the treatment of ischemic heart disease.[433,434]

These approaches are discussed in greater detail under the individual arrhythmias in Chapter 21.

SIGNAL-AVERAGING TECHNIQUES. Signal averaging is a method that improves signal-to-noise ratio when signals occur recurrently and the noise is random, i.e., not synchronous with the signal. In conjunction with other methods of noise reduction, signal averaging can detect cardiac signals of a few microvolts. With this method, potentials generated by the sinus and AV nodes,[435] His-bundle, and bundle branches are detectable at the body surface.[436–438] The duration of the His-Purkinje waveform corresponds to the H-V interval recorded by the catheter technique. A new development permits high amplification, "on-line" His bundle recordings from the skin surface.[436] Signal averaging has also been applied to improve resolution of potentials that are detectable by standard recording techniques. Examples of such application include recording fetal electrocardiograms[439] as well as recording P waves and ST waves during exercise.[440]

Detecting late ventricular activation in patients with intraventricular conduction delay and ventricular tachycardias may become clinically useful.[441] Delayed activation potentials may serve as a portent of serious ventricular arrhythmias,[442,443] a guide to antiarrhythmic therapy, a diagnostic aid in detecting heart disease, or a means of differentiating between reentrant and automatic ectopic beats. It is likely that signal averaging and other techniques of signal conditioning will become increasingly important in the next several years.

References

1. Keith, A., and Flack, M. W.: The form and nature of the muscular connections between the primary divisions of the vertebrate heart. J. Anat. Physiol. 41:172, 1907.
2. James, T. N.: Anatomy of the conduction system of the heart. In Hurst, J. W. (ed.): The Heart. New York, McGraw-Hill Book Co., 1982.
3. Anderson, R. H., and Becker, A. E.: Gross anatomy and microscopy of the conducting system. In Mandel, W. J. (ed.): Cardiac Arrhythmias, Their Mechanisms, Diagnosis and Management. Philadelphia, J. B. Lippincott, 1980.
4. James, T. N.: Anatomy of the Coronary Arteries. New York, Harper and Row, 1961.
5. James, T. N.: The sinus node as a servomechanism. Circ. Res. 32:307, 1973.
6. James, T. N., Sherf, L., Fine, G., and Morales, A. R.: Comparative ultrastructure of the sinus node in man and dog. Circulation 34:139, 1966.
7. Masson-Pevet, M., Bleeker, W. K., and Gas, D.: The plasma membrane of leading pacemaker cells in the rabbit sinus node: A qualitative and quantitative ultrastructural analysis. Circ. Res. 45:621, 1979.
8. Trautwein, W., and Uchizono, K.: Electron microscopic and electrophysiologic study of the pacemaker in the sino-atrial node of the rabbit heart. Z. Zellforsch. Mikrosk. Anat. 61:96, 1963.
9. Bleeker, W. K., Mackaay, A. J., Masson-Pevet, M., Bouman, L. N., and Becker, A. E.: Functional and morphological organization of the rabbit sinus node. Circ. Res. 46(1):11, 1980.
10. Becker, A. E., Bouman, L. N., Janse, M. J., and Anderson, R. H.: Functional anatomy of the cardiac conduction system, Harrison, D. C. (ed.): Cardiac Arrhythmias: A Decade of Progress. Boston, G. K. Hall, 1981, p. 3.
11. Levy, M. N., and Martin, P. J.: Neural control of the heart. In Berne, R. M., et al. (eds.): Handbook of Physiology. Section 2, The Cardiovascular System. Vol. I, The Heart. Bethesda, Md., American Physiological Society, 1979, p. 581.
12. Randall, W. C.: Sympathetic control of the heart. In Randall, W. C. (ed.): Neural Regulation of the Heart. New York, Oxford University Press, 1977.
13. Zipes, D. P., Mihalick, M. J., and Robbins, G. T.: Effects of selective vagal and stellate ganglion stimulation on atrial refractoriness. Cardiovasc. Res. 8:647, 1974.
14. Prystowsky, E. N., Naccarelli, G. V., Jackman, W. M., Rinkenberger, R. L., Heger, J. J., and Zipes, D. P.: Enhanced vagal tone produced by neck collar suction shortens atrial refractoriness in man. Am. J. Cardiol. 47:496, 1981.

15. Takahashi, N., and Zipes, D. P.,: Pre- and postsynaptic modulation of adrenergic effects on canine sinus nodal automaticity and AV nodal conduction by vagal stimulation. Clin. Res. *30*:485A, 1982.

16. James, T. N.: The connecting pathways between the sinus node and the AV node and between the right and left atrium in the human heart. Circulation *53*: 609, 1963.

17. Hogan, P. M., and Davis, L. D.: Electrophysiological characteristics of canine atrial plateau fibers. Circ. Res. *28*:62, 1971.

18. Sherf, L., and James, T. N.: Fine structure of cells and their histologic organization within internodal pathways of the heart: clinical and electrocardiographic implications. Am. J. Cardiol. *44*:345, 1979.

19. Roberts, D. E., Hersch, L. T., and Scher, A. M.: Influence of cardiac fiber orientation on wavefront voltage, conduction velocity, and tissue resistivity in the dog. Circ. Res. *44*:701, 1979.

20. Scher, A. M., and Spach, M. S.: Cardiac depolarization and repolarization and the electrocardiogram. *In* Berne, R. M., et al. (eds.): Handbook of Physiology, The Cardiovascular System. Bethesda, Md., American Physiological Society, 1979, p. 357.

21. Vassalle, M., and Hoffman, B. F.: The spread of sinus activation during potassium administration. Circ. Res. *17*:285, 1965.

22. Waldo, A. L., Bush, H. L., Jr., Gelband, H., Zorn, G. L., Vitikainen, K. J., and Hoffman, B. F.: Effects on the canine P wave of discrete lesions in the specialized atrial tracts. Circ. Res. *29*:452, 1971.

23. Spach, M. S., Lieberman, M., Scott, J. G., Barr, R. C., Johnson, E. A., and Kootsey, J. M.: Excitation sequences of the atrial septum and the AV node in isolated hearts of the dog and rabbit. Circ. Res. *29*:156, 1971.

24. Janse, M. J., and Anderson, R. H.: Specialized internodal atrial pathways—Fact or fiction? Eur. J. Cardiol. *2*:117, 1974.

25. Hoffman, B. F.: Fine structure of internodal pathways. Am. J. Cardiol. *44*:385, 1979.

26. Wagner, M. L., Lazzara, R., Weiss, R. M., and Hoffman, B. F.: Specialized conducting fibers in the interatrial band. Circ. Res. *18*:502, 1966.

27. Childers, R. W., Merideth, J., and Moe, G. K.: Supernormality in Bachmann's bundle: An *in vitro* and *in vivo* study in the dog. Circ. Res. *22*:363, 1968.

28. Becker, A. E., and Anderson, R. H.: Morphology of the human atrioventricular junctional area. *In* Wellens, H. J. J., et al. (eds.): The Conduction System of the Heart. Philadelphia, Lea and Febiger, 1976, p. 263.

29. Hecht, H. H., Kossmann, C. E., Childers, R. W., Langendorf, R., Ler, M., Rosen, K. M., Pruitt, R. D., Truex, R. L., Uhley, H. N., and Watt, T. B.: Atrioventricular and intraventricular conduction. Revised nomenclature and concepts. Am. J. Cardiol. *31*:232, 1973.

30. James, T. N.: Morphology of the human atrioventricular node, with remarks pertinent to its electrophysiology. Am. Heart J. *62*:652, 1961.

31. Jackman, W. M., Prystowsky, E. N., Naccarelli, G. B., Heger, J. J., and Zipes, D. P.: Enhanced AV nodal conduction: Prevalence and anatomic substrate. Circulation *67*:441, 1983.

32. Kulbertus, H. E., and Demoulin, J. C.: Pathological basis of concept of left hemiblock. *In* Wellens, H. J. J., et al. (eds.): Conduction System of the Heart. Philadelphia, Lea and Febiger, 1976, p. 287.

33. Massing, G. K., and James, T. N.: Anatomic configuration of the His bundle and bundle branches in the human heart. Circulation *53*:609, 1976.

34. Rosenbaum, M. B., Elizari, M. V., and Lazzari, J. O.: The Hemiblocks. Oldsmar, Fla., Tampa Tracings, 1970.

35. Gilmour, R. F., Jr., and Zipes, D. P.: Different electrophysiological responses of canine endocardium and epicardium to combined hyperkalemia, hypoxia and acidosis. Circ. Res. *46*:814, 1980.

36. Janse, M. J., van Capelle, F. J. L., Anderson, R. H., Toubone, P., and Billette, J.: Electrophysiology and structure of the atrioventricular node of the isolated rabbit heart. *In* Wellens, H. J. J., et al. (eds.): The Conduction System of the Heart. Philadelphia, Lea and Febiger, 1976, p. 296.

37. Paes de Carvalho, A., and de Almeida, D. F.: Spread of activity through the atrioventricular node. Circ. Res. *8*:801, 1960.

38. Anderson, R. H., Janse, M. J., van Capelle, F. J. L., Billette, J., Becker, A. E., and Durrer, D.: A combined morphological and electrophysiological study of the atrioventricular node of the rabbit heart. Circ. Res. *35*:909, 1974.

39. Weidmann, S.: The diffusion of radiopotassium across intercalated disks of mammalian cardiac muscle. J. Physiol. *187*:323, 1966.

40. James, T. N., and Spence, C. A.: Distribution of cholinesterase within the sinus node and AV node in the human heart. Anat. Rec. *155*:151, 1966.

41. Thaemert, J. C.: Atrioventricular node innervation in ultrastructural three dimensions. Am. J. Anat. *128*:239, 1970.

42. Wallace, A. G., and Sarnoff, S. J.: Effects of cardiac sympathetic nerve stimulation on conduction in the heart. Circ. Res. *14*:86, 1964.

43. Yanowitz, F., Preston, J. B., and Abildskov, J. A.: Functional distribution of right and left stellate innervation to the ventricles: Production of neurogenic electrocardiographic changes by unilateral alteration of sympathetic tone. Circ. Res. *18*:416, 1966.

44. Randall, W. C., and Armour, J. A.: Gross and microscopic anatomy of the cardiac innervation. *In* Randall, W. C. (ed.): Neural Regulation of the Heart. New York, Oxford University Press, 1977, p. 13.

45. Kralios, F. A., Martin, L., Burgess, M. J., and Millar, K.: Local ventricular repolarization changes due to sympathetic nerve branch stimulation. Am. J. Physiol. *228*:1621, 1975.

46. Martins, J. B., and Zipes, D. P.: Epicardial phenol interrupts refractory period responses to sympathetic but not vagal stimulation in canine left ventricular epicardium and endocardium. Circ. Res. *47*:33, 1980.

47. Mueller, T. M., Barber, M. J., David, B., and Zipes, D. P.: Phenol topically applied to left ventricular epicardium interrupts sympathetic but not vagal afferents. Clin. Res. *30*:208A, 1982.

48. Martins, J. B., and Zipes, D. P.: Effects of sympathetic and vagal nerves on recovery properties of the endocardium and epicardium of the canine left ventricle. Circ. Res. *46*:100, 1980.

49. Han, J., and Moe, G. K.: Nonuniform recovery of excitability in ventricular muscle. Circ. Res. *14*:44, 1964.

50. Angelakos, E. T., King, M. P., and Millard, R. W.: Regional distribution of catecholamines in hearts of various species. Ann. NY Acad. Sci. *156*:219, 1969.

51. Dahlstrom, A., Fuxe, K., Mya-tu, M., and Zellerstrom, B. E. M.: Observations on adrenergic innervation of the dog heart. Am. J. Physiol. *209*:689, 1965.

52. Kent, K. M., Epstein, S. E., Cooper, T., and Jacobowitz, D. M.: Cholinergic innervation of the canine and human ventricular conducting system: Anatomic and electrophysiologic correlations. Circulation *50*:948, 1974.

53. Schmidt, P. G., Grief, B. J., Lund, D. D., and Roskowski, R., Jr.: Regional choline acetyltransferase activity in the guinea pig heart. Circ. Res. *42*:657, 1978.

54. Brown, O. M.: Cat heart acetylcholine, structural proof and distribution. Am. J. Physiol. *231*:781, 1966.

55. Fields, J. Z., Roeske, W. R., Morkin, E., and Yamamura, H. I.: Cardiac muscarinic cholinergic receptors. J. Biol. Chem. *253*:3251, 1978.

56. Levy, M. N.: Sympathetic-parasympathetic interactions in the heart. Circ. Res. *29*:437, 1971.

57. Ruffy, R., Lovelace, D. E., Knoebel, S. B., and Zipes, D. P.: Influence of secobarbital and alphachloralose and of vagal and sympathetic interruption on left ventricular activation following acute coronary artery ligation in the dog. Circ. Res. *48*:884, 1981.

58. Prystowsky, E. N., Jackman, W. M., Rinkenberger, R. L., Heger, J. J., and Zipes, D. P.: Effect of autonomic blockade on ventricular refractoriness and atrioventricular conduction in humans: Evidence supporting a direct cholinergic action on ventricular muscle refractoriness. Circ. Res. *49*:511, 1981.

59. Zipes, D. P., Martins, J. B., Ruffy, R., Prystowsky, E. N., Elharrar, V., and Gilmour, R. F., Jr.: Roles of autonomic innervation in the genesis of ventricular arrhythmias. *In* Abboud, F. M., et al. (eds.): Disturbances in Neurogenic Control of the Circulation. Bethesda, Md., American Physiological Society, 1981, pp. 225–250.

60. Thames, M. D., Klopfenstein, H. S., Abboud, F. M., Mark, A. L., and Walker, J. L.: Preferential distribution of inhibitory cardiac receptors with vagal afferents to the inferoposterior wall of the left ventricle activated during coronary occlusion in the dog. Circ. Res. *43*:512, 1978.

61. Katz, A. M., Messineo, F. C., and Herbette, L.: Ion channels in membranes. Circulation *65*(Suppl. 1):2, 1982.

62. Hille, B.: Ionic channels in nerve membranes. Progr. Biophys. Mol. Biol. *21*:1, 1970.

63. Langer, G. A., and Brady, A. J.: The Mammalian Myocardium. New York, John Wiley, 1974.

64. Fozzard, H. A.: Cardiac muscle: Excitability and passive electrical properties. Progr. Cardiovasc. Dis. *19*:343, 1977.

65. Sperelakis, N.: Origin of the cardiac resting potential. *In* Berne, R. M., et al. (eds.): Handbook of Physiology, The Cardiovascular System. Bethesda, Md., American Physiological Society, 1979, p. 187.

66. McNutt, N. S.: Ultrastructure of intercellular junctions in adult and developing cardiac muscle. Am. J. Cardiol. *25*:169, 1970.

67. Lowenstein, W. R., Kanno, U., and Socolar, S. J.: The cell-to-cell channel. Fed. Proc. *37*:2645, 1978.

68. Carmeliet, E., and Vereecke, J.: Electrogenesis of the action potential and automaticity. *In* Berne, R. M., et al. (eds.): Handbook of Physiology. Bethesda, Md., American Physiological Society, 1979, p. 269.

69. Electrophysiology of the heart. *In* Berne, R. M., et al. (eds.): Handbook of Physiology. Bethesda, Md., American Physiological Society, 1979, pp. 187–428.

70. Page, E.: The electrical potential difference across the cell membrane of heart muscle. Circulation *26*:582, 1962.

71. Thomas, R. C.: Electrogenic sodium pump in nerve and muscle cells. Physiol. Rev. *52*:563, 1972.

72. Hoffman, B. F., and Cranefield, P. F.: Electrophysiology of the Heart. New York, McGraw-Hill Book Co., 1960.

73. Vassalle, M.: Cardiac automaticity and its control. *In* Levy, M. N., and Vassalle, M. (eds.): Excitation and Neural Control of the Heart. Bethesda, Md., American Physiological Society, 1982.

74. Goldman, D. E.: Potential, impedance and rectification in membranes. J. Gen. Physiol. *27*:27, 1943.

75. Baker, P. F., Blaustein, M. P., Hodgkin, A. L., and Skinhardt, L. A.: Influence of calcium on sodium efflux in squid axons. J. Physiol. (Lond.) *200*:431, 1969.

76. Reuter, H., and Seitz, N.: Dependence of calcium efflux from cardiac muscle on temperature and external ion composition. J. Physiol. (Lond.) *195*:451, 1968.

77. Weidmann, S.: The effect of the cardiac membrane potential on the rapid availability of the sodium carrying system. J. Physiol. (Lond.) *127*:213, 1955.

78. Hodgkin, A. L., and Huxley, A. F.: Quantitative description of membrane current and its application to conduction and excitation in nerve. J. Physiol. *117*:500, 1952.

79. Cranefield, P. F.: The Conduction of the Cardiac Impulse, Mt. Kisco, N.Y., Futura Publ. Co., 1975.

80. Zipes, D. P., Bailey, J. C., and Elharrar, V.: The Slow Inward Current and Cardiac Arrythmias. The Hague, Martinus Nijhoff, 1980.

81. Reuter, H., and Scholtz, H.: A study of the ion selectivity and the kinetic properties of the calcium dependent slow inward current in mammalian muscle. J. Physiol. (Lond.) 264:17, 1977.

82. Akiyama, T., and Fozzard, H. A.: Ca and Na selectivity of the active membrane of rabbit AV nodal cells. Am. J. Physiol. 236(1):C1, 1979

83. Mary-Rabine, L., Hoffman, B. F., and Rosen, M. R.: Participation of slow inward current in the Purkinje fiber action potential overshoot. Am. J. Physiol. 237:H204, 1979.

84. Coraboeuf, E.: Voltage clamp studies of the slow inward current. In Zipes, D. P., et al. (eds.): The Slow Inward Current and Cardiac Arrhythmias. The Hague, Martinus Nijhoff, 1980. p. 25.

85. Carmeliet, E.: The slow inward current: Nonvoltage clamp studies. In Zipes, D. P., et al. (eds.): The Slow Inward Current and Cardiac Arrhythmias. The Hague, Martinus Nijhoff, 1980, p. 97.

86. Gilmour, R. F., Jr., and Zipes, D. P.: Basic electrophysiology of the slow inward current. In Antman, E., and Stone, P. H.: Calcium Blocking Agents in the Treatment of Cardiovascular Disorders. Futura Publ. Co., Mt. Kisco, N.Y. (in press).

87. Niedergerke, R., and Orkand, R. K.: The dual effect of calcium on the action potential of the frog's heart. J. Physiol. (Lond.) 184:291, 1966.

88. Reuter, H.: Properties of two inward membrane currents in the heart. Ann. Rev. Physiol. 41:413, 1979.

89. Hauswirth, O., and Singh, B. N.: Ionic mechanisms in heart muscle in relation to the genesis and the pharmacological control of cardiac arrhythmias. Pharmacol. Rev. 30:5, 1979.

90. Watanabe, A. M., Lindemann, J. P., Jones, L. R., Besch, H. R., Jr., and Bailey, J. C.: Biochemical mechanisms mediating neural control of the heart. In Abboud, F. M., Fozzard, H. A., Gilmore, J. P., and Leis, D. J. (eds.): Disturbances in neurogenic control of the circulation. Bethesda, Md., American Physiological Society, 1981.

91. Watanabe, A. M., Jones, L. R., Manalan, A. S., and Besch, H. R., Jr.: Cardiac autononic receptors: Recent concepts from radiolabeled ligand binding studies. Circ. Res. 50:161, 1982.

92. Giles, W., and Noble, S. J.: Changes in membrane current in bullfrog atrium produced by acetylcholine. J. Physiol. (Lond.) 261:103, 1976.

93. Zipes, D. P., and Mendez, C.: Action of manganese ions and tetrodotoxin on atrioventricular nodal transmembrane potentials in isolated rabbit hearts. Circ. Res. 32:447, 1973.

94. Irisawa, H., and Yanagihara, K.: The slow inward current of the rabbit sinoatrial nodal cells. In Zipes, D. P., et al. (eds.): The Slow Inward Current and Cardiac Arrhythmias. The Hague, Martinus Nijhoff, 1980, p. 265.

95. Merideth, J., Mendez, C., Mueller, W. J., and Moe, G. K.: Electrical excitability of atrioventricular nodal cells. Circ. Res. 23:69, 1968.

96. Zipes, D. P., Besch, H. R., and Watanabe, A. M.: Role of the slow current in cardiac electrophysiology (editorial). Circulation 51:761, 1975.

97. Nishimura, M., Kokubun, S., Noma, A., Irisawa, H., and Watanabe, Y.: Membrane current systems in the rabbit atrioventricular node. The first voltage clamp study (abstract). Am. J. Cardiol. 47:429, 1981.

98. Gilmour, R. F., Jr., and Zipes, D. P.: Electrophysiological response of vascularized hamster cardiac transplants to ischemia. Circ. Res. 50:599, 1982.

99. Spear, J. F., Horowitz, L. N., and Moore, E. N.: The slow response in human ventricle. Zipes, D. P., et al. (eds.): The Slow Inward Current and Cardiac Arrhythmias. The Hague, Martinus Nijhoff, 1980, p. 309.

100. Singer, D. H., Baumgarten, C. M., and Ten Eick, R. E.: Cellular electrophysiology of ventricular and other dysrhythmias: Studies on diseased and ischemic heart. Progr. Cardiovasc. Dis. 24:97, 1981.

101. Gilmour, R. F., Jr., Heger, J. J., Prystowsky, E. N., and Zipes, D. P.: Cellular electrophysiological abnormalities of diseased human ventricular myocardium. Am. J. Cardiol. (still in press).

102. Kenyon, J. L., and Gibbons, W. R.: Effects of low-chloride solutions on action potentials of sheep cardiac Purkinje fibers. J. Gen. Physiol. 70:635, 1977.

103. Isenberg, G., and Trautwein, W.: Outward current and extracellular sodium pump in Purkinje fibers. In Fleckenstein, A., and Dhalla, N. S. (eds.): Recent Advances in Studies on Cardiac Structure and Metabolism. Vol. 5. Baltimore, University Park Press, 1975, p. 43.

104. Coraboeuf, E., Deroubaix, E., and Coulombe, A.: Effect of tetrodotoxin on action potentials of the conducting system in the dog. Am. J. Physiol. 236:H561,1979.

105. DiFrancesco, D.: A new interpretation of the pacemaker current in calf Purkinje fibers. J. Physiol. (Lond.) 314:359, 1981.

106. Carmeliet, E., and Saikawa, T.: Shortening of the action potential and reduction of pacemaker activity by lidocaine, quinidine, and procainamide in sheep cardiac Purkinje fibers. An effect on Na or K currents? Circ. Res. 50:257,1982.

107. DeMello, W. C.: Some aspects of the interrelationship between ions and electrical activity in specialized tissue of the heart. In Paes de Carvalho, A., et al. (eds.): The Specialized Tissues of the Heart. Amsterdam, Elsevier Publ. Co., 1961.

108. Brown, H. F.: Electrophysiology of the sinoatrial node. Physiol. Rev. 62:505, 1982.

109. Wit, A. L., and Cranefield, P. F.: Effect of verapamil on the sinoatrial and atrioventricular nodes of the rabbit and the mechanism by which it arrests reentrant atrioventricular nodal tachycardia. Circ. Res. 35:413, 1974.

110. Zipes, D. P., and Fischer, J. C.: Effects of agents which inhibit the slow channel on sinus node automaticity and atrioventricular conduction in the dog. Circ. Res. 34:184, 1974.

111. Tse, W. W.: Evidence of presence of automatic fibers in the canine atrioventricular node. Am. J. Physiol. 225:716, 1973.

112. Wit, A. L., and Cranefield, P. F.: Mechanisms of impulse initiation in the atrioventricular junction and the effects of acetylstrophanthidin. Am. J. Cardiol. 49:921, 1982.

113. Vassalle, M.: Electrogenic suppression of automaticity in sheep and dog Purkinje fibers. Circ. Res. 27:361, 1970.

113a. Gaskell, W. H.: On the innervation of the heart with special reference to the heart of the tortoise. J. Physiol. 4:43, 1884.

114. Zipes, D. P., Wallace, A. G., Sealy, W. C., and Floyd, W. L.: Artificial atrial and ventricular pacing in the treatment of arrhythmias. Ann. Intern. Med. 70:885, 1969.

115. Boineau, J., Schuessler, R. B., Wylds, A. C., Miller, C. B., and Autry, L. A.: Response of atrial pacemaker complex to pharmacologic infusion and cardiac nerve stimulation. Circulation 64(Suppl. IV):327, 1981.

116. Peon, J., Ferrier, G. R., and Moe, G. K.: The relationship of excitability to conduction velocity in canine Purkinje tissue. Circ. Res. 43:125, 1978.

117. Zipes, D. P.: New approaches to antiarrhythmic therapy. New Engl. J. Med. 304:475, 1981.

118. Gadsby, D. C., and Wit, A. L.: Normal and abnormal electrophysiology of cardiac cells. In Mandel, W. J. (ed.): Cardiac Arrhythmias. Philadelphia, J. B. Lippincott, 1980, p. 55.

119. Jennings, R. B., Ganote, C. E., and Reimer, K. A.: Ischemic tissue injury. Am. J. Pathol. 81:179, 1975.

120. Hill, J. L., and Gettes, L. S.: Effect of acute coronary artery occlusion on local myocardial extracellular K^+ activity in swine. Circulation 61:768, 1980.

121. Rovetto, M. J.: Energy metabolism in the ischemic heart. Tex. Rep. Biol. Med. 39:397, 1979.

122. Corr, P. B., and Sobel, B. E.: The importance of metabolites in the genesis of ventricular dysrhythmia induced by ischemia. II. Biochemical factors. Mod. Conc. Cardiovasc. Dis. 48:49, 1979.

123. Wit, A. L., Rosen, M. R., and Hoffman, B. F.: Electrophysiology and pharmacology of cardiac arrhythmias. II. Relation of normal and abnormal electrical activity of cardiac fibers to the genesis of arrhythmias. b. Reentry. Sec. II. Am. Heart J. 88:798, 1974.

124. Sasyniuk, B. I., and Mendez, C.: A mechanism for reentry in canine ventricular tissue. Circ. Res. 28:3, 1971.

125. Mendez, C., and Moe, G. K.: Some characteristics of transmembrane potentials of AV nodal cells during propagation of premature beats. Circ. Res. 19:993, 1966.

126. Friedman, P. L., Stewart, J. R., and Wit, A. L.: Spontaneous and induced cardiac arrhythmias in subendocardial Purkinje fibers surviving extensive myocardial infarction in dogs. Circ. Res. 22:612, 1973.

127. Myerburg, R. J., Gelband, H., Nilsson, K., Sung, R. J., Thurer, R. J., Morales, A. R., and Bassett, A. L.: Long-term electrophysiological abnormalities resulting from experimental myocardial infarction in cats. Circ. Res. 41:73, 1977.

128. Barber, M. J., Mueller, T. M., and Zipes, D. P.: Transmural myocardial infarction produces sympathectomy in noninfarcted myocardium apical to the infarct. Am. J. Cardiol. 49:888, 1982.

129. Elharrar, V., and Zipes, D. P.: Cardiac electrophysiologic alterations during myocardial ischemia. Am. J. Physiol. 233:H329, 1977.

130. Zipes, D. P., Watanabe, A. W., and Besch, H. R.: Clinical electrophysiology and electrocardiography. In Willerson, J. T., and Sanders, C. A. (eds.): The Science and Practice of Clinical Medicine: Clinical Cardiology. New York, Grune and Stratton, 1977, p. 235.

131. Hoffman, B. F., and Rosen, M. R.: Cellular mechanisms for cardiac arrhythmias. Circ. Res. 49:1, 1981.

132. Gilmour, R. F., Jr., and Zipes, D. P.: Electrophysiological characteristics of rodent myocardium damaged by adrenaline. Cardiovasc. Res. 14:582, 1980.

133. Rosen, M. R., and Hordof, A. J.: The slow response in human atrium. In Zipes, D. P., et al. (eds.): The Slow Inward Current and Cardiac Arrhythmias. The Hague, Martinus Nijhoff, 1980, p. 295.

134. Ten Eick, R. E., and Singer, D. H.: Electrophysiological properties of diseased human atrium. I. Low diastolic potential and altered cellular response to potassium. Circ. Res. 44:545, 1979.

135. Surawicz, B.: Depolarization-induced automaticity in atrial and ventricular myocardial fibers. In Zipes, D. P., et al. (eds.): The Slow Inward Current and Cardiac Arrhythmias. The Hague, Martinus Nijhoff, 1980, p. 375.

136. Elharrar, V., and Zipes, D. P.: Voltage modulation of automaticity in cardiac Purkinje fibers. In Zipes, D. P., et al. (eds.): The Slow Inward Current and Cardiac Arrhythmias. The Hague, Martinus Nijhoff, 1980, p. 357.

137. Foster, P. R., Elharrar, V., and Zipes, D. P.: Accelerated ventricular escapes induced in the intact dog by barium, strontium and calcium. J. Pharmacol. Exp. Ther. 200:373, 1977.

138. Ferrier, G. R.: Digitalis arrhythmias: Role of oscillatory afterpotentials. Progr. Cardiovasc. Dis. 19:459, 1977.

139. Cranefield, P. F.: Action potentials, afterpotentials and arrhythmias. Circ. Res. 41:415, 1977.

140. Rosen, M. R., Merker, C., Gelband, H., and Hoffman, B. F.: Mechanisms of digitalis toxicity: Effects of ouabain on phase 4 of canine Purkinje fiber transmembrane potentials. Circulation 47:681, 1973.

141. Hashimoto, K., and Moe, G. K.: Transient depolarizations induced by acetylstrophanthidin in specialized tissue of dog atrium and ventricle. Circ. Res. 32:618, 1973.

142. Cranefield, P. F., and Aronson, R. S.: Initiation of sustained rhythmic activity

by single propagated action potentials in canine Purkinje fibers exposed to sodium-free solution or to ouabain. Circ. Res. *34*:477, 1974.

143. Makarycheu, V. A., Kosharskaya, I. L., and Ulyninsky, L. S.: Automatic activity of the pacemaker cells of the atrioventricular valves in the rabbit heart. Bull. Exp. Biol. Med. *81*:646, 1976.

144. Wit, A. L, Fenoglio, J. J., Wagner, B. M., and Bassett, A. L.: Electrophysiological properties of cardiac muscle in the anterior mitral valve leaflet and the adjacent atrium in the dog: Possible implications for the genesis of atrial dysrhythmias. Circ. Res. *32*:771, 1973.

145. Wit, A. L., and Cranefield, P. F.: Triggered activity in cardiac muscle fibers of the simian mitral valve. Circ. Res. *38*:85, 1976.

146. Wit, A. L., Fenoglio, J. J., Hordof, A. J., and Reemtsma, K.: Ultrastructure and transmembrane potentials of cardiac muscle in the human anterior mitral valve leaflet. Circulation *59*:1284, 1979.

147. Bassett, A. L., Fenoglio, J. J., Jr., Wit, A. L., Myerburg, R. J., and Gelband, J.: Electrophysiological and ultrastructural characteristics of canine tricuspid valve. Am. J. Physiol. *230*:1366, 1976.

148. Wit, A. L., and Cranefield, P. F.: Triggered and automatic activity in the canine coronary sinus. Circ. Res. *41*:435, 1977.

149. Saito, T., Otosuro, M., and Matsubara, T.: Electrophysiologic studies on the mechanism of electrically-induced sustained rhythmic activity in the rabbit right atrium. Circ. Res. *42*:199, 1978.

150. Mary-Rabine, L., Hordof, A. J., Danilo, P., Jr., Malm, J. R., and Rosen, M. R.: Mechanisms for impulse initiation in isolated human atrial fibers. Circ. Res. *47*:267, 1980.

151. Zipes, D. P., Arbel, E., Knope, R. F., and Moe, G. K.: Accelerated cardiac escape rhythms caused by ouabain intoxication. Am. J. Cardiol. *33*:248, 1974.

152. Zipes, D. P., Foster, P. R., Troup, P. J., and Pedersen, D. H.: Atrial induction of ventricular tachycardia: Reentry or triggered automaticity. Am. J. Cardiol. *44*:1, 1979.

153. Rosen, M. R., Fisch, C., Hoffman, B. F., Danilo, P., Jr., Lovelace, D. E., and Knoebel, S. B.: Can accelerated atrioventricular junctional escape rhythms be explained by delayed afterdepolarizations? Am. J. Cardiol. *45*:1272, 1980.

154. Wellens, H. J. J., Brugada, P., Vanagt, E. J. D. M., Ross, D. L., and Bär, F. W. H. M.: New studies with triggered automaticity. *In* Harrison, D. C. (ed.): Cardiac Arrhythmias: A Decade of Progress. Boston, G. K. Hall, 1981, p. 601.

155. Zipes, D. P.: A defense of triggered automaticity (symposium). *In* Harrison, D. C. (ed.): Cardiac Arrhythmias: A Decade of Progress. Boston, G. K. Hall, 1981.

156. Rosen, M. R., and Danilo, P.: Effects of tetrodotoxin, lidocaine, verapamil and AHR-2666 on ouabain-induced delayed afterdepolarizations in canine Purkinje fibers. Circ. Res. *46*:117, 1980.

157. Tsien, R. W., and Carpenter, D. O.: Ionic mechanisms of pacemaker activity in cardiac Purkinje fibers. Fed. Proc. *37*:2127, 1978.

158. Elharrar, V., Bailey, J. C., Lathrop, D. A., and Zipes, D. P.: Effects of aprindine HCl on slow channel action potentials and transient depolarizations in canine Purkinje fibers. J. Pharmacol. Exp. Ther. *205*:410, 1978.

159. Vassalle, M., and Mugelli, A.: An oscillatory current in sheep cardiac Purkinje fibers. Circ. Res. *48*:618, 1981.

160. Kass, R., Tsien, R., and Weingert, R.: Ionic basis of transient inward current induced by strophanthidin in cardiac Purkinje fibers. J. Physiol. (Lond.) *281*:209, 1978.

161. Wit, A. L., Cranefield, P. F., and Gadsby, D. C.: Electrogenic sodium extrusion can stop triggered activity in the canine coronary sinus. Circ. Res. *49*:1029, 1981.

162. Vassalle, M., Cummins, M., Castro, C., and Stuckey, J. H.: The relationship between overdrive suppression and overdrive excitation in ventricular pacemakers in dogs. Cir. Res. *38*:367, 1976.

163. Jalife, J., Antzelevitch, C., and Moe, G. K.: Models of parasystole and reflection. *In* Rosenbaum, M. B. (ed.): Cardiac Arrhythmias. Tha Hague, Martinus Nijhoff, 1982.

164. Antzelevitch, C., Moe, G. K., and Jalife, J.: Electrotonic modulation of pacemaker activity. Further biological and mathematical observations in the behavior of modulated parasystole. Circulation *66*:1225, 1982.

165. Moe, G. K., Jalife, J., Mueller, W. J., and Moe, B.: A mathematical model of parasystole and its application to clinical arrhythmias. Circulation *56*:968, 1977.

166. Cohen, H., Langendorf, R., and Pick, A.: Intermittent parasystole: Mechanism of protection. Circulation *48*:761, 1973.

167. Nau, G. J., Aldariz, A. E., Aconzo, R. S., Chiale, P. A., Elizari, M. V., and Rosenbaum, M. B.: Concealed ventricular parasystole uncovered in the form of ventricular escapes of variable coupling. Circulation *64*:199, 1981.

168. Jalife, J., and Antzelevitch, C.: Phase resetting and annihilation of pacemaker activity in cardiac tissue. Science *206*:695, 1979.

169. Nau, G. T., Aldariz, A. E., Aconzo, R. S., Halpern, S., Davidenko, J. M., Elizari, M. V., and Rosenbaum, M. B.: Modulation of parasystolic activity by non-parasystolic beats. Circulation *66*:462, 1982.

170. Hunter, P. J., McNaughton, P. A., Noble, D.: Analytical models of propagation in excitable cells. Progr. Biophys. Mol. Biol. *30*:99, 1975.

171. Singer, D. H., Lazzara, R., and Hoffman, B. F.: Interrelationships between automaticity and conduction in Purkinje fibers. Circ. Res. *21*:537, 1967.

172. Dominguez, G., and Fozzard, H.: Influence of extracellular K^+ concentration on cable properties and excitability of sheep cardiac Purkinje fibers. Circ. Res. *26*:565, 1970.

173. Simson, M. B., Spear, J. F., and Moore, E. N.: The relationship between atrio-

174. Pick, A., and Langendorf, R.: Interpretation of Complex Arrhythmias. Philadelphia, Lea and Febiger, 1979, p. 127.

175. Zipes, D. P., and Noble, R. J.: Assessment of electrical abnormalities. *In* Hurst, J. W. (ed.): The Heart. 5th ed. New York, McGraw-Hill Book Co., 1982, p. 333.

176. Ferrier, G. R., and Rosenthal, J. E.: Automaticity and entrance block induced by focal depolarization of mammalian ventricular tissues. Circ. Res. *47*:238, 1980.

177. Antzelevitch, C., and Moe, G. K.: Electrotonically-mediated delayed conduction and reentry in relation to "slow responses" in mammalian ventricular conducting tissue. Circ. Res. *49*:1129, 1981.

178. Lieberman, M., Kootsey, J. M., and Johnson, E. A.: Low conduction in cardiac muscle. A biophysical model. Biophys. J. *13*:37, 1973.

179. Watanabe, Y., and Dreifus, L. S.: Inhomogeneous conduction in the AV node: A model for reentry. Am. Heart J. *70*:505, 1965.

180. de la Fuente, D., Sasyniuk, B., and Moe, G. K.: Conduction through a narrow isthmus in isolated canine atrial tissue. A model of the WPW syndrome. Circulation *44*:803, 1971.

181. Zipes, D. P.: Second degree atrioventricular block. Circulation *60*:465, 1979.

182. Erlanger, J.: Further studies on the physiology of heart block: The effects of extrasystoles upon the dog's heart and upon strips of terrapin's ventricle in the various stages of block. Am. J. Physiol. *16*:160, 1906.

183. Schmitt, F. O., and Erlanger, J.: Directional differences in the conduction of the impulse through heart muscle and their possible relation to extrasystolic and fibrillatory contractions. Am. J. Physiol. *87*:326, 1929.

184. McWilliam, J. A.: Fibrillar contraction of the heart. J. Physiol. (Lond.) *8*:296, 1897.

185. Mayer, A. G.: Rhythmical pulsation in scyphomedusae. Publ. No. 47 of Carnegie Institution of Washington, 1906.

186. Mines, G. R.: On dynamic equilibrium in the heart. J. Physiol. (Lond.) *46*:349, 1913.

187. Mines, G. R.: On circulating excitations in heart muscles and their possible relation to tachycardia and fibrillation. Trans. Roy. Soc. Canad. (Sec. IV) *8*:43, 1914.

188. Garrey, W. E.: The nature of fibrillary contraction of the heart. Its relation to tissue mass and form. Am. J. Physiol. *33*:397, 1914.

189. Cranefield, P. F., Klein, H. O., and Hoffman, B. F.: Conduction of the cardiac impulse. I. Delay, block and one-way block in depressed Purkinje fibers. Circ. Res. *28*:199, 1971.

190. Wit, A. L., Cranefield, P. F., and Hoffman, B. F.: Slow conduction and reentry in the ventricular conducting system. II. Single and sustained circus movement in networks of canine and bovine Purkinje fibers. Circ. Res. *30*:11, 1972.

191. Rinkenberger, R. L., Prystowsky, E. N., Jackman, W. M., Heger, J. J., and Zipes, D. P.: Conversion of nonsustained ventricular tachycardia to sustained ventricular tachycardia during drug therapy as determined by serial electrophysiology studies. Am. Heart J. *103*:177, 1982.

192. Prystowsky, E. N., Heger, J. J., Jackman, W. M., Naccarelli, G. V., and Zipes, D. P.: Incessant supraventricular tachycardia following myocardial infarction. Am. Heart J. *103*:426, 1982.

193. Antzelevitch, C., Jalife, J., and Moe, G. K.: Frequency-dependent alterations of conduction in Purkinje fibers. A model of phase 4 facilitation and block. *In* Rosenbaum, M. B. (ed.): Cardiac Arrhythmias. The Hague, Martinus Nijhoff, 1982.

194. Antzelevitch, C., Jalife, J., and Moe, G. K.: Characteristics of reflection as a mechanism of reentrant arrhythmias and its relationship to parasystole. Circulation *61*:182, 1980

195. Lewis, T.: Observations upon flutter and fibrillation. Part IV. Impure flutter; theory of circus movement. Heart *7*:293, 1920.

196. Rosenblueth, A., and Garcia Ramos, J.: Studies on atrial flutter and fibrillation. II. The influence of artificial obstacles on experimental auricular flutter. Am. Heart J. *33*:677, 1947.

197. Boineau, J. P., Mowrey, C. R., Hudson, R. D., Hughes, D. G., Erdin, R. A., Jr., and Wilds, A. C.: Observations on reentrant excitation pathways and the refractory period distributions in spontaneous and experimental atrial flutter in the dog. *In* Kulbertus, H. E. (ed.): Reentrant Arrhythmias. Baltimore, University Park Press, 1977, pp. 72–98.

198. Pastelin, G., Mendez, R., and Moe, G. K.: Participation of atrial specialized conduction pathways in atrial flutter. Circ. Res. *42*:386, 1978.

199. Josephson, M. E., and Seides, S. F.: Clinical Cardiac Electrophysiology. Philadelphia, Lea and Febiger, 1979, p. 68.

200. Waldo, A. L., MacLean, W. H., Karp, R. B., Kouchoukos, N. T., and James, T. N.: Entrainment and interruption of atrial flutter with atrial pacing. Studies in man following open heart surgery. Circulation *56*:737, 1977.

201. Zipes, D. P., and DeJoseph, R. L.: Dissimilar atrial rhythms in man and dog. Am. J. Cardiol. *32*:618, 1973.

202. Schecter, D. C.: Flashbacks: Ventricular fibrillation. Part I. PACE *2*:490, 1979.

203. Schecter, D. C.: Flashbacks: Ventricular fibrillation. Part II. PACE *2*:648, 1979.

204. Porter, W. T.: On the results of ligation of the coronary arteries. J. Physiol. (Lond.) *15*:121, 1894.

205. Zipes, D. P., Fischer, J., King, R. M., Nicoll, A., and Jolly, W. W.: Termination of ventricular fibrillation in dogs by depolarizing a critical amount of myocardium. Am. J. Cardiol. *36*:37, 1975.

206. Moe, G. K., and Abildskov, J. A.: Atrial fibrillation as a self-sustaining arrhythmia independent of focal discharge. Am. Heart J. *58*:59, 1969.

207 Moe, G. K.: On the multiple wavelet hypothesis of atrial fibrillation. Arch. Intern. Pharmacodyn. *140*:183, 1962.

208. Han, J., Malozzi, A. M., and Moe, G. K.: Sinoatrial reciprocation in the isolated rabbit heart. Circ. Res. *22*:355, 1968.

209. Wu, D., Amat-y-Leon, F., Denes, P., Dhingra, R. C., Pietras, R. J., and Rosen, K. M.: Demonstration of sustained sinus and atrial reentry as a mechanism of paroxysmal supraventricular tachycardia. Circulation *51*:234, 1975.

210. Weisfogel, G. M., Batsford, W. P., Paulay, K. L., Josephson, M. E., Ogunkelu, J. B., Akhtar, M., Seides, S. F., and Damato, A. N.: Sinus node reentrant tachycardia in man. Am. Heart J. *90*:295, 1975.

211. Allessie, M. A., and Bonke, F. I. M.: Direct demonstration of sinus nodal reentry in the rabbit heart. Circ. Res. *44*:557, 1979.

212. Mandel, W. J., Hayakawa, H., Danzing, R., and Marcus, H. S.: Evaluation of sinoatrial node function in man by overdrive suppression. Circulation *44*:59, 1971.

213. Klein, H. O., Singer, D. H., and Hoffman, B. F.: Effects of atrial premature systoles on the sinus rhythm in the rabbit. Circ. Res. *32*:480, 1973.

214. Prystowsky, E. N., Grant, A. O., Wallace, A. G., and Strauss, H. C.: An analysis of the effects of acetylcholine on conduction and refractoriness in the rabbit sinus node and atrium. Circ. Res. *44*:112, 1979.

215. Steinbeck, G., Allessie, M. A., Bonke, F. I. M., and Lammers, W. J. E. P.: Sinus node response to premature atrial stimulation in the rabbit studied with multiple microelectrode impalement. Circ. Res. *43*:695, 1978.

216. Allessie, M. A., Bonke, F. I. M., and Schopman, F. J. G.: Circus movement in rabbit and atrial muscle as a mechanism of tachycardia. II. The role of nonuniform excitability in the occurrence of unidirectional block, as studied with multiple microelectrodes. Circ. Res. *39*:168, 1976.

217. Allessie, M. A., Bonke, F. I. M., and Schopman, F. J. G.: Circus movement in rabbit atrial muscle as a mechanism of tachycardia. III. The "leading circle" concept: A new model of circus movement in cardiac tissue without the involvement of an anatomical obstacle. Circ. Res. *41*:9, 1977.

218. Boineau, J. P., Schuessler, R. B., Mooney, C. R., Miller, C. B., Wylds, A. C., Hudson, R. D., Borremans, J. M., and Brockus, C. W.: Natural and evoked atrial flutter due to circus movement in dogs. Am. J. Cardiol. *45*:1167, 1980.

219. Coumel, P., and Barold, S. S.: Mechanisms of supraventricular tachycardia. In Narula, O. (ed.): His Bundle Electrocardiography and Clinical Electrophysiology. Philadelphia, F. A. Davis Co., 1975, p. 203.

220. Coumel, P., Flammang, D., Attuel, P., and Leckercq, J. F.: Sustained intraatrial reentrant tachycardia. Electrophysiologic study of 20 cases. Clin. Cardiol. *2*:176, 1979.

221. Wu, D., Denes, P., Amat-y-Leon, F., Dhingra, R., Wyndham, C. R. C., Bauernfeind, R., Latif, P., and Rosen, K. M.: Clinical electrocardiographic and electrophysiologic observations in patients with paroxysmal supraventricular tachycardia. Am. J. Cardiol. *41*:1045, 1978.

222. Hering, H. E.: Ueber die Automatie des Saugethierherzens. Arch. ges. Physiol. *116*:143, 1907.

223. deBoer, S.: Fortgesetzte Untersuchung über Kammerflimmern. Arch. ges. Physiol. *188*:67, 1921.

224. Scherf, D., and Shookoff, C.: Experimentelle Untersuchungen über die "Umkehr-Extrasystole" (reciprocating beat). Wien. Arch. inn. Med. *12*:501, 1926.

225. Scherf, D., and Shookhoff, C.: An experimental study of reciprocating rhythm. Arch. Intern. Med. *67*:372, 1941.

226. Rosenblueth, A., and Rubio, R.: La influencia de la frecuencia de estimulacion sobre los tiempos de propagacion auriculoventricular y ventriculilo-auricular. Arch. Inst. Cardiol. (Mexico) *25*:535, 1955.

227. Mignone, R. J., and Wallace, A. G.: Ventricular echoes: Evidence for dissociation of conduction and reentry within the AV node. Circ. Res. *19*:638, 1966.

228. Moe, G. K., and Mendez, C.: Physiological basis of reciprocal rhythm. Progr. Cardiovasc. Dis. *8*:461, 1966.

229. Mendez, C., Han, J., Garcia de Jalon, P. D., and Moe, G. K.: Some characteristics of ventricular echoes. Circ. Res. *16*:562, 1965.

230. Mendez, C., and Moe, G. K.: Demonstration of dual AV conduction system in the isolated rabbit heart. Circ. Res. *19*:378, 1966.

231. Janse, M. J., Van Capelle, F. J. L., Freud, G. E., and Durrer, D.: Circus movement within the AV node as a basis for supraventricular tachycardia as shown by multiple microelectrode recording in the isolated rabbit heart. Circ. Res. *28*:403, 1971.

232. Wit, A. L., Goldreyer, B. N., and Damato, A. N.: An in vitro model of paroxysmal supraventricular tachycardia. Circulation *43*:862, 1971.

233. White, P. D.: A study of atrioventricular rhythm following auricular flutter. Arch. Intern. Med. *16*:517, 1915.

234. Drury, A. N.: Paroxysmal tachycardia of AV nodal origin, exhibiting retrograde heart block and reciprocal rhythm. Heart *11*:405, 1924.

235. Gallavardin, L., and Veil, P.: Deux cas de nouveaux tachycardie en salves chez de jeunes sujets. Arch. Med. Coeur *20*:1, 1927.

236. Scherf, D., and Cohen, J.: The Atrioventricular Node and Selected Cardiac Arrhythmias. New York, Grune and Stratton, 1964, p. 226.

237. Lewis, T.: Mechanism and Graphic Registration of the Heart Beat. London, Shaw and Son, 1925, p. 396.

238. Kistin, A. D.: Atrial reciprocal rhythm. Circulation *32*:687, 1965.

239. Moe, G. K., Cohen, W., and Vick, R. L.: Experimentally induced paroxysmal AV nodal tachycardia in the dog. Am. Heart J. *65*:87, 1963.

240. Schulienburg, R. N., and Durrer, D.: Atrial echo beats in the human heart elicited by induced atrial premature beats. Circulation *37*:680, 1968.

241. Hunt, N. C., Cobb, F. R., Waxman, M. B., Zeft, H. J., Peter, R. H., and Morris, J. J., Jr.: Conversion of supraventricular tachycardias with atrial stimulation. Evidence for reentry mechanism. Circulation *38*:1060, 1968.

242. Bigger, J. T., and Goldreyer, B. N.: The mechanism of supraventricular tachycardia. Circulation *42*:673, 1970.

243. Goldreyer, B. N., and Damato, A. N.: Essential role of atrioventricular conduction delay in the initiation of paroxysmal supraventricular tachycardia. Circulation *43*:679, 1971.

244. Denes, P., Wu, D., Dhingra, R. C., Chuquimia, R., and Rosen, K. M.: Demonstration of dual AV nodal pathways in patients with paroxysmal supraventricular tachycardia. Circulation *48*:549, 1973.

245. Wu, D.: Dual atrioventricular nodal pathways: A reappraisal. PACE *5*:72, 1982.

246. Wu, D., Denes, P., Amat-y-Leon, F., Wyndham, C. R. C., Dhingra, R., and Rosen, K. M.: An unusual variety of atrioventricular nodal reentry due to retrograde dual atrioventricular nodal pathways. Circulation *56*:50, 1977.

247. Spurrell, R. A. J., Krikler, D. M., and Sowton, E.: Effects of verapamil on electrophysiological properties of anomalous atrioventricular connection in Wolff-Parkinson-White syndrome. Brit. Heart J. *36*:256, 1974.

248. Wellens, H. J. J., Tan, S. L., Bar, F. W. H., Duren, D. R., Lie, K. I., and Dohmen, H. M.: Effects of verapamil studied by programmed electrical stimulation of the heart in patients with paroxysmal reentrant supraventricular tachycardia. Brit. Heart J. *39*:1058, 1977.

249. Rinkenberger, R. L., Prystowsky, E. N., Heger, J. J., Troup, P. J., Jackman, W. M., and Zipes, D. P.: Effects of intravenous and chronic oral verapamil administration in patients with supraventricular tachyarrhythmias. Circulation *62*:996, 1980.

250. Janse, M. J.: Influence of the direction of the atrial wavefront on AV nodal transmission in isolated hearts and rabbits. Circ. Res. *25*:439, 1969.

251. Zipes, D. P., Mendez, C., and Moe, G. K.: Evidence for summation and voltage dependency in rabbit atrioventricular nodal fibers. Circ. Res. *32*:170, 1973.

252. Rahilly, G. T., Zipes, D. P., Naccarelli, G. V., Jackman, W. M., Heger, J. J., and Prystowsky, E. N.: Autonomic blockade in patients with normal and abnormal atrioventricular nodal function. Am. J. Cardiol. *49*:898, 1982.

253. Shenasa, M., Gilbert, C. J., Schmidt, D. H., and Akhtar, M.: Procainamide and retrograde atrioventricular nodal conduction in man. Circulation *65*:355, 1982.

254. Denes, P., Kehoe, R., and Rosen, R. M.: Multiple reentrant tachycardias due to retrograde conduction of dual atrioventricular bundles with atrioventricular nodal-like properties. Am. J. Cardiol. *44*:162, 1973.

255. Langendorf, R., and Pick, A.: Manifestations of concealed reentry in the atrioventricular junction. Eur. J. Cardiol. *1*:11, 1973.

256. Josephson, M. E., and Kastor, J. A.: Paroxysmal supraventricular tachycardia. Is the atrium a necessary link? Circulation *54*:430, 1976.

257. Ko, P. T., Naccarelli, G. V., Gulamhusein, S., Prystowsky, E. N., Zipes, D. P., and Klein, G. J.: Atrioventricular dissociation during paroxysmal junctional tachycardia. PACE *4*:670, 1981.

258. Zipes, D. P., Gaum, W. E., Genetos, B. C., Glassman, R. D., Noble, R. J., and Fisch, C.: Atrial tachycardia without P waves masquerading as an AV junctional tachycardia. Circulation *55*:253, 1977.

259. Schulienburg, R. M., Durrer, D.: Further observations on the ventricular echo phenomenon elicited in the human heart. Is the atrium part of the echo pathway? Circulation *45*:629, 1972.

260. Wolff, L., Parkinson, J., and White, P. D.: Bundle branch block with short P-R interval in healthy young people prone to paroxysmal tachycardia. Am. Heart J. *5*:685, 1950.

261. Durrer, D., Schoo, L., Schulienburg, R. M., and Wellens, H. J. J.: The role of premature beats in the initiation and the termination of supraventricular tachycardia in the Wolff-Parkinson-White syndrome. Circulation *36*:644, 1967.

262. Zipes, D. P., DeJoseph, R. L., and Rothbaum, D. A.: Unusual properties of accessory pathways. Circulation *49*:1200, 1974.

263. Gallagher, J. J., Pritchett, E. L. C., Sealy, W. C., Casell, J., and Wallace, A. G.: The pre-excitation syndromes. Progr. Cardiovasc. Dis. *20*:285, 1978.

264. Kent, A. F. S.: Researches on the structure and function of the mammalian heart. J. Physiol. *14*:233, 1893.

265. Kent, A. F. S.: Observations on the auriculo-ventricular junction of the mammalian heart. Quart. J. Exp. Physiol. *7*:193, 1913.

266. Wellens, H. J. J.: The electrophysiologic properties of the accessory pathway in the Wolff-Parkinson-White syndrome. In Wellens, H. J. J., et al. (eds.): The Conduction System of the Heart. Philadelphia, Lea and Febiger, 1976.

267. Coumel, P., and Attuel, P.: Reciprocating tachycardia in overt and latent preexcitation. Influence of functional bundle branch block on the rate of the tachycardia. Eur. J. Cardiol. *1*:423, 1974.

268. Barold, S. S., Coumel, P.: Mechanisms of atrioventricular junctional tachycardia. Role of reentry and concealed accessory bypass tracts. Am. J. Cardiol. *39*:97, 1977.

269. Hammill, S. C., Pritchett, E. L. C., Klein, G. J., Smith, W. M., and Gallagher, J. J.: Accessory atrioventricular pathways that conduct only in the antegrade direction. Circulation *62*:1335, 1980.

270. Lown, B., Ganong, W. F., and Levine, S. A.: The syndrome of short PR interval, normal QRS complex and paroxysmal rapid heart action. Circulation *5*:693, 1952.

271. James, T. N.: The Wolff-Parkinson-White syndrome: Evolving concepts of its pathogenesis. Progr. Cardiovasc. Dis. *13*:159, 1970.

272. Gallagher, J. J., Smith, W. M., Kasell, J. H., Benson, D. W., Jr., Sterba, R., and Grant, A. O.: Role of Mahaim fibers in cardiac arrhythmias in man. Circulation *64*:176, 1981.

273. Holzmann, M., and Scherf, D.: Über Elektrokardiogramme mit verkürzter Vorhof-Kammer-Distanz und positiven P-Zacken. Klin. Med. *121*:404, 1932.

274. Wolferth, C. C., and Wood, F. C.: Mechanisms of production of short PR intervals and prolonged QRS complexes in patients with presumably undamaged hearts: Hypothesis of accessory pathway of auriculoventricular conduction (bundle of Kent). Am. Heart J. *8*:297, 1933.

275. Wenckebach, K. F., and Winterberg, H.: Die Unregelmässige Herztätigkeit. Leipzig, Engelmann, 1927.

276. Scherf, D., and Schott, A. Extrasystoles and Allied Arrhythmias. New York, Grune and Stratton, 1953.

277. Cranefield, P. F., and Hoffman, B. F.: Conduction of the cardiac impulse. II. Summation and inhibition. Circ. Res. *28*:220, 1971.

278. Wit, A. L., Hoffman, B. F., and Cranefield, P. F.: Slow conduction and reentry in the ventricular conducting system. I. Return extrasystole in canine Purkinje fibers. Circ. Res. *30*:1, 1972.

279. Sasyniuk, B. I., and Mendez, C.: A mechanism for reentry in canine ventricular tissue. Circ. Res. *28*:3, 1973.

280. Friedman, P. L., Stewart, J. R., Fenoglio, J. J., Jr., and Wit, A. L.: Survival of subendocardial Purkinje fibers after extensive myocardial infarction in dogs. In vitro and in vivo correlations. Circ. Res. *33*:597, 1973.

281. Moe, G. K., Mendez, C., and Han, J.: Aberrant AV impulse propagation in the dog heart: A study of functional bundle branch block. Circ. Res. *16*:261, 1965.

282. Zipes, D. P.: Reentry in the ventricles. In Recent Advances in Ventricular Conduction. Advances in Cardiology. Vol. 14. Basel, Karger, 1975, p. 51.

283. Glassman, R. D., and Zipes, D. P.: Site of antegrade and retrograde functional right bundle branch block in the intact canine heart. Circulation *64*:1277, 1981.

284. Akhtar, M., Gilbert, C., Wolf, F. G., and Schmidt, D. H.: Reentry within the His-Purkinje system. Elucidation of reentrant circuit using right bundle branch and His bundle recordings. Circulation *38*:295, 1978.

285. Spurrell, R. A. J., Sowton, E., and Deuchar, D. C.: Ventricular tachycardia in 4 patients evaluated by programmed electrical stimulation of the heart and treated in two patients by surgical division of anterior radiation of left bundle branch. Br. Heart J. *35*:1014, 1973.

286. Josephson, M. E., Horowitz, L. N., Farshidi, A., and Kastor, J. A.: Recurrent sustained ventricular tachycardia. I. Mechanisms. Circulation *57*:431, 1978.

286a. Lloyd, E. A., Zipes, D. P., Heger, J. J., and Prystowsky, E. N.: Sustained ventricular tachycardia due to bundle branch re-entry. Am. Heart J. *104*:1095, 1982.

287. Fontaine, G., Guiraudon, G., Frank, R., Fillette, F., Cabrol, C., and Grosgogeat, Y.: Surgical management of ventricular tachycardia unrelated to myocardial ischemia or infarction. Am. J. Cardiol. *49*:397, 1982.

288. Wallace, A. G., Mignone, R. J.: Physiologic evidence concerning the reentry hypothesis for ectopic beats. Am. Heart J. *72*:60, 1966.

289. Scherlag, B. J., Helfant, R. H., Haft, J. I., and Damato, A. N.: Electrophysiology underlying ventricular arrhythmias due to coronary ligation. Am. J. Physiol. *219*:1665, 1970.

290. Boineau, J. P., and Cox, J. L.: Slow ventricular activation in acute myocardial infarction. A source of reentrant premature ventricular contractions. Circulation *48*:703, 1973.

291. El-Sherif, N., Hope, R. R., Scherlag, B. J., and Lazzara, R.: Reentrant ventricular arrhythmias in the late myocardial infarction period. I. Conduction characteristics in the infarction zone. Circulation *55*:686, 1977.

292. El-Sherif, N., Hope, R. R., Scherlag, B. J., and Lazzara, R.: Reentrant ventricular arrhythmias in the late myocardial infarction period. II. Patterns of initiation and termination of reentry. Circulation *55*:702, 1977.

293. El-Sherif, N., Smith, R. A., and Evans, K.: Canine ventricular arrhythmias in the late myocardial infarction period. 8. Epicardial mapping of reentrant circuits. Circ. Res. *49*:255, 1981.

294. Wit, A. L., Allessie, M. A., Bonke, F. I. M., Lammers, W., Smeets, J., and Fenoglio, J. J., Jr.: Electrophysiologic mapping to determine the mechanism of experimental ventricular tachycardia initiated by premature impulses. Experimental approaches and initial results demonstrating reentrant excitation. Am. J. Cardiol. *49*:166, 1982.

295. Ideker, R. E., Klein, G. J., Harrison, L., Smith, W. M., Kasell, J., Reimer, K. A., Wallace, A. G., and Gallagher, J. J.: The transition to ventricular fibrillation induced by reperfusion after acute ischemia in the dog: A period of organized epicardial activation. Circulation *63*:1371, 1981.

296. Janse, M. J., van Capelle, F. J. L., Morsink, H., Kleber, A. G., Wilms-Schopman, F., Cardinal, R., d'Alnoncourt, C. N., and Durrer, D.: Flow of "injury" current and patterns of excitation during early ventricular arrhythmias in acute regional myocardial ischemia in isolated porcine and canine hearts. Evidence for two different arrhythmogenic mechanisms. Circ. Res. *47*:151, 1980.

297. Furman, S., Parker, B., and Escher. D. J. W.: Transtelephonic pacemaker clinic. J. Thorac. Cardiovasc. Surg. *61*:287, 1971.

298. McHenry, P. L., Fisch, C., Jordan, J. W., and Corya, B. R.: Cardiac arrhythmias observed during maximal treadmill exercise testing in clinically normal men. Am. J. Cardiol. *29*:331, 1972.

299. Blackburn, H., Taylor, H., Hamrell, B., Buskirk, E., Nicholas, W. C., and Thorsen, R. D.: Premature ventricular complexes induced by stress testing. Am. J. Cardiol. *31*:441, 1973.

300. Faris, J. V., McHenry, P. L., Jordan, J. W., and Morris, S. N.: Prevalence and reproducibility of exercise-induced ventricular arrhythmias during maximal exercise testing in normal men. Am. J. Cardiol. *37*:617, 1976.

301. McHenry, P. L., Morris, S. N., Kavalier, M., and Jordan, J. W.: Comparative study of exercise-induced ventricular arrhythmias in normal subjects and patients with documented coronary artery disease. Am. J. Cardiol. *37*:609, 1976.

302. Morris, S. N., and McHenry, P. L.: Cardiac arrhythmias during exercise testing and exercise conditioning. Cardiovasc. Clin. *9*:57, 1978.

303. McHenry, P. L., Morris, S. N., and Kavalier, M.: Exercise-induced arrhythmias — Recognition, classification, and clinical significance. Cardiovasc. Clin. *6*: 245, 1974.

304. Goldschlager, N., Cohn, K., and Goldschlager, A.: Exercise-related ventricular arrhythmias. Mod. Conc. Cardiovasc. Dis. *48*:67, 1979.

305. Goldschlager, N., Cake, D., and Cohn, K.: Exercise-induced ventricular arrhythmias in patients with coronary artery disease. Their relation to angiographic findings. Am. J. Cardiol. *31*:434, 1973.

306. Goldschlager, N., Selzer, A., and Cohn, K.: Treadmill stress tests as indicators of presence and severity of coronary artery disease. Ann. Intern. Med. *85*:277, 1976.

307. Irving, J. B., and Bruce, R. A.: Exertional hypotension and post exertional ventricular fibrillation in stress testing. Am. J. Cardiol. *39*:849, 1977.

308. Helfant, R. H., Pine, R., Kabde, V., and Banka, V. S.: Exercise-related ventricular premature complexes in coronary heart disease. Ann. Intern. Med. *80*:589, 1974.

309. Sheps, D. S., Ernst, J. C., Briese, F. R., Lopez, L. V., Conde, C. A., Castellanos, A., and Myerburg, R. J.: Decreased frequency of exercise-induced ventricular ectopic activity in the second of two consecutive treadmill tests. Circulation *55*:891, 1977.

310. Kennedy, H. L.: Comparison of ambulatory electrocardiography and exercise testing. Am. J. Cardiol. *47*:1359, 1981.

311. Crawford, M., O'Rourke, R. A., Ramakrishna, N., Henning, H., and Ross, J., Jr.: Comparative effectiveness of exercise testing and continuous monitoring for detecting arrhythmias in patients with previous myocardial infarction. Circulation *50*:301, 1974.

312. Holter, N. J.: New method for heart studies: Continuous electrocardiography of active subjects over long periods is now practical. Science *134*:1214, 1961.

313. Kennedy, H. L.: Ambulatory Electrocardiography and Holter Recording Technology. Philadelphia, Lea and Febiger, 1981.

314. Harrison, D. C., Fitzgerald, J. W., and Winkle, R. A.: Ambulatory electrocardiography for diagnosis and treatment of cardiac arrhythmias. N. Engl. J. Med. *294*:373, 1976.

315. Wenger, N. K., Mock, M. B., and Ringquist, I.: Ambulatory Electrocardiographic Recording. Chicago, Year Book Medical Publishers, 1981.

316. Winkle, R. A.: Recent status of ambulatory electrocardiography. Am. Heart J. *102*:757, 1981.

317. Foucachet, Y., Rosier, S. P., Planeix, T., Boisante, L., Delescaut, M. F., Bardet, J., Bourdaris, J. P.: Valeur de l'enregistrement l'electrocardiographique continue par la methode de Holter pour le diagnostic et al surveillance de l'ischemie myocardique. Arch. Mal Coeur, *74*:427, 1981.

317a. Smith, M. S., and Pritchett, E. L. C.: Electrocardiographic monitoring in ambulatory patients with cardiac arrhythmias. Cardiol. Clin. (in press).

318. Barrett, P. A., Peter, C. T., Swan, H. J., Singh, B. N., and Mandel, W. J.: The frequency and prognostic significance of electrocardiographic abnormalities in clinically normal individuals. Progr. Cardiovasc. Dis. *23*:299, 1981.

319. Sobotka, P. A., Mayer, J. H., Bauernfeind, R. A., Kanakis, C., Jr., and Rosen, K. M.: Arrhythmias documented by 24 hour continuous ambulatory electrocardiographic monitoring in young women without apparent heart disease. Am. Heart J. *101*:753, 1981.

319a. Scott, O., Williams, G. J., and Fiddler, G. I.: Results of 24 hour ambulatory monitoring of electrocardiogram in 131 healthy boys aged 10 to 13 years. Brit. Heart J. *44*:304, 1980.

320. Olec, M. D., Smith, N., McNeill, G. P., and Wright, D. S.: Dysrhythmias in apparently healthy subjects. Age-Aging *8*:173, 1979.

321. Abdon, N. J.: Frequency and distribution of long-term ECG recorded cardiac arrhythmias in an elderly population. With special reference to neurological symptoms. Acta Med. Scand. *209*:175, 1981.

322. Mikolich, J. R., Jacobs, W. C., and Fletcher, G. F.: Cardiac arrhythmias in patients with acute cerebrovascular accidents. JAMA *246*:1314, 1981.

323. Lown, B., and Wolf, M.: Approaches to sudden death from coronary heart disease. Circulation *44*:130, 1971.

324. Kennedy, H. L., Chandra, V., Sayther, K. L., and Caralis, D. G.: Effectiveness of increasing hours of continuous ambulatory electrocardiography in detecting maximal ventricular ectopy. Am. J. Cardiol. *42*:925, 1978.

325. Rabkin, S. W., Mathewson, F. A., and Tate, R. B.: Relationship of ventricular ectopy in men without apparent heart disease. Am. Heart J. *101*:135, 1981.

326. Kotler, M. N., Tabatznik, M., Mower, M. M., and Tominagra, S.: Prognostic significance of ventricular ectopic beats with respect to sudden death in the late postinfarction period. Circulation *47*:959, 1973.

327. Moss, A. J., DeCamilla, J., Engstrom, F., Hoffman, W., Odoroff, C., and Davis, H.: The post-hospital phase of myocardial infarction: Identification of patients with increased mortality risk. Circulation *49*:460, 1974.

328. Moss, A. J., DeCamilla, J., Mietlowski, W., Greene, W. A., Goldstein, S., and Locksley, R.: Prognostic grading and significance of ventricular premature beats after recovery from myocardial infarction. Circulation *51*:204, 1975.

329. Vismara, L. A., Amsterdam, E. A., and Mason, D. T.: Relation of ventricular arrhythmias in the late hospital phase of acute myocardial infarction to sudden death after hospital discharge. Am. J. Med. *59*:6, 1975.

330. Ruberman, W., Weinblatt, E., Goldberg, J. D., Frank, C. W., and Shapiro, S.: Ventricular premature beats and mortality after myocardial infarction. N. Engl. J. Med. *297*:750, 1977.

331. Anderson, K. P., DeCamilla, J., and Moss, A. J.: Clinical significance of ven-

tricular tachycardia (3 beats or longer) detected during ambulatory monitoring after myocardial infarction. Circulation 57:890, 1978.

332. Bigger, J. T., Jr., Weld, F. M., and Rolnitzky, L. M.: Prevalence characteristics and significance of ventricular tachycardia (three or more complexes) detected with ambulatory electrocardiographic recording in the late hospital phase of acute myocardial infarction. Am. J. Cardiol. 48:815, 1981.

333. Rozanski, J. J., Castellanos, A., and Myerburg, R. J.: Ventricular ecotopy and sudden death. Cardiovasc. Clin. 11:127, 1980.

334. Ruberman, W., Weinblatt, E., Frank, C. W., Goldberg, J. D., and Shapiro, S.: Repeated one hour of electrocardiograph monitoring of survivors of myocardial infarction at 6 month intervals: Arrhythmia detection and relation to prognosis. Am. J. Cardiol. 47:1197, 1981.

335. Ruberman, W., Weinblatt, E., Goldberg, J. D., Frank, C. W., Chaudhary, B. S., and Shapiro, S.: Ventricular premature complexes and sudden death after myocardial infarction. Circulation 64:297, 1981.

335a. Weaver, W. D., Cobb, L. A., and Hallstrom, A. P.: Ambulatory arrhythimias in resuscitated victims of cardiac arrest. Circulation 66:212, 1982.

335b. Nikolic, G., Bishop, R. L., and Singh, J. B.: Sudden death recorded during Holter monitoring. Circulation 66:218, 1982.

336. Vismara, L. A., Vera, Z., Forester, J. M., Amsterdam, E. A., and Mason, D. T.: Identification of sudden death risk factors in acute and chronic coronary artery disease. Am. J. Cardiol. 39:821, 1977.

337. Fitzgerald, J. W., and DeBusk, R. F.: Early post-infarction ambulatory monitoring and exercise testing in detection of arrhythmias. Am. J. Cardiol. 35:136, 1975.

338. Schulze, R. A., Jr., Strauss, H. W., and Pitt, B.: Sudden death in the year following myocardial infarction. Am. J. Cardiol. 62:192, 1977.

339. Maron, B. J., Savage, D. D., Wolfson, J. K., and Epstein, S. E.: Prognostic significance of 24 hour ambulatory electrocardiographic monitoring in patients with hypertrophic cardiomyopathy: A prospective study. Am. J. Cardiol. 48:252, 1981.

340. McKenna, W. J., England, D., Doi, Y. L., Deanfield, J. E., Oakley, C., and Goodwin, J. F.: Arrhythmia in hypertrophic cardiomyopathy. I. Influence on prognosis. Brit. Heart J. 46:168, 1981.

341. Leichtman, D., Nelson, R., Gobel, F. L., Alexander, C. A., and Cohn, J. N.: Bradycardia with mitral valve prolapse. Ann. Intern. Med. 85:453, 1976.

342. Winkle, R. A., Lopes, M. G., Popp, R. L., and Hancock, E. W.: Life-threatening arrhythmias in the mitral valve prolapse syndrome. Am. J. Med. 60:961, 1976.

343. LeClercq, J. F., Malergue, M. C., Milosevic, D., Rosengarten, M. D., Attuel, P., and Coumel, P.: Ventricular arrhythmias and mitral valve prolapse. A study of 35 cases. Arch. Mal Coeur 73:276, 1980.

344. Greenspon, A. J., and Schaal, S. F.: AV node dysfunction in the mitral valve prolapse syndrome. PACE 3:60, 1980.

345. Shappell, S. D., Marshall, C. E., Brown, R. E., and Bruce, T. A.: Sudden death and the familial occurrence of midsystolic click, late systolic murmur syndrome. Circulation 48:1128, 1973.

346. Lipski, J., Cohen, L., Espinoza, J., Motro, M., Dack, S., and Donoso, E.: Value of Holter monitoring in assessing cardiac arrhythmias in symptomatic patients. Am. J. Cardiol. 37:102, 1976.

347. Tzivoni, D., and Stern, S.: Pacemaker implantation based on ambulatory ECG monitoring in patients with cerebral symptoms. Chest 67:274, 1975.

348. Bigger, J. T., Jr., and Reiffel, J. A.: Sick sinus syndrome. Ann. Rev. Med. 30:91, 1979.

349. Prystowsky, E. N.: The sick sinus syndrome—Diagnosis and treatment. In Donoso, F. (ed.): Advances and Controversies in Cardiology. New York, Grune and Stratton, 1981, p. 93.

350. Crook, B. R. M., Cashman, P. M. M., Stott, F. D., and Raftery, E. B.: Tape monitoring of the electrocardiogram in ambulant patients with sinoatrial disease. Brit. Heart J. 35:1009, 1973.

351. Hindman, M. C., Last, J. H., and Rosen, K. M.: Wolff-Parkinson-White syndrome observed by portable monitoring. Ann. Intern. Med. 79:654, 1973.

352. Bleifer, S. B., Bleifer, D. J., Hansmann, D. R., Sheppard, J. J., and Karpman, H. I.: Diagnosis of occult arrhythmias by Holter electrocardiography. Progr. Cardiovasc. Dis. 16:569, 1974.

353. Winkle, R. A.: Antiarrhythmic drug effect mimicked by spontaneous variability of ventricular ectopy. Circulation 57:1116, 1978.

354. Morganroth, J., Michelson, E., Horowitz, L. N., Josephson, M. E., Pearlman, A. S., and Dunkman, W. B.: Limitations of routine long-term ambulatory electrocardiographic monitoring to assess ventricular ectopy frequency. Circulation 58:408, 1978.

355. Michelson, E. L., Morganroth, J.: How to use Holter monitoring to your patient's best advantage. J. Cardiovasc. Med. 5:119, 1980.

356. Knoebel, S. B., Lovelace, D. E., Rasmussen, S., and Wash, S. E.: Computer detection of premature ventricular complexes: A modified approach. Am. J. Cardiol. 38:440, 1976.

357. Fisher, J. D.: Role of electrophysiologic testing in the diagnosis and treatment of patients with known and suspected bradycardias and tachycardias. Progr. Cardiovasc. Dis. 24:25, 1981.

358. Greene, L. H., Reid, P. R., and Schaeffer, A. H.: The repetitive ventricular response in man: A predictor of sudden death. New Engl. J. Med. 299:729, 1978.

359. Naccarelli, G. V., Prystowsky, E. N., Jackman, W. M., Heger, J. J., Rinkenberger, R. L., and Zipes, D. P.: Repetitive ventricular response. Prevalence and prognostic significance. Brit. Heart J. 46:152, 1981.

360. Nattel, S., Rinkenberger, R. L., Lehrman, L. L., and Zipes, D. P.: Therapeutic blood lidocaine concentration after local anesthesia for cardiac electrophysiologic studies. New Engl. J. Med. 301:418, 1979.

361. Dreifus, L. S.: Clinical judgment is sufficient for the management of conduction defects. Cardiovasc. Clin. 8:195, 1977.

362. Wu, D., and Rosen, K. M.: Clinical judgment is not sufficient for the management of conduction defects. Indications for diagnostic electrophysiologic studies. Cardiovasc. Clin. 8:203, 1977.

363. Langendorf, R., and Pick, A.: Atrioventricular block, type II (Mobitz). Its nature and clinical significance. Circulation 38:819, 1968.

364. Dhingra, R. C., Denes, P., Wu, D., Chuquimia, R., and Rosen, K. M.: The significance of second-degree atrioventricular block and bundle branch block. Observations regarding site and type of block. Circulation 49:638, 1978.

365. Dhingra, R. C., Wyndham, C., Bauernfeind, R., Swiryn, S., Deedwania, P. C., Smith, T., Denes, P., and Rosen, K. M.: Significance of block distal to the His bundle induced by atrial pacing in patients with chronic bifascicular block. Circulation 60:1455, 1979.

366. Strasberg, B., Amat-y-Leon, F., Dhingra, R. C., Palileo, E., Swiryn, S., Bauernfeind, R., Wyndham, C., and Rosen, K. M.: Natural history of chronic second degree atrioventricular nodal block. Circulation 63:1043, 1981.

367. Bonner, A. J., and Zipes, D. P.: Lidocaine and His-bundle extrasystole. His-bundle discharge conducted normally, conducted with functional right or left bundle branch block or blocked entirely (concealed). Arch. Intern. Med. 136:700, 1976.

368. Fisch, C., Zipes, D. P., and McHenry, P. L.: Electrocardiographic manifestations of concealed junctional ectopic impulses. Circulation 53:217, 1976.

368a. Langendorf, R., and Mehlman, J. S.: Block (non-conducted) AV nodal premature systoles imitating first and second degree AV block. Am. Heart J. 34:500, 1947.

368b. Rosen, K. M., Rahimtoola, S. H., and Gunnor, R. M.: Pseudo AV block secondary to non-premature non-propagated His-bundle depolarizations: Documentation by His-bundle electrocardiography, Circulation 42:367, 1970.

369. Dhingra, R. C., Palileo, E., Strasberg, B., Swiryn, S., Bauernfeind, R. A., Wyndham, C. R., and Rosen, K. M.: Significance of the HV interval in 517 patients with chronic bifascicular block. Circulation 64:1265, 1981.

370. Damato, A. N., Varghese, P. J., Caracta, A. R., Akhtar, M., and Lau, S. H.: Functional 2:1 block within the His-Purkinje system: Simulation of type II second degree AV block. Circulation 47:534, 1973.

371. Puech, P., Grolleau, R., and Guimond, L.: Incidence of different types of AV block and their localization by His bundle recordings. In Wellens, H. J. J., et al. (eds.): The Conduction System of the Heart. Philadelphia, Lea and Febiger, 1976, p. 467.

372. McKenna, W. J., Rowland, E., Davies, J., and Krikler, D. M.: Failure to predict development of atrioventricular block with electrophysiological testing supplemented by ajmaline. PACE 3:666, 1980.

373. Wellens, H. J. J., Bar, F. W., and Vanagt, E. J.: Death after ajmaline administration (letters to editor). Am. J. Cardiol. 45:905, 1980.

374. Lie, K. I., Wellens, H. J. J., Schuilenburg, R. M., Becker, A. E., and Durrer, D.: Factors influencing prognosis of bundle branch block complicating acute anteroseptal infarction. The value of His-bundle recordings. Circulation 50:935, 1974.

375. Fisch, G. R., Zipes, D. P., and Fisch, C.: Bundle branch block and sudden death. Progr. Cardiovasc. Dis. 23:187, 1980.

376. Hindman, M. C., Wagner, G. S., JaRo, M., Atkins, J. M., Scheinman, M. M., DeSanctis, R., Hutter, A. H., Jr., Yeatman, L., Rubenfire, M., Pujura, C., Rubin, M., and Morris, J. J.: The clinical significance of bundle branch block complicating acute myocardial infarction. I. Clinical characteristics, determinants of mortality and one-year followup. Circulation 58:679, 1978.

377. Hindman, M. C., Wagner, G. S., JaRo, M., Atkins, J. M., Scheinman, M. M., DeSanctis, R., Hutter, A. H., Jr., Yeatman, L., Rubenfire, M., Pujura, C., Rubin, M., and J. J.: The clinical significance of bundle branch block complicating acute myocardial infarction. II. Indications for temporary and permanent pacemaker insertion. Circulation 58:789, 1978.

378. Solti, F., Szabo, Z., Czako, E., Bodor, E., and Renyi-Vamos, F., Jr.: Adams-Stokes attacks associated with cartoid sinus syncope. Pathogenesis and therapy of the carotid sinus syncope. Kardiologie 69:656, 1980.

379. Beal, M. F., Park, T. S., and Fisher, C. M.: Cerebral atheromatous embolism following carotid sinus pressure. Arch. Neurol. 38:310, 1981.

380. Holden, W., McAnulty, J. H., and Rahimtoola, S. H.: Characterization of heart rate response to exercise in the sick sinus syndrome. Brit. Heart J. 40:923, 1978.

381. Jordan, J. A., Yamaguchi, I., and Mandel, W. J.: Studies on the mechanisms of sinus node dysfunction in a sick sinus syndrome. Circulation 57:217, 1978.

382. Eckberg, D. L., Drabinsky, M., and Braunwald, E.: Defective cardiac parasympathetic control in patients with heart disease. New Engl. J. Med. 285:877, 1971.

383. Cleaveland, C. R., Rangno, R. E., and Shand, D. G.: A standardized isoproterenol sensitivity test: The effects of sinus arrhythmia, atropine and propranolol. Arch. Intern. Med. 130:147, 1972.

384. Stern, S., and Eisenberg, S.: The effect of propranolol (Inderal) on the electrocardiogram of normal subjects. Am. Heart J. 77:192, 1969.

385. Kang, P. S., Gomes, J. A., Kelen, G., and El-Sherif, N.: Role of autonomic regulatory mechanism in sinoatrial conduction and sinus nodal automaticity in sick sinus syndrome. Circulation 64:832, 1981.

386. Desae, J. M., Scheinman, M. M., Strauss, H. C., Massie, B., and O'Young, J.: Electrophysiologic effects of combined autonomic blockade in patients with sinus node disease. Circulation 63:953, 1981.

387. Strauss, H. C., Bigger, J. T., Sardoff, A. C., and Giardina, E. G.: Electrophysiologic evaluation of sinus node function in patients with sinus node dysfunction. Circulation 53:763, 1976.

388. Breidthardt, G., Seipel, L., and Loogen, F.: Sinus node recovery time and calculated sinoatrial conduction time in normal subjects and patients with sinus node dysfunction. Circulation 56:43, 1977.

389. Steinbeck, G., and Luderitz, B.: Comparative study of sinoatrial conduction time and sinus node recovery time. Brit. Heart J. 37:956, 1975.

390. Bigger, J. T., Jr., Cramer, M., and Reid, S.: Ability of Holter electrocardiographic recording and atrial stimulation to detect sinus node dysfunction in symptomatic and asymptomatic patients with sinus bradycardia. Am. J. Cardiol. 40:189, 1977.

391. Rosen, K. M., Loeb, H. S., Sinno, M. Z., Rahimtoola, S. H., and Gunnar, R.: Cardiac conduction in patients with symptomatic sinus node disease. Circulation 43:836, 1971.

392. Narula, O. S.: Atrioventricular conduction disturbances in patients with sinus bradycardia. Circulation 44:1096, 1971.

392a. Kerr, C. R., Grant, A. O., Wenger, T. L., and Strauss, H. C.: Sinus node dysfunction. Cardiol. Clin. (still in press).

393. Narula, D. S., Shanto, N., Vasquez, M., Towne, W. D., and Linhart, J. W.: A new measurement of sino-atrial conduction time. Circulation 58:706, 1978.

394. Hariman, R. J., Krongrad, E., Boxer, R. A., Weiss, M. B., Steeg, C. N., and Hoffman, B. N.: Method for recording electrical activity of the sinoatrial node and automatic atrial foci during cardiac catheterization in human subject. Am. J. Cardiol. 45:775, 1980.

395. Wellens, J. H. H., Bär, F. W. H. M., and Lie, K. I.: The value of the electrocardiogram in the differential diagnosis of a tachycardia with a widened QRS complex. Am. J. Med. 64:27, 1978.

396. Wellens, H. J. J., and Durrer, D.: Supraventricular tachycardia with left aberrant conduction due to retrograde invasion into the left bundle branch. Circulation 38:474, 1968.

397. Wu, D., Amat-y-Leon, F., Simpson, R. J., Jr., Latif, P., Wyndham, C. R. C., Denes, P., and Rosen, K. M.: Electrophysiologic studies with multiple drugs in patients with atrioventricular reentrant tachycardia utilizing an extranodal pathway. Circulation 56:727, 1977.

398. Mason, J. W., and Winkle, R. A.: Electrode-catheter arrhythmia induction in the selection and assessment of antiarrhythmia drug therapy for recurrent ventricular tachycardia. Circulation 58:971, 1978.

399. Horowitz, L. N., Spielman, S. R., Greenspan, A. M., and Josephson, M. E.: Role of programmed stimulation in assessing vulnerability to ventricular arrhythmias. Am. Heart J. 103:604, 1982.

400. Heger, J. J., Prystowsky, E. N., Jackman, W. M., Naccarelli, G. V., and Zipes, D. P.: Comparison between results obtained from electrophysiologic testing, exercise testing and ambulatory ECG recording. In Wenger, N. K., et al. (eds.): Ambulatory Electrocardiographic Recording. Chicago, Year Book Medical Publishers, 1981, p. 379.

401. Gallagher, J. J., Kasell, J. H., Cox, J. L., Smith, W. M., Ideker, R. E., and Smith, W. M.: Techniques of intraoperative electrophysiologic mapping. Am. J. Cardiol. 49:221, 1982.

402. Josephson, M. E., Kastor, J. A., and Horowitz, L. N.: Electrophysiologic management of recurrent ventricular tachycardia in acute and chronic ischemic heart disease. Cardiovasc. Clin. 11:35, 1980.

403. Boineau, J. P., and Cox, J. L.: Rationale for a direct surgical approach to control ventricular arrhythmias. Relation of specific intraoperative techniques to mechanism and location of arrhythmic circuit. Am. J. Cardiol. 49:381, 1982.

404. Ruskin, J. N., DiMarco, J. P., and Garan, H.: Out-of-hospital cardiac arrest: Electrophysiologic observations and selection of long-term antiarrhythmic therapy. N. Engl. J. Med. 303:607, 1980.

405. Mason, J. W.: Repetitive beating after single ventricular extrastimuli: Incidence and prognostic significance in patients with recurrent ventricular tachycardia. Am. J. Cardiol. 45:1126, 1980.

406. Farshidi, A., Michelson, E. L., Greenspan, A. M., Spielman, S. R., Horowitz, L. N., and Josephson, M. E.: Repetitive responses to ventricular extrastimuli: Incidence, mechanism and significance. Am. Heart J. 100:59, 1980.

407. Ruskin, J. N., DiMarco, J. P., and Garan, H.: Repetitive responses to single ventricular stimuli in patients with serious ventricular arrhythmias: Incidence and clinical significance. Circulation 63:767, 1981.

408. Akhtar, M.: The clinical significance of the repetitive ventricular response (editorial). Circulation 63:773, 1981.

409. Gomes, J. A., Kang, P. S., Khan, R., Kelen, G., and El-Sherif, N.: Repetitive ventricular response: Its incidence, inducibility, reproducibility, mechanism and significance. Brit. Heart J. 46:159, 1981.

410. Richards, D. A., Cody, D. V., Denniss, A. R., Russell, P. A., Uther, J. B., and Young, A. A.: Ventricular electrical instability during the first year following myocardial infarction (abstract). Am. J. Cardiol. 49:929, 1982.

410a. Hamer, A., Vohra, J., Hunt, D., and Sloman, G.: Prediction of sudden death by electrophysiologic studies in high risk patients surviving acute myocardial infarction. Am. J. Cardiol. 50:223, 1982.

411. Naccarelli, G. V., Prystowsky, E. N., Jackman, W. M., Heger, J. J., Rahilly, G. T., and Zipes, D. P.: Role of electrophysiologic testing in managing patients who have ventricular tachycardia unrelated to coronary artery disease. Am. J. Cardiol. 50:165, 1982.

412. Robertson, J. F., Cain, M. E., Horowitz, L. N., Spielman, S. R., Greenspan, A. M., Waxman, H. L., and Josephson, M. E.: Anatomic and electrophysiologic correlates of ventricular tachycardia requiring left ventricular stimulation. Am. J. Cardiol. 48:263, 1981.

413. Vandepol, C. J., Farshidi, A., Spielman, S. R., Greenspan, A. M., Horowitz, L. N., and Josephson, M. E.: Incidence and clinical significance of induced ventricular tachycardia. Am. J. Cardiol. 45:725, 1980.

414. DiMarco, J., Garan, H., and Ruskin, J.: Efficacy of quinidine in the treatment of ventricular arrhythmias: The role of electrophysiologic testing. Circulation 64(Suppl. 4):38, 1981.

415. Gulamhusein, S., Naccarelli, G. V., Ko, P. T., Prystowsky, E. N., Zipes, D. P., Barnett, H. J. M., Heger, J. J., and Klein, G. J.: Value and limitations of the clinical electrophysiologic study in the assessment of patients with unexplained syncope. Am. J. Med. 73:700, 1982.

416. DiMarco, J. P., Garan, H., and Ruskin, J. N.: Morbidity associated with electrophysiologic procedures. Am. J. Cardiol. 49:959, 1982.

417. Ross, D. L., Farre, J., Bär, F. W. H. M., Vanagt, E. J., Vassen, W. R. M., Wiener, I., and Wellens, H. J. J.: Comprehensive clinical and electrophysiologic studies in the investigation of documented or suspected tachycardia. Circulation 61:1010, 1980.

418. Jenkins, J. M., Wu, D., and Arzbacher, R. C.: Computer diagnosis of supraventricular and ventricular arrhythmias. A new esophageal technique. Circulation 60:977, 1979.

419. Prystowsky, E. N., Pritchett, E. L. C., and Gallagher, J. J.: Origin of the atrial electrogram recorded from the esophagus. Circulation 61:1017, 1980.

420. Barold, S. S.: Filtered bipolar esophageal electrocardiography. Am. Heart J. 83:431, 1972.

421. Hammill, S. C., and Pritchett, E. L.: Simplified esophageal electrocardiography using bipolar recording leads. Ann. Intern. Med. 95:14, 1981.

422. Gallagher, J. J., Smith, W. M., Kerr, C. R., Kasell, J., Cook, L., Reiter, M., Sterba, R., and Harte, M.: Esophageal pacing: A diagnostic and therapeutic tool. Circulation 65:336, 1982.

423. Spach, M. S., and Barr, R. C.: Physiological correlation and clinical application of isopotential surface maps. In Hoffman, I. (ed.): Vectorcardiography 2: Proceedings of Tenth International Symposium on Vectorcardiography. Amsterdam, North-Holland Publ. Co., 1971.

424. Flowers, N. C., Horan, L. B., Sohi, G. S., Hand, R. C., and Johnson, T. C.: New evidence for inferoposterior myocardial infarction on surface potential maps. Am. J. Cardiol. 38:576, 1976.

425. Holt, H. J., Jr., Barnard, A. C. L., and Kramer, J. O.: Body surface potentials in ventricular hypertrophy: Analysis using a multiple dipole model of the heart. In Alper, T. (ed.): Cardiac Hypertrophy. New York, Academic Press, 1971, p. 611.

426. Mirvis, V. M.: Body surface distributions of repolarization potentials after acute myocardial infarction. II. Relationship between isopotential mapping and ST segment potential summation methods. Circulation 63:623, 1981.

427. Eifler, W. J., Macchi, E., Ritsema van Eck, H. J., Horacek, B. M., and Rautaharju, P. M.: Mechanism of generation of body surface electrocardiographic P waves in normal middle and lower sinus rhythms. Circ. Res. 48:168, 1981.

428. Benson, D. W., Jr., Sterba, R., Gallagher, J. J., Walston, A., and Spach, M. S.: Localization of the site of preexcitation with body surface maps in patients with Wolff-Parkinson-White syndrome. Circulation 65:1259, 1982.

429. Durrer, D., and Roos, J. P.: Epicardial excitation of the ventricles in a patient with Wolff-Parkinson-White syndrome (type B). Circulation 35:15, 1967.

430. Boineau, J. P., Moore, E. N., and Sealy, W. C.: Epicardial mapping in Wolff-Parkinson-White syndrome. Arch. Intern. Med. 135:422, 1975.

431. Waldo, A. L., and James, T. N.: The cardiac conduction system: Electrophysiological studies during open heart surgery. Arch. Intern. Med. 135:411, 1975.

432. Josephson, M. E., Horowitz, L. N., Spielman, S. R., Waxman, H. L., and Greenspan, A. M.: Role of catheter mapping in the preoperative evaluation of ventricular tachycardia. Am. J. Cardiol. 49:207, 1982.

433. Kaiser, G. A., Waldo, A. L., and Bowman, F. O.: The use of ventricular electrograms in operation for coronary artery disease and its complications. Ann. Thorac. Surg. 10:153, 1970.

434. Fontaine, G., Frank, R., and Bonnet, M.: Methode d'etude experimentale et clinique des syndromes de Wolff Parkinson White et d'ischemie myocardique par cartographie de la depolarisation ventriculaire epicardique. Coeur Med. Interne 12:105, 1973.

435. Hombach, V., Braun, V., Hopp, H. W., Gil-Sanchez, D., Scholl, H., Behrenbeck, D. W., Pauchert, M., and Hilger, H. H.: The applicability of the signal-averaging technique in clinical cardiology. Clin. Cardiol. 5:107, 1982.

436. Flowers, N. C., Shvartsman, V., Kennelly, B. M., Sohi, G. S., and Horan, L. G.: Surface recording of His-Purkinje activity on an every-beat basis without digital averaging. Circulation 63:948, 1981.

437. Hishimoto, Y., and Toshitami, S.: Noninvasive recording of His-bundle potential in man: Simplified method. Brit. Heart J. 37:635, 1975.

438. Berbari, E. J., Scherlag, B. J., and El-Sherif, N.: The His-Purkinje electrocardiogram in man: An initial assessment of its uses and limitations. Circulation 54:219, 1976.

439. Hon, E. H., and Lee, S. T.: Noise reduction in fetal electrocardiography. Am. J. Obstet. Gynecol. 87:1086, 1963.

440. Brody, D. A., Arzbacher, R. C., Woosley, M. D., and Sato, T.: The normal atrial electrocardiogram: Morphologic and quantitative variability in bipolar extremity leads. Am. Heart J. 74:4, 1967.

441. Rozanski, J. J., Mortara, D., Myerburg, R. J., and Castellanos, A.: Body surface detection of delayed depolarizations in patients with recurrent ventricular tachycardia and left ventricular aneurysm. Circulation 63:1172, 1981.

442. Simson, M. B.: Use of signals in the terminal QRS complex to identify patients with ventricular tachycardia after myocardial infarction. Circulation 64:235, 1981.

443. Simson, M. B.: Clinical application of signal averaging. Cardiol. Clin. 1:109, 1983.

20
MANAGEMENT OF CARDIAC ARRHYTHMIAS
Pharmacological, Electrical, and Surgical Techniques
by Douglas P. Zipes, M.D.

PHARMACOLOGICAL THERAPY

PRINCIPLES OF CLINICAL PHARMACOKINETICS

Pharmacological treatment of a patient with a cardiac arrhythmia has as its primary objectives to reach an effective and well-tolerated serum drug concentration as rapidly as possible and to maintain this concentration for as long as required without producing adverse effects. In many[1] but not all[2] situations nor with all drugs,[3] serum concentration after equilibration strongly correlates with the antiarrhythmic effect of the drug. Therapeutic serum concentrations for most antiarrhythmic agents are listed in Table 20-1 and are based on concentrations of drugs that exert therapeutic effects without adverse effects in a majority of patients. However, the therapeutic concentration for any individual patient is the amount of drug required *for that patient* to suppress or terminate the cardiac arrhythmia without producing adverse effects. For a specific patient, one must consider the response both of the patient and of the arrhythmia to the drug, and the actual serum concentration of the drug is often of secondary importance. In some patients measured serum concentrations can be useful to establish concentrations needed for prophylaxis, to judge the sensitivity or resistance of the arrhythmia to the drug, and to evaluate symptoms that suggest drug toxicity. Serum concentrations can also be used to determine the effects of changing physiological states on drug concentrations, establish drug compliance or abuse, search for drug interactions, and establish the importance of physiologically active metabolites of the parent compound. Active metabolites may be suspected when the clinical effect of the drug outlasts the therapeutic serum concentration of the drug.

Normally, because antiarrhythmic agents have a narrow toxic-thera-peutic relationship, important complications of therapy may result from amounts of drug that only slightly exceed the amount necessary to produce beneficial effects; lesser concentrations are often subtherapeutic. It is obvious that careful dosing with these agents is essential to maintain adequate but nontoxic amounts of drug in the body, a task facilitated by understanding drug pharmacokinetics, which consists of a quantitative assessment of drug absorption, distribution, metabolism, and excretion. Alterations in the rate of any of these processes may account for significant intra- and interpatient variations in serum concentrations.[4,5] In addition, changes in the functional status of any of the organs involved, primarily the liver and kidneys, may significantly alter dose requirements in a given patient.

Absorption. Drug absorption from the intestinal tract occurs for most drugs with a half-time of absorption in the range of 20 to 30 minutes. Completeness of absorption may vary between 50 and over 90 per cent, depending on the drug, with most absorption occurring in the small intestine. Different preparations of the same drug, e.g., digoxin or phenytoin, may undergo different rates of absorption in the same patient because the tablet preparations have different dissolution rates. Thus, two brands of drug may not result in the same serum concentration.[5] Large amounts of some orally administered drugs, such as propranolol or verapamil, are transformed to inactive metabolites in the liver before they reach the systemic circulation—the so-called first-pass hepatic effect. For such an agent, much more drug must be administered orally than intravenously to achieve the same physiological effect.

Disease states and other factors can alter the rate and completeness of drug absorption. For example, heart failure can cause mucosal edema of the gut and impair the absorption of orally administered drugs, as can decreased intestinal blood flow. Malabsorption syndromes, concomitant use of other drugs, or changes in gut motility caused by diarrheal states or the use of cathartics may alter absorption. Since most antiarrhythmic agents are basic compounds, they are ionized and poorly absorbed at normal gastric pH, and some drugs may decompose at gastric pH. Conditions that delay gastric emptying increase the absorption lag phase between ingestion of these drugs and their arrival in the small intestine, where most absorption takes place, and therefore may decrease absorption. In patients with severe hypotension, shock, or cardiac arrest, impaired tissue perfusion prevents reliable absorption of intramuscularly administered agents; so that these patients should receive all medications by the intravenous (IV) route.

The rate of drug absorption, determined by the time required to achieve maximum serum concentration, and the fraction of drug absorbed influence the drug's *bioavailability*, which is a measure of the amount of drug that reaches the systemic circulation intact. Bioavailability of a drug includes factors such as lack of pill dissolution, metabolism by gut mucosa, hepatic metabolism and binding, and absorption. It is a most important property of the drug. Absorption is thus only one component affecting bioavailability. The fraction of an orally administered drug reaching the systemic circulation intact, or *systemic availability*, can be calculated (assuming equal clearances for IV and oral forms of drug) by comparing the area under the plasma concentration curve achieved with oral and intravenous administrations from the following relationship: systemic availability equals the area under the plasma concentration curve following oral administration/the area under the plasma concentration curve following IV administration times 100 (assuming equal IV and oral doses).

Drug Distribution. Most antiarrhythmic drugs in the therapeutic range are eliminated according to first-order kinetics, which means that the amount of drug eliminated per unit time is directly proportional to the amount (or concentration) of drug in the body. More drug in the body results in more drug excreted by the kidneys or metabolized by the liver, so that the *fraction* of drug eliminated per unit of time remains constant regardless of the amount of drug in the body. For example, one-half the drug may be eliminated in 6 hours whether the total amount of drug in the body is 4 gm or 10 gm, resulting in elimination of 2 gm in the first example and of 5 gm in the second. As a consequence, the elimination half-life, or time required to eliminate half the body load (or to halve the plasma concentration) of such a drug is constant and independent of the total body load. The following discussion will assume first-order kinetics unless otherwise stated.

Generally two models, a *one-compartment open model* and a *two-compartment open model*, are used with relative accuracy to describe and predict serum concentrations at a given time for a variety of dose regimens. Even though these models are oversimplified representations of drug disposition, they provide guidelines for choosing loading doses and maintenance dose schedules for a given patient. In the one-compartment open model, drugs are considered to enter and to be eliminated from a single homogeneous unit that represents the entire body. Drugs entering the compartment are considered to be distributed immediately throughout the compartment, making the concentration of the drug equal to the amount of drug in the compartment divided by the volume of the compartment. The latter equals the amount of the drug in the compartment divided by the drug concentration.

In reality, a one-compartment open model is not entirely appropriate because a certain amount of time is needed to distribute the drug throughout the volume of the compartment. However, the one-compartment model predicts plasma concentration as a function of time and dose, if distribution is significantly faster than the rate of administration or of excretion, which is the case for many antiarrhythmic drugs.

If the rate of drug administration is rapid in relation to drug distribution (e.g., intravenous administration), a two-compartment open model more accurately predicts drug concentrations (Fig. 20–1). In this model the drug enters the system by the central compartment and can leave the system only by distribution into a peripheral compartment or elimination from the central compartment. The central compartment, in dynamic equilibrium with the more slowly equilibrating peripheral compartment, is assumed to consist of the blood volume and extracellular fluid of highly perfused tissues such as heart, lungs, kidneys, and liver, while the peripheral compartment, acting as a reservoir, consists of less well perfused tissue such as muscle, skin, and adipose tissue. The first-order rate constants K_{1-2} and K_{2-1} determine the rate of transfer of drug between the central and peripheral com-

partments or vice versa, with K_e representing the overall elimination rate constant. K_e relates the sum of all methods of irreversible drug elimination from the central compartment to the concentration of drug in that compartment (Fig. 20–1). For antiarrhythmic drugs, the peripheral compartment is generally larger than the central compartment. The concepts of distribution volumes and drug movement are more complex in the two-compartment open model than in the one-compartment open model.[6,7] The two-compartment model may behave similarly to the one-compartment model when drugs are infused slowly or given orally and K_1 approximates K_2, but pronounced differences exist when injections are given rapidly.

Following administration of drugs for which the kinetics are described by a two-compartment model, the curve of plasma drug concentration demonstrates two distinct phases: an early phase (alpha, or distribution phase), characterized by rapidly falling plasma drug concentrations due to distribution between the central compartment and the peripheral compartment, and a second phase (beta, or elimination phase) of slower decline in plasma drug concentration, representing primarily elimination of drugs from the central compartment (Fig. 20–2). *Alpha* is often referred to as the *rate constant for distribution* and *beta* as the *rate constant for elimination*. During the latter beta phase, when the drug is in distribution equilibrium, serum concentrations correlate with the pharmacological effects of the drug. The distribution for quinidine is shown in Figure 20–3.

Several important concepts need to be considered. The extent of extravascular distribution of a drug is obtained by measuring the apparent *volume of distribution*, which is the hypothetical volume into which a dose of drug would have to be diluted to give the observed plasma concentration. It is determined by the dose administered divided by the plasma concentration at time 0. It equals the sum of A and B on the logarithmic plasma concentration axis obtained by extrapolating the alpha and beta phases back to 0 time (Fig. 20–2).[4] A large volume of distribution indicates a wide distribution and extensive tissue uptake of the drug and often exceeds by several times the amount of total body water. The large volume of distribution for most antiarrhythmic agents indicates that they are present in higher concentrations in some tissues than in the plasma. The volume of distribution is dependent on the relative serum and tissue binding characteristics of the drug and may be constricted in some patients, such as those with renal failure, during which a change in serum protein or tissue binding may occur. Quinidine decreases the volume of distribution of digoxin, probably as a result of a decrease in tissue binding of digoxin.

Drug Metabolism and Excretion. Approximately 97 per cent of the dose of any drug is removed from the body in a time equal to five half-lives.[8] *Serum elimination half-life* is defined as the time interval for 50 per cent of the drug present in the body at the beginning of the interval to be eliminated. After one half-life, 50 per cent of the drug remains in the body (assuming no further drug is administered), after two half-lives 25 per cent remains, after three half-lives 12.5 per cent remains, and so forth. Half-life is determined from the relationship $t_{1/2} = 0.693/\text{beta}$ for a two-compartment model (Fig. 20–2). Since changes in drug distribution influence elimination half-life, the equation can be rewritten as $t_{1/2} = 0.693 \times$ volume of distribution/total body clearance.

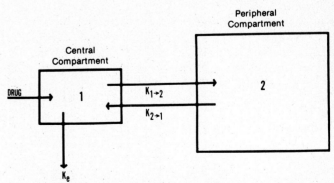

FIGURE 20–1 Two-compartment open model. A smaller central compartment into which drug is administered and from which it is eliminated (K_e) connects in dynamic equilibrium with a larger peripheral compartment.

TABLE 20–1 DOSAGE AND THERAPEUTIC SERUM CONCENTRATIONS FOR ANTIARRHYTHMIC AGENTS

DRUG	USUAL DOSE RANGES — Intravenous (mg) LOADING	Intravenous (mg) MAINTENANCE	Oral (mg) LOADING	Oral (mg) MAINTENANCE	TIME TO PEAK PLASMA CONCENTRATION (ORAL)	EFFECTIVE SERUM OR PLASMA CONCENTRATION (μG/ML)	ELIMINATION HALF-LIFE AFTER ORAL DOSE (HR)	BIOAVAILABILITY (%)	MAJOR ROUTE OF ELIMINATION
Lidocaine	1 to 3 mg/kg at 20 to 50 mg/min	1 to 4 mg/min	N/A	N/A	N/A	1 to 5	1 to 2	N/A	Liver
Quinidine	6 to 10 mg/kg at 0.3 to 0.5 mg/kg/min		600 to 1000	300 to 600 q6h	1.5 to 3.0	3 to 6	5 to 9	60 to 80	Liver
Procainamide	6 to 13 mg/kg at 0.2 to 0.5 mg/kg/min	2 to 6 mg/min	500 to 1000	350 to 1000 q3–6h	1	4 to 10	3 to 5	70 to 85	Kidneys
Disopyramide	1 to 2 mg/kg over 15 min* 1 to 2 mg/kg over 45 min	1 mg/kg/hr*	300 to 400	100 to 400 q6–8h	1 to 2	2 to 5	8 to 9	80 to 90	Kidneys
Phenytoin	100 mg q5min for ≤1000 mg		1000	100 to 400 q12–24h	8 to 12	10 to 20	18 to 36	50 to 70	Liver
Propranolol	0.25 to 0.5 mg, q5min for ≤0.15 to 0.20 mg/kg			10 to 200 q6–8h	2 to 4	0.04 to 0.90	3 to 6	20 to 50	Liver
Bretylium	5 to 10 mg/kg at 1 to 2 mg/kg/min	½ to 2 mg/min					8 to 14	25	Kidneys
Verapamil	10 mg over 1 to 2 min	0.005 mg/kg/min	N/A	4 mg/kg/day*	1 to 2	0.5 to 1.5	3 to 8	10 to 35	Liver
Amiodarone*	5 to 10 mg/kg		800 to 1200 qid for 1 to 4 weeks	80 to 120 q6–8h 200 to 800 qid	4	0.10 to 0.15 1 to 5	30 to 50 days		Liver
Aprindine*	200 mg at 2 mg/min 100 mg at 2 mg/min 30 min later 100 mg at 2 mg/min 6 hr later		100 q6h day 1 75 q6h day 2 50 q6h day 3						
Encainide*	0.6 to 0.9 mg/kg		N/A	25 to 50 q6–12h	2	1 to 2	20 to 30	80 to 90	Liver
Mexiletine*	500 mg	0.5 to 1.0 gm/24 hr	400 to 600	25 to 75 q6–8h	2 to 4	0.5 to 1.0	3 to 4	40	Liver
Tocainide*	750 mg		400 to 600	200 to 300 q6–8h	1 to 2	6 to 12	10 to 17	90	Liver
Ethmozine*			300	400 to 800 q8–12h		0.1		90	Liver
Flecainide*	2 mg/kg			100 to 400 q8h	1.5 to 3.0	0.2 to 0.8	14 to 20	95	Liver
Lorcainide*	1 to 2 mg/kg			100 to 300 q12h 100 q8h	1 to 3	0.3 to 1.0	6 to 20	50	Liver
Propafenone*	1 to 2 mg/kg		600 to 900	150 to 300 q8–12h	1 to 4	2	3 to 4	50 to 75	Liver
Bethanidine*	5 to 20 mg/kg		20 to 30 mg/kg	5 to 10 mg/kg q8h			14	60 to 90	Kidneys
Cibenzoline*	1.0 to 1.2 mg/kg			65 to 81.25 q6h	1 to 2	0.2 to 0.6	7 to 20	100	Kidneys

* Investigational.
Results presented may vary according to doses, disease state, and IV or oral administration.

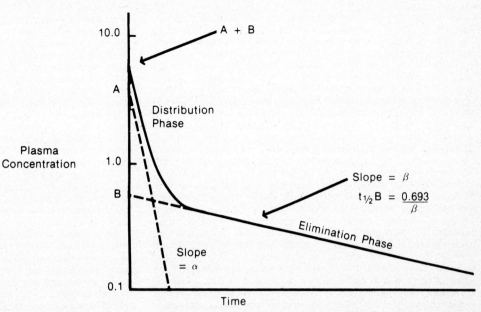

FIGURE 20–2 Schematic diagram of the semilogarithmic plot of drug plasma concentration as a function of time following rapid intravenous injection, according to the principles outlined for a two-compartment open model. (From Gibaldi, M., and Perrier, D.: Drugs and the pharmaceutical sciences. *In* Pharmacokinetics, Vol. I. New York, Marcel Dekker, 1975.)

Drug clearance is analogous to the concept of renal clearance and is the volume of blood totally cleared of drug in unit time. It is the sum of the clearances for each process by which the drug is eliminated and can be calculated from the relationship: clearance = dose of the drug/area under the plasma concentration time curve (AUC). Expressed differently, clearance equals volume of distribution ×

beta, or volume of distribution × 0.693/half-life. A larger volume of distribution increases the elimination half-life at a given clearance. The larger volume of distribution of antiarrhythmic drugs accounts for the relatively long half-life despite their large clearance rates. Quinidine prolongs digitoxin's half-life by decreasing total body clearance.[5] Clearance of drugs with high extraction ratios strongly depends on

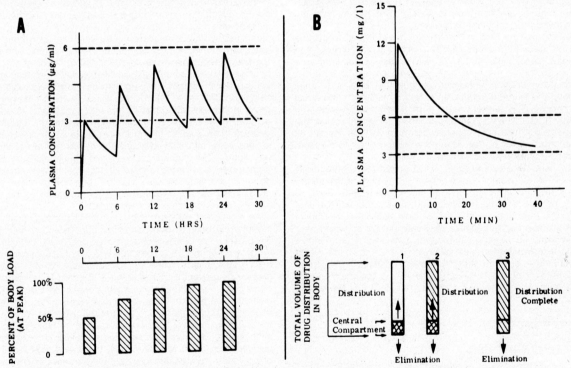

FIGURE 20–3 *A,* Changes in plasma concentration over time after beginning treatment with quinidine. *Top,* Quinidine plasma concentration over time, with the dashed line indicating the therapeutic range. *Bottom,* The hatched bars represent the body load immediately after each dose of quinidine, expressed as a percentage of the load after a dose when a steady state has been achieved. Quinidine is administered every 6 hours (the half-life in this case). Four half-lives, or 24 hours, are required to achieve a body load of quinidine that exceeds 90 per cent of the load at steady state. *B, top,* Plasma concentrations produced by administering a full intravenous loading dose of quinidine as a bolus, with the therapeutic range shown by a dashed line. *Bottom,* The numbered vertical boxes indicate the volume of distribution of quinidine. Just after the drug is given, it is dissolved only in the small central compartment, as in box 1, and very high peak concentrations are achieved (in the toxic range). The drug then distributes throughout the rest of the body. Distribution has a half-life of about 8 minutes and is complete by 30 minutes (box 3). Quinidine concentration is now in the therapeutic range, and further decreases in plasma concentration are due solely to drug elimination. (From Nattel, S., and Zipes, D.P.: Clinical pharmacology of old and new antiarrhythmic drugs. Cardiovasc. Clin. *11:*221, 1980.)

blood flow to the organ from which they are eliminated, such as propranolol, verapamil, or lidocaine in the liver. For antiarrhythmic drugs that have a high renal extraction ratio, such as procainamide and quinidine, reduction of renal flow decreases their clearance.

Function of the organ system that eliminates a given drug from the body determines the elimination half-life. For drugs rapidly metabolized in the liver, hepatic blood flow limits the rate of drug elimination. Disorders that reduce liver blood flow (e.g., low cardiac output, hepatic disease with portacaval shunting) markedly slow the elimination of such drugs. Drugs with a short half-life are convenient to use by intravenous infusion but not by chronic oral dosing, since the short half-life requires frequent oral doses to maintain a fairly constant plasma concentration. Generally, maintenance dosing involves giving a certain amount of the drug at a time interval that equals the elimination half-life. However, with drugs that have very long half-lives, such as 12 hours, this may result in peak values shortly after administration and consequent side effects.[4] Maintaining constant plasma concentrations is necessary because of the narrow toxic-therapeutic ratios exhibited by antiarrhythmic agents. Also, some drugs such as encainide (see p. 667) have active metabolites with half-lives considerably longer than the parent compound, allowing dosing intervals to be more widely spaced than those predicted by the half-life of the parent drug. The rate and extent of metabolism of the same drug may vary greatly from patient to patient owing to a variety of factors, including environment, genetics, age, disease states, and influence of other drugs given concomitantly. A genetically controlled acetyltransferase enzyme system influences the metabolism of some drugs, making about half the American population "rapid" and half "slow acetylators." Rapid acetylators metabolize a greater proportion of a drug dose than do slow acetylators, who may require less drug to achieve any desired serum level or pharmacological effect. Also, rapid acetylators may be more prone to develop reactions from the metabolites of drugs[5] or are less likely to develop side effects from the parent compound for a constant drug dose.

Drugs exist in plasma both in the free form and bound to plasma proteins. Only free drug is capable of distributing into tissues and exerting a pharmacological action. Virtually all assays for drug concentration in the blood measure *both* free and protein-bound drug. For antiarrhythmic drugs, the fraction of drug that is bound varies greatly among the different agents but is fairly constant for individual drugs over the clinically relevant range of plasma concentrations with the exception of phenytoin and disopyramide. Total serum concentrations of a given drug therefore generally correlate well with its clinical effects, and it has not been necessary to develop assays to measure free drug concentrations for antiarrhythmic agents.

When a constant dose of a drug is administered repeatedly (orally or parenterally) at a constant dosing interval, accumulation occurs until drug concentration approaches a constant steady-state level, at which time the rate of drug administration equals the rate of drug elimination. The time it takes to reach steady state is a function of the half-life of the drug; 94 per cent of steady state is achieved after four half-lives and 99 per cent after seven half-lives. A drug with a long half-life takes longer to reach steady state than does one with a short half-life. The average steady-state concentration of a drug equals the fraction of the dose absorbed (F) $\times$ the maintenance dose (dose$_m$) divided by the total body clearance (Cl$_s$) $\times$ the dosing interval (τ):

$$\text{Average steady state concentration} = \frac{F \times \text{dose}_m}{CL_s \times \tau} = \frac{F \times \text{dose}_m t_{\frac{1}{2}}}{0.693 \times V_d \tau}$$

If the drug is given intravenously,[5]

$$\text{Steady state concentration} = \frac{\text{Infusion rate}}{Cl_s} = \frac{\text{Infusion rate } t_{\frac{1}{2}}}{0.693 \ V_d}$$

Finally, it is important to stress that drug pharmacokinetics may differ in normal healthy volunteers compared to patients who have a variety of illnesses. Therefore, information derived from patients as well as normal subjects must be considered when one is planning dosing regimens.

GENERAL CONSIDERATIONS REGARDING ANTIARRHYTHMIC DRUGS

Segregating drugs into various classes, although useful conceptually, will not be emphasized in this chapter.[9] Such classifications* suffer from several inadequacies: (1) all drugs assigned to a single group do not exhibit entirely similar actions, and some drugs exert more than one type of action; (2) classifications are based primarily on the electrophysiological properties exerted by the drugs on normal Purkinje fibers, and the drugs may exert different effects on muscle, on different species, on acutely or chronically damaged tissue, or when the electrolyte milieu is abnormal; in vitro studies on healthy fibers usually establish the properties of antiarrhythmic agents rather than their antiarrhythmic properties;[10] (3) many antiarrhythmic agents produce their effects in vivo not by direct electrophysiological actions on cardiac cells but indirectly by metabolic or anti-ischemic actions, by effects on the central or peripheral autonomic nervous system, by improving circulatory hemodynamics, or by active metabolites; (4) some drugs do not fit neatly into one class, leading to formulation of a variety of classifications; and (5) insights into the mechanisms by which antiarrhythmic agents may affect ion transfer are only recently being gained, and this new knowledge will undoubtedly influence concepts about how antiarrhythmic agents function.

For example, a recently proposed model suggests that antiarrhythmic drugs cross the cell membrane and interact with receptors in the membrane channels when the latter are in the rested, activated, or inactivated states and that each of these interactions is characterized by an association and dissociation rate constant. Transitions among rested, activated, and inactivated states are governed by standard Hodgkin-Huxley-type equations. When the drug is bound (associated) to the channel, the latter cannot conduct, even in the activated state.[11] Some drugs exert greater inhibitory effects at more rapid rates of stimulation, a characteristic called "use-dependence." It is possible that this use-dependence results from preferential interaction of the antiarrhythmic drug with either the open or the inactive channel and little interaction with the resting channels of the unstimulated cell. With increased time spent in diastole (slower rate), a greater proportion of receptors become drug-free and the drug exerts less effect.

Given the fact that enhanced automaticity or reentry can cause cardiac arrhythmias, mechanisms by which antiarrhythmic agents suppress arrhythmias can be postulated. Antiarrhythmic agents can slow the spontaneous discharge frequency of an automatic pacemaker by depressing the slope of diastolic depolarization, shifting the threshold voltage toward zero, or hyperpolarizing the resting membrane potential (Fig. 19-13, p. 618). Mechanisms by which different drugs suppress normal or abnormal automaticity may not be the same. In general, however, most antiarrhythmic agents in therapeutic doses depress the automatic firing rate of spontaneously discharging ectopic sites while minimally affecting the discharge rate of the normal sinus node. Slow-channel blockers like verapamil, beta blockers like propranolol, and some antiarrhythmic agents like amiodarone also depress spontaneous discharge of the normal sinus node, while drugs that exert vagolytic effects, such as disopyramide or quinidine, may increase the sinus discharge rate.

As mentioned earlier (p. 624), reentry depends critically on the timing interrelationships between refractoriness and conduction velocity, the presence of unidirectional block in one of the pathways, and other factors that influence refractoriness and conduction, such as excitability. An antiarrhythmic agent can stop reentry that is already present or prevent it from starting if the drug improves *or* depresses conduction. For example, *improved conduction* can (1) eliminate the unidirectional block so that reentry cannot begin or (2) facilitate conduction in the reentrant loop so that the returning wavefront reenters too quickly, encroaches on fibers still refractory, and becomes extinguished. A drug that *depresses conduction* can transform the unidirectional block to bidirectional block and thus terminate reentry or prevent it from occurring by creating an area of complete block in the reentrant pathway. Finally, most antiarrhythmic agents share the ability to prolong refractoriness relative to their effects on action potential duration, i.e., the ratio of effective refractory period to action potential duration exceeds 1.0. If a drug *prolongs refractoriness* of fibers in the reentrant pathway, the pathway may not recover excitabili-

---

*Classification of antiarrhythmic drugs:

Class I—Drugs that reduce $\dot{V}$max: Lidocaine, quinidine, procainamide, disopyramide, aprindine, encainide, mexiletine, tocainide, ethmozine, flecainide, lorcainide, propafenone, cibenzoline.

Class II—Drugs that inhibit sympathetic activity: Propranolol.

Class III—Drugs that prolong action potential duration: Amiodarone, bethanidine, bretylium, sotalol.

Class IV—Drugs that block the slow inward current: Verapamil.

ty in time to be depolarized by the reentering impulse, and the reentrant propagation ceases. Conversely, a drug that slows conduction without producing block or lengthening refractoriness significantly may promote reentry.

When one is discussing any of the properties of a drug, it is important that the situation and/or model from which conclusions are drawn be defined with care. Electrophysiological, hemodynamic, autonomic, pharmacokinetic, and adverse effects all may differ in normal subjects compared to patients, in normal tissue compared to abnormal tissue, in muscle compared to specialized fibers, and in different species.

LIDOCAINE

Electrophysiological Actions (Tables 20–2 and 20–3). Lidocaine does not affect normal sinus nodal automaticity[12] but does depress both normal[13] and some abnormal forms of automaticity in Purkinje fibers in vitro. External environment significantly influences the effects of lidocaine. At $[K]_o \leq 4.5$ mM/liter, therapeutic concentrations of lidocaine exert little effect on $\dot{V}max$ of phase 0 in normal cardiac Purkinje fibers, while at $[K]_o > 6.0$ mM/liter, therapeutic concentrations of lidocaine reduce $\dot{V}max$ at any level of membrane potential.[14] In the presence of acidosis, lidocaine significantly reduces canine cardiac Purkinje fiber resting membrane potential, action potential amplitude, and $\dot{V}max$ and increases conduction time, at the same concentrations that exert minimal effects when the pH is normal.[15] Therapeutic concentrations of lidocaine depress activity in abnormal ventricular muscle fibers that have survived experimental myocardial infarction.[16–18] The infarct area exhibits elevated $[K]_o$ and reduced pH, and in this environment, lidocaine exaggerates the action potential changes and quickens the time course produced by ischemia, possibly converting areas of unidirectional block into bidirectional block and preventing development of ventricular fibrillation by preventing fragmentation of organized large wavefronts into heterogeneous wavelets.[19] Lidocaine may be arrhythmogenic if it depresses conduction but not to the point of bidirectional block.[12,20] For example, it may create an area of unidirectional block and another area of conduction delay (see p. 623) and promote reentry.

Lidocaine does *not* affect slow-channel–dependent action potentials. In fact, its depressant effect on ischemic potentials and depressed fast responses supports the notion that these ischemic potentials are depressed fast responses rather than slow responses.[19,21] Lidocaine significantly reduces the action potential duration and the effective refractory period of Purkinje fibers and ventricular muscle[13] but not of ordinary or specialized atrial fibers.[12,22] The decrease in action potential duration in Purkinje fibers, thought to relate in large part to an increase in potassium conductance (gk_1), enhancing potassium's loss from the cell, appears to be due to blocking of tetrodotoxin-sensitive sodium channels, decreasing entry of sodium into the cell.[23] In some in vitro preparations, lidocaine can improve conduction by hyperpolarizing tissues depolarized as a result of stretch or low external potassium concentration.[24]

In vivo, lidocaine has a minimal effect on automaticity or conduction except in unusual circumstances. Patients with preexisting sinus nodal dysfunction,[7] abnormal His-Purkinje conduction,[25] or junctional escape rhythms during ischemia[26] may develop depressed automaticity or conduction. This drug may shorten His-Purkinje refractoriness in man.[27] Part of its effects may be to inhibit cardiac sympathetic nerve activity.[28,29]

Hemodynamic Effects. Clinically significant adverse hemodynamic effects are rarely noted unless left ventricular function is severely impaired.

Pharmacokinetics (Table 20–1). Lidocaine is used only parenterally because oral administration results in extensive first-pass hepatic metabolism and unpredictable, low plasma levels with excessive metabolites that may produce toxicity. Hepatic metabolism of lidocaine depends greatly on hepatic blood flow, so that clearance of this drug almost equals (and can be approximated by) measurements of this flow.[30] Severe hepatic disease or reduced hepatic blood flow, as in heart failure or shock, can mark-

TABLE 20–2 IN VIVO ELECTROPHYSIOLOGICAL CHARACTERISTICS

DRUG	ELECTROCARDIOGRAPHIC INTERVALS						ELECTROPHYSIOLOGICAL INTERVALS				
	Sinus Rate	P-R	QRS	Q-T	A-H	H-V	ERP AVN	ERP HPS	ERP A	ERP V	ERP AP
Lidocaine	0	0	0	0	0↓	0↑	0↓	0↑	0	0	0
Quinidine	0↑	↓0↑	↑	↑	↓0↑	0↑	↓0↑	0↑	↑	↑	↑
Procainamide	0	0↑	↑	↑	0↑	0↑	0↑	0↑	↑	↑	↑
Disopyramide	0↑	0	0↑	0↑	0	0↑	0↓	↑	↑	↑	↑
Phenytoin	0	0	0	0↓	0↓	0	0↓	↓	0	0	0
Propranolol	↓	0↑	0	0↓	0↑	0	↑	0	0	0	0
Bretylium	0↓	0↑	0	0↑							0
Verapamil	0↓	↑	0	0	↑	0	↑	0	0	0	0
Amiodarone	↓	0↑	0	↑	↑	0	↑	↑↑	↑	↑	↑
Aprindine	↓	↑	↑	0↑	↑	↑	↑	↑	↑	↑	↑
Encainide	0	↑	↑	↑	↑	↑	↑	↑	↑	↑	↑
Mexiletine	0	0	0	0	0↑	0↑	0↑	0↑	0	0	0
Tocainide	0↓	0	0	0↓	0↑	0	↓	0	0↓	0↓	0
Ethmozine	0↓	0↑	0↑	0					↑	↑	
Flecainide		↑	↑	↑	↑	↑	↑		↑	↑	↑
Lorcainide		0↑	↑	↑	0	↑	0		0	0	↑
Propafenone	0↓	↑	↑	0↑	↑	↑	0↑		0↑	↑	↑
Bethanidine	0↓	0	0	0↑							0
Cibenzoline	↑	↑	↑	0↑	0	↑	0		0	↑	

Results presented may vary according to tissue type, experimental conditions, and drug concentration. ↑ = increase; ↓ = decrease; 0 = no change; 0↑ or 0↓ = slight inconsistent increase or decrease. A = atrium; AVN = AV node; HPS = His-Purkinje system; V = ventricle; AP = accessory pathway (WPW); ERP = effective refractory period—longest S_1-S_2 interval at which S_2 fails to produce a response.

TABLE 20–3 IN VITRO ELECTROPHYSIOLOGICAL CHARACTERISTICS

DRUG	APA	APD	dV/dt	MDP	ERP	CONDUCTION VELOCITY	SINUS NODAL AUTOMATICITY	PF NORMAL PHASE 4	MEMBRANE RESPONSIVENESS	ET	VFT	CONTRACTILITY	SLOW INWARD CURRENT	AUTONOMIC NERVOUS SYSTEM	LOCAL ANESTHETIC EFFECT
Lidocaine	0↓	↓	0↓	0	↓	0↓	0	↓	0↓	0↑	↑	0	0	0	Yes
Quinidine	↓	↑	↓	0	↑	↓	0	↓	↓	↑	↑	0	0	Antivagal alpha blocker	Yes
Procainamide	↓	↑	↓	0	↑	↓	0	↓	↓	↑	↑	↓	0	Slight antivagal	Yes
Disopyramide	↓	↑	↓	0	↑	↓	↑0↓	↓	↓	↑	↑	↓	0	Central: antivagal, antisympathetic	Yes
Phenytoin	0	↓	↑0↓	0	↓	0	0	↓	0↑	0		↓	0	0	Yes
Propranolol	0↑	0↑	0↑	0	↑	0	↓	↓	0↑	0	0↑	↓	0	Antisympathetic	No
Bretylium	0	↑	0	0	↑	0	0↑	0	0	0	↑	0↑	0	Antisympathetic	Yes
Verapamil	0	↓	0	0	0↑	0	↓	0	0	0	0	↓	Inhibit	? Block alpha receptors	Yes
Amiodarone	0	↑	0↓	0	↑		↓	↓	↓	↑			0↑	Antisympathetic	Yes
Aprindine	↓	↓	↓	0	↑		0↑	↓	↓	↑			0↑	0	No
Encainide	↓	↓	↓	0	↑		0	↓	↓	↓			0	0	Yes
Mexiletine	0	↓	↓	0	↓		0	↓	↓	↑	↑	0	0	0	Yes
Tocainide	0	↓	0↓	0	↑		0	↓	↓	↓	↑		0	0	Yes
Ethmozine	↓	↓	↓	0	↑		0	0↓	↓		0	↓	0	0	No
Flecainide	↓	↑	↓	0	↑		0	↓	↓	↑			0	0	Yes
Lorcainide	↓	↑	↓	0	↑		0↑	↓	↓				0	0	Yes
Propafenone			↑			↓	↓	↓	↓	↑	↑	↓	May inhibit	0	Yes
Bethanidine	0	↑	0	0	↑	0		0	↓	0	↑		0	Antisympathetic	Yes
Cibenzoline	↓	↑	↓	0	↑	↓	0	↓	↓	0		↓	0	Slight antivagal	Yes

Key: APA = action potential amplitude; APD = action potential duration; dV/dt = rate of rise of action potential; MDP = maximum diastolic potential; ERP = effective refractory period; PF = Purkinje fibers; ET = excitability threshold; VFT = ventricular fibrillation threshold.

edly decrease the rate of lidocaine metabolism. Prolonged infusion can reduce lidocaine clearance. Its elimination half-life averages about 1 to 2 hours in normal subjects, more than 4 hours in patients after relatively uncomplicated myocardial infarction, more than 10 hours in patients after myocardial infarction complicated by cardiac failure, and even longer in the presence of cardiogenic shock.[31] Maintenance doses should be reduced by one-third to one-half for patients with low cardiac output.

Dosage and Administration (Table 20–1). Although lidocaine may be given intramuscularly, the intravenous route is most commonly used (Fig. 20–4). Intramuscular lidocaine is given in doses of 4 to 5 mg/kg (250 to 350 mg), resulting in effective serum levels at about 15 minutes and lasting for about 90 minutes.[32] Intravenously, lidocaine is given as an initial bolus of 1 to 2 mg/kg body weight at a rate of approximately 20 to 50 mg/min, with a second injection of one-half the initial dose 20 to 40 minutes later.[7] Patients treated with an initial bolus followed by a maintenance infusion may experience transient subtherapeutic plasma concentrations at 30 to 120 minutes after initiation of therapy.[33] A second bolus of about 0.5 mg/kg without increasing the maintenance infusion rate reestablishes therapeutic serum concentrations. If recurrence of arrhythmia appears after a steady state has been achieved (e.g., six to ten hours after starting therapy), a similar bolus should be given and the maintenance infusion rate increased. Increas-

ing the maintenance infusion rate only without an additional bolus results in a very slow increase is plasma lidocaine concentrations, reaching a new plateau in over six hours (four elimination half-lives), and is therefore not recommended.

If the initial bolus of lidocaine is ineffective, up to two more boluses of 1 mg/kg may be administered at 5-minute intervals. Patients who require more than one bolus to achieve a therapeutic effect have arrhythmias that respond only to higher lidocaine plasma concentrations, and a greater maintenance dose may be necessary to sustain these higher concentrations. Patients requiring only a single initial bolus of lidocaine should probably receive a maintenance infusion of 30 μg/kg/min, while those requiring two or three boluses may need infusions at 40 to 50 μg/kg/min.[33] Loading doses may also be administered by rapid infusion and a constant-rate intravenous infusion may be used to maintain an effective concentration. Maintenance infusion rates in the range of 1 to 4 mg/min produce steady-state plasma levels of 1 to 5 μg/ml in patients with uncomplicated myocardial infarction, but these rates must be reduced during heart failure or shock because of concomitant reduced hepatic blood flow.[7]

Clinical Indications. Lidocaine is a very useful antiarrhythmic agent because it demonstrates great efficacy against ventricular arrhythmias of diverse etiology, the ability to achieve effective plasma concentrations rapidly,

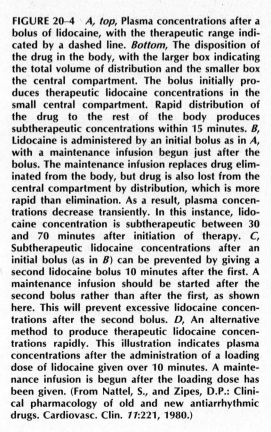

FIGURE 20–4 *A, top,* Plasma concentrations after a bolus of lidocaine, with the therapeutic range indicated by a dashed line. *Bottom,* The disposition of the drug in the body, with the larger box indicating the total volume of distribution and the smaller box the central compartment. The bolus initially produces therapeutic lidocaine concentrations in the small central compartment. Rapid distribution of the drug to the rest of the body produces subtherapeutic concentrations within 15 minutes. *B,* Lidocaine is administered by an initial bolus as in *A,* with a maintenance infusion begun just after the bolus. The maintenance infusion replaces drug eliminated from the body, but drug is also lost from the central compartment by distribution, which is more rapid than elimination. As a result, plasma concentrations decrease transiently. In this instance, lidocaine concentration is subtherapeutic between 30 and 70 minutes after initiation of therapy. *C,* Subtherapeutic lidocaine concentrations after an initial bolus (as in *B*) can be prevented by giving a second lidocaine bolus 10 minutes after the first. A maintenance infusion should be started after the second bolus rather than after the first, as shown here. This will prevent excessive lidocaine concentrations after the second bolus. *D,* An alternative method to produce therapeutic lidocaine concentrations rapidly. This illustration indicates plasma concentrations after the administration of a loading dose of lidocaine given over 10 minutes. A maintenance infusion is begun after the loading dose has been given. (From Nattel, S., and Zipes, D.P.: Clinical pharmacology of old and new antiarrhythmic drugs. Cardiovasc. Clin. *11*:221, 1980.)

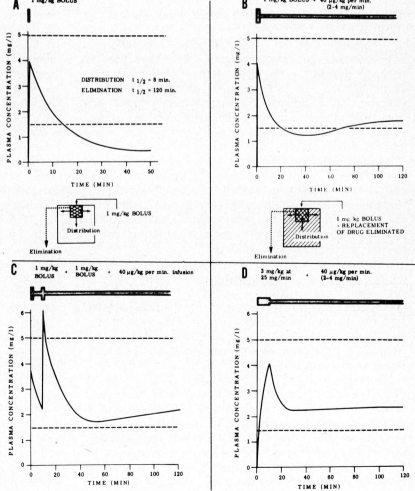

and a fairly wide toxic-to-therapeutic ratio with a low incidence of hemodynamic complications and other side effects. However, its first-pass hepatic effect precludes oral administration, and it is generally ineffective against supraventricular arrhythmias. Although lidocaine has been reported to decrease the ventricular response in patients with atrial fibrillation and Wolff-Parkinson-White syndrome,[34] a recent study demonstrates that when the effective refractory period of the accessory pathway is relatively short, lidocaine generally has no significant effect and may even accelerate the ventricular response during atrial fibrillation.[35]

Lidocaine is used primarily for patients with acute myocardial infarction or recurrent ventricular tachyarrhythmias. In patients resuscitated from out-of-hospital ventricular fibrillation and studied in a randomized, blinded trial,[36] lidocaine was comparable to bretylium in preventing recurrent episodes of ventricular tachyarrhythmia. In patients less than 70 years old who were admitted within six hours of onset of symptoms associated with acute myocardial infarction, lidocaine prophylaxis reduced episodes of ventricular fibrillation compared to results in an untreated control group (p. 1309). However, treated patients had a 15 per cent incidence of lidocaine toxicity, which was greater in older patients, and hospital mortality did not differ between treated and control groups, since in all instancesof lidocaine toxicity, which was greater in older[37] Other studies have not shown a protective effect of lidocaine in preventing ventricular arrhythmias due to infarction,[38] and of 15 randomized trials, most showed no apparent benefit.[39] Yet, evaluation of these data has led to the conclusion that the benefits of prophylactic lidocaine in patients who have acute myocardial infarction probably outweigh the risks[39,40] (p. 1309). Because of conflicting reports, it can be argued that prophylaxis is not indicated for all patients,[7] since death from primary ventricular fibrillation occurs uncommonly in a well-staffed coronary care unit and because of the adverse side effects accompanying lidocaine administration.

Adverse Effects. The most commonly reported adverse effects of lidocaine are dose-related manifestations of central nervous system toxicity: dizziness, paresthesias, confusion, delirium, stupor, coma, and seizures. Occasional sinus node depression and His-Purkinje block have been reported. In patients with atrial tachyarrhythmias, ventricular rate acceleration has been noted.

QUINIDINE

Quinidine and quinine are isomeric alkaloids isolated from the cinchona bark. Although quinidine shares the antimalarial, antipyretic, and vagolytic actions of quinine, the latter lacks the significant electrophysiological and antiarrhythmic effects of quinidine.[41]

Electrophysiological Actions (Tables 20–2 and 20–3). Quinidine exerts little effect on automaticity of the isolated normal sinus node[7] or on the denervated[42] sinus node in vivo but suppresses automaticity in normal Purkinje fibers by decreasing the slope of phase 4 diastolic depolarization and shifting threshold voltage toward zero. It does not affect abnormal automaticity in depolarized Purkinje fibers or delayed afterdepolarizations, and in high doses can cause abnormal automatic discharge in Purkinje fibers.[7] Because of its significant anticholinergic effect[42,43] and reflex sympathetic stimulation resulting from alpha-adrenergic blockade that causes peripheral vasodilation, quinidine may increase sinus nodal discharge rate and may improve AV nodal conduction in the innervated heart in vivo. In patients with the sick sinus syndrome, quinidine can depress sinus nodal automaticity greatly.[7] Direct myocardial effects may prolong AV nodal and His-Purkinje conduction times.[42] Quinidine prolongs duration of action potential of atrial and ventricular muscle and Purkinje fibers slightly (quinine shortens it[41]), while markedly prolonging the effective refractory period without significantly changing resting membrane potential.[44] Action potential amplitude, overshoot, and $\dot{V}$max of phase 0 are reduced. Because of its vagolytic actions, produced through muscarinic blockade,[43] quinidine can shorten Purkinje fiber action potential when the latter has been prolonged by vagal inhibition of beta-adrenergic receptor stimulation.[45] Quinidine appears to bind to inactive sodium channels and unbind from resting channels in a voltage-dependent fashion. This observation helps explain quinidine's greater depressant effects at faster heart rates (when the cells spend a greater percentage of the cardiac cycle in an active state), so-called use-dependence,[46] and predicts that potentially greater toxic effects of quinidine may occur at faster heart rates.

Hemodynamic Effects. Quinidine decreases peripheral vascular resistance and may cause significant hypotension because of its alpha-adrenergic blocking effects. Concomitant administration of vasodilators may exaggerate the potential for hypotension. In some patients, quinidine can increase cardiac output, possibly by reducing afterload. No significant direct myocardial depressant action occurs unless large doses are given rapidly, intravenously. Most of the adverse effects of intravenous quinidine are probably the result of excessive vasodilation.

Pharmacokinetics (Table 20–1). Although orally administered quinidine sulfate and quinidine gluconate exhibit similar degrees of systemic availability, plasma quinidine concentrations peak at about 90 minutes after oral administration of quinidine sulfate and at 3 to 4 hours after oral administration of quinidine gluconate.[7] Intramuscular quinidine produces a higher and an earlier peak plasma concentration[8] but results in incomplete absorption and tissue necrosis. Quinidine may be given intravenously if it is infused slowly. Approximately 80 per cent of plasma quinidine is protein-bound. Both the liver and the kidneys remove quinidine, hepatic metabolism being more important. Approximately 20 per cent is excreted unchanged in the urine.[8] Because congestive heart failure, hepatic disease, or poor renal function may reduce quinidine elimination and increase plasma concentration, dosage probably should be reduced and the drug given cautiously to patients with these disorders while serum quinidine concentration is monitored.

Dosage and Administration (Table 20–1). The usual oral dose of quinidine sulfate for an adult is 300 to 600 mg four times daily, which results in a steady state level within about 24 hours. A loading dose of 600 to 1000 mg produces an earlier effective concentration.[7] Similar doses of quinidine gluconate are used intramuscularly, while the intravenous dose of quinidine gluconate is 6 to 10 mg/kg given at a rate of 0.3 to 0.5 mg/kg/min as blood pressure and ECG parameters are checked frequently.[47] Anticonvulsant drugs may shorten quinidine's half-life and reduce quinidine serum concentration for a given dose.

Clinical Indications. Quinidine is a versatile antiarrhythmic agent, useful for treating both supraventricular and ventricular premature complexes and sustained tachyarrhythmias. It may prevent spontaneous recurrences of AV nodal reentrant paroxysmal supraventricular tachycardia and inhibit tachycardia induced by programmed electrical stimulation by prolonging atrial and ventricular refractoriness and depressing conduction in the retrograde fast pathway.[48] In patients with the Wolff-Parkinson-White syndrome,[49] quinidine prolongs the effective refractory period of the accessory pathway and, by so doing, may prevent reciprocating tachycardias and slow the ventricular response owing to conduction over the accessory pathway during atrial flutter or atrial fibrillation in this disorder. Quinidine and other antiarrhythmic agents may also prevent recurrences of tachycardia by suppressing the "trigger," i.e., the premature atrial or ventricular complex that initiates a sustained tachycardia.

Quinidine successfully terminates atrial flutter or atrial fibrillation in about 10 to 20 per cent of patients, with higher success rates if the arrhythmia is of more recent onset and if the atria are not enlarged. Incremental dosing with quinidine at 2-hour intervals is no longer indicated to terminate atrial flutter or fibrillation. Prior to administering quinidine to these patients, the ventricular response should be slowed sufficiently with digitalis, propranolol, or verapamil, since quinidine-induced slowing of the atrial flutter rate—e.g., from 300 to the range of 200 bpm— plus its vagolytic effect on AV nodal conduction may convert a 2:1 atrioventricular response (two atrial impulses for each QRS complex) to a 1:1 atrioventricular response, with an *increase* in the ventricular rate. Prior to elective cardioversion of patients with atrial fibrillation, quinidine should probably be given for one to two days, since this regimen restores sinus rhythm in some patients, thus obviating DC cardioversion, and helps maintain sinus rhythm once it is achieved.[50] In most patients, quinidine should probably be administered as long as sinus rhythm continues.

Quinidine has prevented sudden death in patients resuscitated because of out-of-hospital cardiac arrest,[51] particularly those who maintained adequate plasma drug levels.[52] In one series, quinidine provided effective long-term control of ventricular tachycardia and ventricular fibrillation in about one-third of patients evaluated by electrophysiological study.[53] The patient population studied probably has a bearing on quinidine's efficacy and may reduce this success rate to less than one-third.

Adverse Effects. The most common adverse effects of chronic oral quinidine therapy are gastrointestinal, including nausea, vomiting, diarrhea, abdominal pain, and anorexia. Central nervous system toxicity includes tinnitus, hearing loss, visual disturbances, confusion, delirium, and psychosis. Cinchonism is the term usually applied to these side effects. Allergic reactions may be manifest as rash, fever, immune-mediated thrombocytopenia, hemolytic anemia, and rarely anaphylaxis. Thrombocytopenia is due to

the presence of antibodies to quinidine-platelet complexes, causing platelets to agglutinate and lyse. In patients receiving oral anticoagulants, quinidine may cause bleeding.[54] Side effects may preclude long-term administration of quinidine in 30 to 40 per cent of patients.

A prominent electrocardiographic feature of quinidine toxicity is slowing of cardiac conduction, sometimes to the point of block. This may become manifest as prolongation of the QRS duration and Q-T interval or SA or AV nodal conduction disturbances. Quinidine-induced cardiac toxicity may be treated with molar sodium lactate.

Quinidine may produce syncope in 0.5 to 2.0 per cent of patients, most often the result of a self-terminating episode of a polymorphic ventricular tachyarrhythmia,[55,56] commonly of a specific variety called *torsades de pointes*[57] (see pp. 725 and 727). Quinidine prolongs the Q-T interval in most patients, whether or not ventricular arrhythmias occur, but significant Q-T prolongation (Q-T interval of 500 to 600 msec) is a general characteristic of quinidine syncope. Many of these patients were also receiving digitalis. Apparently syncope is not related to plasma concentrations of quinidine or duration of therapy.[55] Recently, a diastolic wave following the T wave has been described in patients who experience ventricular arrhythmias while receiving quinidine; however, the significance of this finding needs to be established.[58] Therapy for quinidine syncope requires immediate discontinuation of the drug and avoidance of other drugs that have similar pharmacological effects, such as disopyramide (see p. 659). In spite of the observations regarding "use-dependence," atrial or ventricular pacing may be used to suppress the ventricular tachyarrhythmia and may act by shortening refractoriness at faster rates. For some patients, drugs that do not prolong the Q-T interval, such as lidocaine or phenytoin, may be tried. When pacing is not available, isoproterenol may be given *with caution*.

Drugs that induce hepatic enzyme production, such as phenobarbital or phenytoin, may shorten the duration of quinidine's action by increasing its rate of elimination. Quinidine may elevate serum digoxin[59] and digitoxin[5] concentrations by decreasing total body clearance of digitoxin and by decreasing the clearance, volume of distribution, and affinity of tissue receptors for digoxin[60] (see p. 519).

PROCAINAMIDE

In 1936, Mautz demonstrated that direct application of procaine to the myocardium elevated the threshold of ventricular muscle to electrical stimulation.[61] However, procaine's therapeutic value as an antiarrhythmic agent was limited by its short duration of action and prominent central nervous system effects. A systematic study of procaine congeners and metabolites led to the development of procainamide,[62] which differs from procaine in that it replaces the ester linkage with an amide structure and has a longer duration of action, is effective when given orally, and exhibits increased cardiac effects with decreased central nervous system effects.

Electrophysiological Actions (Tables 20–2 and 20–3). The cardiac actions of procainamide on automaticity, conduction, excitability, and membrane responsiveness resemble those of quinidine and result in depression of excitability in atrium and ventricle, slowing of conduction, and prolongation of the effective refractory period. Like quinidine, procainamide usually prolongs the effective refractory period (ERP) more than it prolongs the action potential duration (APD).[63] When the ERP duration/APD exceeds 1.0, the earliest premature impulse that can be initiated during repolarization arises when the cell has returned to its most negative potential. Premature responses induced at this potential are more likely to have greater $\dot{V}$max and amplitude, presumably establishing better conduction (see p. 618). Thus the antiarrhythmic agent prevents early responses, arising from less negative resting potentials, that might conduct slowly or block, thereby potentiating the development of arrhythmias. A drug that decreases the ratio of ERP duration/APD may allow earlier premature responses to occur at a time when the membrane potential is more positive. Compared to disopyramide and quinidine, procainamide exerts the least anticholinergic effects[43] but does produce more local anesthetic effects than quinidine. It does not affect normal sinus nodal automaticity.

In vitro studies on cat myocardium subjected to acute and chronic myocardial infarction reveal that procainamide decreases differences in refractoriness between tissue types by prolonging action potential duration and refractoriness most markedly in acutely ischemic cells with the shortest action potential duration and refractoriness and least in chronically injured cells with the longest action potential duration and refractoriness; the drug produced intermediate changes in normal cells.[64] In dogs subjected to a previous myocardial infarction, procainamide in vivo decreases excitability and prolongs refractoriness of abnormal myocardium, preventing reinitiation of sustained ventricular tachyarrhythmias in about half the dogs studied and markedly increasing the cycle length of arrhythmias that were still inducible.[65]

The electrophysiological effects of N-acetylprocainamide (NAPA), procainamide's major metabolite, differ from those of the parent compound. NAPA (10 to 40 mg/liter) does not suppress the rate of phase 4 diastolic depolarization of Purkinje fibers and does not alter resting membrane potential, action potential amplitude, or $\dot{V}$max of phase 0 of the action potential of Purkinje fibers or ventricular muscle. However, NAPA prolongs the action potential duration of ventricular muscle and Purkinje fibers in a dose-dependent manner. Toxic doses produce early afterdepolarizations and triggered activity. NAPA given to dogs (50 to 100 mg/kg intravenously) produces single instances as well as salvos of ventricular extrasystoles that at times degenerate to ventricular fibrillation. Doses up to 100 mg/kg intravenously exert slight antiarrhythmic effects in dogs subjected to myocardial infarction 24 hours previously.[66] Procainamide appears to exert greater electrophysiological effects than NAPA.[67]

Hemodynamic Effects. Procainamide may depress myocardial contractility in high doses. It does not produce alpha blockade but may result in peripheral vasodilation via a mild ganglionic blocking action that impairs cardiovascular reflexes.[7]

Pharmacokinetics (Table 20–1). Following intramuscular administration, peak plasma concentrations occur in 15 to 60 minutes, while oral administration produces peak plasma concentration in about one hour. Absorption may be reduced in the first week after myocardial infarction. Approximately 80 per cent of oral procainamide is bioavailable, with 20 per cent bound to serum proteins. The overall elimination half-life for procainamide is three to five hours, with the majority of the drug eliminated unchanged in the urine and 10 to 30 per cent eliminated by hepatic metabolism.[5] A prolonged-release form of procainamide given every 6 hours provides steady-state plasma levels of the drug equivalent to an equal total daily dose of short-acting procainamide given every 3 hours.[68]

The drug is acetylated to NAPA, which is excreted almost exclusively by the kidneys. As renal function decreases and in patients with heart failure, procainamide levels—and particularly NAPA levels—increase and, because of the risk of serious cardiotoxicity, need to be carefully monitored in such situations. NAPA has an elimination half-life of 7 to 8 hours but exceeds 10 hours if high doses are used.[69] Small amounts of procainamide are present in patients receiving NAPA because of deacetylation.[70]

Dosage and Administration (Table 20–1). Procainamide may be given by the oral, intravenous, or intramuscular route to achieve serum concentrations that produce an antiarrhythmic effect in the range of 4 to 10 μg/ml. Occasionally plasma concentrations exceeding 10 μg/ml have been required,[71,72] but the probability of adverse effects may increase with higher plasma concentrations.[73] Several intravenous regimens have been used to administer procainamide. Twenty-five to 50 mg can be given over a one-minute period and then repeated every five minutes until the arrhythmia is controlled, hypotension results, or the QRS complex is prolonged more than 50 per cent. Rather large doses of 6 to 13 mg/kg at a maximum infusion rate of 0.5 mg/kg/min have been used.[47] Another method employs 50 mg/min with the same endpoints.[72] A constant-rate intravenous infusion of procainamide can be given at a dose of 2 to 6 mg/min.[7] The upper limits regarding total dose are flexible and range between 1000 and 2000 mg, depending upon the patient's response.

Oral administration of procainamide requires a 3- or 4-hour dosing interval at a total daily dose of 2 to 6 gm, with a steady state reached within one day. When a loading dose is used, it should be twice the maintenance dose. Frequent dosing is required because of the short elimination half-life in normal subjects. For the prolonged-release form of procainamide, dosing is at 6-hour intervals.[68] A longer half-life may be seen in some cardiac patients, allowing longer intervals between drug administration, but this needs to be documented for the individual patient. Procainamide is well absorbed after intramuscular injection, with virtually 100 per cent of the dose bioavailable.[7]

It has been suggested recently that the plasma concentration of procainamide required to suppress premature ventricular complexes (PVC) in patients who have acute myocardial infarction may be less than the plasma concentration required to prevent spontaneous episodes of symptomatic sustained ventricular tachycardia. Procainamide, 9 μg/ml, suppressed spontaneous episodes of ventricular tachycardia but decreased PVC frequency by only 36 per cent, whereas the mean concentration required to suppress 85 per cent of PVCs was 15 μg/ml. This study raises interesting questions regarding differences in antiarrhythmic thresholds as influenced by the nature of the heart disease as well as by the arrhythmia.[74]

Clinical Indications. Procainamide is used to treat both supraventricular and ventricular arrhythmias and has a spectrum of application comparable to that of quinidine. Although both drugs have similar electrophysiological actions, either drug may effectively suppress a supraventricular or ventricular arrhythmia that is refractory to the other drug.

Procainamide may be used to convert atrial fibrillation of recent onset to sinus rhythm.[75] As with quinidine, prior treatment with digitalis, propranolol, or verapamil is recommended to prevent acceleration of the ventricular response following procainamide therapy. In patients with paroxysmal supraventricular tachycardia, procainamide may inhibit the induction of sustained AV nodal reentrant tachycardia as a result of selective depression of retrograde AV nodal conduction in the fast pathway. In a small number of patients, apparent vagolytic effects of procainamide potentiated the induction of sustained tachycardia.[76] Recently it has been shown that procainamide almost uniformly depresses retrograde AV nodal conduction in patients who do not have tachycardias due to AV nodal reentry or accessory pathways. Therefore, this effect in patients who do have tachycardias cannot be interpreted to indicate the response of a specific tissue type.[77] Procainamide may block conduction in the accessory pathway of patients with the Wolff-Parkinson-White syndrome and has been used intravenously to identify those patients who have a short anterograde effective refractory period of the accessory pathway[78] (p. 712).

Procainamide has been only partially effective in preventing the induction of ventricular tachycardia by programmed stimulation during electrophysiological studies in patients with a history of ventricular tachycardia or ventricular fibrillation. High doses, 500 to 1000 mg orally every 4 hours, resulting in a plasma concentration of up to 13.5 μg/ml may be necessary to suppress ventricular tachycardia in some patients.[71] Most consistently, procainamide slows the rate of the induced ventricular tachycardia.[79] Recently it has been suggested that the response to programmed electrical stimulation of patients receiving procainamide could predict their response to other conventional agents. Failure to induce sustained ventricular tachycardia while patients received procainamide predicted noninducibility while they received other conventional agents. Conversely, the induction of sustained ventricular tachycardia while patients received procainamide predicted the inducibility of ventricular tachycardia when they received other conventional agents and suggested that alternative treatments with investigational drugs, surgery, or electrical therapy be considered. This interesting study requires confirmation.[80] Procainamide may facilitate the induction of ventricular tachycardia, an effect shared by many other antiarrhythmic agents.[81] It can also induce a polymorphic ventricular tachycardia associated with Q-T interval prolongation.[82] NAPA appears to be a less effective antiarrhythmic agent than procainamide, and the antiarrhythmic response to procainamide does not predict the response to NAPA.

Adverse Effects. Multiple adverse noncardiac effects have been reported with procainamide administration and include skin rashes, myalgias, digital vasculitis, and Raynaud's phenomenon. Gastrointestinal side effects are less frequent than with quinidine, and adverse central nervous system side effects are less frequent than with lidocaine. Procainamide may cause giddiness, psychosis, hallucinations, and depression. Toxic concentrations of procainamide can diminish myocardial performance and promote hypotension. A variety of conduction disturbances or ventricular tachyarrhythmias may occur similar to those produced by quinidine, including prolonged Q-T syndrome and polymorphous ventricular tachycardia.[82] However, ventricular tachyarrhythmias do not appear to occur as frequently following procainamide therapy as they do following treatment with quinidine. In the absence of sinus node disease, procainamide does not adversely affect sinus node function. In patients with sinus dysfunction, procainamide tends to prolong corrected sinus node recovery time and may worsen symptoms in some patients who have the bradycardia-tachycardia syndrome.[83] Fever and agranulocytosis may be due to hypersensitivity reactions, and white blood cell and differential blood counts should be performed at regular intervals. Procainamide does not increase the serum digoxin concentration.[7]

Arthralgia, fever, pleuropericarditis, hepatomegaly, and hemorrhagic pericardial effusion with tamponade have been described in a systemic lupus erythematosus (SLE)–like syndrome[84] (p. 1660). The syndrome may occur more frequently and earlier in patients who are "slow acetylators" of procainamide, although this is not entirely clear. The aromatic amino group on procainamide appears important for induction of SLE syndrome, since acetylating this amino group to form NAPA appears to block the SLE-inducing effect.[85] Procainamide-induced SLE syndrome differs from naturally occurring lupus syndrome by sparing the brain and kidney, uncommonly producing hematological complications, and not producing false-positive serological tests for syphilis. Patients who develop drug-induced SLE have antibodies against single-stranded DNA, while those who have naturally occurring SLE develop antibodies against double-stranded DNA. Almost all patients with drug-induced SLE have antibodies to histones, while only one-third of patients with naturally occurring SLE develop antihistone antibodies. Sixty to 70 per cent of patients who receive procainamide develop antinuclear antibodies, with clinical symptoms in 20 to 30 per cent, but this is reversible when procainamide is stopped. When symptoms occur, SLE cell preparations are often positive. Positive serological tests are not necessarily a reason to discontinue drug therapy, but the development of symptoms or a positive anti-DNA antibody is, except for patients whose life-threatening arrhythmia is controlled only by procainamide. Steroid administration in those patients may eliminate the symptoms.[7]

DISOPYRAMIDE

Disopyramide has been approved in the United States for oral but not intravenous adminstration to treat ventricular arrhythmias. Generally, it exerts efficacy comparable to that of quinidine and procainamide against a similar spectrum of arrhythmias but has important side effects including cardiovascular depression, generation of ventricular arrhythmias, and bothersome anticholinergic properties.

Electrophysiological Actions (Tables 20–2 and 20–3). Similar to the in vitro effects of quinidine and procainamide, disopyramide decreases the slope of phase 4 diastolic depolarization in Purkinje fibers. It produces a rate-dependent depression of V̇max of phase 0, prolongs the effective refractory period more than it prolongs the action potential duration,[86] and lengthens conduction time in normal and depolarized Purkinje fibers.[87] Similar to the effects of procainamide in an experimental infarct model studied in vitro,[64] disopyramide reduces the differences in action potential duration between normal and infarcted tissue by lengthening the action potential of normal cells more than it lengthens the action potential of cells from infarcted regions of the heart.[88]

Stereochemical properties influence the effects of disopyramide. Racemic (clinically used) and (+) disopyramide prolong canine Purkinje fiber action potential, while (−) disopyramide shortens it. The (+) isomer exerts approximately three times more vagolytic effects than does the (−) isomer. If Purkinje fibers are treated with isoproterenol (to shorten action potential duration) and then acetylcholine (to antagonize the catecholamine effect and lengthen action potential duration), the vagolytic action of disopyramide eliminates the cholinergic antagonism of beta stimulation, and the action potential shortens.[43] By a similar vagolytic mechanism, disopyramide is capable of speeding up the sinus nodal discharge rate and shortening AV nodal conduction time and refractoriness when the nodes are restrained by cholinergic influences, either in vitro or in vivo.[86,89] Atropine tends to nullify or even reverse this effect. Disopyramide exerts greater anticholinergic effects than quinidine and does not appear to affect alpha- or beta-adrenergic receptors.

Although not a slow-channel blocker, disopyramide can slow the sinus nodal discharge rate by a direct action when given in high concentration[90] and can significantly depress sinus nodal activity in patients with sinus node dysfunction.[91] Atrial and ventricular refractory periods increase. Disopyramide's effect on AV nodal conduction and refractoriness in vivo is not consistent.[89,92,93] AV block may occur occasionally,[94] and since disopyramide can prolong His-Purkinje conduction time, it is possible that infra-His block may result. However, His-Purkinje block did not occur in 22 patients who had bundle branch block and were given disopyramide intravenously.[93] Disopyramide may be administered safely to patients who have first degree or Type I second degree AV block and narrow QRS complexes.[94a] Disopyramide increases the conduction time and effective refractory period of the accessory pathway in Wolff-Parkinson-White syndrome.[95]

Hemodynamic Effects. Maximum hemodynamic effects in patients with left ventricular dysfunction occur immediately after intravenous administration of 2 mg/kg disopyramide and consist of reductions in systemic blood pressure, cardiac index, and stroke index. Right atrial pressure and total peripheral resistance increase. Profound hemodynamic deterioration developed in two of nine patients in this study.[96] Patients who have abnormal ventricular function tolerate the negative inotropic effects of disopyramide quite poorly, and in these patients the drug should be used with extreme caution or not at all.

Pharmacokinetics (Table 20–1). Disopyramide is 80 to 90 per cent absorbed, with a mean elimination half-life of 8 to 9 hours in healthy volunteers but almost 10 hours in patients with heart failure. Total body clearance and volume of distribution decreases in these patients, and mean serum concentration is higher than reported in normal subjects.[97] Renal insufficiency prolongs the elimination time. Thus, in patients who have renal, hepatic, or cardiac insufficiency, loading and maintenance doses need to be reduced. One study of patients who had ventricular arrhythmias showed an elimination half-life of 18 to 19 hours.[98] Peak blood levels after oral administration are seen in 1 to 2 hours, and bioavailability exceeds 80 per cent. The fraction of disopyramide bound to serum protein varies inversely with the total plasma concentration of the drug but may be more stable (30 to 40 per cent) at clinically relevant concentrations of 3 μg/ml.[7,92] About half an oral dose is recovered unchanged in the urine, with about 30 per cent as the mono N-dealkylated metabolite. The metabolites appear to exert less effect than the parent compound.

Dosage and Administration (Table 20–1). Doses are generally 100 to 200 mg orally every six hours with a range of 400 to 1200 mg/day. The intravenous (investigational) dose is 1 to 2 mg/kg as an initial bolus given over 5 to 10 minutes, which may be followed by an infusion of 1 mg/kg/hour.[95]

Clinical Indications. The usefulness of disopyramide in treating multiple categories of atrial and ventricular arrhythmias is still incompletely resolved. Disopyramide appears comparable to quinidine in reducing the frequency of premature ventricular complexes and initial data suggest that it effectively prevents recurrence of ventricular tachycardia in selected patients.[93,99] Its role in preventing arrhythmias and reducing mortality in patients after acute myocardial infarction has not been established[100] and may not be as potent as orally administered aprindine.[101] Disopyramide has been combined safely and effectively with mexiletine to treat patients who had recurrent ventricular tachycardia and/or ventricular fibrillation and were evaluated during electrophysiological study.[102]

Disopyramide terminates attacks of acute paroxysmal supraventricular tachycardia and decreases the frequency of recurrences.[103] It helps prevent recurrence of atrial fibrillation after successful cardioversion as effectively as quinidine[93] and may terminate atrial flutter. In treating patients with atrial fibrillation, and particularly atrial flutter, the ventricular rate must be controlled prior to administering disopyramide, or the atrial rate may decrease sufficiently, aided by the vagolytic effects of disopyramide, to create 1:1 conduction during atrial flutter.[104] Disopyramide prolongs the anterograde and retrograde refractory period of the accessory pathway in patients with the Wolff-Parkinson-White syndrome[95] and may prevent reciprocating tachycardias or slow the ventricular rate during atrial flutter or atrial fibrillation.

Adverse Effects. Three categories of adverse effects are seen following disopyramide administration. The most common adverse effect relates to the drug's potent parasympatholytic properties and includes urinary hesitancy or retention, constipation, blurred vision, closed-angle glaucoma, and dry mouth. Second, disopyramide may produce ventricular tachyarrhythmias that are commonly associated with Q-T prolongation and the ventricular tachycardia called torsades de pointes.[57,93,105,106] Some patients may have "cross sensitivity" to both quinidine and disopyramide and develop torsades de pointes while receiving either drug. When drug-induced torsades de pointes occur, agents that prolong the Q-T interval should be used with great caution. Finally, disopyramide may reduce contractility of the normal ventricle but the depression of ventricular function is much more pronounced in patients with preexisting ventricular failure.[107] Occasionally, cardiovascular collapse can result.[108]

Disopyramide does not appear to alter digitalis metabolism. However, phenytoin may decrease plasma concentration of disopyramide by altering its metabolism.[109]

PHENYTOIN (DIPHENYLHYDANTOIN)

Phenytoin was employed originally to treat seizure disorders and was noted subsequently to abolish ventricular tachycardia in dogs after coronary artery ligation. Although it has been used for many years, phenytoin's value as an antiarrhythmic agent remains limited.

Electrophysiological Actions (Tables 20–2 and 20–3). Therapeutic concentrations of phenytoin do not alter the discharge rate of rabbit sinus nodal tissue but may depress normal automaticity in cardiac Purkinje fibers in vitro[7] or spontaneous ventricular rate in vivo by presumably increasing potassium conductance (the I_{K_1} channel). Phenytoin is very effective in abolishing abnormal automaticity caused by digitalis-induced delayed afterdepolarizations in cardiac Purkinje fibers[110,111] and in suppressing certain digitalis-induced arrhythmias in man.[112] Similar to lidocaine, phenytoin abbreviates Purkinje fiber action potential duration more than it shortens the effective refractory period, thus increasing the ratio of effective refractory period to action potential duration.[7] Phenytoin can cause depolarized cells to repolarize by increasing potassium conductance and, in so doing, may increase the $\dot{V}$max of phase 0 in Purkinje fibers,[113] particularly when these are depressed by digitalis. The rate of rise of action potentials initiated early in the relative refractory period is increased, as is membrane responsiveness, possibly reducing the chance for impaired conduction and block.[63] Phenytoin may slow conduction at high potassium concentrations. Sinus discharge rate and AV conduction in man are minimally affected by phenytoin.

Some of phenytoin's antiarrhythmic effects may be neurally mediated, since phenytoin may reduce the increase in impulse traffic in cardiac sympathetic nerves caused by ouabain toxicity.[114] Injected into the central nervous system, phenytoin protects against digitalis-induced ventricular arrhythmias.[115] The drug may also modulate vagal efferent activity centrally. It has no peripheral cholinergic or beta-adrenergic blocking actions.

Phenytoin exerts minimal *hemodynamic effects*.

Pharmacokinetics (Table 20–1). The pharmacokinetics of phenytoin are less than ideal. Absorption following oral administration is incomplete and delayed and varies with the brand of drug, and plasma concentrations reach their peak 8 to 12 hours later. Ninety per cent of the drug is protein-bound.[8] Phenytoin has limited solubility at physiologic pH, and intramuscular administration is associated with pain, muscle necrosis, sterile abscesses, and variable

absorption. Therapeutic serum concentrations of phenytoin (10 to 20 μg/ml) are similar for treating both cardiac arrhythmias and epilepsy. Lower concentrations may suppress certain digitalis-induced arrhythmias or other arrhythmias when decreased plasma protein binding occurs (as in uremia), since a larger fraction of drug is free and pharmacologically active.

Over 90 per cent of a dose is hydroxylated in the liver to presumably inactive compounds. Some families have a genetically determined inability to hydroxylate phenytoin, while others have a higher than usual capability for hydroxylation.[8] Elimination half-time is about 24 hours and may be slowed in the presence of liver disease or when phenytoin is administered concomitantly with drugs such as phenylbutazone, dicumarol, isoniazid, chloramphenicol, and phenothiazines that compete with phenytoin for hepatic enzymes.[113] Because of the large number of medications that may increase or decrease phenytoin levels during chronic therapy, phenytoin plasma concentration should be determined frequently when changes are made in other medications. In some patients, maintenance dose regimens of phenytoin are difficult to predict because the enzyme system that metabolizes phenytoin becomes saturated at plasma concentrations within the therapeutic range. The half-life then increases with increasing phenytoin load, particularly as plasma concentrations approach the therapeutic range. Above the saturation point, phenytoin elimination follows zero-order kinetics, so that only a fixed amount of drug is eliminated per unit time. These concentration-dependent kinetics for elimination can cause unexpected toxicity, since disproportionately large changes in plasma concentration may follow dose increases.[7]

Dosage and Administration (Table 20–1). To achieve therapeutic plasma concentrations rapidly, 100 mg of phenytoin should be administered intravenously every 5 minutes until the arrhythmia is controlled, adverse side effects result, or about 1 gm has been given. Generally, 700 to 1000 mg will control the arrhythmia. A large vein should be used to avoid pain and development of phlebitis produced by the severely alkalotic (pH 11.0) vehicle in which phenytoin is dissolved.[7] Orally, phenytoin is given as a loading dose of approximately 1000 mg the first day, 500 mg on the second and third days, and 400 mg daily thereafter. All maintenance doses can be given once or twice daily, depending on the brand, because of the long half-life of elimination.

Clinical Indications. Phenytoin has been used successfully to treat atrial and ventricular arrhythmias caused by digitalis toxicity but is much less effective in treating ventricular arrhythmias in patients with ischemic heart disease[7,116] or with atrial arrhythmias not due to digitalis toxicity.[113] The drug has been somewhat more successful in treating ventricular arrhythmias associated with general anesthesia and cardiac surgery.

Adverse Effects. The most common manifestations of phenytoin toxicity are central nervous system effects of nystagmus, ataxia, drowsiness, stupor, and coma. Progression of such symptoms can be correlated with increases in plasma drug concentration. Neurological signs, such as nystagmus on lateral gaze, develop at plasma drug levels of about 20 μg/ml.[7] Nausea, epigastric pain, and anorexia are also relatively common effects of phenytoin. Long-term administration may result in hyperglycemia, hypocalcemia, skin rashes, megaloblastic anemia, gingival hypertrophy, lymph node hyperplasia (a syndrome resembling malignant lymphoma), peripheral neuropathy, and drug-induced systemic lupus erythematosus.[8]

PROPRANOLOL
(See also p. 1349)

Although six beta-adrenergic receptor blocking drugs have been approved for use in the United States (Table 39–5, p. 1350), only propranolol and timolol have been approved to treat arrhythmias or to prevent sudden death after myocardial infarction. It is generally considered that no beta blocker offers distinct advantages over the others and that, when titrated to the proper dose, all can be used effectively to treat cardiac arrhythmias, hypertension, or other disorders.[117] However, differences in pharmacokinetic or pharmacodynamic properties that confer safety, reduce adverse effects, or affect dosing intervals or drug interactions influence the choice of agent.

Beta receptors can be separated into those that affect predominately the heart (beta$_1$) or the bronchi and blood vessels (beta$_2$).[118] In low doses, selective beta blockers can block beta$_1$ receptors more than they block beta$_2$ receptors and might be preferable for treating patients with pulmonary or peripheral vascular diseases. In high doses, the selective beta$_1$ blockers also block beta$_2$ receptors.

Some beta blockers exert intrinsic sympathomimetic activity, i.e., they slightly activate the beta receptor. These drugs appear to be as efficacious as beta blockers without intrinsic sympathomimetic actions and may cause less slowing of heart rate at rest and less prolongation of AV nodal conduction time.[117] Recently, they have been shown to induce less depression of left ventricular function than beta blockers without intrinsic sympathomimetic activity.[119]

The following discussion will concentrate on the use of propranolol as an antiarrhythmic agent.

Electrophysiological Actions. Beta blockers may exert an electrophysiological action by competitively inhibiting catecholamine binding at beta adrenoreceptor sites, an effect almost entirely due to the (−) levorotatory stereoisomer,[117] or by their quinidine-like or direct membrane-stabilizing action. The latter is a local anesthetic effect that depresses I_{Na} and membrane responsiveness in cardiac Purkinje fibers,[120] occurs at concentrations generally 10 times that necessary to produce beta blockade, and most likely plays an insignificant antiarrhythmic role. At low, beta-blocking concentrations, propranolol slows spontaneous automaticity in the sinus node or in Purkinje fibers that are being stimulated by adrenergic tone. In the absence of adrenergic tone, only high concentrations of propranolol slow normal automaticity in Purkinje fibers, probably by a direct membrane action.[121,122] In low concentrations that cause beta-receptor blockade but no local anesthetic effects, beta-blocking drugs do not alter the normal resting membrane potential, maximum diastolic potential, amplitude, $\dot{V}_{max}$, repolarization, or refractoriness of atrial, Purkinje, or ventricular muscle cells[121,122] when these tissues are not being superfused with catecholamines. However, in the presence of isoproterenol, a pure beta-receptor stimulator, beta blockers reverse isoproterenol's accelerating effects on repolarization; in the presence of norepinephrine, beta blockade permits unopposed alpha-adrenergic stimulation to prolong action potential duration in Purkinje fibers.

If values for these action potential parameters were abnormally low to start and were increased by catecholamines, such as a slow response generated in a high-potassium, catecholamine environment, beta-receptor blockade might depress conduction by removing the catecholamine stimulatory effect. At higher concentrations exceeding 3 μg/ml, propranolol depresses $\dot{V}_{max}$, action potential amplitude, membrane responsiveness, and conduction in normal atrial, ventricular, and Purkinje fibers[121,122] without altering resting membrane potential. These effects probably result from depression of sodium conductance. The direct effect of propranolol shortens the action potential duration of Purkinje fibers and, to a lesser extent, of atrial and ventricular muscle fibers.[121,122] Long-term administration of propranolol may lengthen action potential duration. Similar to the effects of lidocaine, acceleration of repolarization of Purkinje fibers is most marked in areas of the ventricular conduction system in which the action potential duration is greatest. The reduction in refractory period is not as great as the reduction in action potential duration (effective refractory period duration/action potential duration > 1.0). At least one beta blocker, sotalol, markedly increases the time course of repolarization in Purkinje fibers and ventricular muscle.

Propranolol slows the sinus discharge rate in humans by 10 to 20 per cent, while severe bradycardia occasionally results if the heart is particularly dependent on sympathetic tone or if sinus node dysfunction is present. The slowing is probably due to beta blockade because D-propranolol does not significantly slow the sinus discharge rate in doses comparable to the racemic mixture. The P-R interval lengthens, as does AV nodal conduction time and refractoriness (if the heart rate is maintained constant), but refractoriness and conduction in the His-Purkinje system remain unchanged even after high doses of propranolol.[123] Therefore, therapeutic doses of propranolol in humans do not exert a direct depressant or "quinidine-like" action but influence cardiac electrophysiology via a beta-blocking action. Beta blockers do not affect conduction in ventricular muscle, as evidenced by their lack of effect on the QRS complex, and they insignificantly prolong the right ventricular effective refractory period[124] and uncorrected Q-T interval.[125,126]

Several observations suggest that the beta-blocking action of propranolol is responsible for its antiarrhythmic effects. The dextrorotatory stereoisomer of beta blockers retains the direct membrane action without beta-blocking properties[127] and does not prevent arrhythmias provoked by catecholamine administration. Also, 1/50th to 1/100th of the plasma concentration necessary to achieve membrane depressant effects on $\dot{V}_{max}$ and overshoot in isolated cardiac muscle possesses antiarrhythmic effects. Thus, beta blockade without direct membrane action prevents many arrhythmias that result from activation of the autonomic nervous system. However, beta blockers with direct membrane action appear necessary to suppress certain experimental arrhythmias, such as those that occur in the dog one to two days after coronary artery ligation or those due to some types of digitalis toxicity.[121,122] In man, the direct membrane effects of beta blockers do not appear necessary for clinical antiarrhythmic actions, and the antiarrhythmic spectrum of clinical effectiveness of beta blockers without direct membrane effects seems to be the same as that of beta blockers with direct membrane effects, including arrhythmias resulting from digitalis intoxication and myocardial infarction. The possible importance of direct membrane effect of some of these drugs cannot be discounted totally because beta blockers with direct membrane actions may affect transmembrane potentials of diseased cardiac fibers at much lower concentrations than are needed to affect normal fibers directly. In addition, the role of important metabolites of propranolol and other beta blockers that may exert electrophysiological actions is not clearly established.

Hemodynamic Effects. Propranolol exerts negative inotropic effects on cardiac contractility and may precipitate or worsen heart failure. By blocking beta receptors, this drug may cause peripheral vasoconstriction.

Pharmacokinetics (Table 20–1). Although various types of beta blockers exert similar pharmacological effects, their pharmacokinetics differ substantially.[117] Propranolol is almost 100 per cent absorbed, but the effects of first-pass hepatic metabolism reduce bioavailability to about 30 per cent and produce significant interpatient variability of plasma concentration for a given dose. Reduction in hepatic blood flow, as in patients with heart failure, decreases the hepatic extraction of propranolol, and in these patients propranolol may further decrease its own elimination rate by reducing cardiac output and hepatic blood flow.[128] Beta blockers eliminated by the kidney tend to have longer half-lives and exhibit less interpatient variability of drug concentration than do those beta blockers metabolized by the liver.

Dosage and Administration (Table 20–1). The appropriate dose of propranolol is best determined by a measure of the patient's physiological response, such as changes in resting heart rate or in the prevention of exercise-induced tachycardia, since wide individual differences exist between the observed physiological effect and plasma concentration. For example, intravenous dosing is best achieved by titrating the dose to a clinical effect, beginning with 0.25 to 0.50 mg and administering doses every five minutes until either a desired effect or toxicity is produced or a total of 0.15 to 0.20 mg/kg has been given. Orally, propranolol is given in four divided doses, usually ranging from 40 to 160 mg a day to more than 1 gram a day. Generally, if one agent in adequate doses proves to be ineffective, other beta blockers will be ineffective also.

Clinical Indications. As an antiarrhythmic agent, propranolol is used most commonly to treat supraventricular tachyarrhythmias. Its effectiveness and mechanism of action vary depending on the arrhythmia. Propranolol may be employed to decrease the rate of persistent sinus tachycardia that results from excessive sympathetic stimulation. Arrhythmias associated with thyrotoxicosis, pheochromocytoma, and anesthesia with cyclopropane or halothane or arrhythmias largely due to excessive cardiac adrenergic stimulation, such as those initiated by exercise or emotion, often respond to propranolol therapy. Beta-blocking drugs usually do not convert chronic atrial flutter or atrial fibrillation to normal sinus rhythm but may be successful if the arrhythmia is of recent onset. The rate of the atrial flutter generally is not changed, but the ventricular response during atrial flutter and atrial fibrillation decreases because beta blockade prolongs AV nodal conduction time and refractoriness. For reentrant supraventricular tachycardias using the AV node as one of the reentrant pathways, such as AV nodal reentrant tachycardia and reciprocating tachycardias in Wolff-Parkinson-White syndrome, or for sinus reentrant tachycardia, propranolol may terminate the tachycardia and be used prophylactically to prevent a recurrence. Combining propranolol with digitalis, quinidine, or a variety of other agents—some of which are investigational—may be effective when propranolol as a single agent fails.

Several other groups of arrhythmias respond particularly well to beta blockade. These include digitalis-induced arrhythmias such as atrial tachycardia, nonparoxysmal AV junctional tachycardia, premature ventricular complexes, or ventricular tachycardia. Part of the effects of propranolol against arrhythmias induced by digitalis results from its action on the central nervous system. If a significant degree of AV block is present during a digitalis-induced arrhythmia, lidocaine or phenytoin may be preferable to propranolol. Propranolol may also be useful to treat ventricular arrhythmias associated with the prolonged Q-T interval syndrome[129] and with mitral valve prolapse.[130] For patients with ischemic heart disease, propranolol generally has not prevented episodes of chronic recurrent ventricular tachycardia that occur in the absence of acute ischemia. However, several clinical trials have demonstrated a reduction in the incidence of overall death and sudden cardiac death after myocardial infarction in patients treated chronically with a variety of beta blockers. The mechanism of this reduction in mortality is not entirely clear and may relate to reduction in the extent of ischemic damage, an antiarrhythmic effect, or both. Survival benefits seem most striking in the first one to two years after myocardial infarction.[131–136, 136a]

Adverse Effects. Adverse cardiovascular effects from propranolol include unacceptable hypotension, bradycardia, or congestive heart failure. The bradycardia may be due to sinus bradycardia or AV block. Uncommonly, propranolol may precipitate left ventricular failure in the absence of previous failure. Sudden withdrawal of propranolol in patients with angina pectoris can precipitate worsening of angina, cardiac arrhythmias, and acute myocardial infarction,[137] possibly owing to heightened sensitivity to beta agonists caused by previous beta blockade. Heightened sensitivity may begin several days after cessation of propranolol therapy and may last five or six days.[138] Other adverse effects of propranolol include worsening of asthma or chronic obstructive pulmonary disease, intermittent claudication, Raynaud's phenomenon, mental depression, increased risk of hypoglycemia among insulin-dependent diabetic patients, easy fatigability, disturbingly vivid dreams or insomnia, and impaired sexual function.

BRETYLIUM TOSYLATE

Bretylium was introduced as an antihypertensive agent in 1959, and its antiarrhythmic potential was recognized several years later.

Electrophysiological Actions (Tables 20–2 and 20–3). Bretylium is selectively concentrated in sympathetic ganglia and their postganglionic adrenergic nerve terminals. After initially *causing* norepinephrine release, bretylium *prevents* norepinephrine release from sympathetic nerve terminals, without depressing pre- or postganglionic sympathetic nerve conduction, impairing conduction across sympathetic ganglia, depleting the adrenergic neuron of norepinephrine, or decreasing the responsiveness of adrenergic receptors.[7] During chronic bretylium treatment, the beta-adrenergic responses to circulating catecholamines are increased. The initial release of catecholamines results in several transient electrophysiological responses such as an increase in the discharge rates of the isolated perfused sinus node and of in vitro Purkinje fibers, often making quiescent fibers automatic. Bretylium initially increases conduction velocity and excitability and decreases refractoriness in the rabbit atrium,[139] and partially depolarized fibers may hyperpolarize. Pretreatment with reserpine or propranolol will prevent these early changes. Initial catecholamine release may aggravate some arrhythmias, such as those caused by digitalis excess[139] or myocardial infarction. Prolonged drug administration lengthens the duration of the action potential and refractoriness of atrial and ventricular muscle and Purkinje fibers.[7,140] The ratio of effective refractory period to action potential duration does not change, nor do membrane responsiveness and conduction velocity. Bretylium exerts little effect on diastolic excitability but increases ventricular fibrillation thresholds significantly.[141] Other adrenergic neuronal blocking agents, such as guanethidine, do not elevate the ventricular fibrillation threshold, while ordinary quaternary ammonium analogs that are not adrenergic neuron blockers can elevate this threshold.[7] Thus, although the chemical sympathectomy-like state may be antiarrhythmic, other factors may be important as well. Recent data obtained from studies of subendocardial Purkinje fibers from infarcted canine hearts indicate that bretylium lengthens the action potential duration most in cells located in proximal areas of the specialized conducting system of normal myocardium and least in cells located within the infarct in which the action potential duration was already lengthened.[142] Perhaps the reduced disparity between action potential duration and refractory period between regions of normal and infarcted myocardium may account for some of the antifibrillatory effects of bretylium in myocardial ischemia. Procainamide[64] and disopyramide[88] exert similar effects. When bretylium was given to conscious dogs subjected to premature electrical stimulation three to six days after myocardial infarction, the drug appeared to prevent the onset of ventricular tachycardia.[143] Bretylium has no effect on vagal reflexes and does not alter the responsiveness of cholinergic receptors in the heart.[7]

Hemodynamic Effects. Bretylium does not depress myocardial contractility, even at high doses.[7] After an initial increase in blood pressure, the drug may cause significant hypotension by blocking the efferent limb of the baroreceptor reflex. Hypotension results most commonly when patients are sitting or standing but may also occur in the supine position in seriously ill patients. Bretylium reduces the extent of the vasoconstriction and tachycardia reflexes during standing. We have noted (unpublished) that orthostatic hypotension may persist for several days after the drug has been discontinued.

Pharmacokinetics (Table 20–1). Bretylium is effective orally as well as parenterally, but it is absorbed poorly and erratically from the gastrointestinal tract. Bioavailability may be less than 50 per cent and elimination almost exclusively by renal excretion without significant metabolism or active metabolites recognized. Elimination half-life is 5 to 10 hours but with fairly wide variability. A recent study of the pharmacokinetics of intravenous and oral bretylium in 12 patients who were survivors of ventricular tachycardia or ventricular fibrillation revealed an elimination half-life of 13.5 hours following single intravenous dosing, which was similar to previous results in normal subjects. Renal clearance accounted for virtually all elimination. Onset of action after intravenous administration occurs within several minutes, but full antiarrhythmic effects may not be seen for 30 minutes to 2 hours. Doses should be reduced in patients with renal insufficiency.[144]

Dosage and Administration (Table 20–1). Bretylium is approved for parenteral administration only and can be given intravenously in doses of 5 to 10 mg/kg body weight diluted in 50 to 100 ml of 5 per cent dextrose in water and administered slowly over 10 to 20 minutes.[145] This dose can be repeated in 1 to 2 hours if the arrhythmia persists. The total daily dose should probably not exceed 30 mg/kg. A similar initial dose, but undiluted, can be given intramuscularly. The maintenance intravenous dose is 0.5 to 2.0 mg/min. Intramuscular injection during cardiopulmonary resuscitation from cardiac arrest and in shock states should be avoided because of unreliable absorption during reduced tissue perfusion. In this situation, bretylium should be given intravenously.

Clinical Indications. Bretylium is currently recommended for use in patients who are in an intensive care setting and who have life-threatening recurrent ventricular tachyarrhythmias that have not responded to lidocaine, quinidine, procainamide, or disopyramide. Bretylium has been remarkably effective in treating some of these patients with drug-resistant tachyarrhythmias.[145,146] In a recent study, bretylium was compared with lidocaine as the initial drug therapy in 46 victims of out-of-hospital ventricular fibrillation in a randomized, blinded trial. No instance of chemical defibrillation was observed with either drug in this study, and bretylium afforded neither significant advantage nor disadvantage compared with lidocaine in the initial management of ventricular fibrillation.[36] However, it can be argued that bretylium was not allowed sufficient time to be effective in this study.

Adverse Effects. Hypotension, most prominently orthostatic but also supine, appears to be the most significant side effect and can be prevented with tricyclic drugs such as protriptyline. Transient hypertension, increased sinus rate, and worsening of arrhythmias,[144] often those due to digitalis excess,[139] may follow initial drug administration and may be due to initial release of catecholamines. Bretylium should be used cautiously or not at all in patients who have a relatively fixed cardiac output, such as those with severe aortic stenosis. Vasodilators or diuretics may enhance these hypotensive effects. Nausea and vomiting may occur following parenteral administration. Parotid pain primarily during meals commonly occurs after 2 to 4 months of oral therapy and is associated with increased salivation without parotid swelling or inflammation.

VERAPAMIL

Verapamil, a synthetic papaverine derivative, was first introduced in 1962 as a smooth muscle relaxant that produced peripheral and coronary vasodilation in animals and man.[92,147] Representing a new class of drugs called "calcium antagonists,"[148–150] oral and intravenous forms of verapamil have recently been approved for clinical use. Oral nifedipine has also been approved for clinical use, but since it exhibits minimal electrophysiological effects at clinically used doses, it will not be discussed here (see p. 1351). Diltiazem has electrophysiological actions similar to verapamil[151,152] but at the time of this writing is approved for use only in the treatment of angina in the United States.

Electrophysiological Actions (Tables 20–2 and 20–3). By blocking the slow inward current (see p. 615) verapamil exhibits electrophysiological effects different from those of other antiarrhythmic agents. In concentrations comparable to those achieved clinically, verapamil, in vitro, does not affect the action potential amplitude, $\dot{V}$max of phase 0, or resting membrane voltage in cells that have fast-response characteristics (atrial and ventricular muscle, the His-Purkinje system). The plateau height of the action potential may be reduced, muscle action potential slightly shortened, and total Purkinje fiber action potential slightly prolonged.[149,153–155] However, in fast-channel cells rendered abnormal by disease, these concentrations of verapamil may suppress electrical activity in atrial[156] or ventricular[157,158] muscle fibers that have reduced resting potentials, suggesting that activity in these cells depends on transmembrane ionic flux through the slow channel. Similarly, verapamil suppresses slow responses elicited by a variety of experimental methods.[148,149] Verapamil also suppresses triggered sustained rhythmic activity and early and late afterdepolarizations (see p. 620). Verapamil and other slow-channel blockers in concentrations that do not affect action potentials of fast-channel dependent cells suppress activity in the normal sinus and AV nodes.[159–165] Verapamil depresses the slope of diastolic depolarization in sinus nodal cells, $\dot{V}$max of phase 0, maximum diastolic potential, and action potential amplitude in the sinus and AV nodal cells and prolongs conduction time and the effective and functional refractory periods of the AV node. The blocking effects of verapamil are more apparent at faster rates of stimulation (use-dependency).

It is important to remember, however, that verapamil does exert some local anesthetic activity[9] because the dextrorotatory stereoisomer of the clinically used racemic mixture exerts slight blocking effects on the fast sodium current. The levorotatory stereoisomer blocks the slow inward current carried by calcium, as well as other ions, traveling through the slow channel. Verapamil does not modify calcium uptake, binding, or exchange by cardiac microsomes nor does it affect calcium-activated ATPase.[166] Verapamil does not block beta receptors, but recent data suggest that it may block alpha receptors. Verapamil may also exert other effects that indirectly alter cardiac electrophysiology, such as decreasing platelet adhesiveness or reducing the extent of myocardial ischemia.[167]

In vivo, both in experimental animals and man, verapamil prolongs conduction time through the AV node (the A-H interval) without affecting the P-A, H-V, or QRS intervals and lengthens the functional and effective refractory periods of the AV node.[168] Spontaneous sinus rate may decrease slightly, an event only partially reversed by atropine. More commonly, the sinus rate does not change significantly in vivo because verapamil causes peripheral vasodilation, transient hypotension, and reflex sympathetic stimulation that mitigates any direct slowing effect verapamil may exert on the sinus node. If verapamil is given to a patient who is also receiving a beta blocker, the sinus nodal discharge rate may slow because reflex sympathetic stimulation is blocked.[169] Verapamil does not exert a direct effect on atrial or ventricular refractoriness or on antegrade or retrograde properties of accessory pathways.[170–172] However, reflex sympathetic stimulation may affect the electrophysiological properties of these fibers and, for example, increase the ventricular response during atrial fibrillation in patients with the Wolff-Parkinson-White syndrome.[171,173] Reflex sympathetic stimulation does not eliminate the direct effects of verapamil on AV nodal properties.

Hemodynamic Effects. Since verapamil interferes with excitation-contraction coupling, it inhibits vascular smooth muscle contraction and causes marked vasodilation in coronary and other peripheral vascular beds.[92] Propranolol does not block the vasodilation produced by verapamil. Reflex sympathetic effects may reduce in vivo the marked negative inotropic action of verapamil on isolated cardiac muscle, but direct myocardial depressant effects of verapamil may predominate when the drug is given in high doses. In patients with well-preserved left ventricular function, combined therapy with propranolol and verapamil appears to be well tolerated,[174] but beta blockade can accentuate the hemodynamic depressant effects produced by oral verapamil.[175] Patients who have reduced left ventricular function may not tolerate the combined blockade of beta receptors and of slow channels and the combined use of verapamil and propranolol in these patients must be undertaken cautiously or not at all. Verapamil decreases myocardial demand for oxygen while decreasing coronary vascular resistance[166] and reduces the extent of ischemic damage in experimental preparations.[176,177] Such changes may be antiarrhythmic.[177,178]

Peak alterations in hemodynamic variables occur 3 to 5 minutes after completion of the verapamil injection, the major effects being dissipated within 10 minutes.[92] Mean arterial pressure decreases and left ventricular end-diastolic pressure increases; systemic resistance decreases and left ventricular dP/dt max decreases. Heart rate, cardiac index, left ventricular minute work, and mean pulmonary artery pressure do not change significantly. Thus, afterload reduction produced by verapamil significantly minimizes its negative inotropic action so that cardiac index may not be reduced. In addition, when verapamil slows the ventricular rate in a patient with a tachycardia, cardiac slowing may also improve hemodynamics. Nevertheless, caution should be exercised when giving verapamil to patients with severe myocardial depression or those receiving beta blockers or disopyramide, because hemodynamic deterioration may progress in some patients.

Pharmacokinetics (Table 20–1).   Following single oral doses of verapamil, measurable effects on AV nodal conduction time occur in 30 minutes and last for as long as six hours.[179] After intravenous administration, the onset of action on AV nodal conduction occurs within 1 to 2 minutes. Changes in the A-H interval are still detectable after six hours[180] and correlate with the plasma concentration of verapamil.[181] Effective plasma concentrations necessary to terminate supraventricular tachycardia are in the range 125 ng/ml following doses of 0.075 mg/kg to 0.150 mg/kg.[182] After oral administration absorption is almost complete, but an overall bioavailability of 10 to 35 per cent suggests substantial first-pass metabolism in the liver. The elimination half-life of verapamil is 3 to 8 hours, with up to 70 per cent of the drug excreted by the kidneys. In patients with atrial fibrillation, an intravenous bolus of 15 mg results in an elimination half-life of 8 hours for verapamil and 10.5 hours for norverapamil, a major metabolite that may contribute to verapamil's electrophysiological actions.[183] Serum protein binding is approximately 90 per cent.[184]

Dosage and Administration (Table 20–1).   The most commonly used intravenous dose is 10 mg infused over 1 to 2 minutes while cardiac rhythm and blood pressure are monitored. A second injection of equal dose may be given 30 minutes later. The initial effect achieved with the first bolus injection, such as slowing of the ventricular response during atrial fibrillation, may be maintained by a continuous infusion of the drug at a rate of 0.005 mg/kg/min. The oral dose is 80 to 120 mg, given three or four times a day.[171]

Clinical Indications.   Intravenous verapamil is the treatment of choice for terminating sustained paroxysmal supraventricular tachycardia that does not terminate following simple vagal maneuvers. Verapamil should definitely be tried prior to attempting termination by digitalis administration, pacing, electrical direct-current cardioversion, or acute blood pressure elevation with vasopressors. This recommendation applies to sinus nodal reentry or to any supraventricular tachycardia, such as AV nodal reentry or reciprocating tachycardias associated with the Wolff-Parkinson-White syndrome, when one of the reentrant pathways is the AV node. Verapamil terminates more than 80 per cent of episodes of paroxysmal supraventricular tachycardias within several minutes.[171,182,185] In patients with AV nodal reentry, the most common mechanism of termination appears to be block in the anterograde or slowly conducting pathway, with block less often in the fast pathway conducting retrogradely.[171,182] In patients who experience reciprocating tachycardias during the Wolff-Parkinson-White syndrome, block terminating the tachycardia almost exclusively occurs in the AV node, not in the accessory pathway.[171]

Verapamil decreases the ventricular response over the AV node in the presence of atrial fibrillation or atrial flutter,[186,187] converting a small number of episodes to sinus rhythm, particularly if the atrial flutter or fibrillation is of recent onset. Some patients who exhibit atrial flutter may develop atrial fibrillation following verapamil administration. Quinidine appears to be more effective than verapamil in establishing and maintaining sinus rhythm in patients with chronic atrial fibrillation.[50] As noted earlier, in patients with atrial fibrillation associated with the Wolff-Parkinson-White syndrome, verapamil may accelerate the ventricular response, and therefore the drug is rela-

tively contraindicated in that situation.[171,173] Less information is available regarding the efficacy of verapamil in treating other types of supraventricular tachycardia. Verapamil may terminate supraventricular tachycardia due to sinus nodal reentry and occasionally may terminate ectopic atrial tachycardias.

Orally, verapamil may prevent the recurrence of AV nodal reentrant and reciprocating tachycardias associated with the Wolff-Parkinson-White syndrome as well as help maintain a decreased ventricular response during atrial flutter or atrial fibrillation.[188] In this regard, the effectiveness of verapamil appears to be enhanced when given concomitantly with digitalis.[171] Verapamil generally has not been effective in treating patients who have recurrent ventricular tachyarrhythmias.[189] However, data from animal models suggest that verapamil may be useful in reducing or preventing ventricular arrhythmias due to acute myocardial ischemia,[177,178] and conceivably, this agent may be useful to help prevent sudden death after acute myocardial infarction.[167]

Adverse Effects.   Verapamil must be used cautiously in patients with significant hemodynamic impairment or in those receiving beta blockers, as previously noted. Hypotension, bradycardia, AV block, and asystole are more likely to occur when the drug is given to patients who are already receiving beta blocking agents. Verapamil should also be used with caution in patients with sinus nodal abnormalities, since marked depression of sinus nodal function or asystole may result in some of these patients.[190] Isoproterenol, calcium, glucagon infusion, or atropine (which may be only partially effective) and temporary pacing may be necessary to counteract some of the adverse effects of verapamil. Isoproterenol may be more effective for treating bradyarrhythmias and calcium for treating hemodynamic dysfunction. Contraindications to the use of verapamil include the presence of advanced heart failure, second- or third-degree AV block without a pacemaker in place, significant sinus node dysfunction, cardiogenic shock, or other hypotensive states. While the drug probably should not be used in patients with manifest heart failure, if the latter is due to a supraventricular tachyarrhythmia, verapamil may restore sinus rhythm or significantly decrease the ventricular rate, leading to hemodynamic improvement. Finally, it is important to note that verapamil may decrease the excretion of digoxin by about 30 per cent. Hepatotoxicity may occur on occasion.

NEW ANTIARRHYTHMIC AGENTS
(Tables 20–1 to 20–3)

In the last several years, many new antiarrhythmic agents have been developed and are now undergoing clinical testing in the United States and other countries. The following discussion will serve as a brief review of selected investigational drugs.

Amiodarone.   Amiodarone is a benzofuran derivative that was introduced more than 15 years ago as a smooth muscle relaxant and coronary vasodilator to treat patients with angina. Subsequently, its antiarrhythmic actions were noted.[92,191,192] Amiodarone prolongs action potential duration and refractoriness in atrial and ventricular muscle and Purkinje fibers,[92,191] decreases the slope of diastolic depolarization of sinus nodal activity, and minimally decreases $\dot{V}$max of phase 0 and resting membrane potential of Purkinje fibers.[192] In vivo, amiodarone suppresses arrhythmias induced experimentally by a variety of means. It slows sinus nodal discharge rate in anesthetized dogs even after pretreatment with propranolol and atropine. In patients, it prolongs the Q-T interval and often produces sinus bradycardia. Right atrial monophasic action potentials are prolonged[193] as is the effective refractory period of atrial and ventricular muscle, accessory pathways, and the AV node following oral administration. Amiodarone given intravenously does not prolong the refractory period of atrial or ventricular muscle. P-R interval and AV nodal conduction time lengthen but the QRS complex does not.[194-196] Amiodarone apparently exerts a moderate antiadrenergic effect that is still incompletely characterized.[92]

When administered intravenously in doses of 2.5 to 10 mg/kg, amiodarone decreases heart rate, systemic vascular resistance, left ventricular contractile force, and left ventricular dP/dt. However, left ventricular output increases.[92] Peak plasma concentrations occur approximately 4 hours after a single oral dose, with an elimination half-life of approximately 5 hours. The onset of action is 5 to 10 minutes after intravenous administration. Steady-state plasma concentrations are reached 2 to 4 weeks after oral therapy is begun, producing therapeutic plasma concentrations ranging from 1 to 3 μg/ml. Suppression of cardiac arrhythmias may require therapy for 10 to 14 days or longer, although some patients respond sooner. Estimated elimination half-life after achieving steady state ranges between 30 and 50 days and amiodarone's antiarrhythmic action may last several weeks after cessation of drug therapy. Thus, based on preliminary data, the drug is cleared rapidly after single doses but slowly after chronic dosing, and it can still be found in the serum one year after cessation of oral therapy.[197] The intravenous dose is 5 to 10 mg/kg and the oral maintenance dose ranges between 200 and 800 mg daily. Higher loading doses have been recommended. To minimize side effects, the maintenance dose should be reduced to the lowest effective amount.

Amiodarone exhibits a broad spectrum of antiarrhythmic efficacy and suppresses a variety of supraventricular and ventricular tachyarrhythmias in adults as well as in children.[195,198-200] Although drug-resistant ventricular tachyarrhythmias can be suppressed, it is of interest that the response of the patient to premature ventricular stimulation during electrophysiological study does not appear to predict the clinical outcome.[195,201] Ventricular tachycardia can still be induced with premature stimulation in many patients who are taking the drug who do not develop a spontaneous recurrence. Even though amiodarone prolongs the Q-T interval, it may suppress arrhythmias in patients with the long Q-T syndrome.[202] Amiodarone may prevent recurrence of AV nodal reentry, reciprocating tachycardias associated with the Wolff-Parkinson-White syndrome, recurrent atrial flutter, and atrial fibrillation.[191]

Adverse effects include corneal microdeposits, bluish skin discoloration, neuromuscular disturbances (particularly at higher doses), elevation (often transient) of hepatic enzymes, hyper- or hypothyroidism, pulmonary alveolitis, and fibrosis.[195,203] Cardiovascular toxicity is minimal, although marked sinus bradycardia requiring pacemaker implantation may occur on occasion.[195] Amiodarone may elevate digitalis levels and may increase the anticoagulant effects of warfarin drugs.

Aprindine. Aprindine exerts prominent local anesthetic effects. In isolated cardiac preparations, aprindine shortens the duration of the action potential more than it shortens the effective refractory period of Purkinje fibers. In cardiac muscle fibers, action potential duration is slightly reduced while the effective refractory period is lengthened.[204-206] Vmax of phase 0 is depressed (more so at rapid rates) at higher extracellular potassium concentrations and to a greater degree than exerted by comparable amounts of lidocaine. Spontaneous phase 4 diastolic depolarization in Purkinje fibers is also depressed or abolished. Aprindine reduces digitalis-induced increases in potassium permeability and suppresses transient depolarizations caused by acetylstrophanthidin in canine Purkinje fibers.[204,207] At slightly elevated concentrations, aprindine depresses slow-channel–dependent membrane oscillations and both the fast and slow inward currents.[206] In intact dogs, aprindine injected into the sinus nodal artery decreases the spontaneous sinus rate; injected into the AV nodal artery, it prolongs the functional refractory period and conduction time of the AV node.[208] Aprindine slows conduction in all cardiac tissues and prolongs the refractory period of the ventricle. It exacerbates ischemia-induced conduction delay and increases the incidence of ventricular arrhythmias induced by acute coronary artery occlusion in dogs[209] when given prior to the occlusion, probably because of increased concentration in the ischemic zone.[2] Therapeutic doses mildly depress myocardial function, slightly decreasing systolic and mean aortic blood pressure during exercise, myocardial contractility, and peak left ventricular dP/dt. Aprindine is well absorbed, has high systemic bioavailability, and is 85 to 95 per cent protein-bound.

Approximately 95 per cent of the hydroxylated metabolites undergo glucuronidation in the liver. Sixty-five per cent of aprindine and its metabolites are found in the urine, with the remaining 35 per cent in the feces. Elimination half-life ranges between 20 and 30 hours. In patients treated chronically with aprindine, the N-desethyl metabolite is present in small amounts in the plasma and exerts some antiarrhythmic actions. Clinically, the full antiarrhythmic effect of aprindine may not occur for several days, even when the drug is administered initially in a loading dose.[147,210] Aprindine is given orally in loading doses of 100 mg every six hours for the first day, 75 mg every six hours the second day, and 50 mg every six hours the third day. The dose is then adjusted, with most patients requiring and tolerating 100 to 150 mg/day, which produces a mean plasma concentration of 1 to 2 μg/ml. Intravenous doses are similar.[211] Response to intravenous aprindine during electrophysiological study in patients who had recurrent ventricular arrhythmias appears to predict the subsequent response to the oral dose.[212]

Aprindine is effective in patients who have both supraventricular and ventricular tachyarrhythmias. Since it prolongs conduction time and refractoriness in the AV node and prolongs the refractory period of the accessory pathway in patients with the Wolff-Parkinson-White syndrome, it may be used to suppress arrhythmias in patients with AV nodal reentry and to produce block in the accessory pathway.[213] Aprindine also suppresses drug-resistant recurrent ventricular tachyarrhythmias[211] and may be useful in patients whose ventricular arrhythmias are associated with mitral valve prolapse[214] or due to digitalis. The toxic-therapeutic ratio for aprindine is narrow, and side effects are common, particularly during the initial loading period and adjustment of the maintenance dose. These side effects, related to the dose and serum concentration of aprindine, include most commonly a tremor of the hand and fingers. As the serum concentration increases, dizziness, intention tremor, ataxia, nervousness, hallucinations, diplopia, memory impairment, or seizures may occur. Neurological side effects are minimal or absent at serum aprindine concentrations less than 1 μg/ml. Cholestatic jaundice and agranulocytosis have been reported to occur generally between the fourth and sixteenth week of aprindine therapy. The estimated incidence of agranulocytosis is approximately 1 per cent, and the condition is reversible if the drug is discontinued in time. Aprindine may cause Q-T prolongation and polymorphous ventricular tachycardia.[215] A derivative, moxaprindine, has undergone preliminary clinical testing, and initial results are encouraging.[216,217]

Encainide. Encainide is a new antiarrhythmic agent that decreases phase 4 diastolic depolarization in Purkinje fibers and decreases action potential duration, Vmax of phase 0, and propagation velocity in atrial, ventricular, and Purkinje fibers without altering resting membrane potential. It does not affect the slow response in vitro. Encainide has several active metabolites, one of which is more potent than the parent compound.[218] In patients, oral encainide prolongs atrial, ventricular, and accessory pathway refractory periods; A-H and H-V intervals; and P-R, QRS, and Q-T intervals.[219] Active metabolites may contribute to its antiarrhythmic efficacy,[219,220] and variation in the conversion of encainide to its active metabolites may be a source of interpatient differences in drug response.[221] Encainide does not alter myocardial contractility or ejection indices in patients with relatively normal ventricular function; in those with markedly reduced ventricular function, as evidenced by elevated left ventricular end-diastolic pressures and reduced cardiac output, encainide further decreases cardiac output slightly.[222]

Encainide exhibits a wide range of bioavailability and a relatively short half-life of 3 to 4 hours. However, the existence of one or more active metabolites permits a long interval between dosing during which the concentration of encainide metabolites exceeds that of the parent compound and is probably responsible for the delayed return (13 hours) of arrhythmias following drug withdrawal.[223] The drug is useful in treating some patients who have supraventricular tachycardias associated with AV nodal reentry or Wolff-Parkinson-White syndrome.[219,224] Encainide suppresses premature ventricular complexes,[225,226] is effective in about 25 to 30 per cent of patients with chronic recurrent ventricular tachyarrhythmias refractory to conventional agents,[227,228] and has a wide therapeutic-to-toxic ratio.[223] Encainide is generally administered orally four times daily in doses of 100 to 300 mg/day. Dose changes should not be made more frequently than every 48 hours. Adverse effects include dizziness, diplopia, vertigo, paresthesia, leg cramps, and a metallic taste in the mouth. Most significant is its potential to cause or exacerbate serious ventricular tachyarrhythmias in approximately 10 per cent of patients treated. Commonly, a polymorphous ventricular tachycardia ensues and may result in hemodynamic collapse. Often, this is not associated with marked Q-T prolongation and may not terminate spontaneously.[229,230]

Mexiletine. Mexiletine, a local anesthetic with anticonvulsant properties, is similar to lidocaine in many of its electrophysiological actions. In vitro, mexiletine shortens the duration of action potential and refractory period, depresses $\dot{V}$max of phase 0, and depresses automaticity of Purkinje fibers but not of the normal sinus node.[92,231] It may result in severe bradycardia and abnormal sinus nodal recovery time in patients with sinus node disease and may depress His-Purkinje conduction in some patients. The effects of mexiletine on sinus and AV nodal properties appear to be variable,[227] possibly because mexiletine may produce different results when tested on abnormal tissue, as may lidocaine. Mexiletine does not appear to affect the refractory period of human atrial and ventricular muscle.

Mexiletine has been reported to be rapidly and almost completely absorbed after oral ingestion by volunteers, with peak plasma concentrations attained in 2 to 4 hours. Elimination half-life in healthy subjects is approximately 10 hours and in patients after myocardial infarction, 17 hours.[92] Therapeutic plasma levels of 1 to 2 μg/ml are maintained by oral doses of 200 to 300 mg every six to eight hours. Absorption is delayed and incomplete in patients who have myocardial infarction and in patients receiving narcotic or analgesic agents that retard gastric emptying.[232] Bioavailability of orally administered mexiletine is approximately 90 per cent, and about 70 per cent of the drug is protein-bound. The apparent volume of distribution is large, reflecting extensive tissue uptake. Normally, mexiletine is eliminated metabolically by the liver, with less than 10 per cent excreted unchanged in the urine. Renal clearance of mexiletine decreases as urinary pH increases.

Several European studies have shown mexiletine to be an effective antiarrhythmic agent for both acute and chronic ventricular arrhythmias.[233,234] Experience in the United States has yielded mixed results. Data from one study of patients who had recurrent ventricular arrhythmias resistant to conventional drugs revealed that only 4 of 19 demonstrated sufficient tolerance of the drug and antiarrhythmic efficacy to continue long-term therapy.[235] However, other studies[236,237] have had more encouraging results, and it seems clear that mexiletine can be effective in some patients with recurrent ventricular tachyarrhythmias. The combinations of mexiletine and amiodarone[238] and mexiletine and disopyramide[102] have been reported to be particularly efficacious. Thirty to 40 per cent of patients may require a change in dose or discontinuation of mexiletine therapy as a result of adverse effects,[239] including tremor, dysarthria, dizziness, paresthesia, diplopia, nystagmus, mental confusion, anxiety, nausea, vomiting, and dyspepsia. Cardiovascular side effects are most often seen after intravenous dosing and include hypotension, bradycardia, and exacerbation of arrhythmia.[240] Adverse effects of mexiletine appear to be dose-related and toxic effects occur at plasma concentrations only slightly higher than therapeutic levels. Therefore, effective use of this antiarrhythmic drug requires careful titration of dose and monitoring of plasma concentration.

Tocainide. Tocainide, a primary amine analog of lidocaine that is effective orally, exerts electrophysiological effects very similar to those of lidocaine.[241] In patients with compensated left ventricular dysfunction, intravenous infusion of tocainide moderately decreases mean arterial pressure and slightly increases pulmonary and systemic vascular resistance and left ventricular end-diastolic pressure without altering heart rate, cardiac index, or left ventricular dP/dt.[242] Bioavailability of tocainide is almost 100 per cent, with virtually no hepatic first-pass effect, which is significantly different from lidocaine. The drug is rapidly and completely absorbed, yielding peak plasma concentrations 1 to 1.5 hours after oral ingestion. Oral regimens of 400 to 600 mg every eight hours produce therapeutic plasma concentrations of 6 to 12 μg/ml. Elimination half-life is approximately 14 hours.

Although tocainide effectively reduces the frequency of premature ventricular complexes,[243,244] it has been less effective in preventing chronic recurrent ventricular tachycardia–ventricular fibrillation in some[227,242,245] but not all[246,247] studies. It did not reduce the incidence

of ventricular fibrillation or symptomatic ventricular tachycardia in a double-blind controlled study of 112 patients after myocardial infarction.[248] Response to lidocaine therapy may help predict an individual's response to tocainide. If lidocaine fails to suppress the ventricular arrhythmia, tocainide has about a 15 per cent chance of being effective. If lidocaine suppresses the ventricular arrhythmia, tocainide has about a 60 per cent chance of being effective.[242,247] Adverse effects are dose-related, similar to those produced by lidocaine, and include nausea, vomiting, anorexia, tremulousness, memory impairment, skin rash, sweating, paresthesia, diplopia, dizziness, anxiety, and tinnitus. Occasionally, tocainide may produce pulmonary fibrosis or induce or aggravate ventricular arrhythmias.[247,249]

Ethmozine. Ethmozine is a phenothiazine derivative that decreases $\dot{V}$max of phase 0, action potential amplitude, and action potential duration in canine Purkinje fibers and decreases the force of Purkinje fiber contraction.[250] Injected into the sinus or AV nodal arteries of dogs, ethmozine does not alter sinus discharge rate or AV nodal conduction at therapeutic concentrations[251] and produces minimal electrophysiological changes in patients.[252] It is well absorbed and extensively metabolized, but little is known about the potential activity of its metabolites. Ethmozine suppresses premature atrial and ventricular arrhythmias but the data from controlled studies are too preliminary at present to draw meaningful conclusions.[253] However, it appears to be well tolerated and offers promise as a new antiarrhythmic agent.

Flecainide. Flecainide exerts electrophysiological effects similar to those of quinidine and procainamide and exhibits a wide spectrum of antiarrhythmic effectiveness. The drug has an elimination half-life of about 20 hours and effectively suppresses premature ventricular complexes[254] and nonsustained episodes of ventricular tachycardia.[255] The effective dose is approximately 200 mg every 12 hours, producing therapeutic plasma concentrations of about 600 ng/ml.[254,255] Side effects in early studies have been minimal and include mild and transient neurological reactions such as blurred vision, lightheadedness, and headache. No significant adverse hemodynamic effects have been noted.[254] Flecainide prolongs conduction time in all cardiac fibers, so that intraatrial, AV nodal, His-Purkinje, and intraventricular conduction times lengthen. High-degree AV block may develop in patients with preexisting bundle branch block.[256] P-R, QRS, and Q-Tc intervals increase at increasing doses, in parallel with antiarrhythmic efficacy.[255] Q-T prolongation and ventricular tachycardia have been reported.[257]

Lorcainide. Lorcainide is an acetanilide derivative with local anesthetic effects that decreases $\dot{V}$max of phase 0 and conduction velocity and slightly prolongs the effective refractory period of Purkinje fibers. It does not affect the slow response and prolongs conduction time in the atria, His-Purkinje system, and ventricles. Elimination half-life ranges in different studies between 5 and 12 hours.[258,259] Important first-pass hepatic effects that reduce bioavailability occur with single 100-mg doses, but bioavailability increases after higher and multiple doses.[258] Lorcainide appears effective against ventricular arrhythmias.[259,260] Insomnia is an important side effect that is effectively treated with diazepam and gradually disappears after continued dosing.

Propafenone. Propafenone appears to be a fairly well tolerated antiarrhythmic agent that prolongs sinus nodal recovery time and lengthens the effective refractory period of the atrium, AV node, ventricle, and accessory pathways.[261] Intraatrial, AV nodal, and His-Purkinje conduction times are prolonged. Elimination half-life is approximately 4 hours, with protein binding exceeding 90 per cent. Preliminary data indicate that this drug is effective against ventricular arrhythmias.[262]

Bethanidine. Bethanidine is a closely related chemical analog of bretylium with similar pharmacological and antifibrillatory actions on the ventricle. Unlike bretylium, bethanidine is rapidly and effectively absorbed after oral administration. Preliminary data demonstrate important antiarrhythmic efficacy.[263]

Other antiarrhythmic agents, such as clofilium,[264] meobentine, cibenzoline, sotalol, and antidepressant drugs such as imipramine and nortriptyline[265] are currently undergoing evaluation.

ELECTRICAL THERAPY OF CARDIAC ARRHYTHMIAS

DIRECT CURRENT CARDIOVERSION

The successful application of external cardioversion[266,267] culminated the research begun in 1899[268] and carried out subsequently by many investigators. Electrical cardioversion offers obvious advantages over drug therapy.[269] Under conditions optimal for close supervision and monitoring, a precisely regulated "dose" of electricity can restore sinus rhythm immediately and safely. The distinction between supraventricular and ventricular tachyarrhythmias—crucial to the proper medical management of arrhythmias—becomes less significant, and the time-consuming titration of drugs with potential side effects is abolished.

MECHANISMS. Electrical cardioversion appears to terminate most effectively those tachycardias presumed to be due to reentry, including atrial flutter and atrial fibrillation, AV nodal reentry, reciprocating tachycardias associated with Wolff-Parkinson-White syndrome, most forms of ventricular tachycardia, ventricular flutter, and ventricular fibrillation. The electric shock, by depolarizing all excitable myocardium, interrupts reentrant circuits, discharges foci, and establishes electrical homogeneity that terminates reentry. A shock that does not end the tachycardia may fail to depolarize critical areas involved in the maintenance of the tachycardia. A tachycardia that terminates and then restarts may be reinitiated by factors provoking the tachycardia in the first place. For example, a tachycardia can be considered according to conditions that initiate it and those that maintain it. A premature depolarization due to enhanced automaticity may initiate a tachycardia that is then maintained by reentrant excitation. Thus, a cardioversion shock may terminate the reentry but not affect the premature systole. The latter may restart the tachycardia after a short period of sinus rhythm. If the precipitating factors are no longer present, interrupting the tachyarrhythmia for only the brief time produced by the shock may prevent its return for long duration even though the anatomical and electrophysiological substrates required for the tachycardia are still present.

Tachycardias thought to be due to disorders of impulse formation (automaticity) include parasystole, some forms of atrial tachycardias with or without AV block, nonparoxysmal AV junctional tachycardia and accelerated idioventricular rhythms. An attempt to cardiovert these tachycardias electrically in most instances is not indicated for several reasons. First, the ventricular rate generally is not very fast and the patient is hemodynamically stable. The tachycardia may terminate spontaneously or with drug therapy. Second, digitalis toxicity may be a cause, in which case electrical countershock would be contraindicated. Third, if these arrhythmias are due to enhanced automaticity, the precipitating and maintaining mechanisms may be the same, i.e., accelerated phase 4 diastolic depolarization. Thus, an electric shock might only "reset" the pacemaker cycle, with the tachycardia continuing after the shock. It is possible that the shock can terminate tachycardias due to enhanced automaticity or triggered activity, but this notion is conjectural at present.

TECHNIQUE. After the procedure has been explained to the patient, a careful physical examination, including palpation of all pulses, should be performed prior to elective cardioversion. A 12-lead electrocardiogram is obtained before and after cardioversion as well as a rhythm strip during the electroshock. The patient should be "metabolically balanced," i.e., blood gases, pH, and electrolytes should be normal with no drug toxicity present. The patient should fast for 6 to 8 hours prior to the shock, if possible. Because patients receiving digitalis without clinical evidence of digitalis toxicity appear to be at low risk for serious postcardioversion ventricular arrhythmias, even when serum digoxin levels are modestly elevated,[270] it does not seem necessary to withhold digitalis for several days prior to elective cardioversion. Maintenance quinidine administration 1 to 2 days before electrical cardioversion of patients with atrial fibrillation may revert 10 to 15 per cent to sinus rhythm and help prevent recurrence of atrial fibrillation once sinus rhythm is restored.

Paddle placement, paddle size, and maximum delivered energy from the external cardioverter have been the subject of some recent controversy.[271-274] A paddle with a 12-cm diameter delivers maximum intracardiac current in dogs. Since the size and configuration of the dog's thorax differ considerably from those of man, the results in dogs may not be applicable to humans. Although 13-cm diameter paddles may not be too large for adult human hearts and should deliver increased intracardiac current,[275] the benefits of a larger paddle size have not been proved for man.[276] The amount of current reaching the heart significantly influences the effectiveness of the shock.[277] For example, an amount of current needed to depolarize a critical mass of excitable myocardial cells appears necessary to terminate fibrillation.[278] Doubling the amount of current that reaches the heart requires a fourfold increase in transthoracic energy.[277] However, it is generally agreed that defibrillators delivering larger energies than those currently commercially available probably are not necessary, even for very large patients,[279] particularly if paddles with large diameters are used. Larger paddles also distribute the intracardiac current over a wider area and may reduce shock-induced myocardial necrosis.

Paddles must be placed in firm contact with the chest wall[273] and are generally positioned in the left infrascapular region (on which the patient lies) and over the upper sternum at the third interspace (Fig. 20–5). A second position is one paddle to the right of the sternum at the level of the first or second rib and the other in the left midclavicular line at the fourth or fifth intercostal space. The effectiveness of these two positions appears fairly comparable.[273]

A synchronized shock, i.e., one delivered during the QRS complex, is used for all cardioversions except for very rapid ventricular tachyarrhythmias, such as ventricular flutter or fibrillation. Because myocardial damage increases directly with increases in applied energy, the minimum effective energy should be used. Therefore, shocks are "titrated" when the clinical situation permits. Except for atrial fibrillation, shocks in the range of 25 to 50 joules successfully terminate most nondigitalis-induced supraventricular tachycardias and should be tried initially. If unsuccessful, a second shock of higher energy may be delivered. The starting level to terminate atrial fibrillation

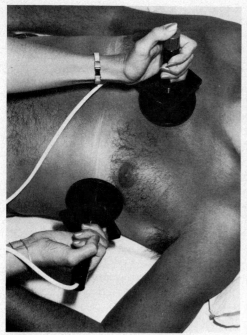
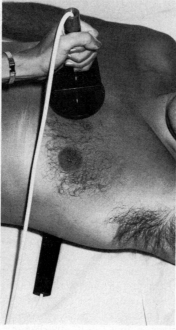

FIGURE 20–5   Paddle position for cardioversion. *Top*, The patient is lying on a flat posterior paddle centered at the tip of the left scapula; the anterior paddle is positioned just below the sterno-manubrial joint. *Bottom*, The anterior paddle is in the same position, while the second paddle is placed over the cardiac apex.

should probably be 50 to 100 joules. For patients with stable ventricular tachycardia, starting levels in the range of 25 to 50 joules may be employed. If there is some urgency to terminate the tachyarrhythmia, one can begin with higher energies. To terminate ventricular fibrillation, 200 to 400 joules are used.

During elective cardioversion, a short-acting barbiturate, such as methohexital in intravenous doses of 25 to 75 mg, or an amnesic, such as diazepam given in incremental intravenous doses of 2.5 to 5 mg at 30-second intervals, may be used. A physician skilled in airway management should be in attendance (preferably an anesthetist, if possible), an intravenous route should be established, and all equipment necessary for emergency resuscitation should be immediately accessible. Before cardioversion, 100 per cent oxygen may be administered for 5 to 15 minutes and is continued throughout the procedure. Manual ventilation of the patient may be necessary to avoid hypoxia during periods of deepest sleep.

INDICATIONS. Before considering electrical cardioversion, the likelihood of establishing and maintaining sinus rhythm using electrical countershock should be weighed against the risks of other forms of therapy. As a rule, any tachycardia that produces complications such as hypotension, congestive heart failure, or angina and does not respond promptly to medical management should be terminated electrically. In almost all instances, the patient's hemodynamic status improves after cardioversion. An occasional patient may develop hypotension, reduced cardiac output, or congestive heart failure following the shock. The reasons for this are not entirely clear but may relate to complications of the cardioversion, such as embolic events, myocardial depression resulting from the anesthetic agent, hypoxia, or lack of restoration of left atrial contraction despite return of electrical atrial systole.[280] Direct-current countershock should not be used in patients with digitalis-induced tachyarrhythmias because electrical cardioversion in that situation may precipitate life-threatening ventricular tachyarrhythmias.

Favorable candidates for electrical cardioversion of atrial fibrillation include those patients who (1) have symptomatic atrial fibrillation and derive significant hemodynamic benefits from sinus rhythm; (2) have embolic episodes; (3) continue to have atrial fibrillation after the precipitating cause has been removed, e.g., following treatment of thyrotoxicosis, pericarditis or myocarditis, myocardial infarction, pneumonia, or pulmonary embolism or after corrective cardiac surgery; (4) have idiopathic atrial fibrillation of less than 12 months' duration; and (5) have a rapid ventricular rate that is difficult to slow. The success rate is high for maintaining sinus rhythm after electrical cardioversion of atrial fibrillation in patients with atria of normal size and in whom atrial fibrillation has been present for less than a year.

Unfavorable candidates for electrical cardioversion of atrial fibrillation include (1) patients with digitalis toxicity, (2) asymptomatic elderly patients who have a well-controlled ventricular rate without therapy, (3) patients with sinus node dysfunction and various unstable supraventricular tachyarrhythmias or bradyarrhythmias (often the bradycardia-tachycardia syndrome) who finally develop and maintain atrial fibrillation (which in essence represents a "cure" of the sick sinus syndrome), (4) those who derive little or no benefit from normal sinus rhythm and promptly revert to atrial fibrillation after cardioversion despite drug therapy, (5) those who have a large left atrium and atrial fibrillation of long standing, (6) those who have infrequent episodes of atrial fibrillation that revert spontaneously to sinus rhythm, (7) those in whom mechanical atrial systole does not accompany the return of electrical atrial systole, (8) those who have atrial fibrillation and advanced heart block, (9) those for whom cardiac surgery is planned in the near future, and (10) those who cannot tolerate antiarrhythmic drugs. Atrial fibrillation is likely to recur after cardioversion in patients who have significant chronic obstructive lung disease, congestive heart failure, or mitral valve disease, particularly mitral insufficiency.

In patients with atrial flutter, slowing the ventricular

rate by administering digitalis or terminating the flutter with quinidine may be difficult, so that electrical cardioversion appears to be the initial treatment of choice. For the patient with a supraventricular tachycardia, electrical cardioversion may be employed when maneuvers to enhance vagal tone or simple medical management have failed to terminate the tachycardia and the clinical setting indicates that fairly prompt restoration of sinus rhythm is desirable because of hemodynamic decompensation or electrophysiological consequences of the tachycardia (e.g., very rapid ventricular rates during atrial fibrillation in a patient with Wolff-Parkinson-White syndrome may progress to ventricular fibrillation). Similarly for patients with ventricular tachycardia, the hemodynamic and electrophysiological consequences of the arrhythmias—e.g., the adequacy of hemodynamic compensation during ventricular tachycardia or the possibility of ventricular tachycardia progressing to ventricular fibrillation—determine the need and urgency for direct current-cardioversion (p. 669). Electrical countershock is the initial treatment of choice for ventricular flutter or ventricular fibrillation.

If, after the first shock, reversion to sinus rhythm does not occur, a higher energy level should be tried. When transient ventricular arrhythmias result after an unsuccessful shock, a bolus of lidocaine may be given prior to delivering a shock at the next energy level. If sinus rhythm returns only transiently and is promptly supplanted by the tachycardia, a repeat shock may be tried, depending on the tachyarrhythmia being treated and its consequences. Administration of an antiarrhythmic agent intravenously may be useful prior to delivering the next cardioversion shock. After cardioversion, the patient should be monitored at least until full consciousness has been restored and preferably for several hours thereafter.

RESULTS. Cardioversion restores sinus rhythm in 70 to over 95 per cent of patients, depending upon the type of tachyarrhythmia.[268] But, as an example, less than one-third to one-half the patients with chronic atrial fibrillation remain in sinus rhythm after 12 months. Thus, maintenance of sinus rhythm once established is the difficult problem, not the immediate termination of the tachycardia, and depends on the particular arrhythmia, the presence of underlying heart disease, and the adequacy of antiarrhythmic drug therapy.

COMPLICATIONS. Arrhythmias after cardioversion may be produced by the clinical conditions that caused the initial tachycardia or the effects of the electrical discharge. Arrhythmias induced by the shock generally are caused by inadequate synchronization, with the shock occurring during the ST segment or T wave. It is important to remember that, occasionally, a properly synchronized shock may produce ventricular fibrillation (Fig. 20–6).[276] Post-shock arrhythmias usually are transient and do not require therapy. A variety of delayed tachyarrhythmias have been described, sometimes associated with quinidine or digitalis therapy, but their nature is not clear. In some instances, post-shock arrhythmias may be related to the significant autonomic discharge of thoracic parasympathetic and sympathetic nerve terminals produced by the transthoracic shock.[281,282] Generally these autonomic imbalances are tran-

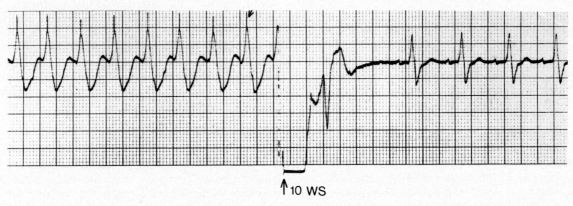

↑10 WS

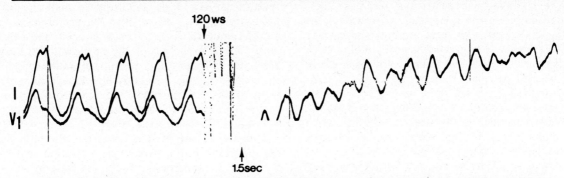

120 ws

I
V₁

1.5sec

FIGURE 20–6 *Top,* A synchronized shock (note synchronization marks in the apex of the QRS complex [↓]) during ventricular tachycardia is followed by a single repetitive ventricular response and then normal sinus rhythm. *Bottom,* A shock synchronized to the terminal portion of the QRS complex in a patient with atrial fibrillation and conduction to the ventricle over an accessory pathway (WPW syndrome) results in ventricular fibrillation that was promptly terminated by a 400-msec shock. Recording was lost for 1.5 sec (↑) owing to baseline drift after the shock.

sient and do not require therapy. Embolic episodes are reported to occur in 1 to 3 per cent of the patients converted to sinus rhythm.[283,284] Prior anticoagulation for 1 to 2 weeks should be considered for patients who have no contraindication to such therapy and who are at high risk for emboli, such as those with mitral stenosis and atrial fibrillation of recent onset, a history of recent or recurrent emboli, a prosthetic mitral valve, enlarged hearts (including left atrial enlargement), or congestive heart failure.[283,284] Anticoagulation with warfarin for several weeks afterward is recommended. However, it must be emphasized that few controlled studies to support this approach have been published.

Although direct-current shock has been demonstrated in animals to cause cardiac injury,[285] studies in man indicate that elevations of myocardial enzymes after cardioversion are not common.[286] ST-segment elevation may occur with elective direct-current cardioversion, although cardiac enzymes and myocardial scintigraphy may be unremarkable.[287]

New Developments.   Ultrasound cardioversion,[288] synchronized transvenous cardioversion by a catheter electrode,[289,290,290a] and defibrillation with implantable devices (see p. 729)[291–293] have all been developed recently. Several of these techniques have undergone clinical testing and offer great promise. Cardioversion of ventricular tachycardia can also be achieved by a chest thump.[294] Its mechanism of termination probably relates to a mechanically induced premature atrial or ventricular complex that interrupts a tachycardia. The thump cannot be timed very well and is probably only effective when delivered during a nonrefractory part of the cardiac cycle. Care must therefore be taken, because the thump can alter a ventricular tachycardia[295] and possibly induce ventricular flutter or fibrillation.[296]

PACEMAKER CONTROL OF CARDIAC ARRHYTHMIAS

Pacing for bradyarrhythmias is well established. More recently, pacing has been shown to terminate effectively a variety of supraventricular tachyarrhythmias. Its use for treating ventricular tachyarrhythmias is limited by its potential for exacerbating the rhythm disturbance (see Chap. 21).

SURGICAL THERAPY OF TACHYARRHYTHMIAS

Use of cardiac surgery to treat patients with recurrent symptomatic tachyarrhythmias has increased in frequency as knowledge about mechanisms of tachycardia and pathways involved in the maintenance of a tachycardia has been gained and new operative approaches have been developed. At present, patient selection remains relatively restricted to severely symptomatic individuals who have had recurrent arrhythmia despite adequate drug therapy. Conceivably, in some instances, such as recurrent tachycardia associated with Wolff-Parkinson-White syndrome, surgery might be considered early for a young person to spare the patient a lifetime of drug therapy, assuming that morbidity, mortality, and chances for surgical cure were acceptable.

The objectives of a surgical approach are to excise or isolate the origin of a tachycardia, to interrupt a reentrant pathway necessary for maintenance of the tachycardia, and to induce AV block in patients with supraventricular tachycardias that cause rapid ventricular responses. AV block also may be produced to interrupt a requisite reentrant pathway associated with reciprocating tachycardias in the Wolff-Parkinson-White syndrome. In addition to these direct surgical approaches, indirect approaches can be useful in selected patients by improving cardiac hemodynamics and myocardial blood flow. Such procedures include aneurysmectomy, coronary artery bypass grafting, or relief of valvular insufficiency or stenosis. Cardiac sympathectomy alters autonomic influences on the ventricle and has been effective in occasional patients who have recurrent ventricular tachycardia with[129] or without the long Q-T syndrome.[297–301]

SUPRAVENTRICULAR TACHYCARDIAS

At the present time, there are primarily three groups of patients who have symptomatic, drug-resistant, recurrent supraventricular tachycardias and are candidates for surgery: (1) those in whom the origin of the tachycardia is confined to a relatively localized area in the atrium; (2) those who have uncontrollably rapid ventricular rates during a supraventricular tachycardia and in whom creation of AV block is desirable; and (3) those with the preexcitation syndrome or one of its variants. Other groups, such as those with AV nodal reentrant tachycardia, may also be candidates in the future owing to the relative ease of creating AV block by means of a new catheter electrode technique.[302,303] Surgery is *not* indicated for eliminating episodes of atrial flutter or atrial fibrillation.

Preoperative assessment of these surgical candidates involves an electrophysiological study to determine whether the tachycardia can be initiated by programmed electrical stimulation to be certain that the initiated tachycardia is identical to that occurring clinically and that the tachycardia can be precipitated so that it can be studied at the time of surgery. It is important to map the tachycardia preoperatively (see below) because general anesthesia, cooling of the heart when the chest is open, and other factors may prevent induction of the tachycardia at surgery and preclude the opportunity for intraoperative mapping. (This is particularly true for ventricular tachycardias.) Also, for tachycardias that cannot be induced electrically, the preoperative electrophysiological study can be performed at a time when the tachycardia has begun spontaneously.

Mapping in the present context is the term applied to the procedure during which the activation sequence—i.e., the origin of and the pathways followed by the electrical impulse as it depolarizes the heart—is determined. Preoperatively, mapping is performed using catheters that bear at their tip electrodes that are several millimeters to one centimeter apart. For a supraventricular tachycardia, the catheter is positioned at various endocardial right atrial sites, around the margin of the tricuspid ring, and along the length of the coronary sinus to obtain recordings of left atrial activity at the region of the AV ring and, at times, through a probe-patent foramen ovale or by a transseptal puncture to map left atrial endocardium. Local activation times recorded with the electrodes at the catheter tip are determined from the rapid component of unipolar electrode recordings or the first peak of the rapid inflection of bipolar recordings. The activation time along with the anatomical position of the electrode establish the site of the earliest area of activation and the subsequent activation sequence.

In patients with the Wolff-Parkinson-White syndrome, mapping can be performed to define both atrial and ventricular insertions of the accessory pathway. The *ventricular insertion* can be determined by locating the earliest site of ventricular activation when the ventricle is depolarized over the accessory pathway during stable sinus rhythm, during atrial pacing from a site near the accessory pathway, or during stable reciprocating tachycardia characterized by anterograde conduction over the accessory pathway and retrograde conduction over the normal pathway. Ventricular mapping of this type is very difficult to do with a catheter electrode and is best done at the time of surgery. Finding the shortest interval between the stimulus applied to various atrial sites and the delta wave of the QRS complex may be helpful, based on the assumption that the shortest interval results when the atrial pacing stimulus is delivered at a site closest to the accessory pathway. The *atrial insertion* of the accessory pathway is determined by locating the earliest site of atrial activation when the atrium is depolarized over the accessory pathway during ventricular pacing or during reciprocating tachycardia characterized by anterograde conduction over the normal pathway and retrograde conduction over the accessory pathway. Atrial mapping during tachycardia is preferable to be certain that the retrograde atrial activation is due solely to conduction over the accessory pathway and is not a fusion P wave. In some patients with multiple accessory pathways, the retrograde P wave may be a fusion of activation from two or more accessory pathways, and one must search carefully for the presence of multiple accessory pathways.[304] Accurate maps obtained in this fashion can localize the atrial and ventricular insertions of the accessory pathway to be opposite each other across the AV groove. Mapping is repeated at the time of operation.[305,306] In patients who have free-wall AV connections, the earliest epicardial activation of the ventricle occurs before or simultaneously with the onset of the delta wave, while in patients with septal connections, the area of earliest epicardial activation of the ventricle occurs after the onset of the surface delta wave.

Various surgical approaches have evolved during which an incision is made at the presumed insertion site of the accessory pathway and the dissection is extended for at least 1 cm on each side of this area. Accessory pathways can be buried in fat pads, can be positioned at the endocardium or epicardium, and may insert in the ventricular septum or free wall of either ventricle. Exceptionally careful dissection is required when the accessory pathway is in a paraseptal location to avoid damaging the AV node or His bundle. After the accessory pathway has been severed, an attempt is made to reinitiate the tachycardia and another map is obtained to be certain that the operation was

successful and that no other accessory pathways exist. Since the first report of successful surgical interruption of an accessory pathway in a patient with the Wolff-Parkinson-White syndrome[307] significant experience has been gained that permits a direct approach to achieve interruption. In addition to cutting the connection, cryosurgery, which involves freezing a portion of the myocardium to interrupt conduction, has been used successfully in some patients.[308] Mortality from the operation is less than 1 to 2 per cent and the success rate for interrupting the AV connection and eliminating the tachycardia exceeds 90 per cent.[309]

Relatively little experience has been acquired with regard to the surgical treatment of supraventricular tachycardias due to abnormalities other than an accessory AV pathway.[310] When the atrial tachycardia is localized to a portion of the atrium, surgical excision of a focal area, such as in the atrial appendage, has effectively removed the tachycardia.[311,312] Of interest, microelectrode studies on the excised tissue in one patient revealed an inducible rhythm localized to a small area of the atrial endocardium, consistent with triggered activity.[311] Electrocautery[313] and cryosurgery[312] have eliminated tachycardia in several patients. In one patient, an encircling incision that contained the earliest point of activation during tachycardia excluded a portion of the left atrium and both pulmonary veins from the remainder of the left atrium[314] and isolated the tachycardia.

Interrupting the AV node–His bundle junction by suture, electrocauterization, incision of the septal portion of the right atrium, and cryothermic ablation have been used in patients with atrial tachycardias with rapid ventricular responses that cannot be slowed by means of drug therapy. Cryothermic ablation appears to represent a preferable technique[315,316] and also has been used to ablate an AV junctional tachycardia arising in the region of the His bundle.[312] Recently, a new technique has been devised to ablate the His bundle by delivering direct-current shocks through a catheter electrode positioned in the His bundle area. In effect, this approach cauterizes the area of His bundle to produce AV block and obviates cardiac surgery.[302,303] It offers a promising, minimally invasive approach to producing AV block and could conceivably be adapted to eliminate sites of ectopic arrhythmia formation or accessory pathways in other parts of the heart.

VENTRICULAR TACHYCARDIA

Surgical therapy for patients with recurrent, drug-resistant, symptomatic ventricular tachycardias is influenced by whether or not patients have ischemic heart disease.

ISCHEMIC HEART DISEASE. In almost all patients who have ventricular tachycardia associated with ischemic heart disease, the arrhythmia, regardless of its configuration on the surface ECG, arises in the left ventricle or on the left ventricular side of the interventricular septum.[317] The contour of the ventricular tachycardia may change either spontaneously or after premature stimulation from a right bundle branch block to a left bundle branch block pattern without a change in the earliest activation site, suggesting that the left ventricular site of origin remains the same, often near a left ventricular aneurysm, but its exit pathway is altered.[318]

Indirect surgical approaches, including cardiac thoracic sympathectomy, coronary artery bypass grafting, and ventricular aneurysm or infarct resection (without mapping) with or without bypass grafting, have been successful in about 60 per cent of reported cases.[319] Better patient selection would probably improve the success rate. For example, coronary artery bypass grafting limited to patients who experience ventricular tachycardia during documented exercise-induced ischemia can prevent recurrence of ventricular tachycardia in almost 100 per cent of patients.[320] However, the number of patients in this group is relatively small compared to the number of patients who have recurrent ventricular tachycardia unrelated to exercise but associated with ischemic heart disease, old myocardial infarction, and scarring. In these latter patients, three types of surgical procedures have been used: isolation, resection, and ablation.

The *encircling endocardial ventriculotomy*[321] involves a transmural ventriculotomy placed perpendicularly or obliquely,[322] relative to the endocardial wall to isolate areas of endocardial fibrosis that are recognized visually. The incision, sparing the epicardium and overlying coronary vessels, is then repaired. When the septum is involved, the ventriculotomy is approximately 1 cm in depth. The rationale for this procedure is to separate arrhythmogenic areas into small islands that become anatomically and electrophysiologically isolated. However, recent animal data suggest that cardiac blood flow to the isolated myocardium may be reduced, adversely affecting myocardial function.[319]

The rationale for the second approach, *endocardial resection*, is based in part on animal data indicating that arrhythmias in dogs subjected to myocardial infarction arise in the subendocardial borders between normal and infarcted tissue.[323] Endocardial resection involves peeling off a layer of endocardium, generally in the rim of an aneurysm, that has been demonstrated by means of mapping proce-

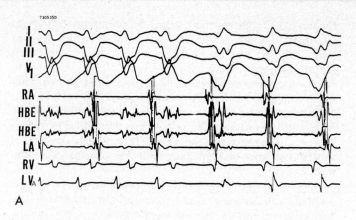

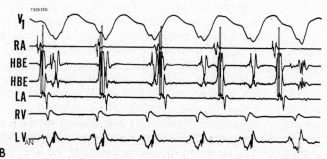

FIGURE 20–8 Spontaneous alteration in QRS contour during ventricular tachycardia. Premature right ventricular stimulation initiated a sustained ventricular tachycardia that initially exhibited a left bundle branch block contour (not shown). The QRS contour during the tachycardia spontaneously changed from left bundle branch block (LBBB) contour to right bundle branch block (RBBB) contour and back again (A). Note that ventricular activation recorded from the left ventricular apex during the RBBB contour tachycardia preceded right ventricular activation (*left*), but that left ventricular activation occurred after right ventricular activation during the LBBB contour tachycardia (*right*). Interpretation of these recordings might suggest that the tachycardia changed its site of origin from the left ventricle during the RBBB contour tachycardia to the right ventricle during the LBBB contour tachycardia. However, repositioning the catheter in the left ventricle to an area near the patient's ventricular aneurysm revealed that even during the LBBB contour tachycardia, an early site of activation in the left ventricle could be located, suggesting that the site of origin remained in the left ventricle and that the impulse simply exited in a different fashion to produce a change in the QRS complex[318] (B). I, II, III, and V_1 = scalar leads; RA = right atrial electrogram; HBE = His bundle electrogram; LA = left atrial electrogram via the coronary sinus; RV = right ventricular apical electrogram; LVA = left ventricular apical electrogram; LVAN = left ventricular electrogram near aneurysm.

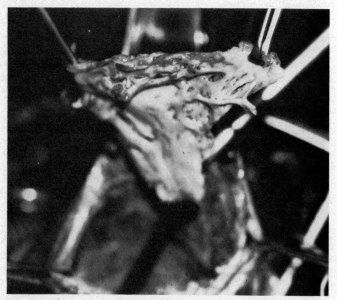

FIGURE 20–7 Endocardial resection. A piece of endocardium resected from the left ventricle in a patient with drug-resistant recurrent ventricular tachycardia. (Surgery was performed by John W. Brown, M.D.)

dures to be the site of earliest activation recorded during the ventricular tachycardia (Fig. 20–7). This resection procedure may cause less disruption to the left ventricular wall than does the encircling endocardial ventriculotomy. Tachycardias arising from the papillary muscles cannot be approached in this fashion,[324] and the papillary muscle may need to be resected if the tachycardia arises in that area. Overall operative mortality for encircling ventriculotomy is slightly higher (13 per cent) than for endocardial resection (7 per cent), and the success rate with endocardial resection is somewhat higher compared to that of encircling endocardial ventriculotomy.[322] However, the number of patients treated with both procedures is still fairly small. Ablative procedures involving ventriculotomy and cryosurgery are mentioned below.

Electrophysiological mapping to find the site of earliest

recorded activation during the ventricular tachycardia is generally used to pinpoint the area to be resected. To obtain a map preoperatively, catheters are positioned at multiple right and left ventricular sites and fluoroscopy directed in several planes establishes their anatomical position. Stable catheter positions are generally at the right ventricular apex, in the His bundle area, and often in the coronary sinus to provide reference electrograms and anatomical reference points to the septum (catheter at the right ventricular apex) and the posterobasal portion of the heart (coronary sinus catheter)[317,325] (Fig. 20–8). Tachycardias that are too rapid, short in duration, or pleomorphic cannot be accurately mapped. In such situations, administering a drug such as procainamide may slow the ventricular tachycardia and transform a nonsustained pleomorphic ventricular tachycardia into a sustained ventricular tachycardia of uniform contour that can be mapped.

Ventricular mapping is also performed at the time of surgery[306] using a handheld electrode moved from site to site. The activation time recorded by this electrode and its anatomical position are compared to the activation time recorded by stationary or reference electrodes fixed at particular positions on the right and left ventricles. The sequence of activation during ventricular tachycardia can then be plotted and the area of earliest activation determined (Figs. 20–9 and 20–10). Using a handheld probe, the ventricular tachycardia must be stable and of uniform configuration, generally for several hundred cycles. Recording from multiple sites simultaneously, coupled with

on-line computer techniques that instantaneously provide an activation map cycle-by-cycle, reduces the time necessary to generate an activation sequence map and will greatly speed and simplify intraoperative mapping. *Cryothermal mapping and ablation* has also been used to confirm the site of origin of a ventricular arrhythmia and then to destroy it. A cryoprobe is cooled to 0°C and its influence on the arrhythmia is noted. If it terminates the tachycardia, the temperature is reduced to −60°C and the area frozen.[326]

Several points are worthy of emphasis. Recording electrical activity in damaged tissue may produce broad, low-amplitude electrograms that may originate from the tissue being sampled or from more distant sites; their onset is difficult to measure accurately. Timing of propagation may be distorted because of changing conduction velocities as the wavefront enters specialized conducting tissue, large muscle bundles, or damaged tissue. During ventricular tachycardia, the origin of the arrhythmia is generally ascribed to electrical activity recorded 25 to 50 msec in advance of the QRS complex. However, that is an arbitrary value, and it is quite clear that such activity may be late following the preceding cycle or early in advance of the next cycle. In addition, when such activity is recorded well after termination of the QRS complex, it becomes difficult to determine with certainty whether the deflections represent depolarization or repolarization. Potentials recorded *prior* to the onset of the surface QRS complex suggest that the origin of the tachycardia is nearby. When the earliest

FIGURE 20–9 Intraoperative mapping for ventricular tachycardia. *A,* One beat of a ventricular tachycardia, as displayed in leads I, II, and III, is shown. Stationary reference electrodes have been sewn on the right ventricular (RV) and left ventricular (LV) epicardium. A handheld exploring electrode reveals that the earliest site of ventricular activation is recorded at site 4, 75 msec in advance of the QRS complex (dotted line). Site 11 (shown below) was activated 27 msec after onset of the QRS complex. Site 4 was resected and the ventricular tachycardia could no longer be initiated. *B,* Postoperatively the patient once again developed ventricular tachycardia but with a different contour (leads II and III). Surgery was repeated and mapping now illustrates that electrical activity was recorded first at site 11, 80 msec in advance of the QRS complex, while activity at site 4 occurred 40 msec after the onset of the QRS complex. Site 11 was resected, and this second form of ventricular tachycardia could no longer be initiated. The patient was discharged without antiarrhythmic drug therapy, with no recurrence of ventricular tachycardia during a follow-up period of one year. (Mapping was performed with the help of John W. Brown, M.D., Eric N. Prystowsky, M.D., and James J. Heger, M.D.)

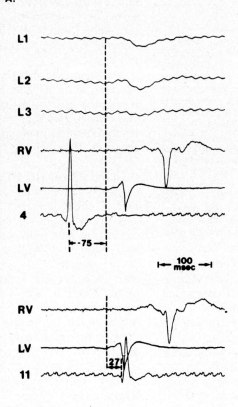

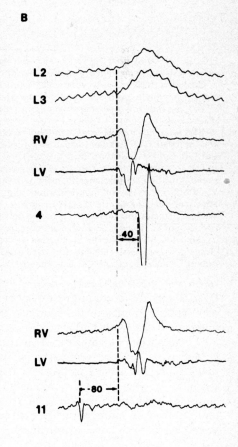

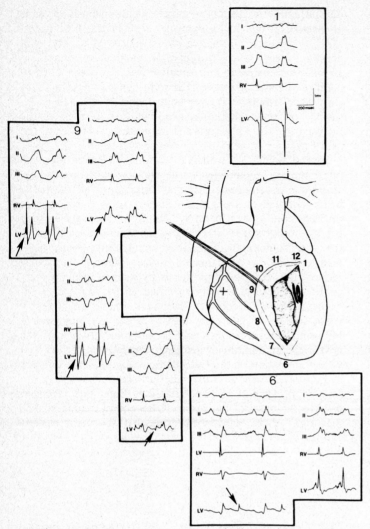

FIGURE 20–10 Partial activation map during ventricular tachycardia. A left ventricular aneurysm has been opened and numbered in a clockwise fashion. Left ventricular endocardial recordings (LV) from a handheld exploring electrode are shown in the inserts for sites 1, 6, and 9. A stationary right ventricular epicardial electrode (RV) has been sewn in place (+ on right ventricle). Ventricular tachycardia with four different contours (see surface leads, insert 9) was initiated. The left ventricular endocardial recordings at site 9 showed earliest activation during each ventricular tachycardia (arrows). Left ventricular recordings at site 6 (right portion of insert 6) show activation starting later than the left ventricular recordings at site 9 but before the left ventricular recording at site 1, which is relatively normal and late in the QRS complex. However, during sinus rhythm (left portion of insert 6), recording at site 6 shows a split, late potential (arrow). Endocardial resection was carried out between sites 6 and 9 with elimination of ventricular tachycardia. (Tracings have been redrawn for clarity.) (Study performed with Robert L. Rinkenberger, M.D., and Robert Kiny, M.D.)

recordable electrical activity occurs *after* the onset of the QRS complex, the site of origin may be in the interventricular septum (similar to the concepts discussed concerning mapping in the Wolff-Parkinson-White syndrome).

It is important to emphasize that the area of earliest recorded activity during ventricular tachycardia may not actually represent the site of origin of the tachycardia, since the latter may originate several centimeters away, for example in a small scarred area, and conduct very slowly until it reaches more normally excitable tissue where it generates a recordable extracellular complex. However,

this area of early activation is probably closely related to the origin of the tachycardia and, based on our present state of knowledge and results from surgery, warrants surgical intervention at that site. Finding an area of "continuous electrical activity"[327] does not necessarily mean that reentry is present or that this is the origin of the tachycardia, since similar activity can be produced by automatically discharging foci; by recording slowly propagating, overlapping, or fragmented wavefronts from several areas;[328,329] or by recording repolarization activity. However, it is likely that the origin of the tachycardia is close by. Of interest is that the site of epicardial breakthrough may be distant from the earliest area of recordable endocardial activity,[317,325,325a] further emphasizing the need for endocardial mapping.

Mapping during sinus rhythm allows one to detect abnormal areas evidenced by delayed activation, fragmentation, abnormal Q waves, delayed potentials, and potentials with decreased voltage and very slow conduction.[325] This technique may also be useful to demonstrate that areas of early activation during ventricular tachycardia represent late activation during sinus rhythm.[319] Whether such abnormal electrograms during sinus rhythm can be used to identify patients prone to tachycardia or whether such areas should be resected is not clear.[330] Delayed epicardial potentials recorded during sinus rythm may not adequately localize the origin of the tachycardia in patients with ventricular tachycardia and ischemic heart disease.[325a]

Pace-mapping[331,332] involves stimulation of various ventricular sites to initiate a QRS contour that duplicates the QRS contour of the ventricular tachycardia, thus establishing the apparent site of origin of the arrhythmia. This technique is limited by several methodological problems and by the possibility that conduction arising from the same site of origin may change and produce a QRS contour with a totally different shape[318] and that stimulating a different site may produce QRS complexes of a similar appearance.

It is not clear whether mapping improves the surgical success rate in patients with ischemic heart disease[333–335] as it appears to do in patients with nonischemic heart disease (see below). However, myocardial resection guided by electrophysiological mapping may reduce the amount of tissue removed, thus helping to preserve myocardial contractile function.

NONISCHEMIC HEART DISEASE. In patients who do not have ischemic heart disease, tachycardias can originate in either the right or the left ventricle, and the type and site of origin of the ventricular tachycardia vary according to the underlying heart disease. In patients who have tetralogy of Fallot, ventricular tachycardia may arise in the region of the right ventricular infundibulectomy scar. Patients with arrhythmogenic right ventricular dysplasia[336] have a right ventricular tachycardia and can be treated by a simple ventriculotomy at the apparent site of origin of the ventricular tachycardia or by isolating portions of the right ventricular free wall from the remainder of the heart.[319,322,337,338] Mapping during sinus rhythm and sustained ventricular tachycardia has been successful in localizing ventricular tachycardia in some patients without ischemic heart disease.[338] The overall surgical success rate and low mortality for this group of patients are promising but still need improvement.[319,337,338] Similarly, mapping may help localize the origin of the ventricular tachycardia in some patients with cardiomyopathies.[326]

Patients who have prolonged Q-T or Q-U syndrome are thought to have arrhythmias due to preponderant left stellate sympathetic tone, and accordingly, left stellate ganglionectomy has been useful therapeutically.[129,339] In some patients with mitral valve prolapse and associated ventricular tachycardia, valve replacement may eliminate the tachycardia.[319]

Acknowledgment

For critical review of Chapters 19 and 20, the author thanks Charles Antzelevitch, Ph.D., Anton Becker, M.D., Robert F. Gilmour, Ph.D., James J. Heger, M.D., Eric N. Prystowsky, M.D., Roger Winkle, M.D., Kevin Browne, M.D., Donald Chilson, M.D., Richard Hauer, M.D., and Elwyn Lloyd, M.D. Unflagging secretarial help was provided by Lee Northcutt and Shirley Myers.

References

1. Giardina, E. G. V., and Bigger, J. T., Jr.: Procainamide against reentrant ventricular arrhythmias: Lengthening RV intervals of coupled ventricular premature depolarization as an insight into the mechanism of action of procainamide. Circulation 48:959, 1973.
2. Nattel, S., Pederson, D. H., and Zipes, D. P.: Alterations in regional myocardial distribution and arrhythmogenic effects of aprindine produced by coronary artery occlusion in the dog. Cardiovasc. Res. 15:80, 1981.
3. Heger, J. J., Prystowsky, E. N., and Zipes, D. P.: Clinical choice of antiarrhythmic drugs. In Josephson, M. E. (ed.): Ventricular Tachycardia— Mechanisms and Management. Mt. Kisco, N.Y., Futura Publishing Co., 1982.
4. Shanks, R. G., and Harrison, D. W.: Pharmacokinetic Principles in Cardiac Arrhythmias: A Decade of Progress. Boston, G. K. Hall, 1981, p. 91.
5. Fenster, P. E., and Perrier, D.: Applications of pharmacokinetic principles to cardiovascular drugs. Mod. Conc. Cardiovasc. Dis. 51:91, 1982.
6. Goldstein, A., Arono, W. L., and Kalman, S. M.: Principles of Drug Action. New York, Harper and Row, 1968.
7. Bigger, J. T., Jr.: Management of arrhythmias. In Braunwald, E. (ed.): Heart Disease: A Textbook of Cardiovascular Medicine. Philadelphia, W. B. Saunders Co., 1980, p. 717.
8. Harrison, D. C., Meffin, P. J., and Winkle, R. A.: Clinical pharmacokinetics of antiarrhythmic drugs. Progr. Cardiovasc. Dis. 20:217, 1977.
9. Singh, B. N., and Vaughn Williams, E. M.: A fourth class of antidysrhythmic action? Effects of verapamil on ouabain toxicity, on atrial and ventricular intracellular potentials and on other features of cardiac function. Cardiovasc. Res. 6:109, 1972.
10. DuPuis, B. A., and Vincent, A. C.: Experimental arrhythmia models. Critical study of correlations with arrhythmias observed in clinical practice. Arch. Mal. Coeur 74:17, 1978.
11. Hondeghem, L., and Katzung, B. G.: Test of a model of antiarrhythmic drug action. Effects of quinidine and lidocaine on myocardial conduction. Circulation 61:1217, 1980.
12. Mandel, W. J., and Bigger, T. J., Jr.: Electrophysiological effects of lidocaine on isolated canine and rabbit atrial tissue. J. Pharmacol. Exp. Ther. 178:81, 1971.
13. Bigger, J. T., Jr., and Mandel, W. J.: Effect of lidocaine on the electrophysiological properties of ventricular muscle and Purkinje fibers. J. Clin. Invest. 49:63, 1970.
14. Singh, B. N., and Vaughn Williams, E. M.: Effect of altering potassium concentration on the action of lidocaine and diphenylhydantoin on rabbit atrial and ventricular muscle. Circ. Res. 29:286, 1971.
15. Nattel, S., Elharrar, V., Zipes, D. P., and Bailey, J. C.: The pH dependent electrophysiological effects of quinidine and lidocaine on canine cardiac Purkinje fibers. Circ. Res. 48:55, 1981.
16. Kupersmith, J., Antman, E. M., and Hoffman, B. F.: In vivo electrophysiological effects of lidocaine in canine acute myocardial infarction. Circulation 36:84, 1975.
17. Kupersmith, J.: Electrophysiological and antiarrhythmic effects of lidocaine in canine acute myocardial ischemia. Am. Heart J. 97:360, 1979.
18. El-Sherif, N., Scherlag, B. J., Lazzara, R., and Hope, R. R.: Reentrant ventricular arrhythmias in the late myocardial infarction period. 4. Mechanism of action of lidocaine. Circulation 56:395, 1977.
19. Cardinal, R., Janse, M. J., vanEeden, I., Werner, G., d'Alnoncourt, C. N., and Durrer, D.: The effects of lidocaine on intracellular and extracellular potentials, activation, and ventricular arrhythmias during acute regional ischemia in the isolated porcine heart. Circ. Res. 49:792, 1981.
20. Patterson, E., Gibson, J. K., and Lucchesi, B. R.: Electrophysiologic actions of lidocaine in a canine model of chronic myocardial ischemic injury. Arrhythmogenic actions of lidocaine. Circulation 64(Suppl. IV):123, 1981.
21. Gilmour, R. F., Jr., and Zipes, D. P.: Electrophysiological response of vascularized hamster cardiac transplants to ischemia. Circ. Res. 50:599, 1982.
22. Rosen, M. R., Merker, C., and Pippenger, C. E.: The effects of lidocaine on the canine ECG and electrophysiologic properties of Purkinje fibers. An effect on steady state sodium currents? Am. Heart J. 91:191, 1976.
23. Colatsky, I.: Mechanisms of action of lidocaine and quinidine on action potential duration in rabbit cardiac Purkinje fibers. Circ. Res. 50:17, 1982.
24. Arnsdorf, M. F., and Bigger, J. T., Jr.: Effect of lidocaine hydrochloride on membrane conductance in mammalian cardiac Purkinje fibers. J. Clin. Invest. 51:2252, 1972.
25. Badui, E., Gracia-Rubi, D., and Estanol, B.: Inadvertent massive lidocaine overdose causing temporary complete heart block in myocardial infarction. Am. Heart J. 102:801, 1981.
26. Kuo, C. S., and Reddy, C. P.: Effect of lidocaine on escape rate in patients with complete atrioventricular block. B. Proximal His bundle block. Am. J. Cardiol. 47:1315, 1981.
27. Ruskin, J. N., Akhtar, M., Damato, A. N., and Foster, J. R.: The effect of lidocaine on reentry within the His-Purkinje system in man. Circulation 62:388, 1980.
28. Miller, B. D., Mark, A. L., and Thames, M. D.: Inhibition of cardiac sympathetic nerve activity with intravenous administration of lidocaine. Circulation 64(Suppl. IV):288, 1981.
29. Gilmour, R. F., Jr., Maesaka, J. F., Morrical, D. G., and Zipes, D. P.: Tetrodotoxin exacerbates ischemia-induced electrogram changes in the dog. Circulation 64(Suppl. IV):192, 1981.
30. Neis, A. S., Shand, D. G., and Wilkinson, G. R.: Altered hepatic blood flow and drug disposition. Clin. Pharmacokinetics 1:135, 1976.
31. Prescott, L. F., Adjepon-Yamoah, K. K., and Talbot, R. G.: Impaired lidocaine metabolism in patients with myocardial infarction and cardiac failure. Br. Med. J. 2:939, 1976.
32. Lie, K. I., Leim, K. L., Louridtz, W. J., Janse, M. J., Willebrands, A. F., and Durrer, D.: Efficacy of lidocaine preventing primary ventricular fibrillation within one hour after a 300 mg intramuscular injection. A double-blind randomized study of 300 hospitalized patients with acute myocardial infarction. Am. J. Cardiol. 43:486, 1978.
33. Nattel, S., and Zipes, D. P.: Clinical pharmacology of old and new antiarrhythmic drugs. Cardiovasc. Res. 11:221, 1980.
34. Josephson, M. E., Kitchen, J. G., III, and Kastor, J. A.: Lidocaine and Wolff-Parkinson-White syndrome with atrial flutter. Ann. Intern. Med. 84:44, 1976.
35. Akhtar, M., Gilbert, C. J., and Shenasa, M.: Effect of lidocaine on atrioventricular response via the accessory pathway in patients with Wolff-Parkinson-White syndrome. Circulation 63:435, 1981.
36. Haynes, R. E., Chinn, T. L., Copass, M. K., and Cobb, L. A.: Comparison of bretylium tosylate and lidocaine in management of out-of-hospital ventricular fibrillation: A randomized clinical trial. Am. J. Cardiol. 48:353, 1981.
37. Lie, K. I., Wellens, H. J., VanCapelle, F. J., and Durrer, D.: Lidocaine in the prevention of primary ventricular fibrillation. A double-blind randomized study of 212 consecutive patients. N. Engl. J. Med. 291:132, 1974.
38. Pentecost, B. L., deGiovanni, J. V., Lamb, P., Cadigan, P. J., Evemy, K. L., and Flint, E. J.: Reappraisal of lignocaine therapy in management of myocardial infarction. Br. Heart J. 45:42, 1981.
39. DeSilva, R. A., Hennekens, C. H., Lown, B., and Casscells, W.: Lignocaine prophylaxis an acute myocardial infarction: An evaluation of randomized trials. Lancet 2:855, 1981.
40. Harrison, D. C.: Should lidocaine be administered routinely to all patients after acute myocardial infarction? Circulation 58:581, 1978.
41. Mirro, M. J., Watanabe, A. M., and Bailey, J. C.: Electrophysiologic effects of the optical isomers of disopyramide and quinidine in the dog: Dependence on stereochemistry. Circ. Res. 48:867, 1981.
42. Mason, J. W., Winkle, R. A., Rider, A. K., Stinson, E. E., and Harrison, D. C.: The electrophysiologic effects of quinidine in the transplanted human heart. J. Clin. Invest. 59:481, 1977.
43. Mirro, M. J., Manalan, A. S., Bailey, J. C., and Watanabe, A. M.: Anticholinergic effects of disopyramide and quinidine on guinea pig myocardium: Mediation by direct muscarinic receptor blockade. Circ. Res. 47:855, 1980.
44. Hoffman, B. F., Rosen, M. R., and Wit, A. L.: Electrophysiology and pharmacology of cardiac arrhythmias. VII: Cardiac effects of quinidine and procainamide. Am. Heart J. 89:804, 1975.
45. Mirro, M. J., Watanabe, A. M., and Bailey, J. C.: Electrophysiological effects of disopyramide and quinidine on guinea pig atria and canine cardiac Purkinje fibers: Dependence on underlying cholinergic tone. Circ. Res. 46:660, 1980.
46. Weld, F. M., Coromilas, J., Rothman, J. N., and Bigger, J. T., Jr.: Mechanisms of quinidine-induced depression of maximum upstroke velocity in bovine cardiac Purkinje fibers. Circ. Res. 50:369, 1982.
47. Mason, J. W., and Winkle, R. A.: Electrode-catheter arrhythmia induction in the selection and assessment of antiarrhythmic drug therapy for recurrent ventricular tachycardia. Circulation 58:971, 1978.
48. Wu, D., Hung, J. S., Kuo, C. T., Hsu, K. S., and Shieh, W. B.: Effects of quinidine on atrioventricular nodal reentrant paroxysmal tachycardia. Circulation 64:823, 1981.
49. Wellens, H. J. J., and Durrer, D.: Effect of procainamide, quinidine and ajmaline in the Wolff-Parkinson-White syndrome. Circulation 50:114, 1974.
50. Rasmussen, K., Wang, H., and Fausa, D.: Comparative efficiency of quinidine

and verapamil in the maintenance of sinus rhythm after DC conversion of atrial fibrillation. A controlled clinical trial. Acta Med. Scand. 645(Suppl.):23, 1981.

51. Ruskin, J. N., DiMarco, J. P., and Garan, H.: Out-of-hospital cardiac arrest: Electrophysiologic observations and selection of long-term antiarrhythmic therapy. N. Engl. J. Med. 303:607, 1980.

52. Myerburg, R. J., Conde, C. A., Sheps, D. S., Appel, R. A., Kiem, I., Sung, R. J., and Castellanos, A.: Antiarrhythmic drug therapy in survivors of pre-hospital cardiac arrest: Comparison of effects on chronic ventricular arrhythmias and recurrent cardiac arrest. Circulation 59:855, 1979.

53. DiMarco, J. P., Garan, H., and Ruskin, J. N.: Efficacy of quinidine in the treatment of ventricular arrhythmias: The role of electrophysiologic testing. Circulation 64(Suppl. IV):38, 1981.

54. Cohen, I. S., Jick, H., and Cohen, S. I.: Adverse reactions to quinidine in hospitalized patients: Findings based on data from the Boston Collaborative Drug Surveillance Program. Progr. Cardiovasc. Dis. 20:151, 1977.

55. Selzer, A., and Wray, H. W.: Quinidine syncope: Paroxysmal ventricular fibrillation occurring during treatment of chronic atrial arrhythmias. Circulation 30:17, 1964.

56. Denes, P., Gabster, A., and Huang, S. K.: Clinical electrocardiographic and followup observations in patients having ventricular fibrillation during Holter monitoring. Role of quinidine therapy. Am. J. Cardiol. 48:9, 1981.

57. Smith, W. M., and Gallagher, J. J.: "Les torsades de pointes": An unusual ventricular arrhythmia. Ann. Intern. Med. 93:578, 1980.

58. Ejvinsson, G., and Orinius, E.: Prodromal ventricular premature beats preceded by a diastolic wave. Acta Med. Scand. 208:445, 1980.

59. Schenck-Gustafsson, K., Jogestrand, T., Nordlander R., and Dahlquis, T. R.: Effect of quinidine on digoxin concentration skeletal muscle and serum in patients with atrial fibrillation. Evidence for reduced binding of digoxin in muscle. N. Engl. J. Med. 305:209, 1981.

60. Ball, W. J., Jr., Tse-Eng, D., Wallick, E. T., Bilezikian, J. P., Schwartz, A., and Butler, V. P., Jr.: Effect of quinidine on the digoxin receptor in vitro. J. Clin. Invest. 68:1065, 1981.

61. Mautz, F. R.: Reduction of cardiac irritability by epicardial and systemic administration of drugs as a protection in cardiac surgery. J. Thorac. Surg. 5:612, 1936.

62. Mark, L. C., Kayden, H. J., Steele, J. M., Cooper, J. R., Berlin, I., Rovenstein, E. A., and Brodie, B. B.: The physiological disposition and cardiac effects of procainamide. J. Pharmacol. Exp. Ther. 102:5, 1951.

63. Moe, G. K., and Abildskov, J. A.: Antiarrhythmic drugs. In Goodman, L. S., and Gilman, A. (eds.): The Pharmacological Basis of Therapeutics. New York, MacMillan, 1975, p. 694.

64. Myerburg, R. J., Bassett, A. L., Epstein, K., Gaide, M. S., Kozlovskis, P., Wong, S. S., Castellanos, A., and Gelband, H.: Electrophysiological effects of procainamide in acute and healed experimental ischemic injury of cat myocardium. Circ. Res. 50:386, 1982.

65. Michelson, E. L., Spear, J. F., and Moore, E. N.: Effects of procainamide on strength interval relations in normal and chronically infarcted canine myocardium. Am. J. Cardiol. 47:1223, 1981.

66. Dangman, K. H., and Hoffman, B. F.: In vivo and in vitro antiarrhythmic and arrhythmogenic effects of N-acetylprocainamide. J. Pharmacol. Exp. Ther. 217:851, 1981.

67. Jaillon, P., and Winkle, R. A.: Electrophysiologic comparative study of procainamide and N-acetylprocainamide in anesthetized dogs: Concentration response relationships. Circulation 60:1385, 1979.

68. Giardina, E. G., Fenster, P., Paul, E., Bigger, J. T., Jr., Mayersohn, M., Perrier, D., and Marcus, F. I.: Efficacy, plasma concentrations and adverse effects of a new sustained release procainamide preparation. Am. J. Cardiol. 46:855, 1980.

69. Roden, D. M., Reele, S. B., Higgins, S. B., Wilkinson, G. R., Smith, R. F., Oates, J. A., and Woosley, R. L.: Antiarrhythmic efficacy, pharmacokinetics and safety of N-acetylprocainamide in human subjects: Comparison with procainamide. Am. J. Cardiol. 46:463, 1980.

70. Kluger, J., Leech, S., Reidenberg, M. M., Lloyd, V., and Drayer, D. E.: Long-term antiarrhythmic therapy with acetylprocainamide. Am. J. Cardiol. 48:1124, 1981.

71. Greenspan, A. M., Horowitz, L. N., Spielman, S. R., and Josephson, M. E.: Large dose procainamide therapy for ventricular tachycardia. Am. J. Cardiol. 46:453, 1980.

72. Horowitz, L. N., Josephson, M. E., Farshidi, A., Spielman, S. R., Michelson, E. L., and Greenspan, A. M.: Recurrent sustained ventricular tachycardia. 3. Role of the electrophysiologic study in selection of antiarrhythmic regimens. Circulation 58:986, 1978.

73. Boccardo, D., Pitchon, R., and Wiener, I.: Adverse reactions and efficacy of high dose procainamide therapy in resistant tachyarrhythmias. Am. Heart J. 102:797, 1981.

74. Myerburg, R. J., Kessler, K. M., Kiem, I., Pefkaros, K. C., Conde, C. A., Cooper, D., Castellanos, A.: Relationship between plasma levels of procainamide, suppression of premature ventricular complexes and prevention of recurrent ventricular tachycardia. Circulation 64:280, 1981.

75. Halpern, S. W., Ellrodt, G., Singh, B. N., and Mandel, W. J.: Efficacy of intravenous procainamide infusion in converting atrial fibrillation to sinus rhythm. Relation to left atrial size. Br. Heart J. 44:589, 1980.

76. Wu, D., Denes, P., Amat-y-Leon, F., Dhingra, R., Wyndham, C. R. C., Bauernfeind, R., Latif, P., and Rosen, K. M.: Clinical electrocardiographic and electrophysiologic observations in patients with paroxysmal supraventricular tachycardia. Am. J. Cardiol. 41:1045, 1978.

77. Shenasa, M., Gilbert, C. J., Schmidt, D. H., and Akhtar, M.: Procainamide and retrograde atrioventricular nodal conduction in man. Circulation 65:355, 1982.

78. Wellens, H. J. J., Braat, S., Brugada, P., Gorgels, A. P. M., and Bar, F. W.: Use of procainamide in patients with the Wolff-Parkinson-White syndrome to disclose a short refractory period of the accessory pathway. Am. J. Cardiol. 50:1087, 1982.

79. Engel, T. R., Meister, S. G., and Luck, J. C.: Modification of ventricular tachycardia by procainamide in patients with coronary artery disease. Am. J. Cardiol. 46:1033, 1980.

80. Waxman, H. L., Sadowski, L. M., and Josephson, M. E.: Response to procainamide during electrophysiologic study for sustained ventricular tachycardia predicts response to other drugs. Circulation 64(Suppl. IV):87, 1981.

81. Prystowsky, E. N., Heger, J. J., Jackman, W. M., Naccarelli, G. V., and Zipes, D. P.: Incessant supraventriculalr tachycardia following myocardial infarction. Am. Heart J. 103:426, 1982.

82. Strasberg, B., Sclarovsky, S., Erdberg, A., Duffy, C. E., Lan, W., Swiryn, S., Agmon, J., and Rosen, K. M.: Procainamide-induced polymorphous ventricular tachycardia. Am. J. Cardiol. 47:1309, 1981.

83. Goldberg, D., Reiffel, J. A., Davis, J. C., Gang, E., Livelli, F., and Bigger, J. T., Jr.: Electrophysiologic effects of procainamide on sinus node function in patients with and without sinus node disease. Am. Heart J. 103:75, 1982.

84. Ladd, A. T.: Procainamide-induced lupus erythematosus. N. Engl. J. Med. 267:1357, 1962.

85. Kluger, J., Drayer, D. E., Reidenberg, M. M., and Lahita, R.: Acetylprocainamide therapy in patients with previous procainamide induced lupus syndrome. Ann. Intern. Med. 95:18, 1981.

86. Danilo, F., Jr., and Rosen, M. R.: Cardiac effects of disopyramide. Am. Heart J. 92:532, 1976.

87. Frame, L. H., and Hoffman, B. F.: Disopyramide's effects are enhanced by fast pacing rates in depolarized tissue. Circulation 64(Suppl. IV):272, 1981.

88. Sasyniuk, B. I., and Kus, T.: Cellular electrophysiologic changes induced by disopyramide phosphate in normal and infarcted hearts. J. Int. Med. 4:20, 1976.

89. Birkhead, J. S., and Vaughan Williams, E. M.: Dual effect of disopyramide on atrial and atrioventricular conduction and refractory periods. Br. Heart J. 39:657, 1977.

90. Katoh, T., Karagueuzian, H., Jordan, J., and Mandel, W.: The cellular electrophysiologic mechanism of the dual actions of disopyramide on rabbit sinus node function. Circulation 66:1216, 1982.

91. LaBarre, A., Strauss, H. C., Scheinman, M. M., Evans, G. T., Bashore, T., Tiedeman, J. S., and Wallace, A. G.: Electrophysiologic effects of disopyramide phosphate on sinus node function in patients with sinus node dysfunction. Circulation 59:226, 1979.

92. Singh, B. N., Collett, J. T., and Chew, C. Y. C.: New perspectives in the pharmacologic therapy of cardiac arrhythmias. Progr. Cardiovasc. Dis. 22:243, 1980.

93. Morady, F., Scheinman, M. M., and Desai, J.: Disopyramide. Ann. Intern. Med. 96:337, 1982.

94. Timins, B. I., Gutman, J. A., and Haft, J. I.: Disopyramide-induced heart block. Chest 79:477, 1981.

94a. Wilkinson, P. R., Desai, J., Hollister, J., Gonzalez, R., Abbott, J. A., and Scheinman, M. M.: Electrophysiologic effects of disopyramide in patients with atrioventricular nodal dysfunction. Circulation 66:1211, 1982.

95. Kerr, C. R., Prystowsky, E. N., Smith, W. M., Cook, L., and Gallagher, J. J.: Electrophysiological effects of disopyramide phosphate in patients with Wolff-Parkinson-White syndrome. Circulation 65:869, 1982.

96. Leach, A. J., Brown, J. E., and Armstrong, P. W.: Cardiac depression by intravenous disopyramide in patients with left ventricular dysfunction. Am. J. Med. 68:839, 1980.

97. Landmark, K., Bredesen, J. E., Thaulow, E., Simonsen, S., and Amlie, J. P.: Pharmacokinetics of disopyramide in patients with imminent to moderate cardiac failure. Eur. J. Clin. Pharmacol. 19:187, 1981.

98. Hulting, J., and Rosenhamer, G.: Hemodynamic and electrocardiographic effects of disopyramide in patients with ventricular arrhythmia. Acta Med. Scand. 199:41, 1976.

99. Heel, R. C., Brogden, R. N., Speight, T. M., and Avery, G. S.: Disopyramide: A review of its pharmacological properties and therapeutic use in treating cardiac arrhythmias. Drugs 15:331, 1978.

100. Wilcox, R. G., Rowley, J. M., Hampton, J. R., Mitchell, J. R., Roland, J. M., and Banks, D. C.: Randomised placebo-controlled trial comparing oxprenolol with disopyramide phosphate in immediate treatment of suspected myocardial infarction. Lancet 2:765, 1980.

101. Pouleur, H., Chaudron, J. M., and Reyns, P.: Effects of disopyramide and aprindine on arrhythmias after acute myocardial infarction. Eur. J. Cardiol. 5:397, 1977.

102. Breithardt, G., Seipel, L., and Abendroth, R. R.: Comparison of the antiarrhythmic efficacy of disopyramide and mexiletine against stimulus induced ventricular tachycardia. J. Cardiovasc. Pharmacol. 3:1026, 1981.

103. Swiryn, S., Bauernfeind, R. A., Wyndham, C. R. C., Dhingra, R. C., Palileo, E., Strasberg, B., and Rosen, K. M.: Effects of oral disopyramide phosphate on induction of paroxysmal supraventricular tachycardia. Circulation 64:169, 1981.

104. Robertson, C. E., and Miller, H. C.: Extreme tachycardia complicating the use of disopyramide in atrial flutter. Br. Heart J. 44:602, 1980.

105. Dhurandhar, R. W., Nademanee, K., and Goldman, A. M.: Ventricular tachy-

cardia flutter associated with disopyramide therapy: A report of three cases. Heart and Lung 7:783, 1978.

106. Tzivoni, D., Keren, A., Stern, S., and Gottlieb, S.: Disopyramide-induced torsades de pointes. Arch. Intern. Med. 141:946, 1981.

107. Podrid, P. J., Schoeneberger, A., and Lown, B.: Congestive heart failure caused by disopyramide. N. Engl. J. Med. 302:614, 1980.

108. Desai, J. M., Scheinman, M. M., Hirschfeld, D., Gonzalez, R., and Peters, R. W.: Cardiovascular collapse associated with disopyramide therapy. Chest 79:545, 1981.

109. Matos, J. A., Fisher, J. D., and Kim, S. G.: Disopyramide-phenytoin interaction. Circulation 64(Suppl. IV):264, 1981.

110. Ferrier, G. R.: Digitalis arrhythmias: Role of oscillatory afterpotentials. Progr. Cardiovasc. Dis. 19:459, 1977.

111. Rosen, M. R., Danilo, P., Jr., Alonso, M. B., and Pippenger, C. E.: Effects of therapeutic concentrations of diphenylhydantoin on transmembrane potentials of normal and depressed Purkinje fibers. J. Pharmacol. Exp. Ther. 197:594, 1976.

112. Fisch, C., Zipes, D. P., and Noble, R. J.: Digitalis toxicity: Mechanism and recognition. Yu, P., and Goodwin, R. (eds.): Progress in Cardiology 4:37, 1975.

113. Wit, A. L., Rosen, M. R., and Hoffman, B. F.: Electrophysiology and pharmacology of cardiac arrhythmias. VIII. Cardiac effects of diphenylhydantoin. Am. Heart J. 90:397, 1975.

114. Gillis, R. A., McClellan, J. R., Sauer, T. S., and Standaert, F. G.: Depression of cardiac sympathetic nerve activity by diphenylhydantoin. J. Pharmacol. Exp. Ther. 179:599, 1971.

115. Garan, H., Ruskin, J. N., and Powell, W. J., Jr.: Centrally mediated effect of phenytoin on digoxin-induced ventricular arrhythmias. Am. J. Physiol. 241: H67, 1981.

116. Peter, T., Ross, D., Duffield, A., Luxton, M., Harper, R., Hunt, D., and Slowman, G.: Effect on survival after myocardial infarction of long-term treatment with phenytoin. Br. Heart J. 40:1356, 1978.

117. Koch-Weser, J., and Frishman, W. H.: Beta-adrenoreceptor antagonists: New drugs and new indications. N. Engl. J. Med. 305:500, 1981.

118. Lands, A. M., Arnold, A., McAuliff, P., Luduena, F. P., and Brown, T. G., Jr.: Differentiation of receptor systems activated by sympathomimetic amines. Nature 214:597, 1967.

119. Taylor, S. H., Silke, B., and Lee, P. S.: Intravenous beta blockade in coronary heart disease. N. Engl. J. Med. 306:631, 1982.

120. Davis, L. D., and Temte, J. V.: Effects of propranolol on the transmembrane potentials of ventricular muscle and Purkinje fibers of the dog. Circ. Res. 22:661, 1968.

121. Wit, A. L., Hoffman, B. F., and Rosen, M. R.: Electrophysiology and pharmacology of cardiac arrhythmias. IX. Cardiac electrophysiologic effects of beta adrenergic receptor stimulation and blockade (Part B). Am. Heart J. 90:665, 1975.

122. Wit, A. L., Hoffman, B. F., and Rosen, M. R.: Electrophysiology and pharmacology of cardiac arrhythmias. IX. Cardiac electrophysiologic effects of beta adrenergic receptor stimulation and blockade (Part C). Am. Heart J. 90:795, 1975.

123. Josephson, M. E., and Seides, S. F.: Clinical Cardiac Electrophysiology. Philadelphia, Lea and Febiger, 1979, p. 68.

124. Prystowsky, E. N., Jackman, W. M., Rinkenberger, R. L., Heger, J. J., and Zipes, D. P.: Effect of autonomic blockade on ventricular refractoriness and atrioventricular conduction in humans: Evidence supporting a direct cholinergic action on ventricular muscle refractoriness. Circ. Res. 49:511, 1981.

125. Ahnve, S., and Vallin, H.: Influence of heart rate and inhibition of autonomic tone on the QT interval. Circulation 65:435, 1982.

126. Browne, K. F., Zipes, D. P., Heger, J. J., and Prystowsky, E. N.: The influence of the autonomic nervous system on the QT interval. Am. J. Cardiol. 49:898, 1982.

127. Alexander, R. W., Williams, L. T., and Lefkowitz, R. T.: Identification of cardiac beta adrenergic receptors by (−) [3H] alprenol binding. Proc. Natl. Acad. Sci. (USA) 72:1564, 1975.

128. Nies, A. S., and Shand, D. G.: Clinical pharmacology of propranolol. Circulation 52:6, 1975.

129. Moss, A. J., and Schwartz, P. J.: Delayed repolarization (QT or QTU prolongation) and malignant ventricular arrhythmias. Mod. Conc. Cardiovasc. Dis. 51:85, 1982.

130. Barlow, J. B., and Pocock, W. A.: Mitral valve prolapse, the specific billowing mitral valve leaflet syndrome, or an insignificant non-ejection systolic click. Am. Heart J. 97:227, 1979.

131. Multicentre International Study: Improvement in prognosis of myocardial infarction by long-term beta-adrenoceptor blockade using practolol: A multicentre international study. Br. Med. J. 3:735, 1977.

132. Ahlmark, G., and Saetre, H.: Long-term treatment with beta blockers after myocardial infarction. Eur. J. Pharmacol. 10:77, 1976.

133. Wilhelmsen, C., Wilhelmsen, L., and Vedin, J. A.: Reduction of sudden death after myocardial infarction by treatment with alprenolol. Lancet 2:1157, 1974.

134. Beta Blocker Heart Attack Study Group: The beta blocker heart attack trial. J.A.M.A. 246:2073, 1981.

135. Hjalmarson, A.: Effect on mortality of metoprolol in acute myocardial infarction: A double-blind randomized trial. Lancet 2:823, 1981.

136. The Norwegian Multicentre Study Group: Timolol-induced reduction in mortality and reinfarction in patients surviving acute myocardial infarction. N. Engl. J. Med. 304:801, 1981.

136a. Gundersen, T., Abrahamsen, A. M., Kjekshus, J., and Rønnevik, P. K. for the Norwegian Multicenter Study Group: Timolol-related reduction in mortality and reinfarction in patients ages 65-75 years surviving acute myocardial infarction. Circulation 66:1179, 1982.

137. Miller, R. R., Olson, H. G., Amsterdam, E. A. L., and Mason, D. T.: Propranolol withdrawal rebound phenomenon. N. Engl. J. Med. 293:416, 1975.

138. Nattel, S., Rango, R. E., and Vanloon, G.: Mechanism of propranolol withdrawal phenomenon. Circulation 59:1158, 1979.

139. Gillis, R. A., Clancy, M. M., and Anderson, R. J.: The deleterious effects of bretylium in cats with digitalis-induced ventricular tachycardia. Circulation 47:976, 1973.

140. Waxman, M. B., and Wallace, A. G.: Electrophysiologic effects of bretylium tosylate on the heart. J. Pharmacol. Exp. Ther. 183:264, 1972.

141. Bacaner, M. B.: Bretylium tosylate for suppression of induced ventricular fibrillation. Am. J. Cardiol. 17:528, 1966.

142. Cardinal, R., Sasyniuk, D. I., Electrophysiological effects of bretylium tosylate in subendocardial Purkinje fibers from infarcted canine hearts. J. Pharmacol. Exp. Ther. 204:159, 1978.

143. Patterson, E., Gibson, J. K., and Lucchesi, B. R.: Prevention of chronic canine ventricular tachyarrhythmias with bretylium tosylate. Circulation 64:1045, 1981.

144. Anderson, J. L., Patterson, E., Wagner, J. G., Johnson, T. A., Lucchesi, B. R., and Pitt, B.: Clinical pharmacokinetics of intravenous and oral bretylium tosylate in survivors of ventricular tachycardia or fibrillation: Clinical application of a new assay for bretylium. J. Cardiovasc. Pharmacol. 3:485, 1981.

145. Holder, D. A., Sniderman, A. D., Fraser, G., and Fallen, E. L.: Experience with bretylium tosylate by a hospital cardiac arrest team. Circulation 55:541, 1977.

146. Cohen, H. C., Gozo, E. G., Jr., Langendorf, R., Kaplan, B. M., Chan, A., Pick, A., and Glick, G.: Response of resistant ventricular tachycardia to bretylium: Relation to site of ectopic focus and location of myocardial disease. Circulation 47:331, 1973.

147. Zipes, D. P., and Troup, P. J.: New antiarrhythmic agents. Am. J. Cardiol. 41:1005, 1978.

148. Cranefield, P. F.: The Conduction of the Cardiac Impulse. Mt. Kisco, N.Y., Futura Publishing Co., 1975.

149. Zipes, D. P., Bailey, J. C., and Elharrar, V.: The Slow Inward Current and Cardiac Arrhythmias. The Hague, Martinus Nijhoff, 1980.

150. Antman, E. M., Stone, P. H., Mueller, J. E., and Braunwald, E.: Calcium channel blocking agents in the treatment of cardiovascular disorders. Ann. Intern. Med. 93:875, 1980.

151. Henry, P. D.: Comparative pharmacology of calcium antagonists: Nifedipine, verapamil, and diltiazem: Am. J. Cardiol. 46:1047, 1980.

152. Lathrop, D. A., Valle-Aguilera, J. R., Millard, R. W., Gaum, W. E., Hannon, D. W., Francis, P. D., Nakaya, H., and Schwartz, A.: Comparative electrophysiologic and coronary hemodynamic effects of diltiazem, nisoldipine and verapamil on myocardial tissue. Am. J. Cardiol. 49:613, 1982.

153. Gilmour, R. F., and Zipes, D. P.: Basic electrophysiology of the slow inward current. In Antman, E. M., and Stone, P. H.: Cardiac Arrhythmias. Mt. Kisco, N. Y., Futura Publishing Co. (in press).

154. Cranefield, P. F., Aaronson, R. S., and Wit, A. L.: Effect of verapamil on the normal action potential and on a calcium dependent slow response of canine cardiac Purkinje fibers. Circ. Res. 34:204, 1974.

155. Rosen, M. R., Wit, A. L., and Hoffman, B. F.: Electrophysiology and pharmacology of cardiac arrhythmias. VI. Cardiac effects of verapamil. Am. Heart J. 89:665, 1975.

156. Hordof, A. J., Edie, R., Malm, J. R., Hoffman, B. F., and Rosen, M. R.: Electrophysiologic properties and response to pharmacologic agents of fibers from diseased human atria. Circulation 54:774, 1976.

157. Spear, J. F., Horowitz, L. N., and Moore, E. N.: The slow response in human ventricle. In Zipes, D. P., Bailey, J. C., and Elharrar, V. (eds.): The Slow Inward Current and Cardiac Arrhythmias. The Hague, Martinus Nijhoff, 1980, p. 309.

158. Gilmour, R. F., Jr., Heger, J. J., Prystowsky, E. N., and Zipes, D. P.: Cellular electrophysiological abnormalities of diseased human ventricular myocardium. Am. J. Cardiol. (in press).

159. Zipes, D. P., and Mendez, C.: Action of manganese ions and tetrodotoxin on atrioventricular nodal transmembrane potentials in isolated rabbit hearts. Circ. Res. 32:447, 1973.

160. Zipes, D. P., and Fischer, J. C.: Effects of agents which inhibit the slow channel on sinus node automaticity and atrioventricular conduction in the dog. Circ. Res. 34:184, 1974.

161. Yamagishi, S.: Effects of tetrodotoxin on the pacemaker action potential of the sinus node. Proc. Jap. Acad. Sci. 42:1194, 1966.

162. Lenfant, J., Mironneau, J., and Gargouil, Y. M.: Analyse de l'activité electrique spontanée de centre de l'automatisme cardiaque de lapin par les inhibiteurs de permeabilités membranaires. CR Acad. Sci. [D] Paris 266:901, 1968.

163. Rougier, O., Vassort, G., and Garnier, D.: Existence and role of the slow inward current during the frog atrial action potential. Pfluegers Arch. 308:91, 1969.

164. Wit, A. L., and Cranefield, P. F.: Effect of verapamil on the sinoatrial and atrioventricular nodes of the rabbit and the mechanism by which it arrests reentrant atrioventricular nodal tachycardia. Circ. Res. 35:413, 1974.

165. Okada, T.: Effect of verapamil on electrical activities of SA node, ventricular muscle and Purkinje fibers in isolated rabbit hearts. Jap. Circ. J. 40:329, 1976.

166. Naylor, W. G., and Szeto, J.: Effect of verapamil on contractility, oxygen utili-

zation, and calcium exchange ability in mammalian heart muscle. Cardiovasc. Res. 6:120, 1972.

167. Zipes, D. P., and Gilmour, R. F.: Calcium antagonists and their potential role in the prevention of sudden coronary death. Ann. NY Acad. Sci. 382:258, 1982.

168. Wellens, H. J. J., Tan, S. L., Bär, F. W. H., Duren, D. R., Lie, K. I., and Dohmen, H. M.: Effects of verapamil studied by programmed electrical stimulation of the heart in patients with paroxysmal reentrant supraventricular tachycardia. Br. Heart J. 39:1058, 1977.

169. Breidthardt, G., Seipel, L., and Wiebringhaus, E.: Dual effect of verapamil on sinus node function in man. In Bonke, F.I.M. (ed.): The Sinus Node. The Hague, Martinus Nijhoff, 1978, p. 129.

170. Spurrell, R. A. J., Krikler, D. M., and Sowton, E.: Effects of verapamil on electrophysiological properties of anomalous atrioventricular connection in Wolff-Parkinson-White syndrome. Br. Heart J. 36:256, 1974.

171. Rinkenberger, R. L., Prystowsky, E. N., Heger, J. J., Troup, P. J., Jackman, W. M., and Zipes, D. P.: Effects of intravenous and chronic oral verapamil administration in patients with supraventricular tachyarrhythmias. Circulation 62:996, 1980.

172. Matsuyama, E., Konishi, T., Okazaki, H., Matsuda, H., Kawai, C.: Effects of verapamil on accessory pathway properties and induction of circus movement tachycardia in patients with the Wolff-Parkinson-White syndrome. J. Cardiovasc. Pharmacol. 3:11, 1981.

173. Gulamhusein, S., Ko, P., Carruthers, S. G., and Klein, G. J.: Acceleration of the ventricular response during atrial fibrillation in the Wolff-Parkinson-White syndrome after verapamil. Circulation 65:348, 1982.

174. Kieval, J., Kirsten, E. B., Kessler, K. M., Mallon, S. M., and Myerburg, R. J.: The effects of intravenous verapamil on hemodynamic status of patients with coronary artery disease receiving propranolol. Circulation 65:653, 1982.

175. Packer, M., Mellen, J., Medina, N., Yushak, M., Smith, H., Holt, J., Guerrero, J., Todd, G. D., McAllister, R. G., and Gorlin, R.: Hemodynamic consequences of combined beta-adrenergic and slow calcium channel blockade in man. Circulation 65:660, 1982.

176. Reimer, K. A., Lowe, J. E., and Jennings, R. B.: The effects of calcium antagonist verapamil on necrosis following temporary coronary artery occlusion in dogs. Circulation 55:581, 1977.

177. Clusin, W. T., Bristow, M. R., Baim, D. S., Schroeder, J. S., Jaillon, P., Brett, P., and Harrison, D. C.: The effects of diltiazem and reduced serum ionized calcium on ischemic ventricular fibrillation in the dog. Circ. Res. 50:518, 1982.

178. Elharrar V., Goum, W. E., and Zipes, D. P.: Effects of various drugs on antiarrhythmias during acute myocardial ischemia. Am. J. Cardiol. 37:134, 1976.

179. Krikler, D. M.: Verapamil in cardiology. Eur. J. Cardiol. 2:3, 1974.

180. Puech, P.: Dissection de la Conduction Sinoventriculaire pour l'Etude du Verapamil Injectable. Montpellier, Centre Hospitalier, 1972.

181. Mangiardi, L. M., Hariman, R. J., McAllister, R. G., Bhargava, V., Surawicz, B., and Shabetai, R.: Electrophysiologic and hemodynamic effects of verapamil. Circulation 57:366, 1978.

182. Sung, R. J., Elser, B., and McAllister, R. G., Jr.: Intravenous verapamil for termination of reentrant supraventricular tachycardias. Intracardiac studies correlated with plasma verapamil concentrations. Ann. Intern. Med. 93:682, 1980.

183. Kates, R. E., Keefe, D. L., Schwartz, J., Harapats, S., Kirsten, E. B., and Harrison, D. C.: Verapamil disposition kinetics in chronic atrial fibrillation. Clin. Pharmacol. Ther. 30:44, 1981.

184. Schomerus, M., Spiegelhalder, B., and Steiren, B.: Physiological disposition of verapamil in man. Cardiovasc. Res. 10:605, 1976.

185. Hamer, A., Peter, T., Platt, M., and Mandel, W. J.: Effects of verapamil on supraventricular tachycardia in patients with overt and concealed Wolff-Parkinson-White syndrome. Am. Heart J. 101:600, 1981.

186. Schamroth, L.: Immediate effects of intravenous verapamil on atrial fibrillation. Cardiovasc. Res. 5:419, 1971.

187. Waxman, H. L., Myerburg, R. J., Appel, R., and Sung, R. J.: Verapamil for control of ventricular rate in paroxysmal supraventricular tachycardia and atrial fibrillation or flutter: A double-blind randomized cross-over study. Ann. Intern. Med. 94:1, 1981.

188. Schwartz, J. B., Keefe, D., Kates, R. E., Kirsten E., and Harrison, D. C.: Acute and chronic pharmacodynamic interaction of verapamil and digoxin in atrial fibrillation. Circulation 65:1163, 1982.

189. Wellens, H. J. J., Farre, J., and Bär, F. W.: The role of the slow inward current in the genesis of ventricular tachycardias in man. In Zipes, D. P., Bailey, J., and Elharrar, V. (eds.): The Slow Inward Current and Cardiac Arrhythmias. The Hague, Martinus Nijhoff, 1980, p. 507.

190. Benaim, M. E.: Asystole after verapamil. Br. Med. J. 2:169, 1972.

191. Rosenbaum, M. B., Chiale, P. A., Ryba, D., and Elizari, M.: Control of tachyarrhythmias associated with Wolff-Parkinson-White syndrome by amiodarone hydrochloride. Am. J. Cardiol. 34:215, 1974.

192. Rosenbaum, M. B., Chiale, P. A., Halpern, M. S., Nau, G. J., Przybylski, J., Levi, R. J., Lazzari, J. O., and Elizari, M. V.: Clinical efficacy of amiodarone as an antiarrhythmic agent. Am. J. Cardiol. 38:934, 1976.

193. Olsson, S. B., Brorson, L., and Varnauskas, E.: Antiarrhythmic action in man. Observations from monophasic action potential recordings in amiodarone treatment. Br. Heart J. 35:1255, 1973.

194. Wellens, H. J. J., Lie, K. I., Bär, F. W., Wesdorf, J. C., Dohmen, H. J., Duren, D. R., and Durrer, D.: Effect of amiodarone in the Wolff-Parkinson-White syndrome. Am. J. Cardiol. 38:189, 1976.

195. Heger, J. J., Prystowsky, E. N., Jackman, W. M., Naccarelli, G. V., Warfel, K. A., Rinkenberger, R. L., and Zipes, D. P.: Amiodarone: Clinical efficacy and electrophysiology during long-term therapy for recurrent ventricular tachycardia. N. Engl. J. Med. 305:539, 1981.

196. Nademanee, K., Hendrickson, J. A., Cannom, D. S., Goldreyer, B. N., and Singh, B. N.: Control of refractory life-threatening ventricular tachyarrhythmias by amiodarone. Am. Heart J. 101:759, 1981.

197. Haffajee, C., Lesko, L., Kanada, A., and Alpert, J. S.: Clinical pharmacokinetics of amiodarone. Circulation 64(Suppl. IV):263, 1981.

198. Podrid, P. J., and Lown, B.: Amiodarone therapy and symptomatic sustained refractory atrial and ventricular tachyarrhythmias. Am. Heart J. 101:374, 1981.

199. Marcus, F. T., Fontaine, G. H., Frank, R., and Grosgogeat, Y.: Clinical pharmacology and therapeutic applications of the antiarrhythmic agent, amiodarone. Am. Heart J. 101:480, 1981.

200. Coumel, P., and Fidelle, J.: Amiodarone in the treatment of cardiac arrhythmias in children: 135 cases. Am. Heart J. 100:1063, 1980.

201. Hamer, A. W., Finerman, W. B., Jr., Peter, T., and Mandel, W. J.: Disparity between clinical and electrophysiologic effects of amiodarone in the treatment of recurrent ventricular tachyarrhythmias. Am. Heart J. 102:992, 1981.

202. Bashour, T., Jokhadar, M., and Cheng, T. O.: Effective management of the long QT syndrome with amiodarone. Chest 79:704, 1981.

203. Sobel, S. M., and Rakita, L.: Pneumonitis and pulmonary fibrosis associated with amiodarone treatment: A possible complication of a new antiarrhythmic drug. Circulation 65:819, 1982.

204. Elharrar, V., Bailey, J. C., Lathrop, D. A., and Zipes, D. P.: Effects of aprindine HCl on slow channel action potentials and transient depolarizations in canine Purkinje fibers. J. Pharmacol. Exp. Ther. 205:410, 1978.

205. Carmeliet, E., and Verdonck, F.: Effects of aprindine and lidocaine on transmembrane potentials and radioactive K-efflux in different cardiac tissues. Acta Cardiol. Suppl. 18:73, 1974.

206. Gilmour, R. F., Chikharev, V. N., Jurevichus, J. A., Zacharov, S. I., Zipes, D. P., and Rozenshtraukh, L. V.: Effect of aprindine on transmembrane currents and contractile force in frog atria. J. Pharmacol. Exp. Ther. 217:390, 1981.

207. Foster, P. R., King, R. M., Nicoll, A. D., and Zipes, D. P.: Suppression of ouabain-induced ventricular arrhythmias with aprindine HCl. A comparison with other antiarrhythmic agents. Circulation 53:315, 1976.

208. Zipes, D. P., Elharrar, V., Gilmour, R. F., Heger, J. J., and Prystowsky, E. N.: Studies with aprindine. Am. Heart J. 100:1055, 1980.

209. Elharrar, V., Gaum, W. E., and Zipes, D. P.: Effect of drugs on conduction delay and the incidence of ventricular arrhythmias induced by acute coronary occlusion in dogs. Am. J. Cardiol. 39:544, 1977.

210. Van Durme, J. P., Rousseau, M., and Mbuyamba, P.: Treatment of chronic ventricular dysrhythmias with a new drug aprindine (AC1802). Acta Cardiol. (Brux) (Suppl.) 18:335, 1974.

211. Fasola, A. F., Noble, R. J., and Zipes, D. P.: Treatment of recurrent tachycardia and fibrillation with aprindine. Am. J. Cardiol. 39:903, 1977.

212. Strassberg, B., Palileo, E., Prechel, D., Bauernfeind, R., Swiryn, S., Wyndham, C. R., Dhingra, R. C., Kehoe, R., and Rosen, K. M.: Ventricular tachycardia: Prediction of response to oral aprindine with intravenous aprindine. Am. J. Cardiol. 47:676, 1981.

213. Zipes, D. P., Gaum, W. E., Foster, P. R., Rosen, K. M., Wu, D., Amat-y-Leon, F., and Noble, R. J.: Aprindine for treatment of supraventricular tachycardias with particular application to WPW syndrome. Am. J. Cardiol. 40:586, 1977.

214. Troup, P. J., and Zipes, D. P.: Aprindine treatment of recurrent ventricular tachycardia in patients with mitral valve prolapse. Am. Heart J. 97:322, 1979.

215. Scagliotti, D., Strasberg, B., Hai, H., Kehoe, R., and Rosen, K. M.: Aprindine-induced polymorphous ventricular tachycardia. Am. J. Cardiol. 49:1297, 1982.

216. Waleffe, A., Guillaume, D., Mary-Rabine, L., and Kulbertus, H.: The efficacy of intravenous moxaprindine on ventricular ectopic activity. Acta Cardiol. (Brux.) 35:257, 1980.

217. Staessen, J., Kesteloot, H.: Moxaprindine in the acute treatment of ventricular arrhythmias in patients with cardiovascular disease. Eur. J. Clin. Pharmacol. 19:167, 1981.

218. Elharrar, V., and Zipes, D. P.: Effects of encainide metabolites (MJ14030 and MJ19444) on canine cardiac Purkinje and ventricular fibers. J. Pharmacol. Exp. Ther. 220:440, 1982.

219. Jackman, W. M., Zipes, D. P., Naccarelli, G. V., Rinkenberger, R. L., Heger, J. J., and Prystowsky, R. H.: Electrophysiology of oral encainide. Am. J. Cardiol. 49:1270, 1982.

220. Winkle, R. A., Peters, F., Kates, R. E., and Harrison, D. C.: The contribution of encainide metabolites to its long-term antiarrhythmic efficacy. Circulation 64(Suppl. IV):264, 1981.

221. Carey, E. L., Duff, H. J., Roden, D. M., Primm, R. K., Oates, J. A., and Woosley, R. L.: Relative electrocardiographic and antiarrhythmic effects of encainide and its metabolites in man. Circulation 64(Suppl. IV):264, 1981.

222. Harrison, D. C., Winkle, R. A., Sami, M., and Mason, J. W.: Encainide: A new and potent antiarrhythmic agent. In Harrison, D. C. (eds.): Cardiac Arrhythmias: A Decade of Progress. Boston, G. K. Hall, 1981, p. 315.

223. Winkle, R. A., Peters, F., Kates, R. E., Tucker, C., and Harrison, D. C.: Clinical pharmacology and antiarrhythmic efficacy of encainide in patients with chronic ventricular arrhythmias. Circulation 64:290, 1981.

224. Prystowsky, E. N., Klein, G., Rinkenberger, R. L., Heger, J. J., Nacarelli, G. V., and Zipes, D. P.: Clinical efficacy and electrophysiologic effects of encainide in patients with Wolff-Parkinson-White syndrome. Circulation (in press).

225. Roden, D. M., Reele, S. B., Higgins, S. B., Mayol, R. F., Gammans, R. E., Oates, J. A., and Woosley, R. L.: Total suppression of ventricular arrhythmias by encainide. N. Engl. J. Med. 302:877, 1980.

226. Sami, M., Harrison, D. C., Kraemer, H., Houston, N., Shimasaki, C., and DeBusk, R. F.: Antiarrhythmic efficacy of encainide and quinidine: Validation of a model for drug assessment. Am. J. Cardiol. 48:147, 1981.

227. Heger, J. J., Prystowsky, E. N., and Zipes, D. P.: Clinical choice of antiarrhythmic drugs. In Josephson, M. E. (ed.): Ventricular Tachycardia—Mechanisms and Management. Mt. Kisko, N.Y., Futura Publishing Co., 1982.

228. Mason, J. W., and Peters, F. A.: Antiarrhythmic efficacy of encainide in patients with refractory recurrent ventricular tachycardia. Circulation 63:670, 1981.

229. Rinkenberger, R. L., Prystowsky, E. N., Jackman, W. M., Heger, J. J., and Zipes, D. P.: Conversion of nonsustained ventricular tachycardia to sustained ventricular tachycardia during drug therapy as determined by serial electrophysiology studies. Am. Heart J. 103:177, 1982.

230. Winkle, R. A., Mason, J. W., Griffin, J. C., and Ross, D.: Malignant ventricular tachyarrhythmias associated with use of encainide. Am. Heart J. 102:857, 1981.

231. Yamaguchi, I., Singh, B. N., and Mandel, W. J.: Electrophysiological action of mexiletine on isolated rabbit atria and canine ventricular muscle and Purkinje fibers. Cardiovasc. Res. 13:288, 1979.

232. Prescott, L. F., Pottage, A., and Clements, J. A.: Absorption, distribution and elimination of mexiletine. Postgrad. Med. J. 53(Suppl. I):50, 1977.

233. Campbell, N. P. S., Pantridge, J. F., and Adjey, A. A. J.: Mexiletine and the management of ventricular dysrhythmias. Eur. J. Cardiol. 6:245, 1977.

234. Talbot, R. G., Julian, D. G., and Prescott, L. F.: Long-term treatment of ventricular arrhythmias with oral mexiletine. Am. Heart J. 91:58, 1976.

235. Heger, J. J., Nattel, S., Rinkenberger, R. L., and Zipes, D. P.: Mexiletine therapy in 15 patients with a drug-resistant ventricular tachycardia. Am. J. Cardiol. 45:627, 1980.

236. Podrid, P. J., and Lown, B.: Mexiletine for ventricular arrhythmias. Am. J. Cardiol. 47:895, 1981.

237. DiMarco, J. P., Garan, H., and Ruskin, J. N.: Mexiletine for refractory ventricular arrhythmias: Results using serial electrophysiologic testing. Am. J. Cardiol. 47:131, 1981.

238. Waleffe, A., Mary-Rabine, L., Legrand, V., Demoulin, J. C., and Kulbertus, H. E.: Combined mexiletine and amiodarone treatment of refractory recurrent ventricular tachycardia. Am. Heart J. 100:788, 1980.

239. Campbell, N. P. S., Pantridge, J. F., and Adgey, A. A. J.: Long-term oral antiarrhythmic therapy with mexiletine. Br. Heart J. 40:796, 1978.

240. Cocco, G., Strozzi, C., Chu, D., and Pansini, R.: Torsades de pointes as a manifestation of mexiletine toxicity. Am. Heart J. 100:878, 1980.

241. Horowitz, L. N., Josephson, M. E., and Farshidi, A.: Human electropharmacology of tocainide, a lidocaine congener. Am. J. Cardiol. 42:276, 1978.

242. Winkle, R. A., Meffin, P. J., and Harrison, D. C.: Long-term tocainide therapy for ventricular arrhythmias. Circulation 57:1008, 1978.

243. Michael, R. A., Neffin, P. J., Fitzgerald, J. W., and Harrison, D. C.: Clinical efficacy and pharmacokinetics of a new orally effective antiarrhythmic, tocainide. Circulation 54:884, 1976.

244. Woosley, R. L., McDivitt, D. G., Nies, A. S., Smith, R. F., Wilkinson, G. R., and Oates, J. A.: Suppression of ventricular ectopic depolarizations by tocainide. Circulation 56:980, 1977.

245. Roden, D. M., Reele, S. B., Higgins, S. B., Carr, R. K., Smith, R. F., Oates, J. A., and Woosley, R. L.: Tocainide therapy for refractory ventricular arrhythmias. Am. Heart J. 100:15, 1980.

246. Young, M. D., Hadidian, Z., Horn, H. R., Johnson, J. L., and Vassalo, H. G.: Treatment of ventricular arrhythmias with oral tocainide. Am. Heart J. 100:1041, 1980.

247. Podrid, P., and Lown, B.: Tocainide for refractory symptomatic ventricular arrhythmias. Am. J. Cardiol. 49:1279, 1982.

248. Ryden, L., Arnman, K., Conradson, T. B., Hofvendahl, S., Mortenson, A., and Smedgard, P.: Prophylaxis of ventricular tachyarrhythmias with intravenous and oral tocainide in patients with and recovering from acute myocardial infarction. Am. Heart J. 100:1006, 1980.

249. Engler, R. L., and LeWinter, M.: Tocainide-induced ventricular fibrillation. Am. Heart J. 101:494, 1981.

250. Danilo, P., Langen, W. B., Rosen, M. R., and Hoffman, B. F.: Effects of the phenothiazine analog, EN 313, on ventricular arrhythmias in the dog. Eur. J. Pharmacol. 45:127, 1977.

251. Ruffy, R., Rozenshtraukh, L. V., Elharrar, V., and Zipes, D. P.: Electrophysiologic effects of ethmozin on canine myocardium. Cardiovasc. Res. 13:354, 1979.

252. Morganroth, J., Michelson, E. L., Kitchen, J. G., and Dreifus, L. S.: Ethmozin: Electrophysiologic effects in man. Circulation 64(Suppl. IV):263, 1981.

253. Podrid, P. J., Lyakishev, A., Lown, B., and Mazur, N.: Ethmozin: A new antiarrhythmic drug for suppressing ventricular premature complexes. Circulation 61:450, 1980.

254. Anderson, J. L., Stewart, J. R., Perry, B. A., vanHamersveld, D. D., Johnson, T. A., Conard, G. J., Chang, S. F., Kvam, D. C., and Pitt, B.: Oral flecanide acetate for the treatment of ventricular arrhythmias. N. Engl. J. Med. 305:473, 1981.

255. Duff, H. J., Roden, D. M., Naffucci, R. J., Vesper, B. S., Conard, G. J., Higgins, S. B., Oates, J. A., Smith, R. F., and Woosley, R. L.: Suppression of resistant ventricular arrhythmias by twice daily dosing with flecainide. Am. J. Cardiol. 48:1133, 1981.

256. Hodges, M., Haugland, J. M., Granrud, G., Conard, G. J., Asinger, R. W., Mikell, F. L., and Krejei, J.: Suppression of ventricular ectopic depolarization by flecainide acetate, a new antiarrhythmic agent. Circulation 65:879, 1982.

257. Lui, H. K., Lee, G., Dietrich, P., Low, R. I., and Mason, D. T.: Flecainide-induced QT prolongation and ventricular tachycardia. Am. Heart J. 103:567, 1982.

258. Ronfeld, R. A.: Pharmacokinetics of new antiarrhythmic drugs in cardiac arrhythmias. Harrison, D. C. (ed.): A Decade of Progress. Boston, G. K. Hall, 1981, p. 135.

259. Somani, P.: Pharmacokinetics of lorcainide, a new antiarrhythmic drug, in patients with cardiac rhythm disorders. Am. J. Cardiol. 48:157, 1981.

260. Somberg, J. C., Willens, S. H., Camilleri, W., Maguire, W., and Miura, D. S.: Effect of lorcainide on suppressing ventricular tachycardia induced by programed stimulation. Circulation 64(Suppl. IV):37, 1981.

261. Waleffe, A., Mary-Rabine, L., de Rijbel, R., Soyeur, D., Legrand, V., and Kulbertus, H. E.: Electrophysiological effects of propafenone studied with programmed electrical stimulation of the heart in patients with recurrent paroxysmal supraventricular tachycardia. Eur. Heart J. 2:345, 1981.

262. Chilson, D. A., Zipes, D. P., Heger, J. J., Browne, F. F., Lloyd, E. A., and Prystowsky, E. N.: Clinical and electrophysiological effeccts of propafenone, a new drug for treating ventricular tachycardia. Clin. Res. 30:706, 1982.

263. Bacaner, M. B., Hoey, M. F., and Macres, M. G.: Suppression of ventricular fibrillation and positive inotropic action of bethanidine sulfate, a chemical analog of bretylium tosylate that is well absorbed orally. Am. J. Cardiol. 49:45, 1982.

264. Greene, H. L., Werner, J. A., Gross, B. W., Kime, G. M., Trobaugh, G. B., and Cobb, L. A.: Selective prolongation of cardiac refractory times in man by clofilium, a new antiarrhythmic agent. Circulation 64(Suppl. IV): 137, 1981.

265. Giardina, E. V., Bigger, J. T., Jr., and Johnson, L. L.: The effect of imipramine and nortriptyline on ventricular premature depolarizations and left ventricular function. Circulation 64(Suppl. IV):316, 1981.

266. Zoll, P. M., Linenthal, A. J., Gibson, W., Paul, M. H., and Norman, L. R.: Termination of ventricular fibrillation in man by externally applied electric countershock. N. Engl. J. Med. 254: 727, 1956.

267. Lown, B., Amarasingham, R., and Newman, J.: New method for terminating cardiac arrhythmias. J.A.M.A. 182:548, 1962.

268. Lown, B.: Electrical reversion of cardiac arrhythmias. Br. Heart J. 29:469, 1967.

269. Zipes, D. P.: The clinical application of cardioversion. Cardiovasc. Clin. 2:239, 1970.

270. Ditchey, R. V., and Karliner, J. S.: Safety of electrical cardioversion in patients without digitalis toxicity. Ann. Intern. Med. 95:676, 1981.

271. Adgey, A. A. J., Patton, J. N., Campbell, N. P. S., and Webb, S. W.: Ventricular defibrillation: Appropriate energy levels. Circulation 60:219, 1979.

272. Tacker, W. A., Jr., and Ewy, G. A.: Emergency defibrillation dose: Recommendations and rationale. Circulation 60:223, 1979.

273. Kerber, R. E., and Sarnat, W.: Factors influencing the success of ventricular defibrillation in man. Circulation 60:226, 1979.

274. Gascho, J. A., Crampton, R. S., Cherwek, M. L., Sipes, J. N., Hunter, F. P., and O'Brien, W. M.: Determinants of ventricular defibrillation in adults. Circulation 60:231, 1979.

275. Ewy, G. A.: Effectiveness of direct current defibrillation. Role of paddle electrode size. Am. Heart J. 93:674, 1977.

276. Kerber, R. E., Jensen, S. R., Grayzel, J., Kennedy, J., and Hoyt, R.: Elective cardioversion: Influence of paddle electrode location and size on success rate and energy requirements. N. Engl. J. Med. 305:658, 1981.

277. Hoyt, R., Grayzel, J., and Kerber, R. E.: Determinants of intracardiac current in defibrillation. Experimental studies in dogs. Circulation 64:818, 1981.

278. Zipes, D. P., Fischer, J., King, R. M., Nicoll, A.deB., and Jolly, W. W.: Termination of ventricular fibrillation in dogs by depolarizing a critical amount of myocardium. Am. J. Cardiol. 36:37, 1975.

279. Lown, B., Crampton, R. S., DeSilva, R. A., and Gascho, J.: The energy for ventricular defibrillation—too little or too much? N. Engl. J. Med. 298:1252, 1978.

280. Mitchell, J. H., and Shapiro, W.: Atrial function and the hemodynamic consequences of atrial fibrillation in man. Am. J. Cardiol. 23:556, 1969.

281. Cobb, F. R., Wallace, A. G., and Wagner, G. S.: Cardiac inotropic and coronary vascular responses to countershock: Evidence for excitation of intracardiac nerves. Circ. Res. 23:731, 1968.

282. Ten Eick, R. E., White, S. R., Ross, S. M., and Hoffman, B. F.: Postcountershock arrhythmia in untreated and digitalized dogs. Circ. Res. 21:375, 1967.

283. Resenkov, L., and McDonald, L.: Complications in 220 patients with cardiac dysrhythmias treated by phased direct current shock and indications for electroconversion. Br. Heart J. 29:926, 1967.

284. Bjerkelund, C. J., and Orning, O. M.: The efficacy of anticoagulant therapy in preventing embolism related to DC electrical conversion of atrial fibrillation. Am. J. Cardiol. 23:208, 1969.

285. DiCola, V. C., Freedman, G. S., Downing, S. E., and Zaret, B. L.: Myocardial uptake of technetium-99m stannous pyrophosphate following direct current transthoracic countershock. Circulation 54:980, 1976.

286. Reiffel, J. A., Gambino, S. R., McCarthy, D. M., and Leahey, E. B., Jr.: Direct current cardioversion: Effect on creatine kinase lactic dehydrogenase and myocardial isoenzymes. J.A.M.A. 239:122, 1977.

287. Chun, P. K., Davia, J. E., and Donohue, D. J.: ST segment elevation with elective DC cardioversion. Circulation 63:220, 1981.

288. Smailys, A., Dulevicius, Z., Muckus, K., and Dauska, K.: Investigation of the possibilities of cardiac defibrillation by ultrasound. Resuscitation 9:233, 1981.

289. Jackman, W. M., and Zipes, D. P.: Transvenous cardioversion—low energy synchronous cardioversion of ventricular tachycardia using a catheter electrode in a canine model of subacute myocardial infarction. Circulation 66:187, 1982.

290. Zipes, D. P., Jackman, W. M., Heger, J. J., Chilson, D. A., Browne, K. F., Naccarelli, G. V., Rahilly, G. T., Jr., and Prystowsky, E. N.: Clinical transvenous cardioversion of recurrent life-threatening ventricular tachyarrhythmias: Low energy synchronized cardioversion of ventricular tachycardia and termination of ventricular fibrillation in patients using catheter electrode. Am. Heart J. 103:789, 1982.

290a. Yee, R., Zipes, D. P., Gulanhusein, Kallok, M. J., and Klein, G. J.: Low energy countershock using an intravascular catheter in acute cardiac care setting. Am. J. Cardiol. 50:1124, 1982.

291. Mirowski, M., Reid, P. R., Mower, M. M., Watkins, L., Gott, V. L., Schauble, J. F., Langer, A., Heilman, M. S., Kolenik, S. A., Fischell, R. E., and Weisfeldt, M. L.: Termination of malignant ventricular arrhythmias with an implantable automatic defibrillator in human beings. N. Engl. J. Med. 303:322, 1980.

292. Mirowski, M., Reid, P. R., Watkins, L., Weisfeldt, M. L., and Mower, M. M.: Clinical treatment of life-threatening ventricular tachyarrhythmias with the automatic implantable defibrillator. Am. Heart J. 102:265, 1981.

293. Deeb, G. M., Griffith, B. P., Thompson, M. E., Langer, A., Heilman, M. S., and Hardesty, R. L.: Lead systems for internal ventricular fibrillation. Circulation 64:242, 1981.

294. Pennington, J. E., Taylor, J., and Brown, B.: Chest thump for reverting ventricular tachycardia. N. Engl. J. Med. 283:1192, 1970.

295. Sclarovsky, S., Kracoff, O., Arditi, A., Strasberg, B., Zafrir, N., Lewin, R. F., and Agmon, J.: Ventricular tachycardia. "Pleomorphism" induced by chest thump. Chest 81:97, 1982.

296. Cotoi, S.: Precordial thump and termination of cardiac reentrant tachyarrhythmias. Am. Heart J. 101:675, 1981.

297. Estes, E. H., and Izlar, H. L.: Recurrent ventricular tachycardia. A case successfully treated by bilateral cardiac sympathectomy. Am. J. Med. 31:493, 1961.

298. Zipes, D. P., Festoff, B., Schaal, S. F., Cox, C., Sealy, W. C., and Wallace, A. G.: Treatment of ventricular arrhythmia by permanent atrial pacemaker and cardiac sympathectomy. Ann. Intern. Med. 68:591, 1968.

299. Nitter-Hauge, S., and Storstein, O.: Surgical treatment of recurrent ventricular tachycardia. Br. Heart J. 35:1132, 1973.

300. Lloyd, R., Okada, R., Stagg, J., Anderson, R., Hattler, B., and Marcus, F.: The treatment of recurrent ventricular tachycardia with bilateral cervico-thoracic sympathetic ganglionectomy. Circulation 50:382, 1974.

301. Schoonmaker, F. W., Carey, T., and Grow, S. B., Sr.: Treatment of tachyarrhythmias and bradyarrhythmias by cardiac sympathectomy and permanent ventricular pacing. Ann. Thorac. Surg. 19:80, 1975.

302. Gonzalez, R., Scheinman, M., Margaretten, W., and Rubinstein, M.: Closed-chest electrode catheter technique for His bundle ablation in dogs. Am. J. Physiol. 10:H283, 1981.

303. Gallagher, J. J., Svenson, R. H., Kasell, J. H., German, L. D., Bardy, G. H., Broughton, A., and Critelli, G.: Catheter technique for closed-chest ablation of the atrioventricular conduction system: A therapeutic alternative for the treatment of refractory supraventricular tachycardia. N. Engl. J. Med. 306:194, 1982.

304. Sealy, W. C., and Gallagher, J. J.: Surgical problems with multiple accessory pathways of atrioventricular conduction. J. Thorac. Cardiovasc. Surg. 81:707, 1981.

305. Gallagher, J. J., Kasell, J., Sealy, W. C., Pritchett, E. L. C., and Wallace, A. G.: Epicardial mapping in the Wolff-Parkinson-White syndrome. Circulation 57:854, 1978.

306. Gallagher, J. J., Kasell, J. H., Cox, J. L., Smith, W. M., Ideker, R. E., and Smith, W. M.: Techniques of intraoperative electrophysiologic mapping. Am. J. Cardiol. 49:221, 1982.

307. Cobb, F. R., Blumenschein, S. D., Sealy, W. C., Boineau, J. P., Wagner, G. S., and Wallace, A. G.: Successful surgical interruption of the bundle of Kent in a patient with Wolff-Parkinson-White syndrome. Circulation 38:1018, 1968.

308. Gallagher, J. J., Sealy, W. C., Anderson, R. W., Kasell, J., Millar, K., Campbell, R. W. F., Harrison, L., Pritchett, E. L. C., and Wallace, A. G.: Cryosurgical ablation of accessory atrioventricular connections. A method for correction of the preexcitation syndrome. Circulation 55:471, 1977.

309. Gallagher, J. J., Sealy, W. C., Cox, J. L., and Kasell, J. H.: Results of surgery for preexcitation in 200 cases. Circulation 64(Suppl. IV):146, 1981.

310. Sealy, W. C., Gallagher, J. J., and Pritchett, E. L.: The surgical approach to supraventricular arrhythmias. Pediatric Cardiovascular Disease. Philadelphia, F. A. Davis, Cardiovascular Clinics 11:365, 1981.

311. Wyndham, C. R. C., Arnsdorf, M. F., Levitsky, S., Smith, T. C., Dhingra, R. C., Denes, P., and Rosen, K. M.: Successful surgical excision of focal paroxysmal atrial tachycardia. Observations in vivo and in vitro. Circulation 62:1365, 1980.

312. Gillett, P. C., Garson, A., Jr., Hesslein, P. S., Karpawich, P. P., Tierney, R. C., Cooley, D. A., and McNamara, D. G.: Successful surgical treatment of atrial, junctional, and ventricular tachycardia unassociated with accessory connections in infants and children. Am. Heart J. 102:984, 1981.

313. Coumel, P., Aigueperse, J., Perrault, M. A., Fantoni, A., Slama, R., and Bouvrain, Y.: Reperage et tentative d'exercise chirurgicale d'un foyer ectopique auriculare gauche avec tachycardia rebelle. Ann. Cardiol. Angiol. 22:189, 1973.

314. Anderson, K. P., Stinson, E. B., and Mason, J. W.: Surgical exclusion of focal paroxysmal atrial tachycardia. Am. J. Cardiol. 49:869, 1982.

315. Klein, G. J., Sealy, W. C., Pritchett, E. L., Harrison, L., Hackel, D. B., Davis, D., Kasell, J., Wallace, A. G., and Gallagher, J. J.: Cryosurgical ablation of the atrioventricular node—His bundle: Long-term followup and properties of the junctional pacemaker. Circulation 61:8, 1980.

316. Sealy, W. C., Gallagher, J. J., and Kasell, J.: His bundle interruption for control of inappropriate ventricular responses to atrial arrhythmias. Ann. Thorac. Surg. 32:429, 1981.

317. Josephson, M. E., Horowitz, L. N., Spielman, S. R., Waxman, H. L., and Greenspan, A. M.: Role of catheter mapping in the preoperative evaluation of ventricular tachycardia. Am. J. Cardiol. 49:207, 1982.

318. Josephson, M. E., Horowitz, L. N., Farshidi, A., Spielman, S. R., Michelson, E. L., and Greenspan, A. M.: Recurrent sustained ventricular tachycardia. 4. Pleomorphism. Circulation 59:459, 1979.

319. Boineau, J. P., and Cox, J. L.: Rationale for a direct surgical approach to control ventricular arrhythmias. Relation of specific intraoperative techniques to mechanism and location of arrhythmic circuit. Am. J. Cardiol. 49:381, 1982.

320. Condini, M. A., Sommerfeldt, L., Eybel, C. E., DeLaria, G. A., and Messer, J. V.: Efficacy of coronary bypass grafting in exercise-induced ventricular tachycardia. J. Thorac. Cardiovasc. Surg. 81:502, 1981.

321. Guiraudon, G., Fontaine, G., Frank, R., Escande, G., Etievent, P., and Cabrol, C.: Encircling endocardial ventriculotomy: A new surgical treatment for life-threatening ventricular tachycardias resistant to medical treatment following myocardial infarction. Ann. Thorac. Surg. 26:438, 1978.

322. Klein, G. J., and Guiraudon, G. M.: Surgical therapy of cardiac arrhythmias. Cardiol. Clin. (in press).

323. Horowitz, L. N., Spear, J. F., and Moore, E. N.: Subendocardial origin of ventricular arrhythmias in 24 hour old experimental myocardial infarction. Circulation 53:56, 1976.

324. Josephson, M. E., Harken, A. H., and Horowitz, L. N.: Endocardial excision. A new surgical technique for the treatment of recurrent ventricular tachycardia. Circulation 60:1430, 1979.

325. Josephson, M. E., Horowitz, L. N., Farshidi, A., Spear, J. F., Kastor, J. A., and Moore, E. N.: Recurrent sustained ventricular tachycardia. 2. Endocardial mapping. Circulation 57:440, 1978.

325a. Josephson, M. E., Simson, M. B., Harken, A. H., Horowitz, L. N., and Falcone, R. A.: The incidence and clinical significance of epicardial late potentials in patients with recurrent sustained ventricular tachycardia and coronary artery disease. Circulation 66:1199, 1982.

326. Gallagher, J. J., Anderson, R. W., Kasell, J., Rice, J. R., Pritchett, E. L. C., Gault, G. H., Harrison, L., and Wallace, A. G.: Cryoablation of drug resistant ventricular tachycardia in a patient with a variant of scleroderma. Circulation 57:190, 1978.

327. Waldo, A. L., and Kaiser, G. A.: Study of ventricular arrhythmias associated with acute myocardial infarction in the canine heart. Circulation 47:1222, 1973.

328. Janse, M. J., vanCapelle, F. J. L., Morsink, H., Kleber, A. G., Wilms-Schopman, F., Cardinal, R., d'Aloncourt, C. N., and Durrer, D.: Flow of "injury" current and patterns of excitation during early ventricular arrhythmias in acute regional myocardial ischemia in isolated porcine and canine hearts. Evidence for two different arrhythmogenic mechanisms. Circ. Res. 47:151, 1980.

329. Wit, A. L., Alessie, M. A., Bonke, F. I. M., Lammers, W., Smeets, J., and Fenoglio, J. J., Jr.: Electrophysiologic mapping to determine the mechanism of experimental ventricular tachycardia initiated by premature impulses. Experimental approaches and initial results demonstrating reentrant excitation. Am. J. Cardiol. 49:166, 1982.

330. Wiener, I., Mindich, B., and Pitchon, R.: Determinants of ventricular tachycardia in patients with ventricular aneurysms: Results of intraoperative epicardial and endocardial mapping. Circulation 65:856, 1982.

331. O'Keefe, D. B., Curry, P. V. L., Prior, A. L., Yates, A. K., Deverall, P. B., and Sowton, E.: Surgery for ventricular tachycardia using operative paced mapping. Br. Heart J. 43:116, 1980.

332. Josephson, M. E., Waxman, H. L., Cain, M. E., Gardner, M. J., and Buxton, A. E.: Ventricular activation during ventricular endocardial pacing. II. Role of pace-mapping to localize origin of ventricular tachycardia. Am. J. Cardiol. 50:11, 1982.

333. Waldo, A. L., Arciniegas, J. G., and Klein, H.: Surgical treatment of life-threatening ventricular arrhythmias: The role of intraoperative mapping and consideration of the presently available surgical techniques. Progr. Cardiovasc. Dis. 23:247, 1981.

334. Kehoe, R., Moran, J., Loeb, J., Sanders, J., Lesch, M., and Michaelis, L.: Visually directed vs. electrically directed endocardial resection in recurrent ventricular tachycardia. Circulation 64(Suppl. IV):89, 1981.

335. Mason, J. W., Stinson, E. B., Winkle, R. A., Oyer, P. E., Griffin, J. C., and Ross, D. L.: Relative efficacy of blind left ventricular aneurysm resection for the treatment of recurrent ventricular tachycardia. Am. J. Cardiol. 49:241, 1982.

336. Marcus, F. I., Fontaine, G. H., Guiraudon, G., Frank, R., Laurenceau, J. L., Malergue, C., and Grosgogeat, Y.: Right ventricular dysplasia: A report of 24 adult cases. Circulation 65:384, 1982.

337. Guiraudon, G. M., Klein, G. J., Gulamhusein, S. S., Painvin, G. A., DelCampo, C., Gonzales, J. C., and Ko, P. T.: Total disconnection of the right ventricular free wall: Surgical treatment of right ventricular tachycardia associated with right ventricular dysplasia. Ann. Thorac. Surg. (in press).

338. Fontaine, G., Guiraudon, G., Frank, R., Fillette, F., Cabrol, C., and Grosgogeat, Y.: Surgical management of ventricular tachycardia unrelated to myocardial ischemia or infarction. Am. J. Cardiol. 49:397, 1982.

339. Moss, A. J., and McDonald, J.: Unilateral cervicothoracic sympathetic ganglionectomy for the treatment of long QT syndrome. N. Engl. J. Med. 285:903, 1971.

21
SPECIFIC ARRHYTHMIAS: DIAGNOSIS AND TREATMENT

by Douglas P. Zipes, M.D.

DIAGNOSTIC AND THERAPEUTIC CONSIDERATIONS

The initial evaluation of the patient suspected of having a cardiac arrhythmia begins by obtaining a careful history, specifically questioning the patient regarding the presence of palpitations, syncope, spells of lightheadedness, chest pain, or symptoms of congestive heart failure. Palpitations, an awareness of the heart beat (p. 9), may result from irregularities in cardiac rate or rhythm or a change in contractility of the heart. Some patients may be able to reproduce this sensation by tapping their hand on their chest, knee, or a table top in a fashion similar to the perceived palpitation or recognize a cadence tapped out by a physician. Such a maneuver may help establish the rate and rhythm of the arrhythmia, narrowing it to a particular rate range, a regular or irregular arrhythmia, or one in which a regular rhythm is interrupted by premature beats. The latter are often perceived only upon the contraction that ends a pause following the premature beat, and the patient may feel as if his heart has stopped for a moment. A rapid irregular tapping may suggest the ventricular re-

sponse to atrial fibrillation while a rapid regular tapping may suggest an atrioventricular (AV) nodal reentrant supraventricular or ventricular tachycardia. Information regarding the nature of onset and termination of the rhythm disturbance is particularly important. Knowing the rate of the arrhythmia is crucial, and a brief demonstration by the physician of how to determine heart rate may yield important dividends. The patient, and sometimes a close relative, should be instructed in how to determine the pulse rate. Answers by the patient to key questions may provide clues to the type of rhythm disturbance, particularly if the physician has some additional information, such as physical findings and a 12-lead electrocardiogram. For example, a young adult with presyncope, normal physical findings, and ECG changes indicating Wolff-Parkinson-White (WPW) syndrome (p. 712) should be asked whether the palpitations are regular or irregular, how fast they are, and how they start and stop. If the tachycardia is regular, with a rate of approximately 200 beats per minute and of sudden onset and termination, it is likely that the patient is experiencing a reciprocating tachycardia (p. 712); on the other hand, if the rhythm is irregular, the patient may have atrial fibrillation, a potentially more serious arrhythmia in the presence of WPW syndrome. In an older patient with presyncope, the physician should suspect ventricular tachycardia (p. 721) if the ventricular rate is fast and atrioventricular (AV) heart block (p. 730) or sinus nodal disease (p. 689) if the rate is slow. The ventricular rhythim may be regular or irregular. Premature atrial or ventricular beats, perceived as dropped or skipped beats by the patient, are probably the most common cause of palpitations.

The physician should inquire about circumstances that may trigger the tachycardia, such as emotionally upsetting events, ingestion of caffeine-containing beverages, cigarette smoking, exercise, excessive alcohol intake, or fatigue. A careful diet and drug history may be useful, for example, in revealing that the patient develops palpitations only after using a nasal decongestant that contains a sympathomimetic vasoconstrictor. States conducive to the genesis of arrhythmias should be considered, such as thyrotoxicosis, pericarditis, mitral valve prolapse, and so forth.

Physical Examination

In addition to recording cardiac rate and rhythm a number of physical findings may be helpful. For example, changes accompanying AV dissociation (p. 735) include variable peak systolic blood pressure as the atria alter their contribution to ventricular filling, variable intensity of the first heart sound as the P-R interval changes despite a regular ventricular rhythm, intermittent cannon *a* waves in the jugular venous pulse as atrial contraction occurs against closed AV valves, and apparent "intermittent" gallop sounds when atrial systole occurs at various times of the cardiac cycle. The *venous pulse* provides a window through which to judge atrial and ventricular rates and relative timing relationships. It is of interest that Wenckebach first noted the two types of second-degree AV block that bear his name (p. 731) by recording the jugular phlebogram before the availability of the electrocardiogram.

Examining the *second heart sound* may be helpful (pp. 31 and 45). A paradoxically split second heart sound may occur during a QRS complex with a left bundle branch block contour that results from ventricular tachycardia or supraventricular tachycardia with aberration. A widely split second heart sound that does not become single during expiration may accompany right bundle branch block. Unfortunately, similar physical findings occur with different cardiac arrhythmias. For example, progressive diminution of the intensity of the first heart sound results as the P-R interval lengthens, which may occur during AV dissociation when the atrial rate exceeds the ventricular rate or during Wenckebach second-degree AV block. Similarly, constant cannon *a* waves may occur with 1:1 atrioventricular relationships during ventricular or supraventricular tachycardia. Since AV dissociation may occur (uncommonly) during a supraventricular tachycardia and VA association may occur during a ventricular tachycardia, the clues provided by physical findings may be only suggestive.

The response to *carotid sinus massage* provides impor-

tant diagnostic information by increasing vagal tone and primarily slowing the rate of sinus nodal discharge and prolonging AV nodal conduction time and refractoriness. Sinus tachycardia slows gradually during carotid massage and then returns to the previous rate when massage is discontinued; AV nodal reentry and reciprocating tachycardias that involve the AV node in one of its pathways sometimes slow slightly, terminate abruptly, or do not change; and the ventricular response to atrial flutter, atrial fibrillation, and some atrial tachycardias usually decreases (Table 21–1). Rarely, carotid sinus massage terminates a ventricular tachycardia.[1,2]

To perform carotid massage, the patient is placed in a supine position, with the neck hyperextended and the head turned away from the side being tested, the sternocleidomastoid muscles relaxed or gently pushed out of the way, and the carotid impulse felt at the angle of the jaw. The carotid bifurcation is touched gently initially with the palmar portion of the fingertips to detect patients who have hypersensitive responses. Then, if no change in cardiac rhythm occurs, pressure is applied more firmly for approximately five seconds first on one side and then on the other (*never* on both sides simultaneously) with a gentle rotating massaging motion. External pressure stimulates baroreceptors in the carotid sinus to trigger a reflex increase in vagal activity and sympathetic withdrawal. Responses may occur with right-sided massage and not left, or vice versa, so that each side should be tested separately. Generally, the maximal response occurs at the first attempt at massage and lesser responses occur with repeated massages performed at short intervals. Some risk is associated with carotid sinus massage,[3] particularly in older patients. Prior to massage, the carotid artery should be auscultated so that massage is not performed in patients who have carotid bruits indicative of carotid arterial disease.

Electrocardiography

The ECG remains the most important and definitive single noninvasive diagnostic test. Initially, a 12-lead electrocardiogram is recorded and a long recording employing the lead that shows distinct P waves is obtained for proper analysis. If P waves are not clearly visible, atrial activity can be recorded by placing the right and left arm leads in various chest positions to discern P waves (so-called Lewis leads), using esophageal electrodes[4-9] or intracavitary right atrial leads (see Fig. 22–17, p. 763).

Each arrhythmia must be approached in a systematic manner to answer the following questions:

Are P waves present?
What are the atrial and ventricular rates?
Are they identical?
Are the P-P and R-R intervals regular or irregular?
If irregular, is it a consistent, repeating irregularity?
Is there a P wave related to each ventricular complex?
Does the P wave precede or follow the QRS complex?
Is the resultant P-R or R-P interval constant?
Are all P waves and QRS complexes identical and normal in contour?
To determine the significance of changes in P-wave or QRS contour, or amplitude, one must know the lead being recorded.
Are P, P-R, QRS, and Q-T durations normal?

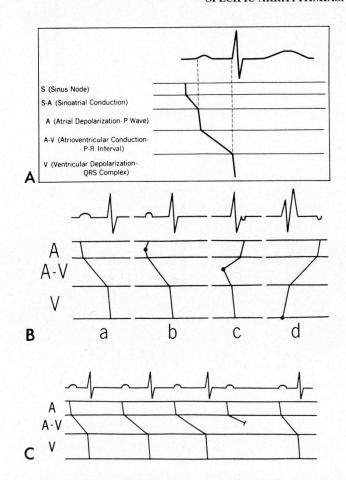

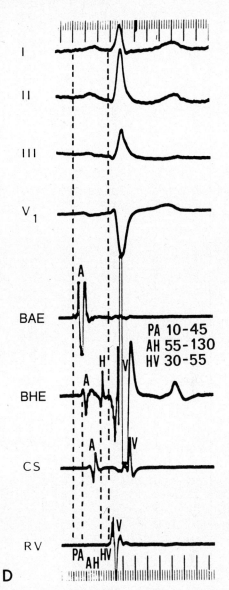

PA 10-45
AH 55-130
HV 30-55

FIGURE 21-1 *A*, Ladder diagram. Straight or slightly sloping lines beginning with the P wave and QRS complex indicate atrial and ventricular depolarization. The time at which the sinus node discharges and the duration of sinoatrial conduction cannot be measured in the surface ECG and are therefore assumed. The sloping line connecting A and V, delimited by the interrupted lines, represents AV conduction.

B, Normal and ectopic beats. a=Normal sinus rhythm; b=ectopic atrial beat; c=AV junctional beat; d=ventricular ectopic beats. All are drawn with appropriate ladder diagrams beneath (T waves omitted). Retrograde atrial conduction is inscribed for the latter two beats. As with the sinus node, the exact discharge time of the AV junctional focus and conduction time from that point to the ventricles and atria are assumed.

C, Second-degree Wenckebach type I AV block. The P-R interval lengthens progressively until finally the fourth P wave fails to reach the ventricles. As the P-R interval is prolonged, note decreasing slope of the line representing AV conduction and the small line perpendicular to the fourth sloping line indicating that the P wave is blocked. (*A* to *C* reproduced with permission from Zipes, D. P., and Fisch, C.: ECG Analysis. 1. Introduction. Premature ventricular complexes. Arch. Intern. Med. *128*:140, 1971.)

D, A single cardiac cycle showing the intervals measured during an electrophysiological study. In this and in similar subsequent figures, BAE indicates bipolar atrial electrogram recording high right atrial activity; BHE indicates the bipolar His electrogram recording low right atrial activity (A), His bundle activity (H), and ventricular septal activity (V); CS indicates bipolar electrogram recording of left atrial activity in coronary sinus lead; RV indicates right ventricular electrogram recording right ventricular activity; I=lead I; II=lead II; III=lead III; V_1=lead V_1; PA=interval representing intraatrial conduction time; AH=interval representing AV nodal conduction time; HV=interval representing His-Purkinje conduction time. All numbers are given in milliseconds. Normal values for P-A, A-H, and H-V intervals are given at the upper right. Paper speed=100 mm/sec unless otherwise stated. Interrupted lines demarcate the various intervals. Note the normal sequence of atrial activation recorded with this technique: high right atrial activity (BAE) precedes low right atrial activity recorded in the BHE lead, which precedes left atrial activity recorded in the CS lead. Large time lines=50 msec.

Considering the clinical setting, what is the signficance of the arrhythmia?

Should it be treated and, if so, how?

The *ladder diagram* is employed to depict depolarization and conduction schematically. Straight or slightly slanting lines drawn on a tiered framework beneath an ECG trace represent electrical events occurring in the various cardiac structures (Fig. 21-1*A* and *B*). Since the ECG and therefore the ladder diagram represent electrical activity against a time base, conduction is indicated by the sloping lines of the ladder diagram in a left to right direction. A less steep line depicts slower conduction. A short bar drawn perpendicular to a sloping line represents blocked conduction (Fig. 21-1*C*). On occasion, activity originating in an ectopic ventricular site may be indicated in another tier drawn beneath the ventricular tier or from the sinus node in a tier drawn above the atrial tier. In general, ectopic atrial, AV junctional, or ventricular activity is diagrammed to begin

TABLE 21–1 ARRHYTHMIA CHARACTERISTICS*

TYPE OF ARRHYTHMIA	P WAVES			QRS COMPLEXES			VENTRICULAR RESPONSE TO CAROTID SINUS MASSAGE	PHYSICAL EXAMINATION			TREATMENT
	Rate	*Rhythm*	*Contour*	*Rate*	*Rhythm*	*Contour*		*Intensity of S₁*	*Splitting of S₂*	*a waves*	
Sinus rhythm	60 to 100	Regular**	Normal	60 to 100	Regular	Normal	Gradual slowing and return to former rate	Constant	Normal	Normal	None
Sinus bradycardia	<60	Regular	Normal	<60	Regular	Normal	Gradual slowing and return to former rate	Constant	Normal	Normal	None, unless symptomatic; atropine
Sinus tachycardia	100 to 180	Regular	May be peaked	100 to 180	Regular	Normal	Gradual slowing† and return to former rate	Constant	Normal	Normal	None, unless symptomatic; treat underlying disease
AV nodal reentry	150 to 250	Very regular except at onset and termination	Retrograde; difficult to see; lost in QRS complex	150 to 250	Very regular except at onset and termination	Normal	Abrupt slowing caused by termination of tachycardia, or no effect	Constant	Normal	Constant cannon *a* waves	Vagal stimulation, verapamil, digitalis, propranolol, DC shock, pacing
Atrial flutter	250 to 350	Regular	Sawtooth	75 to 175	Generally regular in absence of drugs or disease	Normal	Abrupt slowing and return to former rate; flutter remains	Constant; variable if A-V block changing	Normal	Flutter waves	DC shock, digitalis, quinidine, propranolol, verapamil
Atrial fibrillation	400 to 600	Grossly irregular	Baseline undulation, no P waves	100 to 160	Grossly irregular	Normal	Slowing; gross irregularity remains	Variable	Normal	No *a* waves	Digitalis, quinidine, DC shock, verapamil
Atrial tachycardia with block	150 to 250	Regular; may be irregular	Abnormal	75 to 200	Generally regular in absence of drugs or disease	Normal	Abrupt slowing and return to former rate; tachycardia remains	Constant; variable if A-V block changing	Normal	More *a* waves than *c-v* waves	Stop digitalis if toxic; digitalis is if not toxic; possibly verapamil
AV junctional rhythm	40 to 100‡	Regular	Normal	40 to 60	Fairly regular	Normal; may be abnormal but <0.12 second	None; may be slight slowing	Variable§	Normal	Intermittent cannon waves§	None, unless symptomatic; atropine
Reciprocating tachycardias using an accessory (WPW) pathway	150 to 250	Very regular except at onset and termination	Retrograde difficult to see; follow the QRS complex	150 to 250	Very regular except at onset and termination	Normal	Abrupt slowing caused by termination of tachycardia, or no effect	Constant but decreased	Normal	Constant cannon waves	(See AV nodal reentry above)
Nonparoxysmal AV junctional tachycardia	60 to 100‡	Regular	Normal	70 to 130	Fairly regular	Normal; may be abnormal but <0.12 second	None, may be slight slowing	Variable§	Normal	Intermittent cannon waves§	None, unless symptomatic; stop digitalis if toxic
Ventricular tachycardia	60 to 100‡	Regular	Normal	110 to 250	Fairly regular; may be irregular	Abnormal, >0.12 second	None	Variable§	Abnormal	Intermittent cannon waves§	Lidocaine, procainamide, DC shock, quinidine

Arrhythmia										
Accelerated idioventricular rhythm	Regular	60 to 100‡	Normal	50 to 110	Fairly regular; may be irregular	Abnormal, >0.12 second	None	Variable§	Abnormal	Intermittent cannon waves§	None, unless symptomatic; lidocaine, atropine
Ventricular flutter	Regular	60 to 100‡	Normal; difficult to see	150 to 300	Regular	Sine wave	None	Soft or absent	Soft or absent	Cannon waves	DC shock
Ventricular fibrillation	Regular	60 to 100‡	Normal; difficult to see	400 to 600	Grossly irregular	Baseline undulations; no QRS complexes	None	None	None	Cannon waves	DC shock
First-degree AV block	Regular	60 to 100¶	Normal	60 to 100	Regular	Normal	Gradual slowing caused by sinus slowing	Constant, diminished	Normal	Normal	None
Type I second-degree AV block	Regular	60 to 100¶	Normal	30 to 100	Irregular‖	Normal	Slowing caused by sinus slowing and an increase in AV block	Cyclic decrease then increase after pause	Normal	Normal; increasing a-c interval; a waves without c waves	None, unless symptomatic; atropine
Type II second-degree AV block	Regular	60 to 100¶	Normal	30 to 100	Irregular‖	Abnormal, >0.12 second	Gradual slowing caused by sinus slowing	Constant	Abnormal	Normal; constant a-c interval; a waves without c waves	Pacemaker
Complete AV block	Regular	60 to 100‡	Normal	<40	Fairly regular	Abnormal, >0.12 second	None	Variable§	Abnormal	Intermittent cannon waves§	Pacemaker
Right bundle branch block	Regular	60 to 100	Normal	60 to 100	Regular	Abnormal, >0.12 second	Gradual slowing and return to former rate	Constant	Wide	Normal	None
Left bundle branch block	Regular	60 to 100	Normal	60 to 100	Regular	Abnormal, >0.12 second	Gradual slowing and return to former rate	Constant	Paradoxical	Normal	None

*In an effort to summarize these arrhythmias in a tabular form, generalizations have to be made. For example, response to carotid sinus massage may be slightly different from what is listed. Acute therapy to terminate a tachycardia may be different from chronic therapy to prevent a recurrence. Some of the exceptions are indicated in the footnotes; the reader is referred to the text for a more complete discussion.

**P waves initiated by sinus node discharge may not be precisely regular because of sinus arrhythmia.

†Often, carotid sinus massage fails to slow a sinus tachycardia.

‡Any independent atrial arrhythmia may exist or the atria may be captured retrogradely.

§Constant if atria are captured retrogradely.

¶Atrial rhythm and rate may vary, depending on whether sinus bradycardia or tachycardia, etc., is the atrial mechanism.

‖Regular or constant if block is unchanging.

Modified with permission from Zipes, D. P.: Arrhythmias. In Andreoli, K., Fowkes, V., Zipes, D. P., and Wallace, A. G. (Eds.): Comprehensive Cardiac Care. St. Louis, The C. V. Mosby Co., 1983, p. 167.

in the appropriate tier. It is important to remember that sinus nodal discharge and conduction and, under certain circumstances, AV junctional discharge and conduction can only be assumed, since their activity is not recorded on the scalar ECG.

His bundle electrocardiography (p. 634) may be indicated and is performed by introducing multipolar catheter electrodes into the vascular system and positioning them in various parts of the heart. The catheters are used to record local electrical activity and to stimulate the heart. Multiple leads are recorded simultaneously, usually at a paper speed of 50 to 100 mm/sec. (ECGs generally are recorded at a paper speed of 25 mm/sec.) Because of the rigid recording speed, intervals or complexes of normal duration may appear prolonged. An electrode positioned across the septal leaflet of the tricuspid valve records His bundle activity as well as low right atrial activity and high ventricular septal depolarization. Occasionally, a right bundle branch deflection may also be recorded. Three basic measurements are made using the ECG and the His bundle catheter recording: the P-A, A-H, and H-V intervals (Fig. 21–1*D*). The *P-A interval* is the time between the onset of the P wave in the surface tracing (which generally slightly precedes the onset of the high right atrial recording) and the low right atrial deflection, recorded in the His lead. This interval reflects intraatrial conduction and has not proved to be of much clinical value.

The A-H interval is timed from the onset of the first rapid deflection recorded in the atrial electrogram (A) in the His bundle lead to the beginning of the His (H) deflection. Since the low right atrium and His bundle anatomically delimit the boundaries of the atrioventricular (AV) node, the A-H interval closely approximates AV nodal conduction time. The A-H interval is affected importantly by various interventions: atropine and isoproterenol shorten the A-H interval, while vagal maneuvers, digitalis, propranolol, verapamil, and rapid or premature atrial pacing lengthen it. The normal range for the A-H interval is 55 to 130 msec, depending on heart rate, autonomic tone, and other factors.

The H-V interval is the time from the beginning of the H deflection to the earliest onset of ventricular depolarization recorded in *any* lead. This interval represents conduction from the His bundle through the bundle branch–Purkinje system to the point of ventricular muscle activation and is normally constant—between 30 and 55 msec—regardless of heart rate or autonomic tone.

The ventricular rate and duration of an arrhythmia, its site of origin, and the cardiovascular status of the patient primarily determine the electrophysiological and hemodynamic consequences of a particular rhythm disturbance. Electrophysiological consequences, often influenced by the presence of underlying heart disease such as acute myocardial infarction, include the development of serious arrhythmias as a result of rapid or slow rates, initiation of sustained arrhythmias by premature systoles, or the progression of rhythms like ventricular tachycardia to ventricular fibrillation. Circulatory dynamics may be altered by extremes of heart rate or by loss of the atrial contribution to ventricular filling. Rapid rates greatly shorten the diastolic filling time and, particularly in diseased hearts, the increased heart rate may fail to compensate for the reduced stroke output; as a consequence, both arterial pressure and cardiac output decline. Arrhythmias that prevent sequential AV contraction mitigate the hemodynamic benefits of the atrial booster pump, whereas atrial fibrillation causes complete loss of atrial contraction and may reduce cardiac output.[10]

Therapy

The therapeutic approach to a patient with a cardiac arrhythmia begins with an accurate electrocardiographic *interpretation* of the arrhythmia and continues with determination of the *cause* of the arrhythmia (if possible), the nature of the underlying *heart disease* (if any), and the *consequences* of the arrhythmias in the individual patient. Thus, one cannot treat arrhythmias as isolated events without having knowledge of the entire clinical situation. Patients who have arrhythmias, *not* arrhythmias themselves, are treated.

When a patient develops a tachyarrhythmia, slowing the ventricular rate is the initial and often most important therapeutic maneuver. Therapy may differ radically for the same arrhythmia in two different patients because the consequences of tachycardia in individual patients differ. For example, a supraventricular tachycardia at a rate of 200 per minute may produce little or no symptoms in a healthy young adult and therefore requires little or no therapy if it is usually self-limited. The same arrhythmia may precipitate pulmonary edema in a patient with mitral stenosis, syncope in a patient with aortic stenosis, shock in a patient with acute myocardial infarction, or hemiparesis in a patient with cerebrovascular disease. In these situations the tachycardia requires prompt electrical conversion.

The *etiology* of the arrhythmia may influence therapy markedly. Electrolyte imbalance (potassium, magnesium, calcium), acidosis or alkalosis, hypoxemia, and many drugs may produce rhythm disturbances (pp. 236 to 244), and their identification and treatment may abolish or prevent these arrhythmias. Because heart failure may cause arrhythmias, treatment of this condition with digitalis, diuretics, or vasodilators may suppress some of the arrhythmias that accompany cardiac decompensation. Similarly, arrhythmias secondary to hypotension may respond to leg elevation or vasopressor therapy. Mild sedation or reassurance may be successful in treating some arrhythmias related to emotional stress. Precipitating or contributing disease states such as infection, hypokalemia, anemia, and thyroid disorders should be sought and treated. Since therapy always involves some risk, one must be sure—particularly as the therapeutic regimen escalates—that the risks of *not* treating the arrhythmia continue to outweigh the risks of therapy with potentially hazardous antiarrhythmic measures.

INDIVIDUAL CARDIAC ARRHYTHMIAS

SINUS NODAL DISTURBANCES

Normal Sinus Rhythm

Electrocardiographic Recognition. Normal sinus rhythm is arbitrarily limited to impulse formation beginning in the sinus node at frequencies between 60 and 100 beats/min. Infants and children generally have faster heart rates than do adults, both at rest and during exercise. The P wave is upright in leads I, II, and aVf and negative in lead aVr, with a vector in the frontal plane between 0 and +90°. In the horizontal plane, the P vector is directed anteriorly and slightly leftward and therefore may be negative in leads V_1 and V_2 but positive in V_3 to V_6. The P-R interval exceeds 120 msec and may vary slightly with rate. If the pacemaker site shifts, a change in the morphology of the P wave may occur. The rate of sinus rhythm varies significantly and depends on many factors, including age, sex, and physical activity.

The sinus nodal discharge rate responds readily to autonomic stimuli and depends on the effect of the two opposing autonomic influences. Steady vagal stimulation decreases the spontaneous sinus nodal discharge rate and predominates over steady sympathetic stimulation, which increases the spontaneous sinus nodal discharge rate. Single or brief bursts of vagal stimulation may speed, slow, or entrain sinus nodal discharge.[11,12] A given vagal stimulus produces a greater absolute reduction in heart rate when the basal heart rate has been increased by sympathetic stimulation, a phenomenon known as *accentuated antagonism.*[11]

Sinus Tachycardia

Electrocardiographic Recognition (Fig. 21–2*A*). "Tachycardia" is defined as a rate exceeding 100 beats/min. During sinus tachycardia in the adult, the sinus node exhibits a discharge frequency between 100 and 180 beats/min but may be higher with extreme exertion. The maximum heart rate achieved during strenuous physical activity decreases with age from near 200 beats/min to less than 140 beats/min.[13] Sinus tachycardia generally has a gradual onset and termination. The P-P interval may vary slightly from cycle to cycle. P waves have a normal contour but may develop a larger amplitude and become peaked. They appear before each QRS complex with a stable P-R interval unless concomitant AV block ensues.

Accelerated phase 4 diastolic depolarization of sinus nodal cells generally is responsible for sinus tachycardia. Rate changes may result from a shift in pacemaker cells to a different locus within the sinus node. Carotid sinus massage and Valsalva or other vagal maneuvers gradually slow a sinus tachycardia, which then accelerates to its previous rate upon cessation of enhanced vagal tone. More rapid sinus rates may fail to slow in response to a vagal maneuver.

Clinical Features. Sinus tachycardia is common in infancy and early childhood and is the normal reaction to a variety of physiological or pathophysiological stresses such as fever, hypotension, thyrotoxicosis, anemia, anxiety, exertion, hypovolemia, pulmonary emboli, myocardial ischemia, congestive heart failure, or shock. Drugs, such as atropine, catecholamines, thyroid, alcohol, nicotine, or caffeine, or inflammation may produce sinus tachycardia. Persistent sinus tachycardia may be a manifestation of heart failure. In patients with mitral stenosis or severe ischemic heart disease, sinus tachycardia may result in a reduced cardiac output or angina, or may precipitate another arrhythmia, in part related to the abbreviated ventricular filling time and compromised coronary blood flow. *Chronic nonparoxysmal sinus tachycardia* has been described in otherwise healthy persons, possibly owing to increased automaticity of the sinus node or an automatic atrial focus located near the sinus node. The abnormality may result from a defect in either sympathetic or vagal nerve control of sinoatrial automaticity, with or without an abnormality of intrinsic heart rate.[14]

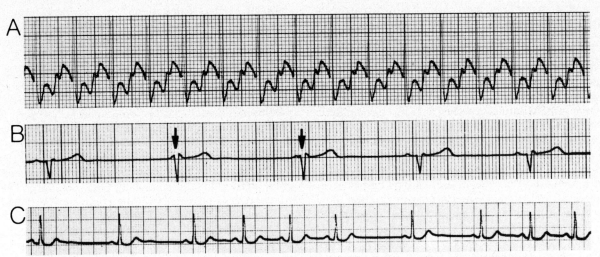

FIGURE 21–2 *A,* Sinoatrial tachycardia (150 beats/min) in a patient during acute myocardial ischemia; note ST-segment depression. *B,* Sinus bradycardia at a rate of 40 to 48 beats/min. The second and third QRS complexes (arrows) represent junctional escape beats. *C,* Nonrespiratory sinus arrhythmia occurring as a consequence of digitalis toxicity. Monitor leads.

Treatment should focus on the *cause* of the sinus tachycardia. Elimination of tobacco, alcohol, coffee, tea, or other stimulants, for example, or the sympathomimetic agents in nose drops may be helpful. Drugs such as propranolol or verapamil may slow the sinus nodal discharge rate. Fluid replacement in a hypovolemic patient or fever reduction in a febrile patient may help slow a sinus tachycardia.

Sinus Bradycardia

Electrocardiographic Recognition (Fig. 21–2*B*). Sinus bradycardia exists in the adult when the sinus node discharges at a rate less than 60 beats/min. P waves have a normal contour and occur before each QRS complex with a constant P-R interval exceeding 120 msec unless concomitant AV block is present. Sinus arrhythmia often coexists.

Clinical Features. Sinus bradycardia may result from excessive vagal or decreased sympathetic tone as well as from anatomical changes in the sinus node (see Sick Sinus Syndrome, p. 693). Sinus bradycardia frequently occurs in healthy young adults, particularly well-trained athletes, and decreases in prevalence with advancing age. During sleep the normal heart rate may fall to 35 to 40 beats/min, especially in adolescents and young adults, with marked sinus arrhythmia sometimes producing pauses of 2 seconds.[15,16] Eye surgery, meningitis, intracranial tumors, increased intracranial pressure, cervical and mediastinal tumors, and certain disease states such as myxedema, hypothermia, obstructive jaundice, fibrodegenerative changes, convalescence from some infections, gram-negative sepsis, and mental depression may produce sinus bradycardia. It also occurs during vomiting or vasovagal syncope (p. 934) and may be produced by carotid sinus stimulation or by administration of parasympathomimetic drugs, amiodarone, beta-adrenergic blocking drugs, clonidine, or calcium-channel blockers (see p. 665). In most instances sinus bradycardia is a benign arrhythmia and actually may be beneficial by producing a longer period of diastole and increasing ventricular filling time. Sinus bradycardia occurs in 10 to 15 per cent of patients with acute myocardial infarction and may be even more prevalent when patients are seen in the early hours of infarction.[17] Unless accompanied by hemodynamic decompensation or arrhythmias, sinus bradycardia generally is associated with a more favorable outcome following myocardial infarction than is the presence of sinus tachycardia and occurs more commonly during inferior than anterior myocardial infarction[18]; it has been noted during reperfusion with thrombolytic agents.[19]

Treatment. Treatment of sinus bradycardia per se is usually not necessary. For example, if the patient with an acute myocardial infarction is asymptomatic, it is probably best not to speed up the sinus rate. If cardiac output is inadequate or if arrhythmias are associated with the slow rate, atropine (0.5 mg IV as an initial dose, repeated if necessary) or, in the absence of myocardial ischemia, isoproterenol (1 to 2 μg/min IV) is usually effective. Lower doses of atropine, particularly when given subcutaneously or intramuscularly, may exert an initial parasympathomimetic effect. Ephedrine or hydralazine may be useful in managing some patients with symptomatic sinus bradycar-

dia.[20] These drugs should be given with caution, so as not to produce too rapid a rate. In some patients who experience congestive heart failure or symptoms of low cardiac output as a result of chronic sinus bradycardia, electrical pacing may be needed. Atrial pacing may be preferable to ventricular pacing in order to preserve sequential atrioventricular contraction and is preferable to drug therapy for long-term management of sinus bradycardia. As a general rule, no available drugs increase the heart rate reliably and safely over long periods without important side effects.

Sinus Arrhythmia (Fig. 21–2*C*)

Sinus arrhythmia is characterized by a phasic variation in sinus cycle length during which the maximum sinus cycle length minus minimum sinus cycle length exceeds 120 msec or the maximum sinus cycle length minus minimum sinus cycle length divided by the minimum sinus cycle length exceeds 10 per cent. It is the most frequent form of arrhythmia and may occur in normal persons. P-wave morphology does not vary, and the P-R interval exceeds 120 msec and remains unchanged, since the focus of discharge remains relatively fixed within the sinus node. Occasionally the pacemaker focus may wander within the sinus node, or its exit to the atrium may change, producing P waves of slightly different contour (but not retrograde) and a slightly changing P-R interval that exceeds 120 msec.

Sinus arrhythmia commonly occurs in the young or aged, especially with slower heart rates or following enhanced vagal tone, such as after the administration of digitalis or morphine. Sinus arrhythmia appears in two basic forms: In the *respiratory* form, the P-P interval cyclically shortens during inspiration, primarily as a result of reflex inhibition of vagal tone, and slows during expiration; breath-holding eliminates the cycle-length variation. *Nonrespiratory* sinus arrhythmia is characterized by a phasic variation in P-P interval unrelated to the respiratory cycle and may be the result of digitalis intoxication.

Symptoms produced by sinus arrhythmia are uncommon, but on occasion, if the pauses between beats are excessively long, palpitations or dizziness may result. Marked sinus arrhythmia can produce a sinus pause sufficiently long to produce syncope if not accompanied by an escape rhythm.

Treatment is usually unnecessary. Increasing the heart rate by exercise or drugs generally abolishes sinus arrhythmia. Symptomatic individuals may experience relief from palpitations with sedatives, tranquilizers, atropine, ephedrine, or isoproterenol administration, as in the treatment of sinus bradycardia.

Ventriculophasic Sinus Arrhythmia. This arrhythmia occurs when the ventricular rate is slow and some atrial (P-P) cycles do not contain a QRS complex. The most common example occurs during complete AV block, when P-P cycles that contain a QRS complex are shorter than P-P cycles without a QRS complex. Similar lengthening may be present in the P-P cycle that follows a premature ventricular complex with a compensatory pause. Alterations in the P-P interval are probably due to the influence of the autonomic nervous system responding to changes in ventricular stroke volume.

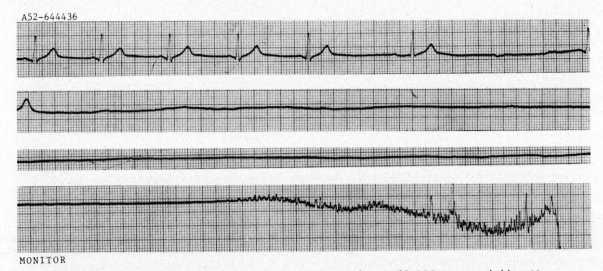

A52-644436

MONITOR

FIGURE 21–3 Sinus arrest, probably as a result of excessive vagal tone. This ECG was recorded in a 16-year-old female admitted because of recurrent syncope. As a nurse approached the patient to draw blood, the sinus rate progressively slowed, the P-R interval lengthened, and almost 40 seconds of asystole ensued. In the terminal portion of this continuous recording, the movement artifacts indicate the beginning of seizure activity. An implanted pacemaker eliminated the syncopal spells.

Sinus Pause or Sinus Arrest (Fig. 21–3)

Sinus pause or sinus arrest is recognized by a pause in the sinus rhythm. The P-P interval delimiting the pause does not equal a multiple of the basic P-P interval. Differentiation of sinus arrest, which is thought to be due to a slowing or cessation of spontaneous sinus nodal automaticity and therefore a disorder of impulse formation (automaticity), from sinoatrial exit block (see below) in patients with sinus arrhythmia may be quite difficult.

Failure of sinus nodal discharge results in absence of atrial depolarization and periods of ventricular asystole if escape beats initiated by latent pacemakers do not occur. Involvement of the sinus node by acute myocardial infarction, degenerative fibrotic changes, effects of digitalis toxicity, or excessive vagal tone all may produce sinus arrest. Transient sinus arrest may have no clinical significance by itself if latent pacemakers promptly escape to prevent ventricular asystole or the genesis of other arrhythmias precipitated by the slow rates.

Treatment is as outlined above for sinus bradycardia. In patients who have a chronic form of sinus node disease (p. 693) characterized by marked sinus bradycardia or sinus arrest, permanent pacing is often necessary.

Sinoatrial (SA) Exit Block (Fig. 21–4)

This arrhythmia is indicated electrocardiographically by the absence of the normally expected P wave, producing a pause, the duration of which is a multiple of the basic P-P interval. SA exit block is due to a conduction disturbance during which an impulse formed within the sinus node fails to depolarize the atria or does so with delay. An interval without P waves that equals approximately two, three, or four times the normal P-P cycle characterizes type II second degree SA exit block. During type I (Wenckebach) second degree SA exit block, the P-P interval progressively shortens prior to the pause, and the duration of the pause is less than two P-P cycles. (See Chapter 7, p. 250, and p. 731 for further explanation of Wenckebach intervals.) First degree SA exit block cannot be recognized electrocardiographically because SA nodal discharge is not recorded. Third degree SA exit block may present as complete absence of P waves and is difficult to diagnose with certainty.

Excessive vagal stimulation, acute myocarditis, infarction, or fibrosis involving the atrium as well as drugs like quinidine, procainamide, or digitalis may produce SA exit block. In contrast to its effects on the AV node, digitalis

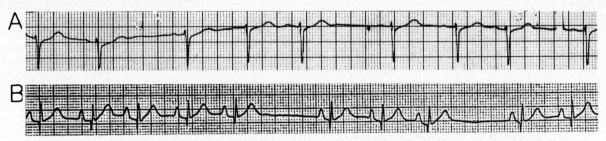

FIGURE 21–4 Sinus nodal exit block. *A,* Type I SA nodal exit block has the following features: the P-P interval shortens from the first to the second cycle in each grouping, followed by a pause. The duration of the pause is less than twice the shortest cycle length, and the cycle after the pause exceeds the cycle before the pause. The P-R interval is normal and constant. Lead V_1. *B,* The P-P interval varies slightly because of sinus arrhythmia. Two pauses in sinus nodal activity occur, equaling twice the basic P-P interval and are consistent with type II 2:1 SA nodal exit block. The P-R interval is normal and constant. Lead III.

B6-550470

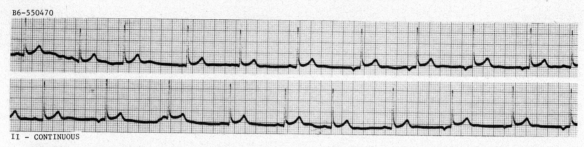

II - CONTINUOUS

FIGURE 21-5   Wandering atrial pacemaker. As the heart rate slows, the P waves become inverted and then gradually revert toward normal when the heart rate speeds up again. The P-R interval shortens to 0.14 sec with the inverted P wave and is 0.16 sec with the upright P wave. This phasic variation in cycle length with varying P-wave contour suggests a shift in pacemaker site and is characteristic of wandering atrial pacemaker.

may produce type II SA exit block. SA exit block is usually transient. It may be of no clinical importance except to prompt a search for the underlying cause. Occasionally, syncope may result if the SA block is prolonged and unaccompanied by an escape rhythm.

Therapy for patients who have symptomatic SA exit block is as outlined for sinus bradycardia.

Wandering Pacemaker (Fig. 21-5)

This variant of sinus arrhythmia, involves the passive transfer of the dominant pacemaker focus from the sinus node to latent pacemakers that have the next highest degree of automaticity located in other atrial sites or in AV junctional tissue. Thus, only one pacemaker at a time controls the rhythm, in sharp contrast to AV dissociation (p. 735). As with other forms of sinus arrhythmia, the change occurs in a gradual fashion over the duration of several beats. The ECG displays a cyclical increase in R-R interval; a P-R interval that gradually shortens and may become less than 120 msec; and a change in the P-wave contour, which becomes negative in lead I or II (depending on the site of discharge) or is lost within the QRS complex. Generally, these changes occur in reverse as the pacemaker shifts back to the sinus node. Rarely the rate may remain unchanged during these P-wave transitions.

Wandering pacemaker is a normal phenomenon that often occurs in the very young or old and particularly in athletes, presumably because of augmented vagal tone. Persistence of an AV junctional rhythm for long periods of time, however, may indicate underlying heart disease. *Treatment* is usually not indicated but, if necessary, is the same as that for sinus bradycardia (see above).

Hypersensitive Carotid Sinus Syndrome
(Fig. 21-6) (See also p. 932)

Electrocardiographic Recognition. This condition is most frequently characterized by cessation of atrial activity due to sinus arrest or SA exit block and ventricular asystole. AV block is observed less frequently, probably in

part because the absence of atrial activity due to sinus arrest precludes the manifestations of AV block. However, if an atrial pacemaker maintained an atrial rhythm (Fig. 22–23, p. 768) during the episodes, a higher prevalence of AV block probably would be noted. In symptomatic patients, AV junctional or ventricular escapes generally do not occur or are present at very slow rates, suggesting that heightened vagal tone can suppress subsidiary pacemakers located in the ventricles as well as supraventricular structures.

Clinical Features. Two types of hypersensitive carotid sinus responses are noted. *Cardioinhibitory* carotid sinus hypersensitivity is defined as ventricular asystole exceeding 3 seconds during carotid sinus stimulation, although it should be emphasized that normal limits have not been carefully established. Asystole exceeding 3 seconds during carotid sinus massage may occur in some normal subjects. *Vasodepressor* carotid sinus hypersensitivity is defined as a decrease in systolic blood pressure of 50 mm Hg or more without associated cardiac slowing or a decrease in systolic blood pressure exceeding 30 mm Hg when the patient's symptoms are reproduced.[21]

Hyperactive carotid sinus reflex is common in older patients, but most are asymptomatic. Even if they complain of syncope or presyncope, the hyperactive reflex elicited with carotid sinus massage may not necessarily be responsible for these symptoms.[22] Direct pressure or extension on the carotid sinus such as head turning, neck tension, and tight collars may reproduce syncope in these patients. However, it must be remembered that such procedures may be a source of syncope by reducing blood flow through the vertebral arteries also.

Because intrinsic sinus nodal dysfunction is generally not the major cause for asystole after carotid sinus stimulation in this syndrome,[23] patients with hypersensitive carotid sinus syndrome may be distinguished from those with sick sinus syndrome (p. 693).[21] Hypersensitive carotid sinus reflex is most commonly associated with coronary artery disease.[24] The mechanism responsible for hypersensitive carotid sinus reflex is not known, but possibilities include a high level of resting vagal tone, hyperrespon-

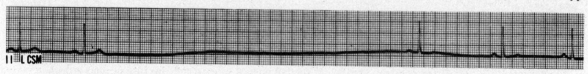

II LCSM

FIGURE 21-6   Hypersensitive carotid sinus syndrome. Gentle left carotid sinus massage (LCSM) produced a prolonged period of asystole. Lead II.

siveness to acetylcholine, excessive release of acetylcholine, and inadequate cholinesterase activity to metabolize the acetylcholine released. Carotid sinus receptors, autonomic centers of the brain stem, and the afferent limb of the reflex have all been incriminated.[21]

TREATMENT. Atropine abolishes cardioinhibitory carotid sinus hypersensitivity. However, the majority of symptomatic patients require pacemaker implantation. It must be stressed that because AV block may occur during the periods of hypersensitive carotid reflex, some form of *ventricular* pacing, with or without atrial pacing, is generally required. Atropine does not prevent the decrease in systemic blood pressure in the vasodepressor form of carotid sinus hypersensitivity, which may result from inhibition of sympathetic vasoconstrictor nerves and possibly activation of cholinergic sympathetic vasodilator fibers. Combinations of vasodepressor and cardioinhibitory types may occur, and vasodepression[25] may account for continued syncope after pacemaker implantation in some patients. Patients who have a hyperactive carotid sinus reflex that does not cause symptoms require no treatment.[22] Drugs such as digitalis, alpha-methyldopa, clonidine,[26] or propranolol may enhance the response to carotid sinus massage and be responsible for symptoms in some patients. Severe vasodepressor or mixed vasodepressor and cardioinhibitory responses may require treatment with either radiation therapy or surgical denervation of the carotid sinus.

Sick Sinus Syndrome

This term[27,28] is applied to a syndrome encompassing a number of sinus nodal abnormalities that include (1) persistent spontaneous sinus bradycardia not caused by drugs, and inappropriate for the physiological circumstance, (2) apparent sinus arrest or exit block, (3) combinations of SA and AV conduction disturbances, or (4) alternation of paroxysms of rapid regular or irregular atrial tachyarrhythmias and periods of slow atrial and ventricular rates (bradycardia-tachycardia syndrome,[29,30] Fig. 21–7). More than one of these conditions can be recorded in the same patient on different occasions, and often their mechanisms can be shown to be causally interrelated and combined with an abnormal state of AV conduction or automaticity.[29,31]

More than one pathophysiological mechanism can produce the clinical manifestations of sick sinus syndrome. The spontaneous clinical arrhythmia and the response to electrophysiological testing (see Chapter 19) depend on the underlying mechanism of sinus nodal dysfunction.[32] Patients who have sinus node disease may be categorized as having intrinsic sinus node disease unrelated to autonomic abnormalities[33,34] or combinations of intrinsic and autonomic abnormalities. Symptomatic patients with sinus pauses and/or SA exit block frequently show abnormal responses on electrophysiological testing and can have a relatively high incidence of life-threatening arrhythmias.[35] In one study of 128 patients diagnosed as having sinus node dysfunction, 33 had sinus bradycardia, 37 had SA block or arrest, and 58 had the bradycardia-tachycardia syndrome. Additional heart disease, predominantly ischemic, was found in 56 per cent. During a followup of about 3 years, nine possible or proven systemic embolic events occurred.[36] In children, sinus node dysfunction most commonly occurs in those with congenital or acquired heart disease, particularly following corrective cardiac surgery. However, it may occur in the absence of other cardiac abnormalities.[37,38] Type I, type II, and complete SA exit block apparently can occur in healthy young boys.[16] Also, excessive training apparently can heighten vagal tone and produce syncope related to sinus bradycardia or AV conduction abnormalities in otherwise normal individuals.[39] The course of the disease is frequently intermittent and unpredictable, influenced by the severity of the underlying heart disease.[39a]

The anatomical basis of sick sinus syndrome may involve total or subtotal destruction of the sinus node, areas of nodal-atrial discontinuity, inflammatory or degenerative changes of the nerves and ganglia surrounding the node, and pathological changes in the atrial wall. Fibrosis and fatty infiltration occur, and the sclerodegenerative processes generally are not limited to the sinus node but involve the AV node or the bundle of His and its branches or distal subdivisions.[40–42] In a study of 111 patients, the amount of nodal cells remaining in the sinus node was found to be inversely proportional to the age of the patient. Chronic SA block was associated with extensive lesions of the approaches to the AV node or of the AV node itself, and the bradycardia-tachycardia syndrome was associated with lesions of the sinus node and atrial muscle. Fibrosis was the main feature of the sinus node lesion.[43]

TREATMENT. For patients with sick sinus syndrome, treatment depends on the basic rhythm problem but generally involves permanent pacemaker implantation when symptoms are manifest (see Chapter 22). Pacing for the bradycardia combined with drug therapy to treat the tachycardia is required in those who fit the bradycardia-tachycardia subset. In these patients, drug therapy without pacing may aggravate the bradycardia. Although some

A30-667201

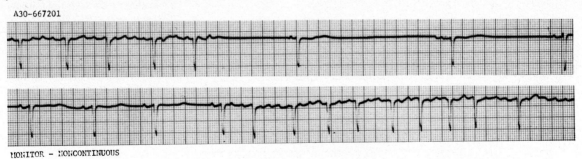

MONITOR - NONCONTINUOUS

FIGURE 21–7 Sick sinus syndrome with bradycardia-tachycardia. Atrial flutter-fibrillation suddenly terminates and is followed by a slow atrial rhythm that gradually increases in rate. Atrial flutter-fibrillation then resumes.

controversy exists about using digitalis, it should be noted that digitalis in therapeutic doses may depress intrinsic sinus nodal function in patients with normal as well as abnormal sinus nodal function. These effects of digitalis are independent of its vagal and antiadrenergic effects, and the drug should be used cautiously in patients with sick sinus syndrome without a pacemaker.[44] Prolonged sinoatrial conduction time in the absence of symptoms is not an indication for prophylactic pacing.[45] Therapy is directed toward control of symptoms.

Sinus Nodal Reentry
(Fig. 21–8) (See also p. 622)

The rate of sinus nodal reentrant tachycardia varies from 80 to 200 beats/min but is generally slower than the other forms of supraventricular tachycardia, with an average rate of 130 to 140 beats/min. Electrocardiographically, P waves are identical or very similar to the sinus P wave morphologically; the P-R interval is related to the tachycardia rate, but generally the R-P interval is long, with a shorter P-R interval (Fig. 21–9D). AV block may occur without affecting the tachycardia, and vagal maneuvers may slow and then abruptly terminate the tachycardia. Electrophysiologically, the tachycardia may be initiated and terminated by premature atrial and, uncommonly, premature ventricular stimulation (Fig. 21–8). Initiation of sinus nodal reentry does not depend on a critical degree of intraatrial or AV nodal conduction delay and the atrial activation sequence is the same as during sinus rhythm. AV nodal Wenckebach block during the tachycardia is common.[46–50] The development of bundle branch block does not affect the cycle length or P-R interval during tachycardia. Prolongation of AV nodal conduction time or development of AV nodal block may occur prior to termination of the tachycardia but does not affect the sinus nodal reentry.

Sinus nodal reentry may account for 5 to 10 per cent of cases of supraventricular tachycardia. It occurs in all age groups without sex predilection. Patients may be slightly older and have a higher incidence of heart disease than do patients with supraventricular tachycardia due to other mechanisms. Many may not seek medical attention because the relatively slow rate of the tachycardia does not result in serious symptoms. On the other hand, sinus nodal reentry may be responsible for apparent "anxiety-related sinus tachycardia" in some patients. Drugs such as propranolol, verapamil, and digitalis may be effective in terminating and preventing recurrences of sinus node reentrant tachycardia.[51]

ATRIAL RHYTHM DISTURBANCES

Premature complexes are one of the most common causes of an irregular pulse. They may originate from any area in the heart, most frequently from the ventricles, less often from the atria and from the AV junctional area, and rarely from the sinus node. Although premature complexes arise in normal hearts, they are more often associated with organic heart disease and increase in frequency with age.

Premature Atrial Complexes

Electrocardiographic Recognition (Fig. 21–10). The electrocardiographic diagnosis of premature atrial complexes is indicated by a premature P wave with a P-R interval exceeding 120 msec (except in WPW syndrome when the P-R interval may be less than 120 msec). Although the contour of the premature P wave may resemble the normal sinus P wave, it generally differs. Variations in the basic sinus rate at times may make the diagnosis of prematurity difficult, but differences in the contour of the P waves are usually apparent and indicate a different focus

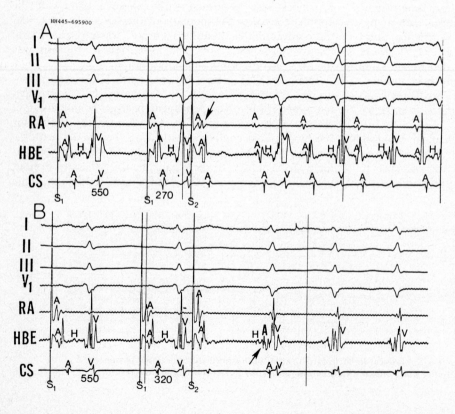

FIGURE 21–8 *A, Sinoatrial nodal reentry.* Premature stimulation of the high right atrium at an S_1-S_2 interval of 270 msec initiates an atrial tachycardia with an activation sequence similar to that occurring during high right atrial pacing. The premature P wave blocks proximal (arrow) to the His bundle but the tachycardia is still initiated. *B, AV nodal reentry.* Premature stimulation of the high right atrium at an S_1-S_2 interval of 320 msec results in a prolonged A-H interval and initiation of *AV nodal reentry.* Retrograde low right atrial activation recorded in the HBE lead occurs before ventricular activation and is followed by left atrial (CS) and high right atrial activation (arrow). This is in sharp contrast to *A,* in which the atrial activation sequence begins in the high right atrium, then the low right atrium (HBE), and then finally the left atrium (CS).

FIGURE 21–9 Diagrammatic representation of various tachycardias. In the top portion of each example, a schematic of the presumed anatomical pathways is drawn; in the bottom half, the ECG presentation and the explanatory ladder diagram are depicted. *A*, AV nodal reentry. In the left example, reentrant excitation is drawn confined to the AV node, with retrograde atrial activity occurring simultaneously with ventricular activity owing to anterograde conduction over the slow AV nodal pathway and retrograde conduction over the fast AV nodal pathway. In the right example, atrial activity occurs slightly later than ventricular activity, owing to retrograde conduction delay. *B*, Atypical AV nodal reentry due to anterograde conduction over a fast AV nodal pathway and retrograde conduction over a slow AV nodal pathway. *C*, Concealed accessory pathway. Reciprocating tachycardia is due to anterograde conduction over the AV node and retrograde conduction over the accessory pathway. Retrograde P waves occur after the QRS complex. *D*, Sinus nodal reentry. The tachycardia is due to reentry within the sinus node, which then conducts to the rest of the heart. *E*, Atrial reentry. Tachycardia is due to reentry within the atrium, which then conducts to the rest of the heart. *F*, Automatic atrial tachycardia. Tachycardia is due to automatic discharge in the atrium, which then conducts to the rest of the heart; it is difficult to distinguish from atrial reentry. *G*, Nonparoxysmal AV junctional tachycardia. Various presentations of this tachycardia are depicted with retrograde atrial capture, AV dissociation with the sinus node in control of the atria, and AV dissociation with atrial fibrillation.

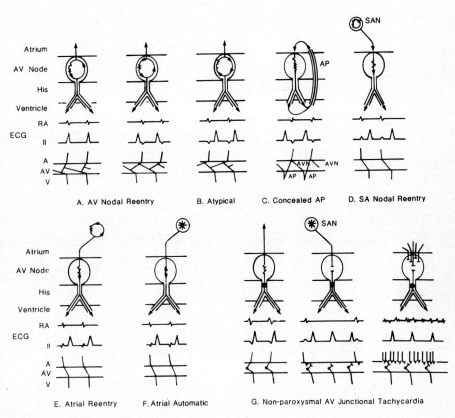

A. AV Nodal Reentry   B. Atypical   C. Concealed AP   D. SA Nodal Reentry

E. Atrial Reentry   F. Atrial Automatic   G. Non-paroxysmal AV Junctional Tachycardia

of origin. When a premature atrial complex occurs early in diastole, conduction may not be completely normal. The AV junction may still be refractory from the preceding beat and prevent propagation of the impulse (blocked or nonconducted premature atrial complex, Fig. 21–10*A*) or cause conduction to be slowed (premature atrial complex with a prolonged P-R interval). As a general rule, the R-P interval is inversely related to the P-R interval: thus, a short R-P interval produced by an early premature atrial complex occurring close to the preceding QRS complex is followed by a long P-R interval. When premature atrial complexes occur early in the cardiac cycle, the premature P waves may be difficult to discern because they are superimposed on T waves. Careful examination of tracings from several leads may be necessary before the premature atrial complex can be recognized as a slight deformity of the T wave. Often such premature atrial complexes may block before reaching the ventricle and may be misinterpreted as a sinus pulse or sinus exit block (Fig. 21–10*A*).

The length of the pause following any premature complex or series of premature complexes is determined by the interaction of several factors. If the premature atrial complex occurs when the sinus node and perinodal tissue are not refractory, the impulse may conduct into the sinus node, discharge it prematurely, and cause the next sinus cycle to begin from that time. The interval between the two normal P waves flanking a premature atrial complex that has reset the timing of the basic sinus rhythm is less than twice the normal P-P interval and the pause after the premature atrial complex is said to be "noncompensa-

tory." Referring to Figure 21–10*E*, reset (noncompensatory pause) occurs when A_1-A_2 interval + A_2-A_3 interval < two times the A_1-A_1 interval, and A_2-A_3 interval > A_1-A_1 interval. The interval between the premature atrial complex (A_2) and the following sinus-initiated P wave (A_3) exceeds one sinus cycle but is less than "fully compensatory" (see below), because the A_2-A_3 interval is lengthened by the time it takes the ectopic atrial impulse to conduct to the sinus node and depolarize it and then for the sinus impulse to return to the atrium. These factors lengthen the return cycle, i.e., the interval between the premature atrial complex (A_2) and the following sinus-initiated P wave (A_3) (Fig. 21–10*E*). Premature discharge of the sinus node by an early premature atrial complex may temporarily depress sinus nodal automatic activity, causing the sinus node to beat more slowly initially[52] (Fig. 21–10*D*). Often when this happens, the interval between the A_3 and the next sinus initiated P wave exceeds the A_1-A_1 interval.

Less commonly, the premature atrial complex may encounter a refractory sinus node or perinodal tissue, in which case the timing of the basic sinus rhythm is not altered, since the sinus node is not reset by the premature atrial complex and the interval between the two normal, sinus-initiated P waves flanking the premature atrial complex is twice the normal P-P interval. The interval following this premature atrial discharge is said to be a "full compensatory pause," i.e., of sufficient duration so that the P-P interval bounding the premature atrial complex is twice the normal P-P interval. However, sinus arrhythmia may lengthen or shorten this pause. Rarely, an *interpolated*

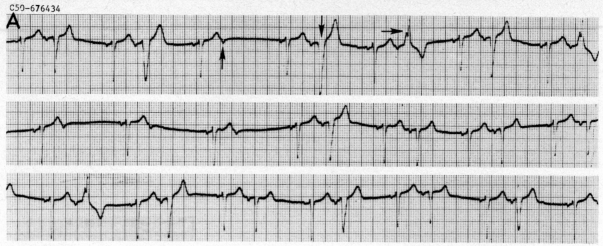

V₁ CONTINUOUS

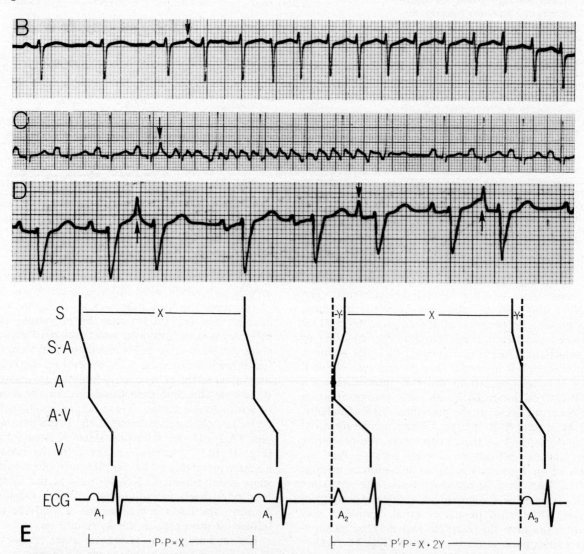

FIGURE 21–10 *A*, Premature atrial complexes that block entirely or conduct with functional right or functional left bundle branch block. Depending on preceding cycle length and coupling interval of the premature atrial complex, the latter blocks entirely in the AV node (↑) or conducts with functional left bundle branch block (↓) or functional right bundle branch block (→).

B, Premature atrial complex (↓) initiates a supraventricular tachycardia probably due to AV nodal reentry.

C and *D*, A premature atrial complex (↓) initiating a short run of atrial flutter (*C*) and a premature atrial complex (↑) depressing the return of the next sinus nodal discharge (*D*). A slightly later premature atrial complex (↓) does not depress sinus nodal automaticity. Panels B=D monitor leads.

E, Diagrammatic example of effects of a premature atrial complex. Sinus interval (A₁ – A₁) equals X. Third P wave represents premature atrial complex (A₂) that reaches and discharges SA node, causing the next sinus cycle to begin at that time. Therefore, the P′–P (A₂–A₃) equals X+2Y msec, assuming no depression of SA nodal automaticity. (Modified from Zipes, D. P., and Fisch, C.: Premature atrial contraction. Arch. Intern. Med. *128*: 453, 1971.)

premature atrial complex may occur. In this case, the pause after the premature atrial complex is very short and the interval bounded by the normal sinus-initiated P waves on each side of the premature atrial complex is only slightly longer than or equals one normal P-P cycle length. The interpolated premature atrial complex fails to affect the sinus nodal pacemaker, and the sinus impulse following the premature atrial complex is conducted to the ventricles, often with a slightly lengthened P-R interval. An interpolated premature complex of any type represents the only type of premature systole that does not actually replace the normally conducted beat. Premature atrial complexes may originate in the sinus node and are identified by premature P waves that have a contour identical to the normal sinus P wave. The cycle after the premature sinus complex equals or is slightly shorter than the basic sinus cycle. Premature sinus complexes are not commonly recognized.[53]

On occasion, when the AV node has had sufficient time to repolarize and conduct without delay, the supraventricular QRS complex initiated by the premature atrial complex may be aberrant in configuration because the His-Purkinje system or ventricular muscle has *not* completely repolarized and conducts with functional delay or block (Fig. 21–10*A*). It is important to remember that the refractory period of cardiac fibers is related directly to heart rate. (In the adult, AV nodal effective refractory period prolongs at shorter cycle lengths.) A slow heart rate (long cycle length) produces a longer refractory period than a faster heart rate. Because of this, a premature atrial complex that follows a long R-R interval (long refractory period) may result in functional bundle branch block (aberrant ventricular conduction, p. 214). Since the right bundle branch has a longer refractory period than the left bundle branch, aberration with a right bundle branch block pattern occurs more commonly than aberration with a left bundle branch block pattern. At shorter cycles, the refractory period of the left bundle branch exceeds that of the right bundle branch[155] and a left bundle branch block pattern may be more likely to occur.

Clinical Features. Premature atrial complexes may occur in a variety of situations, for example, during infection, inflammation, or myocardial ischemia, or they may be provoked by a variety of medications, by tension states, or by tobacco, alcohol, or caffeine. Premature atrial complexes may precipitate or presage the occurrence of sustained supraventricular (Fig. 21–10*B* and *C*) and rarely ventricular tachyarrhythmias.[54-59]

Treatment. Premature atrial complexes generally do not require therapy. In symptomatic patients or when the premature atrial complexes precipitate tachycardias, treatment with digitalis, propranolol, or verapamil may be tried. If these drugs are unsuccessful trials with quinidine, procainamide, or disopyramide should be instituted.

Atrial Flutter (Fig. 21–11) (See also p. 626)

Electrocardiographic Recognition. The atrial rate during atrial flutter is usually 250 to 350 beats/min, although drugs such as quinidine, procainamide, or disopyramide may reduce the rate to the range of 200 beats/min. If this occurs, the ventricles may respond in a 1:1 fashion to the slower atrial rate.[60] Ordinarily the flutter rate is in the range of 300 beats/min, and in untreated pa-

tients, the ventricular rate is half the atrial rate, i.e., 150 beats/min (Fig. 21–11*A*). A significantly slower ventricular rate (in the absence of drugs) suggests abnormal AV conduction. In children, in patients with the preexcitation syndrome (p. 712), occasionally in patients with hyperthyroidism, or in those whose AV nodes conduct rapidly,[61,62] atrial flutter may conduct to the ventricle in a 1:1 fashion, producing a ventricular rate of 300 beats/min.

The ECG reveals identically recurring regular sawtooth flutter waves (Figs. 21–10*C* and 21–11*B*) and evidence of continual electrical activity (lack of an isoelectric interval between flutter waves), often best visualized in leads II, III, aVf, or V_1. The flutter waves are commonly inverted (negative) in these leads and less often are upright (positive). If the AV conduction ratio remains constant, the ventricular rhythm will be regular; if the ratio of conducted beats varies (usually the result of a Wenckebach AV block), the ventricular rhythm will be irregular. Alternation between 2:1 and 4:1 AV conduction often occurs and may be due to two levels of block—2:1 high in the AV node and 3:2 lower down.[63,64] The irregular ventricular response frequently has the structure that results from Wenckebach periodicity. Recurrent alternation of short and long ventricular intervals may be due to concealed conduction (p. 247).[65] Conduction may also be influenced by various degrees of penetration into the AV junction by the flutter impulses, which then affect conduction of subsequent impulses. The ratio of flutter waves to conducted ventricular complexes most often is an even number (e.g., 2:1, 4:1, and so on).[27] Impure flutter (flutter-fibrillation or "flitter"), occurring at a rate faster then pure flutter, shows variability in the contour and spacing of the flutter waves and in some instances may represent dissimilar atrial rhythms, i.e., fibrillation in one atrium and a slower, more regular rhythm resembling atrial flutter in the opposite atrium.[4,66,67] Prolonged atrial conduction time has been found to be a major predisposing factor for the development of atrial flutter.[68]

Clinical Features. Atrial flutter is less common than is atrial fibrillation. Paroxysmal atrial flutter may occur in patients without organic heart disease, while chronic (persistent) atrial flutter is usually associated with underlying heart disease such as rheumatic or ischemic heart disease or cardiomyopathy. It may occur as a result of atrial dilation from septal defects, pulmonary emboli, mitral or tricuspid valve stenosis or regurgitation, or chronic ventricular failure. Toxic and metabolic conditions that affect the heart, such as thyrotoxicosis, alcoholism, or pericarditis, may cause atrial flutter. Occasionally, it may be congenital.[69] Atrial flutter tends to be unstable, reverting to sinus rhythm or degenerating into atrial fibrillation. Uncommonly, the atria may continue to flutter for months or years. In atrial flutter the atria contract, which may, in part, account for less systemic emboli than during atrial fibrillation.

Atrial flutter usually responds to carotid sinus massage with a decrease in ventricular rate in stepwise multiples, returning in a reverse manner to the former ventricular rate at the termination of carotid massage. Very rarely sinus rhythm follows carotid sinus massage. Exercise, by enhancing sympathetic or lessening parasympathetic tone, may reduce the AV conduction delay and produce a doubling of the ventricular rate.

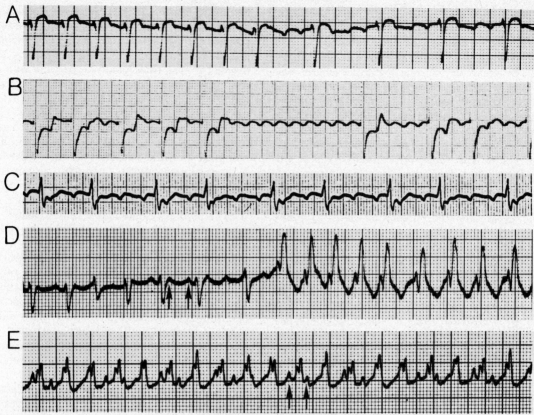

FIGURE 21–11 Various manifestations of atrial flutter. *A*, Atrial flutter at a rate of 300 beats/min conducts to ventricles with 2:1 block. In the midportion of the tracing, carotid sinus massage converts the block to 4:1 and the ventricular rate slows to 75 beats/min. *B*, Carotid sinus massage produces a transient period of AV block clearly revealing the flutter waves. *C*, Quinidine has slowed the atrial flutter rate to approximately 188 beats/min. The block is variable. *D*, Wide QRS complexes with an RSR′ configuration in V$_1$ begin after a short cycle that follows a long cycle in the midportion of the ECG strip. This represents functional right bundle branch block. *E*, the QRS complexes are 0.12 sec in duration and have a regular interval at a rate of 200 beats/min. Atrial activity is also regular at a rate of 300 beats/min and independent from the ventricular activity. Thus, atrial flutter is present with a probable ventricular tachycardia, an example of complete AV dissociation. Flutter waves are indicated by the arrows. Monitor leads in *A, B, C,* and *E*.

Physical examination may reveal rapid flutter waves in the jugular venous pulse. If the relationship of flutter waves to conducted QRS complexes remains constant, the first heart sound will have a constant intensity. Occasionally, sounds caused by atrial contraction may be auscultated.

Treatment. Synchronous direct-current (DC) cardioversion (p. 669) is commonly the initial treatment of choice for atrial flutter, since cardioversion promptly and effectively restores sinus rhythm, often requiring relatively low energies (< 50 joules). If the electrical shock results in atrial fibrillation, a second shock at a higher energy level may be used to restore sinus rhythm or, depending on the clinical circumstances, the atrial fibrillation may be left untreated. The latter will usually revert to atrial flutter or sinus rhythm. If the patient cannot successfully be electrically cardioverted or if electrical cardioversion is contraindicated—for example, after administering large amounts of digitalis—*rapid atrial pacing* can effectively terminate atrial flutter in many patients, producing atrial fibrillation with a slowing of the ventricular rate and concomitant clinical improvement or sinus rhythm.[70-72] Termination of atrial flutter by atrial pacing may be associated with entrainment, whereby at critical rates of overdrive atrial pacing the flutter morphology changes but the flutter does not

terminate.[70] Using such pacing techniques, two types of atrial flutter have been recognized. Both types have uniform beat-to-beat atrial cycle length, morphology, polarity, and amplitude of right atrial electrograms, but one type, slower than the other, is influenced by rapid atrial pacing from the high right atrium while the other is not.[73]

Verapamil (p. 665), given as an initial bolus of 5 to 10 mg IV, followed by a constant infusion at a rate of 5 µg/kg/min to slow the ventricular response, may be tried.[74] Verapamil may restore sinus rhythm in patients with atrial flutter of recent onset but less commonly terminates chronic atrial flutter.

If the flutter cannot be electrically cardioverted or terminated by pacing or by verapamil, or if it recurs at frequent intervals, a *short-acting digitalis preparation* (such as digoxin or deslanoside) can be given. The dose of digitalis necessary to slow the ventricular response varies and at times may result in toxic levels because it is often difficult to slow the ventricular rate during atrial flutter. Frequently, atrial fibrillation develops after digitalis administration and may revert to normal sinus rhythm on withdrawal of digitalis; occasionally, normal sinus rhythm may occur without intervening atrial fibrillation. *Propranolol* (p. 662) effectively diminishes the ventricular response to atrial flutter and may be used together with digitalis in patients whose ventricular rate is not decreased after digitalis. Propranolol does not appear to affect the atrial rate during atrial flutter.

If the atrial flutter persists, *quinidine sulfate* (p. 656), 200 to 400 mg orally every six hours, can be used to restore sinus rhythm. Large doses of quinidine given every 2 hours to terminate atrial flutter or atrial fibrillation prior to the development of DC cardioversion are no longer warranted. If atrial flutter persists after digitalis and quinidine, disopyramide or procainamide administration can be tried empirically. If conversion occurs, the patient is given maintanence doses of digitalis and quinidine, disopyramide, or procainamide. Sometimes treatment of the underlying disorder, such as thyrotoxicosis, is necessary to effect conversion to sinus rhythm. In certain instances atrial flutter may continue, and if the ventricular rate can be controlled with digitalis, conversion may not be indicated. Quinidine maintenance therapy should be discontinued if flutter remains.

It is important to reemphasize that quinidine, procainamide, and disopyramide should *not* be used unless the ventricular rate during atrial flutter has been slowed with digitalis, verapamil, or propranolol. Because of the vagolytic action of quinidine, procainamide, and disopyramide (see Chap. 20) and also their direct effect to slow the atrial rate, AV conduction may be facilitated sufficiently to result in a 1:1 ventricular response to the atrial flutter.[60]

Prevention of recurrent atrial flutter is often difficult to achieve but should be approached as outlined for the prevention of paroxysmal supraventricular tachycardia due to AV nodal reentry (p. 709). If recurrences cannot be prevented, therapy is directed toward controlling the ventricular rate when the flutter does recur, with digitalis alone or combined with propranolol or with oral verapamil.*

Atrial Fibrillation (Fig. 21–12) (See also p. 626)

Electrocardiographic Recognition. This arrhythmia is characterized by totally disorganized atrial depolarizations without effective atrial contraction. Electrical activity of the atrium may be detected electrocardiographically as

---

*At the time of this writing, the use of oral verapamil for this purpose is still investigational, although intravenous verapamil has been approved by the FDA to treat supraventricular tachycardias.

small irregular baseline undulations of variable amplitude and morphology, called F waves, at a rate of 350 to 600 beats/min. At times, small, fine, rapid F waves may occur and are detectable only by right atrial leads, intracavitary, or esophageal electrodes. The ventricular response is grossly irregular ("irregularly irregular") and, in the untreated patient with normal AV conduction, is usually between 100 and 160 beats/min. Atrial fibrillation should be suspected when the ECG shows supraventricular complexes at an irregular rhythm and no obvious P waves. The recognizable F waves probably do not represent total atrial activity but depict only the larger vectors generated by the multiple wavelets of depolarization that occur at any given moment.

Each recorded F wave is not conducted through the AV junction so that a rapid ventricular response comparable to the atrial rate does not occur. Many atrial impulses are canceled, owing to a collision of wavefronts, or are blocked, owing to the varying penetration of many atrial impulses into the AV junction without reaching the ventricles (i.e., concealed conduction [see p. 247]). Such variable penetration affects the conduction of subsequent impulses by delaying or blocking their passage in the AV junction and accounts for the irregular ventricular rhythm during atrial fibrillation. When the ventricular rate is very rapid or very slow, it may appear to be more regular. Even though the conversion of atrial fibrillation to atrial flutter is accompanied by slowing of the atrial rate because of less concealed conduction, an increase in the ventricular response may result, since more atrial impulses are transmitted to the ventricle. Also, it is easier to slow the ventricular rate with drugs during atrial fibrillation than during atrial flutter because the increased concealed conduction makes it easier to produce AV block. A pause in the ventricular rhythm after a premature ventricular complex results from concealed retrograde conduction (p. 247) of the ventricular beat into the AV junction, thus preventing conduction of a number of subsequent atrial impulses.[75] During atrial fibrillation with conduction solely through the AV node, a significant correlation exists between the shortest and mean R-R intervals and the AV nodal functional refractory period, as well as with the shortest ventricular cycle length during atrial pacing that results in 1:1 AV conduction.[61,76]

Clinical Features. Atrial fibrillation may be chronic or intermittent; the former is almost always associated with underlying heart disease, while the latter may occur in apparently normal hearts. Underlying heart disease is more

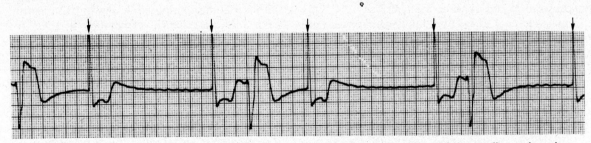

FIGURE 21–12 Atrial fibrillation with a high degree of AV block. Arrows indicate the normally conducted QRS complexes that occur at a very slow rate owing to AV block in the absence of drugs. When the R-R cycle is long, a premature ventricular complex follows, which conforms to the "rule of bigeminy"[27] and indicates that long ventricular cycles tend to be followed by premature ventricular complexes. Monitor lead.

frequent in patients with atrial flutter than in those with atrial fibrillation. The arrhythmia commonly results in patients who have rheumatic heart disease, especially with mitral valve involvement, cardiomyopathy, hypertensive heart disease, pulmonary emboli, pericarditis, and coronary heart disease. Occult or manifest thyrotoxicosis should always be considered in a patient with atrial fibrillation of recent onset.[77] The presence of cardiac failure and rheumatic heart disease are risk factors for the development of atrial fibrillation. Hypertensive cardiovascular disease is the most common antecedent disease, largely because of its frequency in the general population. The development of chronic atrial fibrillation is associated with a doubling of overall mortality and of mortality from cardiovascular disease.[78] Intermittent episodes of atrial fibrillation may recur in some patients only once or twice and in others more frequently. The duration of a single paroxysm may range from less than 24 hours to several weeks. Atrial fibrillation may become permanent in 25 per cent of these patients observed for more than one year.[79]

Mortality is unchanged in patients who have paroxysmal atrial fibrillation with no other identified cardiovascular impairment. However, paroxysmal atrial fibrillation with associated mitral stenosis or coronary disease has been found to be associated with significantly increased mortality. Chronic atrial fibrillation with or without other impairment entails a much higher mortality risk than does paroxysmal atrial fibrillation and is highest in patients with mitral stenosis.[80] Occasionally, patients with long-standing atrial fibrillation may develop spontaneous reversion to sinus rhythm. In the majority of these patients the ECG shows first-degree AV block (see p. 730) after return to sinus rhythm and low-amplitude P waves. Left atrial contraction may not occur in some patients with mitral valve disease, possibly owing to loss of atrial muscle.[81]

Patients with chronic atrial fibrillation are at greatly increased risk of *embolic stroke*. In the absence of rheumatic heart disease, chronic atrial fibrillation is associated with more than a fivefold increase in the incidence of stroke and a seventeenfold increase in patients with rheumatic heart disease. The occurrence of stroke increases directly with the duration of atrial fibrillation.[82] In an autopsy study of patients with atrial fibrillation, embolism was noted in 35 to 40 per cent of patients with mitral valve disease or ischemic heart disease, in 17 per cent of those with other types of heart disease, and in only 7 per cent of a control group of patients with ischemic heart disease without atrial fibrillation. These findings suggest a high risk of embolism from atrial fibrillation of any origin but particularly from that caused by mitral and ischemic heart disease.[83]

Patients who develop atrial fibrillation within one year after acute myocardial infarction are generally older, have a more severe infarction, have higher total mortality at 3 and 12 months after infarction, and have a greater frequency of ventricular tachyarrhythmias and right bundle branch block than do patients who do not develop atrial fibrillation.[84] The presence of atrial fibrillation appears to be related to the type of underlying heart disease, as well as to left atrial size,[85] which can be determined by cardiac echocardiography but not by the amplitude of the F waves on the ECG.[86] The left atrial diameter measured by echocardiography is smaller in patients with paroxysmal atrial fibrillation that terminates spontaneously compared

to that in patients who require DC cardioversion or who have persistent atrial fibrillation.[87] Atrial fibrillation in children is rare and is an indication for a thorough clinical investigation.[88]

The presence or absence of symptoms as a result of atrial fibrillation is determined by multiple factors, the most important of which is cardiac status. The rapid ventricular rate and loss of atrial contraction detrimentally affect cardiac output. Physical findings in patients exhibiting atrial fibrillation include a slight variation in the intensity of the first heart sound, absence of *a* waves in the jugular venous pulse, and an irregularly irregular ventricular rhythm. Often with fast ventricular rates a significant pulse deficit appears, during which the apical rate is faster than the rate palpated at the wrist because each contraction is not sufficiently strong to open the aortic valve or to transmit an arterial pressure wave through the peripheral artery. If the rhythm becomes regular in patients with atrial fibrillation, conversion to one of the following rhythms should be suspected: sinus rhythm, atrial tachycardia, atrial flutter with a constant ratio of conducted beats, or development of junctional or ventricular tachycardia.

Treatment.   When one is treating the patient with atrial fibrillation for the first time, it is important to search for a precipitating cause, such as thyrotoxicosis, mitral stenosis, pulmonary emboli, or pericarditis, and to treat it appropriately, if found. The patient's clinical status determines initial therapy, the objectives being to slow the ventricular rate and to restore atrial systole. If the sudden onset of atrial fibrillation with a rapid ventricular rate results in acute cardiovascular decompensation, electrical cardioversion is the treatment of choice. In the absence of decompensation, the patient may be treated with digitalis to maintain a resting apical rate of 60 to 80 beats/min that does not exceed 100 beats/min after slight exercise. The speed, route, dosage, and type of digitalis preparation administered are determined by the status of the patient. The combined use of digitalis and a beta or calcium-entry blocker[74,89] may be useful in slowing the ventricular rate. Quinidine, given with digitalis, is often necessary to convert to sinus rhythm. The use of large doses of quinidine to produce reversion to normal sinus rhythm is no longer indicated. Prior to electrical cardioversion, maintenance doses of quinidine sulfate in the range of 1.2 to 2.4 grams/day should be administered for a few days. During this time normal sinus rhythm will resume in 10 to 15 per cent of patients. DC cardioversion establishes normal sinus rhythm in over 90 per cent of patients, but sinus rhythm remains for 12 months in only 30 to 50 per cent. Patients with atrial fibrillation of less than 12 months' duration have a greater chance of maintaining sinus rhythm after cardioversion than do those without left atrial enlargement.[90,90a] The role of anticoagulation prior to cardioversion is somewhat controversial because of imperfect studies. Most investigators feel that anticoagulation prior to drug or electrical cardioversion is indicated in patients with a high risk of emboli, i.e., those with mitral stenosis, atrial fibrillation of recent onset, recent or recurrent emboli, a prosthetic mitral valve, or cardiomegaly. Some recommend two weeks of anticoagulation prior to elective cardioversion of atrial fibrillation present for more than about one week, if no contraindications to anticoagulation exist, and continuing anticoagulation for two additional weeks.[90a]

The incidence of embolization during conversion to normal sinus rhythm is 1 to 2 per cent.[91-93] In one noncontrolled study, 454 electrical conversions in 348 patients who had atrial fibrillation, atrial flutter, or atrial tachycardia of long duration resulted in two embolic events in 186 patients who had received anticoagulant therapy over the long term and 11 embolic events in 162 patients who did not receive anticoagulant therapy.[93] Disopyramide or procainamide[94] may be tried in place of quinidine. Serial electrophysiological testing can be used to select appropriate drugs to prevent recurrence of atrial fibrillation in some patients.[95] Rapid atrial pacing will *not* terminate atrial fibrillation.

Many elderly patients tolerate atrial fibrillation well without therapy because the ventricular rate is slow as a result of concomitant AV nodal disease. These patients often have associated sick sinus syndrome, and the development of atrial fibrillation represents a cure of sorts. Such patients may demonstrate serious supraventricular and ventricular arrhythmias or asystole after cardioversion, so that the likelihood of establishing and maintaining sinus rhythm should be weighed against the risks of cardioversion or other forms of therapy.

Atrial Tachycardia With Block (Fig. 21–13)

Electrocardiographic Recognition. In atrial tachycardia, sometimes called atrial tachycardia with block or paroxysmal atrial tachycardia with block (PAT with block), the atrial rate is generally 150 to 200 beats/min. When the tachycardia is due to digitalis excess, the atrial rate may increase gradually as the digitalis is continued (a similar response may occur in nonparoxysmal AV junctional tachycardia) and may be associated with gradual prolongation of the P-R interval. If the atrial rate is not excessive and AV conduction is not significantly depressed by the digitalis, each P wave may conduct to the ventricles. As the atrial rate increases and AV conduction becomes impaired, Wenckebach (Mobitz type I) second-degree AV block may ensue, hence the term atrial tachycardia with block. Frequently, other manifestations of digitalis excess, such as premature ventricular complexes, are present. In nearly half the cases of atrial tachycardia with block, the atrial rate is irregular. Characteristic isoelectric intervals between P waves, in contrast to atrial flutter, are usually present in all leads. However, at rapid atrial rates the distinction between atrial tachycardia with block and atrial flutter may be difficult.

The term "paroxysmal" is used to indicate a tachycardia of sudden onset that changes from sinus rhythm to a tachycardia in one beat—for example, a premature atrial complex precipitating a paroxysmal supraventricular tachycardia (Fig. 21–10*B*). In contrast, the term "nonparoxysmal" refers to a tachycardia that has a gradual onset and termination, similar to the warm-up phenomenon characteristic of automaticity (p. 620). Nonparoxysmal AV junctional tachycardia is such a tachycardia. Because the atrial tachycardia described above appears to be a "nonparoxysmal" variety, the term "paroxysmal atrial tachycardia with block" would be inappropriate.

Clinical Features. Atrial tachycardia with block occurs most commonly in patients with significant organic heart disease, such as coronary artery disease, with or without myocardial infarction, cor pulmonale, or digitalis intoxication. Digitalis toxicity accounts for 50 to 75 per cent of cases of atrial tachycardia with block. Potassium depletion may precipitate the arrhythmia in patients taking digitalis. The signs, symptoms, and prognosis are usually related to underlying cardiovascular status. Because this arrhythmia occurs primarily in patients suffering from serious heart disease, clinical deterioration may result from the arrhythmia.

Physical findings include a variable rhythm and intensity of the first heart sound, owing to the varying AV block and P-R interval. An excessive number of *a* waves may be seen in the jugular venous pulse. Carotid sinus massage increases the degree of AV block by slowing the ventricular rate in a stepwise fashion, as in atrial flutter. It should be performed cautiously in patients who have digitalis toxicity.

Treatment. Atrial tachycardia with block in a patient not receiving digitalis is treated in a manner similar to other atrial tachyarrhythmias. Depending on the clinical situation, digitalis may be administered to slow the ventricular rate and then if atrial tachycardia with block remains, quinidine, disopyramide, or procainamide may be added. If atrial tachycardia with block appears in a patient receiving digitalis, digitalis should initially be assumed to be respon-

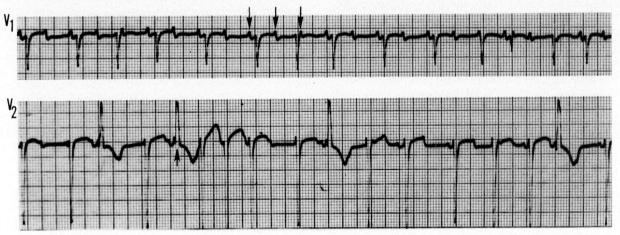

FIGURE 21–13 Atrial tachycardia with varying degrees of AV nodal Wenckebach block. A 3:2 Wenckebach grouping is indicated by the arrows. In V_2, functional right bundle branch block occurs when a short cycle follows a long cycle (arrow).

sible for the arrhythmia. Therapy includes cessation of digitalis and administration of potassium chloride orally or intravenously if serum $[K^+]$ is not abnormally elevated, or drugs such as lidocaine, propranolol, or phenytoin while cardiac rhythm is monitored. Often, the ventricular response is not excessively fast and simply withholding digitalis is all that is necessary.

Two types of atrial tachycardias have been distinguished electrophysiologically: automatic and reentrant atrial tachycardia. While it is likely that one or both of these atrial tachycardias is responsible for atrial tachycardia with block, described above, the relationship, if any, is not clear at present, and these two tachycardias will be discussed separately.

Automatic Atrial Tachycardia
(Fig. 21–9F)

Electrocardiographic Features. Automatic atrial tachycardia is characterized electrocardiographically by a supraventricular tachycardia that generally accelerates after its initiation, with heart rates less than 200 beats/min. The P wave differs from the sinus P wave, the P-R interval is influenced directly by the tachycardia rate, and AV block may exist without affecting the tachycardia. Vagal maneuvers generally do not terminate the tachycardia, even though they may produce AV nodal block. Thus, pharmacological or physiological maneuvers that selectively produce AV block do not affect the automatic focus nor does the development of bundle branch block alter the P-R or R-P interval unless it is associated with prolongation of the H-V interval.

Electrophysiologically, initiation of tachycardia with premature atrial stimulation is generally not possible but is independent of intraatrial or AV nodal conduction delay when it occurs. The atrial activation sequence usually differs from a sinus-initiated P wave, and the A-H interval is related to the tachycardia rate. The rate may gradually accelerate after initiation. The first P wave of the tachycardia is the same as the subsequent P waves of the tachycardia in contrast to most forms of reentrant supraventricular tachycardias, in which the initial and subsequent P waves differ.[96-98] Usually the tachycardia cannot be terminated by pacing; the introduction of premature atrial complexes during tachycardia merely resets the timing of the tachycardia. It is very difficult to differentiate this mechanism from micro-reentry, using the leading circle concept of Allessi (see pp. 622 and 626).

Clinical Features. Many supraventricular tachycardias associated with AV block are probably due to automatic atrial tachycardia, including atrial tachycardia with block due to digitalis intoxication (Fig. 21–13). Automatic atrial tachycardia occurs in all age groups; is thought to be due to enhanced automaticity; and is seen in a setting of myocardial infarction, chronic lung disease (especially with acute infection), acute alcohol ingestion, and a variety of metabolic derangements. Digitalis appears to be a particularly important precipitating agent. Differentiation from other tachycardias such as sinus nodal reentry (if the P waves of the automatic atrial tachycardia resemble the sinus-initiated P waves), atrial reentry (particularly if caused by micro-reentry), and some other mechanisms may be dif-

ficult. In view of the experimental findings of triggered activity from a variety of atrial fibers, including human mitral valve (see p. 620), it is possible that such activity also occurs in man. However, many automatic atrial tachycardias are not suppressed by verapamil.[99]

Therapy is as discussed under atrial tachycardia with block (p. 701).

Atrial Tachycardia due to Reentry
(Fig. 21–9E) (See also p. 626)

Electrocardiographic Recognition. This arrhythmia presents electrocardiographically with a P wave that has a contour different from the sinus P wave, a P-R interval influenced directly by the tachycardia rate, and the ability to develop AV block without interrupting the tachycardia. Electrophysiologically, initiation of the tachycardia occurs with premature stimulation during the atrial relative refractory period, resulting in a critical degree of intraatrial conduction delay, an atrial activation sequence different from that which occurs during sinus rhythm, and an AV nodal conduction time related to the tachycardia rate. Vagal maneuvers generally do not terminate the tachycardia and may produce AV block.[49,100-102]

Clinical Features. The relative infrequency of published reports suggests that atrial reentry is not a commonly recognized cause of supraventricular tachycardia. In a recent report of a group of 20 patients with sustained tachycardia due to intraatrial reentry,[101] the average rate of the tachycardia was 130 beats/min and was started by an atrial extrastimulus, progressively accelerating atrial pacing or an atrial escape beat. In all cases, premature stimulation terminated the tachycardia. Spontaneous termination could be either sudden, with progressive slowing, or alternating long-short cycle lengths.

Chaotic Atrial Tachycardia (Fig. 21–14)

Chaotic (sometimes called multifocal) atrial tachycardia is characterized by atrial rates between 100 and 130 beats/min, with marked variation in P-wave morphology and totally irregular P-P intervals.[103] Generally at least three P-wave contours are noted, with most P waves conducted to the ventricles.[104] This tachycardia occurs commonly in patients with pulmonary disease and in diabetics or older patients and may eventually develop into atrial fibrillation. Digitalis appears to be an unusual cause. Chaotic atrial tachycardia can occur in childhood.[105]

Treatment. Therapy is primarily directed toward the underlying disease. Antiarrhythmic agents are often ineffective in slowing either the rate of the atrial tachycardia or the ventricular response. Empirical trials with standard drugs, with care being taken not to exacerbate the underlying disease (e.g., using verapamil instead of propranolol in patients with bronchospastic pulmonary disease) or to produce drug toxicity, may be warranted in symptomatic patients.

AV JUNCTIONAL RHYTHM DISTURBANCES
AV Junctional Escape Beats

Automatic fibers that are prevented from initiating depolarization by a pacemaker such as the sinus node pos-

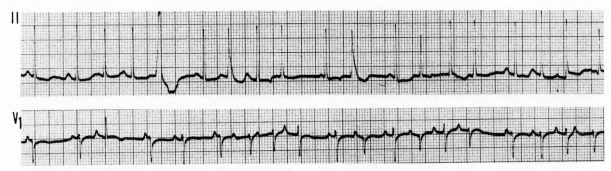

FIGURE 21–14 Chaotic multifocal atrial tachycardia. Premature atrial complexes occur at varying cycle lengths and with differing contours.

sessing a more rapid rate of firing are called *latent pacemakers*. Such latent pacemakers are found in some parts of the atrium, in the AV node–His bundle area, in the right and left bundle branches, and in the Purkinje system. Under usual conditions automatic fibers are *not* found in atrial or ventricular myocardium. It is possible that the N region of the AV node may be automatic, at least in some species.[106,107] A latent pacemaker can become the dominant pacemaker by default or usurpation, that is, by passive or active mechanisms. A decrease in the number of impulses arriving at a latent pacemaker site, the result of slowing of the sinus node or interruption of the propagation of the normal impulse anywhere along its course, allows the latent pacemaker to escape and initiate depolarization passively, by default. An increase in the discharge rate of a latent pacemaker can capture pacemaker control actively, by usurpation. As will be seen, the implication of the two different mechanisms of ectopic impulse formation is important from a therapeutic standpoint.

Electrocardiographic Recognition. An AV junctional escape beat occurs when the rate of impulse formation of the primary pacemaker, generally the sinus node, becomes less than that of the AV junctional region, or when impulses from the primary pacemaker do not penetrate to the region of the escape focus and allow the AV junctional focus to reach threshold and discharge. The interval from the last normally conducted beat to the AV junctional escape beat is a measure of the initial discharge rate of the AV junctional focus and generally corresponds to a rate of 35 to 60 beats/min (Fig. 21–2*B*). Although an AV junctional escape rhythm is usually fairly regular, intervals between subsequent escape beats after the initial escape beat may gradually shorten as the rate of discharge of the escape focus increases, the so-called *rhythm of development* or *warm-up phenomenon*.

The electrocardiogram displays pauses longer than the normal P-P interval, interrupted by a QRS complex of supraventricular configuration with absent, retrograde, fusion, or sinus P waves that do not conduct to the ventricle. If P waves precede the QRS, they have a P-R interval generally less than 0.12 sec. The exact site of impulse formation (i.e., AN, N, or NH regions; low atrium; or His bundle) is not known and may differ from patient to patient and be influenced by the cause of the arrhythmia.

Treatment, if any, lies in increasing the discharge rate of the higher pacemakers and improving AV conduction and may require pacing. Frequently, no treatment is necessary.

Premature AV Junctional Complexes
(Figs. 21–15 to 21–17)

Premature AV junctional complexes are characterized by an impulse that arises prematurely in the AV junction (the exact site—i.e., AN, N, or NH regions; low atrium; or His bundle—is not known and may vary from patient to patient) and that attempts conduction in anterograde and retrograde directions. If unimpeded in its course, the impulse discharges the atrium to produce a premature retrograde P wave and a premature QRS complex with a supraventricular contour. The retrograde P wave may occur before, during, or after the QRS complex (Fig. 21–15). Alterations in conduction time may influence the P-R or R-P relationships without a change in the site of origin of the impulse (Fig. 21–16). Premature AV junctional

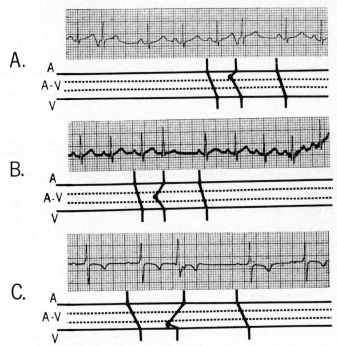

FIGURE 21–15 Premature AV junctional complexes. *A*, The premature AV junctional complex is preceded by a P wave. *B*, The atrial activity associated with this complex cannot be seen but may occur in the terminal portion of the QRS complex. *C*, A retrograde P wave follows the premature AV junctional complex. The ladder diagram indicates the position of the retrograde P wave in relation to the QRS complex by assuming (without adequate basis, see Fig. 21–16) that the premature AV junctional complex arises from upper, mid, and lower regions of the AV node.

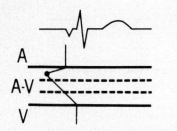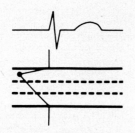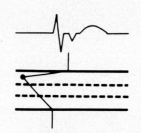

FIGURE 21–16 Diagrammatic representation of premature AV junctional complexes, indicating that the AV junctional focus maintaining a constant site of origin may achieve the P and QRS relationships shown in Figure 21–15 simply by varying conduction time, in this case, to the atrium.

complexes that conduct aberrantly are difficult to distinguish from premature ventricular complexes using the scalar ECG (Fig. 21–17).

Treatment of premature AV junctional complexes is generally not necessary. However, since they may arise distal to the AV node, they may occur early in the cardiac cycle and can initiate a ventricular tachyarrhythmia in some instances. Under these circumstances therapy may be approached as for premature ventricular complexes (see p. 719).

AV Junctional Rhythm (Fig. 21–18)

If the AV junctional escape beats continue for a period of time, the rhythm is called an AV junctional rhythm. Since the inherent rate of the AV junctional tissue is 35 to 60 beats/min, the AV junctional tissue can assume the role of the dominant pacemaker at this rate only by passive default of the sinus pacemaker. The ECG displays a normally conducted QRS complex, which may conduct retrogradely to the atrium or may occur independently of atrial discharge, producing AV dissociation (see p. 735).

An AV junctional escape rhythm may be a normal phenomenon in response to the effects of vagal tone or it may

occur during pathological sinus bradycardia or heart block. The escape beat or rhythm serves as a safety mechanism to prevent the occurrence of ventricular asystole. *Physical findings* vary depending on the P-QRS relationship. Large *a* waves in the jugular venous pulse and a loud, soft, or changing intensity of the first heart sound may be present if atrial contraction occurs when the tricuspid valve is shut.

Therapy is discussed under AV junctional escape beats (see above).

Nonparoxysmal AV Junctional Tachycardia
(Figs. 21–19 and 21–20)

Electrocardiographic Recognition. To usurp dominant pacemaker status, the AV junctional tissue must exhibit enhanced discharge rate such as during nonparoxysmal AV junctional tachycardia. Nonparoxysmal AV junctional tachycardia is usually of gradual onset and termination, hence the modifier "nonparoxysmal." On occasion, nonparoxysmal AV junctional tachycardia may become manifest abruptly because of slowing of the dominant pacemaker that may then allow sudden capture and control of the rhythm by the AV junctional focus.[108] The

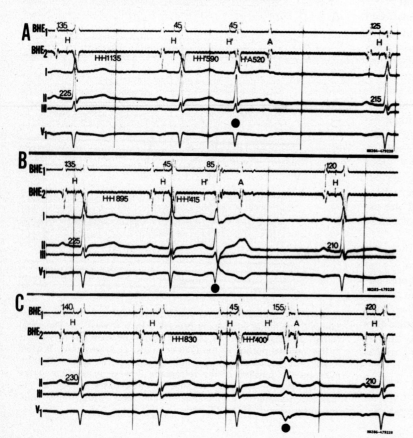

FIGURE 21–17 Premature AV junctional complexes arising in or near the bundle of His (H') conduct normally (A) or with functional right (B) and functional left (C) bundle branch block. The filled circles indicate the premature junctional complex. Anterograde conduction of the premature junctional (H') discharges depends on the coupling interval between the last normal His discharge (H) and (H-H') interval and the spontaneous cycle length (H-H) that preceded H'. When H' follows a shorter preceding cycle length and occurs at longer coupling intervals, a normal QRS complex results. As the preceding H-H cycle lengthens or as the H-H' interval shortens, a zone of functional right bundle branch block occurs, followed by a zone of functional left bundle branch block. Not shown are premature His discharges that fail to conduct entirely (see Fig. 19–30, p. 635). Numbers in milliseconds. Time lines=1 sec in each panel. (Magnification is not the same in all three panels.) (From Bonner, A. J., and Zipes, D. P.: Lidocaine and His bundle extrasystoles. His bundle discharge conducted normally, conducted with functional right or left bundle branch block, or blocked entirely (concealed). Arch. Intern. Med. *136*: 700, 1976.)

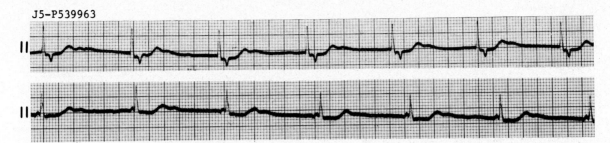

J5-P539963

FIGURE 21–18   AV junctional rhythm. *Top,* AV junctional discharge occurs fairly regularly at a rate of approximately 50 beats/min. Retrograde atrial activity follows each junctional discharge. *Bottom,* Recording made on a different day in the same patient; the AV junctional rate is slightly more variable, and retrograde P waves precede the onset of the QRS complex. The positive terminal portion of the P wave gives the appearance of AV dissociation, which was not present.

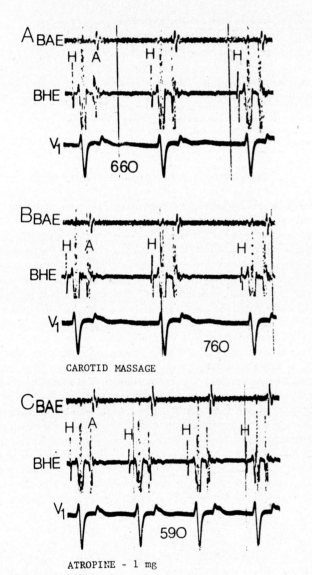

CAROTID MASSAGE

ATROPINE - 1 mg

FIGURE 21–19   Nonparoxysmal AV junctional tachycardia. *A,* Control; *B,* response to carotid sinus massage; *C,* response to atropine, 1 mg intravenously. Note that His bundle depolarization is the earliest recordable electrical activity in each cycle. The atria are depolarized retrogradely (low right atrial activity recorded in BHE precedes high right atrial activity recorded in BAE). Note also that carotid sinus massage slows the junctional discharge rate while atropine speeds it up. From these tracings alone one could not distinguish the rhythm from some other types of supraventricular tachycardias. However, onset and termination of this tachycardia was typical of nonparoxysmal AV junctional tachycardia.

rate of discharge is commonly between 70 and 130 beats/min. Although accepted terminology confers the label of tachycardia to rates exceeding 100 beats/min, this term—although not entirely correct—has generally been accepted, since rates exceeding 60 beats/min represent in effect a tachycardia for the AV junctional tissue.[109,110]

Nonparoxysmal AV junctional tachycardia is recognized by a QRS of supraventricular configuration at a fairly regular rate of 70 to 130 beats/min. Enhanced vagal tone may slow while vagolytic agents may speed up the discharge rate. Although retrograde activation of the atria may occur, the atria commonly are controlled by an independent sinus, atrial, or on occasion a second AV junctional focus resulting in AV dissociation (Fig. 21–9G). The electrocardiographic diagnosis may be complicated by the presence of entrance and exit blocks at the AV junctional tissue level and incomplete forms of AV dissociation.

The cause of this arrhythmia probably is *accelerated automatic discharge* in or near the His bundle. It is possible that nonparoxysmal AV junctional tachycardia originates in atrial fibers without recognition of the latter's role from analysis of the scalar ECG or on intracardiac electrograms, unless a careful search is made.[111] Wenckebach periods may occur (Fig. 7–48, p. 240), but the presence of exit block has not yet been demonstrated by His bundle recording in humans, and the block may be in the AV node with the origin of the nonparoxysmal AV junctional tachycardia proximal to the site of the His bundle recording.[111,112] Accelerated junctional escape beats that have shorter escape intervals when following premature atrial complexes has raised the possibility of *overdrive acceleration* (p. 620) in these fibers.[113]

Clinical Features. Nonparoxysmal AV junctional tachycardia occurs most commonly in patients with underlying heart disease, such as inferior infarction, myocarditis (often the result of acute rheumatic fever), or after open-heart surgery.[114,115] Probably the most important cause is excessive digitalis, which may also produce the ECG manifestations of varying degrees of exit block (usually Wenckebach type) from the accelerated AV junctional focus. Nonparoxysmal AV junctional tachycardia can occur in otherwise healthy individuals without symptoms (Fig. 21–20) or can be a serious and difficult to control tachycardia,[116] occasionally chronic and longlasting.[117]

The clinical features vary depending on the rate of the arrhythmia and the underlying etiology and severity of heart disease. As in most arrhythmias, the physical signs are determined by the relationship of the P wave to the

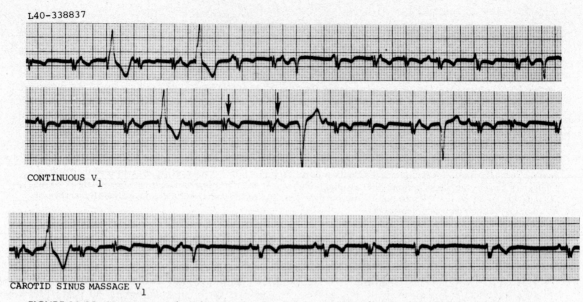

L40-338837

CONTINUOUS V₁

CAROTID SINUS MASSAGE V₁

FIGURE 21–20 Nonparoxysmal AV junctional tachycardia in a healthy young adult. This tachycardia occurs at a fairly regular interval ("W-shaped" complexes) and is interrupted intermittently with atrial captures that produce functional right and left bundle branch block. Two P waves are indicated by arrows. The junctional discharge rate is approximately 120 beats/min (cycle length=500 msec) and the rhythm irregular, sometimes shortened by atrial captures or delayed by concealed conduction that resets and displaces the junctional focus (see Chap. 7). In the bottom strip, carotid sinus massage slows the junctional as well as the sinus discharge rate.

QRS complex and the rate of atrial and ventricular discharge. The first heart sound may therefore be constant or varying, and cannon *a* waves may or may not occur in the jugular venous pulse.

The ventricular rhythm may be regular or irregular, often in a constant fashion. It is especially important to recognize slowing and regularization of the ventricular rhythm in a patient with atrial fibrillation as being a possible early sign of *digitalis intoxication* (p. 239). Initially, during atrial fibrillation, the regular ventricular rhythm may result from an AV junctional escape rhythm because the depressed AV conduction caused by digitalis blocks the passage of impulses from the fibrillating atria (Fig. 21–9G). As digitalis administration is continued, the ventricular rate may then speed because of increased discharge of the AV junctional pacemaker but may still be regular. Further digitalis administration may produce a rate that is slow and irregular because of varying degrees of AV junctional exit block. The rhythm may be misdiagnosed as resumption of conduction from the fibrillating atria. The rate then may increase further because of development of a ventricular tachycardia.

Therapy is directed toward the underlying etiological factor and functional support of the cardiovascular system. If the rhythm is regular, the cardiovascular status is compromised, and the patient is not taking digitalis, digitalis administration should be considered. Cardioversion may be tried if necessary; theoretically, however, if the nonparoxysmal AV junctional tachycardia is due to enhanced automaticity, cardioversion may be ineffective. If the patient tolerates the arrhythmia well, careful monitoring and attention to the underlying heart disease is usually all that is required. The arrhythmia usually will abate spontaneously. If digitalis toxicity is the cause, the drug must be stopped and potassium, lidocaine, phenytoin, or propranolol administered.

Tachycardias Involving the AV Junction

Much confusion exists regarding the nomenclature of tachycardias characterized by a supraventricular QRS complex, a regular R-R interval, and no evidence of ventricular preexcitation. These tachycardias have often been called paroxysmal atrial tachycardia (PAT) if the P wave occurred in front of the QRS complex or paroxysmal nodal or junctional tachycardia (PJT) if the P wave occurred within or just following the QRS complex and exhibited a retrograde contour. Because it is now apparent that a variety of electrophysiological mechanisms can account for these tachycardias (Fig. 21–9), the nonspecific term paroxysmal supraventricular tachycardia (PSVT) has been proposed to encompass the entire group. This term may be inappropriate because tachycardias in patients with accessory pathways (see below) are no more supraventricular than they are ventricular in origin, since they may require participation of both the atria and the ventricles in the reentrant pathway, and they exhibit a QRS complex of normal contour and duration only because anterograde conduction occurs over the normal AV node–His bundle pathways (Fig. 21–9C). If conduction over the reentrant pathway reverses direction and travels in an "antidromic" direction—i.e., to the ventricles over the accessory pathway and to the atria over the AV node–His bundle—the QRS complex exhibits a prolonged duration, although the tachycardia is basically the same. The term *reciprocating tachycardia* has been offered as a substitute for paroxysmal supraventricular tachycardia, but use of such a term presumes the mechanism of the tachycardia to be reentrant (which is probably the case for many supraventricular tachycardias). Reciprocating tachycardia is probably the mechanism of many ventricular tachycardias as well. Thus, no universally acceptable nomenclature exists for these tachycardias. In this chapter, descriptive titles, although

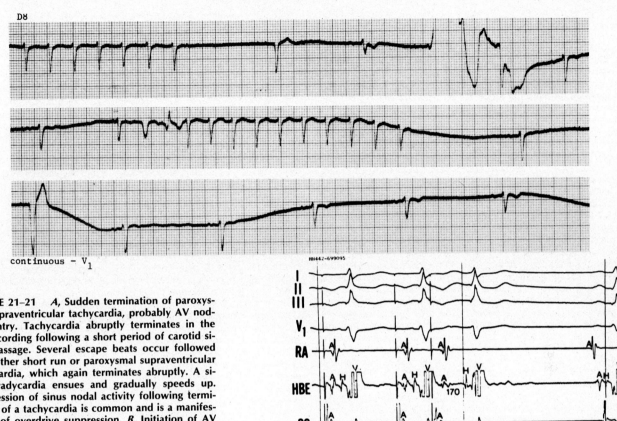

A continuous – V₁

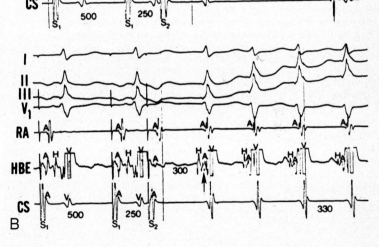

B

FIGURE 21-21 A, Sudden termination of paroxysmal supraventricular tachycardia, probably AV nodal reentry. Tachycardia abruptly terminates in the top recording following a short period of carotid sinus massage. Several escape beats occur followed by another short run or paroxysmal supraventricular tachycardia, which again terminates abruptly. A sinus bradycardia ensues and gradually speeds up. Suppression of sinus nodal activity following termination of a tachycardia is common and is a manifestation of overdrive suppression. B, Initiation of AV nodal reentrant tachycardia in a patient with dual atrioventricular nodal pathways. Upper and lower panels show the last two paced beats of a train of stimuli delivered to the coronary sinus at a pacing cycle length of 500 msec. The results of premature atrial stimulation at an S₁–S₂ interval of 250 msec on two occasions are shown. In the *upper panel*, S₂ was conducted to the ventricle with an AH interval of 170 msec and then was followed by a sinus beat. In the *lower panel*, S₂ was conducted with an AH interval of 300 msec and initiated AV nodal reentry. Note that the retrograde atrial activity occurs (arrow) prior to the onset of ventricular septal depolarization and is superimposed on the QRS complex. Retrograde atrial activity begins first in the low right atrium (HBE lead) and then progresses to the high right atrium (RA) and coronary sinus (CS) recordings.

cumbersome, will be used for the sake of clarity. In addition, the mechanism of reentry will be assumed operative when the weight of evidence supports its presence even though unequivocal proof is lacking (see p. 623).

Atrioventricular (AV) Nodal Reentrant Tachycardia

Electrocardiographic Recognition. Reentrant tachycardia in the AV node is characterized by a tachycardia with a QRS complex of supraventricular origin, with sudden onset and termination generally at rates between 150 and 250 beats/min (commonly 180 to 200 beats/min in adults), and with a regular rhythm. Uncommonly, the rate

may be as low as 110 beats/min and occasionally, especially in children, may exceed 250. Unless functional aberrant ventricular conduction or a previous conduction defect exists, the QRS complex is normal in contour and duration. AV nodal reentry recorded at the onset begins abruptly, usually following a premature atrial complex that conducts with a prolonged P-R interval (see Figs. 21-9A and 21-10B and Fig. 19-24, p. 629). The abrupt termination is sometimes followed by a brief period of asystole or bradycardia (Fig. 21-21A). The R-R interval may shorten over the course of the first few beats at the onset or lengthen over the course of the last few beats preceding termination of the tachycardia. Variation in cycle length is usually caused by variation in AV nodal conduction time. Carotid sinus massage may slow the tachycardia slightly prior to its termination or, if termination does not occur, may produce only slight slowing of the tachycardia (Fig. 21–21*A*).

Electrophysiological Features. An atrial complex that conducts with a critical prolongation of AV nodal conduction time[118-120] generally precipitates AV nodal reentry (Fig. 21–21*B*). Several AV nodal pathways can be diagrammed to explain this tachycardia. In Figure 19–22 (p. 627), the atria are shown as a necessary link in the reentrant pathway, while in Figure 21–9*A* and *B* (p. 695), the atria are not incorporated in the circuit. In most examples, the retrograde P wave occurs at the onset of the QRS complex, clearly excluding the possibility of an accessory pathway. If an accessory pathway in the ventricle were part of the circuit, the ventricles would have to be activated before the accessory pathway and therefore before the atria were depolarized (see Preexcitation Syndrome, p. 712). In approximately 30 per cent of instances, atrial activation begins at the end of, or just after, the QRS complex, giving rise to a discrete P wave on the surface ECG (Fig. 21–9*B*), while in the majority of patients P waves are not seen, since they are buried within the inscription of the QRS complex (Fig. 21–9*A*). In the most common variety of AV nodal reentrant tachycardia, the V-A interval (i.e., between onset of QRS and onset of atrial activity) is less than 50 per cent of the R-R interval and the ratio of A-V to V-A interval exceeds 1.0. Most of these patients during tachycardia have a V-A minimum value of ≤61 msec measured to the earliest recorded atrial activity and of ≤95 msec measured to atrial activity recorded in the high right atrial electrogram. These V-A intervals are longer in patients with tachycardia related to accessory pathways[121] as well as in some other forms of AV nodal reentry (Fig. 21–9*B*). In the majority of patients, anterograde conduction occurs to the ventricle over the slow (alpha) pathway and retrograde conduction over the fast (beta) pathway (see Fig. 19–23, p. 628, and Fig. 21–9*A* and *B*). An atrial complex blocks in the fast pathway anterogradely, travels to the ventricle over the slow pathway, and returns to the atrium over the previously blocked fast pathway. The proximal and distal final pathways for this circus movement appear to be located within the AV node, so that as currently conceived, the circus movement is located totally within the AV node (Fig. 21–9*A* and *B*). The reentrant loop is slow AV nodal pathway → final distal common pathway (probably distal AV node) → retrograde fast AV nodal pathway → final proximal common pathway (probably proximal AV node, possibly a portion of low atrium). The cycle length of the tachycardia generally depends on how well the slow pathway conducts, since the fast pathway usually exhibits excellent capability for retrograde conduction and has the shorter refractory period in the

retrograde direction. Therefore, conduction times in the anterograde slow pathway are a major determinant of the cycle length of the tachycardia. In one study, patients with shorter A-H intervals appeared more likely to have AV nodal reentrant tachycardia because these patients were more likely to have excellent retrogradely conducting fast pathways.[122]

The evidence supporting the dual pathway concept derives from the observation that in these patients, a plot of the A_1-A_2 versus the A_2-H_2 or A_1-A_2 versus the H_1-H_2 intervals shows a discontinuous curve (Fig. 21–22). The explanation is that, at a critical A_1-A_2 interval, the impulse suddenly blocks in the fast pathway and conducts with delay over the slow pathway, with sudden prolongation of the A_2-H_2 (or H_1-H_2) interval. Generally, the A-H interval increases at least 50 msec with only a 10- to 20-msec decrease in the coupling interval of the premature atrial complex. Less commonly, dual pathways may be manifested by different P-R or A-H intervals during sinus rhythm or at identical paced rates or by a sudden jump in the A-H interval during atrial pacing at a constant cycle length. Some patients with AV nodal reentry may not have discontinuous refractory period curves, and some patients who do not have AV nodal reentry may exhibit discontinuous refractory curves. In the latter patients, dual AV nodal pathways may be a benign finding.[123,129] Similar mechanisms of tachycardia can occur in children.[124] Triple AV nodal pathways may be demonstrated in occasional patients.[125]

In less than 5 to 10 per cent of patients with AV nodal reentry, anterograde conduction proceeds over the fast pathway and retrograde conduction over the slow pathway (termed the unusual form of AV nodal reentry), causing atrial activation to begin *after* the QRS complex and producing a long V-A interval and a relatively short A-V interval (generally A-V/V-A < 0.75, Fig. 21–9*B*).[100,102,126-132] Finally, it is possible to have tachycardias that use either the antegrade slow or fast pathways and a retrograde concealed accessory pathway (see below).[133,134]

The ventricles and apparently the atria are not needed to maintain AV nodal reentry in man, and spontaneous AV block has been noted on occasion, particularly at the onset of the arrhythmia. Such block can take place in the AV node distal to the reentry circuit between the AV node and bundle of His, within the bundle of His, or distal to it. Rarely the block may be located between the reentry circuit in the AV node and the atrium.[135,135a] Most commonly when block appears, it is below the bundle of His. Termination of the tachycardia generally results from block in the anterogradely conducting slow pathway ("weak link"), so that a retrograde atrial response is not followed by a His or ventricular response.

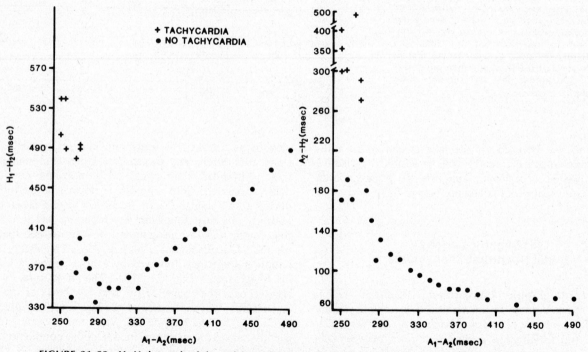

FIGURE 21–22 H_1-H_2 intervals (*left*) and A_2-H_2 intervals (*right*) at various A_1-A_2 intervals. Discontinuous AV nodal curve. At a critical A_1-A_2 interval the H_1-H_2 interval and the A_2-H_2 intervals increase markedly. At the break in the curves, AV nodal reentrant tachycardia is initiated.

The sequence of retrograde atrial activation is normal during AV nodal reentrant supraventricular tachycardia. This means that the earliest site of atrial activation during retrograde conduction over the fast pathway is recorded in the His bundle electrogram followed by electrograms recorded from the os of the coronary sinus and then spreading to depolarize the rest of the right and left atria. During retrograde conduction over the slow pathway in the atypical type of AV nodal reentry, atrial activation recorded in the proximal coronary sinus may precede atrial activation recorded in the low right atrium, suggesting that the slow and fast pathways may enter the atria at slightly different positions.[136] Functional bundle branch block during AV nodal reentrant tachycardia does not modify the tachycardia significantly.

Clinical Features. AV nodal reentry commonly occurs in patients who have no organic heart disease. Symptoms frequently accompany the tachycardia and range from feelings of palpitations, nervousness, and anxiety to angina, heart failure, syncope, or shock, depending on the duration and rate of the tachycardia and the presence of organic heart disease. Tachycardia may cause syncope because of the rapid ventricular rate, reduced cardiac output, and cerebral circulation, or because of asystole when the tachycardia terminates, owing to tachycardia-induced depression of sinus node automaticity (Fig. 21–21). The prognosis for patients without heart disease is usually good.

Hemodynamic consequences of supraventricular tachyarrhythmias in patients with normal ventricular function are due primarily to a marked decrease in left ventricular end-diastolic and stroke volumes with an increase in ejection rate and cardiac output without a significant change in ejection fraction as heart rate is increased and the atrial contribution to ventricular filling is lost.[10] Heart disease or tachycardia may reduce the ejection fraction.[137] Initial hypotension during tachycardia evokes a sympathetic response that increases blood pressure and in turn causes a rise in vagal tone that may terminate the tachycardia.[138]

Treatment. Treatment of the acute attack depends on the underlying heart disease, how well the tachycardia is tolerated, and the natural history of previous attacks in the individual patient. For some patients, rest, reassurance, and sedation may be all that are required to abort an attack. Vagal maneuvers, including carotid sinus massage, Valsalva and Mueller maneuvers, and gagging, serve as the first line of therapy. These maneuvers may slightly slow the tachycardia rate, which then may speed up to the original rate following cessation of the attempt, or they may terminate the tachycardia. Vagal maneuvers should be tried *again* after each pharmacological approach.

Verapamil[99,139–141] (see p. 665), 5 to 10 mg IV, terminates AV nodal reentry successfully in about 2 minutes in over 90 per cent of instances. This drug, or one of the other calcium-entry blockers, such as diltiazem,[142] has become the treatment of choice should simple vagal maneuvers fail. At the time of this writing diltiazem is still an investigational drug for treating arrhythmias.

Cholinergic drugs, particularly edrophonium chloride (Tensilon), a short-acting cholinesterase inhibitor, may terminate AV nodal reentry when administered initially at a trial dose of 3 to 5 mg IV and, if unsuccessful, repeated at a dose of 10 mg IV. Its action is rapid in onset and short in duration, with minimal side effects. Edrophonium should be used cautiously or not at all in patients who are hypotensive or who have lung disease, especially a history of asthma. Treating arrhythmias is not an FDA-approved indication for use of edrophonium.

If these initial approaches are unsuccessful, *intravenous digitalis* administration may be attempted using one of the following short-acting digitalis preparations: ouabain, 0.25 to 0.5 mg IV, followed by 0.1 mg every 30 to 60 minutes, if needed, keeping the total dose less than 1.0 mg within a 24-hour period or 0.01 mg/kg as a single dose over 10 to 15 minutes; digoxin, 0.5 to 1.0 mg IV given over 10 to 15 min, followed by 0.25 mg every 2 to 4 hours, with a total dose less than 1.5 mg within any 24-hour period; or deslanoside, 0.8 mg IV, followed by 0.4 mg every 2 to 4 hours, restricting the total dose to less than 2.0 mg within a 24-hour period. *Oral digitalis* administration to terminate an acute attack is generally not indicated. Vagal maneuvers, previously ineffective, may terminate the tachycardia following digitalis administration and therefore should be repeated.

Propranolol given intravenously at a rate of 0.5 to 1.0 mg/min for a total dose of 0.5 to 3.0 mg may be tried if digitalis administration is unsuccessful. Higher doses may be used in some patients (see Chap. 20). Propranolol must be used cautiously, if at all, in patients with heart failure, chronic lung disease, or a history of asthma because its beta-adrenergic receptor blocking action depresses myocardial contractility and may produce bronchospasm.

Prior to administering digitalis or propranolol, it is advisable to reassess the clinical status of the patient and consider whether DC cardioversion may be advisable. DC shock, administered to patients who have received excessive amounts of digitalis, may be dangerous and may result in serious post-shock ventricular arrhythmias (p. 671). Particularly if signs or symptoms of cardiac decompensation occur, DC electrical shock should be considered early. DC shock, synchronized to the QRS complex to avoid precipitating ventricular fibrillation, successfully terminates AV nodal reentry with energies in the range of 10 to 50 watt-seconds; higher energies may be required in some instances (pp. 626 and 669).

In the event that digitalis has been given in large doses and DC shock is contraindicated, *atrial or ventricular pacing* may restore sinus rhythm. In some instances, esophageal pacing may be useful (p. 756).

Procainamide, quinidine, or disopyramide may be required to terminate AV nodal reentry in some patients. Unless contraindicated, DC cardioversion generally should be employed prior to using these agents, which are more often administered to prevent recurrences. These three drugs selectively depress conduction in the retrograde fast pathway.[143] Disopyramide may at times depress conduction in the slow pathway antegradely.[144] Cardiac glycosides and beta and calcium-entry blockers selectively depress antegrade slow pathway conduction but occasionally may depress conduction in the retrograde fast pathway.

Pressor drugs may terminate AV nodal reentry by inducing reflex vagal stimulation mediated by baroreceptors in the carotid sinus and aorta when the systolic blood pressure is acutely elevated to levels of about 180 mm Hg. One of the following drugs, diluted in 5 to 10 ml of 5 per cent dextrose and water, may be given over 1 to 3 minutes: phenylephrine (Neo-Synephrine), 0.5 to 1.0 mg; methoxamine (Vasoxyl), 3 to 5 mg; or metaraminol (Aramine), 0.5 to 2.0 mg. Pressor drugs should be used cautiously or not at all in the elderly and in patients who have organic heart disease, significant hypertension, hyperthyroidism, or acute myocardial infarction. Today, this potentially dangerous and almost always uncomfortable procedure is rarely needed unless the patient is also hypotensive.

Prevention of recurrences is often more difficult than terminating the acute episode. Initially, one must decide whether the frequency and severity of the attacks warrant long-term drug prophylaxis. If the attacks of paroxysmal tachycardia are infrequent, well tolerated, and either terminate spontaneously or are easily terminated by the patient, no prophylactic therapy may be necessary. If the attacks are sufficiently frequent to necessitate therapy, the patient may be treated with drugs empirically or based on serial electrophysiological testing. Because drug responses are variable, serial electrophysiological testing of multiple drugs appears reasonable in some patients with poorly tolerated tachycardias that recur only sporadically (p. 634).[145]

If empirical testing is desirable, the following choices are recommended: Digitalis is generally the initial drug of choice. It has the advantages of being well- tolerated and requiring administration only once daily. The clinical situation determines the speed of digitalization. Using digoxin, rapid oral digitalization can be accomplished in 24 to 36 hours with an initial dose of 1.0 to 1.5 mg, followed by 0.25 to 0.5 mg every 6 hours for a total dose of 2.0 to 3.0 mg. A less rapid oral regimen digitalizes in 2 to 3 days with an initial dose of 0.75 to 1.0 mg, followed by 0.25 to 0.50 mg every 12 hours for a total dose of 2.0 to 3.0 mg. Alternatively, digoxin administered as a maintenance dose of 0.125 to 0.500 mg achieves digitalization in about one week. Digitoxin, which has a longer duration of action, may be used instead of digoxin. Oral digitalization with digitoxin may be accomplished in 24 to 36 hours with an initial dose of 0.5 to 0.8 mg, followed by 0.2 mg every 6 to 8 hours until a total dose of 1.2 mg is reached. A slower approach involves administering 0.2 mg three times daily for 2 to 3 days. Complete digitalization can also be accomplished in about one month by simply giving a daily maintenance dose of 0.05 to 0.20 mg.

If digitalis alone is unsuccessful, one can then add verapamil, 80 to 120 mg every 6 or 8 hours, quinidine sulfate, 300 to 500 mg every 6 hours, or propranolol, 10 to 40 mg every 6 hours. Procainamide or disopyramide can be used instead of quinidine. In some patients, concomitant administration of digitalis, propranolol, and quinidine or procainamide or disopyramide may be necessary.

For many patients, pacemaker implantation provides acceptable treatment (p. 756). Competitive atrial pacing promptly terminates AV nodal reentry, restoring sinus rhythm immediately or sometimes after a transient episode of atrial flutter or atrial fibrillation, and avoids the necessity of daily drug administration with potential side effects.

Reentry Over a Retrograde Conducting (Concealed) Accessory Pathway

Electrocardiographic Recognition. The presence of an accessory pathway that conducts unidirectionally from the ventricle to the atrium but not in the reverse direction is not apparent in the scalar ECG during sinus rhythm because the ventricle is not preexcited. Therefore, the ECG manifestations of the Wolff-Parkinson-White (WPW) syndrome (see p. 712) are absent and the accessory pathway is said to be "concealed."[146–151] However, since the mechanism responsible for most tachycardias in patients who have the WPW syndrome is probably macro-reentry caused by anterograde conduction over the AV node–His bundle pathway and retrograde conduction over an accessory pathway, the latter, even if it only conducts retrogradely, can still participate in the reentrant circuit. Electrocardiographically, a tachycardia due to this mechanism may be *suspected* when the QRS complex is normal and the retrograde P wave occurs *after* completion of the QRS complex, in the ST segment or early T wave (Fig. 21–9C).

This relationship between P wave and QRS complex results because the ventricle must be activated before the propagating impulse can enter the accessory pathway and excite the atria retrogradely. Therefore, the retrograde P wave must follow ventricular excitation in contrast to AV nodal reentry, in which the atria can be excited during ventricular activation (Fig. 21–9A). Also, the contour of the retrograde P wave may differ from the usual retrograde P wave, since the atria may be activated eccentrically, i.e., in a manner other than the normal retrograde activation sequence, starting at the low right atrial septum as in AV nodal reentry. This occurs because the concealed accessory pathway in most instances is left-sided, i.e., inserts into the left atrium, making the left atrium the first site of retrograde atrial activation and causing the retrograde P wave to be negative in lead I (Fig. 21–23).[152] Finally, since the tachycardia circuit involves the ventricles, if functional bundle branch block occurs in the same ventricle in which the accessory pathway is located, the cycle length of the tachycardia is prolonged.[147] This important change ensues because the bundle branch block lengthens the reentrant circuit (see Preexcitation Syndrome, p. 712). For example, the normal activation sequence for a reciprocating tachycardia circuit with a left-sided accessory pathway without functional bundle branch block progresses from atrium → AV node–His bundle → right and left ventricles → accessory pathway → atrium. However, during functional left bundle branch block, for example, the tachycardia circuit travels from atrium → AV node–His bundle → right ventricle → septum → left ventricle → accessory pathway → atrium. The additional time required for the impulse to travel from the right to the left ventricle before reaching the accessory pathway and atrium lengthens the V-A interval, which lengthens the cycle length of the tachycardia by an equal amount, assuming no other changes in conduction times occur within the circuit. Thus, lengthening of the tachycardia cycle length by more than 35 msec during ipsilateral functional bundle branch block is diagnostic of a free wall accessory pathway if the lengthening can be shown to be due to V-A prolongation only and not to prolongation of the H-V interval (which may develop with the appearance of bundle branch block). In an occasional patient, the increase in cycle length due to prolongation of VA conduction may be nullified by a simultaneous decrease in the P-R (A-H) interval.[153,153a] Patients with septal accessory pathways have VA prolongation of 25 msec or less with functional right or left bundle branch block.[153a] Functional bundle branch block, particularly functional left bundle branch block, during tachycardia occurs much more commonly in patients who have an accessory pathway than in those with AV nodal reentry, probably because in the latter, slow pathway anterograde conduction allows for longer recovery time of the His-Purkinje system, while in tachycardias associated with accessory pathways, anterograde conduction over the AV node may be more rapid.[154] Functional left bundle branch block may occur more commonly during rapid tachycardias, possibly because the refractory period of the right bundle branch appears to be shorter than the left bundle branch at short cycle lengths.[155] Functional bundle branch block in the ventricle contralateral to the accessory pathway does not lengthen the tachycardia cycle if the H-V interval does not lengthen.

An exception to these observations must be noted. If the patient has a septal accessory pathway (see Preexcitation Syndrome, p. 712), retrograde atrial activation will be normal and the cycle length of the tachycardia may not change appreciably with the development of functional bundle branch block. Invasive electrophysiological confirmation may be necessary (see below).

Vagal maneuvers, by acting predominantly on the AV node, produce a response similar to AV nodal reentry, and the tachycardia may transiently slow or transiently slow and then terminate. General-

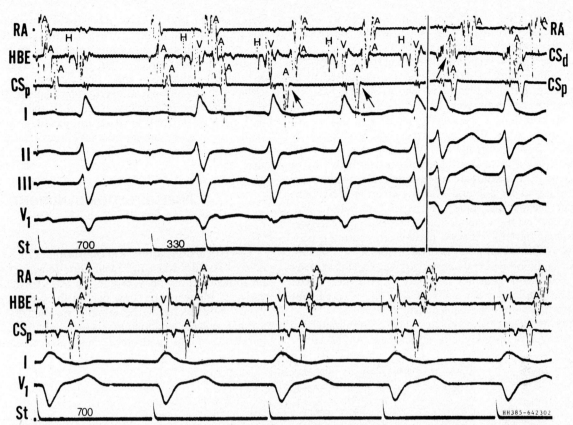

FIGURE 21–23 Retrograde "concealed" accessory pathway and initiation of reciprocating tachycardia in a patient with a left-sided accessory pathway that conducts retrogradely only. The last two stimuli in a train of eight at a cycle length of 700 msec are displayed in the top panel. Premature right atrial stimulation at an interval of 330 msec initiates a reciprocating tachycardia. After the premature stimulus, the A-H interval lengthens slightly and retrograde atrial activity occurs *following* termination of the QRS complex (arrows), beginning first in the CS$_p$ (proximal coronary sinus) electrogram and proceeding to the low right atrial (HBE) and high right atrial (RA) electrograms. Insert at top right indicates that left atrial activity during tachycardia is recorded first in the distal coronary sinus (CS$_d$) electrogram (arrow) consistent with a left lateral accessory pathway. Catheter electrode that is recording CS is at lateral heart border. No evidence of anterograde conduction over an accessory pathway occurred at any cycle length during pacing of the right or left atrium. Right ventricular pacing at a constant cycle length of 700 msec (bottom) initiated the same sequence of retrograde atrial activation seen during the reciprocating tachycardia, thus confirming the presence of retrograde atrial activity over a "concealed" left lateral accessory pathway. (From Zipes, D. P., et al.: Aprindine for treatment of supraventricular tachycardias. Am. J. Cardiol. *40*:586, 1977.)

ly, termination occurs in the anterograde direction, so that the last retrograde P wave fails to conduct to the ventricle.

Electrophysiological features. Electrophysiological criteria supporting the diagnosis of tachycardia involving reentry over a concealed accessory pathway include the fact that initiation of tachycardia depends on a critical degree of atrioventricular delay (necessary to allow time for the accessory pathway to recover excitability), but the delay can be in the AV node or His-Purkinje system, i.e., a critical degree of A-H delay is not necessary. Occasionally, a tachycardia may start with little or no measurable lengthening of AV nodal or His-Purkinje conduction time.[156] The AV nodal refractory period curve is smooth, in contrast to the discontinuous curve found in many patients with AV nodal reentry. Dual AV nodal pathways occasionally may be noted as a concomitant but unrelated finding.

Accessory pathways can be diagnosed by demonstrating that during ventricular pacing premature ventricular stimulation activates the atria prior to retrograde depolarization of the His bundle, indicating that the impulse reached the atria before it depolarized the His bundle and must have traveled a different pathway to do so. Also, if the ventricles can be stimulated prematurely during tachycardia at a time when the His bundle is refractory, and the impulse still conducts to the atrium, this indicates that retrograde propagation traveled to the atrium over a pathway other than the bundle of His.[146] If the premature ventricular complex depolarizes the atria at the same coupling interval at which the premature ventricular complex occurred, one assumes that the stimulation site (i.e., ventricle) is within the reentrant circuit without intervening His-Purkinje or AV nodal tissue that

might increase the V-A and therefore A-A intervals. In addition, if a premature ventricular complex delivered at a time when the His bundle is refractory terminates the tachycardia, an accessory pathway is most likely present.[146,157]

The V-A interval (conduction over the accessory pathway) generally is constant over a wide range of ventricular paced rates and coupling intervals of premature ventricular complexes as well as during the tachycardia in the absence of aberration. Similar short V-A intervals may be observed in patients during AV nodal reentry, but if the VA conduction time or R-P interval is the same during tachycardia *and* ventricular pacing at comparable rates, an accessory pathway is almost certainly present (Fig. 21–23). The V-A interval is usually less than 50 per cent of the R-R interval.[147] The tachycardia can be easily initiated following premature ventricular stimulation that conducts retrogradely in the accessory pathway but blocks in the AV node or His bundle.[157] Atria and ventricles are required components of the macro-reentrant circuit, and therefore continuation of the tachycardia in the presence of AV or VA block excludes an accessory atrioventricular pathway as part of the reentrant circuit.

Clinical Features. The prevalance of concealed accessory pathways is estimated to account for at least 30 per cent of patients with apparent supraventricular tachycardia referred for electrophysiological evaluation. The great majority of these accessory pathways are located between left ventricle and left atrium, uncommonly between right ventricle and right atrium. It is important to be aware of the possibility of a concealed accessory pathway being responsible for apparently "routine" supraventricular tachycardia, since therapeutic response at times may not follow the usual guidelines. Antiarrhythmic targeting may need to be directed toward drugs that affect the accessory pathway such as quinidine, procainamide, or disopyramide. Also, surgical interruption of the accessory pathway may be accomplished (p. 672). The tachycardia rates tend to be faster than those occurring in AV nodal reentry (≥ 200 beats/min), but a great deal of overlap exists between the two groups.[158] Paroxysmal supraventricular tachycardia may be followed by polyuria after termination.[159] Syncope may occur because the rapid ventricular rate fails to provide adequate cerebral circulation or because the tachyarrhythmia may depress the sinus pacemaker, causing a period of asystole when the tachyarrhythmia terminates. Physical examination reveals an unvarying, regular ventricular rhythm with constant intensity of the first heart sound. The jugular venous pressure may be elevated, but the waveform generally remains constant.[160]

Treatment. The therapeutic approach to terminate this form of tachycardia acutely is as outlined for AV nodal re-

entry (see p. 709). It is necessary to achieve block of a single impulse from atrium to ventricle or ventricle to atrium. Generally, the most successful method is to produce transient AV nodal block, and therefore vagal maneuvers, verapamil, digitalis, and propranolol are acceptable choices. Conventional antiarrhythmic agents that prolong activation time or refractory period in the accessory pathway need to be considered as chronic therapy for prophylactic prevention, similar to that discussed for reciprocating tachycardias associated with the preexcitation syndrome.

PREEXCITATION SYNDROME
(Figs. 21–24 and 21–25 and Fig. 19–25, p. 630)

Electrocardiographic Recognition. Preexcitation syndrome[161] occurs when the atrial impulse activates the whole or some part of the ventricle, or the ventricular impulse activates the whole or some part of the atrium, earlier than would be expected if the impulse traveled by way of the normal specific conduction system only.[162] In the Wolff-Parkinson-White syndrome,[163] muscular connections com-

W20-147489

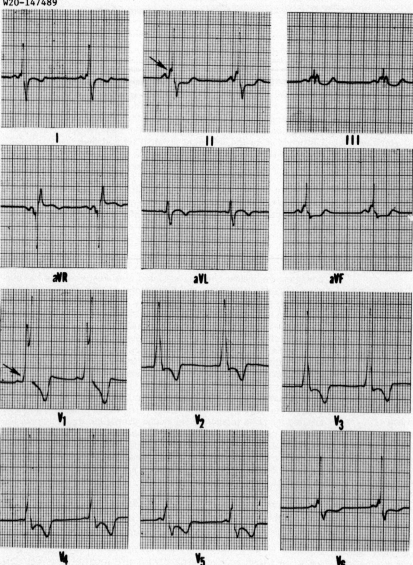

FIGURE 21–24 Wolff-Parkinson-White syndrome due to an accessory pathway, probably located in the left anterior (area 9 in Fig. 21–28) or anterior paraseptal (area 10) position. The delta wave and short P-R intervals can be clearly seen (arrows). The duration of the QRS complex exceeds 120 msec and secondary T-wave changes are present. (From Zipes, D. P., et al.: Preexcitation syndrome. Cardiovasc. Clin. 6:210, 1974.)

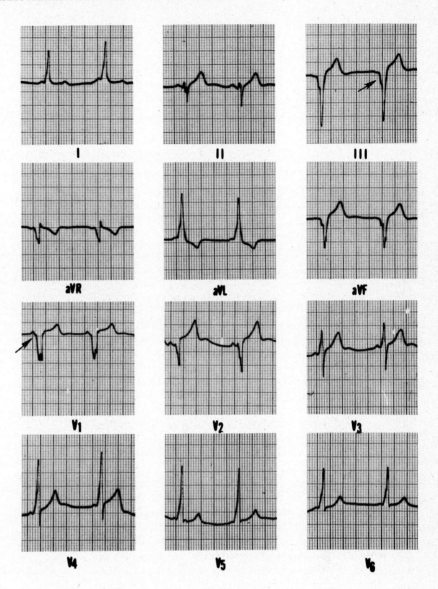

FIGURE 21–25 Wolff-Parkinson-White syndrome probably due to a right lateral accessory pathway (area 3 in Fig. 21–28). The delta wave is indicated by an arrow. (From Zipes, D. P., et al.: Preexcitation syndrome. Cardiovasc. Clin. 6:210, 1974.)

posed of working myocardial fibers exist outside the specialized conducting tissue, in the presence or absence of a well-developed fibrous annulus, and connect atrium and ventricle.[164] They are named *accessory atrioventricular pathways* or connections, commonly called *Kent bundles*,[165,166] and are responsible for the most common variety of preexcitation. Three basic features typify the ECG abnormalities (Figs. 21–24 and 21–25) of patients with the usual form of WPW syndrome caused by an AV connection: (1) P-R interval less than 120 msec during sinus rhythm; (2) QRS complex duration exceeding 120 msec with a slurred, slowly rising onset of the QRS in some leads (delta wave) and usually a normal terminal QRS portion: and (3) secondary ST-T wave changes that are generally directed opposite to the major delta and QRS vectors.

The term *Wolff-Parkinson-White* (WPW) *syndrome* is applied when the patient has symptoms, generally due to tachyarrhythmias. The most common tachycardia is characterized by a normal QRS, by ventricular rates of 150 to 250 beats/min (generally faster than AV nodal reentry), and by sudden onset and termination, behaving in most respects like the tachycardia described for conduction uti-

lizing a concealed pathway (p. 710). The major difference between the two syndromes is the capacity for anterograde conduction over the accessory pathway during atrial flutter or atrial fibrillation (see below).

A variety of other anatomical substrates exist that provide the basis for different ECG manifestations of several variations of the preexcitation syndrome[167] (Fig. 21–26). Fibers from atrium to His bundle bypassing the physiological delay of the AV node are called atriohisian tracts (Fig. 21–26B) and are associated with a short P-R interval and a normal QRS complex. Although demonstrated anatomically[168] (see below), the electrophysiological significance of these tracts in the genesis of tachycardias remains to be established. Indeed, evidence does not support the presence of a specific Lown-Ganong-Levine (LGL) syndrome[169] comprising a short P-R interval, normal QRS complex, and tachycardias related to an atriohisian bypass tract.[170] The short P-R intervals reported in many patients probably represent one end of the spectrum of normal AV conduction.[61] Two varieties of Mahaim fibers[171] include those passing from the AV node to the ventricle, called nodoventricular fibers (Fig. 21–26C), and those arising in

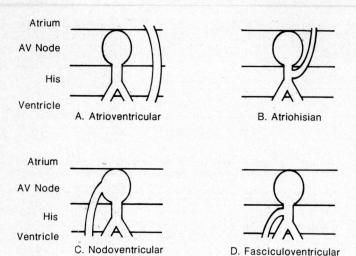

FIGURE 21–26 Schematic representation of accessory pathways.

the His bundle or bundle branches and inserting in the ventricular myocardium, called fasciculoventricular fibers (Fig. 21–26D). For nodoventricular connections, the P-R interval may be normal or short, and the QRS complex is a fusion beat. Fasciculoventricular connections create a normal P-R interval and a fixed, anomalous QRS complex.[172]

Electrophysiological Features (See also pp. 634 and 711). If the Kent bundle accessory pathway is capable of antegrade conduction, two parallel routes of AV conduction are possible, one subject to physiologic delay over the AV node and the other passing directly without delay from atrium to ventricle. This produces the typical QRS complex that is a fusion beat due to depolarization of the ventricle in part by the wavefront traveling over the accessory pathway and in part by the wavefront traveling over the normal AV node–His bundle route. The delta wave represents ventricular activation from input over the accessory pathway. The extent of contribution to ventricular depolarization by the wavefront over each route depends upon their relative activation times. If AV nodal conduction delay occurs, for example, because of a rapid atrial pacing rate or premature atrial complex, more of the ventricle becomes activated over the accessory pathway, and the QRS complex becomes more anomalous in contour. Total activation of the ventricle over the accessory pathway can occur if the AV nodal delay is sufficiently long. In contrast, if the accessory pathway is relatively far from the sinus node, for example, a left lateral accessory pathway, or if AV nodal conduction time is relatively short, more of the ventricle may be activated by conduction over the normal pathway (Fig. 21–27). The normal fusion beat during sinus rhythm has a short H-V interval, or His bundle activation actually begins after the onset of ventricular depolarization, because part of the atrial impulse bypasses the AV node and activates the ventricle early, at a time when the atrial impulse traveling the normal route just reaches the His bundle. This finding of a short or negative H-V interval occurs only during conduction over an accessory pathway or from retrograde His activation during a ventricular tachycardia.

Pacing the atrium at rapid rates, at premature intervals, or from a site close to the atrial insertion of the Kent bundle accentuates the anomalous activation of the ventricles and shortens the H-V interval

even more (His activation may become buried in the ventricular electrogram, Fig. 21–27). The position of the accessory pathway can be determined by a careful analysis of the spatial direction of the delta wave in the 12-lead ECG in maximally preexcited beats[173] (Fig. 21–28) as well as by body surface maps. T-wave abnormalities can occur after disappearance of preexcitation with orientation of the T wave according to the site of preexcitation.[174] In patients who have an atriohisian tract, theoretically the QRS complex would remain normal and the short A-H interval fixed or show little increase during atrial pacing at more rapid rates. Rapid atrial pacing in patients who have

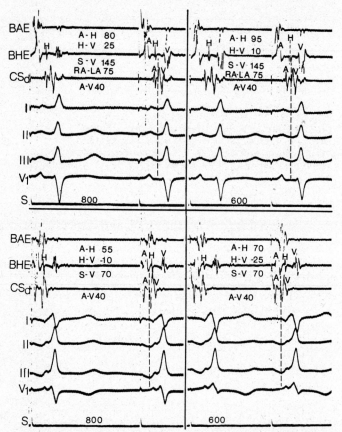

FIGURE 21–27 Influence of pacing site and cycle length on the degree of preexcitation. In this patient with a left anterior accessory pathway (site 9 in Fig. 21–28), pacing the high right atrium at a cycle length of 800 msec (*top left panel*) produced an A-H interval of 80 msec and an H-V interval of 25 msec. The interval from the stimulus to the onset of ventricular activity (S-V) was 145 msec and the right-to-left atrial activation time was 75 msec. The interrupted line indicates the onset of the delta wave. Little preexcitation is seen in the ECG because the fairly rapid AV conduction time over the normal pathway allows much of the ventricle to be activated normally before the impulse traveling from right to left atrium and then over the accessory pathway can depolarize the ventricles. Shortening the pacing cycle length to 600 msec (*top right panel*) without changing the pacing site lengthened the A-H interval by 15 msec and shortened the H-V interval by 10 msec. The other intervals remained the same and the QRS complex changed very slightly. In the *bottom left panel*, the coronary sinus is paced at a cycle length of 800 msec. Even though the A-H interval shortens to 55 msec because of coronary sinus pacing, the S-V shortens to 70 msec, His bundle activation follows the onset of ventricular depolarization by 10 msec, and the QRS complex becomes more aberrant. By pacing at a site near the atrial insertion of the accessory pathway, conduction rapidly reaches the ventricle over the accessory pathway to activate more of the ventricle than when pacing the right atrium at the same cycle length. In the *bottom right panel*, shortening the pacing cycle length to 600 msec lengthens the A-H interval 15 msec, and His bundle activation begins 25 msec after the onset of QRS complex. The S-V and A-V intervals remain unchanged and the QRS complex becomes even more aberrant.

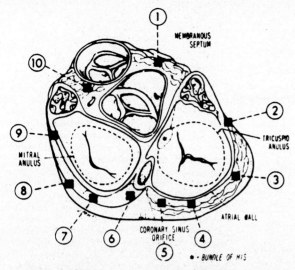

	I	II	III	AVR	AVL	AVF	V₁	V₂	V₃	V₄	V₅	V₆
①	+	+	+(±)	-	±(+)	+	±	±	+(±)	+	+	+
②	+	+	-(±)	-	+(±)	±(-)	±	+(±)	+(±)	+	+	+
③	+	±(-)	-	-	+	-(±)	±	±	±	+	+	+
④	+	-	-	-	+	-	±(+)	±	+	+	+	+
⑤	+	-	-	-(+)	+	-	±	+	+	+	+	+
⑥	+	-	-	-	±(+)	-	+	+	+	+	+	+
⑦	+	-	-	±(+)	+	+	+	+	+	+	+	-(±)
⑧	-(±)	±	±	±(+)	-(±)	±	+	+	+	+	-(±)	-(±)
⑨	-(±)	+	+	-	-(±)	+	+	+	+	+	+	+
⑩	+	+	+(±)	-	±	+	±(+)	+	+	+	+	+

± · Initial 40 msec delta wave isoelectric

+ · Initial 40 msec delta wave positive

- · Initial 40 msec delta wave negative

FIGURE 21–28 In this schematic representation (*top*), sites of the potential position of the accessory pathway are indicated by filled boxes numbered 1 through 10. The delta wave polarity in the 12-lead ECG for each of the 10 sites is depicted in the table at the bottom. (From Gallagher, J. J., et al.: The preexcitation syndromes. Progr. Cardiovasc. Dis. *20*:285, 1978.)

nodoventricular connections shortens the H-V interval and widens the QRS complex but, in contrast to patients who have an atrioventricular connection, (Fig. 21–27) the A-V interval also lengthens. In patients who have fasciculoventricular connections, the H-V interval and QRS complex remain unchanged during rapid atrial pacing.

It is important to remember that, even though the Kent bundle conducts more rapidly than does the AV node (conduction velocity is faster in the accessory pathway), the Kent bundle usually has a longer refractory period during long cycle lengths (e.g., sinus rhythm)— i.e., it takes longer for the accessory pathway to recover excitability than it does for the AV node. Consequently, a premature atrial complex can occur sufficiently early to block anterogradely in the accessory pathway and conduct to the ventricle only over the normal AV node–His bundle (Fig. 21–29). The resultant H-V interval and the QRS complex become normal. Such an event may initiate the most common type of reciprocating tachycardia, which is characterized by anterograde conduction over the normal pathway and retrograde conduction over the accessory pathway (orthodromic)[173,175] (Figs. 21–29

and 21–30). The accessory pathway, blocking in an anterograde direction, recovers excitability in time to be activated following the QRS complex, in a retrograde direction, completing the reentrant loop. Much less commonly, patients can have tachycardias called antidromic tachycardias during which anterograde conduction occurs over the accessory pathway and retrograde conduction over the AV node. The resultant QRS complex is abnormal owing to total ventricular activation over the accessory pathway (Fig. 21–30*C*). In both tachycardias the accessory pathway is an obligatory part of the reentrant circuit.

Rarely, patients may have multiple accessory pathways that maintain the reentrant loop anterogradely over one accessory pathway and retrogradely over the other.[176] Patients who have nodoventricular fibers have tachycardias with a left bundle branch block morphology assumed to be due to a macro-reentrant circuit using the nodoventricular fiber anterogradely and the His-Purkinje system with a portion of the AV node retrogradely[172,177] (Fig. 21–30*F*). This circuit still remains to be established definitively, and it is possible that the nodoventricular pathway is a bystander without participation in the reentrant circuit. No direct relationship between fasciculoventricular fibers and observed arrhythmias has been found.[172] Anatomical-electrophysiological correlative evidence supports the presence and functional significance of nodoventricular fibers.[178]

An incessant form of supraventricular tachycardia has been recognized[179] that generally occurs with a long R-P interval that exceeds the P-R interval (Fig. 21–31) and may be due to an accessory pathway that conducts very slowly, with electrophysiological properties similar to those of the AV node. Tachycardia is maintained by anterograde AV nodal conduction and retrograde conduction over the accessory pathway[180–182] (Fig. 21–30*D*). The long anterograde conduction times over the accessory pathway may prevent ECG manifestations of accessory pathway conduction during sinus rhythm. The QRS is prolonged during sinus rhythm only when conduction times through the AV node–His bundle exceed those in the accessory pathway.[183] Patients can have recurrent, sustained wide QRS tachycardia due to anterograde conduction through the accessory pathway and retrograde conduction over the AV node. Most of these mechanisms found in adults also occur in children.[184]

When retrograde atrial activation during tachycardia occurs over an accessory pathway that connects the left atrium to the left ventricle, the earliest retrograde activity is recorded from a left atrial electrode usually positioned in the coronary sinus (Fig. 21–29). When retrograde atrial activation during tachycardia occurs over an accessory pathway that connects the right ventricle to the right atrium, the earliest retrograde atrial activity generally is recorded from a lateral right atrial electrode. Participation of a septal accessory pathway creates earliest retrograde atrial activation in the low right atrium situated near the septum. These mapping techniques with catheter electrodes and at the time of surgery (pp. 640 and 672) provide the most accurate assessment of the position of the accessory pathway, which can be anywhere in the AV groove except where the ventricles are contiguous (Fig. 21–28). However, it may be difficult to distinguish AV nodal reentry from participation of a septal accessory connection using the retrograde sequence of atrial activation because activation sequences during both tachycardias are similar. Other approaches to demonstrate retrograde atrial activation over the accessory pathway must be tried and can be accomplished by inducing premature ventricular complexes during tachycardia to determine whether retrograde atrial preexcitation can occur at a time when the His bundle is refractory. Since ventriculoatrial conduction cannot occur over the normal conduction system because the His bundle is refractory, an accessory pathway must be present for the atria to become preexcited and must be participating in the tachycardia circuit. No patient with a reciprocating tachycardia due to an accessory AV pathway has a V-A interval less than 70 msec measured from the onset of ventricular depolarization to the onset of the earliest atrial activity recorded on an esophageal lead or less than 95 msec when measured to the high right atrium. In contrast, in the majority of patients with reentry in the AV node, intervals from the onset of ventricular activity to the earliest onset of atrial activity recorded in the esophageal lead are less than 70 msec[185] (see p. 708).

The rhythm of reciprocating tachycardias using an accessory pathway may spontaneously change into atrial flutter or fibrillation.[186] Spontaneous termination of reciprocating tachycardia is common and multiple mechanisms may be involved, with block in the accessory pathway, AV node, or His-Purkinje system.[187]

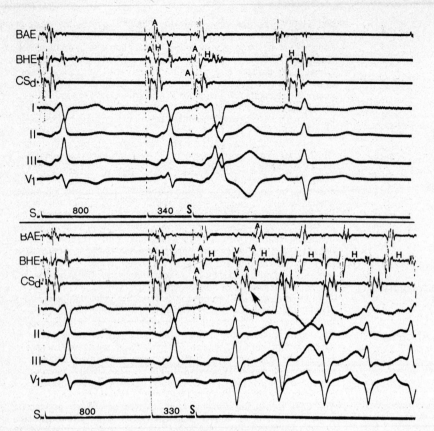

FIGURE 21–29 Initiation of reciprocating tachycardia in Wolff-Parkinson-White syndrome. The last two beats of a regular train at a cycle length of 800 msec and the premature stimulus (S) are shown. *Top*, Premature left atrial stimulation at a cycle length of 340 msec was followed by conduction over the accessory pathway to the ventricle and full preexcitation. *Bottom*, Shortening the premature interval by 10 msec resulted in anterograde block over the accessory pathway, conduction over the normal AV node–His bundle route and loss of ventricular preexcitation (slight functional aberration and H-V prolongation occur). Initiation of a reciprocating tachycardia follows. Note that during reciprocating tachycardia, atrial activation is recorded earliest in the coronary sinus lead, followed by low and high right atrial activation, and is consistent with a left-sided accessory pathway (arrow).

Patients may have other types of tachycardia during which the accessory pathway is an "innocent bystander," i.e., uninvolved in the mechanism responsible for the tachycardia. For example, in patients with atrial flutter or atrial fibrillation, the accessory pathway is not a requisite part of the mechanism responsible for tachycardia, and the latter occurs in the atrium unrelated to the accessory pathway (Fig. 21–30E). Propagation to the ventricle during atrial flutter or atrial fibrillation therefore can occur over the normal AV node–His bundle or accessory pathway. Patients who have paroxysmal atrial fibrillation al-

most always have inducible reciprocating tachycardias as well.[188] Atrial fibrillation presents a potentially serious risk because of the possibility for very rapid conduction over the accessory pathway. At more rapid rates, the refractory period of the accessory pathway may shorten significantly and permit an extremely rapid ventricular response during atrial flutter or atrial fibrillation (Fig. 21–32) that may lead to ventricular fibrillation.[189–191] The rapid ventricular response probably exceeds the ability of the ventricle to follow in an organized fashion, resulting in fragmented disorganized ventricular activation

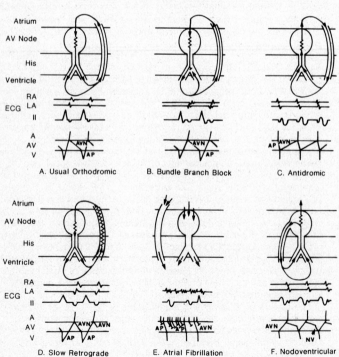

RECIPROCATING TACHYCARDIAS

A. Usual Orthodromic
B. Bundle Branch Block
C. Antidromic
D. Slow Retrograde
E. Atrial Fibrillation
F. Nodoventricular

FIGURE 21–30 Schematic diagram of tachycardias associated with accessory pathways. Format as in Figure 21–9. *A*, Orthodromic tachycardia with anterograde conduction over the AV node–His bundle route and retrograde conduction over the accessory pathway (left-sided for this example as depicted by LA activation preceding RA activation). *B*, Orthodromic tachycardia and ipsilateral functional bundle branch block. *C*, Antidromic tachycardia with anterograde conduction over the accessory pathway and retrograde conduction over the AV node–His bundle. *D*, Orthodromic tachycardia with a slowly conducting accessory pathway. *E*, Atrial fibrillation with the accessory pathway as a bystander. *F*, Anterograde conduction over a portion of the AV node and a nodoventricular pathway and retrograde conduction over the AV node.

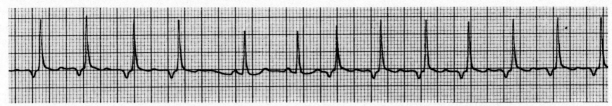

FIGURE 21–31 Scalar ECG appearance of incessant tachycardia due to anterograde conduction over the AV node–His bundle and retrograde conduction over a slowly conducting accessory pathway. Lead II.

and hypotension, and leads to ventricular fibrillation. Alternatively, supraventricular discharge bypassing AV nodal delay may activate the ventricle during the vulnerable period of the antecedent T wave and precipitate ventricular fibrillation.[192] Patients who have had ventricular fibrillation have ventricular cycle lengths during atrial fibrillation in the range of 200 msec or less.[189]

Finally, it is important to remember that patients with preexcitation syndrome may have other causes of tachycardia such as AV nodal reentry,[146] sometimes with dual AV nodal curves,[193] sinus nodal reentry, or even ventricular tachycardia unrelated to the accessory pathway. Accessory pathways may conduct only anterogradely as well as only retrogradely (p. 710).[146,194] If the pathway conducts only anterogradely, it cannot participate in the usual form of reciprocating tachycardia (Fig. 21–30A). It can, however, participate in antidromic tachycardia (Fig. 21–30C) as well as conduct to the ventricle during atrial flutter or atrial fibrillation (Fig. 21–30E). Some data suggest that the accessory pathway demonstrates automatic activity,[27,195] which could conceivably be responsible for some instances of tachycardia.

Clinical Features. The reported incidence of preexcitation syndrome depends in large measure on the population studied, varying from 0.1 to 3.0 per thousand in apparently healthy subjects, with an average of about 1.5 per thousand. The incidence of the electrocardiographic pattern of Wolff-Parkinson-White conduction in 22,500 healthy aviation personnel was 0.25 per cent with a prevalence of documented tachyarrhythmias of 1.8 per cent. However, in a group of referred patients the prevalence of

tachyarrhythmias was 20 per cent.[196] It occurs in all age groups, from the newborn to the elderly, in identical twins, and more often in males (60 to 70 per cent of cases). The majority of adults with preexcitation syndrome have normal hearts,[197] although a variety of acquired and congenital cardiac defects have been reported, including Ebstein's anomaly,[198,199] mitral valve prolapse, and cardiomyopathies. Patients with Ebstein's anomaly (p. 996) often have multiple accessory pathways, right-sided either in the posterior septum or posterolateral wall, with preexcitation localized to the atrialized ventricle. They often have reciprocating tachycardia with a long V-A interval and a right bundle branch block morphology.[199]

Four to 80 per cent of patients with preexcitation syndrome experience recurrent tachyarrhythmias, depending on the patient population, with 80 per cent of these patients having a reciprocating tachycardia, 15 to 30 per cent with atrial fibrillation, and 5 per cent with atrial flutter. Ventricular tachycardia occurs uncommonly. The anomalous complexes may mask or mimic myocardial infarction (p. 230), bundle branch block, or ventricular hypertrophy, and the presence of the preexcitation syndrome may call attention to an associated cardiac defect. Sinus node dysfunction has been reported to be more frequent in patients with the preexcitation syndrome.[200] The prognosis is excel-

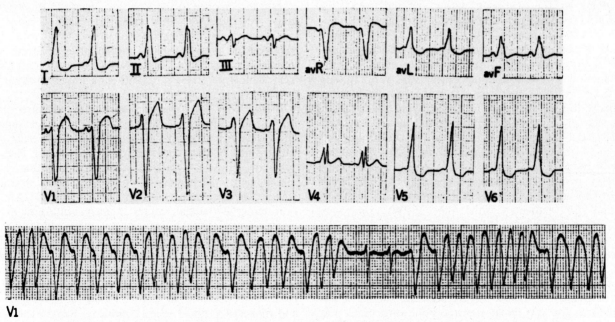

FIGURE 21–32 Preexcitation syndrome is apparent in the 12-lead ECG and may represent a right lateral accessory pathway. During atrial fibrillation the ventricular rate is extremely rapid, at times approaching 350 beats/min. The gross irregularity of the cycle lengths, wide QRS complexes interspersed with normal QRS complexes, and very rapid rate should suggest the diagnosis of atrial fibrillation and an atrioventricular bypass tract.

lent in patients without tachycardia or an associated cardiac anomaly. In patients with recurrent tachycardia the prognosis is good in most, but sudden death occurs rarely, especially when the ventricular rate during tachycardia such as atrial fibillation is rapid or associated congenital defects are present.

It is very likely that acquisition of an accessory pathway occurs congenitally, although its manifestations may present in later years and appear to be "acquired."[156] Some children and adults may lose their tendency to develop tachyarrhythmias as they grow older,[201] possibly owing to fibrotic or other changes at the site of the accessory pathway insertion.[202] The presence or absence of tachycardia associated with the preexcitation syndrome may depend on small changes in activation times in the reentrant loop.

Treatment. Patients with ventricular preexcitation may have no or only occasional tachyarrhythmias unassociated with significant symptoms. These patients do not require electrophysiological evaluation or therapy. However, if a patient has frequent episodes of tachyarrhythmias and/or the arrhythmias cause significant symptoms, therapy should be instituted. Those who suffer significant hemodynamic consequences from the tachycardia should be considered for electrophysiological study (p. 634).

Drugs that increase the refractory period of the accessory pathway or AV node, slow conduction, or cause block in one of the reentry pathways may suppress the reciprocating tachycardia. Verapamil, propranolol, and digitalis prolong conduction time and refractoriness in the AV node. Verapamil[99] and propranolol do not directly affect conduction in the accessory pathway, while digitalis has had variable effects.[203,204] Recently studied, intravenous ouabain had no significant effect on either anterograde or retrograde anomalous pathway refractoriness and did not interfere with the induction of tachycardia in most patients.[205] Because digitalis has been reported to shorten refractoriness in the accessory pathway[204] and speed the ventricular response in some patients with atrial fibrillation,[203] it is advisable *not* to use digitalis as a single drug in patients with the WPW syndrome who have or may develop atrial flutter or atrial fibrillation. Since many patients may develop atrial fibrillation during the reciprocating tachycardia, this caveat probably applies to *all* patients who have tachycardia and the WPW syndrome. Rather, drugs that prolong the refractory period in the accessory pathway such as quinidine, disopyramide, and procainamide should be used. Lidocaine does not prolong refractoriness of the accessory pathway in patients whose effective refractory period ≤ 300 msec.[206] Verapamil[99,207] and lidocaine[206] may increase the ventricular rate during atrial fibrillation in patients with the WPW syndrome. Isoproterenol may expose WPW syndrome and shorten the refractory period of the accessory pathway.[208]

Termination of the acute episode of reciprocating tachycardia, suspected electrocardiographically by a normal QRS complex, regular R-R intervals, a rate of about 200 beats/min, and a P wave in the ST segment, should be approached as for AV nodal reentry. Following vagal maneuvers, verapamil or a similar calcium-entry blocker or edrophonium should be considered as the initial treatment of choice. For atrial flutter or fibrillation, the latter suspected by an anomalous QRS complex and grossly irregular R-R intervals (Fig. 21–32), drugs that prolong

refractoriness in the accessory pathway often coupled with drugs that prolong AV nodal refractoriness (e.g., quinidine and propranolol) must be used. In some patients, particularly with a very rapid ventricular response, electrical cardioversion should be the *initial* treatment of choice.

For long-term therapy to *prevent a recurrence*, it is not always possible to predict which drugs may be most effective for an individual patient. Some drugs actually can increase the frequency of episodes of reciprocating tachycardia by prolonging anterograde and not retrograde refractory periods of the accessory pathway, thereby making it easier for a premature atrial complex to block anterogradely in the accessory pathway. Administration of two drugs, such as quinidine and propranolol or procainamide and verapamil, to decrease conduction capabilities in both limbs of the reentrant circuit may be beneficial. Depending on the clinical situation, empirical drug trials or serial electrophysiological drug testing may be employed to determine optimal drug therapy for patients with reciprocating tachycardia. For patients who have atrial fibrillation with a rapid ventricular response, induction of atrial fibrillation while the patient is receiving therapy is essential to be certain that the ventricular rate is controlled.

Although drugs suppress or modify tachycardia in most patients, an occasional patient may require *surgical ablation* of the accessory pathway (p. 672). Surgical division of the accessory pathway is advisable for patients with frequent symptomatic arrhythmias that are not fully controlled by drugs or with rapid AV conduction over the accessory pathway during atrial flutter or fibrillation and in whom significant slowing of the ventricular response during tachycardia cannot be obtained by drug therapy. Patients who have accessory pathways with very short refractory periods may be poor candidates for drug therapy, since the refractory periods may be prolonged insignificantly in response to the standard agents.[209] *Pacing therapy* may be useful in this syndrome as in many other supraventricular tachyarrhythmias (p. 756), with the exception that precipitation of atrial flutter or atrial fibrillation in a patient with an accessory pathway may result in very rapid ventricular rates and clinical deterioration.[210]

In *summary*, electrocardiographic clues are often present that permit differential diagnosis of the various supraventricular tachycardias.[211] P waves during tachycardia identical to sinus P waves and occurring with a long R-P interval and a short P-R interval are most likely due to sinus nodal reentry. Retrograde (inverted in II, III, and aV$_f$) P waves generally represent reentry involving the AV junction, either AV nodal reentry or reciprocating tachycardia using an accessory pathway. Tachycardia without manifest P waves is probably due to AV nodal reentry (P waves buried in QRS), while a tachycardia with an R-P interval exceeding 60 to 70 msec may be due to an accessory pathway. AV dissociation or AV block during tachycardia excludes the presence of a functioning accessory pathway and makes AV nodal reentry unlikely. Some tachycardias, such as sinus and AV nodal reentry, can occur either simultaneously or at different times in the same patient[99,212] (Fig. 21–8, p. 694). Tachycardia due to intra-His reentry has been described, although the clinical importance of this entity is not established.

VENTRICULAR RHYTHM DISTURBANCES

Premature Ventricular Complexes

Electrocardiographic Recognition. A premature ventricular complex is characterized by the premature occurrence of a QRS complex that is bizarre in shape and has a duration usually more prolonged than the dominant QRS complex, generally exceeding 120 msec. The T wave is commonly large and opposite in direction to the major deflection of the QRS. The QRS complex is not preceded by a premature P wave but may be preceded by a sinus P wave occurring at its expected time. The diagnosis of premature ventricular complex can never be made with unequivocal certainty from the scalar electrocardiogram, since a supraventricular beat or rhythm may mimic the manifestations of ventricular arrhythmia (Figs. 21–17 and 21–33). Retrograde transmission to the atria from the premature ventricular complex occurs fairly frequently but is often obscured by the distorted QRS complex and T wave. If the retrograde impulse discharges and resets the sinus node prematurely, it produces a pause that is not fully compensatory. More commonly, the sinus node and atria are not discharged prematurely by the retrograde impulse, since interference of impulses frequently occurs at the AV junction (see p. 735), establishing a collision between the anterograde impulse conducted from the sinus node and the retrograde impulse conducted from the premature ventricular complex. Therefore, a fully compensatory pause usually follows a premature ventricular complex: the R-R interval produced by the two sinus-initiated QRS complexes on either side of the premature complex equals twice the normally conducted R-R interval. The premature ventricular complex may not produce any pause and may therefore be interpolated (Fig. 21–33), or it may produce a postponed compensatory pause when an interpolated premature complex causes P-R prolongation of the first post-extrasystolic beat to such a degree that the P wave of the second post-extrasystolic beat occurs at a very short R-P interval and is therefore blocked.[213]

Interference within the ventricle may result in *ventricular fusion beats* (see p. 721), which may on occasion be narrower than the dominant beat. For example, a right bundle branch block pattern of a premature ventricular complex arising in the left ventricle of a patient with left bundle branch block may fuse with the dominant left bundle branch block pattern to produce a normally shaped QRS complex. This might also occur when the ventricle with a bundle branch block pattern is paced artificially, producing a narrow ventricular fusion beat between the paced and the sinus-conducted beats. Narrow premature ventricular complexes also have been explained as originating at a point equidistant from each ventricle in the ventricular septum and by arising high in the fascicular system.[214] Whether a compensatory or noncompensatory pause, retrograde atrial excitation, or an interpolated complex, fusion complex or echo beat (p. 627) occurs (Fig. 21–33), it is merely a function of how the AV junction conducts and the timing of the events taking place.

The term *bigeminy* refers to pairs of complexes and indicates a normal and premature complex; *trigeminy* indicates a premature complex following two normal beats; a premature complex following three normal beats is called

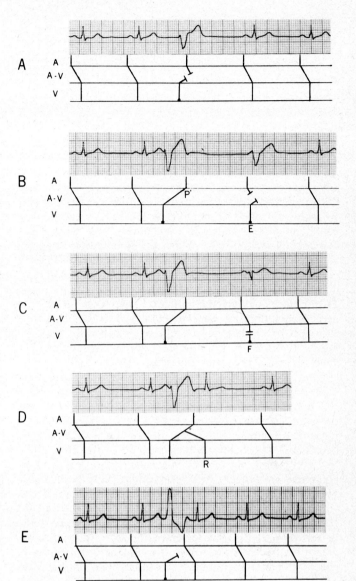

FIGURE 21–33 Premature ventricular complexes. *A* to *D* were recorded in the same patient. *A,* A late premature ventricular complex results in a compensatory pause. *B,* A slower sinus rate and a slightly earlier premature complex result in retrograde atrial excitation (P'). The sinus node is reset, producing a noncompensatory pause. Before the sinus-initiated P wave that follows the retrograde P wave can conduct to the ventricle, a ventricular escape occurs (E). *C,* Events are similar to those in *B* except that a ventricular fusion beat (F) results following the premature ventricular complex owing to a slightly faster sinus rate. *D,* The impulse propagating retrogradely to the atrium reverses its direction after a delay and returns to reexcite the ventricles (R) to produce a ventricular echo. *E,* An interpolated premature ventricular complex is followed by a slightly prolonged P-R interval of the sinus-initiated beat. Lead II.

quadrigeminy, and so on. Two successive premature ventricular complexes are termed a pair or a couplet, while three successive premature ventricular complexes are called a triplet. Arbitrarily, three or more successive premature ventricular complexes are termed ventricular tachycardia. Premature ventricular complexes may have different contours and often are called multifocal (Fig. 21–34). More properly they should be called "multiform," "polymorphic," or "pleomorphic," since it is not known whether multiple foci are discharging or whether conduction of the impulse originating from one site is merely changing.

Premature ventricular complexes may exhibit fixed or

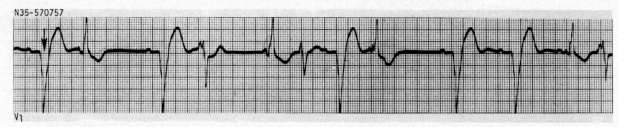

FIGURE 21–34 Multiform premature ventricular complexes. The normally conducted QRS complexes exhibit a left bundle branch block contour (arrow) and are followed by premature ventricular complexes with three different morphologies.

variable coupling, i.e., the interval between the normal QRS complex and the premature ventricular complex may be relatively stable or variable. In the past, fixed coupling has been considered to indicate a reentrant mechanism. We now know that fixed coupling may be due to triggered activity (p. 620) or other possible mechanisms. Variable coupling may be due to parasystole (see Chapter 7, p. 248, and p. 622), to changing conduction in a reentrant circuit, to multiform premature ventricular complexes, or to triggered activity with a varying coupling interval. Usually, it is impossible to determine the precise mechanism responsible for the premature ventricular complex with either constant or variable coupling intervals.

Clinical Features. The prevalence of premature complexes increases with age. Their presence may be manifest by symptoms of palpitations or discomfort in the neck or chest because of the greater than normal contractile force of the post-extrasystolic beat or the feeling that the heart has stopped during the long pause after the premature complex. Long runs of frequent premature ventricular complexes in patients with heart disease may produce angina or hypotension. Frequent interpolated premature ventricular complexes actually represent a doubling of the heart rate and may compromise the patient's hemodynamic status. Activity that increases the heart rate may decrease the patient's awareness of the premature systoles or at times reduce their number. Exercise may increase the number of premature complexes in other patients. Premature systoles may be quite uncomfortable in patients who have aortic regurgitation because of the large stroke volume.

Premature ventricular complexes occur in association with a variety of stimuli and can be produced by direct mechanical, electrical, and chemical stimulation of the myocardium. Often they are seen during infection, in ischemic or inflamed myocardium, or during anesthesia or surgery. They may be provoked by a variety of medications, by tension states, and by excessive use of tobacco, caffeine, or alcohol. Both central and peripheral autonomic stimulation have profound effects on heart rate, which may produce or suppress premature complexes.[215]

Physical examination reveals the presence of a premature beat followed by a pause that is longer than normal. A fully compensatory pause may be distinguished from one that is not fully compensatory, since the former does not change the timing of the basic rhythm. The premature beat is often accompanied by a decrease in intensity of the heart sounds, often with just the first heart sound being heard, which may be sharp and snapping. The relationship of atrial to ventricular systole determines the presence of normal *a* waves or giant *a* waves in the jugular venous pulse, and the length of the P-R interval determines the in-

tensity of the first heart sound. The second heart sound may be abnormally split.

The importance of premature ventricular complexes varies depending on the clinical setting. In the absence of underlying heart disease, the presence of premature ventricular complexes usually has no significance regarding longevity or limitation of activity, and antiarrhythmic drugs are not indicated; the patient should be reassured if he or she is symptomatic. An exception may be middle-aged men, because premature ventricular systoles and complex ventricular arrhythmias occurring in apparently healthy middle-aged men are associated with the presence of coronary heart disease and with a greater risk of subsequent death from coronary heart disease.[216-219] However, it has not been demonstrated that premature ventricular systoles or complex ventricular arrhythmias play a *precipitating* role in the genesis of sudden death in these patients, and the arrhythmias may simply be a marker of heart disease (p. 633). It has not been shown convincingly that antiarrhythmic therapy given to suppress the premature ventricular systoles or complex ventricular arrhythmias reduces the incidence of sudden death in such apparently healthy men. The presence of premature ventricular complexes are thought to reflect an increased risk of cardiac death in patients with hypertrophic cardiomyopathy and mitral valve prolapse. A strong association exists between myocardial infarction size and frequency of premature ventricular complexes found while patients were in the coronary care unit[220] and between poor left ventricular function and frequency of premature ventricular complexes during recovery.[221] In patients suffering from acute myocardial infarction, it has been commonly held that so-called "warning arrhythmias," such as premature ventricular complexes occurring close to the preceding T wave, greater than five or six per minute, bigeminal, multiform, or occurring in salvoes of two, three, or more, may presage or precipitate the occurrence of ventricular tachycardia or fibrillation. However, about half the patients who develop ventricular fibrillation have no "warning arrhythmias" and half who do have "warning arrhythmias" do not develop ventricular fibrillation[222] (p. 728).

Treatment. Extremes of heart rate, both fast and slow, may provoke the development of premature ventricular complexes. Premature ventricular complexes accompanying slow ventricular rates caused by sinus bradycardia or AV block may be abolished by increasing the basic rate with atropine or isoproterenol or by pacing. Conversely, in some patients with sinus tachycardia, slowing the heart rate may eradicate premature ventricular complexes. In the hospitalized patient, lidocaine given intravenously (p. 653) is generally the initial treatment of choice to suppress premature ventricular complexes. Lidocaine can be given intramuscularly in some instances. If maximum dosages of lidocaine are unsuccessful, then procainamide intravenously may be tried. Quinidine may be given intravenously slowly and cautiously. The use of disopyramide intravenously is still investigational. Propranolol or phenytoin may be tried if the other drugs have been unsuccessful. For long-term oral maintenance, quinidine, disopyramide, or procainamide is used, as for the prevention of ventricular tachycardia (p. 723).

Ventricular Tachycardia

Ventricular tachycardia arises in the specialized conduction system distal to the bifurcation of the His bundle, in ventricular muscle, or in combinations of both tissue types. The mechanisms include disorders of impulse formation and conduction (p. 619). The electrocardiographic diagnosis of ventricular tachycardia is suggested when a series of three or more bizarrely shaped premature ventricular complexes occur that exceed 120 msec, with the ST-T vector pointing opposite to the major QRS deflection. The R-R interval may be exceedingly regular or may vary. Atrial activity may be independent of ventricular activity (AV dissociation, p. 735), or the atria may be depolarized by the ventricles retrogradely (VA association). As will be discussed, depending on the particular type of ventricular tachycardia, the rate ranges from 70 to 250 beats/min, and the onset may be paroxysmal (sudden) or nonparoxysmal. QRS contours during the ventricular tachycardia may be unchanging (uniform) or may vary in a random fashion (multiform, polymorphic, or pleomorphic), vary in a more or less repetitive manner (torsades de pointes), vary in alternate complexes (bidirectional ventricular tachycardia), or vary in a stable but changing contour (i.e., right bundle branch contour changing to left bundle branch contour (see Fig. 20–8*A*, p. 674). Ventricular tachycardia may be sustained, defined arbitrarily as lasting longer than 30 seconds or requiring termination because of hemodynamic collapse, or nonsustained when it stops spontaneously in less than 30 seconds.[223,224]

The electrocardiographic distinction between supraventricular tachycardia with aberration and ventricular tachycardia may be extremely difficult at times, since features of

TABLE 21–2 MAJOR FEATURES IN THE DIFFERENTIAL DIAGNOSIS OF WIDE QRS BEATS OR TACHYCARDIA

SUPPORTS SVT	SUPPORTS VT
Slowing or termination by ↑ vagal tone	Fusion beats
Onset with premature P wave	Capture beats
RP interval ≤ 100 msec	AV dissociation
P and QRS rate and rhythm linked to suggest ventricular activation depends on atrial discharge, e.g., 2:1 AV block	P and QRS rate and rhythm linked to suggest atrial activation depends on ventricular discharge, e.g., 2:1 VA block
RSR′ V₁	
Long-short cycle sequence	"Compensatory" pause
	Left axis deviation QRS duration > 140 msec specific QRS contours (see text)

SVT = supraventricular tachycardia;
VT = ventricular tachycardia.

both arrhythmias overlap and under certain circumstances a supraventricular tachycardia can mimic all the criteria established for ventricular tachycardia. Ventricular complexes with bizarre or prolonged configuration indicate only that conduction through the ventricle is abnormal, and they can occur in supraventricular rhythms characterized by preexisting bundle branch block, aberrant conduction during incomplete recovery of repolarization, conduction over accessory pathways, and several other conditions (see p. 244). They do not necessarily indicate the origin of impulse formation or the reason for the abnormal conduction. Conversely, ectopic beats originating in the ventricle uncommonly can have a fairly normal duration and shape.

During the course of a tachycardia characterized by widespread, bizarre QRS complexes, the presence of *fusion beats* and *capture beats* provides maximum support for the diagnosis of ventricular tachycardia (Table 21–2). Fusion beats indicate activation of the ventricle from two different foci, implying that one of the foci had a ventricular origin. Capture of the ventricle by the supraventricular rhythm with a normal configuration of the captured QRS complex at an interval shorter than the tachycardia in question indicates that the impulse has a supraventricular origin (Fig. 21–35). Atrioventricular dissociation (p. 735) has long

018

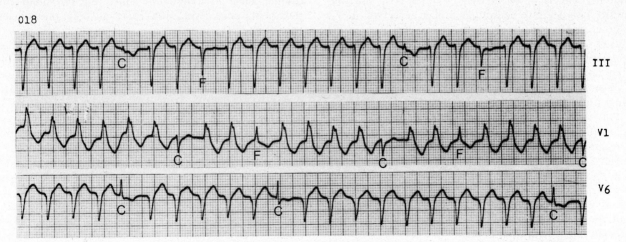

FIGURE 21–35 Fusions and capture beats during a probable ventricular tachycardia. The QRS complex is prolonged, and the R-R interval is regular except for occasional capture beats (C) that have a normal contour and are slightly premature. Complexes intermediate in contour represent fusion beats (F). Thus, even though atrial activity is not clearly apparent, it is likely that AV dissociation is present during a ventricular tachycardia and produces intermittent capture and fusion beats.

been considered a hallmark of ventricular tachycardia. However, retrograde VA conduction to the atria from ventricular beats occurs in a large percentage of patients, and therefore ventricular tachycardia may not exhibit AV dissociation.[225] Atrioventricular dissociation can occur uncommonly during supraventricular tachycardias (see Fig. 19–32*A*, p. 637). Even if a P wave appears to be related to each QRS complex it is at times difficult to determine whether the P wave is conducted anterogradely to the next QRS complex (i.e., supraventricular tachycardia with aberrancy) or retrogradely from the preceding QRS complex (i.e., a ventricular tachycardia). As a general rule, however, AV dissociation during a wide QRS tachycardia is strong presumptive evidence that the tachycardia is of ventricular origin.

Because of the overlapping features of ventricular and supraventricular tachycardias, and because differentiating clues may not be present on a given tracing, it appears best to ascribe a certain probability to the diagnosis that may weigh in favor of its ventricular or supraventricular origin. Some electrocardiographic features characterizing supraventricular arrhythmia with aberrancy include (1) consistent onset of the tachycardia with a premature P wave, (2) a very short R-P interval ($\leq$ 0.1 sec) often requiring an esophageal recording to visualize the P waves, (3) a QRS configuration the same as that which occurs from known supraventricular conduction at similar rates, (4) P and QRS rate and rhythm linked to suggest that ventricular activation depends on atrial discharge (e.g., A-V Wenckebach block), and (5) slowing or termination of the tachycardia by vagal maneuvers.

Analysis of specific QRS contours also may be helpful. For example, QRS contours suggesting a ventricular tachycardia include left-axis deviation in the frontal plane and a QRS duration exceeding 140 msec with a QRS of normal duration during sinus rhythm. During ventricular tachycardia with right bundle branch block appearance, (1) the QRS complex is monophasic or biphasic in V_1 with an initial deflection different from sinus-initiated QRS complex, (2) the amplitude of the R wave in V_1 exceeds the R′, and (3) small R and large S wave or a QS pattern in V_6 may be present. With a ventricular tachycardia having a left bundle branch block contour, (1) the axis may be rightward with negative deflections deeper in V_1 than in V_6, (2) a broad prolonged (> 40 msec) R wave in V_1, and (3) a small Q, large R wave or QS pattern in V_6 may exist. A QRS complex that is similar in V_1 through V_6, either all negative or all positive, favors a ventricular origin as does the presence of 2:1 ventriculoatrial block. Supraventricular beats with aberration often have a triphasic pattern in V_1, an initial vector of the abnormal complex similar to that of the normally conducted beats, and a wide QRS complex that terminates a short cycle length which follows a long cycle (long-short cycle sequence). During atrial fibrillation fixed coupling, short coupling intervals, a long pause after the abnormal beat, and runs of bigeminy rather than a consecutive series of abnormal complexes, all favor ventricular origin of the premature complex rather than supraventricular origin with aberration.[226,227] A grossly irregular, wide QRS tachycardia with ventricular rates faster than 200 beats/min should raise the question of atrial fibrillation with conduction over an accessory pathway (see p. 712 and Fig. 21–32).[226,227] Exceptions exist to all the crite-

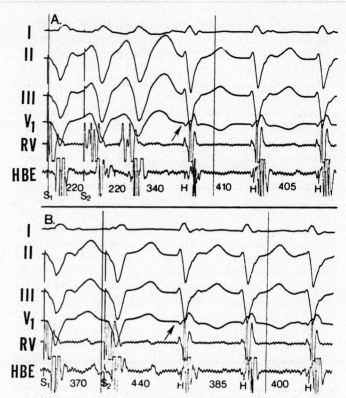

FIGURE 21–36 Precipitation and termination of sustained ventricular tachycardia by premature ventricular stimulation. *A*, The last paced beat (S_1) of a train at a basic cycle length of 550 msec is displayed. Premature ventricular stimulation at an S_1-S_2 interval of 220 msec is followed by a repetitive ventricular response, probably bundle branch reentry (a possible retrograde His depolarization is unlabeled) and then initiation of ventricular tachycardia (arrow). Note that His activation follows the onset of the QRS complex during the ventricular tachycardia. The latter exhibits right bundle branch block and left-axis deviation. *B*, Premature ventricular stimulation at an S_1-S_2 interval of 370 msec initiates the same ventricular tachycardia without a bundle branch reentrant response. (From Zipes, D. P., et al.: Atrial induction of ventricular tachycardia: Reentry versus triggered automaticity. Am. J. Cardiol. *44*:1, 1979.)

ria enumerated above, especially in patients who have preexisting conduction disturbances or preexcitation syndrome; when in doubt, one must rely on sound clinical judgment, considering the ECG as only one of several helpful ancillary tests.

ELECTROPHYSIOLOGICAL FEATURES. Electrophysiologically, ventricular tachycardia can be distinguished by a short or negative H-V interval (i.e., H begins after the onset of ventricular depolarization) because of retrograde activation from the ventricles (see Fig. 19–32, p. 637, and Fig. 21–36). His bundle deflections dissociated from ventricular activation are diagnostic of ventricular tachycardia,[228] with rare exception.[229] His bundle deflections usually are not apparent because they are obscured by simultaneous ventricular septal depolarization or because of inadequate catheter position. The latter must be determined during supraventricular rhythm before the onset or after the termination of the ventricular tachycardia. Ventricular tachycardia may produce QRS complexes of narrow duration and of short H-V interval, most likely when the site of origin is close to the His bundle in the fascicles.[230]

Successful electrical induction of ventricular tachycardia

by premature stimulation of the ventricle (Fig. 21–36)[228,231] depends strongly on the characteristics of the ventricular tachycardia and the anatomic substrate. Sustained ventricular tachycardia and ventricular tachycardia due to coronary artery disease are induced with greater success than are nonsustained ventricular tachycardia and ventricular tachycardia due to noncoronary-related causes.[223] In general, it is more difficult to induce ventricular tachycardia with late premature stimuli compared to early premature stimuli, during sinus rhythm compared to ventricular pacing, and with one premature stimulus compared to two or three. The specificity of ventricular tachycardia induction using more than two premature ventricular stimuli has yet to be established, and preliminary data suggest that nonsustained pleomorphic ventricular tachycardia can be induced in patients who have no history of ventricular tachycardia.[232,233] Occasionally, ventricular tachycardia can be initiated only from the left ventricle[228] or from specific sites in the right ventricle.[234] No clinical, anatomical, electrocardiographic, or electrophysiological features are useful to predict whether left ventricular programmed stimulation will be required to induce ventricular tachycardia in patients.[235] Drugs such as isoproterenol,[236] various antiarrhythmic agents,[237] and alcohol[238] can facilitate the induction of ventricular tachycardia.

The capability of terminating ventricular tachycardia by pacing depends significantly on the rate of the ventricular tachycardia. Slower ventricular tachycardias are more easily terminated and with fewer stimuli than are more rapid ventricular tachycardias. An increasing number of stimuli are required to terminate more rapid ventricular tachycardias, which increases the risks of pacing-induced acceleration of the ventricular tachycardia.[239,240] Following premature stimulation during ventricular tachycardia, a pause may result but the tachycardia continues, suggesting that the origin of the tachycardia is relatively protected.[54,241] Ventricular tachycardia can also be induced and terminated during atrial pacing (see Fig. 19–33, p. 637).[54,59]

With the advent of acceptable surgical techniques to treat some forms of ventricular tachycardia it has become important to localize its origin. The 12-lead electrocardiogram may give misleading information regarding the origin of sustained ventricular tachycardia[242] and extensive endocardial and epicardial mapping studies are generally necessary (see Chapter 19). *Radionuclide phase mapping* of ventricular tachycardia is feasible and appears to provide data consistent with the known electrophysiology of ventricular tachycardia.[243]

CLINICAL FEATURES. Symptoms occurring during ventricular tachycardia depend on the ventricular rate, duration of tachycardia, the presence and extent of the underlying heart disease, and peripheral vascular disease. The location of impulse formation and therefore the way in which the depolarization wave spreads across the myocardium may also be important in some instances of delicate hemodynamic compensation. Physical findings depend in part on the P to QRS relationship. If atrial activity is dissociated from the ventricular contractions, the findings of AV dissociation (p. 735) will be present. If the atria are captured retrogradely, regularly occurring cannon *a* waves appear when atrial and ventricular contractions occur simultaneously and the signs of AV dissociation are absent.

In the author's series of 516 patients treated for symptomatic recurrent ventricular tachycardia, 284 patients have had ischemic heart disease, 74 cardiomyopathy (both congestive and hypertrophic), 75 primary electrical disease, 45 mitral valve prolapse, 20 valvular heart disease, and 18 miscellaneous causes. Primary electrical disease includes patients with ventricular tachycardia and no evidence of structural heart disease. The nature of ischemic heart disease may take various forms including patients with and without a past history of myocardial infarction, angina, congestive heart failure, or left ventricular aneurysm. Coronary artery spasm with normal coronary arteries may cause transient myocardial ischemia with severe ventricular arrhythmias in some patients.[244] In patients resuscitated from sudden cardiac death (Chap. 23) the majority (75 per cent) have severe coronary artery disease and ventricular tachyarrhythmias can be induced by premature ventricular stimulation in approximately 75 per cent.[245,246] When ventricular tachycardia occurs in the ambulatory patient, it is uncommonly induced by R-on-T premature ventricular complexes.[247] Even short runs of ventricular tachycardia consisting of three or four complexes can be important. When detected in the late hospital phase of acute myocardial infarction, ventricular tachycardia identifies a group of patients with a 38 per cent one-year mortality rate compared to 11.6 per cent in a group without tachycardia.[248] Sustained recurrent ventricular tachycardia can also occur in children with or without associated cardiovascular disease.[249,250] In some patients an acute emotional disturbance may be related temporally to the onset of life-threatening ventricular arrhythmias. However, the causal role played by the emotional stress needs to be established.[251]

Termination of a tachycardia by triggering vagal reflexes is considered diagnostic of supraventricular tachycardias. However, ventricular tachycardia uncommonly can be stopped in a similar manner.[1,2] Valsalva may terminate ventricular tachycardia most likely related to an abrupt reduction in cardiac dimension.[252]

TREATMENT. The most important question is deciding which patients should be treated.[252a] The relative risks of symptoms or sudden death for each type of ventricular tachycardia determine the course of therapy. Generally, patients who have sustained ventricular tachycardia with or without structural heart disease and those who have nonsustained ventricular tachycardia with structural heart disease are treated. Patients who have nonsustained ventricular tachycardia without structural heart disease but are symptomatic should be treated while those who are asymptomatic and otherwise healthy may not need therapy but should be followed closely.

Ventricular tachycardia that does not cause hemodynamic decompensation can be treated medically to achieve acute termination by administering lidocaine IV according to the doses indicated on page 657. If lidocaine abolishes the ventricular tachycardia, a continuous IV infusion can be given. If maximum doses of lidocaine are unsuccessful, procainamide or bretylium can be administered IV and, if successful, given as an IV infusion. Although quinidine can be used intravenously, great caution is needed.

If the arrhythmia does not respond to medical therapy, electrical direct-current (DC) cardioversion can be employed. Ventricular tachycardia that precipitates hypotension, shock, angina, or congestive heart failure or symptoms of cerebral hypoperfusion should be treated *promptly* with DC cardioversion (p. 669). Very low energies may terminate ventricular tachycardia, beginning with a synchronized shock of 10 to 50 watt-seconds. Digitalis-induced ventricular tachycardia is best treated pharmacologically. After reversion of the arrhythmia to a normal rhythm, it is essential to institute measures to prevent a recurrence.

Striking the patient's chest, sometimes called "thumpversion," may terminate ventricular tachycardia by mechanically inducing a premature ventricular complex that presumably interrupts the reentrant pathway necessary to support the ventricular tachycardia.[253] Stimulation at the time of the vulnerable period during ventricular tachycardia may accelerate the ventricular tachycardia or possibly provoke ventricular fibrillation.[254]

In patients with recurrent ventricular tachycardia, a pacing catheter can be inserted into the right ventricle and single, double, or multiple stimuli can be introduced competitively to terminate the ventricular tachycardia. This procedure incurs the risk of accelerating the ventricular tachycardia to ventricular flutter or ventricular fibrillation.[240] A new catheter electrode has been developed recently through which synchronized cardioversion can be performed (see Fig. 22–13, p. 759).

Intermittent ventricular tachycardia, interrupted by several supraventricular beats, is generally best treated pharmacologically with lidocaine, quinidine, bretylium, procainamide, or disopyramide. Propranolol or rarely phenytoin may be useful. If these drugs fail, a wide range of investigational antiarrhythmic drugs are available (see Chap. 20).

A search for reversible conditions contributing to the initiation and maintenance of ventricular tachyarrhythmias should be made and the conditions corrected if possible. For example, ventricular arrhythmia related to hypotension or hypokalemia at times may be terminated by vasopressors or potassium, respectively. Slow ventricular rates that are caused by sinus bradycardia or AV block may permit the occurrence of premature ventricular complexes and ventricular tachyarrhythmias that can be corrected by administering atropine, by temporary isoproterenol administration, or by transvenous pacing. (Fig. 22–11, p. 757).

Prevention of recurrences is generally more difficult than is terminating the acute episode. Initial preventive drug therapy for recurrent ventricular arrhythmias in the ambulatory patient should involve quinidine, procainamide, or disopyramide. Propranolol or phenytoin may be tried next, but they are often unsuccessful unless the ventricular tachycardia is related to ischemia, catecholamine stimulation, or digitalis toxicity. Investigational drugs such as amiodarone (p. 666) may be required. Different thresholds for arrhythmic suppression may exist. For example, the serum concentration of procainamide necessary to suppress spontaneous ventricular tachycardia may be lower than the concentration necessary to achieve a significant suppression of premature ventricular complexes.[255] Combinations of drugs with different mechanisms of action may be successful when single drugs fail and allow one to use low doses of both agents rather than high or toxic doses of one drug. Most of the combinations represent empirical trials, but we generally attempt to combine drugs to which the patient has exhibited a partial therapeutic response. A trial

of ventricular or atrial pacing, combined with antiarrhythmic agents if necessary, may be tested; if successful, permanent pacing may be instituted (p. 756). Generally, unless the ventricular tachycardia is initiated by significant bradycardia, such as ventricular rates less than 40 due to complete AV block, attempts at rapid "overdrive" pacing are ineffective over the long term.

Surgery may be used to treat ventricular tachycardia in selected patients. A ventriculotomy in patients who have ventricular tachycardia related to right ventricular dysplasia, encircling endocardial ventriculotomy, or endocardial resection directed by electrophysiological mapping techniques in patients who have ventricular tachycardia related to coronary disease may eliminate recurrences or may make previously ineffective drug regimens efficacious. Coronary bypass surgery alone, without electrophysiological mapping and myocardial resection, in patients who do not have ventricular tachycardia definitely associated with ischemia—e.g., ventricular tachycardia induced by stress testing—has not been very successful (p. 672).

Evaluating the effectiveness of therapy in patients with widely spaced episodes of ventricular tachycardia is a difficult problem because there exists no adequate end point to judge therapy until the patient has another spontaneous recurrence. Because of this, aggressive approaches using programmed electrical stimulation have been used, as described on pages 636 to 638.[256,257]

Specific Types of Ventricular Tachycardia

A variety of fairly specific types of ventricular tachycardia have been identified, related either to a constellation of distinctive electrocardiographic and electrophysiological features or to a specific set of clinical events. While our understanding of electrophysiological mechanisms responsible for clinically occurring ventricular tachycardias is still naïve, being able to identify different kinds of ventricular tachycardias is the first step toward understanding their mechanisms.

Accelerated Idioventricular Rhythm

Electrocardiographic Recognition. The ventricular rate, commonly between 60 and 110 beats/min, usually hovers within 10 beats of the sinus rate, so that control of the cardiac rhythm may be passed back and forth between these two competing pacemaker sites. Consequently, fusion beats often occur at the onset and termination of the arrhythmia as the pacemakers vie for control of ventricular depolarization (Fig. 21–37). Because of the slow rate, capture beats are common. The onset of this arrhythmia is generally gradual (nonparoxysmal) and occurs when the rate of the ventricular tachycardia exceeds the sinus rate because of sinus slowing or SA or AV block. The ectopic mechanism may also begin after a premature ventricular complex, or the ectopic ventricular focus may simply accelerate sufficiently to overtake the sinus rhythm. The slow rate and nonparoxysmal onset avoid the problems initiated by excitation during the vulnerable period and, conse-

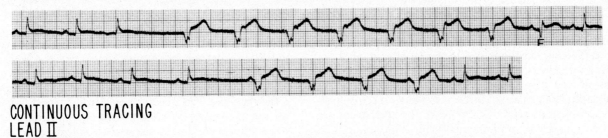

CONTINUOUS TRACING
LEAD II

FIGURE 21-37 Accelerated idioventricular rhythm. *Top,* A premature atrial complex delays the next sinus initiated P wave and allows escape of an accelerated idioventricular rhythm at a rate of about 70 beats/min. The accelerated idioventricular rhythm is again suppressed when the sinus node resumes control of the cardiac rhythm at the end of the tracing. The next to last QRS complex is a fusion beat (F). *Bottom,* Progressive sinus bradycardia allows the escape of the accelerated idioventricular rhythm.

quently, precipitation of more rapid ventricular arrhythmias is rarely seen. Termination of the rhythm generally occurs gradually as the dominant sinus rhythm accelerates or as the ectopic ventricular rhythm decelerates. The ventricular rhythm may be regular or irregular and occasionally may show sudden doubling, suggesting the presence of exit block. Many characteristics suggest enhanced automaticity as the responsible mechanism.

The arrhythmia occurs as a rule in patients who have heart disease, e.g., those with acute myocardial infarction or with digitalis toxicity. It is transient and intermittent, with episodes lasting a few seconds to a minute, and does not appear to affect seriously the course or prognosis of the patient.

Treatment. Suppressive therapy is rarely necessary because the ventricular rate is generally less than 100 beats/min. The following conditions exist during which therapy may be considered: (1) when AV dissociation results in loss of sequential AV contraction and with it the hemodynamic benefits of atrial contribution to ventricular filling; (2) when accelerated idioventricular rhythm occurs together with a more rapid ventricular tachycardia; (3) when accelerated idioventricular rhythm begins with a premature ventricular complex that has a short coupling interval, which causes discharge in the vulnerable period of the preceding T wave; (4) when the ventricular rate is too rapid and produces symptoms; and (5) if ventricular fibrillation develops as a result of the accelerated idioventricular rhythm. This last event appears to be fairly rare.[258] Therapy, when indicated, should be with IV lidocaine, followed by quinidine, bretylium, procainamide, or disopyramide. Often simply increasing the sinus rate with atropine or atrial pacing suppresses the accelerated idioventricular rhythm.[259-261]

Torsades De Pointes

Electrocardiographic Recognition. The term "torsades de pointes" refers to a ventricular tachycardia characterized by QRS complexes of changing amplitude that appear to twist around the isoelectric line and occur at rates of 200 to 250/min (Fig. 21-38A). Originally described in the setting of bradycardia due to complete heart block, torsades de pointes connotes a *syndrome*, not simply an ECG description of the QRS complex of the tachycardia.[262,263] Prolonged ventricular repolarization with Q-T intervals exceeding 500 msec occurs as part of the syn-

drome. The U wave may also become prominent, but its role in this syndrome and in the long Q-T syndrome is not clear. Premature ventricular complexes may discharge during the termination of the T wave, precipitating successive runs of ventricular tachycardia during which the peaks of the QRS complexes appear successively on one side and then on the other of the isoelectric baseline, giving the typical twisting appearance with continuous and progressive

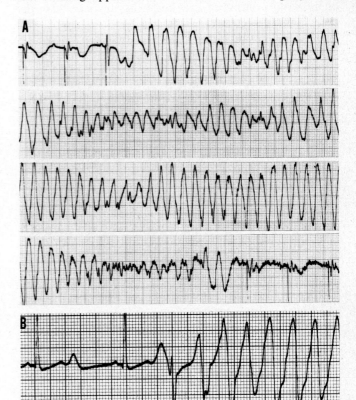

FIGURE 21-38 Torsades de pointes *A,* continuous recording monitor lead. A demand ventricular pacemaker (VVI) had been implanted because of type II second-degree AV block. After treatment with amiodarone for recurrent ventricular tachycardia, the Q-T interval became prolonged (about 640 msec during paced beats), and the patient developed episodes of torsades de pointes. In this recording, the tachycardia spontaneously terminates and a paced ventricular rhythm is restored. Motion artifact is noted at the end of the recording as the patient lost consciousness. *B,* Tracing from a young boy with a congenital long Q-T syndrome. The Q-TU interval in the sinus beats is at least 600 msec. Note TU wave alternans in the first and second complexes. A late premature complex occurring in the downslope of the TU wave initiates an episode of ventricular tachycardia.

changes in QRS contour and amplitude. The tachycardia may terminate with progressive prolongation of cycle lengths and larger and more distinctly formed QRS complexes, ending with a return to the basal rhythm, a period of ventricular standstill, or a new attack of torsades de pointes. Rarely ventricular fibrillation supervenes.[263]

Electrophysiological Features. In recent electrophysiological studies, arrhythmias similar to torsades depointes have been induced by programmed ventricular stimulation in patients who did not have this ventricular tachycardia spontaneously and in whom the Q-T interval of the sinus beats was normal or only slightly prolonged.[264,265] This pleomorphic ventricular tachycardia occurred without the other distinctive features characteristic of the full syndrome of torsades de pointes. The ventricular tachycardia that occurs spontaneously in the *syndrome* is often difficult to initiate by premature stimulation in patients who have it spontaneously.[266] Electrophysiological mechanisms responsible for torsades de pointes are not well understood and may be due to intraventricular reentry. This explanation appears more probable than the original hypothesis, suggesting the presence of an arrhythmia with two variable opposing foci, although data from one animal study support the latter theory.[267]

Clinical Features. Although many predisposing factors have been cited, the most common are severe bradycardia, potassium depletion, or drugs such as quinidine or disopyramide.[268,269] An imbalance between right and left sympathetic innervations may be important in some patients (see The Long Q-T Syndrome, p. 727).[270] When attacks are prolonged, syncope may result.

Management of ventricular tachycardia with a polymorphic pattern depends on whether or not it occurs in the setting of a prolonged Q-T interval. For this practical reason and because the mechanism of the tachycardia may differ depending on whether or not a long Q-T interval is present, it is important to restrict the definition of torsades de pointes to the typical morphology in the setting of a long Q-T and/or a polymorphic U wave[263] in the basal complexes. In all patients with torsades de pointes, administration of antiarrhythmic agents such as quinidine, disopyramide, and procainamide tends to increase the abnormal Q-T interval and worsen the arrhythmia. Temporary ventricular or atrial pacing should be instituted.[263,271,272] Pacing rapidly suppresses the ventricular tachycardia, which often does not recur even after cessation of pacing. Isoproterenol can be tried until pacing is instituted. The cause of the long Q-T should be determined and corrected if possible. When the Q-T interval is normal, polymorphic ventricular tachycardia *resembling* torsades de pointes is diagnosed, and standard antiarrhythmic drugs may be given. In borderline cases, the clinical context may help determine whether treatment should be initiated with antiarrhythmic drugs. In doubtful cases when the Q-T interval is at upper limits of normal, treatment with pacing is preferable.

Bidirectional Ventricular Tachycardia

This is an uncommon ventricular tachycardia characterized by QRS complexes with a right bundle branch block pattern, alternating polarity in the frontal plane from −60 to −90 degrees to +120 to +130 degrees and a regular rhythm (Fig. 21–39). The ventricular rate is between 140 and 200 beats/min. Although the mechanism and site of origin of this tachycardia has remained somewhat controversial,[273] recent evidence supports a ventricular origin.[274-276]

Bidirectional ventricular tachycardia occurs commonly but not exclusively as a manifestation of digitalis excess.[274] When due to the latter, the extent of toxicity is often advanced, with a poor prognosis. Bidirectional ventricular tachycardia occurs typically in older patients and in those with severe myocardial disease but has been noted in an otherwise asymptomatic 18-year-old with mild hyperkalemic periodic paralysis.[275]

Drugs useful to treat digitalis toxicity such as lidocaine, potassium, phenytoin, and propranolol should be considered if excessive digitalis administration is suspected. Otherwise, the usual therapeutic approach to ventricular tachycardia is recommended (p. 723).

032–680921

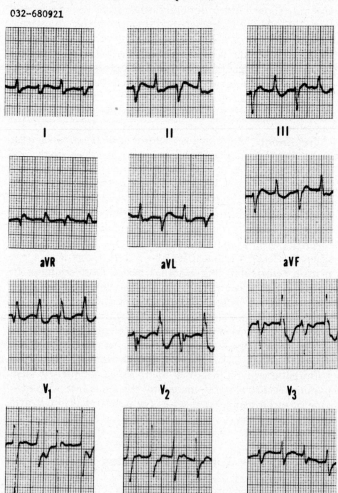

FIGURE 21–39 Bidirectional ventricular tachycardia. The mean frontal plane QRS axis alternates between −60° and +130° in successive beats and all complexes demonstrate a right bundle branch block pattern in V_1. R-R intervals are regular. The tachycardia was shown to be ventricular during an electrophysiological study. (From Morris, S. N., and Zipes, D. P.: His bundle electrocardiography during bidirectional tachycardia. Circulation 48:32, 1973, by permission of the American Heart Association, Inc.)

Repetitive Monomorphic Ventricular Tachycardia

Repetitive monomorphic ventricular tachycardia is defined as three or more consecutive premature ventricular complexes with only brief periods of intervening sinus complexes. Ventricular complexes generally occur in groups of 3 to 15, but occasionally the ventricular tachycardia may be almost continuous. All ventricular complexes have a uniform QRS morphology and interectopic, sinus-conducted complexes have a normal QRS without intraventricular conduction delay or pathologic Q waves (Fig. 21–40). Cycle lengths of the ventricular tachycardia are fairly regular, and the rate ranges between 100 and 150 beats/min, occasionally becoming as rapid as 250 beats/min. Episodes of ventricular tachycardia tend to cluster around certain time periods in an individual patient. Late cycle and variably coupled premature ventricular complexes are common. The tachycardia is difficult to induce with premature ventricular stimulation even though patients may have multiple episodes of spontaneous ventricular tachycardia during the study. Electrophysiological parameters are normal. Abnormal automaticity may be responsible for the tachycardia.[277,277a]

Repetitive monomorphic ventricular tachycardia is often associated with no or minimal structural heart disease and young age and in this setting appears to have an excellent prognosis.[277-281] Arrhythmia-related deaths are reported infrequently.[282] The arrhythmia may disappear with time, perhaps accounting for its reduced prevalence in older populations. The exact prevalence of the tachycardia is difficult to assess, since often it produces no symptoms and may be identified only during routine examination. Of the last 250 patients referred to our hospital for evaluation of ventricular tachycardia, 18 (7 per cent) had this arrhythmia.

When repetitive monomorphic ventricular tachycardia occurs in patients who have normal, sinus-conducted QRS complexes and trivial or no structural heart disease, the ventricular tachycardia appears to be benign and the prognosis favorable. Therapy, as outlined on p. 723, is reserved for patients who are symptomatic from palpitations or have very rapid rates of the ventricular tachycardia.

Bundle Branch Reentrant Tachycardia. Ventricular tachycardia due to bundle branch reentry is characterized by a QRS morphology determined by the circuit established over the bundle branches. Retrograde conduction over the left bundle branch system and anterograde conduction over the right bundle branch will create a QRS complex with a left bundle branch block contour. The frontal plane axis may be about +30 degrees. Electrophysiologically, bundle branch reentrant complexes occur only after a critical S_2-H_2 or S_3-H_3 delay. The H-V interval of the bundle branch reentrant complex equals or exceeds the H-V interval of the spontaneous normally conducted QRS complex.[283,283a]

Although bundle branch reentry has been clearly demonstrated to occur in animals (Fig. 19–27, p. 631) and probably occurs in humans as well, sustained ventricular tachycardia due to bundle branch reentry is a rare event. The long refractory period and rapid conduction velocity of the His-Purkinje system probably prevent sustained circuits of bundle branch reentry from occurring and therefore make it an uncommon mechanism of ventricular tachycardia in man.[283,283a,284]

The therapeutic approach is as for other ventricular tachycardias. Conceivably, creation of bundle branch block might eliminate the tachycardia.

Long Q-T Syndrome (Fig. 21–38B)

Electrocardiographic Recognition. The upper limit for the duration of the normal Q-T interval *corrected* for heart rate (Q-Tc) is 0.44 sec. However, it is possible that the formulas used to correct for heart rate, derived from normal subjects not receiving drugs, are not applicable to patients with abnormal repolarization syndromes or after drugs such as quinidine are administered or after myocardial infarction.[285] Nevertheless, delayed repolarization has been defined as a Q-Tc exceeding 0.44 sec or when the Q-TU pattern appears abnormal in configuration. The nature of the U-wave abnormality and its relationship to the long Q-T syndrome are not clear. Notched bifid and sinusoidal T waves may occur.[286]

Clinical Features. Repolarization abnormalities can be divided into two groups: (1) primary or idiopathic, which is a congenital, often familial disorder (p. 1626) that is sometimes,[58] but not always,[287,288] associated with deafness, and (2) an acquired group caused by various drugs like quinidine,[289,290] disopyramide,[291] phenothiazines, or tricyclic antidepressants; metabolic abnormalities such as hypokalemia; the results of the liquid protein diet[292,293]; central nervous system lesions[294]; autonomic nervous system dysfunction[295]; coronary artery disease with myocardial infarction[295-298]; cardiac ganglionitis[299]; and mitral valve prolapse.[300] The autonomic dysfunction may result from a preponderance of left sympathetic tone.[301-304] Probucol, a

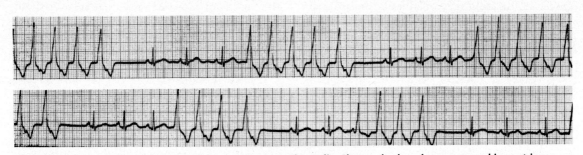

FIGURE 21–40 Repetitive monomorphic ventricular tachycardia. Short episodes of a monomorphic ventricular tachycardia at a rate of 120 to 130 beats/min repeatedly interrupt the normal sinus rhythm. The sinus-initiated QRS complexes are normal in contour with a normal ST segment and T wave.

lipid-lowering agent, has been shown to produce Q-T prolongation and ventricular arrhythmias in dogs and monkeys but not in man.[305]

Symptomatic patients with long Q-T syndrome develop ventricular tachycardias that in many instances are due to torsades de pointes (p. 725). Since sudden death may occur in this group of patients, it is obvious that, in some, the ventricular arrhythmia becomes sustained and probably results in ventricular fibrillation. Patients with congenital long Q-T syndrome who are at increased risk for sudden death include those who have family members who died suddenly at an early age and those who have experienced syncope. Electrocardiograms should be obtained for all family members when the propositus presents with symptoms. Patients should undergo prolonged ECG recording, with various stresses designed to evoke ventricular arrhythmias, such as auditory stimuli,[306] psychological stress,[307] cold pressor stimulation, and exercise. Recently, it has been suggested that the Valsalva maneuver lengthens the Q-T interval and causes T wave alternans and ventricular tachycardia in patients who have prolonged Q-T syndromes with ventricular tachycardia.[308] Catecholamines may be infused in some patients, but this challenge must be performed cautiously, with resuscitative equipment close at hand. Stellate ganglion stimulation and blockade may be useful[304] to provoke or abolish arrhythmias. Premature ventricular stimulation generally does not induce arrhythmias in this syndrome.

Treatment. For patients who have the idiopathic long Q-T syndrome but do not have syncope, complex ventricular arrhythmias, or a family history of sudden cardiac death, no therapy is recommended. In asymptomatic patients with complex ventricular arrhythmias or a family history of premature sudden cardiac death, beta blockers at maximally tolerated doses are recommended. In patients with syncope, beta blockers at maximally tolerated doses, at times combined with phenytoin and phenobarbital, are suggested. For patients who continue to have syncope despite triple drug therapy, left-sided cervicothoracic sympathetic ganglionectomy that interrupts the stellate ganglion and the first three or four thoracic ganglia has been proposed.[286,302]

ARRHYTHMOGENIC RIGHT VENTRICULAR DYSPLASIA

In this infrequently recognized disorder, patients present with ventricular tachycardia that has a left bundle branch block contour, often with right-axis deviation, with T waves inverted over the right precordial leads. Supraventricular arrhythmias may also occur.[309] Premature ventricular stimulation can initiate sustained ventricular tachycardia.

Arrhythmogenic right ventricular dysplasia is a cardiomyopathy with hypokinetic areas involving the wall of the right ventricle. It may be related to Uhl's anomaly (parchment-thin right ventricular wall) in some patients and can be an important cause of ventricular arrhythmias in children and young adults with an apparently normal heart as well as in older patients.[310] Right heart failure or asymptomatic right ventricular enlargement may be present with normal pulmonary vasculature. Males predominate and all patients show an abnormal right ventricle by echo or right

ventricular angiography.[309] ECG during sinus rhythm exhibits complete or incomplete right bundle branch block. Although the conventional pharmacological approaches to therapy may be appropriate, surgical manipulations have been successful in some of these patients[309,311-313] (p. 672).

TETRALOGY OF FALLOT

Chronic serious ventricular arrhythmias may occur in patients some years after repair of tetralogy of Fallot. In one series, almost half of 72 patients had serious ventricular arrhythmias within five years after repair, and four patients had experienced cardiac arrest.[314] Sustained ventricular tachycardia after repair may be caused by reentry at the site of previous operation in the right ventricular outflow tract[315] and may be cured by resection of this area.[316]

CATECHOLAMINE-SENSITIVE VENTRICULAR TACHYCARDIA

Some patients may have ventricular tachycardia due to a sensitivity to the effects of catecholamine stimulation.[317] Stress or exercise may exacerbate these ventricular arrhythmias, which can be suppressed with beta blocker therapy.[318]

Ventricular Flutter
and Ventricular Fibrillation

Electrocardiographic Recognition. These arrhythmias represent severe derangements of the heart beat that usually terminate fatally within 3 to 5 minutes unless corrective measures are undertaken promptly. Ventricular flutter presents as a sine wave in appearance: regular large oscillations occurring at a rate of 150 to 300/min (usually about 200) (Fig. 21-41A). The distinction between rapid ventricular tachycardia and ventricular flutter may be difficult and is usually of academic interest only. Ventricular fibrillation is recognized by the presence of irregular undulations of varying contour and amplitude (Fig. 21-41B). Distinct QRS complexes, ST segments, and T waves are absent.

In an animal model of ischemia, ventricular fibrillation begins as an organized rhythm, with activation occurring in an orderly, rapidly repeating sequence at the border of the ischemic reperfused region. Activation then passes through the nonischemic portion of the ventricles as a single organized wavefront to the opposite side of the heart, with the time between successive activation fronts decreasing. However, the time for each activation front to traverse the ventricles increases, resulting in overlapping cycles in which a new activation front arises before the previous front terminates. This produces totally disorganized electrical activity on the scalar ECG at a time when epicardial electrical activity is still fairly organized.[319]

Clinical Features. Ventricular fibrillation occurs in a variety of clinical situations, most commonly associated with coronary artery disease and as a terminal event. It may occur during antiarrhythmic drug administration, hypoxia, ischemia, atrial fibrillation and very rapid ventricular rates in the preexcitation syndrome, after electric shock administered during cardioversion (Fig. 20-6) or accidentally by improperly grounded equipment, and uncom-

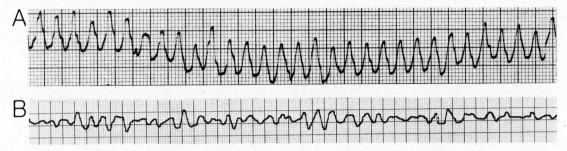

FIGURE 21–41 Ventricular flutter and ventricular fibrillation. *A,* **The sine wave appearance of the complexes occurring at a rate of 300 beats/min is characteristic of ventricular flutter.** *B,* **The irregular undulating baseline typifies ventricular fibrillation.**

monly during competitive cardiac pacing at slow rates (see Chapter 22). Ventricular flutter or ventricular fibrillation results in faintness, followed by loss of consciousness, seizures, and apnea and eventually, if the rhythm continues untreated, death. The blood pressure is unobtainable and heart sounds are usually absent. The atria may continue to beat as an independent rhythm for a time or in response to impulses from the fibrillating ventricles. Eventually, electrical activity of the heart is completely absent.

In patients resuscitated from out-of-hospital cardiac arrest, all but a few have ventricular fibrillation. A nonarrhythmic cause of sudden cardiac death occurs in only a very small number of patients who have acute myocardial infarction.[320] Although 75 per cent of patients resuscitated from sudden cardiac death have significant coronary artery disease, only 20 to 30 per cent evolve acute myocardial infarction. Those who do not evolve a myocardial infarction have a recurrence rate for ventricular fibrillation of approximately 22 per cent in one year and 40 per cent in two years[321] (p. 793). Patients who have ventricular fibrillation and acute myocardial infarction have a recurrence rate at one year of 2 per cent.

The time from warning arrhythmias to development of ventricular fibrillation is short in many patients. In one series, an R-on-T premature ventricular complex occurred in 33 of 48 patients who developed ventricular fibrillation outside the hospital and, along with an increase in heart rate prior to the onset of ventricular fibrillation, appeared to be the most important initiating factor.[322] Another group at high risk for the development of ventricular fibrillation are patients who suffer an anteroseptal myocardial infarction complicated by right or left bundle branch block.[323]

Treatment (See also pp. 672 and 756). Immediate nonsynchronized DC electrical shock using 200 to 400 joules is mandatory treatment for ventricular fibrillation and for ventricular flutter that has caused loss of consciousness. Cardiopulmonary resuscitation is employed only until defibrillation equipment is readied. Time should not be wasted with cardiopulmonary resuscitation if electrical defibrillation can be done promptly. If the circulation is markedly inadequate despite return to sinus rhythm, closed-chest massage with artificial ventilation as needed should be instituted. The use of anesthesia during electric shock is obviously dictated by the patient's condition and is generally not required. After reversion of the arrhythmia to a normal rhythm, it is essential to monitor the rhythm continuously and to institute measures to prevent a recurrence.

Metabolic acidosis quickly follows cardiovascular collapse, and sodium bicarbonate, 1 to 3 ampoules containing 44 mEq of sodium bicarbonate per ampoule, may be needed initially. Additional ampoules judged by results of frequent blood gas and pH determinations may be given every 5 to 8 minutes until adequate cardiorespiratory func-

tion is achieved. If the arrhythmia is terminated within 30 to 60 seconds, significant acidosis does not occur. Also, in this short period of time, artificial ventilation by means of a tightly fitting rubber face mask and an Ambu bag is quite satisfactory and eliminates the delay attending intubation by inexperienced personnel. If such a mask and bag are not available, mouth-to-mouth or mouth-to-nose resuscitation is indicated. It is important to reemphasize that there should be no delay in instituting electrical shock. If the patient is not monitored and it cannot be established whether asystole or ventricular fibrillation caused the cardiovascular collapse, the electric shock should be administered *without* wasting precious seconds attempting to obtain an electrocardiogram. The DC shock may cause the asystolic heart to begin discharging as well as terminate ventricular fibrillation, if the latter is present.

A search for conditions contributing to the initiation of ventricular flutter or fibrillation should be made and the conditions corrected, if possible. A ventricular arrhythmia related to hypotension may at times be terminated by the use of vasopressors. Slow ventricular rates that are due to sinus bradycardia or AV block may permit the occurrence of premature ventricular complexes and ventricular tachyarrhythmias that can be effectively treated by speeding the heart rate. Initial medical approaches to prevent a recurrence of ventricular fibrillation include intravenous administration of lidocaine, bretylium, procainamide, quinidine, or disopyramide. Usually, when ventricular fibrillation occurs, it is irreversible and lethal unless countermeasures are instituted immediately.

HEART BLOCK

Heart block is a disturbance of impulse conduction that may be permanent or transient, owing to anatomical or functional impairment. It must be distinguished from *interference*, a normal phenomenon which is a disturbance of impulse conduction caused by physiological refractoriness due to inexcitability from a preceding impulse. Either interference or block may occur at any site where impulses are conducted, but they are recognized most commonly between the sinus node and atrium (SA block), between the atria and ventricles (AV block), within the atria (intraatrial block), or within the ventricles (intraventricular block). During AV block, the block may occur in the AV node, His bundle, or bundle branches.[324,325] In some instances of bundle branch block, for example, the impulse may only be delayed and not completely blocked in the bundle branch, yet the resulting QRS complex may be indistinguishable from a QRS complex generated by complete bundle branch block.

The conduction disturbance is classified by severity in three categories. During *first-degree heart block*, conduction time is prolonged but all impulses are conducted. *Second-degree heart block* occurs in two forms: Mobitz type I (Wenckebach) and type II. Type I heart block is characterized by a progressive lengthening of the conduction time until an impulse is not conducted. Type II heart block denotes occasional or repetitive sudden block of conduction of an impulse without prior measurable lengthening of conduction time. When no impulses are conducted, *complete or third-degree block is present.* The degree of block may depend in part on the direction of impulse propagation. For unknown reasons, normal retrograde conduction can occur in the presence of advanced anterograde AV block, for example (see Fig. 7–57, p. 252).[326] The reverse can also occur.

Certain features of type I second-degree block deserve special emphasis because when actual conduction times are not apparent in the electrocardiogram, for example, during SA, junctional, or ventricular exit block (see pp. 251 and 691), type I conduction disturbance may be difficult to recognize. During type I block, the increment in conduction time is greatest in the second beat of the Wenckebach group, and the absolute *increase* in conduction time *decreases* progressively over subsequent beats. These two features serve to establish the characteristics of classic Wenckebach group beating: (1) the interval between successive beats progressively decreases, although the conduction time increases (but by a decreasing function); (2) the duration of the pause produced by the nonconducted impulse is less than twice the interval preceding the blocked impulse (which is usually the shortest interval); and (3) the cycle following the nonconducted beat (beginning the Wenckebach group) is longer than the cycle preceding the blocked impulse. Although much emphasis has been placed on this characteristic grouping of cycles, primarily to be able to diagnose Wenckebach exit block, this typical grouping occurs in less than 50 per cent of patients who have type I Wenckebach AV nodal block.

Differences in cycle-length patterns may result from changes in pacemaker rate (e.g., sinus arrhythmia), in neurogenic control of conduction, and changes in the increment of conduction delay. For example, if the P-R increment in the last cycle increases, the R-R cycle of the last conducted beat may lengthen rather than shorten. In addition, since the last conducted beat is often at a critical state of conduction, it may become blocked, producing a 5:3 or 3:1 conduction ratio instead of a 5:4 or 3:2 ratio. During a 3:2 Wenckebach structure, the cycle following the nonconducted beat will be the same as the cycle preceding the nonconducted beat. Finally, *concealed or manifest reentry* (pp. 247 and 250) may alter the P-R interval during Wenckebach block.[327] As the cardiac cycle length is decreased, the AV nodal effective refractory period normally lengthens in adults and the AV nodal functional refractory period shortens slightly.[328,329] In Wenckebach cycles, a progressive increase in AV nodal effective refractory period results.[330]

Atrioventricular (AV) Block

AV block exists when the atrial impulse is conducted with delay or is not conducted at all to the ventricle at a time when the AV junction is not physiologically refractory. **FIRST-DEGREE AV BLOCK.** During first-degree AV block, every atrial impulse conducts to the ventricles, producing a regular ventricular rate, but the P-R interval exceeds 0.20 sec in the adult. P-R intervals as long as 1.0

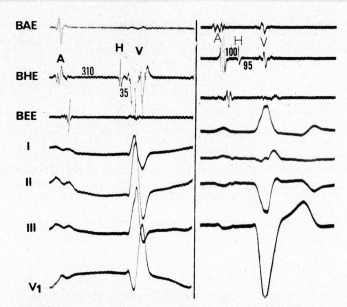

FIGURE 21–42   First-degree AV block. One complex during sinus rhythm is shown. The P-R interval in the left panel measured 370 msec (P-A = 25 msec; A-H = 310 msec; H-V = 35 msec) during a right bundle branch block. Conduction delay in the AV node causes the first-degree AV block. In the panel on the right, the P-R interval is 230 msec (P-A = 35 msec; A-H = 100 msec; H-V = 95 msec) during a left bundle branch block. The conduction delay in the His-Purkinje system causes the first-degree AV block.

sec have been noted and at times may be longer than the P-P interval, a phenomenon known as "skipped" P waves. (Fig. 7–35, p. 227). Clinically important P-R interval prolongation may result from conduction delay in the AV node (A-H interval), in the His-Purkinje system (H-V interval), or at both sites. Equally delayed conduction over both bundle branches uncommonly may produce P-R prolongation without significant QRS complex aberration (Fig. 21–29). Occasionally, intraatrial conduction delay may result in P-R prolongation. If the QRS complex in the scalar ECG is normal in contour and duration, the AV delay almost always resides in the AV node, rarely within the His bundle itself. If the QRS complex shows a bundle branch block pattern, conduction delay may be within the AV node and/or His-Purkinje system (Fig. 21–42). In this latter instance, His bundle electrocardiography is necessary to localize the site of conduction delay. Acceleration of the atrial rate or enhancement of vagal tone by carotid massage may cause first-degree AV nodal block to progress to type I second-degree AV block. Conversely, type I second-

TABLE 21–3   SITE OF SECOND-DEGREE ATRIOVENTRICULAR BLOCK

Type of Block	Normal QRS	BBB
Type I	AVN > > > HPS	AVN > HPS
Type II	HPS > AVN	HPS > > > AVN
1:1 → 2:1: fixed 2:1 or greater	HPS = AVN	HPS > > AVN

Except for the location of type I AV block with a normal QRS and type II AV block with a bundle branch block, quantitative data regarding the other sites of block are not available and these statements must be regarded as the author's impressions.

Abbreviations: AVN = atrioventricular node; HPS = His-Purkinje system; BBB = bundle branch block. Arrows > indicate relative frequency of second-degree AV block at different sites, with one arrow meaning slightly more frequent, and four arrows meaning far more frequent.

From Zipes, D. P.: Second-degree atrioventricular block. Circulation 60:465, 1965, by permission of the American Heart Association, Inc.

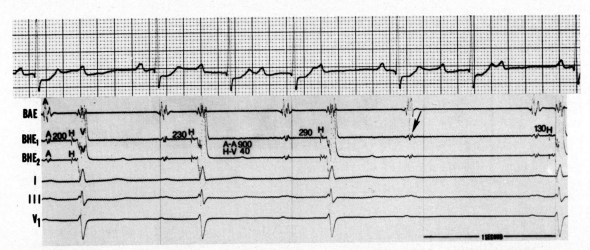

FIGURE 21–43 Type I (Wenckebach) second-degree AV block. In the top strip from a lead II scalar ECG recording, the P-R interval progressively lengthens, and the R-R intervals progressively shorten, culminating in a blocked P wave. The duration of the pause produced by the blocked P wave is less than twice the shortest P-P interval. In the electrophysiological recording shown below, progressive AV nodal conduction delay increases until one P wave (arrow) blocks proximal to the His bundle. The cycle then begins again with marked shortening of the A-H interval to 130 msec. (The first P wave in the electrophysiological recording is not the first P wave of the Wenckebach cycle. Hence, the A-H interval exceeds 130 msec.)

degree AV nodal block may revert to first-degree block with deceleration of the sinus rate.

SECOND-DEGREE AV BLOCK (Table 21–3). Atrial impulses not conducted to the ventricle at a time when physiologic interference is not involved constitutes second-degree AV block. The nonconducted P wave may be intermittent or frequent, at regular or irregular intervals, and may be preceded by fixed or lengthening P-R intervals. A distinguishing feature is that conducted P waves relate to the QRS complex with recurring P-R intervals, i.e., the association of P with QRS is not random. Wenckebach and Hay, by analyzing the *a-c* and *v* waves in the jugular venous pulse, described two types of second-degree AV block. After the introduction of the electrocardiograph, Mobitz classified them as type I and type II.[331] Electrocardiographically, typical type I second-degree AV block is characterized by progressive P-R prolongation culminating in a nonconducted P wave (Fig. 21–43), while in type II second-degree AV block, the P-R interval remains constant prior to the blocked P wave (Fig. 21–44). In both instances the AV block is intermittent and generally repetitive and may block several P waves in a row. Often, the eponyms Mobitz type I and Mobitz type II are applied to the two types of block, while the term "Wenckebach block" refers to type I block only.

Although it has been suggested that type I and type II AV block may be different manifestations of the same electrophysiological mechanism, differing only quantitatively in the size of the increments,[332] clinically separating second-degree AV block into type I and type II serves a useful function and, in most instances, the differentiation can be made easily and reliably from the surface ECG. Type II AV block often antedates the development of Adams-Stokes syncope and complete AV block, while type I AV block with a normal QRS complex is generally more benign and does not progress to more advanced forms of AV conduction disturbance.[333–335]

In the patient with an acute myocardial infarction, type I AV block usually accompanies inferior infarction, is transient, and does not require temporary pacing, whereas type II AV block results in the setting of an acute anterior myocardial infarction, may require temporary or permanent pacing, and is associated with a high rate of mortality, generally due to pump failure[333,336] (p. 1287). A high degree of AV block can occur in patients with acute inferior myocardial infarction and is associated with more myocardial damage and a higher mortality rate compared to those without AV block.[337]

While type I conduction disturbance is ubiquitous and may occur in any tissue in the *in situ* heart, as well as *in vitro,* the site of block for the usual forms of second-degree AV block can be judged with sufficient reliability from the surface ECG to permit clinical decisions without requiring invasive electrophysiological studies in most instances (Table 21–2). Type I AV block with a normal QRS complex almost always takes place at the level of the AV node, proximal to the His bundle.[338] An exception is the uncommon patient with type I intrahisian block.[339] Type II AV block, particularly when it occurs in association with a bundle branch block, is localized to the His-Purkinje system.[338–340] Type I AV block in a patient with a bundle branch block may represent block in the AV node or in the His-Purkinje system.[331,334] Type II AV block in a patient with a normal QRS complex may be due to intrahisian AV block, but the block is likely to be type I AV nodal block, which exhibits small increments in AV conduction time.[341]

The above generalizations encompass the vast majority of patients who present with second-degree AV block. However, certain caveats must be heeded to avoid misdiagnosis because of subtle ECG changes or exceptions:

1. Two:one AV block may be a form of type I or type II AV block (Fig. 21–45). If the QRS complex is normal, the block is more likely to be type I, located in the AV node, and one should search for a transition of the 2:1 block to 3:2 block, during which the P-R interval lengthens in the second cardiac cycle. If a bundle branch block is present, the block may be located either in the AV node or in the His-Purkinje system.

2. AV block may occur simultaneously at two or more levels and may render the distinction between types I and II difficult.

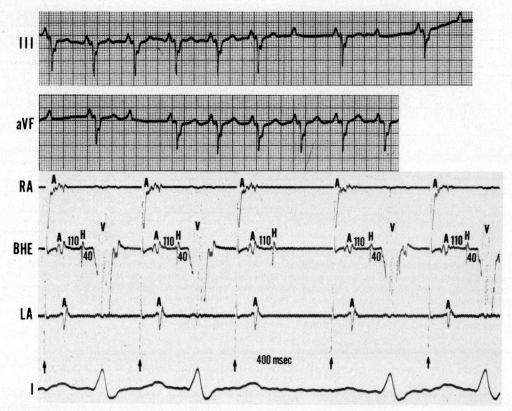

FIGURE 21–44 Type II second-degree AV block. *Top,* The surface electrocardiogram illustrates type II AV block in a patient with right bundle branch block and left anterior hemiblock. *Bottom,* During right atrial pacing at a basic cycle length of 400 msec (pacing spikes indicated by small upright arrows), the A-H and H-V intervals remain constant. Sudden failure of conduction occurs distal to the His bundle recording site following the third P wave.

3. If the atrial rate varies, it may alter conduction times and cause type I AV block to simulate type II or change type II AV block into type I. For example, if the shortest atrial cycle length that just achieved 1:1 AV nodal conduction at a constant P-R interval is decreased by as little as 10 or 20 msec, the P wave of the shortened cycle may block at the level of the AV node without an apparent increase in the antecedent P-R interval.[342] Apparent type II AV block in the His-Purkinje system may be converted to type I in the His-Purkinje system in some patients by increasing the atrial rate.[331]

4. Concealed premature His depolarizations may create electrocardiographic patterns that simulate type I or type II AV block[343,344] (see Fig. 19–30, p. 635, and Figs. 7–51 and 7–52, pp. 245 and 246).

5. Abrupt, transient alterations in autonomic tone may cause sudden block of one or more P waves without altering the P-R interval of the conducted P wave before or after block.[345] Thus, apparent type II AV block would be produced at the AV node. In the absence of atrial pacing, a burst of vagal tone probably lengthens the P-P interval as well as producing AV block.[346]

6. The response of the AV block to autonomic changes, either spontaneous or induced, to distinguish type I from type II AV block may be misleading. Although vagal stimulation generally increases and vagolytic agents decrease the extent of type I AV block,[347,348] such conclusions are based on the assumption that the intervention acts primarily on the AV node and fail to consider rate changes. For example, atropine may minimally improve conduction in the AV node and markedly increase the heart rate, resulting in an increase in AV conduction time and the degree of AV block as a result of the faster atrial rate. Conversely, if an increase in vagal tone minimally prolongs AV conduction time but greatly slows the heart rate, the net effect on type I AV block may be to improve conduction. In general, however, carotid sinus massage improves and atropine worsens AV conduction in patients with His-Purkinje block, while the opposite results are to be expected in patients who have AV nodal block. These two interventions may help differentiate the site of block without invasive study.[349]

7. During type I AV block with high ratios of conducted beats, the increment in P-R interval may be quite small and simulate type II AV block if only the last few P-R intervals prior to the blocked P wave are measured. By comparing the P-R interval of the first beat in the long Wenckebach cycle with that of the beats immediately preceding the blocked P wave, the increment in AV conduction becomes readily apparent.[350]

8. The classic AV Wenckebach structure depends on a stable atrial rate and a maximal increment in AV conduction time for the second P-R interval of the Wenckebach cycle, with a progressive decrease in subsequent beats. Unstable or unusual alterations in the increment or atrial rate, often seen with long Wenckebach cycles, result in atypical forms of type I AV block in which the last R-R interval may lengthen and are common.[351,352]

9. Finally, it is important to remember that the P-R interval in the scalar ECG is made up of conduction through the atrium, the AV node, and the His-Purkinje system. An increment in HV conduction, for example, can be masked in the scalar ECG by a reduction in the A-H interval, and the resulting P-R interval will not reflect the entire increment in His-Purkinje conduction time.[331] Very long P-R intervals (> 200 msec) are more likely to result from AV nodal conduction delay (and block), with or without concomitant His-Purkinje conduction delay.

First-degree and type I second-degree AV block can occur in normal healthy children,[353] and Wenckebach AV block may be a normal phenomenon in well-trained athletes, probably related to an increase in resting vagal tone.[354,355] Occasionally, progressive worsening of the Wenckebach AV conduction disorder may result.[356] In patients who have chronic second-degree AV nodal block (proximal to the His bundle) without organic heart disease, the course is relatively benign, while in those who have organ-

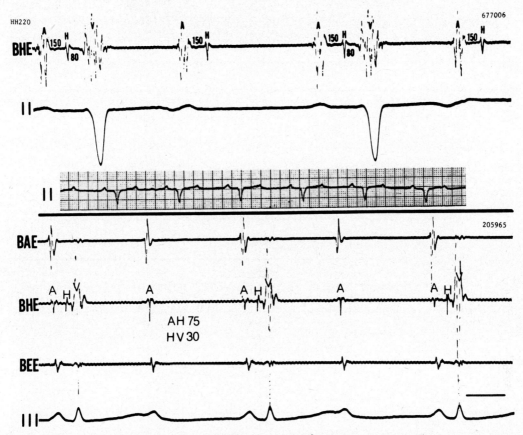

FIGURE 21-45 2:1 AV block proximal and distal to the His bundle deflection in two different patients. *Top,* 2:1 AV block seen in the scalar ECG occurs distal to the His bundle recording site in a patient with right bundle branch block and left anterior hemiblock. The A-H interval (150 msec) and H-V interval (80 msec) are both prolonged. *Bottom,* 2:1 AV block occurs proximal to the bundle of His in a patient with a normal QRS complex. The A-H interval (75 msec) and the H-V interval (30 msec) remain constant and normal.

ic heart disease the prognosis is poor and related to underlying heart disease.[357]

Complete AV Block

Electrocardiographic Recognition. Complete AV block occurs when no atrial activity conducts to the ventricles and therefore the atria and ventricles are controlled by independent pacemakers. Thus, complete AV block is one type of complete AV dissociation (see p. 735). The atrial pacemaker may be sinus or ectopic (tachycardia, flutter, or fibrillation) or may result from an AV junctional focus occurring above the block with retrograde atrial conduction. The ventricular focus is usually located just below the region of block, which may be above or below the His bundle bifurcation. Sites of ventricular pacemaker activity that are in, or closer to, the His bundle appear to be more stable and may produce a faster rate than those located more distally in the ventricular conduction system. The ventricular rate in complete heart block is less than 40 beats/min but may be faster in congenital complete AV block. The ventricular rhythm, usually regular, may vary owing to premature ventricular complexes, a shift in the pacemaker site, an irregularly discharging pacemaker focus, or autonomic influences.

Clinical Features. Complete AV block may result from block at the level of the AV node (usually congenital) (Fig. 21-46), within the bundle of His, or distal to it

in the Purkinje system (usually acquired) (Fig. 21-47). The first two types of block generally exhibit normal QRS complexes and rates of 40 to 60 beats/min because the escape focus that controls the ventricle arises in or near the His bundle. In complete AV nodal block, the P wave is not followed by a His deflection, but each ventricular complex is preceded by a His deflection (Fig. 21-46). His bundle electrocardiography may be useful to differentiate AV nodal from intrahisian block, since the latter may carry a more serious prognosis than the former. Intrahisian block is recognized infrequently without invasive studies. In patients with AV nodal block atropine usually speeds both the atrial and the ventricular rate. Isometric exercise may reduce the extent of AV nodal block.[358] Acquired complete AV block occurs most commonly distal to the bundle of His owing to trifascicular conduction disturbance. Each P wave is followed by a His deflection, and the ventricular escape complexes are not preceded by a His deflection (Fig. 21-47). The QRS complex is abnormal and the ventricular rate is usually less than 40 beats/min.

Unusual forms such as paroxysmal AV block[359,360] or AV block following a period of rapid ventricular rate may occur.[361] Paroxysmal AV block in some instances may be due to hyperresponsiveness of the AV node to vagotonic reflexes.[362] Surgery, electrolyte disturbances, endocarditis, tumors, Chagas' disease, rheumatoid nodules, calcific aortic stenosis, myxedema, polymyositis,[363] infiltrative processes (such as amyloid, sarcoid, or scleroderma), and an

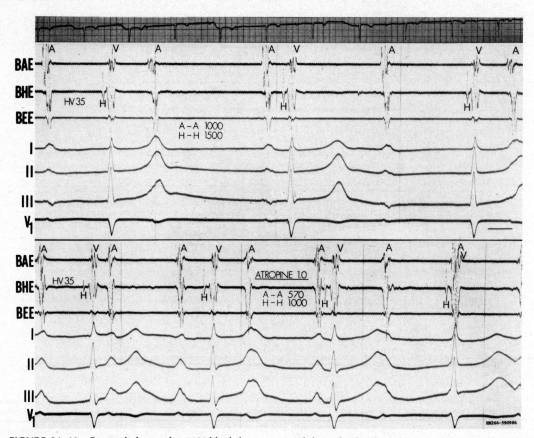

FIGURE 21–46 Congenital complete AV block in a young adult at the level of the AV node. The V₁ surface tracing (*top*) illustrates complete AV block with a normal QRS complex. The top panel of the His bundle recording demonstrates the site of block to be proximal to the His bundle depolarization, at the level of the AV node. The H-V interval is normal (35 msec). The atrial cycles (1000 msec) are completely dissociated from the ventricular cycles (1500 msec). In the bottom panel, after atropine administration (1 mg IV), both the atrial and ventricular rates speed up (A-A interval=570 msec; H-H interval=1000 msec), but complete AV block remains.

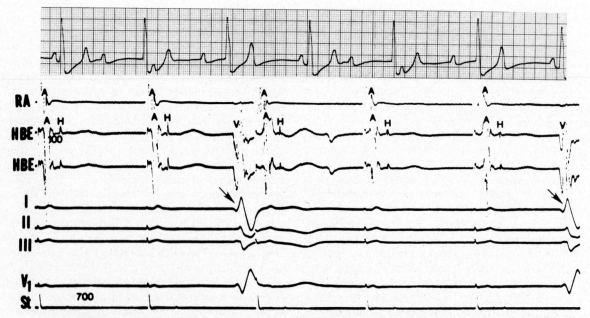

FIGURE 21–47 Acquired complete AV block in a 30-year-old patient with recurrent syncope. In the top monitor strip, complete AV block is evident with a ventricular escape rate of 38 beats/min and an atrial rate of 65 beats/min. In the His bundle recording, left-axis deviation with a right bundle branch block is apparent. The atria are paced at a cycle length of 700 msec and the block is distal to the His bundle recording site. Two ventricular escape beats are seen (arrows) at a rate of approximately 30 beats/min and are not preceded by His bundle activation.

almost endless assortment of common and unusual conditions may produce AV block. In the adult, drug toxicity, coronary disease,[364] and degenerative processes appear to be the most common causes of AV heart block. The degenerative process produces partial or complete anatomical or electrical disruption within the AV nodal region, the AV bundle, or both bundle branches.[365-367]

In children, the most common cause of AV block is congenital (p. 1014). Under such circumstances the AV block may be an isolated finding or associated with other lesions. Children are most often asymptomatic[368]; however, some may develop symptoms that require pacemaker implantation.[369] Mortality from congenital AV block is highest in the neonatal period, is much lower during childhood and adolescence, and increases slowly later in life. Stokes-Adams attacks may occur in patients with congenital heart block at any age. It is difficult to predict the prognosis in the individual patient.[370] A persistent heart rate at rest of 50 beats/min or less correlates with the incidence of syncope, and extreme bradycardia may contribute to the prevalence of Adams-Stokes attacks in children with congenital complete AV block.[371] The site of block may not separate symptomatic children who have congenital or surgically induced complete heart block from those without symptoms. Prolonged recovery times of escape foci following rapid pacing (see discussion of sinus node recovery time, p. 635) and the occurrence of paroxysmal tachycardias may be predisposing factors to the development of symptoms.[372]

Many of the signs of AV block are demonstrated at the bedside. First-degree AV block may be recognized by a long a-c wave interval in the jugular venous pulse and by diminished intensity of the first heart sound as the P-R interval lengthens. In type I second-degree AV block, the heart rate may increase imperceptibly with gradually diminished intensity of the first heart sound, widening of the a-c interval terminated by a pause, and an a wave not followed by a v wave. Intermittent ventricular pauses and

a waves in the neck not followed by v waves characterize type II AV block. The first heart sound maintains a constant intensity. In complete AV block, the findings are the same as those in AV dissociation (see below).

Significant clinical manifestations of first- and second-degree AV block are uncommon and usually consist of palpitations or feelings of the heart "missing a beat." Complete AV block may be accompanied by signs and symptoms of reduced cardiac output, syncope or presyncope, angina, or palpitations due to ventricular tachyarrhythmias.

Treatment. As discussed in detail in Chapter 22, drugs cannot be relied on to increase the heart rate for more than several hours to several days in patients with symptomatic heart block without producing significant side effects. Therefore, temporary or permanent pacemaker insertion is indicated in patients with symptomatic bradyarrhythmias.[373,374] For short-term therapy when the block is likely to be evanescent but still requires treatment or until adequate pacing therapy can be established, vagolytic agents such as atropine are useful for patients who have AV nodal disturbances, while catecholamines such as isoproterenol may be used transiently to treat patients who have heart block at any site (see treatment for Sinus Bradycardia, above). Isoproterenol should be used with extreme caution or not at all in patients who have acute myocardial infarction.

ATRIOVENTRICULAR (AV) DISSOCIATION
(See also pp. 249 and 250)

As the term indicates, dissociated or independent beating of atria and ventricles defines AV dissociation. Pick,[375] proposing a comprehensive classification and consistent terminology, emphasized that AV dissociation is never a *primary* disturbance of rhythm but is a "symptom" of an underlying rhythm disturbance produced by one of three causes or a combination of causes (Fig. 21–48), that pre-

FIGURE 21–48 Diagrammatic illustration of the causes of AV dissociation. A sinus bradycardia that allows the escape of an AV junctional rhythm which does not capture the atria retrogradely illustrates cause I (top panel). Intermittent sinus captures occur (third P wave) to produce incomplete AV dissociation (see Fig. 21–2B, p. 689). For cause II, a ventricular tachycardia without retrograde atrial capture produces complete AV dissociation (see Fig. 21–20, p. 706 and 21–35, p. 721). As the third cause, complete AV block with a ventricular escape rhythm is diagrammed (see Figs. 21–46 and 21–47, p. 734). The combination of causes II and III is shown in panel IV, representing a nonparoxysmal AV junctional tachycardia and some degree of AV block.

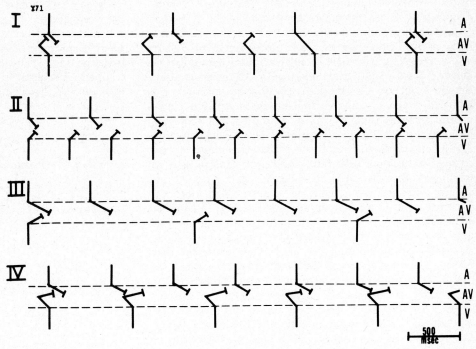

vent the normal transmission of impulses from atrium to ventricle, as follows:

1. Slowing of the dominant pacemaker of the heart (usually the sinus node), which allows escape of a subsidiary or latent pacemaker. AV dissociation by *default* of the primary pacemaker to a subsidiary one in this manner is often a normal phenomenon. It may occur during sinus arrhythmia or sinus bradycardia, permitting an independent AV junctional rhythm to arise (see Fig. 21–2, p. 689).

2. Acceleration of a latent pacemaker that *usurps* control of the ventricles. Abnormally enhanced discharge rate of a usually slower subsidiary pacemaker is pathological and commonly occurs during nonparoxysmal AV junctional tachycardia or ventricular tachycardia without retrograde atrial capture (see Figs. 21–20 and 21–35, pp. 706 and 721).

3. Block, generally at the AV junction, that prevents impulses formed at a normal rate in a dominant pacemaker from reaching the ventricles and allows the ventricles to beat under the control of a subsidiary pacemaker. Junctional or ventricular escape rhythm during AV block, without retrograde atrial capture, are common examples in which block gives rise to AV dissociation. It is important to remember that complete AV block is *not* synonymous with complete AV dissociation: patients who have complete AV block have complete AV dissociation, but patients who have complete AV dissociation may or may not have complete AV block (Figs. 21–46 and 21–47).

4. A combination of causes may exist, for example, when digitalis excess results in the production of a nonparoxysmal AV junctional tachycardia associated with SA or AV block.[109]

With this classification in mind, it is important to emphasize that the term "AV dissociation" is *not* a diagnosis and is analogous to the terms "jaundice" or "fever." One must state that "AV dissociation is present *due to* . . ." and then give the cause. The accelerated rate of a slower, normally subsidiary pacemaker or the slowed rate of a faster, normally dominant pacemaker that prevents conduction due to physiologic collision and mutual extinction of opposing wavefronts (interference), or the manifestations of AV block are the basic disturbances producing AV dissociation. The atria in all these cases beat independently from the ventricles, under control of the sinus node, ectopic atrial, or AV junctional pacemakers, and may exhibit any type of supraventricular rhythms. If a single pacemaker establishes control of both atria and ventricles for one beat (capture) or a series of beats (sinus rhythm, AV junctional rhythm with retrograde atrial capture, ventricular tachycardia with retrograde atrial capture, and so forth), AV dissociation is abolished for that period. Conversely, as stated above, whenever the atria and ventricles fail to respond to a single impulse for one beat (premature ventricular complex without retrograde capture of the atrium) or a series of beats (ventricular tachycardia without retrograde atrial capture), AV dissociation exists for that period. The interruption of AV dissociation by one or a series of beats under the control of one pacemaker, either antegradely or retrogradely, indicates that the AV dissociation is incomplete. Complete or incomplete dissociation may also occur in association with all forms of AV block. Commonly, when AV dissociation occurs as a result of AV block the atrial rate exceeds the ventricular rate. For example, a subsidiary pacemaker with a rate of 40 beats/min may escape in the presence of a 2:1 AV block when the atrial rate is 78. If the AV block is bidirectional, AV dissociation results.

ELECTROCARDIOGRAPHIC AND CLINICAL FEATURES. The electrocardiogram demonstrates the independence of P waves and QRS complexes. The P-wave morphology depends on the rhythm controlling the atria (sinus, atrial tachycardia, junctional, flutter, or fibrillation). During complete AV dissociation both the QRS complex and the P waves appear regularly spaced without a fixed temporal relationship to each other. When the dissociation is incomplete, a QRS complex of supraventricular contour occurs early and is preceded by a P wave at a P-R interval exceeding 0.12 seconds and within a conductable range. This indicates ventricular capture by the supraventricular focus. Similarly, a premature P wave with a retrograde morphology and a conductable R-P interval may indicate retrograde atrial capture by the subsidiary focus.

The physical findings include a variable intensity of the first heart sound as the P-R interval changes, atrial sounds, and *a* waves in the jugular venous pulse lacking a consistent relationship to ventricular contraction. Intermittent large (cannon) *a* waves may be seen in the jugular venous pulse when atrial and ventricular contraction occur simultaneously. The second heart sound may split normally or paradoxically, depending on the manner of ventricular activation. A premature beat representing a ventricular capture may interrupt a regular heart rhythm. When the ventricular rate exceeds the atrial rate, a cyclic increase in intensity of the first heart sound is produced as the P-R interval shortens, climaxed by a very loud sound (bruit de canon). This intense sound is followed by a sudden reduction in intensity of the first heart sound and the appearance of giant *a* waves as the P-R interval shortens and P waves "march through" the cardiac cycle.

TREATMENT. Treatment is directed toward the underlying heart disease and precipitating cause. The individual components *producing the AV dissociation*—not the AV dissociation per se—determine the specific type of antiarrhythmic approaches. Therapy ranges from pacemaker insertion in a patient who has AV dissociation due to complete AV block to lidocaine administration in a patient who has AV dissociation due to a ventricular tachycardia.

Acknowledgments

The author gratefully acknowledges the thoughtful comments of Eric N. Prystowsky, M.D., and James J. Heger, M.D.; also Kevin Brown, M.D., Donald Chilson, M.D., Elwyn Lloyd, M.D., William Miles, M.D., and Brian Skale, M.D. Lee Northcutt and Shirley Myers provided secretarial help.

References

1. Waxman, M. B., and Wald, R.: Termination of ventricular tachycardia by an increase in cardiac vagal drive. Circulation *56*:385, 1977.
2. Hess, D. S., Hanlon, T., Scheinman, M., Budge, R., and Desai, J.: Termination of ventricular tachycardia by carotid sinus massage. Circulation *65*:627, 1982.
3. Beal, M. F., Park, T. S., and Fisher, C. M.: Cerebral atheromatous embolism following carotid sinus pressure. Arch. Neurol. *38*:310, 1981.

4. Zipes, D. P., and DeJoseph, R. L.: Dissimilar atrial rhythms in man and dog. Am. J. Cardiol. 32:618, 1973.

5. Jenkins, J. M., Wu, D., and Arzbacher, R. C.: Computer diagnosis of supraventricular and ventricular arrhythmias. A new esophageal technique. Circulation 60:977, 1979.

6. Prystowsky, E. N., Pritchett, E. L. C., and Gallagher, J. J.: Origin of the atrial electrogram recorded from the esophagus. Circulation 61:1017, 1980.

7. Barold, S. S.: Filtered bipolar esophageal electrocardiography. Am. Heart J. 83:431, 1972.

8. Hammill, S. C., and Pritchett, E. L.: Simplified esophageal electrocardiography using bipolar recording leads. Ann. Intern. Med. 95:14, 1981.

9. Gallagher, J. J., Smith, W. M., Kerr, C. R., Kasell, J., Cook, L., Reiter, M., Sterba, R., and Harte, M.: Esophageal pacing: A diagnostic and therapeutic tool. Circulation 65:336, 1982.

10. Hung, J., Kelly, D. T., Hutton, B. F., Uther, J. B., and Baird, D. K.: Influence of heart rate and atrial transport on left ventricular volume and function: Relation to hemodynamic changes produced by supraventricular arrhythmia. Am. J. Cardiol. 48:632, 1981.

11. Levy, M. N., and Martin, P. J.: Neural control of the heart. In Berne, R. M., et al. (eds.): Handbook of Physiology, The Cardiovascular System. Vol. I. Bethesda, Md., American Physiological Society, 1979, p. 581.

12. Jalife, J., and Moe, G. K.: Phasic effects of vagal stimulation on pacemaker activity of the isolated sinus node of the young cat. Circ. Res. 45:595, 1979.

13. Sheffield, L. T., Holt, J. H., and Reeves, T. J.: Exercise graded by heart rate in electrocardiographic testing for angina pectoris. Circulation 32:622, 1965.

14. Bauernfeind, R. A., Amat-y-Leon, F., Dhingra, R. C., Kehoe, R., Wyndham, C., and Rosen, K. M.: Chronic nonparoxysmal sinus tachycardia in otherwise healthy persons. Ann. Intern. Med. 91:702, 1979.

15. Brodsky, M., Wu, D., Denes, P., Kanakis, C., and Rosen, K. M.: Arrhythmias documented by 24-hour continuous electrocardiographic monitoring in 50 male medical students without apparent heart disease. Am. J. Cardiol. 39:390, 1977.

16. Scott, O., Williams, G. J., and Fiddler, G. I.: Results of 24-hour ambulatory monitoring of electrocardiogram in 131 healthy boys age 10 to 13 years. Br. Heart J. 44:304, 1980.

17. Adgey, A. A. J., Geddes, J. S., Mulholland, H. C., Keegan, D. A. J., and Pantridge, J. F.: Incidence, significance and management of early bradyarrhythmia complicating acute myocardial infarction. Lancet 2:1097, 1968.

18. Norris, R. M., Mercer, C. J., and Yeates, S. E.: Sinus rate in acute myocardial infarction. Br. Heart J. 34:901, 1972.

19. Goldberg, S., Greenspon, A. J., Urban, P. L., Muza, B., Berger, B., Walinsky, P., Maroko, P. R.: Reperfusion arrhythmia: A marker of restoration of antegrade flow during intracoronary thrombolysis for acute myocardial infarction. Am. Heart J. 105:26, 1983.

20. Weiss, A. T., Rod, J. L., Gotsman, M. S., and Lewis, B. S.: Hydralazine in the management of symptomatic sinus bradycardia. Eur. J. Cardiol. 12:261, 1981.

21. Walter, P. F., Crawley, I. S., and Dorney, E. R.: Carotid sinus hypersensitivity and syncope. Am. J. Cardiol. 42:396, 1978.

22. Merx, W., Effert, S., Hanrath, P., Pop, T., Rehder, W., and Schweizer, P.: Hyperactive carotid sinus reflex. Dtsch. Med. Wnschr. 106:135, 1981.

23. Davies, A. B., Stephens, M. R., and Davies, A. G.: Carotid sinus hypersensitivity in patients presenting with syncope. Br. Heart J. 42:583, 1979.

24. Brown, K. A., Maloney, J. D., Smith, C. H., Hartzler, G. O., and Ilstup, D. M.: Carotid sinus reflex in patients undergoing coronary angiography: Relationship of degree and location of coronary artery disease in response to carotid sinus massage. Circulation 62:697, 1980.

25. Wenger, T. L., Dohrmann, M. L., Strauss, H. C., Conley, M. J., Wechsler, A. S., and Wagner, G. S.: Hypersensitive carotid sinus syndrome manifested as cough syncope. PACE 3:332, 1980.

26. Thorman, J., Neuss, H., Schlepper, M., and Mitrovic, V.: Effects of clonidine on sinus node function in man. Chest 80:201, 1981.

27. Pick, A., and Langendorf, R.: Interpretation of Complex Arrhythmias. Philadelphia, Lea and Febiger, 1979, p. 127.

28. Lown, B.: Electrical reversion of cardiac arrhythmias. Br. Heart J. 29:469, 1967.

29. Zipes, D. P., Wallace, A. G., Sealy, W. C., and Floyd, W. L.: Artificial atrial and ventricular pacing in the treatment of arrhythmias. Ann. Intern. Med. 70:885, 1969.

30. Short, D. S.: The syndrome of alternating bradycardia and tachycardia. Br. Heart J. 16:208, 1954.

31. Narula, O. S.: Atrioventricular conduction disturbances in patients with sinus bradycardia. Circulation 44:1096, 1971.

32. Jordan, J. A., Yamaguchi, I., and Mandel, W. J.: Studies on the mechanisms of sinus node dysfunction in a sick sinus syndrome. Circulation 57:217, 1978.

33. Kang, P. S., Gomes, J. A., Kelen, G., and El-Sherif, N.: Role of autonomic regulatory mechanism in sinoatrial conduction and sinus nodal automaticity in sick sinus syndrome. Circulation 64:832, 1981.

34. Desae, J. M., Scheinman, M. M., Strauss, H. C., Massie, B., and O'Young, J.: Electrophysiologic effects of combined autonomic blockade in patients with sinus node disease. Circulation 63:953, 1981.

35. Scheinmann, M. M., Strauss, H. C., Abbott, J. A., Evans, G. T., Peters, R. W., Benditt, D. G., and Wallace, A. G.: Electrophysiologic testing in patients with sinus pauses and/or sinoatrial exit block. Eur. J. Cardiol. 8:51, 1978.

36. Simonsen, E., Nielsen, J. S., and Nielsen, B. L.: Sinus node dysfunction in 128 patients. A retrospective study with followup. Acta Med. Scand. 208:343, 1980.

37. Yabek, S. M., Swensson, R. E., and Jarmakani, J. M.: Electrocardiographic recognition of sinus node dysfunction in children and young adults. Circulation 56:235, 1977.

38. Mackintosh, A. F.: Sinoatrial disease in young people. Br. Heart J. 45:62, 1981.

39. Rasmussen, V., Haunso, S., and Skagen, K.: Cerebral attacks due to excessive vagal tone in heavily trained persons. A clinical and electrophysiologic study. Acta Med. Scand. 204:401, 1978.

39a. Kerr, C. R., Gant, A. O., Wenger, T. L., and Strauss, H. C.: Sinus node dysfunction. Cardiol. Clin. (in press).

40. Rosen, K. M., Loeb, H. S., Sinno, M. Z., Rahimtoola, S. H., and Gunnar, R.: Cardiac conduction in patients with symptomatic sinus node disease. Circulation 43:836, 1971.

41. DeMoulin, J. C., and Kulbertus, H. E.: Histopathological correlates of sinoatrial disease. Br. Heart J. 40:1384, 1978.

42. Bharati, S., Nordenberg, A., Bauernfeind, R., Varghese, J. P., Carvalho, A. G., Rosen, K. M., and Lev, M.: The anatomic substrate for the sick sinus syndrome in adolescents. Am. J. Cardiol. 46:163, 1980.

43. Thery, C., Gosselin, B., Lekieffre, J., and Warembourg, H.: Pathology of the sinoatrial node. Correlation with electrocardiographic findings in 111 patients. Am. Heart J. 93:735, 1977.

44. Gomes, J. A., Kang, P. S., and El-Sherif, N.: Effects of digitalis on the human sick sinus node after pharmacologic autonomic blockade. Am. J. Cardiol. 48:783, 1981.

45. Dhingra, R. C., Amat-y-Leon, F., Wyndham, C., Deedwania, P. C., Wu, D., Denes, P., and Rosen, K. M.: Clinical significance of prolonged sinoatrial conduction time. Circulation 55:8, 1977.

46. Paulay, K. L., Varghese, P. J., and Damato, A. N.: Atrial rhythms in response to an early atrial premature depolarization in man. Am. Heart J. 85:323, 1973.

47. Curry, P. V. L., Evans, T. R., and Krikler, D. M.: Paroxysmal reciprocating sinus tachycardia. Eur. J. Cardiol. 6:199, 1977.

48. Narula, O. S.: Sinus node reentry. A mechanism for supraventricular tachycardia. Circulation 50:1114, 1974.

49. Wu, D., Amat-y-Leon, F., Denes, P., Dhingra, R. C., Pietras, R. J., and Rosen, K. M.: Demonstration of sustained sinus and atrial reentry as a mechanism of paroxysmal supraventricular tachycardia. Circulation 51:234, 1975.

50. Weisfogel, G. M., Batsford, W. P., Paulay, K. L., Josephson, M. E., Ogunkelu, J. B., Akhtar, M., Seides, S. F., and Damato, A. N.: Sinus node reentrant tachycardia in man. Am. Heart J. 90:295, 1975.

51. Fauchier, J. P., Latour, F., Neel, C., Charbonnier, B., and Brochier, M.: Paroxysmal sinoatrial tachycardia. Arch. Mal Coeur 73:165, 1980.

52. Pick, A., Langendorf, R., and Katz, L. N.: Depression of cardiac pacemakers by premature impulses. Am. Heart J. 41:49, 1951.

53. Langendorf, R., and Mintz, S. S.: Premature systoles originating in the sinoauricular node. Br. Heart J. 8:178, 1946.

54. Zipes, D. P., Foster, P. R., Troup, P. J., and Pedersen, D. H.: Atrial induction of ventricular tachycardia: Reentry or triggered automaticity. Am. J. Cardiol. 44:1, 1979.

55. El-Sherif, N., Myerburg, R. J., Scherlag, B. J., Befeler, B., Aranda, J. M., Castellanos, A., Jr., and Lazzara, R.: Electrocardiographic antecedents of primary ventricular fibrillation. Br. Heart J. 38:415, 1976.

56. Myerburg, R. J., Sung, R. J., Gerstenblith, G., Mallon, S. M., Castellanos, A., Jr., and Lazzara, R.: Ventricular ectopic activity after premature atrial beats in acute myocardial infarction. Br. Heart J. 39:1033, 1977.

57. Sakamoto, T., Yamada, T., and Hiejima, K.: Ventricular fibrillation induced by conducted sinus or supraventricular beat. Circulation 48:438, 1973.

58. Jervell, A., and Lange-Nielsen, F.: Congenital deaf-mutism, functional heart disease with prolongation of the QT interval and sudden death. Am. Heart J. 54:59, 1957.

59. Wellens, H. J. J., Bär, F. W., Farre, J., Ross, D. L., Wiener, I., and Vanagt, E. J.: Initiation and termination of ventricular tachycardia by supraventricular stimuli. Am. J. Cardiol. 46:576, 1980.

60. Robertson, C. E., and Miller, H. C.: Extreme tachycardia complicating the use of disopyramide in atrial flutter. Br. Heart J. 44:602, 1980.

61. Jackman, W. M., Prystowsky, E. N., Naccarelli, G. V., Heger, J. J., and Zipes, D. P.: Reevaluation of enhanced AV nodal conduction: Evidence to suggest a continuum of normal nodal physiology. Circulation 67:441, 1983.

62. Moleiro, F., Mendoza, I. J., Medina-Ravell, V., Castellanos, A., and Myerburg, R. J.: One to one atrioventricular conduction during atrial pacing at rates of 300/min in absence of Wolff-Parkinson-White syndrome. Am. J. Cardiol. 48:789, 1981.

63. Besoain-Santander, M., Pick, A., and Langendorf, R.: AV conduction in auricular flutter. Circulation 2:604, 1950.

64. Ashman, R., and Hull, H.: Essentials of Electrocardiography. New York, Macmillan Co., 1947, p. 203.

65. Langendorf, R.: Concealed AV conduction: The effect of blocked impulses on the formation and conduction of subsequent impulses. Am. Heart J. 35:542, 1948.

66. Suarez, L. D., Kretz, A., Alvarez, J. A., Martinez, J. A., and Perosio, A. M.: Dissimilar atrial rhythms. A patient with triple right atrial rhythm. Am. Heart J. 100:678, 1980.

67. Gomes, J. A., Kang, P. S., Matheson, M., Gough, W. B., Jr., and El-Sherif, N.: Coexistence of sick sinus rhythm and atrial flutter-fibrillation. Circulation 63:80, 1981.

68. Simpson, R. J., Foster, J. R., and Gettes, L. S.: Atrial excitability and conduction in patients with interatrial conduction defects. Am. J. Cardiol. 50:1331, 1982.

69. Anderson, K. J., Simmons, S. C., and Hallidie-Smith, K. A.: Fetal cardiac arrhythmia: Antepartum diagnosis of a case of congenital atrial flutter. Arch. Dis. Child. 56:472, 1981.

70. Waldo, A. L., MacLean, W. H., Karp, R. B., Kouchoukos, N. T., and James, T. N.: Entrainment and interruption of atrial flutter with atrial pacing. Studies in man following open heart surgery. Circulation 56:737, 1977.

71. Camm, J., Ward, D., and Spurrell, R.: Response of atrial flutter to overdrive atrial pacing and intravenous disopyramide phosphate, singly and in combination. Br. Heart J. 44:240, 1980.

72. Zipes, D. P.: The contribution of artificial pacemaking to understanding the pathogenesis of arrhythmias. Am. J. Cardiol. 28:211, 1971.

73. Wells, J. L., MacLean, W. A. H., James, T. N., and Waldo, A. L.: Characterization of atrial flutter. Studies in man after open heart surgery using fixed atrial electrodes. Circulation 60:665, 1979.

74. Waxman, H. L., Myerburg, R. J., Appel, R., and Sung, R. J.: Verapamil for control of ventricular rate in paroxysmal supraventricular tachycardia and atrial fibrillation or flutter: A double-blind randomized cross-over study. Ann. Intern. Med. 94:1, 1981.

75. Pritchett, E. L., Smith, W. M., Klein, G. J., Hammill, S. C., and Gallagher, J. J.: The "compensatory pause" of atrial fibrillation. Circulation 62:1021, 1980.

76. Rowland, E., Curry, P., Fox, K., and Krikler, E. R.: Relation between atrioventricular pathways and ventricular response during atrial fibrillation and flutter. Br. Heart J. 45:83, 1981.

77. Forfar, J. C., Miller, H. C., and Toft, A. D.: Occult thyrotoxicosis: A correctable cause of "idiopathic" atrial fibrillation. Am. J. Cardiol. 44:9, 1979.

78. Kannel, W. B., Abbott, R. D., Savage, D. D., and McNamara, P. M.: Epidemiologic features of chronic atrial fibrillation: The Framingham study. N. Engl. J. Med. 306:1018, 1982.

79. Takahashi, N., Seki, A., Imataka, K., and Fujii, J.: Clinical features of paroxysmal atrial fibrillation: An observation of 94 patients. Japn. Heart J. 22:143, 1981.

80. Gajewski, J., and Singer, R. B.: Mortality in an insured population with atrial fibrillation. J.A.M.A. 245:1540, 1981.

81. Olsson, S. B., Orndahl, G., Ernestrom, S., Eskielson, J., Persson, S., Grennert, M. L., and Johanson, B. W.: Spontaneous reversion from longlasting atrial fibrillation to sinus rhythm. Acta Med. Scand. 207:5, 1980.

82. Wolf, P. A., Dawber, P. R., Thomas, H. E., Jr., and Kannel, W. B.: Epidemiologic assessment of chronic atrial fibrillation and risk of stroke: The Framingham study. Neurology 28:973, 1978.

83. Hinton, R. C., Kistler, J. P., Fallon, J. T., Friedlich, A. L., and Fisher, C. M.: Influence of etiology of atrial fibrillation on incidence of systemic embolism. Am. J. Cardiol. 40:509, 1977.

84. Hunt, D., Sloman, G., and Penington, C.: Effects of atrial fibrillation on prognosis of acute myocardial infarction. Br. Heart J. 40:303, 1978.

85. Watson, D. C., Henry, W. L., Epstein, S. E., and Morrow, A. G.: Effects of operation on left atrial size and the occurrence of atrial fibrillation in patients with hypertrophic subaortic stenosis. Circulation 55:178, 1977.

86. Morganroth, J., Horowitz, L. N., Josephson, M. E., and Kastor, J. A.: Relationship of atrial fibrillatory wave amplitude to left atrial size and etiology of heart disease. An old generalization reexamined. Am. Heart J. 97:184, 1979.

87. Ewy, G. A., Ulfers, L., Hager, W. D., Rosenfeld, A. R., Roeske, W. R., and Goldman, S.: Response of atrial fibrillation to therapy: Role of etiology and left atrial diameter. J. Electrocardiol. 13:119, 1980.

88. Radford, D. J., and Izukawa, T.: Atrial fibrillation in children. Pediatrics 59:250, 1977.

89. Stern, E. H., Pitchon, R., King, B. D., Guerrero, J., Schneider, R. R., and Wiener, I.: Clinical use of oral verapamil in chronic and paroxysmal atrial fibrillation. Chest 81:308, 1982.

90. Hansen, J. F., Anderson, E. D., Olesen, K. H., Steiness, E., Lyngborg, K., Anderson, J. D., Efsen, F., Henningsen, P., and Wennevold, A.: DC cardioversion of atrial fibrillation after mitral valve operation. An analysis of long-term results. Scand. J. Thorac. Cardiovasc. Surg. 13:267, 1979.

90a. Mancini, G. B. J., and Goldberger, A. L.: Cardioversion of atrial fibrillation: Consideration of embolization, anticoagulation, prophylactic pacemaker and long term success. Am. Heart J. 104:617, 1982.

91. Lown, B.: Electrical reversion of cardiac arrhythmias. Br. Heart J. 29:469, 1967.

92. Resenkov, L., and McDonald, L.: Complications in 220 patients with cardiac dysrhythmias treated by phased direct current shock and indications for electroconversion. Br. Heart J. 29:926, 1967.

93. Bjerkelund, C. J., and Orning, O. M.: The efficacy of anticoagulant therapy in preventing embolism related to DC electrical conversion of atrial fibrillation. Am. J. Cardiol. 23:208, 1969.

94. Halpern, S. W., Ellrodt, G., Singh, B. N., and Mandel, W. J.: Efficacy of intravenous procainamide infusion in converting atrial fibrillation to sinus rhythm. Relation to left atrial size. Br. Heart J. 44:589, 1980.

95. Bauernfeind, R. A., Swiryn, S. P., Strasberg, B., Palileo, E., Scagliotti, D., and Rosen, K. M.: Electrophysiologic drug testing in prophylaxis of sporadic paroxysmal atrial fibrillation: Technique application and efficacy in severely symptomatic preexcitation patients. Am. Heart J. 103:941, 1982.

96. Goldreyer, B. N., Gallagher, J. J., and Damato, A. N.: The electrophysiologic demonstration of atrial ectopic tachycardia in man. Am. Heart J. 85:205, 1973.

97. Scheinmann, M. M., Basu, D., and Hollenberg, M.: Electrophysiologic studies in patients with persistent atrial tachycardia. Circulation 50:266, 1974.

98. Gillette, P. C., and Garson, A., Jr.: Electrophysiologic and pharmacologic characteristics of automatic ectopic atrial tachycardia. Circulation 56:571, 1977.

99. Rinkenberger, R. L., Prystowsky, E. N., Heger, J. J., Troup, P. J., Jackman, W. M., and Zipes, D. P.: Effects of intravenous and chronic oral verapamil administration in patients with supraventricular tachyarrhythmias. Circulation 62:996, 1980.

100. Coumel, P., and Barold, S. S.: Mechanisms of supraventricular tachycardia. In His Bundle Electrocardiography and Clinical Electrophysiology. Narula, O. S. (ed.): Philadelphia, F. A. Davis Co., 1975, p. 203.

101. Coumel, P., Flammang, D., Attuel, P., and Leclercq, J. F.: Sustained intraatrial reentrant tachycardia. Electrophysiologic study of 20 cases. Clin. Cardiol. 2:176, 1979.

102. Wu, D., Denes, P., Amat-y-Leon, F., Dhingra, R., Wyndham, C. R. C., Bauernfeind, R., Latif, P., and Rosen, K. M.: Clinical electrocardiographic and electrophysiologic observations in patients with paroxysmal supraventricular tachycardia. Am. J. Cardiol. 41:1045, 1978.

103. Schine, K. I., Kastor, J. A., and Yurchak, E. M.: Multifocal atrial tachycardia. Clinical and electrocardiographic features in 32 patients. N. Engl. J. Med. 279:344, 1968.

104. Lipson, M. J., and Naimi, S.: Multifocal atrial tachycardia (chaotic atrial tachycardia). Circulation 42:397, 1970.

105. Bisset, G. S., Siegel, S. F., Gaum, W. E., and Kaplan, S.: Chaotic atrial tachycardia in childhood. Am. Heart J. 101:268, 1981.

106. Tse, W. W.: Evidence of presence of automatic fibers in the canine atrioventricular node. Am. J. Physiol. 225:716, 1973.

107. Wit, A. L., and Cranefield, P. F.: Mechanisms of impulse initiation in the atrioventricular junction and the effects of acetylstrophanthidin. Am. J. Cardiol. 49:921, 1982.

108. Scherf, D., and Cohen, J.: The Atrioventricular Node and Selected Cardiac Arrhythmias. New York, Grune and Stratton, 1964, p. 226.

109. Pick, A., and Dominguez, P.: Nonparoxysmal AV nodal tachycardias. Circulation 16:1022, 1957.

110. Kastor, J. A., and Yurchak, P. M.: Recognition of digitalis intoxication in the presence of atrial fibrillation. Ann. Intern. Med. 67:105, 1967.

111. Zipes, D. P., Gaum, W. E., Genetos, B. C., Glassman, R. D., Noble, R. J., and Fisch, C.: Atrial tachycardia without P wave masquerading as an AV junctional tachycardia. Circulation 55:253, 1977.

112. Castellanos, A., Sung, R. J., and Myerburg, R. J.: His bundle electrocardiography in digitalis-induced atrioventricular junctional Wenckebach periods with irregular HH intervals. Am. J. Cardiol. 43:653, 1979.

113. Rosen, M. R., Fisch, C., Hoffman, B. F., Danilo, P., Jr., Lovelace, D. E., and Knoebel, S. B.: Can accelerated atrioventricular junctional escape rhythms be explained by delayed afterdepolarizations? Am. J. Cardiol. 45:1272, 1980.

114. Zipes, D. P., and Fisch, C.: Atrioventricular dissociation. Arch. Intern. Med. 132:130, 1973.

115. Rosen, K. M.: Junctional tachycardia. Mechanisms, diagnosis, differential diagnosis and management. Circulation 47:654, 1973.

116. Gordon, A., and Gillette, P. C.: Junctional ectopic tachycardia in children: Electrocardiography, electrophysiology and pharmacologic response. Am. J. Cardiol. 44:98, 1979.

117. Palileo, E. V., Bauernfeind, R. A., Swiryn, S. P., Wyndham, C. R., and Rosen, K. M.: Chronic nonparoxysmal junctional tachycardia. Chest 80:106, 1981.

117a. Heddle, B., Brugada, P., Bär, F., and Wellens, H. J. J.: Cycle length change after initiation of reentrant tachycardia. Circulation 66 (Suppl. II): 269, 1982.

118. Bigger, J. T., and Goldreyer, B. N.: The mechanism of supraventricular tachycardia. Circulation 42:673, 1970.

119. Goldreyer, B. N., and Bigger, J. T.: Site of reentry and paroxysmal supraventricular tachycardia in man. Circulation 43:15, 1971.

120. Goldreyer, B. N., and Damato, A. N.: Essential role of atrioventricular conduction delay in the initiation of paroxysmal supraventricular tachycardia. Circulation 43:679, 1971.

121. Benditt, D. G., Pritchett, E. L., Smith, W. M., and Gallagher, J. J.: Ventriculoatrial intervals: Diagnostic use in paroxysmal supraventricular tachycardia. Ann. Intern. Med. 91:161, 1979.

122. Bauernfeind, R. A., Swiryn, S., Strasberg, B., Palileo, E., Wyndham, C., Duffy, C., and Rosen, K. M.: Analysis of anterograde and retrograde fast pathway properties in patients with dual atrioventricular nodal pathways. Observations regarding the pathophysiology of the Lown-Ganong-Levine syndrome. Am. J. Cardiol. 49:283, 1982.

123. Casta, A., Wolff, G. S., Mehta, A. V., Tamer, D., Garcia, O. L., Pickoff, A. S., Ferrer, P. L., Sung, R. H., and Gelband, H.: Dual atrioventricular nodal pathways: A benign finding in arrhythmia-free children with heart disease. Am. J. Cardiol. 46:1013, 1980.

124. Garson, A., Jr., and Gillette, P. C.: Electrophysiologic studies of supraventricular tachycardia in children. I. Clinical-electrophysiologic correlations. Am. Heart J. 102:233, 1981.

125. Swiryn, S., Bauernfeind, R. A., Palileo, E., Strasberg, B., Duffy, C. E., and Rosen, K. M.: Electrophysiologic study demonstrating triple antegrade AV nodal pathways in patients with spontaneous and/or induced supraventricular tachycardia. Am. Heart J. 103:168, 1982.

126. Brugada, P., Bär, F. W., Vanagt, E. J., Friedman, P. L., and Wellens, H. J. J.: Observations in patients showing AV junctional echoes with a shorter PR than RP interval. Am. J. Cardiol. 48:611, 1981.

127. Akhtar, M., Damato, A. N., Ruskin, J. N., Batsford, W. T., Reddy, C. P., Ticzon, A. R., Dhatt, M. S., Gomes, J. A. C., and Calon, A. H.: Antegrade and retrograde conduction characteristics in three patterns of paroxysmal atrioventricular junctional reentrant tachycardia. Am. Heart J. 95:22, 1978.

128. Coumel, P.: Functional reciprocating tachycardias. The permanent and paroxysmal forms of AV nodal reciprocating tachycardias. J. Electrocardiol. 8:79, 1975.

129. Denes, P., Wu, D., Dhingra, R., Amat-y-Leon, F., Wyndham, C., and Rosen, K. M.: Dual atrioventricular nodal pathways: A common electrophysiological response. Br. Heart J. 37:1069, 1975.

130. Denes, P., Wu, D., Dhingra, R. C., Chuquimia, R., and Rosen, K. M.: Demonstration of dual AV nodal pathways in patients with paroxysmal supraventricular tachycardia. Circulation 48:549, 1973.

131. Wu, D.: Dual atrioventricular nodal pathways: A reappraisal. PACE 5:72, 1982.

132. Wu, D., Denes, P., Amat-y-Leon, F., Wyndham, C. R. C., Dhingra, R., and Rosen, K. M.: An unusual variety of atrioventricular nodal reentry due to retrograde dual atrioventricular nodal pathways. Circulation 56:50, 1977.

133. Amat-y-Leon, F., Wyndham, C. R., Wu, D., Denes, P., Dhingra, R. C., and Rosen, K. M.: Participation of fast and slow AV nodal pathways in tachycardias complicating the Wolff-Parkinson-White syndrome. Circulation 55:663, 1977.

134. Rosen, K. M., Bauernfeind, R. A., Swiryn, S., Strasberg, B., and Palileo, E. V.: Dual AV nodal pathways and AV nodal reentrant paroxysmal tachycardia. Am. Heart J. 101:691, 1981.

135. Wellens, H. J. J., Westorp, J. C., Duren, D. R., and Lie, K. I.: Second degree block during reciprocal atrioventricular nodal tachycardia. Circulation 53:595, 1976.

135a. Ko, P. T., Naccarelli, G. V., Gulamhusein, S., Prystowsky, E. N., Zipes, D. P., and Klein, G. J.: Atrioventricular dissociation during paroxysmal junctional tachycardia. PACE 4:670, 1981.

136. Sung, B. J., Waxman, H. L., Saksena, S., and Juma, Z.: Sequence of retrograde atrial activation in patients with dual atrioventricular nodal pathways. Circulation 64:1059, 1981.

137. Swiryn, S., Pavel, D., Byrom, E., Wyndham, C., Pietras, R., Bauernfeind, R., and Rosen, K. M.: Assessment of left ventricular function by radionuclide angiography during induced supraventricular tachycardia. Am. J. Cardiol. 47: 555, 1981.

138. Waxman, M. B., Sharma, A. B., Cameron, D. A., Huerta, F., and Wald, R. W.: Reflex mechanisms responsible for early spontaneous termination of paroxysmal supraventricular tachycardia. Am. J. Cardiol. 49:259, 1982.

139. Sung, R. J., Elser, B., and McAllister, R. G., Jr.: Intravenous verapamil for termination of reentrant supraventricular tachycardias: Intracardiac studies correlated with plasma verapamil concentrations. Ann. Intern. Med. 93:682, 1980.

140. Krikler, D. M.: Verapamil in cardiology. Eur. J. Cardiol. 2:3, 1974.

141. Waxman, H. L., Myerburg, R. J., Appel, R., and Sung, R. J.: Verapamil for control of ventricular rate in paroxysmal supraventricular tachycardia and atrial fibrillation or flutter: A double-blind randomized cross-over study. Ann. Intern. Med. 94:1, 1981.

142. Betriu, A., Chaitman, B. R., Bourassa, M. G., Brévers, G., Scholl, J., Bruneau, P., Gagne, P., and Chabot, M.: Beneficial effect of intravenous diltiazen in the acute management of paroxysmal supraventricular tachyarrhythmias. Circulation 67:88, 1983.

143. Wu, D., Hung, J. S., Kuo, C. T., Hsu, K. S., and Shieh, W. B.: Effects of quinidine on atrioventricular nodal reentrant paroxysmal tachycardia. Circulation 64:823, 1981.

144. Swiryn, S., Bauernfeind, R. A., Wyndham, C. R. C., Dhingra, R. C., Palileo, E., Strasberg, B., and Rosen, K. M.: Effects of oral disopyramide drugs on induction of paroxysmal supraventricular tachycardia. Circulation 64:169, 1981.

145. Bauernfeind, R. A., Wyndham, C. R., Dhingra, R. C., Swiryn, S. P., Palileo, E., Strasberg, B., and Rosen, K. M.: Serial electrophysiologic testing of multiple drugs in patients with atrioventricular nodal reentrant paroxysmal tachycardia. Circulation 62:1341, 1980.

146. Zipes, D. P., DeJoseph, R. L., and Rothbaum, D. A.: Unusual properties of accessory pathways. Circulation 49:1200, 1974.

147. Coumel, P., and Attuel, P.: Reciprocating tachycardia in overt and latent preexcitation. Influence of functional bundle branch block on the rate of the tachycardia. Eur. J. Cardiol. 1:423, 1974.

148. Neuss, H., Schlepper, M., and Thormann, J.: Analysis of reentry mechanisms in the three patients with concealed Wolff-Parkinson-White syndrome. Circulation 51:75, 1975.

149. Spurrell, R. A. J., Krikler, D. M., and Sowton, E.: Concealed bypasses of the atrioventricular node in patients with paroxysmal supraventricular tachycardia revealed by intracardiac electrical stimulation and verapamil. Am. J. Cardiol. 33:590, 1974.

150. Slama, R., Coumel, P., and Bouvrain, Y.: Les syndromes de Wolff-Parkinson-White de type A inapparents ou latents en rythme sinusal. Arch. Mal Coeur 66:639, 1973.

151. Barold, S. S., and Coumel, P.: Mechanisms of atrioventricular junctional tachycardia. Role of reentry and concealed accessory bypass tracts. Am. J. Cardiol. 39:97, 1977.

152. Puech, P., Grolleau, R., and Cinca, J.: Reciprocating tachycardia using a latent left-sided accessory pathway. Diagnostic approach by conventional ECG.

In Kulbertus, H. E. (ed.): Reentrant Arrhythmias. Baltimore, University Park Press, 1977. p. 117.

153. Pritchett, E. L. C., Tonkin, A. M., Dugan, F. A., Wallace, A. G., and Gallagher, J. J.: Ventriculoatrial conduction time during reciprocating tachycardia with intermittent bundle branch block in Wolff-Parkinson-White syndrome. Br. Heart J. 38:1058, 1976.

153a. Kerr, C. R., Gallagher, J. J. and German, L. D.: Changes in ventriculoatrial intervals with bundle branch block aberration during reciprocating tachycardia in patients with accessory atrioventricular pathways. Circulation 66:196, 1982.

154. Prystowsky, E. N., Pritchett, E. L. C., Smith, W. M., Wallace, A. G., Sealy, W. C., and Gallagher, J. J.: Electrophysiologic assessment of the atrioventricular conduction system after surgical correction of ventricular preexcitation. Circulation 59:789, 1979.

155. Chilson, D. A., Zipes, D. P., Heger, J. J., Browne, K. F., Lloyd, E. A., and Prystowsky, E. N.: Functional bundle branch block in man: Evidence of longer refractoriness of left than right bundle branch at faster heart rates. Clin. Res. 30:705A, 1982.

156. Prystowsky, E. N., Heger, J. J., Jackman, W. M., Naccarelli, G. V., and Zipes, D. P.: Postmyocardial infarction incessant supraventricular tachycardia due to concealed accessory pathway. Am. Heart J. 103:426, 1982.

157. Akhtar, M., Shenasa, M., and Schmidt, D. H.: Role of retrograde His-Purkinje block in the initiation of supraventricular tachycardia by ventricular premature stimulation in the Wolff-Parkinson-White syndrome. J. Clin. Invest. 67: 1047, 1981.

158. Farshidi, A., Josephson, M. E., and Horowitz, L. N.: Electrophysiologic characteristics of concealed accessory tracts: Clinical and electrocardiographic correlates. Am. J. Cardiol. 41:1052, 1978.

159. Wood, P.: Polyuria in paroxysmal tachycardia and paroxysmal atrial flutter and fibrillation. Br. Heart J. 25:273, 1963.

160. Harvey, W. P., and Ronan, J. A., Jr.: Bedside diagnosis of arrhythmias. Progr. Cardiovasc. Dis. 8:419, 1966.

161. Oehnell, R. F.: Preexcitation, a cardiac abnormality. Acta Med. Scand. 152 (Suppl.):78, 1944.

162. Durrer, D., Schuilenburg, R. M., and Wellens, H. J.: Preexcitation revisited. Am. J. Cardiol. 25:690, 1970.

163. Wolff, L., Parkinson, J., and White, P. D.: Bundle branch block with short P-R interval in healthy young people prone to paroxysmal tachycardia. Am. Heart J. 5:685, 1950.

164. Becker, A. H., and Anderson, R. H.: The Wolff-Parkinson-White syndrome and its anatomical substrates. Anat. Rec. 201:169, 1981.

165. Kent, A. F. S.: Researches on the structure and function of the mammalian heart. J. Physiol. 14:233, 1893.

166. Kent, A. F. S.: Observations on the auriculo-ventricular junction of the mammalian heart. Quart. J. Exp. Physiol. 7:193, 1913.

167. Anderson, R. H., Becker, A. E., Brechenmacher, C., Davies, M. J., and Rossi, L.: Ventricular preexcitation nomenclature for its substrates. Eur. J. Cardiol. 3: 27, 1975.

168. Brechenmacher, C.: Atrio-His bundle tracts. Br. Heart J. 37:853, 1975.

169. Lown, B., Ganong, W. F., and Levine, S. A.: The syndrome of short PR interval, normal QRS complex and paroxysmal rapid heart action. Circulation 5: 693, 1952.

170. Bauernfeind, R. A., Ayres, B. F., Wyndham, C. C., Dhingra, R. C., Swiryn, S. P., Strasberg, B., and Rosen, K. M.: Cycle length in atrioventricular nodal reentrant paroxysmal tachycardia with observations on Lown-Ganong-Levine syndrome. Am. J. Cardiol. 45:1148, 1980.

171. Mahaim, I.: Kent's fibers and the AV paraspecific conduction through the upper connections of the bundle of His-Tawara. Am. Heart J. 33:651, 1947.

172. Gallagher, J. J., Smith, W. M., Kasell, J. H., Benson, D. W., Jr., Sterba, R., and Grant, A. O.: Role of Mahaim fibers in cardiac arrhythmias in man. Circulation 64:176, 1981.

173. Gallagher, J. J., Pritchett, E. L. C., Sealy, W. C., Casell, J., and Wallace, A. G.: The pre-excitation syndromes. Progr. Cardiovasc. Dis. 20:285, 1978.

174. Nicolai, P., Medevdowsky, J. L., Delaahe, M., Barnay, C., Blache, E., and Pisapia, A.: Wolff-Parkinson-White syndrome: T wave abnormalities during normal pathway conduction. J. Electrocardiol. 14:295, 1981.

175. Durrer, D., Schoo, L., Schuilenberg, R. M., and Wellens, H. J. J.: The role of premature beats in the initiation and the termination of supraventricular tachycardia in the Wolff-Parkinson-White syndrome. Circulation 36:644, 1967.

176. Cinca, J., Valle, V., Gutierrez, L., Figueras, J., and Rius, J.: Reciprocating tachycardia using bilateral anomalous pathways: Electrophysiologic and clinical implications. Circulation 62:657, 1980.

177. Ko, P. T., Naccarelli, G. V., Gulamhusein, S., Prystowsky, E. N., Zipes, D. P., and Klein, G. J.: Atrioventricular dissociation during paroxysmal junctional tachycardia. PACE 4:670, 1981.

178. Motté, G., Brechenmacher, C., Davy, J. M., and Belhassen, B.: Association of nodoventricular and atrioventricular fibers with the origin of reciprocating tachycardia. Electrophysiological and anomal pathological anatomopathological aspect. Arch. Mal Coeur 73:737, 1980.

179. Coumel, P., Attuel, P., and Mugica, J.: Junctional reciprocating tachycardias. In Kulbertus, H. C. (ed.): Reentrant Arrhythmias. Baltimore, University Park Press, 1977.

180. Gallagher, J. J., and Sealy, W. C.: The permanent form of junctional reciprocating tachycardia. Further elucidation of the underlying mechanism. Eur. J. Cardiol. 8:413, 1978.

181. Wellens, H. J. J.: Observations in patients showing AV junctional echoes with a shorter PR than RP interval. Distinction between intranodal reentry or reentry using an accessory pathway with a long conduction time. Am. J. Cardiol. 48:611, 1981.

182. Touboul, P., Atallah, G., and Kirkorian, G.: Role of accessory atrioventricular pathways in the genesis of permanent junctional tachycardia. Arch. Mal Coeur 73:1131, 1980.

183. Gillette, P. C., Garson, A., Cooley, D. A., and McNamara, D. G.: Prolonged and decremental antegrade conduction properties in right anterior accessory connections: Wide QRS antidromic tachycardia of left bundle branch block pattern without Wolff-Parkinson-White configuration in sinus rhythm. Am. Heart J. 103:166, 1982.

184. Gillette, P. C., Garson, A., Jr., and Kugler, J. D.: Wolff-Parkinson-White syndrome in children: Electrophysiologic and pharmacologic characteristics. Circulation 60:1487, 1979.

185. Gallagher, J. J., Smith, W. M., Kasell, J., Smith, W. M., Grant, A. O., and Benson, D. W.: Use of the esophageal lead in the diagnosis of mechanisms of reciprocating supraventricular tachycardia. PACE 3:440, 1980.

186. Sung, R. J., Castellanos, A., Mallon, S. M., Bloom, M. G., Gelband, H., and Myerburg, R. J.: Mechanisms of spontaneous alternation between reciprocating tachycardia and atrial flutter-fibrillation in the Wolff-Parkinson-White syndrome. Circulation 56:409, 1977.

187. Ross, D. L., Farre, J., Bär, F. W., Vanagt, E. J., Brugada, T., Wiener, I., and Wellens, H. J. J.: Spontaneous termination of circus movement tachycardia using an atrioventricular accessory pathway: Incidence, site of block and mechanisms. Circulation 63:1129, 1981.

188. Bauernfeind, R. A., Wyndham, C. R., Swiryn, S. P., Palileo, E. V., Strasberg, B., Lam, W., Westveer, D., and Rosen, K. M.: Paroxysmal atrial fibrillation in the Wolff-Parkinson-White syndrome. Am. J. Cardiol. 47:562, 1981.

189. Klein, G. H., Bashore, T. M., Seller, T. B., Pritchett, E. L. C., and Gallagher, J. J.: Ventricular fibrillation in the Wolff-Parkinson-White syndrome. N. Engl. J. Med. 301:1080, 1979.

190. Dreifus, L. S., Haiat, R., Watanabe, Y., Arriaga, J., and Reitman, N.: Ventricular fibrillation. A possible mechanism of sudden death in patients with Wolff-Parkinson-White syndrome. Circulation 43:520, 1971.

191. Boineau, J. P., and Moore, E. N.: Evidence for propagation of activation across an accessory atrioventricular connection in types A and B preexcitation. Circulation 41:375, 1970.

192. Campbell, R. W., Smith, R. A., Gallagher, J. J., Pritchett, E. L., and Wallace, A. G.: Atrial fibrillation in the preexcitation syndrome. Am. J. Cardiol. 40:514, 1977.

193. Pritchett, E. L., Prystowsky, E. N., Benditt, D. G., and Gallagher, J. J.: "Dual atrioventricular nodal pathways" in patients with Wolff-Parkinson-White syndrome. Br. Heart J. 43:7, 1980.

194. Hammil, S. C., Pritchett, E. L., Klein, G. J., Smith, W. M., and Gallagher, J. J.: Accessory atrioventricular pathways that conduct only in the antegrade direction. Circulation 62:1335, 1980.

195. Bosc, E., Grolleau, R., Puech, P., Latour, H., and Souchon, H.: Automatic activity of the preexcitation pathways. Arch. Mal Coeur 72:359, 1979.

196. Davidoff, R., Schamroth, C. L., and Myerberg, D. P.: The Wolff-Parkinson-White pattern in healthy air crew. Aviat. Space Environ. Med. 52:554, 1981.

197. Newman, D. J., Donoso, E., and Friedberg, C. K.: Arrhythmias in the Wolff-Parkinson-White syndrome. Progr. Cardiovasc. Dis. 9:147, 1966.

198. Bharati, S., Rosen, K., Steinfield, L., Miller, R. A., and Lev, M.: The anatomic substrate for preexcitation in corrected transposition. Circulation 62:831, 1980.

199. Smith, W. M., Gallagher, J. J., Kerr, C. R., Sealy, W. C., Kasell, J. H., Benson, D. W., Jr., Reiter, M. J., Sterba, R., and Grant, A. O.: The electrophysiologic basis and management of symptomatic recurrent tachycardia in patients with Ebstein's anomaly of the tricuspid valve. Am. J. Cardiol. 49:1223, 1982.

200. Hindman, M. C., Last, J. H., and Rosen, K. M.: Wolff-Parkinson-White syndrome observed by portable monitoring. Ann. Intern. Med. 79:654, 1973.

201. Wolff, G. S., Han, J., and Curran, J.: Wolff-Parkinson-White syndrome in the neonate. Am. J. Cardiol. 41:559, 1978.

202. Klein, G. J., Hackel, D. B., and Gallagher, J. J.: Anatomic substrate of impaired antegrade conduction over an accessory atrioventricular pathway in the Wolff-Parkinson-White syndrome. Circulation 61:1249, 1980.

203. Sellers, T. D., Bashore, T. M., and Gallagher, J. J.: Digitalis in the preexcitation syndrome: Analysis during atrial fibrillation. Circulation 56:260, 1977.

204. Wellens, H. J. J., and Durrer, D.: Effect of digitalis on atrioventricular conduction and circus movement tachycardias in patients with Wolff-Parkinson-White syndrome. Circulation 47:1229, 1973.

205. Dhingra, R. C., Palileo, E. V., Strasberg, B., Swiryn, S., Bauernfeind, R., Wyndham, C., and Rosen, K. M.: Electrophysiologic effects of ouabain in patients with preexcitation and circus movement tachycardia. Am. J. Cardiol. 47:139, 1981.

206. Akhtar, M., Gilbert, C. J., and Shenasa, M.: Effect of lidocaine on atrioventricular response via the accessory pathway in patients with Wolff-Parkinson-White syndrome. Circulation 63:435, 1981.

207. Gulamhusein, S., Ko, P., Carruthers, S. G., and Klein, G. J.: Acceleration of the ventricular response during atrial fibrillation in the Wolff-Parkinson-White syndrome after verapamil. Circulation 65:348, 1982.

208. Przybylski, J., Chiale, P. A., Halpern, M. S., Nau, G. J., Elizari, M. V., and

Rosenbaum, M. B.: Unmasking of ventricular preexcitation by vagal stimulation or isoproterenol administration. Circulation 61:1030, 1980.

209. Wellens, H. J. J., Bär, F. W., Dassen, W. R., Brugada, P., Vanagt, E. J., and Farre, J.: Effect of drugs in the Wolff-Parkinson-White syndrome. Importance of initial length of effective refractory period of the accessory pathway. Am. J. Cardiol. 46:665, 1980.

210. Zipes, D. P., Rothbaum, D. A., and DeJoseph, R. L.: Preexcitation syndrome. Cardiovasc. Clin. 1:210, 1974.

211. Josephson, M. E.: Paroxysmal supraventricular tachycardia: An electrophysiologic approach. Am. J. Cardiol. 41:1123, 1978.

212. Paulay, K. L., Ruskin, J. N., and Damato, A. N.: Sinus and atrioventricular nodal reentrant tachycardia in the same patient. Am. J. Cardiol. 36:810, 1975.

213. Langendorf, R.: Ventricular premature systoles with postponed compensatory pause. Am. Heart J. 46:401, 1953.

214. Castillo, C., Castellanos, A., Jr., Agha, A. S., and Myerberg, R.: Significance of His bundle recordings with short H-V intervals. Chest 60:142, 1971.

215. Winkle, R. A.: The relationship between ventricular ectopic beat frequency and heart rate. Circulation 66:439, 1982.

216. Hinkle, L. E., Carver, S. T., and Stevens, M.: The frequency of asymptomatic disturbances of cardiac rhythm and conduction in middle-aged men. Am. J. Cardiol. 24:629, 1969.

217. Chiang, B. N., Perlman, L. V., Ostrander, L. D., and Epstein, F. H.: Relationship of premature systoles to coronary heart disease and sudden death in the Tecumseh epidemiologic study. Ann. Intern. Med. 70:1159, 1969.

218. Moss, A. J., DeCamilla, J., Davis, H., and Bayer, L.: The early post-hospital phase of myocardial infarction: Prognostic stratification. Circulation 54:58, 1976.

219. Ruberman, W., Weinblatt, E., Goldberg, J. D., Frank, C. W., and Shapiro, S.: Ventricular premature beats and mortality after myocardial infarction. N. Engl. J. Med. 297:750, 1977.

220. Ambos, H. D., Roberts, R., Oliver, G. C., Cox, J. R., Jr., and Sobel, B. E.: Infarct size: A determinant of persistence of severe ventricular dysrhythmia. Am. J. Cardiol. 37:116, 1976.

221. Schulze, R. A., Jr., Strauss, H. W., and Pitt, B.: Sudden death in the year following myocardial infarction: Relation to ventricular premature contractions in the late hospital phase and ventricular ejection fraction. Am. J. Med. 62:192, 1977.

222. Lie, K. I., Wellens, H. J. J., and Durrer, D.: Characteristics and predictability of binary ventricular fibrillation. Eur. J. Cardiol. 1:379, 1974.

223. Naccarelli, G. V., Prystowsky, E. N., Jackman, W. M., Heger, J. J., Rahilly, G. T., and Zipes, D. P.: Role of electrophysiologic testing in managing patients who have ventricular tachycardia unrelated to coronary artery disease. Am. J. Cardiol. 50:165, 1982.

224. Rinkenberger, R. L., Prystowsky, E. N., Jackman, W. M., Heger, J. J., and Zipes, D. P.: Conversion of nonsustained ventricular tachycardia to sustained ventricular tachycardia during drug therapy as determined by serial electrophysiology studies. Am. Heart J. 103:177, 1982.

225. Kisten, A. D.: Retrograde conduction to the atria in ventricular tachycardia. Circulation 24:236, 1961.

226. Wellens, J. H. H., Bär, F. W. H. M., and Lie, K. I.: The value of the electrocardiogram in the differential diagnosis of a tachycardia with a widened QRS complex. Am. J. Med. 64:27, 1978.

227. Sandler, I. A., and Marriott, H.: The differential morphology of anomalous ventricular complexes of RBBB type in lead V₁. Ventricular ectopy versus aberration. Circulation 31:551, 1965.

228. Josephson, M. E., Horowitz, L. N., Farshidi, A., and Kastor, J. A.: Recurrent sustained ventricular tachycardia. I. Mechanisms. Circulation 57:431, 1978.

229. Morady, F., Scheinman, M. M., Gonzalez, R., and Hess, E.: His-ventricular dissociation in a patient with reciprocating tachycardia and a nodoventricular bypass tract. Circulation 64:839, 1981.

230. Cohen, H. C., Gozo, E. G., Jr., and Pick, A.: Ventricular tachycardia with narrow QRS complexes (left posterior fascicular tachycardia). Circulation 45:1035, 1972.

231. Wellens, H. J. J.: Value and limitations of programmed electrical stimulation of the heart in the study and treatment of tachycardia. Circulation 57:845, 1978.

232. Gomes, J. A., Kang, P. S., Khan, R., Kelen, G., and El-Sherif, N.: Repetitive ventricular response: Its incidence, inducibility, reproducibility, mechanism and significance. Br. Heart J. 46:159, 1981.

233. Brugada, P., Heddle, B., and Wellens, H. J. J.: Results of a ventricular stimulation protocol using a maximum of four premature stimuli in patients without documented or suspected ventricular arrhythmias. Circulation 66(Suppl. II): 79, 1982.

234. Prystowsky, E. N., Naccarelli, G. V., Rahilly, G. T., Jr., Heger, J. J., and Zipes, D. P.: Electrophysiologic and anatomic characteristics associated with ventricular tachycardia induced at the right ventricular outflow tract but not at the apex. Am. J. Cardiol. 49:959, 1982.

235. Robertson, J. F., Cain, M. E., Horowitz, L. N., Spielman, S. R., Greenspan, A. M., Waxman, H. L., and Josephson, M. E.: Anatomic and electrophysiologic correlates of ventricular tachycardia requiring left ventricular stimulation. Am. J. Cardiol. 48:263, 1981.

236. Reddy, C. P., and Gettes, E. S.: Use of isoproterenol as an aid to electric induction of chronic recurrent ventricular tachycardia. Am. J. Cardiol. 44:705, 1979.

237. Rinkenberger, R. L., Prystowsky, E. N., Jackman, W. M., Heger, J. J., and Zipes, D. P.: Conversion of nonsustained ventricular tachycardia to sustained ventricular tachycardia during drug therapy as determined by serial electrophysiology studies. Am. Heart J. 103:177, 1982.

238. Greenspon, A. J., Stang, J. M., Lewis, R. P., and Schaal, S. F.: Provocation of ventricular tachycardia after consumption of alcohol. N. Engl. J. Med. 301:104, 1979.

239. Wellens, H. J. J., Lie, K. I., and Durrer, D.: Further observations on ventricular tachycardia as studied by electrical stimulation of the heart: Chronic recurrent ventricular tachycardia and ventricular tachycardia during acute myocardial infarction. Circulation 49:647, 1974.

240. Naccarelli, G. V., Zipes, D. P., Rahilly, G. T., Heger, J. J., and Prystowsky, E. N.: Influence of tachycardia cycle length and antiarrhythmic drugs on pacing termination and acceleration of ventricular tachycardia. Am. Heart J. 105:1, 1983.

241. Josephson, M. E., Horowitz, L. N., Farshidi, A., Spielman, S. R., Michaelson, E. L., and Greenspan, A. M.: Sustained ventricular tachycardia: Evidence for protected localized reentry. Am. J. Cardiol. 42:416, 1978.

242. Josephson, M. E., Horowitz, L. N., Waxman, H. L., Cain, M. E., Spielman, S. R., Greenspan, A. M., Marchlinski, F. E., and Ezri, M. D.: Sustained ventricular tachycardia: Role of the 12-lead electrocardiogram in localizing site of origin. Circulation 64:257, 1981.

243. Swiryn, S., Pavel, T., Byrom, M. E., Bauernfeind, R. A., Strasberg, B., Palileo, E., Lam, W., Wyndham, C. R., and Rosen, K. M.: Sequential regional phase mapping of radionuclide gated biventriculograms in patients with sustained ventricular tachycardia: Close correlation with electrophysiologic characteristics. Am. Heart J. 103:319, 1982.

244. Hess, O. M., Graf, C., Frey, R., Dettli, R., and Siegenthaler, W.: Coronary artery spasm with normal coronary arteries as the cause of recurrent ventricular fibrillation. Schweiz. Med. Wnschr. 111:755, 1981.

245. Ruskin, J. N., DiMarco, J. P., and Garan, H.: Out-of-hospital cardiac arrest: Electrophysiologic observations and selection of long-term antiarrhythmic therapy. N. Engl. J. Med. 303:607, 1980.

246. Josephson, M. E., Horowitz, L. N., Spielman, S. R., and Greenspan, A. M.: Electrophysiologic and hemodynamic studies in patients resuscitated from cardiac arrest. Am. J. Cardiol. 46:948, 1980.

247. Winkle, R. A., Derrington, D. C., and Schroeder, J. S.: Characteristics of ventricular tachycardia in ambulatory patients. Am. J. Cardiol. 39:487, 1977.

248. Bigger, J. T., Jr., Weld, F. M., and Rolnitzky, L. M.: Prevalence characteristics and significance of ventricular tachycardia (three or more complexes) detected with ambulatory electrocardiographic recording in the late hospital phase of acute myocardial infarction. Am. J. Cardiol. 48:815, 1981.

249. Pedersen, D. H., Zipes, D. P., Foster, P. R., and Troup, P. J.: Ventricular tachycardia and ventricular fibrillation in a young population. Circulation 60:988, 1979.

250. Vetter, V. L., Josephson, M. E., and Horowitz, L. N.: Idiopathic recurrent sustained ventricular tachycardia in children and adolescents. Am. J. Cardiol. 47:315, 1981.

251. Reisch, P., DeSilva, R. A., Lown, B., and Murawski, B. J.: Acute psychological disturbance preceding life-threatening ventricular arrhythmias. J.A.M.A. 246:233, 1981.

252. Waxman, M. B., Wald, R. W., Finley, J. P., Bonnet, J. F., Downar, E., and Sharma, A. B.: Valsalva termination of ventricular tachycardia. Circulation 62:843, 1980.

252a. Vlay, S. C., and Reid, P. R.: Ventricular ectopy: Etiology, evaluation and therapy. Am. J. Med. 73:899, 1982.

253. Pennington, J. E., Taylor, J., and Brown, B.: Chest thump for reverting ventricular tachycardia. N. Engl. J. Med. 283:1192, 1970.

254. Sclarovsky, S., Kracoff, O., Arditi, A., Strasberg, B., Zafrir, N., Lewin, R. F., and Agmon, J.: Ventricular tachycardia. "Pleomorphism" induced by chest thump. Chest 81:97, 1982.

255. Myerburg, R. J., Kessler, K. M., Kiem, I., Pefkaros, K. C., Conde, C. A., Cooper, D., and Castellanos, A.: Relationship between plasma levels of procainamide, suppression of premature ventricular complexes and prevention of recurrent ventricular tachycardia. Circulation 64:280, 1981.

256. Horowitz, L. N., Spielman, S. R., Greenspan, A. M., and Josephson, M. E.: Role of programmed stimulation in assessing vulnerability to ventricular arrhythmias. Am. Heart J. 103:604, 1982.

257. Josephson, M. E., Kastor, J. A., and Horowitz, L. N.: Electrophysiologic management of recurrent ventricular tachycardia in acute and chronic ischemic heart disease. Cardiovasc. Clin. 11:35, 1980.

258. Zipes, D. P., and Fisch, C.: Accelerated ventricular rhythm. Arch. Intern. Med. 129:650, 1972.

259. Rothfeld, E. L., Zucker, I. R., Parsonnet, V., and Alinsonorin, C. A.: Idioventricular rhythm in acute myocardial infarction. Circulation 37:203, 1968.

260. DeSoyza, N., Bissett, J. K., Kane, J. J., Murphy, M. L., and Doherty, J. E.: Association of accelerated idioventricular rhythm and paroxysmal ventricular tachycardia in acute myocardial infarction. Am. J. Cardiol. 34:667, 1974.

261. Lichstein, E., Riebas-Meneclier, C., Guptka, P. K., and Chadda, K. D.: Incidence and description of accelerated idioventricular rhythm complicating acute myocardial infarction. Am. J. Med. 58:192, 1975.

262. Dessertenne, F.: Considerations sur l'electrocardiogramme de la fibrillation ventriculaire. Arch. Mal Coeur 57:1421, 1964.

263. Fontaine, G., Frank, R., and Grosgogeat, Y.: Torsades de pointes: Definition and management. Mod. Conc. Cardiovasc. Dis. 51:103, 1982.

264. Krikler, D. M., and Curry, P. V. L.: Torsades de pointes, an atypical ventricular tachycardia. Br. Heart J. 38:117, 1976.

265. Horowitz, L. N., Greenspan, A. M., Spielman, S. R., and Josephson, M. E.: Torsades de pointes: Electrophysiologic studies in patients without transient pharmacologic or metabolic abnormalities. Circulation 63:1120, 1981.

266. Wellens, H. J. J., and Lie, K. I.: Ventricular tachycardia: The value of programmed electrical stimulation. In Krikler, D., and Goodwin, J. F. (eds.): Cardiac Arrhythmias. London, Saunders, 1975.

267. Baroy, J. H., Ungerleider, R. M., Smith, W. M., and Ideker, R. E.: A mechanism of torsades de pointes in a canine model. Circulation 67:52, 1983.

268. Smith, W. M., and Gallagher, J. J.: "Les torsades de pointes": An unusual ventricular arrhythmia. Ann. Intern. Med. 93:578, 1980.

269. Keren, A., Tzivoni, D., Gavish, D., Levi, J., Gottlieb, S., Benhorin, J., and Stern, S.: Etiology warning signs and therapy of torsades de pointes—a study of ten patients. Circulation 64:1167, 1981.

270. Schwartz, P. J., Periti, M., and Malliani, A.: The long Q-T syndrome. Am. Heart J. 89:378, 1975.

271. Khan, M. M., Logan, K. R., McComb, J. M., and Adgey, A. A.: Management of recurrent ventricular tachyarrhythmias associated with QT prolongation. Am. J. Cardiol. 47:1301, 1981.

272. Kastor, J. A., Horowitz, L. N., Harken, A. H., and Josephson, M. E.: Clinical electrophysiology of ventricular tachycardia. N. Engl. J. Med. 304:1004, 1981.

273. Rosenbaum, M. B., Elizari, M. V., and Lazzari, L. D.: The mechanism of bidirectional tachycardia. Am. Heart J. 78:4, 1979.

274. Morris, S. N., and Zipes, D. P.: His bundle electrocardiography during bidirectional tachycardia. Circulation 48:32, 1973.

275. Kastor, J. A., and Goldreyer, B. N.: Ventricular origin of bidirectional tachycardia: Case report of a patient not toxic from digitalis. Circulation 48:897, 1973.

276. Cohen, S. I., Deisseroth, A., and Hecht, H. S.: Infra-His bundle origin of bidirectional tachycardia. Circulation 47:1260, 1973.

277. Rahilly, G. T., Prystowsky, E. N., Zipes, D. P., Naccarelli, G. V., Jackman, W. M., and Heger, J. J.: Clinical and electrophysiologic findings in patients with otherwise normal electrocardiograms. Am. J. Cardiol. 50:459, 1982.

277a. Coumel, P., Leclercq, J. F., Attuel, P., Rosengarten, M., Milosevic, D., Slama, P., and Sourrain, Y.: Tachycardies ventriculaires in salves. Etude electrophysiologique et therapeutique Arch. Mal Coeur 73:153, 1980.

278. Froment, R., Gallavardin, L., and Cahen, P.: Paroxysmal ventricular tachycardia: A clinical classification. Br. Heart J. 15:172, 1953.

279. Gallavardin, L., and Veil, P.: Deux nouveaux cas d'extrasystolie-ventriculaire avec salves tachycardiques. Arch. Mal Coeur 22:738, 1929.

280. Parkinson, J., and Papp, C.: Repetitive paroxysmal tachycardia. Br. Heart J. 9:241, 1947.

281. Lesch, M., Lewis, E., Humphries, J. O., and Ross, R.: Paroxysmal ventricular tachycardia in the absence of organic heart disease. Ann. Intern. Med. 66:950, 1967.

282. Steffens, T. G., Pierce, P. L., and Zegerius, R. J.: Multiple ventricular premature beats in 5 adolescents. Eur. J. Cardiol. 8:177, 1978.

283. Lloyd, E. A., Zipes, D. P., Heger, J. J., and Prystowsky, E. N.: Sustained ventricular tachycardia due to bundle branch reentry. Am. Heart J. 104:1095, 1982.

283a. Welch, W. J., Strasberg, B., Coelho, A., and Rosen, K. M.: Sustained macroreentrant ventricular tachycardia. Am. Heart J. 104:166, 1982.

284. Reddy, C. P., and Slack, J. D.: Recurrent ventricular tachycardia: Report of a case with His bundle branch reentry as the mechanism. Eur. J. Cardiol. 11:23, 1980.

285. Browne, K. F., Zipes, D. P., Heger, J. J., and Prystowsky, E. N.: The influence of the autonomic nervous system on the QT interval. Am. J. Cardiol. 49:898, 1982.

286. Moss, A. J., and Schwartz, P. J.: Delayed repolarization (QT or QTU prolongation) and malignant ventricular arrhythmias. Mod. Conc. Cardiovasc. Dis. 51:85, 1982.

287. Romano, C., Gemme, G., and Pongiglione, R.: Aritmie cardiache rare dell'eta pediatrica. II. Accessi sincopali per fibrillazione ventricolare parossistica. La Clinic. Paed. 45:656, 1963.

288. Ward, O. C.: New familial cardiac syndrome in children. J. Irish Med. Assoc. 54:103, 1964.

289. Selzer, A., and Wray, H. W.: Quinidine syncope: Paroxysmal ventricular fibrillation occurring during treatment of chronic atrial arrhythmias. Circulation 30:17, 1964.

290. Reynolds, E. W., and Vander Ark, C. R.: Quinidine syncope and delayed repolarization syndromes. Mod. Conc. Cardiovasc. Dis. 55:117, 1976.

291. Tzivoni, D., Keren, A., Stern, S., and Gottlieb, S.: Disopyramide-induced torsades de pointes. Arch. Intern. Med. 141:946, 1981.

292. Singh, B. N., Gaardner, T. D., Kanegae, T., Goldstein, M., Montgomerie, J. Z., and Mills, H.: Liquid protein diets and torsades de pointes. J.A.M.A. 240:115, 1978.

293. Siegel, R. J., Cabeen, W. R., Jr., and Roberts, W. C.: Prolonged QT interval-ventricular tachycardia syndrome from massive rapid weight loss utilizing the liquid protein modified fast diet. Sudden death with sinus node ganglionitis and neuritis. Am. Heart J. 102:121, 1981.

294. Burch, G. E., Myers, R., and Abildskov, J. A.: New electrocardiographic pattern observed in cerebrovascular accidents. Circulation 9:719, 1954.

295. Schwartz, P. J., and Wolf, S.: QT interval prolongation as predictor of sudden death in patients with myocardial infarction. Circulation 57:1074, 1978.

296. Ahnve, S., Lundman, T., and Shoaleh-var, M.: The relationship between QT interval and ventricular arrhythmias in acute myocardial infarction. Acta Med. Scand. 204:17, 1978.

297. Taylor, G. J., Crampton, R. S., Gibson, R. S., Stebbins, P. T., Waldman, M. T., and Beller, G. A.: Prolonged QT interval at onset of acute myocardial infarction in predicting early phase ventricular tachycardia. Am. Heart J. 102:16, 1981.

298. Haynes, R. E., Hallstrom, A. P., and Cobb, L. A.: Repolarization abnormalities in survivors of out-of-hospital ventricular fibrillation. Circulation 57:654, 1978.

299. James, T. N., Zipes, D. P., Finegan, R. E., Eisele, J. W., and Carter, J. E.: Cardiac ganglionitis associated with sudden unexpected death. Ann. Intern. Med. 91:727, 1979.

300. Bekheit, S., and Ali, A.: QT interval in idiopathic prolapsed mitral valve. Am. J. Cardiol. 41:374, 1978.

301. Yanowitz, F., Preston, J. B., and Abildskov, J. A.: Functional distribution of right and left stellate innervation to the ventricles: Production of neurogenic electrocardiographic changes by unilateral alteration of sympathetic tone. Cir. Res. 18:416, 1966.

302. Moss, A. J., and McDonald, J.: Unilateral cervicothoracic sympathetic ganglionectomy for the treatment of long QT syndrome. N. Engl. J. Med. 285:903, 1971.

303. Schwartz, P. J.: The long QT syndrome. In Kulbertus, H. E., and Wellens, H. J. J. (eds.): Sudden Death. The Hague, Martinus Nijhoff, 1980, pp. 358–378.

304. Crampton, R.: Preeminence of left stellate ganglion in the long QT syndrome. Circulation 59:769, 1979.

305. Zipes, D. P., Martins, J. B., Ruffy, R., Prystowsky, E. N., Elharrar, V., and Gilmour, R. F., Jr.: Roles of autonomic innervation in the genesis of ventricular arrhythmias. In Abboud, F. M., et al. (eds.): Disturbances in Neurogenic Control of the Circulation. Bethesda, Md., American Physiological Society, 1981, pp. 225–250.

306. Wellens, H. J. J., Vermeulen, A., and Durrer, D.: Ventricular fibrillation occurring on arousal from sleep by auditory stimuli. Circulation 46:661, 1972.

307. Lown, B., Temte, J. V., Reich, P., Gaughan, C., Regestein, Q., and Hai, H.: The basis for recurring ventricular fibrillation in the absence of coronary heart disease and its management. N. Engl. J. Med. 294:623, 1976.

308. Mitsutake, A., Takeshita, A., Kuroiwa, A., and Nakamura, M.: Usefulness of the Valsalva maneuver in management of the long QT syndrome. Circulation 63:1029, 1981.

309. Marcus, F. I., Fontaine, G. H., Guiraudon, G., Frank, R., Laurenceau, J. L., Malergue, C., and Grosgogeat, Y.: Right ventricular dysplasia: A report of 24 adult cases. Circulation 65:384, 1982.

310. Dungan, W. T., Garson, A., Jr., and Gillette, P. C.: Arrhythmogenic right ventricular dysplasia. A cause of ventricular tachycardia in children with apparently normal hearts. Am. Heart J. 102:745, 1981.

311. Guiraudon, G. M., Klein, G. J., Gulamhusein, S. S., Painvin, G. A., DelCampo, C., Gonzales, J. C., and Ko, P. T.: Total disconnection of the right ventricular free wall: Surgical treatment of right ventricular tachycardia associated with right ventricular dysplasia. Ann. Thorac. Surg. (in press).

312. Fontaine, G., Guiraudon, G., Frank, R., Fillette, F., Cabrol, C., and Grosgogeat, Y.: Surgical management of ventricular tachycardia unrelated to myocardial ischemia or infarction. Am. J. Cardiol. 49:397, 1982.

313. Klein, G. J., and Guiraudon, G. M.: Surgical therapy of cardiac arrhythmias. In Zipes, D. P. (ed.): Cardiology Clinics. Philadelphia, W. B. Saunders Co., 1983, in press.

314. Kavey, R. E., Blackman, M. S., and Sondheimer, H. M.: Incidence and severity of chronic ventricular dysrhythmias after repair of tetralogy of Fallot. Am. Heart J. 103:342, 1982.

315. Horowitz, L. N., Vetter, V. L., Harken, A. H., and Josephson, M. E.: Electrophysiologic characteristics of sustained ventricular tachycardia occurring after repair of tetralogy of Fallot. Am. J. Cardiol. 46:446, 1980.

316. Harken, A. H., Horowitz, L. N., and Josephson, M. E.: Surgical correction of recurrent sustained ventricular tachycardia on complete repair of tetralogy of Fallot. J. Thorac. Cardiovasc. Surg. 80:779, 1980.

317. Coumel, P., Fidelle, J., Lucet, V., Attuel, P., and Bouvrain, Y.: Catecholamine induced severe ventricular arrhythmias with Adams-Stokes syndrome in children: Report of four cases. Br. Heart J. 40(Suppl.):37, 1978.

318. Coumel, P., Rosengarten, M. D., Leclercq, J. F., and Attuel, P.: Role of sympathetic nervous system in nonischemic ventricular arrhythmias. Br. Heart J. 47:137, 1982.

319. Ideker, R. E., Klein, G. J., Harrison, L., Smith, W. M., Kasell, J., Reimer, K. A., Wallace, A. G., and Gallagher, J. J.: The transition to ventricular fibrillation induced by reperfusion after acute ischemia in the dog: A period of organized epicardial activation. Circulation 63:1371, 1981.

320. Raizes, G., Wagner, G. S., and Hackel, D. B.: Instantaneous nonarrhythmic cardiac death in acute myocardial infarction. Am. J. Cardiol. 39:1, 1977.

321. Cobb, L. A., Werner, J. A., and Trobaugh, G. B.: Sudden cardiac death. I. A decade's experience with out-of-hospital resuscitation. Mod. Conc. Cardiovasc. Dis. 49:31, 1980.

322. Adgey, A. A., Devlin, J. E., Webb, S. W., and Mulholland, H. C.: Initiation of ventricular fibrillation outside hospital in patients with acute ischemic heart disease. Br. Heart J. 47:55, 1982.

323. Lie, K. I., Liem, K. L., Schuilenburg, R. M., David, G. K., and Durrer, D.: Early identification of patients developing late in-hospital ventricular fibrilla-

tion after discharge from the coronary care unit: A 5½ year retrospective and prospective study of 1,897 patients. Am. J. Cardiol. 41:674, 1978.

324. Watanabe, Y., and Dreifus, L. S.: Atrioventricular block. Basic concepts. In Mandel, W. J., (ed.): Cardiac Arrhythmias. Philadelphia, J. B. Lippincott Co., 1980, p. 406.

325. Narula, O., and Shantha, N.: Atrioventricular block: Clinical concepts and His bundle electrocardiography. In Mandel, W. J. (ed.): Cardiac Arrhythmias. Philadelphia, J. B. Lippincott Co., 1980, p. 437.

326. Winternitz, M., and Langendorf, R.: Auriculo-ventricular block with ventriculoauricular response. Am. Heart J. 27:301, 1944.

327. Damato, A. N., Varghese, P. J., Lau, S. H., Gallagher, J. J., and Bobb, G. A.: Manifest and concealed reentry: A mechanism of AV nodal Wenckebach phenomenon. Circ. Res. 30:283, 1972.

328. Denes, P., Wu, D., Dhingra, R., Pietras, R., and Rosen, K. M.: The effects of cycle length on cardiac refractory periods in man. Circulation 49:32, 1974.

329. Wiener, I., Kunkes, S., Rubin, D., Kupersmith, J., Packer, M., Pitchon, R., and Schweitzer, P.: Effects of sudden change in cycle length on human atrial, atrioventricular, nodal and ventricular refractory periods. Circulation 64:245, 1981.

330. Simson, M. B., Spear, J. F., and Moore, E. N.: Electrophysiologic studies on atrioventricular nodal Wenckebach cycles. Am. J. Cardiol. 41:244, 1978.

331. Zipes, D. P.: Second degree atrioventricular block. Circulation 60:465, 1979.

332. El-Sherif, N., Scherlag, D. J., and Lazzara, R.: Pathophysiology of second degree atrioventricular block: A unified hypothesis. Am. J. Cardiol. 35:421, 1975.

333. Langendorf, R., and Pick, A.: Atrioventricular block, type II (Mobitz). Its nature and clinical significance. Circulation 38:819, 1968.

334. Dhingra, R. C., Denes, P., Wu, D., Chuquimia, R., and Rosen, K. M.: The significance of second-degree atrioventricular block and bundle branch block. Observations regarding site and type of block. Circulation 49:638, 1978.

335. Donoso, E., Adler, L. N., and Friedberg, C. K.: Unusual forms of second degree atrioventricular block, including Mobitz type II block, associated with the Morgagni-Adams-Stokes syndrome. Am. Heart J. 67:150, 1964.

336. Rosen, K. M., Loeb, H. S., Chuquimia, R., Sinno, M. Z., Rahimtoola, S. H., and Gunnar, R. M.: Site of heart block in acute myocardial infarction. Circulation 42:925, 1970.

337. Tans, A. C., Lie, K. I., and Durrer, D.: Clinical setting and prognostic significance of high degree atrioventricular block in acute inferior myocardial infarction: A study of 144 patients. Am. Heart J. 99:4, 1980.

338. Damato, A. N., Lau, S. H., Helfant, R. H., Stein, E., Patton, R. D., Scherlag, B. J., and Berkowitz, W. D.: A study of heart block in man using His bundle recordings. Circulation 39:297, 1969.

339. Narula, O. S., and Samet, P.: Wenckebach and Mobitz type II AV block due to block within the His bundle and bundle branches. Circulation 41:947, 1970.

340. Schuilenburg, R. M., and Durrer, D.: Observations on atrioventricular conduction in patients with bilateral bundle branch block. Circulation 41:967, 1970.

341. Rosen, K. M., Loeb, H. S., Gunnar, R. M., and Rahimtoola, S. H.: Mobitz type II block without bundle branch block. Circulation 44:1111, 1971.

342. Spear, J. F., and Moore, E. N.: Electrophysiologic studies on Mobitz type II second degree heart block. Circulation 44:1087, 1971.

343. Langendorf, R., and Mehlman, J. S.: Block (non-conducted) AV nodal premature systoles imitating first and second degree AV block. Am. Heart J. 34:500, 1947.

344. Rosen, K. M., Rahimtoola, S. H., and Gunnar, R . M.: Pseudo AV block secondary to nonpremature nonpropagated His-bundle depolarizations: Documentation by His bundle electrocardiography. Circulation 42:367, 1970.

345. Spear, J. F., and Moore, E. N.: Influence of brief vagal and stellate nerve stimulation on pacemaker activity and conduction within the atrioventricular conduction system of the dog. Circ. Res. 32:27, 1973.

346. Massie, B., Scheinman, M. M., Peters, R., Desai, J., Hirschfield, D., and O'Young, J.: Clinical and electrophysiologic findings in patients with paroxysmal slowing of the sinus rate and apparent Mobitz type II atrioventricular block. Circulation 58:305, 1978.

347. Wenckebach, K. F., and Winterberg, H.: Die Unregelmässige Herztätigkeit. Leipzig, Engelmann, 1927.

348. Gilchrist, A. R.: Clinical aspects of high-grade heart block. Scott. Med. J. 3: 53, 1958.

349. Mangiardi, L. M., Bonamini, R., Conte, M., Gaita, F., Orzan, F., Presbitero, P., and Brusca, A.: Bedside evaluation of atrioventricular block with narrow QRS complexes: Usefulness of carotid sinus massage and atropine administration. Am. J. Cardiol. 49:1136, 1982.

350. El-Sherif, N., Aranda, J., Befeler, B., and Lazzara, R.: Atypical Wenckebach periodicity simulating Mobitz II AV block. Br. Heart J. 40:1376, 1978.

351. Simson, M. B., Spear, J. F., and Moore, E. N.: Electrophysiologic studies on atrioventricular nodal Wenckebach cycles. Am. J. Cardiol. 41:244, 1978.

352. Denes, P., Levy, L., Pick, A., and Rosen, K. M.: The incidence of typical and atypical AV Wenckebach periodicity. Am. Heart J. 89:26, 1975.

353. Southall, D. P., Johnston, F., Shinebourne, E. A., and Johnston, P. G.: 24-hour electrocardiograph study of heart rate and rhythm patterns in population of healthy children. Br. Heart J. 45:281, 1981.

354. Zeppilli, P., Fenici, R., Sassara, M., Pirrami, M. M., and Caselli, G.: Wenckebach second degree AV block in top ranking athletes: An old problem revisited. Am. Heart J. 100:281, 1980.

355. Vitasalo, M. T., Kala, R., and Eisalo, A.: Ambulatory electrocardiographic recording in endurance athletes. Br. Heart J. 47:213, 1982.

356. Young, D., Eisenberg, R., Fish, B., and Fisher, J. D.: Wenckebach atrioventricular block (Mobitz I) in children and adolescents. Am. J. Cardiol. 40:393, 1977.

357. Strasberg, B., Amat-y-Leon, F., Dhingra, R. C., Palileo, E., Swiryn, S., Bauernfeind, R., Wyndham, C., and Rosen, K. M.: Natural history of chronic second degree atrioventricular nodal block. Circulation 63:1043, 1981.

358. Ferrari, I., Bonazzi, O., Gardumi, M., Gregorini, L., Perondi, R., and Mancia, G.: Modulation of atrioventricular conduction by isometric exercises in human subjects. Circ. Res. 49:265, 1981.

359. Coumel, P., Fabiato, A., Wayneberger, M., Motte, G., Slama, R., and Bouvrain, Y.: Bradycardia-dependent atrioventricular block. J. Electrocardiol. 4:168, 1971.

360. Rosenbaum, M. B., Elizari, M. V., Levi, R. J., and Nau, G. J.: Paroxysmal atrioventricular block related to hypotension and spontaneous diastolic depolarization. Chest 63:678, 1973.

361. Wald, R. W., and Waxman, M. B.: Depression of distal AV conduction following ventricular pacing. PACE 4:84, 1981.

362. Strasberg, B., Lam, W., Swiryn, S., Bauernfeind, R., Scagliotti, D., Palileo, E., and Rosen, K. M.: Symptomatic spontaneous paroxysmal AV nodal block to localized hyperresponsiveness of the AV node to vagotonic reflexes. Am. Heart J. 103:795, 1982.

363. Kehoe, R. F., Bauernfeind, R., Tommaso, C., Wyndham, C., and Rosen, K. M.: Cardiac conduction defects in polymyositis: Electrophysiological studies in four patients. Ann. Intern. Med. 94:41, 1981.

364. Ginks, W., Sutton, R., Siddons, H., and Leatham, A.: Unsuspected coronary artery disease as a cause of chronic atrioventricular block in middle age. Br. Heart J. 44:699, 1980.

365. Ohkawa, S., Sugiura, M., Itoh, Y., Kitano, K., Hiraoka, K., Ueda, J., and Murakama, M.: Electrophysiologic and histologic correlates in chronic complete atrioventricular block. Circulation 64:215, 1981.

366. Lev, M.: The pathology of complete atrioventricular block. Progr. Cardiovasc. Dis. 6:317, 1964.

367. Lenegre, J.: Bilateral bundle branch block. Cardiologia 48:134, 1966.

368. Ayres, C. R., Boineau, J. P., and Spach, M. S.: Congenital complete heart block in children. Am. Heart J. 72:381, 1966.

369. Besley, D. C., McWilliams, G. J., Moodie, D. S., and Castle, L. W.: Long-term followup of young adults following permanent pacemaker placement for complete heart block. Am. Heart J. 103:332, 1982.

370. Esscher, E.: Congenital complete heart block. Acta Pediat. Scand. 70:131, 1981.

371. Karpawich, P. P., Gillette, P. C., Garson, A., Jr., Hesslein, P. S., Porter, C. B., and McNamara, D. G.: Congenital complete atrioventricular block: Clinical and electrophysiologic predictors of need for pacemaker insertion. Am. J. Cardiol. 48:109, 1981.

372. Benson, D. W., Jr., Spach, M. S., Edwards, S. B., Sterba, R., Serwer, G. A., Armstrong, B. E., and Anderson, P. A.: Heart block in children. Evaluation of subsidiary ventricular pacemaker recovery times and ECG tape recordings. Pediat. Cardiol. 2:39, 1982.

373. Mond, H. G.: The bradyarrhythmias: Current indications for permanent pacing (Part I). PACE 4:432, 1981.

374. Mond, H. G.: The bradyarrhythmias: Current indications for permanent pacing (Part II). PACE 4:538, 1981.

375. Pick, A.: AV dissociation: A proposal for a comprehensive classification and consistent terminology. Am. Heart J. 66:147, 1963.

22 CARDIAC PACEMAKERS

by Douglas P. Zipes, M.D., and Edwin G. Duffin, Ph.D.

The artificial cardiac pacemaker is an electronic device that delivers electrical stimuli to the heart to treat bradycardias and tachycardias. Essential elements include a power source, usually a battery, which supplies energy for the stimuli and circuitry; an electronic circuit to regulate the timing and characteristics of the stimuli; and a lead composed of electrodes on a catheter or wire to connect the battery and circuit to the heart. The electrode is the uninsulated portion of the lead in contact with the body. At first, pacemakers were external units that provided temporary pacing by delivering stimuli to the skin[1] or to the heart through a lead, with the electronics and power source remaining outside the body. For many clinical situations, temporary pacemakers are still needed. The first totally implantable devices were reported in the late 1950s.[2,3] Today, an estimated one million patients worldwide have implanted pacemakers (500,000 in the United States). Advances in technology have been applied rapidly to pacemaker systems, and pacemakers themselves have changed dramatically from the 250-gram, asynchronous devices of the early 1960s. Present-day systems provide noninvasively programmable single- and dual-chamber pacemakers, which weigh typically 40 to 50 grams, last an estimated six to ten years, and are highly reliable.

INDICATIONS FOR PACING

Pacemakers are employed to treat patients who have symptomatic bradycardias and tachycardias. (The use of pacing as a diagnostic tool is discussed in Chapter 20.) The nature of the arrhythmia and how likely it will persist or recur determine whether pacing, either temporary or permanent, is indicated (Table 22-1). As a general rule, drugs do not successfully and reliably speed up the heart rate or improve atrioventricular (AV) conduction for longer than several hours to several days in patients who have symptomatic bradycardias, without producing intolerable side effects. Therefore, regardless of the arrhythmia causing the bradycardia (e.g., sinus bradycardia or AV block), pacing may be indicated in such cases. In addition, pacing may be used both to terminate and to prevent a recurrence of some forms of tachycardia. The type of tachycardia and clinical setting determine whether pacing should be employed. Most often, other therapeutic approaches, particularly drugs and electrical cardioversion, are tried before pacing is instituted. The choice between temporary and permanent pacing is based on whether the rhythm disturbance is likely to be transient or permanent.

TEMPORARY PACING FOR BRADYCARDIAS. Temporary pacing is indicated in a variety of circumstances in which a symptomatic bradycardia is present or is likely to occur, such as after cardiac surgery,[4] during right heart catheterization in patients with preexisting left bundle branch block, during administration of some drugs that might inappropriately slow the heart rate, and prior to implanting a permanent pacemaker in patients with symptomatic bradycardia. Temporary pacing may also be useful in some patients who have symptoms of heart failure associated with reduced cardiac output secondary to a slow rate (Table 22-1).

Temporary Pacing During Acute Myocardial Infarction (See also p. 1306). The role of temporary pacing during acute myocardial infarction (MI) in patients who develop *AV conduction disturbances* is controversial because the risk-to-benefit ratio is unclear. For untreated patients who develop AV block in this situation the mortality rate is not well established, often because reported studies are spuriously influenced by forms of AV block that do not require pacing. For example, patients who develop an inferior wall MI may have first-degree or type I second-degree AV block combined with an accelerated AV junctional rhythm, giving rise to complete AV dissociation (p. 735). These patients are commonly misclassified as having complete AV block. Since the second-degree AV block and junctional rhythm are usually transient and do not require therapy,[5] this group is considered erroneously to have recovered from complete AV block, a classification that favorably biases the results regarding the natural history of complete AV block during acute MI. Furthermore, causes of death not directly related to the conduction disturbance, such as ventricular fibrillation, may lead to sudden death of these patients.[6] Such a death may be reported incorrectly as being due to complete heart block. However, it seems fairly clear, that the extent of myocardial involvement and resultant degree of heart failure are the most important prognostic factors in patients who develop AV conduction disturbances during acute MI.[7,8]

P-R interval prolongation during acute MI has been reported to be associated with an increased incidence of progression to high-degree AV block.[6,7,9,10] Although P-R prolongation often occurs in patients in whom high-degree AV block follows, the significance of this finding in any given patient is obscure. In the setting of bundle branch block, it may reflect block at the AV nodal level, combined AV nodal and His-Purkinje system conduction delay, or His-Purkinje delay alone. Abrupt complete heart block frequently occurs without demonstrable prior P-R prolongation. Therefore, although P-R interval prolongation and the development of high-degree AV block may be related statistically, they may not be causally related. For example, P-R interval delay may be due to preexistent AV nodal disturbance, while sudden complete heart block may be due to an acute His-Purkinje block. Thus, first-degree AV block that develops before or during acute MI as an isolated finding is not an indication for temporary pacing.

Type I second-degree AV block (p. 731) most commonly occurs during acute *inferior* MI, presumably owing to transient ischemia or increased vagal tone in the region of the AV node, while *type II second-degree AV block* (p. 731) commonly occurs during acute *anterior* MI, resulting from a large infarction that includes the interventricular septum.[11-13] Type I second-degree AV block generally is transient, blocks in the AV node, is not associated with symptoms, and does not require pacing. On the other hand, type II second-degree AV block is most commonly due to block in the His-Purkinje system, occurs in the setting of a bundle branch block, may progress to complete AV block, and requires temporary pacing.[14,15] Whether or not pacing is attempted, type II AV block is associated with a high mortality because of the concomitant large MI.[16]

Patients who develop first-degree or type I second-degree AV block with a normal QRS complex and only axis deviation generally do not require prophylactic pacing. Uncommonly, acute inferior MI results in a bradycardia that does require pacing. This may be a sinus bradycardia, or second-degree or complete AV block that is not transient and does not respond satisfactorily to atropine.[10]

Available data on the significance of *H-V interval prolongation* as an indicator of progression to high-degree AV block in acute MI have led to controversial conclusions. Most patients studied who progress to complete heart block do demonstrate H-V interval prolongation during acute MI.[6] However, this finding does not necessarily imply that complete heart block is imminent, particularly if the H-V interval prolongation preceded the onset of acute MI—a fact not always known. Thus, the clinical usefulness of recording the H-V interval to predict subsequent development of complete AV block as well as survival during acute MI is still not settled.[7]

Development of *complete AV block* should be considered in the same manner as type II second-degree AV block. As mentioned earlier, it is important not to confuse the diagnosis of complete AV dissociation with complete AV block (see Chapter 21). Mortality is influenced in large measure by the severity of the underlying heart disease. However, patients who develop type II second-degree or complete AV block without pulmonary edema or shock still have a higher mortality rate than patients who do not have advanced AV block, with many deaths due to the abrupt development of AV block.[16] Therefore, temporary pacing is clearly indicated in this group of patients.

Temporary pacing is warranted in patients who develop *bifascicular block* (defined as alternating right and left bundle branch block), right bundle branch block with left axis deviation, right bundle branch block with right axis deviation, and perhaps left bundle branch block with P-R interval prolongation when they appear to be at increased risk of developing high-degree AV block.[7,10,15,16] Left bundle branch block with P-R prolongation is included in this group, because while these findings may represent bifascicular block in association with AV nodal disease, the majority of these patients have a prolonged H-V interval and probably trifascicular disease.

The role of prophylactic pacing in the setting of acute anterior MI with new right bundle branch block and a normal axis or with new left bundle branch block and a normal P-R interval is more controversial; however, some evidence of decreased morbidity associated with pacing seems to justify its use in patients who do not have heart failure, provided that the complication rate of inserting a temporary pacing catheter is low.[7] It would appear that *preexisting, stable* right bundle branch block or left bundle branch block with or without axis deviation is *not* an indication for prophylactic pacing, whether the block is present in a patient who has an acute infarction or in other situations, such as in patients undergoing surgery. While the development of bifascicular block is associated with a higher incidence of progression to advanced AV block, the mortality among patients who develop new bundle branch block and acute MI is similar to that among patients who had bundle branch block prior to the infarction.[17,19]

In summary, prophylactic temporary pacing appears warranted in patients who have an acute MI and who develop type II second- or third-degree AV block or bifascicular block of recent onset.[7] Bundle branch block complicating acute MI identifies the individual at significant risk of developing congestive heart failure, with mortality often secondary to myocardial failure or refractory ventricular arrhythmias. The presence of high-degree AV block per se appears to increase mortality in patients without pump failure, and immediate survival may be enhanced by prophylactic pacing in patients at high risk for developing abrupt complete heart block complicating acute

TABLE 22–1   PACING INDICATIONS

	DEFINITELY INDICATED	PROBABLY INDICATED	PROBABLY NOT INDICATED	DEFINITELY NOT INDICATED
Complete AV Block				
Congenital (AV nodal)				
Asymptomatic				X
Symptomatic	T,P			
Acquired (His-Purkinje)				
Asymptomatic		T,P		
Symptomatic	T,P			
Surgical (persistent)				
Asymptomatic	T	P		
Symptomatic	T,P			
Second-degree AV Block				
Type I (AV nodal)				
Asymptomatic				X
Symptomatic	T,P			
Type II (His-Purkinje)				
Asymptomatic		T,P		
Symptomatic	T,P			
First-degree AV Block				
AV Nodal				
Asymptomatic				X
Symptomatic			X	
His-Purkinje				
Asymptomatic				X
Symptomatic			X	
Bundle Branch Block				
Asymptomatic				X
Symptomatic				
Normal H-V		P‡		
Prolonged H-V	P			
Distal His block at paced atrial rates <130/min	P			
LBBB during right heart catheterization	T			
Acute Myocardial Infarction				
Newly acquired bifascicular BBB	T			
Preexisting BBB				X
Newly acquired BBB plus transient complete AV block	T	P		
Second-degree AV block				
Type I (asymptomatic)				X
Type II	T	P		
Complete AV block	T	P		
Atrial Fibrillation with Slow Ventricular Response				
Asymptomatic				X
Symptomatic	T,P			
Sick Sinus Syndrome				
Asymptomatic			X	
Symptomatic	T,P			
Hypersensitive Carotid Sinus Syndrome				
Asymptomatic			X	
Symptomatic	T,P			
Bradycardia-Tachycardia Syndrome				
Asymptomatic			X	
Symptomatic	T,P			
Bradycardia-Miscellaneous				
Asymptomatic			X	
Symptomatic	T,P			
Tachycardia Prevention△				
Associated with bradycardia	T,P			
Associated with long Q-T, torsades de pointes	T	P		
Not associated with bradycardia, long Q-T, torsades de pointes (after drug failure)		T	P**	

TABLE 22–1 PACING INDICATIONS (*Continued*)

	DEFINITELY INDICATED	PROBABLY INDICATED	PROBABLY NOT INDICATED	DEFINITELY NOT INDICATED
Tachycardia Termination (after drug failure)**△				
Atrial flutter	T,P			
Atrial fibrillation				X
AV nodal reentry	T,P			
Reciprocating tachycardia in WPW syndrome	T,P^{II}			
Ventricular tachycardia	Tss	Pss		

T = Temporary pacing; P = permanent pacing; X = pacing not indicated
BBB = Bundle branch block; LBBB = left bundle branch block
HV = Measure of His-Purkinje conduction time
△ = Site and rate of stimulation may influence success
II = Atrial fibrillation with a rapid ventricular response may be a complication
** = Prove efficacy with temporary pacing
ss = May accelerate VT
‡ = No other cause found for symptoms

MI but who do not manifest evidence of heart failure. The assumption that prophylactic pacing improves the survival of patients who have bundle branch block and significant heart failure complicating acute MI remains speculative. Finally, patients who develop symptomatic bradycardia of any type that responds poorly to drug therapy should be considered as candidates for pacing.

TEMPORARY PACING FOR TACHYCARDIAS (See also p. 672 and Chapter 21). Temporary pacing may be useful to *terminate* a variety of tachycardias, including atrial flutter (p. 697), reciprocating tachycardias involving the sinus or AV node or an accessory pathway (p. 707), and some sustained ventricular tachycardias (p. 724). Isolated examples of other tachycardias terminated by pacing have been reported. Pacing does *not* terminate atrial or ventricular fibrillation. It is used generally when drug therapy has been ineffective and/or electrical cardioversion is contraindicated (suspicion of digitalis toxicity, for example), when cardioversion is required repeatedly owing to frequent recurrence of the tachycardia, or when a pacing catheter is already in place.[20]

Pacing can *prevent* several types of tachycardias, such as those associated with significant bradycardias like complete AV block or with a prolonged Q-T interval that result in torsades de pointes[21,22] (see Fig. 21–38, p. 725). Patients who have the bradycardia-tachycardia syndrome may require pacing after termination of the tachycardia to prevent the bradycardia (p. 693). Use of rapid pacing rates may suppress premature beats and prevent some tachycardias from recurring. Paired or coupled atrial pacing may reduce the ventricular rate if the premature atrial complex blocks in the AV junction; paired or coupled ventricular stimulation may reduce the effective ventricular rate if the premature ventricular complex results in electrical without mechanical systole. However, such premature stimulation risks precipitation of fibrillation. Finally, temporary atrial pacing has been used as a stress test in patients suspected of having coronary artery disease.[23]

PERMANENT PACING FOR BRADYCARDIAS. As with temporary pacing, permanent pacing is indicated in patients who have *symptomatic bradycardia*, regardless of the nature of the arrhythmia, as long as the bradycardia is likely to be permanent or recurrent; i.e., it is not associated with a transient condition such as acute MI or drug toxicity. The most common indication for permanent pacing—responsible for 50 percent of all implants—is fixed or intermittent complete third-degree AV block,[24] with sclerotic degeneration of the AV conducting system being the primary etiology. An additional 26 percent of pacemaker implants are to treat patients who have the sick sinus syndrome,[24] manifest as sinus arrest or block, severe sinus bradycardia, or alternating periods of bradycardia and supraventricular tachycardia (brady-tachy syndrome, see p. 693). In these patients, drugs used to treat the tachycardia may aggravate the bradycardia, requiring permanent pacing for the latter. Patients symptomatic from sinus bradycardia or AV block caused by hypersensitive carotid sinus syndrome[25] or slow ventricular rates during chronic atrial fibrillation[26] are also candidates for pacemakers. Sometimes asystole or bradycardia occurs only at the termination of a tachycardia and may be responsible for the patient's symptoms.

Major questions arise when one is considering prophylactic permanent pacing. There is general—although not complete—agreement that permanent pacing is indicated in *asymptomatic* patients who have acquired complete AV block or well-documented, type II second-degree AV block, since their natural history appears to progress to the point of symptoms. Although patients with documented transient high-degree AV block are at a substantial risk of sudden death, one could argue against permanently pacing a sedentary elderly individual who has complete AV block but has been completely asymptomatic.

The prognosis for patients who have *chronic bundle branch block* depends to a large extent on the presence and etiology as well as the severity of the associated heart disease. In most patients, the terminal event is usually one of heart failure or the complications of coronary artery disease. In the absence of clinically detectable heart disease, the long-term prognosis for this group of patients is good without pacing. Ventricular arrhythmias occur more often in patients who have chronic bundle branch block than in the normal population, but the mechanism of sudden death in any given patient is speculative. Most patients who die suddenly, especially those who have coronary artery disease, probably develop ventricular fibrillation. No clinical variable (such as age, syncope, angina, or shortness of breath), physical finding (such as an S_3 gallop, cardiomegaly, or heart failure), or electrocardiographic finding (such as right bundle branch block with left axis deviation, right bundle branch block with right axis deviation, or P-R interval prolongation) is useful in predicting progression to complete heart block. All the above variables occur frequently in patients who have bundle branch block, yet the progression to complete heart block is relatively infrequent.

A recent study indicates that more patients who have chronic bifascicular block with a prolonged H-V interval develop AV block than do patients who have a normal H-V interval (0.6 vs. 4.5 per cent), but the risk of developing trifascicular block is still small, and routine permanent pacing is not warranted in patients with chronic bifascicular block with a prolonged H-V interval.[27] Development of His-Purkinje block during atrial pacing at rates less than 130 ppm appears to be a possible marker for development of complete heart block.[28] However, the opposite—namely a normal H-V interval—does not exclude progression to complete heart block. Data for patients with unexplained recurrent syncope or presyncope and bundle branch block suggest that permanent pacing is reasonable therapy only after an effort has been made to exclude noncardiac and other cardiac causes for the symptoms. Some observers believe that documentation of bradyarrhythmia or measurement of the H-V interval is essential prior to institution of pacing in these patients.

Finally, several studies indicate that permanent prophylactic pacing reduces sudden death in survivors of acute MI complicated by bundle branch block and transient high-degree AV block. However, the number of patients studied is small and the data are not conclusive.[10,16]

PERMANENT PACING FOR TACHYCARDIAS.
Preventing tachycardia has become an important therapeutic application of pacing, for which several approaches are available. Tachycardias that occur only in the setting of bradycardias can be prevented by pacing at normal rates. In general, pacing at accelerated rates to prevent recurrences of tachycardias in patients who otherwise have normal heart rates and rhythms is not successful over the long term. Therefore, except for bradycardia-related tachycardia, the most successful application of antitachycardia pacing in this area is to *terminate* tachycardias after they start[4,29–31] rather than to *prevent* their occurrence.[29,32–34]

PACEMAKER MODALITIES

Pacemakers perform basically two functions: they all stimulate the heart, and most can sense impulses as well, i.e., they are equipped with amplifiers that register or recognize (sense) a spontaneous cardiac electrical event and then use that information to modulate the timing of the electrical stimulus delivered (pace). These two functions can be carried out in the atrium or ventricle, or in both chambers.[35,36] Sensing and stimulation are accomplished with electrode pairs directly contacting the myocardium (a bipolar system) or with one electrode located at the heart and a second electrode, usually the pacemaker case, located remotely (a unipolar system).

Because pacemakers operate in a variety of complex combinations, a letter code—originally three positions[37] and now five[38]—has been devised as a shorthand notation to identify the different types of pacemakers (Table 22–2). Symbols placed in the first two positions indicate the chambers in which the pacemaker paces (first position) and in which it senses (second position). "A" or "V" indicates that the device paces or senses the atrium or the ventricle; "D" indicates that it paces or senses in both chambers. "S" indicates a single-chamber unit designed to be suitable for either atrial or ventricular pacing, depending on how its parameters are programed. The third position signifies in what manner the pacemaker responds to spontaneous electrical activity. "O" indicates that the pacemaker does not sense spontaneous electrical activity and therefore discharges at a fixed rate and is not influenced by cardiac events. "I" indicates that the pacemaker is inhibited from delivering a stimulus for a certain period of time in response to sensed electrical activity; i.e.,

TABLE 22–2　FIVE-POSITION PACEMAKER CODE

I. CHAMBER PACED	II. CHAMBER SENSED	III. MODE OF RESPONSE	IV. PROGRAMMABILITY	V. TACHYARRHYTHMIA FUNCTIONS*
V = Ventricle	V = Ventricle	I = Inhibited	P = Programmable rate and/or output	B = Burst
A = Atrium	A = Atrium	T = Triggered	M = Multiprogrammable	N = Normal rate competition
D = Atrium and ventricle	D = Atrium and ventricle	D = Atrial triggered and ventricular inhibited	O = None	S = Scanning
	O = None	R = Reverse		E = Externally activated
S = single chamber	S = single chamber	O = None		O = None

This table provides a "shorthand" description of pacemaker operation. Symbols placed in the first two positions indicate chambers in which the pacemaker functions; a symbol in the third position, the mode of operation of the pacemaker; in the fourth position, its programmable characteristics; and in the fifth position, its antitachycardia features. For example, if the pacing lead were inserted into the ventricle and the pulse generator were a ventricular demand inhibited unit, the chamber paced would be ventricle and the first letter in the five position code would be "V." The chamber sensed would be ventricle and, therefore, the second letter in the five-position code would also be "V." The mode of response of the pacemaker would be to inhibit a pacing spike when spontaneous electrical activity were sensed and, therefore, "I" would be in the third position. If only the rate and/or output of the pulse generator could be programed externally, "P" would be in the fourth position. If the pacemaker were used to treat tachycardias, the tachyarrhythmia function would be indicated in the fifth position. Pulse generators that pace or sense in both atrium and ventricle are indicated by the designation "D," meaning dual. If the pacemaker does not have a function in one of the classifications, "O" is used. Finally, some pacemakers have a "reverse" function in that they discharge when the rate becomes too fast (and are thus used to terminate tachycardias). These pacemakers are indicated by the letter "R" in the third position. The different types of tachyarrhythmia functions are discussed in the chapter. Recently, the letter "C" has been suggested for the fourth position to indicate a "communicating" function, i.e., telemetry, with programmable features assumed.

An "S" may be used as a manufacturer's designation to label multiprogrammable single-chamber pacemakers adaptable for either atrial or ventricular use.

* The fourth and fifth positions are optional, as is a comma separating the third and fourth positions.

its discharge cycle is "reset" by the spontaneous event. "T" indicates that a stimulus is discharged in response to sensed activity, while "D" in the third position indicates that the pacemaker responds to sensed atrial activity by delivering a stimulus to the ventricle; i.e., it acts as an artificial AV node but responds to sensed ventricular activity by inhibiting its ventricular stimulus (it is reset). "R" indicates the response mode of a special type of pacemaker used to treat patients who have certain kinds of tachycardias. It discharges stimuli when the sensed heart rate *exceeds* a preset value and is quiescent at normal heart rates. Thus, it functions in reverse relative to most pacemakers, which are usually quiescent when the heart rate exceeds a particular value and discharge when the patient's rate falls below that preset value.

The fourth and fifth positions have been newly added. Position four indicates whether and to what extent pacemaker function can be reversibly changed noninvasively ("programed"). "P" indicates that only the rate and/or output can be altered, while "M" designates that other functions—such as sensitivity, duration of amplifier refractoriness, and so forth—can also be programed. Recently, a "C" has been added to indicate a "communicating" feature, i.e., telemetry, with programmable functions assumed to be present. The fifth position is reserved for pacemakers used to treat tachycardias. Stimuli may be delivered as a burst, "B" (a short train of generally rapid sequential stimuli); at a normal rate, "N," in fixed-rate competition with the tachycardia; or at various intervals that automatically scan the cardiac cycle, "S," in an effort to find the

TABLE 22–3 SENSING AND PACING CAPABILITIES OF AVAILABLE PACING MODALITIES

PACEMAKER TYPE	ICHD CODE	SENSES		PACES	
		Atrium	*Ventricle*	*Atrium*	*Ventricle*
Atrial asynchronous	AOO			X	
Ventricular asynchronous	VOO				X
Atrial demand	AAI, AAT	X		X	
Ventricular demand	VVI, VVT		X		X
Atrial synchronous	VAT	X			X
Atrial synchronous ventricular inhibited	VDD	X	X		X
AV sequential	DVI		X	X	X
Optimal sequential	DDD	X	X	X	X

appropriate premature interval that will successfully terminate the tachycardia.

The most commonly implanted pacemaker today is the demand ventricular pacemaker. It paces the ventricle (V), senses ventricular activity (V), and is inhibited from discharging (I) by sensed ventricular events—hence, the VVI pacemaker. If its rate and output only were programmable (P) and it delivered a burst of stimuli (B) in response to a tachycardia, it would be designated VVIPB.

Each of the pacing modalities has different functional capabilities (Table 22–3) and therefore specific indications and contraindications, which will be reviewed (Table 22–4).

TABLE 22–4 INDICATIONS AND CONTRAINDICATIONS FOR AVAILABLE PACING MODES

MODE	INDICATIONS	CONTRAINDICATIONS	ADVANTAGES	DISADVANTAGES
AOO	• Obsolete			
VOO	• Obsolete			
AAI, AAT	• SSS with normal AV conduction	• Atrial inexcitability • High atrial threshold • Abnormal AV conduction	• Simplest system providing properly timed sequential AV contraction; requires only one lead	• Ventricle not paced should AV block develop
VVI, VVT	• SSS without retrograde AV conduction • SSS with no hemodynamic benefit of atrial pacing • Chronic atrial fibrillation or flutter with AV block and a slow ventricular rate	• Hemodynamic insufficiency due to loss of AV synchrony ("pacemaker syndrome")	• Historical inertia • Relative simplicity	• Does not provide AV synchronous contraction • Rate does not change in response to external demands
VAT, VDD	• Normal sinus node function with impaired AV conduction	• Inappropriate atrial tachycardia or bradycardia • Retrograde atrial activation following ventricular stimulation or PVCs	• Maintains atrial transport and normal sinus control of ventricular rate when atrial rate is within tracking limits of pacemaker	• Does not maintain synchronous contractions during atrial bradycardia, since it does not pace the atria • Requires two leads
DVI	• Atrial bradyarrhythmias with or without impaired AV conduction	• Extended periods of atrial fibrillation/flutter	• Maintains sequential AV contraction during sinus bradycardia	• Does not alter rate in response to physiological demands • Does not maintain AV synchronous contractions during periods of normal sinus rhythm and AV block • Competitive atrial pacing during normal sinus rhythm • Requires two leads
DDD	• Atrial bradyarrhythmias with or without impaired AV conduction • Normal sinus node function with impaired AV conduction	• Retrograde atrial activation following ventricular stimulation or PVCs • Extended periods of atrial fibrillation/flutter • Frequent atrial tachycardias	• Maintains sequential AV contraction and sinus control of ventricular rate during normal sinus rhythm and during sinus bradycardia	• Requires two leads

SSS = Sick sinus syndrome

ATRIAL ASYNCHRONOUS

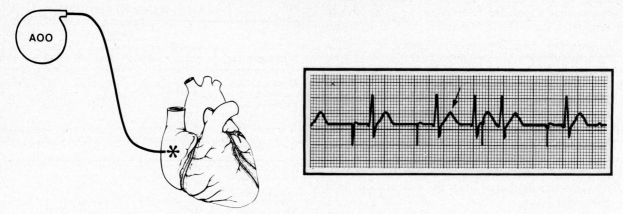

FUNCTION: PACES ATRIUM

FIGURE 22–1   Atrial asynchronous pacemaker (AOO). *Left,* Schematic diagram of heart with an asynchronous atrial pacemaker connected to the right atrium. Asterisk at atrial lead termination indicates that the device stimulates in the atrium. Letters labeling the pacemaker conform to the first three positions of the pacemaker code, as indicated in Table 22–2. *Right,* Representative ECG produced by atrial asynchronous pacing. The first, second, fourth, and fifth ventricular complexes are normally conducted following atrial paced complexes. The third ventricular complex was normally conducted following a spontaneous atrial depolarization (arrow). Pacemaker timing was not reset by this spontaneous atrial event because the pacemaker has no sensing capability.

ATRIAL AND VENTRICULAR ASYNCHRONOUS PACEMAKERS (AOO, VOO).   The original pacemakers simply stimulated the myocardium at a constant rate independent of the underlying cardiac rhythm; used for pacing only, these pacemakers could not sense any spontaneous activity. Placed in the atrium, the pacemaker is called an asynchronous atrial pacemaker (AOO) (Fig. 22–1); in the ventricle, it is a ventricular asynchronous pacemaker (VOO) (Fig. 22–2). Asynchronous pacemakers are rarely used today.

ATRIAL AND VENTRICULAR DEMAND PACEMAKERS (AAI, AAT, VVI, VVT).   In the early 1970s, sensing circuits were added to pacemakers so that they

stimulated only on demand when they could sense no appropriate underlying spontaneous rhythm. This sensing function prevented both competitive pacing and the attendant risk of inducing ventricular fibrillation. *Demand pacemakers* may operate in inhibited (I) and triggered (T) modes. Inhibited devices withhold the stimulus and reset their timing upon sensing spontaneous cardiac activity. *Triggered devices* are designed to deliver a stimulus immediately upon sensing spontaneous depolarization, into the absolute refractory period of the tissue, and simultaneously to reset their timing. Both types deliver a stimulus at the end of their timing cycle (pacemaker escape interval) if no spontaneous cardiac activity is detected (Figs. 22–3

VENTRICULAR ASYNCHRONOUS

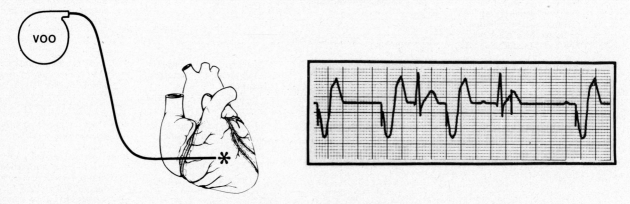

FUNCTION: PACES VENTRICLE

FIGURE 22–2   Ventricular asynchronous pacemaker (VOO). *Left,* Schematic diagram showing a VOO pacemaker connected to the right ventricle, with an asterisk at the lead termination to indicate that the pacemaker stimulates in the ventricle. *Right,* Representative ECG produced by ventricular asynchronous pacing. The first, second, fourth, and sixth ventricular complexes are produced by ventricular pacing. The third and fifth complexes result from conduction of normal sinus atrial activity and do not alter the pacemaker timing, since this device has no sensing capability. The stimulus in the T wave of the next-to-last QRS complex is ineffective because it occurs during the ventricular refractory period.

ATRIAL DEMAND

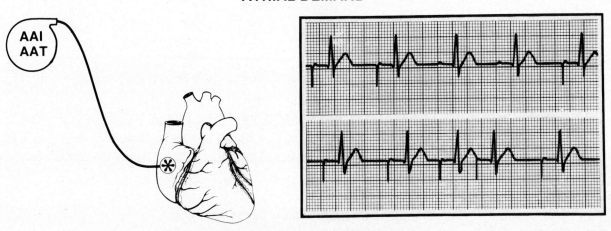

FUNCTION: PACES, SENSES ATRIUM

FIGURE 22–3 Atrial demand pacemakers (AAI, AAT). *Left,* Schematic diagram showing an atrial demand pacemaker connected to the right atrium. The lead termination is marked with a circle to indicate that the pacemaker senses atrial cardiac activity and an asterisk to indicate that the pacemaker stimulates in the atrium. *Right,* Representative ECGs produced by atrial inhibited (AAI, upper tracing) and atrial triggered (ATT, lower tracing) pacing. In the upper tracing, the first, second, and fifth atrial complexes are pacemaker-induced; the third and fouth atrial complexes are spontaneous and reset the pacemaker timing while inhibiting delivery of the stimulus. In the lower tracing, the first, second, and fifth atrial complexes are pacemaker-induced; the third and fourth atrial complexes are spontaneous and reset the pacemaker timing while triggering delivery of the stimulus into refractory atrial tissue. Note that the stimulus is delivered *after* the onset of the third and fourth P waves but initiates the other P waves.

and 22–4). The sensing circuits of these pacemakers are turned off for a period of time following delivery of a stimulus or sensing of spontaneous activity to avoid recognition of inappropriate signals such as T waves. This time interval is called the *pacemaker refractory period.*

The triggered mode was proposed to address concerns

that unipolar inhibited devices might allow a patient to become asystolic if extracardiac signals were sensed (e.g, pectoral muscle potentials, electrical signals from radio transmitters or power lines) and were erroneously interpreted to be cardiac signals and thus inhibited pacemaker output. Modern circuitry has reduced the likelihood

VENTRICULAR DEMAND

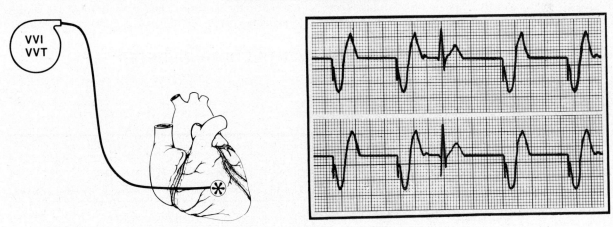

FUNCTION: PACES, SENSES VENTRICLE

FIGURE 22–4 Ventricular demand pacemakers (VVI, VVT). *Left,* Schematic diagram showing a ventricular demand pacemaker connected to the right ventricle, with a circle and an asterisk at the lead termination to indicate that the pacemaker senses ventricular cardiac activity and stimulates in the ventricle. *Right,* Representative ECGs produced by ventricular inhibited (VVI, upper tracing) and ventricular triggered (VVT, lower tracing) pacing. In the upper tracing, the first, second, fourth, and fifth ventricular complexes are pacemaker-induced; the third ventricular complex results from normally conducted sinus activity. This ventricular complex resets the pacemaker timing and inhibits delivery of the ventricular stimulus. In the lower tracing, the first, second, fourth, and fifth ventricular complexes are pacemaker-induced; the third ventricular complex is the result of normally conducted sinus activity. This ventricular complex resets the pacemaker timing and triggers delivery of the stimulus into the refractory ventricular tissue. Note that the stimulus is delivered *after* the onset of the third QRS complex but initiates the other QRS complexes.

ATRIAL SYNCHRONOUS

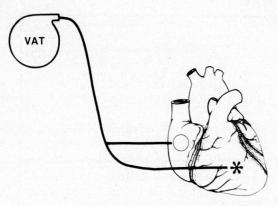

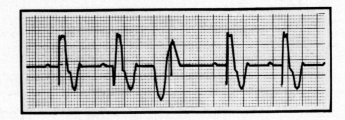

FUNCTION: SENSES ATRIUM; PACES VENTRICLE

FIGURE 22–5   Atrial synchronous pacemaker (VAT). *Left,* Schematic diagram showing a VAT pacemaker with leads connected to the right atrium and ventricle. The circle at the atrial lead termination indicates that the pacemaker senses atrial activity and the asterisk at the ventricular lead termination indicates that the pacemaker stimulates in the ventricle. *Right,* Representative ECG produced by atrial synchronous ventricular pacing. The first, second, fourth, and fifth ventricular complexes are stimulated by the pacemaker in response to pacemaker sensing of the spontaneous atrial activity. The third ventricular complex is a PVC that occurs simultaneously with a sinus-initiated atrial event. Since the pacemaker does not sense ventricular activity, it is triggered by the P wave (obscured by the PVC) and delivers a ventricular stimulus into the ST segment of the PVC.

of such occurrences. The disadvantages of stimulating when not really necessary, such as distorting the ECG waveform and draining more power from the pacemaker, have resulted in relatively little use of the triggered mode. However, the triggered mode can be valuable in terminating some tachycardias. For example, since the implanted unit senses electrical activity, it can be triggered to pace the heart in response to a series of stimuli delivered to the patient's chest wall from an external source. Also, triggered units are helpful diagnostically to be certain when or if the pacemaker sensed a spontaneous event, since in essence it "marks" that event by delivering a stimulus. Triggered function, therefore, is generally available in modern

programmable pacemakers as an option for either permanent or temporary (diagnostic) purposes.

ATRIAL SYNCHRONOUS VENTRICULAR PACEMAKERS (VAT, VDD).   To approximate normal cardiac function more closely, sophisticated dual-chamber (atrium and ventricle) "physiologic" pacemakers were developed. The *atrial synchronous ventricular pacemaker* (VAT) (Fig. 22–5) was designed for use in patients with normal sinus node function but impaired AV conduction.[39] This device senses atrial activity by means of an electrode in the atrium and, after a suitable delay, paces the ventricles; it does not pace the atrium. This method of atrial sensing and ventricular pacing preserves the atrial contribution to ven-

ATRIAL SYNCHRONOUS VENTRICULAR INHIBITED

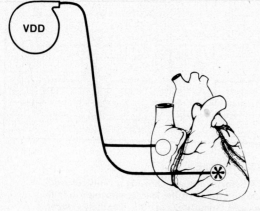

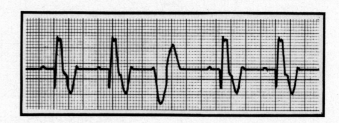

FUNCTION: SENSES ATRIUM; PACES, SENSES VENTRICLE

FIGURE 22–6   Atrial synchronous ventricular inhibited pacemaker (VDD). *Left,* Schematic diagram showing a VDD pacemaker with leads connected to the right atrium and ventricle. The circle at the atrial lead termination indicates that the pacemaker senses atrial activity and the circle and asterisk at the ventricular lead termination indicate that the pacemaker senses spontaneous ventricular activity and stimulates in the ventricle. *Right,* Representative ECG produced by VDD pacing. This recording is identical to the VAT pacemaker ECG shown in Figure 22–5 except that the PVC is sensed by the ventricular amplifier and prevents the pacemaker from synchronizing to the sinus P wave (obscured by the PVC) and pacing into the ST segment of the PVC.

tricular filling and maintains sinus control over the ventricular rate. Thus, exercise that stimulates acceleration of the sinus rate concomitantly increases the paced ventricular rate. Rate limitation is one design feature of this pacemaker, so that during atrial bradycardia the unit paces as an asynchronous ventricular pacemaker at a predetermined back-up rate. During atrial tachycardia the pacemaker paces no faster than its upper rate limit, yielding an AV response to sensed atrial activity that is 2:1, or similar to type I second-degree AV block. The VAT device has been refined by the addition of a ventricular sense amplifier, resulting in a new type of pacemaker called the *atrial synchronous ventricular inhibited pacemaker*[40] (VDD) (Fig. 22-6). Addition of the ventricular sense amplifier is important because it provides a demand mode for back-up pacing during bradycardia. It also prevents the atrial amplifier from triggering a ventricular stimulus in the event that a premature ventricular complex (PVC) produces a strong enough signal to be detected at the atrial electrode. To prevent such undesirable triggering, the system is designed to ensure that ventricular amplifer sensing takes precedence. Finally, ventricular sensing prevents competitive pacing when a PVC occurs during the A-V interval while the device is tracking normal sinus activity.

Like the VAT pacemaker, the VDD pacemaker still does not pace the atrium, but it does sense and pace the ventricle. During sinus bradycardia, VAT and VDD pacemakers function in the VOO and VVI modes, respectively, and therefore, under such circumstances, do not maintain sequential AV contraction. Contraindications to VDD pacing include the presence of atrial tachycardias and bradycardias and the occurrence of retrograde conduction to the atria with a long V-A interval during ventricular pacing or PVCs. Such retrograde activation will be sensed by a VDD pacemaker, triggering a ventricular stimulus and initiating a pacemaker-induced tachycardia.

AV SEQUENTIAL PACEMAKERS (DVI). For patients with abnormal sinus node function (sinus bradycardia, sinus arrest, and so forth) as well as impaired AV conduction, the atrial contribution to ventricular filling can be preserved by means of an AV sequential pacemaker[41] (DVI) (Fig. 22-7). This pacemaker senses only ventricular activity but is capable of stimulating both the atrium and the ventricle. Following ventricular sensed or paced events, this device monitors the ventricular electrogram. If ventricular activity is not detected within a prescribed pacemaker escape interval, the device stimulates the atrium. The pacemaker then waits long enough to allow passage of a normal AV interval and, if no ventricular activity occurs, paces in the ventricle. Some AV sequential pacemakers are of the committed type, i.e., they do not wait for normal AV conduction to occur but, instead, always deliver a stimulus to the ventricles following delivery of an atrial stimulus.[42,43] Sensed spontaneous ventricular activity inhibits the ventricular stimulus and resets all pacemaker timing. If the ventricular rate is sufficiently rapid, atrial stimuli from the pacemaker are also inhibited. It is important to reemphasize that the DVI pacemaker does *not* sense spontaneous atrial activity and therefore cannot alter the paced rate in response to physiologic needs.

OPTIMAL SEQUENTIAL PACEMAKERS (DDD). The optimal sequential pacemaker[44] (DDD) combines features of the AAI, VDD, and DVI pacemakers by functioning as an atrial demand pacemaker (AAI) during normally conducted sinus bradycardia, as an atrial synchronous pacemaker (VDD) during normal sinus rates that block or conduct with delay to the ventricle, and as an AV sequential pacemaker (DVI) during sinus bradycardia character-

AV SEQUENTIAL

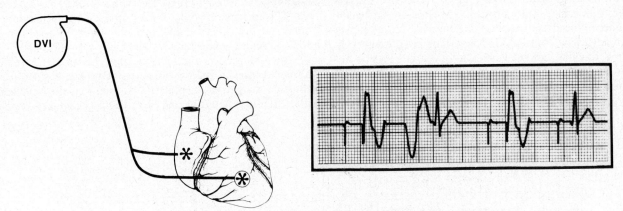

FUNCTION: PACES ATRIUM; PACES, SENSES VENTRICLE

FIGURE 22-7 AV sequential pacemaker (DVI). *Left*, Schematic diagram showing a DVI pacemaker with leads connected to the right atrium and ventricle. The asterisk at the atrial lead termination indicates that the pacemaker paces the atrium, and the asterisk and circle at the ventricular lead termination indicate that the pacemaker senses ventricular activity and stimulates in the ventricle. *Right*, A representative ECG produced by AV sequential pacing. The first two stimulus artifacts are the result of atrial and ventricular sequential pacing, which produces paced atrial and ventricular complexes. The second and third ventricular complexes are a PVC and a normally conducted QRS following spontaneous atrial activity. These ventricular complexes (sensed only by the ventricular amplifier) inhibit both the atrial and ventricular stimuli. The third and fourth stimulus artifacts are again atrial and ventricular sequential pacing, occurring because no additional spontaneous ventricular activity took place within the pacemaker's escape interval. The final stimulus artifact, an atrial stimulus, produced an atrial complex that conducted normally to the ventricles. This conducted ventricular activity inhibited the ventricular stimulus and reset all pacemaker timing.

OPTIMAL SEQUENTIAL

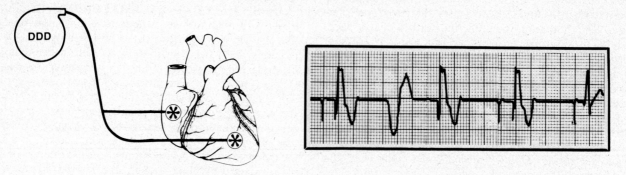

FUNCTION: PACES, SENSES ATRIUM; PACES, SENSES VENTRICLE

FIGURE 22–8 Optimal sequential pacemaker (DDD). *Left*, Schematic diagram of a DDD pacemaker with leads connected to the right atrium and ventricle. Asterisks and circles at the atrial and ventricular lead terminations indicate that the pacemaker paces and senses in both atrium and ventricle. *Right*, A representative ECG produced by DDD pacing. The first and fourth cardiac cycles, each preceded by two stimulus artifacts, are produced by atrial and ventricular sequential stimulation. The second QRS complex is a PVC, which resets all pacemaker timing and inhibits pacing. The third QRS complex is the result of ventricular pacing triggered by the pacemaker's sensing of the preceding sinus atrial event. The fifth QRS complex is the normally conducted result of atrial pacing.

ized by blocked or prolonged AV conduction. During normally conducted sinus impulses, the pacemaker is totally inhibited (Fig. 22–8). Thus, this pacemaker most closely approaches the normal electrophysiology of the heart in order to preserve the optimal hemodynamic relationships between atrial and ventricular contraction.

Current contraindications to its use are (1) the presence of atrial tachycardias that are inappropriate for governing ventricular rate (since the DDD pacemaker senses the atrial rate and paces the ventricle accordingly), and (2) as with the VDD units, retrograde conduction to the atrium with a long V-A conduction time following paced ventricular beats (the retrograde atrial response is sensed, triggers a paced ventricular beat, and thus creates an iatrogenic pacemaker-induced tachycardia). Ultimately, the latter will be eliminated as a contraindication as improved designs allow atrial tracking devices to handle retrograde signals appropriately. Except for these circumstances, in which a DVI pacemaker might be preferred, the DDD pacemaker can be substituted for all existing pacemakers.

HYSTERESIS. Pacemakers with hysteresis are designed to operate as follows: the pacemaker escape interval (interval between the last sensed spontaneous activity and the first paced beat) exceeds the interval between subsequent consecutive pacing cycles, so that normal sinus rhythm can be maintained over a wide range of rates (pacemaker-inhibited) while ensuring an adequate pacing rate when needed. This type of operation is displayed in Figure 22–9.

It is important to recognize the different rate capabilities offered by different pacemakers. AAI, AAT, VVI, VVT, and DVI pacemakers have a fixed rate that can be changed by reprograming the pacemaker. The AAI and AAT pacemakers (assuming normal AV conduction) ensure that both atrial and ventricular rates do not drop below a minimal constant value while the VVI and VVT devices maintain a minimal constant ventricular rate. The DVI pacemaker behaves like the AAI pacemaker except that it also paces the ventricle to maintain the ventricular rate equal to the atrial rate. The VDD pacemaker "tracks"

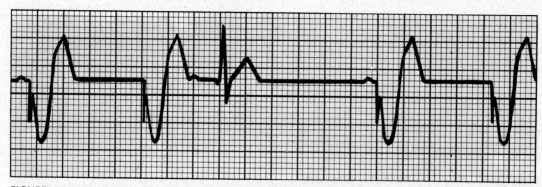

FIGURE 22–9 Operation of a VVI pacemaker incorporating hysteresis. Following two paced ventricular complexes, a sinus beat conducts to the ventricles and inhibits the pacemaker. When no additional spontaneous ventricular activity occurs, the pacemaker "escapes" at an interval of 1200 msec, with subsequent pacing intervals of 857 msec. Thus, the escape interval of the pacemaker exceeds the pacing interval, thereby allowing the patient to remain in a normally conducted rhythm for as much time as possible.

the atrial rate between the lower escape interval of the pacemaker, at which it functions at a constant rate in the VVI mode, and an upper rate limit at which the pacemaker creates second-degree AV block to maintain a fairly constant ventricular rate. The DDD pacemaker functions as a VDD pacemaker through the normal and fast rates but maintains a constant rate for atria and ventricles in the lower range by functioning in the AAI or DVI mode. Naturally, each of these pacemakers can be inhibited by changes in the spontaneous rhythm that alters the heart rate.

HEMODYNAMIC CONSEQUENCES OF SEQUENTIAL AV CONTRACTION

Ventricular (VVI) pacing provides symptomatic improvement for the vast majority of patients who have sick sinus syndrome or impaired AV conduction by establishing a basal ventricular rate that ensures adequate cardiac output. Increasing evidence suggests that some patients are not well served by ventricular pacing,[45-49] either because this pacing mode does not restore sufficient cardiac function to meet the demands of normal daily activity, or because the unnatural cardiac activation sequence associated with VVI pacing interferes with effective cardiac pumping. During ventricular pacing, atrial contractions may be absent, dissociated from ventricular activity, or improperly coupled to ventricular events by retrograde conduction. Inappropriately timed atrial systole effectively eliminates the booster pump action of the atrium present during normal sinus rhythm and impairs valve function.[50]

A consistent ventriculoatrial activation sequence may be associated with even greater hemodynamic compromise than is random AV dissociation because of significant decreases in systemic and left ventricular blood pressure and cardiac output, with concomitant increases in right atrial, ventricular, and pulmonary pressures.[51] In some patients, congestive heart failure may result.[46] Numerous acute studies have shown gains in cardiac output that vary from 2% to 67% after substitution of AV sequential[52-55] or atrial synchronous ventricular pacing[56] for ventricular pacing. Maintenance of hemodynamic gains chronically has been shown in more recent studies in which ventricular demand and atrial synchronous ventricular pacing were compared using measurements obtained by invasive means from exercising patients.[57,58] Patients were first paced for three-month intervals in either the VDD or the VVI mode and were then switched to the other mode. Invasive hemodynamic studies at rest and during exercise after each three-month interval revealed that during the heaviest workload, VDD pacing increased cardiac output 3.8 liters/min (mean) compared to VVI pacing despite a substantial compensatory increase in stroke volume that occurred with VVI pacing. Arteriovenous oxygen concentration differences during the heaviest workload and arterial lactate levels were lower during VDD pacing. Mean working capacity increased 23% and was statistically the same in patients both below and above 65 years of age. A progressive decrease in long-term performance with VVI pacing was evidenced by decreased work capacity, increased heart size, and increased pulmonary artery pressure, while the significant gains seen with VDD pacing were maintained chronically.

Thus, it seems clear that appropriately timed atrial systole has an important influence on cardiac performance. One question remains unresolved: whether dual-chamber devices should be considered for all patients or only for selected groups, such as those whose cardiovascular function is impaired and those who require significant increases in cardiac output (e.g., youngsters or athletically active people).

MODE SELECTION

Selection of an appropriate pacemaker modality for a given patient can be rather complex, requiring knowledge of the electrophysiological performance of the sinus node, AV conduction pathways and hemodynamic status. When available, these data can be used with the algorithm illustrated in Figure 22–10 to select the most suitable type(s) of device. We begin by considering whether sinus node function is normal or abnormal. If it is normal (right branch, Fig. 22–10) and the patient does not suffer angina at elevated rates, an atrial tracking pacemaker (VDD, DDD) may be appropriate, provided that the patient does not have prolonged retrograde conduction time to the atrium following ventricular paced beats. Such retrograde conduction would produce a pacemaker-mediated tachycardia if combined with an atrial tracking device. If there is retrograde conduction, or if there is need to control the upper pacing rate either to limit it in order to prevent angina or to ensure AV synchrony via atrial overdrive, an AV sequential (DVI) pacemaker would be selected. If sinus node function is abnormal (left branch, Fig. 22–10), with frequent periods of atrial fibrillation or flutter, a ventricular demand pacemaker (VVI, VVT) would be chosen. If atrial flutter or fibrillation is not present and AV conduction is normal, an atrial demand pacemaker (AAI, AAT) can be implanted unless the patient has *hypersensitive carotid sinus syndrome*. An atrial pacemaker is inappropriate therapy for patients with this syndrome, since AV conduction is frequently blocked by the excessive vagal tone (although this response is often veiled by concomitant sinus arrest). In patients with hypersensitive carotid sinus syndrome, a DVI pacemaker is the preferred type. If the predominant atrial rhythm is normal with infrequent or brief episodes of atrial bradyarrhythmia, it is likely that an atrial tracking pacemaker (VDD, DDD) may be suitable. The considerations cited above (potential for angina, retrograde conduction) should be reviewed before proceeding with selection of a tracking pacemaker. Finally, if sinus function

TABLE 22–5 CONCISE SUMMARY OF INDICATIONS FOR AVAILABLE PACING MODES

AV CONDUCTION	Normal	Bradycardia	Bradycardia-Tachycardia
Normal	O	AAI	AAI
AV block without prolonged retrograde conduction time	VDD,DDD	DDD,DVI	DVI,VVI
AV block with prolonged retrograde conduction time	DVI	DVI	DVI

O = No pacemaker indicated

It is given that the patient needs a pacemaker and that it is desirable to maintain atrial transport and rate control. Select the appropriate pacing mode.

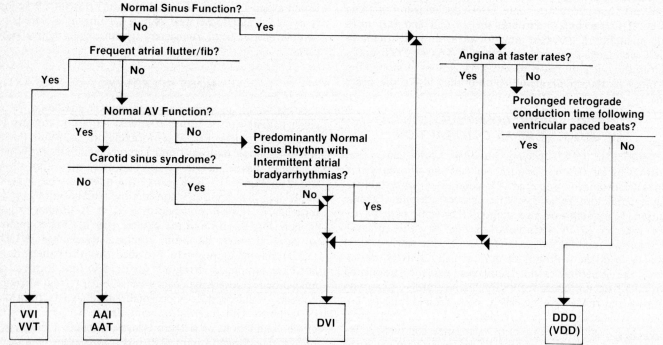

FIGURE 22–10   A flow chart providing an algorithm for selection of an appropriate pacemaker modality. This decision tree is described in detail in the text.

and AV conduction are both abnormal, atrial flutter or fibrillation is infrequent or absent, and the patient has extended periods of bradycardia, a DVI pacemaker should be selected.

A concise summary of the resultant pacemaker mode selection produced by the algorithm of Figure 22-10 is presented in Table 22-5.

PACING FOR TACHYCARDIAS[20,29,59-61]

Pacing to treat patients with tachycardias can be divided into four categories: (1) the need to maintain a normal rate when a required antiarrhythmic regimen produces bradycardia, (2) slowing the ventricular rate, (3) prevention of recurrence of tachycardia, and (4) termination of tachycardia already present.[29]

In the first category, drugs such as digitalis, propranolol, clonidine, and amiodarone (see Chapter 21) may result in symptomatic bradycardias that require some form of pacing to maintain normal heart rates. Similarly, His-bundle ablation to interrupt AV conduction in a patient with drug-refractory supraventricular tachycardia with a rapid ventricular rate results in a bradycardia (due to the AV block) that requires pacing.[62,63] Classically, VVI pacemakers have been used for this purpose, although dual-chamber devices may be more desirable under specific circumstances in which the patient may be capable of achieving sustained periods of AV synchrony.

An infrequently used alternative approach to patients with uncontrollable supraventricular tachycardia is the use of rapid atrial stimulation, which may initiate atrial fibrillation and/or AV block and thus reduce ventricular rate.[64,65]

Coupled atrial pacing has also been used to reduce ventricular rate in drug-resistant atrial tachycardia.[66] These approaches reduce the ventricular rate if atrial impulses block in the AV junction. Paired or coupled ventricular pacing for supraventricular or ventricular tachycardias reduces the *effective* ventricular rate by producing an electrical but not a mechanical response. The required closely coupled premature ventricular stimulation may produce ventricular fibrillation.

Pacing successfully prevents recurrence of tachycardia only in selected circumstances. In 1960 Linenthal and Zoll demonstrated that ventricular pacing at slightly elevated but generally normal rates usually eliminated ventricular tachyarrhythmias in patients with advanced AV block and slow heart rates punctuated by bouts of ventricular tachycardias.[67] The occurrence of ventricular tachyarrhythmias in association with bradycardia may be related in part to a greater disparity between action potential duration and refractory period at slow heart rates (p. 619). This temporal dispersion of recovery of excitability may be accentuated by a premature extrasystole, causing inhomogeneous areas of conduction delay and block that may lead to reentry. Pacing at faster rates in the absence of ischemia may improve the synchrony of recovery and alleviate the ventricular arrhythmias (Fig. 22-11).

It is important to note that accelerating the heart rate in the presence of ischemia may increase the degree of conduction delay occurring in the ischemic area and increase the temporal dispersion of refractoriness. These changes may result in ventricular tachycardia and ventricular fibrillation.[68] When one is pacing patients who have had a myocardial infarction, care should be taken to find an optimal heart rate that will alleviate the arrhythmias but will not exacerbate the ischemia or provoke new arrhythmias.

In some cases simply improving the patient's hemodynamic status[32] or restoring normal AV synchrony by means of an appropriate standard pacemaker[33,69] will prevent the development of tachycardia. In others, pacing at moderately elevated rates suppresses ectopy and the recurrence of tachycardias. This effect must be well documented before a permanent pacemaker is implanted, because permanent pacing often fails to prevent recurrence of tachycardia over the long term. Also, the site of pacing—atrial or ventricular—may make a difference in efficacy. Short-term, temporary rapid pacing may effectively suppress ventricular tachycardias associated with torsades de pointes and Q-T prolongation. The mechanism by which this pacing mode is successful in some instances may relate to the phenomenon of overdrive suppression (p. 620). In patients who have accessory pathways, an atrial synchronous or DDD pacemaker with a suitably short A-V interval may preclude development of a reciprocating tachycardia while preserving normal sinus control of ventricular rate.[70]

Selected drug-resistant tachycardias, not amenable to surgical therapy, can sometimes be terminated by a pacemaker designed to produce an appropriate sequence of electrical stimuli. Some of the pacemakers are activated by the *patient* when he perceives the presence of a tachyarrhythmia,[31,71–73] while others automatically discharge when the *pacemaker* senses that a tachycardia is present.[74,75] Various cadences of stimuli can be delivered, including short bursts at high rates (Fig. 22-12), stimuli that scan the cardiac cycle and automatically change rate[76] or shift the timing of one or more premature stimuli,[77] and coupled or paired stimuli. A "dual-demand" pacemaker automatically delivers stimuli at a fixed but relatively slow (e.g., 70 bpm) rate when it senses the presence of a bradycardia (e.g., rates less than 70 bpm) or tachycardia (e.g., rates greater than 150 bpm).[78] The tachycardia is terminated when an appropriately timed stimulus occurs during a particular part of the tachycardia cycle; this is called "underdrive termination." Dual-chamber (DVI) pacemakers can be made to operate in the dual-demand mode and pace with short A-V intervals for patients who have accessory pathways.[79,80] Unique custom-built devices with characteristics tailored for specific patients can also be applied.

Although a tachycardia that could be terminated by pacing stimuli was previously believed to be due to reentry, we now know this is not necessarily so, in view of the phenomenon of triggered activity, discussed on p. 620. Nevertheless, assuming reentry to be the mechanism sustaining a tachycardia, we can consider certain principles of

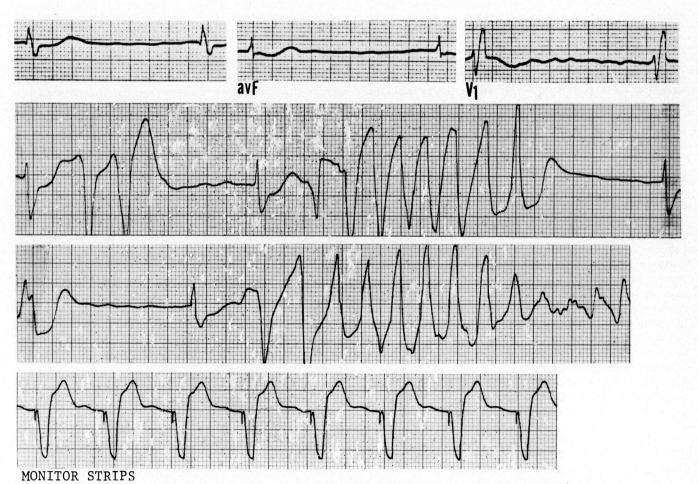

MONITOR STRIPS

FIGURE 22–11 Electrocardiogram showing runs of ventricular tachycardia consequent to an inadequate ventricular escape rate in a patient with chronic atrial fibrillation and complete AV block (upper panels). Ventricular pacing at a rate of 85 ppm abolished the ventricular arrhythmia (lower panel).

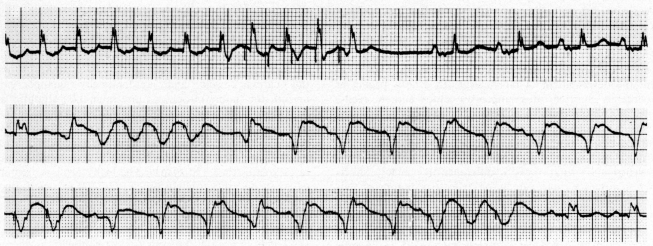

FIGURE 22–12   In the top tracing, a burst of pacing stimuli delivered from a patient-activated radiofrequency transmitter-receiver pacemaker terminates an episode of paroxysmal supraventricular tachycardia. In the middle tracing, a burst from a similar unit initiates an episode of a rather slow ventricular tachycardia, which is then terminated by a second burst of three stimuli (bottom tracing).

pacing. The mechanism by which a pacemaker stimulus terminates the tachycardia is invasion of the reentrant circuit (Fig. 19–23, p. 628) and making a portion of it refractory to the reentrant impulse, which then expires. To accomplish this, the paced impulse must propagate from its site of stimulation to the reentrant pathway in time to depolarize a part of the pathway. Factors that favorably influence this accomplishment are short refractory periods and rapid conduction, anatomically large reentrant circuits (e.g., Wolff-Parkinson-White syndrome reciprocating tachycardia rather than a micro-reentry circuit), tachycardia with slow rates, and pacemaker electrode positioning close to the reentrant circuit.[61]

The following serves as a simple example (based on certain assumptions about the reentrant circuit). An anatomically determined reentrant tachycardia with a cycle length of 500 msec (rate 120/min) and tissue in the pathway with a refractory period of 250 msec, can be depolarized during an interval of 250 msec when the fibers have recovered excitability from the previous cycle and have not yet been depolarized by the next cycle (excitable gap = 500 msec − 250 msec). A tachycardia with a cycle length of 300 msec (rate 200/min) and tissue with a refractory period of 280 msec has an excitable gap of only 20 msec. Since the paced impulse must reach the circuit before the spontaneous impulse from the circuit has a chance to propagate to the pacing site and make the intervening path refractory, the time available for this to occur is one-half the duration of the excitable gap, assuming equal conduction time from the circuit to the pacing site and vice versa. This would be 125 msec for the first example and 10 msec for the second. Knowing this, we can calculate how far away the pacing electrodes can be placed from the reentrant circuit and still terminate the tachycardia. Distance (d) equals velocity × time. Assuming propagation in muscle of 100 cm/sec, the electrode must be within 12.5 cm (d = 0.1 cm/msec × 125 msec) for the first tachycardia and within 1.0 cm (d = 0.1 cm/msec × 10 msec) for the second.

Single stimuli often fail to terminate a tachycardia because they fail to invade the circuit during the excitable gap, and pairs or bursts of stimuli must be used. While the use of multiple stimuli increases the success rate for termination, it also increases the likelihood of accelerating the tachycardia to flutter or fibrillation. Naturally, this is not acceptable for a ventricular tachycardia, so that pacing in this situation must be used conservatively. Also, initiation of atrial fibrillation in patients who have an accessory pathway with a short refractory period may result in unacceptably fast ventricular rates.

To solve some of these problems, the principles of transthoracic cardioversion have been adapted for use with a device that can deliver synchronized cardioversion shocks with energies of 0.075 to 2.000 joules via a catheter electrode to terminate sustained ventricular tachyarrhythmias successfully and safely[81-83] (Fig. 22–13). This system can also terminate supraventricular tachyarrhythmias (Fig. 22–14). In addition, an implantable defibrillator has been developed and used successfully in patients to terminate ventricular fibrillation.[84,85] These latter two advances may significantly increase the application of electrical devices for long-term treatment of tachycardias. Currently, pacing for tachycardia control accounts for less than 3 per cent of all pacemaker implantations.

PROGRAMMABILITY OF PACEMAKERS

Almost all permanent pacemaker implants today employ a programmable pacemaker. Programmability can be defined as noninvasive, reversible alteration of the electronically controlled performance of an implantable device such as a pacemaker. Use of a simple magnet to convert a demand pacemaker to its asynchronous mode is generally excluded from this definition, although it is in reality a simple form of programming. In the most advanced pacemakers, many performance characteristics are programmable, including rate, stimulus output amplitude or duration, amplifier sensitivity, amplifier refractory period, hysteresis, pacing mode (e.g., unipolar/bipolar, VVI/VVT/VOO), and operation of special information transfer channels (telemetry of intracardiac electrograms, programmed settings,

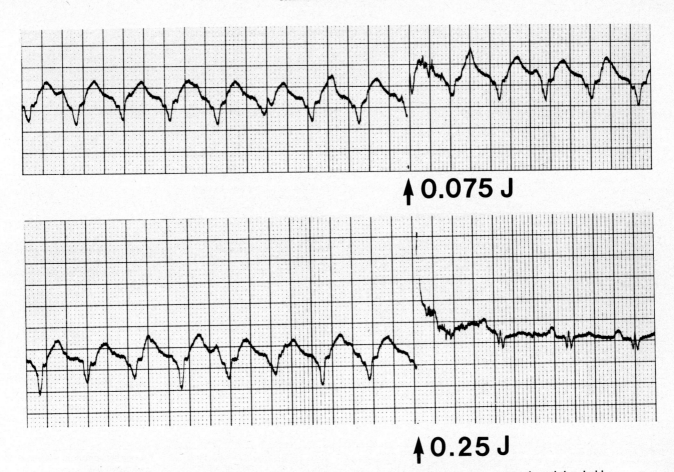

↑ 0.075 J

↑ 0.25 J

FIGURE 22–13 Electrocardiogram of a patient with ventricular tachycardia. In the upper panel a subthreshold shock of 0.075 joule is delivered synchronously into the QRS complex through a transvenous catheter. In the lower panel a transvenous synchronous shock of 0.25 joule successfully terminates the tachycardia. II = Lead II.

FIGURE 22–14 Electrocardiogram of a patient with ventricular tachycardia. A, A 0.25-joule shock is delivered synchronously into the QRS complex through a transvenous catheter. The stimulus fails to convert the ventricular rhythm but induces atrial fibrillation. B, A shock of 1.0 joule is delivered synchronously into the QRS complex, and the atrial fibrillation and ventricular tachycardia are both terminated to restore normal sinus rhythm. I, II, III, V_1 = scalar leads; esop = esophageal lead. (Study performed with the help of Eric N. Prystowsky, M.D., and James J. Heger, M.D.)

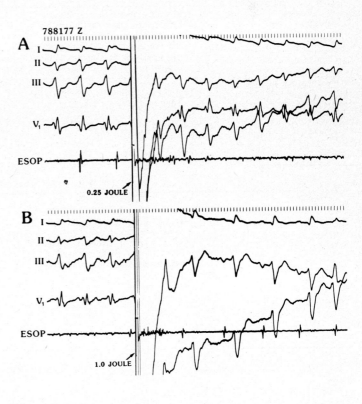

TABLE 22–6   APPLICATIONS OF PROGRAMMABLE PACEMAKER PARAMETERS

PARAMETER	PATIENT/PACEMAKER OPTIMIZATION	DIAGNOSTIC APPLICATIONS	CORRECTION OF MALFUNCTIONS
• Rate	• Improve cardiac output by allowing greater range of conducted sinus activity • Minimize angina by keeping the rate below that which produces pain • Suppress arrhythmias • Adapt pulse generator to pediatric needs (faster rates) • Terminate tachycardias with short rapid bursts of stimuli • Minimize "pacemaker syndrome" due to AV dissociation by selecting low rate	• Suppress pacing to assess underlying rhythm by ECG • Test AV conduction with an atrial pacemaker by determining rates at which AV block occurs • Test sinus function with an atrial pacemaker by using periods of rapid pacing to determine sinus node recovery times • Confirm atrial capture by altering pacemaker rate and observing concomitant ventricular rate change	
• Output Amplitude or Duration	• Maximize pulse generator longevity by selecting output energy that provides the minimal level of stimulation consistent with reliable maintenance of pacing • Provide increased energy for high-threshold patients • Avoid extracardiac stimulation (pectoral muscle, phrenic nerve)	• Evaluate pacing threshold	• Regain capture following threshold increases due to effects of infarcts, electrolyte disturbances, drugs • Eliminate diaphragmatic and pectoral muscle stimulation
• Amplifier Sensitivity	• Establish appropriate sensitivity to detect intracardiac electrogram while avoiding sensing of extraneous signals (pectoral muscle potentials, electromagnetic interference) • Increase sensitivity for atrial sensing applications	• Alter sensitivity to evaluate possible sources of oversensing or undersensing	• Compensate for changes in intracardiac electrogram amplitude • Resolve oversensing of T waves, muscle potentials, electromagnetic interference
• Refractory Period	• Extend duration for atrial pacing to avoid sensing conducted QRS complex • Shorten duration in ventricular pacing to detect closely coupled ventricular complexes	• Alter duration to evaluate possible causes of over- or undersensing	• Lengthen duration to avoid T-wave sensing • Shorten duration to eliminate failure to sense closely coupled ventricular complexes • Lengthen duration of atrial amplifier refractory period in VDD or DDD device to avoid sensing retrogradely conducted atrial activity
• Hysteresis	• Minimize pacemaker syndrome by allowing sinus rhythm to be maintained over widest possible rate range while establishing adequately high pacing rate when needed		
• Unipolar/Bipolar		• Evaluate lead fracture (bipolar, unipolar) • Enhance stimulus artifact visibility on ECG (bipolar, unipolar) • Evaluate oversensing (unipolar, bipolar)	• Convert to unipolar function to regain capture in case of lead fracture • Change mode to adapt to altered electrogram causing sensing failure • Convert to bipolar to eliminate sensing of myopotentials • Convert to bipolar to avoid extracardiac stimulation
• Mode	• Select optimum mode (e.g., VDD for patients who have normal sinus function and impaired AV conduction) • Alter mode if patient's needs change (e.g., VDD to DVI if patient develops sinus bradycardia)	• Establish triggered mode to enable external control of pacemaker from chest electrodes and external stimulator to perform noninvasive electrophysiological studies of sinus function, AV conduction, tachycardia initiation, efficacy of antiarrhythmic agents, and so forth; tachycardias can be terminated in a similar fashion • Confirm oversensing signal source by selecting triggered mode	• Change to backup mode (e.g., VVI) if atrial portion of dual-chamber system is nonfunctional (e.g., lead displacement) • Prevent oversensing by selecting asynchronous mode

TABLE 22–6   APPLICATIONS OF PROGRAMMABLE PACEMAKER PARAMETERS (*continued*)

PARAMETER	PATIENT/PACEMAKER OPTIMIZATION	DIAGNOSTIC APPLICATIONS	CORRECTION OF MALFUNCTIONS
• AV Delay	• Maximize hemodynamic efficacy • Control/prevent tachyarrhythmias		
• Atrial Rate Tracking Limit	• Maintain widest range of sinus rate control without incurring angina • Control ventricular response to atrial arrhythmias • Prevent synchronization to atrial activity at short R-P intervals during ventricular escape pacing in VDD mode that results in AV dissociation with pacemaker captures • Reduce the long delay between the sensed P wave and the resultant rate limit-delayed stimulus in the ventricle to minimize the occurrence of retrograde atrial activity	• Select high rate limit for stress testing	• Reduce tracking rate limit if pectoral muscle activity triggers rapid pacing
• Telemetry		• Compare programed settings to actual device operation • Use marker channel indicators to determine which events pacemaker is causing and which events are being sensed • Use electrogram to evaluate causes of under- or oversensing • Use electrogram to evaluate drug effects on myocardium	

device operation indicators such as a "marker channel," battery status, lead impedance). In addition, in dual-chamber pacemakers it is frequently possible to program A-V intervals, atrial rate tracking limits, and the pacing mode (e.g., DDD to DVI or VVI).

Programmability benefits the patient by optimizing pacemaker function for specific patient needs, minimizing the need for invasive procedures to correct malfunctions or to revise the system to meet changing patient needs,[86-88] and facilitating troubleshooting procedures. Table 22–6 indicates applications for many of the commonly available programmable parameters. It should be emphasized that programmability must be used with care, since it presents the risk of establishing inappropriate parameter settings (e.g., insufficient output energy to maintain capture, dangerously high or low rates), and imposes a greater need for maintaining accurate records to prevent erroneous decisions when a clinician is unfamiliar with the rationale for the current programmed settings in a given patient.

POWER SOURCES

Nearly all pacemakers are battery-powered. External pacemakers typically have standard alkaline or mercury batteries of the type used in common household appliances (e.g., transistor radios, flashlights), although an occasional external device employs a rechargeable or lithium battery. Implantable pacemakers are generally powered by one of five energy sources: mercury-zinc batteries, rechargeable batteries, nuclear batteries, lithium batteries, or radiofrequency energy broadcasted to the pacemaker from an external device called a transmitter.[89]

Mercury-zinc batteries were the standard power source for nearly all pacemakers manufactured during the 1960s and early 1970s. These batteries are heavy, lose a significant amount of their capacity to internal intrinsic losses ("self-discharge"), so that pacemaker longevity is limited typically to 24 to 42 months; and they produce hydrogen gas making it impractical to seal the pacemaker hermetically and protect it from damaging body fluids. Virtually no modern pacemaker uses mercury-zinc cells.

Rechargeable batteries have functioned successfully in pacemakers but have not achieved wide acceptance because they require frequent attention from the patient or his family to maintain the battery in a charged state and, more importantly, because the lithium battery (described below) has proven so effective and trouble-free that it has become the present power source of choice. In the early 1970s nuclear batteries were developed for implantable pacemakers. The most commonly employed nuclear battery converted the heat generated by the decay of radioisotopic plutonium into electrical energy. Pacemakers using these batteries have demonstrated the greatest actual longevity of any pacemaker to date, surpassing in performance even the lithium battery as a pacemaker power source. However, regulatory requirements associated with the use of nuclear systems made them inconvenient for the implanting physicians, and unattractive from a commercial standpoint.

Virtually all current pacemakers are powered by one of the many varieties of the lithium battery. These batteries share certain characteristics that make them especially suitable for implantation, yet they exhibit significant differences.[90] Each of the lithium systems offers high-energy density and low internal losses due to self-discharge. Most of the systems can be hermetically sealed to prevent ingress of body fluids and egress of damaging battery materials. Each system offers unique electrical characteristics and varying degrees of reliability.[91-93] The most commonly used lithium batteries are the lithium iodide, lithium cupric sulfide, and lithium silver chromate.

Reported performance characteristics of the major power sources clearly show the substantial progress made toward creating a pacemaker that will have sufficient longevity to obviate replacement in the majority of patients. In 1981, survival probabilities were reported for large groups of pacemakers using the power sources described. A series of approximately 2000 mercury-zinc pacemakers showed a cumulative survival probability of 35 per cent at four years. Six thousand lithium pacemakers showed a cumulative survival probability of 79 per cent at 7.3 years and a small series of 143 nuclear pacemakers exhibited a survival probability of 94 per cent at 7.3 years. These data reflect actual clinical results and clearly demonstrate the longevity advantages of nuclear and lithium power sources.

A small group of special-purpose antitachycardia pacemakers is powered by radiofrequency energy transmitted through the body to the implantable device.[31] This is practical because these pacemakers are not required to pace constantly but are used to generate short bursts of rapid asynchronous stimuli to terminate episodes of tachycardia. These devices are manually activated by the patient who, when experiencing the symptoms induced by tachycardia, places a small battery-powered transmitter over the receiver unit and presses a button, causing the transmitter to energize the implanted stimulator. This technique eliminates the need for pacemaker replacement due to power-source depletion and makes it possible to reduce the size and weight of the implanted stimulator.

PACEMAKER ELECTRODE SYSTEMS ("LEADS")[94,95]

The pulse generator is electrically connected to the heart by means of a wire and electrode system referred to as a lead. Electrodes may be unipolar or bipolar. In bipolar systems the positive (anode) and negative (cathode) electrodes are both located within the cardiac chamber and are in contact with the endocardium or are on the heart. Unipolar systems place only the cathode at the heart and use a large area anode electrode, usually the metallic housing of the pulse generator, at a remote location. Either approach is clinically acceptable. There is a common misconception that unipolar leads provide larger signals for sensing purposes. There is, in fact, no statistical difference in signal amplitude or slew rate of electrograms generated from unipolar or bipolar recordings.[96] Pacing thresholds are also similar. However, bipolar systems are less susceptible to extraneous electromagnetic interference (e.g., electrical signals generated by nearby power lines, automobile spark plugs, radio transmitters), extracardiac myopotential interference, unwanted extracardiac stimulation, or threshold changes due to defibrillatory currents.

Permanent pacing leads are designed either for transvenous or for epicardial placement. Probably more than 90 per cent of implants are by the transvenous route. Transvenous leads are usually implanted within the right ventricular apex for ventricular pacing and in the right atrial appendage or coronary sinus for atrial application. Leads are typically inserted via the cephalic, subclavian, or external jugular veins, using fluoroscopy for visualization and stiff wires (stylets) inserted within the lumen of the lead to facilitate control during positioning. The stylets must be removed following lead placement to avoid damaging the lead. A rapid technique for lead placement in the subclavian vein with minimal trauma employs a single venipuncture using a special percutaneous lead introducer.[97] This approach is gaining favor and involves minimal risk, although there is the possibility of inadvertently entering the pleural cavity or the arterial system. The newly introduced urethane insulated leads have reduced diameters and a decreased coefficient of friction, making it possible to pass an atrial and a ventricular lead through a single vein, facilitating the use of dual-chamber pacemakers.[98,99]

Transvenous leads come in a variety of designs, each

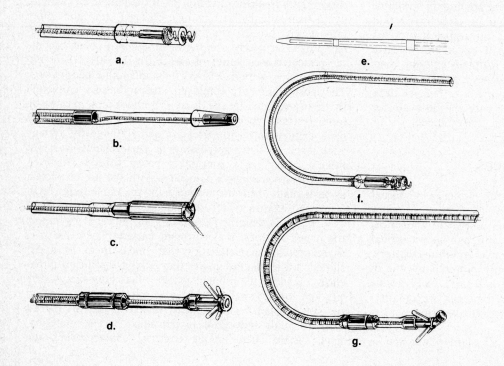

FIGURE 22–15 Examples of atrial and ventricular transvenous pacemaker electrodes. *a*, Unipolar endocardial urethane lead with a screw-in tip electrode for active fixation to the atrial or ventricular endocardial surface. *b*, Bipolar ventricular electrode utilizing flanged Silastic tip for positioning stability. *c*, Unipolar ventricular electrode with extensible metallic barb that provides active fixation to the ventricular myocardium. *d*, Bipolar urethane ventricular electrode with flexible tines adjacent to the ring tip electrode. The tines provide passive lead fixation by lodging within the trabecular structure of the ventricle. *e*, Bipolar Silastic lead designed for stable placement in the coronary sinus. The electrodes are shaped for atrial pacing applications. *f*, Unipolar urethane lead with J shape and screw-in tip electrode for active fixation to the atrial endocardial surface. *g*, Bipolar urethane atrial lead with J shape and flexible tines adjacent to the tip electrode. The J shape and tines provide passive fixation of the electrode within the atrium.

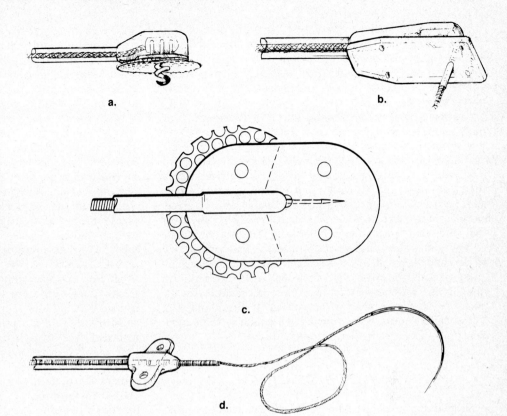

FIGURE 22–16 Examples of atrial and ventricular epicardial electrodes. *a*, Silastic sutureless unipolar ventricular electrode with corkscrew tip. Positive fixation is achieved by screwing the electrode into the myocardium. *b*, Silastic unipolar epicardial electrode designed to be sutured to either atrial or ventricular myocardium. *c*, Urethane unipolar epicardial barbed hook electrode providing positive fixation (without sutures) to either atrial or ventricular myocardium. *d*, Silastic unipolar electrode for atrial or ventricular use. The needle and suture material extending from the exposed stainless-steel electrode are used to fasten the electrode directly to the myocardium.

purporting to ensure stable permanent positioning of the electrodes[100–106] (Fig. 22–15). Many atrial leads also incorporate a "J" shape to aid in proper positioning within the atrial appendage. The transvenous approach is associated with very low morbidity and, with current lead designs, a very low rate of displacement.[102,103] Epicardial leads are used less frequently than transvenous systems, although they are of particular benefit in problem patients with smooth dilated right ventricles or in those with truncated right atrial appendages. The placement approach depends on the type of epicardial electrode used. A transthoracic approach (thoracotomy) is used to apply electrodes that are sutured to the myocardium. More commonly, for ventricular applications a sutureless corkscrew electrode is used, since this device can be applied via a transmediastinal approach, avoiding entrance into the pleural cavity and reducing morbidity and discomfort[107] (Fig. 22–16).

Temporary pacing leads include transvenous catheter electrodes, wire electrodes, and—in extreme circumstances—precordial skin electrodes. The technique for placing temporary transvenous catheter electrodes is similar to

that used for permanent leads. Placement is facilitated by designing the catheters stiffer than would be acceptable for permanent use and by sometimes incorporating additional aids such as inflatable balloons or cuffs that "float" the catheter in the blood stream to the right ventricle. In the absence of fluoroscopy, ECG recordings from the catheter enable the user to determine the location of the electrodes (Fig. 22–17). Wires frequently are placed in the atria and ventricles of patients at the time of open-heart surgery. These stainless-steel wires are used during the surgical procedure and during the postoperative recovery phase to help control the cardiac rhythm. Electrograms recorded from these electrodes aid in diagnosing complex arrhythmias.[4] In emergency situations, wire electrodes can be inserted percutaneously into the heart using a pericardiocentesis (or similar) needle. Also, during emergencies, surface skin electrodes placed on the chest wall can be stimulated with very high (and quite painful) voltages to achieve cardiac pacing transthoracically. Such an approach should be used only until a transvenous catheter electrode can be positioned. An improved technique for noninvasive pacing, re-

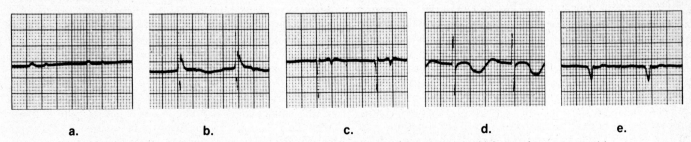

FIGURE 22–17 Electrograms obtained when bipolar electrode is located in the high superior vena cava (*a*), superior vena cava/right atrium (*b*), right atrium (*c*), right ventricle (*d*), and pulmonary artery (*e*). All tracings were calibrated at 1 mV/cm except *d*, which is recorded at one-half standard.

ported to cause minimal discomfort and to be suitable for prolonged use, requires special large-surface area electrodes and external pulse generators that provide stimuli of very long duration (about 40 msec).[108] This may offer a viable alternative approach if such equipment can be readily obtained.

For temporary and permanent pacing it is important to place the electrodes in a position that provides acceptably low stimulation thresholds and sufficiently large intracardiac signals to be sensed by the pulse generator. Generally this requires acute thresholds for atrium or ventricle of less than 2mA and 1.25 V, with stimuli 0.5 msec in duration, and ventricular electrograms greater than 4 mV or atrial electrograms exceeding 2 mV. Thresholds generally rise following acute positioning of the leads, reach a peak two to four times the acute values within the first two to six weeks, and then fall to intermediate values.[109] The electrogram typically decreases in amplitude by 15 per cent; its rate of rise with respect to time (slew rate) decreases as much as 50 per cent with maturation of the implant.[110] These factors must be considered when one is evaluating the appropriateness of a given lead position.

PACEMAKER FOLLOW-UP

Despite the reliability of modern pacemakers, it is important to examine the patient and the pacemaker system regularly after implantation. Such follow-up has four major goals: (1) evaluation of the electrical function of the pacing system to detect malfunctions or imminent power-source depletion; (2) inspection of the implant site for possible difficulties, such as erosion or infection; (3) evaluation of the patient's cardiac status so that reprogramming or revision of the pacing system or of the concomitant drug regimen can be accomplished; and (4) maintenance of the physician-patient interaction to evaluate other problems or health needs, provide reassurance of progress, and offer an opportunity to discuss concerns that may arise.

The follow-up schedule should be arranged to allow close monitoring during the immediate postimplant period, moderately frequent observation during the routine service life of the system, and increased surveillance as the system nears completion of its service life. A suggested schedule is as follows: six and twelve weeks postimplant, twice annually, beginning six months postimplant, and monthly once the initial signs of power-source depletion are observed. (In almost all pacemakers, power-source depletion appears as a rate decrease when the system is monitored by passing a magnet over the pulse generator.) Given the longevity of modern systems, it may be counterproductive to attempt to stretch out the last few months of service through frequent monitoring, since this will probably add only 5 to 10 per cent to the total service life while increasing monitoring costs by 30 to 40 per cent.

Follow-up visits should be scheduled in the physician's office or in a special pacemaker clinic[111] where the patient can be seen in person. Telephone monitoring of the patient's ECG, pacing rate, and duration of the pulse generator stimulus carried out between personal evaluations can be of value as a supplement but should not replace office visits. Each visit should include a 12-lead ECG recording

with a rhythm strip showing that the pacemaker appropriately captures and senses; measurement of pacemaker parameters using appropriate rate and pulse width measurement equipment; and a general physical examination, including careful scrutiny of the pacemaker pocket. Results of the follow-up procedure should be carefully recorded,[112] since much of the required analysis depends on *changes* in operation rather than absolute values of measured parameters. This record is especially important when following patients who have programmable pacemakers[113] in which changes may be totally innocuous if intentional (e.g., rate change programed to improve cardiac output) or may signify device performance problems (e.g., rate decrease due to battery depletion).

Care should be exercised in selecting follow-up equipment, and data must be analyzed with full understanding and knowledge of the idiosyncrasies of the equipment used. For example, digital monitoring and recording systems frequently do not register the pacemaker stimulus or artifact reliably and reproducibly because of its extremely short duration. As a result, the artifact may not always be recorded even though present, or its polarity and amplitude may vary markedly throughout the recording. Alternatively, such systems may substitute a standardized artifact for the real signal and eliminate diagnostic information in the process. As another example, some follow-up clinics perform waveform analysis using an oscilloscope or special ECG machine to display the waveshape of the pacemaker stimulus. One must be fully aware of the correct stimulus waveshape for each pacemaker to be evaluated. Modern pacemakers frequently produce much more complex stimulus pulse shapes than the traditional "square wave," and it is not unusual for such waveforms to be misread as signs of malfunction.

An often underestimated benefit of follow-up is a reduction in patient anxiety. A clear answer to a simple question can be extremely important to a patient's quality of life. In recognition of this, some clinics have formed pacemaker clubs that allow patients to meet periodically to compare notes and provide mutual support.

PACEMAKER MALFUNCTION

Complex systems involving electrical, mechanical, and physiological interactions inevitably malfunction, and pacemakers are no exception. Fortunately, the detection and correction of such problems are relatively straightforward when one uses the appropriate equipment.[114,115]

EQUIPMENT.   To start with, accurate patient records that include full descriptions of the pacemaker, the implantation procedure, and follow-up information are mandatory. Next, the most useful troubleshooting tool is a 12-lead ECG machine. This permits evaluation of pacemaker sensing, capture, and approximate rate; evaluation of electrode positioning by vectorial analysis of the stimulus artifact and of the pacemaker-generated QRS complex or P wave[116]; and confirmation of appropriate function for the mode of pacing employed. A digital counter is necessary to evaluate accurately changes in pacing rate and pulse width due to battery depletion, component failure, or reprogramming. A magnet placed over the pacemaker converts nearly all units to asynchronous operation, which enables evaluation of capture when the patient's intrinsic rhythm inhibits the pacemaker, and can be useful in diagnosing oversensing by disabling all sensing function. Magnets should be employed with care, since some pacemakers can be programed by application of a suitable magnet, and there is always a slight risk of inducing tachyarrhythmias when one is pacing asynchronously.

Carotid sinus massage or the Valsalva maneuver may slow a patient's intrinsic rhythm and induce pacing, while exercise may be used to speed the patient's spontaneous rate to evaluate sensing capability. Chest-wall stimulation with an external stimulator connected to precordial surface electrodes can be utilized to test sensing function and to determine rate tracking limits for atrial tracking pacemakers (VAT, VDD, DDD). Manipulation of the pulse generator in its pocket can sometimes elicit electrocardiographic signs of a loose connection or damaged lead close to the generator site. X-ray or fluoroscopy of the chest and pacemaker system in multiple views helps determine lead position, gross lead fractures, and disconnections at the generator. An overpenetrated baseline chest x-ray (PA and lateral) following implantation should be obtained to establish lead configuration before the patient is discharged. An oscilloscope or special ECG recorder designed to display the waveshape of the pacemaker stimulus is used by some centers to evaluate lead problems or unusual component failures.

A pacemaker programmer, by allowing the user to vary stimulus strength, amplifier sensitivity, rates, refractory period, and pacing modes, enables noninvasive evaluation of multiple functions. In some of the newer systems, such a programmer permits the user to obtain noninvasive intracardiac electrograms to evaluate sensing operation. Many systems include digital telemetry of the programed settings of the pacemaker allowing actual performance to be compared with expected performance. The most sophisticated systems provide a "marker channel," a noninvasively telemetered tracing that, in conjunction with a surface ECG, clearly identifies pacemaker sensing and pacing operations (Fig. 22–18).

Invasive procedures are necessary if noninvasive approaches should fail. A pacing system analyzer is used to analyze the implantable pulse generator function (sensitivities, refractory periods, rates, pulse widths, and amplitudes), to evaluate lead integrity and positioning, and to provide electrophysiological data such as stimulation thresholds, electrogram amplitudes, or responses to pacing. Pacemaker-related problems fall into five broad categories: failure to pace, failure to sense, oversensing, pacing at an altered rate, and undesirable patient/pacemaker interactions.

FAILURE TO PACE. Failure to pace is inappropriate nondelivery of a stimulus or delivery of an ineffective stimulus that fails to depolarize the myocardium at a time when the myocardium is fully excitable. *Failure to deliver a stimulus* can result from the following: improper connection of the lead to the generator (e.g., set screws not tightened); broken lead wires with no insulation defect; "cross talk" between atrial and ventricular portions of dual-chamber pacemakers (discussed below); pulse generator component failure; power-source depletion or oversensing (discussed below). *Delivery of an ineffective stimulus*, with resultant loss of capture, may be due to lead dislodgment (the most common cause); myocardial perforation with lead migration to an extracardiac position; failure of lead insulation and/or wire fracture; increased stimulation threshold due to infarct, drug effects, electrolyte imbalances, or fibrosis at the electrode site; or inappropriate programming of pacemaker stimulus strength. Lack of capture when a stimulus is delivered during the myocardial refractory period is a frequent source of misdiagnosis.

FAILURE TO SENSE. Failure to sense intracardiac signals may be due to lead dislodgment (the most common cause); inadequate amplitude or waveshape of the intracardiac electrogram due to inappropriate lead placement, fibrosis, infarct, drugs, or electrolyte disturbances; inappropriate programming of amplifier sensitivity, refractory periods, or mode (e.g., AOO, VOO); lead fracture or insulation defect; connector defect; or component failure (e.g., stuck magnetic reed switch).

Occasionally, sensing failure is misdiagnosed when spontaneous activity occurs simultaneously with delivery of the pacemaker stimulus and results in fusion beats. The reason for this is as follows: electrical activity may occur within the myocardium and be visible on the surface ECG record before it reaches the pacemaker electrode site. Concurrently with initial spontaneous depolarization, the pacemaker escape interval may elapse with resultant stimulation just prior to arrival of the spontaneous depolarization. This apparent failure to sense is, in fact, perfectly normal operation. Similar electrocardiographic patterns occur when stimuli are delivered into refractory tissue, as in AAT or VVT pacing. These events are termed "pseudo-fusion," since they do not alter the electrical activation sequence of the tissue and are characterized on the ECG by a stimulus that merely distorts inscription of the P-wave or QRS-complex.

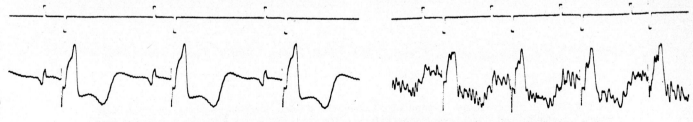

FIGURE 22–18 Lower tracings are lead III surface electrocardiograms from patient with normally functioning atrial synchronous ventricular inhibited pacemaker. Upper tracings are marker channels transmitted by the implanted pacemaker, indicating detection of atrial activity (small positive deflection) and pacing in ventricles (larger negative deflection). Right half of panel was recorded during exercise to show utility of marker channel in identifying atrial activity in presence of interference.

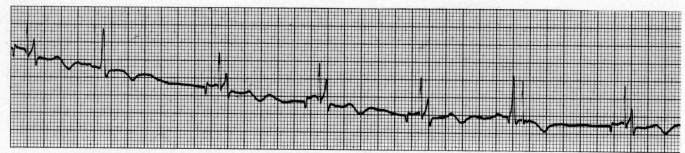

FIGURE 22–19 Surface ECG demonstrating an example of a "committed" mode DVI pacemaker. Note that the first, third, fourth, fifth, and seventh complexes are initiated by an atrial spike (small negative deflection) that paces the atrium and then a ventricular spike (large upright deflection) that paces the ventricle. The second QRS complex occurs sufficiently early to inhibit pacemaker discharge. However, the sixth QRS complex occurs early but not early enough to inhibit the atrial discharge. Following the atrial spike (seen as the initial negative deflection preceding the onset of the QRS complex, after the P wave), a conducted QRS complex occurs. However, this complex is not sensed by the pacemaker, which is, by design, committed to deliver a ventricular stimulus (large upright spike following the QRS complex in the ST segment) after stimulating the atrium, regardless of spontaneous ventricular activity. (Monitor lead.)

Another cause of apparent sensing failure is reversion to asynchronous operation in the presence of electromagnetic interference—also a normal mode of operation for many pacemakers. Finally, closely coupled intracardiac signals may occur within the pacemaker refractory period and not be sensed. This is frequently seen with certain AV-sequential (DVI) pacemakers that initiate the ventricular sense amplifier refractory period upon stimulating in the atrium. If the atrial response propagates to the ventricles, the pacemaker will not sense this conducted ventricular activity, but will stimulate into the refractory tissue. This is normal operation of such "committed" DVI devices (Fig. 22–19).

OVERSENSING. Occasionally, a pacemaker senses signals other than the cardiac signals it is designed to detect—a phenomenon referred to as "oversensing." Ventricular sensing pacemakers (DVI, VVI, VVT, VDD, DDD) may sense T waves if the pacemaker amplifier is too sensitive or if its refractory period is too short, or if the patient has unusually large or delayed T waves, as in hyperkalemia or hypocalcemia. A dislodged ventricular lead resting near the right ventricular outflow tract may cause inappropriate sensing of atrial activity. Conversely, atrial sensing pacemakers (AAI, AAT, VAT, VDD, DDD) may inappropriately sense ventricular activity if the atrial amplifier refractory period is too short or if the atrial signals are too small to be sensed, with consequent failure to initiate appropriate atrial refractory periods. The ventricular amplifier in some AV sequential pacemakers (DVI) may sense delivery of an atrial stimulus and inhibit the ventricular stimulus ("cross talk") if the pacemakers are used with incorrectly spaced bipolar electrodes or if the atrial and ventricular electrodes are not separated by a suitable distance (typically 4 cm minimum). Unipolar pacemakers may sense skeletal muscle potentials generated by contraction of the major pectoralis muscles, resulting in inappropriate inhibition (AAI, VVI, DVI, VDD, DDD) or triggering (AAT, VVT, VDD, VAT, DDD) of stimuli.

All pacemakers, except asynchronous devices, sense voltage changes that are produced when a lead with a hairline fracture or loose connection makes intermittent contact (make-break signals) (Fig. 22–20), or when two endocardial leads come into contact. Electromagnetic interference (EMI) from power lines, radio or television

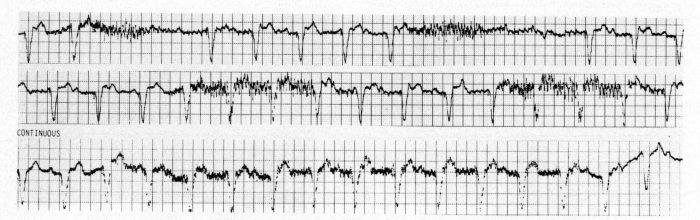

FIGURE 22–20 Electrocardiograms demonstrating inhibition of a bipolar demand pacemaker by make-break potentials created by intermittent contact at the pulse generator/lead connection. Make-break potentials were generated when the patient flexed the pectoralis major muscles ("noisy" portions of recordings). *Top,* Pacemaker in demand mode. Pulse generator discharge inhibited during isometric pectoralis muscle activity. *Middle,* Pacemaker converted to continuously discharging (asynchronous) mode by external application of magnet. Pulse generator discharges at normal rate during isometric exercise. *Bottom,* Pacemaker in demand mode following correction of improperly seated electrode terminal at the pulse generator connector block. Isometric pectoralis exercise has no effect on pulse generator discharge rate. (Monitor leads, 25 mm/sec paper speed.)

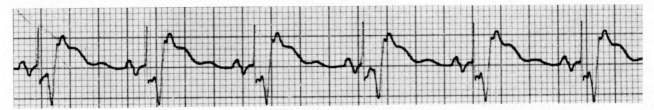

FIGURE 22–21 Electrocardiogram of a patient with a normally functioning noncommitted DVI pacemaker. In this recording, the pacemaker's atrial escape interval is completed shortly after the occurrence of spontaneous atrial activity (which is not sensed because DVI pacemakers have no atrial sensing circuits). The atrial stimulus, therefore, occurs immediately prior to the ventricular complex, which results from normal conduction of atrial activity. The pacemaker's ventricular stimulus is appropriately inhibited by sensing the conducted ventricular complex. Such records sometimes lead to a misdiagnosis of ventricular pacing at an accelerated rate when, in fact, the record indicates normal DVI pacemaker operation with delivery of atrial stimuli only. (Monitor lead.)

transmitters, and other electrical noise sources may occasionally be sensed, especially by unipolar pacemakers, because the large separation between electrodes enhances EMI detection. Sometimes this results in inhibition or triggering, but more commonly it produces reversion to the asynchronous mode that provides the patient with continued pacing support. Microwave ovens and weapons detection equipment no longer pose significant threats because of pacemaker design changes. Very rarely, a pacemaker may sense the afterpotentials remaining on a lead after delivery of a stimulus. Most often this is the result of using very wide pulse widths or excessively short refractory periods. Intrinsic EMI sources from muscle artifacts present more troublesome clinical problems than do extrinsic EMI sources from the environment.

In all cases of suspected oversensing, placing the pacemaker in an asynchronous mode (with application of a magnet when the pacemaker is permanent or turning off the sensitivity if it is an external device) will abolish the symptoms caused by the pacemaker malfunction and confirm the diagnosis (Fig. 22–20).

PACING AT AN ALTERED RATE. Causes of unexpected pacing at an altered rate include oversensing that induces rate slowing due to inhibition or rate acceleration due to triggering; rate drift, a gradual benign shift of the pacing rate due to component aging or temperature effects (most commonly found in older pacemakers that do not use digital timing circuits); rate reduction built into most pacemakers to indicate approaching power-source depletion; and component failure (usually causing either no stimulus output or a rapid stimulation that is typically limited to less than 150 ppm by "runaway" protection circuits).

Frequent misdiagnoses of pacing at an altered rate include presence of rate hysteresis that produces a long escape interval following sensed activity; reprogramming a programmable pacemaker without proper recording of the change in the patient records; tracking spontaneous intrinsic cardiac rate accelerations with VVT, AAT, VAT, VDD, or DDD pacemakers; misinterpretation of nonpacemaker artifacts such as rapid spike potentials generated by muscle fasciculation[117] or electrical noise in the ECG recording system. Lack of familiarity with operation of the device may lead to misdiagnosis. For example, a DVI pacemaker perceived to be pacing the ventricles at a rate equivalent to its V-A interval may, in fact, be delivering stimuli to the atrium and appropriately inhibiting ventricular stimuli in response to conducted ventricular activity (Fig. 22–21).

UNDESIRABLE PATIENT/PACEMAKER INTERACTIONS. Occasionally, undesirable patient/pacemaker system interactions develop. The pacemaker pocket may become infected or develop a hematoma, or the generator may erode through the pocket site. These problems occur less frequently with the current small, light-weight generators. Some patients exhibit "twiddler's syndrome," toying with their pulse generators and rotating them in their pockets, which could result in lead retraction and total system failure.

Some forms of therapy may adversely affect the operation of a pacemaker system. For example, defibrillation with the paddles placed too near the pulse generator may damage pacemaker components or may induce large currents in the pacing lead sufficient to elevate pacing thresholds or impair electrogram characteristics. Similarly, therapeutic amount of radiotherapy may adversely affect pacing function. Direct contact between an electrocautery probe and the pulse generator may damage pacemaker circuits.

Extracardiac stimulation of the pectoralis muscles or diaphragm may be observed. These problems generally are restricted to unipolar pacemakers, although they have been reported to occur rarely with bipolar systems. Decreasing the pulse width, voltage, or current of the stimulus usually eliminates or reduces such extracardiac stimulation.

Incorrect pacing mode selection for a given patient or changes in a patient's status postimplant can have serious consequences. For example, atrial tracking pacemakers (VAT, VDD, DDD) may detect retrograde atrial activity conducted with a long R-P interval following ventricular stimulation, and may induce "pacemaker tachycardia" with a rate equal to the pacemaker's upper rate limit (Fig. 22–22). Patients with an AAI pacemaker implanted to treat sinus node dysfunction or a hypersensitive carotid sinus syndrome may develop AV block (Fig. 22–23). Patients may respond poorly to other specific pacing modes depending on their underlying hemodynamic and electrophysiological substrates. In many such cases, multiprogrammable pacemakers allow alteration of pacing system characteristics without resorting to invasive procedures.

ILLUSTRATIVE APPROACHES. The following examples demonstrate how to approach problems of pacemaker malfunction. In the first case, we consider intermittent loss of capture and failure to sense spontaneous ventricular activity (Fig. 22–24). The atient had a ventricular-demand (VVI) pacemaker implanted one year ago.

The first step in troubleshooting is to list the likely causes of the symptoms. Since there are two malfunctions

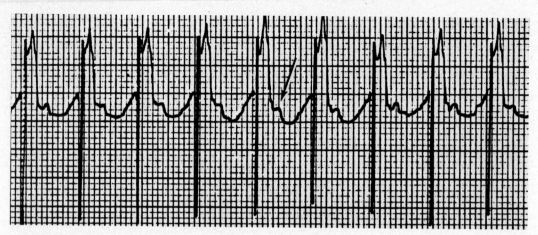

FIGURE 22–22 Electrocardiogram of a patient with a DDD pacemaker demonstrating pacemaker-induced tachycardia due to retrograde atrial activation. Each ventricular stimulus produces a retrograde P wave, which in turn triggers the pacemaker to produce yet another ventricular stimulus. This process usually repeats at a rate equal to the pacemaker's maximum tracking rate, which in this example is 135 ppm. Retrograde P wave indicated by arrow. (Lead I.)

in this example (failure to sense and failure to pace), it is highly probable—although not absolutely certain—that there is a common cause. The most likely etiologies are as follows:

Lack of Capture:
Lead dislodgment, perforation.
Lead wire fracture.
Lead insulation failure.
Pulse generator failure.
Inappropriate programming of output energy.
High threshold.
Misread ECG ("loss of capture" seen only when stimulus occurs during cardiac refractory period).

Lack of Sensing:
Lead dislodgment, perforation.
Lead wire fracture.
Lead insulation failure.
Pulse generator failure.
Inappropriate programming of amplifier sensitivity or refractory period.

Inadequate electrogram amplitude (due to infarct, electrolyte disturbance, myocardial disease).
Electromagnetic interference induced reversion to asynchronous mode.
Stuck reed switch.
Misread ECG (fusion beats).

Analysis should begin by comparing a recent 12-lead ECG to a baseline tracing that predates occurrence of the problem. The current tracing should be carefully reviewed to exclude misinterpretation of fusion beats as sensing failure or of pacing stimuli occurring during the cardiac refractory period as lack of capture. Reversion to the asynchronous mode due to electromagnetic interference usually can be eliminated as a cause of nonsensing if a 12-lead ECG shows no signs of electrical interference. Comparing the current and baseline ECGs establishes the presence or absence of lead position changes, including perforation, as evidenced by shifts in the vectors of the paced QRS complexes and pacing artifacts. It is important to remember that digital ECG systems with low sampling rates can-

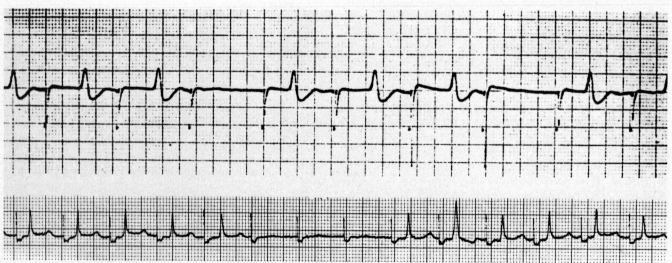

FIGURE 22–23 The top electrocardiogram illustrates inappropriate use of an atrial demand pacemaker (AAI) in a patient with type I second-degree AV block. P waves cannot be seen clearly in this lead (monitor) but follow each atrial pacing stimulus. In the lower recording, carotid sinus massage during atrial pacing in a patient with hypersensitive carotid sinus syndrome results in a series of nonconducted P waves. (Monitor lead.)

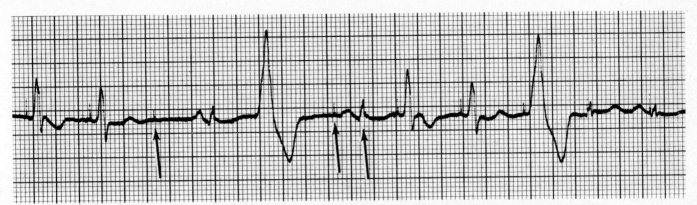

FIGURE 22-24 Failure of a VVI pacemaker. Note that pacing stimuli occasionally fail to elicit a paced QRS complex (first and second arrows), and the pacemaker occasionally fails to sense spontaneous ventricular activity (third arrow) even though it occurs after completion of the ventricular amplifier's refractory period. (Monitor lead.)

not be used to determine the vector of the pacemaker stimulus reliably. An x-ray or fluoroscopy is used to help diagnose lead dislodgment. Insulation defects in the lead result in vector changes in the pacing artifact, but not in the paced QRS complex.

Applying a magnet results in pacing without sensing. In most pacemakers, magnet application alters the pacing rate (sometimes by only a few milliseconds) to confirm that the reed switch is functioning and to eliminate the possibility of nonsensing due to a jammed reed switch.

Inappropriate programming can be evaluated by reprogramming the amplifier sensitivity and refractory period to restore sensing and to increase the stimulus intensity to restore capture. If such reprogramming failed to resolve the problem, or if the parameter settings required are not within normally accepted values, inappropriate programming can be excluded.

Wire fracture can produce nonsensing and lack of capture, but it is generally accompanied by random resetting of the escape interval as the broken wire ends touch intermittently. An x-ray pinpoints some but not all fractures. In this example (Fig. 22-24) the regularity of the escape intervals probably eliminates wire fractures as the cause of the problem.

At this point, noninvasive procedures have been explored to evaluate most potential causes for the reported malfunctions. Threshold elevation, inadequate electrogram characteristics, and pulse generator failure all require invasive evaluation, although some noninvasive determinations can be obtained if the patient has a sophisticated multiprogrammable pulse generator. Some of these devices can telemeter the intracardiac electrogram, facilitating evaluation of sensing problems. They also allow the user to obtain noninvasive threshold measurements. Nevertheless, correction of sensing and pacing failures due to any of these causes will require invasive procedures.

In the example cited, ECG evidence, shown in Figure 22-25, is most consistent with a lead dislodgment. Note the axis shift in the pacemaker-stimulus artifact and in the paced QRS complexes. Lead displacement is the most common cause of sensing and capture failures.

To extend the troubleshooting process to dual-chamber systems, the electrocardiograms of Figure 22-26 are analyzed. These records are taken from a patient who has a bipolar noncommitted atrioventricular sequential pacemak-

er (DVI), which was programed to an A-V interval of 150 msec. The patient's electrocardiogram exhibited variable A-V intervals up to 200 msec. (Fig. 22-26, upper panel) with no evidence of ventricular pacing. If the pacing system were functioning normally, no A-V interval would exceed the programed 150 msec. Potential causes for failure to pace include broken lead, defective pacemaker/lead connection, "cross talk" between atrial and ventricular channels of dual-chamber pacemakers, component failure, battery depletion, or oversensing. Oversensing could be due to sensing of P or T waves, myopotentials, electromagnetic interference, lead polarization after potentials, and cross talk (sensing of the atrial stimulus by the ventricular amplifier of a dual-chamber device) as well as detection of make-break potentials created by intermittent contact of broken electrode wires or loose connections at the pulse generator (Fig. 22-20).

As shown in the lower tracing of Figure 22-26, placement of the magnet over the pulse generator restored normal AV sequential pacing. This strongly suggests a problem due to oversensing. Myopotential inhibition can be excluded, since the generator is bipolar (muscle inhibition of bipolar generators is exceedingly rare) and because the atrial stimuli continue to occur without prolonged pauses. Electromagnetic interference is also eliminated because the generator is bipolar and there is no evidence of interference in the ECG. T-wave sensing is not a possible cause because the T waves occur after the point in the pacemaker timing cycle when a ventricular stimulus should have been generated. A loose connection is eliminated by manipulating the generator in the pocket while recording the ECG. Lead fractures are relatively uncommon, there was no evidence of pacing failure with the magnet in place, and x-ray examination showed no evidence of conductor failure. Measurement of the A-V intervals in the upper panel of Figure 22-26 reveals that the third, fifth, seventh, and ninth atrial stimuli were timed from the preceding QRS complexes (the V-A interval for this pacemaker is programed to 600 msec). The remaining stimuli were timed from their preceding occurrence rather than from the preceding QRS complexes. Thus, it is fairly evident that this pacemaker is being affected by "cross-talk" between its atrial and ventricular channels. Each atrial stimulus is sensed by the ventricular amplifier that inhibits delivery of a ventricular stimulus. When the spontaneous

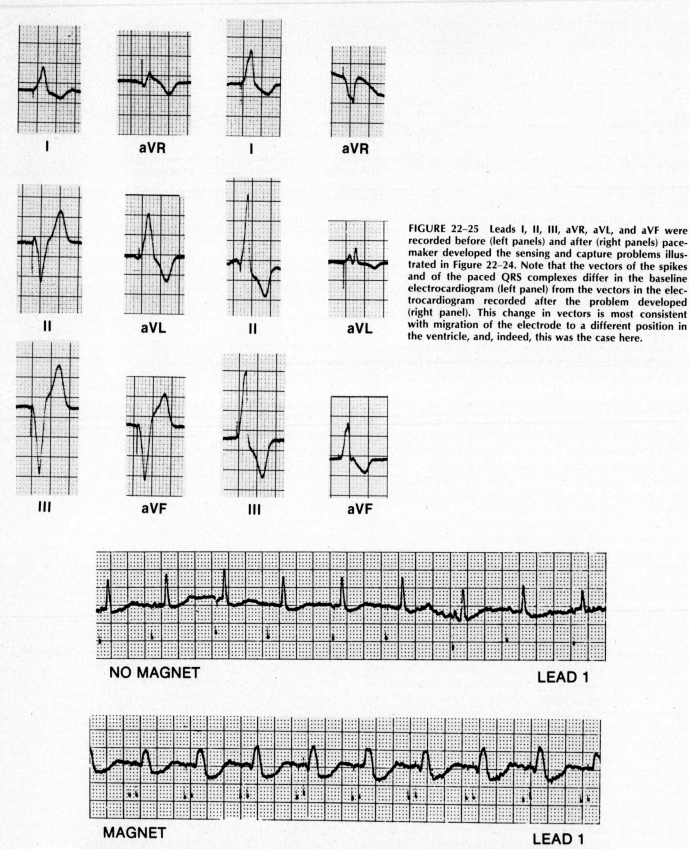

FIGURE 22–25 Leads I, II, III, aVR, aVL, and aVF were recorded before (left panels) and after (right panels) pacemaker developed the sensing and capture problems illustrated in Figure 22–24. Note that the vectors of the spikes and of the paced QRS complexes differ in the baseline electrocardiogram (left panel) from the vectors in the electrocardiogram recorded after the problem developed (right panel). This change in vectors is most consistent with migration of the electrode to a different position in the ventricle, and, indeed, this was the case here.

FIGURE 22–26 Electrocardiogram of a patient with a bipolar noncommitted AV sequential (DVI) pacemaker programed to a V-A interval of 600 msec and an A-V interval of 150 msec. The upper tracing, recorded without a magnet over the generator, shows A-V intervals as long as 200 msec with no evidence of ventricular pacing. Placement of a magnet over the generator converts it to asynchronous pacing and restores the ventricular pacing function (lower panel). This is an example of "cross talk," a malfunction in which the ventricular stimulus is inhibited by inappropriate ventricular sensing of the atrial stimulus. In this case the cause was current leakage from damaged insulation on the atrial lead. (Lead I.)

QRS complex occurs sufficiently late after the atrial stimulus so that the QRS falls outside the ventricular amplifier refractory period (200 msec), the pacemaker timing is reset for a second time by the ventricular complex. Consequently, the atrial pacing rate is variable and the A-V interval is not controlled by the pacemaker. The patient's ventricular escape rhythm maintains the cardiac rhythm.

After the pacemaker pocket was opened it was found that a 4.5-volt pacing stimulus delivered to the atrial lead reset the ventricular amplifier, thus confirming the diagnosis. Lead impedance measurements indicated a defect in the atrial lead insulation, which was found at the curvature on its J portion after removal of the lead. The insulation break allowed leakage currents from the atrial stimulus to create sufficient voltage at the ventricular lead to inhibit ventricular output. Replacement of the atrial lead corrected the problem.

These two examples are chosen to illustrate that pacing problems cover the range from being fairly simple to quite complex. Very sophisticated knowledge is required to deal with selection, implantation, and management of modern, multiprogrammable dual-chamber pacing devices.

PATIENT CONCERNS

A pacemaker can extend the patient's longevity and may greatly improve his quality of life. Yet the patient's psychological needs must be considered as well if therapy is to provide maximal benefit. The patient should understand why he has a pacemaker, how it works (in simple terms), and what it will and will not do for him (many patients think that a pacemaker cures or makes the heart stronger). He should be told what, if any, lifestyle restrictions must be observed. If this is not explained, patients may become excessively apprehensive to the point of even avoiding bathing lest they "short-circuit" their pacemakers. The patient will be greatly concerned about his dependency on the pacemaker, the risks of its failing, the anticipated longevity of the system, and the severity of the replacement procedure. If these issues are addressed with clear concise answers in lay terms, the patient with a pacemaker can fully enjoy the extension and better quality of life that this device makes possible.

Acknowledgment

The authors thank Serge Barold, M.D., for critical comments.

References

1. Zoll, P.: Resuscitation of the heart in ventricular standstill by external electric stimulation. N. Engl. J. Med. 247:768, 1952.
2. Elmquist, R., and Senning, A.: An implantable pacemaker for the heart. Proc. 2nd Int. Conf. Med. Elec. Eng., London, Iliffe and Sons, Ltd. 1959.
3. Zoll, P., and Linenthal, A.: Long-term electrical pacemakers for Stokes-Adams disease. Circulation 22:341, 1960.
4. Waldo, A., Wells, J., Cooper, T., and MacLean, W.: Temporary cardiac pacing: Applications and techniques in the treatment of cardiac arrhythmias. Prog. Cardiovasc. Dis. 23(6):451, 1981.
5. Lev, M., Kinare, S., and Pick, A.: The pathogenesis of atrioventricular block in coronary artery disease. Circulation 42:409, 1970.
6. Lie, K., Wellens, H., Schulienburg, R., Becker, A., and Durrer, D.: The factors influencing prognosis of bundle branch block complicating acute anteroseptal infarction. The value of His-bundle recordings. Circulation 50:935, 1974.
7. Fisch, G., Zipes, D., and Fisch, C.: Bundle branch block and sudden death. Prog. Cardiovasc. Dis. 23:187, 1980.
8. Nimitz, A., Shubrooks, S., Hutter, A., and DeSanctis, R.: The significance of bundle branch block during acute myocardial infarction. Am. Heart J. 90:439, 1975.
9. Atkins, J., Leshin, S., Blomqvist, G., et al.: Ventricular conduction blocks and sudden death in acute myocardial infarction. N. Engl. J. Med. 288:281, 1973.
10. Hindman, M. C., Wagner, G. S., JaRo, M., Atkins, J., DeSanctis, R., Hutter, A., Morris, J., Rubenfire, M., Scheinman, M., and Yeatman, L.: The clinical significance of bundle branch block complicating acute myocardial infarction. II. Indications for temporary and permanent pacemaker therapy. Circulation 58:689, 1978.
11. Langendorf, R., and Pick, A.: Atrioventricular block type II (Mobitz)—Its nature and clinical significance. Circulation 38:819, 1968.
12. McNally, E., and Benchimol, A.: Medical and physiological considerations in the use of artificial cardiac pacing. Part 1. Am. Heart J. 75:380, 1968.
13. Zipes, D.: Second degree atrioventricular block. Circulation 60:465, 1979.
14. Dhingra, R., Denes, P., Wu, D., Chuquimia, R., and Rosen, K.: The significance of second degree atrioventricular block and bundle branch block. Observations regarding site and type of block. Circulation 49:638, 1974.
15. Rosen, K., Lobe, M., Chuquimia, R., Sinno, M., Rahimtoola, S., and Gunnar, R.: Site of heart block in acute myocardial infarction. Circulation 42:925, 1970.
16. Hindman, M., Wagner, G., JaRo, M., Atkins, J., Scheinman, M., DeSanctis, R., Hutter, H., Yeatman, L., Rubenfire, M., Pujura, C., Rubin, M., and Mars, J.: The clinical significance of bundle branch block complicating acute myocardial infarction. I. Clinical characteristics, hospital mortality, and one year follow-up. Circulation 58:679, 1978.
17. Gann, D., Balachandran, P., El-Sherif, N., and Samet, P.: Prognostic significance of chronic versus acute bundle branch block in acute myocardial infarction. Chest 67:298, 1975.
18. Godman, M., Lassers, B., and Julian, D.: Complete bundle branch block complicating acute myocardial infarction. N. Engl. J. Med. 282:237, 1970.
19. Gould, L., Venkataraman, K., Mohammad, N., and Gomprecht, R.: Prognosis of right bundle branch block in acute myocardial infarction. J.A.M.A. 219:502, 1972.
20. Batchelder, J., and Zipes, D. P.: Treatment of tachyarrhythmias by pacing. Arch. Intern. Med. 135:1115, 1975.
21. Keren, A., Tzivoni, D., Gavish, D., Levi, J., Gottlieb, S., BenHorin, J., and Stern, S.: Etiology, warning signs and therapy of Torsade de Pointes. Circulation 64:1167, 1981.
22. Smith, W., and Gallagher, J.: "Les Torsade de Pointes": An unusual ventricular arrhythmia. Ann. Intern. Med. 93:578, 1980.
23. Robson, R. H., Pridie, R., and Fluck, D. C.: Evaluation of rapid atrial pacing in diagnosis of coronary artery disease. Br. Heart J. 38:986, 1976.
24. Goldman, B. S., and Parsonnet, V.: World survey on cardiac pacing. PACE 2(5):W1, 1979.
25. Sutton, R., Perrins, J., and Citron, P.: Physiological cardiac pacing. PACE 3:207, 1980.
26. Furman, S.: Cardiac pacing and pacemakers. I. Indications for pacing bradyarrhythmias. Am. Heart J. 93(4):523, 1977-B.
27. Dhingra, R., Palileo, E., Strasberg, B., Swiryn, S., Bauernfeind, R., Wyndham, C., and Rosen, K.: Significance of the HV interval in 517 patients with chronic bifascicular block. Circulation 64:1265, 1981.
28. Dhingra, R., Wyndham, C., Bauernfeind, R., Swiryns, S., Deedwania, P., Smith, T., Senes, P., and Rosen, K.: Significance of block distal to the His bundle induced by atrial pacing in patients with chronic bifascicular block. Circulation 60:1455, 1979.
29. Citron, P., and Duffin, E.: Implantable pacemakers for management of tachyarrhythmias. Herz 4(3):269, 1979.
30. Cooper, T., MacLean, W., and Waldo, A.: Overdrive pacing for supraventricular tachycardia: A review of theoretical implications and therapeutic techniques. PACE 1(2):196, 1978.
31. Kahn, A., Morris, J., and Citron, P.: Patient-initiated rapid atrial pacing to manage supraventricular tachycardia. Am. J. Cardiol. 38:200, 1976.
32. Hyman, A.: Permanent programmable pacemakers in the management of recurrent tachycardias. PACE 2(1):28, 1979.
33. Khan, M., Logan, K., McComb, J., and Adgey, A.: Management of recurrent ventricular tachyarrhythmias associated with QT prolongation. Am. J. Cardiol. 47(6):1301, 1981.
34. Leclercq, J., Rosengarten, M., Delcourt, P., Attuel, P., Coumel, P., and Slama, R.: Prevention of intraatrial reentry by chronic atrial pacing. PACE 3:163, 1980.
35. Harthorne, J.: Indications for pacemaker insertion: Types and modes of pacing. Prog. Cardiovasc. Dis. 23(6):393, 1981.
36. Sutton, R., and Citron, P.: Electrophysiological and hemodynamic basis for application of new pacemaker technology in sick sinus syndrome and atrioventricular block. Br. Heart J. 41:600, 1979.
37. Parsonnet, V., Furman, S., and Smyth, N. P. D.: Implantable cardiac pacemakers: Status report and resource guideline. Circulation 50:A21, 1974.
38. Parsonnet, V., Furman, S., and Smyth, N. P. D.: A revised code for pacemaker identification. PACE 4(4):400, 1981-B.
39. Nathan, D., Center, S., and Wu, C.: An implantable synchronous pacemaker for the long-term correction of complete heart block. Am. J. Cardiol. 11:362, 1963.

40. Kruse, I., Ryden, L., and Duffin, E.: Clinical evaluation of atrial synchronous ventricular inhibited pacemakers. PACE 3:641, 1980.

41. Berkovits, B., Castellanos, A., and Lemberg, L.: Bifocal demand pacing. Circulation 39:44, 1969.

42. Barold, S., Falkoff, M., Ong, L., and Heinle, R.: Committed and uncommitted AV sequential DVI pulse generators. Arrhythmias and electrocardiographic manifestations of normal function. Stimucoeur 9:353, 1981.

43. Barold, S., Falkoff, M., Ong, L., and Heinle, R.: Characterization of pacemaker arrhythmias due to normally functioning AV demand (DVI) pulse generators. PACE 3(6):712, 1980.

44. Funke, H. D.: Three years' experience in optimized sequential cardiac pacing. Stimucoeur 9(1):26, 1981.

45. Alicandri, C., Fouad, F., Tarazi, R., Castle, L., and Morant, V.: Three cases of hypotension and syncope with ventricular pacing: Possible role of atrial reflexes. Am. J. Cardiol. 42:137, 1978.

46. Davidson, D., Braak, C., Preston, T., and Judge, R.: Permanent ventricular pacing: Effect on long-term survival, congestive heart failure, and subsequent myocardial infarction and stroke. Ann. Intern. Med. 77:345, 1972.

47. Gamal, M., and Van Gelder, L.: Chronic ventricular pacing with ventriculo-atrial conduction versus atrial pacing in three patients with symptomatic sinus bradycardia. PACE 4:100, 1981.

48. Miller, M., Fox, S., Jenkins, R., Schwartz, J., and Toonder, F.: Pacemaker syndrome: A noninvasive means to its diagnosis and treatment. PACE 4:503, 1981.

49. Patel, A., Yap, V., and Thomsen, J.: Adverse effects of right ventricular pacing in a patient with aortic stenosis. Chest 72:103, 1977.

50. Samet, P., Bernstein, W., and Levine, S.: Significance of the atrial contribution to ventricular filling. Am. J. Cardiol. 15:195, 1965-B.

51. Ogawa, S., Dreifus, L., Shenoy, P., Brockman, S., and Berkovits, B.: Hemodynamic consequences of atrioventricular and ventriculoatrial pacing. PACE 1:8, 1978.

52. Chamberlain, D., Leinbach, R., Vassaux, C., Kastor, J., DeSanctis, R., and Sanders, C.: Sequential atrioventricular pacing in heart block complicating acute myocardial infarction. N. Engl. J. Med. 282:577, 1970.

53. Hartzler, G., Maloney, J., and Curtis, J., and Barnhorst, D.: Hemodynamic benefits of atrioventricular sequential pacing after cardiac surgery. Am. J. Cardiol. 40:232, 1977.

54. Samet, P., Castillo, C., and Bernstein, W.: Hemodynamic consequences of sequential atrioventricular pacing. Am. J. Cardiol. 21:207, 1968.

55. Samet, P., Castillo, C., and Bernstein, W.: Hemodynamic sequelae of atrial, ventricular, and sequential atrioventricular pacing in cardiac patients. Am. Heart J. 72:725, 1966.

56. Karlof, I.: Hemodynamic effect of atrial triggered versus fixed rate pacing at rest and during exercise in complete heart block. Acta Med. Scand. 197:195, 1975.

57. Kruse, I., Arnman, K., Conradson, T., and Ryden, L.: A comparison of acute and long-term hemodynamic effects of ventricular inhibited and atrial synchronous ventricular inhibited pacing. Circulation 65:846, 1982.

58. Kruse, I., and Ryden, L.: A comparison of physical work capacity and systolic time intervals with ventricular inhibited and atrial synchronous ventricular inhibited pacing. Br. Heart J. 46:129, 1981.

59. Haft, J.: Treatment of arrhythmias by intracardiac electrical stimulation. Prog. Cardiovasc. Dis. 16(6):539, 1974.

60. Wellens, H., Bar, F., Gorgels, A., and Muncharaz, J.: Electrical management of arrhythmias with emphasis on the tachycardias. Am. J. Cardiol. 41:1025, 1978-A.

61. Wellens, H.: Value and limitations of programmed electrical stimulation of the heart in the study and treatment of tachycardias. Circulation 57:845, 1978-B.

62. Gallagher, J., Svenson, R., Kasell, J., German, L., Bardy, G., Broughton, A., and Critelli, G.: Catheter technique for closed-chest ablation of the atrioventricular conduction system: A therapeutic alternative for the treatment of refractory supraventricular tachycardia. N. Engl. J. Med. 306:194, 1982.

63. Giannelli, S., Ayres, S. M., Gomprecht, R. F., Conklin, E. F., and Kennedy, R. J.: Therapeutic surgical division of the human conduction system. J.A.M.A. 199:123, 1967.

64. Davidson, R., Wallace, A., Sealy, W., and Gordon, M.: Electrically induced atrial tachycardia with block; a therapeutic application of permanent radio frequency atrial pacing. Circulation 44:1014, 1971.

65. Preston, T., Haynes, R., Gavin, W., and Hessel, E.: Permanent rapid atrial pacing to control supraventricular tachycardia. PACE 2:331, 1979.

66. Arbel, E., Cohen, H., Langendorf, R., and Glick, G.: Successful treatment of drug-resistant atrial tachycardia and intractable congestive heart failure with permanent coupled atrial pacing. Am. J. Cardiol. 41:336, 1978.

67. Zoll, P. M., Linenthal, A. J., and Zarsky, L. R.: Ventricular fibrillation: Treatment and prevention by external electric currents. N. Engl. J. Med. 262:105, 1960.

68. Zipes, D., and Knoebel, S.: Rapid rate-dependent ventricular ectopy. Adverse responses to atropine induced rate increase. Chest 62:255, 1972.

69. Levy, S., Gerard, R., Jausseran, J., Boyer, C., Clementy, J., Baudet, E., and Bricaud, H.: Long-term results of permanent atrioventricular sequential demand pacing. PACE 2:175, 1979.

70. Leclercq, J. F., Attuel, P., and Coumel, P.: Les stimulateurs cardiaques destines à traiter les tachycardies paroxystiques. Stimucoeur 7(1):8, 1979.

71. Hartzler, G., Holmes, D., and Osborn, M.: Patient-activated transvenous cardiac stimulation for the treatment of supraventricular and ventricular tachycardia. Am. J. Cardiol. 47:903, 1981.

72. Hartzler, G.: Treatment of recurrent ventricular tachycardia by patient-activated radio frequency ventricular stimulation. Mayo Clin. Proc. 54:75, 1979.

73. Ruskin, J., Garan, H., Poulin, F., and Harthorne, J.: Permanent radiofrequency ventricular pacing for management of drug-resistant ventricular tachycardia. Am. J. Cardiol. 46:317, 1980.

74. Griffin, J., Mason, J., and Calfee, R.: Clinical use of an implantable automatic tachycardia-terminating pacemaker. Am. Heart J. 100:1093, 1980.

75. Neumann, G., Funke, H. D., Bakels, N., Kirchoff, P. G., and Schaede, A.: A new atrial demand pacemaker for the management of supraventricular tachycardias. Proc. VIth World Symp. Cardiac Pacing, 27-7, 1979.

76. Mandel, W. J., Laks, M. M., Yamaguchi, I., Fields, J., and Berkovits, B.: Recurrent reciprocating tachycardias in the Wolff-Parkinson-White syndrome. Chest 69:769, 1976.

77. Camm, A., Nathan, A., Hellestrand, K., Ward, D., and Spurrell, R.: The clinical evaluation of tachycardia termination by utilizing autodecremental atrial pacing. PACE 4(3):A-84, 1981.

78. Curry, P., Rowland, E., and Krikler, D.: Dual-demand pacing for refractory atrioventricular reentry tachycardia. PACE 2(2):137, 1979.

79. Castellanos, A., Waxman, M., Maleiro, F., Berkovits, B., and Sung, R.: Preliminary studies with an implantable multimodal AV pacemaker for reciprocating atrioventricular tachycardias. PACE 3:257, 1980.

80. Maloney, J., Medina-Ravell, V., Pieretti, O., Portillo, B., Maduro, C., Castellanos, A., and Berkovits, B.: Follow-up assessment of dual-demand, dual-chamber DVI-DVO pacing for automatic conversion, control, and prevention of refractory paroxysmal supraventricular tachycardia. PACE 4(3):A-57, 1981.

81. Jackman, W. M., and Zipes, D. P.: Low energy synchronous cardioversion of ventricular tachycardia using a catheter electrode in a canine model of subacute myocardial infarction. Circulation 66:187, 1982.

82. Zipes, D., Jackman, W., Heger, J., Chilson, D., Browne, K., Nacarelli, G., Rahilly, G., and Prystowsky, E.: Clinical transvenous cardioversion of recurrent life-threatening ventricular tachyarrhythmias: Low energy synchronized cardioversion of ventricular tachycardia and termination of ventricular fibrillation in patients using a catheter electrode. Am. Heart J., 103:789, 1982.

83. Zipes, D., Prystowsky, E., Browne, K., Chilson, D., and Heger, J.: Additional observations on transvenous cardioversion of recurrent ventricular tachycardia. Am. Heart J., 104:163, 1982.

84. Mirowski, M., Reid, P. R., Watkins, L., Weisfeldt, M. L., and Mower, M. M.: Clinical treatment of life-threatening ventricular tachyarrhythmias with the automatic implantable defibrillator. Am. Heart J. 102:265, 1981.

85. Mirowski, M., Reid, P. R., Mower, M. M., Watkins, L., Gott, V., Schauble, J., Langer, A., Heilman, M., Kolenik, S., Fischell, R., and Weisfeldt, M.: Termination of malignant ventricular arrhythmias with an implanted automatic defibrillator in human beings. N. Engl. J. Med. 303(6):322, 1980.

86. Furman, S., and Pannizzo, F.: Output programmability and reduction of secondary intervention after pacemaker implantation. J. Thorac. Cardiovasc. Surg. 81(5):713, 1981-A.

87. Hayes, D. L., Maloney, J. D., Merideth, J., Holmes, D. R., Gersh, B., Broadbent, J. C., Osborn, M. J., and Fetter, J.: Initial and early follow-up assessment of the clinical efficacy of a multiparameter-programmable pulse generator. PACE 4(4):417, 1981.

88. Parsonnet, V., and Rodgers, T.: The present status of programmable pacemakers. Prog. Cardiovasc. Dis. 23(6):401, 1981-C.

89. Parsonnet, V.: Cardiac pacing and pacemakers. VII. Power sources for implantable pacemakers. Part 1. Am. Heart J. 94(4):517, 1977.

90. Owens, B.: The role of solid electrolytes in lithium pacemaker batteries. Solid State Ionics 3:273, 1981-B.

91. Bilitch, M., Hauser, R. G., Goldman, B.S., Furman, S., and Parsonnet, V.: Performance of cardiac pacemaker pulse generators. PACE 5(1):139, 1982.

92. Hurzeler, P., Morse, D., Leach, C., Sands, B.S., Milton, J., Pennock, R., and Zinberg, A.: Longevity comparisons among lithium anode power cells for cardiac pacemakers. PACE 3:555, 1980.

93. Owens, B., Brennen, K., and Kim, J.: Lithium pacemaker reliability. Stimucoeur 9:371, 1981-A.

94. Greatbatch, W.: Metal electrodes in bioengineering. CRC Crit. Rev. Bioeng. 5(1):1, 1981.

95. Smyth, N. P. D.: Techniques of implantation: Atrial and ventricular, thoracotomy and transvenous. Prog. Cardiovasc. Dis. 23(6):435, 1981.

96. DeCaprio, V., Hurzeler, P., and Furman, S.: A comparison of unipolar and bipolar electrograms for cardiac pacemaker sensing. Circulation 56:750, 1977.

97. Littleford, P., Parsonnet, V., and Spector, S.: Method for the rapid and atraumatic insertion of permanent endocardial pacemaker electrodes through the subclavian vein. Am. J. Cardiol. 43:980, 1979.

98. Parsonnet, V.: Routine implantation of permanent transvenous pacemaker electrodes in both chambers. A technique whose time has come. PACE 4(1):109, 1981-A.

99. Parsonnet, V., Werres, R., Atherley, T., and Littleford, P.: Transvenous insertion of double sets of permanent electrodes. J.A.M.A. 243:62, 1980.

100. Bisping, H., Kreuzer, J., Birkenheier, H.: Three years' clinical experience with a new endocardial screw-in lead with introduction protection for use in the atrium and ventricle. PACE 3(4):424, 1980.

101. El Gamal, M., vanGelder, B.: Preliminary experience with the helifix electrode for transvenous atrial implantation. PACE 2(4):444, 1979.

102. Furman, S., Pannizzo, F., and Campo, I.: Comparison of active and passive adhering leads for endocardial pacing. II. PACE 4(1):78, 1981-B.

103. Furman, S., Pannizzo, F., and Campo, I.: Comparison of active and passive adhering leads for endocardial pacing. PACE 2(4):417, 1979.

104. Messenger, J., Castellanet, M., Ellestadt, M., Greensberg, P., Wilson, W., and Stephenson, N.: New permanent endocardial atrial J lead: Implantation techniques and clinical performance. PACE 4(3):A-59, 1981.

105. Mond, H., and Sloman, G.: Small tined ventricular pacemaker leads — reduction of lead complications. PACE 4(3):A-60, 1981.

106. Smyth, N. P. D., Citron, P., Keshishian, J. M., Garcia, J. M., and Kelly, L. C.: Permanent pervenous atrial sensing and pacing with a new J shaped lead. J. Thorac. Cardiovasc. Surg. 72:565, 1976.

107. deFeyter, P., Majid, P., Hoitsma, H., Stroes, W., and Roos, J.: Permanent cardiac pacing with sutureless myocardial electrodes: Experience in first one hundred patients. PACE 3(2):144, 1980.

108. Zoll, P., Zoll, R., and Belgard, A.: External noninvasive electric stimulation of the heart. Crit. Care Med. 9(5):393, 1981.

109. Furman, S., Hurzeler, P., and Mehra, R.: Cardiac pacing and pacemakers. IV. Threshold of cardiac stimulation. Am. Heart J. 94(1):115, 1977-E.

110. Furman, S., Hurzeler, P., and DeCaprio, V.: Cardiac pacing and pacemakers. III. Sensing the cardiac electrogram. Am. Heart J. 93(6):794, 1977-D.

111. Furman, S.: Cardiac pacing and pacemakers. VIII. The pacemaker follow-up clinic. Am. Heart J. 94(6):795, 1977-C.

112. MacGregor, D., Correy, H., Noble, E., Smardon, S., Wilson, G., Goldman, B., and Wigle, E.: Computer assisted reporting system for the follow-up of patients with cardiac pacemakers. PACE 3(5):568, 1980.

113. Zipes, D. P.: Pacing 1980. PACE 4(2):182, 1981.

114. Cook, A. M., and Webster, J. G.: Therapeutic Medical Devices. Englewood Cliffs, N.J., Prentice Hall, Inc., 1981.

115. Furman, S.: Cardiac pacing and pacemakers. VI. Analysis of pacemaker malfunction. Am. Heart J. 94(3):378, 1977-A.

116. Kaul, J., Macfarlane, P., Thomson, R., and Bain, W.: An analysis of electrocardiographic, radiographic, and vector cardiographic findings in patients with implanted cardiac pacemakers. Am. Heart J. 99:686, 1980.

117. Williams, D., and Thomas, D.: Muscle potentials simulating pacemaker malfunction. Br. Heart J. 38:1096, 1976.

23 CARDIOVASCULAR COLLAPSE AND SUDDEN CARDIAC DEATH

by Bernard Lown, M.D.

HISTORICAL BACKGROUND

The problem of sudden cardiac death has been recognized since the dawn of recorded history, yet it now looms as a major problem in contemporary cardiology. In the industrially developed world, its sheer magnitude is compelling, constituting 15 to 20 per cent of all natural fatalities. In the United States, as many as 450,000 persons succumb to this condition annually. About 60 to 65 per cent of the more than 700,000 deaths from coronary heart disease every year are sudden and occur outside the hospital while the victim is attending to normal, routine activities. Although multiple causes of this phenomenon have been identified, in the majority of cases the essential pathophysiological factors relate to myocardial ischemia—the consequence of coronary atherosclerosis.

Until the advent of the coronary care unit (CCU) for treating acute myocardial infarction in the early 1960's, a sense of futility prevailed in dealing with the problem of sudden cardiac death. Its occurrence was unpredictable—the seemingly healthy subject was afflicted outside the hospital—and the pathological findings almost invariably implicated far-advanced coronary atherosclerosis. Therefore it was not illogical to deem it a stage in the inexorable advance of coronary disease, thereby generating an attitude of inevitability, irreversibility, and helplessness. However, the growth of experience in the CCU made clear that sudden death, which was most likely to occur at the inception of a myocardial ischemic episode, was reversible and could be prevented (Chap. 37).[1] An outgrowth of the CCU was the initiation of mobile coronary units to expedite treatment of the victim of myocardial infarction within the community.[2-7] These developments, as well as the widespread popularization of cardiopulmonary resuscitation techniques among nonmedical personnel, have shed new light on the syndrome of sudden cardiac death and have demonstrated decisively that this problem can be contained.

DEFINITION OF SUDDEN DEATH

The term *sudden death* is subject to wide-ranging interpretations, depending on whether it is employed by the epidemiologist, the pathologist, the clinician, the medical examiner, or the nonmedical public.[8] Customarily, the medical designation encompasses only death from natural causes and therefore excludes homicide, accidents, poisoning, or suicide. An essential element of the definition is its unanticipated occurrence. Differences in the definition of sudden death relate to the meaning imparted to "sudden" in the temporal sense. The problem is frequently compounded by the fact that the death may not have been witnessed. Death may be instantaneous or may be a process of intermediate duration, not exceeding 24 hours. Thus there are three essential elements: (1) a natural process, (2) an unexpected occurrence, and (3) a rapid development.

Sudden death can thus be defined as an unexpected, nontraumatic, non–self-inflicted fatality in patients with or without preexisting disease who die within 1 hour of the onset of the terminal event. In the case of unwitnessed death, the victim has been seen to be well within the preceding 24 hours.

DIFFERENTIAL DIAGNOSIS OF CARDIOVASCULAR COLLAPSE

Sudden cardiovascular collapse does not invariably denote a cardiac catastrophe leading to death. Most often it is a benign condition in which a quick recovery can be expected without therapeutic intervention. However, when the collapse is due to inadequate cardiac output, dire consequences ensue. Since cerebral metabolism is aerobic and depends on an uninterrupted blood supply, more than 4 minutes of asystole result in brain damage. Moreover, as little as 2 minutes of elapsed time of cardiac arrest affect the ease and outcome of resuscitation attempts, a fact probably related to the rapid development of acidosis in the hypoxic heart.[9] Prompt action is therefore mandatory, but before appropriate action is initiated, it is exigent to distinguish between simple syncope and cardiovascular collapse. A brief examination of the differential diagnosis of cardiovascular collapse is therefore in order; yet even a list as seemingly comprehensive as that shown in Table 23-1 is hardly exhaustive. As is frequently the case with clinical classifications such as this one, diverse mechanisms preclude physiological logic in developing the schematization. Necessarily more than one mechanism is involved in any of the conditions listed.

Syncope, also discussed in Chapter 28, is an abrupt, transient loss of consciousness which is the consequence of impaired cerebral metabolism due to deprivation of essential substrates such as oxygen and glucose. Four levels of possible derangements may contribute to the cerebral abnormality[10]: (1) diminution or interruption of the cerebral circulation; (2) inadequacy of cardiac output; (3) compromise of systemic blood pressure; and (4) insufficiency of oxygen and/or energy substrates in the blood delivered to the brain. In each of the clinical conditions listed in Table 23-1, various combinations of these four factors are implicated. For example, when there is loss of consciousness due to rapid tachyarrhythmia, all four factors are involved. The rapid heart action is associated with a low cardiac output that necessarily leads to reduced blood pressure, impaired cerebral circulation, and diminished oxygen tension in the blood.

The physician encountering a patient in *cardiovascular collapse* must determine whether the problem (1) relates to a self-terminating functional derangement or (2) is the result of an organic condition. The former circumstance is benign and ephemeral and resolves with time; the latter is serious and major, jeopardizes survival, and requires prompt and precisely defined measures. Up to 30 per cent of apparently healthy adults will report having experienced at least a single syncopal attack.[11] A second consideration is whether the cause is cardiac or noncardiac. Although cardiac causes are implicated in the vast majority of instances of cardiovascular collapse, the most common basis for loss of consciousness is *vasodepressor syncope*. When observed at its onset, vasodepressor syncope is preceded by symptoms of autonomic hyperactivity, including marked pallor and profuse sweating; during the collapse itself, a pulse is generally present, though faint. In contrast, *cardiac arrest* is characterized by deepening cyanosis of rapid onset, absence of heart sounds, and a lack of detectable pulses in the major vessels. These findings are sufficient to diagnose cardiac arrest.

TABLE 23-1   DIFFERENTIAL DIAGNOSIS OF CARDIOVASCULAR COLLAPSE

I. *Cardiovascular Factors*
  A. Arrhythmias
    1. Tachyarrhythmias
      a. Ventricular
      b. Supraventricular, including junctional
    2. Bradyarrhythmias
      a. Sinus node failure
      b. AV nodal disease
      c. His-Purkinje conduction impairment and Adams-Stokes syndrome
    3. Asystole
  B. Low-output states
    1. Acute myocardial infarction
      a. Congestive heart failure
      b. Cardiogenic shock
    2. Cardiomyopathy
    3. Acquired valvular stenosis
      a. Aortic stenosis
      b. Mitral stenosis
      c. Tricuspid stenosis
    4. Pericardial tamponade
    5. Hypovolemia
      a. Diuretic drugs
      b. Vasodilator drugs
    6. Postural hypotension
  C. Rupture of the heart (intracardiac or extracardiac)
  D. Aortic dissection
  E. Miscellaneous cardiac conditions
    1. Coronary embolism
    2. Cardiac tumors
    3. Subacute bacterial endocarditis
    4. Primary pulmonary hypotension
II. *Respiratory Factors*
  A. Pulmonary embolism
  B. Sudden infant death syndrome
  C. Pneumonitis
  D. Bronchial asthma
  E. "Café coronary"
  F. Asphyxia
  G. Exposure to volatile hydrocarbons ("sniffing death")
  H. Tussive syncope
  I. Pickwickian syndrome
III. *Central Nervous System Factors*
  A. Vasodepressor syncope (common faint)
  B. Carotid sinus sensitivity
  C. Stroke
    1. Cerebrovascular hemorrhage
    2. Thrombosis or embolism
  D. Pulseless disease (Takayasu's disease)
  E. Epilepsy
  F. Post micturition
  G. Infection (meningitis and encephalomyelitis)
  H. Psychologically initiated syncope
    1. Hyperventilation syndrome
    2. Hysteria
IV. *Metabolic Factors*
  A. Hypoxia
  B. Hypoglycemia
  C. Adrenal insufficiency
  D. Hypercalcemia
V. *Miscellaneous Conditions*
  A. Drugs
  B. Alcoholism
  C. Cirrhosis of the liver
  D. Hemorrhage
  E. Allergic reactions
  F. Trauma (air and fat embolism)
  G. Poisoning
  H. Electrical shock
  I. Stings and bites
  J. Overwhelming sepsis

It is essential to consider briefly the important non-cardiac conditions associated with cardiovascular collapse and to differentiate them from sudden cardiac death.

PULMONARY DISEASE

Although a multiplicity of pulmonary conditions may be associated with cardiovascular collapse, only those that present problems in the differential diagnosis of sudden cardiac death, as defined earlier, will be briefly considered.

Pulmonary Embolism (See also Chap. 46). Though extremely common, pulmonary embolism is frequently an elusive diagnostic entity. When it occurs in the absence of pulmonary infarction, the classic triad indicative of pulmonary embolism with infarction, i.e., hemoptysis, pleuritic chest pain, and dyspnea, is present in only a minority of patients. Pulmonary embolism should be suspected when there is dyspnea of sudden onset in an elderly patient with congestive heart failure or in patients who have undergone recent surgical procedures, especially orthopedic, or who have been immobilized for whatever reason. The possibility of pulmonary embolism should also be entertained in cases in which young women taking oral contraceptives experience unexplained dyspnea. When embolism is massive, obstructing at least two main pulmonary arteries as identified by angiographic studies, sudden unexplained dyspnea is the most characteristic initial symptom. There is often little else in the history, physical examination, or chest roentgenogram to lend credence to the diagnosis.

Tachypnea and tachycardia were the most commonly observed signs, occurring in 88 per cent and 63 per cent of patients, respectively.[12] Unexpected cardiovascular collapse and death in presumably normal subjects as a result of pulmonary embolism is most unusual.

Syncope may be the initial manifestation of pulmonary embolism.[13] Of 132 patients with angiographically documented pulmonary embolism, 14 per cent[14] experienced syncope, and in two-thirds of these patients, syncope was the initial symptom which caused them to seek medical attention. There were no differences between the group with syncope and that without with regard to age, associated heart disease, or the presence of congestive heart failure. However, the majority of the patients were women exhibiting severe hypotension, which was observed in 76 per cent of the patients with syncope. By contrast, only 12 per cent of the 115 patients with pulmonary embolism who did not have syncope exhibited hypotension. Nearly all the patients with syncope had evidence of right ventricular failure, were strikingly hypoxemic, and demonstrated obstruction of more than 50 per cent of the pulmonary circulation. Pulmonary infarction was uncommon among them. Some electrocardiographic evidence of acute cor pulmonale (new S_I-Q_{III}-T_{III} pattern) or new incomplete right bundle branch block was present in 60 per cent of the patients with syncope as opposed to only 12 per cent of those without syncope.

The problem of diagnosis is less difficult when syncope is caused by pulmonary embolism in the hospitalized patient. Considering the possibility of pulmonary embolism in the differential diagnosis of syncope is not an academic exercise, for the majority of patients survive when appropriately treated with heparin.[15] Rarely, pulmonary embolism, when massive, may cause electromechanical dissociation, as shown in Figure 23–1, and little else may be present to indicate the correct diagnosis. Acute rhythm disorders secondary to transient increases in pulmonary arterial pressure may also result from pulmonary arteriolar constriction. Such arterial narrowing may be secondary to the release of vasoactive substances following embolization of small pulmonary arteries in which direct mechanical factors cannot be responsible for the cardiac collapse.

Sudden Infant Death Syndrome (SIDS). Crib death is the leading cause of fatality in the first year of life and occurs with a frequency of 1 to 3 per 1000 live births. It has been estimated to claim 8,000 to 10,000 infants annually. It is defined as the sudden infant death syndrome (SIDS) and is diagnosed after autopsy by the exclusion of inherently lethal pathologic findings.[16] Death occurs during quiet sleep in infants between 1 and 6 months of age. There is significant association of SIDS with winter months, lower socioeconomic class, and a history of prematurity.[17] Eighty per cent of the affected infants, however, are not premature. An upper respiratory infection may have been recognized for a day or more.

The paucity of autopsy findings in SIDS has suggested a cardiac arrhythmia as the underlying mechanism. The abnormalities implicated have included progressive bradycardia cured by selective thoracic vagotomy[18] and ventricular fibrillation.[19,20] Schwartz has suggested that asymmetrical sympathetic innervation of the heart is the basis for the long Q-T syndrome and that this results from congenital underdevelopment of the right stellate ganglion.[20] He proposed that there may be a similar asymmetrical condition during maturation of the normal infant; the stress of hypoxia may then stimulate the left stellate ganglion and favor ventricular fibrillation.

A number of observations argue *against* the preeminence of a cardiac factor in SIDS. Among infants the age of frequent arrhythmias is the first month of life and does not correspond with the age of vulnerability to SIDS, which spares the first month and peaks during the third or fourth month.[16] A careful study of electrocardiograms of families of SIDS victims has failed to corroborate the presence of Q-T prolongation as reported by Maron et al.[19] When 108 first-degree relatives of 26 patients with SIDS were compared with 99 subjects from 22 control families, there were no demonstrable differences in Q-T interval duration.[21] The postresuscitation electrocardiograms of 21 aborted SIDS infants showed *no* prolongation of the Q-T interval.[22] Furthermore, in postmortem studies of SIDS the oxygen tension in the left heart has been found to be consistently low, suggesting that the heart beat continued *after* respiration ceased.[23] In a separate autopsy study, Beckwith found a high percentage of completely unclotted blood in SIDS, thought to be due to continued perfusion of tissues under profoundly hypoxic conditions with attendant release of fibrinolysins.[24]

It seems likely that the majority of crib deaths are not related to arrhythmia or a primary cardiac factor. A more probable explanation is that the condition is due to apnea, with a defect in regulation of alveolar ventilation.[25] Postmortem histological findings in many victims of SIDS indicate a history of chronic hypoxemia. These include pulmonary arteriolar hypertrophy, retention of brown fat, prolonged extramedullary hematopoiesis, hypertrophy of carotid bodies, and an enlarged right ventricle.[26] No doubt some infant fatalities are related to a cardiac mechanism, but these constitute a minority, perhaps accounting for less than 10 per cent of all such deaths.

Café Coronary. This condition is often confused with sudden death from coronary disease, since it typically afflicts the middle-aged man with dentures who is partaking of a hearty meal. An incidence of 0.66 per 100,000 population has remained constant over the past two decades.[27] Invariably, alcoholic beverages have been imbibed. While talking heatedly, he will take a large morsel of beef which will stick in the oropharynx and cause tracheal obstruction. The patient rapidly becomes blue, clutching at the throat and upper chest in desperate attempts at ventilation; the futile struggle merely augments the cyanosis. These symptoms are frequently misinterpreted as being due to a heart attack. Rather than maneuvers to dislodge the impacted bolus, futile attempts at chest pressure and mouth-to-mouth ventilation prove to be of no avail, and the patient succumbs unnecessarily from asphyxiation.

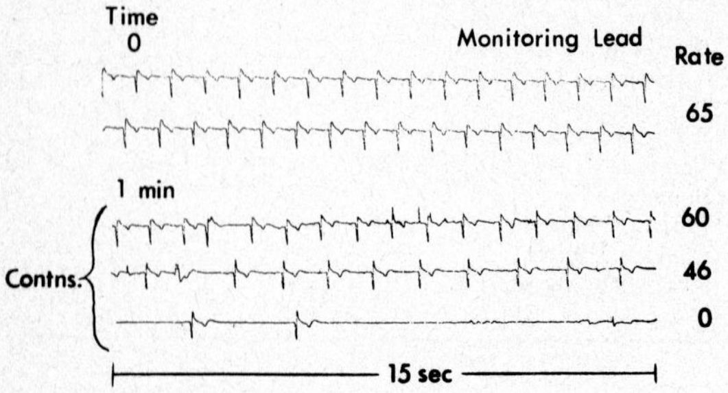

FIGURE 23–1 Electrocardiogram of patient with coronary artery disease and congestive heart failure. During trendscription, loss of blood pressure, pulse, consciousness, and pupil dilation occurred. One minute later cardiac rhythm was still regular, but within the ensuing 60 seconds, bradycardia became marked, terminating in asystole. Resuscitation was unavailing. On postmortem examination, massive embolism was found to have obstructed the main pulmonary artery. Pulse was lost at the inception of this recording, at a time when the electrocardiographic tracing was unaltered.

Volatile Hydrocarbon Inhalation. More and more ecological hazards are emerging as new products with uncertain effects on the cardiovascular system become available. An epidemic of 110 sudden deaths has been described among American youngsters, primarily on the West Coast and predominantly in white males ages 11 to 23, which resulted from sniffing airplane glue or hairsprays.[28] Severe cardiac arrhythmias intensified by hypercapnia and stress of activity are presumed to have caused the almost instantaneous fatality. Generally, after inhaling these toxic substances, the subjects will start running and will suddenly drop dead. The volatile hydrocarbons most frequently involved in deaths caused by aerosol sniffing are trichlorofluoromethane, dichlorodifluoromethane, and cryofluorane. It has long been known that the release of catecholamines that accompanies exercise and exertion potentiates the cardiac effects of volatile hydrocarbons.

CENTRAL NERVOUS SYSTEM FACTORS (see also Chap. 28)

Vasodepressor Syncope. The most common form of syncope is ascribable to a vasodepressor syndrome with vagal activation. It is primarily related to peripheral arteriolar vasodilatation with or without attendant bradycardia. Unfortunately, such collapse mimics a cardiac arrest, and the inexperienced bystander may institute cardiopulmonary resuscitation, resulting in serious visceral injury as well as rib fractures.

Carotid Sinus Syndrome. Although Weiss and Baker first emphasized that a hypersensitive carotid sinus may be responsible for syncopal episodes, appreciation of this possibility probably antedates its more recent description.[29] The Greeks may have been aware that compression of the carotid artery affected cerebral function, for the term "carotid" derives from *karos*, a Greek word meaning "heavy sleep." The earliest medical report is that of Parry in 1799, who noted that pressure on the bifurcation of the common carotid artery produced dizziness and slowing of the heart.[30] The episode, whether occurring spontaneously or induced deliberately, depends upon marked slowing of the heart rate, reduction in arterial pressure, or both.

Syncopal attacks due to carotid sinus sensitivity can be distinguished from seizures of other etiology in that they occur predominantly while the patient is standing, their onset is rapid and duration short, the postictal sensorium is clear, and they can be reproduced by means of brief carotid sinus massage.

Attacks may be precipitated by any factor that exerts direct pressure or tension on the carotid sinus. When carotid sinus sensitivity exists, it can usually be elicited on both sides, albeit to unequal degrees. This syndrome is due to sensitization not of the efferent outflow of the vagus as it enters the heart muscle but rather of the afferent nerve endings within the carotid sinus itself. It must be borne in mind that the carotid sinus in some individuals is quite sensitive, even to the extent that massage will precipitate loss of consciousness, and yet no spontaneous symptoms have ever occurred. Sensitization to carotid sinus stimulation is afforded by digitalis drugs, aging, and coronary artery disease; thus, carotid sinus syndrome represents merely an accentuation of the normal baroreflex.

Stroke. It is generally believed that stroke accounts for 10 to 20 per cent of sudden deaths.[31-33] Much of the literature on this subject derives from reports of medical examiners in metropolitan areas. These data are somewhat limited in value in that the types of cases reported include many that are medically unattended; significant numbers are also missed because they do not fall under the purview of the medical examiner. Furthermore, many patients who survive long enough will die in the hospital.

A recent prospective study conducted in a defined population is relevant to the problem of sudden death in victims of cerebrovascular accidents.[34] Among 993 new cases of strokes of all types occurring in residents of Rochester, Minnesota, during a 15-year period there were 255 deaths due to a first stroke. Fifty-two patients (30 women and 22 men) died within 24 hours, and in each case, this was the first clinically apparent stroke. The median age was 65 years, and the median time from onset to death was 10 hours. Only three deaths were virtually instantaneous, and all were due to subarachnoid hemorrhage. Most of these sudden deaths, unlike in the case of cardiac death, occurred *after* the patient had reached a hospital. All but 10 of the patients survived to reach the hospital, and in all but a few of the cases the nature of the illness was known before death occurred.

Epilepsy. Unexpected sudden death unrelated to status epilepticus has been described in epileptics in the absence of accident or concomitant natural disease. Lancisi, who wrote the first treatise on sudden death in Rome in 1707, already mentioned such a termination in victims who had a history of "fits."[35] In a careful study of eight fatal episodes by Hirsch and Martin, patients ranged from 6 to 30 years of age, and death occurred suddenly without manifestations of a motor seizure except for a brief tonic phase.[36] No satisfactory anatomical cause of death was established at autopsy in any case. Death has been ascribed to a pathophysiological mechanism in which seizure discharge in the brain stem leads to acute disruption of cardiac or respiratory function or both.

DRUGS. Only a fraction of the possible associated factors implicated in sudden cardiovascular collapse are listed in Table 23–1. Of these the most important etiological factor relates to the use or abuse of drugs.

A few key drugs of cardiovascular significance will be considered here. The most important group of agents includes the digitalis glycosides, quinidine, and psychotropic drugs.

Digitalis Glycosides (see also p. 523). It is well appreciated that these drugs can cause a profusion of diverse arrhythmias. There is veritably no abnormal cardiac mechanism that has not been reported at one time or another to have been precipitated by an excess of digitalis or by sensitization of glycoside action by potassium deficit.[37] An unusual recent epidemic of digitalis intoxication provided the first opportunity for studying the epidemiology of digitalis overdosage in a community.[38] Because of an error in manufacture, a large number of patients mistakenly received 0.20 mg of digitoxin and 0.05 mg of digoxin instead of 0.25 mg of digoxin. One hundred and seventy-nine patients were studied, 125 of whom had taken the faulty tablets for more than 3 weeks. There were six sudden deaths. Extreme fatigue and major disturbances in vision were observed in 95 per cent of the patients. A sense of "deadly tiredness or miserable feeling," a diminution in muscular strength, and difficulty in walking were common prodromes to the occurrence of major arrhythmias. Psychic disturbances such as bad dreams, restlessness, nervousness, agitation, listlessness, drowsiness, and fainting as well as pseudohallucination and delirium were noted in 65 per cent of the patients. Of the visual disturbances, most had hazy vision and had difficulty reading. Nearly all patients experienced a disturbance in red-green color perception.[38] Death that results from excessive digitalis is invariably due to ventricular fibrillation rather than to complete heart block.

Quinidine (see also p. 656). Almost since the introduction of quinidine, reports have appeared of syncopal episodes and sudden death during the course of treatment. Quinidine-induced syncope is heralded by few or no prodromes. Ventricular fibrillation is invariably demonstrated as the cause (Fig. 23–2). Attacks are characteristically sudden, are seldom preceded by warning symptoms, and consist of an abrupt loss of consciousness with cessation of respiration and involuntary muscle contractions. Occasionally grand mal seizures occur, in which case there is usually rapid and complete but possibly transient recovery. Syncopal attacks usually occur within 1 to 3 hours after the last dose of quinidine and are generally not observed with high doses of the drug. In most cases, the syncope occurs while the patient is receiving maintenance doses of quinidine. Blood levels at the time of the episode have invariably been within a low therapeutic range.[39] A majority of patients do not have prolongation of the Q-T interval,

Quinidine Syncope   Monitor Lead

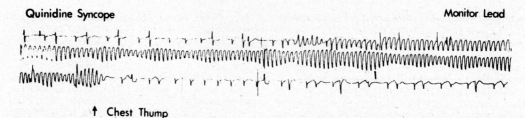

↑ Chest Thump

FIGURE 23–2 Within 48 hours following cardioversion for atrial fibrillation, the patient began to experience ventricular bigeminy while receiving 1.2 gm of quinidine in divided doses daily. Ventricular fibrillation ensued and was terminated by means of a chest thump. Numerous such bouts recurred over the next 3 hours. Blood quinidine level was 2.8 μcg/ml.

though hypokalemia may be an important predisposing factor. Nonsustained ventricular fibrillation is the basis for the syncope. Generally, these patients have also been receiving digitalis drugs. It may be that in the presence of hypokalemia, digitalis evokes ventricular ectopic activity, and quinidine, by lengthening the refractory period in the conduction system, promotes reentrant arrhythmias.

Phenothiazines and Tricyclic Antidepressants (see also pp. 1838 and 1891). With introduction of the phenothiazines and tricyclic antidepressant drugs, sudden death had been ascribed to these psychotropic agents. However, in Massachusetts more than a century ago, Dr. Luther Bell reported sudden death in schizophrenic patients in whom autopsy revealed no adequate explanation.[40] This has been referred to as "Bell's mania," "lethal catatonia," or "exhaustion death." Thus, although sudden, unexplained death in the mentally ill is a phenomenon that has been described for over a century, in the past two decades it has been largely attributed to phenothiazines. Whether the so-called phenothiazine deaths are due to the drug itself or to the syndrome of "lethal catatonia" or whether they merely reflect the increasing recognition of the widespread occurrence of sudden death in the community is not certain.[41]

There appears to be an increased risk of sudden death in cardiac patients receiving amitriptyline. In a hospital-based drug information survey, Coull and coworkers have investigated unexpected death in patients diagnosed as having disease and who were receiving this drug.[42] Of 53 patients with cardiac disease, 6 died suddenly after receiving the drug compared with none of 53 control patients matched for sex and age, diagnosis, and length of stay in the hospital. This high frequency of unexpected death was not found in patients receiving imipramine nor in patients receiving amitriptyline who did not have cardiac disease.

SUDDEN CARDIAC DEATH

The prevailing point of view is that sudden cardiac death in the United States is most frequently due to coronary heart disease. Scars of prior myocardial infarction are common, and coronary atherosclerosis is extensive. The problem resides not in the hospital but within the community. The prospective pooled epidemiological studies in Framingham and Albany have confirmed that sudden, unexpected death observed to occur within 1 hour of collapse is the initial and terminal expression of coronary heart disease in over half of the decedents.[43]

SOME EPIDEMIOLOGICAL CONSIDERATIONS. Among patients with ischemic heart disease, the incidence

of sudden death increases with age. Indeed, when all known risk factors are combined, age continues to be a potent predictor of a coronary event. This is particularly true among individuals with high-risk coronary profiles.[44] The incidence of sudden death from ischemic heart disease in the age range of 50 to 60 has been estimated to be approximately 2.0 per thousand per year for white men, 1.3 for black men, 1.1 for black women, and 0.5 for white women.[43,45,46] In these retrospective studies of sudden death, up to half the decedents have had known heart disease, they are predominantly male, and risk of sudden death increases with age, hypertension, heavy cigarette smoking, and diabetes mellitus. It is therefore pertinent to examine whether there exists a particular risk-factor profile predisposing to sudden cardiac death.

Role of Coronary Risk Factors. In the pooled prospective study cited above, the question of whether certain characteristics define a coronary population more susceptible to sudden death was carefully examined.[43,47] The population studied involved 4120 men ages 45 to 74. With 1 hour serving as the cutoff point to define sudden death, 109 coronary deaths were adjudged sudden and 125 nonsudden. The classic risk factors (Chap. 35) evaluated were hypercholesterolemia, hypertension, and smoking. No combination of risk factors permitted identification of patients destined to die suddenly. In some population subsets, however, the presence of certain risk factors isolated enhanced susceptibility to sudden death according to sex or race. For example, there was a high prevalence (55 per cent) of hypertension among black women who died suddenly, white women who were heavy smokers had a fourfold higher risk of sudden death, and a higher risk was also noted for divorced and single women, regardless of race.[48]

There are no persuasive data to show that correcting hyperlipidemia will protect against sudden death; however, lowering of blood pressure may exert a beneficial effect, and there is a suggestion that cessation of smoking may be salutary. Wilhelmson et al. have shown that among patients who stopped smoking after suffering myocardial infarction, the risk of sudden death appeared to be reduced in the succeeding 2 years.[49] From the point of view of the clinician who might wish to institute prophylactic measures, the risk factors at present identified define enhanced susceptibility to coronary heart disease, but no combination of currently recognized risk factors uniquely selects out a subset of the population prone to sudden cardiac death. It must be emphasized, however, that death, though often unexpected, is not entirely unpredictable, since three-fourths of those dying suddenly have been recognized previously as having hypertension, heart disease, or diabetes mellitus.[50]

Prodromes to Sudden Cardiac Death. In the second and third decades of this century when myocardial infarction was first recognized as a distinctive syndrome, pioneers such as Herrick[51] and Levine[52] were already aware of the presence in some patients of a symptomatic phase antedating the acute attack. The incidence of such symptoms was not appreciated until Feil[53] and Sampson and Eliaser[54] reported the presence of premonitory pains in the period prior to hospitalization in patients with myocardial infarction. Since the advent of the coronary care unit in the late 1960's, it has been found that two-thirds of the patients experiencing myocardial infarction develop prodromal symptoms in the period prior to infarction.[55,56] (See also Chapter 37.)

Pain is the most common premonitory symptom and has been noted in 70 to 100 per cent of the patients having prodromes. Other symptoms were much less common and include weakness, dyspnea, fatigue, nausea, nervousness, palpitation, and depression. The problem is more complex when one attempts to assess the occurrence of prodromes among victims of sudden cardiac death, because in this case, the only knowledgeable witness is not available to provide testimony. However, the fact that many patients who present with myocardial infarction have experienced worsening angina has suggested that sudden cardiac death might also be preceded by such warnings which, if heeded, could permit institution of prophylactic measures.[50,57]

It is therefore pertinent to examine prospective studies that have focused on prodromes in the hope of identifying patients susceptible to myocardial infarction and sudden death. In a defined population of 25,000 men between the ages of 35 and 69 living in Edinburgh, Scotland, complete information on all acute heart attacks was obtained from general practitioners.[58] During a 6-month period, 87 patients died suddenly within 1 hour of the onset of symptoms and 104 patients sustained myocardial infarction. Only 10 (12 per cent) of those who died suddenly had recently consulted their doctor because of new or worsening anginal pain compared with the 34 (33 per cent) who subsequently sustained infarction. A further point of interest was that of the 87 patients who died suddenly, 40 (46 per cent) had seen a doctor within the preceding 4 weeks. However, of these, only 10 patients had referred to symptoms of angina pectoris; the majority saw their physicians for a variety of reasons unrelated to the heart. This study was then extended to a period of 2½ years involving 251 patients with unstable angina referred by general practitioners from their communities.[59] Of those patients enrolled during this period, only 10 per cent progressed to definite myocardial infarction; an additional 2 per cent had a possible myocardial infarction; and 3 per cent died suddenly. It is therefore evident that only a small proportion of sudden cardiac deaths in the community could be identified by means of a change in or new occurrence of cardiac symptoms.

From these facts a number of epidemiologists have concluded that the risk factors for sudden death are identical to those factors predisposing to coronary artery atherosclerosis, with similar therapeutic and prophylactic implications.[60] The long-held view that sudden cardiac death is the consequence of acute myocardial infarction has been the basis for its use as a model in the experimental laboratory; however, since an acute myocardial lesion is not necessarily the basis for sudden cardiac death, and it is possible that a wrong model has been selected, an entirely different set of risk factors may require investigation.

PATHOLOGY OF SUDDEN CARDIAC DEATH. In the large majority of patients with sudden cardiac death, severe occlusive atherosclerotic disease of major epicardial coronary vessels is present.[61,62] In nearly two-thirds of cases, three vessels showed more than 75 per cent luminal stenosis.[63] The particular arteries involved in victims of sudden cardiac death were the left anterior descending (96 per cent), right coronary (79 per cent), left circumflex (66 per cent), and left main coronary (34 per cent) arteries. The vascular obstruction was generally found in both proximal and distal segments of epicardial arteries.[64-66] Surprisingly, left main coronary artery involvement is rare. Davies[65] found this lesion in only 4 of 194 victims of sudden cardiac death (2 per cent), whereas Baroldi et al.[62] noted it in 10 of 208 cases (5 per cent).

Acute coronary arterial events such as thrombosis of the diseased vessel, hemorrhage into a plaque, or rupture of a plaque have been sought as possible explanations for sudden death. Such vascular lesions are, in fact, observed in only a minority of cases.[62] The incidence of acute occlusive thrombosis is related to the length of survival. Fewer than one-third of patients will exhibit such a lesion when survival is 1 hour.[67,68] However, in nearly 90 per cent of patients dying from acute transmural myocardial infarction, fresh thrombotic lesions will be evident in one or more coronary arteries when death is long delayed, leading to the observation that thrombosis may be the *consequence* rather than the *cause* of myocardial infarction.[65,68] (See also Chap. 37 for a discussion of this subject.)

Abnormalities of intramyocardial arteries are rarely the principal vascular lesion in sudden cardiac death and virtually never exist apart from significant involvement of the epicardial vessels.[62,63,69] Coronary microembolism may play a role in the pathologic conditions of a small percentage of patients dying suddenly and may be of platelet, thrombotic, or atheromatous origin.[70] Platelet aggregates have been found in small coronary vessels in a majority of cases of sudden cardiac death studied by Haerem[70] but not by Lie and Titus[69] or by Davies.[65] Pertinent in this context is the observation of Folts and coworkers that cyclic reductions in flow to zero occurred when the lumen of a canine coronary artery was obstructed by 60 to 80 per cent.[71] Periodic cessation of flow was due to platelet aggregates, and this process was prevented by aspirin administration. It may well be that by the time ventricular fibrillation supervenes, the provocative platelet nidus has disaggregated, thereby explaining its absence on postmortem study. Specific lesions in the vessels of the sinoatrial or atrioventricular nodes are, as a rule, absent.[62] Lie and Titus found discrete infarctions or hemorrhage in the atrioventricular junction or peripheral bundle branches in only 2 of 49 victims of sudden cardiac death.

Selective myocardial necrosis, characterized by widely scattered myofibrillar degeneration, is found in about 80 per cent of cases of sudden cardiac death.[61] Changes typical of myocardial infarction are unusual. Cardiomegaly of moderate degrees is observed in about one-half to two-thirds of cases.[62,69]

Thus, it can be concluded that sudden cardiac death does not exhibit a *distinctive* constellation of pathomorphological lesions. Advanced degrees of coronary atherosclerosis and its myocardial consequences are the rule, and the spectrum of lesions extends from the minor and trivial to the most severe. Acute thrombosis is noted in about 10 per cent of cases and recent myocardial infarction in about 5 per cent.[61,62] That the underlying cardiac disease is not the exclusive variable is indicated by the fact that when subjects afflicted with cardiac arrest are promptly resuscitated, they survive for prolonged periods and frequently without significant limitations due to the underlying heart disease.

Pertinent new data relating to coronary pathology and myocardial impairment are now being derived from angiographic and hemodynamic studies of patients resuscitated from imminent sudden cardiac death. Weaver and coworkers have examined coronary anatomy and left ventricular function in 64 patients with ischemic heart disease who were successfully resuscitated after out-of-hospital ventricular fibrillation.[72] The majority (72 per cent) had a previous history of cardiovascular disease, and in the remaining 28 per cent ventricular fibrillation was the first indication of the presence of a cardiac problem. In 60 of the 64 patients the diameter of at least one major coronary artery was reduced 70 per cent or more. Severe stenosis of two coronary arteries was observed in 28 per cent, and 33 per cent had triple-vessel disease. Distribution of coronary lesions showed nearly equal involvement of the left anterior descending, circumflex, and right coronary arteries. The left main coronary artery showed moderate stenosis in only four patients and severe narrowing in only one. In 20 patients (30 per cent) more than half the left ventricular wall circumference contracted abnormally, and only 19 patients (30 per cent) were free of left ventricular contraction abnormalities. Mitral regurgitation was present in nine patients and was judged to be moderate in four and mild in five. Of these 64 resuscitated patients, 14 subsequently died suddenly or had recurrent episodes of ventricular fibrillation and showed more extensive abnormalities of the coronary artery and myocardium.

The studies of Cobb and coworkers, however, lend support to the view that while coronary artery disease is extensive, myocardial infarction is not usual.[73] Thus, only 57 of 305 patients resuscitated from ventricular fibrillation showed sequential electrocardiographic changes consistent with acute transmural infarction (Fig. 23–3). Even this low incidence of 20 per cent may be an excessive figure with regard to the precipitation of sudden cardiac death by acute myocardial infarction. It is possible that in patients with extensive coronary vascular disease, cessation of myocardial perfusion during ventricular fibrillation as well as the attendant stresses of cardiopulmonary resuscitation is the cause of infarction.

CLINICAL BACKGROUNDS FOR NONISCHEMIC SUDDEN CARDIAC DEATH.

Although coronary heart disease plays a preeminent role and accounts for over 75 per cent of sudden cardiac deaths, other cardiac conditions are implicated in about 20 per cent. Table 23–2 lists a number of these conditions, but is not intended to be ex-

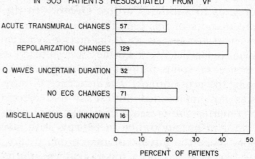

OCCURRENCE OF ELECTROCARDIOGRAPHIC CHANGES OF ACUTE MYOCARDIAL INFARCTION IN 305 PATIENTS RESUSCITATED FROM VF

	PERCENT OF PATIENTS
ACUTE TRANSMURAL CHANGES	57
REPOLARIZATION CHANGES	129
Q WAVES UNCERTAIN DURATION	32
NO ECG CHANGES	71
MISCELLANEOUS & UNKNOWN	16

FIGURE 23–3 This tabulation of electrocardiographic changes of acute myocardial infarction after resuscitation from ventricular fibrillation derives from the Seattle experience. (From Cobb, L. A., et al.: Clinical predictors and characteristics of the sudden cardiac syndrome. *In* Proceedings of the First U.S.–U.S.S.R. Symposium on Sudden Death, Yalta, October 3–5, 1977. U.S. Department of Health, Education, and Welfare, Public Health Service, National Institutes of Health, D.H.E.W. Publication No. NIH78-1470, 1978.)

haustive. Those conditions in which there is particular interest will now be considered briefly.

Mitral Valve Prolapse Syndrome (see also p. 1089). The wide clinical application of echocardiography has emphasized the prevalence of abnormal mitral valve motion syndromes. Arrhythmias associated with this syndrome include ventricular premature beats, ventricular tachycardia, paroxysmal atrial tachycardia, and atrial fibrillation.[74-78] In the majority of patients, the ventricular premature beats decrease during sleep.[79]

Despite the ubiquity of ventricular arrhythmias among patients with prolapse of the mitral valve, sudden cardiac death is uncommon.[80,81] When it does occur, sudden death has been presumed to be due to ventricular fibrillation. A composite clinical profile emerges: a woman in her thirties or forties, with significant prolapse of the mitral valve, advanced grades of ventricular ectopic activity, and a history

TABLE 23–2   CAUSES OF SUDDEN CARDIAC DEATH IN ABSENCE OF CORONARY ARTERY DISEASE

I. *Congenital Heart Disease*
  A. Structural anomalies
  B. Electrical derangements due to
    1. Sinoatrial disease
    2. Atrioventricular nodal disease
    3. Accessory bypass tracts
    4. Hereditary Q-T prolongation syndromes
      a. Jervell and Lange-Nielsen syndrome
      b. Romano-Ward syndrome
II. *Acquired Heart Disease*
  A. Acute pericardial tamponade
  B. Myocardial disease
    1. Obstructive and nonobstructive cardiomyopathy
    2. Myocarditis
    3. Infiltrative disease (e.g., amyloid, sarcoid, hemochromatosis, scleroderma, and so on)
    4. Primary degeneration of conduction system
    5. Metastatic malignant disease
    6. Cardiac tumors (e.g., atrial myxomas)
  C. Valvular disease
    1. Subacute bacterial endocarditis
    2. Mitral valve prolapse syndrome
    3. Aortic stenosis
    4. Displacement of valve prosthesis
  D. Coronary embolism
  E. Cardiac rupture and dissection
III. *Apparently Normal Heart*

of syncopal or presyncopal attacks. Rarely, bradycardia and asystole are demonstrated to be the mechanisms for syncope.[82] Among patients with prolapse of the mitral valve and syncope, as in syncope of any etiology, there is need to define the causative mechanism precisely before launching into a prophylactic program against recurrent cardiovascular collapse.

Hereditary Q-T Prolongation Syndromes (see also pp. 727 and 1626). Two syndromes have been related to hereditary prolongation of the Q-T interval. These are characterized by a family history of syncopal episodes and sudden death due to paroxysmal ventricular arrhythmias. When associated with autosomal recessive inheritance and congenital deafness, it has been designated the *Jervell and Lange-Nielsen syndrome.*[83] When the pattern of inheritance is autosomal dominant and no deafness is present, it has been termed the *Romano-Ward syndrome.*[84,85] Asymmetrical activation of the peripheral sympathetic nervous system had been suggested as the factor possibly responsible for the Q-T prolongation.[86,87] This may result in a reduction in neural activity of the right cardiac sympathetic nerves and/or enhanced activity of the left. Schwartz and colleagues have recently called attention to multiple reports of low resting heart rates in affected individuals and to failure of exercise to increase the rate appropriately.[87] Stimulation of the left stellate ganglion prolongs the Q-T interval, reduces the threshold for ventricular fibrillation, and enhances ventricular excitability.[88] Changes in the Q-T interval and T wave analogous to those found in the hereditary Q-T interval prolongation syndromes have been produced in experimental animals by means of right stellate ganglion section and left stellate ganglion stimulation.[89,90] Indeed, unilateral cervicothoracic sympathetic ganglionectomy has been reported to eliminate recurrent malignant arrhythmias.[91] However, some investigators have failed to demonstrate clearcut sympathetic imbalance to account for the Q-T prolongation.[92] The Q-T interval reflects the duration of myocardial electrical refractoriness. When this interval is prolonged, disparity in recovery of excitability is increased in myocardial fibers. Thus, an impulse discharged prematurely is more likely to encounter varying degrees of recovery and will traverse an erratic path favoring reentrant depolarization and self-sustaining electrical activity.

Preexcitation Syndromes (see also pp. 628 and 712). Accelerated conduction from atrium to ventricle, usually engaging accessory pathways that either bridge the atrioventricular groove or merely bypass atrioventricular junction nodal tissue, is usually a benign congenital disorder. Disabling arrhythmias afflict only a minority of these patients. Sudden death, however, has been reported in the Wolff-Parkinson-White syndrome.[93,94] Two mechanisms are believed to be implicated in the precipitation of ventricular fibrillation. The first involves the development of an early premature atrial depolarization which traverses the bypass tract and captures the ventricle during its vulnerable period. The second mechanism is due to ultrarapid tachycardia as a consequence of atrial fibrillation and the antegrade conduction of the impulse down the anomalous pathway. The rapid ventricular rate may cause inadequate coronary artery flow and lead to ischemia, cardiac hypoxia, and ventricular fibrillation. At

times digitalis glycosides may shorten the refractory period in the anomalous pathway and thus, in the presence of atrial fibrillation, paradoxically accelerate the ventricular response. In the presence of rates of 300 beats/min or more, ventricular ischemia ensues and fibrillation may be precipitated. Among 25 patients with Wolff-Parkinson-White syndrome who experienced ventricular fibrillation, in all the mechanism was atrial fibrillation with rapid ventricular response from antegrade conduction over the accessory pathway.[94]

Left Ventricular Outflow Tract Obstruction, Obstructive and Nonobstructive Cardiomyopathy, and Aortic Valvular Stenosis (see also Chaps. 30, 32, and 41). The association of aortic stenosis with sudden cardiac death has been appreciated in children as well as in adults of all ages, including patients with bicuspid valves irrespective of etiology (i.e., of congenital, rheumatic, or calcific origin).[95-97] Syncope and sudden death have also been reported to have occurred in patients with subvalvular stenosis. The predisposing factors for syncope and sudden death in patients with aortic valvular stenosis include (1) a large left ventricle, (2) a high systolic gradient across the aortic valve with a markedly reduced valve area, and (3) replacement of myocardium by fibrosis. In a hemodynamic study of 29 patients with aortic stenosis, near syncope was found to be associated with a fall in cardiac output, without significant arrhythmias.[96] Sudden death is also a problem among long-term survivors of aortic valve replacement. Sixteen such patients were distinguished from a control group of 52 survivors by the occurrence of ventricular arrhythmias (44 per cent vs. 10 per cent, p < 0.05) and the greater incidence of congestive heart failure (62 per cent vs. 8 per cent, p < 0.05).[98] Late sudden death has also been reported after surgical repair of *coarctation of the aorta.* Among 343 such patients followed for an average of 12 years, there were 38 late fatalities, of which 16 were sudden and unexpected, an incidence of 47 per cent.[99] The incidence of sudden death was much higher in patients operated on after puberty than in children and may relate to the duration of the hypertensive stress on the aorta, since rupture of an aortic aneurysm is not uncommon.

Sudden death is observed not uncommonly in various forms of hypertrophic obstructive cardiomyopathy. It has been estimated that this condition accounts for 1 in every 200 sudden deaths, occurring most often in those under age 30.[100] The comprehensive studies of this syndrome by Frank and Braunwald showed that among 126 patients for whom the natural history of their disease was fully described, 10 died as a consequence of their disease, and 6 of these deaths were sudden and unexpected.[101]

Chronic Bifascicular Block (see also page 219). It has been presumed that sudden death in patients with chronic bifascicular block is due to progression to complete heart block, and therefore the insertion of a pacemaker has been deemed the proper prophylactic measure. However, current studies indicate that the incidence of spontaneous progression to complete heart block is relatively low.[102,103] There is, on the other hand, a high incidence of sudden cardiac death in patients with bifascicular block. Among 277 patients with bifascicular block, 60 had complete left bundle branch block, 196 had complete right bundle branch block with left anterior fascicular block, and 21 had complete right bundle branch block with left posterior fascicular block. Sixty-eight of these patients died (24.5 per cent), 30 of whom died suddenly during a mean follow-up of 555 ± 24 days. There was a significantly higher incidence of left bundle branch block, a significantly lower incidence of right bundle branch block, and a greater prevalence of ventricular premature beats in those who died suddenly. Electrophysiological studies showed no significant differences in the atrial-His (A-H) and His-ventricular (HV) intervals between the groups who died and those who survived. Ten of the deaths were instantaneous and were not preceded by any symptoms. In four cases in which death was documented electrocardiographically, ventricular fibrillation was the terminal event. These investigators believe that ventricular fibrillation rather than progression to complete heart block constitutes the basis for sudden cardiac death among patients with advanced degrees of intraventricular conduction impairment.[102,103]

Subjects with Normal Hearts. Any review of the literature concerning sudden cardiac death reveals a small percentage of individuals in whom, after the most careful pathomorphological search, no explanation is found for the unexpected fatality[104,105]; this is a more common finding among the young. In 18 patients who experienced recurrent ventricular fibrillation or ventricular tachycardia, 6 had no demonstrable cardiac abnormalities by extensive noninvasive and invasive studies.[106] As the practice of out-of-hospital resuscitation becomes more widespread and effective, increasing numbers of individuals with few demonstrable structural cardiovascular abnormalities will probably be found. It is conceivable that the lethal derangements in rhythm in these individuals are due to neurochemical as well as electrophysiological malfunction that cannot be identified with the use of present techniques. It has been suggested that ventricular fibrillation triggered by higher neural activity accounts for these sudden fatalities.[107,108] However, in a group of 29 highly conditioned athletes who died suddenly, Maron et al.[109] found structural cardiovascular abnormalities in 28. The most common cause of death, which was overlooked during life, was hypertrophic cardiomyopathy, which was present in 14 athletes. An additional rare cause of unheralded sudden death in previously healthy persons has been attributed to intramural bridging of the left anterior descending coronary artery.[110] In each of three subjects, death occurred during strenuous exercise.

Miscellaneous Causes. The list of unusual causes of sudden death is extensive and variegated. These causes alter with the fashion of the times. With popularization of liquid protein diets for rapid weight reduction, there have been numerous healthy people, especially young women, who have suddenly died. Isner et al.[111] reported on 17 such patients who were free of cardiovascular disease prior to dieting. All but one were severely obese women. In an average of 5 months of rigorous caloric restrictions, they lost 35 per cent of their predicted body weight. Electrocardiograms made during dieting were available in 10 patients; 9 of these showed Q-T interval prolongations and all 10 exhibited paroxysmal ventricular tachycardia. A detailed prospective study of the effects of a liquid protein diet was conducted by Lantigua et al.[112] in six grossly obese sub-

jects. In three of the six, life-threatening arrhythmias were documented by means of 24-hour Holter monitoring. These developed within 4 weeks of initiating the reducing diet. The arrhythmias were unrelated to changes in body potassium balance. Prolongation of the Q-T interval present in many of these patients predisposes to malignant ventricular arrhythmias. But the basis for the Q-T alteration remains obscure and is not accounted for by hypokalemia, hypocalcemia, or hypomagnesemia. Unkown deficiencies of proteins, trace elements, and micronutrients may be the critical factor; on the other hand, starvation induces pathological alteration in the hypothalamic-pituitary axis, which may account for both the Q-T interval changes and the arrhythmia.[183]

SUDDEN CARDIAC DEATH RELATED TO ISCHEMIC HEART DISEASE. The overwhelming majority of sudden deaths are related to impaired coronary perfusion of the myocardium in patients with extensive atherosclerotic vascular disease. When sudden cardiac death develops as a consequence of myocardial infarction, prodromal symptoms are usually present and frequently lead to hospitalization. In the absence of myocardial infarction, death is frequently instantaneous. Sudden cardiac death therefore may be considered in these two circumstances and may occur either in the hospital or in the community.

Death in the Hospital. In hospitalized patients with acute myocardial infarction, sudden cardiac death is due to one of three mechanisms: (1) ventricular fibrillation; (2) bradyarrhythmia, including complete heart block; or (3) electromechanical dissociation. The tendency for ventricular fibrillation to occur, both in experimental animals following coronary artery ligation and in humans, is strikingly enhanced at the very inception of an acute ischemic episode. In humans, it has been estimated that ventricular fibrillation is 25 times more frequent during the initial 4 hours after the onset of symptoms than in the following 24 hours.[113] If resuscitation is promptly effected, the fact that ventricular fibrillation had occurred may not in itself alter the prognosis of patients with myocardial infarction. Indeed, life expectancy is essentially the same as in those patients with comparable infarcts who had not experienced ventricular fibrillation.[114,115]

Bradyarrhythmias with hypotension and asystole or complete heart block are responsible for a small percentage of cases of sudden cardiac death in patients with acute myocardial infarction. These disorders are more common when the transmural lesion is in an inferior position than when it is located elsewhere. Indeed, 61 per cent of patients with inferior infarction exhibit such disorders within 1 hour after onset of symptoms.[3,114]

A small group of patients with acute myocardial infarction who die suddenly present a most unusual sequence of events:[1] There is loss of consciousness, pulse, and blood pressure; heart sounds are inaudible; respiration is gasping; and yet the electrocardiographic pattern is seemingly unaltered. Rapidly the rate of ventricular depolarization decreases; P waves flatten and then disappear; and the QRS widens progressively until it becomes broad and deformed, eventuating in a completely asystolic straight line. Resuscitation and cardiac pacing are unavailing. This stage has been termed electromechanical dissociation.[1,115] Possible explanations include cardiac rupture, reflex sympathetic inhibition, and massive extension of infarction.

A small number of sudden deaths due to arrhythmia occur among patients convalescing from acute myocardial infarction after discharge from the coronary care unit.[116,117] Post CCU in-hospital sudden cardiac death has been reported to afflict 3 to 20 per cent of patients who succumb during the hospitalization.[118] Certain clinical features during this convalescence period help identify those at increased risk for in-hospital sudden cardiac death and include the following:

1. Persistent sinus tachycardia.
2. Anterior location of transmural infarct.
3. High incidence of complex ventricular arrhythmias at the onset of acute infarction.
4. Development of recent fascicular or bundle branch block.
5. High prevalence of arrhythmias associated with pump failure, such as atrial tachycardia, atrial flutter, and atrial fibrillation.
6. Presence of significant left ventricular failure.

There is no correlation between the occurrence of ventricular arrhythmia at the onset of myocardial infarction and the prevalence of ectopic activity during later in-hospital convalescence.[119] By contrast, occurrence of significant ventricular arrhythmias in the late hospital phase following recovery from acute myocardial infarction is associated with an increased incidence of sudden cardiac death during the 7 months after hospitalization.[118] This association is especially striking in those patients who, in addition to having an arrhythmia, had a reduced left ventricular ejection fraction.[118]

Death Outside the Hospital. The advent of coronary care units and their success in resuscitating patients with ventricular fibrillation have led to the development of mobile life support units to help alleviate the problem of sudden cardiac death occurring outside the hospital setting. Especially instructive has been the broadly based, ongoing community effort in Seattle, Washington.[6,72,73,120,121] During a 6-year period, over 400 patients with ventricular fibrillation have been resuscitated before admission to the hospital and were ultimately discharged as long-term survivors. An important aspect of this program is the extensive system of public education in cardiopulmonary resuscitation. In approximately 35 per cent of cases of cardiac arrest, resuscitation is initiated by 1 of the 125,000 citizens who have completed a specialized training program. In those instances in which resuscitation was initiated by bystanders, the frequency of long-term survival doubled in comparison with those in which resuscitation was delayed until the arrival of specialized emergency teams.

Cobb and coworkers made the important observation that there is a very high rate of recurrence of ventricular fibrillation among survivors of cardiopulmonary resuscitation.[73,120,121] The mortality rate at 1 year was 26 per cent; at 2 years it was 36 per cent. Among the 305 patients successfully resuscitated who had ischemic heart disease, there were 112 deaths, of which 86 (77 per cent) were due to repeated episodes of ventricular fibrillation or sudden cardiac death. Interestingly, when ventricular fibrillation had resulted from acute myocardial infarction, the mortality at 1 year was only 4 per cent and at 2 years 11 per cent. These figures are consistent with the experience in coronary care units already discussed, i.e., that ventricular fibrillation at the inception of an ischemic coronary attack may not adversely affect prognosis.[114,115]

At present two syndromes of sudden cardiac death can be distinguished (Table 23-3).[122] A minority of patients experience myocardial infarction with prodromes of chest pain during the preceding several weeks, and death is delayed during this terminal episode. In the majority of those dying suddenly (about 80 per cent) primary electrical failure occurs, prodromes are absent, the predisposition to recurrent ventricular fibrillation following successful resuscitation continues, and death is usually instantaneous. The precipitating factors in this latter group remain to be defined. Exercise and undue exertion are unusual provocative factors; indeed, nearly 75 per cent of all sudden deaths occur at home and 8 to 12 per cent at work.[32,123] In fewer than 5 per cent of the victims, sudden cardiac death has been preceded by diverse strenuous physical exertion. Although the incidence of sudden cardiac death increases with age, there is a suggestion that death outside the hospital is more likely to occur in the young.

The underlying mechanism in the majority of those who die suddenly and who have been monitored is ventricular fibrillation. The mechanism of this arrhythmia is considered on p. 626.

APPROACHES TO CONTAINING THE PROBLEM OF SUDDEN CARDIAC DEATH

There are essentially two approaches now being considered for containing the problem of sudden cardiac death. The first is a community-wide program of cardiopulmonary resuscitation. The major limitations of this approach relate first to the fact that the patient is reached only *after* the event and even a trivial delay in the initiation of cardiopulmonary support or minor errors in technique can often spell failure. In the second place, even the most successful outcome provides no assurance against recurrence, and the victim may not be fortunate enough to have a witness to his cardiac arrest.

The second approach is identification of the patient susceptible to ventricular fibrillation *before* the event and initiation of a prophylactic antiarrhythmic program. How is the patient predisposed to sudden cardiac death to be recognized? An essential hypothesis has been that certain types of ventricular premature beats (VPB's) in patients with ischemic heart disease are indicators of enhanced risk.[124-127]

VPB's AS RISK INDICATORS. Increasingly, medical attention is being directed to ventricular ectopic activity, an interest which derives from experience in the coronary care unit.[1] The hypothesis relating VPB's to electrical instability of the heart and to a predisposition to ventricular fibrillation led to a corollary formulation that suppression of ventricular extrasystoles in patients with ischemic heart disease may protect against sudden cardiac death.[124-127] These hypotheses derive from experience with acute myocardial infarction. However, it does not necessarily follow that the presence of VPB's is a risk indicator for

TABLE 23–3   SUDDEN CARDIAC DEATH SYNDROMES

CHARACTERISTIC FINDINGS	MYOCARDIAL INFARCTION	ELECTRICAL FAILURE
Prodromes	Present	Absent
Duration of final episode	Minutes to hours	Seconds
Pathological findings		
Thrombotic or atheromatous coronary artery occlusion	Frequently present	Absent
Acute myocardial infarction	Present	Absent
Post resuscitation (changes of myocardial infarction)		
ECG	Present	Absent
Enzymes	Sequential	Absent
Monitoring (VPB's)	Present	Advanced grades
Recurrence of ventricular fibrillation (1-year follow-up)	Low ($<5\%$)	High ($=30\%$)

instantaneous death in the absence of an overt myocardial ischemic event. Obviously this question is of critical importance and must be answered.

Prevalence of VPB's. A routine electrocardiogram recorded in healthy men, which provides about 45 seconds of monitoring information, generally detects few, if any, VPB's. Thus, among 67,375 asymptomatic men in the military services, Hiss and coworkers noted a prevalence rate of ectopic beats of only 0.6 per cent.[128] Complex forms of VPB's were even more unusual. Heart rate did not correlate with the presence of arrhythmia.

The advent of monitoring technology has permitted surveillance of ambulatory subjects while they are engaged in usual activities. Brodsky and coworkers examined 50 normal male medical students who ranged in age from 23 to 27 years.[129] All were free of the stigmata of cardiovascular disease. The subjects participated in routine daily activities. Fifty-six per cent had one or more atrial premature beats, and 50 per cent exhibited one or more VPB's. However, the frequency of ectopic beats per hour was low, and only one subject had more than 50 VPB's during the 24-hour monitoring period. Multiform VPB's were noted in six, and early ectopic beats interrupting the T wave were observed in three. In one subject an episode of ventricular tachycardia consisting of five consecutive cycles at a rate of 136 beats/min occurred during sleep. These observations lend support to the view that the mere presence of VPB's does not necessarily imply a diseased heart and, furthermore, that frequent or complex forms of ventricular ectopic beats are unusual in young, healthy adult males.

Individuals without demonstrable heart disease as determined by current techniques may, however, exhibit multiform and repetitive ventricular ectopic arrhythmias without suffering adverse effects and without experiencing a dire prognosis. Thus, Kennedy and Underhill studied 25 asymptomatic and apparently healthy subjects who exhibited such multiple ventricular arrhythmias.[130] In 18, no cardiac abnormalities were discovered by means of cardiac catheterization and coronary angiography. In seven, mild heart derangements, if any, were suspected. The ar-

rhythmias had been known to be present for an average of 6 years (range 1 to 30 years). In 19 of the 24 patients VPB's were predominantly of right ventricular origin, and in 21 of 23 they disappeared during maximal exercise testing. Antiarrhythmic drug regimens were generally ineffective.

Hinkle and coworkers monitored for 6 hours 811 employed men ranging in age from 35 to 65 years.[131] Of these, 325 were judged to be at high risk for coronary heart disease. Occurrence of VPB's was found to be a function of age. The frequency of multiform VPB's correlated with VPB prevalence, whereas early VPB's interrupting the T waves were found in 5.5 per cent and were associated with multiformity. All men having greater than 10 VPB's per 1000 beats exhibited coronary heart disease, hypertension, or chronic lung disease.[132] Eighty-eight per cent of 184 patients with ischemic heart disease who were monitored for 24 hours exhibited VPB's.[133] As might be anticipated, the occurrence of VPB's in a population with ischemic heart disease is directly related to the duration of monitoring (Table 23–4).

Patterns of VPB's. The ubiquity of VPB's among patients with coronary heart disease would make their mere presence an unlikely risk indicator for sudden cardiac death. It may well be that risk resides in some specific attribute of the VPB, such as the degree of prematurity, QRS complex morphology, site of origin, or repetitive pattern.

Degree of Prematurity. Even before the era of the coronary care unit, Smirk and Palmer suggested that extrasystoles which interrupt T waves, the so-called "R-on-T phenomenon," predispose to sudden death.[134] It has long been appreciated that the presence of a prolonged Q-T interval, which places the vulnerable period later in the cardiac cycle, is associated with sudden fatality. Han and Goel have emphasized that ventricular fibrillation is more readily induced by early VPB's in the presence of clinical or electrocardiographic evidence of myocardial infarction, bradycardia, Q-T prolongation, and increased T-wave duration.[135] Experimental studies indicate that very early

TABLE 23–4   EXTENT OF EXPOSURE OF VPB'S IN PATIENTS WITH CORONARY HEART DISEASE AND DURATION OF MONITORING

	PATIENTS WITH VPB'S (%)	DURATION OF MONITORING (MIN)
ECG recording	10 to 14	$\simeq 1$
Trendscription	40	30
Sedentary monitoring	50	60
Exercise testing	56	15 to 20
Ambulatory monitoring	85 to 88	24 hours

VPB's which interrupt the T wave occur during the ventricular vulnerable period. This period of enhanced susceptibility to fibrillation may be approximated by the ratio between the onset of the QRS complex of the VPB (QR') as related to the QRS of the preceding normal cycle and the Q-T interval. Thus, when the QR'/QT ratio is less than 1.0, the VPB is likely to depolarize the heart during the vulnerable period with a high risk of ventricular fibrillation.[1,136] In dogs with acute myocardial infarcts, Epstein and associates demonstrated that ventricular fibrillation occurred only in those animals exhibiting ectopic beats within 0.43 sec of the preceding QRS complex, though not in all of them.[137] In contrast, ventricular ectopy beyond 0.43 sec was never associated with fibrillation.

The significance of the R-on-T phenomenon has been questioned.[138] When local bipolar electrocardiograms were recorded in the acutely infarcted heart, isolated areas of fractionation and increased duration of refractoriness with delayed epicardial activation were noted. These sustained areas of excitation apparently functioned as a source for reentrant ectopic beats.[139–141] In fact, in the presence of ischemia, the duration of the vulnerable period cannot be defined precisely from the Q-T interval of the surface electrocardiogram. Williams and coworkers observed that spontaneous tachyarrhythmias, as well as the ectopic mechanism induced by paced beats, were almost invariably initiated by pulses with long coupling intervals.[142] Ventricular tachycardia always followed the ectopic beat with the greatest fractionation and delay recorded in the electrogram of the ischemic zone.

Some clinical studies indicate that the onset of ventricular tachycardia or repetitive ventricular activity does not require an early ectopic beat. Thus, DeSoyza and coworkers found that the mean coupling interval of ectopic beats initiating ventricular tachycardia in patients with acute myocardial infarction was not different from that of isolated ectopic beats in the same patient.[143] In fact, only 12 per cent of episodes of ventricular tachycardia were initiated by VPB's with T-wave interruptions. In these same patients 16 per cent of such early VPB's were not followed by repetitive activity. On the other hand, Rothfeld and colleagues found that in patients with acute myocardial infarction, 25 per cent of the paroxysms of ventricular tachycardia were initiated by VPB's with T-wave interruption; furthermore, they emphasize that these episodes were more resistant to lidocaine and more often degenerated into fibrillation.[144] Wellens and colleagues, employing programmed stimulation of the myocardium, scanned the entire period of diastole, including the Q-T interval.[145] They were unable to induce ventricular tachyarrhythmias in patients with acute myocardial infarction who had had ventricular tachycardia. El-Sherif and associates found that the R-on-T phenomenon initiated 10 of 20 episodes of primary ventricular fibrillation.[146] However, 200 of 430 patients with acute myocardial infarction exhibited such early VPB's without developing repetitive ventricular arrhythmias.

It is of course possible that the pathophysiology of ventricular tachycardia is different from that of ventricular fibrillation. Furthermore, it has already been emphasized that out-of-hospital sudden cardiac death is, in a majority of instances, unrelated to acute myocardial infarction. Ear-

ly VPB's interrupting T waves probably have prognostic significance for sudden death. Thus, Ruberman and associates have found an increased mortality among coronary heart disease patients who exhibit the R-on-T phenomenon.[147] Similarly, Oliver et al., who monitored patients in the late hospital phase and early post-hospital period after recovery from myocardial infarction, found evidence suggesting that R-on-T is associated with augmented risk for sudden cardiac death.[148] Indeed, they maintain that this is the single most reliable VPB characteristic for identifying those individuals predisposed to sudden death. Campbell and coworkers,[149] in a comprehensive study of this issue, examined the continuously recorded electrocardiographic recording of 1787 patients admitted to a coronary care unit within 12 hours of acute myocardial infarction. Of 17 patients with primary ventricular fibrillation, the arrhythmia was initiated by R-on-T VPB complex in 16 (QR'/QT ≤ 0.85), whereas only 4 of 265 of ventricular tachycardia episodes were so initiated.

Morphology of the QRS Complex. It has been suggested that the QRS complex of the VPB widens with age and with the severity of heart disease.[150] Soloff studied 411 patients and categorized VPB's into classic forms (i.e., those having smooth depolarization and smooth, oppositely directed repolarization) and bizarre forms (i.e., those having variable deformities of the QRS complex and T wave).[151] Of the 169 with classic morphologic findings, 71 (42 per cent) had no heart disease; by contrast, only 18 (7 per cent) of the 242 with bizarre forms were free of cardiac illness. To date no data have been presented ascribing prognostic implications for sudden cardiac death to differing QRS configurations of the VPB.

Site of Origin. Hiss and coworkers observed in normal individuals a 3:1 ratio of VPB's originating in the right ventricle (left bundle branch block pattern) compared with those originating in the left ventricle (right bundle branch block pattern).[128] Manning et al. noted that the majority of VPB's in patients with ischemic heart disease originated in the left ventricle.[152] Rosenbaum has asserted that VPB's in normal individuals possess a characteristic morphology, since they nearly always arise in the area approximating the anterior papillary muscle of the right ventricle.[153] Our experience does not support such a differentiation between VPB's in relation to the presence or absence of heart disease. Brodsky and coworkers also found both morphologic types among normal medical students.[129]

Repetitive Activity. As early as 1929, Esler and White pointed out that VPB's in bigeminal patterns or in pairs, especially when multiform or bidirectional, were evidence of serious heart disease.[154] Such forms are unusual in the young and in those with normal hearts. Thus, Hiss et al. observed only 3 subjects with multiform VPB's among 952 exhibiting ectopic activity, and only 6 had brief repetitive salvos.[128] Bigger et al.[155] have reported that occurrence of even a single episode of ventricular tachycardia of three or more beats during 24-hour monitoring inordinately increases late mortality in patients surviving acute myocardial infarction. In 50 patients exhibiting this finding, overall 1-year mortality was 38.0 per cent compared with 11.6 per cent in a control group without tachycardia (p < 0.001). Multiple logistic regression analysis showed the presence

TABLE 23–5   A GRADING SYSTEM FOR VPB'S

VPB CHARACTERISTICS

Grade		
	0	No ventricular beats
	1A	Occasional, isolated VPB's (less than 30/hr) less than 1/min
	1B	Occasional, isolated VPB's (less than 30/hr) more than 1/min
	2	Frequent VPB's (more than 30/hr)
	3	Multiform VPB's
	4A	Repetitive VPB's couplets
	4B	Repetitive VPB's salvos
	5	Early VPB's (i.e., abutting or interrupting the T wave)

This grading system is applied to a 24-hour monitoring period and indicates the number of hours within that period during which a patient has VPB's of a particular grade, expressed as superscripts in the resulting "equation." Subscripts indicate particular aspects of the VPB's of a given grade. For example, in the equation below, the subscript for grade 2 indicates the approximate total number of grade 2 VPB's over the 24-hour period; for grade 3 it denotes the number of different forms observed in any single hour; for grade 4B the two subscripts indicate the largest number of paroxysms of tachycardia in a single hour and the maximum number of successive cycles, respectively; for grade 5 the subscript represents the largest number of early ectopic beats in any single hour. A complete translation of this particular equation is as follows:

$$0^3 \quad 1A^0 \quad 1B^4 \quad 2_{760}^6 \quad 3_2^6 \quad 4A_3^2 \quad 4B_{4-7}^2 \quad 5_3^1$$

Grade		
	0	Occurred during 3 hours
	1A	No infrequent VPB's
	1B	Infrequent VPB's but more than 1/min observed during 4 hours
	2	Occurred during 6 hours (with a total of 760 VPB's)
	3	Occurred during 6 hours; exhibited two forms
	4A	Occurred during 2 hours; greatest frequency in any single hour was 3
	4B	Occurred during 2 hours; there were 4 paroxysms, and the longest duration was 7 cycles
	5	An early VPB observed 3 times during a single hour in the 24-hour monitoring session

of paroxysms of tachycardia to be an independent predictor of high risk.

Our experimental findings have indicated that repetitive ectopic cycles reduce the threshold for ventricular fibrillation in the vulnerable period. The triggering of fibrillation is enhanced when salvos of ectopic beats tend to accelerate with progressive abbreviation in cycle length.[156,157] Therefore, evidence to date suggests that it is not the mere presence of VPB's but their type, frequency, and repetitive form that have prognostic implications for sudden cardiac death.

Grading of VPB's.   The mere presence of simple VPB's in 1 hour of monitoring has little prognostic significance.[158] The fact that VPB's are noted in 85 per cent of patients with ischemic heart disease argues that if VPB's are risk predictors for sudden cardiac death, this property inheres not in their mere occurrence but rather in some specific attributes. These considerations impelled us to devise a grading system based on clinical experience, intuition, and common sense (Table 23–5).[126] Implicit in this categorization of VPB's is the fact that some grades carry a higher risk for sudden cardiac death.

Support for the VPB hypothesis has been provided in two large epidemiological studies.[147,158,159] The Coronary Drug Project Study was a long-term, randomized, double-blind trial to evaluate the safety of drugs that lower lipid levels in an attempt to prolong the life of survivors of one or more documented myocardial infarctions.[159] Eligible men were between the ages of 30 and 65 years at the time of enrollment, had survived their most recent infarction for at least 3 months, and were free of cardiac manifestations of their disease. Of the 8342 recruited survivors of infarction, one-third (2789) were randomly assigned to a placebo-treated group. Complete, edited baseline data for all measured variables were available from 2035 men who had composed the cohort that was subsequently followed up for 3 years. Among these, the resting baseline electrocardiogram in 235 men (11.5 per cent) showed one or more

VPB's. During the follow-up period, there were 256 deaths. These were twice as frequent among those with any VPB's (21.7 per cent) compared with those with none (11.4 per cent). Excess, long-term risk of death, including sudden death, was associated with frequent VPB's, with couplets and runs (grade 4), and possibly with early-cycle VPB's. The excess risk associated with these grades of VPB's was independent of 28 other variables related to baseline electrocardiographic and clinical characteristics.

The second investigation involved 1739 men with prior myocardial infarctions selected from the New York Health Insurance Plan study of 120,000 men, ages 35 to 74 years.[147,158] These patients were monitored for 1 hour while sedentary. The average follow-up was 24.4 months. Sudden cardiac death was defined as occurring within minutes of a patient's usual state of health and in the absence of symptoms or findings, suggesting acute myocardial infarction. Analysis of survival data that take account of other important prognostic variables established that the presence of complex VPB's (e.g., R-on-T, runs of two or more, multiform or bigeminal VPB's) in the monitoring hour was asso-

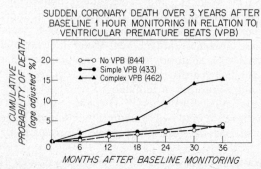

FIGURE 23–4   The mere presence of VPB's, even when they are frequent, does not increase the risk for sudden cardiac death. However, complex forms are associated with a more than threefold increase in mortality. (From Ruberman, W., et al.: Ventricular premature beats and mortality after myocardial infarction. N. Engl. J. Med. 279:750, 1977.)

ciated with a risk of sudden cardiac death that was three times greater than that observed in men free of complex VPB's (Fig. 23–4).

VPB's and Severity of Heart Disease. It may be argued that advanced grades of VPB's carry adverse prognostic implications, because they reflect the severity of the underlying ischemic heart disease.[160] CCU studies have already indicated a correlation between infarct size, as estimated by creatinine phosphokinase and isoenzymes, and the frequency and grade of ventricular arrhythmias.[161] Epidemiological studies have related the prevalence of VPB's to the extent of myocardial damage. A number of clinical studies have shown an association between the degree of ventricular functional impairment and the occurrence of advanced grades of VPB's.[162–164]

Calvert et al. monitored the electrocardiograms of 124 patients for 24 hours prior to catheterization and coronary angiography.[165] VPB's were demonstrated in 83 per cent. Patients exhibiting only one-vessel disease did not differ from normal persons in the frequency or grade of VPB's; however, those with multivessel disease had a significantly higher incidence of VPB's of advanced grade. Similarly, the presence of elevated left ventricular end-diastolic pressure of asynergy was associated with increased ventricular ectopy. Persistence of VPB's of advanced grade, namely, their recurrence over 3 or more hours, was found only in the presence of multivessel involvement.[165] Among 15 patients with both asynergy and significantly elevated left ventricular end-diastolic pressures (>19 mm Hg), paroxysms of ventricular tachycardia were noted in 40 per cent and coupled beats in 67 per cent compared with 6 and 12 per cent, respectively, in the 34 patients without these hemodynamic abnormalities ($p < 0.005$).

Similar findings have been reported by Schulze and coworkers, who monitored a small number of patients subjected to cardiac catheterization during the late hospital phase following recovery from acute myocardial infarction.[163,164] Patients with complicated arrhythmias (multiform, coupled, or ventricular premature beats with T-wave interruption or ventricular tachycardia) had a greater number of proximally obstructed major coronary arteries and more extensive atherosclerotic disease than those who demonstrated infrequent or no ectopic activity. Equally persuasive are the studies of Cobb and coworkers.[73] Coronary arteriography and left ventriculography were performed in 64 patients with ischemic heart disease who had been successfully resuscitated from ventricular fibrillation. The majority had extensive abnormalities in left ventricular contraction and stenotic lesions involving two or more vessels. Advanced pathological impairment in coronary flow as well as in asynergy of left ventricular wall motion was the most ominous finding predictive of recurrent ventricular fibrillation.[72]

On the basis of these data, it may be argued that prognostic implications do not reside in the VPB but rather in the extent of cardiac disease, for the grade of ectopic activity is largely an expression of the severity of the ischemic process. A corollary inference may be adduced regarding the futility of attempting to control ventricular arrhythmia when the ultimate outcome is determined by the extent of the heart disease. A recent study by Schulze et al. counters such a conclusion.[118] Although advanced grades of VPB's were limited to those patients with ejection fractions of

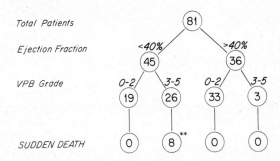

FIGURE 23–5 Among 81 patients who recovered from acute myocardial infarction, 45 had reduced ejection fraction, and those who died suddenly were only a subset of patients with VPB's of grades 3 to 5. (From Schultze, R. A., et al.: Sudden death in the year following myocardial infarction. Am. J. Med. *62*:192, 1977.)

** p <0.02.

less than 40 per cent, sudden, out-of-hospital death was encountered only in those with advanced grades of ectopic beats (Fig. 23–5). Thus, among 45 patients with impaired ejection, 19 did not have significant grades of VPB's, and in a 7-month follow-up period none died. By contrast, among 26 patients with similar hemodynamic deficit but with advanced grades of VPB's, 8 died suddenly ($p < 0.02$). It may well be that extensive cardiac disease predisposes to advanced grades of oft-recurring ventricular arrhythmia, but the presence of these ectopic beats increases the chances of sequential VPB's discharging during the vulnerable period and thereby precipitating ventricular fibrillation.

DIRECT EXPOSURE OF CARDIAC ELECTRICAL INSTABILITY. Reliance on VPB's as an indicator of electrical instability presents a number of limitations. First, it is an elusive target—sporadic and random in occurrence. Second, advanced grades of VPB's have a reproducibility of only about 40 per cent.[165] Third, VPB's may represent the wrong target. In any one individual there is no certainty that the presence of VPB's is synonymous with an electrically unstable myocardium. Although we aim at ventricular ectopic activity, the target is actually ventricular fibrillation. It may well be that in a particular patient the two are disparate electrophysiological phenomena. Fourth, there is no certainty that controlling VPB's will prevent sudden cardiac death. Finally, exposing the presence of VPB's is time-consuming and costly. Direct measurements of electrical instability are therefore necessary, and the following are a number of electrophysiological approaches that are now being applied clinically with increasing frequency.

Repetitive Ventricular Ectopic Activity. Massive electrical currents delivered outside the vulnerable period of the cardiac cycle fail to provoke arrhythmias other than standstill. Even during the vulnerable period, impulses of as much as 50,000 microjoules, which greatly exceed threshold, are required to elicit repetitive activity. This is seven orders of magnitude above the threshold for inducing a single propagated response in diastole, for which as little as 1 microjoule may suffice. We have found in animal experiments that the cardiac glycosides predispose the heart to repetitive ventricular response with threshold energies, i.e., energies just sufficient to induce a single depolarization in diastole.[166–168] This has been designated as the repetitive ventricular response (RVR) phenomenon. The most sensitive part of the cardiac cycle for the repetitive ventricular response follows immediately after inscription of the T wave, well beyond the vulnerable period of the cardiac cycle. It was found to be due to digitalis-induced enhancement of Purkinje fiber automaticity and required transient suppression of sinus rhythm and therefore was not dependent on an initiating impulse.[167,168] Elicitation of the repetitive ventricular response was facilitated by abbreviating cycle length[168]; as little as three short, paced cycles sufficed to reinduce the response after its subsidence in the unpaced heart.

The unmasking of enhanced Purkinje fiber automaticity following digitalization has been employed by Jenzer and coworkers to assess the presence of electrical instability in the ischemic myocardium.[169] Following acute coronary occlusion and the development of myocardial ischemia, a single stimulus delivered early in diastole elicited the repetitive ventricular ectopic activity. Green and coworkers have demonstrated that in patients this phenomenon can be used to expose the presence of electrical instability.[170] They studied 50 patients with recurrent and refractory symptomatic ventricular tachycardia, 18 of whom had been resuscitated from cardiac arrest, and an additional 12 normal patients referred for various chest pain syndromes. Forty-four of the 50 patients with recurrent ventricular tachycardia demonstrated the repetitive ventricular response, whereas such a response was observed in none of the 12 normal patients ($p < 0.001$). During the ensuing year of follow-up, symptomatic ventricular tachycardia or sudden cardiac death occurred in 73 per cent with the repetitive ventricular response compared with only 14 per cent who did not show the response ($p < 0.001$). A "Lown Class 4B and 5A" arrhythmia on Holter monitoring prior to hospital discharge was more frequent among patients with subsequent sudden cardiac death or ventricular tachycardia[170] compared with those free of these arrhythmias ($p < 0.02$).

Repetitive Extrasystole. A different approach to exposing the presence of electrical instability is the use of sequential pulsing during the vulnerable period. It has been postulated that electrical instability is present when a stimulus of just threshold intensity induces repetitive electrical activity when discharged during the ventricular vulnerable period.[171] In animals with coronary artery occlusion, salvos of extrasystoles precede the emergence of ventricular fibrillation.[156,157] By altering the intensity and timing of the third pulse in a sequence of triple pulsing, one can probe for changes in cardiac electrical stability. This technique has been designated sequential R-on-T pulsing.[157,172]

To study alterations in electrical stability in the presence of acute myocardial infarction, an animal model was employed in which a 10-minute period of coronary artery occlusion was followed by abrupt release.[157] Two minutes after abrupt, closed-chest occlusion of the left anterior descending coronary artery in dogs, sequential R-on-T pulsing demonstrates a striking drop in the threshold for ventricular fibrillation[157] and a lengthening in duration of the vulnerable period (Fig. 23–6). Thus, whereas the control threshold for ventricular fibrillation averaged 56 mA, with occlusion it fell to 1.6 mA, returned to control levels, and immediately upon release was reduced to 3.6 mA. During both occlusion and release, there was a material lengthening in the duration of the vulnerable period as well. The time course of these changes in cardiac vulnera-

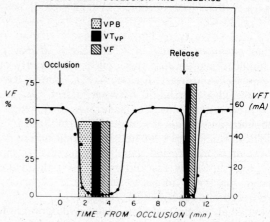

FIGURE 23–6 Measurement of ventricular fibrillation threshold (VFT) (i.e., ventricular vulnerability) during 10-minute coronary artery occlusion and release. The threshold is strikingly reduced within 2 minutes of occlusion, only to rebound within 5 minutes. A sharp drop then recurs with reperfusion. The time course of vulnerability is analogous to the emergence and recession of ventricular arrhythmia.

bility paralleled the emergence and recession of arrhythmias and the altered susceptibility to ventricular fibrillation after coronary artery occlusion and release. If the coronary occlusion was maintained beyond the point of spontaneous arrhythmias, sequential pulsing elicited ventricular fibrillation with pulses within the physiological range of intensity. Unlike the repetitive ventricular response phenomenon, in which an extrasystole occurs after a pause following the stimulus, in repetitive extrasystole the response is early. Thus, at a time when the animal appeared fully recovered and free of ventricular ectopic activity, a tendency toward repetitive electrical activity could still be demonstrated. The objective of this technique is not to induce tachyarrhythmia but to elicit repetitive ventricular ectopic activity.

Electrical Stimulation. Durrer et al.[173] and Coumel et al.[174] in 1967 independently reported on the use of programmed electrical stimulation of the heart for provoking and terminating supraventricular tachyarrhythmias in patients afflicted with these disorders. One or more extrastimuli are delivered to the endocardium at various sites and at variable pacing rates. Stimulation close to the pathway with the longest refractory period facilitates induction of the tachycardia. Arrhythmias can be reproducibly initiated as well as terminated (p. 634).

The recent development of electrophysiological *mapping techniques* for determining the site of origin of the potentially lethal ventricular tachyarrhythmias has promoted insight into the mechanism of ventricular fibrillation in humans and has provided methods for medical as well as surgical management.[175-180] Ventricular tachyarrhythmias could be induced by programmed electrical stimulation in 40 of 59 patients who had been resuscitated from out-of-hospital cardiac arrest.[181] In 23 patients the arrhythmia was sustained ventricular tachycardia, in 10 the mechanism was *torsades de pointes* (p. 725), and in 7 it was ventricular fibrillation. In the 19 patients with noninducible arrhythmia, 9 had coronary artery disease (48 per cent), compared with 34 of 40 (85 per cent) in whom an arrhythmia could be provoked. This initiation of arrhythmia was dependent upon the emergence of fragmented systolic and diastolic electrical activity.[182]

These invasive procedures, though proving invaluable in facilitating the management of refractory ventricular tachyarrhythmias, are unlikely to prove practicable in the detection of patients predisposed to sudden death among those who are free of malignant arrhythmias, who constitute the overwhelming majority of the victims of sudden death.

TRANSIENT RISK FACTORS FOR VENTRICULAR FIBRILLATION. If electrical instability is an abnormal electrophysiological condition of prolonged duration, a pertinent question relates to the possible trigger factors that provoke ventricular fibrillation at the particular time when it does occur. Since no structural lesions have been shown to precipitate the catastrophic arrhythmia, one must turn to transient functional inputs to the heart sufficient to derange its electrophysiological properties. Among the transient risk factors that should be considered are those originating in higher nervous centers.

It has long been appreciated that stimulation of the brain can provoke a variety of arrhythmias and can lower the ventricular vulnerable threshold. In the animal with acute myocardial ischemia, such central nervous system stimulation suffices to provoke ventricular fibrillation.[108,183] Vagal neural traffic or adrenal catecholamines are not the conduits for this brain-heart linkage nor are accompanying increases in heart rate or blood pressure prerequisites for the changes in cardiac excitability.

Sympathetic Neural Activity. Electrical instability of the heart can also be induced by stimulating the stellate ganglia, way stations of sympathetic neural traffic from brain to heart.[183] R-on-T pulsing of the right ventricle with twice threshold currents does not provoke ventricular fibrillation unless either the right or the left stellate ganglion is stimulated simultaneously.[184] Control of heart rate by pacing and prevention of the rise in blood pressure by controlled exsanguination do not decrease the incidence of ventricular fibrillation during R-on-T pulsing and peripheral sympathetic stimulation. When efferent fibers to the stellate ganglion are sectioned or when the animal is pretreated with reserpine, these changes in cardiac vulnerability are prevented.

Quantitative as well as qualitative differences between the right and left stellate ganglia have been defined.[185–187] The left ganglion exerts its influence predominantly on the posterior ventricular surface, whereas the right ganglion affects mainly the anterior ventricular wall.[89] Left stellate stimulation produces exclusively inotropic effects, whereas right stellate stimulation results in both chronotropic and inotropic changes.[188] Brown has shown that there is a surge of sympathetic discharge during the onset of acute myocardial infarction.[189] Malliani and colleagues have recorded increased firing from sympathetic preganglionic fibers at the level of the third thoracic vertebra during acute myocardial ischemia.[190] If sympathetic neural discharge is a factor in determining the heart's vulnerability to ventricular fibrillation, pharmacologic adrenergic ablation should protect the acutely ischemic heart from arrhythmias. In closed-chest dogs, pretreatment with propranolol prevents the reduction in threshold for ventricular fibrillation attendant to occlusion of the left anterior descending coronary artery.[191] However, beta-adrenergic blockade does not prevent the lowering in threshold that follows coronary reperfusion. These findings indicate that activation of the sympathetic nervous system is largely responsible for the enhanced predisposition to fibrillation during the early period of coronary artery occlusion but is not a factor in the genesis of arrhythmia immediately upon reestablishment of flow.

It has also been demonstrated that reflex lessening of sympathetic activity decreases cardiac vulnerability.[192] Since acute increases in blood pressure reduce cardiac sympathetic tone, pharmacologic and mechanical measures were employed to induce hypertension and determine neural effects on the heart. Injection of the alpha-adrenergic–stimulating drug phenylephrine or constriction of the thoracic aorta, which resulted in a rise of blood pressure, increased the threshold for ventricular fibrillation.[192] Cervical vagotomy did not prevent the protection from acute hypertension, but carotid denervation did. A protective effect resulting from an increase in blood pressure was also demonstrated in dogs during acute myocardial ischemia.[193] These findings indicate that reflex diminution of sympathetic tone such as that evoked by elevations in arterial blood pressure may decrease the susceptibility to ventricular fibrillation in animals subjected to coronary artery occlusion. Blood pressure manipulation during reperfusion, however, produces no changes in vulnerability.

Vagal Nerve Activity. A prevailing attitude among physiologists and clinicians until recently has been that vagus innervation is limited to supraventricular structures with only negligible, if any, effects on the ventricles. Persuasive evidence has now been amassed demonstrating parasympathetic influences on both inotropic and chronotropic properties of the ventricular myocardium.[194] There is also anatomical evidence indicating a rich cholinergic network juxtaposed to ventricular conduction tissue; this indicates that vagal nerve activity might modify ventricular excitability as well.[195,196] These recent findings are in accord with an observation made more than a century ago. In 1859 Einbrodt, a Russian investigator working in Karl Ludwig's laboratory, found that vagal stimulation raised the threshold for ventricular fibrillation in open-chest dogs.[197] Kent and coworkers[195] and Myers et al.[198] confirmed and extended this observation. They showed that stimulation of the vagus increases the threshold of the vulnerable period in normal as well as in ischemic dogs. When, instead of open-chest dogs, intact animals were studied by Kolman and colleagues, no salutary effect could be attributed to the vagus.[199] Under conditions of reduced sympathetic discharge, intense vagal stimulation had only slight effects on ventricular vulnerability. However, when sympathetic activity was augmented by thoracotomy or by direct stimulation of cardiac sympathetic fibers, a definite antifibrillatory vagal effect was demonstrated. Similar findings were observed when ventricular excitability was the object of investigation.[200]

The effect of the vagus nerve in opposing vulnerability changes induced by sympathetic neural discharge applies equally to neurohumoral adrenergic release.[201] Vagal stimulation restores the fibrillation threshold, which is reduced by norepinephrine administration, but the restoration is only to the control level. The action of the vagus nerve on cardiac vulnerability is related to its muscarinic properties and can be abolished by atropine.[202] The principal locus of vagal projection in the ventricle is the His-Purkinje system, which is also richly endowed with sympathetic neuroeffector terminals.[196] This provides the anatomical substrate for sympathetic-parasympathetic interactions on ventricular excitability. There is also evidence of such interactions at the molecular level.[203-205]

Psychological Factors.   A crucial question is whether behavioral and psychological variables can alter cardiac vulnerability and thereby predispose to ventricular fibrillation. Until recently no such experimental data were available.

It has long been appreciated that when the intensity of electrical discharge during the vulnerable period is increased progressively, repetitive extrasystoles frequently precede the emergence of ventricular fibrillation (Fig. 23–7).[206] In order for the threshold for repetitive extrasystoles to be used as a marker for fibrillation, it was necessary to demonstrate (1) a constant quantitative relationship between the current for repetitive extrasystole and the current for ventricular fibrillation, namely, a fixed coincidence of the two indices within the cardiac cycle; and (2) a constant relationship under diverse experimental conditions, especially those involving neural intervention. Experimental observations suggested that repetitive extrasystole and ventricular fibrillation share a common electrophysiological basis and that the threshold for repetitive extrasystoles *can* be used as a reliable endpoint for assessing susceptibility to fibrillation.[207] The psychological paradigm consisted of exposing the animal to two environments, one of which was stressful. The latter consisted of a Pavlovian sling in which the dog received a single 5-joule transthoracic shock at the end of each experimental period on 3 successive days.[208] In the sling, the dogs were restless, salivated excessively, exhibited somatic tremor, and had a mean heart rate of 136 beats/min. In the cage, the stimulus current for repetitive extrasystoles averaged 43 mA, whereas in the sling, the mean threshold was markedly reduced to 14 mA (p < 0.001). These findings indicate that psychological stress can profoundly lower the cardiac threshold for ventricular fibrillation. That this reduction was mediated by

sympathetic neural activity is further supported by the fact that the cardiospecific, beta-adrenergic–blocking drug tolamolol hydrochloride completely eliminated the stress-induced alteration in cardiac vulnerability.[209]

Psychological stress can also provoke spontaneous arrhythmias in animals with coronary artery occlusion. When animals conditioned in both cage and sling environments later underwent coronary artery ligation, they consistently developed arrhythmias, including ventricular tachycardia and R-on-T extrasystoles,[210] when returned to the sling environment. The arrhythmias promptly disappeared once the animals were returned to the nonaversive cage.

Animal experiments thus demonstrate that different environmental stresses may alter the vulnerability of the heart to ventricular fibrillation. In animals with acute coronary occlusion, psychological stress is a sufficient factor for provoking malignant arrhythmias. Although these effects are mediated by neurophysiological inputs to the heart, remaining to be defined are the precise neural pathways and neurochemical processes that integrate psychological activity and determine the specific neural traffic within the sympathetic nervous system that alters cardiac electrical stability.

Neurochemical Studies.   If central neural traffic traversing the sympathetic nervous system modulates cardiac predisposition to arrhythmias, it is reasonable to surmise that neural outflow may be affected centrally. It has indeed been found that intravenous administration of the biochemical precursor of serotonin, either L-tryptophan or 5-hydroxy-L-tryptophan, inhibits sympathetic neural outflow.[211-213] Pretreatment with the decarboxylase inhibitor carbidopa, which circulates peripherally without crossing the blood-brain barrier, tends to restrict the formation of serotonin to the central nervous system. Because the serotonin thus formed would rapidly oxidize, the systemic monoamine oxidase inhibitor phenelzine is given to protect central serotonin from degradation. This results in accumulation of serotonin within the central nervous system but not in the periphery. When dogs are given the serotonin precursor L-tryptophan or 5-hydroxy-L-tryptophan in conjunction with the monoamine oxidase inhibitor phenelzine and the selective peripheral L–amino acid decarboxylase inhibitor carbidopa, ventricular vulnerability is markedly elevated.[214] These findings, though preliminary, nonetheless suggest that we are at the threshold of an era of neurochemical discoveries promising profound insights concerning brain-heart interactions.

Psychological Stress and Sudden Cardiac Death.   It is widely believed that emotions can profoundly alter cardiac function and may predispose to sudden cardiac death. Engel has provided a compendium of anecdotal reports gleaned from the daily press relating the occurrence of sudden death to intense emotions such as grief, fear, frustration, rage, joy, and so forth.[215] Wellens and coworkers have described a 14-year-old girl who experienced syncopal attacks on being awakened from sleep by auditory stimuli.[216] Hemodynamic and electrophysiological studies failed to identify structural cardiac abnormalities, and the coronary angiogram was also normal. During these episodes, the electrocardiogram registered prolongation of the Q-T interval followed by ventricular ectopic activity and spon-

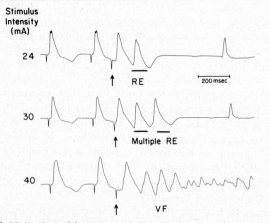

FIGURE 23–7 Repetitive extrasystoles (RE) emerge before the induction of ventricular fibrillation (VF) with increasing stimulating currents delivered during the vulnerable period. Thus, a single stimulus at currents less than 24 milliamperes (mA) elicits but a single response. However, with higher currents, dual and multiple repetitive extrasystoles emerge, and finally, with 40 mA, ventricular fibrillation is provoked.

taneously terminating attacks of ventricular fibrillation. Objective evidence from clinical studies has shown that emotional stress occasioned by public speaking,[217] automobile driving,[218] and spectator sports[219] results in significant ST-segment and T-wave alterations and in increases of ventricular ectopic beats and of serum catecholamines. These changes can be suppressed by beta-adrenergic blockade.[217,218] Sleep, during which sympathetic tone is reduced, usually causes diminution in VPB's. In 45 patients who had VPB's while awake during 24-hour monitoring, 78 per cent exhibited a reduction in both frequency and grade of ectopic activity during sleep.[220]

Although it can be documented in humans that stress increases both sympathetic neural traffic and ventricular ectopy, the possibility of a direct relationship between psychological factors and sudden cardiac death is subject to considerable speculation and does not lend itself to precise documentation.[221] Epidemiological studies indicate an increased prevalence of sudden death during bereavement[222] and following significant life changes (p. 1834).[223] In the first 6 months after loss of a spouse, the death rate among 4486 widows and widowers, 55 years of age or older, increased 40 per cent above the expected rate for a married population matched for age.[222] Rahe and coworkers retrospectively interviewed the families of 226 victims of sudden cardiac death in Helsinki, Finland, and noted that significant life changes such as divorce, grief, and altered work patterns had occurred during the 6 months preceding death compared with status in the same interval 1 year earlier (see Table 57–2, p. 1834).[223] Among patients recovering from acute myocardial infarction, one risk factor for sudden cardiac death proved to be ward rounds.[224] A fivefold greater incidence of sudden death occurred during medical daily ward rounds than would have been anticipated had these deaths been random. The physician-in-chief's rounds, held only once weekly, accounted for half the sudden fatalities. Increasing experience with patients resuscitated from non–infarct-related, out-of-hospital sudden cardiac death is proving instructive with regard to the possible role of psychological factors. In one such patient, a 39-year-old man who had twice experienced ventricular fibrillation, extensive studies, including coronary angiography, showed no evidence of cardiovascular disease.[107] However, data were amassed indicating a role for higher nervous activity in the genesis of the ventricular arrhythmia. These included the psychiatric make-up of the patient, the emotional stress attending the first cardiac arrest, the provocation of advanced grades of VPB's and ventricular tachycardia during ward rounds, the prevalence of arrhythmia during the rapid eye movement (REM) stage of sleep when he had violent dreams, the occurrence of the second episode of ventricular fibrillation during a similar period of sleep, and finally the observations that meditation and cardioselective beta-adrenergic–blocking drugs decreased the ventricular arrhythmia.

The studies cited above sanction the view that higher nervous activity may constitute a transient risk factor for sudden cardiac death. So far, a major role can be ascribed to the sympathetic limb of the autonomic nervous system; the cardiac mechanism involves reduction in the vulnerable period threshold for ventricular fibrillation. In patients with ischemic heart disease and electrical instability, such

neural traffic primarily engaging the adrenergic system may suffice to provoke lethal ventricular arrhythmias.

ALTERNATIVE HYPOTHESES FOR THE MECHANISM OF SUDDEN CARDIAC DEATH. So far, the major thrust of the discussion has related sudden cardiac death to the occurrence of cardiac arrhythmias triggered by transient risk factors and predisposed to by electrical instability. In the experimental animal, ventricular fibrillation can be induced by two different mechanisms, namely, obstruction of coronary flow and its release, with resulting reperfusion. The latter is unrelated to neural factors and is the more likely to provoke ventricular fibrillation.[157,191] Occlusion for as brief an interval as 4 to 6 minutes activates those factors responsible for inducing ventricular fibrillation on release. It may well be that transient interference with coronary flow is critical for the genesis of ventricular fibrillation. In this context it is possible that platelet aggregates and coronary vasospasm may transiently infringe on coronary blood flow. These two mechanisms therefore deserve consideration.

Platelet Function. Hughes and Tonks were the first to demonstrate that microemboli of platelet aggregates can lodge in the microcirculation of the rabbit heart and cause multiple myocardial necrotic lesions.[225,226] Later, Jorgensen et al. conducted studies in swine in which the direct coronary infusion of adenosine diphosphate (ADP) caused rapid onset of transient circulatory collapse accompanied by electrocardiographic changes of myocardial ischemia; in some animals ventricular fibrillation developed.[227] At the time of these cardiac effects the concentration of platelets in coronary venous blood was reduced to 70 to 75 per cent of the pre-ADP infusion values. These effects abated within 10 minutes. Numerous platelet aggregates were noted in the coronary microcirculation of animals sacrificed during the height of this phenomenon. When these swine were made thrombocytopenic by administering ^{32}P, ADP infusion was unaccompanied by myocardial changes. Folts and coworkers demonstrated a cyclic disappearance of coronary flow in vessels that had been narrowed externally.[71] During these cycles of myocardial ischemia, ventricular arrhythmia emerged. Platelet aggregates were identified in the partially obstructed arteries. This phenomenon of cyclic reduction in coronary flow was prevented by pretreatment with aspirin. Haerem found platelet aggregates in the intramyocardial vessels of patients dying suddenly of coronary artery disease, but these lesions were absent in those that died from other causes.[70]

In addition to their capacity for mechanical obstruction by aggregation, platelets release humoral factors that may contribute to impairment of blood flow. It has been established that the vasoactive amines, released by thrombin from the platelets coating the emboli, contribute to the magnitude of the vascular response in pulmonary embolism.[228,229] The platelet humoral factors are responsible for vascular and airway constriction and contribute to the mortality rate caused by such embolisms.[230,231] As early as 1953, Comroe and coworkers suggested that serotonin (5-hydroxytryptophan) might be the responsible agent for the reflex and direct cardiopulmonary changes associated with pulmonary embolism.[232] Zervas et al. have also shown that pretreatment with reserpine prevented vasospasm in animals subjected to experimental subarachnoid hemorrhage.[233] The protective effect was related to marked reduction in blood serotonin. The feeding of kanamycin to monkeys inhibited cerebrovascular vasospasm.[234] The effect was again associated with and seemingly related to a marked reduction of blood serotonin concentration.

Additional evidence that platelets may be implicated in the mechanism of sudden cardiac death was provided by Ellis and coworkers, who found that when human platelets are aggregated by thrombin, material is released that causes strips of tissue cut from the porcine coronary artery to contract.[235] Peak contraction occurred within 1 minute and dissipated within 4 to 8 minutes. Indomethacin, which inhibits prostaglandin synthesis, prevented the shortening of the coronary artery strip, suggesting that the contractile substance was a prostaglandin. These investigators adduced evidence that thromboxane A_2, one of the principal biologically active prostaglandins released from aggregated platelets, was the contractile factor.[235]

Pertinent to the platelet hypothesis in relation to sudden cardiac death is the fact that infusion of catecholamines such as norepinephrine induces subendocardial necrosis, which is associated with platelet aggregates in the myocardial microcirculation.[236,237] Stress itself may initiate such platelet aggregation in the coronary circulation. Total vascular occlusion occurred in rats subjected to such stressful stimuli as heat or electric shock.[238] The cardiac lesions produced by stress are similar to those observed following catecholamine administration and have also been reported in patients dying from pheochromocytoma.[239] Barr and coworkers have noted an association between thrombocythemia and the occurrence of ventricular arrhythmias.[240] The patient, a young woman with angiographically normal coronary arterial vessels, experienced recurring episodes of Prinzmetal's variant angina pectoris and episodes of nocturnal ventricular tachycardia. The only abnormality was a blood platelet count of 1,000,000/mm³. Symptoms as well as arrhythmia abated after the initiation of salicylate therapy.

The following hypothesis appears to be supported by substantial evidence: Given a myocardium with electrical instability due to extensive coronary atherosclerosis, psychophysiological stress or enhanced neural sympathetic tone favors formation of platelet aggregates in regions of plaques and turbulent flow; there follows release of biogenic amines and prostaglandins, which induce spasm of large vessels, leading to major coronary artery obstruction as well as to impaired flow in tributaries. Ventricular fibrillation is triggered on platelet disaggregation and the abrupt onset of reperfusion.

Coronary Arterial Spasm (see also p. 1360). The reality of coronary arterial spasm is better appreciated since the description by Prinzmetal et al. of a variant form of angina pectoris.[241] The absence of significant coronary atherosclerosis among a number of patients with this syndrome has been widely reported.[242-244] The role of vasospasm was first conclusively demonstrated by Dhurandhar et al.[245] and by Oliva et al.[246] and has been amply confirmed.[247-250] Especially persuasive are the observations of Maseri and coworkers, who have found that coronary vasospasm is not only limited to variant angina but also is an initiating event in myocardial infarction.[248,249] The concept of vascular spasm in the coronary circulation

has profound implications. The investigations of Mudge and coworkers are especially relevant.[251] They measured coronary vascular resistance before and during the initial portion of a cold pressor test in patients with normal and with diseased coronary arteries. Although coronary resistance did not change in the former group, it rose in those with ischemic heart disease. The alpha-adrenergic–blocking drug phentolamine abolished reflex coronary vasoconstriction in several patients who experienced angina pectoris. In patients with Prinzmetal's angina, coronary arterial spasm can also be induced by ergot alkaloids[252,253] as well as by the vagotonic agent methacholine.[254,255]

Relevant to the problem of sudden cardiac death is the fact that Prinzmetal's angina is associated with a ubiquity of VPB's, which may be of advanced grade. It is well appreciated that the current of injury as well as coronary spasm may occur without the patient feeling any discomfort, and one may therefore surmise that in the electrically unstable heart, diverse neural traffic to the heart may provoke coronary vascular spasm, which enhances myocardial ischemia and triggers arrhythmia, which in turn may culminate in ventricular fibrillation at the onset of impaired flow or upon reperfusion. There may also be platelet aggregates and release of diverse biogenic amines, prostaglandins as well as bradykinins, which participate in varying degrees and contribute to the final denouement.

CLINICAL APPROACHES TO SUDDEN CARDIAC DEATH

Patients with Acute Myocardial Infarction. Among those dying suddenly, a major problem is delay in seeking medical attention (Chap. 57).[256] Patients' denial of the gravity of their condition or misinterpretation of symptoms is a significant reason for delayed hospitalization.[7,257-259] Curiously, patients with previous myocardial infarction or with preexisting angina pectoris delay the longest in seeking help.[258] In the pre-hospital phase of myocardial infarction, the most important component of patient delay relates to self-treatment and seeking advice from family, friends, and neighbors.[259] Arrival at the hospital is invariably delayed well beyond the critical first hour, when about 60 per cent of all sudden cardiac deaths occur. Clearly, part of the problem is lack of education on the part of both the medical profession and the lay public about the need for expeditious hospitalization with the advent of symptoms that suggest a heart attack. However, one cannot be overly optimistic that education alone, no matter how intensive, will overcome entrenched habit and fear. Experience with physicians who have heart attacks is sadly instructive; they frequently procrastinate longer than laymen. Certainly this is not due to ignorance of the consequences.

The physician can, however, shorten delay by advising patients with ischemic heart disease to proceed immediately to an appropriate health care facility if there is an abrupt onset of chest pain or if preexisting angina changes in quality or duration. The patient should be instructed to contact an emergency ambulance service directly and bypass calling a physician if symptoms are disabling. When the physician is in the presence of a patient having an acute coronary episode, the first therapeutic objective is to allay anxiety and to assuage pain. The former requires a reassuring demeanor and encouragement; the latter is readily controlled by parenteral morphine. The next objective is to protect against fatal arrhythmia. Monitoring is not required for the initiation of appropriate measures. Even if the heart rate is regular on auscultation or even if an electrocardiographic monitor shows an absence of VPB's, an unheralded outburst of ventricular fibrillation is not precluded.[146,260] The administration of a bolus of 75 mg of lidocaine intravenously followed by 300 mg intramuscularly will prevent malignant ventricular arrhythmia in a large majority of patients. Double-blind studies have demonstrated the protective effect of lidocaine at the very inception of a coronary ischemic event.[261,262] If symptomatic bradycardia is present and heart rates are less than 50 per minute, the judicious use of small doses of atropine may prove salutary. Self-administration of either of these drugs by the patient places an unwarranted burden on the victim. The precise guidelines for the proper use of these medications require medical appraisal and sound clinical judgment.

Patients with Primary Electrical Failure. This syndrome usually lacks prodromes, and death is frequently instantaneous. When time does elapse, the patient may find symptoms difficult to interpret properly and is unlikely to summon help. When help is summoned, it may be too late. As already noted, there are essentially two distinct strategies: (1) reach the patient at the inception of the terminal event and provide emergency cardiopulmonary resuscitative care; and (2) identify the potential victim and initiate prophylactic measures against fatal arrhythmia.

Emergency Care. Current medical efforts for coping with sudden death place major reliance upon cardiopulmonary resuscitation, the intent being to reach the patient expeditiously at the very onset of the potentially lethal attack in order to terminate the ventricular fibrillation and stabilize the heart rhythm. Community-based ambulance services are beginning to incorporate the expertise and facilities found in the coronary care unit and are now gaining popularity. The essential concepts and guidelines for resuscitation were enunciated during the first National Conference on Standards for Cardiopulmonary Resuscitation and Emergency Cardiac Care, held in May, 1973.[263] Two essential strategies were defined and have been recently updated:[264,264a] basic life support and advanced life support.

Emergency first aid procedures, consisting of the recognition of airway obstruction and of respiratory and cardiac arrest and the proper application of cardiopulmonary resuscitation (CPR), constitute the elements of *basic life support.* CPR involves opening and maintaining a patent airway, providing artificial ventilation by means of rescue breathing, and maintaining artificial circulation by means of external cardiac compression. Paramount among the goals of CPR is to restore a cardiac mechanism as expeditiously as possible. The interval between the onset of cardiac arrest and the restoration of a normal cardiac rhythm will determine the success of defibrillation, the capacity to maintain an effective rhythm, the extent of neurologic damage as well as the achievement of long-term survival. Therefore the objectives in cardiac resuscitation are the prompt delivery of oxygenated blood to vital organs by means of cardiac massage and the reestablishment of a

heartbeat by means of defibrillation. The priority given to these two procedures depends upon the conditions under which cardiac arrest occurs. Thus, if the arrest is witnessed and a defibrillator is close at hand, one aims first to restore a cardiac mechanism. If, however, the event is unwitnessed, or the area is not equipped with a defibrillator, routine cardiopulmonary efforts are initiated and defibrillation is deferred.

Advanced life support includes, in addition to the basic life support outlined above, a number of adjunctive procedures, including intravenous fluid and drug administration, cardiac defibrillation, stabilization of blood pressure, rhythm monitoring, control of arrhythmias, and postresuscitation care.

CARDIOPULMONARY RESUSCITATION (CPR)

THUMPVERSION At the very inception of ventricular fibrillation, there is frequently observed an ultrarapid regular rhythm designated as ventricular tachycardia of the vulnerable period—$VT_{(vp)}$.[136] This mechanism is believed to result from a self-sustained reentrant wavefront of depolarization circulating around the perimeter of an infarct or of an ischemic area. This view is supported by the observation that one or more threshold pulses delivered directly to the endocardium may terminate this arrhythmia. $VT_{(vp)}$ can also be abolished by one hundredth of the energy required to defibrillate the heart transthoracically. This fact is of profound clinical significance, since such low energies can be delivered to the heart by means of a chest thump.[265] If thumping of the lower sternum is delayed, even momentarily, ventricular fibrillation emerges and is resistant to this maneuver. Effectiveness of the chest thump is due to transduction of the mechanical input to an electrical pulse, i.e., an extrasystole, which depolarizes part of the pathway traversed by the abnormal reentrant excitation.[266] This technique is especially valuable in the patient who is being monitored and when the arrest has been witnessed.

In utilizing the precordial thump, the following guidelines must be observed:

1. One should deliver a sharp, quick blow to the midportion of the sternum, hitting with the lower, fleshy portion of the fist from a distance of 8 to 12 inches above the chest.

2. It must be administered during the first minute after onset of the cardiac arrest.

3. If there is no cardiac response on repeating the chest thump, basic life support must not be further delayed.

Artificial Ventilation. An important factor in successful resuscitation is the immediate establishment of a patent airway (Fig. 23–8). This requires examination of the mouth to assure that no obstruction is present, such as loosely fitting dentures, vomitus, or any other foreign body. The most common cause of airway obstruction in the unconscious person is the tongue, which recedes to the posterior pharyngeal wall. Patency of the airway is assured by tilting the victim's head backward as far as possible. This simple maneuver may suffice for the resumption of spontaneous respiration. With the victim lying on his back, his neck fully extended, so that the base of the tongue no longer obstructs the upper end of the trachea, the rescuer

Summary of Basic Life Support

Airway

Is victim unconscious?

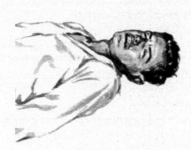

Head-tilt maneuver

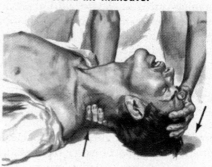

Breathing

Is victim breathing?

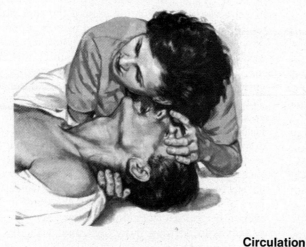

If not, quickly give 4 full mouth-to-mouth ventilations

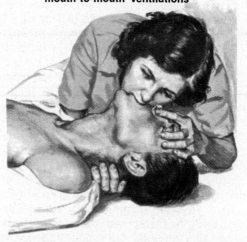

Circulation

Is carotid pulse present?

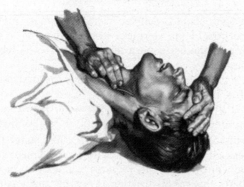

If not, give external cardiac compression

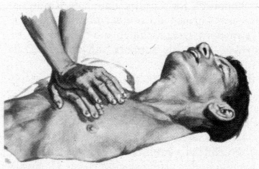

One rescuer: 15 compressions / 2 ventilations
every 15 seconds

Two rescuers: 5 compressions / 1 ventilation
every 5 seconds

FIGURE 23–8   Emergency maneuvers in a patient with cardiac or cardiorespiratory arrest. (© Copyright 1974 CIBA Pharmaceutical Company, Division of CIBA-GEIGY Corporation. Reprinted with permission from Clinical Symposia, illustrated by Frank H. Netter, M.D. All rights reserved.)

accomplishes the head tilt maneuver by placing one hand beneath the victim's neck and the other hand on the forehead and then lifting the neck while pressing the head backward. The head must be maintained in this position throughout resuscitation. Thereupon, mouth-to-mouth or mouth-to-nose breathing is initiated. A plastic airway can be used if available. With one hand behind the victim's neck, holding the victim's head in a position of maximum backward tilt, the rescuer pinches the victim's nostrils together with the thumb and index finger of the other hand, opens his mouth widely, takes a deep breath, places his mouth over the victim's mouth to create a tight seal, and exhales completely.

This is a simple and effective means of delivering oxygenated air by untrained personnel. The cycle should be repeated every 5 seconds for as long as respiratory inadequacy persists. By observing the rise and fall of the chest and by noting the escape of air during exhalation as well as the resistance encountered during inspiration as the victim's lungs expand, the rescuer can determine whether ventilation is adequate. Often much valuable time is wasted by medical or paramedical personnel in attempting to insert an endotracheal tube as the initial measure in management of cardiac arrest. In the majority of instances, endotracheal intubation is not required. Mouth-to-nose ventilation is preferred and is recommended when it is impossible to open the victim's mouth, when there is injury to the mouth, or when it is difficult to achieve a tight seal.

Artificial Circulation. Cardiac arrest is recognized by the absence of a pulse in the large arteries of an unconscious victim who is not breathing. Having rapidly ventilated the subject four times, one instantly checks for a carotid pulse. While maintaining the head tilt with one hand on the forehead, the rescuer now initiates external cardiac compression, which consists of rhythmic application of pressure to the lower half of the sternum but not over the xiphoid process. External cardiac compression is always accompanied by artificial ventilation. This method is relatively simple and can be used successfully by personnel who have had only a minimum of training. It involves compression of the heart between sternum and spine; lateral cardiac motion is limited by the pericardium. The patient must be in a horizontal position on a hard surface, preferably the floor, if one is indoors. Elevation of lower extremities while the rest of the body remains horizontal may promote venous return and augment artificial circulation during external cardiac compression. The pressure required must be of a magnitude to depress the lower sternum by a minimum of 3 to 5 cm. The long axis of the heel of one's hand is placed parallel to and over the long axis of the lower half of the sternum, and the heel of the other hand is placed on the dorsum of the first. If applied too high, the massage will prove ineffective and may cause multiple rib fractures. The arms are kept straight at the elbow to allow pressure to be applied almost vertically. The shoulders of the resuscitator should be directly above the victim's sternum, so that compression can be carried out by forceful movements of the back and shoulders with elbows fully extended rather than by flexion and extension of the arm at the elbow. Compressions must be regular, uninterrupted, and carried out at a frequency of 60 per minute; relaxation should be abrupt and equal to compression in duration. A ratio of 5:1 is maintained between ventilation and cardiac compression.

Cardiopulmonary resuscitation is best accomplished by two rescuers, one on either side of the patient, who can then switch positions when necessary without any significant interruption of the 5:1 rhythm. If the rescuer is alone, 18 compressions should be applied, and the lungs should be ventilated two times, and this cycle should be continued until help arrives. To attain proficiency one must practice these resuscitative maneuvers using mannequins and under the direction of skilled instructors.

The effectiveness of CPR has been ascribed to compression of the arrested heart between the sternum and the vertebral column. However, early observations indicated that similar intrathoracic arterial and venous pressure levels prevailed during chest compression.[267] Weisfeldt and associates[268] have questioned whether the pumping action of the heart during CPR is a critical factor in maintaining blood flow. They have noted that the effectiveness of CPR correlates with the rise of intrathoracic pressure; for example, in patients with flail chest, no arterial blood pressure is generated until paradoxical thoracic expansion is prevented by binding the chest. Furthermore, by transiently preventing expiration or by maintaining pressure on the AMBU bag in intubated patients, arterial pressure is increased with the greater intrathoracic pressure. In extensive studies, these workers[268] failed to find a pressure gradient across the heart during chest compression. However, they did observe an extrathoracic arteriovenous gradient. Flow occurs because of a rise in intrathoracic pressure, which generates an extrathoracic arteriovenous gradient. These observations are in accord with the demonstration by Criley et al.[269] that continuous coughing can maintain consciousness in the arrested patient.

ADVANCED LIFE SUPPORT. Advanced life support does not imply abandoning cardiopulmonary resuscitation but rather supplementing it with more definitive measures as additional resources and personnel reach the scene. It entails the use of supplemental oxygen as soon as it becomes available. Exhaled air ventilation delivers generally about 16 to 17 per cent oxygen to the victim. This may produce an alveolar oxygen tension of 80 torr. However, because of the low cardiac output associated with external cardiac compression, the presence of intrapulmonary shunting, and ventilation-perfusion abnormalities, marked discrepancies will occur between alveolar and arterial oxygen tension, and hypoxemia will invariably be present. Monitoring for arrhythmia defines the cardiac mechanism and permits the institution of defibrillation. However, blind defibrillation is preferred if time is to be wasted in gaining an adequate electrocardiographic signal.

Defibrillation. The electrode paddles to be applied to the chest as well as the chest areas involved must be adequately covered with electrode paste in order to lower electrical impedance. One electrode is placed in the right 2nd intercostal space rather than over the sternum. The other electrode is either placed in the midaxillary line in the 5th interspace or, if a flat paddle is available, positioned posteriorly at the angle of the left scapula. An energy setting of 400 wsec suffices to revert all patients with primary ventricular fibrillation. With currently used defibrillators, the energy delivered at such a setting is generally about 320 wsec. Recommendations have been made that the energy output of defibrillators currently in use be increased above this limit.[270,271] These suggestions are based on experimental studies in animals and have presumed that the energy of defibrillation is largely a function of body weight. It has been stated that a maximal setting of 400 wsec is inadequate for defibrillating 35 per cent or more of patients who weigh in excess of 50 kg.[271] However, clinical experience is at variance with these opinions. Indeed, Pantridge et al.[272] and Crampton[273] have maintained the contrary, namely, that the maximum energies currently employed for defibrillation are excessive. A single 200-wsec shock reverted 73 of 82 (89 per cent) patients with ventricular fibrillation; a second discharge at the same setting restored sinus rhythm in an additional 7 per cent, resulting in a total success rate of 96 per cent.[272] There was no correlation between ease of reversion and body weight. In one recent clinical experience a man weighing 190 kg (418 lb) was successfully resuscitated with a single 400-wsec shock after a prolonged episode of ventricular fibrillation.[274]

Kerber and Sarnat[275] found no difference in body weight in patients successfully defibrillated compared with those in whom the procedure failed. Nor was there a difference of energy per body weight in the two groups. Patients who were defibrillated were less acidotic and were younger in age.

The question of the energy to be employed is not a minor issue, since electrical discharge can prove injurious even when delivered transthoracically, and these injuries are directly related to the energy content of the shock.[276] Such myocardial injury may prevent successful resuscitation. It needs to be emphasized that when a single discharge fails to revert, repeating the discharge at the same energy level will frequently prove successful. This is due to the fact that the initial discharge lowers skin impedance and thus more current is being delivered with the second discharge.

Intravenous Medications.   Once ventilation and cardiac massage are being well sustained, an intravenous route must be established. If circulation is not restored, sodium bicarbonate, 1 mEq/kg, should be injected to combat metabolic acidosis and is repeated after 10 minutes. Once an effective rhythm is restored, further drug administration is governed by arterial blood gas and pH measurements. Epinephrine is an essential drug that proves of great value at times. Although this catecholamine theoretically predisposes to ventricular fibrillation, in practice it has been shown to enhance defibrillation, especially when fine-wave arrhythmia prevails. If, after defibrillation, an ineffectual contraction is restored, the ensuing myocardial hypoxia predisposes to recurrence of the arrhythmia. Since epinephrine increases myocardial contractility and elevates perfusion pressure, it not only lowers the threshold for defibrillation but may also prevent electromechanical dissociation. A dose of 0.5 ml of a 1/1000 solution diluted to 10 ml should be administered intravenously every 5 minutes during the resuscitation effort. When an intravenous route cannot be established, intracardiac administration of this drug may be essential.

When reversion results in profound bradycardia and there is resumption of fibrillation, the intravenous administration of 0.5 mg of atropine may prove salutary. Such a bolus can be repeated in 5 minutes to accelerate the heart rate above 60 per minute. Another essential drug to be used early in resuscitation is lidocaine. This drug raises the fibrillation threshold and has minimal deleterious effects on myocardial contractility, systemic arterial pressure, and venous return. It also diminishes or entirely eliminates advanced grades of VPB's and may thereby reduce recurrence of tachyarrhythmias. Lidocaine is to be given as a 75-mg bolus intravenously, repeated in 2 minutes, and then followed by a continuous infusion of 2 to 3 mg/min but not exceeding 4 mg/min. Bretylium tosylate, an adrenergic-blocking agent, raises the threshold for ventricular fibrillation in experimental animals and may cause spontaneous defibrillation in humans. In a randomized blind trial comparing bretylium with lidocaine in 146 victims of out-of-hospital ventricular fibrillation, no advantage or disadvantage was noted for either drug.[276a]

Two other drugs may be useful. If the resuscitated patient experiences chest pain, *morphine sulfate* will both relieve pain and assuage anxiety. It is especially valuable when pulmonary edema attends the onset of acute myocardial infarction, which was the cause of the cardiac arrest. The intravenous administration of 5 to 8 mg generally suffices. At times it may be necessary to use *calcium chloride*, which increases myocardial contractility, prolongs systole, and enhances ventricular automaticity. Again, this should be used when defibrillation has been repeated several times or when the heart cannot be defibrillated because of fine, rapid oscillations of the fibrillatory wave pattern. The usual recommended dose of calcium chloride is 2.5 ml to 5 ml of a 10 per cent solution providing 3.4 to 6.8 mEq of calcium. When calcium gluconate is infused, the dose is 10 ml of a 10 per cent solution providing 4.8 mEq of calcium.

The initial management of cardiac arrest is crucial. One frequently encounters a patient with a badly damaged brain who lingers as a tragic reminder of belated, inadequate, or improper CPR. Unfortunately during such emergencies there are no adequate records kept to provide insight into precisely what went wrong. In many hospitals cardiac arrest teams do not exist, and the responsibility for CPR devolves on those in the immediate vicinity of the victim. The multitude of bystanders tend to impede the resuscitative effort, which is neither well coordinated nor well directed, thereby jeopardizing survival.

MANAGEMENT OF THE PATIENT AT RISK FOR SUDDEN CARDIAC DEATH

Basically three approaches are available for preventing sudden cardiac death: (1) mass prophylaxis with antiarrhythmic drugs, (2) implanted defibrillators, or (3) individualized antiarrhythmic therapy.

MASS PROPHYLAXIS.   The most logical approach is to initiate a prophylactic program with some effective antiarrhythmic measure for those deemed to be at risk for sudden cardiac death. The target population is large, including not only patients with overt manifestations of ischemic heart disease but also those having high-risk profiles for coronary disease. The latter population represents two-thirds of the victims. Currently available antiarrhythmic measures are not suitable for wide prophylactic use, because of the potential of serious adverse reactions. The following calculation makes clear the poor trade-off in employing antiarrhythmic drugs. Patients who have recovered from acute myocardial infarction constitute a high-risk group for sudden cardiac death. In such a group, one may anticipate an annual mortality of 4 per cent, with a 3 per cent incidence of sudden cardiac death. Assuming the availability of an antiarrhythmic drug that would reduce mortality by 30 per cent, sudden death could be prevented in 1 patient per 100 survivors of myocardial infarction per year. However, 99 patients would be burdened with the inconvenience of taking daily medications, at significant psychological and economic costs. Furthermore current antiarrhythmic drugs generally induce toxic reactions in about 30 per cent of recipients. Thus, although one patient might be saved, 30 others certainly might suffer adverse reactions. Until safe and highly effective measures are found, employment of prophylactic antiarrhythmic drugs requires precise identification of the potential victim.

SURVIVORS OF OUT-OF-HOSPITAL CARDIAC ARREST. Ample experience has now been gained with out-of-hospital cardiac arrest to permit definition of the decisive variables determining survival. Eisenberg et al.[277] have shown that survival relates to four factors: (1) whether cardiac arrest was witnessed, (2) the cardiac rhythm at the time of arrest, (3) whether or not CPR was initiated by lay bystanders, and (4) speed in arrival time of paramedic unit. In 611 patients with out-of-hospital cardiac arrest, these variables were predictive of outcome (Table 23–6). Among 22 patients with favorable findings on all four predictive factors, 15, or 70 per cent, were discharged alive. This contrasts with only 1 survivor among 97 patients with all four unfavorable findings. Myerburg et al.[278] have also ascribed critical importance to the cardiac arrest rhythm. Among 352 consecutive victims of out-of-hospital cardiac arrest, of 24 patients presenting with ventricular tachycardia, 16, or 67 per cent, were ultimately discharged alive. When the arrhythmia was ventricular fibrillation, 55, or 23 per cent, recovered. However, when a bradyarrhythmia was the initial mechanism, of 108 such patients only 9 were resuscitated and none survived. Another helpful predictor is the heart rate immediately after defibrillation. Only 5 per cent survived when the rate was less than 60 beats/min, and 17 per cent when it ranged from 60 to 100 beats/min; of these 43 per cent were long-term survivors.[278]

TABLE 23–6 OUTCOME AMONG 611 PATIENTS WITH OUT-OF-HOSPITAL CARDIAC ARREST

EVENT WITNESSED	NUMBER OF PATIENTS	DISCHARGED ALIVE (%)
+	380	28*
−	231	3
ARRYTHMIA OF CARDIAC ARREST		
VT or VF	389	28*
Asystole	222	3
BYSTANDER-INITIATED CPR		
+	168	32*
−	443	14
RESPONSE TIME (MIN)		
<4.0	39	56
4.0–8.0	139	35
>8.0	186	17

*p <0.01.
From Eisenberg, M., et al.: The ACLS score: Predicting survival from out-of-hospital cardiac arrest. J.A.M.A. *246*:50, 1981.

Improvement in results of resuscitation following out-of-hospital cardiac arrest has been progressive. In the period from 1971 to 1973, overall survival was 14 per cent, whereas from 1973 to 1978, it had increased to 23 per cent.[278] At present, the hospital discharge rate from out-of-hospital ventricular fibrillation is up to 30 per cent.[279] However, long-range survival has been poor. In a prospective follow-up of 276 resuscitated patients who were discharged alive from the hospital, the probability of remaining alive at 4 years was only 49 per cent, compared with 80 per cent of a normal population adjusted for age and sex and 66 per cent for a population of patients discharged after myocardial infarction.[280] But even those surviving are not spared major neurologic and intellectual impairments. In a prospective study of 63 survivors, seizure activity was observed in 30 per cent.[281] Most commonly, it began within 12 hours, usually occurring either as partial seizures or as myoclonic activity and rarely as a tonic-clonic type of "shivering." A good prognosis for survival and sound neurologic outcome was related to the presence, at the time of admission to hospital, of pupillary responses to light, oculocephalic reflexes, purposeful responses to pain, and spontaneous respiration.

Promise of reducing the inordinate toll of sudden death is being provided by the beta-adrenergic–blocking drugs that result in a low incidence of adverse reactions. Numerous studies have reported favorable results in long-term treatment of patients with ischemic heart disease, and these have been recently reviewed.[282] The most persuasive report is the Norwegian Multicenter Study with timolol in patients surviving acute myocardial infarction.[283] The number of sudden deaths was reduced by about 50 per cent among 1884 randomized to either placebo or timolol groups and followed an average of 17 months.

IMPLANTATION OF DEFIBRILLATORS. For the patient who is greatly threatened by the possibility of recurring ventricular fibrillation, Mirowski et al.[284,285] have suggested the intriguing approach of implanting in the chest a standby automatic defibrillator system. Such a completely implanted defibrillator unit can reverse ventricular fibrillation in dogs. Compared with transthoracic delivery of the shock, intracardiac defibrillation requires only a fraction of the energy. Though this method is fraught with technical difficulties, on first examination it is impressive in its seeming logic. However, difficult problems remain to be surmounted, such as sensing the onset of ventricular fibrillation, prevention of electrical injury, and absence of methods for determining operational readiness and efficacy of an implanted unit.[286] It is our view that placing an electronic device in the chest does not appear to be the answer to the problem of sudden cardiac death. For the immediate future, the potential victim will need to be identified and protected by an individualized antiarrhythmic program.

SELECTION OF PATIENTS FOR ANTIARRHYTHMIC TREATMENT. At present, antiarrhythmic drugs are to be employed largely for those individuals identified as being at high risk for sudden cardiac death. The following constitute the essential subgroups of patients for whom therapy is indicated:

1. Patients who previously experienced primary ventricular fibrillation without associated evidence of acute myo-

cardial infarction. These patients are at highest risk of sudden cardiac death; nearly one-third will succumb within a year of their initial resuscitation.

2. Patients with ischemic heart disease who on monitoring or exercise stress testing exhibit ventricular tachycardia of more than three successive cycles and with rates in excess of 180 beats/min. The risk of sudden cardiac death is greater if the arrhythmia is ventricular tachycardia of the vulnerable period, or $VT_{(vp)}$, or if the salvos consist of accelerating cycles.

3. Patients within the first 6 months after recovery from acute myocardial infarction who have angina pectoris of recent onset or who demonstrate grade 4 or 5 VPB's.

4. Patients who are being subjected to profound psychological stress or are in a state of bereavement because of loss of spouse and have developed grade 4 or 5 VPB's for the first time.

5. Patients with prolonged Q-T intervals who have experienced unexplained syncope and have VPB's of grade 2 or higher.

6. Young women with prolapse of the mitral valve who on monitoring show episodic Q-T interval prolongation and VPB's. Treatment is even more essential if they have experienced syncope or if there is a history of sudden death among close family members.

7. Patients in whom exercise stress induces both ST-segment depression ≥ 2 mm and grade 4 and 5 VPB's either at peak exercise or immediately upon recovery.

8. Patients who develop ventricular ectopic activity when they experience angina pectoris.

9. Patients who are severely disabled because of frequent VPB's.

Patients are generally unaware that they are experiencing VPB's. Often the physician's well-meaning but misguided concern over the presence of cardiac irregularities cues the patient to the abnormal pulse and provokes undue anxiety and psychological disquiet, which may then stimulate further arrhythmia. The mere appearance of VPB's does not portend a dire prognosis and should not be a cause for alarm. The vast majority of individuals with VPB's require little more than reassurance from the physician about the benign nature of this condition. Treatment of sporadic VPB's is directed only at the symptomatic individual in whom simple conservative measures fail to allay anxiety. In these patients, continued and oft-repeated reassurance, instruction in relaxation techniques, encouragement of adequate participation in recreation, initiation of an aerobic exercise program, discontinuation of caffeine-containing beverages and of cigarette smoking, and the judicious use of minor doses of beta-adrenergic–blocking agents (propranolol, 10 to 20 mg three to four times daily; metoprolol, 50 mg twice daily; or atenolol, 25 mg once daily) will suffice for allaying symptoms. In many cases the use of medications may be tailored to the patient's individual problem, e.g., if arrhythmia occurs primarily with exercise, solely at night, or only during periods of intense turmoil, then the beta-blocking agent or some other drug is administered only during or in anticipation of these specific situations.

STRATEGY OF MANAGEMENT. Physicians increasingly encounter patients who either have been resuscitated from ventricular fibrillation or experience oft-

recurring bouts of ventricular tachycardia which result in either syncope or profound hemodynamic compromise leading to rapid deterioration of cardiac function. These groups of rhythm disorders have been labeled *malignant ventricular arrhythmias*.[105] To date, there is a paucity of clinical guidelines for managing these patients. Therapeutic measures have been empirical and haphazard. Our experience over the past decade with patients who have had malignant ventricular arrhythmias suggests the following elements for a successful management program.[105,287]

1. Thorough evaluation of the cardiac as well as the human problem is required. There is need to focus attention on the psychological stresses that not infrequently predispose to or cause the arrhythmia.[107] Although the physician may be unable to alter the complex social and psychological milieu, merely the expression of interest and sympathy is profoundly therapeutic.

2. In order to define the prevalence and type of ventricular arrhythmia, 24-hour monitoring as well as exercise stress testing is required.

3. Acute drug testing employing programmed trendscription (i.e., a compressed recording of heart rhythm [p. 799] is a prerequisite for the expeditious screening of drugs for efficacy as well as for appropriate dosage. It also indicates which drug or drugs may aggravate rather than lessen arrhythmia.

4. If advanced grades of VPB's are infrequent or nonreproducible, as is true in 15 per cent of patients with malignant arrhythmias, repetitive ventricular response (RVR) testing is employed to assess drug efficacy.

5. An antiarrhythmic drug should be tried for 48 to 72 hours at each selected dosage. Exercise testing and 24-hour monitoring must be conducted with every dose level.

6. The therapeutic objective is to suppress grades 4 and 5 ventricular arrhythmias. This goal may not be readily achieved; a reduction in frequency of these grades may be the only option. However, if rapid ventricular tachyarrhythmias are provoked during exercise, drugs must be manipulated until the rhythm disturbances are completely suggested. If extrastimulus testing is employed, the endpoint is abolition of nonsustained ventricular tachycardia consisting of three or more cycles.

7. The use of drug combinations is indicated in all instances of ventricular fibrillation. A "fail-safe" system of drug protection, namely, the employment of two or more agents that have proved effective is mandated by the risk of recurrence. In other disorders physicians may have an opportunity to remedy therapeutic error, but this is infrequently the case with ventricular fibrillation.

8. The digitalis glycosides may contribute to suppression of ventricular arrhythmia. The benefit of digitalis drugs is best judged by the use of acetylstrophanthidin.[288]

9. Psychological stress testing may expose advanced grades of ventricular ectopy and may thereby provide useful insights into the factors contributing to the genesis of arrhythmia. This type of provocation also defines the adequacy of a selected antiarrhythmic program.

10. Psychiatric support for the patient and the use of relaxation techniques such as meditation facilitate management of the so-called intractable ventricular arrhythmias.

11. Accurate and meticulous record keeping, as already emphasized by Winkle et al., is mandatory.[289] Daily tabula-

tion of data, including precise time of drug administration, dosage, trendscription findings, and monitoring and exercise results as well as any untoward reactions, is essential to the development of an effective drug program.

Our experience indicates that the majority of patients with recurrent malignant ventricular arrhythmias can be protected by a combination of medical measures.

Ambulatory 24-Hour Electrocardiographic Monitoring. The most effective method for recognizing rarely occurring arrhythmic events is to monitor a patient equipped with a portable recorder for 24 hours while the individual is performing usual daily activities. As already indicated, nearly 90 per cent of patients with ischemic heart disease will demonstrate VPB's and 41 per cent will exhibit repetitive ectopic beats of grade 4 as their maximal grade during at least 1 monitoring hour. It should be emphasized that advanced grades are nonpersistent, sporadic, and relatively rare events. Thus, among 100 men with ischemic heart disease (mean age 57), grade 4 arrhythmia was present in 40 patients during at least 1 hour, but only half these patients demonstrated this grade of VPB's during 2 monitored hours and only 7 (17.5 per cent) exhibited this grade during 12 of the 24 hours.[133] There is an additional problem of reproducibility in successive monitoring sessions.

Monitoring for VPB's by means of 24-hour recordings presents additional problems. It is costly, it is difficult to correlate occurrence of arrhythmia precisely with life events, and there is a variable time lag between monitoring tape interpretation and transmittal of data to the physician. Furthermore, interpretation of the record must rely on sample selection by a third party, the technician reading the tapes, who is generally unfamiliar with the clinical problem. Nonetheless, this technique remains for the present the foundation for defining the patient at risk for sudden cardiac death as well as assessing the therapeutic efficacy of various drug regimens.

Trendscription. This method provides an immediate print-out that permits the physician to examine all the data and then interpret these within the context of clinical circumstances.[290] It fills the gap between the limited arrhythmia information provided by the recording of a routine electrocardiogram and the veritable deluge of output derived from 24-hour monitoring (Fig. 23–9). Thirty minutes of information is presented in a compressed form, recorded on a rotating drum. This method of data condensation is coupled with statistical time sampling and instantaneously provides the physician with significant trends of ectopic activity by means of a print-out that can be easily visualized and readily interpreted. Its greatest value is its use in judging the efficacy and safety of antiarrhythmic drugs.[291]

Exercise Stress Testing to Expose VPB's. In the experimental animal as well as in humans, the frequency of ventricular ectopic beats increases as a function of the presence and extent of myocardial ischemia. Exercise burdens the myocardium with accelerated heart rate, rise in blood pressure, preloading of the ventricle, enhanced sympathetic nervous activity, augmented catecholamine excretion, and, in patients with restricted coronary flow, tissue hypoxia and acidosis. Jelinek and Lown have demonstrated that maximal exercise stress is an effective method for exposing ventricular premature beats in patients with ischemic heart disease.[292] These VPB's are observed primarily during the peak of exercise and in the immediate postexercise recovery period. Whereas normal subjects may develop arrhythmia with exercise, advanced grades of VPB's are more common in those subjects with ischemic heart disease. Indeed, several studies have correlated the occurrence and grade of ectopic activity with the severity of angiographically demonstrated coronary artery disease and with the extent of abnormalities in the motion of the left ventricular wall.[293–295] In some patients with severe ischemic heart disease and recurrent ventricular fibrillation, 24-hour monitoring does not expose the presence of high grades of VPB's, which are demonstrated only with exercise.

Psychological Stress Testing. As with exercise testing, the objective of psychological stress testing has been to devise a method that will reproducibly precipitate ventricular arrhythmias. The basis for this method derives from clinical observations as well as earlier cited investigations. The fact that a 24-hour monitoring period consistently shows a greater frequency of advanced grades of VPB's compared with maximal exercise stress argues for a psychological rather than a hemodynamic trigger for the ectopic beats. At no time during such a 24-hour monitoring period does the patient achieve peak heart rates as high as those that occur during the exercise stress. To date, we have been only episodically successful in precipitating VPB's in about 25 per cent of patients by means of psychological stress. This is a promising but as yet unexplored area.[296]

Problems in Managing Patients with Malignant Ventricular Arrhythmias. The mainstay of prevention of sudden cardiac death consists of the use of antiarrhythmic drugs to subdue advanced grades of VPB's or electrophysi-

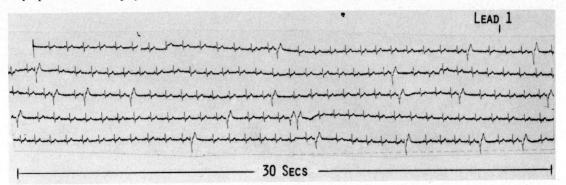

LEAD 1

|— 30 SECS —|

FIGURE 23–9 Part of a trendscription, presenting half the width of the usual record, which inscribes an entire minute of information in a single line. The ease of recognizing VPB's is evident.

ologically provoked ventricular repetitive activity. However, merely administering an antiarrhythmic drug in the hope of preventing fatality is an exercise in futility. Schaffer and Cobb found that 73 per cent of 64 patients who had recurrent ventricular fibrillation were receiving antiarrhythmic therapy at the time of sudden death.[120]

Therapy must be individualized. When an antiarrhythmic drug fails to prevent a recurrence, there is no certainty about whether an improper drug had been chosen or whether an incorrect dose had been administered. Generally, when an antiarrhythmic agent is used, the physician gauges therapeutic efficacy by abatement of symptoms or prevention of recurrence of sustained and demonstrable arrhythmia. When a disordered mechanism of the heartbeat is devoid of symptoms, repeated Holter monitoring sessions are required to determine whether a drug is of value. When ectopic beats are infrequent and sporadic, there is no certainty—even with longer or more frequent periods of monitoring—that the selected drug is effective. Clearly, new techniques are needed to determine drug effectiveness as well as proper dosage for the individual patient with VPB's.

We have therefore attempted to streamline drug therapy by introducing the method of *acute drug testing.*[291] The essential principle is based on the conception that the effectiveness of most antiarrhythmic drugs is related to the establishment of a so-called significant therapeutic blood concentration (see Chap. 20). This can be achieved rapidly by administering a single large oral dose. The purpose of acute drug testing is thus to establish therapeutic blood levels during a brief period of time in order to define during the course of drug action its effects on arrhythmia and to observe immediately whether any possible toxic complication ensues. Since only a single dose is used, drug effects are short-lived and any risk to the patient is of brief duration. After performing a series of such tests with different drugs, one can establish within a relatively short period of time which drugs are optimally effective in any given patient. This is referred to as "phase-one" study.

Quinidine is generally the first drug tested. This is followed by procainamide, diphosphopyramide, and propranolol. The doses employed are 600 mg for quinidine, 1.5 gm for procainamide, 300 mg for diphosphopyramide, and 80 mg for propranolol. These are administered as single oral doses. Then a number of newer drugs, such as mexiletine, tocainide, aprindine, ethmozine, encainide, lorcainide, propafonone, and amiodarone, are tested. Whether further study of any particular agent is undertaken is determined by its efficacy as well as by the occurrence of any untoward effects.

Once the most effective drug is defined, a "phase-two" study is initiated. The patient is given maintenance therapy with the selected drug for a period of 48 to 72 hours. Drug efficacy is then determined by means of 24-hour ambulatory monitoring as well as maximum exercise stress testing on a motorized treadmill and in a small percentage by repetitive ventricular response (RVR) testing. Psychological stress testing is also employed to provoke arrhythmia and thereby to provide additional certainty about adequacy of a particular drug program. Such a systematic approach removes much of the guesswork in antiarrhythmic management and permits tailoring of the drug to the particular response of the individual patient.

Use of Digitalis Glycosides. It has been shown that acetylstrophanthidin may reduce or abolish VPB's.[288] Testing with this drug therefore identifies those patients who may profit from glycoside administration.[297] The reduction of ventricular premature beats by acetylstrophanthidin is not due to the positive inotropic effect of this drug. Only 15 of 65 patients in whom acetylstrophanthidin reduced or abolished ventricular arrhythmia were in cardiac decompensation at the time the test was performed. An alternative explanation relates the salutary effect on VPB's to the vagotonic action of the cardiac glycosides.[298,299] It has long been appreciated that digitalis increases carotid sinus sensitivity and thereby augments vagal action.[299] Evidence was presented earlier indicating that the vagus nerve has a profound indirect effect on cardiac excitability by opposing heightened adrenergic tone. Relevant are the findings that parasympathetic maneuvers such as carotid sinus massage [298] or administration of agents with vagotonic actions[300-302] decrease the frequency of VPB's or abolish ventricular tachycardia. The findings related to acetylstrophanthidin have been replicated in some patients by maintenance digitalis therapy. Our experience indicates, however, that glycosides are *adjunctive* but cannot serve as the sole therapeutic agent against malignant ventricular arrhythmias.

Psychiatric Support and Relaxation Techniques. The patient who has experienced ventricular fibrillation or who is threatened with sudden cardiac death is subjected to inordinate emotional tension. In many instances the anxiety is of such enormity that it can be controlled by the patient only by a demeanor of quietude and complete insouciance. These feelings are blanketed by profound depression manifested in somatic and psychological symptoms at times completely unrelated to the heart. Insomnia and impotence are frequent problems. Loss of concentration and seeming indifference to current events or earlier ambitions are part of the psychological state. Unless the physician addresses the emotional dimension boldly and judiciously with sympathy and understanding, there is little likelihood of successfully managing the patient with an arrhythmia. A therapeutic objective is to promote confidence and incorrigible optimism about the future.

Patients are also encouraged to meditate for brief periods each day in order to foster inner relaxation. The practice is noncultic, and no mantra is employed. Psychological equanimity is also promoted by an aerobic exercise program adapted to the particular experience, aptitudes, and predilections of the individual patient. Again, fetishism and overindulgence are discouraged. Open discussion of the subject of sudden death and the fact that it now can be controlled helps assuage the burden of uncertainty, which, like a veritable Damoclean sword, haunts the patient who has once experienced malignant ventricular arrhythmia.

Effectiveness of the Therapeutic Program. A key question is whether diminution of advanced grades of VPB's affords any protection against sudden cardiac death. This question can be resolved most expeditiously by determining whether patients who have recurrent ventricular fibrillation are protected from this lethal arrhythmia when VPB's are suppressed. We examined this question in 114 consecutive patients referred for management of intractable malignant ventricular arrhythmias.[303] Of this group 72 per cent had experienced primary ventricular fibrillation, and the remainder had symptomatic recurrent ventricular tachycardia associated either with syncope or with hemodynamic compromise. Seventy-three patients (64 per cent) had coronary heart disease, 24 (21 per cent) had miscellaneous forms of heart disease, and 17 (14.9 per cent) were free of demonstrable cardiac disease; the average age was 53 years. Of the 114 patients, 88 (77 per cent) were controlled, as evidenced by elimination of grades 4B and 5 VPB's on both 24-hour Holter monitoring as well as during maximum symptom-limited treadmill exercise stress testing. Twenty-six patients were not controlled. Among the group deemed to have been controlled, only 4 experienced sudden cardiac death over an average follow-up of 21.5 months. However, 13 of the 26 not controlled died suddenly after an average follow-up of 155 months.

The evidence presented indicates that in patients with ischemic heart disease the occurrence of VPB's is associated with an increased risk of sudden cardiac death. Such risk is further enhanced when the VPB's are of advanced grade. Although abolition of arrhythmia appears to reduce susceptibility to ventricular fibrillation, it is not clear whether protection results from reduction in VPB's or as a consequence of changes in the fibrillation threshold quite apart from the ectopic suppressive action. The above-mentioned experience suggests that a majority of patients having recurrent malignant arrhythmias can be protected by medical measures. This subset of patients, however, represents but a small minority of those at risk from sudden death. Newer methods are needed for identifying the large groups that are threatened. A noninvasive screening test for electrical instability of the myocardium must now be developed.

VALUE OF CARDIAC OPERATIONS FOR CONTROL OF MALIGNANT ARRHYTHMIAS
(See also Chap. 20)

Coronary artery bypass grafting and ventricular aneurysmectomy have been the surgical procedures most commonly employed for managing drug-resistant, oft-recurrent ventricular tachyarrhythmias. Successful suppression of arrhythmia by such blind approaches is achieved in fewer than 30 per cent of patients.[304] Although the majority of patients with these arrhythmias do have multivessel coronary artery disease as well as ventricular aneurysms, electrophysiological mapping techniques (p. 640) have demonstrated that the sites of origin of the reentrant mechanisms are at or near the subendocardium at the border of infarction and/or aneurysm.[176,177,180–182] These areas are generally not resected during standard aneurysmectomy. The fact that these arrhythmias often have a precisely localizable anatomical basis invites resection of the nidus for the arrhythmia. The most extensive experience with intraoperative mapping has been reported by Josephson and coworkers.[305] Endocardial resection was carried out in 60 patients with recurrent ventricular tachyarrhythmias; 52 had concomitant aneurysmectomies, whereas 40 received in addition an average of 1.6 grafts per patient. There were 5 operative deaths. Of the remaining 55, in 42 ventricular tachycardia was not inducible, and they were discharged without medication. In 13 patients, arrhythmias could be induced during electrophysiological testing. In a follow-up period of 2 to 41 months, there have been 9 late deaths among the 55 patients surviving operation. At follow-up of 40 months, the predicted actuarial survival curve on patients who had endocardial resection is 62 per cent. In the absence of a medically treated control group, the significance of these results remains uncertain.

With the advent of new and more effective antiarrhythmic drugs, there will be less need to resort to complex and costly operative procedures. In the above-cited study of Josephson et al.,[305] only 10 patients had received experimental drugs. In any case surgery cannot be the strategy of care for the multitudes who are predisposed to sudden cardiac death.[306]

CONCLUDING COMMENTS

Sudden cardiac death continues to exact an inordinate toll in premature and preventable fatalities. In the brief decade since this phenomenon has received increased medical attention, there have been a number of substantial advances. The mechanism has been decisively identified as being due to ventricular fibrillation. Acute anatomical lesions have been shown to be absent. Fatality has been proved to be due to an electrical accident. Resuscitation has been often accomplished, and long survival has been assured for many. Community CPR programs have evolved which have resulted in many lives being saved. VPB's have been established as indicators of increased susceptibility to sudden cardiac death, and advanced grades of ectopic beats have been shown to be largely implicated. Increasingly, patients at risk are being identified. Methodological approaches have been developed which permit tailoring of antiarrhythmic drugs to individual needs. Newer and more effective antiarrhythmic drugs are becoming available to the clinician. Electrophysiological techniques have emerged that permit identification of the precise site of initiation of the reentrant mechanism. The role of higher nervous factors in the genesis of ventricular arrhythmias and ventricular fibrillation has been demonstrated. Finally, the long-prevalent attitude of pessimism and futility is being replaced by a sense of challenge and opportunity. One can be hopeful that it will not require the passage of still another decade before this problem will be largely controlled.

References

1. Lown, B., Fakhro, A. M., Hood, W. B., Jr., and Thorn, G. W.: The coronary care unit: New perspectives and directions. J.A.M.A. 199:188, 1967.
2. Pantridge, J. F., and Geddes, J. S.: A mobile intensive care unit in the management of myocardial infarction. Lancet 2:271, 1967.
3. Pantridge, J. F., and Adgey, A. A. J.: Prehospital coronary care: The mobile coronary care unit. Am. J. Cardiol. 24:666, 1969.
4. Nagel, E. L., Hirschman, J. C., Nussenfeld, S. R., Rankin, D., and Lunbland, E.: Telemetry-medical command in coronary and other mobile emergency care systems. J.A.M.A. 214:332, 1970.
5. Grace, W. J.: The mobile coronary care unit and the intermediate coronary care unit in the total systems approach to coronary care. Chest 58:363, 1970.
6. Cobb, L. A., Conn, R. D., Samson, W. E., and Philbin, J. E.: Prehospital coronary care: The role of rapid response mobile intensive coronary care system. Circulation 43:II-139, 1971.
7. Liberthson, R. R., Nagel, E. L., Hirschman, J. C., and Nussenfeld, S. R.: Prehospital ventricular defibrillation. Prognosis and followup course. N. Engl. J. Med. 291:317, 1974.
8. Paul, O., and Schatz, M.: On sudden death. Circulation 43:7, 1971.
9. Chazan, J. A., Stevson, R., and Kurland, G. S.: The acidoses of cardiac arrest. N. Engl. J. Med. 278:360, 1968.
10. Noble, J. R.: The patient with syncope. J.A.M.A. 237:1372, 1977.
11. Murdoch, B. D.: Loss of consciousness in healthy South African men: Incidence, causes and relationship to EEG abnormality. S. Afr. Med. J. 57:771, 1980.
12. Wenger, N. K., Stein, P. D., and Willis, P. W.: Massive acute pulmonary embolism: The deceivingly nonspecific manifestations. J.A.M.A. 220:843, 1972.
13. Levine, S. A.: Clinical Heart Disease. Philadelphia, W. B. Saunders Co., 1958, p. 297.
14. Thames, M. D., Alpert, J. S., and Dalen, J. E.: Syncope in patients with pulmonary embolism. J.A.M.A. 238:2509, 1977.
15. Alpert, J. S., Smith, R., Carlson, C. J., Ockéne, I. S., Dexter, L., and Dalen, J.

E.: Mortality in patients treated for pulmonary embolism. J.A.M.A. *236*:1477, 1976.

16. Gutheroth, W. G.: Sudden infant death syndrome (crib death). Am. Heart J. *93*:784, 1977.

17. Valdes-Dapena, M. A.: Sudden unexpected death in infancy. A review of the world literatures. 1954–1966. Pediatrics *39*:123, 1967.

18. Coryllos, E.: Vagal dysfunction and sudden infant death syndrome: One possible cause and its management. N. Y. State J. Med. *82*:731, 1982.

19. Maron, B. J., Clark, C. E., Goldstern, R. E., and Epstein, S. E.: Potential role of Q-T interval prolongation in sudden infant death syndrome. Circulation *54*: 423, 1976.

20. Schwartz, P. J.: Cardiac sympathetic innervation and the sudden infant death syndrome. Am. J. Med. *60*:167, 1976.

21. Kukolich, M. K., Telsey, A., Ott, J., and Motulsky, A. G.: Sudden infant death syndrome: Normal QT interval on ECG relatives. Pediatrics *60*:51, 1977.

22. Kelly, D. H. R., Shannon, D. C., and Liberthson, R. R.: The role of the QT interval in the sudden infant death syndrome. Circulation *55*:633, 1977.

23. Patrick, J. R.: Cardiac or respiratory death. *In* Bergman, A. B., Beckwith, J. B., and Ray, C. J. (eds.): Sudden Infant Death Syndrome. Seattle, University of Washington Press, 1970, p. 130.

24. Beckwith, J. B.: Observations on the pathological anatomy of sudden infant death syndrome. *In* Bergman, A. B., Beckwith, J. B., and Ray, C. J. (eds.): Sudden Infant Death Syndrome. Seattle, University of Washington Press, 1970, pp. 83–132.

25. Shannon, D. C., Kelly, D. H., and O'Connell, K.: Abnormal regulation of ventilation in infants at risk for sudden infant death syndrome. N. Engl. J. Med. *297*:747, 1977.

26. Naeye, R. L.: Pulmonary arterial abnormalities and the sudden infant death syndrome. N. Engl. J. Med. *289*:1167, 1973.

27. Mittleman, R. E., and Wetli, C. V.: The fatal cafe coronary: Foreign-body airway obstruction. J.A.M.A. *247*:1285, 1982.

28. Bass, M.: Sudden sniffing death. J.A.M.A. *212*:2075, 1970.

29. Weiss, S., and Baker, J. P.: The carotid sinus reflex in health and disease. Its role in the causation of fainting and convulsions. Medicine *12*:297, 1933.

30. Parry, C. H.: An inquiry into symptoms and causes of syncope anginosa, commonly called angina pectoris. Bath, England, Cruttwell, 1799.

31. Burch, G. E., and DePasquale, N. P.: Sudden, unexpected, natural death. Am. J. Med. Sci. *249*:86, 1965.

32. Kuller, L.: Sudden and unexpected nontraumatic deaths in adults: A review of epidemiologic and clinical studies. J. Chron. Dis. *19*:1165, 1966.

33. Spain, D. M., Brades, V. A., and Mohr, C.: Coronary atherosclerosis as a cause of unexpected and unexplained death: An autopsy study from 1949–1959. J.A.M.A. *174*:384, 1960.

34. Phillips, L. H., Whisnant, J. P., and Reagan, T. J.: Sudden death from stroke. Stroke *8*:392, 1977.

35. Lancisi, G. M.: De Subitaneis Mortibus. Rome, Buagnai, 1707. Translated by P. D. White and A. V. Boursy. New York, St. John's University Press, 1971.

36. Hirsch, C. S., and Martin, D. L.: Unexpected death in young epileptics. Neurology *21*:682, 1971.

37. Lown, B., and Levine, S. A.: Current Advances in Digitalis Therapy. Boston, Little, Brown and Co., 1954.

38. Lely, A. H., and Van Enter, H. J.: Large scale digitoxin intoxication. Br. Med. J. *2*:734, 1970.

39. Selzer, A., and Wray, H. W.: Quinidine syncope: Paroxysmal ventricular fibrillation occurring during treatment of chronic atrial arrhythmias. Circulation *30*: 17, 1964.

40. Bell, L. V.: On a form of disease resembling mania and fever. Am. J. Insanity *6*:97, 1849.

41. Peele, R., and Von Loetzen, I. S.: Phenothiazine deaths: A critical review. Am. J. Psychiatry *130*:306, 1973.

42. Coull, D. C., Crooks, J., Dingwall-Fordyce, I., Scott, A. M., and Weir, R. D.: Amitriptyline and cardiac disease: Risk of sudden death identified by monitoring system. Lancet *2*:590, 1970.

43. Kannel, W. B., Doyle, J. T., McNamara, P. M., Quickenton, P., and Gordon, T.: Precursors of sudden coronary death. Factors related to incidence of sudden death. Circulation *51*:608, 1975.

44. Kannel, W. B., and Thomas, H., Jr.: Sudden coronary death: The Framingham Study. Ann. N. Y. Acad. Sci. *382*:3, 1982.

45. Weinblatt, E., Shapiro, S., Frank, C., and Sager, R.: Prognosis of men after the first myocardial infarction. Am. J. Pub. Health *58*:1329, 1968.

46. Kuller, L. H., Lilienfeld, A., and Fisher, R.: An epidemiologic study of sudden and unexpected deaths in adults. Medicine *48*:341, 1968.

47. Doyle, J. T., Kannel, W. B., McNamara, R. M., Quickenton, P., and Gordon, T.: Factors related to the suddenness of death from coronary disease: Combined Albany-Framingham Studies. Am. J. Cardiol. *37*:1073, 1976.

48. Kuller, L. H., Perper, J., and Cooper, M.: Demographic characteristics and trends in arteriosclerotic heart disease mortality: Sudden death and myocardial infarction. Circulation *52*:III–1, 1975.

49. Wilhelmson, C., Vedin, J. A., Elmfeldt, E., Tibblin, G., and Wilhelmsen, L.: Smoking and myocardial infarction. Lancet *1*:415, 1975.

50. Kuller, L. H., Cooper, M., and Perper, J.: Epidemiology of sudden death. Arch. Intern. Med. *129*:714, 1972.

51. Herrick, J. B.: Clinical features of sudden obstruction of the coronary arteries. J.A.M.A. *59*:2015, 1912.

52. Levine, S. A.: Coronary thrombosis: Its various clinical features. Medicine *8*: 245, 1929.

53. Feil, H.: Preliminary pain in coronary thrombosis. Am. J. Med. Sci. *193*:42, 1937.

54. Sampson, J. J., and Eliaser, M.: The diagnosis of impending acute coronary artery occlusion. Am. Heart J. *13*:675, 1937.

55. Solomon, H. A., Edwards, A. L., and Killip, T.: Prodromata in acute myocardial infarction. Circulation *40*:463, 1969.

56. Stowers, M., and Short, D.: Warning symptoms before major myocardial infarction. Br. Heart J. *32*:833, 1970.

57. Feinleib, M., Simon, A. B., Gillum, R. F., and Margolis, J. R.: Prodromal symptoms—signs of sudden death. Circulation *52*:III–155, 1975.

58. Fulton, M., Lutz, W., Donald, K. W., Kirby, B. J., Duncan, B., Morrison, S. L., Kerr, F., Julian, D. G., and Oliver, M. F.: Natural history of unstable angina. Lancet *1*:860, 1972.

59. Duncan, B., Fulton, M., Morrison, S. L., Lutz, W., Donald, K. W., Kerr, F., Kirby, B. J., Julian, D. G., and Oliver, M. F.: New and worsening angina. Br. Med. J. *1*:981, 1976.

60. Doyle, J. T.: Profile of risk of sudden death in apparently healthy people. Circulation *52*:III–176, 1975.

61. Reichenback, D. D., Moss, N. S., and Meyer, E.: Pathology of the heart in sudden cardiac death. Am. J. Cardiol. *39*:865, 1977.

62. Baroldi, G., Falzi, G., and Mariani, F.: Sudden coronary death: A postmortem study in 208 selected cases compared to 97 "control" cases. Am. Heart J. *98*: 20, 1979.

63. Titus, J. L., Oxman, H. A., Connolly, D. C., and Nobrega, F. T.: Sudden unexpected death as the initial manifestation of coronary heart disease. Clinical and pathologic observations. Singapore Med. *14*:291, 1973.

64. Roberts, W. C.: Coronary arteries in fatal acute myocardial infarction. Circulation *45*:215, 1972.

65. Davies, J. M.: Pathological view of sudden cardiac death. Br. Heart J. *45*:88, 1981.

66. Roberts, W. C., and Jones, A. A.: Quantification of coronary arterial narrowing at necropsy in sudden coronary death: Analysis of 31 patients and comparison with 25 control subjects. Am. J. Cardiol. *44*:39, 1979.

67. Schwartz, C., and Gerrity, R. G.: Anatomical pathology of sudden unexpected cardiac death. Circulation *52*:III–18, 1975.

68. Spain, D. M., and Brades, V. A.: Sudden death from coronary heart disease. Chest *58*:107, 1970.

69. Lie, J. T., and Titus, J. L.: Pathology of the myocardium and the conduction system in sudden coronary death. Circulation *52*:III–41, 1975.

70. Haerem, J. W.: Platelet aggregates in intramyocardial vessels of patients dying suddenly and unexpectedly of coronary artery disease. Atherosclerosis *15*:199, 1972.

71. Folts, J. D., Crowell, E. R., and Rowe, G. G.: Platelet aggregation in partially obstructed vessels and its elimination with aspirin. Circulation *54*:365, 1976.

72. Weaver, D. W., Lorch, G. S., Alvarez, H. A., and Cobb, L. A.: Angiographic findings and prognostic indicators. Circulation *54*:895, 1976.

73. Cobb, L. A., Hallstrom, A. P., Weaver, D. W., Copass, M. K., and Haynes, R. E.: Clinical predictors and characteristics of the sudden cardiac death syndrome. *In* Proceedings of the First U.S.–U.S.S.R. Symposium on Sudden Death, Yalta, October 3–5, 1977. U.S. Department of Health, Education, and Welfare, Public Health Service, National Institutes of Health, D.H.E.W. Publication No. NIH 78–1470, 1978.

74. Criley, J. M., Lewis, K. B., Humphries, J. O., and Ross, R.: Prolapse of the mitral valve: Clinical and cine-angiographic findings. Br. Heart J. *28*:488, 1966.

75. Hancock, E. W., and Cohn, K.: The syndrome associated with midsystolic click and late systolic murmur. Am. J. Med. *41*:183, 1966.

76. Shell, W. E., Walton, J. A., Clifford, M. E., and Willis, P. W.: The familial occurrence of the syndrome of mid-late systolic click and late systolic murmur. Circulation *39*:327, 1969.

77. Stannard, M., Sloman, J. G., Hare, W. S. C., and Goble, A. J.: Prolapse of the posterior leaflet of the mitral valve: A clinical, familial and cineangiographic study. Br. Med. J. *3*:71, 1967.

78. DeMaria, A. N., Amsterdam, E. A., Vismara, L. A., Markson, W., Broochini, R., and Mason, D. T.: The variable spectrum of rhythm disturbances in the mitral valve prolapse syndrome (abstract). Circulation *50*:III–222, 1974.

79. Winkle, R. A., Lopes, M. G., Fitzgerald, J. W., Goodman, D. J., Schroeder, J. S., and Harrison, D. C.: Arrhythmias in patients with mitral valve prolapse. Circulation *52*:73, 1975.

80. Jeresaty, R. M.: Sudden death in the mitral valve prolapse-click syndrome. Am. J. Cardiol. *37*:317, 1976.

81. Allen, H., Harris, A., and Leatham, A.: Significance and prognosis of an isolated late systolic murmur: a nine to 22 year follow up. Br. Heart J. *36*:525, 1974.

82. Leichtman, D., Nelson, R., Gobel, F. L., Alexander, C. S., and Cohn, J. N.: Bradycardia with mitral valve prolapse: A potential mechanism of sudden death. Ann. Intern. Med. *85*:453, 1976.

83. Jervell, A., and Lange-Nielsen, F: Congenital deaf mutism, functional heart disease with prolongation of Q-T interval and sudden death. Am. Heart J. *54*: 59, 1957.

84. Romano, C., Gemme, G., and Pongiglione, R.: Aritmie cardiache rare dell'eta pediatrica. La Clinic Paed. *45*:656, 1963.

85. Ward, O. C.: A new familial cardiac syndrome in children. J. Irish Med. Assoc. *54*:103, 1964.

86. Vincent, G. M., Abildskov, J. A., and Burgess, M. J.: Q-T internal syndromes. Progr. Cardiovasc. Dis. 16:527, 1974.

87. Schwartz, P. J., Periti, M., and Malliani, A.: The long QT syndrome. Am. Heart J. 89:378, 1975.

88. Han, J., and Moe, G. K.: Nonuniform recovery of excitability in ventricular muscle. Circ. Res. 14:44, 1964.

89. Yanowitz, F., Preston, J. B., and Abildskov, J. A.: Functional distribution of right and left stellate innervation to the ventricles: Production of neurogenic electrocardiographic changes by unilateral alteration of sympathetic tone. Circ. Res. 18:416, 1966.

90. Schwartz, P. J., and Malliani, A.: Electrical alternation of the T wave: Clinical and experimental evidence of its relationship with the sympathetic nervous system and the long Q-T syndrome. Am. Heart J. 89:45, 1975.

91. Moss, A., and McDonald, J.: Unilateral cervicothoracic sympathetic ganglionectomy for the treatment of long Q-T interval syndrome. N. Engl. J. Med. 285:903, 1971.

92. Curtiss, E. I., Heibel, R. H., and Shaver, J. A.: Autonomic maneuvers in hereditary Q-T interval prolongation (Romano-Ward syndrome). Am. Heart J. 95:420, 1978.

93. Dreifus, L. S., Haiat, R., Watanabe, Y., Arriaga, J., and Reitman, N.: Ventricular fibrillation. A possible mechanism of sudden death in patients with Wolff-Parkinson-White syndrome. Circulation 43:520, 1971.

94. Klein, G. J., Bashere, T. M., Sellers, T. D., Pritchett, E. L. C., Smith, W. M., and Gallagher, J. J.: Ventricular fibrillation in the Wolff-Parkinson-White syndrome. N. Engl. J. Med. 301:1080, 1979.

95. Braunwald, E., Goldblatt, A., Aygen, M., Rockoff, S. D., and Morrow, A. G.: Congenital aortic stenosis: Clinical and hemodynamic findings in 100 patients. Circulation 27:426, 1963.

96. Flann, M. D., Braniff, B. A., Kimball, R., and Hancock, E. W.: Mechanism of effort syncope in aortic stenosis. Circulation 26:II–109, 1967.

97. Schwartz, L. S., Goldfischer, J., Sprague, G., and Schwartz, S. P.: Syncope and sudden death in aortic stenosis. Am. J. Cardiol. 23:647, 1969.

98. Santinga, J. T., Marvin, M., Kirsh, M. D., Flora, J. D., and Brymer, J. F.: Factors relating to late sudden death in patients having aortic valve replacement. Ann. Thorac. Surg. 29:249, 1980.

99. Forfang, K., Rostad, H., Sörland, S., and Levorstad, K.: Late sudden death after surgical correction of coarctation of the aorta. Acta Med. Scand. 206:375, 1979.

100. Editorial: A cause of sudden death. Br. Med. J. 1:129, 1971.

101. Frank, S., and Braunwald, E.: Idiopathic hypertrophic subaortic stenosis: clinical analysis of 126 patients with emphasis on the natural history. Circulation 37:759, 1968.

102. Dhingra, R. C., Denes, P., Wu, D., Wyndham, C. R., Amat-y-Leon, F., Towne, W. D., and Rosen, K. M.: Prospective observations in patients with chronic bundle branch block and marked H-V prolongation. Circulation 53: 600, 1976.

103. Denes, P., Dhingra, R. C., Wu, D., Wyndham, C. R., Amat-y-Leon, F., and Rosen, K. M.: Sudden death in patients with chronic bifascicular block. Arch. Intern. Med. 137:1005, 1977.

104. Moritz, A. R., and Zamcheck, N.: Sudden and unexpected deaths of young soldiers: Disease responsible for such deaths during World War II. Arch. Pathol. 42:459, 1946.

105. Lown, B., and Graboys, T. B.: Management of patients with malignant ventricular arrhythmias. Am. J. Cardiol. 39:910, 1977.

106. Pederson, D. H., Zipes, D. P., Foster, P. R., and Troup, P. J.: Ventricular tachycardia and ventricular fibrillation in a young population. Circulation 60: 988, 1979.

107. Lown, B., Temte, J. V., Reich, P., Gaughan, C., Regestein, Q., and Hai, H.: Basis for recurring ventricular fibrillation in the absence of coronary heart disease and its management. N. Engl. J. Med. 294:623, 1976.

108. Lown, B., and Verrier, R. L.: Neural activity and ventricular fibrillation. N. Engl. J. Med. 294:1165, 1976.

109. Maron, B. J., Roberts, W. C., McAlister, H. A., Rosing, D. R., and Epstein, S. E.: Sudden death in young athletes. Circulation 62:218, 1980.

110. Morales, A. R., Romanell, R., and Boucek, R. J.: The mural left anterior descending coronary artery, strenuous exercise and sudden death. Circulation 62: 230, 1980.

111. Isner, J. M., Sours, H. E., Paris, A. L., Ferman, V. J., and Roberts, W. C.: Sudden, unexpected death in avid dieters using the liquid protein fast diet: Observation in 17 patients and role of the prolonged QT interval. Circulation 60: 1401, 1979.

112. Lantigua, R. A., Amatruda, J. M., Biddle, T. L., Forbes, G. B., and Lockwood, D. H.: Cardiac arrhythmias associated with a liquid protein diet for the treatment of obesity. N. Engl. J. Med. 303:735, 1980.

113. Lawrie, D. M., Higgins, M. R., Godman, M. J., Oliver, M. F., Julian, D. G., and Donald, K. W.: Ventricular fibrillation complicating acute myocardial infarction. Lancet 2:523, 1968.

114. Geddes, J. S., Adgey, A. A. J., and Pantridge, J. F.: Prognosis after recovery from ventricular fibrillation complicating ischemic heart disease. Lancet 2:273, 1967.

115. Lown, B., Klein, M. D., and Hershberg, P. I.: Coronary and precoronary care. Am. J. Med. 46:705, 1969.

116. Thompson, P., and Sloaman, G.: Sudden death in hospital after discharge from coronary care unit. Br. Med. J. 2:136, 1971.

117. Graboys, T. B.: In-hospital sudden death after coronary care unit discharge. Arch. Intern. Med. 135:512, 1975.

118. Schultze, R. A., Strauss, H. W., and Pitt, B.: Sudden death in the year following myocardial infarction. Am. J. Med. 62:192, 1977.

119. Vismara, L. A., DeMaria, A. N., Hughes, J. L., Mason, D. T., and Amsterdam, E. A.: Evaluation of arrhythmias in the late hospital phase of acute myocardial infarction compared to coronary care unit ectopy. Br. Med. J. 37: 598, 1975.

120. Schaffer, W. A., and Cobb, L. A.: Recurrent ventricular fibrillation and modes of death in survivors of out-of-hospital ventricular fibrillation. N. Engl. J. Med. 293:260, 1975.

121. Cobb, L. A., Baum, R. S., Alvarez, H., and Schaffer, W. A.: Resuscitation from out of hospital ventricular fibrillation: 4 years follow-up. Circulation 52: III–223, 1975.

122. Lown, B., and Graboys, T. B.: Sudden death: An ancient problem newly perceived. Cardiovasc. Med. 2:219, 1977.

123. Wikland, B.: Death from arteriosclerotic heart disease outside hospitals. Acta Med. Scand. 184:129, 1968.

124. Lown, B., and Ruberman, W.: The concept of precoronary care. Mod. Concepts Cardiovasc. Dis. 39:97, 1970.

125. Lown, B.: Sudden death from coronary artery disease. In Waldenstrom, J., Larson, T., and Ljungestedt, N. (eds.): Early Phases of Coronary Heart Disease: The Possibility of Prediction (Skandia International Symposia). Stockholm, Nordiska Bokhandelns Forlag, 1973, pp. 255–277.

126. Lown, B., Vassaux, C., Hood, W. B., Jr., Fakhro, A. M., Kaplinsky, E., and Roberge, G.: Unresolved problems in coronary care. Am. J. Cardiol. 20: 494, 1967.

127. Lown, B., and Wolf, M.: Approaches to sudden death from coronary heart disease. Circulation 44:130, 1971.

128. Hiss, R., Averill, K., and Lamb, L.: EKG findings in 67,375 asymptomatic subjects. Am. J. Cardiol. 6:96, 1960.

129. Brodsky, M., Wu, D., Denes, P., Kanakis, C., and Rosen, K. M.: Arrhythmias documented by 24 hour continuous electrocardiographic monitoring in 50 male medical students without apparent heart disease. Am. J. Cardiol. 39:390, 1977.

130. Kennedy, J., and Underhill, S. J.: Frequent or complex ventricular ectopy in apparently healthy subjects: A clinical study of 25 cases. Am. J. Cardiol. 38: 141, 1976.

131. Hinkle, L. E., Jr., Carver, S. T., and Argyros, D. C.: The prognostic significance of ventricular premature beats in healthy people and in people with coronary heart disease. Acta Cardiol. 18 (Suppl.):5, 1974.

132. Hinkle, L. E., Jr., Carver, S. T., and Stevens, M.: Frequency of asymptomatic disturbances of cardiac rhythm and conduction in middle-aged men: Study of 301 active American men with 6 hour monitoring. Am. J. Cardiol. 24:629, 1969.

133. Lown, B. Calvert, A. F., Armington, R., and Ryan, M.: Monitoring for serious arrhythmias and high risk of sudden death. Circulation 52:189, 1975.

134. Smirk, F. H., and Palmer, D. G.: A myocardial syndrome: With particular reference to the occurrence of sudden death and of premature systoles interrupting antecedent T-waves. Am. J. Cardiol. 6:620, 1960.

135. Han, J., and Goel, B.: Electrophysiologic precursors of ventricular arrhythmia. Arch. Intern. Med. 129:749, 1972.

136. Wolff, G. A., Veith, F., and Lown, B.: A vulnerable period for ventricular tachycardia following myocardial infarction. Cardiovasc. Res. 2:111, 1968.

137. Epstein, S. E., Beiser, G. D., Rosing, D. R., Talano, J. V., and Karsh, R. B.: Experimental acute myocardial infarction. Characterization and treatment of the malignant premature ventricular contractions. Circulation 47:446, 1973.

138. Engel, R. T., Meister, S. G., and Frankl, W. S.: The "R on T" phenomenon: an update and critical review. Ann. Intern. Med. 88:221, 1978.

139. Scherlag, B. J., El-Sherif, N., Hope, R., and Lazzara, R.: Characterization and localization of ventricular arrhythmias resulting from myocardial ischemia and infarction. Circ. Res. 35:372, 1974.

140. Waldo, A. L., and Kaiser, G. A.: A study of ventricular arrhythmias associated with acute myocardial infarction in the canine heart. Circulation 47:1222, 1973.

141. Boineaux, J. P., and Cox, J. T.: Slow ventricular activation in acute myocardial infraction: A source of re-entrant premature ventricular contractions. Circulation 48:702, 1973.

142. Williams, D. O., Scherlag, B. J., Hope, R. R., El-Sherif, N., and Lazzara, R.: The pathophysiology of malignant ventricular arrhythmias during acute myocardial ischemia. Circulation 50:1163, 1974.

143. DeSoyza, N., Bissett, J. K., Kane, J. J., Murphy, M. L., and Doherty, J. E.: Ectopic ventricular prematurity and its relationship to ventricular tachycardia in acute myocardial infarction in man. Circulation 50:529, 1974.

144. Rothfeld, E. L., Parsonnet, J., McGorman, W., and Linden, S.: Harbingers of paroxysmal ventricular tachycardia in acute myocardial infarction. Chest 71: 142, 1977.

145. Wellens, H. J. J., Durrer, D. R., and Lie, K. I.: Observations on mechanisms of ventricular tachycardia in man. Circulation 54:237, 1976.

146. El-Sherif, N., Myerburg, R. J., Scherlag, B. J., Befeler, R., Aranda, J. M., Castellanos, A., and Lazzara, R.: Electrocardiographic antecedents of primary ventricular fibrillation. Value of R on T phenomenon in myocardial infarction. Br. Heart J. 38:415, 1976.

147. Ruberman, W., Weinblatt, E., Goldberg, J. D., Frank, C. W., Chaudhary, B. S., and Shapiro, S.: Ventricular premature complexes and sudden death after myocardial infarction. Circulation 64:297, 1981.

148. Oliver, G. C.: Ventricular arrhythmias in coronary artery disease and their relationship to sudden death. in Proceedings of the First U.S.–U.S.S.R. Sympo-

sium on Sudden Death, Yalta, October 3–5, 1977. U. S. Department of Health, Education, and Welfare, Public Health Service, National Institutes of Health, D.H.E.W. Publication No. NIH 78–1470, 1978.

149. Campbell, R. W. F., Murray, A., and Julian, D. G.: Ventricular arrhythmias in the first 12 hours of acute myocardial infarction: Natural history study. Br. Heart J. 46:351, 1981.

150. Huppert, B., and Berliner, K.: The intraventricular conduction time of ventricular premature systoles. Cardiologica 27:87, 1955.

151. Soloff, L.: Ventricular premature beat—diagnostic of myocardial disease. Am. J. Med. Sci. 242:289, 1969.

152. Manning, G., Ahuja, A., and Gutierrea, M. R.: Electrocardiographic differentiation between ventricular premature beats from subjects with normal and diseased hearts. Cardiologia 23:462, 1968.

153. Rosenbaum, M.: Classification of ventricular extrasystoles according to form. J. Electrocardiol. 2:289, 1969.

154. Estler, J., and White, P. D.: Clinical significance of ventricular premature beats with reference to heart rate. Arch. Intern. Med. 43:606, 1929.

155. Bigger, T. J., Weld, F. M., Rolnitzky, M. L.: Prevalence, characteristics and significance of ventricular tachycardia (three or more complexes) detected with ambulatory electrocardiographic recording in the late hospital phase of acute myocardial infarction. Am. J. Cardiol. 48:815, 1981.

156. Thompson, P., and Lown, B.: Sequential R/T pacing to expose electrical instability in the ischemic ventricle. Clin. Res. 20 (Abstr.):401, 1972.

157. Axelrod, P. J., Verrier, R. L., and Lown, B.: Vulnerability to ventricular fibrillation during acute coronary arterial occlusion and release. Am. J. Cardiol. 36:776, 1976.

158. Ruberman, W., Weinblatt, E., Goldberg, J. D., Frank, C. W., and Shapiro, S.: Ventricular premature beats and mortality after myocardial infarction. N. Engl. J. Med. 279:750, 1977.

159. The Coronary Drug Project Research Group: Prognostic importance of premature beats following myocardial infarction. Experience in the Coronary Drug Project. J.A.M.A. 223:1116, 1973.

160. Moss, A. J., Davis, H. T., DeCamilla, J., and Bayer, L. W.: Ventricular ectopic beats and their relation to sudden and nonsudden cardiac death after myocardial infarction. Circulation 60:998, 1979.

161. Roberts, R., and Sobel, B.: Relationship between infarct size and ventricular arrhythmia. Br. Heart J. 37:1169, 1975.

162. Sharma, S. D., Ballantyne, F., and Goldstein, S.: The relationship of ventricular asynergy in coronary artery disease to ventricular premature beats. Chest 66:358, 1974.

163. Schulze, R. A., Jr., Rouleau, J., Rigo, P., Bowers, S., Strass, H. W., and Pitt, B.: Ventricular arrhythmias in late hospital phase of acute myocardial infarction; relation to left ventricular function detected by gated cardiac blood pool scanning. Circulation 52:1006, 1975.

164. Schulze, R. A., Jr., Humphries, J. O., Griffith, L. S. C., Ducci, H., Achuff, S., Baird, M. G., Mellits, E. D., and Pitt, B.: Left ventricular and coronary angiographic anatomy: Relationship to ventricular irritability in the late hospital phase of acute myocardial infarction. Circulation 55:839, 1977.

165. Calvert, A., Lown, B., and Gorlin, R.: Ventricular premature beats and anatomically defined coronary heart disease. Am. J. Cardiol. 39:627, 1977.

166. Lown, B., Cannon, R. L., III, and Ross, M. A.: Electrical stimulation and digitalis drugs. Repetitive response in diastole. Proc. Soc. Exp. Biol. Med. 126:698, 1967.

167. Lown, B., and Cannon, R. L., III: Electrical stimulation to estimate the degree of digitalization: Experimental studies. Am. J. Cardiol. 22:251, 1968.

168. Hagemeijer, F., and Lown, B.: Effect of heart reate on electrically induced repetitive ventricular responses in the digitalized dog. Circ. Res. 27:333, 1970.

169. Jenzer, H., Lohrbauer, L., and Lown, B.: Response to single threshold stimuli following acute myocardial infarction. Proc. Soc. Exp. Biol. Med. 141:606, 1972.

170. Green, L. H., Reid, P. R., and Schaeffer, A. H.: The repetitive ventricular response in man: an index of ventricular electrical instability. Am. J. Cardiol. 41 (Abstr.):400, 1978.

171. Lown, B.: New concepts and approaches to sudden cardiac death. Schweiz. Med. Wschr. 106:1522, 1976.

172. Lown, B., Verrier, R. L., and Blatt, C. M.: Precordial mechanical stimulation for exposing electrical instability of the heart. Am. J. Cardiol. 42:425, 1978.

173. Durrer, D., Schoo, L., Schuilenburg, R. M., and Wellens, H. J. J.: The role of premature beats in the initiation and termination of supraventricular tachycardia in Wolff-Parkinson-White syndrome. Circulation 36:644, 1967.

174. Coumel, P. H., Cabrol, C., Fabiato, A., Gourgon, R., and Slama, R.: Tachycardia permanente par rhythme reciproque. Arch. Mal Coeur 60:1830, 1967.

175. Wellens, H. J. J.: Value and limitations of programmed electrical stimulation of the heart in the study and treatment of tachycardias. Circulation 57:845, 1978.

176. Josephson, M. E., Horowitz, L. N., Farshidi, A., and Kastor, J. A.: Recurrent sustained ventricular tachycardia: Mechanism. Circulation 57:431, 1978.

177. Horowitz, L. N., Josephson, M. E., and Kastor, A. J.: Intracardiac electrophysiologic studies as method for the optimization of drug therapy in chronic ventricular arrhythmias. Prog. Cardiovasc. Dis. 23:81, 1980.

178. Fontaine, G., Guiraudon, G., Frank, R., Gerbaux, A., Cousteau, J. P., Varillon, A., Gay, J., Cabral, C., and Focquet, J.: La cartographie épicardique et le traitement chirurgical par simple ventriculotomie de certaines tachycardies ventriculaires rebelles par réentrée. Arch. Mal Coeur 68:113, 1975.

179. Ruskin, J. N., DiMarco, J. P., and Garan, H.: Out-of-hospital cardiac arrest. N. Engl. J. Med. 303:607, 1980.

180. Horowitz, L. N., Josephson, M. E., Kastor, J. A., and Harken, A. H.: Ventricular resection guided by epicardial and endocardial mapping for treatment of recurrent ventricular tachycardia. N. Engl. J. Med. 302:589, 1980.

181. Horowitz, L. N., Spielman, S. R., Greenspan, A. M., and Josephson, M. E.: Mechanism in the genesis of recurrent ventricular tachycardia as revealed by clinical electrophysiologic studies. Ann. N. Y. Acad. Med. 382:116, 1982.

182. Josephson, M. E., Horowitz, L. N., and Farshidi, A.: Continuous local electrical activity: A mechanism of recurrent ventricular tachycardia. Circulation 57:659, 1978.

183. Lown, B., Verrier, R. L., and Rabinowitz, S. H.: Neural psychologic mechanisms and the problem of sudden cardiac death. Am. J. Cardiol. 39:890, 1977.

184. Verrier, R. L., Thompson, P., and Lown, B.: Ventricular vulnerability during sympathetic stimulation: role of heart rate and blood pressure. Cardiovasc. Res. 8:602, 1974.

185. Schwartz, P. J., Verrier, R., and Lown, B.: Effect of stellectomy and vagotomy on ventricular refractoriness in dogs. Circ. Res. 40:536, 1977.

186. Schwartz, P. J., Snebold, N. G., and Brown, A. M.: Effects of unilateral cardiac sympathetic denervation on the ventricular fibrillation threshold. Am. J. Cardiol. 37:1036, 1976.

187. Schwartz, P. J., Stone, H. L., and Brown, A. M.: Effects of unilateral stellate ganglion blockade on the arrhythmias associated with coronary occlusion. Am. Heart J. 92:589, 1976.

188. Randall, W. C., and Rohse, W. G.: The augmentor action of the sympathetic cardiac nerves. Circ. Res. 4:470, 1956.

189. Brown, A. M.: Excitation of afferent cardiac sympathetic nerve fibers during myocardial ischaemia. J. Physiol. (Lond.) 190:703, 1969.

190. Malliani, A., Schwartz, P. J., and Zanchetti, A.: A sympathetic reflex elicited by experimental coronary occlusion. Am. J. Physiol. 217:703, 1969.

191. Corbalan, R., Verrier, R. L., and Lown, B.: Differing mechanisms for ventricular vulnerability during coronary artery occlusion and release. Am. Heart J. 92:223, 1976.

192. Verrier, R., Calvert, A., Lown, B., and Axelrod, P.: Effect of acute blood pressure elevation on the ventricular fibrillation threshold. Am. J. Physiol. 226:893, 1974.

193. Blatt, C. M., Verrier, R. L., and Lown, B.: Acute blood pressure elevation and ventricular fibrillation threshold during coronary artery occlusion and reperfusion in the dog. Am. J. Cardiol. 39:523, 1977.

194. Higgins, C. B., Vatner, S. F., and Braunwald, E.: Parasympathetic control of the heart. Pharmacol. Rev. 25:119, 1974.

195. Kent, K. M., Smith, E. R., Redwood, D. R., and Epstein, S. E.: Electrical stability of the acutely ischemic myocardium: Influences of heart rate and vagal stimulation. Circulation 47:291, 1973.

196. Kent, K. M., Epstein, S. E., Cooper, T., and Jacobowitz, D. M.: Cholinergic innervation of the canine and human ventricular conducting system: anatomic and electrophysiologic correlations. Circulation 50:948, 1974.

197. Einbrodt, E.: Über Herzreizung und ihr Verhältnis zum Blutdruck. Vienna, Akademie der Wissenschaften Sitzungsberichte 38:345, 1859.

198. Myers, R. W., Pearlman, A. S., Hyman, R. M., Goldstein, R. A., Kent, K. M., Goldstein, R. E., and Epstein, S. E.: Beneficial effects of vagal stimulation and bradycardia during experimental acute myocardial ischemia. Circulation 49:943, 1974.

199. Kolman, B. S., Verrier, R. L., and Lown, B.: The effect of vagus nerve stimulation upon vulnerability of the canine ventricle: Role of sympathetic-parasympathetic interactions. Circulation 52:578, 1975.

200. Kolman, B. S., Verrier, R. L., and Lown, B.: The effect of vagus nerve stimulation upon excitability of the canine ventricle: Role of sympathetic-parasympathetic interactions. Am. J. Cardiol. 37:1041, 1975.

201. Verrier, R. L., Rabinowitz, S. H., and Lown, B.: Vagal and adrenergic interactions and ventricular electrical stability. Clin. Res. 23:212A, 1975.

202. Rabinowitz, S. H., Verrier, R. L., and Lown, B.: Muscarinic effects of vagosympathetic trunk stimulation on the repetitive extrasystole threshold. Circulation 53:622, 1976.

203. Murad, F., Chi, Y. M., and Rall, T. W.: Adenylcyclase. III. The effect of catecholamines and choline esters on the formation of adenosine-3',5'-phosphate by preparations from cardiac muscle and liver. J. Biol. Chem. 237:1233, 1962.

204. LaRaia, P. J., and Sonnenblick, E. H.: Autonomic control of cardiac C-AMP. Circ. Res. 28:377, 1971.

205. Watanabe, A. M., and Besch, H. R., Jr.: Interaction between cyclic adenosine monophosphate and cyclic guanosine monophosphate in guinea pig ventricular myocardium. Circ. Res. 37:309, 1975.

206. Wiggers, C. J., and Wegria, R.: Ventricular fibrillation due to single, localized induction and condenser shocks applied during the vulnerable phase of ventricular systole. Am. J. Physiol. 128:520, 1940.

207. Matta, R. J., Verrier, R. L., and Lown, B.: The repetitive extrasystole as an index of vulnerability to ventricular fibrillation. Am. J. Physiol. 230:1469, 1976.

208. Lown, B., Verrier, R. L., and Corbalan, R.: Psychologic stress and threshold for repetitive ventricular response. Science 182:834, 1973.

209. Matta, R. J., Lawler, J. E., and Lown, B.: Ventricular electrical instability in the conscious dog: Effects of psychologic stress and beta adrenergic blockade. Am. J. Cardiol. 38:594, 1976.

210. Corbalan, R., Verrier, R., and Lown, B.: Psychologic stress and ventricular arrhythmias during myocardial infarction in the conscious dog. Am. J. Cardiol. 34:692, 1974.

211. Antonaccio, M. J., and Robson, R. D.: Cardiovascular effects of 5-hydroxytryptophan in anesthetized dogs. J. Pharm. Pharmacol. 25:495, 1973.

212. Antonaccio, M. J., and Robson, R. D.: Centrally mediated cardiovascular effects of 5-hydroxytryptophan in MAO-inhibited dogs: modification by autonomic antagonists. Arch. Int. Pharmacodyn. Ther. 231:200, 1975.

213. Baum, T., and Shropshire, A. T.: Inhibition of efferent sympathetic nerve activity by 5-hydroxytryptophan and centrally administered 5-hydroxytryptamine. Neuropharmacology 142:227, 1975.

214. Rabinowitz, S. H., and Lown, B.: Central neurochemical factors related to serotonin metabolism and cardiac ventricular vulnerability for repetitive electrical activity. Am. J. Cardiol. 41:516, 1978.

215. Engel, G. L.: Sudden and rapid death during psychologic stress. Folk lore or folk wisdom? Ann. Intern. Med. 74:771, 1971.

216. Wellens, J. J. H., Vermeulen, A., and Durrer, D.: Ventricular fibrillation occurring on arousal from sleep by auditory stimuli. Circulation 46:661, 1972.

217. Taggart, P., Carruthers, M., and Somerville, W.: Electrocardiograms, plasma catecholamines and lipids, and their modification by oxyprenolol, when speaking before an audience. Lancet 2:341, 1973.

218. Taggart, P., Gibbons, D., and Somerville, W.: Some effects of motor-car driving on the normal and abnormal heart. Br. Med. J. 4:130, 1969.

219. Rose, K. D.: The post-coronary patient as a spectator sportsman, In Eliot, R. S. (ed.): Stress and the Heart. New York, Futura Publishing Co., 1974, p. 207.

220. Lown, B., Tykocinski, M., Garfein, A., and Brooks, P.: Sleep and ventricular premature beats. Circulation 48:691, 1973.

221. Lown, B., DeSilva, R. A., Reich, P., and Murawski, B. J.: Psychophysiologic factors in sudden cardiac death. Am. J. Psychiatry 137:1325, 1980.

222. Parkes, C. M., Benjamin, B., and Fitzgerald, R.: Broken heart: Statistical study of increased mortality among widowers. Br. Med. J. 1:740, 1969.

223. Rahe, R. H., Bennett, L., Romo, M., Siltanen, P., and White, R. J.: Subjects' recent life changes and coronary heart disease in Finland. Am. J. Psychiatry 130:1222, 1973.

224. Jarvinen, K. A. J.: Can ward rounds be a danger to patients with myocardial infarction? Br. Med. J. 1:318, 1955.

225. Hughes, A., and Tonks, R. S.: Experimental embolic carditis. J. Pathol. Bacteriol. 72:497, 1956.

226. Hughes, A., and Tonks, R. S.: The role of microemboli in the production of carditis in hypersensitivity experiments. J. Pathol. Bacteriol. 77:207, 1959.

227. Jorgensen, L., Roswell, H. C., Hovig, T., Glynn, M. F., and Mustard, J. F.: Adenosine diphosphate–induced platelet aggregation and myocardial infarction in swine. Lab. Invest. 17:616, 1967.

228. Halmagyi, D., Starzechi, B., and Horner, G.: Humoral transmission of cardiorespiratory changes in experimental lung embolism. Circ. Res. 14:546, 1964.

229. Thomas, D., Gurewich, V., and Ashford, T.: Platelet adherence to thromboemboli in relation to the pathogenesis and treatment of pulmonary embolism. N. Engl. J. Med. 274:953, 1966.

230. Gurewich, V., Thomas, D., Stem, M., and Wessler, S.: Bronchoconstriction in the presence of pulmonary embolism. Circulation 27:339, 1963.

231. Smith, G., and Smith, A.: The role of serotonin in experimental pulmonary embolism. Surg. Gynecol. Obstet. 101:691, 1955.

232. Comroe, J., VanLingen, B., Stroud, B., and Roncoroni, A.: Reflex and direct cardiopulmonary effects of 5-OH-tryptamine (serotonin). Am. J. Physiol. 173:379, 1953.

233. Zervas, N. T., Kuwayama, A., Rosoff, C. B., and Salzman, E. W.: Modification by inhibition of platelet function. Arch. Neurol. 28:400, 1973.

234. Zervas, N. T., Hori, H., and Rosoff, C. B.: Experimental inhibition of serotonin by antibiotic: prevention of cerebral vasospasm. J. Neurosurg. 41:259, 1974.

235. Ellis, E. L., Oelz, O., Roberts, L. J., II, Payne, N. A., Sweetman, B. J., Nies, A. S., and Oates, J. A.: Coronary arterial smooth muscle contraction by a substance released from platelets: Evidence that it is thromboxane A2. Science 193:1135, 1976.

236. Hoak, J. C., Warner, E. D., and Connor, W. E.: New concepts of levarterenol-induced acute myocardial necrosis. Arch. Pathol. 87:332, 1969.

237. Haft, J. I., Krantz, P. D., Albert, F. J., and Fani, K.: Intravascular platelet aggregation in the heart by norepinephrine. Microscopic studies. Circulation 46:698, 1972.

238. Haft, J. I., and Fani, K.: Stress and the induction of intravascular platelet aggregation in the heart. Circulation 48:164, 1973.

239. VanVliet, P. D., Burchell, H. B., and Titus, J. L.: Focal myocarditis associated with pheochromocytoma. N. Engl. J. Med. 274:1102, 1966.

240. Barr, I., Cohen, P., Berken, A., and Lown, B.: Thrombocythemia and myocardial ischemia with normal coronary angiogram. Arch. Intern. Med. 134:528, 1974.

241. Prinzmetal, M., Ekmekci, A., Kennamer, R., Kwoczynski, J. K., Shubin, H., and Toyoshima, H.: Variant form of angina pectoris: Previously undelineated syndrome. J.A.M.A. 174:1794, 1960.

242. Whiting, R. B., Klein, M. D., VanderVeer, J., and Lown, B.: Variant angina pectoris. N. Engl. J. Med. 282:709, 1970.

243. MacAlpin, R. N., Kattus, A. A., and Alvaro, A. B.: Angina pectoris at rest with preservation of exercise capacity: Prinzmetal's variant angina. Circulation 47:946, 1973.

244. Endo, M., Kanda, L., Hosoda, S., Hayashi, H., Kirosawa, K., and Konno, S.: Prinzmetal's variant form of angina pectoris: re-evaluation of mechanism. Circulation 52:33, 1975.

245. Dhurandhar, R. W., Watt, D. L., Silver, M. D., Trimble, A. S., and Adelman, A. S.: Prinzmetal's variant form of angina with arteriographic evidence of coronary arterial spasm. Am. J. Cardiol. 30:902, 1972.

246. Oliva, P. B., Potts, D. E., and Pluss, R. G.: Coronary arterial spasm in Prinzmetal's angina: Documentation by coronary arteriography. N. Engl. J. Med. 288:745, 1973.

247. Cheng, T. O., Bashour, T., Kelsar, G. A., Weiss, L., and Bacos, J.: Variant angina of Prinzmetal with normal coronary arteriograms. A variant of the variant. Circulation 47:476, 1973.

248. Maseri, A., L'Abbate, A., Baroldi, G., Chierchia, S., Marzilli, M., Ballestra, A. M., Severi, S., Parodi, O., Biagini, A., Distante, A., and Pesola, P.: Coronary vasospasm as a possible cause of myocardial infarction: A conclusion derived from the study of "preinfarction" angina. N. Engl. J. Med. 299:1271, 1978.

249. Maseri, A., Severi, S., and Marzullo, P.: Role of coronary arterial spasm in sudden coronary ischemic death. Ann. N. Y. Acad. Sci. 382:204, 1982.

250. Hillis, D., and Braunwald, E.: Coronary arterial spasm. N. Engl. J. Med. 299:695, 1978.

251. Mudge, F. H., Jr., Grossman, W., Mills, R. M., Jr., Lesch, M., and Braunwald, E.: Reflex increase in coronary vascular resistance in patients with ischemic heart disease. N. Engl. J. Med. 295:1333, 1976.

252. Clark, D. A., Quint, R. A., Bolen, J., and Schroeder, J. S.: The angiographic demonstration of coronary artery spasm in patients with suspected variant angina: Method and therapeutic implications. Am. J. Cardiol. 35(Abstr.):127, 1975.

253. Huepler, F., Proudfit, W., Siegel, W., Shirey, E., Razavi, M., and Sones, M. F.: The ergonovine maleate test for the diagnosis of coronary artery spasm. Circulation 52 (Abstr.):II-11, 1975.

254. Yasue, H., Touyama, M., and Shimamoto, M.: Role of autonomic nervous system in the pathogenesis of Prinzmetal's variant form of angina. Circulation 50:534, 1974.

255. Athanasopoulos, C., and Maroutsos, C.: Prinzmetal's angina. Br. Heart J. 39:911, 1977.

256. Hackett, T., and Cassem, N.: Factors contributing to delay in responding to the signs and symptoms of acute myocardial infarction. Am. J. Cardiol. 24:651, 1969.

257. Whipple, G.: Physician-induced treatment delays in the pre-CCU period. In Proceedings of the National Conference on Standards for CPR and Emergency Cardiac Care, 1975, p. 139.

258. Goldstein, S., Moss, A. J., and Greene, W.: Sudden death in acute myocardial infarction. Arch. Intern. Med. 129:720, 1972.

259. Gillum, R., Feinleib, M., Margolis, J. R., Fabsitz, R. R., and Brasch, R. C.: Delay in the hospital phase of acute myocardial infarction. Arch. Intern. Med. 136:649, 1976.

260. Lie, K. I., Wellens, H. J., Downar, E., and Durrer, D.: Observations on patients with primary ventricular fibrillation complicating acute myocardial infarction. Circulation 52:755, 1975.

261. Lie, K. I., Wellens, H. J., VanCapelle, F. J., and Durrer, D.: Lidocaine in the prevention of primary ventricular fibrillation. N. Engl. J. Med. 291:1324, 1974.

262. Valentine, P. A., Frew, J. L., Mashford, M. L., and Sloman, J. G.: Lidocaine in the prevention of sudden death in the pre-hospital phase of acute infarction: A double-blind study. N. Engl. J. Med. 291:1327, 1974.

263. American Heart Association and National Resuscitation Council: Standards for cardiopulmonary resuscitation (CPR) and emergency cardiac care (ECC). J.A.M.A. 277:836, 1974.

264. Standards and guidelines for cardiopulmonary resuscitation (CPR) and emergency cardiac care (ECC). J.A.M.A. 244:453, 1980.

264a. Silverberg, R. A., and Weil, M. M.: Changing concepts in cardiac resuscitation. McIntosh, M. D. (ed.): Baylor College of Medicine, Cardiology Series, Vol. 5, No. 2, 1982, 27 pp.

265. Pennington, J. E., Taylor, J., and Lown, B.: Chest thump for reverting ventricular tachycardia. N. Engl. J. Med. 283:1192, 1970.

266. Lown, B., and Taylor, J.: "Thump-version." N. Engl. J. Med. 283:1223, 1970.

267. Weale, F. E., and Rothwell-Jackson, R. L.: The efficiency of cardiac massage. Lancet 1:990, 1982.

268. Weisfeldt, M. I., Chandra, N., Tsitlik, J. E., and Rudikoff, M.: New attempts to improve blood flow during CPR. In Schluger, J., and Lyon, F. E. (eds.): CPR and Emergency Cardiac Care. New York, EM Books, 1980, p. 29.

269. Criley, J. M., Blaufuss, A. N., and Kissel, G. L.: Cough-induced cardiac resuscitation. J.A.M.A. 236:1246, 1976.

270. Geddes, L. A., Tacker, W. A., Rosborough, J. P., Moore, A. G., and Geddes, P.: Electrical dose for ventricular defibrillation of large and small animals using precordial electrodes. J. Clin. Invest. 53:310, 1974.

271. Tacker, W. A., Galioto, F., Guitiani, E., Geddes, L. A., and McNamara, D.: Energy dosage for human defibrillation. N. Engl. J. Med. 290:214, 1974.

272. Pantridge, J. F., Adgey, A. A. J., and Geddes, J. S.: The Acute Coronary Attack. New York, Grune and Stratton, 1975, pp. 66–78.

273. Crampton, R. S.: Low-energy ventricular defibrillation and miniature defibrillators. J.A.M.A. 235:2284, 1976.

274. DeSilva, R. A., and Lown, B.: Energy requirements for defibrillation of a markedly overweight patient. Circulation 57:827, 1978.

275. Kerber, R. E., and Sarnat, W.: Factors influencing the success of ventricular defibrillation in man. Circulation 60:226, 1979.

276. Lown, B., Crampton, R. S., and DeSilva, R. A.: The energy for ventricular fibrillation defibrillation—Too little or too much? N. Engl. J. Med. 298:1252, 1978.

276a. Haynes, R. E., Chin, T. L., Copass, M. K., and Cobb, L. A.: Comparison of bretylium tosylate and lidocaine in management of out of hospital ventricular fibrillation: A randomized clinical trial. Am. J. Cardiol. 48:353, 1981.

277. Eisenberg, M., Hallstrom, A., and Bergner, L.: The ACLS score: Predicting survival from out-of-hospital cardiac arrest. J.A.M.A. *246*:50, 1981.
278. Myerburg, R. J., Kessler, K. M., Zaman, L., Conde, C. A., and Castellanos, A.: Survivors of prehospital cardiac arrest. J.A.M.A. *247*:1485, 1982.
279. Cobb, L. A., Werner, J. A., and Trobough, G. B.: Sudden cardiac death. I. A decade's experience with out-of-hospital resuscitation. Mod. Concepts Cardiovasc. Dis. *49*:31, 1980.
280. Eisenberg, M., Hallstrom, A., and Bergner, L.: Long-term survival after out-of-hospital cardiac arrest. N. Engl. J. Med. *306*:1340, 1982.
281. Snyder, B. D., Hauser, W. A., Loewenson, R. B., Leppik, I. E., Ramirez-Lassepas, M., and Gummit, R. J.: Neurologic prognosis after cardiopulmonary arrest. III. Seizure activity. Neurology *30*:1292, 1980.
282. Hjalmarsen, A.: Beta blocking agents, current status in the prevention of sudden coronary death. Ann. N. Y. Acad. Sci. *382*:805, 1982.
283. Norwegian Multicenter Study Group: Timolol-induced reduction in mortality and reinfarction in patients surviving acute myocardial infarction. N. Engl. J. Med. *304*:801, 1981.
284. Mirowski, M., Mower, M., Staewen, W. S., Tabatznik, B., and Mendeloff, A. I.: Standby automatic defibrillator: An approach to prevention of sudden coronary death. Arch. Intern. Med. *126*:158, 1970.
285. Mirowski, M., Mower, M. M., Reid, P. P., and Watkins, L., Jr.: Implantable automatic defibrillators—Their potential in prevention of sudden coronary death. Ann. N.Y. Acad. Sci. *382*:371, 1982.
286. Lown, B., and Axelrod, P.: Implanted stand-by defibrillators. Circulation *46*:637, 1972.
287. Lown, B., Podrid, P. J., DeSilva, R. A., and Graboys, T. B.: Sudden cardiac death—Management of the patient at risk. Curr. Prob. Cardiol. *4*:1, 1980.
288. Lown, B., Graboys, T. B., Podrid, P. J., Cohen, B. H., Stockman, M. B., and Gaughan, C. E.: Effect of a digitalis drug on ventricular premature beats (VPB's). N. Engl. J. Med. *296*:301, 1977.
289. Winkle, R. A., Alderman, E. L., Fitzgerald, J. W., and Harrison, D. C.: Treatment of recurrent symptomatic ventricular tachycardia. Ann. Intern. Med. *85*:1, 1976.
290. Lown, B., Matta, R. J., and Besser, H. W.: Programmed "Trendscription:" A new approach to electrocardiographic monitoring. J.A.M.A. *232*:39, 1975.
291. Gaughan, C. E., Lown, B., Lanigan, J., Voukydis, P., and Besser, H. W.: Acute oral testing for determining antiarrhythmic drug efficacy. I. Quinidine. Am. J. Cardiol. *38*:677, 1976.
292. Jelinek, M. V., and Lown, B.: Exercise stress testing for exposure of cardiac arrhythmias. Prog. Cardiovasc. Dis. *16*:497, 1974.
293. Zaret, B. L., and Conti, C. R., Jr.: Exercise-induced ventricular irritability: hemodynamic and angiographic correlations. Am. J. Cardiol. *29*:298, 1972.
294. Helfant, R. H., Pine, R., Kalde, V., and Banka, V.: Exercise related ventricular premature complexes in coronary heart disease: Correlation with ischemia and angiographic severity. Ann. Intern. Med. *80*:589, 1974.
295. Goldschlager, N., and Selzer, A.: Treadmill test as an indicator of presence and severity of coronary artery disease. Ann. Intern. Med. *85*:277, 1976.
296. Lown, B., and DeSilva, R. A.: Roles of psychologic stress and autonomic nervous system changes in provocation of ventricular premature beats. Am. J. Cardiol. *41*:979, 1978.
297. Lown, B., Klein, M. D., Barr, I., Hagemeijer, F., Kosowsky, B. D., and Garrison, H.: Sensitivity to digitalis drugs in acute myocardial infarction. Am. J. Cardiol. *30*:388, 1972.
298. Lown, B., and Levine, S. A.: The carotid sinus: Clinical value of its stimulation. Circulation *23*:776, 1961.
299. Nichol, A. D., and Strauss, H.: The effects of digitalis, urginin, congestive cardiac failure and atropine on the hyperactive carotid sinus. Am. Heart J. *25*:746, 1943.
300. Nalhauson, M. H.: Action of acetylbetamethylcholine on ventricular rhythm induced by adrenalin. Proc. Soc. Exp. Biol. Med. *32*:1297, 1943.
301. Waxman, M. B., Downar, E., Berman, N. D., and Felderhof, D. H.: Phenylephrine (neosynephrine) terminated ventricular tachycardia. Circulation *50*:656, 1974.
302. Weiss, T., Lattin, G. M., and Engelman, K.: Vagally mediated suppression of premature ventricular contractions in man. Am. Heart J. *89*:700, 1975.
303. Lown, B., and Graboys, T. B.: Ventricular premature beats and sudden cardiac death. *In* McIntosh, H. (ed.): Baylor Coll. Med. Card. Series *3*:4, 1980.
304. Harken, A. H., Horowitz, R. M., and Josephson, M. E.: Comparison of standard aneurysmectomy with directed endocardial resection for treatment of recurrent sustained ventricular tachycardia. J. Thorac. Cardiovasc. Surg. *80*:527, 1980.
305. Josephson, M. E., Horowitz, L. N., and Harken, A. H.: Surgery for recurrent sustained ventricular tachycardia associated with coronary artery disease: The role of subendocardial resection. Ann. N. Y. Acad. Sci. *382*:381, 1982.
306. Lown, B.: Sudden cardiac death: The major challenge confronting contemporary cardiology. Am. J. Cardiol. *43*:313, 1979.

24
HIGH–CARDIAC OUTPUT STATES

by William Grossman, M.D., and Eugene Braunwald, M.D.

METABOLIC DETERMINANTS OF CARDIAC OUTPUT

Discussion of high–cardiac output states should begin with a definition of normal cardiac output and a brief review of the factors that determine cardiac output. The quantity of blood delivered to the systemic circulation per unit of time is termed the *cardiac output*, generally expressed in liters per min. For a normal adult weighing 70 kg, resting cardiac output is approximately 6.25 liters/min.[1] Since the total volume of blood contained in the vascular system is approximately 75 ml/kg body weight in normal subjects,[2] or 5.2 liters in a 70-kg man, it is apparent that the total blood volume is moved around the circulation in a little less than 1 minute. Transient but substantial increases in cardiac output normally occur in response to changing metabolic demands, such as with exercise. However, a sustained increase in cardiac output—the subject of this chapter—is distinctly abnormal and contributes significantly to the symptoms and clinical presentation of several disease states.

The blood pumped by the heart delivers oxygen and a variety of substrates to the metabolizing tissues and removes carbon dioxide and other products of metabolism. In addition, blood transfers the heat generated by metabolic activity from the internal organs to the cutaneous bed, where it is dissipated. Derangement of any of the homeostatic mechanisms by which these functions are regulated can result in sustained deviations of the cardiac output (either increases or decreases) from its normal value.

Oxygen Requirements of the Tissues

The average normal adult consumes 130 ml/sq meter of oxygen each minute, delivered by the blood to metabolically active tissues. If arterial blood normally contains 19 ml O_2/dl (95 per cent saturation if oxygen carrying capacity equals 20 ml O_2/dl), and if cardiac output equals 3.25 liters/min/sq meter, then by Fick's principle (p. 289) the mixed venous blood returning from metabolically active tissue will have an oxygen content of approximately 15 ml/dl, i.e., an oxygen saturation of 75 per cent. The arteriovenous oxygen difference of 4 ml/dl represents the average normal extraction of oxygen by the body's tissues in the basal state. This average extraction represents a heterogeneity of metabolic activities, with skin, kidney, and skeletal muscle extracting relatively little oxygen in the basal state, whereas the heart extracts approximately 12 ml O_2/dl at rest.

As tissue metabolism increases, the arteriovenous oxygen difference rises and is limited at constant flow by a factor termed the *extraction reserve*. The normal extraction reserve for oxygen is 3, which means that given the augmented metabolic demand, the tissues can extract three times the normal quantity of oxygen, i.e., 3×4 ml O_2/dl $= 12$ ml O_2/dl.[3] Thus, if arterial saturation remains constant at 95 per cent, full utilization of the extraction reserve results in a mixed venous oxygen content of 7 ml/dl $(19 - 12$ ml/dl), or 35 per cent saturation, which corresponds to the pulmonary arterial oxygen saturation found in normal subjects studied at maximal exercise.

It is of interest that this value of 3 for the extraction reserve of oxygen predicts that in progressive cardiac decompensation, in order to meet the basal oxygen requirements of the body, oxygen extraction will increase until the arteriovenous oxygen difference has tripled, i.e., until the limit of extraction reserve has been reached and cardiac output has fallen to one-third its normal value. Further reduction of cardiac output results in systemic hypoxia, anaerobic metabolism, metabolic acidosis, and eventually circulatory collapse. It has been observed repeatedly that a persistent fall in resting cardiac output to below one-third of normal resting values is incompatible with life. However, long before the cardiac output has declined to this low level, the heart will be unable to meet the augmented requirements of the metabolizing tissues during activity or in resting patients with a hyperkinetic state, such as pregnancy or hyperthyroidism.

Under basal or near-basal conditions in the intact subject, most changes in cardiac output can be accounted for by changes in the capacity of the peripheral vascular bed to return blood to the heart, which, in turn, causes alterations in the preload. Conditions that lower peripheral vascular resistance are among the most important factors augmenting the venous return and therefore elevating cardiac output. These include anemia, arteriovenous fistulas, beriberi, thyrotoxicosis, pregnancy, and Paget's disease. A reduction in vascular resistance also occurs in (1) muscular exercise, in which dilatation occurs in the arterioles supplying the exercising muscles; (2) fever, in which there is reduced vascular resistance as a consequence of dilated cutaneous vessels; and (3) severe anoxia, in which generalized vascular dilatation also often occurs. These reductions in vascular resistance increase cardiac output not only by lowering ventricular afterload but also by reducing the impedance to venous return, thus tending to increase ventricular preload.

Guyton has properly emphasized the significance of venous return in the regulation of cardiac output.[3] He has pointed out that the ratio of blood volume to capacitance of the systemic circulation determines the level of peripheral venous pressure and that this ratio is a prime determinant of the venous pressure gradient (i.e., the pressure difference between the small veins and the right atrium), which is closely related to the force that returns blood to the heart. According to this formulation, an augmentation of blood volume or reduction of venous capacitance will raise this gradient, augment venous return, and, in the presence of normal cardiac function, increase cardiac output.

As pointed out in Chapters 13 and 14, cardiac output depends upon the interactions of intrinsic myocardial contractility with the prevailing conditions of myocardial loading. Figure 24–1 describes this interaction in terms of the resting and active left ventricular pressure-volume relationships. According to this formulation,[4–6] ACDE represents the control cardiac cycle (Fig. 24–1). End-diastolic pressure and volume are indicated by point A, isovolumetric contraction by line ABC, ejection by line CD, isovolumetric relaxation by line DE, and diastolic filling by segment EA. This type of construction is based on the concept that at constant contractility, ventricular pressure and volume at end systole (point D) always return to the active pressure-volume relationship (upper curve) (Fig. 12–26, p. 432). When left ventricular afterload is decreased, as occurs with the reduction of systemic vascular resistance and blood viscosity (characteristic of most of the conditions discussed in this chapter[7]), the resultant cardiac cycle is denoted by ABFG, which has a considerably larger stroke volume (SV_Y) than the control stroke volume for cycle ABCDE (SV_X). If left ventricular preload now rises, as occurs with an arteriovenous fistula and many of the other conditions to be discussed, the resultant cardiac cycle would be denoted by HIFG, with stroke volume SV_Z rising further still. Thus, the reduction of afterload and increase in preload act in concert to augment stroke volume, in some instances quite strikingly. With no change in heart rate or preload, this lowering of afterload will be translated into an increase in cardiac output.

Increases in contractility, not illustrated in Figure 24–1, would cause the active pressure-volume relationship curve to shift upward and to the left, so that at any given preload and afterload left ventricular ejection would proceed to a smaller end-systolic volume, thereby delivering a larger stroke volume. Since the minute cardiac output is the product of stroke volume and heart rate, the latter is also an important determinant of the cardiac output.

Left ventricular afterload is influenced by a number of variables, including the tone of the systemic arterioles, elasticity of the aorta and large arteries, viscosity of the blood, presence of aortic stenosis, and size and thickness of the left ventricle (Chap. 14). Left ventricular preload is a function of the condition of the mitral valve, compliance of the left ventricle, blood volume, venous tone, and vigor and timing of left atrial contraction. Most importantly, it

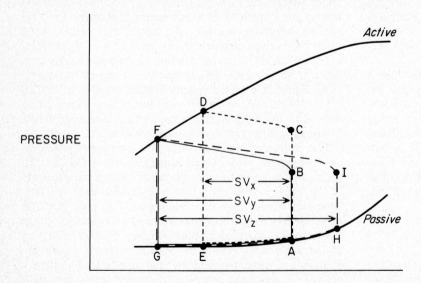

FIGURE 24–1 Influence of alterations in preload and afterload on left ventricular stroke volume. Reduction in afterloads leads to augmentation of stroke volume if preload is held constant, whereas augmentation of preload increases stroke volume if afterload is constant. In most conditions associated with a high–cardiac output state, both afterload reduction and preload augmentation are present. The control cardiac cycle is inscribed by points ABCDE; pure afterload reduction leads to cycle ABFG; a cycle demonstrating both afterload reduction and preload augmentation is indicated by HIFG. SV_X represents the stroke volume of the control cycle, SV_Y the augmented stroke volume effected by afterload reduction alone, and SV_Z the stroke volume with combined afterload reduction and preload augmentation, as might be seen with an arteriovenous fistula.

is a function of the venous return to the left atrium; this in turn is determined by the pressure gradient responsible for the return of blood from the systemic veins to the right atrium and, of course, by the function of the right side of the heart as well as pulmonary vascular resistance. When the latter two parameters are normal, the venous return pressure gradient becomes the principal determinant of left ventricular preload.

Heat Dissipation and Conservation

Body temperature and its regulation are important determinants of cardiac output. Hypothermia lowers cardiac output and hyperthermia raises it in an exponential relationship.[8,9] Temperature elevation raises cardiac output by means of two distinct mechanisms: (1) Cellular metabolism, and therefore oxygen consumption, and the production of vasodilator metabolites are a function of body temperature. With increased oxygen consumption and production of vasodilator metabolites, cardiac output rises as a consequence of reduced afterload and increased venous return, as described above. (2) Cutaneous blood flow is the principal means available to the body for temperature regulation. When total body metabolism is augmented or body temperature rises or both, marked increases in cutaneous blood flow to dissipate heat may be sufficient to increase total cardiac output substantially. The importance of this mechanism is evident in patients with the common forms of low-output congestive heart failure who are unable to increase cardiac output, cannot augment cutaneous blood flow, and therefore exhibit considerable difficulty with heat dissipation.

Substantial increases in cardiac output normally occur in response to increased environmental heat and humidity. Burch and associates have reported that in the humid tropical summer weather of New Orleans, measurements of cardiac output were 57 per cent greater than in an air-conditioned ward.[8,9] Since oxygen consumption was higher in the hot, humid environment, it was not possible to determine whether the increased output was simply a response to increased metabolic demand. However, the arterial–mixed venous oxygen difference either remained unchanged or fell, suggesting that the rise in cardiac output exceeded the oxygen requirement and reflected the body's attempt to increase the effectiveness of heat dissipation. Systemic arteriolar resistance falls in a hot and humid environment,[8] presumably reflecting dilatation of the cutaneous bed, and the resultant reduction in ventricular afterload and augmentation of venous return may be an important mechanism in mediating cardiac output.

CARDIAC RESPONSE TO INCREASES IN OUTPUT LOAD

Just as the normal cardiovascular system can increase its activity to meet the augmented peripheral demands imposed by muscular exertion, the normal heart can tolerate the higher demands imposed by hypermetabolic states (e.g., fever, pregnancy, and hyperthyroidism) and hyperkinetic, nonhypermetabolic conditions (e.g., anemia, arteriovenous fistula, and beriberi) in which reduction of afterload and augmentation of venous return and preload lead to increased flow load. Relying on dilatation and hypertrophy as its principal compensatory mechanisms, the

heart can maintain normal tissue oxygenation for many years. On the other hand, when imposed on a heart whose function is intrinsically impaired, these increased demands cannot be met, and the physiological and clinical manifestations of heart failure appear.

Obviously there are exceptions to these basic principles. Extreme anemia (hematocrit < 15 per cent); the combination of severe anemia (hematocrit = 15 to 20 per cent) and arteriovenous fistula, as occurs in patients with renal failure with placement of an external shunt for hemodialysis (p. 1756); and the rapid development of severe hyperthyroidism (e.g., thyroid storm) or a large arteriovenous fistula (e.g., aortocaval) may overwhelm even a normal heart and result in heart failure.

Adaptation of the heart to an abnormal burden depends not only on the baseline state of myocardial function when the additional burden is imposed and on the magnitude of the burden, but also on the *rate* at which the new burden is added. Thus, severe anemia, thyrotoxicosis, and an arteriovenous fistula are far more likely to lead to cardiac decompensation when they develop suddenly rather than slowly. For this reason, conditions such as Paget's disease or Albright's syndrome, in which volume overload develops slowly, rarely, if ever, cause heart failure.

HIGH-OUTPUT HEART FAILURE. Cardiac output that was markedly elevated before the development of heart failure tends to remain high afterward, a condition termed *high-output heart failure*. The mechanisms responsible for the development of heart failure in these patients are complex and depend on the underlying disease process. In most of these conditions the heart is called upon to pump an abnormally large volume, and the effect on the myocardium is similar to that which occurs with regurgitant valvular lesions (Chap. 32). In addition, as discussed below, thyrotoxicosis and beriberi may impair myocardial metabolism directly, and severe anemia may interfere with myocardial function by producing myocardial hypoxia.

Clinically, it is sometimes difficult to distinguish between low-output and high-output heart failure. The normal range of cardiac output in the basal state is wide (2.6 to 4.0 liters/min/sq meter), and in many patients with so-called low-output heart failure, the cardiac output *at rest* may actually be within normal limits. On the other hand, in patients with high-output failure, cardiac output may not be excessive but rather is close to the upper limit of normal, particularly when heart failure is severe. Regardless of the absolute level of output, however, cardiac failure may be said to be present when the characteristic clinical manifestations are accompanied by a depression of the curve relating ventricular end-diastolic volume to cardiac performance or by a depression in the end-systolic or active ventricular pressure-volume relation (Figure 14–11, p. 477).

In the usual forms of low-output heart failure, the characteristically inadequate delivery of oxygen to the metabolizing tissues is reflected in an abnormally widened arterial–mixed venous oxygen difference (Chap. 14). In mild cases, this abnormality may become evident only during the stress of increased activity. In patients with high-output heart failure, the arterial–mixed venous oxygen difference is usually normal or may even be abnormally low, as in arteriovenous fistula, because the mixed venous oxygen saturation is raised by the admixture of blood that has been shunted away from some of the metabolizing tissues. In such cases delivery of oxygen to these tissues is reduced, despite the low arterial–mixed venous oxygen difference. When heart failure occurs in patients with high cardiac output, the arterial–mixed venous oxygen difference still exceeds the level that existed after the level of cardiac output rose but *prior* to the development of heart failure, and therefore the cardiac output, although high in the normal range or elevated, is nonetheless lower than it was before heart failure developed.

CONDITIONS ASSOCIATED WITH SUSTAINED INCREASES IN CARDIAC OUTPUT

Anemia

Physiological Mechanisms. Anemia is most commonly responsible for a sustained increase in cardiac output, which occurs consistently when the hematocrit falls below 25 per cent.[10] When the anemia is associated with a condition that produces a marked rise in blood viscosity (which increases afterload), such as multiple myeloma or macroglobulinemia, cardiac output may fail to rise even in the absence of heart disease. Studies by Richardson and Guyton have supported a role for the lowered viscosity of blood in the high cardiac output of anemia.[7] In addition, Murray and Escobar found that when exchange transfusions were carried out in dogs with methemoglobinemia using blood in which viscosity was unaltered, cardiac output remained unchanged.[11] However, when a reduction of oxygen carrying capacity similar to that in methemoglobinemia was produced by an exchange transfusion with low-viscosity dextran, cardiac output rose. Fowler and Holmes produced acute anemia in dogs by exchange transfusion with low molecular weight (70,000 daltons) or high molecular weight (500,000 daltons) dextran.[12] The former produced a 93 per cent increase in cardiac output and the latter only a 43 per cent increase. Since the severity of the anemia was the same in both groups (hematocrit = 18 per cent), they concluded that the difference in cardiac output probably reflected the substantial differences in viscosity. Since an increase in cardiac output still occurred in the dogs with normal blood viscosity who received high molecular weight dextran, it is clear that lowered viscosity, although important, cannot be the sole cause of increased cardiac output. The reduced left ventricular afterload in anemia results from a reduction not only in blood viscosity but in systemic arteriolar tone as well. The mechanism responsible for the latter change is unclear, but local tissue hypoxia, lactic acidemia, and the accumulation of vasodilator metabolites such as adenosine and possibly of bradykinin may all play a role.

To investigate the adjustment of the peripheral circulation to severe anemia, Vatner et al. induced anemia in conscious dogs by progressive phlebotomy and volume replacement over a period of 2 to 4 weeks.[13] At a hematocrit of 22 per cent, heart rate was elevated and resistance to flow in the coronary and iliac beds was strikingly reduced, whereas resistance in the mesenteric and renal beds remained essentially constant. In the presence of more severe anemia (hematocrit = 14 per cent), resistance in the mesenteric and renal beds also declined. On exercise, both

coronary and iliac blood flow rose further, but, in contrast to nonanemic dogs, in which mesenteric and renal flow remained constant during exercise, both the mesenteric and the renal blood flow fell markedly (Fig. 24–2). Thus in resting, conscious dogs, reduction in visceral flow is *not* a feature of the cardiovascular response to severe anemia, although some redistribution of blood flow does occur; however, the added stress of exercise during severe anemia results in substantial reductions in flow in at least the mesenteric and renal vascular beds.

There is evidence that the autonomic nervous system plays a key role in the circulatory adaptation to anemia. The responses to severe isovolemic anemia in intact dogs were compared with those in dogs subjected to chronic cardiac denervation. The elevation of cardiac output was significantly greater in the intact animals than in the denervated ones. In intact dogs, the increase in cardiac output stemmed predominantly from a rise in heart rate, whereas elevations in stroke volume played a less important role. In contrast, in the cardiac denervated dogs, the increase in cardiac output tended to be the result of an augmented stroke volume.[14] In this connection the finding of Liang and Huckabee that tissue hypoxia can lead to an autonomic reflex response resulting in reduced arteriolar resistance is of considerable interest.[15] Thus, it may be concluded that an intact autonomic nervous system is necessary for mediation of the normal circulatory response to acutely induced anemia.

Duke and Abelmann studied 24 patients with chronic

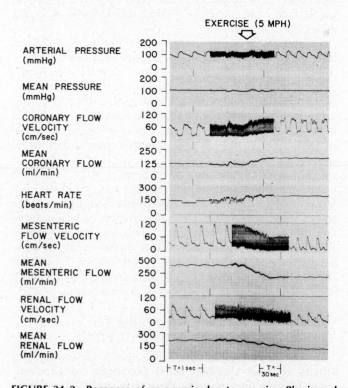

FIGURE 24–2 Response of an anemic dog to exercise. Phasic and mean arterial pressures and phasic and mean blood flows in the coronary, mesenteric, and renal beds are shown along with heart rate. In each case regional flow was initially recorded simultaneously with arterial pressure. (From Vatner, S. F., et al.: Regional circulatory adjustments to moderate and severe chronic anemia in conscious dogs at rest and during exercise. Circ. Res. *30*:731, 1972, by permission of the American Heart Association, Inc.)

anemia (iron deficiency or megaloblastic) and found that with corrective treatment, the cardiac index fell to normal (from 4.7 to 3.4 liters/min/sq meter), heart rate decreased (from 83 to 70 beats/min), and systemic vascular resistance rose (from 1017 to 1526 dynes-sec-cm^{-5}).[16] These changes could be reproduced acutely while the subjects were still anemic by infusion of methoxamine or assumption of the upright posture, suggesting that a combination of vasodilatation and a redistribution of blood volume might be responsible for mediating the hyperkinetic circulatory response to chronic anemia.

Clinical Findings. The consequences of anemia depend to an important extent on its rate of development. When it occurs rapidly, as in hemorrhage, blood volume is not maintained, and the picture of hypovolemic shock predominates (Chap. 18). If anemia develops more slowly, so that blood volume is maintained, cardiac output rises—predominantly as a result of tachycardia—with little change in stroke volume. In chronic severe anemia, heart rate is usually normal or only minimally elevated, and cardiac output is therefore elevated principally as a consequence of augmented stroke volume; the latter is associated with cardiac dilatation and hypertrophy. Not only is the cardiac output elevated at rest, but the augmentation of output during exercise tends to be excessive, often exceeding 1000 ml/100 ml increase in oxygen consumption per minute (normal = 550 to 800 ml).[17] This excessive response is sometimes seen in patients with only mild anemia (hematocrit = 30 per cent) who have normal resting cardiac outputs.[18] Since cardiac output is elevated while pulmonary artery pressure is normal, calculated pulmonary vascular resistance (like calculated systemic vascular resistance) is often reduced, and this variable declines further during exercise.[19] Left ventricular end-diastolic pressure remains within normal limits even in severe anemia, unless heart failure supervenes.[20]

The effect of *acute* anemia on cardiac function was studied by Case et al., who found that in normal dogs left ventricular function became depressed when the hematocrit was reduced below 24 per cent.[21] However, the otherwise normal human heart can tolerate moderately severe anemia (hematocrit = 20 to 25 per cent) for many years without showing any impairment of function; when heart failure occurs in patients with this degree of anemia, *it usually signifies the presence of underlying heart disease that had been compensated until the burden of an augmented cardiac output was added.* Similar considerations apply to the development of angina pectoris and other manifestations of myocardial ischemia. However, two important exceptions should be noted: (1) patients with severe anemia (hematocrit ≤ 15 per cent), in whom clinical evidence of impaired cardiac function can exist even in the absence of apparent underlying heart disease; and (2) patients with sickle cell anemia (p. 1678), who do *not* exhibit a reduction of viscosity and therefore lose this hemodynamic benefit imparted by other forms of anemia. Also, in these patients small thrombi characteristically develop in the pulmonary and coronary vessels, thereby impairing both systemic and cardiac oxygenation and leading to pulmonary hypertension, cor pulmonale, and perhaps even myocardial fibrosis secondary to ischemia. In addition, there may be arterial oxygen unsaturation secondary to pulmonary venous-arte-

rial shunting. These patients exhibit hyperventilation, an increased alveolar-arterial oxygen tension gradient, abnormal ventilation of the dead space during exercise, and a disturbance of pulmonary perfusion with venous-arterial shunting. The most likely basis for these changes is the sickling phenomenon within the pulmonary vascular bed.[22] Arterial hypoxemia, produced by the pulmonary shunt, probably accounts for some of the exercise hyperpnea, partly by increasing chemoreceptor drive and by augmenting lactic acidemia.[23]

History. Chronic anemia produces surprisingly few symptoms, which may consist of easy fatigability, mild exertional dyspnea, and occasionally palpitations and cardiac awareness (Chap. 49). If heart failure or angina pectoris is present, it is likely that the high cardiac output is superimposed on some specific cardiac abnormality, such as valvular stenosis or regurgitation, or coronary artery obstruction. Patients with sickle cell anemia and hemoglobin sickle cell (SC) disease may complain of chest pain and unexplained dyspnea due to in situ pulmonary thrombosis and infarction.[22]

Physical Examination. The anemic patient generally has a pale "pasty" appearance; in black, brown, or tanned persons in whom examination of the skin color is of little help, a finding of paleness of the conjunctivae, mucous membranes, and palmar creases is helpful. Arterial pulses are bounding, "pistol shot" sounds can be heard over the femoral arteries (Duroziez's sign), and subungual capillary pulsations (Quincke's pulse) are present as in patients with aortic regurgitation. A medium-pitched, midsystolic murmur along the left sternal border, generally Grade 1/6 to 3/6 in intensity (rarely accompanied by a thrill), is common. Heart sounds are accentuated, and the pulmonic component of the second heart sound may be particularly prominent in patients with sickle cell anemia and pulmonary hypertension; in these patients a right ventricular lift can usually be palpated. Elevation of cardiac output and the physical findings characteristic of anemia are present in patients with sickle cell anemia and hemoglobin SC disease at *higher* hemoglobin levels than in patients with other forms of anemia.[20] A mid-diastolic flow murmur secondary to augmented blood flow across the mitral value orifice, holosystolic murmurs resulting from tricuspid and mitral regurgitation secondary to ventricular dilatation, and, rarely, diastolic murmurs resulting from aortic and pulmonic value incompetence secondary to dilatation of these vessels may be heard. Occasionally, a third heart sound is audible at the cardiac apex. Jugular venous distention is uncommon, and although peripheral edema and hepatomegaly are occasionally present, they may be due not only to heart failure but also to accompanying abnormalities such as hypoproteinemia and nutritional deficiency.

Laboratory findings in patients with severe anemia usually include mild or moderate cardiomegaly on chest roentgenogram. The electrocardiogram usually does not show any specific changes but may show T-wave inversions in lateral precordial leads. The echocardiogram generally shows a modest and symmetrical increase in size of all chambers, with large systolic excursions of the septal and posterior left ventricular walls and a normal ejection fraction. Hematological and blood chemical findings reflect the specific type of anemia present.

Treatment.   Treatment of heart failure associated with severe anemia should be specific for the anemia (e.g., iron, folate, vitamin B_{12}, and so forth). When congestive heart failure is present, diuretics and cardiac glycosides are advisable, although some clinicians feel that the latter drugs are not helpful in this condition. It is our opinion that since most patients with heart failure and anemia have significant underlying heart disease, the administration of glycosides is desirable, because these drugs augment the depressed contractility on which the anemia is superimposed.

When both heart failure and anemia are severe, treatment must be carried out on an urgent basis and presents a difficult challenge. On the one hand, correction of the anemia is desirable to reduce the heart's workload; on the other hand, a too rapid expansion of the blood volume could intensify the manifestations of heart failure. The diagnostic steps for determining the etiology of the anemia should be taken immediately (e.g., blood withdrawn for serum iron, folate, and vitamin B_{12} measurements). *Packed red blood cells* should then be transfused slowly (250 to 500 ml/24 hr), preceded or accompanied by vigorous diuretic therapy (e.g., furosemide, 20 to 40 mg IV immediately followed by 40 mg orally every 8 hours), and the patient should be observed *closely* for the development or exacerbation of dyspnea and pulmonary rales, so that the transfusion can be discontinued immediately to avoid precipitating pulmonary edema. Vasodilator therapy is rarely helpful, since impedance to left ventricular emptying is already markedly reduced in most cases.

Hyperthyroidism (See also p. 1727)

Physiological Mechanisms.   Substantial increases in cardiac output commonly occur in hyperthyroidism, and cardiac indexes of 5 to 7 liters/min/sq meter are common,[24-26] generally resulting from both increased stroke volume and increased heart rate. At least four mechanisms appear to contribute to this high-output state:

1. Augmented metabolic rate that causes vasodilation as seen with muscular exercise. It has been well documented that systemic vascular resistance is decreased in hyperthyroidism.[24-26]

2. Increased heat production consequent to the augmented metabolism characteristic of hyperthyroidism results in elevation of cardiac output owing to cutaneous dilatation. This latter mechanism is particularly important in patients with thyroid storm in whom hyperthermia—with temperatures occasionally as high as 106°F (41°C)—is associated with an intense cardiac drive to maintain an elevated cardiac output,[27,28] occasionally resulting in high-output failure and circulatory collapse.

3. Thyroid hormone has a direct, stimulating effect on myocardial contractility,[29-32] which augments stroke volume at any preload and afterload. This effect has been clearly documented in animal experiments[29,31,33] as well as in humans[30,32] and may involve a fundamental alteration in myocardial contractile proteins, such as increased activity of myosin ATPase.[33-36]

4. There is still an undefined relationship between the hyperthyroid state and the sympathoadrenal system, characterized by suppression of the manifestations of the hyperthyroid state by administration of antiadrenergic agents. The tachycardia, widened pulse pressure, and shortened circulation time all return toward normal with beta-receptor blockade,[24-26,30] indicating that adrenergic influences play a role in maintaining the high-output state in hyperthyroid patients. However, it should be noted that the tachycardia of thyrotoxicosis is due not only to the *direct* effects of thyroid hormone and adrenergic influences on the sinoatrial node but also to a reduction in the cholinergic restraint. This does not appear to result from decreased responsiveness of the end organ or impaired release of the cholinergic nerve transmitter but rather from a reduction in cholinergic discharge in the thyrotoxic state, which may result from an abnormality in central or afferent mechanisms.[37] Beta-adrenergic stimulation potentiates certain biochemical changes induced at the cell membrane level by triiodothyronine.[38]

Clinical Findings.   Symptoms may include nervousness, personality disorder, heat intolerance, or weight loss with increased appetite and fatigue. Palpitations are common, and atrial fibrillation is occasionally the presenting manifestation. Symptoms of congestive heart failure are rare and, as discussed below, suggest underlying cardiac disease of a different nature.

The principal *physical findings* of hyperthyroidism include tremor; widened palpebral fissures with resultant "stare"; lid lag; exophthalmos; warm, moist, smooth skin; and hyperactive deep tendon reflexes. Cardiovascular examination often reveals tachycardia, a widened pulse pressure, and brisk carotid and peripheral arterial pulsations. The cardiac apex is hyperkinetic on palpation. The first heart sound is loud, and third and fourth sounds are occasionally present. A midsystolic murmur along the left sternal border, secondary to increased flow, is common; occasionally this murmur has an unusual scratchy component (the so-called Means-Lerman scratch) thought to be due to the rubbing together of normal pleural and pericardial surfaces as a consequence of hyperkinetic heart action. Rarely, systolic murmurs of mitral and tricuspid regurgitation, presumably secondary to papillary muscle dysfunction, may occur in thyrotoxicosis and disappear with the establishment of the euthyroid state.

Laboratory findings are those of hyperthyroidism and include elevated levels of thyroxine or triiodothyronine, mild normochromic normocytic anemia, occasional relative lymphocytosis, low serum cholesterol levels, and occasional elevation of serum alkaline phosphatase.

The *chest roentgenogram* is usually normal, although the echocardiogram may show increased left ventricular wall thickness and chamber dimensions and a normal or increased ejection fraction and velocity of shortening.[32] Systolic time intervals may show a low value for the ratio of the preejection period to left ventricular ejection time (PEP/LVET ratio), consistent with increased myocardial contractility (Chap. 3).

The *electrocardiogram* shows widespread but nonspecific ST-segment elevation and upward coving, with terminal T-wave inversion in about one-fourth of patients and shortening of the Q-T interval.[39] ST-segment depression is uncommon in the absence of coronary artery disease. Varying degrees of atrioventricular block,[40] presumably owing to inflammatory changes in the atrioventricular node induced by hyperthyroidism, are occasional manifestations. Atrial fibrillation may occur and is often associated with an unusually rapid ventricular response (i.e., 170 to 220 beats/min) as a consequence of the markedly shortened refractory period of the atrioventricular conduction system. There is relative resistance to slowing of the ventricular rate with digitalis.[41] Spontaneous reversion to sinus rhythm is common.

Treatment. Management of the cardiovascular manifestations of hyperthyroidism depends primarily on treatment of the endocrine abnormality, as outlined in Chapter 51. However, the elevated heart rate, systolic pressure, pulse pressure, and cardiac output, palpitations, and other manifestations of cardiac hyperactivity, as well as tremor, lid lag, hyperreflexia, and widened palpebral fissures can be reduced by administering antiadrenergic agents.[42] The rapid ventricular rate of atrial fibrillation responds particularly well to intravenous propranolol, which may be administered in 1-mg increments every 5 minutes until the ventricular rate is controlled; sometimes sinus rhythm is restored. *Thyroid storm* with hyperpyrexia, marked tachycardia, and pulmonary edema also responds to propranolol, 1 to 2 mg administered intravenously as above, together with sodium iodide (to prevent further release of stored thyroid hormones), and diuretics, adrenal glucocorticoids, cooling blankets, aspirin, and intravenous fluids.[43] Oral propranolol in divided doses ranging from 160 to 400 mg/day (or equivalent doses of another beta blocker [p. 1349]) is also usually effective in controlling many of the cardiovascular manifestations of hyperthyroidism described above. It must be appreciated, however, that despite the salutary effects of beta-blocking agents, they are only adjunctive measures and do not affect the underlying disease process. Indeed, they do not reduce the elevated metabolic rate.

THYROTOXIC HEART DISEASE. As in many other high-output states, the hyperkinetic state of hyperthyroidism does not usually lead to heart failure or angina pectoris in the absence of underlying cardiac or coronary artery disease; the normal heart appears capable of tolerating the burden imposed by hyperthyroidism simply by means of dilatation and hypertrophy. A rare exception is the development of heart failure in patients with neonatal thyrotoxicosis without underlying heart disease.[44] However, when the elevated flow load of hyperthyroidism is superimposed on a reduced cardiovascular reserve (i.e., asymptomatic or only mildly symptomatic heart disease), congestive heart failure is likely to ensue. Similarly, in a patient with obstructive coronary artery disease who is asymptomatic or who has only mild evidence of ischemia in the euthyroid state, the demand for increased coronary blood flow with hyperthyroidism frequently leads to an exacerbation of angina.

Beta-adrenergic blockade may be both helpful and harmful in patients with thyrotoxic heart disease and *heart failure*. Although it may be beneficial by lowering the ventricular rate, particularly by prolonging the refractory period of the atrioventricular conduction system in patients with atrial fibrillation, it may also diminish myocardial contractility by blocking the adrenergic support of the heart. Therefore it must be administered cautiously to the patient with thyrotoxic heart disease and heart failure and only after treatment with glycosides, with the patient at rest and under careful observation. The initial dose should be small (e.g., propranolol, 0.5 mg IV or 10 mg orally), and the patient should be observed after the administration to assure that heart failure is not intensified. Propranolol is particularly useful in the management of angina pectoris associated with hyperthyroidism, and in this condition larger doses are usually well tolerated.

The association of thyrotoxicosis and anginal pain has been demonstrated in the presence of normal coronary vessels on arteriography.[45] These patients showed ischemia in that pacing resulted in lactate production. The possibility of thyrotoxicosis should therefore be considered in the differential diagnosis of patients having anginal pain and normal coronary arteriograms (Chap. 39).

It is particularly important to recognize so-called *apathetic hyperthyroidism*, a condition in which the usual clinical manifestations of hyperthyroidism (i.e., palpitations, tachycardia, and moist skin) are not present. In these patients the first clinical signs of thyrotoxicosis may be unexplained heart failure, an exacerbation of angina pectoris, or unexplained atrial fibrillation, usually but not always with a rapid ventricular rate. Hence it is important to consider the diagnosis of hyperthyroidism in all patients, particularly those over the age of 55 years, who present in this fashion.

Systemic Arteriovenous Fistulas

Systemic arteriovenous fistulas may be congenital or acquired; the latter are either post-traumatic or iatrogenic. Increased cardiac output associated with such fistulas depends on the size of the communication and the magnitude of the resultant reduction in systemic vascular resistance. An increased right atrial pressure does not seem to be necessary to maintain the high-output state, although plasma volume is generally increased.

An experimental model of chronic high-output heart failure due to an arteriovenous fistula has been developed in the rat.[46] At 2 months after creation of an aortocaval fistula, cardiac output and left ventricular end-diastolic pressure were increased, and there was significant biventricular hypertrophy. Blood flow to the splanchnic bed was decreased, but flow to the heart, brain, and kidneys was preserved. Many other physiological characteristics in this model resemble findings in the clinical situation.

The *physical findings* depend in part on the underlying disease and the location of the shunt. In general, a widened pulse pressure, brisk carotid and peripheral arterial pulsations, and mild tachycardia are present. *Branham's sign* (also called Nicaladoni-Branham's sign), which consists of slowing of the heart following manual compression of the fistula,[47,48] is present in the majority of cases; this maneuver also raises arterial and lowers venous pressure. The tachycardia associated with arteriovenous fistula has been studied in an experimental preparation,[49] and the results suggest the operation of a cardioaccelerator reflex with both afferent and efferent pathways in the vagus nerves.

The skin overlying the fistula is warmer than normal, and a "machinery" murmur and thrill are usually present over the lesion. Third and fourth heart sounds are commonly heard, as well as a precordial midsystolic murmur. The electrocardiographic changes of left ventricular hypertrophy are often seen. Rarely, the fistula may become infected, leading to bacterial endarteritis.

CONGENITAL ARTERIOVENOUS FISTULAS. Congenital arteriovenous fistulas result from arrest of the normal embryonic development of the vascular system and are structurally similar to embryonic capillary networks. They range from barely noticeable strawberry birthmarks to enormous clusters of engorged vascular channels that may deform an entire extremity. Most frequently, the vessels of the lower extremities are involved (i.e., femoral, iliac, and popliteal), and the resultant clinical manifestations vary enormously.[50] When fistulas are large, patients generally complain of disfigurement as well as of swelling and pain in the limb (Table 24–1). Left heart failure occurs, particularly in patients with larger lesions that involve the pelvis as well as the extremities.[51,52] Physical examination shows hemangiomatous changes associated with venous distention, deformity, and increased limb length. The fistulous connection may involve any vascular bed, including the internal mammary artery–pulmonary artery connection. Angiography is useful in confirming the diagnosis and in determining the physical extent of the anomaly.

Surgical excision is the ideal treatment, but in many instances the lesions are not sufficiently localized to permit this. The results of ligation and excision have been unsatisfactory in the majority of cases, since the congenital arteriovenous communications are usually not confined to a single anatomical segment or to a circumscribed anatomical region. Complete cure of these lesions is possible in only a few instances. Embolization of Gelfoam pellets delivered through a catheter has been reported to obliterate multiple systemic arteriovenous fistulas and thereby diminish high-output heart failure.[53]

Hereditary hemorrhagic telangiectasia (Osler-Weber-Rendu disease) may be associated with arteriovenous fistulas, particularly in the lungs and liver; the latter condition can produce a hyperkinetic circulation as well as hepatomegaly with abdominal bruits. Because of the presence of oxygenated blood in the inferior vena cava and right atrium, this condition may be misdiagnosed as atrial septal defect.[54]

The congenital arteriovenous communication resulting from *hemangioendothelioma of the liver* is commonly associated with marked increases in cardiac output, sometimes as high as 10.5 liters/min/sq meter, and congestive heart failure.[55,56] These lesions, which are extremely difficult to treat surgically, may be quite large, increase in size with time, and lead to heart failure even in infancy. They are often associated with sizable cutaneous hemangiomas, which

should alert the clinician to the possibility of their presence. Hepatic hemangioendotheliomas have been reported to respond to prednisone in the newborn[55] or to hepatic artery ligation.[56]

ACQUIRED ARTERIOVENOUS FISTULAS. Naturally acquired arteriovenous fistulas occur most frequently following injuries such as gunshot wounds and may involve any part of the body, most frequently the thigh.[57] Blood flow in the affected limb distal to the fistula diminishes after the creation of the fistula but then returns to normal and often increases with the passage of time. The affected limb is usually larger than its opposite member, and the overlying skin is warmer; cellulitis, venostasis, edema, and dermatitis with pigmentation frequently occur, in part as a consequence of chronically elevated venous pressure. Surgical repair or excision is generally advisable in fistulas that develop following gunshot wounds or trauma. An arteriovenous fistula may be produced by inadvertent damage to blood vessels during an operation, most frequently in nephrectomy, laminectomy, or cholecystectomy.

A rare form of acquired arteriovenous fistula results from spontaneous rupture of an aortic aneurysm into the inferior vena cava. This usually produces an enormous arteriovenous shunt and rapidly progressive left ventricular failure. On physical examination a pulsating mass can be readily palpated superficially in the abdomen, and a continuous bruit is audible.

Massive fistulas may be associated with Wilms' tumor of the kidney, and these have, on rare occasions, caused high-output cardiac failure in children.[58]

Several reports have appeared describing high-output congestive heart failure resulting from the arteriovenous shunts surgically constructed for vascular access in patients on chronic hemodialysis.[59-62] Cardiac outputs as high as 10 liters/min/sq meter, which decrease substantially during temporary occlusion of the shunt, have been found in such patients. These values undoubtedly also reflect the chronic anemia present in many of these patients, but it is clear that it is the added hemodynamic burden imposed by the shunt that precipitates heart failure in patients who had previously tolerated chronic anemia without apparent impairment of cardiac function. It is usually possible to revise or band the fistula to reduce it to the appropriate size for dialysis without compromising cardiac function (Fig. 24–3).[61]

As is the case with other hyperkinetic lesions, the rapidity of the onset of the load and its size, as well as the presence and severity of the underlying heart disease, determines whether or not heart failure will develop.

Beriberi Heart Disease

Pathogenesis and Clinical Considerations. This condition is due to severe thiamine deficiency persisting for at least 3 months. Clinical beriberi is found most frequently in the Far East, although even in that part of the world it is far less prevalent now than in the past. It occurs predominantly in those individuals whose staple diet consists of polished rice, which is deficient in thiamine but high in carbohydrates. The presence of thiamine in the enriched flour used in white bread has virtually eradicated this disease in the United States and Western Europe, where beriberi is found most commonly in diet faddists and

---

TABLE 24–1 CONGENITAL ARTERIOVENOUS ANOMALIES

Common Complaints	
Disfigurement	20%
Swelling	19%
Pain	15%
Other (pulsation, ulceration, increased length of limb)	20%
Physical Signs	
Hemangioma, varices, bruit, or swelling, alone or in combination	100%
Color changes	
Erythema	40%
Cyanosis	12%

Adapted from Szilagyi, D. E., et al.: Congenital arteriovenous anomalies of the limbs. Arch. Surg. *111*:423, 1976. Copyright 1976, American Medical Association.

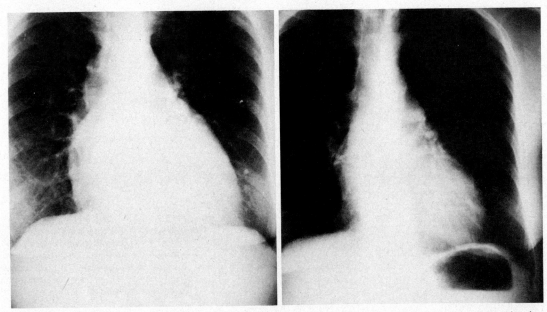

FIGURE 24–3 *Left,* Chest roentgenogram demonstrating cardiomegaly and pulmonary vascular congestion in patient with high-output cardiac failure attributable to end-to-side cephalic vein–radial artery fistula in wrist. *Right,* One month after banding of vein, cardiomegaly has decreased and pulmonary vascular congestion has improved. (From Anderson, C. B., et al.: Cardiac failure and upper extremity arteriovenous dialysis fistulas. Arch. Intern. Med. *136*:292, 1976. Copyright 1976, American Medical Association.)

alcoholics; like polished rice, alcohol is low in vitamin B$_1$ but has a high carbohydrate content. In the West, alcoholics become thiamine-deficient not only because of a low intake of the vitamin but also because they eat "junk" foods or drink large quantities of beer, with their high carbohydrate content and therefore their great demand for thiamine. A reappearance of beriberi heart disease has been reported in Japan, mainly in teenagers, and has been attributed to the recent tendency for teenagers to ingest excessive amounts of sweet carbonated drinks, instant noodles, and polished rice.[62a] Most cases presented in the summer months and were believed to be precipitated by strenuous physical exercise with a resultant sudden increase in thiamine requirements. All of the patients presented with edema ("wet beriberi") with general malaise and fatigue. Neurological manifestations were uncommon. Hemodynamic findings in those studied before and after treatment with thiamine are presented in Figure 24–4. Since their original description by Wenckebach,[63,64] the hemodynamic abnormalities associated with beriberi heart disease have gained considerable attention.[65–68] The elevation of cardiac output is presumably secondary to the reduced systemic vascular resistance, and it is suspected that the latter is caused by lesions of the sympathetic nuclei.

The role of thiamine diphosphate as a coenzyme is well established. In mammals, thiamine diphosphate is required for a variety of reactions that have in common the cleavage of carbon-carbon bonds—the oxidative decarboxylation of alpha-keto acids (pyruvate and alpha-ketoglutarate) and keto analogs of leucine, isoleucine, and valine and the transketolase reaction in the pentose phosphate pathway. Thiamine triphosphate is important in the binding of thiamine diphosphate to its various apoenzymes. The entire spectrum of changes in thiamine deficiency can be explained by the inhibition of these key enzymatic reactions and, in some instances, by the accumulation of proximal metabolites.

Physical findings in most cases presenting in Western countries are those of the high-output state and usually of severe generalized malnutrition and vitamin deficiency. Evidence of peripheral neuropathy with sensory and motor deficits is common (so-called dry beriberi), as is the presence of nutritional cirrhosis characterized by paresthesias of the extremities, decreased or absent knee and ankle jerks, painful glossitis, the anemia of combined iron and folate deficiency, and hyperkeratinized skin lesions. However, the recent cases in Japanese teenagers[62a] were not characterized by other signs of vitamin or nutritional deficiency, and it is possible that similar cases (wet beriberi above) may present in Western teenagers indulging in similar dietary fads.

Beriberi heart disease[69–71] is characterized by evidence of biventricular failure, sinus rhythm, and marked edema (so-called wet beriberi). There is arteriolar vasodilatation, and the cutaneous vessels may be dilated, or in later cases with congestive heart failure, they may be constricted. Therefore, the absence of warm hands does not discount the diagnosis of beriberi. A third heart sound and an apical systolic murmur are heard almost invariably, and there is a wide pulse pressure characteristic of the hyperkinetic state.

The electrocardiogram characteristically exhibits low voltage of the QRS, prolongation of the Q-T interval, and low voltage or inversion of T waves. The chest roentgenogram usually shows biventricular enlargement, pulmonary congestion, and pleural effusions. In alcoholics with beriberi heart disease, the left ventricular ejection fraction and peak left ventricular dP/dt are usually reduced.[69] The role played by alcoholic cardiomyopathy (p. 1406) in this hemodynamic picture is not clear. The cardiac output falls, and the peripheral resistance rises acutely when thiamine is administered in the catheterization laboratory.[69]

Laboratory diagnosis can be made by demonstration of increased serum pyruvate and lactate levels in the presence

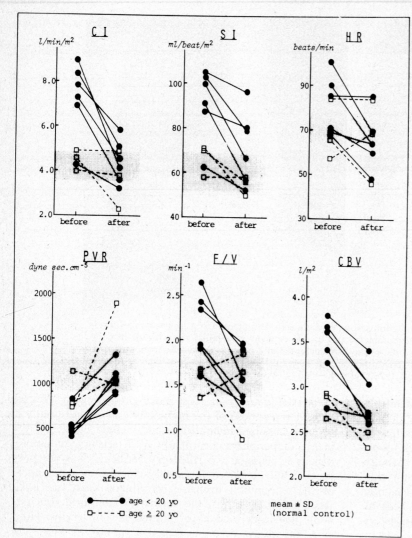

FIGURE 24-4 Changes in cardiac index (CI), stroke index (SI), heart rate (HR), peripheral vascular resistance (PVR), blood turnover rate (F/V), and circulatory blood volume (CBV) in patients treated for beriberi in Kyoto, Japan. (Reprinted with permission from Kawai, C., et al.: Reappearance of beriberi heart disease in Japan. Am. J. Med. *69*:383, 1980.)

of a low transketolase level.[72] Thiamine concentration may be determined in biological fluids,[73-75] and the blood thiamine level furnishes an index of thiamine availability, whereas transketolase activity indicates the ability to convert thiamine into metabolically active forms. The most reliable test of thiamine deficiency is the augmentation of whole blood or erythrocyte transketolase (ETK) activity with treatment (the absolute levels being of little aid). Thiamine functions as a coenzyme for transketolase in the pentose phosphate pathway of glucose metabolism. An increase of circulating ETK activity with treatment or when thiamine diphosphate is added to the patient's blood in vitro (the so-called TPP [thiamine pyrophospate] effect) is helpful in the diagnosis. In the in vitro test, the normal TPP effect is a 0 to 14 per cent increase of ETK activity; a 15 to 24 per cent increase is a borderline response, and a 25 per cent or more increase is evidence of clinical thiamine deficiency.[76] Leukocyte transketolase activity may prove to be a more sensitive index of the thiamine deficiency than the erythrocyte activity.

At *postmortem examination* the heart usually shows simple dilation without other changes. On microscopic examination, there is sometimes edema and hydropic degeneration of the muscle fibers. Nonspecific but abnormal histological and electron microscopic changes have been found in cardiac biopsy specimens.

Heart failure may develop explosively in beriberi, and some patients succumb to the illness within 48 hours of the onset of symptoms. So-called "Shoshin" beriberi, seen most frequently in the Orient, is a fulminating form of the disease[77] characterized by hypotension, tachycardia, and lactic acidosis; if left untreated, the patients die in pulmonary edema. Thus, since the course of the disease may advance rapidly, treatment must be begun immediately once the diagnosis has been established. In the Western world this fulminant form of the disease is quite uncommon.

Treatment. Akbarian and coworkers have reported careful hemodynamic studies which suggest that vasomotor depression or paralysis may be responsible for the depressed vascular resistance.[68] They studied four patients in whom ethanol excess was responsible for the thiamine deficiency. All had increased heart rate and cardiac output (averaging 6 liters/min/sq meter) and reduced arterial–mixed venous oxygen difference and systemic vascular resistance. Right and left ventricular filling pressure and blood volume were also elevated. In one patient intravenous thiamine led to a decrease in cardiac output (from 8.0 to 3.9 liters/min) and an elevation of systemic vascular resistance (from 969 to 1863 dynes-sec-cm^{-5}). Since ouabain then led to substantial improvement, the investigators concluded that the thiamine had converted high-output failure to low-output failure. In other studies, they found that the low systemic vascular resistance did not respond to methoxamine infusion until after correction of the thiamine deficiency.

Patients with beriberi heart disease fail to respond adequately to digitalis and diuretics alone. However, improvement after the administration of thiamine (up to 100 mg IV followed by 25 mg per day orally for 1 to 2 weeks) may be dramatic. Marked diuresis, decrease in heart rate and size, and clearing of pulmonary congestion may occur within 12 to 48 hours.[68,78] However, the acute reversal of the vasodilatation induced by correction of the deficiency may cause the unprepared left ventricle to go into low-output failure. Therefore, patients should receive a glycoside and diuretic therapy along with thiamine.

Latent beriberi deficiency may occur in conditions such as alcoholic cardiomyopathy and in other forms of refractory congestive heart failure. The possibility of thiamine deficiency should be considered in many patients with heart failure of obscure origin. It should be pointed out that the development of thiamine deficiency has been reported in patients receiving prolonged treatment with furosemide.[78a] Thus, patients with heart failure from other etiologies could develop superimposed beriberi heart disease unless adequate thiamine intake is maintained.

Paget's Disease

Pathogenesis. Paget's disease of bone is an asymmetrical process characterized by extremely rapid bone formation and resorption of the involved areas. Histologically, this excessive formation and resorption of bone is mediated by osteoblasts and is followed by replacement of normal marrow by vascular fibrous connective tissue, increases in the vascularity of the diseased bones, and an increase in the size of the vessels originating from the periosteal plexus with an augmentation of periosteal vascularity. Increased blood flow occurs through extremities involved by Paget's disease and may be as high as nine times the normal level.[79,80] Because of the increased vascularity of bone affected by Paget's disease, it has been assumed that this high flow occurred through the involved bone.[79,81,82] However, studies with radioactive technetium-labeled microspheres injected into the femoral arteries of patients with Paget's disease have shown no evidence of arteriovenous shunting.[83] Instead, it appears that the additional blood flow through an affected, resting limb passes through the *cutaneous tissue* overlying the involved bone, possibly secondary to local heat production resulting from the increased metabolic activity of affected bone.[80]

Clinical Findings. These are a function of the extent of the disease and the specific bones involved. Involvement of at least one-third of the skeleton by Paget's disease in an active stage, accompanied by a high alkaline phosphatase level, is necessary before a clinically significant augmentation of cardiac output is observed. The physical findings are those of Paget's disease of bone with swelling or deformity of one or more long bones, enlargement of the skull, facial pain, headache, backache or pain, and an elevated blood alkaline phosphatase level. The cardiovascular findings are not distinguishable from those in other conditions with high-output states. In addition, metastatic calcifications are characteristic. If they involve the heart, they may lead to sclerosis and calcification of the valve rings, with extension into the interventricular septum, and may produce abnormalities of atrioventricular or interventricular conduction.

Treatment. Treatment is generally unsatisfactory, although the long-term use of salmon calcitonin may be beneficial; however, the reported effects of such treatment on the high-output state are mixed.[82,84] Recently oral etidronate disodium has been introduced. This diphosphonate is similar in structure to pyrophosphate, which modifies the crystal growth of calcium hydroxyapatite by adsorption onto the crystal surface, where it inhibits either crystal resorption or crystal growth. There is suppression of rapid turnover of bone, as reflected in bone scans, as well as reduction of urinary hydroxyproline and serum alkaline phosphatase. Etidronate disodium provides symptomatic relief, including reduced bone pain, in many patients. In two-thirds of patients the elevated cardiac output returns to normal within 3 months.[85]

Cytotoxic drugs, including actinomycin D and mithramycin, have also been found to be useful in lowering the elevated cardiac output in Paget's disease, but these potent agents have serious toxic side effects.

Fibrous Dysplasia (Albright's Syndrome)

This condition, in which there is proliferation of fibrous tissue in bone, may also be associated with an elevated cardiac output.[86–89] Fibrous dysplasia has the appearance typical of fibromas, in which are embedded areas of coarse fiber bone with wide osteoid seams, prominent cement lines, and many thin-walled sinusoids; it has been postulated that these sinusoids act as multiple minute arteriovenous fistulas, leading to deformity and fractures. There is abnormal cutaneous pigmentation (i.e., dark brown macules) on one side of the midline and sexual precocity in females. Multiple bones are involved, and the cardiac output may be elevated, as in patients with Paget's disease of bone.

Pregnancy

The effects of pregnancy on the normal circulation and the relationship between pregnancy and cardiovascular disease are discussed in detail in Chapter 53. Here it should be pointed out that in pregnancy cardiac output rises slowly to a peak averaging 40 per cent above control and is accompanied by an increase in blood volume and a reduction in systemic vascular resistance. The elevation of cardiac output is related only in part to the augmented total metabolism characteristic of pregnancy, because the output reaches a peak between the twentieth and twenty-fourth weeks of gestation, yet the combined oxygen needs of mother and fetus continue to climb to reach a peak at term; hormonal effects appear to be responsible in part. This physiological increase in cardiac output does not lead to congestive failure, except when the pregnancy is superimposed on underlying cardiac disease or is added to another major cardiovascular burden.

Hyperkinetic Heart Syndrome

Gorlin and coworkers described a group of patients with increased cardiac output of no discernible cause; cardiac indices averaged 6.4 liters/min/sq meter, with slightly elevated systolic and pulse pressures, normal mean arterial pressure, and low systemic vascular resistance.[90,91] Most were young men with a hyperkinetic precordium, often with third and fourth heart sounds, systolic ejection clicks, midsystolic murmurs along the left sternal border, electrocardiograms suggestive of left ventricular hypertrophy, and radiological evidence of plethoric lung fields. The high value for oxygen consumption (177 ml/min/sq meter) in Gorlin's early report suggested that anxiety contributed to the elevated cardiac output. Indeed, it had been pointed out earlier by Hickam et al. that anxiety can lead to significant increases in oxygen consumption and cardiac output.[92] However, it is now clear that in some patients with this syndrome cardiac output is elevated even after sedation and in the presence of normal oxygen consumption (Fig. 24–5).

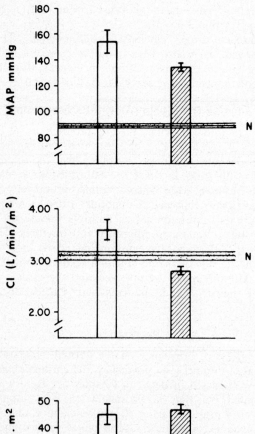

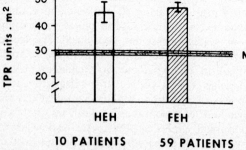

FIGURE 24–5 Hemodynamic characteristics of hyperkinetic essential hypertension. Both mean arterial pressure (MAP) and cardiac index (CI) were significantly higher in the 10 hypertensive patients with hyperkinetic circulation than in the 59 patients with fixed essential hypertension. HEH and FEH = hyperkinetic and fixed essential hypertension, respectively; N = normal values for laboratory; TPR = total peripheral resistance. Bars indicate standard error. (From Ibrahim, M. M., et al.: Hyperkinetic heart in severe hypertension: A separate clinical hemodynamic entity. Am. J. Cardiol. 35:667, 1975.)

TABLE 24–2   IDIOPATHIC HYPERKINETIC HEART SYNDROME: PRESENTING MANIFESTATIONS

Clinical Findings

Young males
Generally asymptomatic
Systolic cardiac murmurs
Overactivity of heart and pulses
Labile hypertension in 50% of patients
LVH by ECG in most patients

Hemodynamic Findings

Increased cardiac index
Decreased A − V O₂ difference
Normal O₂ consumption
Normal heart rate
Increased LV ejection rate
Increased pulse pressure
Decreased SVR

LVH = left ventricular hypertrophy; SVR = systemic vascular resistance. (Modified from Gillum, R. F., Teichholz, L. E., Herman, M. V., et al.: The idiopathic hyperkinetic heart syndrome: Clinical course and long-term prognosis. Am. Heart J. *102*:728, 1981.)

These patients generally receive medical attention because of palpitations, tachycardia, cardiac awareness, atypical chest pain, an unconvincing history of fatigue, dyspnea, or tachypnea. Various diagnoses have been attached to these patients, including neurasthenia, anxiety neurosis, Da Costa syndrome, effort syndrome, and soldier's heart.[93] A similar condition has been described by Frohlich and coworkers as "hyperdynamic beta-adrenergic circulatory state," since treatment with propranolol resulted in improvement.[94]

The elevated systolic arterial pressure and cardiac output and lowered systemic vascular resistance characteristic of this condition are restored to normal by beta-adrenergic blockade. Therapy with a beta-adrenergic blocking agent has been effective in some patients; indeed, cardiac output has been maintained at normal levels for 2 years with doses of 80 to 160 mg/day and promptly returned to the previously elevated levels when the drug was discontinued (Fig. 24–6 and Table 24–2).[95]

There has been some speculation that the hyperkinetic heart syndrome is related to hypertrophic obstructive cardiomyopathy, in that a hyperkinetic precordium, systolic murmur, and elevated cardiac output are present in both conditions (Chap. 41). However, the resemblance between these two conditions is superficial, and no definitive link between them has been proved. Although it has been proposed that hypertrophic obstructive cardiomyopathy may be a complication of the hyperkinetic syndrome, the authors have not encountered any patient in whom this transition occurred, nor has it been satisfactorily documented by others.

Recently, two studies have been reported describing the long-term follow-up of patients who had been diagnosed as having the hyperkinetic heart syndrome.[96,97] In one study,[96] 14 patients were observed for 5 years. Half the group received propranolol, and the remaining 7 patients received placebo. There was symptomatic improvement in the treated group, and symptoms recurred when propranolol was stopped. However, neither propranolol-treated nor placebo-treated patients developed echocardiographic evidence of left ventricular hypertrophy. In the second study,[97] 19 patients initially diagnosed as having hyperkinetic heart syndrome were followed for periods of 11 to 25 years. One

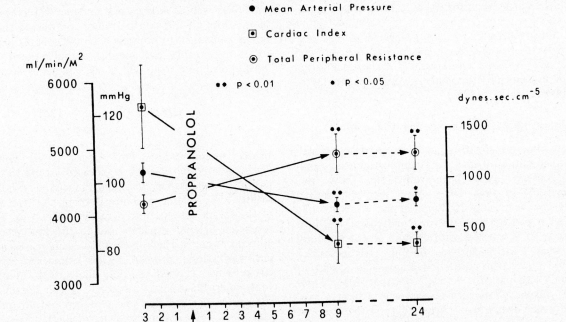

FIGURE 24–6 Average changes in mean arterial pressure, cardiac index, and total peripheral resistance induced by short-term (9 days) and long-term (24 months) treatment with propranolol in hyperkinetic patients. Statistical comparison is made between values in the control and in the treated state. (From Guazzi, M., et al.: Long-term treatment of the hyperkinetic heart syndrome with propranolol. Am. J. Med. Sci. *270*:465, 1975.)

patient died of complicating severe mitral stenosis. Of the remaining patients, in general, the initial physical findings had disappeared or decreased. Two patients developed sustained hypertension. It was concluded that the long-term prognosis of the condition is excellent, and beta blockade was recommended only for those with significant symptoms or hypertension.

An abnormally elevated cardiac output at rest may be responsible for the elevation of arterial pressure in some patients with essential hypertension (Chap. 26). Although this is generally associated with early or labile hypertension,[98] an elevated cardiac output has been observed in some patients with fixed, severe hypertension as well.[99] Presumably, the augmented sympathetic drive to the heart and vascular bed is responsible for both elevated cardiac output and elevated vascular resistance in this subset of patients.

Hepatic Disease

Increased cardiac output has been reported to occur in patients with cirrhosis of the liver,[100–103] and it has been speculated that it may represent the effect of arteriovenous shunting (e.g., vascular spiders) within the liver and other organs. Microarteriovenous fistulas in the lung are usually responsible for arterial hypoxemia and the shunting in the lung[101,102,104–106]; less commonly, collateral vessels between the portal and pulmonary veins are responsible for the right-to-left shunting and cyanosis. In some cases pulmonary arteriovenous shunting may result in 10 to 20 per cent of mixed venous blood traversing the lungs without gas exchange.[101]

Hepatocellular failure, regardless of etiology, increases the cardiac output and induces systemic vasodilatation. The increase in cardiac output may be striking, with eleva-

tions of two to four times the normal value at rest.[100] In patients with acute hepatitis the hyperkinetic state reverses when the hepatitis subsides. The mechanism responsible for the widespread arteriolar dilatation and the resulting hyperkinetic state is not clear. Hypoxemia can contribute to the high cardiac output, as in patients with severe anemia, but does not appear to be a sufficient explanation. Diminished deactivation of vasodilator substances and estrogens may be important.

Renal Disease (See also Chap. 52)

Cardiac output has been reported to increase in some[107–109] but not all[110] patients with acute glomerulonephritis. In a report of six patients with acute glomerulonephritis,[107] cardiac output was increased to an average of 5.4 liters/min/sq meter. Oxygen consumption also increased, as did mean arterial and pulmonary wedge pressures, whereas systemic vascular resistance was normal and the arterial–mixed venous oxygen difference was reduced. Since the patients were in the oliguric stage of their disease, it appears that the combination of hypervolemia, resulting from abnormal salt and water retention, and the increased metabolic rate (high oxygen consumption) was responsible for the high–cardiac output state.

The *pulmonary edema* that occurs in some patients with acute nephritis is not usually a reflection of left ventricular failure, but rather it may be a consequence of the hypervolemia. In addition, left ventricular work may be strikingly elevated as a consequence of the augmentation of cardiac output and arterial pressure; this is associated with an elevation of left ventricular end-diastolic pressure as the ventricle moves to the steep portion of its diastolic pressure-volume curve (Chap. 14). This condition has been termed the *congested state* by Eichna to contrast it with heart failure, in which a true abnormality of cardiac function occurs.[111]

As has already been pointed out, elevated cardiac output secondary to anemia is quite common in chronic renal failure; the arteriovenous fistula created for a vascular access site in patients on hemodialysis often contributes to this high-output state (p. 1756).

Pulmonary Disease (See also Chap. 46)

Although some investigators have reported elevated values for cardiac output at rest in patients with chronic pulmonary disease,[112] most have failed to show this consistently;[113–117] in fact, some have reported finding unexplained left ventricular dysfunction and a low cardiac output in such patients.[116,117] Burrows and coworkers, in a detailed study of 50 patients with chronic obstructive lung disease, found that cardiac output averaged 2.5 liters/min/sq meter with values exceeding 4 liters/min/sq meter in only two patients.[113] It appears that in some patients with chronic pulmonary disease who exhibit a predominance of obstructive bronchitis with marked hypoxemia (Type B, "blue bloaters"), cardiac output is normal or increased, probably reflecting a response to the lowered arterial oxygen tension and the augmented blood volume resulting from secondary polycythemia. Cardiac output is generally depressed in patients with classic cor pulmonale.

Polycythemia Vera (See also Chap. 49)

This condition is also frequently associated with increased cardiac output,[118] despite the added resistance to ventricular ejection imposed by the increased viscosity; right and left atrial pressures are usually normal, and the elevated cardiac output returns to normal with appropriate treatment of the polycythemia. Cobb et al. have speculated that the marked hypervolemia in this condition is responsible for the high output despite elevated viscosity.[118] The most serious cardiovascular consequence of polycythemia vera is the high risk of developing intravascular thromboses.

Carcinoid Syndrome (See also page 1430)

This syndrome, characterized by cutaneous flushing, telangiectasia, diarrhea, and bronchial constriction, results from the release of serotonin and other mediators by carcinoid tumors.[119] These tumors vary in their synthesis of indoles and may elaborate chemically unrelated agents, including histamine, bradykinin, and adrenocorticotropic hormone. In addition to the endocardial disease, described in Chapter 41, an elevated cardiac output in the resting state accompanied by a reduced arterial–mixed venous oxygen difference is quite common.[120] It results from the reduction of vascular resistance, presumably owing to continuous release of mediator(s) and/or to excessive blood flow through metastatic tumors, the latter producing an arteriovenous fistula–like effect.

Dermatological Disorders

Cardiac output is increased in certain erythrodermic skin diseases such as psoriasis and exfoliative dermati-

tis[121,122] as well as in Kaposi's sarcoma.[123] Increased flow of blood through the skin or tumor, producing the hemodynamic equivalent of multiple arteriovenous fistulas, appears to be responsible, and cardiac output returns to normal with appropriate treatment of the cutaneous disorder.

Obesity (See also p. 1741)

Massive obesity is characterized by marked increases in blood volume, cardiac output, and stroke volume. Left ventricular filling pressure is elevated, owing to the combination of increased preload and reduced ventricular distensibility.[124,125] Arterial pressure is often elevated as a result of the raised cardiac output in the presence of a relatively restricted arterial capacity due to the low vascularity of adipose tissue.[126] The combination of increased stroke volume and arterial pressure results in marked elevations of stroke work. The left ventricle dilates (Fig. 24–6), and left ventricular function, as reflected in the relation between left ventricular end-diastolic pressure and stroke work, as well as in V_{max}, is depressed, particularly in the extremely obese person.[124]

Weight loss results in normalization of oxygen consumption, cardiac output, and systemic arterial pressure, but ventricular filling pressures may remain elevated.[127] When obesity persists, as is usually the case, systemic hypertension often becomes severe, and the combination of excessive preload and afterload and the resultant left ventricular hypertrophy and dilatation may lead to congestive heart failure[126] (Fig. 24–7).

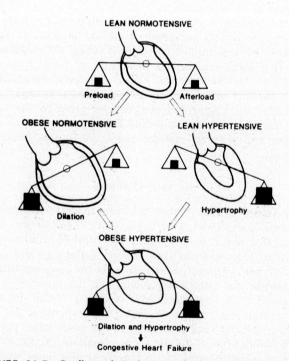

FIGURE 24–7 Cardiac adaptation to obesity and hypertension. Obesity produces dilation (and hypertrophy) of the left ventricle, and hypertension produces only concentric hypertrophy. (Reproduced with permission from Messerli, F. H.: Cardiovascular effects of obesity and hypertension. Lancet 1:1165, 1982.)

References

1. Barratt-Boyes, B. G., and Wood, E. H.: Cardiac output and related measurements and pressure values in the right heart and associated vessels together with an analysis of the hemodynamic response to the inhalation of high oxygen mixtures in healthy subjects. J. Lab. Clin. Med. 51:72, 1958.

2. Sjostrand, T.: Blood volume. In Hamilton, S. F., and Dow, P. (eds.): Handbook of Physiology. Section 2. Circulation. Volume II, Washington, D.C., American Physiological Society, 1962, p. 53.

3. Guyton, A. C.: The relationship of cardiac output to arterial pressure control. Circulation 64:1079, 1981.

4. Sagawa, K.: The end-systolic pressure-volume relation of the ventricle: Definition, modifications, and clinical use. Circulation 63:1223, 1981.

5. Mahler, G., Covell, J. R., and Ross, J., Jr.: Systolic pressure-diameter relations in the normal conscious dog. Cardiovasc. Res. 9:447, 1975.

6. Weber, K. T.: Seminar on the mechanics of ventricular contraction. Physiologic and clinical correlations. Am. J. Cardiol. 40:739, 1977.

7. Richardson, T. Q., and Guyton, A. C.: Effects of polycythemia and anemia on cardiac output and other circulatory factors. Am. J. Physiol. 197:1167, 1959.

8. Burch, G. E., and Hyman, A.: Influence of a hot and humid environment upon cardiac output and work in normal man and in patients with congestive heart failure at rest. Am. Heart J. 53:665, 1957.

9. Burch, G. E., DePasquale, N., Hyman, A., and DeGraff, A. C.: Influence of tropical weather on cardiac output, work, and power of right and left ventricles of man resting in hospital. Arch. Intern. Med. 104:553, 1959.

10. Clarke, T. N. S., Prys-Roberts, C., Biro, G., Foex, P., and Bennett, M. J.: Aortic input impedance and left ventricular energetics in acute isovolemic anaemia. Cardiovasc. Res. 12:49, 1978.

11. Murray, J. F., and Escobar, E.: Circulatory effects of blood viscosity: Comparison of methemoglobinemia and anemia. J. Appl. Physiol. 25:594, 1968.

12. Fowler, N. O., and Holmes, J. C.: Blood viscosity and cardiac output in acute experimental anemia. J. Appl. Physiol. 39:453, 1975.

13. Vatner, S. F., Higgins, C. B., and Franklin, D.: Regional circulatory adjustments to moderate and severe chronic anemia in conscious dogs at rest and during exercise. Circ. Res. 30:731, 1972.

14. Glick, G., Plauth, W. H., Jr., and Braunwald, E.: Role of the autonomic nervous system in the circulatory response to acutely induced anemia in unanesthetized dogs. J. Clin. Invest. 43:2112, 1964.

15. Liang, C., and Huckabee, W. E.: Mechanisms regulating the cardiac output response to cyanide infusion: A model of hypoxia. J. Clin. Invest. 52:3115, 1973.

16. Duke, M., and Abelmann, W. H.: The hemodynamic response to chronic anemia. Circulation 39:503, 1969.

17. Sproule, B. J., Mitchell, J. H., and Miller, W. F.: Cardiopulmonary physiological responses to heavy exercise in patients with anemia. J. Clin. Invest. 39:378, 1960.

18. Graettinger, J. S., Parsons, R. L., and Campbell, J. A.: A correlation of clinical and hemodynamic studies in patients with mild and severe anemia with and without congestive failure. Ann. Intern. Med. 58:617, 1963.

19. Kumar, A. E., Gupta, G. D., Kumar, R., and Singh, M. M.: Pulmonary vascular adaptation to the hyperkinetic state of severe anemia. Clin. Res. 17:578, 1969.

20. Varat, M. A., Adolph, R. J., and Fowler, N. O.: Cardiovascular effects of anemia. Am. Heart J. 83:415, 1972.

21. Case, R. B., Berglung, E., and Sarnoff, S. J.: Ventricular function. VII. Changes in coronary resistance and ventricular function resulting from acutely induced anemia and the effect thereon of coronary stenosis. Am. J. Med. 18:397, 1955.

22. Moser, K. M., and Shea, J. G.: The relationship between pulmonary infarction, cor pulmonale and the sickle states. Am. J. Med. 22:561, 1957.

23. Miller, G. J., Serjeant, G. R., Sivapraqasam, S., and Petch, M. C.: Cardiopulmonary responses and gas exchange during exercise in adults with homozygous sickle-cell disease. Clin. Sci. 44:113, 1973.

24. Pietras, R. J., Real, M. A., Poticha, G. S., Bronsky, D., and Waldstein, S. S.: Cardiovascular response to hyperthyroidism. Arch. Intern. Med. 129:426, 1972.

25. Wilson, W. R., Theilen, E. D., and Fletcher, F. W.: Pharmacologic effects of beta adrenergic receptor blockage in patients with hyperthyroidism. J. Clin. Invest. 43:1697, 1964.

26. Wiener, L., Stout, B. D., and Cox, J. W.: Influence of beta sympathetic blockade on the hemodynamics of hyperthyroidism. Am. J. Med. 46:227, 1969.

27. Das, G., and Krieger, M.: Treatment of thyrotoxic storm with intravenous administration of propranolol. Ann. Intern. Med. 70:985, 1969.

28. Dillon, P. T., Babe, J., Meloni, C. R., and Canary, J. J.: Reserpine in thyrotoxic crises. N. Engl. J. Med. 283:1020, 1970.

29. Buccino, R. A., Spann, J. F., Jr., Pool, P. E., Sonnenblick, E. H., and Braunwald, E.: Influence of thyroid state on intrinsic contractile properties and energy stores of the myocardium. J. Clin. Invest. 46:1669, 1967.

30. Grossman, W., Robin, N. I., Johnson, L. W., Brooks, H. L., Selenkow, H. A., and Dexter, L.: The enhanced myocardial contractility of thyrotoxicosis. Ann. Intern. Med. 74:869, 1971.

31. Taylor, R. R., Covell, J. W., and Ross, J., Jr.: Influence of thyroid state on left ventricular tension velocity relations in the intact, sedated dog. J. Clin. Invest. 48:775, 1969.

32. Lewis, B. S., Ehrenfelk, E. N., Lewis, N., and Gotsman, M. S.: Echocardiographic left ventricular function in thyrotoxicosis. Am. Heart J. 97:460, 1979.

33. Goodkind, M. J., Dambach, G. E., Thyrum, P. T., and Luchi, R. J.: Effect of thyroxine on ventricular myocardial contractility and ATPase activity in guinea pigs. Am. J. Physiol. 226:66, 1974.

34. Banerjee, S. K., Flink, I. L., and Morkin, E.: Enzymatic properties of native and N-ethylmaleimide modified cardiac myosin from normal and thyrotoxic rats. Circ. Res. 39:319, 1976.

35. Rovetto, M. J., Hjalmarson, A. C., Morgan, H. E., Barrett, M. J., and Goldstein, R. A.: Hormonal control of cardiac myosin ATPase in the rat. Circ. Res. 31:397, 1972.

36. Yazaki, Y., and Raben, M. S.: Effect of thyroid state on the enzymatic characteristics of cardiac myosin. Circ. Res. 36:208, 1975.

37. White, C. W., and Zimmerman, T. J.: Reduced cholinergic sinus node restraint in hyperthyroidism. Circulation 54:890, 1976.

38. Etzkorn, J., Hopkins, P., Gray, J., Segal, J., and Ingbar, S. H.: Beta-adrenergic potentiation of the increased in vitro accumulation of cytoleucine by rat thymocytes induced by triiodothyronine. J. Clin. Invest. 63:1172, 1979.

39. Hoffman, I., and Lowrey, R. D.: The electrocardiogram in thyrotoxicosis. Am. J. Cardiol. 8:893, 1960.

40. Muggia, A. L., Stjernholm, M., and Houle, T.: Complete heart block with thyrotoxic myocarditis. N. Engl. J. Med. 283:1099, 1970.

41. Braunwald, E., Mason, D. T., and Ross, J., Jr.: Studies on the cardiocirculatory actions of digitalis. Medicine (Balt) 44:233, 1965.

42. Gaffney, T. E., Braunwald, E., and Kahler, R. L.: Effects of guanethidine on tri-iodothyroxine induced hyperthyroidism in man. N. Engl. J. Med. 265:16, 1961.

43. Newmark, S. R., Himathonekum, T., and Shane, J. M.: Hyperthyroid crises. J.A.M.A. 230:592, 1974.

44. Shapiro, S., Steiner, M., and Dimich, I.: Congestive heart failure in neonatal thyrotoxicosis. A curable cause of heart failure in the newborn. Clin. Pediatr. 14:1155, 1975.

45. Resnekov, L., and Falicov, R. E.: Thyrotoxicosis and lactate-producing angina pectoris with normal coronary arteries. Br. Heart J. 39:51, 1977.

46. Flaim, S. F., Minteer, W. J., Nellis, S. H., and Clark, D. P.: Chronic arteriovenous shunt: Evaluation of a model for heart failure in the rat. Am. J. Physiol. 236:H398, 1979.

47. Nicoladoni, C.: Phlebarteriectasie der rechten oberen Extremitat. Arch. Klin. Chir. 18:252, 1875.

48. Branham, H. H.: Aneurysmal varix of the femoral artery and vein following a gunshot wound. Int. J. Surg. 3:250, 1890.

49. Gupta, P. D., and Singh, M.: Neural mechanism underlying tachycardia induced by non-hypotensive A-V shunt. Am. J. Physiol. 236:H35, 1979.

50. Szilagyi, D. E., Smith, R. F., Elliott, J. P., and Hageman, J. H.: Congenital arteriovenous anomalies of the limbs. Arch. Surg. 111:423, 1976.

51. Becker, D. G., Fish, C. R., and Juergen, S. J. L.: Arteriovenous fistulas of the female pelvis. Obstet. Gynecol. 31:799, 1968.

52. Price, A. C., Coran, A. G., and Mattern, A. L.: Hemangio-endothelioma of the pelvis: A cause of cardiac failure in the newborn. N. Engl. J. Med. 286:647, 1972.

53. Coel, M. N., and Alksne, J. F.: Embolization to diminish high output failure secondary to systemic angiomatosis (Ullman's syndrome). Vasc. Surg. 12:336, 1978.

54. Radtke, W. E., Smith, H. C., Fulton, R. E., and Adson, M. R.: Misdiagnosis of atrial septal defect in patients with hereditary telangiectasis (Osler-Weber-Rendu disease) and hepatic arteriovenous fistulas. Am. Heart J. 95:235, 1978.

55. Rocchini, A. P., Rosenthal, A., Issenberg, H. J., and Nadas, A. S.: Hepatic hemangioendothelioma: Hemodynamic observations and treatment. Pediatrics 57:131, 1976.

56. DeLorimer, A. A., Simpson, E. B., Baum, R., and Carlsson, E.: Hepatic artery ligation for hepatic hemangiomatosis. N. Engl. J. Med. 277:333, 1967.

57. Dorney, E. R.: Peripheral AV fistula of fifty-seven years' duration with refractory heart failure. Am. Heart J. 54:778, 1957.

58. Sanyal, S. K., Saldivar, V., Coburn, T. P., Wrenn, E. L., Jr., and Kumar, M.: Hyperdynamic heart failure due to A-V fistula associated with Wilms' tumor. Pediatrics 57:564, 1976.

59. Anderson, C. B., Codd, J. R., Graff, R. A., Groce, M. A., Harter, H. R., and Newton, W. T.: Cardiac failure and upper extremity arteriovenous dialysis fistulas. Arch. Intern. Med. 136:292, 1976.

60. Ahearn, D. J., and Maher, J. F.: Heart failure as a complication of hemodialysis arteriovenous fistula. Ann. Intern. Med. 77:201, 1972.

61. Anderson, C. B., and Groce, M. A.: Banding of arteriovenous dialysis fistulas to correct high-output cardiac failure. Surgery 78:552, 1975.

62. Fee, H. J., Levisman, J., Doud, R. B., and Golding, A. L.: High output congestive failure from femoral arteriovenous shunts for vascular access. Ann. Surg. 183:321, 1976.

62a. Kawai, C., Wakabayashi, A., Matsumura, T., and Yui, Y.: Reappearance of beriberi heart disease in Japan; a study of 23 cases. Am. J. Med. 69:383, 1980.

63. Aalsmeer, W. C., and Wenckebach, K. F.: Herz und Kreislauf, bei der Beriberi Krankheit. Wien. Arch. Int. Med. 16:193, 1929.

64. Wenckebach, K. F.: Das Beriberi-Herz. Berlin, Julius Springer-Verlag, 1934.

65. Keefer, C. S.: The beriberi heart. Arch. Intern. Med. 45:1, 1930.

66. Weiss, S., and Wilkinson, R. W.: The nature of the cardiovascular disturbances in nutritional deficiency states (beriberi). Ann. Intern. Med. 11:104, 1937.

67. Burwell, C. S., and Dexter, L.: Beriberi heart disease. Trans. Assoc. Am. Phys. 60:59, 1947.

68. Akbarian, M., Yankopoulos, N. A., and Abelmann, W. H.: Hemodynamic studies in beriberi heart disease. Am. J. Med. *41*:197, 1966.

69. Akram, H., Maslowski, A. H., Smith, B. L., and Nichols, M. G.: The haemodynamic, histopathological and hormonal features of alcoholic beriberi. Q. J. Med. *50*:359, 1981.

70. Carson, P.: Alcoholic cardiac beriberi. Br. Med. J. *284*:1817, 1982.

71. Editorial: Cardiovascular beriberi. Lancet *1*:1287, 1982.

72. Akbarian, M., and Dreyfus, P. M.: Blood trans-ketolase activity in beriberi heart disease. J.A.M.A. *20*:77, 1968.

73. Baker, H., and Frank, O.: Clinical Vitaminology: Methods and Interpretation. New York, Wiley Interscience, 1968.

74. Baker, H., quoted in Sauberlich, H. E.: Biochemical alterations in thiamine deficiency—their interpretation. Am. J. Clin. Nutr. *20*:543, 1967.

75. Brin, M.: Erythrocyte transketolase in early thiamine deficiency. Ann. N.Y. Acad. Sci. *98*:528, 1962.

76. Brin, M.: The use of the erythrocyte in the functional evaluation of vitamin adequacy. *In* Bishop, L., and Surgenor, D. M. (eds.): The Red Blood Cell. New York, Academic Press, 1964, p. 45.

77. Jeffrey, F. E., and Abelmann, W. H.: Recovery of proved Shoshin beriberi. Am. J. Med. *50*:123, 1971.

78. Whittemore, R., and Caddell, J. L.: Metabolic and nutritional diseases. *In* Moss, A. J., et al. (eds.): Heart Disease in Infants, Children and Adolescents. 2nd ed. Baltimore, Williams and Wilkins Co., 1977, pp. 590 and 591.

78a. Yui, Y., Fujiwara, H., Mitsui, H., et al.: Furosemide-induced thiamine deficiency. Jpn. Circ. J. *42*:744, 1978.

79. Edholm, O. G., and Howarth, S.: Studies on the peripheral circulation in osteitis deformans. Clin. Sci. *12*:277, 1953.

80. Heistad, D. D., Abboud, F. M., Schmid, P. G., Mark, A. L., and Wilson, W. R.: Regulation of blood flow in Paget's disease of the bone. J. Clin. Invest. *55*:69, 1975.

81. DeDeuxchaisnes, C. N., and Krane, S. M.: Paget's disease of bone: Clinical and metabolic observations. Medicine (Balt.) *43*:233, 1964.

82. Woodhouse, N. J. Y., Crosbie, W. A., and Mohamedally, S. M.: Cardiac output in Paget's disease: Response to long-term salmon calcitonin therapy. Br. Med. J. *4*:686, 1975.

83. Rhodes, B. A., Gregson, N. D., and Hamilton, C. R., Jr.: Absence of anatomic arteriovenous shunts in Paget's disease of bone. N. Engl. J. Med. *287*:686, 1972.

84. Crosbie, W. A., Mohamedally, S. M., and Woodhouse, N. J. Y.: Effect of salmon calcitonin on cardiac output, oxygen transport, and bone turnover in patients with Paget's disease. Clin. Sci. Molec. Med. *48*:537, 1975.

85. Henley, J. W., Croxson, R. S., and Ibbertson, H. K.: The cardiovascular system in Paget's disease of bone—the response to therapy with calcitonin and diphosphonate. N. Z. Med. J. *84*(Abstr.):161, August, 1976.

86. Howarth, S.: Cardiac output in osteitis deformans. Clin. Sci. *12*:271, 1953.

87. Rutishauser, E., Veyrat, R., and Rouiller, C.: La vascularization de l'os pagétique, étude anatomo-pathologique. Presse Méd. *62*:654, 1954.

88. Lequime, J., and Denolin, H.: Circulatory dynamics in osteitis deformans. Circulation *12*:215, 1955.

89. McIntosh, H. D., Miller, D. E., Gleason, W. L., and Goldner, J. L.: The circulatory dynamics of polyostotic fibrous dysplasia. Am. J. Med. *32*:393, 1962.

90. Gorlin, R., Brachfeld, N., Turner, J. O., Messer, J. V., and Salazar, E.: The idiopathic high cardiac output state. J. Clin. Invest. *38*:2144, 1959.

91. Gorlin, R.: The hyperkinetic heart syndrome. J.A.M.A. *182*:823, 1962.

92. Hickam, J. B., Cargill, W. H., and Golden, A.: Cardiovascular reactions to emotional stimuli. Effect on cardiac output, arteriovenous oxygen difference, arterial pressure, and peripheral resistance. J. Clin. Invest. *27*:290, 1947.

93. Editorial: The hyperkinetic heart. Lancet *2*:967, 1982.

94. Frohlich, E. D., Tarazi, R. C., and Dustan, H. P.: Hyperdynamic beta adrenergic circulatory state: Increased beta receptor responsiveness. Arch. Intern. Med. *123*:1, 1969.

95. Guazzi, M., Polese, A., Magrini, F., Fiorentini, C., and Olivari, M. T.: Long-term treatment of the hyperkinetic heart syndrome with propranolol. Am. J. Med. Sci. *270*:465, 1975.

96. Fiorentini, C., Olivarai, M. T., Moruzzi, P., and Guazzi, M. D.: Long-term follow-up of the primary hypertrophic heart. Am. J. Med. *71*:221, 1981.

97. Gillum, R. F., Teicholz, L. E., Herman, M. V., and Gorlin, R.: The idiopathic hyperkinetic heart syndrome: Clinical course and long-term prognosis. Am. Heart J. *102*:728, 1981.

98. Julius, S., and Esler, M.: Autonomic nervous cardiovascular regulation in borderline hypertension. Am. J. Cardiol. *36*:685, 1975.

99. Ibrahim, M. M., Tarazi, R. C., Dustan, H. P., Bravo, E. L., and Gifford, R. W.: Hyperkinetic heart in severe hypertension: A separate clinical hemodynamic entity. Am. J. Cardiol. *35*:667, 1975.

100. Kowalski, J. J., and Abelmann, W. H.: The cardiac output at rest in Laennec's cirrhosis. J. Clin. Invest. *32*:1025, 1953.

101. Wechsler, R. L., Myers, J. D., Dekker, A., Carey, L., and Stilley, J. W.: Cardiovascular effects of severe liver disease. Am. J. Dig. Dis. *21*:114, 1976.

102. Wolfe, J. D., Tashkin, D. P., Holly, F. E., Brachman, M. B., and Genovesi, M. G.: Hypoxemia of cirrhosis. Am. J. Med. *63*:746, 1977.

103. Murray, J. F., Dawson, A. M., and Sherlock, S.: Circulatory changes in chronic liver disease. Am. J. Med. *24*:358, 1958.

104. Karlish, A. J., Marshall, R., Reid, L., and Sherlock, S.: Cyanosis with cirrhosis: A case with pulmonary arteriovenous shunting. Thorax *22*:555, 1967.

105. Hales, M.: Multiple small arteriovenous fistulae of the lungs. Am. J. Pathol. *32*:927, 1956.

106. Berthelot, P., Walker, M. B., Sherlock, S., and Reid, L.: Arterial changes in the lungs in cirrhosis of the liver: Lung spider nevi. N. Engl. J. Med. *274*:291, 1966.

107. Binak, K., Sirmaci, N., Ucak, D., and Harmanci, N.: Circulatory changes in acute glomerulonephritis at rest and during exercise. Br. Heart J. *37*:833, 1975.

108. McCrary, W. W.: The heart in glomerulonephritis. Pediatrics *69*:1176, 1966.

109. DeFanzio, V., Christensen, R. C., Regan, T. J., Baer, L. M., Morita, Y., and Hellems, H. K.: Circulatory changes in acute glomerulonephritis. Circulation *20*:190, 1959.

110. Eichna, L. W., Farber, S. T., Berger, A. R., Rader, B., Smith, W. W., and Albert, R. E.: Non-cardiac circulatory congestion simulating congestive heart failure. Trans. Assoc. Am. Phys. *67*:72, 1954.

111. Eichna, L. W.: Circulatory congestion and heart failure. Circulation *22*:864, 1960.

112. Harvey, R. M., Ferrer, M. I., Richards, D. W., and Cournand, A.: Influence of chronic pulmonary disease on the heart and circulation. Am. J. Med. *10*:719, 1951.

113. Burrows, B., Kettel, L. J., Niden, A. H., Rabinowitz, M., and Diener, C. F.: Patterns of cardiovascular dysfunction in chronic obstructive lung disease. N. Engl. J. Med. *286*:912, 1972.

114. Fowler, N. O., Westcott, R. N., Scott, R. C., and Hess, E.: The cardiac output in chronic cor pulmonale. Circulation *6*:888, 1952.

115. Williams, J. F., Childress, R. H., Boyd, D. L., Higgs, L. M., and Behnke, R. H.: Left ventricular function in patients with chronic obstructive pulmonary disease. J. Clin. Invest. *47*:1143, 1968.

116. Baum, G. L., Schwartz, A., Llamas, R. M., and Castillo, C.: Left ventricular function in chronic obstructive lung disease. N. Engl. J. Med. *285*:361, 1971.

117. Frank, M. J., Weisse, A. B., Moschos, C. B., and Levinson, G. E.: Left ventricular function, metabolism, and blood flow in chronic cor pulmonale. Circulation *47*:798, 1973.

118. Cobb, L. A., Kramer, R. J., and Finch, C. A.: Circulatory effects of chronic hypervolemia in polycythemia vera. J. Clin. Invest. *39*:1722, 1960.

119. Grahame-Smith, D. G.: The carcinoid syndrome. *In* Bondy, P. K., and Rosenberg, L. E. (eds.): Metabolic Control and Disease. 8th ed. Philadelphia, W. B. Saunders Co., 1980, p. 1703.

120. Schwaber, J. R., and Lukas, D. S.: Hyperkinemia and cardiac failure in the carcinoid syndrome. Am. J. Med. *32*:846, 1962.

121. Voight, G. C., Kronthal, H. L., and Crounse, R. G.: Cardiac output in erythroderma skin disease. Am. Heart J. *72*:615, 1966.

122. Shuster, S.: High output cardiac failure from skin disease. Lancet *1*:1338, 1963.

123. Hecht, H. H., Candiolo, B. M., Malkinson, F. D., Nair, K. G., and Saqueton, A. C.: On cardio-cutaneous syndromes. Trans. Assoc. Am. Phys. *80*:91, 1967.

124. DeVitiis, O., Fazio, S., Petito, M., Maddalena, G., Contaldo, F., and Mancini, M.: Obesity and cardiac function. Circulation *64*:477, 1981.

125. Masserli, F. H., Ventura, H. O., Reisin, E., Dreslinski, G. R., Dunn, F. G., MacPhee, A. A., and Frohlich, E. D.: Borderline hypertension and obesity: Two prehypertensive states with elevated cardiac output. Circulation *66*:55, 1982.

126. Masserli, F. H.: Cardiovascular effects of obesity and hypertension. Lancet *1*:1165, 1982.

127. Backman, L., Freyschuss, U., Hallberg, D., and Melcher, A.: Reversibility of cardiovascular changes in extreme obesity. Acta Med. Scand. *205*:367, 1979.

25 PULMONARY HYPERTENSION

by William Grossman, M.D., Joseph S. Alpert, M.D.,
and Eugene Braunwald, M.D.

NORMAL PULMONARY CIRCULATION

During the passage of blood through the lungs, hemoglobin molecules are normally oxygenated to nearly their full capacity and the blood is cleansed of much particulate matter and bacteria. The lung, in addition to functioning as a blood oxygenator and filter, plays a dominant role in achieving acid-base balance by excreting carbon dioxide, thereby helping to maintain an optimum blood pH.[1] Normally, the pulmonary vascular bed offers remarkably little resistance to flow. Pulmonary hypertension results when reductions in the caliber of the pulmonary vessels or increases in pulmonary blood flow occur.

PULMONARY BLOOD FLOW, PRESSURE, AND RESISTANCE

NORMAL ADULT CIRCULATION. *Pulmonary blood flow* refers to the volume of blood per unit of time that passes from the pulmonary artery through the alveolar capillaries and into the pulmonary veins. However, it must be remembered that the lungs have a dual circulation and receive both systemic venous blood (the "pulmonary blood flow") through the pulmonary artery and arterial blood through the bronchial circulation. The bronchial arteries ramify normally into a capillary network drained by bronchial veins, some of which empty into the pulmonary veins, whereas the remainder empty into the systemic venous bed. Therefore the bronchial circulation constitutes a physiological "right-to-left" shunt. The function of the bronchial circulation is to provide nutrition to the airways. Normally blood flow through this system is quite low, amounting to approximately 1 per cent of cardiac output[2]: the resulting desaturation of left atrial blood is usually trivial. However, in some forms of pulmonary disease, e.g., advanced bronchiectasis or cystic fibrosis, and in the presence of congenital cardiovascular malformations that cause cyanosis, the blood flow through the bronchial circulation can increase significantly and account for nearly 30 per cent of the cardiac output.[3] In pulmonary disease, significant right-to-left shunting through the bronchial circulation may result in arterial desaturation. In cyanotic congenital heart disease, bronchial blood flow may participate in gas exchange and improve systemic oxygenation.

The normal pulmonary artery pressure in an individual living at sea level has a peak systolic value of 18 to 25 mm Hg, an end-diastolic value of 6 to 10 mm Hg, and a mean value ranging from 12 to 16 mm Hg (Chap. 9).* Definite pulmonary hypertension is present when pulmonary artery systolic and mean pressures exceed 30 and 20 mm Hg, respectively. Mean pulmonary venous pressure is usually 6 to 10 mm Hg; therefore, the normal arteriovenous pressure

---

*All pressures discussed here are in reference to atmospheric pressure at the level of the heart. True transmural pressures are more physiologically meaningful, especially when pulmonary parenchymal disease is present, but these are rarely measured.

difference, which moves the entire cardiac output across the pulmonary vascular bed, ranges from 2 to 10 mm Hg. This small pressure gradient is all the more remarkable when one considers that to move the same amount of blood per minute through the systemic vascular bed a pressure differential of approximately 90 mm Hg (sytemic arterial mean pressure minus right atrial mean pressure) is required.

Thus, the normal pulmonary vascular bed offers less than one-tenth the *resistance* to flow offered by the systemic bed. *Vascular resistance* is generally quantified, by analogy to Ohm's law, as the ratio of pressure drop (ΔP in mm Hg) to mean flow (Q in liters/min) (p. 292). The ratio is commonly multiplied by 79.9 (or 80 for simplification) to express the results in dynes-seconds-centimeters^{-5}. This conversion to metric units may be avoided, i.e., resistance may be expressed in units of mm Hg/liter/min, which are sometimes referred to as hybrid units, PRU (peripheral resistance units), or Wood units. The calculated pulmonary vascular resistance in normal adults[4] is 67 ± 23 (S.D.) dynes-sec-cm^{-5}.

Vascular resistance reflects a composite of variables that includes, but is not limited to, the cross-sectional area of small muscular arteries and arterioles. Other determinants are blood viscosity, the total mass of lung tissue (i.e., resistance is higher in infants and children than in adults), proximal vascular obstruction (e.g., pulmonary coarctation, pulmonary embolism, peripheral pulmonic stenosis), and extramural compression of vessels (perivascular edema).

Because the pulmonary vascular bed contains considerable elastic tissue, the cross-sectional area of the bed varies directly with transmural pressure and flow. Therefore, pulmonary vascular resistance decreases passively with increases in flow, as illustrated in Figure 46–15, p. 1591. The fall in resistance results in part from the increase in the radius of distensible vessels secondary to increased flow. From a consideration of the Poiseuille relationship—in which $R = \Delta P/Q = 8\eta\ell/\pi r^4$, where R = resistance, ΔP = pressure drop, Q = flow, η = viscosity of fluid, and ℓ and r = length and radius of the vessel, respectively—it is apparent that resistance can be effectively influenced by even small changes in the radius of the vessel. Recruitment of additional vascular channels will also contribute to the fall in resistance that characterizes increased flow through the pulmonary circuit. This phenomenon is particularly prominent in the upright position, when vessels in the upper parts of the lungs are in a partially collapsed state owing to low hydrostatic pressure (p. 1576).

The reduction in resistance in a distensible vascular bed which occurs with increased flow has been offered as the explanation for the absence of pulmonary hypertension in many patients with large left-to-right intracardiac shunts, particularly of the pretricuspid variety (e.g., atrial septal defect). However, it must be pointed out that the increased distensibility of pulmonary vessels in such situations has developed over years and that this principle is not necessarily applicable to acute increases in pulmonary blood flow.[5] In this regard, the results of studies with unilateral occlusion of a pulmonary artery using a balloon catheter are relevant.[6] Figure 25–1 illustrates the relationship between the flow and pressure drop, ΔP, across the left lung

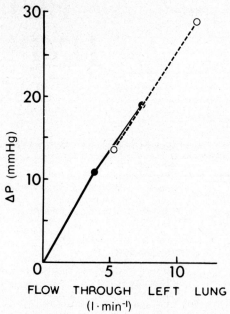

FIGURE 25–1 The relation between the drop in pressure (ΔP) and blood flow across the left lung in a supine normal human subject studied with and without occlusion of one pulmonary artery during rest (●—●) and exercise (○—○). In both states, rest and exercise, the lower circles indicate flow through both lungs and the upper circles flow through one lung. (From Harris, P., and Heath, D.: The Human Pulmonary Circulation. 2nd ed. New York, Churchill Livingstone, 1977.)

during balloon occlusion of the right pulmonary artery, at rest and during exercise, and under both conditions together. It is apparent that acute increases in flow in the supine position were associated with increases in ΔP, so that vascular resistance of the lung (the slope of the line relating ΔP to flow) remained unchanged. In the upright position, however, blood vessels in the upper part of the lung are usually in a partially or fully collapsed state (Fig. 17–4, p. 564) and with an increase in flow, these vessels may be expanded, thereby reducing vascular resistance.[5]

The influence of blood viscosity on pulmonary vascular resistance is also important, particularly in cyanotic patients with hematocrits in excess of 60 per cent or in severely anemic patients with hematocrits less than 20 per cent. In experiments in dogs in which pulmonary pressure-flow curves were constructed at varying hematocrits and rates of flow, ΔP doubled when the hematocrit was increased from 43 per cent to 64 per cent at a normal flow, indicating a doubling of effective pulmonary vascular resistance.[7] Interestingly, at higher hematocrits (54 per cent and greater) ΔP did not increase linearly with flow, i.e., resistance decreased with increased flow, indicating an increase in distensibility and/or recruitment of previously collapsed vessels.

FETAL AND NEONATAL CIRCULATIONS (see also p. 946). In the fetus, oxygenated blood enters the heart from the inferior vena cava and streams across the foramen ovale to the left atrium, left ventricle, ascending aorta, and cranial vessels. Desaturated blood returns from the superior vena cava and passes through the tricuspid valve into the right ventricle and pulmonary artery. Since the resistance of the pulmonary vascular bed in the collapsed fetal lung is extremely high, only 10 to 30 per cent of the total right ventricular output passes through the lungs, the remainder being shunted across the ductus arteriosus to the descending aorta and thence back to the placenta. At birth, there is an abrupt change in the pulmonary circulation. With the first breath of extrauterine life, expansion of the lungs and the abrupt rise in the pO_2 of blood lead to a release of pulmonary arteriolar vasoconstriction and a stretching and dilatation of muscular pulmonary arteries and arterioles, with a marked drop in vascular resistance.[8-10] This facilitates a large increase in pulmonary blood flow and results in an augmented left atrial volume and pressure. The latter closes the flap valve of the foramen ovale, so that interatrial right-to-left shunting ordinarily ceases within the first hour of life. Normally, the ductus arteriosus closes over the next 10 hours as a result of contraction of the thick smooth muscle bundles within its wall in response to a rising arterial oxygen tension and a change in the prostaglandin milieu.[11] Following the initial dramatic fall in pulmonary vascular resistance at birth, there is a continuous decline over the first few months of life associated with thinning of the media of muscular pulmonary arteries and arterioles until the normal adult pattern is achieved.[2,12]

RESPONSE TO METABOLIC, NEURAL, HORMONAL, AND PHARMACOLOGICAL FACTORS

It is well established that acute *hypoxia* elicits pulmonary vasoconstriction[13-16,16a] (Fig. 25–2), and there is general agreement that this response is part of a self-regulatory mechanism for adjusting capillary perfusion to alveolar ventilation. There appears to be an age dependency and a considerable species variability in the magnitude of this vasoconstrictor response, which is quite intense in cattle, intermediate in humans and the pig, and comparatively mild in dogs and sheep[17]; hypoxic vasoconstriction is more pro-

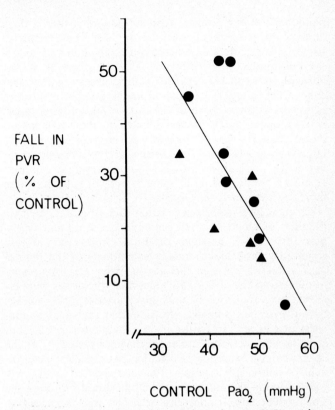

FIGURE 25–3 Fall in pulmonary vascular resistance (PVR) at 1 hour after administration of 20 mg of nifedipine in 13 patients with acute respiratory failure, expressed as a percentage of control value and related to control arterial partial pressure of oxygen (PaO_2). Triangles indicate patients with lung restriction; circles represent patients without restriction. Patients with the most severe resting hypoxemia showed the greatest reduction in pulmonary vascular resistance with nifedipine. (Reprinted with permission from Simoneau, C. T., et al.: Inhibition of hypoxic pulmonary vasoconstriction by nifedipine. N. Engl. J. Med. *304*:1592, 1981.)

found in the infant or young mammal than in the adult. Variability exists within a given species as well, and there is strong evidence for a genetic determination of individual reactivity to hypoxia in animals.[17,18] This finding, if it is applicable to humans, may be relevant to the occasional familial occurrence of primary pulmonary hypertension in humans (p. 839).

The mechanism of the acute pulmonary vasoconstriction that occurs in response to hypoxia is uncertain (Fig. 25–2). There is some evidence that hypoxia-induced local release of histamine may play an important role, with pulmonary vasoconstriction secondary to stimulation of pulmonary vascular H_1-receptors (cf. discussion of histamine below). A role of increased slow-channel calcium entry into vascular smooth muscle in mediating hypoxic pulmonary vasoconstriction is suggested by the observation that the Ca^{++} blocking agent verapamil inhibits hypoxic pulmonary vasoconstriction.[19] The clinical relevance of this observation is supported by a study of the pulmonary vascular effects of nifedipine in 13 patients with acute respiratory failure, studied in a respiratory care unit.[20] In this study, the Ca^{++} channel blocking agent nifedipine produced a reduction in pulmonary vascular resistance dependent on the severity of hypoxia (Fig. 25–3).

The effects of chronic hypoxia on pulmonary hemodynamics and histology have been studied in the rat.[21] Mean

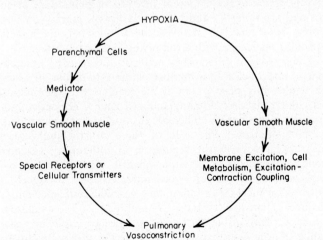

FIGURE 25–2 Alternate hypotheses to explain pulmonary vasoconstriction during hypoxia. *Left,* Indirect mechanism—mediator released by nonmuscle (parenchymal) cells of the lungs diffuses to vascular smooth muscle, where it engages cellular receptors and mechanisms to activate the contractile process. *Right,* Direct mechanism—the effects of hypoxia are exerted directly on vascular smooth muscle by affecting one or more stages in the contractile process; excitation, contraction, or the coupling of the two. (From Fishman, A. P.: Hypoxia on the pulmonary circulation; how and where it acts. Circ. Res. *38*:221, 1976, by permission of the American Heart Association, Inc.)

pulmonary artery pressure rose substantially after 3 days of hypoxia and had doubled by day 14. These hemodynamic changes were associated with (1) abnormal extension of muscle into peripheral arteries where it is not normally present, (2) increased wall thickness of the muscular arteries, and (3) reduction in the number of arteries expressed as an increase in the ratio of alveoli to arteries. In a follow-up study,[22] it was found that these hypoxia-induced chronic vascular changes were more extensive in infants than in adult rats. Furthermore, after recovery under normoxic conditions for 3 months, residual vascular changes were present in all animals studied, but again were more severe in the younger rats.

Changes in alveolar oxygenation directly affect the oxygenation of blood in small pulmonary arteries and arterioles by direct gaseous diffusion from the alveoli, respiratory bronchioles, and alveolar ducts in the pulmonary arterioles,[23–25] even though the latter are "upstream" in relation to the alveoli. This fact, taken together with evidence for a reduction in pulmonary arterial blood volume during hypoxia,[26] supports the view that the small pulmonary arteries and arterioles are the main sites of vasoconstriction and increased resistance during hypoxia.[26,27] While alveolar oxygen tension is a major physiological determinant of pulmonary arteriolar tone, a reduction in the oxygen tension in the mixed venous blood flowing through the small pulmonary arteries and arterioles may also lead to pulmonary arterial vasoconstriction.[15,28]

Acidemia appears to potentiate the effects of hypoxemia (Fig. 46–6, p. 1577), whereas alkalosis may be protective.[29–31] Thus, two potent stimuli for vasodilatation in the systemic arteriolar bed cause vasoconstriction of pulmonary arteries and arterioles. Although *hypercapnia* can be shown to increase pulmonary vascular resistance in some experimental preparations, the effects are variable and probably not important in humans.[15]

With regard to *neural regulation* of pulmonary vascular resistance, it should be pointed out that morphological studies have demonstrated that the media and adventitia of the large elastic pulmonary arteries and of the large pulmonary veins are supplied by nerve fibers that may influence the distensibility of these capacitance vessels.[2,13] Although neural regulation of pulmonary vascular resistance can be demonstrated[32] and may be particularly important in fetal life, its importance in the normal human adult is uncertain.

Chemical and hormonal regulation of pulmonary vascular resistance is a complex and as yet incompletely understood subject, with roles having been reported for catecholamines, acetylcholine, prostaglandins, histamine, bradykinin, serotonin, and angiotensin.[2,13,23,33–60] The exact site of action of these agents within the pulmonary vascular tree (i.e., arterioles, venules, capillaries, and so on) is uncertain at present.

There is controversy concerning the effects of *alpha-adrenergic agonists* on the pulmonary vascular bed. Several studies have shown that norepinephrine causes increases in pulmonary arterial and wedge pressures with no change in pulmonary blood flow or pulmonary vascular resistance.[48–51] Systemic arterial pressure increases markedly, and this presumably accounts for the increase in pulmonary venous pressure. In one study an increase in pulmonary vascular resistance with norepinephrine was reported,[52] and there is experimental evidence for alpha-adrenergic–mediated constriction of small pulmonary arteries and veins induced by either the injection of norepinephrine or the stimulation of sympathetic nerves.[53]

The alpha blocker phentolamine has been shown to lower pulmonary vascular resistance.[54] In addition, tolazoline (Priscoline), which also exhibits alpha-adrenergic blocking action, may exert a strong pulmonary vasodilating effect in some patients. Tolazoline was first reported in the pharmacological literature as a vasodepressor agent having effects comparable to those of histamine. Subsequently, it was shown to antagonize the actions of alpha-adrenergic agonists. Like phentolamine, it is an imidazoline compound, and both these agents have vasodepressor effects independent of their alpha-adrenergic antagonistic properties. In fact, there is some evidence that the pulmonary vasodilator effect of tolazoline is mediated through histamine-2 receptors.[55] Tolazoline has been reported to produce a transient fall in pulmonary vascular resistance in patients with pulmonary hypertension having a major reversible component.[56] Dresdale et al. described a patient with primary pulmonary hypertension in whom mean pulmonary arterial pressure fell from 70 to 31 mm Hg after administration of tolazoline.[57] The wedge pressure was not measured, but cardiac output rose. When 1 mg/kg of tolazoline is injected into the pulmonary artery of patients with pulmonary hypertension, a reduction of pulmonary resistance identifies a vasoconstrictive component of the elevated pulmonary artery pressure.[58]

Beta-adrenergic stimulation with isoproterenol has been shown repeatedly to cause pulmonary *vasodilatation*.[6] In contrast, beta-adrenergic blockade does not produce any change in pulmonary vascular resistance, suggesting that there is no tonic activation of beta receptors for maintenance of the normal low pulmonary vascular resistance. *Acetylcholine* is also a potent relaxant of pulmonary arteries and arterioles[33–35] and transiently lowers pulmonary vascular resistance in patients with elevated pulmonary vascular resistance with a major reversible component.

Lung tissue is particularly active in the synthesis, metabolism, and release of a number of the *prostaglandins*, some of which may play a role in the regulation of pulmonary vascular resistance. Prostaglandins I_2 and E are active pulmonary vasodilators, whereas $F_{2\alpha}$ and A_2 are pulmonary vasoconstrictors.[36] The role of these prostaglandins and their precursors in the regulation of pulmonary vascular tone in humans is uncertain at present. However, the prostaglandin synthesis inhibitor (indomethacin) produced a substantial increase in pulmonary vascular resistance and a decline in cardiac output.[37] If inhibition of prostaglandin synthesis leads to an *increase* in pulmonary vascular resistance, it might be expected that specific prostaglandin infusion might have a vasodilatory effect on the pulmonary vasculature. This was examined in two studies of patients with pulmonary hypertension (primary in nine cases and secondary to thromboembolism and obstructive airway disease in the other two cases) who received an intravenous infusion of PGI_2 (prostacyclin).[38,39] Pulmonary arterial pressure and pulmonary vascular resistance fell toward normal; however, systemic vascular resistance decreased as well (with resultant systemic hypotension in three of the four cases), and the ratio of pulmonary to systemic vascular resistance remained unchanged or increased in all cases. This suggests that PGI$_2$ acted as a general vasodilator, without selective pulmonary vascular action.

Histamine, a vasodilator in the systemic circulation, is primarily a vasoconstrictor in the pulmonary vascular bed. Since large doses of chlorpheniramine and other antihistamines or histamine depletors attenuate the hypoxia-induced pulmonary vasoconstrictor response, it has been suggested that histamine may actually be the chemical mediator of hypoxia-induced vasoconstriction in animals.[40-44] This suggestion is supported by the observation that the periarterial mast cells in the rat and guinea pig lung lose their granules and apparently release histamine during hypoxia.[27] However, other experimental findings are contradictory,[13] and as a consequence, the role of histamine in the regulation of the pulmonary circulation in man remains unclear. Perhaps this confusion can be resolved by the recent finding that histamine may have both pulmonary vasoconstrictor (H$_1$-receptor) and vasodilator (H$_2$-receptor) actions.[59-61] In at least one study, histamine acted as a pulmonary vasoconstrictor in the presence of normal oxygenation and as a vasodilator under hypoxic conditions.[59] As mentioned above, tolazoline may act through stimulation of the H$_2$-receptors.[55]

Serotonin is a potent pulmonary vasoconstrictor in experimental animals[46] but apparently has little or no effect in humans.[47] In this regard, it should be noted that in patients with hepatic metastases of malignant carcinoid of the bowel, large quantities of serotonin are produced and changes in the endocardium and valves of the right side of the heart may occur (p. 1430), but these patients do not exhibit pulmonary hypertension. *Angiotensin II*, generated in the lung by means of enzymatic conversion of angiotensin I, is thought to be a potent pulmonary vasoconstrictor.[27] However, its role in the normal regulation of pulmonary vascular resistance in humans is unknown.

RESPONSE TO ENVIRONMENTAL FACTORS

Life at *high altitude* is associated with pulmonary hypertension of variable severity, reflecting the range of reactivities of different persons to the pulmonary vasoconstrictive effect of hypoxia.[15,62-64] As discussed earlier, pulmonary arterial pressure normally declines rapidly following birth at sea level. However, the fall in pulmonary artery pressure of infants born at high altitude may be slower in onset and of lesser magnitude.[65] Mean pulmonary arterial pressure in normal adults living 10,000 feet above sea level is approximately 25 mm Hg[66] and increases to over 50 mm Hg with exercise. The relationship between *cigarette smoking* and chronic obstructive lung diseases is clear.[67-69] Since many patients with chronic obstructive lung diseases exhibit pulmonary hypertension (Chap. 46),[70,71] cigarette smoking may be considered an indirect stimulus to the development of pulmonary hypertension.

SECONDARY PULMONARY HYPERTENSION

A classification of conditions associated with pulmonary hypertension is given in Table 25–1. As can be seen, pulmonary hypertension results when there is increased resistance to blood flow at any of a number of sites within the circulation, the pulmonary vascular bed itself representing only one of these potential sites. In addition to increased resistance to blood flow (Table 25–1, I–III), markedly increased flow alone may cause pulmonary hypertension, even when resistance to flow is normal at every point in the circulation. Hypoventilation and its various causes (Table 25–1, IV) have been listed as a separate category of conditions associated with pulmonary hypertension, although this is somewhat arbitrary, and it might well be argued that these conditions all produce pulmonary hypertension by hypoxic pulmonary vasoconstriction and thus represent a subcategory of increased resistance to flow through the pulmonary vascular bed (Table 25–1, II).

Increased Resistance to Pulmonary Venous Drainage

PATHOPHYSIOLOGY. Increased resistance to pulmonary venous drainage is a mechanism common to several conditions of diverse etiology in which pulmonary arterial hypertension occurs. Altered resistance to pulmonary venous drainage may be the result of diseases affecting the left ventricle or pericardium, mitral or aortic valvular disease, or rare entities such as cor triatriatum, left atrial myxoma, or pulmonary veno-occlusive disease (see below).

The magnitude of pulmonary hypertension depends, in part, on the performance of the right ventricle. In response to an acute stress, such as pulmonary embolism, the normal right ventricle of an adult living at sea level can tolerate systolic pulmonary pressures of 45 to 50 mm Hg, above which right ventricular failure supervenes. Systolic pressures of 80 to 100 mm Hg can be generated only by a hypertrophied right ventricle that undergoes normal perfusion. If right ventricular infarction or ischemia has occurred,[72-74] or if the right and left ventricles are both affected by a myopathic process, right ventricular failure will occur at lower levels of pulmonary vascular pressures, and significant pulmonary hypertension may not develop despite an increase in pulmonary vascular resistance.

In the presence of a healthy, nonischemic right ventricle, an increase in left atrial pressure from subnormal levels up to 7 mm Hg results in a fall in both pulmonary vascular resistance and the pressure gradient across the lungs.[5] These reductions may reflect distention of a population of compliant small vessels or recruitment of additional vascular channels or both. With further increases in left atrial pressure, pulmonary arterial pressure rises pari passu with pulmonary venous pressure, i.e., at a constant pulmonary blood flow, the pressure gradient between the pulmonary artery and veins and the pulmonary vascular resistance remains constant.[5] Finally, when pulmonary venous pressure

TABLE 25–1   CLASSIFICATION OF PULMONARY HYPERTENSION

I. Increased Resistance to Pulmonary Venous Drainage
   A. Elevated left ventricular diastolic pressure
      1. Left ventricular failure
      2. Reduced left ventricular compliance
      3. Constrictive pericarditis
   B. Left atrial hypertension
      1. Mitral valve disease
      2. Cor triatriatum
      3. Left atrial myxoma
   C. Pulmonary venous obstruction
      1. Congenital stenosis of pulmonary veins
      2. Anomalous pulmonary venous connection with obstruction
      3. Pulmonary veno-occlusive disease
II. Increased Resistance to Flow Through Pulmonary Vascular Bed
   A. Decreased cross-sectional area of pulmonary vascular bed secondary to parenchymal diseases
      1. Chronic obstructive pulmonary disease
      2. Restrictive lung disease
      3. Collagen-vascular diseases (scleroderma, systemic lupus erythematosus [SLE], rheumatoid arthritis)
      4. Fibrotic reactions (Hamman-Rich syndrome, desquamative interstitial pneumonitis, pulmonary hemosiderosis)
      5. Sarcoidosis
      6. Neoplasm
      7. Pneumonia
      8. Status postpulmonary resection
   B. Decreased cross-sectional area of pulmonary vascular bed secondary to Eisenmenger's syndrome
   C. Other conditions associated with decreased cross-sectional area of the pulmonary vascular bed
      1. Primary pulmonary hypertension
      2. Hepatic cirrhosis and/or portal thrombosis
      3. Chemically induced—aminorex fumarate, *Crotalaria* alkaloids
      4. Persistent fetal circulation in the newborn
III. Increased Resistance to Flow Through Large Pulmonary Arteries
   A. Pulmonary thromboembolism
   B. Peripheral pulmonic stenosis
   C. Unilateral absence or stenosis of a pulmonary artery
IV. Hypoventilation
   A. Obesity-hypoventilation syndromes
   B. Pharyngeal-tracheal obstruction
   C. Neuromuscular disorders
      1. Myasthenia gravis
      2. Poliomyelitis
      3. Damage to central respiratory center
   D. Disorders of the chest wall
   E. Pulmonary parenchymal disorders associated with hypoventilation
V. Miscellaneous Causes of Pulmonary Hypertension
   A. High-altitude pulmonary edema
   B. Isolated partial anomalous pulmonary venous drainage
   C. Tetralogy of Fallot
   D. Hemoglobinopathies
   E. Intravenous drug abuse
   F. Alveolar proteinosis
   G. Takayasu's disease

approaches or exceeds 25 mm Hg on a chronic basis, a disproportionate elevation of pulmonary artery pressure occurs, i.e., the pressure gradient between the pulmonary artery and pulmonary vein rises while pulmonary blood flow remains constant or falls, indicating an elevation in pulmonary vascular resistance that is due, in part, to pulmonary vasoconstriction. The latter occurs to a variable extent in response to passive elevations of pulmonary venous pressure and probably reflects the reactivity of the pulmonary vasculature, which may be variable between and within species.

In the dog, for example, experimental production of pulmonary venous hypertension rarely results in vasoconstrictive pulmonary hypertension.[75,76] This probably reflects the low reactivity of the canine vascular bed, since in this species even acute hypoxia fails to elicit a consistent substantial pulmonary vasoconstrictor response. In contrast, the bovine pulmonary vascular bed is more reactive; pulmonary venous constriction in the calf results in substantial and progressive pulmonary arterial vasoconstriction.[77] In the human there is considerable variability in pulmonary arterial vasoconstriction in response to pulmonary venous hypertension. Marked reactive pulmonary hypertension, with pulmonary artery systolic pressures in excess of 80 mm Hg, occurs in somewhat less than one-third of patients with pulmonary venous pressures elevated chronically in excess of 25 mm Hg. The fact that less than one-third of patients with severe mitral stenosis develop severe reactive pulmonary hypertension also argues in favor of a spectrum of variability in pulmonary vascular reactivity to chronic increases in pulmonary venous pressure. This is similar to the marked variability in pulmonary vascular reactivity to hypoxia, discussed earlier. The mechanism involved in elevating pulmonary vascular resistance is unclear. There may be a neural component; also, an elevation of pulmonary venous pressure may narrow or close airways, which may diminish ventilation and lead to hypoxia and, in turn, elevate pulmonary artery pressure. Finally, interstitial pulmonary edema secondary to pulmonary venous hypertension may encroach on the vascular lumen and contribute to the pulmonary arterial hypertension.

Transient, unilateral balloon occlusion of one pulmonary artery in patients with increased pulmonary venous pressure and disproportionate pulmonary arterial hypertension increases the flow through the contralateral lung and produces a substantial fall in vascular resistance.[78] This finding is in contrast to that in normal subjects, in whom increased flow through one lung is not associated with a fall in resistance[5] (Fig. 25–1), and indicates that the increased resistance in patients with pulmonary venous hypertension and markedly elevated pulmonary vascular resistance cannot be due entirely to fixed anatomical changes. Finally, pulmonary vasodilatation in response to the injection of acetylcholine into the pulmonary arteries in some patients with mitral stenosis and severe pulmonary hypertension also supports the concept of a pulmonary arterial vasoconstrictor contribution to the pulmonary hypertension in these patients with chronic increases in pulmonary venous pressure.[33,35,79]

The *pulmonary blood volume* is an additional determinant of pulmonary artery pressure in patients with increased resistance to pulmonary venous drainage. The volume of blood in the lungs obviously reflects a balance between inflow and outflow and is therefore influenced by the output of the two ventricles and the relative distensibilities of the pulmonary vascular bed and the left side of the heart. If the output of the left ventricle decreases transiently while that of the right ventricle remains constant, pulmonary blood volume and therefore pulmonary vascular pressures will tend to rise until the outputs of the two ventricles again equalize. Similarly, if the distensibility of the left heart decreases (as may occur in left ventricular hypertrophy, fibrosis, acute ischemia, or constrictive pericarditis) relative to that of the pulmonary vascular bed, pulmonary vascular pressures and blood volume will increase. Obviously, recruitment (i.e., opening of previously unperfused vessels by increasing vascular distensibility) will limit the rise in pulmonary vascular pressure for any given increase in pulmonary blood volume.

PATHOLOGY. *Structural changes* in the pulmonary vascular bed develop in association with chronic pulmonary venous hypertension, irrespective of its etiology. At the ultrastructural level, these changes include swelling of the pulmonary capillary endothelial cells, thickening of their basal lamina, and wide separation of groups of connective tissue fibrils, indicative of interstitial edema. With persistence of the edema, there is proliferation of reticular and elastic fibrils, so that the alveolar capillaries become embedded in dense connective tissue.[6] The permeability of interendothelial junctions is dependent on pulmonary capillary pressure, with leakage of large molecules (40,000 to 60,000 daltons) occurring at capillary pressures in excess of approximately 30 mm Hg.[80,81]

Light microscopic examination of the lungs of patients with pulmonary venous hypertension shows distention of pulmonary capillaries, thickening and rupture of the basement membranes of endothelial cells, and transudation of erythrocytes through these ruptured membranes into the alveolar spaces, which contain fragments of disintegrating erythrocytes. Pulmonary hemosiderosis is commonly observed (Fig. 6–26A, p. 165), and may progress to extensive fibrosis. In the late stages of pulmonary venous hypertension, areas of hemorrhage may be scattered throughout the lungs, edema fluid and coagulum may collect in the alveolar spaces, and there may be widespread organization and fibrosis of pulmonary alveoli. Membranous pneumocytes are absent from the alveolar walls, having been replaced by granular pneumocytes and giving rise to what is termed "cuboidal metaplasia." Occasionally, particularly in patients with chronic pulmonary venous hypertension due to mitral valve disease, ossification of alveolar spaces will occur[82,83] (Fig. 6–26B, p. 165). Pulmonary lymphatics may become markedly distended, giving the appearance of lymphangiectasis, particularly when the pulmonary venous pressure chronically exceeds 30 mm Hg.

Anatomical changes in the pulmonary arteries in pulmonary hypertension secondary to increased resistance to pulmonary venous drainage depend on whether the pulmonary venous hypertension is the result of a congenital malformation (in which case the alterations are present at birth) or acquired. When pulmonary venous (and therefore arterial) hypertension is *congenital*, the elastic tissue in the main pulmonary artery resembles that of the fetal pulmonary artery and the adult aorta, i.e., the elastic fibrils are long, uniform, unbranched, and parallel to one another. When the pulmonary hypertension is acquired, the elastic tissue in the pulmonary trunk is of the adult pulmonary variety, i.e., the elastic fibrils are short, irregular, and branched and form a loosely arranged network. Structural alterations in the small pulmonary arteries and arterioles include medial hypertrophy and intimal fibrosis and, rarely, necrotizing arteritis. However, vasodilatation and plexiform lesions are not seen. As discussed later (p. 833) the latter lesions characterize the "irreversible" forms of pulmonary arterial hypertension, and their absence in that form of pulmonary hypertension associated with chronic pulmonary venous pressure elevation correlates with the reversibility of the pulmonary hypertension.

Morphological changes in pulmonary blood vessels have correlated with the hemodynamic findings in patients with mitral stenosis who underwent both hemodynamic assessment and lung biopsy. Medial hypertrophy in the small muscular pulmonary arteries and muscularization of arterioles occurred only when pulmonary vascular resistance exceeded 260 dynes-sec-cm$^{-5} \cdot$ m^2,[84] but a linear relationship did not exist between the degree of medial hypertrophy and the level of pulmonary vascular resistance, suggesting that factors in addition to medial hypertrophy caused the pulmonary hypertension. Pulmonary lymphangiectasis occurred only with marked elevations of pulmonary venous pressure, and the presence of pulmonary hemosiderosis did not correlate well with the level of the pulmonary artery wedge pressure.

PULMONARY HYPERTENSION SECONDARY TO ELEVATION OF LEFT VENTRICULAR DIASTOLIC PRESSURE

Left ventricular failure resulting from ischemic heart disease, hypertension, left-sided valvular heart disease, or cardiomyopathy will result in increased left ventricular end-systolic volume; higher ventricular end-diastolic pressure; and passive elevations of left atrial, pulmonary venous, and pulmonary arterial pressures. Since chronic increases in mean left ventricular filling pressure exceeding 25 mm Hg are uncommon, the resultant pulmonary arterial hypertension will be only moderate, unless increases in pulmonary vascular resistance occur. In the absence of an increase in the latter, a normal pulmonary artery mean pressure of 15 mm Hg rises to approximately 30 mm Hg as a result of severe left ventricular failure, characterized by an increase of 15 mm Hg in left ventricular mean diastolic pressure (e.g., from 10 to 25 mm Hg). Since cardiac output is usually reduced in such patients, the mean pulmonary artery pressure would be considerably less than 30 mm Hg if pulmonary vascular resistance remained unchanged. However, many patients with left ventricular failure exhibit increased pulmonary vascular resistance (i.e., in the range of 200 to 300 dynes-sec-cm^{-5}) and moderately severe pulmonary hypertension (pulmonary artery systolic and mean pressures exceeding 60 and 40 mm Hg, respectively).

Decreased left ventricular compliance resulting from a variety of causes may be associated with increased resistance to left ventricular filling and passive increase in left atrial, pulmonary venous, and pulmonary arterial pressures. Specific conditions associated with decreased left ventricular compliance include concentric left ventricular hypertrophy from a variety of causes,[85–87] diffuse fibrosis as a consequence of ischemic disease,[88] and restrictive cardiomyopathy of various etiologies.[89–91] These causes of pulmonary arterial hypertension should be distinguished from those secondary to left ventricular contractile failure, since they do not respond to digitalis or other inotropic drugs. Usually, the levels of pulmonary hypertension in such patients are only moderate, and increases in pulmonary vascular resistance are less marked than with other causes of elevated pulmonary venous pressure.

Constrictive pericarditis (Chap. 43) is also associated with increased pulmonary artery pressures as a result of an increase in the resistance to pulmonary venous drainage into the left side of the heart. Pulmonary artery systolic pressure is usually only mildly increased in this condition, ranging from 35 to 45 mm Hg at rest,[91] but commonly exceeds 50 to 60 mm Hg in such patients during exertion.[92]

PULMONARY HYPERTENSION SECONDARY TO LEFT ATRIAL HYPERTENSION

Mitral stenosis (Chap. 32) represents an important cause of pulmonary hypertension.[93] Although the increased pulmonary artery pressure in this condition is initially a result of an increase in resistance to pulmonary venous drainage, many patients subsequently exhibit marked pulmonary vasoconstriction and anatomical changes in vessels, so that the pulmonary hypertension is "reactive" as well as "passive." The elevation of pulmonary vascular resistance and the associated pulmonary hypertension may come to dominate the clinical picture in mitral stenosis (Fig. 25–4).[94–97] Thus, patients with mitral stenosis often develop what might be considered to be a more proximal obstruction at the level of the pulmonary arterioles and small muscular arteries (the "second stenosis"), with resultant pulmonary hypertension equal to or exceeding systemic arterial pressure. The clinical picture in such patients is characterized by right ventricular failure with distended neck veins, hepatomegaly, and ascites (p. 1067). Patients exhibit marked fatigue, occasionally a more serious complaint than dyspnea. The murmur of mitral stenosis may be soft or even inaudible, and the opening snap of the stenotic mitral valve may be indistinguishable from a loud pulmonic component of S_2, owing to narrowing of the S_2–opening snap interval. Pulmonary congestion and edema may not be prominent clinically. Cardiac output is usually markedly reduced. This constellation of findings may obscure the underlying diagnosis of mitral stenosis and suggest instead either primary pulmonary hypertension or pulmonary hypertension secondary to some other disorder, such as chronic recurrent pulmonary embolism.

Diagnostic studies permit identification of the cause of the severe pulmonary hypertension. The echocardiogram shows features characteristic of mitral stenosis (pp. 109 and 1071), although an echocardiographic pattern mimicking mitral stenosis can, on rare occasions, be seen in patients with pulmonary hypertension.[98] At cardiac catheterization, the pulmonary arterial hypertension is associated with substantial elevations of the pulmonary wedge pressure, and there is generally a sizable (> 10 mm Hg) pressure gradient between pulmonary capillary wedge and left ventricular diastolic pressures. The latter finding is of key importance in distinguishing mitral stenosis from primary pulmonary hypertension, a condition in which the wedge pressure is normal and in which there is no diastolic pressure gradient between the wedge and left ventricular pressures (p. 841).

In general, acute elevations of pulmonary venous pressure to ≥ 25 mm Hg result in the formation of pulmonary edema. However, pulmonary venous pressure may rise gradually to levels of 35 mm Hg or more without the development of gross pulmonary edema.[95,99–101] At least three mechanisms that tend to protect against pulmonary edema formation are operative in patients with mitral stenosis and chronic elevations of pulmonary venous pressure in excess of 25 mm Hg (Chap. 17). First, lymphatic drainage of the pulmonary interstitium increases abruptly when pulmonary venous pressure is increased to 25 mm Hg.[102,103] Acute increases in pulmonary lymph flow of up to eight times the resting level will occur when pulmonary venous pressure is raised to 30 mm Hg for a 10-minute interval, and the increased lymphatic flow will persist at high levels for 30 to 60 minutes after pulmonary venous pressure has returned to normal.[102] In models of *chronic* pulmonary venous pressure elevation, increases in pulmonary lymph flow of up to 28 times normal have been observed.[103] Histological evidence of marked dilatation of the pulmonary lymphatics has been observed in some patients with chronic left atrial pressure overload.[2,104] Thus, despite the imbalance of Starling forces at the capillary level, the edema fluid may be drained away as rapidly as it is formed, and as a result chronic elevation of pulmonary venous pressure to levels exceeding 30 to 35 mm Hg may not lead to clinical evidence of pulmonary edema.

Diminished permeability of the capillary alveolar barrier is a second protective mechanism that might be operative in patients with *chronic* pulmonary venous hypertension in excess of 25 mm Hg. There is morphological evidence of thickening of the layer between the capillary lumen and the alveolar space.[105–108]

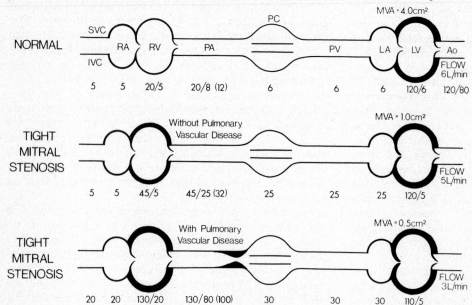

FIGURE 25–4 Schematic diagram of cardiopulmonary circulation in patients with tight mitral stenosis with and without pulmonary vascular disease. Pressures (in mm Hg) are listed for the superior and inferior venae cavae (SVC and IVC), right atrium (RA), right ventricle (RV), pulmonary arteries (PA), capillaries (PC), veins (PV), left atrium (LA), left ventricle (LV), and aorta (Ao) for the normal circulation (*upper panel*) and for the two types of mitral stenosis (*middle and lower panels*). Note that with pulmonary vascular disease (the "second stenosis") severe pulmonary hypertension occurs, and right ventricular failure develops. (Modified from the data of Dexter[94–96] and Schlant.[183])

A third mechanism operating in patients with mitral stenosis and other conditions characterized by chronic increased resistance to pulmonary venous drainage is the reactive constriction of small muscular pulmonary arteries and arterioles. This constriction, which results in considerable elevation of pulmonary artery pressure, is usually associated with a significant decline in right ventricular output (and therefore pulmonary blood flow). The lower pulmonary blood flow tends to diminish the formation of pulmonary edema, since it results in substantially lower left atrial and pulmonary venous pressures at any given size of the mitral valve orifice[109] or for any given impairment of left ventricular function. Despite this protective effect of pulmonary vasoconstriction, pulmonary hypertension is often tolerated poorly in these patients, who commonly show prominent signs of right ventricular failure. Thus, the patient trades pulmonary for peripheral edema and the symptom of dyspnea for the fatigue and lethargy of low cardiac output.

After corrective surgery on the mitral valve, both pulmonary vascular resistance and pulmonary hypertension decline,[110–112] the major extent of which is noted within the first postoperative week. Factors involved in this improvement include reduction of reactive vasoconstriction resulting from (1) distention of the pulmonary vascular bed (i.e., from relief of myogenic vasoconstriction); (2) the resolution of edema within the walls of small arteries and arterioles; and (3) reversal of the morphological changes in Heath-Edwards Grades I to III (p. 833) seen commonly in mitral stenosis.

PULMONARY HYPERTENSION SECONDARY TO PULMONARY VENOUS OBSTRUCTION

Obstruction to pulmonary venous drainage also occurs in association with unusual conditions, such as cor triatriatum, stenosis of pulmonary veins, obstructive forms of anomalous pulmonary venous connection (p. 1008), and pulmonary veno-occlusive disease.

Cor triatriatum is a malformation in which partitioning of the left atrium creates two left atrial subchambers (p. 984). The posterior subchamber receives the pulmonary venous inflow, which then drains through an opening in the partition into the anterior subchamber and thence through the mitral orifice into the left ventricle. When the opening in the partition separating the two left atrial subchambers is small, severe pulmonary venous and pulmonary arterial hypertension result.[113] The diagnosis is established by angiocardiography, and operative correction may be curative.

Pulmonary veno-occlusive disease is an uncommon condition characterized by progressive fibrotic obstruction of the veins and particularly the venules of both lungs. Histological examination may reveal intimal fibrosis in many veins resembling organization of a thrombus, with a central luminal channel surrounded by a rim of collagenous tissue or with recanalization of a number of wide luminal channels, separated by septa. The lungs show pulmonary edema with congestion and areas of interstitial fibrosis and hemosiderosis. The involvement of veins and lungs may be diffuse, but in some instances the most severe lesions are focal and not equally distributed. The condition usually affects children or young adults and is characterized clinical-

ly by exertional dyspnea, orthopnea, and cyanosis. The pulmonary artery pressure is usually markedly elevated (frequently $\geq$ 70 mm Hg systolic), and right ventricular failure may be present.

The pathogenesis of the obstructive changes is unknown, and it is debated regarding whether this condition represents a distinct entity or a syndrome of various causes.[114] Since it has been observed that a febrile, influenza-like illness sometimes precedes pulmonary veno-occlusive disease, it has been proposed that a viral infection may deplete the pulmonary venous endothelium of its plasminogen activator, thus leading to in situ thrombosis.[115] In pulmonary veno-occlusive disease, in contrast to primary pulmonary hypertension, the radiographic changes are suggestive of pulmonary venous hypertension with Kerley B lines (p. 173) and sometimes interstitial and alveolar pulmonary edema. If the pulmonary veno-occlusive disease affects large veins, the wedge pressure will be elevated, and this measurement will then serve to distinguish this condition from primary pulmonary hypertension. However, if the disease affects primarily the smaller veins, the wedge pressure may not reflect the level of the pressure within the pulmonary capillaries and may even be normal.[5]

Increased Resistance to Flow Through the Pulmonary Vascular Bed

PULMONARY PARENCHYMAL DISEASE

Pulmonary hypertension is a common sequel to chronic bronchitis and emphysema (Chap. 46).[70,116] It had long been believed that the elevated pulmonary artery pressures in patients with emphysema resulted from destruction of the pulmonary vascular bed. Current views minimize this pathogenic pathway, since no direct correlation exists between the severity of the emphysema and the degree of right ventricular hypertrophy.[117,118]

PATHOPHYSIOLOGY. Hypoxia-induced vasoconstriction probably plays a major role in producing pulmonary hypertension in patients with chronic bronchitis and emphysema.[2,119–121] There is also evidence for a pulmonary vasoconstrictive action by hydrogen ions, particularly in the presence of hypoxia. In this regard, in patients with chronic obstructive lung disease, pulmonary artery pressure correlates inversely with arterial oxygen saturation and directly with arterial pCO_2,[122–125] providing indirect evidence for a role for hypoxia and hypercapnia in the production of pulmonary hypertension. When patients with chronic bronchitis and emphysema inspire high concentrations of oxygen acutely, there is only a modest decrease in pulmonary artery pressure and vascular resistance,[123,126–128] both of which remain considerably elevated. This suggests that muscular hypertrophy of pulmonary arterioles may in itself be of importance in maintaining the hypoxic pulmonary hypertension. In patients with chronic bronchitis and emphysema, the administration of 30 per cent oxygen for 4 to 8 weeks results in more substantial relief of pulmonary hypertension than do brief periods of oxygen inhalation,[109] indicating that its basis is multifactorial (Chap. 46).

Blood volume and red cell mass, in particular, increase during acute respiratory failure and may contribute to the development of elevated pulmonary arterial pressures. By increasing blood viscosity, increases in hematocrit to within the range commonly seen in chronic bronchitis and emphysema (i.e., 50 to 55 per cent) result in 30 to 50 per cent increases in the transpulmonary arteriovenous pressure gradient at constant blood flow.

SPECIFIC DISORDERS. In patients with *chronic obstructive lung disease*, the extent of destruction of alveoli and the accompanying reductions in alveolar surface area do not correlate closely with the degree of pulmonary hypertension. Thus, the decrease in the cross-sectional area of the pulmonary capillary bed in such patients plays a minor role in elevating pulmonary vascular resistance. A particular association exists between centrilobular (as opposed to panacinar) emphysema and pulmonary hypertension. Right ventricular hypertrophy may occur when only 10 to 15 per cent of the lung is involved in centrilobular emphysema, in contrast to 40 to 70 per cent involvement in patients with panacinar emphysema. This difference may reflect poorer gas exchange in the former circumstance. In patients with advanced bullous emphysema, physical compression of or encroachment on pulmonary capillary beds may play a role, and reduction of pulmonary artery pressure following resection of bullae has been reported;[129] this may be related to reduced compression of the vessel and in part to the associated improvement of gas exchange.

Progressive interstitial pulmonary fibrosis may be associated with pulmonary hypertension. The latter occurs particularly in patients with *scleroderma*, in whom the fibrotic process leads to major reduction in the cross-sectional area of the pulmonary vascular bed due to obliteration of alveolar capillaries and narrowing and obliteration of many small arteries and arterioles.[2,130–132] Moreover, a marked elevation of pulmonary artery pressure (≥ 100 mm Hg systolic) and resistance (≥ 2000 dynes-sec-cm^{-5}) in patients with a variant of scleroderma, the *CREST syndrome* (calcinosis, Raynaud's phenomenon, sclerodactyly, and telangiectasia), has been reported[133] (p. 1663).

Fibrous obliteration of the pulmonary vascular bed and pulmonary hypertension have also been described in patients with isolated Raynaud's phenomenon,[134–136] dermatomyositis,[137] systemic lupus erythematosus,[136,138,139,139a] and rheumatoid arthritis.[140] Pulmonary hypertension is a rare accompaniment of the Hamman-Rich syndrome,[141] desquamative interstitial pneumonia, idiopathic pulmonary hemosiderosis,[142] and sarcoidosis.[143] It is not clear whether significant pulmonary hypertension may result from pulmonary fibrosis due to radiation therapy.

Diffuse lymphatic spread of carcinoma may cause pulmonary hypertension and right heart failure.[144,145] In many cases tumor microemboli and the attendant thrombotic and fibrotic reaction lead to vascular obstruction. Lastly, obstruction of the major pulmonary arteries by tumor (usually sarcoma) may be a cause of right ventricular and main pulmonary artery hypertension.[2,146]

EISENMENGER'S SYNDROME (See also Chap. 29 and 30)

Decreased cross-sectional area of the pulmonary arteriolar bed with irreversible pulmonary hypertension characterizes the so-called Eisenmenger's syndrome. This term was used by Wood[147] to refer to patients with congenital

cardiac lesions and severe pulmonary hypertension in whom reversal of a left-to-right shunt has occurred. Left-to-right shunts are due usually to congenital cardiovascular malformations[148] (e.g., atrial and ventricular septal defects, patent ductus arteriosus). Much less commonly they result from acquired lesions (e.g., ventricular septal defect secondary to acute myocardial infarction).

PATHOPHYSIOLOGY. Pulmonary hypertension in congenital heart disease may occur simply because of increased pulmonary blood flow. When chronic, the increased pulmonary flow is often associated with a passive reduction in pulmonary resistance and little elevation of pulmonary vascular pressures. In a normal adult with a pulmonary blood flow (PBF) of 5 liters/min, a pulmonary vascular resistance (PVR) of 60 dynes-sec-cm^{-5}, and a mean left atrial pressure (LA) of 6 mm Hg, the pulmonary artery mean pressure (PA) may be calculated from the expression

$$PVR = \frac{(PA - LA)80}{PBF} = \frac{(PA - 6)80}{5} = 60 \text{ dynes-sec-cm}^{-5}$$

$$PA = \frac{60 \times 5}{80} + 6 = 10 \text{ mm Hg}$$

If PBF is doubled, a reduction in PVR to 30 dynes-sec-cm^{-5} will maintain PA mean pressure at a normal level of 10 mm Hg. However, if PBF is increased four- to sixfold, the reserve capacity of the pulmonary vascular bed will be exceeded, and pulmonary artery pressure will rise. Thus, if the PVR is 30 dynes-sec-cm^{-5}, a PBF of 30 liters/min will be associated with a mean PA pressure that is only minimally elevated at 17 mm Hg, although the high right ventricular stroke volumes associated with the augmentation in pulmonary blood flow result in considerably higher values (40 to 45 mm Hg) for pulmonary artery and right ventricular systolic pressures. If the capacity of the pulmonary vascular bed to accommodate extra blood flow is diminished owing to mild parenchymal lung disease that results in a higher, albeit normal, PVR of 90 dynes-sec-cm^{-5}, the mean PA pressure in the patient with a PBF of 30 liters/min will approximate 40 mm Hg; systolic PA and right ventricular pressures may exceed 60 mm Hg. If no underlying arteriolar vascular disease exists, abolition of the shunt by corrective operation restores pulmonary blood flow and PA pressure to normal.

Commonly, an increase in pulmonary vascular resistance makes a variable contribution to the pulmonary hypertension associated with congenital heart disease. The increase in vascular resistance may have both a functional and a fixed component. The former—the "Bayliss" or myogenic theory—is thought to be related to pulmonary arteriolar vasoconstriction stimulated by distention of muscular pulmonary arteries and arterioles. According to this concept, distention of the vessel acts as a stimulus to vasoconstriction, which then leads to increased work of the vascular smooth muscle and in turn to hypertrophy of the smooth muscle in the vessel wall.[5]

If a congenital cardiovascular defect causes pulmonary hypertension from the time of birth, the small, muscular arteries of the fetal lung may undergo delayed or only partial involution, resulting in persistently high levels of pulmonary vascular resistance (p. 950). This is true especially of those lesions in which a left-to-right shunt directly enters the right ventricle or pulmonary artery (i.e., a post–tricuspid valve shunt, such as ventricular septal defect or patent ductus arteriosus); these patients experience a higher incidence of severe and irreversible pulmonary vascular damage than those in whom the shunt is proximal to the tricuspid valve (pretricuspid shunts, as in atrial septal defect and partial anomalous pulmonary venous drainage). In the latter category, pulmonary pressures fall after birth, and the fetal vascular pattern usually regresses; later in life, however, pulmonary hypertension may result from a large pretricuspid left-to-right shunt, which enhances the risk of pulmonary vascular damage.

PATHOLOGY. Pulmonary vascular obstructive disease in the presence of a congenital cardiovascular anomaly may be reversible or irreversible. From an anatomical point of view, reversible conditions are those in which the decreased pulmonary arteriolar cross-sectional area is the result of medial hypertrophy and vasoconstriction; irreversibility is associated with the presence of necrotizing arteritis and plexiform lesions in these small vessels.[2,148a] The classification by Heath and Edwards[149] of six grades of structural change is widely employed to assess the potential reversibility of pulmonary vascular disease and is summarized as follows: *Grade I* is characterized by hypertrophy of the media of small muscular pulmonary arteries and arterioles. In *Grade II*, intimal cellular proliferation is added to the medial hypertrophy. *Grade III* is characterized by advanced medial thickening with hypertrophy and hyperplasia, together with progressive intimal proliferation and concentric fibrosis that results in obliteration of many arterioles and small arteries. In *Grade IV*, dilatation and so-called "plexiform lesions" of the muscular pulmonary arteries and arterioles are observed (Fig. 25–5). The latter consist of a plexiform network of capillary-like channels within a dilated segment of a muscular pulmonary artery. The channels are separated by proliferating endothelial cells, which often contain thrombi; indeed, the network of capillary channels may constitute recanalization of a thrombus. *Grade V* changes include complex plexiform, angiomatous, and cavernous lesions and hyalinization of intimal fibrosis. Finally, *Grade VI* is characterized by the presence of necrotizing arteritis.

The Heath and Edwards classification implies that the morphological alterations are sequential, with Grade I being the earliest stage and Grade VI being the "end stage"

of pulmonary vascular obliterative disease. That such an orderly progression may not in fact occur is suggested by the findings of Wagenvoort and Wagenvoort, which indicate that plexiform lesions develop gradually in areas affected by necrotizing arteritis. They have suggested that fibrinoid necrosis of a small segment of a pulmonary arterial branch leads to medial destruction and subsequent aneurysmal dilatation of the vessel as well as the formation of a fibrin clot in the lumen, often with admixture of platelets.[2,148a,150,151] Organization of the fibrin clot by strands of intimal cells leads to formation of the plexus; the small capillary-like channels within the plexus (Fig. 25–5) provide continuity to the distal portion of the artery, which undergoes poststenotic dilatation. With time, the inflammatory component of the process subsides, fibrin disappears, and the strands of intimal cells become fibrotic. Wagenvoorts' view is supported by animal experiments in which end-to-end systemic-pulmonary anastomoses resulted in arteritis and fibrinoid necrosis prior to the appearance of plexiform lesions.[152–159] Thus, although Heath-Edwards Grades I, II, and III may represent chronological progression, evidence exists that Grade VI (necrotizing arteritis) changes appear next, followed by Grades IV and V end-stage alterations.

CLINICAL CONSIDERATIONS. As mentioned above, *Eisenmenger's syndrome* is the term used by Wood to refer to patients with congenital central communications with severe pulmonary hypertension, in whom reversal of a left-to-right shunt has occurred across the pulmonary-systemic communication.[147] The patients described originally by Eisenmenger had ventricular septal defects, and the term *Eisenmenger's complex* is applied to patients with severe pulmonary hypertension and right-to-left shunt through such a defect. The term *Eisenmenger's syndrome* is applied to any anomaly in which the pathophysiological process leads to obliterative pulmonary vascular disease, including pretricuspid and post-tricuspid shunts. Heath-Edwards Grades IV to VI changes are usual in these patients; occasionally, lesser anatomical changes predominate and may be reversible after successful corrective operation.

Two examples will serve to illustrate these points:

The first is the infant with a large left-to-right shunt through a ventricular septal defect. Pulmonary artery pressure is elevated both because the large defect allows equilibration of pressures between the two ventricles and because pulmonary blood flow is excessive in the face of the reduced lumen/wall ratios of the neonatal pulmonary arteries and arterioles. Widening of the lumen and thinning of the me-

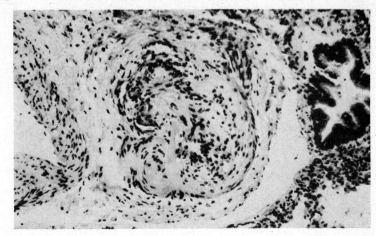

FIGURE 25–5 Histological section from the lung of a 3-year-old boy with a common atrioventricular canal and severe pulmonary hypertension. A muscular pulmonary artery with an early plexiform lesion is seen as well as fibrinoid necrosis of the media and active proliferation of intimal cells. (From Wagenvoort, C. A., and Wagenvoort, N.: Pathology of Pulmonary Hypertension. 2nd ed. New York, John Wiley and Sons, 1977.)

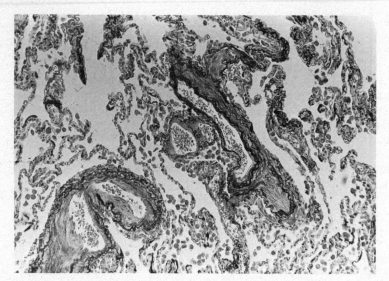

FIGURE 25–6   Photomicrograph of a lung biopsy specimen from a 35-year-old man with a patent ductus arteriosus and systemic pulmonary hypertension. A predominance of advanced changes is seen, including plexiform and dilatation lesions.

dia are delayed or only partial in these vessels as a consequence of the distention and increased wall tension. With time, additional hypertrophy of vascular smooth muscle may result in further elevation in pulmonary vascular resistance. The latter has both a functional and an anatomical component; the former is due to increased vascular smooth muscle tone whereas early in life the latter consists of medial hypertrophy and intimal cellular proliferation and fibrosis. The functional component may be intensified by hypoxia and relieved transiently by infusion of acetylcholine or tolazoline or by breathing 100 per cent oxygen. If corrective surgery is performed at this stage, an *immediate* reduction toward normal in pulmonary artery pressure may be anticipated owing to the reduction in pulmonary blood flow and release of the vasoconstrictor stimulus. A more *gradual* reduction in pulmonary artery pressure may then ensue with regression of the reversible anatomical changes (medial hypertrophy, intimal cellular proliferation, and fibrosis). If corrective surgery is not performed, there may be further anatomical obliterative changes, with the development of necrotizing arteritis and plexiform lesions. The more extensive the fixed vascular lesions, the higher the risk of corrective operation and the poorer the clinical result even if the patient survives. However, it should be recognized that despite increased pulmonary vascular resistance an immediate reduction in pulmonary artery pressure may occur following surgical interruption of the shunt as long as pulmonary blood flow exceeds systemic flow (i.e., if a net left-to-right shunt exists) (Chaps. 29 and 30). The higher the preoperative pulmonary vascular resistance, the less likely is regression of the pulmonary vascular changes.

The second example illustrates the favorable changes resulting from cardiac surgery in a 35-year-old man with patent ductus arteriosus who presented with symptoms of right heart failure, polycythemia (hematocrit of 60 per cent), and cyanosis of the lower extremities. Cardiac catheterization revealed pulmonary artery pressure equal to systemic levels (110/55 mm Hg) and markedly elevated pulmonary vascular resistance (982 dynes-sec-cm^{-5}). Flow across the ductus arteriosus was bidirectional, but the net shunt was left-to-right (pulmonary/systemic flow ratio of 1.8:1.0). Lung biopsy at operation showed advanced vascular obliterative changes (Fig. 25–6). A hemodynamic study immediately following ligation of the ductus arteriosus showed a decline in pulmonary artery pressure commensurate with the reduction in pulmonary blood flow. Repeat study 6 months later showed a substantial fall in pulmonary vascular resistance (464 dynes-sec-cm^{-5}) and pulmonary artery pressure (65/20 mm Hg) possibly due to regression of some of the pathological changes and to improved oxygenation of arterial blood as congestive failure and postoperative pulmonary dysfunction resolved. An additional factor may have been resolution of the polycythemia. A final postoperative evaluation of this patient 9 months later (15 months postoperatively) showed a further reduction in pulmonary vascular resistance (337 dynes-sec-cm^{-5}) and pulmonary artery pressure (50/24 mm Hg).

When the pulmonary vascular resistance has increased to equal (or exceed) systemic resistance, and the anatomical changes of the pulmonary vessels are predominantly those of Grades IV to VI, surgical closure of the intracardiac communication will fail to relieve pulmonary hypertension and will be associated with a prohibitive immediate risk. Operation will, in fact, hasten death in most survivors who had either balanced shunts or predominant right-to-

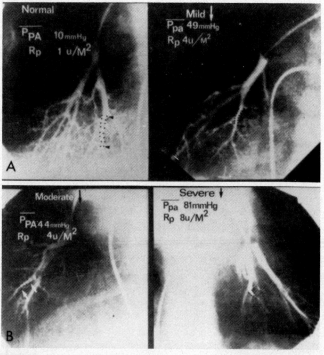

FIGURE 25–7   *A,* The left panel is a wedge angiogram from a patient with normal mean pulmonary artery pressure ($\overline{P}_{pa}$). There is gradual tapering of the arteries (arrows indicate luminal diameters of 2.5 mm and 1.5 mm) and dense background haze. The right-hand panel is a wedge angiogram from a patient with elevated $\overline{P}_{pa}$ and mild elevation of pulmonary vascular resistance (Rp); the arteries taper more abruptly (see arrows), and the background haze is mildly decreased. *B,* The left panel is a wedge angiogram from a patient with elevated Rp in whom the arteries taper (see arrows at luminal diameters of 2.5 mm and 1.5 mm), and the background haze is moderately decreased. The right-hand panel is a wedge angiogram from a patient with severe elevation in Rp in whom the arteries taper very abruptly (see arrows), and the background haze is severely reduced. (Reproduced with permission from Rabinovitch, M., Keane, J. F., Fellows, K. E., et al.: Quantitative analysis of the pulmonary wedge angiogram in congenital heart defects. Circulation *63:*152, 1981.)

left shunts, since closure of the right-to-left communication merely increases the load on an already overburdened right ventricle. Structural changes in the pulmonary vascular bed can be evaluated by means of quantitative analysis of the pulmonary wedge angiogram.[155] This technique has been employed successfully by Rabinovitch, Reid, and coworkers, who have demonstrated progressively more abrupt tapering of the pulmonary arteries in patients with increasingly abnormal hemodynamics and increasingly severe structural changes in lung biopsy tissue (Fig. 25–7).[156]

OTHER CONDITIONS ASSOCIATED WITH DECREASED CROSS-SECTIONAL AREA OF THE PULMONARY VASCULAR BED

Primary pulmonary hypertension has been more recently called "unexplained pulmonary hypertension" by a working committee of the World Health Organization[157] (p. 836).

Hepatic cirrhosis and portal vein thrombosis have been occasionally associated with pulmonary hypertension and obliterative changes in the pulmonary arteriolar bed.[158-160] Fishman has speculated that there is a common pathophysiological mechanism to these cases and others where pulmonary hypertension is associated with ingestion of a variety of substances (*Crotalaria* alkaloids,[161] aminorex[162]), and he has termed this "dietary pulmonary hypertension."[163] According to this concept, certain metabolites of ingested foods or drugs may induce pulmonary hypertension if they gain access to the pulmonary circulation or, if by damaging the liver, they lead to release of vasoactive substances that subsequently reach the lungs and injure pulmonary vessels.

Persistent fetal circulation in the newborn has been reported as a cause of severe pulmonary hypertension.[164-166] Affected infants exhibit cyanosis, tachypnea, acidemia, normal pulmonary parenchymal markings on chest x-ray, and anatomically normal hearts. Cyanosis is the result of right-to-left shunting across the foramen ovale and through a patent ductus arteriosus.[164] The condition may be due to persistence of extremely muscular small pulmonary arteries, a diminution in the absolute number of these resistance vessels, or a combination of the two.[166]

INCREASED RESISTANCE FLOW THROUGH LARGE PULMONARY ARTERIES

Pulmonary thromboembolism (Chap. 46) may cause pulmonary hypertension by impeding blood flow through the major pulmonary arteries and their branches. Generally, a single episode of pulmonary embolism resolves with treatment, and follow-up studies reveal normal pulmonary vasculature and pressure in the majority of patients.[167,168]

Peripheral pulmonic stenosis is a congenital lesion that occurs particularly in association with supravalvular aortic stenosis or as a sequela of the rubella syndrome (p. 985). Hypertension in the proximal pulmonary arteries depends on the extent, location, and severity of the stenotic lesions.[2,169,170]

Unilateral absence of either the right or the left pulmonary artery is a rare congenital anomaly.[171] Often the condition is associated with a ventricular septal defect or patent ductus arteriosus, and the incidence of pulmonary hypertension is high. Pulmonary hypertension may also be observed in the absence of associated abnormalities, pre-

sumably because the thick-walled fetal pulmonary arterial bed is stimulated to constrict and undergo anatomical obliterative changes when the total cardiac output flows through only one lung from birth onward. The same mechanism may operate in patients with unilateral pulmonary artery stenosis in whom elevated pressure is observed in the main and uninvolved pulmonary arteries. Relief of the obstructive lesion by operation has been associated with marked improvement.[172]

HYPOVENTILATION

As discussed earlier in this chapter, conditions associated with hypoxia may cause pulmonary hypertension, particularly if there is associated acidemia[29-31] (Figure 46–6, p. 1577). A number of disorders that affect the upper airways, neuromuscular control, or pulmonary parenchyma lead to hypoventilation and (in the setting of a reactive pulmonary vascular bed) pulmonary hypertension.

The obesity-hypoventilation syndrome[173,174] (p. 1596), also called the pickwickian syndrome, may lead to substantial pulmonary hypertension (mean pulmonary artery pressure ≥ 50 mm Hg), which correlates with the presence of hypoxemia and acidosis. *Pharyngeal-tracheal obstruction* occurs in the presence of hypertrophied tonsils and adenoids[175,176] and may cause reversible pulmonary hypertension (p. 1597).

Neuromuscular disorders such as myasthenia gravis, poliomyelitis, and damage to the central respiratory center[177] may cause hypoventilation of sufficient severity to result in pulmonary hypertension (p. 1596). *Disorders of the chest wall* (kyphoscoliosis, pectus excavatum) may also cause hypoventilation and pulmonary hypertension (p. 1596).

The pulmonary hypertension in all of these conditions subsides with restoration of normal respiration and correction of the hypoxia. It should also be recognized that hypoxia may intensify pulmonary hypertension of other causes. For example, severe pulmonary hypertension occurring in children with a left-to-right shunt who reside at high altitude is often due to the combination of high pulmonary blood flow and superimposed hypoxic pulmonary vasoconstriction; pulmonary pressures may fall rapidly toward normal when residence is established at sea level.

OTHER CAUSES OF PULMONARY HYPERTENSION

High-altitude pulmonary edema (p. 568) is an entity associated with reversible pulmonary hypertension. It is observed particularly in individuals acclimatized to high altitudes who, after a stay of some days or weeks at sea level, return to high altitude.[178] The finding of high-altitude pulmonary edema in four persons without a right pulmonary artery has been reported,[179] giving support to speculation concerning the combined role of hypoxia and hyperperfusion in patients with this anomaly.[180]

Severe pulmonary hypertension is an occasional but unusual finding in patients with *isolated partial anomalous pulmonary venous drainage.*[181] Speculation exists that the cause may be the increase in pulmonary blood flow associated perhaps with a reflex pulmonary arterial vasoconstriction secondary to distention of the right atrium.

The cause of the pulmonary hypertension that occasionally develops following surgical correction of *tetralogy of Fallot* is unclear. In the patient with tetralogy of Fallot, pulmonary vascular thrombotic lesions are common and, if extensive, may predispose to pulmonary hypertension when operation—either complete correction or creation of a left-to-right shunt—causes a sudden increase in pulmonary blood flow.[2,182]

Sickle cell anemia may be complicated by in situ pulmonary thrombosis and infarction, although, as discussed in Chapter 49, this does not usually lead to pulmonary hypertension. There are two case reports of cor pulmonale associated with hemoglobin SC disease,[184,185] but the prevalence of pulmonary hypertension in individuals with this condition is unknown.

Intravenous drug abuse may lead to diffuse pulmonary vascular occlusion and pulmonary hypertension, as in the case of a 25-year-old man who injected himself with crushed, dissolved pentazocine intravenously has been reported.[186] After 1 month he developed chest pain, shortness of breath, and fatigue and was found to have a pulmonary artery pressure of 72/30 mm Hg (mean 46 mm Hg) with a right atrial pressure of 14 mm Hg. Analysis of lung biopsy material implicated embolization of the cellulose filter material in the tablet with subsequent severe tissue reaction and granuloma formation. Prednisone therapy led to improvement in the clinical state and gradual lowering of the pulmonary artery pressure.

A patient in whom moderately severe pulmonary hypertension developed in association with *alveolar proteinosis* has been reported.[187] Hypoxemia seemed to be the mediating factor, and the patient showed substantial reduction in pulmonary artery pressure (60/25 mm Hg to 32/14 mm Hg) in response to oxygen inhalation. Pulmonary arte-

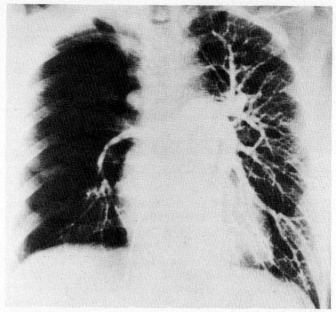

FIGURE 25–8 Pulmonary angiogram from a 27-year-old Japanese woman with Takayasu's disease and pulmonary hypertension. There is marked narrowing of the right pulmonary artery and no appearance of its branches. (Reprinted with permission from Kawai, C.: Pulmonary pulseless disease: Pulmonary involvement in so-called Takayasu's disease. Chest *73*:651, 1978.)

rial involvement with pulmonary hypertension has been reported to occur in approximately 25 per cent of patients with *Takayasu's disease*.[188,189] The pulmonary pressure elevations are usually only moderate, but striking abnormalities may be present on lung scan or pulmonary angiogram (Fig. 25–8).

PRIMARY (UNEXPLAINED) PULMONARY HYPERTENSION

In some patients with pulmonary hypertension, no cause is discernible, in which case the pulmonary hypertension is termed idiopathic, essential, unexplained,[157] or, most frequently, *primary*. In contrast to systemic hypertension, in which the etiology is primary (essential) in a large percentage of patients (Chap. 26), primary hypertension in the pulmonary circuit is uncommon. Primary pulmonary hypertension (PPH) is often readily suspected on clinical examination, but the diagnosis should be made only after detailed examination of the heart and lungs, i.e., ordinarily after cardiac catheterization and pulmonary angiography have revealed no specific cause for the pulmonary hypertension.

ETIOLOGY

Although a number of theories have been advanced to explain the origin of PPH, none has as yet gained clear ascendancy. Indeed, were the etiology of the pulmonary hypertension clear, the designation "primary" would not be appropriate.

Recurrent occult venous thrombosis with pulmonary embolism may be extremely difficult to exclude as the cause of pulmonary hypertension. A number of patients with chron-

ic, recurrent thromboembolic disease develop pulmonary hypertension and cor pulmonale slowly, with no overt clinical manifestation of pulmonary embolism (p. 1597). Early in the course such patients may exhibit pulmonary angiographic findings characteristic of emboli, but late in the course such findings may be absent. Therefore, it has been argued that PPH may result from recurrent episodes of asymptomatic pulmonary embolism.[190] In support of this theory is the common autopsy finding of clinically unrecognized organizing or recanalizing pulmonary emboli in patients considered during life to have had PPH.[190–192] Moreover, one can produce experimental pulmonary arterial lesions in animals resembling those seen in patients with PPH by intravenous injection of autologous thrombi or other material (e.g., plant spores or polystyrene beads).[193–197] The fact that PPH occasionally develops or worsens post partum also supports a thromboembolic or an amniotic fluid embolic etiology.[192,193]

An alternative explanation relates the development of PPH to *thrombosis* in situ in small pulmonary arteries, with resultant widespread pulmonary vascular obstruction. In support of this theory, various defects in coagulation, including abnormal platelet function and defective fibrinolysis, have been demonstrated in patients with

PPH.[191,193,198–203] A relationship between microangiopathic hemolytic anemia, thrombocytopenia, and PPH has also been suggested.[201] The development of PPH in young women taking contraceptive pills has been thought to be related to the hypercoagulable state that these agents induce.

On the other hand, numerous pathological studies have demonstrated clear-cut morphological differences in the pulmonary vascular bed of patients with thromboembolic or thrombotic pulmonary hypertension, compared with changes noted in patients with PPH. These findings argue *against* recurrent pulmonary thromboembolism or in situ thrombosis as the etiology of PPH.[191–193,199,200] In patients with thromboembolic or thrombotic pulmonary hypertension, thrombi of varying sizes and in various stages of organization can generally be demonstrated in pulmonary arteries and arterioles. By contrast, in patients with PPH, pulmonary arterioles exhibit intimal fibrosis of the onion-skin type, medial hypertrophy, fibrinoid necrosis and arteritis, dilatation, and plexiform lesions (Figs. 25–9 and 25–10); thrombi in pulmonary arteries and arterioles, when present, are small and of recent origin. It seems, therefore, that despite their similar clinical and hemodynamic features, PPH and recurrent silent venous thromboembolism can be distinguished pathologically. Although it is possible that a fraction of patients considered on clinical grounds to be suffering from PPH may be found at autopsy to have had chronic thromboembolism, this does not provide a clue to the etiology of PPH; instead, it suggests that PPH may occasionally be falsely diagnosed during life. Obviously, it is of great clinical importance to differentiate these two conditions, since effective treatment for chronic pulmonary thromboembolism is available.

Several *congenital defects* have been proposed as causes of PPH. A deficiency in the media of the pulmonary arterial bed resulting in intimal thickening and proliferation with consequent obstruction of small pulmonary vessels has been suggested as the underlying defect.[204] Persistence of the fetal pulmonary arterial architecture,[205] increased systemic-pulmonary arterial collaterals,[206–208] and a generalized degenerative pulmonary arteriopathy[209] have also been proposed, although the latter two lesions are felt to be secondary to the pulmonary hypertension itself,[192,199,200] and none has been found in the systemic arteries of patients with PPH.

The occurrence of an arteritis and of fibrinoid necrosis in the walls of the smaller pulmonary arteries, and the frequent presence of Raynaud's phenomenon in patients with PPH, has led some authorities to suggest that PPH may be a form of *collagen-vascular or autoimmune disease.*[210,211] Since Raynaud's phenomenon is an expression of vasospasm in digital arteries, its presence in 10 to 30 per cent of patients with PPH suggests that vasospasm in pulmonary arteries may be present as well. Interestingly, in families of patients with PPH, other members not affected by the disease may exhibit Raynaud's phenomenon. Pulmonary hypertension occurs frequently in patients with the so-called CREST syndrome, a variant of scleroderma (calcinosis, Raynaud's phenomenon, esophageal dysfunction, sclerodactyly, and telangiectasia). The histological changes in the pulmonary vessels in patients with this syndrome resemble those seen in patients with PPH and are similar to those seen in the pulmonary vessels of about 10 per cent of patients with the more usual forms of scleroderma.[133]

Takayasu's arteritis (giant cell) frequently involves the pulmonary vessels (Fig. 25–8), but the pathological changes resemble those seen in systemic arteries (p. 1558). In the vast majority of these patients, the aorta and major arch vessels are involved as well. This condition can also be distinguished from PPH by virtue of the fact that the occlusive changes occur in the large and intermediate vessels rather than in the more distal vessels characteristic of PPH.[189]

A number of cases of PPH coexisting with postnecrotic *hepatic cirrhosis* have been reported, suggesting that a vasculitis might be responsible for the pulmonary hypertension.[212–216] *Polyarteritis nodosa* and *hypersensitivity to a variety of drugs*, including penicillin, chloramphenicol, and the sulfonamides, have also been suggested as etiologies for PPH,[200,217] although allergic vasculitis is unlikely to affect only the pulmonary vasculature.[192] Occasionally a patient with PPH has been erroneously diagnosed as suffering from polyarteritis nodosa limited to the lungs.[192,218]

Pulmonary hypertension has developed in a number of individuals who had ingested the anorexigenic drug *aminorex fumarate.*[219–221] The clinical course of these patients was similar to that of patients with PPH, although in some instances regression of pulmonary hypertension upon withdrawal of the drug was reported.[222] Although causation has not been demonstrated definitively, the circumstantial evidence in favor of this relationship is impressive.[193] Since only 0.2 per cent of individuals ingesting the drug develop pulmonary hypertension, some other factor such as a genetic predisposition or an idiosyncratic reaction must be involved.

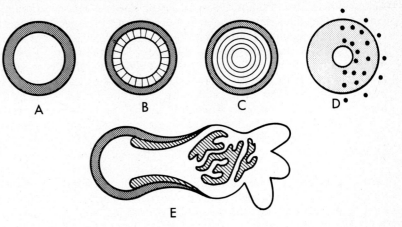

FIGURE 25–9 Plexogenic pulmonary arteriopathy. Arteries with (A) medial hypertrophy, (B) cellular intimal proliferation, (C) concentric-laminar intimal fibrosis, (D) fibrinoid necrosis with or without arteritis, and (E) plexiform lesions. (From Wagenvoort, C. A., and Wagenvoort, N.: Pathology of Pulmonary Hypertension. New York, copyright 1977, reprinted by permission of John Wiley and Sons, Inc.)

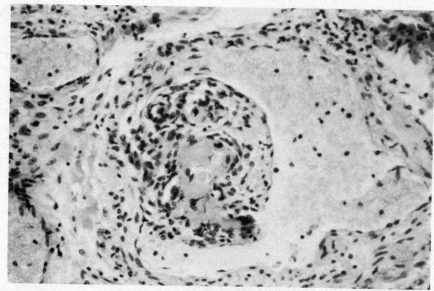

A

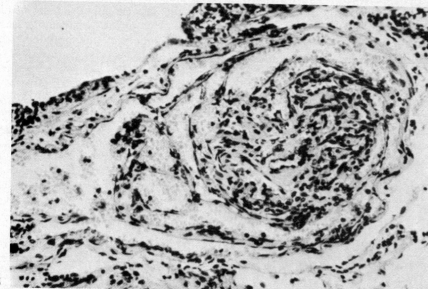

B

FIGURE 25–10   *A*, Early plexiform lesion of muscular pulmonary artery in a 13-year-old girl with unexplained plexogenic pulmonary arteriopathy. There is active proliferation of cells in a fibrin clot (hematoxylin and eosin, ×225). *B*, Full-grown plexiform lesion in muscular pulmonary artery in a 28-year-old woman with unexplained plexogenic pulmonary arteriopathy (hematoxylin and eosin, ×225). (From Wagenvoort, C. A., and Wagenvoort, N.: Pathology of Pulmonary Hypertension. New York, copyright 1977, reprinted by permission of John Wiley and Sons, Inc.)

Severe pulmonary hypertension can be produced in rats by the administration of *monocrotaline* or other pyrrolizidine alkaloids derived from the seeds of the plant *Crotalaria spectabilis* or of *fulvine*, an alkaloid derived from *Crotalaria fulva*.[193,223,224] Severe necrotizing pulmonary arteritis and luminal obstruction in small venules develops in these animals. Pyrrolizidine alkaloids appear not to act directly on the pulmonary circulation but are converted in the liver to metabolites that exhibit a hepatotoxic effect before they affect the pulmonary vascular bed.[225] Although natives of the West Indies who ingest *Crotalaria fulva* in "bush tea" may develop veno-occlusive disease of the liver,[193,226] no instances of pulmonary hypertension in humans have been attributed to *Crotalaria*.

The following observations suggest that *female hormones* may be involved in the genesis of PPH: (1) This condition occurs most frequently in pubertal females, (2) there is a tendency for exacerbations to occur in the postpartum period, (3) there may be an association between the use of oral contraceptives and the development of PPH,[227] and (4) the pulmonary vascular bed of the female

rat is more susceptible to hypoxia than is that of the male rat.[35] The manner in which this endocrine effect may operate on the pulmonary vascular bed is obscure.

Thus, in most patients considered on clinical grounds to have PPH, no evidence can be adduced to support the etiological importance of thromboembolism, congenital or immunological abnormalities, collagen-vascular disease, or drug ingestion. Although pulmonary hypertension can truly be said to be primary in such patients, a number of factors have been identified that may shed some light on the mechanisms underlying the development of pulmonary hypertension, even in these patients. It is well known that there is considerable interindividual variation in the reactivity of the pulmonary vascular bed. Vasoconstrictive stimuli, such as hypoxia or acidosis, can produce marked pulmonary hypertension in one person and be essentially without effect in another. The pulmonary arterial pressor response to hypoxia is particularly great in individuals with blood group A.[35] This variability in the responsivity of the pulmonary vascular bed undoubtedly accounts for the fact that only a minority of individuals develop pulmonary edema on exposure to high altitude (p. 568). In addition, the severity of pulmonary hypertension and the level of pulmonary vascular resistance vary considerably among individuals with congenital heart disease and comparably sized ventricular septal defects. Presumably, there is a *genetic basis for these differences in pulmonary vascular reactivity*, just as there appears to be a genetic basis for the increased reactivity of the systemic vascular bed in essential systemic hypertension (pp. 863 and 1636).

The finding of increased pulmonary vascular reactivity and pulmonary vasoconstriction in patients with PPH, suggests that a marked *vasospastic or constrictive tendency* underlies the development of PPH in predisposed individuals.[192,193,228,229] The autonomic nervous system has been considered a factor in the development of PPH through stimulation of the pulmonary vascular bed by either neuronally released or circulating catecholamines. In some patients with PPH, the response to pulmonary vasodilators such as tolazoline, acetylcholine, or isoproterenol is a reduction in both pulmonary artery pressure and pulmonary vascular resistance,[228–236] supporting the notion of the importance of the autonomic nervous system in maintaining an elevated level of pulmonary vascular resistance. Other patients, however, are unresponsive to pulmonary vasodilating agents.[56,237] Samet and Bernstein reported an interesting case of a patient with PPH who, when examined initially, exhibited marked pulmonary vasodilatation in response to an infusion of acetylcholine.[238] Three years later, on repeat catheterization, the pulmonary hypertension was more severe, and the patient did not respond to acetylcholine infusion. This observation suggests that patients with PPH initially may have increased pulmonary vasomotor tone. As the disease progresses, functional changes give way to fixed, anatomical lesions unaffected by pharmacological intervention.

Familial cases of PPH have been reported with autosomal dominant inheritance;[203,235,239–241] other than from a positive family history, there is no way to distinguish these patients from those with the sporadic form of the disease. They may represent instances of the genetic transmission of extreme pulmonary vascular reactivity. The interplay between certain environmental factors such as hypoxia and a genetic predisposition for pulmonary vascular reactivity may also underlie the development of PPH. The reactivity of the pulmonary vascular bed of cattle to hypoxia has been shown clearly to be genetically determined.[18] In addition, it has been reported that the incidence of PPH increases at high altitude and that children with this condition improve when they move to lower altitudes;[192] conversely, patients with PPH may deteriorate if they ascend to higher altitudes.[3]

PATHOLOGICAL FINDINGS

Several pathological findings are common to almost all patients with PPH: (1) intimal thickening of the smaller pulmonary arteries and arterioles with fibrosis, producing a characteristic "onionskin" configuration (Fig. 25–11); (2) increased thickness of the media of muscular pulmonary arteries and muscularization of arterioles; (3) necrotizing arteritis in the walls of muscular pulmonary arteries with fibrinoid necrosis of the media of such vessels[191–194, 242]; and

(4) *plexiform lesions*, i.e., dilated, thin-walled side branches of muscular pulmonary arteries probably resulting from endothelial proliferation (Figs. 25–9 and 25–10). These lesions are responsible for the term *plexogenic pulmonary arteriopathy*, which was accepted by a working party of the World Health Organization[193] and which is now frequently used to characterize the pathological changes in this condition. Although characteristic of PPH, these anatomical changes are not pathognomonic of the disease and are also found in patients with pulmonary hypertension secondary to cardiac shunts (p. 833).

The pathological diagnosis of PPH can be made when the above-mentioned features, particularly the plexiform lesions, occur in the absence of congenital cardiac shunts and when there is no evidence of old or fresh pulmonary emboli, such as eccentric intimal proliferation, recanalizing channels, and intraluminal fibrous webs. The pattern of elastic tissue of the pulmonary trunk is of the adult variety in PPH, consistent with the belief that the pulmonary hypertension was acquired during adult life.[243] A number of pathological findings are *secondary* to the pulmonary hypertension itself, i.e., in situ thromboses in small pulmonary arteries, atherosclerosis of the major pulmonary arterial trunks, and marked right ventricular hypertrophy.

Recently, Reid and coworkers examined the lungs of a number of patients with PPH using quantitative pathological techniques and electron microscopy.[199,244] These investigators noted thickening of the basement membranes and of the endothelial cells of small ($< 40 \mu m$), nonmuscular pulmonary arterioles. The endothelial cells also contained increased numbers of organelles and pinocytotic vesicles, suggesting heightened metabolic activity; indeed, in some

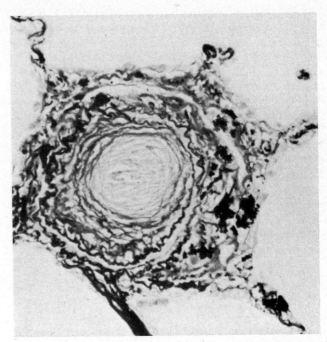

FIGURE 25–11 Transverse section of muscular pulmonary artery from a case of primary pulmonary hypertension in a man 50 years of age. There is intimal fibroelastosis of the "onionskin" type, with atrophy and disruption of the underlying media (elastic/van Gieson, ×375.) (From Harris, P., and Heath, D.: The Human Pulmonary Circulation. 2nd ed. New York, Churchill Livingstone, 1977.)

nonmuscular pulmonary arterioles, proliferation of endo-thelial cells obliterated the vascular lumen.[244] Quantitative analysis of the vessel population in patients with PPH demonstrated a distinct reduction in the number of small, nonmuscular pulmonary arterioles. Residual, non-functioning "ghost vessels" seemed to remain in place of these small arterioles. At more proximal levels of the pul-monary vascular bed, there was considerable hypertrophy of smooth muscle of the media of small muscular pulmo-nary arteries.[199]

A *tentative* pathophysiological scheme for PPH consis-tent with the observed findings, but not yet firmly estab-lished, is presented in Figure 25–12. In an individual who is susceptible—whether on a genetic or an acquired basis —stimuli for pulmonary vasoconstriction result in exces-sive responses and transient pulmonary hypertension. Fre-quent episodes of pulmonary vasoconstriction and the resultant pulmonary hypertension eventually cause hyper-trophy of the smooth muscle in the media of these vessels and perhaps thickening and proliferation of the endothelial cells in the nonmuscular vessels. Ultimately, the vessels are reduced in number, and the residua of these destroyed ves-sels can be seen histologically as "ghost vessels." Destruc-tion of large numbers of pulmonary arterioles reduces the cross-sectional area of the pulmonary vascular bed, thus producing a permanent increase in pulmonary vascular re-sistance and fixed pulmonary hypertension. The latter, in turn, damages other blood vessels and initiates a vicious cycle, with progressively rising pulmonary arterial pres-sure.

CLINICAL FEATURES

NATURAL HISTORY AND SYMPTOMATOLOGY.
In one large series, patients ranged from 16 to 69 years of age (average 33 years),[192] and the female-to-male ratio was 4:1. However, cases have also been described in infants and young children, and in these younger individuals, a fe-male preponderance is not evident. Most patients with PPH come to medical attention relatively late in the course of the disease, after symptoms have developed and after a latent, asymptomatic phase with progressive pulmonary hypertension has passed. Since there is currently no conve-nient way to identify such individuals, the duration of this asymptomatic phase is unknown.

Some patients with PPH, followed by means of serial

Vasoconstriction or vasospasm in susceptible individuals
↓
Decreased flow in small pulmonary arterioles and reactive pulmonary hypertension
↓
Damage to and eventual loss of small pulmonary arterioles (replaced by ghost vessels)
↓   ↑
Pulmonary hypertension
↓
Decreased cross-sectional area in pulmonary vascular bed at level of small pulmonary arterioles
↓
Development of plexiform lesions with further reduction of vascular cross-sectional area

FIGURE 25–12   Possible pathogenesis of primary pulmonary hyper-tension.

catheterization over a number of years, exhibit some hemo-dynamic improvement if they are given pulmonary vasodilating agents when they are first seen.[228,229] During later stages of the disease, however, such drugs have no ef-fect on the pulmonary vascular bed.[229,238] Late in the course of the disease, patients develop right ventricular failure, and exertional syncope may occur, presumably because of a low fixed cardiac output and hypoxemia. PPH is a fatal disease in almost all instances; the duration of symptoms varies, but on the average death occurs approximately 3 years after the onset of symptoms. The course may be more precipitous in some patients, particularly in children, whereas a few patients have lived for as long as 30 years after the onset of symptoms.[2,245] In one reported case, PPH appeared to regress.[246]

Patients with PPH commonly complain of exertional dyspnea, syncope, precordial chest pain, weakness, and, later, dyspnea at rest.[191,233,242,247] These symptoms probably all result from low cardiac output or hypoxemia or both. Precordial chest pain may also be secondary to ischemia of the right ventricular subendocardium or distention of the pulmonary artery or both.[248–250] The pain may radiate to the neck but not characteristically to the arms. Palpita-tions are also common and may be caused by ventricular tachyarrhythmias, which occur not infrequently in the late stages of PPH. Occasionally, cough and hemoptysis occur. These latter symptoms may be due to rupture of dilated plexiform lesions, to in situ pulmonary arterial thrombo-ses, or to episodes of pulmonary embolism occurring late in the course of the disease. Pulmonary embolism occurs frequently as a *result* of severe right ventricular failure, and it may intensify the pulmonary hypertension. Howev-er, as has already been pointed out, the clinical distinction between these two pathogenetic sequences—(1) PPH → right ventricular failure → pulmonary thrombotic and/or embolic disease → further pulmonary hypertension → more severe right ventricular failure as opposed to (2) pul-monary thrombotic and/or embolic disease → secondary pulmonary hypertension → right ventricular failure—may be difficult to make.

PHYSICAL EXAMINATION.
Examination of pa-tients with PPH discloses findings consistent with pulmo-nary hypertension and right ventricular pressure overload: a large *a* wave in the jugular venous pulse; a low-volume, carotid arterial pulse with a normal upstroke; a left para-sternal (right ventricular) heave; a systolic pulsation pro-duced by a dilated, tense pulmonary artery in the second left interspace; an ejection click and flow murmur in the same area; a closely split second heart sound with a prom-inent pulmonic component; a fourth heart sound of right ventricular origin; and, late in the course, signs of right ventricular failure (hepatomegaly, peripheral edema, and ascites) may be present. Patients with severe pulmonary hypertension may also have prominent *v* waves in the jug-ular venous pulse, owing to tricuspid regurgitation; a third heart sound of right ventricular origin; a high-pitched early diastolic murmur of pulmonic regurgitation; and a holo-systolic murmur of tricuspid regurgitation.[191,242,247] Cyanosis is a late finding in PPH and may be due to a patent fora-men ovale with a right-to-left shunt occurring secondary to elevation of right atrial pressure. Other causes for cyanosis include a markedly reduced cardiac output with systemic

vasoconstriction, intrapulmonary right-to-left shunting via vascular anastomoses, and ventilation-perfusion mismatches in the lung itself.[247] Rarely, the left laryngeal nerve becomes paralyzed as a consequence of compression by a dilated pulmonary artery.[232]

LABORATORY FINDINGS

Hematological and Chemical Studies. Results of these studies are usually normal in patients with PPH. If there is arterial oxygen desaturation, polycythemia may be present. A number of investigators have reported hypercoagulable states, abnormal platelet function, defects in fibrinolysis, and other abnormalities of coagulation in patients with PPH.[191,193,198,200] Abnormal liver function tests can indicate right ventricular failure with resultant systemic venous hypertension.

Electrocardiography. The electrocardiogram in PPH will exhibit right atrial and right ventricular enlargement, and a direct correlation between the magnitude of the QRS-T angle and the level of pulmonary arterial pressure has been reported.[191]

Roentgenography. X-ray examination of the chest in patients with PPH shows enlargement of the main pulmonary artery and its major branches, with marked tapering of peripheral arteries.[251] The right ventricle and atrium may also be enlarged. Fluoroscopic examination may disclose exaggerated pulsations of secondary pulmonary arterial branches, reflecting an elevation in pulmonary arterial pulse pressure. However, in contrast to the plethoric peripheral lung fields in patients with left-to-right shunts, oligemia is noted in these lung regions in patients with PPH (Fig. 25-13). It has been suggested that survival in PPH correlates inversely with the size of the main pulmonary artery[252]—a reasonable suggestion, since the latter correlates with the height of the pulmonary arterial pressure.

Pulmonary Function Tests. Pulmonary function tests are usually normal; rarely, a defect in diffusion capacity is present and may be the result of increased capillary-to-alveolar distance secondary to hypertrophy of vascular endothelial cells.[244] Some patients have increased residual volumes and reduced maximum voluntary ventilation.[191,232,232a] Arterial blood gas analysis usually reveals evidence of hyperventilation with low pCO_2 and elevated pH, whereas arterial pO_2 is normal or slightly reduced.

Echocardiography. This technique demonstrates enlarged right ventricular dimensions, small or normal left ventricular dimensions, and a thickened interventricular septum; the septal/posterior left ventricular wall ratio may be abnormally increased, as in hypertrophic obstructive cardiomyopathy (Chap. 5), but the other echocardiographic signs characteristic of that condition are not present. The E-F slope of the anterior mitral valve leaflet is reduced, presumably because of the diminished flow rate across the mitral valve, whereas the diastolic motion of the posterior mitral leaflet is normal. Systolic prolapse of the mitral valve is frequently present, as is abnormal septal motion of the ventricular septum, presumably due to right ventricular dilatation or tricuspid and pulmonic regurgitation or both.[253]

Lung Scan. Perfusion lung scans in patients with PPH are usually either normal or demonstrate small, nonspeci-

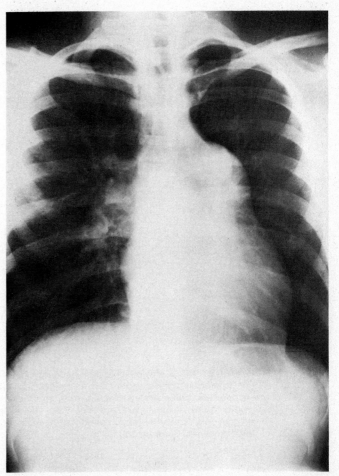

FIGURE 25-13 Frontal chest roentgenogram of a 15-year-old boy with PPH. Note the enlarged main pulmonary artery and the radiolucent lung fields. (Courtesy of Dr. Lloyd E. Hawes.)

fic, subsegmental defects. Lung scanning may be hazardous late in the course of the disease because the macroaggregated albumin particles employed in scanning may significantly reduce the already critically narrowed cross-sectional area of the pulmonary vascular bed.[254]

Catheterization and Angiography. The diagnosis of PPH cannot be confirmed without performing catheterization and pulmonary angiography. Some patients may be too ill for one or both of these procedures (see below), and in such individuals, the diagnosis must remain tentative and be based primarily on exclusion, following clinical evaluation and noninvasive tests. Right-heart catheterization reveals elevated pulmonary arterial and right-ventricular systolic pressures that may approach, equal, or sometimes even exceed systemic arterial levels; right atrial pressure may also be increased. The calculated pulmonary vascular resistance is extremely high, approaching or sometimes even exceeding systemic vascular resistance. When tricuspid regurgitation is absent, the *a* wave in the right atrial pressure tracing is predominant; when it is present, the height of the *v* wave may equal or exceed that of the *a* wave. Left ventricular, left atrial, and pulmonary capillary wedge pressures are low or normal, but it is often difficult to record the pulmonary capillary wedge pressure. A patent foramen ovale with a small right-to-left shunt is frequently present.

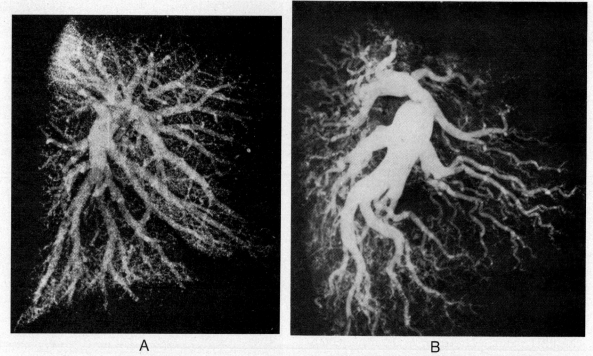

A   B

FIGURE 25–14   *A*, Postmortem pulmonary arteriogram of a normal lung in a 22-year-old man. The caliber of the pulmonary arteries tapers down gradually, and there is a rather dense background filling of vessels. *B*, Postmortem pulmonary arteriogram from an 18-year-old man with unexplained plexogenic pulmonary arteriopathy (primary pulmonary hypertension). The main branches are dilated. (From Wagenvoort, C. A., and Wagenvoort, N.: Pathology of Pulmonary Hypertension. New York, copyright 1977, reprinted by permission of John Wiley and Sons, Inc.)

Pulmonary angiography demonstrates large central pulmonary arteries with marked peripheral tapering. Postmortem arteriograms demonstrate absence of "background haze" secondary to the loss of small, nonmuscular pulmonary arterioles (Fig. 25–14).[199] Right ventriculography usually demonstrates a thick-walled chamber, sometimes with delayed emptying, i.e., elevated right ventricular end-diastolic and end-systolic volumes and a reduced ejection fraction, a result of the markedly elevated pulmonary vascular resistance.

DIAGNOSIS

It is essential that diagnostic efforts be vigorously pursued in patients with severe pulmonary hypertension in order to insure that no patient with secondary pulmonary hypertension is erroneously classified as having PPH. Secondary pulmonary hypertension is frequently treatable in that the cause can often be attacked directly, and the prognosis is usually not as grave as it is in PPH. However, it must be appreciated that patients with PPH tolerate diagnostic procedures poorly. These individuals can experience sudden cardiovascular collapse and even death during or shortly after the induction of general anesthesia for surgical procedures, during cardiac catheterization and angiography, and even following arterial puncture or radioisotopic lung scanning.[192] Angiography appears to be particularly hazardous in advanced cases. Although the mechanism responsible for the cardiovascular collapse and sudden death has not been clearly defined, it may be presumed that these interventions act as stimuli to further

constriction of the already narrowed pulmonary vascular bed, followed by the sudden development or exacerbation of right heart failure or arrhythmias or both.

The *differential diagnosis* of PPH includes a number of causes of secondary pulmonary hypertension. Indeed, a definitive diagnosis of PPH can be established post mortem only after careful histological examination of the pulmonary vasculature. Exclusion of mitral stenosis, congenital cardiac defects (including cor triatriatum), pulmonary embolism, and pulmonary venous obstruction by means of catheterization and angiography is imperative. *"Silent" mitral stenosis*, i.e., without the characteristic diastolic murmur, can be excluded by means of echocardiographic visualization of the motion of the mitral valve and the absence of a transvalvular pressure gradient (Chap. 32). *Congenital heart defects* with Eisenmenger's syndrome can be ruled out if significant left-to-right or right-to-left shunts are absent. The use of indicator-dilution curves (p. 290) and angiography is useful in this regard. *Cor triatriatum* (p. 948) is recognized by angiographic visualization of the left atrial membrane. This entity presents a characteristic left atrial echo with normal echocardiographic mitral valve motion. Cardiac catheterization reveals the hemodynamic pattern of mitral stenosis, i.e., a diastolic pressure gradient between the left ventricle and the chamber proximal to the membrane. *Pulmonary embolism* (Chap. 46) can be excluded by means of pulmonary angiography, and *sickle cell disease with in situ pulmonary vascular thrombosis* (Chap. 49) can be evaluated by hemoglobin electrophoresis. The presence of severe *pulmonary parenchymal disease* can be recognized by the characteristic physical findings, chest roentgenogram, and pulmonary function tests (Chap. 46).

Collagen vascular disease is suggested by the involvement of other organ systems or the presence of abnormal immunological phenomena, such as antinuclear antibodies and LE cells. *Pulmonary veno-occlusive disease* is characterized by progressive narrowing of nearly all small pulmonary veins and venules, many of which exhibit complete occlusion by fibrous tissue.

TREATMENT OF PULMONARY HYPERTENSION

Treatment of pulmonary hypertension (Table 25–2) will be most successful when it is possible to identify the inciting cause and remove it before irreversible damage has been done to the pulmonary vasculature. Thus, closure of central shunts while they are still predominantly left-to-right, and before extensive plexiform and angiomatoid lesions have developed in the lungs, will usually correct pulmonary hypertension in the setting of congenital heart disease with central left-to-right shunt. Patients with hypoventilation secondary to hypertrophied tonsils and adenoids will experience cure of associated pulmonary hypertension with tonsillectomy.[176]

In patients in whom removal of the inciting cause is not possible (e.g., where the cause is unknown, as in primary pulmonary hypertension), therapy for pulmonary hypertension is directed at decreasing resistance to pulmonary blood flow and improving the cardiocirculatory response to right ventricular pressure overload.

Decreasing resistance to pulmonary blood flow can be accomplished only when the site of the increased resistance (Table 25–1) is identified. Thus, when left ventricular failure with secondary left atrial hypertension is the cause of increased resistance to pulmonary blood flow, improvement of left ventricular failure (Chap. 12) will lead to lowering of pulmonary artery pressure. When decreased cross-sectional area of the pulmonary vascular bed is causing pulmonary hypertension, *pulmonary vasodilators* may be tried; it is likely that they will be effective only in cases in which active vasoconstriction of small muscular arteries or arterioles is contributing significantly to the pulmonary hypertension.[254a]

PRIMARY PULMONARY HYPERTENSION. In recent years, there has been considerable interest in the use of pulmonary vasodilators as chronic therapy for primary pulmonary hypertension.[37–39,255–272,272a] This approach is based on the observation that muscular hypertrophy, rather than intimal hyperplasia, is the earliest finding in patients developing primary pulmonary hypertension.[255] Because of the difficulty in predicting or interpreting the results of vasodilator therapy in patients with unexplained pulmonary hypertension, lung biopsy has been recommended whenever possible before starting pulmonary vasodilator therapy.[157,264] There is much to recommend this approach, including the possibility of uncovering a specific but unexpected cause of the pulmonary hypertension, such as pulmonary thromboembolism or collagen-vascular disorder, as well as assessing the reversibility or irreversibility of the vascular changes prior to treatment.[264] This latter point is all the more important, since vasodilator therapy may be hazardous in some patients with advanced pulmonary hypertension.[37,263] Vasodilator agents that have been used for either the acute or the chronic treatment of pulmonary hypertension include oxygen,[71,120,121,265] hydralazine,[256,257,269,271] phentolamine,[258,273] sublingual isoproterenol,[259,260,272] diazoxide,[262,263] nifedipine,[20,267–270,270a] prostacyclin,[38,39,266] and tolazoline.[56,231,232] Effectiveness of these agents has been quite variable. In one report of 10 women with acute primary pulmonary hypertension, only sublingual isoproterenol (alone or combined with isosorbide dinitrate) produced a fall in pulmonary vascular resistance: Diazoxide, hydralazine, phentolamine, and tolazoline were ineffective.[37] In contrast, hydralazine was found to be effective in each of 4 patients with primary pulmonary hypertension by one group[256] and in 6 of 12 patients with primary pulmonary hypertension by a second group.[257] Similar conflicting results have been reported for diazoxide.[37,261–263] Prostacyclin (PGI2) has been reported to reverse completely the pulmonary vasoconstriction in a neonate with persistent fetal circulation[266] but was less impressive in four adult patients with pulmonary hypertension of diverse etiology.[38] Nifedipine has been reported to prevent the acute pulmonary vasoconstriction associated with hypoxia,[20] and preliminary reports suggest that it may have therapeutic value in pulmonary hypertension of various etiologies.[267–269]

Conflicting results are not surprising, since most institutions have been able to study only small numbers of patients, and the underlying pathologic condition (reversible vs. irreversible pulmonary vascular changes) has been unknown for the majority of patients in nearly all published reports on vasodilation therapy for pulmonary hypertension. Despite these shortcomings, there appears to be a heterogeneity in individual responsiveness to various pulmonary vasodilators, and there is evidence that the findings on acute drug testing predict long-term results of treatment for individual patients.[256–258,265,270] Accordingly, it seems reasonable to assess the acute hemodynamic response to a variety of agents in the patient with severe pulmonary hypertension and to use the results of this assessment to design chronic therapy. As already mentioned, it is essential to determine the underlying cause of the patient's pulmonary hypertension whenever possible, since this may affect therapy in a fundamental way: An aggressive diagnostic approach, including lung biopsy, may be necessary in many cases.

Heart-lung transplantation has been performed as therapy for advanced pulmonary vascular disease[274] and was successful in a 45-year-old woman with primary pulmonary hypertension and a 30-year-old man with Eisenmenger's syndrome. With advances in immunosuppressive therapy (e.g., cyclosporin A) and surgical technique, it is likely that additional numbers of patients will be treated with lung or combined heart-lung transplantation.

Antiinflammatory agents (steroids) have been used in the treatment of pulmonary hypertension in specific disorders in which vasculitis or arteritis or both may play a role in causing the pulmonary hypertension,[138,139,143,188] although their effectiveness in these conditions is difficult to assess.

Anticoagulation is clearly indicated in pulmonary hypertension associated with recurrent pulmonary emboli.[167] Its role in other forms of pulmonary hypertension (e.g., veno-occlusive disease) is conjectural and rests on postmortem or biopsy studies showing thrombi in large and small pulmonary veins or arteries.[2,5,114,148,182,184,185,264,275] Whether these

TABLE 25–2   TREATMENT OF PULMONARY HYPERTENSION

I. Removal of Inciting Cause (when possible)
 Examples: Surgical correction of mitral stenosis[110–112] or cor triatriatum,[113] closure of anatomical site of predominant left-to-right shunt, removal of massively hypertrophied tonsils and adenoids,[175] avoidance of offending drug or agent (aminorex, *Crotalaria* alkaloids, intravenous drug abuse)

II. Decrease Resistance to Pulmonary Blood Flow
 A. Lower left atrial or left ventricular diastolic pressure, when these are elevated
 B. Pulmonary vasodilators
  1. Oxygen[71,120,121,265]
  2. Hydralazine[256,257,269,271]
  3. Phentolamine[258]
  4. Isoproterenol[259,260,272]
  5. Diazoxide[261–263]
  6. Nifedipine[20,267–270]
  7. Prostaglandins[37–39,266]
  8. Tolazoline[56–58]
 C. Lung transplantation[274]
 D. Antiinflammatory agents in specific disorders: Takayasu's disease,[188] SLE, and other collagen-vascular disorders[138,139,143]
 E. Anticoagulation: recurrent pulmonary embolism,[167] pulmonary veno-occlusive disease

III. Improving Cardiocirculatory Response to Right Ventricular Pressure Overload
 A. Appropriate pulmonary toilet to maximize alveolar ventilation and oxygenation
 B. Prophylaxis (vaccines) for influenza and pneumonia; prompt, vigorous treatment of any pulmonary infection
 C. Diuretics (spironolactone and furosemide or a thiazide) with low-salt diet
 D. Pulmonary vasodilators (see II B)
 E. Inotropic agents (digitalis glycosides, newer oral beta agonists, and so on)

changes are causative (or at least contributory) to pulmonary hypertension in individual patients is highly conjectural, and no general recommendation can be given regarding whether long-term anticoagulation therapy should or should not be used with such patients.

Even when pulmonary hypertension can be neither cured nor improved, the cardiocirculatory response to right ventricular pressure overload can usually be improved with amelioration of right heart failure and an increase in forward cardiac output. The elements of a program designed to accomplish these goals is given in Table 25–2, III, A to E.

References

1. Comroe, J. H., Jr.: The main functions of the pulmonary circulation. Circulation *33*:146, 1966.
2. Wagenvoort, C. A., and Wagenvoort, N.: Pathology of Pulmonary Hypertension. 2nd ed. New York, John Wiley and Sons, 1977.
3. Fritts, H. W., Harris, P., Chidsey, C. A., Clauss, R. H., and Cournand, A.: Estimation of flow rate through bronchial-pulmonary vascular anastomoses with use of T-1824 dye. Circulation *23*:390, 1961.
4. Barratt-Boyes, B. G., and Wood, E. H.: Cardiac output and related measurements and pressure values in the right heart and associated vessels, together with an analysis of the hemodynamic response to the inhalation of high oxygen mixtures in healthy subjects. J. Lab. Clin. Med. *51*:72, 1958.
5. Harris, P., and Heath, D.: The Human Pulmonary Circulation. 2nd ed. New York, Churchill Livingstone, 1977, 684 pp.
6. Harris, P., Segel, N., and Bishop, J. M.: The relation between pressure and flow in the pulmonary circulation in normal subjects and in patients with chronic bronchitis and mitral stenosis. Cardiovasc. Res. *1*:73, 1968.
7. Nihill, M. R., McNamara, D. G., and Vick, R. L.: The effects of increased blood viscosity on pulmonary vascular resistance. Am. Heart J. *92*:65, 1976.
8. Dawes, G. S., Mott, J. C., Widdicombe, J. G., and Wyatt, D. G.: Changes in the lungs of the newborn lamb. J. Physiol. *121*:141, 1953.
9. Adams, F. H., and Lind, J.: Physiologic studies on the cardiovascular status of normal newborn infants. Pediatrics *19*:431, 1957.
10. Rudolph, A. M.: The changes in the circulation after birth. Their importance in congenital heart disease. Circulation *41*:343, 1970.
11. Friedman, W. F., Molony, D. A., and Kirkpatrick, S. E.: Prostaglandins: Physiological and clinical correlations. Adv. Pediatr. *25*:151, 1978.
12. Naeye, R. L.: Arterial changes during the perinatal period. Arch. Pathol. *71*:121, 1961.
13. Fishman, A. P.: Hypoxia on the pulmonary circulation: How and where it acts. Circ. Res. *38*:221, 1976.
14. Von Euler, U. S., and Liljestrand, G.: Observations on the pulmonary arterial blood pressure in the cat. Acta Physiol. Scand. *12*:301, 1946.
15. Fishman, A. P.: Respiratory gases in the regulation of the pulmonary circulation. Physiol. Rev. *41*:214, 1961.
16. Silove, E. D., Inoue, T., and Grover, R. F.: Comparison of hypoxia, pH, and sympathomimetic drugs on bovine pulmonary vasculature. J. Appl. Physiol. *24*:355, 1968.
16a. Haneda, T., Nakajima, T., Shirato, K., Onodera, S., and Takisima, T.: Effects of oxygen breathing on pulmonary vascular input impedance in patients with pulmonary hypertension. Chest *83*:520, 1983.
17. Grover, R. F., Vogel, J. H. K., Averill, K. H., and Blount, S. G.: Pulmonary hypertension. Individual and species variability relative to vascular reactivity. Am. Heart J. *66*:1, 1963.
18. Weir, E. K., Tucker, A., Reeves, J. T., and Will, D. H.: Pulmonary hypertension in cattle at high altitude. Cardiovasc. Res. *8*:745, 1975.
19. McMurty, I. F., Davidson, A. B., Reeves, J. T., and Grover, R. F.: Inhibition of hypoxic pulmonary vasoconstriction by calcium antagonist in isolated rat lungs. Circ. Res. *38*:99, 1960.
20. Simonneau, G., Escourron, P., Duroux, P., and Lockhart, A.: Inhibition of hypoxic pulmonary vasoconstriction by nifedipine. N. Engl. J. Med. *304*:1582, 1981.
21. Rabinovitch, M., Gamble, W., Nadas, A. S., Miettinen, O. S., and Reid, L.: Rat pulmonary circulation after chronic hypoxia: Hemodynamic and structural features. Am. J. Physiol. *236*:H818, 1979.
22. Rabinovitch, M., Gamble, W. J., Miettinen, O. S., and Reid, L.: Age and sex influence on pulmonary hypertension of chronic hypoxia and on recovery. Am. J. Physiol. *240*:H62, 1981.
23. Sobel, B. J., Bottex, G., Emirgil, C., and Gissen, H.: Gaseous diffusion from alveoli to pulmonary vessels of considerable size. Circ. Res. *13*:71, 1963.
24. Staub, N. C.: Gas exchange vessels in the cat lung. Fed. Proc. *20*:107, 1961.
25. Jameson, A. G.: Gaseous diffusion from alveoli into pulmonary arteries. J. Appl. Physiol. *19*:448, 1964.
26. Glazier, J. B., and Murray, J. F.: Sites of pulmonary vasomotor reactivity in the dog during alveolar hypoxia and serotonin and histamine infusion. J. Clin. Invest. *50*:2550, 1971.
27. Bergofsky, E. H.: Mechanisms underlying vasomotor regulation of regional pulmonary blood flow in normal and disease states. Am. J. Med. *57*:378, 1974.
28. Hauge, A.: Hypoxia and pulmonary vascular resistance: The relative effects of pulmonary arterial and alveolar PO_2. Acta Physiol. Scand. *76*:121, 1969.
29. Liljestrand, G.: Chemical control of the distribution of the pulmonary blood flow. Acta Physiol. Scand. *44*:216, 1958.
30. Enson, Y., Giuntini, C., Lewis, M. L., Morris, T. Q., Ferrer, M. I., and Harvey, R. M.: The influence of hydrogen ion concentration and hypoxia on the pulmonary circulation. J. Clin. Invest. *43*:1146, 1964.
31. Vogel, J. G. K., and Blount, G., Jr.: The role of hydrogen ion concentration in the regulation of pulmonary arterial pressure: Observations in a patient with hypoventilation and obesity. Circulation *32*:788, 1965.
32. Kadowitz, P. J., Joiner, P. D., and Hyman, A. L.: Effect of sympathetic nerve stimulation on pulmonary vascular resistance in the intact spontaneously breathing dog. Proc. Soc. Exp. Biol. Med. *147*:68, 1974.
33. Harris, P.: Influence of acetylcholine on the pulmonary arterial pressures. Br. Heart J. *29*:272, 1957.
34. Fritts, H. W., Harris, P., Clauss, R. H., Odell, J. E., and Cournand, A.: The effect of acetylcholine on the human pulmonary circulation under normal and hypoxic conditions. J. Clin. Invest. *37*:99, 1958.
35. Wood, P., Besterman, E. M., Towers, M. K., and McIlroy, M. B.: The effect of acetylcholine on pulmonary vascular resistance and left atrial pressure in mitral stenosis. Br. Heart J. *19*:279, 1957.
36. Kadowitz, P. J., and Hyman, A. L.: Differential effects of prostaglandins A_1 and A_2 on pulmonary vascular resistance in the dog. Proc. Soc. Exp. Biol. Med. *149*:282, 1975.
37. Hermiller, J. B., Bambach, D., Thompson, M. J., Huss, P., Fontana, M. E., Magorien, M. D., Unverferth, D. V., and Leier, C. V.: Vasodilators and prostaglandin inhibitors in primary pulmonary hypertension. Ann. Intern. Med. *97*:480, 1982.
38. Guadagni, D. N., Ikram, H., and Maslowski, A. H.: Haemodynamic effects of prostacyclin (PGI_2) in pulmonary hypertension. Br. Heart J. *45*:385, 1981.
39. Rubin, L. J., Groves, B. M., Reeves, J. T., Frosdono, M., Handel, F., and Cato, A. E.: Prostacyclin-induced acute pulmonary vasodilation in primary pulmonary hypertension. Circulation *66*:334, 1982.
40. Kay, J. M., Waymire, J. C., and Grover, R. F.: Lung mast cell hyperplasia and pulmonary histamine forming capacity in hypoxic rats. Am. J. Physiol. *226*:178, 1974.
41. Haas, F., and Bergofsky, E. H.: Role of the mast cell in the pulmonary pressor response to hypoxia. J. Clin. Invest. *51*:3154, 1972.
42. Hauge, A.: Role of histamine in hypoxic pulmonary hypertension in the rat. I. Blockade or potentiation of endogenous amines, kinins, and ATP. Circ. Res. *22*:371, 1968.
43. Hauge, A., and Melmon, K. L.: Rise of histamine in hypoxic pulmonary hypertension in the rat. II. Depletion of histamine, serotonin, and catecholamines. Circ. Res. *22*:385, 1968.
44. Susmano, A., and Carleton, R. A.: Prevention of hypoxic pulmonary hypertension by chlorpheniramine. J. Appl. Physiol. *31*:531, 1971.

45. Altura, B. M., and Zweifach, B. W.: Pharmacologic properties of antihistamines in relation to vascular reactivity. Am. J. Physiol. 209:550, 1965.

46. Shepherd, J. T., Donald, D. E., Linder, E., and Swan, H. J. C.: Effect of small doses of 5-hydroxytryptamine (serotonin) on pulmonary circulation in the closed chest dog. Am. J. Physiol. 197:963, 1959.

47. Harris, P., Fritts, H. W., and Cournand, A.: Some circulatory effects of 5-hydroxytryptamine in man. Circulation 21:1134, 1960.

48. Luchsinger, P. C., Seipp, H. W., and Patel, D. V.: Relationship of pulmonary artery wedge pressure to left atrial pressure in man. Circulation 11:315, 1962.

49. Regan, T. J., DeFazio, V., Binak, K., and Hellems, H. K.: Norepinephrine induced pulmonary congestion in patients with aortic valve regurgitation. J. Clin. Invest. 38:1564, 1959.

50. Fowler, N. O., Westcott, R. N., Scott, R. C., and McGuire, J.: The effect of norepinephrine upon pulmonary arteriolar resistance in man. J. Clin. Invest. 30:517, 1951.

51. Goldring, R. M., Turino, G. M., Cohen, G., Jameson, A. G., Bass, B. G., and Fishman, A. P.: The catecholamines in the pulmonary arterial pressor response to acute hypoxia. J. Clin. Invest. 41:1211, 1962.

52. Patel, D. J., Lange, R. L., and Hecht, H. H.: Some evidence for active constriction in the human pulmonary vascular bed. Circulation 18:19, 1958.

53. Kadowitz, P. J., Joiner, P. D., and Hyman, A. L.: Influence of sympathetic stimulation and vasoactive substances on the canine pulmonary veins. J. Clin. Invest. 56:354, 1975.

54. Yoshida, Y.: Studies on the pathologic physiology of pulmonary hypertension in mitral valve disease. I. The role of sympathetic nervous system on the increment of pulmonary vascular resistance. Jpn. Circ. J. 33:359, 1969.

55. Sanders, J., Miller, D. D., and Patil, P. N.: Alpha adrenergic and histaminergic effects of tolazoline-like imidazolines. J. Pharmacol. Exp. Ther. 195:362, 1975.

56. Rudolph, A. M., Paul, M. H., Sommer, L. S., and Nadas, A. S.: Effects of tolazoline hydrochloride (Priscoline) or circulatory dynamics of patients with pulmonary hypertension. Am. Heart J. 55:424, 1958.

57. Dresdale, D. T., Michton, R. J., and Schultz, M.: Recent studies in primary pulmonary hypertension including pharmacodynamic observations on pulmonary vascular resistance. Bull. N.Y. Acad. Med. 30:195, 1954.

58. Vogel, J. H. K., Grover, R. F., Jamieson, G., and Blount, S. G., Jr.: Long-term physiologic observations in patients with ventricular septal defect and increased pulmonary vascular resistance. Adv. Cardiol. 11:108, 1974.

59. Tucker, A., Hoffman, E. A., and Weir, E. K.: Histamine receptor antagonism does not inhibit hypoxic pulmonary vasoconstriction in dogs. Chest 71 (Suppl):261, 1977.

60. Okpako, D. T.: A dual action of histamine on guinea pig lung vessels. Br. J. Pharmacol. 45:311, 1972.

61. Tucker, A., Weir, E. K., Reeves, J. T., and Grover, F.: Histamine H_1 and H_2 receptors in pulmonary and systemic vasculature of the dog. Am. J. Physiol. 229:1008, 1975.

62. Moret, P., Covarrubias, E., Coudert, J., and Duchosall, F.: Cardiocirculatory adaptation to chronic hypoxia. Acta Cardiol. (Brux.) 27:596, 1972.

63. Penazola, D., Sime, F., Banchero, N., Gamboa, R., Cruz, J., and Marticorena, E.: Pulmonary hypertension in healthy men born and living at high altitudes. Am. J. Cardiol. 11:150, 1963.

64. Hecht, H. H., and McClement, J. H.: A case of chronic mountain sickness in the United States: Clinical, physiologic, and electrocardiographic observations. Am. J. Med. 25:470, 1968.

65. Penazola, D., Sime, F., Banchero, N., and Gamboa, R.: Pulmonary hypertension in healthy men born and living at high altitudes. Med. Thorac. 19:449, 1962.

66. Vogel, J. H. K., Weaver, W. F., Rose, R. L., Blount, S. G., Jr., and Grover, R. F.: Pulmonary hypertension on exertion in normal men living at 10,150 feet (Leadville, Colorado). Med. Thorac. 19:461, 1962.

67. Niewoehner, D. E., Kleinerman, J., and Rice, D. B.: Pathologic changes in the peripheral airways of young cigarette smokers. N. Engl. J. Med. 291:755, 1974.

68. United States Department of Health, Education, and Welfare: The health consequences of smoking: A report of the Surgeon General, 1972. DHEW publication #(HSM) 72-7516. Washington, D.C., Government Printing Office, 1972.

69. Spain, D. M., Siegel, H., and Bradess, V. A.: Emphysema in apparently healthy adults: smoking, age, and sex. J.A.M.A. 224:322, 1973.

70. Burrow, B., Fletcher, C. M., Niden, A. H., Rabinowitz, M., and Diener, C. F.: Patterns of cardiovascular dysfunction in chronic obstructive lung disease. N. Engl. J. Med. 286:912, 1972.

71. Neff, T. A., and Petty, T. L.: Long-term continuous oxygen therapy in chronic airway obstruction. Ann. Intern. Med. 72:621, 1970.

72. Brooks, H. L., Kirk, E. S., Vokonas, P. S., Urschel, C. W., and Sonnenblick, E. H.: Performance of the right ventricle under stress. J. Clin. Invest. 50:2176, 1971.

73. Berman, J. L., Green, L. G., and Grossman, W.: Right ventricular diastolic pressure in coronary artery disease. Am. J. Cardiol. 44:1263, 1979.

74. Lorell, B. H., Leinbach, R. C., Pohost, G. M., Gold, H. K., Dinsmore, R. E., Hutter, A. M., Jr., Pastore, J. D., and DeSanctis, R. W.: Right ventricular infarction. Am. J. Cardiol. 43:463, 1979.

75. Vasco, J. S., Elkins, R. C., Fogarty, T. J., and Morrow, A. G.: The experimental production of chronic mitral valvular obstruction. J. Thorac. Cardiovasc. Surg. 53:875, 1967.

76. Haddy, F. J., Ferrin, A. L., Hannon, D. W., Alden, J. F., Adams, W. L., and Baronofsky, I. D.: Cardiac function in experimental mitral stenosis. Circ. Res. 1:219, 1953.

77. Silove, E. D., Tavernor, W. D., and Berry, C. L.: Reactive pulmonary arterial hypertension after pulmonary venous constriction in the calf. Cardiovasc. Res. 6:36, 1972.

78. Charms, B. L., Brofman, B. L., and Adicoff, A.: Differential pulmonary artery occlusion in patients with chronic pulmonary disease. Am. J. Med. 26:527, 1959.

79. Soderholm, B., and Werko, L.: Acetylcholine and the pulmonary circulation in mitral valvular disease. Br. Heart J. 21:1, 1959.

80. Kay, J. M., and Edwards, F. R.: Ultrastructure of the alveolar-capillary wall in mitral stenosis. J. Pathol. 111:239, 1973.

81. Szidon, J. P., Pietra, G. G., and Fishman, A. P.: The alveolar-capillary membrane and pulmonary edema. N. Engl. J. Med. 286:1200, 1972.

82. Hicks, J. D.: Acute arterial necrosis in the lungs. J. Pathol. Bacteriol. 65:333, 1953.

83. Whitaker, W., Black, A., and Warrack, A. J. N.: Pulmonary ossification in patients with mitral stenosis. J. Fac. Radiol. (Lond.) 7:29, 1955.

84. Jordan, S. C., Hicken, P., Watson, D. A., Heath, D., and Whitaker, W.: Pathology of the lungs in mitral stenosis in relation to respiratory function and pulmonary haemodynamics. Br. Heart J. 28:101, 1966.

85. Grossman, W., and Barry, W. H.: Diastolic pressure-volume relations in the diseased heart. Fed. Proc. 39:148, 1980.

86. Grossman, W., McLaurin, L. P., and Stefadouros, M. A.: Left ventricular stiffness associated with chronic pressure and volume overloads in man. Circ. Res. 35:793, 1974.

87. Grossman, W., McLaurin, L. P., Moos, S. P., Stefadouros, M. A., and Young, D. T.: Wall thickness and diastolic properties of the left ventricle. Circulation 49:129, 1974.

88. Dodek, A., Kassebaum, D. G., and Bristow, J. D.: Pulmonary edema in coronary artery disease without cardiomegaly: Paradox of the stiff heart. N. Engl. J. Med. 286:1347, 1972.

89. Benotti, J. R., Grossman, W., and Cohn, P. F.: The clinical profile of restrictive cardiomyopathy. Circulation 61:1206, 1980.

90. Kern, M. J., Lorell, B. H., and Grossman, W.: Cardiac amyloidosis masquerading as constrictive pericarditis. Cathet. Cardiovasc. Diagn. 8:629, 1982.

91. Shabetai, R., and Grossman, W.: Profiles in constrictive pericarditis, cardiac tamponade, and restrictive cardiomyopathy. In Grossman, W. (ed.): Cardiac Catheterization and Angiography. 2nd ed. Philadelphia, Lea and Febiger, 1980.

92. Sawyer, C. G., Burwell, C. S., Dexter, L., Eppinger, E. C., Goodale, W. T., Gorlin, R., Harken, D. E., and Haynes, F. W.: Chronic constrictive pericarditis: Further consideration of the pathologic physiology of the disease. Am. Heart J. 44:207, 1952.

93. Alpert, J. S., Irwin, R. S., and Dalen, J. E.: Pulmonary hypertension. Curr. Probl. Cardiol. 5:39H, 1981.

94. Dexter, L., and Grossman, W.: Profiles in valvular heart disease. In Grossman, W. (ed.): Cardiac Catheterization and Angiography. 2nd ed. Philadelphia, Lea and Febiger, 1980.

95. Dexter, L.: Physiologic changes in mitral stenosis. N. Engl. J. Med. 254:829, 1956.

96. Lewis, B. M., Gorlin, R., Houssay, H. E. J., Haynes, F. W., and Dexter, L.: Clinical and physiological correlations in patients with mitral stenosis. Am. Heart J. 43:2, 1952.

97. Wood, P.: An appreciation of mitral stenosis. I. Clinical features; II. Investigation and results. Br. Med. J. 1:1051 and 1131, 1954.

98. McLaurin, L. P., Gibson, T., Waider, W., Grossman, W., and Craige, E.: An appraisal of mitral valve echocardiograms mimicking mitral stenosis in conditions with right ventricular pressure overload. Circulation 48:801, 1973.

99. Araujo, J., and Lukas, D. S.: Interrelationships among pulmonary capillary pressure, blood flow and valve size in mitral stenosis: Limited regulatory effects of the pulmonary vascular resistance. J. Clin. Invest. 31:1082, 1952.

100. Wood, P.: Pulmonary hypertension with special reference to the vasoconstrictive factor. Br. Heart J. 20:557, 1958.

101. Davies, L. G., Goodwin, J. F., and VanLeuven, B. D.: The nature of pulmonary hypertension in mitral stenosis. Br. Heart J. 16:440, 1954.

102. Robin, E. R., and Meyer, E. C.: Cardiopulmonary effects of pulmonary venous hypertension with special reference to pulmonary lymphatic flow. Circ. Res. 8:324, 1960.

103. Uhley, H. N., Leeds, S. E., Sampson, J. J., and Friedman, M.: Role of pulmonary lymphatics in chronic pulmonary edema. Circ. Res. 11:966, 1962.

104. Parker, F., and Hicken, P.: The relation between left atrial hypertension and lymphatic distention in lung biopsies. Thorax 15:54, 1960.

105. Parker, F., and Weiss, S.: The nature and significance of the structural changes in the lungs in mitral stenosis. Am. J. Pathol. 12:573, 1936.

106. Coalson, J. J., Jacques, W. E., Campbell, G. S., and Thompson, W. M.: Ultrastructure of the alveolar capillary membrane in congenital and acquired heart disease. Arch. Pathol. 83:377, 1967.

107. Kay, J. M., and Edwards, F. R.: Ultrastructure of the alveolar capillary wall in mitral stenosis. J. Pathol. 111:239, 1973.

108. Heath, D., and Edwards, J. E.: Histological changes in the lung in diseases associated with pulmonary venous hypertension. Br. J. Dis. Chest 53:8, 1959.

109. Gorlin, R., Lewis, B., Haynes, F. W., Spiegel, R. J., and Dexter, L.: Factors regulating pulmonary capillary pressure in mitral stenosis. Am. Heart J. 41:834, 1951.

110. Braunwald, E., Braunwald, N. S., Ross, J., Jr., and Morrow, A. G.: Effects of mitral valve replacement on pulmonary vascular dynamics of patients with pulmonary hypertension. N. Engl. J. Med. 273:509, 1965.

111. Dalen, J. E., Matloff, J. M., Evans, G. L., Hoppin, F. G., Bhardwaj, P., Harken, D. E., and Dexter, L.: Early reduction of pulmonary vascular resistance after mitral valve replacement. N. Engl. J. Med. 277:387, 1967.

112. Zener, J. C., Hancock, E. W., Shumway, N. E., and Harrison, D. C.: Regression of extreme pulmonary hypertension after mitral valve surgery. Am. J. Cardiol. 30:820, 1972.

113. Magidson, A.: Cor triatriatum. Severe pulmonary arterial hypertension and pulmonary venous hypertension in a child. Am. J. Cardiol. 9:603, 1962.

114. Wagenvoort, C. A.: Pulmonary veno-occlusive disease: Entity or syndrome. Chest 69:82, 1976.

115. Liebow, A. A., McAdam, A. J., Carrington, C. B., and Vigmonte, M.: Intrapulmonary veno-obstructive disease. Circulation 36 (Suppl. II):172, 1967.

116. Ferrer, M. I.: Disturbances in the circulation in patients with cor pulmonale. Bull. N.Y. Acad. Med. 41:942, 1965.

117. Cromie, J. B.: Correlation of anatomic pulmonary emphysema and right ventricular hypertrophy. Am. Rev. Respir. Dis. 84:657, 1961.

118. Hicken, P., Heath, D., and Brewer, D.: The relation between the weight of the right ventricle and the percentage of abnormal air space in the lung in emphysema. J. Pathol. Bacteriol. 92:519, 1966.

119. Harvey, R. M., Ferrer, M. I., Richards, D. W., and Cournand, A.: Influence of chronic pulmonary disease on the heart and circulation. Am. J. Med. 10:719, 1951.

120. Abraham, A. S., Cole, R. B., Green, I. D., Hedworth-Whitty, R. B., Clarke, S. W., and Bishop, J. M.: Factors contributing to the reversible pulmonary hypertension in patients with acute respiratory failure studied by serial observation during recovery. Circ. Res. 24:51, 1969.

121. Abraham, A. S., Cole, R. B., and Bishop, J.: Effects of prolonged oxygen administration on the pulmonary hypertension of patients with chronic bronchitis. Circ. Res. 23:147, 1968.

122. Segel, N., and Bishop, J. M.: The circulation in patients with chronic bronchitis and emphysema at rest and during exercise with special reference to the influence of changes in blood viscosity and blood volumes on the pulmonary circulation. J. Clin. Invest. 45:1555, 1966.

123. Horsfield, K., Segel, N., and Bishop, J. M.: The pulmonary circulation in chronic bronchitis at rest and during exercise breathing air and 80% oxygen. Clin. Sci. 34:473, 1968.

124. Harvey, R. M., Ferrer, M. I., Richards, D. W., Jr., and Cournand, A.: Influence of chronic pulmonary disease on the heart and circulation. Am. J. Med. 10:719, 1951.

125. Yu, P. N., Lovejoy, F. W., Joos, H. A., Nye, R. E., and McCann, W. S.: Studies of pulmonary hypertension. I. Pulmonary circulatory dynamics in patients with pulmonary emphysema at rest. J. Clin. Invest. 32:130, 1953.

126. Kitchin, A. H., Lowther, C. P., and Matthews, M. B.: The effect of exercise and of breathing oxygen-enriched air on the pulmonary circulation in emphysema. Clin. Sci. 21:93, 1961.

127. Wilson, R. H., Hoseth, W., and Dempsey, M. E.: The effects of breathing 99.6% oxygen on pulmonary vascular resistance and cardiac output in patients with pulmonary emphysema and chronic hypoxia. Ann. Intern. Med. 42:629, 1955.

128. Aber, G. M., Harris, A. M., and Bishop, J. M.: The effect of acute changes in inspired oxygen concentration on cardiac, respiratory and renal function in patients with chronic obstructive airways disease. Clin. Sci. 26:133, 1964.

129. Foreman, S., Weill, H., Duke, R., George, R., and Ziskind, M.: Bullous disease of the lung: Physiologic improvement after surgery. Ann. Intern. Med. 69:757, 1968.

130. Connor, P. K., and Bashour, F. A.: Cardiopulmonary changes in scleroderma. A physiologic study. Am. Heart J. 61:494, 1961.

131. Oram, S., and Stokes, W.: The heart in scleroderma. Br. Heart J. 23:243, 1961.

132. Naeye, R. L.: Pulmonary vascular lesions in systemic scleroderma. Dis. Chest 44:368, 1963.

133. Salerni, R., Rodnan, G. P., Leon, D. F., and Shaver, J. A.: Pulmonary hypertension in the CREST syndrome variant of progressive systemic sclerosis (scleroderma). Ann. Intern. Med. 86:394, 1977.

134. Seldin, D. W., Ziff, M., and DeGraff, A. V., Jr.: Raynaud's phenomenon associated with pulmonary hypertension. Tex. State J. Med. 58:654, 1962.

135. Winters, W. L., Jr., Joseph, R. R., and Lerner, N.: "Primary" pulmonary hypertension and Raynaud's phenomenon. Arch. Intern. Med. 114:821, 1964.

136. Kanemoto, N., Gonda, N., Katsu, M., and Fukada, J.: Two cases of pulmonary hypertension with Raynaud's phenomenon: Primary pulmonary hypertension and systemic lupus erythematosus. Jpn. Heart J. 16:354, 1975.

137. Caldwell, I. W., and Aitchison, J. D.: Pulmonary hypertension in dermatomyositis. Br. Heart J. 18:273, 1956.

138. Aitchison, J. D., Williams, A. W.: Pulmonary changes in disseminated lupus erythematosus. Ann. Rheum. Dis. 15:26, 1956.

139. Sack, K. E., Bekheit, S., Fadem, S. Z., and Bedrossian, C. W. M.: Severe pulmonary vascular disease in systemic lupus erythematosus. South. Med. J. 72:1016, 1979.

139a. Santini, D., Fox, D., Kloner, R. A., Konstam, M., Rude, R. E., and Lorell, B. H.: Pulmonary hypertension in systemic lupus erythematosis: Hemodynamics and effects of vasodilator therapy. Clin. Cardiol. 3:406, 1980.

140. Walker, W. C., and Wright, V.: Pulmonary lesions and rheumatoid arthritis. Medicine 47:501, 1968.

141. Muschenheim, C.: Some observations on the Hamman-Rich disease. Am. J. Med. Sci. 241:279, 1961.

142. Soergel, K. H., and Sommers, S. C.: Idiopathic pulmonary hemosiderosis and related syndromes. Am. J. Med. 32:499, 1962.

143. Michaels, L., Brown, N. J., and Cory-Wright, M.: Arterial changes in pulmonary sarcoidosis. Arch. Pathol. 69:741, 1960.

144. Altemus, L. R., and Lee, R. E.: Carcinomatosis of the lung with pulmonary hypertension. Arch. Intern. Med. 119:32, 1967.

145. Kane, R. D., Hawkins, H. K., Miller, J. A., and Noce, P. S.: Microscopic pulmonary tumor emboli associated with dyspnea. Cancer 36:1473, 1975.

146. Jacques, J. E., and Barclay, R.: The solid sarcomatous pulmonary artery. Br. J. Dis. Chest 11:123, 1974.

147. Wood, P.: The Eisenmenger syndrome, or pulmonary hypertension with reversed central shunt. Br. Med. J. 2:755, 1958.

148. Hoffman, J. J. E., Rudolph, A. M., and Heymann, M. A.: Pulmonary vascular disease with congenital heart lesions: Pathologic features and causes. Circulation 64:873, 1981.

148a. Wagenvoort, C. A., and Wagenvoort, N.: Pathology of the Eisenmenger syndrome and primary pulmonary hypertension. Adv. Cardiol. 11:123, 1974.

149. Heath, D., and Edwards, J. E.: The pathology of hypertensive pulmonary vascular disease. A description of six grades of structural changes in the pulmonary arteries with special reference to congenital cardiac septal defects. Circulation 18:533, 1958.

150. Wagenvoort, C. A.: The morphology of certain vascular lesions in pulmonary hypertension. J. Pathol. Bacteriol. 78:503, 1959.

151. Wagenvoort, C. A.: Hypertensive pulmonary vascular disease complicating congenital heart disease: A review. Cardiovasc. Clin. 5:43, 1973.

152. Downing, S. E., Pursel, S. E., Vidone, R. A., Brandt, H. M., and Liebow, A. A.: Studies on pulmonary hypertension with special reference to pressure-flow relationships in chronically distended and undistended lobes. Med. Thorac. 19:76, 1962.

153. Harley, R. A., Friedman, P. J., Saldana, M., Liebow, A. A., and Carrington, C. B.: Sequential development of lesions in experimental extreme pulmonary hypertension. Am. J. Pathol. 52:52A, 1968.

154. Saldana, M. E., Harley, R. A., Liebow, A. A., and Carrington, C. B.: Extreme experimental pulmonary hypertension in relation to polycythemia. Am. J. Pathol. 52:935, 1968.

155. Rabinovitch, M., and Reid, L. M.: Quantitative structural analysis of the pulmonary vascular bed in congenital heart defects. In Engle, M. E. (ed.): Pediatric Cardiovascular Disease. Philadelphia, F. A. Davis, 1981, pp. 149–169.

156. Rabinovitch, M., Keane, J. F., Fellows, K. E., Castaneda, A. R., and Reid, L.: Quantitative analysis of the pulmonary wedge angiogram in congenital heart defects. Circulation 63:152, 1981.

157. Fishman, A. P.: Unexplained pulmonary hypertension. Circulation 65:651, 1982.

158. Senior, R. M., Britton, R. C., Turino, G. M., Wood, J. A., Langer, G. A., and Fishman, A. P.: Pulmonary hypertension associated with cirrhosis of the liver and portacaval shunts. Circulation 37:88, 1968.

159. Levine, O. R., Harris, R. C., Blanc, W. A., and Mellins, R. B.: Progressive pulmonary hypertension in children with portal hypertension. J. Pediatr. 83:964, 1973.

160. Segel, N., Kay, J. M., Bayley, T. J., and Paton, A.: Pulmonary hypertension with hepatic cirrhosis. Br. Heart J. 30:575, 1968.

161. Kay, J. M., and Heath, D.: Crotalaria spectabilis: Pulmonary Hypertension Plant. Springfield, Ill., Charles C Thomas, 1969, pp. 1–136.

162. Kay, J. M., Smith, P., and Heath, D.: Aminorex and the pulmonary circulation. Thorax 26:262, 1971.

163. Fishman, A. P.: Dietary pulmonary hypertension. Circ. Res. 35:657, 1974.

164. Levin, D. E., Heymann, M. A., Kitterman, J. A., Gregory, G. A., Phibbs, R. H., and Rudolph, A. M.: Persistent pulmonary hypertension of the newborn infant. J. Pediatr. 89:626, 1976.

165. Finn, M. C., Williams, L. C., and King, T. D.: Persistent fetal circulation in the newborn. J. La. State Med. Soc. 129:169, 1977.

166. Haworth, S. G., and Reid, L.: Persistent fetal circulation: Newly recognized structural features. J. Pediatr. 88:614, 1976.

167. Paraskos, J. A., Adelstein, S. J., Smith, R. E., Rickman, F. D., Grossman, W., Dexter, L., and Dalen, J. E.: Late prognosis of acute pulmonary embolism. N. Engl. J. Med. 289:55, 1973.

168. Dalen, J. E., Banas, J. S., Jr., Brooks, H. L., and Dexter, L.: Resolution rate of acute pulmonary embolism in man. N. Engl. J. Med. 280:1194, 1969.

169. Delaney, T. B., and Nadas, A. S.: Peripheral pulmonic stenosis. Am. J. Cardiol. 13:451, 1964.

170. McCue, C. M., Robertson, L. W., Lester, R. G., and Mauck, H. P.: Pulmonary artery coarctations. J. Pediatr. 67:222, 1965.

171. Pool, P. E., Vogel, J. H. K., and Blount, S. G., Jr.: Congenital unilateral absence of a pulmonary artery. Am. J. Cardiol. 10:706, 1962.

172. Cohn, L. H., Sanders, J. H., Jr., and Collins, J. J., Jr.: Surgical treatment of congenital unilateral pulmonary arterial stenosis with contralateral pulmonary hypertension. Am. J. Cardiol. 38:257, 1976.

173. Burwell, C. S., Robin, E. D., Whaley, R. D., and Bickelmann, A. G.: Extreme obesity associated with alveolar hypoventilation. Am. J. Med. 21:811, 1956.

174. James, T. N., Frame, B., and Coates, E. D.: De subitaneis mortibus. III. Pickwickian syndrome. Circulation 48:1311, 1973.

175. Noonan, A. J.: Reversible cor pulmonale due to hypertrophied tonsils and adenoids: Studies in two cases. Circulation 32 (Suppl. II):164, 1965.

176. Menashe, V. D., Farrchi, C., and Miller, M.: Hypoventilation and cor pulmonale due to chronic upper airway obstruction. J. Pediatr. 57:198, 1965.

177. Naeye, R. L.: Alveolar hypoventilation and cor pulmonale secondary to damage to the respiratory center. Am. J. Cardiol. 8:416, 1961.

178. Hultgren, H. N., Lopez, C. E., Lundberg, E., and Miller, H.: Physiologic studies of pulmonary edema at high altitude. Circulation 29:393, 1964.

179. Hackett, P. H., Creagh, C. E., Grover, R. F., Honigman, B., Houston, C. S., Reeves, J. T., Sophocles, A. M., and Van Hardenbroek, M.: High altitude pulmonary edema in persons without the right pulmonary artery. N. Engl. J. Med. 302:1070, 1980.

180. Staub, N. C.: Pulmonary edema—Hypoxia and overperfusion. N. Engl. J. Med. 302:1085, 1980.

181. Saaluke, M. G., Shapiro, S. R., Perry, L. W., and Scott, L. P.: Isolated partial anomalous pulmonary vascular obstructive disease. Am. J. Cardiol. 39:439, 1977.

182. Heath, D., DuShane, J. W., Wood, E. H., and Edwards, J. E.: The etiology of pulmonary thrombosis in cyanotic congenital heart disease with pulmonary stenosis. Thorax 13:213, 1958.

183. Schlant, R. C.: Altered cardiovascular function of rheumatic heart disease and other acquired valvular disease. In Hurst, J. L., and Logue, R. B. (eds.): The Heart. 4th ed. New York, McGraw-Hill Book Co., 1978, p. 971.

184. Durant, J. R., and Cortes, F. M.: Occlusive pulmonary vascular disease associated with hemoglobin SC disease. Am. Heart J. 71:100, 1966.

185. Rowley, P. T., and Enlander, D.: Hemoglobin SC disease presenting as acute cor pulmonale. Am. Rev. Respir. Dis. 98:494, 1968.

186. Houck, R. J., Bailey, G. L., Daroca, P. J., Brazda, F., Johnson, F. B., and Klein, R. C.: Pentazocine abuse: Report of a case with pulmonary arterial cellulose granulomas and pulmonary hypertension. Chest 77:2, 1980.

187. Oliva, P. B., and Vogel, J. H. K.: Reactive pulmonary hypertension in alveolar proteinosis. Chest 58:167, 1970.

188. Kawai, C., Ishikawa, K., Kato, M., Ishii, Y., and Nakao, K.: Pulmonary pulseless disease: Pulmonary involvement in so-called Takayasu's disease. Chest 73:651, 1978.

189. Lande, A., and Bard, R.: Takayasu's arteritis: An unrecognized cause of pulmonary hypertension. Angiography 27:114, 1976.

190. Rosenberg, S. A.: A study of the etiological basis of primary pulmonary hypertension. Am. Heart J. 68:484, 1964.

191. Trell, E., and Lindstrom, C.: Primary and chronic thromboembolic pulmonary hypertension. Acta Med. Scand. 534 (Suppl.):1, 1972.

192. Wagenvoort, C. A., and Wagenvoort, N.: Primary pulmonary hypertension. A pathologic study of the lung vessels in 156 clinically diagnosed cases. Circulation 42:1163, 1970.

193. Hatano, S., and Strasser, T. (eds.): Primary pulmonary hypertension. Report on a WHO meeting. Geneva, World Health Organization, 1975.

194. Edwards, W. D., and Edwards, J. E.: Clinical primary pulmonary hypertension—three pathological types. Circulation 56:884, 1977.

195. Harrison, C. V.: Experimental pulmonary arteriosclerosis. J. Pathol. Bacteriol. 60:289, 1948.

196. Bernard, P. J.: Pulmonary arteriosclerosis and cor pulmonale due to recurrent-thromboembolism. Circulation 10:343, 1954.

197. Bernard, P. J.: Thrombo-embolic primary pulmonary hypertension. Br. Heart J. 16:93, 1954.

198. Inglesby, T. V., Singer, J. W., and Gordon, D. S.: Abnormal fibrinolysis in familial pulmonary hypertension. Am. J. Med. 55:5, 1973.

199. Anderson, E. G., Simon, G., and Reid, L.: Primary and thrombo-embolic pulmonary hypertension: a quantitative pathological study. J. Pathol. 110:273, 1973.

200. Trell, E.: Primary and chronic thromboembolic pulmonary hypertension. Angiology 23:558, 1972.

201. Stuard, I. D., Heusinkveld, R. S., and Moss, A. J.: Microangiopathic hemolytic anemia and thrombocytopenia in primary pulmonary hypertension. N. Engl. J. Med. 287:869, 1972.

202. Franz, R. C., Ziady, F., Coetzee, W. J. C., and Hugo, N.: A possible causal relationship between defective fibrinolysis and pulmonary hypertension. S. Afr. Med. J. 55:170, 1979.

203. Tubbs, R. R., Levin, R. D., Shirey, E. K., and Hoffman, G. C.: Fibrinolysis in familial pulmonary hypertension. Am. J. Clin. Pathol. 71:384, 1979.

204. Evans, W., Short, D. S., and Bedford, D. E.: Solitary pulmonary hypertension. Br. Heart J. 19:93, 1957.

205. Goodale, F., Jr., and Thomas, W. A.: Primary pulmonary arterial disease. Arch. Pathol. 58:568, 1954.

206. Wade, G., and Ball, J.: Unexplained pulmonary hypertension. Q. J. Med. 26:83, 1957.

207. Wood, D. A., and Miller, M.: The role of the dual pulmonary circulation in various pathologic conditions of the lungs. J. Thorac. Surg. 7:649, 1938.

208. Brinton, W. D.: Primary pulmonary hypertension. Br. Heart J. 12:305, 1950.

209. James, T. N.: Degenerative arteriopathy with pulmonary hypertension: a revised concept of so-called primary pulmonary hypertension. Henry Ford Hosp. Med. Bull. 9:271, 1961.

210. Walcott, G., Burchell, H. B., and Brown, A. L.: Primary pulmonary hypertension. Am. J. Med. 49:70, 1970.

211. Farrar, J. F., Reye, R. D. K., and Stuckey, D.: Primary pulmonary hypertension in childhood. Br. Heart J. 23:605, 1961.

212. Naeye, R. L.: "Primary" pulmonary hypertension with coexisting portal hypertension. A retrospective study of six cases. Circulation 22:376, 1960.

213. Segel, N., Kay, J. M., Bayley, T. J., and Paton, A.: Pulmonary hypertension with hepatic cirrhosis. Br. Heart J. 30:575, 1968.

214. Lal, S., and Fletcher, E.: Pulmonary hypertension and portal venous system thrombosis. Br. Heart J. 30:723, 1968.

215. Senior, R. M., Britton, R. C., Turino, G. M., Wood, J. A., Langer, G. A., and Fishman, A. P.: Pulmonary hypertension associated with cirrhosis of the liver and with portacaval shunts. Circulation 37:88, 1968.

216. Chun, P. K. C., San Antonio, R. P., and Davia, J. E.: Laennec's cirrhosis and primary pulmonary hypertension. Am. Heart J. 99:779, 1980.

217. Barnard, P. J., and Davel, J. G. A.: Primary pulmonary vascular disease with cor pulmonale: Report of three cases in children, one with congenital hypertension and two siblings with allergic vasculitis and disorders of skeletal epiphyses. Am. J. Dis. Child. 92:115, 1956.

218. Braunstein, H.: Periarteritis nodosa limited to the pulmonary circulation. Am. J. Pathol. 31:837, 1955.

219. Gurtner, H. P., Gertsch, M., Salzmann, C., Scherrer, M., Stucki, P., and Wyss, F.: Häufen sich die primär vaskulären Forem des Cor Pulmonale? Schweiz. Med. Wschr. 98:1579, and 1695; 1968.

220. Gahl, von K., Fabel, H., Freiser, E., Harmjanz, D., Ostertag, H., and Stender, H. S.: Primäre vaskuläre pulmonale Hypertonie. Z. Kreislaufforsch. 59:868, 1970.

221. Gurtner, H. P.: Pulmonary hypertension, "plexogenic pulmonary arteriopathy" and the appetite depressant drug aminorex: Post or propter? Bull. Eur. Physiopathol. Resp. 15:897, 1979.

222. Gertsch, M., and Stucki, P.: Weitgehend reversibele primär vaskuläre pulmonale Hypertonie bei einem Patienten mit Menocil-Einnahme. Z. Kreislaufforsch. 59:902, 1970.

223. Meyrick, B., and Reid, L.: Development of pulmonary arterial changes in rats fed Crotalaria spectabilis. Am. J. Pathol. 94:37, 1979.

224. Wagenvoort, C. A., Wagenvoort, N., and Dijk, H. J.: Effect of fulvine on pulmonary arteries and veins of the rat. Thorax 29:522, 1974.

225. Mattocks, A. R.: Toxicity of pyrrolizidin alkaloids. Nature 217:723, 1968.

226. Stuart, K. L., and Bras, G.: Veno-occlusive disease of the liver. Q. J. Med. 26:291, 1957.

227. Kleiger, R. E., Boxer, M., Ingham, R. E., and Harrison, D. C.: Pulmonary hypertension in patients using oral contraceptives. A report of six cases. Chest 69:143, 1976.

228. Lee, D. T., Roveti, G. C., and Ross, R. S.: The hemodynamic effects of isoproterenol on pulmonary hypertension in man. Am. Heart J. 65:361, 1963.

229. Daoud, F. S., Reeves, J. T., and Kelly, D. B.: Isoproterenol as a potential pulmonary vasodilator in primary pulmonary hypertension. Am. J. Cardiol. 42:817, 1978.

230. Shepherd, J. T., Edwards, J. E., Burchell, H. B., Swan, H. J. C., and Wood, E. H.: Clinical, physiological and pathological considerations in patients with idiopathic pulmonary hypertension. Br. Heart J. 19:70, 1957.

231. Gardiner, J. M.: The effect of "priscol" in pulmonary hypertension. Aust. Ann. Med. 3:59, 1954.

232. Yu, P. N.: Primary pulmonary hypertension: Report of six cases and review of literature. Ann. Intern. Med. 49:1138, 1958.

232a. Fernandez-Bonetti, P., Lupi-Herera, E., Martinez-Guerra, M. L., Barrios, R., Seoane, M., and Sandoval, J.: Peripheral airway obstruction in idiopathic pulmonary artery hypertension (primary). Chest 83:732, 1983.

233. Marshall, R. J., Helmholz, H. F., and Shepherd, J. T.: Effect of acetylcholine on pulmonary vascular resistance in a patient with idiopathic pulmonary hypertension. Circulation 20:391, 1959.

234. Charms, B. L.: Primary pulmonary hypertension: Effect of unilateral pulmonary artery occlusion and infusion of acetylcholine. Am. J. Cardiol. 8:94, 1961.

235. Robertson, B., Rosenhamer, G., and Lindberg, J.: Idiopathic pulmonary hypertension in two siblings. Acta Med. Scand. 186:569, 1969.

236. Rao, B. N. S., Moller, J. H., and Edwards, J. E.: Primary pulmonary hypertension in a child: Response to pharmacologic agents. Circulation 40:583, 1969.

237. Yu, P. N.: Pulmonary Blood Volume in Health and Disease. Philadelphia, Lea and Febiger, 1969.

238. Samet, P., and Bernstein, W. H.: Loss of reactivity of the pulmonary vascular bed in primary pulmonary hypertension. Am. Heart J. 66:197, 1963.

239. Melmon, K. L., and Braunwald, E.: Familial pulmonary hypertension. N. Engl. J. Med. 269:770, 1963.

240. Rogge, J. D., Mishkin, M. E., and Genovese, P. D.: The familial occurrence of primary pulmonary hypertension. Ann. Intern. Med. 65:672, 1966.

241. Kingdon, H. S., Cohen, L. S., Roberts, W. C., and Braunwald, E.: Familial occurrence of primary pulmonary hypertension. Arch. Intern. Med. 118:422, 1966.

242. Kuida, H., Dammin, G. J., Haynes, F. W., Rapaport, E., and Dexter, L.: Primary pulmonary hypertension. Am. J. Med. 23:166, 1957.

243. Heath, D., and Edwards, J. E.: Configuration of elastic tissue of pulmonary trunk in idiopathic pulmonary hypertension. Circulation 21:59, 1960.

244. Meyrick, B., Clarke, S. W., Symons, C., Woodgate, D. J., and Reid, L.: Primary pulmonary hypertension—A case report including electron microscopic study. Br. J. Dis. Chest 68:11, 1974.

245. Suarez, L. D., Sciandro, E. E., Llera, J. J., and Perosio, A. M.: Long-term followup in primary pulmonary hypertension. Br. Heart J. 41:702, 1979.

246. Bourdillon, P. D. V., and Oakley, C. M.: Regression of primary pulmonary hypertension. Br. Heart J. 38:264, 1976.

247. Sleeper, J. C., Orgain, E. S., and McIntosh, H. D.: Primary pulmonary hyper-

tension. Review of clinical features and pathologic physiology with a report of pulmonary hemodynamics derived from repeated catheterization. Circulation 26:1358, 1962.

248. Lasser, R. P., and Genkins, G.: Chest pain in patients with isolated pulmonic stenosis. Circulation 15:258, 1957.

249. Ross, R. S.: Right ventricular hypertension as a cause of precordial pain. Am. Heart J. 61:134, 1961.

250. Viar, W. N., and Harrison, T. R.: Chest pain in association with pulmonary hypertension; its similarity to the pain of coronary disease. Circulation 5:1, 1952.

251. Kanemoto, N., Furuya, H., Etoh, T., Sasamoto, H., and Matsuyama, S.: Chest roentgenograms in primary pulmonary hypertension. Chest 76:45, 1979.

252. Anderson, G., Reid, L., and Simon, G.: The radiographic appearances in primary and in thromboembolic pulmonary hypertension. Clin. Radiol. 24:113, 1973.

253. Goodman, D. J., Harrison, D. C., and Popp, R. L.: Echocardiographic features of primary pulmonary hypertension. Am. J. Cardiol. 33:438, 1974.

254. Child, J. S., Wolfe, J. D., Tashkin, D., Nakano, F.: Fatal lung scan in a case of pulmonary hypertension due to obliterative pulmonary vascular disease. Chest 67:308, 1975.

254a.Rich, S., Martinez, J., Lam, W., Levy, P. S., and Rosen, K. M.: Reassessment of the effects of vasodilator drugs in primary pulmonary hypertension: Guidelines for determining a pulmonary vasodilator response. Am. Heart J. 105:119, 1983.

255. Reeves, J. T.: Hope in primary pulmonary hypertension? N. Engl. J. Med. 302: 112, 1980.

256. Rubin, L. J., and Peter, R. H.: Oral hydralazine therapy for primary pulmonary hypertension. N. Engl. J. Med. 302:69, 1980.

257. Lupi-Herrera, E., Sandoval, J., Seoane, M., and Bialostozky, D.: The role of hydralazine therapy for pulmonary arterial hypertension of unknown cause. Circulation 65:645, 1982.

258. Ruskin, J. N., and Hutter, A. M.: Primary pulmonary hypertension treated with oral phentolamine. Ann. Intern. Med. 90:772, 1979.

259. Shettigar, U. R., Hultgren, H. N., Specter, M., Martin, R., and Davies, D. H.: Primary pulmonary hypertension: favorable effect of isoproterenol. N. Engl. J. Med. 295:1414, 1978.

260. Daoud, F. S., Reeves, J. T., and Kelly, D. B.: Isoproterenol as a potential pulmonary vasodilator in primary pulmonary hypertension. Am. J. Cardiol. 42: 817, 1978.

261. Wang, S. W. S., Pohl, J. E. F., Rowlands, D. J., and Wade, E. G.: Diazoxide in the treatment of primary pulmonary hypertension. Br. Heart J. 40:572, 1978.

262. Klinke, W. P., and Gilbert, J. A. L.: Diazoxide in primary pulmonary hypertension. N. Engl. J. Med. 302:91, 1980.

263. Buch, J., and Wennevold, A.: Hazards of diazoxide in pulmonary hypertension. Br. Heart J. 46:401, 1981.

264. Fishman, A. P.: Primary pulmonary hypertension: More light or more tunnel? Ann. Intern. Med. 94:815, 1981.

265. Nagasaka, Y., Akuisu, H., Lee, Y. S., Fugimoto, S., and Chikamori, J.: Long-term favorable effects of oxygen administration on a patient with primary pulmonary hypertension. Chest 74:299, 1978.

266. Lock, J. E., Olley, P. M., Coceani, P. M., Swyer, P. R., and Rowe, R. D.: Use of prostacyclin in persistent fetal circulation. Lancet 1:1343, 1979.

267. DeFeyter, P. J., Kerkkamp, H. J. J., and deJong, J. P.: Sustained beneficial effect of nifedipine in primary pulmonary hypertension. Am. Heart J. 105:333, 1983.

268. Melot, C., Naeije, R., Mols, P., Vandenbossche, J-L., and Denolin, H.: Effects of nifedipine on ventilation/perfusion matching in primary pulmonary hypertension. Chest 83:203, 1983.

269. Olivari, M. T., Cohn, J. N., Carlyle, P., and Levine, T. B.: Beneficial hemodynamic and exercise response to nifedipine in primary pulmonary hypertension. J. Am. Coll. Cardiol. 1:735, 1983.

270. Rubin, L. J., Nicod, P., Hillis, L. D., and Firth, B. G.: Hemodynamic effects of nifedipine in primary pulmonary hypertension. J. Am. Coll. Cardiol. 1:735, 1983.

270a.Packer, M., Medina, N., and Yushak, M.: Adverse hemodynamic and clinical effects of nifedipine in patients with primary pulmonary hypertension. J. Am. Coll. Cardiol. 1:270, 1983.

270b.Wise, J. R., Jr.: Nifedipine in the treatment of primary pulmonary hypertension. Am. Heart J. 105:693, 1983.

271. Packer, M., Meller, J., Medina, N., Yushak, M., Goldstein, M., and Teirstein, A.: Verapamil therapy for primary pulmonary hypertension: Initial results and comparison to hydralazine. Circulation 66:II, 1982 (abstract).

272. Lupi-Herrera, E., Bialostozky, D., and Sobrino, A.: The role of isoproterenol in pulmonary artery hypertension of unknown etiology (primary). Chest 79: 292, 1981.

272a.Fyler, D. C.: Can vasodilators ameliorate pulmonary hypertension? J. Cardiovasc. Med. 8:237, 1983.

273. Cohen, M. L., and Kronzon, I.: Adverse hemodynamic effects of phentolamine in primary pulmonary hypertension. Ann. Intern. Med. 95:591, 1981.

274. Reitz, B. A., Wallwork, J. L., Hunt, S. A., Pennock, J. L., Billingham, M. E., Oyer, P. E., Stinson, E. B., and Shumway, N. E.: Heart-lung transplantation: Successful therapy for patients with pulmonary vascular disease. N. Engl. J. Med. 306:557, 1982.

275. Steele, P. M., Fuster, V., and Ewards, W. D.: Idiopathic pulmonary hypertension: Correlation of pathological type, anticoagulant therapy and outcome in 120 patients. J. Am. Coll. Cardiol. 1:735, 1983.

26 SYSTEMIC HYPERTENSION: MECHANISMS AND DIAGNOSIS

by Norman M. Kaplan, M.D.

Hypertension is the leading cause of death and disability among adults living today in nonprimitive societies. Despite significant advances in the recognition and control of hypertension, it remains the major risk factor for coronary, cerebral, and renal vascular diseases, the causes of over half of all deaths in the United States. More than half of all heart attacks and two-thirds of all strokes occur in individuals who were previously hypertensive.[1]

In the past 15 years, significant decreases in mortality—and probably in morbidity as well—associated with both heart attacks and strokes have been recorded in the U.S.[2] These decreases likely reflect a combination of factors that

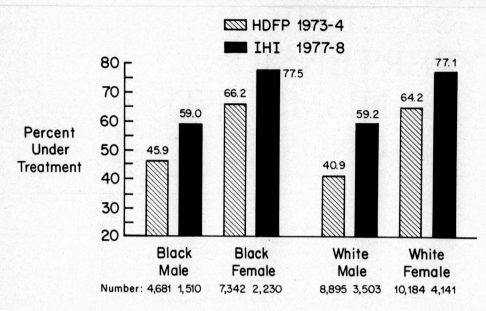

FIGURE 26–1 Percentage of hypertensives in three U.S. communities whose blood pressure was under treatment in 1973–74 (HDFP) and in 1977–78 (IHI). (From Apostolides, A. Y., et al.: Impact of hypertension information on high blood pressure control between 1973 and 1978. Hypertension *2*:708, 1980, by permission of the American Heart Association, Inc.)

have reduced the overall cardiovascular risk status of the American population, including declines in smoking, in consumption of saturated fats, and in physical inactivity.[3] In addition, a significant part of this reduction likely reflects improvements in the management of millions of patients with hypertension[4] (Fig. 26–1).

As impressive as these improvements are, major problems persist: (1) many hypertensive individuals are at risk because their disease remains undiagnosed and untreated; (2) most hypertension remains idiopathic, primary, or "essential," and without knowledge of causes, prevention of the disease is not possible; (3) in most cases, it is difficult for patients to comply with antihypertensive therapy indefinitely. This and the succeeding chapter attempt to provide guidance for the clinician in handling these problems of management. In this chapter, the mechanisms most likely responsible for primary and secondary hypertension are presented so that diagnostic evaluation can be more sharply focused. In Chapter 27, therapy will be systematically presented, with emphasis on nonpharmacological approaches as well as the rational use of drugs, with the goal of improving patient compliance with lifelong management.

GENERAL CONSIDERATIONS

To provide the background for the physician to deal efficiently and effectively with hypertensive patients, the following general questions will be examined initially:
— At what level is blood pressure considered to be abnormally high?
— How common is hypertension?
— What are the frequencies of various hypertensive diseases?
— What are the risks of uncontrolled hypertension?

Thereafter, the pathophysiology of the primary as well as the major forms of secondary hypertensive diseases will be discussed. Although Chapter 27 deals exclusively with therapy, the coverage of secondary diseases in this chapter will be accompanied by brief descriptions of their specific therapies.

Definition of Hypertension

More and more people are having their blood pressure taken. As more asymptomatic people are being found to have elevated blood pressure, the need to identify those with sufficiently elevated levels to justify therapy has become an increasing problem in clinical practice. The problem largely revolves around the wide variation in blood pressure throughout the day and night, both in persons whose levels remain normal and in those with high levels[5] (Fig. 26–2). In some cases, this variation accompanies physical activity and emotional stress, but in others it is without obvious cause. In a few patients, markedly high readings clearly indicate serious disease requiring immediate treatment. But in most, initial readings are not so high as to indicate immediate danger, and the diagnosis should be substantiated by repeated readings. The reason for such care is obvious: the diagnosis of hypertension imposes heavy psychological and socioeconomic burdens and implies a commitment to lifelong therapy.

DOCUMENTATION OF HYPERTENSION

In deciding what is normal or abnormal for an individual, these guidelines should be followed:

1. Multiple readings should be taken using appropriate techniques (Table 26–1). These guidelines complement the recommendations made in 1980 by an American Heart Association expert committee.[6]
2. Although the logical approach is to average the multiple readings in deciding whether hypertension is or is not present, even a single high reading should not be disre-

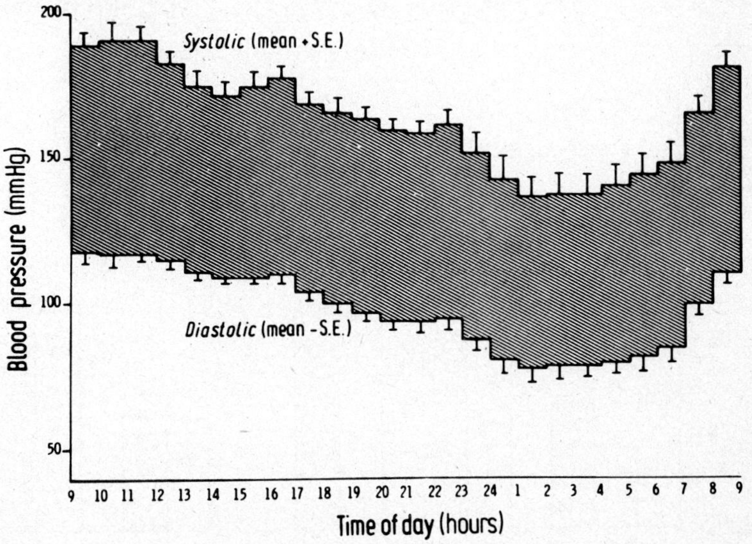

FIGURE 26–2 The hourly mean systolic and diastolic blood pressures of 20 previously untreated ambulant hypertensive subjects recorded continuously by means of intraarterial cannulation. (From Millar-Craig, M. W., et al.: Circadian variation of blood pressure. Lancet *1*:795, 1978.)

garded. Single, casual readings have been found to relate closely to the subsequent development of cardiovascular disease, both in the Framingham Study[7] and by actuarial analysis.[8]

3. Relatively small elevations, if left untreated, are associated with significant morbidity and mortality. The data shown in Figure 26–3 from life insurance actuarial experience were based on one set of readings obtained under rather uncontrolled conditions, but they are supported by the more careful observations from Framingham, showing increases in cardiovascular morbidity and mortality with each increment in blood pressure.[7]

4. As clearly shown by the Framingham data, systolic elevations pose a risk equal to or greater than diastolic elevations.[7] Even isolated systolic hypertension is a risk, particularly for stroke[9] (Table 26–2), but we remain uncertain about both the value of and the techniques for its treatment. The need for greater certainty with regard to the management of such patients is obvious, since as many as one-third of people over 65 have isolated systolic hypertension.[10]

A particular problem may cause falsely high readings in the elderly. Markedly sclerotic vessels may not be occluded until very high pressures are exerted by sphygmoma-

TABLE 26–1   GUIDELINES IN MEASURING BLOOD PRESSURE

I. Conditions for the patient
  A. Posture
    1. For initial reading, patient should be supine for 5 minutes; take blood pressure in both arms and, in patients below age 20, one leg. Thereafter take readings immediately and 2 minutes after the patient stands.
    2. For routine follow-up, patient should sit quietly for 5 minutes and the arm should be supported at the level of the heart.
    3. For patients receiving therapy, occasionally check for postural changes.
  B. Circumstances
    1. No caffeine for preceding hour.
    2. No smoking for preceding 15 minutes.
    3. No exogenous adrenergic stimulants, e.g., phenylephrine in nasal decongestants or eye drops for pupillary dilation.
    4. A quiet, warm setting.
    5. Home readings under varying circumstances, may be preferable and more accurate in predicting subsequent cardiovascular morbidity.*
II. Equipment
  A. Cuff size: preferably the bladder should encircle and cover two thirds of the length of the arm; if not, place the bladder over the brachial artery; if bladder is too small, spuriously high readings may result.†
  B. Manometer: anaeroid gauges should be calibrated every 6 months against a mercury manometer.
  C. For infants, use equipment employing ultrasound, e.g., the Doppler method.
III. Technique
  A. Number of readings
    1. Initially, take three readings, separated by as much time as is practical, on three different days.
    2. Thereafter, or with higher initial readings, take at least two readings.
    3. Anticipate considerable variability; readings must vary by at least 10 mm Hg to be significantly different; if variation exceeds 10 mm Hg, take additional readings.
  B. Performance
    1. Inflate the bladder quickly to a pressure of 20 mm Hg above the systolic, as recognized by disappearance of the radial pulse.
    2. Deflate the bladder 3 mm Hg every second.
    3. Record the Korotkoff phase V (disappearance) except in children, in whom use of phase IV (muffling) is advocated
    4. If Korotkoff sounds are weak, have the patient raise the arm and open and close the hand 5 to 10 times, after which the bladder should be inflated quickly.

*Ibrahim, M. M., et al.: Electrocardiogram in evaluation of resistance of antihypertensive therapy. Arch. Intern. Med. *137*:1125, 1977. Copyright 1977, American Medical Association.
†Nielsen, P. E., and Janniche, H.: The accuracy of auscultatory measurement of arm blood pressure in very obese subjects. Acta Med. Scand. *195*:403, 1974.

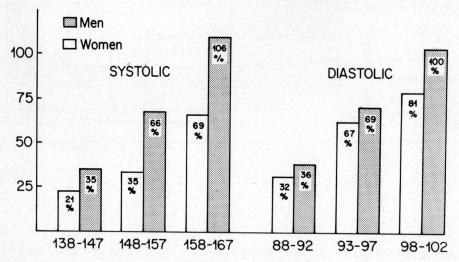

FIGURE 26-3 Excess mortality observed over 20 years by initial systolic and diastolic blood pressures among 4.5 million men and women who obtained life insurance. (From Society of Actuaries: Blood Pressure Study, 1979. Recording and Statistical Corp., 1980.)

nometry, so that indirect readings may be considerably higher than those found on direct intraarterial measurement.[11] In patients with high readings but no hypertensive retinopathy, cardiac hypertrophy, or other evidence of longstanding hypertension, "pseudohypertension" should be suspected before treatment is begun.

5. If the pressures taken repeatedly are coming down, home recordings may be particularly useful to document the course of changes in blood pressure. Home readings will likely be 5 to 10 mm Hg lower than those taken in the office and often show a progressive fall with time.[12]

6. For the individual patient, the diagnosis of definite hypertension should be made when most readings are at a level known to be associated with a significantly higher cardiovascular risk without treatment. Life insurance actuarial data indicate that mortality is increased significantly when blood pressure levels are above the following:

Men below age 45	140/90 mm Hg
Men above age 45	140/95 mm Hg
Women at any age	150/95 mm Hg

Although these limits are below the "official" level designated by the World Health Organization, i.e., 160/95, they may, in fact, be too high: in Framingham, persons with casual blood pressure measurements between 140/90 and 160/95 had a doubled risk of cardiovascular disease over the subsequent 18 years.[7]

Even lower levels may, in the future, be used to define

hypertension. When the risk for major coronary events by the level of diastolic blood pressure was determined for over 7000 white American men ages 40 to 59, a 52 per cent increase in relative risk was noted for those in the middle quintile, whose diastolic pressures were between 80 and 87, compared to patients with diastolic pressures below 80 mm Hg[13] (Table 26-3). These men had no clinical evidence of heart disease at entry and were followed for 8.6 years. On the basis of these findings, those with diastolic pressures above 85 mm Hg should be advised that they may be at increased risk and counseled to follow better health habits, hopefully to lessen the progression toward definite hypertension.

BORDERLINE HYPERTENSION

In view of the usual changeability of the blood pressure, the term "labile" is inappropriate for describing diastolic pressures that exceed 90 mm Hg only occasionally. Instead, the term "borderline" should be used. In many patients, initial diastolic readings are above 90 mm Hg but subsequent readings, taken soon after, will be well below this value. In the Hypertension Detection and Follow-up Program, 29 per cent of blacks and 39 per cent of whites displayed this pattern.[14] In a screening program, 52 per cent of the adults whose initial readings were over 90 mm Hg had subsequent readings below this value, with such lability most prevalent in young white men.[15] Even a larger number of children with initially high readings will be nor-

TABLE 26-2 RISK OF STROKE OVER 24 YEARS OF FOLLOW-UP IN FRAMINGHAM (MEN AND WOMEN, AGES 50 TO 79, WITH DIASTOLIC BLOOD PRESSURE BELOW 95 MM HG)

| | MEN | | WOMEN | |
SYSTOLIC BP	Population at Risk (Person-Years)	Age Adjusted Rate/1000 in 2 Years	Population at Risk (Person-Years)	Age Adjusted Rate/1000 in 2 Years
140	6,735	5.3	7,827	3.8
140 to 159	1,816	7.4	2,894	6.6
160	544	21.0	1,295	9.6

Data from Kannel, W. B., et al.: Systolic blood pressure, arterial rigidity and risk of stroke. J.A.M.A. 245:1225, 1981.

TABLE 26–3   THE 8.6-YEAR RISK FOR MAJOR CORONARY EVENTS IN 7054 WHITE MEN BY DIASTOLIC BLOOD PRESSURE AT ENTRY

DIASTOLIC BP AT ENTRY*	ADJUSTED RATE OF MAJOR CORONARY EVENTS PER 1000	RELATIVE RISK	ABSOLUTE EXCESS RISK PER 1000
Below 80 (Quintiles 1 and 2)	66.0	1.0	—
80 to 87 (Quintile 3)	100.6	1.52	34.6
88 to 95 (Quintile 4)	109.4	1.66	43.4
Above 95 (Quintile 5)	143.3	2.17	77.3

*The blood pressure ranges varied slightly for various 5-year age groups: 40 to 44, 45 to 49, and so on.

Data from The Pooling Project Research Group. J. Chron. Dis. *31:*201, 1978.

mal on repeat examinations. One large survey found fewer than 1 per cent with persistent elevations, although 13 per cent had high readings initially.[16]

It is probably best to advise such patients that their blood pressure level is "borderline" and should be checked annually while they follow general hygienic measures. Long-time tracking of patients with such transient hypertension has not been sufficient to provide firm data regarding the likelihood that persistent hypertension will develop. The available evidence suggests that this likelihood is greater, but long-term followup studies have shown that persistently elevated blood pressure develops in only about 20 per cent of such cases.[17]

HYPERTENSION IN CHILDREN AND ADOLESCENTS
(See also pp. 891 and 1055)

The caution advised in handling adults with transient or borderline hypertension is even more necessary in dealing with children. Now that the blood pressure of large numbers of normal children have been measured and the data have been made available,[18] those with single readings above the 95th percentile might be considered abnormal. However, the Task Force on Blood Pressure Control in Children has wisely warned against premature labeling of such children as hypertensive, since long-time tracking of those with such levels is only now being carried out.[19] Those with levels above the 95th percentile on at least three separate occasions are considered to have "sustained elevated blood pressure," whereas those with only one such reading are said to have "high normal blood pressure."[18] Appropriate management for asymptomatic children with sustained elevated blood pressure has not been settled. Although most maintain similarly high readings over three- to four-year periods, many become normotensive.[20] Such patients should be carefully followed, with particular emphasis placed on weight reduction in the hope of preventing progression of the disease.

Frequency of Hypertension

As we have come to recognize the usual—and often considerable —variability of blood pressure, we also recognize the wisdom of the late Sir George Pickering, who repeatedly warned against artificially classifying patients as "normotensive" or "hypertensive" on the basis of a single reading.[21] Obviously, the level chosen to divide the population greatly affects the number of people considered hypertensive. In a large screening program of a representative population, the per-

centage of hypertensive individuals was 18 per cent using 160/95 mm Hg as the dividing line but rose to 38 per cent if the level 140/90 was used.[22]

Most surveys have assigned 160/95 mm Hg as the minimum blood pressure level denoting hypertension for adults. The levels used to define hypertension in the previous section are lower, but this diagnosis should be based on multiple readings taken under more controlled circumstances. Even using the higher number, which is likely to underestimate the number of younger people at risk, hypertension is common, and its frequency increases with the age of the population (Fig. 26–4). The incidence of hypertension among blacks is greater at every age beyond adolescence and a given level of hypertension tends to induce more vascular damage in blacks than in whites, even though systemic hemodynamics are similar in the two races.[23]

Among the large number of people with hypertension, it is helpful to know whether some secondary process, hopefully curable by operation or more easily controlled by a specific drug, is likely to be present. In this way, the clinician can determine whether more definitive diagnostic testing is in order (Table 26–4). In many of the secondary forms, the hypertension is often obviously related to the underlying disease and therefore of little diagnostic or therapeutic concern. Our attention will be directed toward those forms that more often enter into the differential diagnosis of hypertension because of their frequency or their lack of readily apparent distinguishing features.

Most surveys to determine the relative proportion of various secondary diseases are biased by the prior selection process, with only the increasingly suspect population "funneled" to an investigator interested in that disease. By this means, estimates as high as 20 per cent for certain secondary forms of hypertension have been published, but these should not be applied to the population at large.

Two surveys highlight the problem: Among 236 patients referred to a medical center for an extensive evaluation to detect secondary diseases, 16 per cent were found to have renovascular hypertension and 12 per cent primary aldosteronism.[24] On the other hand, markedly lower figures were obtained when an estimate was made of the total number of hypertensive patients seen at the Mayo Clinic and related to the number of surgical procedures performed over a three-year period.[25] Only 0.18 per cent underwent surgery for renovascular hypertension, and 0.01 per cent for primary aldosteronism. Although these figures are too low, since not all patients were adequately tested and not all those identified underwent surgery, they may be closer

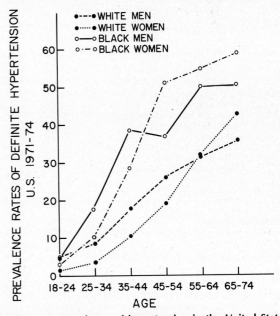

FIGURE 26–4 Prevalence of hypertension in the United States defined as the percentage of people with systolic blood pressure of at least 160 mm Hg or diastolic blood pressure of at least 95 mm Hg. (Data from the Health and Nutrition Examination Survey, 1971–1974. Source: Advance Data, Vital and Health Statistics of the National Center for Health Statistics, No. 1, October 18, 1976.)

TABLE 26–4   TYPES OF HYPERTENSION

I. Systolic and diastolic hypertension
  A. Primary, essential, or idiopathic
  B. Secondary
    1. Renal
      a. Renal parenchymal disease
        (1) Acute glomerulonephritis
        (2) Chronic nephritis
        (3) Polycystic disease
        (4) Connective tissue diseases
        (5) Diabetic nephropathy
        (6) Hydronephrosis
      b. Renovascular
      c. Renin-producing tumors
      d. Renoprival
      e. Primary sodium retention (Liddle's syndrome,
        Gordon's syndrome)
    2. Endocrine
      a. Acromegaly
      b. Hypothyroidism
      c. Hypercalcemia
      d. Hyperthyroidism
      e. Adrenal
        (1) Cortical
          (a) Cushing's syndrome
          (b) Primary aldosteronism
          (c) Congenital adrenal hyperplasia
        (2) Medullary: pheochromocytoma
      f. Extraadrenal chromaffin tumors
      g. Carcinoid
      h. Exogenous hormones
        (1) Estrogen
        (2) Glucocorticoids
        (3) Mineralocorticoids: licorice, carbenexolone
        (4) Sympathomimetics
        (5) Tyramine-containing foods and MAO
          inhibitors
    3. Coarctation of the aorta
    4. Pregnancy-induced hypertension
    5. Neurological disorders
      a. Increased intracranial pressure
        (1) Brain tumor
        (2) Encephalitis
        (3) Respiratory acidosis: lung or CNS disease
      b. Quadriplegia
      c. Acute porphyria
      d. Familial dysautonomia
      e. Lead poisoning
      f. Guillain-Barré syndrome
    6. Acute stress, including surgery
      a. Psychogenic hyperventilation
      b. Hypoglycemia
      c. Burns
      d. Pancreatitis
      e. Alcohol withdrawal
      f. Sickle cell crisis
      g. Postresuscitation
      h. Postoperative
    7. Increased intravascular volume
    8. Drugs and other substances
II. Systolic hypertension
  A. Increased cardiac output
    1. Aortic valvular regurgitation
    2. AV fistula, patent ductus
    3. Thyrotoxicosis
    4. Paget's disease of bone
    5. Beriberi
    6. Hyperkinetic circulation
  B. Rigidity of aorta

---

to what primary care practitioners might expect to find among their patients.

Estimates more likely to be indicative of the numbers of cases usually seen in clinical practice are shown in Table 26–5.[26–28] Berglund et al.[26] surveyed a random sample of the 47- to 54-year-old men in Göteborg, Sweden, who were found to have a blood pressure above 175/115 mm Hg, so that both women and milder hypertensives were excluded. Even though secondary forms are more common among those with more severe hypertension, 94 per cent of these patients with diastolic readings above 115 mm Hg had primary (essential) hypertension.

TABLE 26–5   FREQUENCY OF VARIOUS DIAGNOSES IN HYPERTENSIVE SUBJECTS

DIAGNOSIS	BERGLUND	RUDNICK	DANIELSON
Essential hypertension	94%	94%	95.3%
Chronic renal disease	4%	5%	2.4%
Renovascular disease	1%	0.2%	1.0%
Coarctation	0.1%	0.2%	
Primary aldosteronism	0.1%		0.1%
Cushing's syndrome		0.2%	0.1%
Pheochromocytoma			0.2%
Oral contraceptive–induced	(Men only)	0.2%	0.8%
Number of patients	689	665	1000

From Berglund, G., et al.: Br. Med. J. 2:554, 1976; Rudnick, K. V., et al.: Can. Med. Assoc. J. *117*:492, 1977; Danielson, M., and Dammström, B.: Acta Med. Scand. *209*:451, 1981.

A closer approximation of usual medical practice is the survey by Rudnick et al.[27] in which the patients were middle-class whites seen in a family practice in Hamilton, Canada, from 1965 to 1974. As in all three of these surveys, many of the patients underwent intravenous pyelography in addition to a history, physical examination, and routine urine and blood tests. Although a few with secondary diseases may have been missed in each of these surveys, the closeness of these data strongly support the view that in 95 per cent of all hypertensives there will be no recognizable cause.

The Changing Nature of Childhood Hypertension. Even among children, secondary hypertension is less common than indicated by previous surveys of hospital-based populations. As more apparently normal children are being screened and more are found to be hypertensive, the clinical presentation of childhood hypertension is changing from that of a rare and serious disease, usually related to renal damage, to a fairly common and usually asymptomatic process, in most cases without recognizable cause.[19] Many prepubertal hypertensive children do not have underlying secondary diseases, whereas most recognized after puberty have idiopathic hypertension.

The Need for Selectivity in Screening Tests. Because of the relatively low frequency of these various secondary diseases, selectivity in performing the various screening and diagnostic tests is warranted. The presence of features "inappropriate" for hypertension (Table 26–6) indicates the need for additional tests. However, for 9 of the 10 hypertensive patients in whom these features are absent, a hematocrit, urine analysis, automated blood biochemical profile (including plasma glucose, potassium, creatinine, and cholesterol), and an electrocardiogram are all that is required.

Although some would include other tests, the greater the number of screening tests done for relatively rare diseases, the more likely a false-positive result will arise. Based on Bayes' theorem (p. 273), which relates the predictive value of tests to their sensitivity and specificity of detection and the prevalence of the disease, and using a prevalence rate of 2 per cent for renovascular hypertension, an intravenous pyelogram (IVP) suggestive of renal hypertension has only a 10 per cent predictive value for that diagnosis.[29]

The practitioner is well-advised to limit the application of the IVP and other screening tests to those relatively few patients with suspicious features on initial history, physical examination, and laboratory testing, so that the predictive value of a positive test will justify its

TABLE 26–6   FEATURES OF "INAPPROPRIATE" HYPERTENSION

1. Onset before age 20 or after age 50 years
2. Level of blood pressure > 180/110 mm Hg
3. Organ damage
  a. Funduscopic findings of Grade 2 or higher
  b. Serum creatinine > 1.5 mg/100 ml
  c. Cardiomegaly (on x-ray or echocardiogram) or left ventricular hypertrophy (on electrocardiogram)
4. Features indicative of secondary causes
  a. Unprovoked hypokalemia
  b. Abdominal bruit
  c. Variable pressures with tachycardia, sweating, tremor
  d. Family history of renal disease
5. Poor response to therapy that is usually effective

use. Thus, among children, in whom renal hypertension is much more prevalent, addition of the IVP to "routine" testing enabled recognition of all those cases due to secondary causes.[30] However, in adults without features suggestive of renovascular hypertension (i.e., young age, severe hypertension, abdominal bruit), an abnormal IVP is more likely to be a false-positive result rather than a true-positive, indicative of a specific diagnosis.[4]

Natural History of Untreated Hypertension

Knowledge about the natural history of the disease must be gleaned from what has already been reported. Since the efficacy of antihypertensive therapy has been proved, simply observing large numbers of hypertensives for prolonged periods without instituting suitable therapy is no longer ethical. However, useful information about the shorter-term effects of untreated hypertension (3 to 5 years) has been obtained from the placebo-treated controls in recently completed trials of therapy for mild hypertension.

SYMPTOMS AND SIGNS

Because uncomplicated hypertension is almost always asymptomatic, people may be unaware for as long as 10 to 20 years that their elevated blood pressure is causing progressive cardiovascular damage. Only if blood pressure measurements are made frequently and people are made aware that, even if they are asymptomatic, hypertension is harmful will the remaining 50 per cent of Americans with hypertension that is unrecognized or inadequately treated be managed effectively.

Symptoms often attributed to hypertension, i.e., headache, nosebleed, tinnitus, dizziness, and fainting, may be seen just as commonly among normotensive people.[31] Headache is usually considered the most frequent and bothersome symptom. Some believe it to be related to the disease,[32] while others believe that it is largely nonspecific, often psychogenic, and more likely to be identified among hypertensive patients because they are more likely to be asked about the symptom. In a survey among people still unaware that they had hypertension, 16 per cent had headaches; among patients aware of their hypertension, receiving no therapy, and otherwise similar to those who were unaware, 74 per cent had headaches, mostly attributable to anxiety.[33] After reviewing the literature and his own experience in Australia, Bauer concludes that "headache appears to be a signal of a sociopsychological disorder rather than a truly hypertensive symptom. It is often precipitated or aggravated by the recognition of hypertension. . . . Symptomatic relief does not relate to blood pressure lowering, but to reassurance, suggestion, and cessation of analgesic abuse."[34]

Nocturia and postural unsteadiness were the only other symptoms more commonly noted among untreated hypertensives in the British series.[32]

COURSE OF THE DISEASE WITHOUT TREATMENT

As noted in Table 26–3, the presence of even minimal hypertension is accompanied by significant increases in coronary disease and mortality. Careful observations of the Framingham cohort clearly portray the increased risks for various types of cardiovascular diseases over many years among those with hypertension (Fig. 26–5).

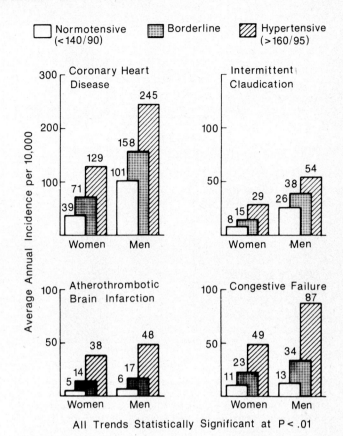

All Trends Statistically Significant at P < .01

Source: The Framingham Study Monograph, Section 30

FIGURE 26–5 Risks of coronary heart disease, intermittent claudication, atherothrombotic brain infarction, and congestive failure for women and men ages 45 to 74 in the Framingham cohort, based upon the blood pressure status at each biennial exam over an 18-year follow-up (From Kannel, W. B., and Sorlie, P.: Hypertension in Framingham. *In* Paul, O. (ed.): Epidemiology and Control of Hypertension. Miami, Symposia Specialists, 1975, p. 558.)

But these figures may be misleading, since they seem to imply that most hypertensives, including those with minimally elevated pressures, will get into trouble, and rather quickly. Remember that the actuarial data shown in Figure 26–3 are percentages of *excess* mortality, relative to the experiences of the entire insured population. The fact that men whose initial diastolic pressure was in the range of 88 to 92 mm Hg had a 36 per cent increased mortality does not mean that 36 per cent of these men died, from hypertension or any other cause. Similarly, the data shown in Table 26–3, which includes part of the Framingham cohort, indicate that those white men with diastolic pressures of 80 to 87 mm Hg had a 52 per cent greater relative risk of having a major coronary event over an 8.6-year period but not that 52 per cent did, in fact, have such an event. A large majority of hypertensives portrayed in both sets of data did not die or suffer a coronary event.

Nonetheless, because there are so many people with hypertension, the fact that even a minority of them will suffer a premature cardiovascular catastrophe in the course of their disease makes hypertension a major societal problem. In fact, when the death rates for various levels of diastolic blood pressure are multiplied by the proportion of people in the population who have these various levels, the majority of excess deaths attributable to hypertension are clearly

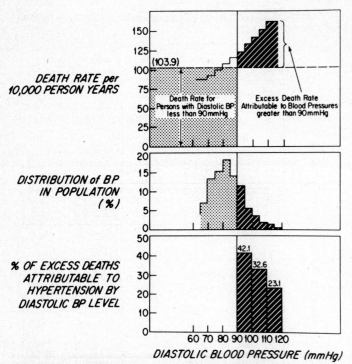

DEATH RATE per 10,000 PERSON YEARS

DISTRIBUTION of BP IN POPULATION (%)

% OF EXCESS DEATHS ATTRIBUTABLE TO HYPERTENSION BY DIASTOLIC BP LEVEL

DIASTOLIC BLOOD PRESSURE (mmHg)

FIGURE 26–6 Percentage of excess deaths attributable to hypertension by diastolic blood pressure level (*bottom*), based on the death rate observed in Framingham (*top*) and the distribution of the blood pressure found in the HDFP population (*middle*). (From The Hypertension Detection and Follow-up Program. Circ. Res. *40*:I–106, 1977, by permission of the American Heart Association, Inc.)

shown to occur among those with the minimally elevated pressures[35] (Fig. 26–6).

As the public and the medical profession have become aware of the overall societal consequences of even "mild" hypertension, enthusiasm for its early recognition and aggressive treatment has been generated. This enthusiasm for therapy was apparent even before definitive evidence was available that treatment would relieve some of these risks. In 1978, prior to publication of the results of any large-scale trials of therapy for mild hypertension, 92 per cent of physicians surveyed in New York indicated that they prescribed antihypertensive drugs for asymptomatic patients with a diastolic pressure of 90 to 104 mm Hg.[36]

A closer look at the issue of deciding upon the need for therapy will be provided in the next chapter. However, further consideration of the natural course of hypertension— as it applies to the individual patient—is needed in order to answer a basic question: Is the blood pressure high enough to justify medical intervention? Unless the risk is high enough to mandate some form of intervention there seems no need to identify and label the person as hypertensive, since psychological and socioeconomic burdens accompany this label; unless risks clearly outweigh these burdens, caution is obviously advised. A cogent view of this issue has been offered by Geoffrey Rose[37]:

As doctors we are trained to feel responsible for patients— that is, to care for the sick; and from that position accepting responsibility for those with major risk factors is not too difficult a transition. They are almost patients. A general practitioner, say, makes a routine measurement of a man's blood pressure and finds it raised. Thereafter both the man and the doctor will say

that he 'suffers' from high blood pressure. He walked in a healthy man but he walks out a patient, and his newfound status is confirmed by the giving and receiving of tablets. An inappropriate label has been accepted because both public and professional feel that if the man were not a patient the doctor would have no business treating him. In reality the care of the symptomless hypertensive person is preventive medicine, not therapeutics.

Rose would certainly not deny the benefits of preventive medicine but he goes on to emphasize the need for great caution in applying preventive measures to large groups of people:

If a preventive measure exposes many people to a small risk, the harm it does may readily—as in the case of clofibrate—outweigh the benefits, since these are received by relatively few. . . . We may thus be unable to identify that small level of harm to individuals from long-term intervention that would be sufficient to make that line of prevention unprofitable or even harmful. Consequently we cannot accept long-term mass preventive medication.[37]

We are thus left with a dilemma: for the mass of hypertensives, even those with the least elevated pressures, there is an increased risk; for the individual hypertensive, the risk may not justify the labeling or treatment of the condition.

ASSESSMENT OF INDIVIDUAL RISK

Guidelines to help the practitioner resolve this dilemma in dealing with the individual patient are available, based upon the overall assessment of cardiovascular risk and the biological aggressiveness of the hypertension. These guidelines are intended to apply only to those with "mild" hypertension, as defined in the HDFP as diastolic pressure between 90 and 104 mm Hg; those with diastolic levels persistently above 105 mm Hg have been shown to be at high enough risk from the hypertension per se to justify immediate intervention.[38]

Overall Cardiovascular Risk. The Framingham study and other epidemiological surveys have clearly defined certain risk factors for premature cardiovascular disease beyond hypertension (see Chap. 35). For varying levels of blood pressure, the Framingham data show the increasing likelihood of a vascular event over the next eight years for both men and women at various ages as more and more risk factors are added (Fig. 26–7). Notice that a 40-year-old man with a systolic blood pressure of 195 mm Hg who is otherwise at low risk would have a 4.6 per cent chance of developing a vascular event in the next eight years. A man of the same age with the same pressure but with all the additional risk factors has a 70.8 per cent chance. Obviously the higher the overall risk, the more intensive the interventions should be.

Target Organ Damage. The biological aggressiveness of a given level of hypertension varies between individuals. This inherent propensity to induce vascular damage can be ascertained best by examination of the eyes, heart, and kidney.

Funduscopic Examination. As described by Keith, Wagener, and Barker in 1939, vascular changes in the fundus reflect both hypertensive neuroretinopathy and arteriosclerotic retinopathy.[39] The two processes first induce narrowing of the arteriolar lumen (Grade 1) and then sclerosis of the adventitia and/or thickening of the arteriolar

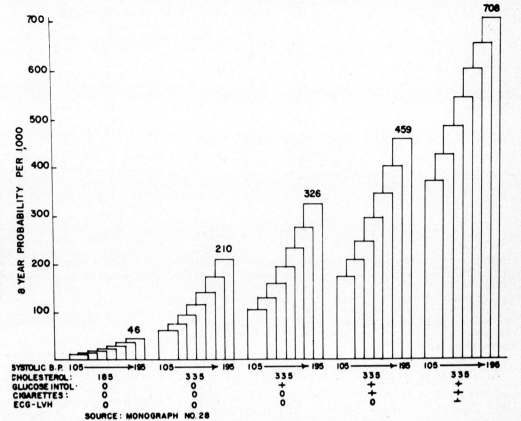

FIGURE 26–7 The 8-year risk of cardiovascular disease for 40-year-old men in Framingham according to progressively higher systolic blood pressure at specified levels of other risk factors. (From Kannel, W. B.: *In* Genest, J., et al. (eds.): Hypertension: Physiopathology and Treatment. Copyright © 1977 McGraw-Hill Book Company. Used with the permission of McGraw-Hill Book Company.)

wall, visible as arteriovenous nicking (Grade 2). With progressive arteriosclerosis, the vein becomes invisible below the arteriole and then completely obstructed. Progressive hypertension induces rupture of small vessels, seen as hemorrhages and exudates (Grade 3) and eventually papilledema (Grade 4) (see Fig. 2–2, p. 18).

Among 855 50-year old men followed for 12.5 years, attenuated arterioles and focal narrowing were found to be closely related to the presence of hypertension and subsequent mortality from strokes, whereas crossing defects were more predictive of mortality from arteriosclerotic diseases.[40]

Cardiac Involvement. Evidence of cardiac involvement includes the following:

1. Left ventricular hypertrophy on electrocardiography, based on increased voltage of QRS complexes, intrinsicoid deflection over V_5 or V_6 greater than 0.06 sec, and ST-segment depression greater than 0.5 mm (Chap. 7).

2. Left ventricular enlargement on x-ray (Chap. 6) or echocardiography (Chap. 5). Echocardiograms are more sensitive in recognizing early cardiac involvement; in 234 patients with mild to moderate hypertension (mean BP = 150/95 mm Hg), 61 per cent had an echocardiographic abnormality.[41]

3. Changes indicative of coronary artery disease.

4. Manifestations of left ventricular failure.

In Framingham, electrocardiographic evidence of left ventricular hypertrophy was a serious prognostic sign: 32 per cent of men with this finding succumbed to a cardiovascular catastrophe within five years, and congestive failure occurred 10 times more commonly.[7]

Renal Function. Renal dysfunction, too subtle to be recognized, is likely responsible for the development of most hypertension. As will be discussed, increased renal retention of salt and water may be a mechanism initiating idiopathic hypertension, but the increase is so small that it escapes detection. With detailed study, including arteriography[42] and biopsy,[43] both structural damage and functional derangement can be found in almost all hypertensive individuals, even in those with apparently early, mild disease. In patients with longstanding hypertension, creatinine clearance may be decreased, albumin may be found in the urine, and a loss of concentrating ability may be manifested by nocturia. As hypertension-induced nephrosclerosis proceeds, the plasma creatinine level begins to rise, and eventually renal insufficiency with uremia develops in 10 to 20 per cent of patients. Prognosis can be closely related to the degree of renal damage[44] (Fig. 26–8).

Renin as a Prognostic Guide. In 1972, data were published showing that a group of hypertensives with low levels of plasma renin activity (PRA) had a more benign course, with no heart attacks or strokes uncovered on retrospective analysis.[45] Subsequently, many investigators have examined the relationship between renin levels and cardiovascular complications, and with very few exceptions, patients with low PRA have been found to have no more benign a course than do those with normal PRA.[46] Indeed, in a five-year prospective study, patients with initially low renin levels suffered as many heart attacks and strokes as those with normal levels, but when a cardiovascular complication appeared, initially low renin levels tended to rise.[47] This sequence may provide a rational explanation for the finding in the retrospective study of Brunner et al.,[45] since patients whose initially low renin levels rose after a complication would not have been recognized retrospectively.

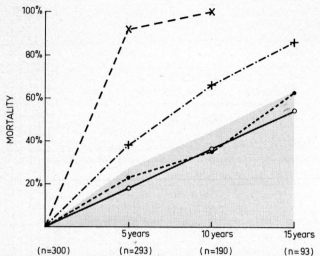

FIGURE 26–8 Mortality graph of hypertensive patients with normal and impaired renal function, all followed and treated in a single clinic. The shaded area is the mortality curve for all 300 patients. ◯——◯ = Normal renal function; ●- - -● = proteinuria; X----X = BUN of 21 to 44 mg/100 ml; X- - -X = BUN above 45 mg/100 ml. (From Bauer, G. E., and Humphrey, T. J.: The natural history of hypertension with moderate impairment of renal function. Clin. Sci. Molec. Med. 45:191s, 1973.)

Based on these various assessments of overall cardiovascular risk and the severity of the hypertension, it should be possible to determine the approximate status and prognosis for individual patients.

The Short-Term Course of Low-Risk Hypertension. The data on the four-year experiences of over 1600 "low-risk" hypertensives who served as the controls in the Australian Therapeutic Trial document the validity of this assessment.[48] For patients to enter this placebo-versus-drug trial—the largest yet reported—the second set of diastolic pressures had to be between 95 and 109 mm Hg and they had to be free of all identifiable cardiovascular disease. They can therefore be considered "low-risk" hypertensives.

Over the next four years, in the majority of these patients, who were given placebo tablets but neither nondrug nor drug therapy, blood pressures dropped progressively, from an average of 157/102 to 144/91 mm Hg. The diastolic pressure was below 95 mm Hg in 47.5 per cent at the end of the trial. The fall in blood pressure was not related to any recognizable change in the patient's status. Similar decreases occurred in those whose weight went up or down or stayed the same.[49] It is of great interest that no excess morbidity or mortality occurred among those whose diastolic pressures stayed below 100 mm Hg.

These results strongly support the view that certain patients can be characterized as being at relatively low risk and can therefore safely do without drug therapy long enough to allow one to observe the course of their blood pressure and, if indicated, the effectiveness of nondrug therapies. The large number of patients whose pressures fell and the large average degree of fall may seem surprising, but unlike most other trials, none of these patients started with any identifiable cardiovascular disease or complications of their hypertension. Moreover, placebo may be more effective than no therapy. Similar results were observed in a smaller trial of male patients free of target organ damage who had diastolic pressures below 110 mm Hg and were followed for three years and given no placebo pills.[50] About half the nontreated group exhibited a fall in diastolic pressure, and relatively little trouble developed in those with pressures initially below 100 mm Hg.

The Potential for Progression. As comforting as these data are about the short-term benignity of "low-risk" hypertension, it should be noted that the diastolic blood pressure rose above 110 mm Hg in 12.2 per cent of the nondrug-treated patients in the Australian trial[48] and in 17.2 per cent of those in the Oslo trial.[50] Levels above 110 mm

Hg demand immediate attention, so that continual monitoring of the blood pressure levels is obviously needed for all patients with even the mildest "low-risk" hypertension.

A Synthesis of Risk. Taken altogether, the data indicate that the degree of risk from hypertension can be categorized with reasonable accuracy, taking into account the level of the blood pressure, the biological nature of the hypertension as assessed from target organ function, and the coexistence of other risks. Although there is increased risk for the hypertensive population as a whole, most of the trouble will develop in those with higher levels of pressure, considerable target organ damage, and other risk factors. For them, immediate and "aggressive" reduction of pressure seems indicated. But for the majority, who are at relatively low risk, the more reasonable approach is to continue to monitor the blood pressure while encouraging healthy habits, i.e., weight control, moderate sodium restriction, isotonic exercise, and relaxation, in hopes of slowing progression of the disease (Chap. 27).

This approach justifies the screening and identification of all persons with elevated blood pressure. Since there is no certain way to predict the course of the blood pressure, all hypertensives should be followed and the recognition of their hypertension used as motivation to follow good health habits. In this way, no harm should be done and a potentially considerable benefit gained, if progression of the disease can be slowed by nondrug therapies.

COMPLICATIONS OF HYPERTENSION

For those with "high-risk" hypertension, premature development of various cardiovascular diseases is engendered by the acceleration of atherosclerosis, the pathological hallmark of uncontrolled hypertension. If untreated, about half of hypertensive patients die of coronary heart disease, a third of stroke, and 10 to 15 per cent of renal failure. Those with rapidly accelerating hypertension die more frequently of renal failure.[4]

It is easy to underestimate the role of hypertension in producing the underlying vascular damage that leads to these cardiovascular catastrophes. Hypertension as a cause of death is recorded on fewer than 20 per cent of death certificates even though the physician is aware of its presence.[51] Death is attributed to stroke or myocardial infarction instead of to the hypertension that was largely responsible. Moreover, hypertension may not persist after a myocardial infarction or stroke.

In general, the vascular complications of hypertension can be considered to be either "hypertensive" or "atherosclerotic" (Table 26–7). Those listed as "hypertensive" are more directly caused by the increased level of the blood pressure per se and can be prevented by lowering this level. Those listed as "atherosclerotic" have more multiple causations (Chap. 35), and although hypertension may represent quantitatively the most significant of the known risk factors, lowering the blood pressure may not, by itself, prevent progression of the atherosclerotic process. As shown in Figure 26–9, the translation of elevated pressure into vascular damage may proceed by numerous pathways, some well defined (shown as solid lines) and others still uncertain (shown as dotted lines).[52]

The path from hypertension to vascular disease likely involves two interrelated processes: pulsatile flow and smooth muscle cell replication. Applying the physical principles of stress, O'Rourke[53] concludes that "one would expect that pulse pressure and maximal dP/dt would be more important in causing arterial degeneration and damage than mean arterial pressure. . . . Structural damage to the aortic media can be attributed to increases in mean pressure, pulse pressure and

TABLE 26–7   VASCULAR COMPLICATIONS OF HYPERTENSION

HYPERTENSIVE	ATHEROSCLEROTIC
Malignant phase	Coronary heart disease
Hemorrhagic stroke	Sudden death
Congestive heart failure	Other arrhythmias
Nephrosclerosis	Atherothrombotic stroke
Aortic dissection	Peripheral vascular disease

From Smith, W. M.: Treatment of mild hypertension. Results of a ten-year intervention trial. Circ. Res. 25(Suppl. I):98, 1977, by permission of the American Heart Association, Inc.

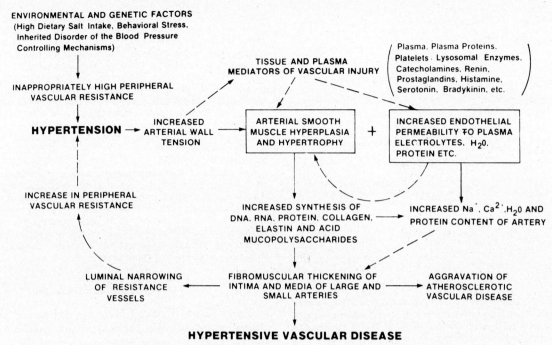

FIGURE 26-9 A unified concept of the causes and results of hypertensive vascular disease. (From Hollander, W.: Role of hypertension in atherosclerosis and cardiovascular disease. Am. J. Cardiol. *38*:786, 1976.)

dP/dt. These changes can be held responsible for medionecrosis, aneurysm formation, and for the later complications of aortic dissection and cerebral hemorrhage. Pulsatile stresses on the aortic wall are also responsible for the early intimal and subintimal changes of atheroma so that the same factors operating in hypertension can explain the increased incidence of atheroma in hypertension."

The critical importance of pulsatile flow in causing damage to vessel walls has been shown by Palmer in studies of hypertensive turkeys susceptible to aortic dissection.[54] A specific connection between these mechanical forces and the reaction by the arterial wall, which may lead to the development of atheroma, has been demonstrated in tissue taken from patients with coarctation of the aorta: arterial smooth muscle cells previously exposed to high pressure in vivo have a shorter in vitro life span, suggesting that they have already undergone an increased number of replications in response to the high pressure.[55]

Regardless of how the damage occurs, hypertension is a major factor in cardiovascular disease, as is most clearly shown in the data from Framingham (Fig. 26-5). Let us examine more closely these various cardiovascular diseases, the incidence of which is so clearly increased by hypertension.

Ischemic Heart Disease (See also p. 1216). Hypertension increases left ventricular wall tension, leading to structural, biochemical, and physiological changes in the myocardium (Fig. 26-10). These, in concert with accelerated atherosclerosis in coronary vessels, lead to ischemic heart disease manifested as angina, myocardial infarction, and sudden death. Left atrial and ventricular enlargement and dysfunction are recognized in most patients with uncomplicated hypertension, particularly by means of echocardiography.[41,56] When such overt abnormalities appear, risk of a coronary event sharply increases, as is clearly shown by the Framingham study.[7] In the 26-year Manitoba study, a rise in the level of systolic blood pressure was even more strongly associated with the incidence of ischemic heart disease than was an initially high level.[57] Moreover, survival after infarction was related to the preexisting level of the blood pressure[58] (Fig. 26-11). The improved prognosis offered by beta-adrenergic blocking drugs after myocardial infarction[59] may in part reflect their antihypertensive effects.

After myocardial infarction, hypertension may recede and never return to its previous level. In 58 hypertensive patients, blood pressure returned to normal in 37 after infarction and remained normal for up to eight weeks.[60] On the other hand, if hypertension persists, it poses a major risk of death.[61]

Congestive Heart Failure. The relationships between hypertension and congestive heart failure were clearly demonstrated in the Framingham study[62]: Hypertension was present in 75 per cent of all patients with congestive heart failure; the incidence of failure increased in both men and women at all ages as systolic or diastolic pressure increased; despite treatment, 50 per cent of those who developed congestive heart failure died within five years.

The bases for these relationships are shown in Figure 26-10. Heart

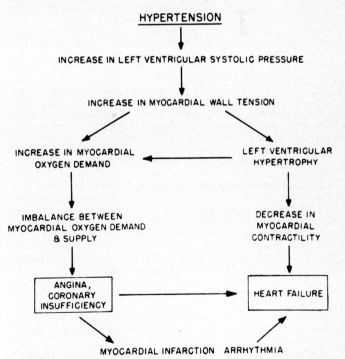

FIGURE 26-10 Adverse effects of hypertension on myocardial function. (From Hollander, W.: Role of hypertension in atherosclerosis and cardiovascular disease. Am. J. Cardiol. *38*:786, 1976.)

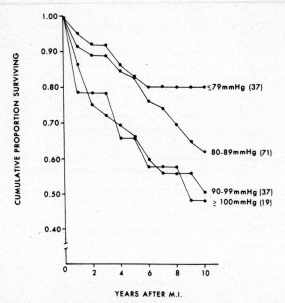

FIGURE 26–11 Survival curves after myocardial infarction according to the last diastolic blood pressure before infarction. (Number of patients shown in parentheses.) (From Rabkin, S. W., et al.: Prognosis after acute myocardial infarction: Relation to blood pressure values before infarction in a prospective cardiovascular study. Am. J. Cardiol. *40*:604, 1977.)

failure is preceded by left ventricular hypertrophy and functional impairment, with a decreased ejection rate and a prolonged tension-time index.[63] After heart failure occurs, aggressive reduction of blood pressure may be lifesaving[64]; however, the presence of hypertension in severe heart failure may be masked by the fall in blood pressure that accompanies a markedly reduced cardiac output. This sequence may be mistaken for idiopathic congestive cardiomyopathy, usually with concentric hypertrophy.[65]

Large-Vessel Disease. Occlusive vascular disease of both proximal and peripheral arteries is increased in patients with hypertension (Fig. 26–5). Presumably by accentuating atherosclerosis and medial necrosis, hypertension is also a predisposing factor in aneurysm and dissection of the aorta.[66] If the pressure is high with aortic dissection, therapy should include rapid lowering of systolic blood pressure to 100 to 120 mm Hg with a parenteral antihypertensive agent (Chap. 44).

Cerebral Vascular Disease. Hypertension is an even more potent risk factor for cerebrovascular accidents than for coronary or renal vascular disease. In Framingham, brain infarcts occurred 5 to 30 times more commonly in hypertension than in normotensive subjects[67] (Fig. 26–5). Systolic pressures are even more predictive than are diastolic pressures,[68] and isolated systolic hypertension, so commonly seen in the elderly, is associated with a two to four times greater incidence of strokes compared with normotensive people of the same age.[9]

In hypertensive patients, strokes most commonly arise from atherothrombotic infarcts of smaller penetrating branches of the middle cerebral and basilar arteries. Intracerebral hemorrhage, although less common, is more lethal. Subarachnoid bleeding also occurs more commonly in hypertensives. Transient ischemic attacks (TIA), temporary episodes of focal cerebral dysfunction, develop more commonly on the background of hypertension and, in concert with carotid bruits, are indicative of an increased risk of stroke.[69]

More subtle defects in cerebral function may accompany hypertension. When 20 men with newly discovered, untreated diastolic blood pressures above 105 mm Hg were compared to 20 normotensive subjects matched for age, educational level, and occupational status, those with hypertension were significantly slower in reaction time and in performance of other tests of attention span.[70]

Lowering the blood pressure prevents initial and recurrent strokes.[71] Unless the pressure is very high and causing immediate damage, a gradual reduction of longstanding hypertension is wise, allowing cerebral autoregulation to maintain normal perfusion. As shown by Strandgaard and coworkers, rapid reduction of chronically elevated pressures to levels well tolerated by normal individuals may invoke cerebral hypoperfusion,[72] which may cause ischemic brain damage.[73] Elderly patients are particularly susceptible because the mechanism of cerebral autoregulation becomes sluggish with age.[74]

Renal Damage. Hypertension is the most common cause of progressive renal insufficiency, and some evidence of renal damage is common in patients with hypertension. This evidence, reflecting nephrosclerosis, includes an elevated serum uric acid level, present in one-third of untreated hypertensives.[75] Levels of a lysosomal enzyme, N-acetyl-β-D-glucosaminidase, thought to be of renal origin, are frequently elevated in both serum and urine of patients with mild hypertension.[76]

The course of the relationship between hypertension and the kidneys is often uncertain: as they progress, primary renal diseases, frequently cause hypertension. As we shall see, renal dysfunction, although clinically not bothersome, may be the basic defect of primary hypertension, and the degree of renal dysfunction is closely related to the prognosis[44] (Fig. 26–8). Antihypertensive treatment will protect the kidneys, allowing some patients with even far-advanced renal insufficiency to survive for many years.[77]

HYPERTENSION IN BLACKS

Blacks have hypertension more frequently than do whites, and they suffer more morbidity and mortality from it.[78] In particular, they suffer more renal damage, leading to a significantly greater prevalence of end-stage renal disease requiring chronic dialysis.[79]

Hypertension seen in blacks has been characterized as having a relatively greater component of fluid volume excess, including a higher prevalence of low levels of plasma renin activity[80] and their greater responsiveness to diuretic therapy.[81] These and other features suggestive of volume excess may reflect larger degrees of one or more of the abnormalities in sodium transport across cell membranes that will be described in the next section, Mechanisms of Primary Hypertension. Black hypertensives have been found to have greater suppression of ouabain-insensitive Na-K pump activity than white hypertensives[82]—a defect which, if generalized, would result in higher intracellular sodium concentrations.

Perhaps blacks, who originally lived in hot, arid climates in which avid sodium conservation was necessary for survival, have evolved the physiological machinery that offers protection in their original habitat, in which the diet was relatively low in sodium, but that makes them susceptible to "sodium overload" when they migrate to areas where sodium intake is excessive. This view is supported by the experience of the Xhosa people in Southern Africa: when they migrated to urban areas, their blood pressures began to rise in association with their increased dietary intake of sodium.[83]

A complete annotated bibliography through late 1981 relative to hypertension among blacks has recently been published.[84]

HYPERTENSION IN WOMEN

Unlike blacks, women in general suffer less cardiovascular morbidity and mortality than men for any degree of hypertension (Fig. 26–5). Moreover, hypertension is less common in women than in men before the age of menopause (Fig. 26–4). Perhaps the lower frequency and severity of hypertension reflect the lower blood volume and viscosity afforded women by their monthly menses.

HYPERTENSION IN THE ELDERLY

We have previously noted the high frequency and risks of systolic hypertension among the elderly. As more people live longer, more predominantly systolic and combined systolic and diastolic hypertension will be seen among people over age 65. These individuals may have certain special needs:

— To a large extent, the progressive rise in systolic pressure reflects a loss of compliance within the major arteries due to permanent sclerosis; therapy may be either ineffectual, since vasodilation may not be possible, or poorly tolerated, since a shrinkage of fluid volume or decrease in cardiac output may diminish blood flow to the brain.

— Baroreceptor sensitivity often decreases with age, so that the buffering provided by this reflex with changes in posture and the like may be lost; old people may experience a greater rise in blood pressure upon standing[85] as well as the propensity for postural hypotension.[74]

— More elderly patients with significant hypertension of recent onset will have chronic renal disease or atherosclerotic renovascular disease as a cause of their hypertension.[86]

Now that we have reviewed the background of hypertension, let us examine what is known about the causes of the form of this condition responsible for 95 per cent of all cases, idiopathic or primary hypertension, in which the cause is unknown. At least some new clues have come to light.

MECHANISMS OF PRIMARY (ESSENTIAL) HYPERTENSION

Without knowledge of the specific cause, we can begin by considering those factors known to affect the blood pressure (Fig. 26–12). Although other forces may be involved, *cardiac output* and *peripheral resistance* are the primary determinants. The interplay of various derangements in factors affecting cardiac output and peripheral resistance may precipitate the disease; these may differ in both type and degree in different patients. Looking for a single defect in all patients with essential hypertension may be a mistake. Note the sage advice presented in an editorial in *Lancet*:

Blood pressure is a measurable end-product of an exceedingly complex series of factors including those which control blood-vessel caliber and responsiveness, those which control fluid volume within and outside the vascular bed, and those which control cardiac output. None of these factors is independent; they interact with each other and respond to changes in blood pressure. It is not easy, therefore, to dissect out cause and effect. Few factors which play a role in cardiovascular control are completely normal in hypertension: indeed, normality would require explanation since it would suggest a lack of responsiveness to increased pressure.[87]

The search for such defects to unravel the pathogenesis of essential hypertension may be misguided for another reason—it may not be a distinct disease caused by specific abnormalities. George Pickering was the most persistent and eloquent advocate of the concept that essential hypertension was only a quantitative deviation from the norm, so that people were rather arbitrarily called "hypertensive" if they were on the higher portion of a unimodal distribution curve, rather than being a separate portion of a biomodal curve.[21] The distribution of large populations is unimodal (Fig. 26–6), but such curves do not exclude the possiblity that those who become hypertensive are, in fact, qualitatively different.

Before presenting a specific hypothesis that includes such qualitative differences, let us examine the hemodynamic patterns of cardiac output and peripheral resistance that have been measured in patients with hypertension. One caution is needed: the pathogenesis of the disease is likely a slow and gradual process. By the time the blood pressure is high, the initiating faults may no longer be apparent, since they may have been "normalized" by the compensatory interactions alluded to in the *Lancet* editorial.

Nonetheless, when a group of untreated, young hypertensive patients was initially studied, cardiac output was normal or slightly increased and peripheral resistance was normal[88] (Fig. 26–13). Over the next 10 years, cardiac output fell and peripheral resistance rose. A similar conversion from initially high cardiac output to increased peripheral resistance has been found by others.[89]

Although this "traditional" pattern is found in some patients, it may not be usual or obligatory. On the one hand, in a few patients a high-output state may be present even

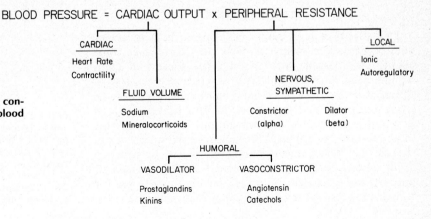

FIGURE 26–12 Some of the factors involved in the control of blood pressure that affect the basic equation: blood pressure = cardiac output × peripheral resistance.

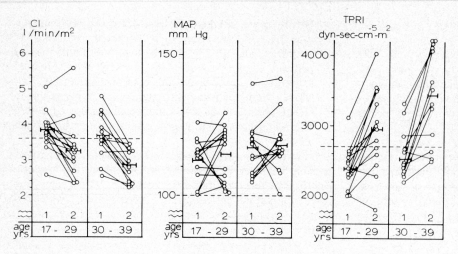

FIGURE 26–13 A 10-year follow-up study of the hemodynamics at rest in 28 untreated patients with essential hypertension. Cardiac index (CI), mean arterial pressure (MAP), and total peripheral resistance index (TPRI) at first (1) and second (2) study. Values between brackets (I___I) are mean values. The broken horizontal lines represent the upper limits of normal. (From Lund-Johansen, P.: Hemodynamic alterations in hypertension—spontaneous changes and effects of drug therapy. Acta Med. Scand. Suppl. *603*:1, 1977.)

after 20 years[90]; on the other, peripheral resistance is often abnormally high, even in those patients with initially high outputs. The expected response to increased cardiac output is vasodilation with a fall in peripheral resistance. Thus, "normal" resistance in the presence of a high cardiac output is actually abnormally elevated, constituting the primary mechanism of the hypertension.[91] Those patients with persistently expanded blood volume who would be expected to have relatively low peripheral resistance have an even higher resistance than those with greatly reduced volumes.[92] In short, Tarazi advises that "the spectrum of hemodynamic changes associated with volume disturbances in hypertension is too wide to be forced under one hypothesis alone."[92]

The eventual primacy of the factor of increased peripheral resistance can be shown in both human and animal models of hypertension with an initial increase in fluid volume and cardiac output. Patients with primary aldosteronism, completely controlled with spironolactone, were followed after administration of the aldosterone antagonist was discontinued, and the syndrome was allowed to recur in its natural manner.[93] The initial overexpansion of plasma volume returned toward normal while peripheral resistance progressively rose.

In another hypertensive syndrome thought to be related mainly to excess blood volume, i.e., the administration of salt loads to both humans and animals with reduced renal mass, there is again an initial increase in cardiac output, but within a few weeks the output returns to near the control level and peripheral resistance rises[94] (Fig. 26–14).

AUTOREGULATION

The pattern of high output changing to high resistance does occur in some instances. How does the change come about? One possible mechanism is the process of autoregulation, a property intrinsic to resistance vessels, in which an increase in blood flow beyond the needs of the tissue leads to vasoconstriction. As this decreases blood flow and brings supply and demand into balance, it results in an increase in peripheral resistance.[94] Folkow has shown that this functional change is followed quickly by structural alterations that thicken the vessel walls.[95] In concert or independently, an increase in vascular reactivity to pressor stimuli may also be involved. In experimental models, the

increased sensitivity of vascular smooth muscle to pressor stimuli appears before the blood pressure rises and may thus be a primary mechanism for increased peripheral resistance.[96]

To summarize the observational data, cardiac output and fluid volume may be elevated initially, but the hypertension is maintained by an increased peripheral resistance that may reflect, first, functional tightening and, then, structural thickening of vessel walls.

Before looking for specific causes for this hemodynamic

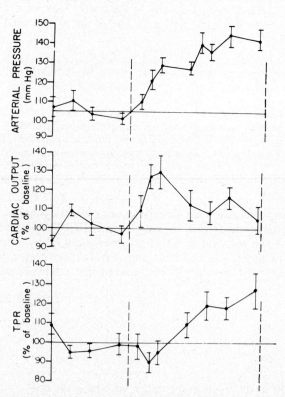

FIGURE 26–14 Arterial pressure, cardiac output, and total peripheral resistance in six partially nephrectomized dogs infused with 0.9 per cent saline. After an 8-day control period, partial nephrectomy was performed, indicated by the broken vertical line. Saline was infused continuously for the next 13 days. (From Coleman, T. G., et al.: Whole-body circulatory autoregulation and hypertension. Circ. Res. *29*(Suppl. II):76, 1971, by permission of the American Heart Association, Inc.)

pattern, the genetic predisposition for hypertension should be recognized.

GENETIC PREDISPOSITION (See also p. 1636)

Familial correlations relative to blood pressure levels have been found in infants as young as 6 months of age, supporting a genetic mechanism.[97] In studies of twins and family members in which the degree of familial aggregation of the blood pressure is compared to the closeness of genetic sharing, the genetic contribution has been estimated to be as low as 30 per cent to as high as 60 per cent.[98] The blood pressure of parents was much more closely related to that of their natural children than to that of their adopted children.[99] Since both the natural and the adopted children shared the same environment, these data support a predominant role for heredity in the familial resemblance regarding blood pressure.

The debate concerning the roles of heredity and environment may be largely academic, but it could have important practical implications. First, the children and siblings of hypertensives should be more carefully screened. Second, they should be vigorously advised to avoid environmental factors known to aggravate hypertension and increase cardiovascular risks, i.e., obesity, smoking, inactivity, and sodium.

The Inherited Defect. If heredity does indeed play a role, what is inherited? Children of hypertensive parents have shown a greater blood pressure response to psychological stress, which was further accentuated after they ingested 10 additional grams of sodium chloride for two weeks.[100] Although exposure to high levels of stress may induce hypertension regardless of the genetic substrate, it is obvious that not all who are exposed to stress develop hypertension. A genetically determined heightened response to stress and sodium would be in keeping with the findings of Falkner et al.[100]

Enhancement of stress-mediated rises in blood pressure by extra dietary sodium noted in these studies is in keeping with the accentuation of pressor responsiveness to exogenous norepinephrine[101] and angiotensin[102] after increased sodium intake. The enhanced pressor sensitivity to these hormones may reflect an increase in their vascular receptors induced by high sodium intake.[103]

The evidence for a role of excessive dietary sodium intake in the pathogenesis of hypertension is summarized in Table 26–8. We are all consuming more sodium than we

---

TABLE 26–8   EVIDENCE FOR A ROLE OF SODIUM IN PRIMARY (ESSENTIAL) HYPERTENSION

1. In large populations, the prevalence of hypertension tends to increase with increasing levels of sodium intake.
2. Multiple, scattered groups who consume little sodium (less than 50 mmol/day) have little or no hypertension. When they consume more sodium, hypertension appears.
3. Animals given sodium loads, if genetically predisposed, develop hypertension.
4. Some people, when given large sodium loads over short periods, develop an increase in vascular resistance and blood pressure.
5. An increased concentration of sodium is present in the vascular tissue and blood cells of most hypertensives.
6. Sodium restriction, to a level of 60 to 90 mmol per day, will lower blood pressure in most people. The antihypertensive action of diuretics requires an initial natriuresis.

TABLE 26–9   ABNORMAL ERYTHROCYTE NA+/K+ FLUX TEST IN NORMOTENSIVE CHILDREN OF NORMOTENSIVE OR HYPERTENSIVE PARENTS

| | PARENTS' BLOOD PRESSURE | | |
	Both Normotensive	One Hypertensive	Both Hypertensive
Number of children	86	97	19
Number with + test	3	52	14
Per cent + test	3.5%	53.6%	73.6%
Per cent expected with autosomal dominant gene	0	50.0%	75.0%

Data from Meyer, P., et al.: Inheritance of abnormal erythrocyte cation transport in essential hypertension. Br. Med. J. *282*:1114, 1981.

---

need and likely a great deal more than our ancestors consumed up until fairly recent times. The increase in sodium probably occurred when food sources began to be harvested, stored, and processed instead of grown or caught and eaten fresh.[104]

Before proceeding with this hypothesis, note should be taken of perhaps the most provocative and far-reaching evidence of a genetic defect that may interact directly with excess dietary sodium intake. This comes from studies on the movement (or flux) of sodium and potassium across red blood cell membranes.[105] These studies have shown an abnormal Na-K flux in half the normotensive children with one parent hypertensive and in three-fourths of the children with both parents hypertensive (Table 26–9), closely fitting an autosomal dominant mode of inheritance. As we shall see, such a defect in sodium transport could lead directly to hypertension.

But the primary hypothesis to be developed here involves additional steps. The hypothesis proposes that a genetic abnormality exposes some of the population to the pro-hypertensive effects of one or more environmental factors. The person predisposed by an inherited defect might not develop hypertension if the environmental factor were avoided. Both the genetic defect and the environmental factor are needed. Similarly, the degree of hypertension that develops could reflect varying degrees of exposure to the environmental factor(s). Homozygotes might also develop more hypertension than heterozygotes, or there may be more than one genetic defect, so that the end result could vary markedly with the interplay of multiple genetic and environmental factors.

As complicated as the eventual situation may be, the hypothesis to be developed will propose only one of two possible genetic defects involving sodium transport and two major environmental factors. The genetic defects involve the renal excretion of sodium and the transport of sodium across cell membranes; the environmental factors are excess dietary sodium intake and stress. This hypothesis, based on evidence still incomplete, may turn out to be wrong or incomplete, but at this time it seems both logical and parsimonious.

Let us go back, then, to the idea that the effects of stress plus excess dietary sodium are responsible for activation of the sympathetic nervous system in people somehow genetically predisposed to develop hypertension. Evidence for an increased degree of sympathetic nervous activation in hypertensives is summarized in Table 26–10.

TABLE 26–10 EVIDENCE FOR SYMPATHETIC NERVOUS ACTIVATION IN PRIMARY (ESSENTIAL) HYPERTENSION

1. In animals, acute hypertension can be induced by the release of catecholamines in response to discrete brain lesions.
2. In rats bred to become hypertensive spontaneously, alerting stimuli invoke greater discharges from central autonomic centers.
3. Some hypertensive people have high plasma catecholamine levels that correlate with the blood pressure.
4. Hypertensives with high plasma catechols (and high plasma renin levels) display greater suppressed hostility on psychometric testing.
5. Some hypertensives overrespond to stress; and people exposed to high levels of psychogenic stress develop more hypertension.
6. Drugs that inhibit adrenergic nervous activity lower the blood pressure.

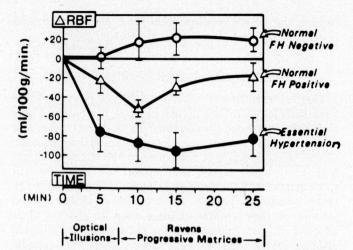

FIGURE 26–16 The response of renal blood flow (RBF) to the mild emotional stress provoked by performing a nonverbal IQ test, Ravens Progressive Matrices, in normotensives with either a negative or a positive family history and in patients with essential hypertension. (From Hollenberg, N. K., et al.: Essential hypertension: Abnormal renal vascular and endocrine responses to a mild psychological stimulus. Hypertension 3:11, 1981, by permission of the American Heart Association, Inc.)

SYMPATHETIC NERVOUS ACTIVATION

Increased sympathetic nervous activity could raise blood pressure in a number of ways—alone or in concert with catecholamine stimulation of renin release—by causing arteriolar and venous constriction, by increasing cardiac output or by altering the normal renal pressure-volume relationship.[106] Renin release is directly stimulated by sympathetic discharge. Although plasma renin activity is usually normal in patients early in the course of hypertension, such "normal" levels may be inappropriately high, since both the higher level of blood pressure and the relatively overfilled vascular bed should serve to shut off the release of renin. The combination of high catecholamines and renin-angiotensin levels may then result in a disturbed pressure-natriuresis.

PRESSURE-NATRIURESIS

When the normal kidney is exposed to higher arterial pressure, it quickly excretes extra sodium and water, the process of pressure-natriuresis. Guyton and coworkers have long argued that this process must be defective in a hypertensive, because if it were normal, whatever caused the pressure to rise would be countered by enhanced natriuresis, which would shrink fluid volume and restore normal pressure.[107] This resetting of the pressure-natriuresis curve has been explained by increased resistance within the renal efferent arterioles[108] (Fig. 26–15), which could arise from exposure to increased amounts of or increased sensitivity to angiotensin II or catecholamines.[109] The greater

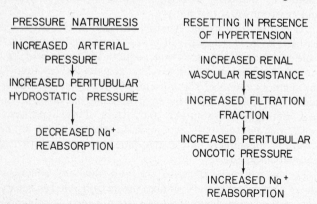

FIGURE 26–15 Origin of pressure natriuresis (*left*) and its resetting in the presence of essential hypertension (*right*). (From Brown, J. J., et al.: Renal abnormality of essential hypertension. Lancet 2:320, 1974.)

degree of efferent arteriolar constriction would increase the fraction of blood filtered (filtration fraction), increasing the peritubular oncotic pressure and thereby exerting a greater force for reabsorption of tubular sodium.

Both human[110] and animal[111] data have shown increased renal efferent arteriolar constriction early in the course of hypertension. Studies in humans by Hollenberg et al.,[110] using radioxenon to measure renal blood flow, have shown excessive sympathetically mediated, reversible intrarenal vasoconstriction in early hypertension and, to a lesser degree, in normotensives with a positive family history for hypertension (Fig. 26–16). In animal studies by Click et al.,[111] direct visualization of renal tissue in hypertensive hamsters demonstrated a greater degree of constriction of efferent than of afferent arterioles upon exposure to either norepinephrine or angiotensin.

Plasma Volume. The reset pressure-natriuresis curve would eventuate in a relatively greater volume within the circulation for the level of blood pressure. A relatively expanded plasma volume has been measured in at least 80 per cent of hypertensive patients compared with the expected and observed progressive decrease in volume with increasing blood pressure among normotensive subjects[112] (Fig. 26–17).

This relatively increased plasma volume, inappropriately high for the level of blood pressure, would overfill the vascular bed. Although there may be an absolute increase in plasma or extracellular fluid volume, the vascular bed is also likely to be somewhat smaller in response to the vasoconstrictive action of the increased levels of catecholamines and angiotensin.

Natriuretic Hormone. When plasma volume is expanded, renal excretion of sodium is increased, in part by the action of a circulating natriuretic hormone, which has still not been identified as to structure but is widely recognized as to function.[113] Natriuretic substances have been shown to be present in the blood and urine of both normal subjects and hypertensives whose blood volume is

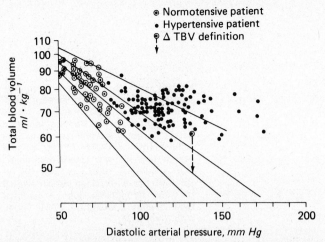

FIGURE 26–17 The relation between diastolic blood pressure and total blood volume (TBV) in 48 normotensive (open circles) and 106 hypertensive (solid circles) subjects. Only 20 per cent of the hypertensive patients fell within the 95 per cent confidence limits of the normal curve. The ΔTBV represents the degree of the pressure-volume disturbance. (Reprinted from London, G. M., et al.: Volume-dependent parameters in essential hypertension. Kidney Int. *11*:204, 1977, with permission.)

expanded.[114,115] In animals, the hormone appears to come from the hypothalamus.[116] Increased circulating levels of an endogenous inhibitor of NaK-ATPase, which shares immunological determinants with the cardiac glycoside digoxin and which has been called "endoxin," have been measured in both volume-expanded dogs[117] and hypertensive monkeys.[118] This may well be the putative natriuretic hormone. Another natriuretic factor has been extracted from cardiac atrial tissue.[118a]

The hormone increases natriuresis by inhibiting NaK-ATPase activity in the kidney, thereby reducing active sodium reabsorption. Plasma levels of an inhibitor of renal NaK-ATPase were 25 times higher when normal subjects were on a high-sodium diet (when increased amounts of a natriuretic hormone are expected) than when they were on a low-sodium diet.[119] In the plasma of patients with essential hypertension the concentration of an inhibitor of renal NaK-ATPase activity is raised.[120] The natriuresis provoked by the inhibition of renal NaK-ATPase would counter the forces that initially increased renal sodium reabsorption at the onset of the process, which eventually leads to hypertension, so that the tendency toward continually expanding fluid volume would be thwarted. Such an enhanced natriuresis has long been recognized to accompany human hypertension.[4]

Beyond its renal site of action, there is mounting evidence that natriuretic hormone acts upon NaK-ATPase activity elsewhere, such as in leukocytes[121] and, most importantly, vascular smooth muscle.[122] This inhibition of extrarenal NaK-ATPase would diminish the active extrusion of sodium from cells by the Na-K pump mechanism. Evidence for reduced NaK-ATPase activity includes the following four observations: (1) Hypertensives have been found to have a reduced rate constant for active sodium efflux from white blood cells (WBCs), a process that is ouabain-sensitive and therefore considered to reflect NaK-ATPase activity.[121] (2) The active sodium efflux rate was reduced most in those with the lowest plasma renin levels,

who might be expected to have the greatest effective expansion of vascular volume (and the highest levels of natriuretic hormone).[123] (3) After therapy with diuretics, which should shrink vascular volume and diminish the stimulus for natriuretic hormone, the abnormality in active sodium efflux from hypertensives' WBCs was corrected.[124] (4) Moreover, a decrease in sodium efflux rate was induced in the WBCs of normotensives by incubation of their cells in the serum from hypertensives.[125]

Until now, these observations in human hypertensive subjects in support of an extrarenal site of impaired sodium efflux by natriuretic hormone–induced inhibition of NaK-ATPase activity have been limited to WBCs, since it has not been possible to examine vascular tissue. In dogs and rats with nongenetic volume-expanded hypertension, suppression of Na-K pump activity has been measured in the blood vessels and heart,[126] and the suppression appears to arise from a circulating, heat-stable, ouabain-like agent evoked from the brain by volume expansion[127]—all characteristics that fit what is known about natriuretic hormone.

On the other hand, Overbeck and associates, using ouabain-sensitive rubidium uptake as a measure of Na-K pump activity have repeatedly found *increased* Na-K pump activity in the arterial tissue of rats with various forms of hypertension, including both nongenetic and genetic volume-expanded models.[128] These investigators conclude that the increased pump activity may reflect a compensatory increase in the number of active sarcolemmal pumps, perhaps in response to increased passive permeability of vascular smooth muscle to sodium, which develops in various experimental models.[129] This sequence has been shown to occur in rat aortic smooth muscle cells in culture after exposure to angiotensin II: sodium uptake increased about threefold, and presumably as a consequence of the increased intracellular sodium, Na-K pump activity almost doubled.[130] Thus, whenever intracellular sodium concentration is increased, Na-K pump activity may be stimulated in a compensatory manner, thereby obscuring the effect of a pump inhibitor such as natriuretic hormone, which previously blocked sodium efflux and was responsible for the initial rise in intracellular sodium.

Effects on Blood Pressure. Despite this possible sidetrack, the mounting evidence for the presence of a natriuretic hormone that inhibits NaK-ATPase in volume-expansion forms of hypertension fulfills the prediction made in 1969 by Dahl and coworkers, based upon their studies on parabiotic rats.[131] A logical connection between the suppression of NaK-ATPase and the development of hypertension involves an increase in intracellular sodium, an increase previously recognized in the arteries[132] and red[133] and white[121] blood cells of hypertensive patients.

INTRACELLULAR SODIUM AND CALCIUM

The next step in this sequence was provided by Blaustein[134] when he showed that an increase in intracellular sodium enhances a sodium-calcium exchange mechanism and thereby increases intracellular calcium. Blaustein calculated that a rise of 0.5 mmol/liter in intracellular sodium could give rise to an increase in intracellular calcium of 4 to 40 μmol/liter—enough to increase the resting tone of vascular smooth muscle by 50 per cent.

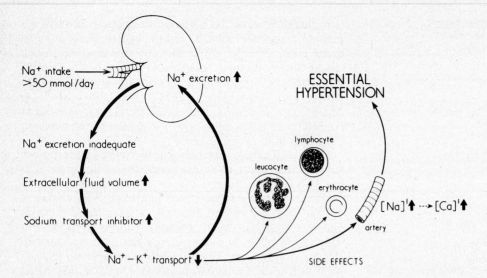

FIGURE 26–18 Hypothesis for the pathogenesis of essential hypertension, starting with a dietary sodium intake above 50 mmol/day and an inherited defect in renal sodium excretion. (Reprinted from deWardener, H. E., and MacGregor, G. A.: Dahl's hypothesis that a saluretic substance may be responsible for a sustained rise in arterial pressure: Its possible role in essential hypertension. Kidney Int. 18:1, 1980, with permission.)

The increase in intracellular calcium is translated into an increase in vascular resistance by its binding to a myofilament regulatory protein and stimulation of myosin phosphorylation.[135] Indirect support for such calcium-mediated vasoconstriction in primary hypertensives comes from the lowering of their blood pressure, but not that of normotensives, by calcium entry–blocking drugs.[136] In the same study, the blood pressure of both normotensives and hypertensives was lowered by nitroprusside, which is thought not to inhibit calcium entry.

THE COMPLETE HYPOTHESIS

The complete hypothesis incorporates a great deal of what is known about experimental and clinical primary hypertension. The major portion of this hypothesis was formulated by deWardener and MacGregor (Fig. 26–18). They proposed that the increased fluid volume that stimulates natriuretic hormone was induced by an inherited defect in sodium excretion, acting in concert with excessive dietary sodium intake. The basis for their proposal for an inherited decrease in renal sodium excretion was the experimental evidence from kidney transplantation involving both the Dahl[137] and the Milan[138] hypertensive rats, which showed that the blood pressure "follows the kidney": When a kidney is taken from a hypertensive donor rat and transplanted into a normotensive host rat, the blood pressure of the host rises. The reverse also occurs, i.e., a kidney implanted from a normotensive rat lowers the blood pressure of a hypertensive host.

This proposal, however, skips the rather convincing evidence of a resetting of the pressure-natriuresis curve and does not require the mediation of stress-induced activation of the sympathetic nervous system. Therefore, although it is less parsimonious, the scheme portrayed in Figure 26–19 is presented as a more complete representation of the currently available clinical and experimental evidence for the pathogenesis of essential hypertension.

Additional Sodium Transport Defects. Most of this hypothesis (and deWardener's as well) can be bypassed by the direct insertion in the scheme of a defect in membrane permeability to sodium, as shown in the bottom right corner of Figure 26–19. Such a defect was proposed by Losse et al. in 1960,[133] but the current enthusiasm for its role

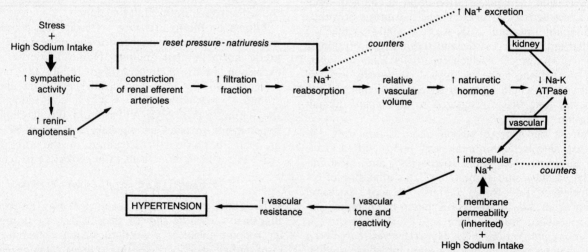

FIGURE 26–19 Hypothesis for the pathogenesis of primary (essential) hypertension, starting from two points, shown as heavy arrows. One, starting on the top left, is the combination of stress and high sodium intake, which induces an increase in natriuretic hormone and thereby inhibits sodium transport. The other, starting at the bottom right, invokes an inherited defect in sodium transport plus a high sodium intake to induce an increase in intracellular sodium.

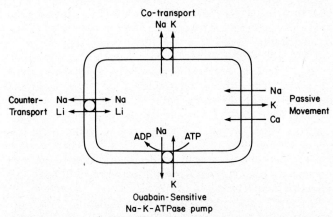

FIGURE 26–20 Schematic representation of four sodium transport mechanisms that have been demonstrated in red blood cells.

arose from the demonstration of alterations in transport mechanisms other than the active, ouabain-sensitive NaK-ATPase pump that is suppressed by natriuretic hormone. The four transport systems shown in Figure 26–20 are only some of those which may be involved in maintaining the marked concentration gradient of sodium between extracellular fluid (with 140 mmol/liter of sodium) and intracellular fluid (with 7 to 10 mmol/liter).[139] The NaK-ATPase pump is likely the primary physiological regulator, whereas the others may operate mainly in the presence of a sodium load.[140] Defects in the other three transport mechanisms in red blood cells shown in Figure 26–20 have been found in the majority of hypertensives tested: passive movement was shown to be increased by Wessels in 1967,[141] the Na-K cotransport mechanism was first found to be suppressed by Garay and Meyer in 1979,[142] and the Na-Li countertransport system was first reported to be increased by Canessa et al. in 1980.[143] About three-fourths of patients have been reported to have either reduced Na-K cotransport or increased Na-Li countertransport[144]; however, the two are often not found together,[145] and they are thought to reflect two different transport proteins.[146]

The decreased Na-K cotransport could result in an increased intracellular sodium concentration and thereby lead into the remainder of the scheme shown at the bottom of Figure 26–19. Moreover, a preliminary report has indicated that a similar cotransport mechanism exists in vascular smooth muscle cells.[147]

These defects may be specifically responsible for the pathogenesis of hypertension or may simply be in vitro markers for another process. Of considerable interest is the evidence that they are inherited, being present in about half the normotensive children of hypertensive parents[148] (Table 26–9). Support for a genetic connection comes from the finding of similar reductions in sodium efflux (i.e., the cotransport mechanism) in the red blood cells of three types of genetically hypertensive rats.[149] Moreover, a higher proportion of black Africans than white Frenchmen have the defect, in keeping with the different frequency of hypertension in the two populations.[150]

Problems with the Sodium Transport Concept. Although the preceding evidence for an inherited defect that could so easily interact with dietary sodium intake to in-

duce hypertension is attractive, discrepancies have already begun to appear. Thus, although countertransport was increased in the red blood cells of hypertensives in both Paris and Boston, the cotransport was reduced in the Parisians but increased in the Bostonians.[146] Other investigators have been unable to find alterations in cotransport in the red cells of patients with essential hypertension compared to normotensives.[151,152] The considerable overlap in cotransport noted by some has brought the use of the test as a genetic marker into question.[153] Moreover, an increased passive influx of Na+ into ouabain-treated red cells was found in 19 of 21 American white hypertensives but no such defect was found in the cells of 32 American black hypertensives.[153a]

Some of these discrepancies may be methodological in origin as well as reflections of variability in drug intake, plasma potassium levels and one or more of a host of factors, such as obesity, that may alter red cell sodium transport.[154] Moreover, the human may be similar to the rat[149] in having multiple genetically determined defects in sodium transport.

Beyond these discrepancies, the applicability of what goes on in the non-nucleated red cell under the highly artificial conditions of the assays used to measure cotransport to what is happening in human vascular tissue obviously remains to be proved, and it will take years to show that the defect serves as a genetic marker by foretelling the appearance of hypertension among normotensives with the defect. But as techniques to measure sodium transport become simpler, we may find one or another that will provide, at the least, a readily available marker of an individual's predisposition to hypertension and, hopefully, an insight into what causes this condition.

Other Hypotheses

At present, the "sodium transport" hypothesis is the most attractive unifying hypothesis for the pathogenesis of hypertension. As shown in Figure 26–19, it encompasses most of the other hypotheses given currency in the recent past—autoregulation, renal pressure-natriuresis, sympathetic-stress, and renin-angiotensin. But before leaving the mechanisms of primary hypertension, let us look at other possible mechanisms and associations with other conditions. In view of the probable role of the renin-angiotensin system both in primary and in some cases of secondary hypertension, further discussion of this system is in order.

THE RENIN-ANGIOTENSIN-ALDOSTERONE SYSTEM

The proteolytic enzyme renin cleaves a substrate protein in plasma to liberate the decapeptide angiotensin I. This inactive prohormone is in turn converted into the potent octapeptide hormone angiotensin II by a converting enzyme. Angiotensin II performs two major related roles: one involves control of blood pressure by constricting arterial vessels, the other control of body fluid volume by increasing renal retention of salt and water (Fig. 26–21). The two effects are the result of multiple actions. In addition, recall the evidence for a direct connection between angiotensin and the previously described sodium transport hypothesis shown in cultured rat aortic smooth muscle cells.[130] When angiotensin II was added to these cells, their perme-

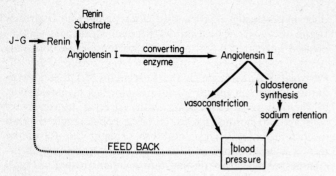

FIGURE 26–21 Overall scheme of the renin-angiotensin mechanism.

ability to sodium was increased threefold and intracellular sodium concentration rose proportionally. Angiotensin may thereby short-circuit part of the scheme shown in Figure 26–19 and induce hypertension by a direct effect on sodium transport.

Increases in renin-angiotensin are directly responsible for renovascular hypertension and are associated with a variety of other hypertensive diseases to be considered subsequently. As noted earlier, inappropriately high levels of angiotensin may be one of the switches that turns on the pathogenetic mechanism. Measuring plasma renin activity (PRA) may also provide a marker for different elements of the hypertensive spectrum.

THE NATURE OF RENIN. Although recognized in 1898, the various forms of renin remain poorly characterized:

1. The human kidney contains at least two forms of renin, most with a molecular weight (MW) of 40,000 but some with a higher MW, around 55,000.[155] Some renal renin is inactive and is biochemically similar to the inactive renin in plasma.[156]

2. In plasma, there appear to be at least three forms of renin: normal, active (MW $\simeq$ 40,000); big, active (MW $\simeq$ 54,000); and big, inactive (MW $\simeq$ 54,000). The third, inactive form can be activated in vitro by acidification or exposure to cold or proteolytic enzymes such as kallikrein.[157,158] The active component is measured by assays using a pH of 5.5 to 7.4, whereas both active and inactive forms are measured by assays using a pH below 4.0. The latter are preferably called assays of plasma renin concentration or total renin activity.

3. Tissue isorenins have also been described, particularly in the brain,[159] where all the components of the system have been identified.[160] A protein having the molecular weight of renin and that is immunologically cross-reactive with renal renin has been said to be synthesized by arterial smooth muscle cells in culture.[161]

4. Another protease enzyme, tonin, purified from rat submaxillary glands, cleaves angiotensin II directly from renin substrate.[162]

Why bother with all these forms of renin, particularly since some are found only after extreme and unphysiological manipulations? Although they may be largely laboratory curiosities, certain hints as to their possible clinical importance have surfaced, suggesting that big or inactive forms of renin may be physiologically potent as precursors

of normal or active renin.[163] Furthermore, this information indicates the need for care in performing renin assays and in interpreting results from different laboratories.[164]

USE OF RENIN ASSAYS. Beyond these methodological considerations, clinicians using renin assays must be aware that various physiological or pharmacological maneuvers may affect the level of plasma renin activity (PRA) (Table 26–11). Since renin release is under multiple controls, these various conditions may influence renin levels by means of more than one mechanism. Thus, upright posture may increase renin by decreasing effective plasma volume, decreasing renal perfusion pressure, and increasing catecholamine levels.

A few of these conditions deserve elucidation:

Age. In both normotensive[165] and hypertensive[80] people, renin levels progressively decline with advancing age, an important factor in the choice of normal controls for comparison with hypertensive patients.

Race. Blacks, both normotensive and hypertensive, have lower renin levels than whites.[80] Values obtained from nor-

TABLE 26–11 CLINICAL CONDITIONS AFFECTING RENIN LEVELS

DECREASED PRA	INCREASED PRA
Expanded fluid volume	*Shrunken fluid volume*
Salt loads, oral or IV	Salt deprivation
Primary salt retention	Fluid losses
(Liddle's syndrome,	Diuretic-induced
Gordon's syndrome)	GI losses
Mineralocorticoid excess	Hemorrhage
Primary aldosteronism	Salt-wasting renal disease
Congenital adrenal hyperplasia	Decreased effective plasma volume
Cushing's syndrome	Upright posture
Licorice excess	Adrenal insufficiency
Deoxycorticosterone (DOC),	Cirrhosis with ascites
18-hydroxy-DOC excess	Nephrotic syndrome
Catecholamine deficiency	*Decreased renal perfusion pressure*
Autonomic dysfunction	Therapy with peripheral
Therapy with adrenergic	vasodilators
neuronal blockers	Renovascular hypertension
Therapy with beta-adrenergic	Accelerated-malignant hypertension
blockers	sion
	Chronic renal disease (renin-dependent)
Hyperkalemia	dent)
	Juxtaglomerular hyperplasia
Decreased renin substrate (?)	(Bartter's syndrome)
Androgen therapy	
	Catecholamine excess
Decrease of renal tissue	Pheochromocytoma
Hyporeninemic hypoaldosteronism	Stress: hypoglycemia, trauma
Chronic renal disease (volume-dependent)	Exercise
Anephric state	Hyperthyroidism
Increasing age	Caffeine
Unknown	*Hypokalemia*
Low-renin essential hypertension	
	Increased renin substrate
	Pregnancy
	Estrogen therapy
	Autonomous renin hypersecretion
	Renin-secreting tumors
	Acute damage to juxtaglomerular cells
	Acute renal failure
	Acute glomerulonephritis
	Unknown
	High-renin essential hypertension

From Kaplan, N. M.: Clinical Hypertension. 3rd ed. Baltimore, Williams and Wilkins Co., 1982, p. 220.

mal blacks should probably be used when defining the renin status of hypertensive blacks.

Posture. A few minutes of standing will markedly elevate renin levels.[166] Posture can conveniently be used as a stimulus for renin testing and must be taken into account in clinical use of the procedure. If "basal" levels are being examined, patients should be supine for at least an hour.

Dietary sodium intake. Renin levels will increase in patients ingesting less that 75 mEq of sodium per day.

Natural variation. Without any obvious cause, renin secretion varies from minute to minute and displays a diurnal rhythm.[167]

Exogenous factors. Some drugs affect renin levels by means of obvious effects on the blood pressure and body fluid volume. Estrogens routinely increase PRA by their activation of the hepatic synthesis of renin substrate, so that more angiotensin is generated for any given level of renin. Inhibitors of prostaglandin synthesis (e.g., aspirin and indomethacin) will blunt the renin response to diuretic stimulation.[168] The amount of caffeine in two or three cups of coffee will increase PRA, presumably by activation of catecholamine release.[169]

The patient's *sex* and the *level of the blood pressure* may also affect renin responsiveness; women and patients with higher diastolic levels responded less well to diuretics and upright posture.[170]

The lesson to be learned from all this is that renin secretion and PRA levels can be altered by a multitude of factors, some easily recognized and avoided and others still not identified. Even when the same assay procedure and testing conditions are used in the same patients without any recognizable changes in their conditions, renin status may change. Twenty-two of 85 patients initially found to have a low renin level in response to a low-salt diet plus upright posture had a normal renin level when retested.[171] Differences in renin status appear when different stimuli are used. When nine different stimuli were used in the same 47 hypertensive patients, only 28 per cent had consistently normal levels, and none of the testing procedures provided maximal detection of both low- and high-renin states.[172] The prudent clinician will take as many of the known variables into account as possible and recognize the vagaries of PRA, taking care neither to ascribe more certainty to a given level than is justified nor to make important diagnostic, prognostic, or therapeutic decisions based upon small differences.

RENIN LEVELS IN ESSENTIAL HYPERTENSION. Many studies have reaffirmed Helmer's original findings[173] that among patients with uncomplicated essential hypertension, about 30 per cent have low values, 60 per cent normal, and 10 per cent high.

The percentage of cases of low-renin hypertension progressively increases as the age of the population increases. Although this may represent a different underlying hypertensive process, more likely it simply reflects a progressive decline in functioning juxtaglomerular cells or in their responsiveness, a process that occurs in normal subjects as well but is accentuated in hypertensive individuals, in whom nephrosclerosis is usually more advanced.[174]

The separation of patients into low, normal, and high categories is in large part artifactual. The dividing line between low and normal is arbitrary and depends upon the type of analysis applied to the data. Renin levels in essential hypertension follow a continuous distribution curve, with a predominance of lower values because of the larger proportion of blacks and older people in the hypertensive population[175] (Fig. 26–22). As shown in this schematic view, PRA measurements can be useful for recognizing certain hypertensive syndromes with distinctly low or high levels. For the majority of patients with essential hypertension, little is to be gained from a determination of their renin status.

The concept that renin profiling could identify the relative contributions of vasoconstriction and volume to the underlying hypertensive process has been proposed.[176] According to this bipolar vasoconstriction-volume analysis of hypertension, arteriolar vasoconstriction by angiotensin II is predominantly responsible for the hypertension in patients with "high renin," and volume expansion is predominantly responsible in those with "low renin." When renin levels and the relative proportions of volume and vasoconstriction have actually been measured, no such relation has been found.[92,177] In fact, as renin levels increased, peripheral resistance progressively decreased—the reverse effect of that predicted by this proposal.[177]

THE ROLE OF RENIN IN ESSENTIAL HYPERTENSION. Foregoing the confusion as to the actual significance of renin levels, let us reexamine the question whether or not the renin-angiotensin-aldosterone mechanism plays a role in the pathogenesis of essential hypertension. The available evidence suggests a limited role at most. As an example, renin levels were *lower* in a group of "pre-hypertensive" young adults with sustained higher levels of blood pressure.[178] However, some argue that the role for renin is much greater.[176]

As we have seen, most patients with essential hypertension have normal levels of PRA. Since high pressure in the renal afferent arterioles should suppress the release of re-

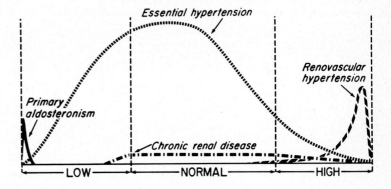

FIGURE 26–22 Schematic representation of plasma renin activity in various hypertensive diseases. The expected number of patients with each type of hypertension is indicated along with their proportion of low, normal, or high renin levels. (From Kaplan, N. M.: Renin profiles: The unfulfilled promises. *J.A.M.A. 238*:611, 1977. Copyright 1977, American Medical Association.)

nin from the juxtaglomerular cells through the baroreceptor mechanism, the presence of normal renin levels may be considered inappropriate. Thus, the normal negative feedback between blood pressure and renin release may be imperfect in hypertension, resulting in inappropriately high renin levels, which may contribute to the hypertension. Support for a possible role of renin in such patients comes from the fall in their blood pressure when they are given an inhibitor of the enzyme that converts the inactive angiotensin I to the active angiotensin II.[179] This same enzyme is also responsible for the inactivation of the vasodepressor bradykinin, so the fall in blood pressure could reflect bradykinin accumulation and not necessarily indicate a role for renin.

A number of possible explanations for these "inappropriately" normal renin levels have been provided:

1. Renin release cannot be normally turned off: When exogenous angiotensin II was infused into normal-renin and high-renin hypertensives, their plasma renin levels were not suppressed normally.[180]

2. Renin release is being driven by heightened adrenergic stimulation: Esler et al.[181] found increased neural stimulation of renin release in patients with high-renin hypertension, as reflected in higher basal levels of plasma norepinephrine, greater responsiveness of PRA to the adrenergically mediated stimulus of upright posture, and a greater degree of suppression by beta-adrenergic blockade.

3. Renin release is abnormally sensitive to adrenergic stimulation: Morganti et al.[182] found that patients with high renin levels had normal plasma levels of norepinephrine and similar rises after the head-up tilt test. They conclude, therefore, that the degree of neural stimulation is not different but rather that the sensitivity of renin responsiveness is increased.

4. The adrenal aldosterone response to angiotensin II is decreased: Some patients with either normal or high renin levels show a subnormal rise in plasma aldosterone in response to endogenous and exogenous angiotensin II.[183] If aldosterone and the body fluid volume that it regulates are poorly responsive to angiotensin, it would require higher levels to "close the volume-renin-aldosterone feedback loop, potentially resulting in greater vasoconstrictor activity."[184]

On the other hand, those with low renin levels, which seem more appropriate to primary hypertension, may owe their low levels to increased sensitivity of adrenal receptors to angiotensin, so that less renin-angiotensin would be needed to maintain fluid volume; when given exogenous angiotensin, low-renin patients show a supernormal rise in plasma aldosterone.[185]

We are left with no clear definition of the role of renin-angiotensin in essential hypertension. In patients with natural or induced high renin levels, renin-angiotensin probably has a considerable influence. In the majority of hypertensive patients, with normal or low renin levels, the effect of renin-angiotensin on hypertension is probably only minimal.

LOW-RENIN ESSENTIAL HYPERTENSION. The presence of low or suppressed renin levels in 30 per cent of the hypertensive population, as previously argued, most likely represents a Gaussian distribution curve that is shifted toward the low side by the larger proportion of blacks and older people and not indicative of a peculiar form of hypertension. Nonetheless, the known presence of low renin levels in other hypertensive diseases associated with mineralocorticoid excess or volume expansion (Table 26–12) has prompted an extensive search for such a mechanism in low-renin essential hypertension. In addition, some believe that patients with low renin levels may have a better prognosis and special therapeutic needs.

Diagnosis. The possible mechanisms for low-renin hypertension go beyond volume expansion with or without mineralocorticoid excess (Table 26–12), although an expanded body fluid volume is a logical explanation for

---

TABLE 26–12   LOW-RENIN HYPERTENSION

POSSIBLE MECHANISMS	CLINICAL EXPRESSION
I. "Physiologic" inhibition of renin release	
A. Increased pressure at the juxtaglomerular apparatus and/or increased sodium at macula densa	
1. Elevated perfusion pressure	Primary hypertension
2. Expanded effective plasma volume	
a. Renal sodium retention	
(1) Primary	Liddle's syndrome
(2) Secondary to increased mineralocorticoid activity	
(a) Aldosterone	Primary aldosteronism
(b) Deoxycorticosterone (DOC)	Congenital adrenal hyperplasia, adrenal tumors
(c) 18-OH-DOC and other steroids	
(d) Glycyrrhizinic acid	Licorice, carbenoxolone toxicity
b. Prolonged excessive salt intake in genetically predisposed	
c. Decreased natiuretic hormone	
3. Decreased capacity of vascular bed	
B. Decreased sympathetic nervous system activity	Diabetes mellitus, adrenergic blocking drugs
C. Increased potassium intake	
D. Increased systemic or intrarenal angiotensin II	
II. Derangement of juxtaglomerular apparatus	
A. Inability to produce or release renin	Chronic renal disease, (?) primary hypertension
B. Defect in sensing mechanism	(?) Primary hypertension
III. Interference with generation of angiotensin II in vitro or enhanced generation of angiotensin II in vivo	
IV. Increased sensitivity to angiotensin II	(?) Primary hypertension

From Kaplan, N. K.: Clinical Hypertension. 3rd ed. Baltimore, Williams and Wilkins Co., 1982.

low-renin hypertension. Even though such expansion has been reported, the majority of careful analyses have failed to indicate any abnormality. In one of the better studies, total exchangeable sodium was shown to be the same in low-renin hypertensives as in normal-renin hypertensives and normotensive controls, whereas it was appropriately expanded in untreated primary aldosteronism.[186]

If volume expansion were responsible for low-renin hypertension, a logical mechanism would be an excess in mineralocorticoid hormone. Despite initial claims that an excess of one or another mineralocorticoid is present, subsequent study has failed to document either the excess or the mineralocorticoid potency of the putative hormone.[187] Perhaps most meaningful is the observation that the plasma in low-renin hypertension, unlike that of patients with known mineralocorticoid excess, displays no excessive competition for binding to mineralocorticoid receptors,[188] suggesting that the search for such a hormone may prove to be futile.

Prognosis. As noted earlier in this chapter, one retrospective study showed that patients with low-renin hypertension had no myocardial infarcts or strokes over a 7-year interval, whereas 11 per cent of normal-renin and 14 per cent of high-renin patients had experienced one of these cardiovascular complications.[45] A number of subsequent studies have failed to document an improved prognosis in low-renin hypertension.[46] The only prospective study has found equal numbers of myocardial infarcts and strokes among those with initially low renin levels as among those with initially normal levels.[47] A rise in renin levels was noted after a vascular complication, providing a plausible explanation for those few retrospective studies which have reported a lower incidence of complications in low-renin hypertensives.

Therapy. In keeping with their presumed volume excess, patients with low-renin essential hypertension have been found to have a greater fall in blood pressure when given diuretics than do normal-renin patients.[189] However, others report no difference between the response to diuretics in the two groups.[190]

If low-renin hypertensive patients do respond better to diuretics, the response does not necessarily indicate a greater volume load. By definition, patients with low renin are less responsive to stimuli that increase renin levels, including diuretics, so that they experience a lower rise in PRA with diuretic therapy. Less renin and angiotensin could result in less compensatory vasoconstriction and aldosterone secretion, so that volume depletion would proceed and the blood pressure would fall further in low-renin hypertensive patients given a diuretic.

In the aggregate, the evidence that patients with low renin are unique in the spectrum of essential hypertension seems slim. For now, the prudent clinician should assume that the determination of renin status has little to offer in deciding on the management of patients with essential hypertension.

VASOPRESSIN

High endogenous levels of this hormone have been incriminated in certain experimental models of hypertension, but measurements in humans do not substantiate a relation between even very high plasma levels and hypertension.[191]

VASODEPRESSOR DEFICIENCY

In addition to an excess of the various pressor hormones, a deficiency of one or more vasodepressor hormones may be involved in experimental and clinical hypertension.

Bradykinin. This nonapeptide is cleaved from a protein substrate, kininogen, by the action of the enzyme kallikrein. It is difficult to measure bradykinin levels, and its role remains undefined. Decreased urinary excretion of kallikrein was found in some patients with essential hypertension.[192] However, subsequent study has found no evidence of systemic deficiency of kallikrein or bradykinin in patients with essential hypertension.[193]

Prostaglandins. These ubiquitous fatty-acid derivatives have profound pharmacological effects, but their involvement in human disease remains unproved. Recently, prostaglandins that act at their site of synthesis have been shown to produce physiologically important effects, so that the search for circulating prostaglandins may be futile. Prostacyclin, synthesized within the vessel wall, is vasodilatory; thromboxane A, released from platelets, is vasoconstrictive.[194]

The major site of prostaglandin action relative to hypertension may be in the kidney. PGE_2 is synthesized mainly in the renal medulla by medullary interstitial cells. When PGE_2 or the precursor, arachidonic acid, is infused into the renal artery, renal vasodilation, increased renal blood flow, and natriuresis follow. Thus, PGE_2 may protect against ischemia. When renal blood flow is compromised, both renin and prostaglandins are released. By this mechanism the kidney can raise systemic blood pressure via renin-angiotensin without diminishing renal blood flow, since intrarenal prostaglandins would counteract the effects of intrarenal angiotensin.[195] A deficiency of PGE_2 might then lead to hypertension by impairing renal function and permitting fluid retention as well as by accentuating the ill effects of renin-angiotensin. Decreased levels of urinary PGE_2 have been measured in hypertensive patients and have been related to decreased renal blood flow and urinary sodium excretion.[196]

Renomedullary Lipids. In addition to the acidic prostaglandins, two lipids from renomedullary interstitial cells have been identified which exert definite antihypertensive effects in animals.[196a] One is neutral, the other highly polar. The polar vasodepressor substance appears to be an alkyl ether analog of phosphatidylcholine. The role of these renomedullary lipids in human pathophysiology is not yet known.

OTHER POSSIBLE MECHANISMS

The preceding does not exhaust the list of suggested mechanisms for essential hypertension. Excesses or deficiencies of various minerals and changing ratios among dietary sodium, calcium, and potassium have also been postulated. Of these various claims, the evidence for a lower dietary calcium intake among hypertensives is most impressive.[197] Yet the blood pressure has been found to correlate directly with both serum and urinary levels of calcium.[198] Hypertensives may have a renal leak of calcium, compensated for by increased secretion of parathyroid hormone. A possible role of endogenous opioid peptides in the regulation of blood pressure has been noted in animals,[199] but there are no data pertaining to humans. Support for these and other postulated mechanisms is meager, and the overall scheme shown in Figure 26–19 seems more than adequate to explain the pathogenesis of essential hypertension. However, a number of associations between essential hypertension and other conditions have been noted and may offer additional insights into the potential causes and possible prevention of the disease.

Associations With Other Conditions

OBESITY.   Despite the possible overestimation of blood pressure levels in the obese because of the use of small sphygmomanometer cuffs, true hypertension is more common among these individuals and adds to their risk of developing ischemic heart disease.[200] The association of excessive weight gain with the development of hypertension has been particularly obvious in children and young adults.[19] It is hoped that the prevention of obesity will reduce the incidence of hypertension.

The manner in which obesity causes hypertension likely involves the mass of fat per se.[201] In terms of hemodynamics, overweight hypertensives may have an inappropriately increased cardiac output and a relatively restricted arterial capacity.[202] It is of interest that the red cells of a group of obese *normotensive* Pima Indians showed reduced NaK-ATPase activity[203] in a manner analogous to that shown in Figure 26–19 to be possibly involved in the pathogenesis of hypertension.

Weight reduction as a means of treating established hypertension is discussed in Chapter 27.

ALCOHOL INTAKE.   In the Framingham cohort, the prevalence of hypertension in those who drank more than an average of two ounces of ethanol or three mixed drinks a day was higher than in those who drank less[204] (Fig. 26–23). In other studies, a linear correlation between alcohol consumption and blood pressure has been observed, which is independent of age, adiposity, and smoking.[205] Despite their increased propensity for developing hypertension, those who drink one or two ounces of alcohol a day have less coronary heart disease than either teetotalers or heavier drinkers.[206]

SMOKING.   Cigarette smoking raises the blood pressure, probably through the nicotine-induced release of norepinephrine from adrenergic nerves.[207] Yet when smokers quit, a trivial rise in blood pressure may occur, probably reflecting a gain in weight.[208]

DIABETES MELLITUS (See also p. 1738).   Hypertension is present in about two-thirds of longstanding diabetics with the intercapillary glomerulosclerosis described by Kimmelstiel and Wilson, and the prevalence of essential hypertension in the overall diabetic population is somewhat increased.[209] This may be related to an exaggerated pressor responsiveness to norepinephrine observed in a group of diabetics without renal insufficiency.[210]

When hypertensive, diabetics may confront some interesting problems. With progressive renal insufficiency and autonomic neuropathy, they may have few functioning juxtaglomerular cells and a reduced ability to stimulate the release of renin. As a result, very low renin levels are frequently observed, with a tendency toward the syndrome of hyporeninemic hypoaldosteronism. If hypoglycemia develops because of too much insulin or other drugs, severe hypertension may occur as a result of stimulated sympathetic nervous activity.

When treated for hypertension, diabetics are also susceptible to some special problems. Diuretics may exacerbate their carbohydrate intolerance, probably by inducing potassium deficiency. Those who are brittle and prone to hypoglycemia may have problems if they are given beta blockers, since their protective catecholamine response would be blunted, and severe hypoglycemia might develop without warning.

POLYCYTHEMIA (See also p. 1684).   Polycythemia vera is frequently associated with hypertension. More common is a "pseudo" or "stress" polycythemia with a high hematocrit and increased blood viscosity but contracted plasma volume as well as normal red cell mass and serum erythropoietin levels.[211] Such patients may also have elevated plasma fibrinogen levels.[212] Cerebral blood flow was reduced in patients with hematocrits between 47 and 58 per cent and rose significantly after venesection.[213] Reduction of the blood pressure may normalize the hematocrit and blood viscosity.[211]

GOUT.   Hyperuricemia is present in 25 to 50 per cent of individuals with untreated essential hypertension—about five times the frequency among normotensive persons.[214] In 71 male hypertensives, asymptomatic hyperuricemia was associated with decreased renal blood flow, presumably a reflection of nephrosclerosis.[75] When diuretics are used, the uric acid level rises further; however, even after prolonged exposure, patients with diuretic-induced hyperuricemia do not seem to develop urate deposition, so that treatment for the elevated uric acid level is usually unnecessary.[215] Nonetheless, gout may be precipitated in those who are genetically susceptible.

OTHER DISEASES.   Cancer mortality has been found to be increased among hypertensives without relation to therapy or other known risk factors.[216] On the other

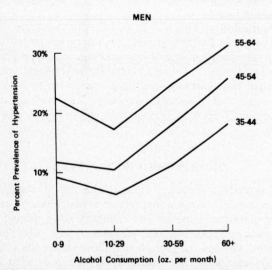

FIGURE 26–23   Prevalence of hypertension in various age groups in Framingham study plotted against their average alcohol consumption. (From Kannel, W. B., and Sorlie, P.: Hypertension in Framingham. *In* Paul, O. (ed.): Epidemiology and Control of Hypertension. Miami, Symposia Specialists, 1975.)

hand, a lower death rate from cancer among hypertensives was reported from England.[217]

Other diseases and conditions have been found more commonly in patients with essential hypertension, including uterine fibromyoma, color blindness, and increased intraocular pressure.[4] In addition, a number of diseases themselves induce hypertension, and these will now be discussed.

SECONDARY FORMS OF HYPERTENSION

These will be considered in the approximate order of their frequency based on the data shown in Table 26–5: oral contraceptive use, renal parenchymal disease, renovascular hypertension (and renin-secreting tumors), adrenal causes of hypertension (primary aldosteronism, Cushing's syndrome, pheochromocytoma, and congenital adrenal hyperplasia), and a miscellaneous group. Of the less common forms listed in Table 26–4, only those recently elucidated will be discussed.

Oral Contraceptive Use

The use of estrogen-containing oral contraceptive pills may be the most common cause of secondary hypertension. Most women who take them experience a slight rise in blood pressure, and about 5 per cent will develop hypertension (i.e., a blood pressure above 140/90 mm Hg) within five years of pill use—more than twice the incidence seen among women of the same age who do not use the pill.[218] Although the hypertension is usually mild, it may persist after the pill is discontinued, may be severe, and is almost certainly a factor in the increased cardiovascular mortality seen in young women who take oral contraceptives. Despite these facts, the pill has provided effective and safe birth control for millions of women and the need for oral contraceptives remains.[219]

The dangers of the pill need to be put into proper perspective. While it is true that use of the pill is associated with increased morbidity and mortality, overall mortality from cardiovascular diseases has been progressively declining among women in the United States, at a rate equal to that noted among American men. Although the relative rates of coronary and cerebral vascular diseases are increased three- to seven fold among users of the pill—and much of this effect persists even after the pill is stopped— the absolute number of women affected is small, particularly among those below age 35 who do not smoke.[220] The excess annual death rate attributable to pill use for women under 35 who do not smoke is one per 77,000, whereas for women 35 to 44 who smoke the excess is one per 2,000. Thus, for most, the pill—particularly the currently used low-estrogen and progestogen forms—seems safe for the purposes of temporary birth control.

Hypertension is likely one of the major contributors to the cardiovascular complications from the pill, in concert with an increased tendency for the blood to clot, changes in lipid and carbohydrate metabolism, an increase in coronary artery smooth muscle tone, and proliferation of fibroblasts and smooth muscle cells in vessel walls.[221] The propensity toward a rise in blood pressure is accentuated by heavy alcohol intake: among women taking the pill, consumption of more than 10 ounces of ethanol a week was associated with a systolic blood pressure 8 mm Hg higher than that among those drinking 0.1 to 1.1 ounces a week.[222]

INCIDENCE. The best data on the incidence of pill-induced hypertension have come from a large, ongoing study by the Royal College of General Practitioners. They found a 2.6 times greater incidence of hypertension among 23,000 pill-users compared to 23,000 nonusers, resulting in a 5 per cent incidence over five years of pill use.[218] The incidence of hypertension increased with long duration of pill use, being only slightly higher than that among the controls during the first year but rising to almost three times higher by the fifth year.

Similar data have come from a survey of 13,358 American women, with new cases of hypertension occurring over a three-year period at a rate of 6.8 per 1,000 among pill-users compared to 1.2 per 1,000 among nonusers.[223] In a much smaller but more carefully performed prospective study of 186 Scottish women, during the first two years of pill use the systolic pressure rose in 164 (by more than 25 mm Hg in 8) and the diastolic pressure rose in 150 (by more than 20 mm Hg in two).[224] After three years, the mean rise in 83 of these women was 9.2 mm Hg (Fig. 26–24). Use of smaller amounts of estrogen than the 50 μg taken by most of these women may induce less hypertension: In six women whose blood pressure returned to normal when they were not on oral contraceptives, mean blood pressure was considerably higher (172/112) with the 50-μg estrogen pill than the level of 155/95 recorded with a 30-μg estrogen pill.[225] Obviously more data are needed to document the possibility that lower-dose pills are safer.

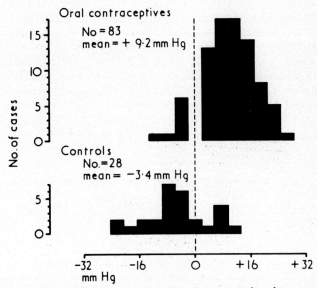

FIGURE 26–24 Changes in systolic blood pressure after three years in 83 women taking oral contraceptives and in 28 controls using mechanical methods of contraception. (Weir, J. R., et al.: Blood pressure in women taking oral contraceptives. Br. Med. J. 7:533, 1974.)

CLINICAL FEATURES

Predisposing Factors. Any woman taking estrogens may develop hypertension, but the likelihood is much greater among those over age 35 and in those who are obese. A positive family history of hypertension is present in about half. The presence of hypertension during a prior pregnancy increases the likelihood but not enough to preclude pill use in such women who require contraception. One in 20 women with prior pregnancy-induced hypertension became hypertensive while on the pill over a three-year period—twice the rate among nulliparous women taking the same contraceptive.[226] Interestingly, women with sustained hypertension did not experience a further rise in blood pressure during a one-year period of pill use.[227]

Course of the Hypertension. In most women, the hypertension is mild, but in some it may accelerate rapidly and cause severe renal damage. When the pill is discontinued, blood pressure falls to normal within three to six months in about one-half of cases. Whether the pill caused permanent hypertension in the other half or just uncovered essential hypertension at an earlier time remains unknown. Among 14 women whose hypertension receded when the pill was discontinued, seven developed spontaneous hypertension during the subsequent six years.[228] In a few patients, the hypertension rapidly accelerates and causes extensive renal damage, very rarely a full-blown hemolytic uremic syndrome.[229] Even when the hypertension recedes after the pill is stopped, considerable renal damage may persist.[230]

MECHANISMS OF HYPERTENSION. The pill likely causes hypertension by renin-aldosterone–mediated volume expansion. Increases in body weight, plasma volume, and cardiac output were measured in 30 women given an oral contraceptive for two to three months, even though their blood pressure rose very little over this short interval.[231]

Estrogens and the synthetic progestogens used in oral contraceptive pills both cause sodium retention. This likely results from the following sequence (Fig. 26–25). (1) Estrogen increases the hepatic synthesis of renin substrate. (2) In the presence of increased substrate, more angiotensin is generated from whatever level of renin is present in the circulation. As a result of the increased level of angiotensin II, renin release is partially inhibited, so that its concentration in peripheral blood is lowered. Nonetheless, overall plasma renin activity and angiotensin II levels remain elevated. (3) The increased levels of angiotensin stimulate ad-renal synthesis of aldosterone. (4) Aldosterone causes sodium retention. At the same time, systemic and renal vasoconstriction is induced by the angiotensin, and renal blood flow is shifted downward.[232] Significant elevations of blood pressure may occur only in those with the greatest degree of vascular sensitivity to the increased levels of angiotensin.

When women with pill-induced hypertension are given the angiotensin antagonist saralasin, blood pressure falls in those whose blood pressure subsequently becomes normal when the pill is stopped.[233] Thus, the overall evidence strongly supports a renin-angiotensin-aldosterone mechanism in pill-induced hypertension, with a greater sensitivity to this mechanism in the 5 per cent of women who develop overt hypertension.

The amount of progestogen may also influence the development of vascular disease: In the original Royal College data, more hypertension was seen with higher doses of progestogen.[218] Subsequently, more vascular disease has been noted with the use of 250 μg of levonorgestrel than with 150 μg of this progestogen.[234]

MANAGEMENT. The use of estrogen-containing oral contraceptives should be restricted in women over age 35, particularly if they are already hypertensive, smoke, have hypercholesterolemia, and are obese. Women given the pill should be properly monitored as follows: (1) the supply should be limited initially to three months and thereafter to six months; (2) the patient should be required to return for a blood pressure check before an additional supply is provided; and (3) if blood pressure has risen, an alternative contraceptive should be offered.[235]

If the pill remains the only acceptable contraceptive, the elevated blood pressure can be reduced with appropriate therapy. In view of the probable role of aldosterone, use of a diuretic-spironolactone combination seems appropriate. In those who stop taking the pill, evaluation for secondary hypertensive diseases should be postponed for at least three months to allow the renin-aldosterone changes to remit. If the hypertension does not recede, additional workup and therapy may be needed.

POSTMENOPAUSAL ESTROGEN USE. Millions of women use estrogen for its potential benefits after menopause. These "replacement" doses do not induce hypertension as often as in those who use estrogen for contraception,[236] even though they do induce the various changes in the renin-aldosterone mechanism seen with the pill.[237] In fact, lower blood pressures have been reported

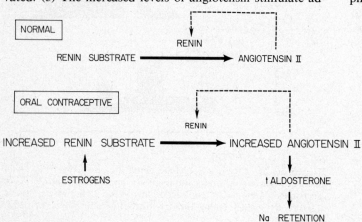

FIGURE 26–25 Schematic representation of the changes in the renin-angiotensin system induced by oral contraceptives containing estrogen. The dotted lines show the feedback inhibition of renin release by angiotensin II.

among postmenopausal estrogen users.[238] Moreover, two case-control studies have shown a significantly *lower* mortality rate from coronary heart disease among postmenopausal estrogen users than nonusers.[239,240]

Renal Parenchymal Disease
(See also Chapter 52)

Beyond the oral contraceptive pill, renal parenchymal disease, mainly chronic glomerulonephritis, is the most common form of secondary hypertension, responsible for 2 to 4 per cent of cases of hypertension seen in unselected adult populations (Table 26–5). As chronic renal disease worsens, hypertension usually appears and contributes further to the deterioration of renal function. In addition, primary hypertension is a common *cause* of progressive renal damage. In the United States, it is responsible for at least one of every six patients with end-stage renal disease (ESRD) entering chronic dialysis or renal transplantation programs.[79] Their higher prevalence of hypertension is likely responsible for the significantly higher rate of ESRD among American blacks; with hypertension as the underlying cause in one-third to one-half of these cases.

Not only does hypertension cause renal failure and renal failure cause hypertension, but more subtle renal dysfunction may be involved in the 95 per cent of patients with primary (essential) hypertension. As discussed earlier (pp. 864 to 867), the kidneys may initiate the hemodynamic cascade that eventuates in primary hypertension. As that disease progresses, some renal dysfunction is demonstrable in most patients, and progressive renal damage is the end result and the cause of death in at least 10 per cent of hypertensives. As we have already seen, and shall document further in Chapter 27, early therapy will protect against nephrosclerosis, so that there is hope that the control of hypertension will slow the progression and reduce the frequency of end-stage renal disease.

In considering hypertension with renal parenchymal disease, we shall follow a sequence of progressively worsening renal damage:

1. Acute renal diseases that are often reversible.
2. Unilateral and bilateral diseases without renal insufficiency.
3. Chronic renal disease with renal insufficiency.
4. Hypertension in the anephric state and after renal transplantation.

ACUTE RENAL DISEASES

Hypertension may appear with any sudden, severe insult to the kidneys that markedly impairs either the excretion of salt and water, leading to volume expansion, or the reduction of renal blood flow, setting off the renin-angiotensin mechanism. Bilateral ureteral obstruction is an example of the former; sudden bilateral renal artery occlusion, as by emboli, is an example of the latter. Relief of either may dramatically reverse severe hypertension. Some of the collagen diseases may also produce rapidly progressive renal damage. The more common acute processes are glomerulonephritis and oliguric renal failure.

Acute Glomerulonephritis. The classic syndrome of type-specific poststreptococcal nephritis appearing after pharyngitis has become much less common, but acute glomerulonephritis is involved in a variety of diseases of diverse causes and courses. Moreover, although the epidemic poststreptococcal disease is still usually self-limited,[241] recent reports have documented a progressive smoldering course in some patients that may lead to renal insufficiency.[242] Patients with sporadic disease may have underlying, previously unrecognized chronic renal disease, and they frequently have progressive renal disease with hypertension.[243] Typically, hypertension accompanies the oliguria and fluid retention of the acute injury. Renal damage is usually obvious based on urinary findings, but these may be minimal, and hypertension of a severe nature may be the overriding feature. Although the hypertension probably reflects fluid expansion, peripheral resistance has been found to be increased.[244] Absolute renin levels are usually not very high but may be inappropriately elevated in the presence of overexpansion of fluid volume and hypertension.[245]

Regardless of the mechanism, the hypertension is best relieved by fluid and sodium restriction and by appropriate doses of potent diuretics such as furosemide. Dialysis and parenteral antihypertensive drugs may be needed if encephalopathy supervenes. In milder cases, the hypertension recedes as the edema is relieved. However, some patients have a rapidly progressive course, often with prolonged anuria.

Acute Oliguric Renal Failure. More commonly, acute renal failure appears after shock develops in patients in whom renin levels are already high, such as cirrhotics with ascites or at the end of pregnancy. The release of even more renin by decreased blood pressure and effective circulating blood volume may flood the renal vasculature and cause such intense renal vasoconstriction that renal function shuts down.[246] A hemolytic-uremic syndrome may accompany the acute renal failure.[247]

Hypertension in this setting is usually not an important problem and can be controlled by preventing volume overload. High doses of furosemide may be helpful, but dialysis is often needed. Although this may allow recovery even after prolonged oliguria, up to 50 per cent of patients with acute renal failure die, usually from complications of the underlying disease responsible for the renal failure.[248]

Vasculitis. Rapidly progressive renal deterioration with severe hypertension occurs not infrequently in the course of scleroderma and other forms of vasculitis (see Chap. 47). Therapy with antihypertensives, particularly angiotensin-converting enzyme inhibitors, may reverse the process.[249]

RENAL DISEASE WITHOUT RENAL INSUFFICIENCY

Although an entire kidney may be removed without obvious effect and no rise in blood pressure, hypertension may be associated with unilateral and bilateral renal parenchymal diseases in the absence of significant renal insufficiency. Such hypertension may reflect other unrecognized processes, but most likely it is caused by activation of the renin-angiotensin mechanism. However, in some patients whose hypertension has been relieved by correction of a renal defect, the levels of renin have not been found to be high.

Unilateral Renal Parenchymal Disease. Congenital hypoplasia and acquired infections may affect only one kidney, causing a reduction in size and function. Most of these small kidneys do not cause hypertension, and when they are indiscriminately removed, hypertension is relieved in only about 25 per cent of patients.[250] Of that 25 per cent, most have arterial occlusive disease, either as the primary cause of the renal atrophy or secondary to irregular scarring of the parenchyma.[251] In many of these cases, high levels of renin can be found in the venous blood from the shrunken kidney,[252] while in some, renal vein renin tests have been falsely negative.[253]

Renal tumors, including rare juxtaglomerular cell tumors, Wilms' tumors, and hypernephromas, may be accompanied by renin-induced hypertension.[254]

Hydronephrosis. Either unilateral or bilateral ureteral obstruction may cause hypertension, and relief of the obstruction may also relieve the hypertension. In most patients with curable hypertension from hydronephrosis, renin levels are increased.[255]

Polycystic Kidney Disease. Although patients with adult polycystic kidney disease usually progress to renal insufficiency, some retain reasonably normal glomerular filtration rates (GFR) and display no azotemia during their course. Hypertension, although more common in those with renal failure, is present in perhaps half of those with a normal GFR and likely reflects variable degrees of both renin excess and fluid retention.[256]

Chronic Pyelonephritis. The relationship between pyelonephritis and hypertension is multifaceted: pyelonephritis, either unilateral or bilateral, may cause hypertension[257]; hypertensive individuals may be more susceptible to renal infection.[258] In patients with hypertension but fairly normal renal function, renin levels are usually high,[259] probably from interstitial scarring with obstruction of intrarenal vessels.

CHRONIC RENAL DISEASES WITH RENAL INSUFFICIENCY

As dialysis and transplantation prolong the lives of more patients with renal insufficiency, their hypertension must be dealt with over much longer periods. Hypertension in most patients with renal insufficiency is predominantly caused by volume overload. With proper attention to salt and water intake and adequate dialysis, control of the blood pressure is usually not particularly difficult. Unfortunately, some patients are much more fragile, alternating between low and high pressures, and some are much more resistant, presumably because of a greater contribution of high renin levels to their hypertension. With judicious use of available therapy, hypertension should not be a major problem for most patients with renal insufficiency. However, in concert with various mechanisms for vascular damage,[260] hypertension remains a major risk factor for the increasing prevalence of cardiovascular disease in these patients.

Mechanisms for Hypertension. Volume excess is the predominant mechanism for hypertension, and this may involve increases in pressor sensitivity to sodium,[261] redistribution of more fluid into the intravascular space,[261] and inhibition of sodium transport via NaK-ATPase pumps.[262] Some degree of renin-mediated vasoconstriction is probably involved in many and may be unmasked by therapy with angiotensin-converting enzyme inhibitors.[263] In addition, adrenergic hyperactivity may contribute, although this too may be apparent only after therapy.[264]

This admixture of mechanisms for the clinical syndrome has also been observed in experimental studies of renal hypertension. However, confusion has arisen largely because models appropriate for renovascular hypertension have been used inappropriately to study the "renoprival" hypertension of chronic renal disease. When appropriate models are used, *volume* is the predominant mechanism for the hypertension of renal insufficiency and *renin* the predominant mechanism for renovascular hypertension. In Figure 26–26, the effects of removing sodium and water and their reinfusion are shown in four groups of rats, including a normal group and a group without kidneys.[265] The anephric animals are exquisitely sensitive to volume changes. In the next group, animals with one kidney removed and the artery to the other partially clamped (the one kidney–one clip Goldblatt model), the pressure is also responsive to volume, but it remains above normal even after excess volume is removed, presumably reflecting the persistence of excess renin. This is a model for *renovascular hypertension plus renal insufficiency*. In the fourth group, one renal artery is clamped and the other kidney is intact (two kidney–one clip Goldblatt model). This is the model for *renovascular hypertension* most frequently seen in humans. When volume is initially reduced, blood pressure rises even further, probably because even more renin is secreted. After volume is restored, the blood pressure changes little.

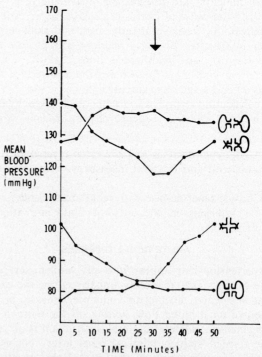

FIGURE 26–26 Effects on blood pressure in four different groups of rats by removal of sodium by peritoneal dialysis at time zero and the reinfusion of an equal amount of saline at the time indicated by the arrow. The symbols at the right (from the top) define the groups of animals studied as follows: one renal artery clipped and the other left untouched; one renal artery clipped and the other kidney removed; both kidneys removed; sham bilateral nephrectomy. (From Swales, J. D., et al.: Dual mechanism for experimental hypertension. Lancet 2:1181, 1971.)

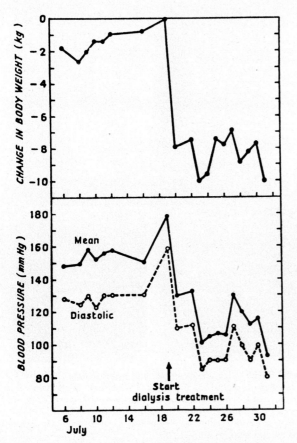

FIGURE 26–27 Effect of decrease in body fluid volume because of dialysis upon the blood pressure of a patient with chronic renal disease. (From Blumberg, A., et al.: Extracellular volume in patients with chronic renal disease treated for hypertension by sodium restriction. Lancet 2:69, 1967.)

In the typical patient with chronic renal failure, as in the one kidney–one clip Goldblatt model, the decreased functioning renal mass is unable to handle the usual sodium and water intake, so that intravascular volume progressively expands and raises the blood pressure. When the excess volume is removed by dialysis, blood pressure falls promptly and impressively[266] (Fig. 26–27).

In a few—perhaps 10 per cent of the total group of hypertensives with chronic renal failure—hypersecretion of renin is the predominant mechanism[267]; while most of these patients may respond to treatment with antihypertensive agents, a few require nephrectomy.[268] The predominant role of excess renin may be identified by the blood pressure reduction with the angiotensin antagonist saralasin or the converting enzyme inhibitor captopril.[263] Even in those individuals with mainly volume-dependent or controllable hypertension, renin almost certainly plays some role. Their renin levels, although not inordinately high, cannot be suppressed by volume expansion to the low levels observed in normal controls.[269]

SPECIAL CIRCUMSTANCES. A few special circumstances relating to hypertension in chronic renal disease will now be considered. Use of antihypertensive therapy for patients with renal disease is covered in Chapters 27 and 51.

Diabetic Nephropathy. Hypertension often accompanies the syndrome of diabetic nephropathy caused by in-

tercapillary glomerulosclerosis. The hypertension may reflect both advancing renal insufficiency with the inability to handle volume loads and extensive structural narrowing of the peripheral vasculature—the hallmark of long-standing diabetes. Moreover, intrarenal hypertension may accelerate the progress of the glomerulosclerosis.[270] As common as it is, hypertension may not be as severe or as likely to progress to an accelerated-malignant phase in diabetics with nephropathy for two reasons: first, these patients often have a diminished intravascular volume due to the hypoalbuminemia of the nephrotic syndrome; second, they have low renin levels, presumably due to hyalinization of juxtaglomerular cells.[271]

Hyporeninemic Hypoaldosteronism. Renin levels may become so low that the syndrome of hyporeninemic hypoaldosteronism develops. Although this pattern may accompany other forms of chronic renal disease, it is found most commonly among diabetics, since they are unable to mobilize either the aldosterone or the insulin needed to transfer potassium from the blood to the tissues and are thus particularly vulnerable to hyperkalemia.[272]

Whether diabetic or not, patients with this syndrome are usually recognized by a degree of hyperkalemia out of proportion to the degree of renal damage. The low renin levels are inadequate to stimulate aldosterone, and renal potassium excretion falls. Renin suppression in these patients may also reflect the expansion of fluid volume so common in advanced renal disease. Caution is obviously needed in treating such patients with either supplemental potassium or potassium-sparing diuretics.

Hypercalcemia. Whenever blood calcium is above normal, blood pressure usually rises; however, patients with chronic renal disease are particularly vulnerable to this condition. Marked hypertensive reactions have occurred when these patients are inappropriately given "therapeutic" calcium loads to offset the low plasma levels commonly seen in renal insufficiency or as a test for hyperparathyroidism.[273]

Analgesic Nephropathy. Permanent renal damage may supervene after prolonged exposure to analgesics, particularly phenacetin. In some countries, notably Australia, this is a common form of chronic renal disease.[274] Until late in their course, these patients have a greater propensity for salt-wasting and therefore may have less severe hypertension. However, in Australians, severe hypertension has been noted in 50 to 86 per cent of patients with analgesic nephropathy. Among those with malignant hypertension, a higher prevalence of renal artery stenosis and, at times, of active sloughing of renal papillae was observed.[274] Although aspirin alone seems to cause renal dysfunction rarely, it may reversibly depress glomerular filtration if given to patients with underlying renal disease or during sodium restriction, presumably because of the increased dependency of renal perfusion upon renal prostaglandins under these circumstances.[275]

HYPERTENSION IN THE ABSENCE OF RENAL TISSUE. In the absence of functioning renal tissue, blood pressure is mainly dependent upon body fluid volume. Without either the vasoconstrictor effects of renal renin or the vasodepressor actions of various renal hormones, blood pressure may be particularly labile and sensitive to changes in adrenergic activity. When the kidneys are removed for control of severe hypertension, blood pressure becomes normal, but hypertension may return with excess fluid loads or, as described below, after renal transplantation. The sympathetic nerves may be important in controlling the blood pressure; high levels of catecholamines may be responsible for hypertension in patients without renal tissue, and autonomic insufficiency may be a cause for dialysis-related hypotension.[276]

HYPERTENSION AFTER RENAL TRANSPLANTATION. A variety of problems may give rise to hypertension after renal transplantation, including stenosis of the renal artery at the site of anastomosis, rejection reactions, high doses of adrenal steroids, and excess renin derived from the retained diseased kidneys. Even when these causes were excluded, hypertension was found in 20 per cent of patients one year after transplantation.[277] Higher blood pressures correlated with older age, heavier body weight, and higher serum creatinine levels. Less hypertension was found in those receiving higher doses of prednisone, suggesting that glucocorticoids play a minimal role in posttransplant hypertension but not excluding their role in individual patients. More hypertension was observed when the kidney came from a cadaver than from a living related donor.

Unfortunately, renin measurements in these patients may not always reflect the ischemia, probably because volume expansion is also present and tends to suppress renin release. The response to the angiotensin antagonist saralasin may be a better indicator of the role of the renin-angiotensin system.[278] Whatever the mechanism, the hypertension that occurs in both chronic dialysis and renal transplant patients adds to their considerable susceptibility to accelerated cardiovascular disease, so that the elevated blood pressure in these patients should be treated intensively.

Renovascular Hypertension
(See also Chapter 52)

PREVALENCE. Fewer than 2 per cent of adults with hypertension have renovascular hypertension, the prevalence in different series varying from less than 1 to as high as 20 per cent, depending on the extent of patient selection.[4] Higher prevalence figures sometimes reflect the inclusion of patients with renovascular disease in whom the hypertension is not caused by renal ischemia. As people grow older, atherosclerotic disease of the renal arteries becomes increasingly common, in both normotensive and hypertensive patients.[279] Obviously, the diagnosis must be based upon evidence that the renovascular lesion is the cause of the hypertension.

Renovascular hypertension is seen in children, usually as a result of congenital dysplasia of the renal arteries. Infants have been found to develop the syndrome from thrombosis of the renal artery following catheterization of the umbilical artery.[280] In adults, the two major types of renovascular disease tend to appear at different times in different sexes. Atherosclerotic disease (Fig. 26–28) affecting mainly the proximal third of the main renal artery is seen mostly in men ages 40 to 70. Fibroplastic disease (Fig. 26–29) involving mainly the distal two-thirds and branches of the renal arteries appears most commonly in women ages 20 to 50. Overall, about two-thirds of cases

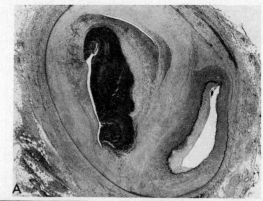
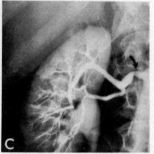
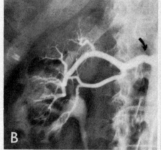

FIGURE 26–28 Cross section (A) and arteriograms (B and C) of an atherosclerotic plaque in the right renal artery. Progression from B to C occurred over a one-year period. (From Stewart, B. H., et al.: Correlation of angiography and natural history in evaluation of patients with renovascular hypertension. J. Urol. *104*:231, Baltimore, Williams and Wilkins Co., 1970.)

are caused by atherosclerotic disease and one-third by fibroplastic disease. The nonatherosclerotic stenoses involve all layers of the renal artery, but the most common is medial fibroplasia.[281] In addition, there are a number of other intrinsic and extrinsic causes of renovascular hypertension.[4] An interesting association between increased mobility of the right kidney and fibroplastic involvement of the right renal artery has been noted.[282] With repeated stretching of the renal artery, structural changes might be produced, leading to renal artery stenosis sufficient to cause renovascular hypertension.

Among blacks, less atherosclerosis develops in the main renal arteries and the incidence of renovascular hypertension is lower.[283] Among diabetic hypertensive individuals, despite their greater propensity for vascular disease, the incidence of atherosclerotic renal artery stenosis is not increased.[284] The sudden onset or worsening of hypertension among elderly patients may represent renovascular hypertension.

MECHANISMS

Since Goldblatt, in searching for the mechanism underlying essential hypertension, produced renovascular hypertension in the dog in 1934, the pathophysiology of this disease has been studied extensively. Confusion was introduced by the use of one-kidney models, which, as previously noted (p. 876), are more appropriate to the study of renoprival hypertension. Although some controversy remains, the sequence of changes in the two-kidney (one-clip) model and in patients with renovascular hypertension almost certainly starts with the release of increased amounts of renin when enough ischemia is induced to di-

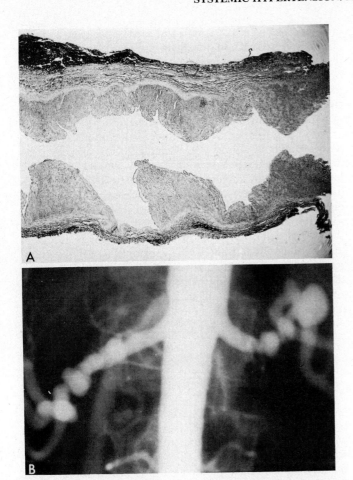

FIGURE 26–29 Fibromuscular dysplasia with medial fibroplasia. *A*, Longitudinal section of the vessel with multiple stenoses and mural aneurysms. *B*, The arteriogram shows bilateral multifocal stenoses with mural aneurysms. (From Harrison, E. G., and McCormack, L. J.: Pathologic classification of renal arterial disease in renovascular hypertension. Mayo Clin. Proc. *46*:161, 1971.)

minish pulse pressure in the renal afferent arterioles (Fig. 26–30). In people, as in animals, reduction of renal perfusion pressure by 50 per cent leads to an immediate and persistent increase in renin secretion from the ischemic kidney with suppression of secretion from the contralateral one.[285] Not only are renin levels markedly elevated but blockade of angiotensin activity with the antagonist

saralasin or the converting enzyme inhibitor will correct the hypertension.[286] With time, renin levels fall, blood pressure fails to respond to short infusions of angiotensin antagonists, and the hemodynamic pattern changes to include an expanded volume and increased cardiac output.

The sequence shown in Figure 26–30 is most likely responsible: the increased angiotensin stimulates aldosterone, causing volume expansion, and partially inhibits renin release. Despite the changed pattern, renin is almost certainly still responsible, although its chronic effects may involve more of its secondary stimulation of aldosterone and, thereby, volume expansion. In addition, angiotensin acts centrally to increase thirst and exert pressor actions. Lesions in the third ventricle of rats blocked the induction of renovascular hypertension.[287]

In patients with proved renovascular hypertension of many years' duration, excess renin secretion persists,[288] so that the experimental data are confirmed clinically. However, more than simply renin excess and its consequences may be involved: experimentally, the sympathetic nervous system is activated,[289] although catecholamine levels are not measurably higher in patients with unilateral renal hypertension.[290] When hypertension in rats is reversed by removal of the renal artery clip, the blood pressure drops further than if the ischemic kidney is removed, suggesting that vasodepressors may be involved.[291] In dogs, inhibition of prostaglandin synthesis does not alter the development of renovascular hypertension,[292] but renal prostaglandins may be responsible for the increase in sodium and water excretion that follows the initial volume retention.

In both animals and man, when renovascular hypertension induces extensive nephrosclerosis in the contralateral kidney, a different picture may evolve. Relief of the stenosis may not relieve the hypertension; rather, the contralateral kidney becomes the culprit, with the stenotic kidney's vessels having been protected from the high pressure. With removal of the contralateral kidney, the hypertension may recede.[293]

Variants. Most renovascular hypertension appears as partial obstruction of one main renal artery. However, only a branch need be involved, and segmental disease was found in 11 per cent of cases in one series.[294] On the other hand, apparent complete occlusion of the renal artery, if slow in developing, will allow development of enough col-

FIGURE 26–30 Stepwise hemodynamic changes in development of renovascular hypertension. The circled numbers represent the likely sequence of hemodynamic and hormonal changes in each phase of the disease: 1 = the immediate consequences of renal ischemia, 2 = changes that occur in a few days, and 3 and 4 = changes that eventually develop as the disease becomes chronic.

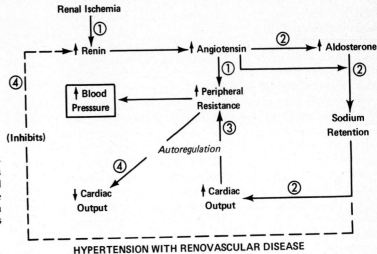

HYPERTENSION WITH RENOVASCULAR DISEASE

lateral flow to preserve the viability of the kidney. Thereby, the seemingly nonfunctioning kidney may be responsible for continued renin secretion and hypertension. If recognized, such totally occluded vessels can sometimes be repaired, with return of renal function and relief of hypertension.[295]

The process is often bilateral, although usually one side is clearly predominant. In the Cooperative Study, 25 per cent of the subjects had bilateral atherosclerotic or fibroplastic disease.[296] The possibility should be suspected, particularly if rapidly progressive oliguric renal failure develops without evidence of obstructive uropathy.

DIAGNOSIS

The presence of certain clinical features indicates the need for a screening test for renovascular hypertension in perhaps 10 per cent of all hypertensives. A positive screening test—or very strong clinical features—calls for more definitive confirmatory tests.

Clinical Features. Renovascular hypertension may be suspected on the following clinical grounds:

— The presence of an abdominal bruit, particularly if a diastolic component is present and if the bruit is heard lateral to the midline. Bruits confined to systole and heard mostly in older patients and that are loudest in the epigastrium and in the middle usually reflect atherosclerosis in the abdominal aorta.

— Onset of hypertension before age 30, particularly in white women who are slender.

— Sudden onset of hypertension after age 50, particularly in white men.

— Onset of hypertension after renal trauma.

— Severe, rapidly accelerating hypertension that is difficult to control.

— Evidence of rapidly deteriorating renal function.

The clinical picture of the two major forms of renovascular disease differ, as confirmed by the Cooperative Study on Renovascular Hypertension[297]: "Patients with atherosclerotic lesions were older, had a higher systolic blood pressure and more frequent arterial disease in areas outside of the kidney, and were more likely to develop target-organ damage than patients with essential hypertension. By contrast, patients with fibromuscular hyperplasia were young, predominantly female, more likely to have no family history of hypertension, and less prone to develop cardiomegaly."

Some patients have renovascular hypertension but may have none of these clinical features and clinically resemble patients with mild idiopathic hypertension. Nonetheless, these features should be used to exclude the majority of hypertensives from additional work-up and to identify the 10 per cent or so who should undergo a complete evaluation. As described earlier, the routine performance of an intravenous pyelogram (IVP) or other screening test on all hypertensives would result in more false-positive than true-positive results,[29] mandating even more unnecessary examinations, with their attendant costs and risks. However, those who present with rapidly accelerating hypertension with Grade 3 or 4 retinopathy should be highly suspect; among 123 such patients, at least 23 per cent had renovascular hypertension.[298] Once again, this was less common among blacks, but in at least 4 per cent this curable cause was found for their severe hypertension. The high frequency of renovascular hypertension in this series may reflect a greater propensity for the development of hypertensive encephalopathy on the background of renovascular hypertension than with other forms of hypertension in patients, as has been noted in animals.[299]

Screening Tests. No additional work-up need be done if the patient is clearly not a candidate for surgical treatment or transluminal angioplasty. This should be decided before, not after, subjecting the patient to either screening or confirmatory tests for renovascular hypertension. The diagnosis need not be made if therapy will be medical, since the same treatment protocol will be followed whether the hypertension is idiopathic or renovascular in origin. It may turn out that transluminal angioplasty will be an alternative to surgery for poor-risk patients, so that more of the latter will deserve evaluation.

Patients who are *less* likely candidates for surgical treatment include those with the following features:

— Hypertension of over 2 years' duration.

— Age over 55.

— Coexisting diseases (particularly atherosclerosis) that increase operative mortality.

— Relatively mild hypertension that is easily manageable with drugs.

— Inconclusive diagnostic studies.

On the other hand, patients with many of these features who are unwilling or unable to follow medical therapy, whose blood pressure level does not respond to adequate therapy, or who have marked stenosis of a renal artery or rapidly advancing renal damage may be considered for surgery and should be subjected to further study.

For screening among populations with an expected prevalence of perhaps 5 per cent (taking only those with clinical features suggestive of renovascular hypertension), an easy and safe procedure that results in very few false-negatives is needed. A certain number of false-positive results must be expected; considering that about 20 per cent of all adults will have primary (essential) hypertension, at least 20 per cent of patients with renovascular hypertension would be expected to have positive screening tests but would not be cured through repair of the stenosis, and these are therefore classified as "false-positives."

The four procedures commonly used as screening tests for renovascular hypertension were compared in a large population of hypertensives, 64 of whom turned out to have surgically reversible renovascular hypertension[300] (Table 26–13). Based upon this and numerous other published series, including the Cooperative Study, the following guidelines seem appropriate.

TABLE 26–13 SCREENING TESTS FOR RENAL VASCULAR HYPERTENSION

	ESSENTIAL HYPERTENSION	RENOVASCULAR HYPERTENSION
Number of patients	199	64
Systolic/diastolic bruit	1%	39%
Abnormal IVP	2%	76%
Upright PRA > 30 ng/ml/3 hr	5%	27%
Depressor response to saralasin	2 of 13	12 of 23

From Grim, C. E., et al.: Sensitivity and specificity of screening tests for renal vascular hypertension. Ann. Intern. Med. *91*:617, 1979.

Bruit. Almost half of patients with renovascular hypertension have a systolic and diastolic bruit. If one is heard, additional evaluation is indicated; if one is not heard, the diagnosis is certainly not excluded.

Intravenous Pyelography. Rapid-sequence IVP should be performed when clinical features suggest renovascular hypertension. Based on the three major criteria for features suggestive of renal ischemia (Table 26–14), results were false-positive in 11.4 per cent of 771 patients with essential hypertension and false-negative in 17 of 138 patients with proved renovascular hypertension.[301]

If the rates of sensitivity and specificity of the IVP from the Cooperative Study on Renovascular Hypertension are used and a prevalence of renovascular hypertension of 2 per cent in the general population is assumed (i.e., 10 per cent of all hypertensives), an abnormal IVP would be only 10 per cent predictive of the diagnosis, according to Bayes' theorem[29] (p. 273). However, if prior screening had increased the prevalence of the disease in the population tested to 10 per cent, a positive IVP would now be 40 per cent predictive. A negative IVP offers greater than 99 per cent assurance that renovascular hypertension is not present.

The IVP is readily available and provides additional information concerning renal parenchymal disease. As digital subtraction angiography becomes more readily available (p. 191), it will be possible to view the renal arteries and the IVP simultaneously, so there may be better reason to do the procedure in more patients.[302] The IVP is usually safe; 1.7 per cent of 33,000 patients had an adverse reaction, of which only 5 per cent were severe and there was one death.[303] However, the elderly who have severe hypertension, renal insufficiency, or diabetes are at much greater risk of incurring acute renal failure.[304]

Renography and Split-Function Studies. Isotopic renography can be substituted for the IVP, although it is somewhat less accurate. If the expensive equipment and skilled personnel are available, the renogram provides data concerning renal blood flow quickly and with less discomfort and risk to the patient but with less discrimination between vascular and parenchymal disease than is obtained with the IVP.

Split-function tests have been virtually abandoned, since the other procedures provide equally satisfactory evidence of the functional significance of renovascular disease with much less inconvenience and discomfort to the patient.

Peripheral Blood Renin Assays. By themselves, peripheral blood PRA levels are of only limited value in screening for renovascular hypertension. Most hypertensives with high PRA do not have renovascular hypertension (Table 26–15), and at least one-third of patients with proved

TABLE 26–14 FEATURES OF IVP SUGGESTIVE OF RENOVASCULAR HYPERTENSION

1. Disparity in renal size > 1.5 cm
2. Delayed appearance time of contrast medium of one or more minutes
3. Late hyperconcentration of contrast medium
4. Suggestive but less specific features:
   a. Ureteral and pelvic notching
   b. Decreased volume of the collecting system
   c. Parenchymal atrophy
   d. Nonfunctioning kidney, with normal retrograde pyelogram
   e. Defect in renal silhouette suggestive of segmental infarction
   f. Renal ptosis > 7.5 cm

TABLE 26–15 HIGH-RENIN HYPERTENSION

I. Increased renin substrate
   A. Estrogen intake, pregnancy-induced
   B. Cortisol excess
II. Increased renal renin secretion
   A. Renal artery stenosis
   B. Renin-secreting tumors
   C. Intrarenal ischemia
     1. Accelerated-malignant hypertension
     2. Renal parenchymal disease
III. Unknown—Essential hypertension (10 per cent)

renovascular hypertension have normal peripheral blood PRA.[252] Better discrimination may be provided by obtaining the blood after the patient has been upright for one or more hours and by relating the PRA level to the 24-hour urine sodium determination. Thirteen of 14 patients with high PRA detected by this technique were cured by operation; of 10 with normal PRA, five failed to respond to corrective surgery.[305] If the peripheral blood PRA is elevated, when obtained under appropriate conditions, additional work-up for renovascular hypertension is indicated. However, if the criterion for abnormality is set high enough to exclude most false-positives, as in the series of Grim et al. (Table 26–13), many false-negatives will be noted and the procedure becomes a poor screening test.

Blood Pressure Response to Saralasin. Renin-mediated hypertension may be easier to identify by observing the blood pressure response to infusion of the angiotensin antagonist saralasin. In a series of 1036 hypertensive patients, Streeten and Anderson found false-positive responses in about 5 per cent and false-negative responses in about 12 per cent.[306] Note, however, the much lower discrimination achieved in the study by Grim et al. (Table 26–13).

The procedure must be done carefully. In order to accentuate the differences between patients with high and normal renin, a mild state of volume contraction is required. This can be achieved with 40 mg of intravenous furosemide followed by 2 hours of upright posture. The same volume contraction minimizes the pressor response seen if saralasin is given to patients with low renin levels, since this antagonist also has agonist effects. To prevent both marked pressor responses in those with low renin and marked depressor responses in those with high renin, the infusion of saralasin should begin with a low dose, 0.05 to 0.10 μg/kg/min, and gradually be increased until a response occurs, to a maximum of 10 μg/kg/min.

The other available blocker of angiotensin activity, the converting-enzyme inhibitor captopril, lacks the discriminatory power of saralasin as a testing agent, since it lowers the blood pressure of most hypertensives with normal as well as high renin levels.[179]

Confirmatory Tests. If renovascular hypertension is suspected, from either an abnormal screening test or a strongly suggestive clinical setting, the diagnosis must be established and the nature of the disease defined before operation, regardless of the outcome of screening tests. Some perform renal arteriography first, others determine the renal vein renin ratio. If the degree of clinical suspicion is high, both tests may be performed at the same time; however, patients should not receive renin-suppressing antihypertensive drugs, including all adrenergic blocking agents, for at least a few days before the renal vein catheter study, whereas these drugs may be needed to lower blood pressure enough to minimize the risks of arteriography. Therefore, if the patient is on effective therapy, arteriography may be done first. If results are negative, renal vein renin levels need not be determined. On the other hand, arteriography is a more dangerous procedure and may not be needed if the renin ratio is normal. These guidelines are further beclouded by the increasing recognition that some patients without lateralizing renin ratios may be cured by surgery (see later).

As digital subtraction angiography becomes more readily available and accurate, it may be possible to visualize the renal arteries (and obtain an IVP) with much less morbidity. However, at the present time, it is not possible to exclude or completely define renovascular disease—particularly branch lesions—by using this procedure. Renal arteriography still has a place. One could argue that in patients for whom definitive examination of the renal arterial architecture is needed, a transfemoral arteriogram remains the procedure of choice.

Renal Vein Renin Ratio. This procedure has been used widely since Helmer and Judson showed in 1960 that functionally significant renovascular disease could be recognized by the finding of high levels of renin activity in blood obtained by percutaneous catheterization of the renal veins[307] (Fig. 26–31). According to a survey of published data, 93 per cent of patients with a lateralizing ratio—i.e., greater than 1.5 to 2.0 between the abnormal

TABLE 26–16 OPERATIVE RESULTS IN HYPERTENSIVE PATIENTS WITH UNILATERAL STENOSIS OF A MAIN RENAL ARTERY WITH RESPECT TO RENAL VEIN RENIN RATIOS

	NUMBER OF PATIENTS	PATIENTS WITH LATERALIZING RENAL VEIN RENIN RATIOS		PATIENTS WITHOUT LATERALIZING RENAL VEIN RENIN RATIOS	
		Cured or Improved	Failed	Cured or Improved	Failed
Summary of literature review	412	267	19	64	62
Present data	56	24	3	24	5
Totals	468	291 (93%)	22 (7%)	88 (57%)	67 (43%)

Data from Marks, L. S., et al.: Renovascular hypertension: Does the renal vein renin ratio predict operative results? J. Urol. *115*:365, 1976. Copyright 1976, The Williams and Wilkins Co., Baltimore.

and contralateral sides—were cured or improved by operation[308] (Table 26–16). However, when patients who had other features suggestive of renovascular hypertension but who did not have a lateralizing ratio greater than 2.0 were subjected to operation, 57 per cent were also cured or improved. Use of a ratio of 1.5 would decrease the number of false-negatives but would increase the number of false-positive tests. When patients with essential hypertension were tested, 19 per cent had a renal vein renin ratio of 1.5 or higher.[309] Although this may reflect asymmetrical nephrosclerosis, it probably results from the common practice of using a single catheter and sequentially sampling the renal veins. Renin secretion is episodic, and by the time the catheter is switched, significantly more or less renin may be coming from one renal vein than from the other.

To enhance the reliability of the procedure and accentuate the difference between the two sides, renin secretion should be stimulated by prior volume contraction using a low-salt diet and diuretics or converting enzyme inhibitor.[310] To insure further that surgical cure is probable, renin secretion from the contralateral kidney should be completely suppressed, as shown by a renin level identical to that in the inferior caval blood (Fig. 26–31).

Renovascular disease is bilateral in 25 per cent of patients, but usually one side is more involved, and an abnormal renin ratio is usually found.[311] Care should be taken to obtain blood draining any area in which segmental or branch arterial disease may be present.

Renal Arteriography. Ultimately the renal vasculature must be visualized to prove the diagnosis and to decide upon the feasibility and type of operation. The transfemoral approach is preferred, allowing selective visualization of each artery and its branches. Films can be taken with the patient upright to unravel vessels involved with medial fibroplasia that are often long and curled. Care must also be taken not to miss atherosclerotic lesions in the renal artery where it originates from the aorta. Sometimes arterial spasm from irritation by the catheter may give the false appearance of a lesion.

Although the arteriogram is needed to diagnose renovascular disease, it provides little help in deciding upon surgical curability. In the Cooperative Study, neither the degree of stenosis, the presence of poststenotic dilatation, nor the presence of collateral circulation was of much value in predicting the success of operation for individual pa-

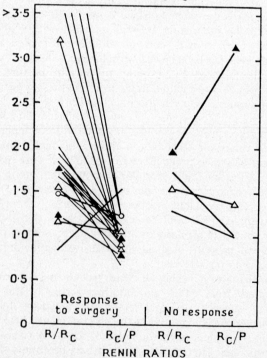

FIGURE 26–31 Relation between renal vein renin ratio (R/R_c) and R_c/P in 25 patients with renovascular hypertension, classified according to response to surgery. R_c = nonstenotic or less involved renal vein; P = peripheral blood PRA. (From Stockigt, J. R., et al.: Renal-vein renin in various forms of renal hypertension. Lancet *1*: 1194, 1972.)

tients.[296] Patients with stenosis of greater than 90 per cent may require operation to prevent complete occlusion.

THERAPY

Unfortunately, little is known about the natural history of untreated renovascular disease so it is difficult to assess the results of therapy. No properly controlled study comparing medical versus surgical treatment is available, although one is in progress at Vanderbilt Medical School.[312] Advances in medical therapy have made it easier to control the hypertension and the availability of transluminal angioplasty offers another "curative" approach, but current evidence supports surgical repair as being more likely to provide relief of hypertension and preserve renal function. Among 41 patients randomly allocated to medical therapy in the ongoing Vanderbilt trial, 17 showed deterioration of renal function or loss of renal size, despite acceptable blood pressure control in 15 of the 17.[312]

Operation should be considered in patients with proved, functionally significant renovascular disease if their general status and life expectancy are reasonably good. Better results follow repair of fibroplastic disease, in part because these patients tend to be younger and healthier. In various series, about 5 per cent of patients die during or after surgery; about 90 per cent of those with fibroplastic disease are cured or improved after one year, and about 70 per cent of those with atherosclerotic disease are similarly helped.[313,314] Vascular repair should always be attempted. Although initial results with nephrectomy may be as good, the other renal artery is obviously susceptible to the same process.[315]

The response to surgery may be predicted based on the response to the angiotensin-converting enzyme inhibitor captopril, which also provides effective medical therapy for those unable to undergo an operation.[316]

More and more patients may be subjected to transluminal angioplasty as cumulative experience seems to document its safety and effectiveness.[317] In patients with marked renal insufficiency from stenosis of a solitary kidney or bilateral disease, vessels have been successfully dilated.[318] On the other hand, most patients above 60 years of age who are subjected to surgical treatment improve,[319] so this remains the preferable approach for most patients.

We have, then, easier ways to recognize renovascular disease and more effective ways to relieve renovascular hypertension. As our sights are focused on the 5 to 10 per cent of patients likely to have this condition, we should be able to diagnose and treat many of them, with the expectation of relieving a considerable burden of severe hypertension.

Renin-Secreting Tumors

Made up of juxtaglomerular cells or hemangiopericytomas, these tumors have been found mostly in young patients with severe hypertension, very high renin levels both in peripheral blood and in the kidney harboring the tumor, and secondary aldosteronism manifested by hypokalemia.[320] The tumor can usually be recognized by selective renal angiography, usually done because of the suspicion of renovascular hypertension. More commonly, children with Wilms' tumors may have hypertension and high renin levels that revert to normal after nephrectomy.[321]

Adrenal Causes of Hypertension
(See also Chapter 51)

Three adrenal causes of hypertension will now be considered—primary excesses of aldosterone, cortisol, and catecholamines—which together constitute less than 1 per cent of all hypertensive diseases. In addition, congenital adrenal hyperplasia will be discussed. Each can usually be recognized with relative ease, and patients suspected of having these disorders can be screened by means of readily available tests. However, specific identification of the particular adrenal disease responsible for each type of hormonal excess, which is necessary before decisions concerning therapy can be made, can be difficult.

PRIMARY ALDOSTERONISM (See also p. 1733)

First recognized almost 30 years ago, this disease is relatively rare (Table 26–5), although it may be found fairly often in selected populations.[24,322,323]

Pathophysiology. Primary aldosterone excess usually arises from solitary benign adenomas. As diagnostic tests improve and become more readily available, larger numbers of patients with minimal features are recognized and found to have bilateral adrenal hyperplasia, the number varying from one-fifth[323] to more than half[322] of the cases of aldosteronism. The validity of defining the condition in these patients with bilateral hyperplasia as "idiopathic hyperaldosteronism" has been strongly denied by investigators from the MRC Blood Pressure Unit.[324,325] Their argument is persuasive, and I agree with their conclusion that "idiopathic hyperaldosteronism is at the upper end of a wider-than-normal distribution of aldosterone in essential hypertension, from which it has been separated wrongly."[325] Nonetheless, there is evidence that such patients may be responding to an unknown stimulus to aldosterone secretion, including suppression of their high aldosterone levels by the serotonin antagonist cyproheptadine.[326]

Some other variants are seen: a few patients have familial glucocorticoid-suppressible hyperaldosteronism[327]; a few extraadrenal tumors may hypersecrete aldosterone[328]; exogenous mineralocorticoids may cause "pseudoaldosteronism," including the glycyrrhizinic acid in licorice from candy[329] or chewing tobacco[330] and nasal sprays mistakenly containing mineralocorticoid instead of glucocorticoid.[331]

Whatever the source, excess aldosterone causes hypertension and hypokalemia, here defined as a plasma potassium level below 3.2 mEq/liter (Fig. 26–32). Very rarely, the syndrome has been recognized in normotensive individuals.[332] Not so rarely, hypokalemia may be absent or only intermittent, but in most patients with adenomas, persistent hypokalemia is almost invariable.[328]

The hypertension begins as a volume overload but soon converts, as do apparently all forms of hypertension, to increased peripheral resistance.[93] The degree of hypertension can be significant, with a mean pressure in one group of 136 patients of 205/123 mm Hg.[328] Malignant hypertension may supervene,[333] and in the large series from Scotland, four of the 136 patients had histological evidence of malignant hypertension on renal biopsy.[328] Furthermore, 23 per cent of their patients had a serious vascular complication

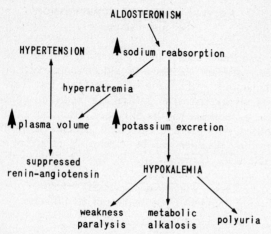

FIGURE 26–32 Pathophysiology of primary aldosteronism. (From Kaplan, N. M.: Primary aldosteronism. *In* Astwood, E. B., and Cassidy, C. E. (eds.): Clinical Endocrinology. Vol. II. New York, 1968, p. 468, by permission of Grune and Stratton.)

such as stroke or myocardial infarction. Thus, the hypertension can be serious.

In association with the increased pressure and expanded volume, renin secretion is suppressed. This finding has been almost invariable with the syndrome, but the overwhelming majority of hypertensive patients with suppressed renin do not have primary aldosteronism (Table 26–12).

Hypokalemia results from the aldosterone-mediated increase in renal potassium wastage. Although hypokalemia may not be recognized until diuretics or salt loads are ingested, the effects may be striking, with muscular weakness, polyuria, metabolic alkalosis, impaired carbohydrate tolerance, and blunting of circulatory reflexes.

Diagnosis.   No serious consideration need be given the diagnosis of primary aldosteronism unless hypertension and hypokalemia coexist. If the rare normokalemic patient with the disease is thereby missed, little will be lost as long as the patient is protected by appropriate treatment for the hypertension. Since this will likely include a diuretic, significant hypokalemia will soon become manifest, making the diagnosis obvious.

Potassium-Wasting.   The first step in evaluating the hypokalemic hypertensive should be the determination of potassium excretion in a 24-hour urine sample collected while the patient is hypokalemic, receiving no supplemental potassium or diuretic, and ingesting a normal sodium intake (i.e., urinary sodium excretion is above 100 mEq/day) (Fig. 26–33). If urinary potassium under these circumstances is less than 30 mEq/day, mineralocorticoid excess is highly unlikely, and the work-up can be aborted; if the value is above 30, further evaluation is warranted.

In most hypertensive patients hypokalemia is caused by the prior use of diuretics. Losses may be large and may require prolonged potassium supplementation. On the other hand, severe hypokalemia appearing soon after the initiation of diuretic therapy may presage primary aldosteronism.

Renin Suppression.   If urinary potassium-wasting has been documented, the patient should receive potassium supplementation for a period of 3 to 6 weeks to bring the plasma potassium level within the normal range and maintain it, so that subsequent studies will be unaffected by hypokalemia. One or another mild stimulus to renin secretion should be applied to demonstrate suppression. By whatever technique, renin levels are almost invariably and significantly suppressed in patients with primary aldosteronism.

Aldosterone Excess.   Increased levels of aldosterone can be found in urine or blood. When urine is used, the

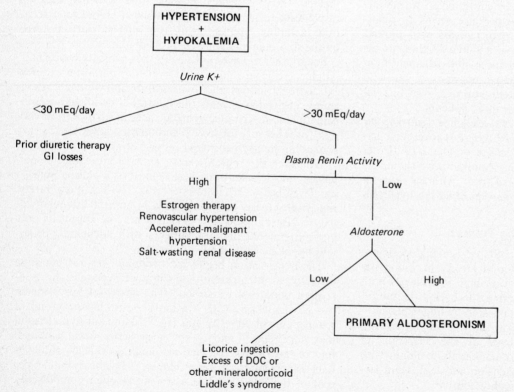

FIGURE 26–33 Flow diagram for the differential diagnosis of hypertension with hypokalemia. (From Kaplan, N. M.: Clinical Hypertension. 3rd ed. Baltimore, Williams and Wilkins Co., 1982, p. 306.)

24-hour collection should contain over 100 mEq of sodium to insure that high aldosterone levels are not simply secondary to sodium restriction. Various techniques to suppress endogenous aldosterone secretion have been used to insure further that the aldosterone excess is primary. These include infusions of saline, injections of DOCA, and oral administration of fludrocortisone (Florinef).

One of the easiest and most reliable procedures is the saline suppression test of plasma aldosterone[334] in which 2 liters of normal saline are infused over a four-hour interval. The plasma aldosterone level remains high in those with primary aldosteronism but is suppressed to below 6 ng/100 ml in patients with essential hypertension or secondary aldosteronism.

Once the diagnosis is established, a less direct approach may be used to document the diagnosis and to prepare the patient for surgery, i.e., the response to high doses of the aldosterone antagonist spironolactone.[335] It may also be useful in predicting the response to operation; in one study the decrease in blood pressure with spironolactone was closely correlated to the subsequent response to operation in 44 patients tested.[336]

Bilateral Adrenal Hyperplasia. Various maneuvers are available to differentiate patients with apparent aldosterone excess due to bilateral adrenal hyperplasia from those with an adrenal adenoma.[4] The differential diagnosis should be made, and only those patients with a tumor should be subjected to operation, since it may not be possible to determine the type of pathologic condition at operation without removing both adrenal glands.

Now that computerized axial tomography (CAT) is capable of identifying adrenal lesions as small as 1.0 cm, this procedure has become the best initial test to identify the type of adrenal disease.[337] If it fails to define an adrenal adenoma when the clinical situation is strongly suggestive, bilateral adrenal vein catheterization with venography and analysis of venous steroid levels should be attempted.[323] Rather than false-negative tests, there will likely be more problems with false-positive CAT scans, i.e., finding nonfunctioning adrenal tumors, which are present in a considerable number of normotensive and hypertensive people.[338]

Therapy. Once the diagnosis of primary aldosteronism is made and the type of adrenal disorder has been established, the choice of therapy is fairly easy: patients with a solitary adenoma require resection of the tumor; those with bilateral hyperplasia should be treated with spironolactone and a thiazide diuretic.[336] Fortunately, the doses of spironolactone required for chronic therapy are usually low enough to avoid bothersome side effects. Triamterene[339] and amiloride[340] (p. 533) will also control the disease if spironolactone is poorly tolerated. When an adenoma is resected, about 75 per cent of patients will become normotensive, while the other 25 per cent remain hypertensive, either from preexisting essential hypertension or from renal damage due to prolonged secondary hypertension.[341]

CUSHING'S SYNDROME (See also p. 1732)

Hypertension occurs in about 80 per cent of patients with Cushing's syndrome. If left untreated, it can cause congestive heart failure and death.[342] As with hypertension of other endocrine causes, the longer hypertension is present, the less likely it will be to disappear when the disease is cured.[341]

Mechanism of Hypertension. Blood pressure may increase for a number of reasons:

1. The secretion of a mineralocorticoid, DOC or aldosterone, may also be increased along with cortisol.

2. The excess cortisol exerts a sufficient intrinsic salt-retaining effect to expand volume and lead to hypertension.

3. Cortisol stimulates the synthesis of renin substrate, which in turn causes more angiotensin to be generated. The angiotensin antago-

nist saralasin lowered the blood pressure of seven of nine patients with Cushing's syndrome.[343]

4. Vascular reactivity to pressor substances, including norepinephrine, increases.

Diagnosis. The syndrome should be suspected in patients with central obesity, thin skin, muscle weakness, and osteoporosis. If clinical features are suggestive, the diagnosis can be either ruled out or virtually assured by the simple, overnight *dexamethasone suppression test.*[344] In normal subjects, the level of plasma cortisol in a sample drawn at 8 A.M. after a bedtime dose of 1 mg of dexamethasone should be below 7 μg/100 ml. If the level is higher, additional workup is in order to establish both the diagnosis of cortisol excess and the pathological type. Patients who are under stress or depressed may fail to show suppression. Measurement of urine free cortisol levels is almost as good a screening test: most patients who do not have Cushing's syndrome excrete less than 100 μg/24 hours.

The next procedure should be a longer dexamethasone suppression test, using 0.5 mg every 6 hours and then 2.0 mg every 6 hours, each for 2 days. Urinary 17-hydroxycorticoid (17-HOCS) or free cortisol excretion should be measured on the second day of each dose. Patients with Cushing's syndrome will fail to suppress urinary 17-HOCS to below 2.5 mg/day on the 0.5-mg dose; if Cushing's syndrome is caused by an excess pituitary ACTH drive with bilateral adrenal hyperplasia, urinary 17-HOCS will be suppressed to below 50 per cent of the control value on the 2.0 mg dose.[344] As plasma ACTH assays become more reliable, they provide additional differentiation between pituitary and ectopic ACTH excess on the one hand and adrenal tumors with ACTH suppression on the other.

If hormonal excess is documented, the source of the adrenal disease should be documented further by CAT scans of the pituitary, chest, and abdomen.[345]

Therapy. In about two-thirds of patients with Cushing's syndrome, the process begins with overproduction of ACTH by the pituitary, which leads to bilateral adrenal hyperplasia. Although pituitary hyperfunction may reflect a hypothalamic disorder, the majority of patients have discrete pituitary adenomas that can usually be resected by selective transsphenoidal microsurgery.[346] In children with fairly mild disease, conventional high-voltage pituitary irradiation is often curative.[347] High-energy proton-beam irradiation has also been used. Only rarely is bilateral adrenalectomy necessary. Medical therapy is almost never curative.

If an adrenal tumor is present, it should be surgically removed. With earlier diagnosis and more selective surgical therapy, it is hoped that more patients with Cushing's syndrome will be cured without the need for lifelong glucocorticoid replacement therapy and with permanent relief of their hypertension.

Pheochromocytoma (See also p. 1734)

The wild fluctuations in blood pressure and dramatic symptoms of pheochromocytoma usually alert both the patient and the physician to the possibility of this diagnosis. However, the fluctuations may be missed or, as occurs in half the patients, the hypertension may be persistent. The symptoms may be ascribed to psychoneurosis by practitioners desensitized to "spells," which usually represent menopausal hot flushes or anxiety-induced hyperventilation. Unfortunately, if the diagnosis is missed, severe complications may arise from very high blood pressure and damage to the heart by catecholamines. Stroke and hypertensive crises with encephalopathy and retinal hemorrhages occur most commonly, probably because extremely high levels of pressure develop suddenly in vessels unprepared by chronic hypertension. Fortunatey, a simple and inexpensive test will detect the disease with virtual certainty, so that diagnostic indecision may be minimized.

PATHOPHYSIOLOGY. Pheochromocytomas may arise wherever the sympathogonia from the primitive neural crest come to lie. These cells differentiate into ganglion cells, neuroblasts, and chromaffin cells. Tumors develop from each of these cell types; ganglioneuromas and neuroblastomas usually occur in children and are recognized by the excretion of large amounts of homovanillic acid (HVA), which is a metabolite of dopamine, the immediate precursor of norepinephrine. Paragangliomas may arise in chemoreceptor tissue, where they are called chemodectomas; along the sympathetic chain, including the organ of Zuckerkandl; and in the urinary bladder. A pheochromocytoma was found in 10 of 18 patients with neurofibromatosis and hypertension.[347a]

The majority of pheochromocytomas, about 90 per cent, arise in the adrenal medulla; 10 per cent of these are bilateral and another 10 per cent are malignant. Multiple adrenal tumors are particularly common in patients with simple familial pheochromocytoma and multiple endocrine adenomatosis, Type II, in association with medullary carcinoma of the thyroid (Sipple's syndrome); or with mucosal ganglioneuromas in addition (Type IIB or III). Diffuse medullary hyperplasia may precede the development of tumors, and the tumors may, in fact, reflect extreme degrees of nodular hyperplasia.[348]

Secretion from nonfamilial pheochromocytomas varies considerably, with small tumors tending to secrete larger proportions of active catecholamines. If the predominant secretion is epinephrine, which is formed only in the adrenal medulla, the symptoms reflect its effects—mainly systolic hypertension due to increased cardiac output, tachycardia, sweating, flushing, and apprehension. If norepinephrine is predominantly secreted, as from some of the adrenal tumors and from almost all the extraadrenal tumors, the symptoms include both systolic and diastolic hypertension from peripheral vasoconstriction but less tachycardia, palpitations, and anxiety.

DIAGNOSIS. Many more hypertensive patients have variable blood pressures and "spells" than the 0.2 per cent or so who harbor a pheochromocytoma. A number of stresses and some rather rare diseases may involve transient catecholamine release (Table 26–17). Other causes of

TABLE 26–17 DIFFERENTIAL DIAGNOSIS OF PHEOCHROMOCYTOMA

Recurrent spells
  Anxiety with hyperventilation
  Menopause
  Hypoglycemia*
  Angina
  Paroxysmal tachycardia
  Lead poisoning
  Migraine and cluster headaches
  Diencephalic seizures
  Familial dysautonomia
  Acrodynia*
  Porphyria*
  Carcinoid*
Paroxysmal hypertension
  Acute pulmonary edema
  Acute myocardial infarction
  Stroke
  Brain tumor*
  Rebound after abrupt cessation of clonidine and other antihypertensives*
  Hypertensive crises associated with MAO inhibitors*
  Intake of sympathomimetic drugs*
  Autonomic dysreflexia (quadriplegia)*
Hypertension and hypermetabolism
  Thyrotoxicosis
  Diabetes mellitus
  Eclampsia

*Reported to cause increased levels of catecholamines.

TABLE 26–18 CONDITIONS IN WHICH PATIENTS SHOULD BE SCREENED FOR PHEOCHROMOCYTOMA

Paroxysmal hypertension
  OR
Persistent hypertension, if accompanied by
  Headache
  Sweating
  Palpitations
  Nervousness
  Weight loss
  Hypermetabolism
  Orthostatic hypotension
Severe pressor response in association with
  Induction of anesthesia
  Pregnancy or delivery
  Surgery
  Histamine for gastric analysis
  Intake of phenothiazines, tricyclic antidepressants, or adrenal glucocorticoids
  Saralasin testing for angiotensin-mediated hypertension
Family history of pheochromocytoma, medullary carcinoma of the thyroid, or hyperparathyroidism
Neurocutaneous lesions

recurrent spells of paroxysmal hypertension may not be related to increased sympathetic nervous activity.

A pheochromocytoma should be suspected in patients with hypertension that is either paroxysmal or persistent and accompanied by certain symptoms and signs, as listed in Table 26–18. In addition, children and patients with rapidly accelerating hypertension should be screened. Those whose tumors secrete predominantly epinephrine are prone to postural hypotension from a contracted blood volume and blunted sympathetic reflex tone. Suspicion should be heightened if activities such as bending over, exercise, or palpation of the abdomen cause repetitive spells that begin abruptly, advance rapidly, and subside within minutes.

High levels of catecholamines may induce acute myocarditis, which may progress to cardiomyopathy and left ventricular failure.[349] In the patient described by Baker et al., the decreased cardiac output that resulted from myocardial damage kept the blood pressure normal.[349] Acute myocardial infarction also occurs with increased frequency.[350] Opiates given to such patients may raise the pressure through release of catecholamines.[351]

LABORATORY CONFIRMATION

Screening. The easiest and best procedure is either a 24-hour or spot urine assay for total metanephrines.[352] This catecholamine metabolite is least affected by various interfering substances including antihypertensive drugs. Among 50 patients seen at the Mayo Clinic, the metanephrine test gave the lowest number of false-negatives (4 per cent) when compared with vanillylmandelic acid (VMA) assays (29 per cent), urinary catecholamines (21 per cent), or basal plasma catecholamines (47 per cent).[353] The ranges for these three urinary tests are shown in Table 26–19.

Urinary metanephrine excretion will be increased if patients are taking sympathomimetic drugs or MAO inhibitors and will be decreased for the next few days after use of x-ray contrast media containing methylglucamine (e.g., Renografin, Hypaque). Therefore, the urine should be collected before an IVP or other such procedure is done.

Plasma catecholamine assays are now becoming available and may provide a way to confirm the diagnosis but will not serve as a screening test, since they result in too

TABLE 26–19 URINARY TESTS FOR PHEOCHROMOCYTOMA

COMPOUND	URINARY EXCRETION (MG/DAY OR µG/MG CREATININE)	
	Normal Adults	*Pheochromocytoma*
Free catecholamines	<0.1	0.1 to 10.0
Metanephrine + normetanephrine	<1.2	1.0 to 100.0
Vanillylmandelic acid	<6.5	5 to 600

many false-positive values.[345] If plasma levels are equivocal, measurement of a plasma norepinephrine level 3 hours after a single 0.3-mg oral dose of the adrenergic inhibitor clonidine has been shown to separate the nonpheochromocytoma patients, whose levels are suppressed, from those with the disease, who do experience suppression.[355]

Localization of the Tumor. Once the diagnosis has been made, medical therapy should be given and the tumor localized, if possible, by CAT scan, which usually demonstrates the typically large tumors with ease. It is hoped that radioisotopes that localize in chromaffin tissue will become available to be of additional help in those few patients in whom localization is not possible by current techniques.[348]

THERAPY. Once diagnosed and localized, pheochromocytomas should be resected. Great care should be taken in preparing patients for operation and managing them through the procedure.[356] The most important part of their preoperative management is adequate adrenergic blockade over enough time to overcome vasoconstriction and allow the reduced blood volume to reexpand. If the tumor is unresectable, chronic medical therapy with the alpha blocker phenoxybenzamine (Dibenzyline) or the inhibitor of catechol synthesis α-methyl-tyrosine (Demser) can be used.

Congenital Adrenal Hyperplasia

Two distinct enzymatic defects may induce hypertension: (1) 11-hydroxylase deficiency, which leads to virilization (from excessive androgens) and hypertension with hypokalemia (from excessive DOC), which may not become manifest until adult life[357]; and (2) 17-hydroxylase deficiency, which causes similar hypertension from excess DOC but also failure of secondary sexual development because sex hormones are also deficient.[358] Affected children are hypertensive, but the defect in sex hormone synthesis may not become obvious until after puberty. Thereafter, affected males display ambiguity of sexual development and females fail to mature or menstruate.

Miscellaneous Causes of Hypertension

A host of other causes of hypertension are known (see Table 26–4). One that is likely becoming more common is ingestion of various drugs[359]—prescribed (e.g., Danazol[360]), over-the-counter (e.g., phenylpropanolamine[361]), and illicit (e.g., cocaine).

Coarctation of the Aorta
(See also Chapters 29 and 30)

Congenital narrowing of the aorta may occur at any level of the thoracic or abdominal aorta. It is usually found just beyond the origin of the left subclavian artery or distal to the insertion of the ligamentum arteriosum. The coarctation may be localized or more diffuse. Other cardiac anomalies usually accompany the latter, and over half

of those afflicted die during the first year of life, although operative treatment of both the coarctation and associated anomalies may reduce this mortality rate.[362] With less severe postductal lesions, damage is more insidious, and symptoms may not appear until the teens or later. To diminish the development of congestive failure, endocarditis, and stroke, the obstruction should be recognized and corrected before the age of 5 years.[363] The pathogenesis of the hypertension may be more complicated than simple mechanical obstruction: the renin-angiotensin levels may be inappropriately high-normal[364] and the sympathetic nervous system may be activated.[365] Hypertension in the arms and weak or absent femoral pulses are the classic features of coarctation. The lesion may be detected by cross-sectional echocardiography[366] (p. 975). Aortography proves the diagnosis. Immediately after surgical repair, the blood pressure may transiently rise even further, and mesenteric arteritis may develop. These changes may reflect very high levels of renin-angiotensin[367] and catecholamines.[368] The latter may persist for up to six months after operation.

HYPERPARATHYROIDISM

Hypertension occurs in one-fourth to one-half of patients with hyperparathyroidism and is found commonly in patients with other hypercalcemic states.[369] As more and more patients are found to be hypertensive and undergo routine testing of serum calcium, asymptomatic hypercalcemia associated with hyperparathyroidism is not infrequently recognized. Moreover, thiazide diuretics—the most frequently used drugs in the treatment of hypertension—may accentuate previously borderline hypercalcemia. Hypercalcemia was found in 1.9 per cent of patients receiving thiazides compared to 0.6 per cent in the remainder in a community screening program.[370] Of 15 persistently hypercalcemic hypertensive individuals, 14 turned out to have hyperparathyroidism.

The mechanism by which hypercalcemia elevates the blood pressure is unknown. Calcium directly increases the contractility of vascular smooth muscle and may activate the sympathetic nervous system.[369] Interestingly, parathyroid function may be enhanced in essential hypertension, as a homeostatic response to a urinary calcium leak.[371]

HYPERTENSION AFTER CARDIAC SURGERY

Transient hypertension may develop postoperatively for various reasons: pain, physical and emotional excitement, hypoxia, hypercapnia, and excessive volume loads[372] (Table 26–20). More severe hypertension has been noted following various cardiovascular surgical procedures:
— *Coronary bypass surgery*. The incidence, exceeding 33 per cent, is far higher than after other major cardiac or noncardiac surgery. The problem appears more commonly on the background of

TABLE 26–20 HYPERTENSION ASSOCIATED WITH CARDIAC SURGERY

Preoperative
  Anxiety, angina, and the like
  Discontinuation of antihypertensive therapy
  "Rebound" from discontinuing beta-blocking agents in patients with coronary artery disease
Intraoperative
  Induction of anesthesia
    Specific drugs
    Hypertension due to tracheal intubation and nasopharyngeal, urethral, or rectal manipulation
  Precardiopulmonary bypass (during sternotomy and chest retraction)
  Cardiopulmonary bypass
  Postcardiopulmonary bypass (during surgery)
Postoperative
  Early—within 2 hours
    Obvious cause: Hypoxia, hypercarbia, ventilatory difficulties, hypothermia, shivering, arousal from anesthesia
    No obvious cause: After myocardial revascularization; less frequently after valve replacement; early (Sealy type I) hypertension after resection of aortic coarctation
  Intermediate—12 to 36 hours after surgery: Sealy type II after repair of aortic coarctation
  Late—weeks to months: After aortic valve replacement by homografts

From Estafanous, F. G., and Tarazi, R. C.: Systemic arterial hypertension associated with cardiac surgery. Am. J. Cardiol. *46*:685, 1980.

preexisting hypertension, greater than 50 per cent obstruction of the left main coronary artery, or the preoperative use of beta blockers.[373] The hemodynamic pattern of increased peripheral resistance could be explained by the markedly high plasma catecholamine and renin activity measured in such patients. Since many of these patients will have been receiving beta-blocker therapy that has been discontinued, the postoperative hypertension may to some extent reflect a rebound phenomenon. Therapy is often required, and intravenous nitroprusside and stellate ganglion or thoracic epidural block are effective.[372]

— *Aortic valve replacement*. Transient hypertension may give way to more permanent hypertension. In one series, 53 per cent of 116 patients were hypertensive five years after surgery, and hypertension was a major determinant of late failure of the homograft valve.[374]

— *Closure of an atrial septal defect*.[375]

PREGNANCY-INDUCED HYPERTENSION
(See also Chapter 53)

A small percentage of women enter pregnancy with hypertension. A larger number develop hypertension during pregnancy. With a diastolic blood pressure exceeding 84 mm Hg at any time during gestation, fetal mortality increases, even more so if accompanied by proteinuria[376] (Fig. 26–34). About 10,000 fetal deaths in the United States every year are attributable to hypertension.[377] Although the cause of pregnancy-induced hypertension is unknown, it can be recognized early and managed with relative ease, to the advantage of both mother and baby.

DEFINITIONS

Blood pressure falls during the course of normal pregnancy to levels lower than those found in nonpregnant women[378] (Fig. 26–35), so that different criteria are needed for the diagnosis of hypertension. In most cases, these involve a rise in blood pressure of 30/15 mm Hg or more, or an absolute level greater than 140/90 on two or more occasions taken at least 6 hours apart. As with other forms of hypertension, the blood pressure may vary by 20 to 40 mm Hg within short intervals for no apparent reason.[379]

The types of hypertension seen include the following:

1. *Preeclampsia*: Hypertension with proteinuria and/or edema developing after the 20th week of gestation.

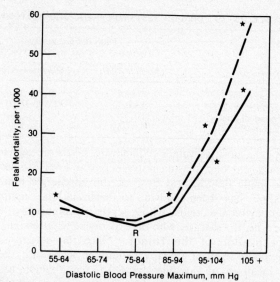

FIGURE 26–34 Fetal mortality in relation to the maximal diastolic blood pressure recorded during 38,636 pregnancies by the Collaborative Perinatal Project. The solid line represents the total series; the broken line represents the patients with concomitant proteinuria of any degree. Asterisks designate mortality significantly higher than in patients with normal maximal diastolic values (R). (From Friedman, E. A., and Neff, R. K.: Hypertension–hypotension in pregnancy. Correlation with fetal outcome. J.A.M.A. *239*:2249, 1978.)

2. *Eclampsia*: The above, plus convulsions not caused by coincidental neurological disease.

3. *Chronic hypertension of whatever cause*: Most of these patients turn out to have essential hypertension that may not have been recognized prior to pregnancy and that is often masked by the usual fall in blood pressure during the midtrimester. Women with pressures above 110/75 at weeks 17 to 20 have a greater chance of developing pregnancy-induced hypertension.[380]

4. *Preeclampsia superimposed on chronic hypertension*.

MECHANISMS

The hemodynamic changes of normal pregnancy are described in Chapter 53. When preeclampsia begins, peripheral resistance rises, vascular reactivity to pressor agents

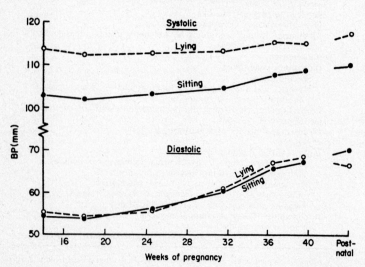

FIGURE 26–35 Mean blood pressures of 226 primigravidas seen at St. Mary's Hospital, London. Included are all the patients seen at or before 20 weeks of pregnancy over an 18-month interval. (From MacGillivray, I., et al.: Blood pressure survey in pregnancy. Clin. Sci. *37*:395, 1969.)

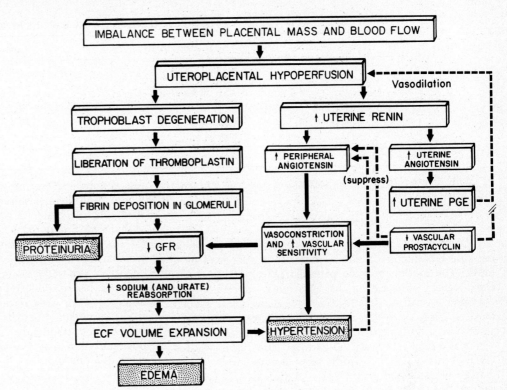

FIGURE 26-36 A unified working hypothesis for the pathophysiology of pregnancy-induced hypertension. The solid lines lead to the three primary manifestations: proteinuria, edema, and hypertension. The dotted lines indicate attempts to counteract the underlying defect of uteroplacental hypoperfusion. (From Kaplan, N. M.: Clinical Hypertension. 3rd ed. Baltimore, Williams and Wilkins Co., 1982, p. 367).

increases, plasma volume falls, and renal function diminishes.[381] Although the hypoperfused uterus may produce more renin, the levels of renin, angiotensin, and aldosterone in the maternal circulation all fall when the syndrome is full-blown. A unified working hypothesis has been constructed to explain these changes (Fig. 26–36); although parts of this scheme remain unproved, it serves as a useful model. The basic problem seems to be an imbalance between placental mass and blood flow.[382] In some women predisposed to preeclampsia, placental blood flow is impaired, as in those with diabetes or preexisting chronic hypertension. In others, placental mass is increased, as in those with multiple births and hydatidiform moles. In those with the greatest predisposition, young primigravidas, both a relatively greater placental mass and an inadequately developed blood supply may be involved.[383]

Whatever the basic reason, when the uteroplacental structure is hypoperfused, the cascade of events shown in Figure 26–36 is set into motion. Events shown on the left are well documented; those on the right are less so, but they have received support from recent investigations.

When the uterus is hypoperfused, it secretes more renin, which generates more angiotensin within the placental circulation. In response to moderately increased levels of angiotensin, uteroplacental blood flow increases,[384] possibly as a result of the action of angiotensin to liberate increased amounts of vasodilatory prostaglandins,[385] in particular prostacyclin.[386] The vasodilation provides an appropriate compensatory response to hypoperfusion, but this compensation may be inadequate in the preeclamptic patient: prostacyclin levels in amniotic fluid,[387] urine,[388] and fetal and maternal blood vessels[389] are lower in those with preeclampsia than in normal pregnancy. If an inability to synthesize prostaglandins is involved, it may also explain another aspect of developing preeclampsia—increased pressor sensitivity to exogenous angiotensin.[390]

Normal pregnant women are relatively resistant to the pressor effects of angiotensin. High levels of prostaglandins could explain this resistance in normal pregnancy.[391] Decreased prostaglandin (PG) levels, as would be expected after administration of the inhibitor of PG synthesis indomethacin, caused normal pregnant women to become much more sensitive to angiotensin.[390] Women who develop preeclampsia show increased pressor sensitivity to angiotensin well before their blood pressure rises.[390] Thus, uteroplacental prostaglandins, including prostacyclin, which enters the systemic circulation,[392] may mediate the vasodilated, low-pressure state of normal pregnancy and a decrease in these vasodepressor hormones may be involved in the pathogenesis of preeclampsia. Prostaglandins may be involved in another manner: plasma levels of free-radical oxidation products generated during prostaglandin biosynthesis are increased in preeclampsia; these free radicals may induce tissue injury.[393]

OTHER THEORIES

As attractive as this scheme appears, other theories are favored by some, including (1) a primary alteration in platelet function leading to slow intravascular coagulation with fibrin deposition[394]; and (2) an immunological basis, which could explain the increased incidence of preeclampsia in first pregnancies, its familial tendency, and its association with an enlarged placenta.[395] The familial tendency is compatible with a single recessive gene.[396]

Clinical Features

The distinction between preeclampsia and chronic hypertension should be made, since the former is a self-limited disease that is a threat only to the first pregnancy and should be treated more conservatively, with less pharmacological intervention. In most patients, the distinction can

TABLE 26–21   DIFFERENCES BETWEEN PREECLAMPSIA AND CHRONIC HYPERTENSION

	PREECLAMPSIA	CHRONIC HYPERTENSION
Age	Young (<20)	Older (>30)
Parity	Primigravida	Multipara
Onset	After 20 weeks of pregnancy	Before 20 weeks of pregnancy
Weight gain and edema	Sudden	Gradual
Systolic blood pressure	<160	>160
Funduscopic findings	Spasm, edema	Arteriovenous nicking, exudates
Proteinuria	Present	Absent
Plasma uric acid	Increased	Normal
Blood pressure after delivery	Normal	Elevated

be made (Table 26–21), but sometimes this can be done only after delivery.

HYPERTENSION

As previously noted, the absolute level of the blood pressure elevation need not be great to increase fetal mortality. The mother may be particularly vulnerable to encephalopathy because of her previously normal blood pressure. As will be described in more detail under Hypertensive Crises (p. 892), cerebral blood flow is kept constant over a fairly narrow range of mean arterial pressure, which is roughly between 60 and 110 mm Hg in normotensive individuals. A previously normotensive young woman whose blood pressure rises acutely to 150/100 may exceed the upper limit of autoregulation, resulting in a breakthrough of cerebral blood flow that leads to cerebral edema, convulsions, and all the clinical manifestations of eclampsia.

OTHER FEATURES

Proteinuria and Renal Damage. Even traces of proteinuria add significantly to the seriousness of the clinical situation (Fig. 26–34). Renal damage may be reflected in a falling creatinine clearance rate and a rising plasma uric acid concentration.

Edema. Some pedal edema is seen in over half of normal pregnant women, but a sudden weight gain of more than 2 pounds in one week and the subsequent appearance of more generalized edema commonly forewarns of preeclampsia.

Additional Features. On funduscopic examination, sequential constriction of the retinal arterioles is seen first, followed by retinal edema causing a retinal sheen. The presence of arteriovenous nicking and exudates suggests a chronic hypertensive process. If any of the following clinical features is present and does not improve, delivery within 24 hours should be considered: diastolic blood pressure above 110 mm Hg, headaches, visual scotomas, proteinuria 2+ or greater, or epigastric pain.

Management

PREVENTION. The only sure preventative against the syndrome of pregnancy-induced hypertension is prevention of pregnancy among teenagers. Once pregnant, primigravidas should be watched carefully, particularly if they are young or diabetic or have a family history of preeclampsia.

A simple test to predict subsequent preeclampsia has been described[397] and has been found to have fair specificity and sensitivity.[398] The supine pressor test, or "roll-over" test, involves measuring the blood pressure first in the left lateral recumbent position and then in the supine position. A rise in the diastolic pressure of 20 mm Hg or greater within 2 to 5 minutes is considered positive and predicts a 70 to 90 per cent chance of subsequent preeclampsia; women with a negative test have a greater than 90 per cent chance of remaining normotensive.

If the test is done on a normotensive primigravida at about the 28th week of pregnancy and if the result is positive, the patient should be instructed to restrict her activity, be seen frequently, and be warned that immediate hospitalization may be necessary if early features of preeclampsia develop.

TREATMENT

Once the blood pressure rises, the patient's physical activity should be restricted, preferably through admission to a high-risk pregnancy unit where she can be carefully observed. Remarkable results have been achieved in such a low-cost hospital setting.[399] Most women became normotensive without medication and safely carried their fetus to maturity. As a result, perinatal mortality fell to 9 per 1000—lower than that noted among infants born to women without preeclampsia on the general obstetric ward at the same hospital.[399]

ANTIHYPERTENSIVE THERAPY. Only if the diastolic pressure does not fall below 110 mm Hg on modified bedrest is antihypertensive drug therapy used. Diuretics and salt restriction are avoided, particularly since there is increasing evidence that preeclampsia is associated with a shrunken plasma volume.[381] Methyldopa (Aldomet) or hydralazine (Apresoline) has been usually chosen, the former for more chronic oral use and the latter for more acute parenteral use. In a randomly controlled trial, half of a group of hypertensive women, most with chronic, preexisting hypertension, received methyldopa, while the other half were left untreated. Their children were closely followed for 7½ years and the following differences were noted: the treated sons were lighter and shorter; sons whose mothers were started on methyldopa between 16 and 20 weeks' gestation had smaller heads but no difference in intelligence quotients.[400] Thus, there may be some developmental problems, particularly if methyldopa is started during the midtrimester. Since methyldopa acts centrally to influence the metabolism of the neurotransmitter dopamine, the safety of other drugs has been investigated.

Beta blockers initially received a bad press, with scattered reports of fetal hypoglycemia, bradycardia, and respiratory depression.[401] However, a properly controlled comparison showed that therapy with oxprenolol was equally effective as methyldopa and was associated with fewer fetal difficulties.[402] Another, less well controlled study of metoprolol had similar results.[403]

If the patient enters pregnancy while receiving antihypertensive drugs, including diuretics, the medications are usually continued, based on the idea that the mother should be protected and that the fetus will not suffer from any sudden hemodynamic shifts such as occur when therapy is first begun. Among women with chronic hypertension but who were not undergoing treatment, therapy with either hydralazine or methyldopa significantly reduced the incidence of preeclampsia compared to the course among a placebo-treated group.[404] Thus, those with chronic hypertension should probably be started on therapy early in their pregnancy.

MANAGEMENT OF ECLAMPSIA. With appropriate care of preeclampsia, eclampsia hardly ever supervenes; when it does, however, maternal mortality may reach 14 per cent and fetal mortality 27 per cent.[405] Among those women who die, contraction band necrosis of the myocardium, indicative of coronary artery spasm, is frequently noted and may be a contributing factor.[406]

Susceptible patients are given magnesium sulfate ($MgSO_4$) prophylactically, and blood pressure is brought under control with antihypertensive agents. Diazoxide, although favored by some, will cause labor to cease, since it relaxes uterine muscles. If convulsions have already occurred, they can be halted with $MgSO_4$, and delivery should be delayed until the blood pressure is controlled and fluid and electrolyte balance is achieved. With this approach, there have been no maternal deaths and fetal survival has been excellent in 154 consecutive cases.[399]

CONSEQUENCES. The long-term prognosis of women with pregnancy-induced hypertension is excellent. When some 200 women who had had eclampsia were followed for up to 44 years, the distribution of blood pressures was identical to that in the general population.[396] Chesley concludes that "eclampsia neither is a sign of latent essential hypertension nor causes hypertension."

POSTPARTUM HYPERTENSION

After delivery, women may develop transient or persistent hypertension. In many, early essential hypertension may have been masked by the hemodynamic changes of pregnancy. However, some women develop postpartum heart failure that may be related to hypertension or may be a primary cardiomyopathy[407] (see Chapter 52). A small number of others develop rapidly progressive acute oliguric renal failure associated with severe hypertension.[408]

HYPERTENSION IN CHILDREN AND ADOLESCENTS
(See also Chapter 31)

The linkage between hypertension in children and adolescents and that in adults is being strengthened, but long-term tracking studies are not available to document the natural history of the process. As an example, taken from the description of abnormal sodium transport in the pathogenesis of primary hypertension earlier in this chapter, half of the normotensive children of hypertensive parents have the abnormality but it will take another 20 or more years to determine whether the abnormality presages the development of hypertension.

Regardless, a great deal of work is being done to define the frequency, mechanisms, natural history, and treatment of hypertension in childhood. Many of these aspects are covered in Chapter 31, and only a few will be highlighted here.

BLOOD PRESSURE MEASUREMENTS

The grids shown on page 1057, published in 1977 by a task force of the NHLBI, have been widely accepted as the "official" new standards for the distribution of blood pressure levels in normal male and female children, ages 2 to 17 years. However, other surveys have found the normal levels to be lower by an average of 5 to 10 mm Hg and few children to be definitely hypertensive.[409] The most obvious reason for these lower levels is the use of more than one blood pressure measurement in most of these studies.

The need to take more than one reading was shown as follows: in the Muscatine survey, 13 per cent of the 6,622 schoolchildren had elevated blood pressure on the first examination but less than 1 per cent had persistent elevations[410]; in Dallas, 8.9 per cent of 10,641 eighth-graders had levels at or above the 95th percentile on the first screening but only 1.2 per cent had hypertension on reexamination.[411]

In a number of studies, repeated measurements are being taken to assess the tracking of blood pressure levels. Correlations as high as 0.7 are noted over one year. Although lesser degrees of correlation are noted over long periods of time, the tracking of both systolic and diastolic pressures does persist for up to eight years.[412] Thus, the long-term course of blood pressure can be predicted with increasing confidence during early childhood. The need for repeated blood pressure measurements for all children is now established, with particular emphasis on families with hypertension, premature deaths, or other risk factors for cardiovascular disease.

ESSENTIAL OR PRIMARY HYPERTENSION

The studies by Zinner et al., in addition to providing long-term tracking data, reconfirm their previous findings of familial aggregation of both blood pressure and the excretion of kallikrein in the urine.[412] Low levels of this vasodilator could represent a causal mechanism for primary (essential) hypertension.

As noted before, about half the normotensive children of hypertensive parents have a rate of Na^+/K^+ flux within the range seen in patients with established, primary hypertension.[105] Whether those children will develop hypertension remains to be seen. If so, a new tool of great value in unraveling the mechanisms of hypertension may be available.

In the meantime, the levels of blood pressure in children have been shown to be related to various factors (Table 26–22). Perhaps the most important, beyond prior levels of blood pressure, is body weight, shown in various studies to be more closely related than age. In hopes of preventing subsequent hypertension, prevention of childhood obesity is being increasingly advocated, along with a reduction in the high levels of sodium intake. Of interest, the blood pressures of healthy black children are not higher—and may be lower—than those seen in white children.[413,414] Thus, the reasons for the much greater incidence of hypertension in black adults must be sought among factors

TABLE 26–22 EPIDEMIOLOGICAL FACTORS RELATED TO BLOOD PRESSURE LEVELS IN CHILDREN AND ADOLESCENTS

Genetic

  Parental and sibling blood pressure levels
  Erythrocyte sodium flux
  Urinary kallikrein level

Environmental

  Socioeconomic status
  Rural vs. urban residence
  Migration from developing to developed area
  Pulse rate

Mixed genetic and environmental

  Body mass and muscular development
  Salt
  Stress

From Lieberman, E.: *In* Kaplan, N. M. (ed.): Clinical Hypertension. 3rd ed. Baltimore, Williams and Wilkins Co., 1982, p. 420.

with long "incubation" or which are active mainly beyond adolescence. When asymptomatic children with persistently elevated pressures are studied, most turn out to have no recognizable secondary cause. In Muscatine, 23 of the 41 with high pressures were obese; of the 18 lean subjects, 13 had essential hypertension.[410]

The hemodynamic profile in children with primary hypertension is complex and variable. In a study of the cardiac output, fluid volumes, and intraarterial blood pressure in 42 young hypertensives (ages 15 to 25), there was no clear relation of the blood pressure to either cardiac output or blood volume.[415] Thus, hypertension in children does not usually fit a "hyperdynamic" pattern with high cardiac output and fast pulse rates.

The role of the sympathetic nervous and angiotensin mechanisms in blood pressure elevation among children remains unknown. Plasma renin and aldosterone levels tend to be *low* in those with the higher levels of blood pressure,[416] particularly among blacks.[417] Plasma catecholamine levels are usually normal,[416] but they may show a greater cardiovascular response to mental and other types of stress.[418]

The potential harm of even relatively small elevations in blood pressure may be found in careful studies of heart size and function. In 114 hypertensive high school students, heart size and contractile functions as determined by echocardiography were significantly increased in comparison to findings in normotensives of the same age.[419]

SECONDARY HYPERTENSION

As more experience is gained, the need for extensive laboratory work-up for the majority of postpubertal children with relatively mild hypertension continues to be deemphasized.[19] Only those with fairly severe hypertension or an abnormality on initial screening laboratory studies need to undergo additional testing, including an IVP. As shown years ago by Londe and coworkers,[419] most hypertension in children has no apparent cause but, when the diastolic is above 120 mm Hg, perhaps 95 per cent will have secondary hypertension. Thus, it may be appropriate to investigate more thoroughly only those with abnormalities on the physical examination or on urine analysis and those with a blood pressure that is 10 mm Hg or more above the 95th percentile.

THERAPY

The proper therapy for children with hypertension remains uncertain. In general, the guidelines for adult hypertension provided in Chapter 27 seem appropriate for the young, although a longer trial of weight reduction and sodium restriction seems indicated before drug treatment is begun. The long-term effects of various antihypertensive agents need to be more carefully assessed.

HYPERTENSIVE CRISES

Having considered the various forms of hypertension—both idiopathic and secondary—in children and adults, we will now turn to the life-threatening complication of all hypertensive diseases, hypertensive crisis.

Definitions

A number of clinical circumstances may require rapid reduction of the blood pressure (Table 26–23).

Hypertensive crisis: The presence of a blood pressure level so high that immediate vascular necrosis threatens. A mean arterial pressure above 150 mm Hg is enough to produce vascular damage within hours in experimental animals.[420] In humans, a diastolic pressure above 140 mm Hg is usually associated with acute vascular damage, although some may suffer seriously from lower levels and others manage to withstand even higher levels without apparent harm. As we shall see, the rapidity of the rise may be more important than the degree in producing acute vascular damage.

TABLE 26–23   CIRCUMSTANCES REQUIRING RAPID REDUCTION OF BLOOD PRESSURE

1. Hypertensive encephalopathy from any cause
    a. Essential hypertension
    b. Renal parenchymal diseases: acute and chronic glomerulonephritis
    c. Renal vascular disease
    d. Toxemia of pregnancy
2. Uncontrolled hypertension
    a. Malignant hypertension
    b. Pheochromocytoma
    c. Intake of catecholamine precursors in patients taking MAO inhibitors
    d. Head injuries
    e. Severe burns
    f. Rebound hypertension after cessation of antihypertensive drugs
3. Severe to moderate hypertension accompanying
    a. Acute left ventricular failure
    b. Intracranial hemorrhage
    c. Dissecting aneurysm of the aorta
    d. Postoperative bleeding at vascular suture lines
    e. Severe epistaxis

From Kaplan, N. M.: Clinical Hypertension. 3rd ed. Baltimore, Williams and Wilkins Co., 1982, p. 194.

Hypertensive encephalopathy: The association of headache, irritability, alterations in consciousness, and other manifestations of central nervous dysfunction with sudden and marked elevations in blood pressure. Symptoms can be reversed by a reduction in the pressure.

Accelerated hypertension: Retinal hemorrhages and exudates, usually with diastolic pressures above 140 mm Hg. This usually represents a sudden increase in chronically elevated blood pressure.

Malignant hypertension: Papilledema and diastolic pressures usually above 140 mm Hg. Accelerated hypertension usually precedes malignant hypertension. Without reduction of the pressure, death rapidly ensues, usually because of destruction of the kidneys.

Incidence

In about 1 per cent of patients with essential hypertension, the disease progresses to an accelerated or malignant phase. Presumably, if left untreated, many more patients would follow this pattern, since the incidence had been higher before effective therapies became available,[421] and it seems to be decreasing steadily. Ten per cent of patients with diastolic pressure below 115 mm Hg experienced a rise in pressure to above 125 when given placebos over a 5-year period[38]; if therapy had not been started, some would likely have progressed to malignant hypertension.

Any hypertensive disease can initiate malignant hypertension. Some, including pheochromocytoma and renovascular hypertension, do so at a higher rate than does essential hypertension. However, since hypertension is idiopathic in over 90 per cent of all patients, the largest number of hypertensive crises appear when there is preexisting essential hypertension.

Pathophysiology

Two distinct but usually concurrent processes are involved. One is functional, i.e., the dilatation of cerebral arterioles, allowing excessive cerebral blood flow that leads to hypertensive encephalopathy. The other is structural, i.e., acute damage to the arteriolar wall, resulting in fibri-

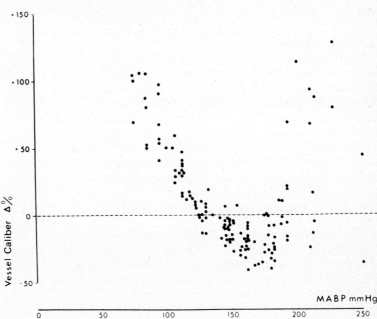

FIGURE 26–37 Change observed in the caliber of pial arterioles with a caliber less than 50 μ in 8 cats when blood pressure was raised by intravenous infusion of angiotensin II. Calculation is based on the percentage of change from the caliber at a mean arterial blood pressure (MABP) of 135 mm Hg. (From MacKenzie, E. T., et al.: Effects of acutely induced hypertension in cats on pial arteriolar caliber, local cerebral blood flow, and the blood-brain barrier. Circ. Res. *39*:33, 1976, by permission of the American Heart Association, Inc.)

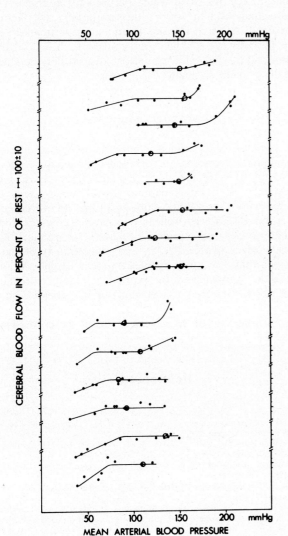

FIGURE 26–38 Curves of cerebral blood flow with varying levels of blood pressure in 14 patients: 8 hypertensive (*top*) and 6 normotensive (*bottom*). Each patient's habitual pressure is indicated by the open circle. The curves reflect autoregulation, with a shift upward or to the right in the hypertensives. Both lower and upper limits of autoregulation are shown. Note the breakthrough of CBF when the upper limit is exceeded. (From Johansson, B., et al.: On the pathogenesis of hypertensive encephalopathy. Circ. Res. *35*(Suppl.):I–167, 1974, by permission of the American Heart Association, Inc.)

noid necrosis. Both processes are most likely the consequences of very high blood pressure and may develop without apparent involvement of the renin-angiotensin or other hormonal mechanisms.[420]

Studies done in animals and man by Strandgaard and associates have elucidated the mechanism of encephalopathy. First, they directly measured the caliber of pial arterioles over the cerebral cortex in cats whose blood pressures were varied over a wide range by infusion of vasodilators or angiotensin II[422] (Fig. 26–37). As the pressure fell, the arterioles became dilated; as the pressure rose, the arterioles became constricted. Thus a constant cerebral blood flow was maintained by means of autoregulation. However, when mean arterial pressure rose above 180 mm Hg, the tightly constricted vessels could no longer withstand the pressure and suddenly became dilated. This began in an irregular manner, first in areas with less muscular tone and then diffusely, producing generalized vasodilatation. This breakthrough of cerebral blood flow hyperperfuses the brain under high pressure, causing leakage of fluid into the perivascular tissue, and resulting in cerebral edema and the syndrome of hypertensive encephalopathy.

In human subjects, they repetitively measured cerebral blood flow by an isotopic technique while lowering or raising the blood pressure with vasodilators or vasoconstrictors in a manner similar to that in the animal studies.[423] Curves depicting cerebral blood flow demonstrate autoregulation with a constancy of flow over mean pressures in normotensive persons from about 60 to 120 mm Hg and in hypertensive patients from about 110 to 180 mm Hg (Fig. 26–38). This shift to the right in the hypertensive patients is the result of structural thickening of the arterioles as an adaptation to the chronically elevated pressures.[424]

When pressures were raised beyond the upper limit of autoregulation, the same "breakthrough" with hyperperfusion occurred as was seen in the animal studies (Fig. 26–38). In previously normotensive people, whose vessels have not been altered by prior exposure to high pressure, breakthrough occurred at about 120 mm Hg mean arterial pressure; in hypertensive patients, the breakthrough occurred at about 180 mm Hg.

These studies confirm clinical observations. In previously normotensive people, severe encephalopathy occurs with relatively little hypertension. In children with acute glomerulonephritis and in women with eclampsia, convulsions may occur owing to hypertensive encephalopathy with blood pressures as low as 150/100 mm Hg. Obviously, chronically hypertensive patients withstand such pressures without duress. However, when pressures increase sufficiently, they too may develop encephalopathy.

Manifestations and Course

The symptoms and signs of hypertensive crises are usually dramatic (Table 26–24). However, some may be relatively asymptomatic, despite markedly elevated pressures and extensive organ damage. Young black men are particularly prone to experience a hypertensive crisis with severe renal insufficiency but little obvious prior distress.

When the blood pressure is so high as to induce encephalopathy or accelerated-malignant hypertension, the following clinical features are frequently seen:

1. Renal insufficiency with protein and red cells in the urine and azotemia. Acute oliguric renal failure may develop.

2. Elevated levels of plasma renin activity from the diffuse intrarenal ischemia, resulting in secondary aldosteronism, often manifested by hypokalemia. Although not causal, the secondarily elevated renin and aldosterone levels most likely exacerbate the hypertensive process, so that a vicious cycle is established: severe hypertension → intrarenal vascular damage → increased renin secretion → increased hypertension by the vasoconstrictor action of angiotensin II and by its stimulation of aldosterone, causing additional volume overload.

3. Microangiopathic hemolytic anemia with red cell fragmentation and intravascular coagulation.

If left untreated, patients die quickly from brain damage or more gradually from renal damage. Before effective therapy was available, fewer than 25 per cent of patients with malignant hypertension were alive after one year and only 1 per cent after five years.[425] With therapy, over 70 per cent survive for one year and about 50 per cent for five years.[426] Death in patients with severe hypertension is usually from stroke or renal failure if it occurs in the first few years after onset.[426] If therapy keeps patients alive for longer than five years, death will likely be caused by coronary disease. Although this could reflect some ill effect of anti-

TABLE 26–24   CLINICAL CHARACTERISTICS OF HYPERTENSIVE CRISIS

Blood pressure: Usually > 140 mm Hg diastolic
Funduscopic findings: Hemorrhages, exudates, papilledema
Neurological status: Headache, confusion, somnolence, stupor,
   visual loss, focal deficits, seizures, coma
Cardiac findings: Prominent apical impulse, cardiac enlargement,
   congestive failure
Renal: Oliguria, azotemia
Gastrointestinal: Nausea, vomiting

From Kaplan, N. M.: Clinical Hypertension. 3rd ed. Baltimore, Williams and Wilkins Co., 1982.

TABLE 26–25   DISEASES TO BE DIFFERENTIATED FROM A HYPERTENSIVE CRISIS

Acute left ventricular failure
Uremia from any cause, particularly with volume overload
Cerebral vascular accident
Subarachnoid hemorrhage
Brain tumor
Head injury
Epilepsy (postictal)
Collagen diseases, particularly lupus, with cerebral vasculitis
Encephalitis
Overdose and withdrawal from narcotics, amphetamines, and so on
Acute anxiety with hyperventilation syndrome

From Kaplan, N. M.: Clinical Hypertension. 3rd ed. Baltimore, Williams and Wilkins Co., 1982, p. 200.

hypertensive therapy on the coronary vessels, it is likely that high pressure per se plays an important role in causing strokes and renal damage and a lesser role in causing coronary artery disease in which the primary mechanism is atherosclerosis and in which other important risk factors are involved. Antihypertensive treatment is particularly effective in reducing deaths from congestive heart failure, providing additional evidence against any cardiotoxic effect of the drugs or the reduction in pressure.

Differential Diagnosis

The presence of hypertensive encephalopathy or accelerated-malignant hypertension demands immediate, aggressive therapy to lower the blood pressure effectively. Except in pregnancy or in catecholamine excess, therapy may be instituted before the specific cause is known. However, certain serious diseases as well as one psychogenic problem, i.e., acute anxiety with hyperventilation, can mimic a hypertensive crisis (Table 26–25), and management of these conditions may obviously require different diagnostic and therapeutic approaches. In particular, blood pressure should not be lowered too abruptly in a patient with a stroke.

Specific therapy of hypertensive crises is covered in Chapter 27.

References

1. Roberts, W. C.: The hypertensive diseases. Evidence that systemic hypertension is a greater risk factor to the development of other cardiovascular diseases than previously suspected. Am. J. Med. 59:523, 1975.
2. National Center for Health Statistics: Births, marriages, divorces, and deaths for 1981. Monthly Vital Statistics Report 30 (12):1, 1982.
3. Kannel, W. B.: Meaning of the downward trend in cardiovascular mortality. J.A.M.A. 247:877, 1982.
4. Kaplan, N. M.: Clinical Hypertension. 3rd ed. Baltimore, Williams and Wilkins Co., 1982.
5. Pickering, T. G., Harshfield, G. A., Kleinert, H. D., Blank, S., and Laragh, J. H.: Blood pressure during normal daily activities, sleep and exercise. Comparison of values in normal hypertensive subjects. J.A.M.A. 247:992, 1982.
6. Kirkendall, W. M., Feinleib, M., Freis, E. D., and Mark, A. L.: Recommendations for human blood pressure determination by sphygmomanometers. Hypertension 3:510A, 1981.
7. Dawber, T. R.: The Framingham Study. The Epidemiology of Atherosclerotic Disease. Cambridge, Massachusetts, Harvard University Press, 1980.
8. Society of Actuaries and Association of Life Insurance Medical Directors of America: Blood Pressure Study, 1979. Recording and Statistical Corp., 1980.
9. Kannel, W. B., Wolf, P. A., McGee, D. L., Dawber, T. R., McNamara, P., and Castelli, W. P.: Systolic blood pressure, arterial rigidity and risk of stroke. The Framingham study. J.A.M.A. 245:1225, 1981.
10. Gifford, R. W., Jr.: Isolated systolic hypertension in the elderly. J.A.M.A. 247:781, 1982.

11. Spence, J. D., Sibbald, W. J., and Cape, R. D.: Pseudohypertension in the elderly. Clin. Sci. Molec. Med. 55:399s, 1978.
12. Laughlin, K. D., Fisher, L., and Sherrard, D. J.: Blood pressure reductions during self-recording of home blood pressure. Am. Heart J. 298:629, 1979.
13. The Pooling Project Research Group: Relationship of blood pressure, serum cholesterol, smoking habit, relative weight and ECG abnormalities to incidence of major coronary events: Final report of the pooling project. J. Chron. Dis. 31:201, 1978.
14. Hypertension Detection and Follow-up Program Cooperative Group: Blood pressure studies in 14 communities. A two-stage screen for hypertension. J.A.M.A. 237:2385, 1977.
15. Carey, R. M., Reid, R. A., Ayers, C. R., Lynch, S. S., McLain, W. L., III, and Vaughan, E. D., Jr.: The Charlottesville blood-pressure survey. Value of repeated blood-pressure measurements. J.A.M.A. 236:847, 1976.
16. Rames, L. K., Clarke, W. R., Connor, W. E., Reiter, M. A., and Lauer, R.M.: Normal blood pressures and the evaluation of sustained blood pressure elevation in childhood. The Muscatine (Iowa) study. Pediatrics 61:245, 1978.
17. Julius, S., Hansson, L., Andren, L, Gudbrandsson, T., Sivertsson, R., and Svensson, A.: Borderline hypertension. Acta Med. Scand. 208:481, 1980.
18. National Heart, Lung, and Blood Institute: Report of the Task Force on Blood Pressure Control in Children. Pediatrics 59 (Suppl.):797, 1977.
19. Lieberman E.: Hypertension in childhood and adolescence. In Kaplan, N. M. (ed.): Clinical Hypertension. 3rd ed. Baltimore, Williams and Wilkins Co., 1982, p. 411.
20. Voors, A. W., Webber, L. S., and Berenson G. S.: Time course study of blood pressure in children over a three-year period. Bogalusa heart study. Hypertension 2 (Suppl. I):I–202, 1980.
21. Pickering, G.: Hypertension: Definitions, natural histories and consequences. Am. J. Med. 52:570, 1972.
22. Itskovitz, H. S., Kochar, M. S., Anderson, A. J., and Rim, A. A.: Patterns of blood pressure in Milwaukee. J.A.M.A. 238:864, 1977.
23. Messerli, F. H., DeCarvalho, J. G. R., Christie, B., and Frohlich, E. D.: Essential hypertension in black and white subjects. Am. J. Med. 67:27, 1979.
24. Grim, C. E., Weinberger, M. H., Higgins, J. T., and Kramer, N. J.: Diagnosis of secondary forms of hypertension. A comprehensive protocol. J.A.M.A. 237:1331, 1977.
25. Tucker, R. M., and Labarthe, D. R.: Frequency of surgical treatment for hypertension in adults at the Mayo Clinic from 1973 through 1975. Mayo Clin. Proc. 52:549, 1977.
26. Berglund, G., Andersson, O., and Wilhelmsen, L.: Prevalence of primary and secondary hypertension: Studies in a random population sample. Br. Med. J. 2:554, 1976.
27. Rudnick, K. V., Sackett, D. L., Hirst, S., and Holmes, C.: Hypertension in family practice. Canad. Med. Assoc. J. 3:492, 1977.
28. Danielson, M., and Dammström, B.: The prevalence of secondary and curable hypertension. Acta Med. Scand. 209:451, 1981.
29. Fagan, T. J.: Nomogram for Bayes theorem. N. Engl. J. Med. 293:257, 1975.
30. Aschinberg, L. C., Zeis, P. M., Miller, R. A., John, E. G., and Chan, L. L.: Essential hypertension in childhood. J.A.M.A. 238:322, 1977.
31. Weiss, N. S.: Relation of high blood pressure to headache, epistaxis, and selected other symptoms. N. Engl. J. Med. 287:631, 1972.
32. Bulpitt, C. J., Dollery, C. T., and Carne, S.: Change in symptoms of hypertensive patients after referral to hospital clinic. Br. Heart J. 38:121, 1976.
33. Stewart, I. McD. G., and Lond, M. D.: Headache and hypertension. Lancet 1:1261, 1953.
34. Bauer, G. E.: Hypertension and headache. Aust. N.Z.J. Med. 6:492, 1976.
35. Hypertension Detection and Follow-Up Program Cooperative Group: The Hypertension Detection and Follow-Up Program. A progress report. Circ. Res. 40:I–106, 1977.
36. Thompson, G. E., Alderman, M. H., Wassertheil-Smoller, S., Rafter, J. G., and Samet, R.: High blood pressure diagnosis and treatment: Consensus recommendations vs. actual practice. Am. J. Public Health 71:413, 1981.
37. Rose, G.: Strategy of prevention: Lessons from cardiovascular disease. Br. Med. J. 282:1847, 1981.
38. Veterans Administration Cooperative Study Group on Antihypertensive Agents: Effects of treatment on morbidity in hypertension. II. Results in patients with diastolic blood pressure averaging 90 through 114 mm Hg. J.A.M.A. 213:1143, 1970.
39. Keith, N. M., Wagener, H. P., and Barker, N. W.: Some different types of essential hypertension: Their course and prognosis. Am. J. Med. Sci. 268:336, 1974.
40. Svardsudd, K., Wedel, H., Aurell, E., and Tibblin, G.: Hypertensive eye ground changes. Acta Med. Scand. 204:159, 1978.
41. Savage, D. D., Drayer, J. I. M., Henry, W. L., Mathews, E. C., Ware, J. H., Gardin, J. M., Cohen, E. R., Epstein, S. E., and Laragh, J. H.: Echocardiographic assessment of cardiac anatomy and function in hypertensive subjects. Circulation 59:623, 1979.
42. Hollenberg, N. K., and Adams, D. F.: The renal circulation in hypertensive disease. Am. J. Med. 60:773, 1976.
43. Wollam, G. L., and Gifford, R. W., Jr.: The kidney as a target organ in hypertension. Geriatrics 31:71, 1976.
44. Bauer, G. E., and Humphrey, T. J.: The natural history of hypertension with moderate impairment of renal function. Clin. Sci. Molec. Med. 45:191s, 1973.
45. Brunner, H. R., Laragh, J. H., Baer, L., Newton, M. A., Goodwin, F. T., Krakoff, L. R., Bard, R. H., and Buhler, F. R.: Essential hypertension: Renin and aldosterone, heart attack and stroke. N. Engl. J. Med. 286:441, 1972.

46. Kaplan, N. M.: The prognostic implications of plasma renin in essential hypertension. J.A.M.A. 231:167, 1975.
47. Birkenhager, W. H., Kho, T. L., Schalekamp, M.A.D.H., Kolsters, G., Wester, A., and De Leeuw, P. W.: Renin levels and cardiovascular morbidity in essential hypertension. A prospective study. Acta Clin. Belg. 32:168, 1977.
48. Management Committee: The Australian therapeutic trial in mild hypertension. Lancet 1:1261, 1980.
49. Management Committee: Untreated mild hypertension. Lancet 1:185, 1982.
50. Helgeland, A.: Treatment of mild hypertension: A five year controlled drug trial. The Oslo Study. Am. J. Med. 69:725, 1980.
51. Schweitzer, M. D., Gearing, F. R., and Perera, G. A.: The epidemiology of primary hypertension. J. Chron. Dis. 18:847, 1965.
52. Hollander, W.: Role of hypertension in atherosclerosis and cardiovascular disease. Am. J. Cardiol. 38:786, 1976.
53. O'Rourke, M. D.: Pulsatile arterial hemodynamics in hypertension. Aust. N.Z.J. Med. 6:40, 1976.
54. Palmer, R. F.: Vascular compliance and pulsatile flow as determinants of vascular injury. In Laragh, J. H., Buhler, F. R., and Seldin, D. W. (eds.): Frontiers in Hypertension. New York, Springer-Verlag, 1981.
55. Bierman, E. L., Brewer, C., and Baum, D.: Hypertension decreases replication potential of arterial smooth muscle cells: Aortic coarctation in humans as model. Proc. Soc. Exp. Biol. Med. 166:335, 1981.
56. Dunn, F. G., Chandraratna, P., DeCarvalho, J. G. R., Basta, L. L., and Frohlich, E. D.: Pathophysiologic assessment of hypertensive heart disease with echocardiography. Am. J. Cardiol. 39:789, 1977.
57. Rabkin, S. W., Mathewson, F. A. L., and Tate, R. B.: Longitudinal blood pressure measurements during a 26-year observation period and the risk of ischemic heart disease. Am. J. Epidemiol. 109650, 1979.
58. Rabkin, S. W., Mathewson, F. A. L., and Tate, R. B.: Prognosis after acute myocardial infarction: Relation to blood pressure values before infarction in a prospective cardiovascular study. Am. J. Cardiol. 40:604, 1977.
59. Beta-Blocker Heart Attack Trial Research Group: A randomized trial of propranolol in patients with acute myocardial infarction. I. Mortality results. J.A.M.A. 247:1707, 1982.
60. Astrup, J., Bisgaard-Frantzen, H. O., Nielsen, S. L., and Rossing, N.: Blood pressure–lowering effect of acute myocardial infarction. Lancet 2:903, 1976.
61. Kannel, W. B., Sorlie, P. Castelli, W. P., and McGee, D.: Blood pressure and survival after myocardial infarction: The Framingham study. Am. J. Cardiol. 45:326, 1980.
62. McKee, P. A., Castelli, W. P., McNamara, P. M., and Kannel, W. B.: The natural history of congestive heart failure: The Framingham study. N. Engl. J. Med. 285:1441, 1971.
63. Tarazi, R. C., and Levy, M. N.: Cardiac responses to increased afterload. Hypertension 4 (Suppl. II):II-8, 1982.
64. Breckinridge, A.: Vasodilators in heart failure. Br. Med. J. 284:765, 1982.
65. Goodwin, J. D.: Congestive and hypertrophic cardiomyopathies. A decade of study. Lancet 1:731, 1970.
66. Roberts, W. C.: Aortic dissection: Anatomy, consequences, and causes. Am. Heart J. 101:195, 1981.
67. Kannel, W. B., Dawber, T. R., Sorlie, P., and Wolf, P. A.: Components of blood pressure and risk of atherothrombotic brain infarction: The Framingham study. Stroke 7:327, 1976.
68. Rabkin, S. W., Mathewson, F. A. L., and Tate, R. B.: Predicting risk of ischemic heart disease and cerebrovascular disease from systolic and diastolic blood pressures. Ann. Intern. Med. 88:342, 1978.
69. Wolf, P. A., Kannel, W. B., Sorlie, P., and McNamara, P.: Asymptomatic carotid bruit and risk of stroke. The Framingham study. J.A.M.A. 245:1442, 1981.
70. Boller, F., Vrtunski, P. B., Mack, J. L., and Kin, Y.: Neuropsychological correlates of hypertension. Arch. Neurol. 34:701, 1977.
71. Whisnant, J. P., Cartlidge, N. E. F., and Elveback, L. R.: Carotid and vertebral-basilar transient ischemic attacks: Effect of anticoagulants, hypertension, and cardiac disorders on survival and stroke occurrence—A population study. Ann. Neurol. 3:107, 1978.
72. Strandgaard, S.: Autoregulation of cerebral blood flow in hypertensive patients. The modifying influence of prolonged antihypertensive treatment on the tolerance to acute, drug-induced hypotension. Circulation 53:720, 1976.
73. Ledingham, J. G. G., and Rajagopalan, B.: Cerebral complications in the treatment of accelerated hypertension. Quart. J. Med. 48:25, 1979.
74. Wollner, L., McCarthy, S. T., Soper, N. D. W., and Macy, D. J.: Failure of cerebral autoregulation as a cause of brain dysfunction in the elderly. Br. Med. J. 1:1117, 1979.
75. Messerli, F. H., Frohlich, E. D., Dreslinski, G. R., Suarez, D. H., and Aristimuno, G. G.: Serum uric acid in essential hypertension: An indicator of renal vascular involvement. Ann. Intern. Med. 93:817, 1980.
76. Simon, and Altman, S.: Increased serum N-acetyl-β-D-glucosaminidase activity in human hypertension. Clin. Exp. Hyper. Theory Practice A4 (3):355, 1982.
77. Woods, J. W., Blythe, W. B., and Huffines, W. D.: Management of malignant hypertension complicated by renal insufficiency. N. Engl. J. Med. 241:10, 1974.
78. Cruickshank, J. D., and Beevers, D. G.: Epidemiology of hypertension: Blood pressure in blacks and whites. Clin. Sci. 62:1, 1982.
79. Rostand, S. G., Kirk, K. A., Rutsky, E. A., and Pate, B. A.: Racial differences in the incidence of treatment for end-stage renal disease. N. Engl. J. Med. 306:1276, 1982.

80. Kaplan, N. M., Kem, D. C., Holland, O. B., Kramer, N. J., Higgins, J., and Gomez-Sanchez, C. E. The intravenous furosemide test: A simple way to evaluate renin responsiveness. Ann. Intern. Med. *84*:639, 1976.

81. Holland, O. B., and Fairchild, C.: Renin classification for diuretic and beta-blocker treatment of black hypertensive patients. J. Chron. Dis. *35*:179, 1982.

82. Woods, K. O., Beevers, D. G., and West, M.: Familial abnormality of erythrocyte cation transport in essential hypertension. Br. Med. J. *282*:1186, 1981.

83. Sever, P. S., Peart, W. S., Gordon, D., and Beighton, P.: Blood-pressure and its correlates in urban and tribal Africa. Lancet *2*:60, 1980.

84. Gibson, G. S., and Gibbons, A.: Hypertension among blacks. An annotated bibliography. Hypertension *4* (1):I-1, 1982.

85. Berkman, M., Magnier, J. P., Tran, M. D., and Thillaud, P.: Orthostatic increase in blood pressure in the elderly. Am. Heart J. *97*:131, 1979.

86. Maxwell, M. H., Bleifer, K. H., Franklin, S. S., and Varady, P. D.: Cooperative study of renovascular hypertension: Demographic analysis of the study. J.A.M.A. *220*:1195–1204, 1972.

MECHANISMS OF PRIMARY HYPERTENSION

87. Editorial: Catecholamines in essential hypertension. Lancet *1*:1088, 1977.

88. Lund-Johansen, P.: Hemodynamic alterations in hypertension—spontaneous changes and effects of drug therapy. Acta Med. Scand. Suppl. *603*:1, 1977.

89. Weiss, Y. A., Safar, M. E., London, G. M., Simon, A. C., Levenson, J. A., and Milliez, P. M.: Repeat hemodynamic determinations in borderline hypertension. Am. J. Med. *64*:382, 1978.

90. Ibrahim, M. M., Tarazi, R. C., Dustan, H. P., Bravo, E. L., and Gifford, R. W., Jr.: Hyperkinetic heart in severe hypertension: A separate clinical hemodynamic entity. Am. J. Cardiol. *35*:667, 1975.

91. Korner, P. H.: Circulatory regulation in hypertension. Br. J. Clin. Pharmacol. *13*:95–105, 1982.

92. Tarazi, R. C.: Hemodynamic role of extracellular fluid in hypertension. Circ. Res. *38* (Suppl. II):73, 1976.

93. Wenting, G. J., Man In'T Veld, A. J., and Schalekamp, M. A. D. H.: Time-course of vascular resistance changes in mineralocorticoid hypertension of man. Clin. Sci. *61*:97, 1981.

94. Coleman, T. J., Samar, R. E., and Murphy, W. R.: Autoregulation versus other vasoconstrictors in hypertension. Hypertension *1*:324, 1979.

95. Folkow, B.: Physiological aspects of primary hypertension. Physiol. Rev. *62*:347–504, 1982.

96. Hermsmeyer, K., Abel, P. W., and Trapani, A. J.: Norepinephrine sensitivity and membrane potentials of caudal arterial muscle in DOCA-salt, Dahl, and SHR hypertension in the rat. Hypertension *4* (Suppl. II):II-49–II-51,1982.

97. Levine, R. S., Hennekens, C. H., Duncan, R. C., Robertson, E. G., Gourley, J., Cassady, J. C., and Gelband, H.: Blood pressure in infant twins: Birth to 6 months of age. Hypertension *2* (Suppl. I):I-29, 1980.

98. Havlik, R. J., and Feinleib, M.: Epidemiology and genetics of hypertension. Hypertension *4* (Supp. III):III-121–III-127, 1982.

99. Biron, P., Mongeau, J. G., and Bertrand, D.: Familial aggregation of blood pressure in 558 adopted children. Canad. Med. Assoc. J. *115*:773, 1976.

100. Falkner, B., Onesti, G., and Hayes, P.: The role of sodium in essential hypertension in genetically hypertensive adolescents. *In* Onesti, G., and Kim, K. E., (eds.): Hypertension in the Young and the Old. New York, Grune and Stratton, 1981, p. 29.

101. Johansson, B.: Vascular smooth muscle reactivity. Ann. Rev. Physiol. *43*:359, 1981.

102. Kaplan, N. M., and Silah, J. G.: Effect of angiotensin II on blood pressure in humans with hypertensive disease. J. Clin. Invest. *43*:659, 1964.

103. Wright, G. B., Alexander, R. W., Ekstein, L. S., and Gimbrone, M. A., Jr.: Sodium, divalent cations, and guanine nucleotides regulate the affinity of the rat mesenteric artery angiotensin II receptor. Circ. Res. *50*:462, 1982.

104. Blackburn, H., and Prineas, R.: Diet and hypertension: Anthropology, epidemiology and public health implications. *In* Paoletti, R., and Gotto, A. (eds.): Advances in Cardiovascular Diseases (*in press*).

105. Meyer, P., Garay, R. P., Nazaret, C., Dagher, G., Bellet, Z. M., Broyer, M., and Feingold, J.: Inheritance of abnormal erythrocyte cation transport in essential hypertension. Br. Med. J. *282*:1114, 1981.

106. Abboud, F. M.: The sympathetic system in hypertension. Hypertension *4* (Suppl. II):II-208, 1982.

107. Guyton, A. C., Coleman, T. G., Cowley, A. W., Jr., Scheel, K. W., Manning, R. D., Jr., and Norman, R. A., Jr.: Arterial pressure regulation. Overriding dominance of the kidneys in long-term regulation and in hypertension. Am. J. Med. *52*:584, 1972.

108. Brown, J. J., Lever, A. F., Robertson, J. I. S., and Schalekamp, M. A. D. H.: Renal abnormality of essential hypertension. Lancet *2*:320, 1974.

109. Kaplan, N. M.: The Goldblatt Memorial Lecture. Part II: The role of the kidney in hypertension. Hypertension *1*:456, 1979.

110. Hollenberg, N. K., Williams, G. H., and Adams, D. F.: Essential hypertension: Abnormal renal vascular and endocrine responses to a mild psychological stimulus. Hypertension *3*:11, 1981.

111. Click, R. L., Joyner, W. L., and Gilmore, J. P.: Reactivity of glomerular afferent and efferent arterioles in renal hypertension. Kidney Int. *15*:109, 1979.

112. London, G. M., Safer, M. E., Weiss, Y. A., Corvol, P. L., Lehner, J. P., Menard, J. M., Simon, A. C., and Milliez, P. L.: Volume-dependent parameters in essential hypertension. Kidney Int. *11*:204, 1977.

113. de Wardener, H. E., and MacGregor, G. A.: The natriuretic hormone and essential hypertension. Lancet *1*:1450–1454, 1982.

114. Sealey, J. E., Kirshma, D., and Laragh, J. H.: Natriuretic activity in plasma and urine of salt-loaded man and sheep. J. Clin. Invest. *48*:2210, 1969.

115. Licht, A., Stein, S., McGregor, C. W., Bourgoignie, J. J., and Bricker, N. S.: Progress in isolation and purification of an inhibitor of sodium transport obtained from dog urine. Kidney Int. *21*:339, 1982.

116. Clarkson, E. M., Koutsaimanis, K. G., Davidman, M., Du Bois, M., Penn, W. P., and deWardener, H. E.: The effect of brain extracts on urinary sodium excretion of the rat and the intracellular sodium concentration of renal tubule fragments. Clin. Sci. Molec. Med. *47*:201, 1974.

117. Plunket, W. C., Hutchins, P. M., Gruber, K. A., and Buckalew, V. M.: Evidence for a vascular sensitizing factor in plasma of saline-loaded dogs. Hypertension *4*:581–589, 1982.

118. Gruber, K. A., Rudel, L. L., and Bullock, B. C.: Increased circulating levels of an endogenous digoxin-like factor in hypertensive monkeys. Hypertension *4*:348, 1982.

118a.Keeler, R.: Atrial natriuretic factor has a direct, prostaglandin-independent action on kidneys. Can. J. Physiol. Pharmacol. *60*:1078–1082, 1982.

119. deWardener, H. E., Clarkson, E. M., Bitensky, L., MacGregor, G. A., Alaghband-Zadeh, J., and Chayen, J.: Effect of sodium intake on ability of human plasma to inhibit renal Na^+-K^+ adenosine triphosphatase in vitro. Lancet *1*:411, 1981.

120. Hamlyn, J. M., Ringel, R., Schaeffer, J., Levinson, P. D., Hamilton, B. P., Kowarski, A. A., and Blaustein, M. P.: A circulating inhibitor of (Na$^+$K)-ATPase associated with essential hypertension. Nature (in press) 1983.

121. Edmondson, R. P. S., Thomas, R. D., Hilton, P. J., Patrick, J., and Jones, N. F.: Abnormal leucocyte composition and sodium transport in essential hypertension. Lancet *2*:1003, 1975.

122. Haddy, F. J., Pamnani, M., Clough, D., and Huot, S.: Role of a humoral sodium-potassium pump inhibitor in experimental low renin hypertension. Life Sci. *30*:571, 1982.

123. Edmondson, R. P. S., and MacGregor, G. A.: Leucocyte cation transport in essential hypertension: Its relation to the renin-angiotensin system. Br. Med. J. *282*:1267, 1981.

124. Poston, L., Jones, R. B., Richardson, P. J., and Hilton, P. J.: The effect of antihypertensive therapy on abnormal leucocyte sodium transport in essential hypertension. Clin. Exp. Hypertension *3*:693, 1981.

125. Poston, L., Sewell, R. B., Wilkinson, S. P., Richardson, P. J., Williams, R., Clarkson, E. M., MacGregor, G. A., and de Wardener, H. E.: Evidence for a circulating sodium transport inhibitor in essential hypertension. Br. Med. J. *282*:847, 1981.

126. Pamnani, M. B., Clough, D. L., Huot, S. J., and Haddy, F. J.: Sodium-potassium pump activity in experimental hypertension. In Vanhoutte, P. M., and Leusen, I. (eds.) Vasodilation. New York, Raven Press, 1981.

127. Songu-Mize, E., Bealer, S. T., and Caldwell, R. W.: Effect of AV3V lesions on development of DOCA-salt hypertension and vascular Na$^+$-pump activity. Hypertension *4*:575–580, 1982.

128. Brock, T. A., Smith, J. F., and Overbeck, H. W.: Relationship of vascular sodium-potassium pump activity to intracellular sodium in hypertensive rats. Hypertension *4* (Suppl. II):II-43, 1982.

129. Friedman, S. M.: Evidence for an enhanced transmembrane sodium (Na$^+$) gradient induced by aldosterone in the incubated rat tail artery. Hypertension *4*:230, 1982.

130. Brock, T. A., Lewis, L. J., and Smith, J. B.: Angiotensin increases Na$^+$ entry and Na$^+$/K$^+$ pump activity in cultures of smooth muscle from rat aorta. Proc. Natl. Acad. Sci. USA *79*:1438, 1982.

131. Dahl, L. K., Knudsen, K. D., and Iwai, J.: Humoral transmission of hypertension: Evidence from parabiosis. Circ. Res. *25*:I-21, 1969.

132. Tobian, L., Jr., and Binton, J. T.: Tissue cations and water in arterial hypertension. Circulation *5*:754, 1952.

133. Losse, H., Wermeyer, H., and Wessels, F.: The water and electrolyte content of erythrocytes in arterial hypertension. Klin. Wschr. *38*:393, 1960.

134. Blaustein, M. P.: Sodium ions, calcium ions, blood pressure regulation, and hypertension: A reassessment and a hypothesis. Am. J. Physiol. *232*:C165–C173, 1977.

135. Murphy, R. A.: Myosin phosphorylation and crossbridge regulation in arterial muscle. Hypertension *4* (Suppl. II):II-3, 1982.

136. Hulthen, U. L., Bolli, P., Amann, F. W., Kiowski, W., and Bühler, F. R.: Enhanced vasodilation in essential hypertension by calcium channel blockade with verapamil. Hypertension *4* (Suppl. II):II-31, 1982.

137. Dahl, L. K., and Heine, M.: Primary role of renal homografts in setting chronic blood pressure levels in rats. Circ. Res. *36*:692, 1975.

138. Bianchi, G., Baer, P. G., Fox, U., and Guidi, E.: The role of the kidney in the rat with genetic hypertension. Postgrad. Med. J. *53*(Suppl. 2):123, 1977.

139. Tosteson, D. C.: Cation countertransport and cotransport in human red cells. Fed. Proc. *40*:1429, 1981.

140. Meyer, P., and Garay, R. P.: Hypertension as a membrane disease. Eur. J. Clin. Invest. *11*:337, 1981.

141. Wessels, F., Junge-Hulsing, G., and Losse, H.: Untersuchungen zur Natriumpermeabilität der Erythrozyten bei Hypertonikern mit familiärer Hochdruckbelastung. Z. Kreislaufforsch. *56*:374, 1967.

142. Garay, R. P., and Meyer, P.: A new test showing abnormal net Na$^+$and K$^+$ fluxes in erythrocytes of essential hypertensive patients. Lancet *1*:349, 1979.

143. Canessa, M., Adragna, N., Solomon, H. S., Connolly, T. M., and Tosteson, D.

C.: Increased sodium-lithium countertransport in red cells of patients with essential hypertension. N. Engl. J. Med. *302*:772, 1980.

144. Garay, R. P.: Cation transport in essential hypertension. Lancet *1*:501, 1982.

145. Cusi, D., Barlassina, C., Ferrandi, M., Lupi, P., Ferrari, P., and Bianchi, G.: Familial aggregation of cation transport abnormalities and essential hypertension. Clin. Exp. Hypertens. *3*:871, 1981.

146. Canessa, M., Bize, I., Solomon, H., Adragna, N., Tosteson, D. C., Dagher, G., Garay, R. P., and Meyer, P.: Na countertransport and cotransport in human red cells: Function, dysfunction, and genes in essential hypertension. Clin. Exp. Hypertens. *3*:783, 1981.

147. Tuck, M. L., Garay, R. P., and Meyer, P.: Identification of the Na+, K+ cotransport system in vascular smooth muscle cells: Effects of catecholamines on cation transport. Clin. Res. *30*:340A, 1982 (abstr).

148. Woods, J. W., Falk, R. J., Pittman, A. W., Klemmer, P. J., Watson, B. S., and Namboodiri, K.: Increased red-cell sodium-lithium countertransport in normotensive sons of hypertensive parents. N. Engl. J. Med. *306*:592, 1982.

149. De Mendonca, M., Knorr, A., Grichois, M., Ben-Ishay, D., Garay, R. P., and Meyer, P.: Erythrocytic sodium ion transport systems in primary and secondary hypertension of the rat. Kidney Int. *21*:11(S-69), 1982.

150. Garay, R. P., Nazaret, C., Dagher, G., Bertrand, E., and Meyer, P.: A genetic approach to the geography of hypertension: Examination of Na+-K+ cotransport in Ivory Coast Africans. Clin. Exp. Hypertens. *3*:861, 1981.

151. Swarts, H. G. P., Bonting, S. L., de Pont, J. J. H. H. M., Stekhoven, F. M. A. H. S., Thien, T. A., and Van't Laar, A.: Cation fluxes and Na+-K+-activated ATPase activity in erythrocytes of patients with essential hypertension. Hypertension *3*:641, 1981.

152. Walter, U., and Distler, A.: Abnormal sodium efflux in erythrocytes of patients with essential hypertension. Hypertension *4*:205, 1982.

153. Davidson, J. S., Opie, L. H., and Keding, B.: Sodium-potassium cotransport activity as genetic marker in essential hypertension. Br. Med. J. *284*:539, 1982.

153a. Etkin, N. L., Mahoney, J. R., Forsthoefel, M. W., Gillum, R. F., and Eaton, J. W.: Racial differences in hypertension-associated red cell sodium permeability. Nature *297*:588, 1982.

154. Cumberbatch, M., and Morgan, D. B.: Relations between sodium transport and sodium concentration in human erythrocytes in health and disease. Clin. Sci. *60*:555, 1981.

155. Inagami, T.: Renin. In Soffer, R. L. (ed.): Biochemical Regulation of Blood Pressure. New York, John Wiley & Sons, 1981.

156. Atlas, S. A., Sealey, J. E., Hesson, T. E., Kaplan, A. P., Menard, J., Corvol, P., and Laragh, J. H.: Biochemical similarity of partially purified inactive renins from human plasma and kidney. Hypertension *4* (Suppl. II):II–86, 1982.

157. Sealey, J. E., Atlas, S. A., and Laragh, J. H.: Prorenin and other large molecular weight forms of renin. Endocr. Rev. *4*:365, 1980.

158. Hsueh, W. A.: Inactive renin in human plasma. Is it prorenin? Mineral Electrolyte Metab. *7*:169, 1982.

159. Ganten, D., and Speck, G.: The brain renin-angiotensin system: A model for the synthesis of peptides in the brain. Biochem. Pharmacol. *27*:2379, 1978.

160. Fishman, M. C., Zimmerman, E. A., and Slater, E. E.: Renin and angiotensin: The complete system within the neuroblastoma X glioma cell. Science *214*:921, 1981.

161. Re, R., Fallon, J. T., Dzau, V., Quay, S., and Haber, E.: Renin synthesis by canine aortic smooth muscle cells in culture. Life Sciences *30*:99, 1982.

162. Ikeda, M., Gutkowska, J., Thibault, G., Boucher, R., and Genest, J.: Purification of tonin by affinity chromatography. Hypertension *3*:81, 1981.

163. Day, R. P., Luetscher, J. A., and Zager, P. G.: Big renin: Identification, chemical properties and clinical implications. Am. J. Cardiol. *37*:667, 1976.

164. Preibisz, J. J., Sealey, J. E., Aceto, R. M., and Laragh, J. H.: Plasma renin activity measurements: An update. Cardiovasc. Rev. Rep. *3*:787, 1982.

165. Crane, M. G., and Harris, J. J.: Effect of aging on renin activity and aldosterone excretion. J. Lab. Clin. Med. *87*:947, 1976.

166. Sassard, J., Vincent, M., Annat, G., and Bizollon, C. A.: A kinetic study of plasma renin and aldosterone during changes of posture in man. J. Clin. Endocrinol. Metab. *42*:20, 1976.

167. Katz, F. H., Romfh, P., and Smith, J. A.: Episodic secretion of aldosterone in supine man: Relationship to cortisol. J. Clin. Endocrinol. Metab. *35*:178, 1972.

168. Rumpf, K. W., Frenzel, S., Lowitz, H. D., and Scheler, F.: The effect of indomethacin on plasma renin activity in man under normal conditions and after stimulation of the renin-angiotensin system. Prostaglandins *10*:611, 1975.

169. Robertson, D., Frolich, J. C., Carr, R. K., Watson, J. T., Hollifield, J. W., Shand, D. G., and Oates, J. A.: Effects of caffeine on plasma renin activity, catecholamines and blood pressure. N. Engl. J. Med. *298*:181, 1978.

170. McDonald, R. H., Jr., Corder, C. N., Vagnucci, A. H., and Shuman, J.: The multiple factors affecting plasma renin activity in essential hypertension. Arch. Intern. Med. *138*:557, 1978.

171. Crane, M. G., Harris, J. J., and Johns, V. J., Jr.: Hyporeninemic hypertension. Am. J. Med. *52*:457, 1972.

172. Holle, R., Levy, S. B., and Stone, R. A.: A composite analysis of renin classification methods. Arch. Intern. Med. *138*:1514, 1978.

173. Helmer, O. M.: Renin activity in blood from patients with hypertension. Canad. Med. Assoc. J. *90*:221, 1964.

174. Swales, J. D.: Low-renin hypertension: Nephrosclerosis? Lancet *1*:75, 1975.

175. Kaplan, N. M.: Renin profiles: The unfulfilled promises. J.A.M.A. *238*:611, 1977.

176. Laragh, J. H., Letcher, R. L., and Pickering, T. G.: Renin profiling for diagnosis and treatment of hypertension. J.A.M.A. *241*:151, 1979.

177. Fagard, R., Amery, A., Reybrouck, T., Lijnen, P., Billiet, L., and Joossens, J. V.: Plasma renin levels and systemic hemodynamics in essential hypertension. Clin. Sci. Molec. Med. *52*:591, 1977.

178. Kotchen, T. A., Guthrie, G. P., Jr., Cottrill, C. M., McKean, H. E., and Kotchen, J. M.: Low renin-aldosterone in "prehypertensive" young adults. J. Clin. Endocrinol. Metab. *54*:808, 1982.

179. Case, D. B., Wallace, J. M., Keim, H. J., Weber, M. A., Sealey, J. E., and Laragh, J. H.: Possible role of renin in hypertension as suggested by renin-sodium profiling and inhibition of converting enzyme. N. Engl. J. Med. *296*:641, 1977.

180. Williams, G. H., Hollenberg, N. M., Moore, T. J., Dluhy, R. G., Bavli, S. Z., Solomon, H. S., and Mersey, J. H.: Failure of renin suppression by angiotensin II in hypertension. Circ. Res. *42*:46, 1978.

181. Esler, M., Zweifler, A., Randall, O., Julius, S., and DeQuattro, V.: The determinants of plasma-renin activity in essential hypertension. Ann. Intern. Med. *88*:746, 1978.

182. Morganti, A., Pickering, T. G., Lopez-Ovejero, J. A., and Laragh, J. H.: High and low renin subgroups in essential hypertension: Differences and similarities in their renin and sympathetic responses to neural and nonneural stimuli. Am. J. Cardiol. *46*:306, 1980.

183. Dluhy, R. G., Bavli, S. Z., Leung, F. K., Solomon, H. S., Moore, T. J., Hollenberg, N. K., and Williams, G. H.: Abnormal adrenal responsiveness and angiotensin II dependence in high renin essential hypertension. J. Clin. Invest. *64*:1270, 1979.

184. Williams, G. H., Hollenberg, N. K., Moore, T. J., Swartz, S. L., and Dluhy, R. G.: The adrenal receptor for angiotensin II is altered in essential hypertension. J. Clin. Invest. *63*:419, 1979.

185. Wisgerhof, M., and Brown, R. D.: Increased adrenal sensitivity to angiotensin II in low-renin essential hypertension. J. Clin. Invest. *61*:1456, 1978.

186. Lebel, M., Brown, J. J., Kremer, D., Robertson, J. I. S., Schalekamp, M., Davies, D. L., Lever, A. F., Tree, M., Beevers, D. G., Frazier, R., Morton, J. J., and Wilson, A.: Sodium and the renin-angiotensin system in essential hypertension and mineralocorticoid excess. Lancet *2*:308, 1974.

187. Gomez-Sanchez, C. E.: The role of steroids in human essential hypertension. Biochem. Pharmacol. *31*:893, 1982.

188. Baxter, J. D., Schambelan, M., Matulich, D. T., Spindler, B. J., Taylor, A. A., and Bartter, F. C.: Aldosterone receptors and the evaluation of plasma mineralocorticoid activity in normal and hypertensive states. J. Clin. Invest. *58*:579, 1976.

189. Vaughan, E. D., Jr., Laragh, J. H., Gavras, I., Buhler, F. E., Gavras, H., Brunner, H. R., and Baer, L.: Volume factor in low and normal renin essential hypertension. Am. J. Cardiol. *32*:523, 1973.

190. Holland, O. B., Gomez-Sanchez, C., Fairchild, C., and Kaplan, N. M.: Role of renin classification for diuretic treatment of black hypertensive patients. Arch. Intern. Med. *139*:1365, 1979.

191. Padfield, P. L., Brown, J. J., Lever, A. F., Morton, J. J., and Robertson, J. I. S.: Blood pressure in acute and chronic vasopressin excess. N. Engl. J. Med. *304*:1067, 1981.

192. Margolius, H. S., Horwitz, D., Pisano, J. J., and Keiser, H. R.: Relationships among urinary kallikrein, mineralocorticoids and human hypertensive disease. Fed. Proc. *35*:203, 1976.

193. Holland, O. B., Chud, J. M., and Braunstein, H.: Urinary kallikrein excretion in essential and mineralocorticoid hypertension. J. Clin. Invest. *65*:347, 1980.

194. Moncada, S., and Vane, J. R.: Arachidonic acid metabolites and the interactions between platelets and blood vessel walls. N. Engl. J. Med. *300*:1142, 1979.

195. Romero, J. C., and Strong, C. G.: The effect of indomethacin blockade of prostaglandin synthesis on blood pressure of normal rabbits and rabbits with renovascular hypertension. Circ. Res. *40*:35, 1977.

196. Weber, P. C., Siess, W., Sherer, B., Held, E., Witzgall, H., and Lorenz, R.: Arachidonic acid metabolites, hypertension and arteriosclerosis. Klin. Wochenschr. *60*:479–488, 1982.

196a. Muirhead, E. E., Byers, L. W., Desiderio, D. M., Brooks, B., and Brosius, W. M.: Antihypertensive lipids from the kidney: Alkyl ether analogs of phosphatidylcholine. Fed. Proc. *40*:2285–2290, 1981.

197. McGarron, D. A., Morris, C. D., and Cole, C.: Dietary calcium in human hypertension. Science *217*:267–269, 1982.

198. Kesteloot, H., and Geboers, J.: Calcium and blood pressure. Lancet *1*:813, 1982.

199. Lang, R. E., Bruckner, U. B., Kempf, B., Rascher, W., Sturm, V., Unger, T., Speck, G., and Ganten, D.: Opioid peptides and blood pressure regulation. Clin. Exper. Hyper. Theory and Practice *A4*:249–269, 1982.

200. Rabkin, S. W., Mathewson, F. A. L., and Hsu, P. H.: Relation of body weight to development of ischemic heart disease in a cohort of young North American men after a 26 year observation period: The Manitoba study. Am. J. Cardiol. *39*:452, 1977.

201. Siervogel, R. M., Roche, A. F., Chumlea, W. C., Morris, J. G., Webb, P., and Knittle, J. L.: Blood pressure, body composition, and fat tissue cellularity in adults. Hypertension *4*:382, 1982.

202. Messerli, F. H.: Cardiovascular effects of obesity and hypertension. Lancet *1*:1165, 1982.

203. Klimes, I., Nagulesparan, M., Unger, R. H., Aronoff, S. L., and Mott, D. M.: Reduced Na+,K+ -ATPase activity in intact red cells and isolated membranes from obese man. J. Clin. Endocrinol. Metab. *54*:721, 1982.

204. Kannel, W. B., and Sorlie, P.: Hypertension in Framingham. In Paul, O. (ed.):

Epidemiology and Control of Hypertension. Miami, Symposia Specialists, 1975, p. 553.

205. Cooke, K. M., Frost, G. W., Thornell, I. R., and Stokes, G. S.: Alcohol consumption and blood pressure. Med. J. Aust. *1*:65, 1982.

206. Klatsky, A. L., Friedman, G. D., and Siegelaub, A. B.: Alcohol and mortality. Ann. Intern. Med. *95*:139, 1981.

207. Cryer, P. E., Haymond, M. W., Santiago, J. V., and Shah, S. D.: Norepinephrine and epinephrine release and adrenergic mediation of smoking-associated hemodynamic and metabolic events. N. Engl. J. Med. *295*:573, 1976.

208. Gordon, T., Kannel, W. B., Dawber, T. R., and McGee, D.: Changes associated with quitting cigarette smoking: The Framingham study. Am. Heart J. *90*:322, 1975.

209. Christlieb, A. R., Warram, J. H., Krolewski, A. S., Busick, E. J., Ganda, O. M. P., Asmal, A. C., Soeldner, J. S., and Bradley, R. F.: Hypertension: The major risk factor in juvenile-onset insulin-dependent diabetics. Diabetes *30* (Suppl. 2):90, 1981.

210. Beretta-Piccoli, C., and Weidmann, P.: Exaggerated pressor responsiveness to norepinephrine in nonazotemic diabetes mellitus. Am. J. Med. *71*:829, 1981.

211. Chrysant, S. G., Frohlich, E. D., Adamopoulos, P. N., Stein, P. D., Whitcomb, W. H., Allen, E. W., and Neller, G.: Pathophysiologic significance of "stress" or relative polycythemia in essential hypertension. Am. J. Cardiol. *37*:1069, 1976.

212. Letcher, R. L., Chien, S., Pickering, T. G., Sealey, J. E., and Laragh, J. H.: Direct relationship between blood pressure and blood viscosity in normal and hypertensive subjects. Role of fibrinogen and concentration. Am. J. Med. *70*:1195, 1981.

213. Humphrey, P. R. D., Marshall, J., Russell, R. W. R., Wetherley-Mein, G., DuBoulay, G. H., Pearson, T. C., Symon, L., and Zilkha, E.: Cerebral bloodflow and viscosity in relative polycythaemia. Lancet *2*:873, 1979.

214. Breckenridge, A.: Hypertension and hyperuricaemia. Lancet *1*:15, 1966.

215. Editorial: Hypertension and uric acid. Lancet *1*:365, 1981.

216. Raynor, W. J., Jr., Shekelle, R. B., Rossof, A. H., Maliza, C., and Paul, O.: High blood pressure and 17-year cancer mortality in the Western Electric Health Study. Am. J. Epidemiol. *113*:371, 1981.

217. Gillis, G. R., Hole, D., MacLean, D. S., Hawthorne, V. M., Watt, H. D., and Watkinson, G.: High blood-pressure and cancer? Lancet *2*:612, 1975.

SECONDARY FORMS OF HYPERTENSION

218. Oral Contraceptive Study of the Royal College of General Practitioners: Hypertension. *In* Oral Contraceptives and Health. New York, Pitman Publishing Corp., 1974, p. 37.

219. Zelnik, M., Kim, Y. J., and Kantner, J. F.: Probabilities of intercourse and conception among U.S. teenage women, 1971 and 1976. Fam. Plan. Perspect. *11*:177, 1979.

220. Royal College of General Practitioners Oral Contraception Study: Further analyses of mortality in oral contraceptive users. Lancet *1*:541, 1981.

221. Stadel, B. V.: Oral contraceptives and cardiovascular disease. N. Engl. J. Med. *305*:672, 1981.

222. Wallace, R. B., Barrett-Connor, E., Criqui, M., Wahl, P., Hoover, J., Hunninghake, D., and Heiss, G.: Alteration in blood pressures associated with combined alcohol and oral contraceptive use—the Lipid Research Clinics Prevalance Study. J. Chron. Dis. *35*:251, 1982.

223. Fisch, I. R., and Frank, J.: Oral contraceptives and blood pressure. J.A.M.A. *237*:2499, 1977.

224. Weir, R. J.: When the pill causes a rise in blood pressure. Drugs *16*:522, 1978.

225. Weir, R. J.: Effect on blood pressure of changing from high to low dose steroid preparation in women with oral contraceptive induced hypertension. Scott. Med. J. *27*:212–215, 1982.

226. Pritchard, J. A., and Pritchard, S. A.: Blood pressure response to estrogen-progestin oral contraceptive after pregnancy-induced hypertension. Am. J. Obstet. Gynecol. *129*:733, 1977.

227. Spellacy, W. N., and Birk, S. A.: The effects of mechanical and steroid contraceptive methods on blood pressure in hypertensive women. Fertil. Steril. *25*:467, 1974.

228. Woods, J. W.: Oral contraceptives and hypertension. Lancet *2*:653, 1967.

229. Hauglustaine, B., VanDamme, B., Vanrenterghem, Y., and Michielsen, P.: Recurrent hemolytic uremic syndrome during oral contraception. Clin. Nephrol. *15*:148, 1981.

230. Boyd, W. N., Burden, R. P., and Aber, G. M.: Intrarenal vascular changes in patients receiving oestrogen-containing compounds—A clinical, histological, and angiographic study. Quart. J. Med. (n.s.) *44*:415, 1975.

231. Walters, W. A. W., and Lim, Y. L.: Haemodynamic changes in women taking oral contraceptives. J. Obstet. Gynecol. Brit. Commonw. *77*:1007, 1970.

232. Hollenberg, N. K., Williams, G. H., Burger, B., Chenitz, W., Hooshmand, I., and Adams, D. F.: Renal blood flow and its response to angiotensin II. Circ. Res. *38*:35, 1976.

233. Streeten, D. H. P., Anderson, G. H., Jr., and Dalakos, T. G.: Angiotensin blockade: Its clinical significance. Am. J. Med. *60*:817, 1976.

234. Kay, C. R.: Progestogens and arterial disease—Evidence from the Royal College of General Practitioners' study. Am. J. Obstet. Gynecol. *142*:762, 1982.

235. Kaplan, N. M.: Complications of the birth control pill. *In* Isselbacher, K. J., Adams, R. D., Braunwald, E., Martin, J. P., Petersdorf, R. G., and Wilson, J. D. (eds.): Update I. Harrison's Principles of Internal Medicine. New York, McGraw-Hill Book Co., 1981, p. 57.

236. Pfeffer, R. I., Kurosaki, T. T., and Charlton, S. K.: Estrogen use and blood pressure in later life. Am. J. Epidemiol. *110*:469, 1979.

237. Pallas, K. G., Holzwarth, G. J., Stern, M. P., and Lucas, C. P.: The effect of conjugated estrogens on the renin-angiotensin system. J. Clin. Endocrinol. Metab. *44*:1061, 1977.

238. Barrett-Connor, E., Brown, W. V., Turner, J., Austin, M., and Criqui, M. H.: Heart disease risk factors and hormone use in postmenopausal women. J.A.M.A. *241*:2167, 1979.

239. Bain, C., Willett, W., Hennekens, C. H., Rosner, B., Belanger, C., and Speizer, F. E.: Use of postmenopausal hormones and risk of myocardial infarction. Circulation *64*:42, 1981.

240. Ross, R. K., Mack, T. M., Henderson, B. E., Paganini-Hill, A., and Arthur, M.: Menopausal oestrogen therapy and protection from death from ischaemic heart disease. Lancet *1*:858, 1981.

241. Kurtzman, N. A.: Does acute poststreptococcal glomerulonephritis lead to chronic renal disease? N. Engl. J. Med. *298*:795, 1978.

242. Garcia, R., Rubio, L., and Rodriguez-Iturbe, B.: Long-term prognosis of epidemic poststreptococcal glomerulonephritis in Maracaibo: Follow-up studies 11 to 12 years after the acute episode. Clin. Nephrol. *15*:291, 1981.

243. Schact, R. G., Gallo, G. R., Gluck, M. C., Iqbal, M. S., and Baldwin, D. S.: Irreversible disease following acute poststreptococcal glomerulonephritis in children. J. Chron. Dis. *32*:515, 1979.

244. Birkenhager, W. H., Schalekamp, M. A. B. H., Schalekamp-Kuyken, M., Kolsters, P. A., Kolsters, G., and Krauss, X. H.: Interrelations between arterial pressure, fluid-volume, and plasma-renin concentration in the course of acute glomerulonephritis. Lancet *1*:1086, 1970.

245. Rodriguez-Iturbe, B., Baggio, B., Colina-Chourio, J. J., Favaro, S., Garcia, R., Sussana, F., Castillo, L., and Borsatti, A.: Studies on the renin-aldosterone system in the acute nephritic syndrome. Kidney Int. *19*:445, 1981.

246. Levinsky, N. G.: Pathophysiology of acute renal failure. N. Engl. J. Med. *296*:1453, 1977.

247. Ponticelli, C., Rivolta, E., Imbasciati, E., Rossi, E., and Mannucci, P. M.: Hemolytic uremic syndrome in adults. Arch. Intern. Med. *140*:353, 1980.

248. Harrington, J. T., and Cohen, J. J.: Current concepts. Acute oliguria. N. Engl. J. Med. *292*:89, 1975.

249. Traub, Y. M., Shapiro, A. P., Osial, T. A., Jr., Rodnan, G. P., Medsger, T. A., Leb, D. E., and Christy, W. C.: Response of patients with renal involvement by progressive systemic sclerosis to antihypertensive therapy. Clin. Sci. *61*:395a, 1981.

250. Smith, H. W.: Unilateral nephrectomy in hypertensive disease. J. Urol. *76*:685, 1956.

251. Gifford, R. W., Jr., McCormack, L. J., and Poutasse, E. F.: The atrophic kidney: Its role in hypertension. Mayo Clin. Proc. *40*:834, 1965.

252. Stockigt, J. R., Noakes, C. A., Collins, R. D., Schambelan, M., and Biglieri, E. G.: Renal-vein renin in various forms of renal hypertension. Lancet *1*:1194, 1972.

253. Lamberton, R. P., Noth, R. H., and Glickman, M.: Frequent falsely negative renal vein renin tests in unilateral renal parenchymal disease. J. Urol. *125*:477, 1981.

254. Dahl, T., Eide, I., and Fryjordet, A.: Hypernephroma and hypertension. Acta Med. Scand. *209*:121, 1981.

255. Weidmann, P., Beretta-Piccoli, C., Hirsch, D., Reubi, F. C., and Massry, S. G.: Curable hypertension with unilateral hydronephrosis. Studies on the role of circulating renin. Ann. Intern. Med. *87*:437, 1977.

256. Nash, D. A., Jr.: Hypertension in polycystic kidney disease without renal failure. Arch. Intern. Med. *137*:1571, 1977.

257. Meyer, P., Luscher, T., Rufener, J., Pouliadis, G., Vetter, H., Greminger, P., Siengenthaler, W., and Vetter, W.: Prävalenz der Hypertonie bei Röntgenologischen Zeichen der Pyelonephritis im intravenosen Pyelogramm. Schweiz. Med. Wschr. *111*:482, 1981.

258. Shapiro, A. P., Sapira, J. D., and Scheib, E. T.: Development of bacteriuria in hypertensive population. A 7-year follow-up study. Ann. Intern. Med. *74*:861, 1971.

259. Holland, N. H., Kotchen, T., and Bhathena, D.: Hypertension in children with chronic pyelonephritis. Kidney Int. *8*:S-43, 1975.

260. Ayus, J. C., Frommer, J. P., and Young, J. B.: Cardiac and circulatory abnormalities in chronic renal failure. Semin. Nephrol. *1*:112, 1981.

261. Koomans, H. A., Roos, J. C., Boer, P., Geyskes, G. G., and Mees, E. J. D.: Salt sensitivity of blood pressure in chronic renal failure. Evidence for renal control of body fluid distribution in man. Hypertension *4*:190, 1982.

262. Swaminathan, R., Glegg, G., Cumberbatch, M., Zareian, Z., and McKenna, F.: Erythrocyte sodium transport in chronic renal failure. Clin. Sci. *62*:489, 1982.

263. Brunner, H. R., Wauters, J., McKinstry, D., Waeber, B., Turini, G., and Gavras, H.: Inappropriate renin secretion unmasked by captopril (SQ 14 225) in hypertension of chronic renal failure. Lancet *2*:704, 1978.

264. Henrich, W. L., Mitchell, H., Anderson, S., Cronin, R., and Pettinger, W. A.: Effect of antihypertensive therapy on plasma catecholamines in renal failure patients. Clin. Nephrol. *16*:131, 1981.

265. Swales, J. D., Queiroz, F. P., Thurston, H., Medina, A., and Holland, J.: Dual mechanism for experimental hypertension. Lancet *2*:1181, 1971.

266. Blumberg, A., Hegstrom, R. M., Nelp, W. B., and Scribner, B. H.: Extracellular volume in patients with chronic renal disease treated for hypertension by sodium restriction. Lancet *2*:69, 1967.

267. Weidmann, P., and Maxwell, M. H.: The renin-angiotensin-aldosterone system in terminal renal failure. Kidney Int. *8*:S-219, 1975.

268. Lee, C., Neff, M. S., Slifkin, R. F., and Leiter, E.: Bilateral nephrectomy for hypertension in patients with chronic renal failure on a dialysis program. J. Urol. *119*:20, 1978.

269. Warren, D. J., and Ferris, T. F.: Renin secretion in renal hypertension. Lancet *1*:159, 1970.

270. Hostetter, T. H., Rennke, H. G., and Brenner, B. M.: The case for intrarenal hypertension in the initiation and progression of diabetic and other glomerulopathies. Am. J. Med. *72*:375, 1982.

271. Christlieb, A. R.: Nephropathy, the renin system, and hypertensive vascular disease in diabetes mellitus. Cardiovasc. Med. *3*:417, 1978.

272. Perez, G. O., Lespier, L., Knowles, R., Oster, J. R., and Vaamonde, C. A.: Potassium homeostasis in chronic diabetes mellitus. Arch. Intern. Med. *137*:1018, 1977.

273. Weidmann, P., Massry, S. G., Coburn, J. W., Maxwell, M. H., Atleson, J., and Kleeman, C. R.: Blood pressure effects of acute hypercalcemia. Studies in patients with chronic renal failure. Ann. Intern. Med. *76*:741, 1972.

274. Kincaid-Smith, P.: Analgesic abuse and the kidney. Kidney Int. *17*:250, 1980.

275. Muther, R. S., Potter, D. M., and Bennett, W. M.: Aspirin-induced depression of glomerular filtration rate in normal humans: Role of sodium balance. Ann. Intern. Med. *94*:317, 1981.

276. Textor, S. C., Gavras, H., Tifft, C. P., Bernard, D. B., Idelson, B., and Brunner, H.: Norepinephrine and renin activity in chronic renal failure. Evidence for interacting roles in hemodialysis hypertension. Hypertension *3*:294, 1981.

277. Jacquot, C., Idatte, J. M., Bedrossian, J., Weiss, Y., Safar, M., and Bariety, J.: Long-term blood pressure changes in renal homotransplantation. Arch. Intern. Med. *138*:233, 1978.

278. Zawada, E. T., Maxwell, M. H., Marks, L. S., Lee, D. B. N., and Kaufman, J. J.: The diagnostic and therapeutic uses of saralasin in renal transplant hypertension. J. Urol. *123*:148, 1980.

279. Eyler, W. R., Clark, M. D., Garman, J. E., Rian, R. L., and Meininger, D.: Angiography of the renal areas including a comparative study of renal arterial stenoses in patients with and without hypertension. Radiology *78*:879, 1962.

280. Plumer, L. B., Kaplan, G. W., and Mendoza, S. A.: Hypertension in infants — a complication of umbilical arterial catheterization. J. Pediat. *89*:802, 1976.

281. Harrison, E. G., Jr., and McCormack, L. J.: Pathologic classification of renal arterial disease in renovascular hypertension. Mayo Clin. Proc. *46*:161, 1971.

282. de Zeeuw, D., Burema, J., Donker, A. J. M., van der Hem, G. K., and Mandema, E.: Nephroptosis and hypertension. Lancet *1*:213, 1977.

283. Keith, T. A., III: Renovascular hypertension in black patients. Hypertension *4*:438, 1982.

284. Munichoodappa, C., D'Elia, J. A., Libertino, J. A., Gleason, R. E., and Christlieb, A. R.: Renal artery stenosis in hypertensive diabetics. J. Urol. *121*:555, 1979.

285. Fiorentini, C., Guazzi, M. D., Olivari, M. T., Bartorelli, A., Necchi, G., and Magrini, F.: Selective reduction in renal perfusion pressure and blood flow in man: Humoral and hemodynamic effects. Circulation *63*:973, 1981.

286. Barger, A. C.: The Goldblatt Memorial Lecture. Part I: Experimental renovascular hypertension. Hypertension *1*:447, 1979.

287. Buggy, J., Fink, G. D., Johnson, A. K., and Brody, M. J.: Prevention of the development of renal hypertension by anteroventral third ventricular tissue lesions. Circ. Res. *40*(Suppl. I):110, 1977.

288. Winer, B. M., Lubbe, W. F., Simon, M., and Williams, J. A.: Renin in the diagnosis of renovascular hypertension. J.A.M.A. *202*:139, 1967.

289. Katholi, R. W., Whitlow, P. L., Winternitz, S. R., and Oparil, S.: Importance of the renal nerves in established two-kidney, one clip Goldblatt hypertension. Hypertension *4* (Suppl. II):II–166, 1982.

290. Weidmann, P., Schiffl, H., Ziegler, W. H., Glück, Z., Meier, A., and Keusch, G.: Catecholamines, sodium and renin in unilateral renal hypertension in man. Mineral Electrolyte Metab. *7*:97, 1982.

291. Russell, G. I., Bing, R. F., Thurston, H., and Swales, J. D.: Surgical reversal of two-kidney one-clip hypertension during inhibition of the renin-angiotensin system. Hypertension *4*:69, 1982.

292. Dietz, J. R., Davis, J. O., DeForrest, J. M., Freeman, R. H., Echtenkamp, S. F., and Seymour, A. A.: Effects of indomethacin in dogs with acute and chronic renovascular hypertension. Am. J. Physiol. *240*:H533, 1981.

293. Thal, A. P., Grage, T. B., and Vernier, R. L.: Function of the contralateral kidney in renal hypertension due to renal artery stenosis. Circulation *27*:36, 1963.

294. Bookstein, J. J.: Segmental renal artery stenosis in renovascular hypertension. Radiology *90*:1073, 1968.

295. Zinman, L., and Libertino, J. A.: Revascularization of the chronic totally occluded renal artery with restoration of renal function. J. Urol. *118*:517, 1977.

296. Bookstein, J. J., Abrams, H. L., Buenger, R. E., Reiss, M. D., Lecky, J. W., Franklin, S. S., Bleifer, K. W., Varady, P. D., and Maxwell, M. H.: Radiologic aspects of renovascular hypertension. Part 3. Appraisal of arteriography. J.A.M.A. *21*:368, 1972.

297. Simon, N., Franklin, S. S., Bleifer, K. W., and Maxwell, M. H.: Clinical characteristics of renovascular hypertension. J.A.M.A. *220*:1209, 1972.

298. Davis, B. A., Crook, M. E., Vestal, R. E., and Oates, J. A.: Prevalence of renovascular hypertension in patients with grade III or IV hypertensive retinopathy. N. Engl. J. Med. *301*:1273, 1979.

299. Mueller, S. M., and Luft, F. C.: The blood-brain barrier in renovascular hypertension. Stroke *13*:229, 1982.

300. Grim, C. E., Luft, F. C., Weinberger, M. H., and Grim, C. M.: Sensitivity and specificity of screening tests for renal vascular hypertension. Ann. Intern. Med. *91*:617, 1979.

301. Bookstein, J. J., Abrams, H. L., Buenger, R. E., Lecky, J., Franklin, S. S., Reiss, M. D., Bleifer, K. H., Klatte, E. C., Varady, P. D., and Maxwell, M. H.: Radiologic aspects of renovascular hypertension. Part 2. The role of urography in unilateral renovascular disease. J.A.M.A. *220*:1225, 1972.

302. Hillman, B. J., Ovitt, T. W., Capp, M. P., Prosnitz, E. H., Osborne, R. W., Goldstone, J., Zukoski, C. F., and Malone, J. M.: The potential impact of digital video substraction angiography on screening for renovascular hypertension. Radiology *142*:577, 1982.

303. Witten, S. M.: Reactions to urographic contrast media. J.A.M.A. *231*:974, 1975.

304. Teruel, J. L., Marcen, R., Onaindia, J. M., Serrano, A., Quereda, C., and Ortuno, J.: Renal function impairment caused by intravenous urography. A prospective study. Arch. Intern. Med. *141*:1271, 1981.

305. Vaughan, E. D., Jr., Buhler, F. R., Laragh, J. H., Sealey, J. E., Baer, L., and Bard, R. H.: Renovascular hypertension: Renin measurements to indicate hypersecretion and contralateral suppression, estimate renal plasma flow, and score for surgical curability. Am. J. Med. *55*:402, 1973.

306. Streeten, D. H. P., and Anderson, G. H., Jr.: Outpatient experience with saralasin. Kidney Int. *15*:S–44, 1979.

307. Helmer, O. M., and Judson, W. E.: The presence of vasoconstrictor and vasopressor activity in renal vein plasma of patients with arterial hypertension. *In* Skelton, F. R. (ed.): Hypertension: Proceedings of the Council for High Blood Pressure Research, Vol. 8. New York, American Heart Association, 1960, p. 38.

308. Marks, L. S., Maxwell, M. H., Varady, P. D., Lupu, A. N., and Kauffman, J. J.: Renovascular hypertension: Does the renal vein renin ratio predict operative results? J. Urol. *115*:365, 1976.

309. Maxwell, M. H., Marks, L. S., Varady, P. D., Lupu, A. N., and Kauffman, J. J.: Renal vein renin in essential hypertension. J. Lab. Clin. Med. *86*:901, 1975.

310. Re, R., Novelline, R., Escourrou, M. T., Athanasoulis, C., Burton, J., and Haber, E.: Inhibition of angiotensin-converting enzyme for diagnosis of renal-artery stenosis. N. Engl. J. Med. *298*:582, 1978.

311. Foster, J. H., Dean, R. H., Pinkerton, J. A., and Rhamy, R. K.: Ten years' experience with the surgical management of renovascular hypertension. Ann. Surg. *177*:755, 1973.

312. Dean, R. H., Kieffer, R. W., Smith, B. M., Oates, J. A., Nadeau, J. H. J., Hollifield, J. W., and DuPont, W. D.: Renovascular hypertension. Arch. Surg. *116*:1408, 1981.

313. Kaufman, J. J.: Renovascular hypertension: The UCLA experience. J. Urol. *121*:139, 1979.

314. Novick, A. C., Straffon, R. A., Stewart, B. H., Gifford, R. W., and Vidt, D.: Diminished operative morbidity and mortality in renal revascularization. J.A.M.A. *246*:749, 1981.

315. Jones, E. O. P., Wilkinson, R., and Taylor, R. M. R.: Contralateral renal artery fibromuscular dysplasia after nephrectomy for renal artery stenosis. Br. Med. J. *1*:825, 1978.

316. Atkinson, A. B., Brown, J. J., Cumming, A. M. M., Fraser, R., Lever, A. F., Leckie, B. J., Morton, J. J., and Robertson, J. I. S.: Captopril in renovascular hypertension: Long-term use in predicting surgical outcome. Br. Med. J. *284*:689, 1982.

317. Mahler, F., Probst, P., Haertel, M., Weidmann, P., and Krneta, A.: Lasting improvement of renovascular hypertension by transluminal dilatation of atherosclerotic and nonatherosclerotic renal artery stenoses. Circulation *65*:611, 1982.

318. Madias, N. E., Kwon, Q. J., and Millan, V. G.: Percutaneous transluminal renal angioplasty. A potentially effective treatment for preservation of renal function. Arch. Intern. Med. *142*:693, 1982.

319. Delin, K., Aurell, M., Granerus, G., Holm, J., and Schersten, T.: Surgical treatment of renovascular hypertension in the elderly patient. Acta Med. Scand. *211*:169, 1982.

320. Conn, J. W., Cohen, E. L., Lucas, C. P., McDonald, W. J., Mayor, G. H., Blough, W. M., Jr., Eveland, W. C., Bookstein, J. J., and Lapides, J.: Primary reninism. Hypertension, hyperreninemia, and secondary aldosteronism due to renin-producing juxtaglomerular cell tumors. Arch. Intern. Med. *130*:682, 1972.

321. Sheth, K. J., Tang, T. T., Blaedel, M. E., and Good, T. A.: Polydipsia, polyuria, and hypertension associated with renin-secreting Wilms' tumor. J. Pediat. *92*:921, 1978.

322. Streeten, D. H. P., Tomycz, N., and Anderson, G. H., Jr.: Reliability of screening methods for the diagnosis of primary aldosteronism. Am J. Med. *67*:403, 1979.

323. Weinberger, M. H., Grim, C. E., Hollified, J. W., Kem, D. C., Ganguly, A., Kramer, N. J., Yune, H. Y., Wellman, H., and Donohue, J. P.: Primary aldosteronism. Ann. Intern. Med. *90*:386, 1979.

324. Davies, D. L., Beevers, D. G., Brown, J. J., Cumming, A. M. M., Fraser, R., Lever, A. F., Mason, P. A., Morton, J. J., Robertson, J. I. S., Titterington, M., and Tree, M.: Aldosterone and its stimuli in normal and hypertensive man: Are essential hypertension and primary hyperaldosteronism without tumour the same condition? J. Endocrinol. *81*:12, 1979.

325. Padfield, P. L., Davies, D., Lever, A. F., Robertson, J. I. S., Brown, J. J., Fraser, R., and Morton, J. J.: The myth of idiopathic hyperaldosteronism. Lancet *2*:83, 1981.

326. Gross, M. D., Grekin, R. J., Gniadek, T. C., and Villareal, J. Z.: Suppression of aldosterone by cyproheptadine in idiopathic aldosteronism. N. Engl. J. Med. *305*:181, 1981.

327. Ganguly, A., Grim, C. E., Bergstein, J., Brown, R. D., and Weinberger, M.

H.: Genetic and pathophysiologic studies of a new kindred with glucocorticoid-suppressible hyperaldosteronism manifest in three generations. J. Clin. Endocrinol. Metab. *53*:1040, 1981.

328. Ferriss, J. B., Beevers, D. G., Brown, J. J., Davies, D. L., Fraser, R., Lever, A. F., Mason, P., Neville, A. M., and Robertson, J. I. S.: Clinical, biochemical and pathological features of low renin ("primary") hyperaldosteronism. Am. Heart J. *95*:375, 1978.

329. Ibsen, K. K.: Liquorice consumption and its influence on blood pressure in Danish school-children. Dan. Med. Bull. *28*:124, 1981.

330. Blachley, J. D., and Knochel, J. P.: Tobacco chewer's hypokalemia: Licorice revisited. N. Engl. J. Med. *302*:784, 1980.

331. Mantero, F., Armanini, D., Opocher, G., Fallo, F., Sampieri, L., Cuspidi, B., Ambrosi, C., and Faglia, G.: Mineralocorticoid hypertension due to a nasal spray containing 9α-fluoroprednisolone. Am. J. Med. *71*:352, 1981.

332. Kono, T., Ikeda, F., Oseko, F., Imura, H., and Tanimura, H.: Normotensive primary aldosteronism: Report of a case. J. Clin. Endocrinol. Metab. *52*:1009, 1981.

333. Kaplan, N. M.: Primary aldosteronism with malignant hypertension. N. Engl. J. Med. *269*:1282, 1963.

334. Kem, D. C., Weinberger, M. H., Mayes, D. M., and Nugent, C. A.: Saline suppression of plasma aldosterone in hypertension. Arch. Intern. Med. *128*:380, 1971.

335. Spark, R. F., and Melby, J. C.: Aldosteronism in hypertension. The spironolactone response test. Ann. Intern. Med. *69*:685, 1968.

336. Ferriss, J. B., Beevers, D. G., Brody, M. J., Brown, J. J., Davies, D. L., Fraser, R., Kremer, D., Lever, A. F., and Robertson, J. I. S.: The treatment of low-renin ("primary") hyperaldosteronism. Am. Heart J. *96*:97, 1978.

337. Abrams, H. L., Siegelman, S. S., Adams, D. F., Sanders, R., Feinberg, H. J., Hessel, S. J., and McNeil, B. J.: Computed tomography versus ultrasound of the adrenal gland: A prospective study. Radiology *143*:121, 1982.

338. Kaplan, N. M.: The steroid content of adrenal adenomas and measurements of aldosterone production in patients with essential hypertension and primary aldosteronism. J. Clin. Invest. *46*:728, 1967.

339. Ganguly, A., and Weinberger, M. H.: Triamterene-thiazide combination: Alternative therapy for primary aldosteronism. Clin. Pharmacol. Ther. *30*:246, 1981.

340. Griffing, G. T., Cole, A. G., Aurecchia, S. A., Sindler, B. A., Komanicky, P., and Melby, J. C.: Amiloride in primary hyperaldosteronism. Clin. Pharmacol. Ther. *31*:56, 1982.

341. O'Neal, L. W., Kissane, J. M., and Hartroft, P. M.: The kidney in endocrine hypertension. Arch. Surg. *100*:498, 1970.

342. Ross, E. J., and Linch, D. C.: Cushing's syndrome—killing disease: Discriminatory value of signs and symptoms aiding early diagnosis. Lancet *2*:646–649, 1982.

343. Dalakos, T. G., Elias, A. N., Anderson, G. H., Jr., Streeten, D. H. P., and Schroeder, E. T.: Evidence for an angiotensinogenic mechanism of the hypertension of Cushing's syndrome. J. Clin. Endocrinol. Metab. *46*:114, 1978.

344. Crapo, L.: Cushing's syndrome: A review of diagnostic tests. Metabolism *28*:955, 1979.

345. White, F. E., White, M. C., Drury, P. L., Fry, I. K., and Besser, G. M.: Value of computed tomography of the abdomen and chest in investigation of Cushing's syndrome. *284*:771, 1982.

346. Bigos, S. T., Somma, M., Rasio, E., Eastman, R. C., Lanthier, A., Johnston, H. H., and Hardy, J.: Cushing's disease: Management by transsphenoidal pituitary microsurgery. J. Clin. Endocrinol. Metab. *50*:348, 1980.

347. Jennings, A. S., Liddle, G. W., and Orth, D. N.: Results of treating childhood Cushing's disease with pituitary irradiation. N. Engl. J. Med. *297*:957, 1977.

347a. Kalff, V., Shapiro, B., Lloyd, R., Sisson, J. C., Holland, K., Nakajo, M., and Beierwaltes, W. H.: The spectrum of pheochromocytoma in hypertensive patients with neurofibromatosis. Arch. Intern. Med. *142*:2092–2098, 1982.

348. Valk, T. W., Frager, M. S., Gross, M. D., Sisson, J. C., Wieland, D. M., Swanson, D. P., Mangner, T. J., and Beierwaltes, W. H.: Spectrum of pheochromocytoma in multiple endocrine neoplasia. A scintigraphic portrayal using ^{131}I-metaiodobenzylguanidine. Ann. Intern. Med. *94*:762, 1981.

349. Baker, G., Zeller, N. H., Weitzner, S., and Leach, J. K.: Pheochromocytoma without hypertension presenting as cardiomyopathy. Am. Heart J. *83*:688, 1972.

350. Gupta, K. K.: Phaeochromocytoma and myocardial infarction. Lancet *1*:281, 1975.

351. Chaturvedi, N. C., Walsh, M. J., Boyle, D. M., and Barber, J. M.: Diamorphine-induced attack of paroxysmal hypertension in phaeochromocytoma. Br. Med. J. *2*:538, 1974.

352. Kaplan, N. M., Kramer, N. J., Holland, O. G., Sheps, S. G., and Gomez-Sanchez, C.: Single-voided urine metanephrine assays in screening for pheochromocytoma. Arch. Intern. Med. *137*:190, 1977.

353. Remine, W. H., Chong, G. C., Van Heerden, J. A., Sheps, S. G., and Harrison, E. G., Jr.: Current management of pheochromocytoma. Ann. Surg. *179*:740, 1974.

354. Bravo, E. L., Tarazi, R. C., Gifford, R. W., Jr. and Stewart, B. H.: Circulating and urinary catecholamines in pheochromocytoma. N. Engl. J. Med. *301*:682, 1979.

355. Bravo, E. L., Tarazi, R. C., Fouad, F. M., Vidt, D. G., and Gifford, R. W., Jr.: Clonidine-suppression test. A useful aid in the diagnosis of pheochromocytoma. N. Engl. J. Med. *305*:623, 1981.

356. Manger, W. M., and Gifford, R. W., Jr.: Hypertension secondary to pheochromocytoma. Bull. N.Y. Acad. Med. *58*:139, 1982.

357. Cathelineau, G., Brerault, J., Fiet, J., Julien, R., Dreux, C., and Canivet, J.: Adrenocortical 11β-hydroxylation defect in adult women with postmenarchial onset of symptoms. J. Clin. Endocrinol. Metab. *51*:287, 1980.

358. Biglieri, E. G., Herron, M. A., and Brust, N.: 17-Hydroxylation deficiency in man. J. Clin. Invest. *45*:1946, 1966.

359. Messerli, F. H., and Frohlich, E. D.: High blood pressure. A side effect of drugs, poisons, and food. Arch. Intern. Med. *139*:682, 1979.

360. Bretza, J. A., Novey, H. S., Vaziri, N. D., and Warner, A. S.: Hypertension. A complication of danazol therapy. Arch. Intern. Med. *140*:1379, 1980.

361. Horowitz, J. D., Howes, L. G., Christophidis, N., Louis, W. J., Lang, W. J., Fennessy, M. R., and Rand, M. J.: Hypertensive responses induced by phenylpropanolamine in anorectic and decongestant preparations. Lancet *1*:60, 1980.

362. Shinebourne, E. A., Tam, A. S. Y., Elsee, A. M., Paneth, M., Lennox, S. C., Cleland, W. P., Lincoln, C., Joseph, M. C., and Anderson, R. H.: Coarctation of the aorta in infancy and childhood. Br. Heart J. *38*:375, 1976.

363. Liberthson, R. R., Pennington, D. G., Jacobs, M. L., and Daggett, W. M.: Coarctation of the aorta: Review of 234 patients and clarification of management problems. Am. J. Cardiol. *43*:835, 1979.

364. Alpert, B. S., Bain, H. H., Balfe, J. W., Kidd, B. S. L., and Olley, P. M.: Role of the renin-angiotensin-aldosterone system in hypertensive children with coarctation of the aorta. Am. J. Cardiol. *43*:828, 1979.

365. Warren, D. J., and Smith, R. S.: Inappropriate renin secretion and abnormal cardiovascular reflexes in coarctation of the aorta. Br. Heart J. *45*:733, 1981.

366. Weyman, A. E., Caldwell, R. L., Hurwitz, R. A., Girod, D. A., Dillon, J. C., Feigenbaum, H., and Green, D.: Cross-sectional echocardiographic detection of aortic obstruction. Part 2. Coarctation of the aorta. Circulation *57*:498, 1978.

367. Rocchini, A. P., Rosenthal, A., Barger, A. C., Castaneda, A. R., and Nadas, A. S.: Pathogenesis of paradoxical hypertension after coarctation resection. Circulation *54*:382, 1976.

368. Benedict, C. R., Grahame-Smith, D. G., and Fisher, A.: Changes in plasma catecholamines and dopamine beta-hydroxylase after corrective surgery for coarctation of the aorta. Circulation *57*:598, 1978.

369. Vlachakis, N. D., Frederics, R., Velasquez, M., Alexander, N., Singer, F., and Maronde, R. F.: Sympathetic system function and vascular reactivity in hypercalcemic patients. Hypertension *4*:452, 1982.

370. Christensson, T., Hellstrom, K., and Wengle, B.: Hypercalcemia and primary hyperparathyroidism. Arch. Intern. Med. *137*:1138, 1977.

371. McCarron, D. A., Pingree, P. A., Rubin, R. J., Gaucher, S. M., Molitch, M., and Krutzik, S.: Enhanced parathyroid function in essential hypertension: A homeostatic response to a urinary calcium leak. Hypertension *2*:162, 1980.

372. Estafanous, F. G., and Tarazi, R. C.: Systemic arterial hypertension associated with cardiac surgery. Am. J. Cardiol. *46*:685, 1980.

373. Whelton, P. K., Flaherty, J. T., MacAllister, N. P., Watkins, L., Potter, A., Johnson, D., Russel, R. P., and Walker, W. G.: Hypertension following coronary artery bypass surgery. Role of preoperative propranolol therapy. Hypertension *2*:291, 1981.

374. Layton, C., Brigden, W., McDonald, L., Monro, J., McDonald, A., and Weaver, J.: Systemic hypertension after homograft aortic valvar replacement. A cause of late homograft failure. Lancet *2*:1343, 1973.

375. Cockburn, J. S., Benjamin, I. S., Thompson, R. M., and Bain, W. H.: Early systemic hypertension after surgical closure of atrial septal defect. J. Thorac. Cardiovasc. Surg. *16*:1, 1975.

376. Friedman, E. A., and Neff, R. K.: Hypertension-hypotension in pregnancy. Correlation with fetal outcome. J.A.M.A. *239*:2249, 1978.

377. Chesley, L. C.: Hypertensive Disorders in Pregnancy. New York, Appleton-Century-Crofts, 1978.

378. MacGillivray, I., Rose, G. A., and Rowe, B.: Blood pressure survey in pregnancy. Clin. Sci. *37*:395, 1969.

379. Sawyer, M. M., Lipshitz, J., Anderson, G. D., Dilts, P. V., and Halperin, L.: Diurnal and short-term variation of blood pressure: Comparison of pre-eclamptic, chronic, hypertensive, and normotensive patients. Obstet. Gynecol. *58*:291, 1981.

380. Gallery, E. D. M., Hunyor, S. N., Ross, M., and Gyory, A. Z.: Predicting the development of pregnancy-associated hypertension: The place of standard blood-pressure measurement. Lancet *1*:1273, 1977.

381. Gallery, E. D. M.: Pregnancy-associated hypertension: Interrelationships of volume and blood pressure changes. Clin. Exper. Hyper.—Hyper. in Pregnancy *B1*:39, 1982.

382. Lunnell, N. O., Nylund, L. E., Lewander, L. E., and Sarby, B.: Uteroplacental blood flow in pre-eclampsia measurements with indium-113m and a computer-linked gamma camera. Clin. Exper. Hyper.—Hyper. in Pregnancy *B1*:105, 1982.

383. Gant, N. F., Madden, J. D., Chand, S., Worley, R. J., Strong, J. D., and MacDonald, P. C.: Metabolic clearance rate of dehydroisoandrosterone sulfate. V. Studies of essential hypertension complicating pregnancy. Obstet. Gynecol. *47*: 319, 1976.

384. Ferris, T. F., Stein, J. H., and Kauffman, J.: Uterine blood flow and uterine renin secretion. J. Clin. Invest. *51*:2827, 1972.

385. Terrango, N. A., Terrango, D.A., Pacholczyk, D., and McGiff, J. C.: Prostaglandins and the regulation of uterine blood flow in pregnancy. Nature *249*:57, 1974.

386. Downing, I., Shepherd, G. L., and Lewis, P. J.: Kinetics of prostacyclin synthetase in umbilical artery microsomes from normal and pre-eclamptic pregnancies. Br. J. Clin. Pharmac. *13*:195, 1982.

387. Bodzenta, A., Thompson, J. M., Poller, L., Burslem, R. W., and Wilcox, F. L.:

Prostacyclin-like and kallikrein activity of amniotic fluid in pre-eclampsia. Br. J. Obstet. Gynecol. 88:1217, 1981.

388. Goodman, R. P., Killam, A. P., Brash, A. R., and Branch, R. A.: Prostacyclin production during pregnancy: Comparison of production during normal pregnancy and pregnancy complicated by hypertension. Am. J. Obstet. Gynecol. 142:817, 1982.

389. Remuzzi, G., Marchesi, D., Zoja, C., Muratore, D., Mecca, G., Misiani, R., Rossi, E., Barbato, M., Capetta, P., Donati, M. B., and de Gaetano, G. Reduced umbilical and placental vascular prostacyclin in severe pre-eclampsia. Prostaglandins 20:105, 1980.

390. Gant, N. F., Worley, R. J., Everett, R. B., and MacDonald, P. C.: Control of vascular responsiveness during human pregnancy. Kidney Int. 18:253, 1980.

391. Pipkin, F. B., Hunter, J. C., Turner, S. R., and O'Brien, P. M. S.: Prostaglandin E₂ attenuates the pressor response to angiotensin II in pregnant subjects but not in nonpregnant subjects. Am. J. Obstet. Gynecol. 142:168, 1982.

392. Gerber, J. G., Payne, N. A., Murphy, R. C., and Nies, A. S.: Prostacyclin produced by the pregnant uterus in the dog may act as a circulating vasodepressor substance. J. Clin. Invest. 67:632, 1981.

393. Wickens, D., Wilkins, M. H., Lunec, J., Ball, G., and Dormandy, L. T.: Free-radical oxidation (peroxidation) products in plasma in normal and abnormal pregnancy. Ann. Clin. Biochem. 18:158, 1981.

394. Whigham, K. A. E., Howie, P. W., Drummond, A. H., and Prentice, C. R. M.: Abnormal platelet function in pre-eclampsia. Br. J. Obstet. Gynecol. 85:28, 1978.

395. Scott, J. S., Jenkins, D. M., and Need, J. A.: Immunology of pre-eclampsia. Lancet 1:704, 1978.

396. Chesley, L. C.: Hypertension in pregnancy: Definitions, familial factor, and remote prognosis. Kidney Int. 18:234, 1980.

397. Gant, N. D., Chand, S., Worley, R. J., Whalley, P. J., Crosby, U. D., and MacDonald, P. C.: A clinical test useful for predicting the development of acute hypertension in pregnancy. Am. J. Obstet. Gynecol. 120:1, 1974.

398. Kuntz, W. D.: Supine pressor (roll-over) test: An evaluation. Am. J. Obstet. Gynecol. 137:764, 1980.

399. Pritchard, J. A.: Management of preeclampsia and eclampsia. Kidney Int. 18:259, 1980.

400. Cockburn, J., Ounsted, M., Moar, V. A., and Redman, C. W. G.: Final report of study on hypertension during pregnancy: The effects of specific treatment on the growth and development of the children. Lancet 1:647, 1982.

401. Habib, A., and McCarthy, J. S.: Effects on the neonate of propranolol administered during pregnancy. J. Pediatr. 91:808, 1977.

402. Gallery, E. D. M., Saunders, D. M., Hunyor, S. N., and Gyory, A. Z.: Randomized comparison of methyldopa and oxprenolol for treatment of hypertension in pregnancy. Br. Med. J. 1:1591, 1979.

403. Sandstrom, B.: Adrenergic beta-receptor blockers in hypertension of pregnancy. Clin. Exper. Hyper.—Hyper. in Pregnancy. B1:127, 1982.

404. Welt, S. I., Dorminy, J. H., Jelovsek, F. R., Crenshaw, M. C., and Gall, M. D.: The effect of prophylactic management and therapeutics on hypertensive disease in pregnancy: Preliminary studies. Obstet. Gynecol. 57:557, 1981.

405. Lopez-Llera, M.: Complicated eclampsia. Fifteen years' experience in a referral medical center. Am. J. Obstet. Gynecol. 142:28, 1982.

406. Bauer, T. W., Moore, G. W., and Hutchins, G. M.: Morphologic evidence for coronary artery spasm in eclampsia. Circulation 65:255, 1982.

407. Brockington, I. F.: Postpartum hypertensive heart failure. Am. J. Cardiol. 27:650, 1971.

408. Strauss, R. G., and Alexander, R. W.: Postpartum hemolytic uremic syndrome. Obstet. Gynecol. 47:169, 1976.

409. Fixler, D. E., Kautz, J. A., and Dana, K.: Systolic blood pressure differences among pediatric epidemiological studies. Hypertension 2 (Suppl. I):I-3, 1980.

410. Rames, L. K., Clarke, W. R., Connor, W. E., Reiter, M. A., and Lauer, T. M.: Normal blood pressures and the evaluation of sustained blood pressure elevation in childhood: the Muscatine study. Pediatrics 61:245, 1978.

411. Fixler, D. E., Laird, W. P., Fitzgerald, V., Stead, S., and Adams, R.: Hypertension screening in schools: Results of the Dallas study. Pediatrics 63:32, 1979.

412. Zinner, S. H., Margolius, H. S., Rosner, B., and Kass, E. H.: Stability of blood pressure rank and urinary kallikrein concentration in childhood: An eight year follow-up. Circulation 58:908, 1978.

413. Harlan, W. R., Coroni-Huntley, J., and Leaverton, P. E.: Blood pressure in childhood. The National Health Examination Survey. Hypertension 1:559, 1979.

414. Reed, W. L.: Racial differences in blood pressure levels of adolescents. Am. J. Public Health 71:1165, 1981.

415. Fouad, F. M., Tarazi, R. C., Dustan, H. P., and Bravo, E. L.: Hemodynamics of essential hypertension in young subjects. Am. Heart J. 96:646, 1978.

416. Sinaiko, A. R., Gillum, R. F., Jacobs, D. R., Sopko, G., and Prineas, R. J.: Renin-angiotensin and sympathetic nervous system activity in grade school children. Hypertension 4:299, 1982.

417. Voors, A. W., Webber, L. S., and Berenson, G. S.: Racial contrasts in cardiovascular response tests for children from a total community. Hypertension 2:686, 1980.

418. Falkner, B., Kushner, H., Onesti, G., and Angelakos, E. T.: Cardiovascular characteristics in adolescents who develop essential hypertension. Hypertension 3:521, 1981.

419. Goldring, D., Hernandez, A., Choi, S., Lee, J. Y., Londe, S., Lindgren, F. T., and Burton, R. M.: Blood pressure in a high school population. II. Clinical profile of the juvenile hypertensive. J. Pediatr. 95:298, 1979.

420. Beilin, L. J., and Goldby, F. S.: High arterial pressure versus humoral factors in the pathogenesis of the vascular lesions of malignant hypertension. Clin. Sci. Molec. Med. 52:111, 1977.

421. Lee, T. H., and Alderman, M. H.: Malignant hypertension: Declining mortality rate in New York City, 1958 to 1974. N.Y. State J. Med. 78:1389, 1978.

422. MacKenzie, E. T., Strandgaard, S., Graham, D. I., Jones, J. V., Harper, A. M., and Farrar, J. K.: Effects of acutely induced hypertension in cats on pial arteriolar caliber, local cerebral blood flow, and the blood-brain barrier. Circ. Res. 39:33, 1976.

423. Strandgaard, S., Olesen, J., Skinhoj, E., and Lassen, N. A.: Autoregulation of brain circulation in severe arterial hypertension. Br. Med. J. 1:507, 1973.

424. Jones, J. V., Fitch, W., Mackenzie, E. T., Strandgaard, S., and Harper, A. M.: Lower limit of cerebral blood flow autoregulation in experimental renovascular hypertension in the baboon. Circ. Res. 39:555, 1976.

425. Hodge, J. V., McQueen, E. C., and Smirk, F. H.: Results of hypotensive therapy in arterial hypertension. Br. Med. J. 1:1, 1961.

426. Barnett, A. J., and Silberberg, F. G.: Long-term results of treatment of severe hypertension. Med. J. Aust. 2:960, 1973.

27

SYSTEMIC HYPERTENSION: THERAPY

by Norman M. Kaplan, M.D.

INTRODUCTION

In the United States, the general attitude toward the therapy of hypertension has rapidly swung, like a pendulum, from overly conservative to one that is likely too liberal. Occurring over the past 10 years, this dramatic change has come about through the confluence of a number of factors, including (1) increasing awareness in the medical community and among the public of the dangers of untreated hypertension—the "silent killer;" (2) the availability of effective, safe, and easily tolerated medications; and (3) the documentation of protection against cardiovascular damage through reduction of blood pressure with drug therapy. Protection by therapy was shown first for malignant hypertension in the late 1950s,[1] then, in 1967, for diastolic levels between 115 and 129 mm Hg,[2] for diastolic levels between 104 and 115 in 1970,[3] and, most recently, for levels above 90[4] or 95.[5] As noted in Chapter 26 (see Fig. 26–6, p. 856), the proportion of the hypertensive population brought under the therapeutic umbrella has increased markedly as the criterion for the acceptable lower limit for treatment has been reduced: over 70 per cent of the total hypertensive population is in the "mild" category, with diastolic blood pressure between 90 and 104 mm Hg, and this group comprises about 30 million Americans.

The high degree of risk associated with diastolic pressures above 105 and the marked protection against that risk afforded by antihypertensive drug therapy demonstrated in the Veterans Administration Cooperative Study[3] strongly support the validity of active pharmacotherapy for persons with pressures at that level—assuming that such pressures have been shown to persist after the initial observation. Recall the tendency for many such high readings to fall upon repeat measurements.[6] Although only diastolic levels are being referred to, an even closer relation to eventual risk has been shown for systolic levels in the Framingham study.[7] Specific coverage of therapy for pre-

dominantly systolic hypertension is provided later in this chapter. For now, the focus is on the majority of patients, i.e., those with diastolic pressures between 90 and 104 mm Hg.

CURRENT ENTHUSIASM TOWARD THERAPY

As we shall see, the evidence that drug therapy is needed to protect an individual against mild hypertension is neither as conclusive nor as encompassing as many have assumed.[8] Even so, the medical community has been more than willing to accept the evidence in support of treatment for a larger proportion of the hypertensive population: In a survey of physicians in New York carried out in 1978, *before* publication of the results of any large-scale trials showing that treatment was of value in mild hypertension, 92 per cent indicated that they would treat patients whose diastolic pressure was 90 to 104 mm Hg.[9]

Two reasons have been given to explain this enthusiastic acceptance of the need for active drug therapy in mild hypertension, even in advance of proof of its efficacy.[10] First is the belief that such an approach would be *preventive*, based on the demonstrated benefits of therapy for more severe hypertension. The second is a *sociological* premise, based on two widely held attitudes: (1) "technological optimism—the disposition to employ technologies in the belief that the benefits that flow from them will outweigh whatever unforeseen and undesirable effects ensue, and that these effects will themselves be manageable by existing or potential technological means"; and (2) "therapeutic activism—physicians prefer to take the risk of treating when intervention may not be called for to the potential error of not treating when treatment is needed."[10]

This enthusiasm to treat may involve almost 60 million Americans, if all those with diastolic pressures above 90 mm Hg are included.[11] Over 27 million new prescriptions for antihypertensive drugs were

TABLE 27–1   GUIDE TO THERAPY
WHEN DIASTOLIC BLOOD PRESSURE IS 90 TO 104 mm Hg*

Under 45 years of age 1	Target organ damage 2
Black 1	Parent with major
	cardiovascular event 1
Male 1	Hypercholesterolemia 1
All diastolic pressures >95 1	Smoker 1
Systolic pressures >165 1	

Drug therapy if diastolic blood pressure is:
100 to 104 with 2 points or more
95 to 99 with 3 points or more
90 to 94 with 4 points or more

*Recommended by Dr. Edward Freis.

written in 1981; with regard to sales in the United States, seven of the top 20 drugs were antihypertensive agents. It should be noted that this enthusiasm—referred to as "early and aggressive treatment" in widely seen advertisements—is not shared by physicians elsewhere; in England, most physicians withhold therapy until diastolic pressures exceed 100 mm Hg.[12]

A MORE MODERATE VIEW

Based upon a careful analysis of evidence available as of late 1982, a more moderate position than that currently taken by most American physicians would seem to be warranted. Results of another large therapeutic trial now being conducted in England[13] may provide more evidence in favor of earlier and more aggressive therapy, but the results of the Hypertension Detection and Follow-up Program (HDFP)[4] and of the Australian trial[5] do not prove the need for routine drug therapy for all those with mild hypertension. Let us examine the evidence in support of a more moderate position: "that such therapy should be provided selectively, quickly to those at high risk, but only after a period of observation plus non-drug therapy for the majority. Hopefully, such selectivity in using drug therapy will protect those in immediate need while at the same time postponing or perhaps removing the need for such therapy in many more patients."[14]

THE DEGREE OF RISK

The overall increase in long-term cardiovascular risk from even a mild degree of hypertension has been amply documented (see Fig. 26–3, p. 852). But, as noted in the preceding chapter, the majority of patients with mild hypertension do not suffer apparent harm over a few years. Recall the experience of the 1600 patients who served as controls in the Australian trial[5]: the majority of those patients who entered the trial with diastolic pressures between 95 and 109 mm Hg experienced a lowering of blood pressures over the next four years, and those whose pressures stayed below 100 mm Hg had no excess morbidity or mortality (Fig. 27–1). On the other hand, remember that in 12.2 per cent of this placebo-treated group, blood pressures progressed to 110 mm Hg or higher, indicating the *need for continued surveillance* of all patients identified as hypertensive. These Austra-

lian patients were free of identifiable cardiovascular damage at the time of entry into the trial. Therefore, their relatively benign short-term experience should not be extrapolated to those patients with more biologically aggressive disease, evidenced by target organ damage.

The need to consider factors other than blood pressure that contribute to cardiovascular risk has been cogently demonstrated by Alderman and Madhavan.[15] Using the risk factors found in the Framingham study to be major predictors of the development of cardiovascular disease, they calculated the likelihood of such complications appearing over a 15-year interval in men and women aged 35 who had similar blood pressure levels but were at varying degrees of overall risk (Fig. 27–2). Note that a "high-risk" man with a systolic blood pressure of 195 has an 86 per cent likelihood of developing cardiovascular disease, whereas a "low-risk" man of the same age and with the same blood pressure has a 15 per cent chance and a similar "low-risk" woman only a 6 per cent chance.

The Framingham data can be used to calculate the probable risk for adults with any combination of factors, to provide some objective evidence for each individual as to the urgency of the need for active intervention. Some years ago, Dr. Edward Freis formulated a simple guide to drug therapy for patients with diastolic pressures of 90 to 104, assigning points to many of the known factors associated with increased risk and choosing therapy based on total score (Table 27–1). The purpose of these assessments is to limit the immediate use of drug therapy to that part of the population with mild hypertension who are most in need, i.e., taking more precise aim rather than scatter-shooting at many to protect a few.

This rationale is based on two more assumptions: (1) drug therapy may not be needed for many whose blood pressure responds to time and nondrug therapies and (2) drug therapy may invoke its own inherent risks. Following this line of reasoning, we will next examine the evidence that drug therapy offers protection to such patients.

PROTECTION BY THERAPY

The drug-treated half of the Australian patients had 30 per cent less morbidity and mortality than did the placebo-treated half over the three years of the trial, associated with an average 6 mm Hg lower diastolic blood pressure (88 versus 94).[5]

FIGURE 27-1 Average diastolic blood pressure levels during the four years of the Australian therapeutic trial of the 1617 patients randomly assigned to placebo therapy. Patients were divided into three groups based on their initial diastolic blood pressure upon entry into the trial. The excess morbidity and mortality observed in the placebo group occurred in those whose diastolic BP averaged 100 mm Hg or higher (noted by asterisks). (Drawn from Report of the Management Committee. Lancet *1*:1261, 1980.)

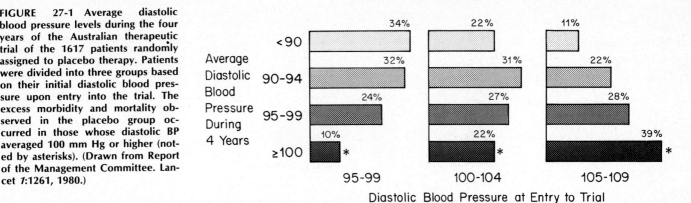

PLACEBO TREATMENT
OF HYPERTENSION IN 1617 PATIENTS

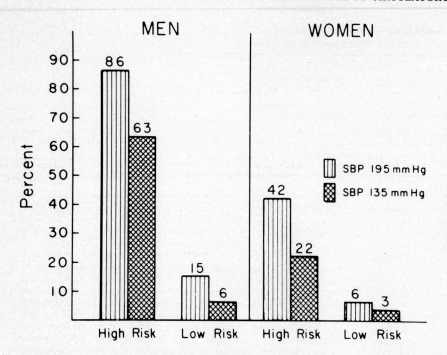

FIGURE 27-2 Risk of developing cardiovascular disease in 15 years for 35-year-old men and women, according to systolic blood pressure (SBP) level and risk status in the Framingham cohort. High risk = Left ventricular hypertrophy (LVH) by ECG, cigarette smoker, blood cholesterol level of 310 mg/100 ml, and glucose intolerance. Low risk = No LVH by ECG, nonsmoker, blood cholesterol of 235 mg/100 ml, and no glucose intolerance. (From Alderman, M.H., and Madhaven, S.: Management of the hypertensive patient: A continuing dilemma. Hypertension 3:192, 1981, by permission of the American Heart Association, Inc.)

In the HDFP, the 11,000 patients whose initial pressures were between 90 and 104 were all offered therapy, but half were more intensively treated (the Stepped-Care group) than the other half (the Referred-Care group). At the end of the five-year study, the Stepped-Care group had a 20 per cent lower overall mortality rate than did the Referred-Care group, associated with a 5 mm Hg lower average diastolic blood pressure (83 versus 88 mm Hg).[4] These results, along with similar data from a smaller study done in Oslo,[16] have been considered definitive proof of the value of "early and aggressive" therapy of all patients with mild hypertension. However, closer examination of these results suggests that they should not be applied to the universe of mild hypertensives.

The HDFP Data. As for the HDFP data, the 20 per cent reduction in overall and cardiovascular mortality was accompanied by a 13 per cent reduction in mortality from noncardiovascular diseases. This decrease likely reflects the more intensive overall medical care provided the Stepped-Care group and suggests that the program was "as much a trial of medical care as of antihypertensive drugs."[17] Some

may assume that the 20 per cent difference in mortality rates means that 20 per cent of the less actively treated group died and could have been protected by further reduction in their blood pressure. In fact, the 20 per cent reduction in mortality represents an actual difference in survival of less than 1.5 per cent between the two groups, with 94 per cent of the Stepped-Care and 92.5 per cent of the Referred-Care alive at the end of the five years. The 1.5 per cent difference is a 20 per cent relative difference in the rates for the two groups, but the smaller number is a more accurate representation of the actual number of people who would benefit from therapy.

The Australian Trial. In the Australian trial, the development of cardiovascular disease, referred to as trial end points, was continually monitored, and when a statistically significant difference of 30 per cent was noted, the trial was stopped, providing strong evidence for the value of drug therapy. When the data are closely scrutinized, two additional conclusions can be reached. First, as noted earlier, the overall 30 per cent excess in morbidity occurred only among the placebo-treated patients whose diastolic blood pressure averaged above

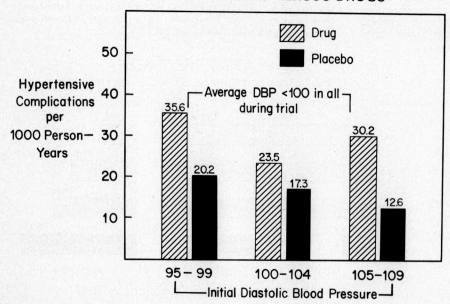

FIGURE 27-3 Cardiovascular complications per 1000 person-years among those receiving drugs and those receiving placebo during the Australian therapeutic trial. Note that for those whose average diastolic blood pressure (DBP) was below 100, regardless of the initial DBP range, complication rates were lower in those not on drugs. More of those from each initial DBP group who were on drugs achieved an end DBP below 100. (Drawn from Report of the Management Committee. Lancet 1:1261, 1980.)

100 mm Hg. When the average diastolic pressures of the entire placebo-treated population throughout the trial is portrayed (Fig. 27–1), the majority (78 per cent) are shown to be below 100 mm Hg, even among those who started with pressure readings between 105 and 109 mm Hg. Thus the excess complications occurred in the 22 per cent of the placebo-treated group whose average diastolic pressure was above 100 mm Hg throughout the four years of the study.

Second, for those whose DBP was below 100 mm Hg, there were *fewer* complications among those on placebo than among those on drug therapy. As shown in Figure 27–3, the patients are again divided into three groups based on their initial level of diastolic pressure and only those whose average pressure was below 100 during the four years of the trial are portrayed. Since more of the drug-treated patients in each subdivision had an average diastolic pressure below 100 during the trial, there are more of them in each set. Since the numbers of patients and their duration of exposure to risk differ between the two groups, the obvious interpretation may be misleading, but it is hard to deny that interpretation: those given drugs had *more* cardiovascular complications than those with comparable blood pressures who were not receiving antihypertensive drugs. This interpretation, in turn, can be explained in various ways: (1) More of the drug-treated patients who averaged the same diastolic blood pressure during the trial as the placebo-treated group started with higher pressures; even though all patients were free of identifiable cardiovascular disease at the start of the trial, those with higher initial pressures might have been more likely to experience clinical complications despite the lowering of their pressure. (2) Although drugs are effective in protecting against complications, they are not able to remove the excess risk entirely. (3) Drugs are inherently toxic and patients with uncomplicated hypertension whose diastolic pressure stays below 100 are better off not receiving drug therapy.

The third interpretation may not be valid, but it cannot be dismissed. As we shall see, every group of antihypertensive drugs may adversely affect one or more cardiovascular risk factors, thereby diminishing, if not ablating, the potential benefits of the reductions of blood pressure. For example, diuretics tend to raise plasma cholesterol levels by 15 mg/dl—an effect recognized only after they had been used in the treatment of millions of hypertensives for almost 20 years.[18] Recall the warning by Geoffrey Rose, quoted in Chapter 26, (p. 856) that "if a preventive measure exposes many people to a small risk, the harm it does may readily . . . outweigh the benefits since those are received by relatively few."[19]

Overall Guidelines for the Use of Drug Therapy

The preceding discussion has attempted to establish three premises: (1) the relative risk for cardiovascular disease is based upon more than just the blood pressure, and by using simple clinical tools, it is possible to establish each individual's relative risk status; (2) for most mild hypertensives, the short-term risk is minimal, and the use of nondrug therapies (plus the spontaneous fall in pressure observed in some) may be adequate to relieve even that small degree of risk; and (3) drug therapy may pose inherent long-term risks along with the bother of more obvious and immediate side effects.

Based upon these premises, the author believes that the following guidelines are appropriate for deciding upon the institution of therapy, once the presence of hypertension has been confirmed by multiple blood pressure readings:

1. Patients with diastolic blood pressure above 100 mm Hg, particularly if it is accompanied by target organ damage or other major cardiovascular risks, should begin drug therapy immediately.

2. Patients with diastolic levels below 100 mm Hg who are otherwise at low risk should be encouraged to lose weight if obese, reduce sodium intake, exercise regularly, relax, and drink alcohol only in moderation. (More specific

details about these nondrug therapies are provided later in this chapter.)

3. Patients whose diastolic pressure remains below 100 mm Hg should not be given drugs and should be observed at least every six months. If the diastolic pressure rises to and remains above 100, the patient should be treated with appropriate drugs.

4. When drug therapy is given, the diastolic blood pressure should be reduced to the low 80s, if that goal can be reached without bothersome side effects.

OTHER VIEWPOINTS

This more cautious approach is similar to that espoused by many outside the United States. A committee representing the World Health Organization and the International Society of Hypertension, after analyzing the published data from trials of the treatment of mild hypertension, offered this conclusion in early 1982: "The first line of treatment for people with mild hypertension should be observation, perhaps combined with general health measures such as weight reduction and restriction of salt intake."[13]

Although this viewpoint may reflect the consensus of most experts outside the U.S., many in the U.S. would argue for more widespread and earlier use of drug therapy.[20] Their arguments include the following: the assessment of relative risk is by no means certain, and most patients fall into an intermediate risk group; various nondrug therapies have not been shown to be either practical or effective for large groups of patients over prolonged periods; drug therapy will lower blood pressure, and providing it to most patients will avoid errors based on incorrect assessments of risk and will satisfy the widespread assumption that if their problem is not serious enough to be treated with medication, it is not serious enough to mandate changes in longstanding habits of life style. Furthermore, the HDFP found that patients with mild hypertension and no evidence of target organ damage achieved significant protection from stroke morbidity and mortality,[21] supporting the view that the overall benefit of more intensive drug therapy outweighs the potential hazards.

THE QUESTION OF PROTECTION FROM CORONARY DISEASE

Amid these arguments, an additional factor has given some authorities pause in advocating drug therapy for mild hypertension; i.e., an apparent lack of protection from the major cardiovascular risk, coronary artery disease. In the earlier trials, including those by the VA[2,3] and USPHS,[22] the reduction in the incidence of coronary disease offered by therapy was not statistically significant. In the Australian trial, fewer cases of fatal coronary artery disease occurred in the drug-treated group than in those treated with placebo (2 versus 8), but the difference in nonfatal coronary events (70 versus 89) was, once again, not statistically significant. In the HDFP, deaths from myocardial infarction were reduced by 46 per cent but deaths from "ischemic heart disease" were 9 per cent higher in the more actively treated Stepped-Care group.

The difficulty in showing protection from coronary artery disease likely reflects several factors: the advanced age of the study populations and the early age of onset of coronary atherosclerosis, the relatively short duration of the studies, and the multiple etiologies of coronary artery disease. Hypertension probably plays a less direct role in causing coronary artery disease than in causing heart failure, stroke, and renal damage. Coronary atherosclerosis is accentuated by high blood lipid levels, smoking, stress, and a sedentary life style.

Nonetheless, a noncontrolled study involving men with more severe hypertension, i.e., diastolic pressures above 115 mm Hg, did show a significant decrease in nonfatal and fatal coronary artery disease among 635 treated patients compared to 391 untreated ones.[23] Moreover, preliminary data from the HDFP report a "substantial" decrease in four indices of coronary artery disease among the Stepped-Care group compared to the less intensively treated Referred-Care group.[24] These include a lower incidence of angina by history and of myocardial infarction by history, Rose Questionnaire, and electrocardiography.

Further evidence comes from a study of left ventricular hypertrophy, which may accelerate the clinical appearance of coronary artery disease. With echocardiography, reduction of left ventricular mass index has been demonstrated in patients whose blood pressure was successfully lowered by the use of antihypertensive drugs for a year or longer.[25]

Thus, evidence is mounting that antihypertensive therapy will protect against coronary artery disease. Some assume that the impressive protection against the recurrence of myocardial infarction afforded by various beta blockers administered after an initial infarction may apply to the primary prevention of coronary artery disease as a result of their blood pressure–lowering effect. Caution is advised, since a number of factors related to a prior myocardial infarction differentiate the two circumstances. Proof of specific protection against the development of coronary artery disease has not been shown for beta blockers or any other drug used in the treatment of hypertension. In the studies in which primary protection has been shown — the HDFP, the Australian trial, and the series reported by Wilhelmsen[23] — a multiplicity of drugs was used, diuretics being the most common.

WHOM TO TREAT WITH DRUGS

Based on all this evidence, there appears to be no single answer to the question of whom to treat with drugs for mild hypertension. Each patient must be considered separately, taking various factors into account. However, the foregoing discussion should indicate the wisdom of withholding drug therapy from many of these patients, at least until the effects of time and nondrug therapies have been given a chance.

Having advocated the use of nondrug therapies, I will now examine the evidence that these approaches may be of help and provide practical guidelines for their use.

NONDRUG THERAPY

Interest in the use of various nondrug therapies for the treatment of hypertension, particularly diet and exercise, has risen markedly in the past few years. Yet, many practitioners either do not use them or use them in a casual, perfunctory manner. This hesitant attitude can be attributed both to the sparsity of firm evidence indicating that these therapies succeed and to the difficulty many have faced in convincing patients to adhere to them. However, this situation is likely to change: evidence for the effectiveness of these approaches is growing, techniques for improving adherence are being popularized, and patients seem increasingly willing to adopt changes in life style. These changes come at a propitious time, when many more people are being identified as hypertensive and are considered in need of lowering their blood pressure. Although most have turned first to drugs, the evidence presented in the previous section suggests that these can be safely withheld from many hypertensives to allow nondrug therapies a chance to be effective.

In part, the underuse of nondrug therapies is due to the excitement over newly available drugs and the massive advertising campaigns to promote their use. Without commercial advocates, nondrug therapies have been unable to compete. Moreover, when physicians decide to treat a condition, they expect immediate results with virtual certainty. Certainly these expectations were justified when the majority of patients had fairly severe hypertension; however, as the large number of patients with mild hypertension enter the picture, a more relaxed, gradual approach to their management seems likely to be adopted.

An awareness and concern about the problem of patients' adherence to drug therapy have increased, and considerable efforts to improve compliance are being made. Similarly, attention toward adherence to nondrug therapies will likely improve their acceptance and effectiveness. These measures should be introduced gradually and gently. Too many and too drastic changes in life style will discourage patients from accepting needed care. Eventually, however, all hypertensive patients should benefit from mild restriction of dietary salt, reduction of excess body weight, and regular isotonic exercise. Although high blood lipid levels and cigarette smoking have little, if any, direct effect on blood pressure, patients with hypertension should be encouraged to eliminate these risk factors that predispose to cardiovascular disease.

DIETARY SODIUM RESTRICTION

In Chapter 26, evidence was presented incriminating the typically high sodium content of the diet of people living in acculturated, industrialized societies as a cause of hypertension. Once hypertension is present, modest salt restriction will help lower the blood pressure. One of the best demonstrations of this effect was seen among 19 unselected patients with mild hypertension (average blood pressure after 2 months of no treatment = 156/98).[26] The patients were all placed on a diet moderately restricted in sodium for 2 weeks and then entered into a double-blind randomized crossover study of two 4-week intervals when either a placebo or matching sodium chloride tablets were given (Fig. 27-4). Patients were given the number of tablets estimated to restore their sodium intake to the usual level. At the end of the placebo period, when daily sodium excretion averaged 86 mmol, supine blood pressure fell an average of 12/6 mm Hg; when sodium intake was restored to an average of 162 mmol per day, the average blood pressure rose to within 1 mm Hg of its level at the beginning of the study.

We observed a similar reduction of blood pressure in a group of patients whose dietary sodium intake was reduced so that they achieved a decrease in daily sodium excretion from 195 mmol to 72 mmol.[27] In addition, the amount of diuretic-induced potassium wastage was halved during the periods of lower sodium intake, providing another rationale for sodium restriction.

Both these studies utilized a moderate reduction of dietary sodium intake, to levels of 2 grams of sodium (88 mmol) per day. More rigid restriction, although possibly more effective in reducing blood pressure, is both impractical and, perhaps, counterproductive with regard to potassium conservation if diuretic therapy is used concomitantly. When patients were given only 17 mmol of sodium per day along with a daily diuretic, they wasted more potassium,[28] probably because the rigid sodium restriction activated the renin-aldosterone system, which, in the presence of diuretic-induced sodium delivery to the distal parts of the renal tubule, caused more potassium to be swept into the urine. Such rigid sodium restriction also activates the sympathetic nervous system,[29] so that the antihypertensive potential may be further limited.

The desired moderate degree of sodium restriction can

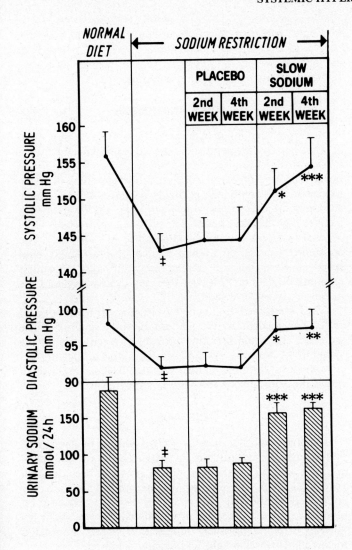

be easily accomplished by having the patient follow these guidelines:

1. Salt should not be added to food during cooking or at the table.

2. If a salty taste is desired, use a half sodium and half potassium chloride preparation such as Morton's Lite Salt® or a pure KCl substitute.

3. Avoid or minimize the use of processed foods, to which excess sodium has been added (Table 27-2).

4. Recognize the sodium content of some antacids and proprietary medications. Whereas Alka-Seltzer® contains over 500 mg of sodium, Rolaids® are virtually salt-free.

In order to ensure adherence to the diet, measuring the sodium content of an occasional overnight urine collection will be helpful, particularly if the patient is given immediate feedback as to its content so that, if additional instruction is needed, it can be provided at that visit.[30]

The Question of Potassium. Some of the advantages of a lower sodium intake may relate to its tendency to increase body potassium content, both by a coincidental increase in dietary potassium intake and by a decrease in diuretic-induced potassium wastage. Although potassium deficiency clearly exerts multiple effects that may increase the blood pressure,[31,32] evidence that correction of hypoka-

FIGURE 27-4 Average systolic and diastolic blood pressure and urinary sodium excretion on a normal diet, 2 weeks after dietary sodium restriction, and at 2-week intervals during the randomized crossover trial of placebo or sodium chloride tablets (Slow Sodium). (*p < 0.05, **p < 0.01, and ***p < 0.001 comparing equivalent measurement on Slow Sodium to placebo; ‡p < 0.001 comparing measurement on normal diet to 2 weeks of dietary sodium restriction.) (From MacGregor, G. A., et al.: Double-blind randomised crossover trial of moderate sodium restriction in essential hypertension. Lancet 1:351, 1982.)

TABLE 27–2 SODIUM CONTENT OF SOME AMERICAN FOODS*

Comparable foods with either low or high sodium content:

Low	High
Shredded Wheat®: 1 mg/oz	Corn Flakes®: 305 mg/oz
Green beans, fresh: 5 mg/cup	Green beans, canned: 925 mg/cup
Orange juice: 2 mg/cup	Tomato juice: 640 mg/cup
Turkey, roasted: 70 mg/3 oz	Turkey dinner: 1,735 mg
Ground beef: 57 mg/3 oz	Frankfurter, beef: 425 mg each
Pork, uncooked: 65 mg/3 oz	Bacon, uncooked: 1,400 mg/3 oz

Some foods with very high sodium content:
Catsup, 1 Tbs: 156 mg
Olive, one: 165 mg
Cinnamon roll, one: 630 mg
Soup (chicken noodle), one cup: 1,050 mg
Dill pickle, one large: 1,928 mg

The sodium content of some "fast foods":
Kentucky Fried Chicken®
  (3 pieces of chicken,
  mashed potatoes and gravy,
  cole slaw, and roll)   2,285 mg
McDonald's Big Mac®   962 mg
Burger King Whopper®   909 mg
Dairy Queen Chili Dog®   939 mg
Taco Bell Enchirito®   1,175 mg

*1000 mg sodium = 44 mEq sodium.

lemia or addition of dietary potassium will lower the blood pressure is skimpy.[33,34] Nonetheless, as we shall see, diuretic-induced hypokalemia may be more of a danger than many suspect, so that, for various reasons, hypertensive patients should be protected from potassium depletion.

WEIGHT REDUCTION

After a critical review of 21 published studies on the effects of weight loss on hypertension, it was concluded that weight loss is effective in reducing the blood pressure.[35] In one report from Israel, 81 moderately overweight hypertensive patients were placed on a diet restricted to 800 to 1200 calories a day; over a 2-month period, all lost at least 3 kg, with a mean weight loss of 10.5 kg.[36] During this interval, all but two experienced a significant reduction in blood pressure related to the degree of weight loss. The mean fall in blood pressure with weight reduction was 26/20 mm Hg among the subgroup receiving no antihypertensive drugs and was 37/23 mm Hg among those receiving drugs. In order to ensure that the decrease in blood pressure was not attributable to concomitant salt restriction, the patients on the diet were asked to increase their sodium intake; the 24-hour urinary sodium excretion in these patients turned out to be even higher than that of the control group.

This study is among the best published to document the antihypertensive efficacy of weight reduction; however, follow-up was for only two months, and the rate of recidivism among obese people is so high that few may receive long-term benefit. Certainly an attempt at weight reduction in obese hypertensive patients should be made, again, in a gentle and gradual manner. The discovery that they have hypertension may be a strong motivation for patients to reduce. A further incentive may be the knowledge that, if weight reduction succeeds in lowering blood pressure, the need for taking medications may be delayed or avoided. However, the physician should not rely on weight reduction alone to control hypertension.

ALCOHOL AND COFFEE

Moderate alcohol consumption, less than 2 ounces of ethanol per day, does not increase the prevalance of hypertension or exert any significant pressor effects.[37] Other than being a source of extra calories, moderate alcohol intake need not be prohibited, particularly since it may reduce coronary events,[38] perhaps by increasing the level of protective high-density lipoproteins.[39] Such protection from coronary disease was demonstrable in subjects who consumed a moderate amount of alcohol in a regular, consistent pattern but not among binge drinkers of similar amounts of alcohol.[40] Heavier drinking clearly increases the likelihood of hypertension.[37]

When consumed by noncoffee drinkers, the ingestion of caffeine equivalent to the amount in three cups of coffee will raise the blood pressure, probably by activation of the sympathetic nervous system.[41] Even in those who are accustomed to drinking coffee, a 5 to 10 mm Hg rise in blood pressure for one to two hours may occur.[41a]

EXERCISE

Isometric exercise such as weight-lifting, pushing, and pulling may be harmful to the hypertensive patient. During an isometric contraction, blood pressure rises often to very high levels by a reflex mechanism.[42] There are few controlled studies of the effect of isotonic exercise on blood pressure. Those that are available show a slight reduction in blood pressure,[43] but the effect may be related to the coincidental weight loss usually achieved.

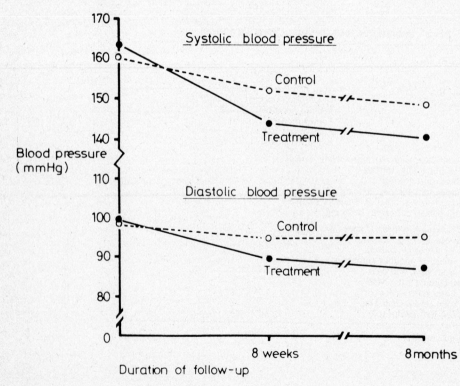

FIGURE 27-5 Average systolic and diastolic blood pressures in 99 hypertensives who received biofeedback-aided relaxation therapy (Treatment) and 97 who did not (Control) at 8 weeks (the completion of the active training) and at 8 months. (From Patel, C., et al.: Controlled trial of biofeedback-aided behavioural methods in reducing mild hypertension. Br. Med. J. *282*:2005, 1981.)

One of the better studies involved a group of 27 Chilean women who undertook three 30-minute sessions per week of calisthenics and jogging for three months, during which they reached 70 per cent of their maximal heart rate.[44] Average resting blood pressure fell from 181/113 to 161/97 mm Hg. Thereafter, they stopped exercising for three months, and their average blood pressure rose back to 179/113. When they resumed the exercise program, pressures fell again and remained lower for the next 24 months while they continued to exercise.

RELAXATION TECHNIQUES

Although relaxation of skeletal muscles has long been known to lower the blood pressure,[45] most studies have failed to show sustained effects of various types of relaxation therapies.[43] However, an impressive effect was observed by Patel et al.[46] They randomly assigned half of a group of newly identified hypertensives to a biofeedback-aided relaxation program for 8 weeks, while the other half served as controls, being seen as often but not given the relaxation therapy. Both at the end of the active program and six months later (during which time the subjects had been asked to continue to practice relaxation but had not been seen), blood pressures among the treated group were significantly lower (Fig. 27-5).

THE POTENTIAL OF NONDRUG THERAPY

Part of the antihypertensive effect reported with these and other nondrug therapies may be attributable to the nonspecific fall in blood pressure so often seen when repeated readings are taken.[6] Such decreases may reflect a statistical regression toward the mean, a placebo effect, or a relief of anxiety and stress with time. (The same phenomenon is probably also responsible for much of the initial response to drug therapy, so that success may be attributed to both drugs and nondrugs when it is deserved by neither.)

Few long-term studies of the effectiveness of nondrug therapies have been carried out. In one organized program, 67 obese hypertensive men were given nutritional advice about calories, fat, and sodium and were encouraged to exercise and to stop smoking, but they received no medications.[47] After five years, they had lost an average of 10 pounds, showed a mean decrease in blood pressure of 12/9 mm Hg, and had reduced their mean serum cholesterol level by 25 mg/dl.

Whether such success can be achieved by individual practitioners is uncertain. However, since help is available, including various educational materials for patients, professional assistants such as dietitians and psychologists, and groups organized for weight reduction, exercise, and relaxation therapies, the effort would appear to be worthwhile.

ANTIHYPERTENSIVE DRUG THERAPY

If the nondrug therapies outlined above are not followed or turn out to be ineffective, or if the level of hypertension at the outset is so significant that immediate drug therapy is deemed necessary, the general guidelines listed in Table 27-3 should be helpful in improving patient adherence to lifelong treatment. More detailed guidance is also available.[48]

GENERAL GUIDELINES

Most of the points listed in Table 27-3 are rather obvious, but a few deserve additional comment. Item 5d, "Use the fewest daily doses needed," has been shown to affect patient compliance.[49] Unfortunately, prescriptions for most antihypertensive drugs often call for more daily doses than are necessary. The recommended frequency of administration of many antihypertensive drugs has been based on their concentration in and disappearance from the blood. As a result, most manufacturers of antihypertensive drugs recommend that the drug be given three or four times a day. But these drugs work at various intracellular and membrane sites, and their concentration in the plasma may be largely irrelevant relative to their antihypertensive action.

Now that prolonged monitoring of blood pressure is technically feasible, the duration of antihypertensive effectiveness can be used as the basis for the timing of therapy. When this more appropriate basis is used, surprising results have been noted. In a study involving therapy with methyldopa, blood pressure was at least as well controlled by a single bedtime dose as when the same total dose was given in the traditional regimen of three times a day.[50] Similar results have been noted with twice-a-day therapy with clonidine,[51] propranolol,[52] and hydralazine.[53] In moderately

TABLE 27-3   GENERAL GUIDELINES TO IMPROVE PATIENT ADHERENCE TO ANTIHYPERTENSIVE THERAPY

1. Be aware of the problem of nonadherence and be alert to signs of patient noncompliance
2. Establish the goal of therapy: To reduce blood pressure to normotensive levels with minimal or no side effects
3. Educate the patient about the disease and its treatment
4. Maintain contact with the patient
   a. Encourage visits and calls to allied health personnel
   b. Use home blood pressure readings
   c. Allow the pharmacist to monitor therapy
   d. Make contact with patients who do not return
5. Keep care inexpensive and simple
   a. Do the least work-up needed to rule out secondary causes
   b. Obtain follow-up data from laboratory only yearly unless indicated more often
   c. Use nondrug, no-cost therapies
   d. Use the fewest daily doses needed
   e. If appropriate, use combination tablets
6. Prescribe according to pharmacological principles
   a. Add one drug at a time
   b. Start with small to medium doses, aiming for 5 to 10 mm Hg reductions at each stage
   c. Prevent volume overload with adequate diuretic and salt restriction
   d. Anticipate side effects
   e. Adjust doses or drugs to ameliorate significant side effects that do not disappear spontaneously
   f. Continue to add drugs, step-wise, in sufficient doses to achieve the goal of therapy

Modified from Kaplan, N. M.: Clinical Hypertension, 3rd ed. Baltimore, Williams and Wilkins Co., 1982.

large amounts, single doses of propranolol continue to be effective for 24 hours.[54] At present, most antihypertensive medications can be given to most patients either once a day (reserpine, guanethidine, nadolol, atenolol) or twice a day (clonidine, methyldopa, prazosin, propranolol, metoprolol, hydralazine). A few patients may be better controlled with more frequent doses.

PHARMACOLOGICAL PRINCIPLES. The second item under 6 in Table 27-3 suggests starting with small doses of medication, aiming for a reduction of 5 to 10 mm Hg in blood pressure at each step. Some physicians, by nature and training, desire to control a patient's hypertension rapidly and completely. However, regardless of which drugs are used, this approach often leads to easy fatigability, weakness, and postural dizziness or a feeling of being washed out, which many patients find intolerable, particularly when they felt well before therapy was begun. Although hypokalemia and other electrolyte abnormalities may be responsible for some of these symptoms, a more likely explanation has been provided by the studies of Strandgaard and coworkers.[55] As shown in the top half of Figure 27-6, they reconfirmed the constancy of cerebral blood flow by autoregulation over a range of mean arterial pressures from about 60 to 120 mm Hg in normal subjects and 110 to 180 mm Hg in patients with hypertension. This shift to the right protects the hypertensive patient from a

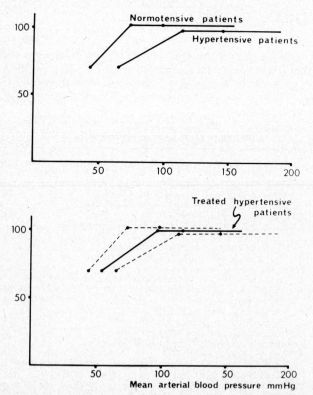

CEREBRAL BLOOD FLOW percent of rest

FIGURE 27-6 Idealized curves of cerebral blood flow showing the range of autoregulation in normotensive and hypertensive patients (upper graph) and the shift back toward normal after antihypertensive therapy (lower graph). The lower limit of autoregulation maintaining a normal cerebral blood flow is a mean arterial blood pressure of about 60 mm Hg in normotensive and 110 in hypertensive individuals. (From Strandgaard, S.: Autoregulation of cerebral blood flow in hypertensive patients. Circulation *53*:720, 1976, by permission of the American Heart Association, Inc.)

surge of blood flow, which could cause cerebral edema. However, the shift also predisposes the hypertensive patient to cerebral ischemia when blood pressure is lowered.

Note that the lower limit of autoregulation necessary to preserve a constant cerebral blood flow in hypertensive patients is about 110 mm Hg. Thus, acutely lowering the pressure from 160/110 (mean = 127) to 140/85 (mean = 102) may induce cerebral hypoperfusion, although hypotension in the accepted sense has not been produced. This provides an explanation for what many patients experience at the start of antihypertensive therapy, i.e., manifestations of cerebral hypoperfusion, even though blood pressure levels do not seem inordinately low.

These observations suggest the need for a gentle, gradual approach to antihypertensive therapy in order to avoid symptoms related to overly aggressive blood pressure reduction. Fortunately, as shown in the bottom half of Figure 27-6, if therapy is continued for a period of time, the curve of cerebral autoregulation does shift back toward normal, allowing patients to tolerate greater reductions in blood pressure without experiencing symptoms.

STEPPED CARE. The last item in Table 27-3 refers to the addition of drugs, stepwise, in sufficient doses to achieve the goal of therapy. Over the past 30 years the purely empirical basis for the use of antihypertensive drugs has gradually been replaced by a more rational and effective stepped-care approach,[56] which involves use of a diuretic initially followed by an adrenergic blocking drug and, if necessary, a vasodilator.

As pointed out earlier (p. 909), attempts have been made to provide a more scientific basis for selecting the drug that most closely fits a patient's hemodynamic disturbance.[57] This approach, based on the renin profile, divides hypertension into either a predominantly "volume" or a predominantly "vasoconstriction" mechanism and advocates the use of a diuretic initially in the former and a beta blocker initially in the latter. The concept is attractive, but, as detailed in Chapter 26, the actual measurements of volume and vasoconstriction do not uphold use of the plasma renin level as an appropriate index for these hemodynamic variables. As we have seen, almost all hypertension is related to increased peripheral resistance. Moreover, a single renin measurement cannot be considered a certain indication of a patient's long-term status. Therefore, the renin profile does not appear to offer a more rational guide to therapy.

As it has turned out, the stepped-care approach makes good scientific sense as well as providing effective therapy, and none who follows it need apologize for its empirical beginnings. Use of a diuretic first controls about half of all hypertensive patients with less expense and fewer side effects than any other regimen. Moreover, the diuretic enhances the effectiveness of whatever second drug is used, preventing the "pseudotolerance" that develops because of the fluid retention that frequently follows the use of all adrenergic blocking drugs and vasodilators.[58] In addition, supplemental use of a vasodilator as the third drug, required in about 10 per cent of patients whose hypertension is not controlled by a diuretic and adrenergic blocking drug, has been shown to be eminently sound on pharmacological grounds as well.[59] However, problems with diuretics continue to surface. These problems may explain the higher mortality rate observed in those with the mildest level of hypertension and with preexisting ECG abnormalities who were more intensively treated in the Multiple Risk Factor Intervention Trial (MRFIT).[59a] Therefore, the use of one or another adrenergic blocking drugs as an alternative to a diuretic as the first step in therapy may be appropriate.

Having considered the general guidelines, let us now examine each type of antihypertensive drug, starting with the one used first for most patients—a diuretic.

DIURETICS (See also pp. 527 to 534)

Diuretics useful in the treatment of hypertension may be divided into four major groups: (1) thiazides, (2) related sulfonamide compounds, (3) loop diuretics, and (4) potassium-sparing agents (Table 27-4).

MODE OF ACTION. All diuretics initially lower the blood pressure by increasing urinary sodium excretion and by reducing plasma volume, extracellular fluid volume, and cardiac output.[60] Within 6 to 8 weeks, the lowered plasma and extracellular fluid volumes are maintained but cardiac output returns to normal. At this point and beyond, the lower blood pressure is related to a fall in peripheral resistance, thereby correcting the underlying hemodynamic defect of hypertension.

The mechanism responsible for the lowered peripheral resistance is unknown. It occurs despite increased renin-aldosterone levels, resulting from a lower blood pressure and decreased plasma volume, as well as increased plasma norepinephrine levels.[61] On the other hand, plasma levels of the hydrolysis product of the vasodilator prostacyclin are elevated, both after 3 days and 10 weeks of thiazide therapy.[62] Even though the chronic effect of diuretics involves a fall in peripheral resistance, the need for an initial diuresis in the antihypertensive action of these drugs has been shown by their failure to lower the blood pressure in chronic dialysis patients with nonfunctioning kidneys.[63]

The diuretic-induced rise in renin secretion stimulates aldosterone, which retards the continued sodium diuresis. Both the renin-induced vasoconstriction and the aldosterone-induced sodium retention prevent continued diminution of body fluids and a fall in blood pressure while diuretic therapy is continued. The extent of decrease in blood pressure has been found to relate closely to the degree of secondary aldosterone excess: in patients treated with chlorthalidone whose pressures fell more than 10 per cent, aldosterone rose less than 10 per cent; in those whose pressures fell less, excretion of aldosterone almost doubled.[64]

CLINICAL EFFECTS. With continuous diuretic therapy, blood pressure usually falls about 15/10 mm Hg, although the degree depends upon various factors, including the initial height of the pressure, the amount of salt ingested, the adequacy of renal function, and the intensity of the counterregulatory renin-aldosterone response. The reduction of pressure may be much greater in more severe than in milder hypertension: in 227 hypertensive patients treated for up to 12 years with diuretics alone, mean blood pressure fell from 203/121 to 162/97, and in 50 per cent diastolic pressure was reduced to below 100 mm Hg and in another 35 per cent to below 110 mm Hg.[65] As shown in this study, the antihypertensive effect of the diuretic persists indefinitely, although it may be overwhelmed by dietary sodium intake above 15 to 20 grams per day.

If other drugs are needed, the diuretic should be continued. Without a concomitant diuretic, most other antihypertensive drugs will cause sodium retention. This mechanism probably reflects the success of the drugs in lowering pressure and may involve the abnormal renal pressure–natriuresis relationship in hypertension (see Fig. 26-15, p. 864). Just as it takes more pressure to excrete a given load of sodium in the hypertensive individual, so does a lowering of pressure to normal incite sodium retention. The hypertensive kidney is consistent: for normal sodium excretion, normal pressure is too low just as high pressure is adequate.

The critical need for adequate diuretic therapy to keep intravascular volume diminished has been repeatedly documented.[58] Therefore, diuretics will likely continue to be the foundation of antihypertensive therapy.

DOSAGE AND CHOICE OF AGENT. Most patients with mild to moderate hypertension and reasonably intact renal function, i.e., serum creatinine below 2.0 mg/dl, will

TABLE 27–4   DIURETICS USEFUL IN THE TREATMENT OF HYPERTENSION

	DAILY DOSE (MG)	DURATION OF ACTION (HR)
Thiazides		
Chlorothiazide (Diuril)	500 to 1000	6 to 12
Hydrochlorothiazide (Esidrix, HydroDiuril, Oretic)	25 to 200	12 to 18
Benzthiazide (Aquatag, Exna)	25 to 200	12 to 18
Hydroflumethiazide (Saluron)	25 to 50	18 to 24
Bendroflumethiazide (Naturetin)	5 to 20	More than 18
Methyclothiazide (Enduron)	2.5 to 10.0	More than 24
Trichlormethiazide (Metahydrin, Naqua)	2 to 4	More than 24
Polythiazide (Renese)	1 to 4	24 to 48
Cyclothiazide (Anhydron)	1 to 2	18 to 24
Related sulfonamide compounds		
Chlorthalidone (Hygroton)	25 to 100	24 to 72
Quinethazone (Hydromox)	50 to 200	18 to 24
Metolazone (Zaroxolyn)	1.0 to 10.0*	24
Loop diuretics		
Furosemide (Lasix)	40 to 120*	4 to 6
Ethacrynic acid (Edecrin)	50 to 400	12
Potassium-sparing diuretics		
Spironolactone (Aldactone)	25 to 100	8 to 12
Triamterene (Dyrenium)	100 to 300	12
Amiloride (Midamor)	5 to 10	24

*Larger doses may be useful in patients with renal insufficiency.

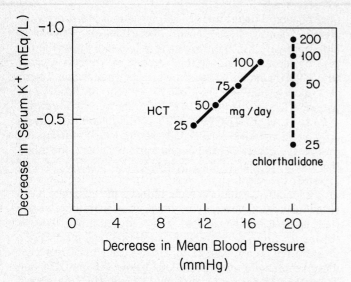

FIGURE 27-7 Effects of varying doses of hydrochlorothiazide (HCT) and chlorthalidone on the blood pressure and serum potassium in two groups of hypertensives. The different doses of chlorthalidone and HCT were given for 6- to 8-week periods in random order. (Data on HCT from Degnbol, B., et al.: The effect of different diuretics on elevated blood pressure and serum potassium. Acta Med. Scand. *193*:407, 1973; data on chlorthalidone from Tweeddale, M. G., et al.: Antihypertensive and biochemical effects of chlorthalidone. Clin. Pharmacol. Ther. *22*:519, 1977.)

respond to the lower doses of the various diuretics listed in Table 27-4, an amount equivalent to 25 mg of hydrochlorothiazide. Larger doses will have some additional antihypertensive effect but at the price of additional potassium wastage[66] (Fig. 27-7). With chlorthalidone, maximal antihypertensive effectiveness is achieved with 25 mg a day.[67] For uncomplicated hypertension, a moderately long-acting thiazide is a logical choice and a single morning dose of hydrochlorothiazide will provide a 24-hour antihypertensive effect.[68] When a short-acting drug (furosemide, 40 mg given twice daily) was compared to a longer acting drug (hydrochlorothiazide, 50 mg given twice daily), blood pressure was lowered significantly only with the longer acting drug.[69]

With renal insufficiency, manifested by a serum creatinine level above 2.5 mg/100 ml or creatinine clearance be-

low 25 ml/min, thiazides are usually not effective, and multiple doses of furosemide or a single dose of metolazone will be needed.[70]

SIDE EFFECTS (Fig. 27-8). A number of biochemical changes often accompany successful diuresis, including a decrease in plasma potassium and increases in uric acid and cholesterol.

Hypokalemia. Serum potassium falls an average of 0.6 mmol/liter after institution of continuous, daily diuretic therapy for hypertension.[71] Among 158 hypertensives given diuretics for two years, plasma potassium levels fell to between 3.0 and 3.3 mmol/liter in 29 per cent and to between 2.6 and 2.9 mmol/liter in 7 per cent.[72] Although this fall in serum concentration may not reflect a significant decrease in total body potassium,[73] it may precipitate potentially hazardous ventricular ectopic activity, even in patients not known to be susceptible because of concomitant digitalis therapy or myocardial irritability.[74] The arrhythmogenic effect of diuretic-induced hypokalemia may become manifest only at times of stress, when catecholamines may lower the plasma potassium level another 0.5 to 1.0 mMol/liter.[74a] Acute myocardial infarction is one such stress wherein a high frequency of ventricular arrhythmias has been noted in patients with diuretic-induced hypokalemia.[74b] The degree of diuretic-induced hypokalemia may diminish with time despite continued therapy.[75] This may reflect a decrease in the secretion of potassium after the higher initial rate of tubular fluid flow down the nephron, which sweeps more potassium into the urine.[76]

Most patients are unaware of mild diuretic-induced hypokalemia, although it may contribute to leg cramps, polyuria, and muscle weakness. But subtle interference with antihypertension therapy may accompany even mild hypokalemia; volume retention and a rise in plasma angiotensin are seen experimentally.[77] In addition to increasing the propensity to ventricular ectopic activity, hypokalemia may precipitate serious arrhythmias in patients receiving digitalis (see Chap. 16). The occasional loss of carbohydrate tolerance and the frequent rise in plasma lipids seen with diuretic use may reflect a suppression of insulin secretion by hypokalemia.

Prevention of hypokalemia is preferable to correction of

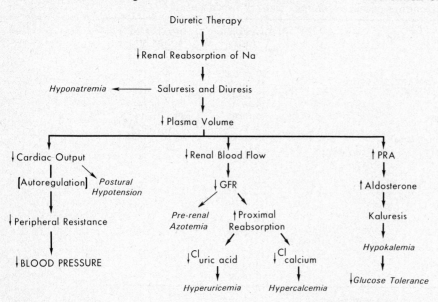

FIGURE 27-8 Desired antihypertensive action and various side effects of diuretics are shown to arise from the changes induced by a reduction in plasma volume.

potassium deficiency. The following maneuvers should help prevent diuretic-induced hypokalemia.

— Use the smallest amount of diuretic needed (Fig. 27–7).
— Use a moderately long-acting (12- to 18-hour) diuretic, since longer acting drugs (e.g., chlorthalidone) may increase potassium loss.[27]
— Restrict sodium intake to 60 to 100 mEq a day (i.e., 2 sodium).
— Increase dietary potassium intake.
— Restrict concomitant use of laxatives.
— Use a combination of a thiazide with a potassium-sparing agent. If the latter is prescribed, avoid supplemental potassium, since dangerous hyperkalemia may supervene if these drugs are given together.
— The concomitant use of a beta blocker may diminish potassium loss, presumably by blunting the diuretic-induced rise in renin-aldosterone, but hypokalemia may still occur with the combination.[78]

If hypokalemia is to be treated, the above maneuvers should be instituted along with some form of supplemental potassium. Potassium chloride is preferred for correction of the associated alkalosis. Despite the occasional appearance of mucosal lesions by gastroscopy after very large doses,[78a] a resin-matrix, slow-release tablet of KCl is both safe and effective, and most patients prefer it to liquid preparations. If tolerated, KCl can be given as a salt substitute; thereby, extra potassium will be provided at little expense while sodium intake is reduced.[79] Caution is necessary when supplemental KCl is given to older patients with borderline renal function in whom hyperkalemia may be induced.

In some patients, concomitant diuretic-induced magnesium deficiency will prevent the restoration of intracellular deficits of potassium[80] so that hypomagnesemia should be corrected.

Hyperuricemia. The serum uric acid level is elevated in as many as one-third of untreated hypertensive patients, particularly in those who are obese.[81] With chronic diuretic therapy, hyperuricemia appears in another third of patients, probably as a consequence of increased proximal tubular reabsorption accompanying volume contraction.[82] Even more marked hyperuricemia may develop when an adrenergic blocking drug is added to the diuretic.[81]

Diuretic-induced hyperuricemia only rarely precipitates acute gout or chronic nephropathy, but, based on observation of patients with idiopathic hyperuricemia, the potential for such complications remains. Assuming that urate excretion is diminished, patients with serum uric acid levels persistently above 10 mg/dl should probably be treated with a uricosuric drug such as probenecid. Although allopurinol is often used, it is more likely to cause side effects and seems a less rational choice, since the problem is a failure to excrete uric acid and not its overproduction.

Hyperlipidemia. Serum triglyceride and, to a lesser degree, serum cholesterol levels often rise after diuretic therapy.[18,83] Fortunately, the rise in lipids can be prevented by a "prudent" low-saturated fat diet.[84]

Hypercalcemia. A slight rise in serum calcium, less than 0.5 mg/dl, is frequently seen with effective diuretic therapy, at least in part because increased calcium reabsorption accompanies the increased sodium reabsorption in the proximal tubule induced by contraction

of extracellular fluid volume. The rise is of little clinical importance except in patients with previously unrecognized hyperparathyroidism, who may experience a much more marked rise.

Hyperglycemia. Diuretics may impair glucose tolerance[85] and rarely may precipitate diabetes, perhaps by direct suppression of insulin secretion from the diuretic-induced hypokalemia.

Other Problems. A surprisingly high rate of impotence (22.6 per cent) was found among men taking 10 mg a day of bendrofluazide, compared to a rate of 10.1 per cent among those on placebo and 13.2 per cent among those on propranolol in the large Medical Research Council (MRC) trial.[86] This high rate may reflect the rather large dose of diuretic, perhaps through hypokalemia. Although inhibitors of prostaglandin synthesis (e.g., indomethacin) will blunt the diuretic effect of loop diuretics, no such interference occurs with thiazides.[87]

OTHER DIURETICS

Loop Diuretics. As described in Chapter 26, loop diuretics are usually needed in the treatment of hypertensive patients with renal insufficiency, defined as a serum creatinine above 2.5 mg/dl. Furosemide has been most widely used, although metolazone may work as well and requires only a single daily dose.[70] Many use furosemide in the management of uncomplicated hypertension, but, as noted earlier, this drug seems to provide less antihypertensive effect when given once or twice a day than do longer acting diuretics.

Potassium-Sparing Agents. These drugs are not diuretics but are usually employed in combination with a diuretic. Of the three currently available, one (spironolactone) is an aldosterone antagonist, while the other two (dyrenium and amiloride) are direct inhibitors of potassium secretion. In combination with a thiazide diuretic, they will diminish the amount of potassium wasting; although they are more expensive than thiazides alone, they may decrease the total cost of therapy by reducing the need to monitor and treat potassium depletion.

Diuretics Under Investigation. Of a number of diuretics currently under investigation, most are similar to agents now available. Indapamide may also inhibit calcium entry.[88]

AN OVERVIEW OF DIURETICS IN HYPERTENSION

Diuretics have been effective for the treatment of millions of hypertensive patients during the past 25 years. They will reduce diastolic pressure and maintain it below 90 mm Hg in about half of all hypertensive patients, providing the same degree of effectiveness as beta blockers and most other antihypertensive drugs.[89] In two groups that constitute a rather large portion of the hypertensive population, the elderly[90] and blacks,[91] diuretics alone are more effective than beta blockers. One diuretic tablet per day is usually all that is needed, minimizing cost and maximizing adherence to therapy.

The side effects of diuretic therapy are usually benign and, except for the potential hazards of hypokalemia, are of little clinical significance. Patients tolerate them better than[92] or as well as[86] the other drugs: in the large MRC trial in which patients were randomly given either a diuretic or a beta blocker, the percentage of patients who withdrew from therapy because of side effects during the first two years was almost identical for the two drugs.[86]

Some investigators view the hemodynamic changes induced by diuretic therapy as hazards.[57] However, objective evidence does not support the potential vasculotoxic effects of diuretic-induced increases in plasma renin activity.[93] Unless the patient undergoes excessive diuresis and is dehydrated, the hemodynamic changes incurred with chronic diuretic therapy are exactly what is needed, i.e., little, if any, fall in cardiac output and a reduction in peripheral and renal vascular resistance.[60] Thus the recommendation that a diuretic be the first drug in the therapy of virtually all hypertensive patients seemed logical.[56] However, the disquieting evidence that diuretics may be associated with additional risks for coronary disease[59a] has led to the idea that adrenergic blocking drugs be considered as initial therapy.[59b] If an adrenergic blocking drug is chosen for initial therapy, a tendency for volume retention should be recognized and moderate sodium restriction strongly encouraged. If fluid retention occurs or the blood pressure is inadequately controlled, the addition or substitution of a diuretic should be considered.

ADRENERGIC BLOCKING DRUGS

A number of adrenergic blocking drugs are available including some that act centrally upon vasomotor center activity, peripherally upon neuronal catecholamine discharge, or by blocking alpha and/or beta receptors (Table 27–5); some act at multiple sites. Figure 27–9, a schematic view of the ending of an adrenergic nerve and the effector cell with its receptors, depicts how some of these drugs act. When the nerve is stimulated, norepinephrine, which is synthesized and stored in granules, is released into the synaptic cleft. It binds to postsynaptic alpha and beta receptors and thereby initiates various intracellular processes. In the vascular smooth muscle, alpha stimulation causes constriction and beta stimulation causes relaxation. In the central vasomotor centers, sympathetic outflow is inhibited

TABLE 27–5 ADRENERGIC BLOCKERS

Drugs that Act Within the Neuron
 Reserpine
 Guanethidine (Ismelin)
 Bethanidine (Tenathan)
 Debrisoquine
Drugs that Act Upon Receptors
 Predominantly Central Agonists
  Methyldopa (Aldomet)
  Clonidine (Catapres)
  Guanabenz (Wytensin)
  Lofexidine
 Predominantly Peripheral Antagonists
 Alpha
  Pre- and postsynaptic:
   Phenoxybenzamine (Dibenzyline)
   Phentolamine (Regitine)
  Postsynaptic: Prazosin (Minipress)
 Beta
  Atenolol (Tenormin)
  Metoprolol (Lopressor)
  Nadolol (Corgard)
  Pindolol (Visken)
  Propranolol (Inderal)
  Timolol (Blocadren)
  Acebutolol, sotalol, etc.
 Alpha and Beta: Labetolol

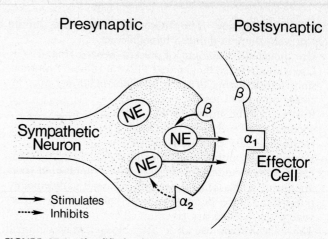

FIGURE 27-9 Simplified schematic view of the adrenergic nerve ending showing that norepinephrine (NE) is released from its storage granules when the nerve is stimulated and enters the synaptic cleft to bind to alpha$_1$ and beta receptors on the effector cell (postsynaptic). In addition, a short feedback loop exists, in which NE binds to alpha$_2$ and beta receptors on the neuron (presynaptic), either to inhibit or to stimulate further release.

by alpha stimulation; the effect of beta stimulation is unknown.

An important aspect of sympathetic activity involves the feedback of norepinephrine to alpha and beta receptors located on the neuronal surface, i.e., presynaptic receptor.[94] Presynaptic alpha-receptor activation inhibits further norepinephrine release, whereas presynaptic beta-receptor activation stimulates further norepinephrine release. These presynaptic receptors probably play a role in the action of some of the drugs to be discussed.

Elucidation and quantitation of the various actions of these drugs remain incomplete. The listing in Table 27–5 is based upon the predominant site of action according to currently available data. The beta-adrenergic receptor blockers almost certainly act upon central vasomotor mechanisms, but most of their effect probably depends on peripheral actions.

Drugs That Act Within the Neuron

Reserpine, guanethidine, and related compounds act to inhibit the release of norepinephrine from peripheral adrenergic neurons, each in a different manner, totally unlike the feedback suppression of norepinephrine release that may be involved in the effects of the alpha-agonists methyldopa, clonidine, and guanabenz.

RESERPINE. Reserpine, the most active and widely used of the derivatives of the rauwolfia alkaloids, depletes the postganglionic adrenergic neurons of norepinephrine by inhibiting its uptake into storage vesicles, exposing it to degradation by cytoplasmic monoamine oxidase. The peripheral effect is predominant, although the drug enters the brain and depletes central catecholamine stores as well. This probably accounts for the sedation and depression seen with reserpine use.

The drug has certain advantages; only one dose a day is needed; in combination with a diuretic, the antihypertensive effect is significant, with a mean decrease in diastolic pressure of 16.7 mm Hg noted in one study[95] and an effect equal to or greater than that noted with methyldopa or propranolol in another;[96] little postural hypotension is noted; and many patients experience no side effects. The drug has a flat dose-response curve, so that a dose of only 0.05 mg a day will give almost as much antihypertensive effect as 0.125 or 0.25 mg a day but fewer side effects.[97]

The psychological depression that occurs in perhaps 2 per cent of patients may be severe but difficult to recognize and treat. The specter of breast cancer associated with reserpine raised in 1974 has not been substantiated.[98] Although it remains popular in some places, the use of reserpine has declined progressively.

GUANETHIDINE. Guanethidine and a series of related guanidine compounds, including bethanidine and debrisoquine, act by inhibiting the release of norepinephrine from the adrenergic neurons, perhaps by a local anesthetic-like effect on the neuronal membrane. In order to act, the drug must be actively transported into the nerve through an amine pump. Various drugs, in particular tricyclic antidepressants, amphetamines, and ephedrine, will competitively block the uptake of guanethidine into the nerves and thereby antagonize its effects.

Its low lipid solubility prevents guanethidine from entering the brain, so that sedation, depression, and other side effects on the central nervous system are not seen. Initially, the predominant hemodynamic effect is to decrease cardiac output; after continued use, peripheral resistance declines. Blood pressure is reduced further when the patient is upright, owing to gravitational pooling of blood in the legs, since compensatory sympathetic nervous system-mediated vasoconstriction is blocked. This results in the most common side effect, postural hypotension. Patients should be advised to arise slowly, sleep with the head of the bed elevated, and wear elastic hose to minimize this potential problem.

Unlike reserpine, guanethidine has a steep dose-response curve, so that it can be successfully used in treating hypertension of any degree in daily doses of 10 to 300 mg. Like reserpine, it has a long biological half-life and may be given once daily. As other drugs have become available, guanethidine has been relegated mainly to the treatment of severe hypertension. Now that the combination of beta blockers and vasodilator drugs has become the most widely prescribed treatment for severe hypertension, the use of guanethidine will probably decline further.

Bethanidine and debrisoquine are similar to guanethidine but have a shorter duration of action and, perhaps, fewer side effects.[99]

Drugs That Act Upon Receptors

PREDOMINANTLY CENTRAL AGONISTS

METHYLDOPA (ALDOMET). Since the late 1960's, methyldopa had been the most widely used of the adrenergic blockers, but its use has fallen off as beta blockers have become more popular. At first it was thought that methyldopa entered the catecholamine biosynthetic pathway by inhibiting dopa-decarboxylase. Later it was believed to act by inducing the synthesis of alpha-methylnorepinephrine in peripheral sympathetic nerves, which would serve as a weak or false neurotransmitter. Finally, the primary site of action has been found to be within the central nervous system, where alpha-methylnorepinephrine is released from adrenergic neurons and stimulates central alpha receptors, reducing the sympathetic outflow from the central nervous system.[100]

The blood pressure falls mainly from a decrease in peripheral resistance with little effect upon cardiac output. However, as is true with all adrenergic blockers, patients with borderline cardiac function may be thrown into congestive failure by removal of adrenergic support. On the other hand, when 10 hypertensives were treated with methyldopa, the degree of left ventricular hypertrophy as seen by echocardiography was reduced in four patients within 12 weeks, although blood pressure was not significantly altered.[101] Renal blood flow is well maintained, and significant postural hypotension is unusual. Therefore, the drug has been widely used in hypertensive patients with renal insufficiency or cerebral vascular disease; smaller doses are needed in the presence of renal insufficiency. Renin levels usually decrease, but the reduction in blood pressure is dependent neither upon initially high plasma renin activity nor upon a subsequent fall in this level.

On the basis of pharmacokinetic data, the drug has been prescribed in three or four doses a day. However, it need be given no more than twice daily.[50] The dosage range is from 250 to 3000 mg a day, with most patients responding to 750 to 1500 mg. As in the case of the other adrenergic blockers and peripheral vasodilators, methyldopa is best used in combination with a diuretic.

Side effects include some that are common to centrally acting drugs that reduce sympathetic outflow: sedation, dry mouth, orthostatic hypotension, impotence, and galactorrhea. However, methyldopa causes some unique side effects that are probably of an autoimmune nature, since a positive antinuclear antibody test is seen in about 10 per cent of patients who take the drug, a positive Coombs' test in about 25 per cent, and abnormal liver function tests in about 8 per cent. Less commonly, these laboratory abnormalities presage serious trouble: myocarditis;[102] hemolytic anemia in about 0.2 per cent; and acute hepatitis or chronic hepatic injury,[103] which may be related to the binding of a reactive metabolite with liver cell macromolecules.[104]

CLONIDINE (CATAPRES). Although they differ in structure, clonidine shares many features with methyldopa: it most likely acts in the same central sites, has similar antihypertensive efficacy, and causes many of the same bothersome but less serious side effects (e.g., sedation, dry mouth) but does not induce the autoimmune side effects.

This imidazoline derivative acts as an alpha-adrenergic receptor agonist and lowers blood pressure by stimulating the postsynaptic alpha receptors in the vasomotor centers of the brain.[100] Sympathetic outflow from the brain is thereby reduced, resulting in a decrease in basal heart rate and cardiac output and a fall in peripheral resistance. Since the baroreceptor reflex is left intact, blood pressure responds appropriately to upright posture and exercise, so that hypotension is rarely a problem. Renal blood flow is well maintained, and renin secretion is reduced. The decrease in renin is not necessary for the decrease in blood pressure but may be responsible for an immediate effect in patients with high renin levels.[105]

As an alpha-receptor agonist, the drug also acts upon presynaptic alpha receptors and inhibits norepinephrine release (Fig. 27-9), and plasma catecholamine levels fall.[106] The drug has a fairly short biological half-life, so that when it is discontinued, the inhibition of norepinephrine release disappears within about 12 to 18 hours, and plasma catecholamine levels rise. This is probably responsible for a rapid rebound of the blood pressure to pretreatment levels and the occasional appearance of withdrawal symptoms, including tachycardia, restlessness, and sweating. Rarely, the blood pressure increases beyond the pretreatment level. Similar overshoots have been reported after the discontinuation of a variety of other antihypertensives,[107] including methyldopa, but since that drug has a longer biological half-life, the blood pressure does not usually rise until about 48 hours later and then more gradually. If the rebound requires treatment, clonidine may be reintroduced or alpha-receptor antagonists may be given.

By itself, clonidine will often induce fluid retention, so that it should generally be used with a diuretic and be given in two doses a day. After control has been achieved with two daily doses of clonidine and a diuretic, it may be maintained with a single bedtime dose.

GUANABENZ. This drug differs in structure but shares many characteristics with both methyldopa and clonidine, acting primarily as a central alpha-agonist. However, it may differ in *not* causing reactive fluid retention,[108] so that it may turn out to be effective without the need for a concomitant diuretic.

LOFEXIDINE AND GUANFACINE. These drugs, similar to clonidine, are under clinical investigation.[109,109a]

Predominantly Peripheral Antagonists

ALPHA-RECEPTOR ANTAGONISTS. Prior to 1977, the only alpha blockers used to treat hypertension were *phenoxybenzamine* (Dibenzyline) and *phentolamine* (Regitine). These drugs are effective in acutely lowering blood pressure, but their effects are offset by an accompanying increase in cardiac output, and side effects are frequent and bothersome. Their limited effect may reflect their blockade of presynaptic alpha receptors, which interferes with the feedback inhibition of norepinephrine release (Fig. 27–9). Increased catecholamine release would then blunt the action on postsynaptic alpha receptors. Their use has largely been limited to the treatment of patients with pheochromocytoma.

Prazosin (Minipress) is a selective antagonist of the postsynaptic alpha receptors. Although this drug was introduced as a peripheral vasodilator, subsequent study has clearly shown its primary effect to be that of a postsynaptic alpha blocker.[110] By blocking alpha-mediated vasoconstriction, prazosin induces a fall in peripheral resistance. Since the presynaptic alpha receptor is left unblocked, the feedback loop for the inhibition of norepinephrine release is intact, an action which is almost certainly responsible for the greater antihypertensive effect of the drug and the absence of concomitant tachycardia, tolerance, and renin release. The inhibition of norepinephrine release may also account for the propensity toward postural hypotension. However, this is noted mainly with the first dose, and a greater initial effect on receptors in the veins, leading to an abrupt loss of sympathetic venous tone with venous pooling, has been invoked to explain this first-dose hypotension.[111] This problem can be mitigated by limiting the first dose to 0.5 mg to 1.0 mg.

Prazosin is about as effective as methyldopa and is similarly aided by concomitant use of a diuretic. It can be safely and effectively used in patients with renal insufficiency. The addition of small doses of prazosin has been found to be particularly effective in the management of severe hypertension refractory to other medications.[112] The ability of the drug to dilate the venous capacitance bed and reduce preload while also lowering systemic resistance has prompted its successful use in the treatment of severe congestive heart failure[113] (see Chap. 16).

Side effects, beyond first-dose hypotension, include persistent postural hypotension, dizziness, weakness, fatigue, and headaches. However, most patients find the drug easy to take, with little (if any) sedation, dry mouth, or impotence.

BETA-RECEPTOR ANTAGONISTS (see also pp. 1349–1350). In the past few years, beta blockers have been used increasingly, becoming the most popular form of antihypertensive therapy, after diuretics. Their popularity reflects their relative effectiveness and freedom from bothersome side effects. However, they are no more effective in lowering blood pressure than are other adrenergic blocking agents such as reserpine,[95] and side effects occur in up to 25 per cent of hypertensive patients who take them.[14] Some of these side effects, including bradycardia, bronchospasm, and peripheral vasospasm, may be quite bothersome. However, for the majority of patients who do not develop such side effects, beta blockers are usually easier to take than are other adrenergic blocking drugs, since somnolence, dry mouth, and impotence are rarely encountered. Moreover, more cardioselective beta blockers are now available, and their use will reduce, although not eliminate, some of the serious side effects.[114]

Beta blockers may have an important advantage over other antihypertensives, i.e., protection from coronary disease and the risk of angina, myocardial infarction, and sudden death. Such protection has been shown in patients, both hypertensive and normotensive, after an initial myocardial infarction with a variety of beta blockers (see Chap. 38). However, no data are available regarding the prevention of initial episodes of coronary disease, except for the results of the HDFP and Australian trials described earlier in this chapter, which involved a variety of antihypertensive drugs. Beta blockers may provide protection beyond their antihypertensive effects: their antianginal and antiarrhythmic actions are well documented, and they inhibit both the aggregation of platelets and their synthesis of the vasoconstrictor thromboxane.[115] Whether or not beta blockers provide clinically important primary cardioprotection, they can be used for their known antihypertensive effects, with the possibility of protection from coronary events viewed as a bonus—greatly desired but not yet proved.

The Variety of Beta Blockers. The beta blockers now being used in the United States are listed in Table 39–5 (p. 1350). Among the first to be widely used was practolol, which has since been withdrawn because it resulted in an oculomucocutaneous syndrome that caused blindness and peritoneal fibrosis. This reaction appears to be a hypersensitivity response[116] and may be unique to practolol, the only beta blocker to possess an acetanilid side chain. Similar reactions to the other beta blockers have been extremely unusual.

Propranolol was first used in the treatment of hypertension in 1964, and as many as 15 beta blockers are now available in some European countries. Pharmacologically, these beta blockers differ considerably with respect to degree of absorption, protein binding, and bioavailability. But the three most important differences affecting their clinical use are cardioselectivity, intrinsic sympathomimetic activity, and lipid solubility. Despite all these differences, they all seem to be effective antihypertensives, and about equally so.[117]

Cardioselectivity. As seen in Table 39–5 (p. 1350), atenolol and metoprolol are relatively cardioselective, having a greater blocking effect on the beta$_1$-receptors in the heart than on the beta$_2$-receptors in the bronchi, peripheral blood vessels, and elsewhere. Such cardioselectivity can be easily shown using small doses in acute studies; with the rather high doses used to treat hypertension, part of this effect is lost. Nonetheless, atenolol and metoprolol cause less clinically bothersome beta$_2$-mediated side effects.[114] Two randomized crossover trials demonstrate the advantages: the rise in plasma triglyceride and fall in HDL-cholesterol levels were less with atenolol and metoprolol than with propranolol[118]; metoprolol did not impair glucose metabolism in noninsulin-dependent diabetes but propranolol did.[119]

Intrinsic Sympathomimetic Activity (ISA). Pindolol has the greatest ISA, interacting with beta receptors to cause a measurable agonist response, but at the same time, blocking the greater agonist effects of endogenous catecholamines. As a result, while in usual doses pindolol lowers the blood pressure to about the same degree as other beta blockers, it causes a smaller decline in heart rate, cardiac output, and renin levels.[120] However, with higher doses, less antihypertensive effect and even a paradoxical rise in blood pressure may be noted, presumably because of the considerable agonist effect. Although the clinical relevance of this difference remains to be proved, a drug with high ISA may prove useful when a beta blocker is needed for patients in whom bradycardia or peripheral vascular disease is a problem.

Lipid Solubility. Atenolol and nadolol are the least lipid-soluble of the beta blockers listed in Table 39–5 (p. 1350). This translates into some clinically important advantages: (1) because they are not taken up and metabolized in the liver, they reach and maintain stable plasma concentrations quickly, requiring fewer dose titrations; (2) since they escape hepatic inactivation, they remain as active drugs in the plasma much longer, allowing once-a-day dosage; and (3) because they do not enter the brain as readily, they may cause fewer central nervous system (CNS) side effects. When 33 patients who experienced such side effects (depression, insomnia, nightmares) while on propranolol were switched to atenolol, the symptoms were relieved in 24.[121] On the other hand, since these drugs are removed mainly through renal excretion, high blood levels may accumulate in patients with renal insufficiency.

Mode of Action. Despite these and other differences, the various beta blockers now available seem about equipotent as antihypertensive agents.[117] How they lower the blood pressure remains uncertain, although a number of possible mechanisms are likely to be involved (Fig. 27–10). Cardiac output falls 15 to 20 per cent, renin release is reduced about 60 per cent, and central nervous beta-adrenergic blockade may reduce sympathetic discharge. Recall, too, that blockade of presynaptic beta receptors should in-

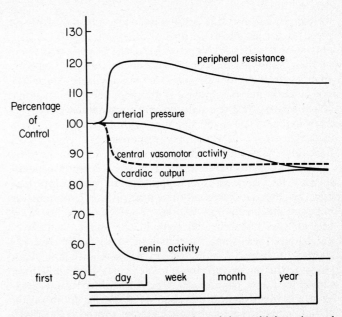

FIGURE 27-10 Schematic representation of the multiple actions of beta-blocker therapy over variable periods of time. The solid lines have been measured; the dotted line of central vasomotor activity has not. (Adapted from Birkenhager, W. H., et al.: Therapeutic effects of β-adrenoceptor blocking agents in hypertension. *In* Frick, P., et al.: Advances in Internal Medicine and Pediatrics. No. 39. Berlin, Springer-Verlag, 1977, pp. 117–134.)

hibit catechol release (Fig. 27–9). Although propranolol decreases plasma clearance of norepinephrine and thereby raises plasma norepinephrine levels,[122] no obvious inhibition of sympathetic nervous function has been demonstrable.[123] On the other hand, in rats, propranolol antagonizes the enhancement of sympathetic nerve transmission by angiotensin II, apparently through the release of prostaglandins.[124] Other CNS effects may also be involved; again in rats, brain serotonergic activity was reduced after treatment with metoprolol.[125]

At the same time that beta blockers are lowering blood pressure through various means, their blockade of peripheral beta receptors inhibits vasodilation, leaving alpha receptors open to catechol-mediated vasoconstriction. As a result, peripheral resistance rises and stays up.[126] Although evidence for a parallel decrease in alpha-mediated vasoconstriction has been found,[127] a decrease in peripheral blood flow is a common problem with beta-blocker therapy in cold climates.

Clinical Effects. Even in small doses, beta blockers begin to lower the blood pressure within a few hours, although their maximal effect may not be noted for some weeks.[128] Even though progressively higher doses have usually been given, careful study has shown a near-maximal effect from smaller doses: in a double-blind crossover study involving 24 patients, 40 mg of propranolol twice a day provided the same antihypertensive effects as 80, 160, or 240 mg twice a day.[129] The degree of blood pressure reduction is at least comparable to that noted with other antihypertensive drugs. By itself, a beta blocker will lower the diastolic blood pressure to below 90 mm Hg in about half the patients with mild to moderate hypertension; when combined with a diuretic, the percentage rises to about 80 per cent.[95] Duration of action is well beyond the drug's plasma half-life. With propranolol, which has a 3-

to 6-hour half-life, the antihypertensive effect of 240 mg given once daily persisted for up to 28 hours.[54]

One of the attractions of these drugs is the consistency of their antihypertensive action, which is altered little by changes in activity, posture, or temperature. Since the sympathetic nervous system is blocked, the hemodynamic responses to stress are reduced, but most patients can perform ordinary physical activities without difficulty. With maximal stress, however, the response may be blunted, probably enough to interfere with athletic performance.[130]

Beta blockers have been proposed as initial monotherapy for most cases of hypertension.[131] This approach may be effective for many younger, white hypertensives but may not be suitable for the majority of older or black patients. As noted before, both blacks and patients over age 50 have been found to respond less well to beta-blocker monotherapy.[90,91] Moreover, in patients with low renin levels at the outset, propranolol alone has sometimes been shown to induce paradoxical *hypertension*.[132] This unexpected rise in blood pressure probably reflects the combination of fluid retention and alpha-adrenergic–mediated peripheral and renal vasoconstriction that occurs in the face of blockade of beta$_2$-receptors in the vascular bed. In patients with normal or high renin, the inhibition of renin by propranolol probably counteracts both these antagonistic actions. If beta-blocker therapy is given with a diuretic, the potential problems of fluid retention and paradoxical hypertension will be avoided without the need to determine a patient's renin status.

Special Uses for Beta Blockers

Coexisting Coronary Disease. Even without proof that beta blockers protect patients from initial coronary events, the antiarrhythmic and antianginal effects of the drug make them especially valuable in hypertensive patients with coexisting coronary disease.

Patients Needing Antihypertensive Vasodilator Therapy. If a diuretic and an adrenergic blocker are inadequate to control blood pressure, the addition of a vasodilator is a logical third step. When used alone, vasodilators induce reflex sympathetic stimulation of the heart. The simultaneous use of beta blockers prevents this undesirable increase in cardiac output, which not only bothers the patient but also dampens the antihypertensive effect of the vasodilator.

Patients With Hyperkinetic Hypertension. Some hypertensive patients have increased cardiac output that may persist for many years. Beta blockers should be particularly effective in such patients, but a reduction in exercise capacity may restrict their use in young athletes.[130]

Patients With Marked Anxiety. The somatic manifestations of anxiety—tremor, sweating, and tachycardia—can be helped. In one controlled study, the performance of 24 musicians was found to improve when they took 40 mg of oxprenolol before the concert.[133] The undesirable effects of methods commonly used to control anxiety, i.e., alcohol and tranquilizers, were not observed.

Patients Taking Tricyclic Antidepressants and Antipsychotic Agents. The effects of guanethidine, clonidine, and other adrenergic neuronal blocking drugs may be blunted by these agents; beta blockers should not be affected. Moreover, they may counteract the tachycardia and ar-

rhythmias sometimes seen with the tricyclics (see Chap. 56). Sedation and depression rarely develop as side effects of beta blockers and other central nervous system problems are rare except with very high doses.

Patients in Whom Diuretics are Contraindicated. Diuretics can exacerbate diabetes and gout. Although these problems can be managed, use of a beta blocker without a diuretic is rational and will likely be effective. As previously described, fluid retention and a subsequent loss of antihypertensive efficacy less commonly follow betablocker therapy than they do therapy with other nondiuretic antihypertensive drugs.

Side Effects. Most of the side effects of beta blockers relate to their major pharmacological action, the blockade of beta receptors. Those which are less cardioselective are likely to cause more of the beta$_2$-mediated side effects. The experience of a group of English clinicians in treating a large number of hypertensives with either a nonselective drug (propranolol) or a more selective one (atenolol) documents this difference[114] (Table 27–6). With propranolol, 9.7 per cent of patients had to discontinue the drug, whereas with atenolol, only 2.2 per cent had to discontinue its use.

If patients with preexisting bronchospasm are excluded, the most common problem is peripheral vasospasm. Fatigue likely reflects the decrease in cerebral blood flow that may accompany successful lowering of the blood pressure by any drug[55] (see Figure 27–6). More direct effects on the central nervous system—depression, insomnia, bad dreams, and hallucinations—occur in some patients. Of all the side effects, these are most dose-dependent. The remainder are likely to develop, if at all, with small doses and do not tend to increase in frequency with higher doses, presumably because smaller doses provide as much beta blockade as will occur in most tissues. The more frequent side effects of other adrenergic blocking drugs—sedation, depression, dry mouth, impotence, and postural hypotension—are very rare. Thus, if patients escape the rather serious side effects, they are likely to tolerate the drugs well, and most prefer these to all others.[128]

The reduction in cardiac output, one of the pharmacological effects of beta blockers, might be expected to induce *congestive heart failure* rather frequently. However, with the reduction in arterial pressure the demands upon

TABLE 27–6   ADVERSE EFFECTS WITH PROPRANOLOL
(390 PATIENTS, 10 YEARS) AND ATENOLOL (543 PATIENTS, 4 YEARS)

	PERCENTAGE OF PATIENTS	
	Propranolol	*Atenolol*
Heart failure	0.8	0.4
Peripheral vascular disturbances:		
Cold extremities	2.5	2.8
Worsening claudication	2.8	1.3
Bronchospasm	5.1	3.3
Central nervous system disturbances:		
Vivid dreams, hallucinations	2.5	0.9
Dizziness, ataxia	0.4	1.1
Depression	0.8	0.7
Fatigue	3.9	3.9
Impotence	0.2	0.2
Total adverse effects	24.1	16.9

From Zacharias et al.: Atenolol in hypertension: A study of long-term therapy. Postgrad. Med. J. *53* (Suppl. 3):102, 1977.

the heart are lowered even more, so that failure was noted in only 0.8 per cent of Zacharias' patients during their 10 years on propranolol (Table 27–6), a number below that expected in patients with hypertension for this length of time.

Diabetics may have additional problems with nonselective beta blockers such as propranolol. The responses to hypoglycemia, both the symptoms and the counterregulatory hormonal changes that raise blood sugar levels, are partially dependent upon sympathetic nervous activity. Diabetics susceptible to hypoglycemia may have more serious reactions when taking propranolol. However, the majority of more stable diabetics can take the drug without difficulty, while the more cardioselective beta blockers, such as metoprolol, are preferable for diabetics with more brittle disease.[119]

When propranolol is discontinued suddenly, *angina pectoris* may appear for the first time or, if present previously, may be intensified (p. 1350).[134] Patients with hypertension are more susceptible to coronary disease, so they should be weaned gradually. Blood pressure may also rebound to high levels.[107] These effects may reflect a state of supersensitivity or an increase in the number of beta receptors induced during the prior beta blockade, leading to augmented responsiveness to normal levels of endogenous catecholamines. The withdrawal syndrome can be prevented by use of a small dose (30 mg a day) for 2 weeks before complete withdrawal.[135] If patients require immediate cessation of oral therapy, they can be protected by continuous propranolol infusion.[136]

Patients with *renal insufficiency* may take beta blockers without additional hazard, although a 20 per cent fall in renal blood flow and glomerular filtration rate has been measured with noncardioselective beta blockers, presumably from beta$_2$-mediated renal vasoconstriction.[137] Dosage of the lipid-insoluble atenolol and nadolol should be reduced in patients with renal insufficiency.

Caution is advised in patients suspected of having *pheochromocytoma*, since unopposed alpha-adrenergic action may precipitate a serious hypertensive crisis if this disease is present. The use of beta blockers during *pregnancy* has been beclouded by scattered case reports of various fetal problems. However, two prospective studies found that the use of beta blockers to treat hypertension during pregnancy did not lead to an increase in fetal morbidity.[138,139]

Perturbations of *lipoprotein metabolism* may accompany the use of beta blockers. After 8 weeks of propranolol therapy, serum HDL-cholesterol was reduced by 13 per cent and total triglycerides increased by 24 per cent.[140] Less marked changes were noted with the cardioselective agents atenolol and metoprolol than with propranolol.[118]

Impotence has been reported only rarely. In the large MRC trial, the frequency of impotence, as determined by questionnaire, was 10.1 per cent among those on placebo and 13.2 per cent among those on propranolol.[86]

The metabolism and bioavailability of beta blockers—particularly the lipid-soluble ones, such as propranolol, which are metabolized in the liver—may be affected by various factors that alter liver blood flow and enzymatic activity. As examples, decreases in hepatic extraction and/or metabolism, leading to higher blood levels of propranolol, have been reported with concomitant cimetidine therapy[141]; increases in liver metabolism, leading to lower

blood levels of active drug, have been found after consumption of alcohol.[142] Moreover, some people (about 10 per cent of those tested in England) have a genetically determined deficiency in drug oxidation, which leads to unusually high concentrations of lipid-soluble beta blockers and may be responsible for a greater propensity to develop side effects when usual doses are given.[143]

An Overview of Beta Blockers in Hypertension. Beta blockers will likely continue to be the most popular of the adrenergic inhibitors in the treatment of hypertension. They may be particularly effective in those with high-renin states, such as renovascular hypertension. In some with ordinary hypertension, they may be effective when used alone. If a beta blocker is chosen, a more cardioselective, lipid-insoluble one (see Table 39–5, p. 1350) offers the likelihood of greater patient adherence to therapy, since only one dose a day will be needed and side effects will likely be minimized.

ALPHA- AND BETA-RECEPTOR ANTAGONISTS. The combination of an alpha and a beta blocker may often prove to be effective for patients resistant to one drug alone. There are promising reports of a drug, labetolol, which combines both alpha- and beta-blocking actions, in a ratio of approximately 1:3. The fall in pressure results mainly from a decrease in peripheral resistance, with little or no fall in cardiac output.[144] Side effects have been minimal, although 9 of 47 patients developed a positive antinuclear factor. Intravenous labetolol has been used successfully to treat hypertensive emergencies, particularly those resulting from catecholamine excess.[145]

VASODILATORS

If a diuretic and adrenergic blocker do not control the blood pressure, a peripheral vasodilator is an appropriate third drug. Hydralazine (Apresoline) is the only agent of this type now available for routine use. Minoxidil is even more potent but is usually reserved for patients with severe, refractory hypertension associated with renal insufficiency. Diazoxide and nitroprusside are given intravenously for hypertensive crises and will be discussed at the end of this chapter.

HYDRALAZINE. First introduced in 1953, hydralazine has regained popularity since it was recognized that beta blockers could be used to prevent its side effects and enhance its efficacy[59] (Fig. 27–11). Since the early 1970's, hydralazine in combination with a diuretic and a beta blocker has been used increasingly to treat more severe hypertension. The drug acts directly to relax the smooth muscle in precapillary resistance vessels with little or no effect on postcapillary venous capacitance vessels. As a result, blood pressure falls but, in doing so, a number of reactive processes are activated that blunt the decrease in pressure and cause side effects. However, when a diuretic is used to overcome the tendency for fluid retention and a beta blocker is used to prevent the reflex increase in sympathetic activity and rise in renin, the vasodilator is more effective and causes few, if any, side effects (Fig. 27–12).

The drug need be given only twice a day,[53] and its daily dosage should be kept below 400 mg to prevent the lupuslike syndrome that appears in 10 to 20 per cent of patients who receive more. This reaction, although uncomfortable to the patient, is completely reversible and does not cause

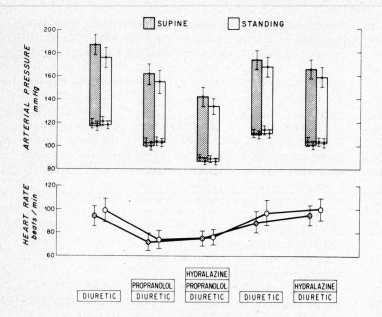

FIGURE 27-11 Arterial pressures and heart rates of 23 hypertensive patients treated with four drug regimens. The combination of hydralazine and propranolol provided the greatest effect on blood pressure without a rise in heart rate. (From Zacest, R., et al.: Treatment of essential hypertension with combined vasodilatation and beta-adrenergic blockade. N. Engl. J. Med. *286*:617, 1972, by permission of the New England Journal of Medicine.)

permanent injury. In fact, *lower* subsequent blood pressure and improved survival has been noted among 42 patients with this toxic reaction when compared to matched-patients given hydralazine but who did not experience the reaction.[146] The reaction is very rare with daily doses of 200 mg or less and is more common in slow acetylators of the drug.

Without the protection conferred by concomitant use of an adrenergic blocker, numerous other side effects—tachycardia, flushing, headache, and precipitation of angina—are seen; with the combination, most patients experience few or no side effects.

MINOXIDIL. This drug, unrelated to other vasodilators, acts in a manner similar to hydralazine but is even more effective. It has been found to be particularly useful in managing patients with severe hypertension and renal insufficiency.[147] Even more than with hydralazine, diuretics and adrenergic blockers must be used with minoxidil to prevent the reflex increase in cardiac output and fluid retention. Unfortunately, the drug also causes hair to grow profusely, and the facial hirsutism discourages some women from taking the drug. Previous concerns that the drug

leads to pulmonary hypertension and causes right atrial lesions, as it does in dogs, have been shown to be unfounded.[147] However, pericardial effusions have appeared in about 3 per cent of those given minoxidil and are likely related to the renal insufficiency that is usually present but are sometimes seen in patients without renal or cardiac failure.[148]

CALCIUM-ENTRY BLOCKERS
(See also p. 1350–1353)

One or more of these agents will probably be approved for use in the treatment of hypertension. Of those currently available for treatment of coronary disease, nifedipine has the most attractive hemodynamic profile: it has the greatest peripheral vasodilatory action with little effect on cardiac conduction. Initial trials have shown nifedipine to be effective, both by sublingual and by oral routes.[149,149a,149b] Verapamil is also effective,[150] and both agents tend to reduce blood pressure significantly only in those patients with hypertension.[151]

The antihypertensive effect of these agents may be so fast and so marked as to precipitate coronary ischemic

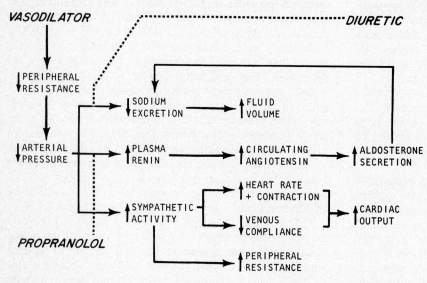

FIGURE 27-12 The primary and secondary effects of vasodilator therapy in essential hypertension and the manner by which diuretic and beta-adrenergic blocker therapy can overcome the undesirable secondary effects. (Adapted from Koch-Weser, J.: Vasodilator drugs in the treatment of hypertension. Arch. Intern. Med. *133*:1017, 1974. Copyright 1974, American Medical Association.)

changes on ECG.[152] But of potentially greater concern are the possible diffuse effects of these agents on various secretory processes that involve calcium entry.[153] Verapamil has been found to dampen the release of gonadotropin and thyrotropin from the pituitary,[154] but the clinical significance of these hormonal changes remains uncertain.

As the basic mechanisms of action of various antihypertensive agents are being unraveled, inhibition of calcium entry may turn out to be common to many: both beta-[155] and alpha-adrenergic[156] blocking drugs may work in this manner, as may direct-acting vasodilators.[157]

RENIN-ANGIOTENSIN BLOCKERS

Activity of the renin-angiotensin system may now be inhibited in four ways (Fig. 27–13), three of which can be applied clinically. The first, use of adrenergic blockers to inhibit the release of renin, was discussed earlier in this chapter. The second, direct inhibition of renin activity by antirenin antibodies, is not now clinically feasible. The fourth, blockade of angiotensin's actions by a competitive blocker, is used, in the form of saralasin, as a diagnostic test for renovascular hypertension and was described on page 881. The third, inhibition of the enzyme that converts the inactive decapeptide angiotensin I to the active octapeptide angiotensin II, is now feasible with the use of the orally effective converting enzyme inhibitor (CEI) *captopril* (Capoten).[158] Captopril is likely the first of a family of CEI's, the second of which (MK-421) is already being investigated.[159] Introduced for use only in patients resistant or intolerant to other medications, captopril has now been found to be both effective in and well tolerated by patients with mild hypertension.[160] In these patients, as in those with more severe hypertension, a diuretic is usually needed to achieve an adequate response.

MODE OF ACTION. Captopril was synthesized as a specific inhibitor of the converting enzyme that breaks the peptidyldipeptide bond in angiotensin I. It binds to three sites on the converting enzyme, thereby preventing the enzyme from attaching to and splitting the angiotensin I structure. Since angiotensin II cannot be formed and angiotensin I is inactive, the CEI paralyzes the workings of the renin-angiotensin system, thereby removing the effects of endogenous angiotensin II as both a vasoconstrictor and a stimulant to aldosterone synthesis. In about 70 per

cent of hypertensives, the blood pressure falls and, in almost all, the levels of aldosterone are reduced.[161]

The same enzyme which converts angiotensin I to angiotensin II is also responsible for inactivation of the vasodepressor hormone bradykinin. By inhibiting the breakdown of bradykinin, CEI may increase the concentration of a vasodepressor hormone while it decreases the concentration of a vasoconstrictor hormone.[162] At the same time, levels of vasodilatory prostaglandins may also be increased. However it works, captopril lowers blood pressure mainly by reducing peripheral resistance, with little if any effect upon heart rate, cardiac output, or body fluid volumes.

CLINICAL USE. The antihypertensive response to captopril is greatest in those patients whose hypertension is being generated by high levels of angiotensin II, such as those with renovascular hypertension or scleroderma. Similarly, the response in those with lesser contributions by angiotensin II will be enhanced by concomitant use of a diuretic, which will raise endogenous angiotensin II levels.

In multiple clinical trials, the mean decrease in blood pressure was 11 per cent in those who started with low renin, 14 per cent in those with normal renin, and 19 per cent in those with high renin.[163] Among 40 patients with an average initial blood pressure of 174/110 mm Hg, captopril alone lowered the blood pressure by 23/14 mm Hg; captopril plus hydrochlorothiazide lowered it by 51/20 mm Hg.[164]

The initial dose of captopril may precipitate a rather dramatic but transient fall in blood pressure, but the full effect may not be seen for 7 to 10 days.[161] The initial dosage is usually 25 mg three times a day, which is then gradually increased to a maximum of 150 mg three times a day. Since much of the drug is excreted by the kidneys, smaller doses are usually adequate in patients with renal insufficiency. The response to captopril is usually well maintained, perhaps because its marked suppression of aldosterone mitigates the tendency toward volume expansion that often antagonizes the effects of other hypertensives. However, half the patients in one series[165] required larger doses or more diuretic to maintain long-term control.

Captopril has been found to be effective in reducing afterload in the treatment of severe congestive heart failure (see p. 539).

SIDE EFFECTS. Among 81 patients, captopril caused

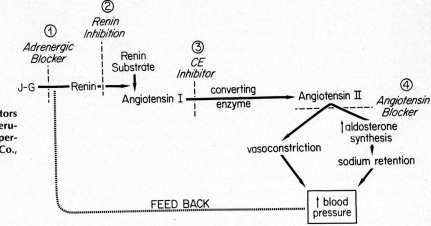

FIGURE 27-13 The four sites of action of inhibitors of the renin-angiotensin system. (J-G = juxtaglomerular apparatus.) (From Kaplan, N. M.: Clinical Hypertension, 3rd ed. Baltimore, Williams and Wilkins Co., 1982, p. 223.)

side effects in 47 per cent, necessitating withdrawal in 23 per cent.[166] About 20 per cent develop a skin rash or some disturbance in taste. Fortunately, two more serious complications are much less common: membranous glomerulopathy (in about 1 per cent) and bone marrow suppression with leukopenia (in perhaps 0.3 per cent). Changes in renal biopsy specimens similar to those found after captopril have been observed in hypertensives who have never taken the drug,[167] but a cause-and-effect relationship with overt renal damage has been clearly demonstrated.[168] Leukopenia has occurred within three months of the onset of therapy but has been slowly progressive and is reversible if recognized and the drug discontinued.[169]

SPECIAL CONSIDERATIONS IN THERAPY

CHOICE OF DRUGS. The stepped-care approach has used a diuretic first, an adrenergic blocker second, and a vasodilator third. As previously discussed, an adrenergic blocker may be as effective as and safer than a diuretic for initial therapy. Whether used as first or second drug, effectiveness differs little among the adrenergic blockers: along with a diuretic, all these agents will lower blood pressure to below 90 mm Hg in about 80 per cent of hypertensive patients. The choice is then logically made based on ease of administration and freedom from side effects. Certain trade-offs may be required: reserpine and guanethidine may be given in only one dose per day, but the side effects may be intolerable; methyldopa, despite its efficacy, may cause some unique and serious problems; if poor patient compliance is anticipated, clonidine should be avoided; prazosin may provide more "physiological" control of the blood pressure but may cause bothersome postural hypotension; beta blockers are probably most convenient for most patients but may cause serious side effects even after careful exclusion of patients known to be susceptible. Although the evidence for protection from coronary events afforded by beta blockers is not yet conclusive, the possibility of this advantage, added to the relative freedom from bothersome side effects, makes a beta blocker—preferably one that is cardioselective—the usual choice for the second drug. Patients who cannot take a beta blocker can be given clonidine or prazosin.

If a third drug is needed, hydralazine will usually be added, although prazosin or clonidine may also be effective if a beta blocker is the second drug. The combination of a beta blocker and either of these adrenergic drugs, which have mechanisms of action that differ from those of the beta blocker, is logical and effective.

REASONS FOR INADEQUATE RESPONSE. Often patients do not respond well because they do not take their medications. On the other hand, what appears to be a poor response based upon office readings of blood pressure may turn out to be an adequate response (as corroborated by improvements in the ECG) when home readings are evaluated.[170] However, a number of factors may be responsible for a poor response even if the appropriate medication is taken regularly (Table 27–7). Perhaps most common is volume overload due to either inadequate diuretic or excessive dietary sodium intake. If the latter is suspected, the sodium content in an overnight or 24-hour urine sample should be measured. If this level exceeds 100

TABLE 27–7 CAUSES OF POOR RESPONSE TO ANTIHYPERTENSIVE DRUGS

1. Inadequate drugs (? poor adherence)
   a. Doses too low
   b. Inappropriate combinations
   c. Rapid inactivation (hydralazine, propranolol)
   d. Antagonism from other drugs
      (1) Sympathomimetics
      (2) Antidepressants
      (3) Adrenal steroids
      (4) Estrogens
2. Associated diseases
   a. Renal insufficiency
   b. Renovascular hypertension
   c. Pheochromocytoma
3. Volume overload
   a. Inadequate diuretic
   b. Excessive sodium intake
   c. Fluid retention from reduction of blood pressure
   d. Progressive renal damage
4. Volume depletion → increased renin → vasoconstriction
   a. Renal salt-wasting
   b. Overly aggressive diuretic therapy

mEq/day, some restriction of dietary salt should be prescribed. Larger doses or more potent diuretics may bring resistant hypertension under control.[171] However, there are a few patients whose blood pressure is resistant to therapy because of overly vigorous diuresis, which contracts vascular volume and activates both renin and catecholamines.[172] This is most likely to occur in patients with obligatory salt-wasting due to interstitial renal disease.

ANESTHESIA IN HYPERTENSIVE PATIENTS. Most anesthesiologists suggest that hypertensive patients be well controlled by means of medications prior to anesthesia and surgery. On the basis of careful hemodynamic measurements in patients receiving various antihypertensive medications, Prys-Roberts et al. found "no evidence that any antihypertensive drugs other than reserpine in any way predisposed to adverse circulatory changes, either in the patient's response to anesthesia or during recovery."[173] Patients receiving beta blockers may have slightly higher blood pressures during anesthesia but fewer problems with tachycardia, increases in pressure during intubation, or electrocardiographic evidence of myocardial ischemia.[174]

TREATMENT OF CHILDREN. Almost nothing is known about the effects of various antihypertensive medications given to children over long periods of time. Since most of the adrenergic blockers act upon the central nervous system, their effects upon growth hormone, gonadotropins, and other hormones involved in maturation and growth should be ascertained. However, in the absence of adequate data, a stepped-care approach similar to that advocated for adults is advised.[175] The doses of drugs are largely interpolated from those used in adults on a mg/kg basis. Emphasis has been placed upon the need for weight reduction in hypertensive children who are obese, thereby attempting to control hypertension without the need for drug therapy.

HYPERTENSION DURING PREGNANCY. (See pages 888 to 891.)

THE ELDERLY WITH SYSTOLIC HYPERTENSION. Here again, almost no data are available as to the indications for therapy and the appropriate choice of drugs. If both systolic and diastolic pressures are elevated, elderly patients should be handled in a manner similar to that for younger persons; they seem to respond as well and have no more problems with medications.[176] In view of the reduced effectiveness of the baroreceptor reflex and the failure of cerebral autoregulation that may occur in the elderly,[177] drugs with a propensity to cause postural hypotension should be avoided, and all drugs should be given in slowly increasing doses to prevent excessive lowering of the pressure.

Isolated systolic hypertension presents a risk, particularly of strokes.[178] It is likely that judicious lowering of the pressure will protect against and not precipitate cardiovascular catastrophes. Admittedly, most systolic pressure elevations are due to structural hardening of the arterial walls, and the vessels may not be able to dilate as well as the constricted, more compliant vessels of young people. The goal of therapy should be relaxed; a systolic pressure of 160 mm Hg seems reasonable for people over 60 years of age. It is hoped that data on the effectiveness of therapy for isolated systolic hypertension will be forthcoming.

Some elderly people may have very high blood pressure as measured by the sphygmomanometer but may have less or no hypertension when direct intraarterial readings are made.[179] Presumably the pseudohypertension is related to the failure of the sphygmomanometer cuff to collapse the rigid artery beneath the cuff. For those patients with vessels that feel rigid and who have few retinal or cardiac findings of hypertension, as would be expected with high sphygmomanometer readings, direct intraarterial measurements should be made before therapy is begun.

Prescription of a thiazide diuretic plus moderate sodium restriction seems the logical first step. As a second step, small doses of methyldopa or clonidine seem preferable to beta blockers, which appear to be less effective in the elderly, or prazosin, which may cause postural hypotension. Hydralazine may be tolerated as a second step, presumably because of reduced baroreceptor reflex sensitivity to vasodilation.

HYPERTENSION WITH RENAL INSUFFICIENCY.

In the presence of renal insufficiency, hypertension is usually predominantly caused by volume excess, and most patients can be successfully treated with salt restriction and diuretics.[180] When serum creatinine exceeds 2.5 mg/dl, thiazides are usually relatively ineffective, and either metolazone or high doses of furosemide are required.[70] A few patients with chronic renal disease have a more resistant form of hypertension, usually associated with—and perhaps caused by—high levels of plasma renin activity. Although a few of these patients will require bilateral nephrectomy to control their hypertension, medical therapy with beta blockers, minoxidil,[147] or captopril[158] has been increasingly effective, not only in controlling the hypertension but in halting the deterioration of renal function.[181] With appropriate therapy, hypertension can be controlled in most patients, and even in some patients with far-advanced renal insufficiency, long-term therapy can halt the deterioration.

HYPERTENSION WITH CONGESTIVE HEART FAILURE.

Cardiac output may fall so markedly in hypertensive patients who are in heart failure that their blood pressure is reduced, obscuring the degree of hypertension; often, however, the diastolic pressure is raised by intense vasoconstriction while the systolic pressure falls as a result of the reduced stroke volume. Lowering the blood pressure may, by itself, relieve the heart failure, but often diuretics and digitalis are needed. Antihypertensive drugs that primarily decrease cardiac output, particularly beta blockers, which remove the heart's needed sympathetic support, may be dangerous in the presence of heart failure. Prazosin has been found to be particularly effective,[113] presumably because it dilates veins and reduces preload as well.

HYPERTENSION WITH ISCHEMIC HEART DISEASE.

The coexistence of coronary artery disease makes antihypertensive therapy even more essential, since relief of the hypertension may ameliorate the coronary disease. Beta blockers are particularly useful if angina or arrhythmias are present, and calcium-entry blockers will probably also find a major use in such patients.

HYPERTENSION WITH DIABETES MELLITUS.

Diuretics may worsen diabetic control, probably because they induce potassium depletion.[71] Brittle diabetics on insulin should not be given nonselective beta blockers, since these drugs may prevent the outpouring of catecholamines that counteracts a precipitous fall in blood sugar levels, thereby preventing the recognition of impending hypoglycemia and delaying the rebound rise in the blood sugar.

HYPERTENSION WITH PSYCHIATRIC ILLNESS.

Patients who are anxious and emotionally labile may benefit from the calming effects of beta blockers upon the somatic manifestations of anxiety.[133] However, caution is advised in using high doses of beta blockers, which may induce nightmares and hallucinations. If antidepressant or antipsychotic medications are needed, they will not blunt the effects of beta blockers as they may those of guanethidine, methyldopa, or clonidine.

THERAPY FOR HYPERTENSIVE CRISES

When diastolic blood pressure exceeds 140 mm Hg, rapidly progressive damage to the arterial vasculature is demonstrable experimentally, and a surge of cerebral blood flow may rapidly lead to encephalopathy[55] (see Fig. 27–6). Since previously normotensive patients may develop encephalopathy at much lower levels of blood pressure, such an elevated pressure must be quickly lowered.

A number of drugs for this purpose are now available (Table 27–8), and others, such as labetolol[145] are under investigation. If diastolic pressure exceeds 140 mm Hg, and the patient has any complications such as a stroke or congestive failure, a constant infusion of nitroprusside is most effective and will almost always lower the pressure to the desired level. Constant monitoring, preferably with an intraarterial line, is mandatory; a slightly excessive dose may abruptly lower the pressure to levels that will induce shock. The potency and rapidity of action of nitroprusside make it the treatment of choice for life-threatening hypertension. Cyanide toxicity from prolonged therapy can be prevented by intravenous hydroxycobalamin.[182] Occasionally, as in therapy for aortic dissection, beta-adrenergic blockade with propranolol may enhance the efficacy and safety of nitroprusside.[183]

With less serious hypertension, intravenous diazoxide is effective and usually safe. The use of 300-mg doses given by rapid bolus injection may lower the pressure too much

TABLE 27–8 DRUGS FOR TREATMENT OF HYPERTENSIVE CRISIS (IN ORDER OF RAPIDITY OF ONSET OF ACTION)

	ADULT DOSAGE	TIME COURSE OF ACTION			ADVANTAGES	DISADVANTAGES	SIDE EFFECTS
		Onset	*Maximum*	*Duration*			
Nitroprusside (Nipride)	50 mg/500 ml 5% glucose in water IV	< 1 min	1 to 2 min	2 to 5 min	Effective instantly, continuously, and consistently	Requires constant monitoring of BP and dose	Nausea
Diazoxide (Hyperstat)	150 to 300 mg by rapid IV injection	1 min	2 to 4 min	4 to 12 hr	Effective rapidly and consistently	Fixed dosage; occasional hypotension	Tachycardia, nausea, flushing
Hydralazine (Apresoline)	10 to 50 mg IM	10 to 20 min	20 to 40 min	3 to 6 hr	Ease of administration; maintains renal blood flow	Increases cardiac output	Tachycardia, nausea, headache
Reserpine (Serpasil)	0.5 to 5.0 mg IM	1½ to 3 hr	3 to 4 hr	6 to 24 hr	Gradual and prolonged effect	Delayed onset of action; sedative; cumulative effect may cause hypotension	Sedation, nasal congestion
Methyldopa (Aldomet)	250 to 1000 mg IV	2 to 3 hr	3 to 5 hr	6 to 12 hr	Gradual and prolonged effect	Not always effective; delayed onset of action	Sedation, lack of effect

and cause cerebral or myocardial ischemia. Such excessive hypotension can be avoided by either repeated injections of 150 mg each or slow infusions, with little delay in reducing the pressure to safe levels.[184]

The other drugs listed in Table 27–8 are less satisfactory for rapid reduction of very high blood pressure. However, in less emergent situations oral therapy may be adequate.[185] Intramuscular hydralazine is widely used to treat preeclampsia. With any of these agents, intravenous furosemide is often needed to lower the blood pressure further and prevent retention of salt and water.

Once the patient is out of immediate danger, oral therapy, usually consisting of a combination of diuretic, beta blocker, and hydralazine, should be initiated. Under these circumstances, the gradual, gentle approach toward lowering the pressure, advocated earlier in this chapter for most hypertensive patients, seems inappropriate. Fortunately, fewer patients in a hypertensive crisis are being seen, presumably because more hypertensive patients are being recognized and treated before the disease enters this malignant course. It is hoped that the continued successful treatment of many more hypertensives will lead to similar increases in prevention of the other, more subtle, but more frequent, long-range sequelae of hypertension.

References

1. Dustan, H. P., Schneckloth, R. E., Corcoran, A. C., and Page, I. H.: The effectiveness of long-term treatment of malignant hypertension. Circulation 18:644, 1958.
2. Veterans Administration Cooperative Study Group on Antihypertensive Agents: Effects of treatment on morbidity in hypertension. Results in patients with diastolic blood pressures averaging 115 through 129 mm Hg. J.A.M.A. 202:116, 1967.
3. Veterans Administration Cooperative Study Group on Antihypertensive Agents: Effects of treatment on morbidity in hypertension. II. Results in patients with diastolic blood pressure averaging 90 through 114 mm Hg. J.A.M.A. 213:1143, 1970.
4. Hypertension Detection and Follow-up Program Cooperative Group: Five-year findings of the Hypertension Detection and Follow-up Program. I. Reduction in mortality of persons with high blood pressure, including mild hypertension. J.A.M.A. 242:2562, 1979.
5. Report of the Management Committee: The Australian therapeutic trial in mild hypertension. Lancet 1:1261, 1980.
6. Laughlin, K. D., Fisher, L., and Sherrard, D. J.: Blood pressure reductions during self-recording of home blood pressure. Am. Heart J. 98:629, 1979.
7. Kannel, W. B., Dawber, T. R., and McGee, D. L.: Perspectives on systolic hypertension. Circulation 61:1179, 1980.
8. Kaplan, N. M.: Whom to treat: The dilemma of mild hypertension. Am. Heart J. 101:867, 1981.
9. Thomson, G. E., Alderman, M. H., Wassertheil-Smoller, S., Rafter, J. G., and Samet, R.: High blood pressure diagnosis and treatment: Consensus recommendations vs actual practice. Am. J. Public Health 71:413, 1981.
10. Guttmacher, S., Teitelman, M., Chapin, G., Garbowski, G., and Schnall, P.: Ethics and preventive medicine: The case of borderline hypertension. Hastings Center Reports 11:12, 1981.
11. Frohlich, E. D.: Continued gains in hypertension. Am. J. Cardiol. 47:375, 1981.
12. Taylor, L., Foster, M. C., and Beevers, D. G.: Divergent views of hospital staff on detecting and managing hypertension. Br. Med. J. 1:715, 1979.
13. W.H.O./I.S.H. Mild Hypertension Liaison Committee. Trials of the treatment of mild hypertension. Lancet 1:149, 1982.
14. Kaplan, N. M.: The therapy of hypertension. In Clinical Hypertension. 3rd ed. Baltimore, Williams and Wilkins Co., 1982, p. 108.
15. Alderman, M. H., and Madhavan, S.: Management of the hypertensive patient: A continuing dilemma. Hypertension 3:192, 1981.
16. Helgeland, A.: Treatment of mild hypertension: A five year controlled drug trial. Am. J. Med. 69:725, 1980.
17. Peart, W. S., and Miall, W. E.: M.R.C. mild hypertension trial. Lancet 1:104, 1980.
18. Ames, R. P., and Hill, P.: Increases in serum-lipids during treatment of hypertension with chlorthalidone. Lancet 1:721, 1976.
19. Rose, G.: Strategy of prevention: Lessons from cardiovascular disease. Br. Med. J. 282:1847, 1981.
20. Moser, M.: On the management of "mild hypertension." Arch. Intern. Med. 141:1587, 1981.
21. Hypertension and Follow-up Program Cooperative Group: Five-year findings of the hypertension detection and follow-up program. III. Reduction in stroke incidence among persons with high blood pressure. J.A.M.A. 247:633, 1982.
22. Smith, W. M.: Treatment of mild hypertension. Results of a ten-year intervention trial. Circ. Res. 40 (Suppl. I):I-98, 1977.
23. Wilhelmsen, L., Berglund, G., Sannerstedt, R., Hansson, L., Andersson, O., Sievertsson, R., and Wikstrand, J.: Effect of treatment of hypertension in the primary preventive trial, Göteborg, Sweden. J. Clin. Pharmacol. 7 (Suppl. 2):261, 1979.
24. Hypertension Detection and Follow-up Program Cooperative Group: Beneficial effect of the hypertension detection and follow-up program stepped care regime on indices of coronary artery and myocardial disease. Am. J. Cardiol. 49:912, 1982 (abstract).
25. Rowlands, D. B., Glover, D. R., Ireland, M. A., McLeay, R. A. B., Stallard, T. J., Watson, R. D. S., and Littler, W. A.: Assessment of left-ventricular mass and its response to antihypertensive treatment. Lancet 1:467, 1982.

NONDRUG THERAPY

26. MacGregor, G. A., Markandu, N. D., Best, F. E., Elder, D. M., Cam, J. M., Sagnella, G. A., and Squires, M.: Double-blind randomised crossover trial of moderate sodium restriction in essential hypertension. Lancet 1:351, 1982.
27. Ram, C. V. S., Garrett, B. N., and Kaplan, N. M.: Moderate sodium restriction and various diuretics in the treatment of hypertension. Arch. Intern. Med. 141:1015, 1981.
28. Landmann-Suter, R., and Struyvenberg, A.: Initial potassium loss and hypokalemia during chlorthalidone administration in patients with essential hyperten-

sion: The influence of dietary sodium restriction. Eur. J. Clin. Invest. 8:155, 1978.

29. Warren, S. E., Vieweg, W. V. R., and O'Connor, D. T.: Sympathetic nervous system activity during sodium restriction in essential hypertension. Clin. Cardiol. 3:348, 1980.

30. Kaplan, N. M., Simmons, M., McPhee, C., Carnegie, A., Stefanu, C., and Cade, S.: Two techniques to improve adherence to dietary sodium restriction in the treatment of hypertension. Arch. Intern. Med. 42:1638, 1982.

31. Linas, S. L.: Mechanism of hyperreninemia in the potassium-depleted rat. J. Clin. Invest. 68:347, 1981.

32. Knochel, J. P.: Neuromuscular manifestations of electrolyte disorders. Am. J. Med. 72:521, 1982.

33. MacGregor, G. A., Smith, S. J., Markandu, N. D., Banks, R. A., and Sagnella, G. A.: Moderate potassium supplementation in essential hypertension. Lancet 2:567–570, 1982.

34. Iimura, O., Kijima, T., Kikuchi, K., Miyama, A., Ando, T., Nakao, T., and Takigami, Y.: Studies on the hypotensive effect of high potassium intake in patients with essential hypertension. Clin. Sci. 61:77s, 1981.

35. Hovell, M. F.: The experimental evidence for weight-loss treatment of essential hypertension: A critical review. Am. J. Public Health 72:359, 1982.

36. Reisin, E., Abel, R., Modan, M., Silverberg, D. S., Eliahou, H. E., and Modan, B.: Effect of weight loss without salt restriction on the reduction of blood pressure in overweight hypertensive patients. N. Engl. J. Med. 298:1, 1978.

37. Cooke, K. M., Frost, G. W., Thornell, I. R., and Stokes, G. S.: Alcohol consumption and blood pressure. Med. J. Aust. 1:65, 1982.

38. Klatsky, A. L., Friedman, G. D., and Siegelaub, A. B.: Alcohol and mortality. Ann. Intern. Med. 95:139, 1981.

39. Castelli, W. P., Gordon, T., Hjortland, M. C., Kagan, A., Doyle, J. T., Hames, C. G., Hulley, S. B., and Jukel, W. J.: Alcohol and blood lipids. Lancet 2:153, 1977.

40. Gruchow, H. W., Hoffmann, R. G., Anderson, A. J., and Barboriak, J. J.: Effects of drinking patterns on the relationship between alcohol and coronary occlusion. Atherosclerosis 43:393, 1982.

41. Robertson, D., Frölich, J. C., Carr, R. K., Watson, J. T., Hollifield, J. W., Shand, D. G., and Oates, J. A.: Effects of caffeine on plasma renin activity, catecholamines and blood pressure. N. Engl. J. Med. 298:181, 1978.

41a. Freestone, S., and Ramsay, L. E.: Effect of coffee and cigarette smoking on the blood pressure of untreated and diuretic-treated hypertensive patients. Am. J. Med. 73:348–353, 1982.

42. Hoel, B. L., Lorensten, E., and Lund-Larsen, P. G.: Hemodynamic responses to sustained hand-grip in patients with hypertension. Acta Med. Scand. 188:491, 1970.

43. Black, H. R.: Nonpharmacologic therapy for hypertension. Am. J. Med. 66:837, 1979.

44. Roman, O., Camuzzi, A. L., Villalon, E., and Klenner, C.: Physical training program in arterial hypertension. Cardiology 67:230, 1981.

45. Jacobson, E.: Variation of blood pressure with skeletal muscle tension and relaxation. Ann. Intern. Med. 12:1194, 1939.

46. Patel, C., Marmot, M. G., and Terry, D. J.: Controlled trial of biofeedback-aided behavioural methods in reducing mild hypertension. Br. Med. J. 282:2005, 1981.

47. Stamler, J., Farinaro, E., Mojonnier, L. M., Hall, Y., Moss, D., and Stamler, R.: Prevention and control of hypertension by nutritional-hygienic means. J.A.M.A. 243:1819, 1980.

ANTIHYPERTENSIVE DRUG THERAPY

48. Haynes, R. B., Mattson, M. E., Chobanian, A. V., Dunbar, J. M., Engebretson, T. O., Jr., Garrity, T. F., Leventhal, H., Levine, R. J., and Levy, R. L.: Management of patient compliance in the treatment of hypertension. Hypertension 4:415, 1982.

49. Haynes, R. B., Sackett, D. L., Taylor, D. W., Roberts, R. S., and Johnson, A. L.: Manipulation of the therapeutic regimen to improve compliance: Conceptions and misconceptions. Clin. Pharmacol. Ther. 22:125, 1977.

50. Wright, J. M., Orozco-Gonzalez, M., Polak, G., and Dollery C. T.: Duration of effect of single daily dose methyldopa therapy. Br. J. Clin. Pharmacol. 13:847–854, 1982.

51. Jain, A. K., Ryan, J. R., Vargas, R., and McMahon, F. G.: Efficacy and acceptability of different dosage schedules of clonidine. Clin. Pharmacol. Ther. 21:382, 1977.

52. Wilkinson, P. R., Dixon, N., and Hunter, K. R.: Twice-daily propranolol treatment for hypertension. J. Intern. Med. Res. 2:220, 1974.

53. Silas, J. H., Ramsay, L. E., and Freestone, S.: Hydralazine once daily in hypertension. Br. Med. J. 284:1602, 1982.

54. Watson, R. D. S., Stallard, T. J., and Littler, W. A.: Influence of once-daily administration of β-adrenoceptor antagonists on arterial pressure and its variability. Lancet 1:1210, 1979.

55. Strandgaard, S.: Autoregulation of cerebral blood flow in hypertensive patients. Circulation 53:720, 1976.

56. The Joint National Committee on Detection, Evaluation, and Treatment of High Blood Pressure: The 1980 report of the Joint National Committee on detection, evaluation, and treatment of high blood pressure. Arch. Intern. Med. 140:1280, 1980.

57. Laragh, J. H.: Vasoconstriction-volume analysis for understanding and treating

hypertension: The use of renin and aldosterone profiles. Am. J. Med. 55:261, 1973.

58. Dustan, H. P., Tarazi, R. C., and Bravo, E. L.: Dependence of arterial pressure on intravascular volume in treated hypertensive patients. N. Engl. J. Med. 286:861, 1972.

59. Zacest, R., Gilmore, E., and Koch-Weser, J.: Treatment of essential hypertension with combined vasodilation and beta-adrenergic blockade. N. Engl. J. Med. 286:617, 1972.

59a. Multiple Risk Factor Intervention Trial Research Group: Multiple risk factor intervention trial. Risk factor changes and mortality results. J.A.M.A. 248:1465–1477, 1982.

59b. Kaplan, N. M.: Mild hypertension: When and how to treat. Arch. Intern. Med. 1983 (in press).

60. Freis, E. D.: Salt in hypertension and the effects of diuretics. Ann. Rev. Pharmacol. Toxicol. 19:13, 1979.

61. Lake, C. R., Ziegler, M. G., Coleman, M. D., and Kopin, I. J.: Hydrochlorothiazide-induced sympathetic hyperactivity in hypertensive patients. Clin. Pharmacol. Ther. 26:428, 1979.

62. Webster, J., Dollery, C. T., Hensby, C. N., and Friedman, L. A.: Antihypertensive action of bendroflumethiazide: Increased prostacyclin production? Clin. Pharmacol. Ther. 28:751, 1980.

63. Bennett, W. M., McDonald, W. J., Kuehnel, E., Hartnett, M. N., and Porter, G. A.: Do diuretics have antihypertensive properties independent of natriuresis? Clin. Pharmacol. Ther. 22:499, 1977.

64. Weber, M. A., Drayer, J. I. M., Rev, A., and Laragh, J. H.: Disparate patterns of aldosterone response during diuretic treatment of hypertension. Ann. Intern. Med. 87:558, 1977.

65. Beevers, D. G., Hamilton, M., and Harpur, J. E.: The long-term treatment of hypertension with thiazide diuretics. Postgrad. Med. J. 47:639, 1971.

66. Degnbol, B., Dorph, S., and Marner, T.: The effect of different diuretics on elevated blood pressure and serum potassium. Acta Med. Scand. 192:407, 1973.

67. Tweeddale, M. G., Ogilvie, R. L., and Ruedy, J.: Antihypertensive and biochemical effects of chlorthalidone. Clin. Pharmacol. Ther. 22 (Part 1):519, 1977.

68. Lutterodt, A., Nattel, S., and McLeod, P. J.: Duration of antihypertensive effect of a single daily dose of hydrochlorothiazide. Clin. Pharmacol. Ther. 27:324, 1980.

69. Anderson, J., Godfrey, B. E., Hill, D. M., Munro-Faure, A. D., and Sheldon, J.: A comparison of the effects of hydrochlorothiazide and of furosemide in the treatment of hypertensive patients. Quart. J. Med. 40:541, 1971.

70. Dargie, H. J., Allison, M. E. M., Kennedy, A. C., and Gray, M. J. B.: High dosage metolazone in chronic renal failure. Br. Med. J. 4:196, 1972.

71. Morgan, D. B., and Davidson, C.: Hypokalaemia and diuretics: An analysis of publications. Br. Med. J. 280:905, 1980.

72. Sandor, F. F., Pickens, P. T., and Crallan, J.: Variations of plasma potassium concentrations during long-term treatment of hypertension with diuretics without potassium supplements. Br. Med. J. 284:711, 1982.

73. Kassirer, J. P., and Harrington, J. T.: Diuretics and potassium metabolism: A reassessment of the need, effectiveness and safety of potassium therapy. Kidney Int. 11:505, 1977.

74. Holland, O. B., Nixon, J. V., and Kuhnert, L.: Diuretic-induced ventricular ectopic activity. Am. J. Med. 70:762, 1981.

74a. Struthers, A. D., Reid, J. L., Lawrie, C. B., and Rodger, J. C.: β-adrenoceptor–linked Na/K ATPase. Drugs, 1983 (in press).

74b. Nordrehaug, J. E.: Malignant arrhythmias in relation to serum potassium values in patients with an acute myocardial infarction. Acta Med. Scand. (Suppl.) 647:101–107, 1981.

75. Lemieux, G., Beauchemin, M., Vinay, P., and Gougoux, A.: Hypokalemia during the treatment of arterial hypertension with diuretics. Can. Med. Assoc. J. 122:905, 1980.

76. Good, D. W., and Wright, F. S.: Luminal influences on potassium secretion: Sodium concentration and fluid low rate. Am. J. Physiol. 236:F192, 1979.

77. Hollenberg, N. K., Williams, G., Burger, B., and Hooshmand, I.: The influence of potassium on the renal vasculature and the adrenal gland, and their responsiveness to angiotensin II in normal man. Clin. Sci. Molec. Med. 49:527, 1975.

78. Skehan, J. D., Barnes, J. N., Drew, P. J., and Wright, P.: Hypokalaemia induced by a combination of a beta-blocker and a thiazide. Br. Med. J. 284:83, 1982.

78a. McMahon, F. G., Ryan, J. R., Akdamar, F., and Ertan, A.: Upper gastrointestinal lesions after potassium chloride supplements: A controlled clinical trial. Lancet 2:1059–1061, 1982.

79. Sopko, J. A., and Freeman, R. M.: Salt substitutes as a source of potassium. J.A.M.A. 238:608, 1977.

80. Sheehan, J., and White, A.: Diuretic-associated hypomagnesaemia. Br. Med. J. 285:1157–1159, 1982.

81. Helgeland, A., Hjermann, I., Holme, I., and Leren, P.: Serum triglycerides and serum uric acid in untreated and thiazide-treated patients with mild hypertension. Am. J. Med. 64:34, 1978.

82. Weinman, E. J., Eknoyan, G., and Suki, W. N.: The influence of the extracellular fluid volume on the tubular reabsorption of uric acid. J. Clin. Invest. 55:283, 1975.

83. Goldman, A. I., Steele, B. W., Schnaper, H. W., Fitz, A. E., Frolich, E. D., and Perry, H. M., Jr.: Serum lipoprotein levels during chlorthalidone therapy. J.A.M.A. 244:1691, 1980.

84. Grimm, R. H., Leon, A. S., Hunninghake, D. B., Lenz, K., Hannan, P., and Blackburn, H.: Effects of thiazide diuretics on plasma lipids and lipoproteins in mildly hypertensive patients. Ann. Intern. Med. 94:7, 1981.

85. Amery, A., Berthaux, P., Bulpitt, C., Deruyttere, M., de Schaepdryver, A., Dollery, C., Fagard, R., Forette, F., Hellermans, J., Lund-Johansen, P., Mutsers, A., and Tuomilehto, J.: Glucose intolerance during diuretic therapy. Lancet 1:681, 1978.

86. Medical Research Council Working Party on Mild to Moderate Hypertension: Adverse reactions to bendrofluazide and propranolol for the treatment of mild hypertension. Lancet 2:539, 1981.

87. Williams, R. L., Davies, R. O., Berman, R. S., Holmes, G. I., Huber, P., Gee, W. L., Lin, E. T., and Benet, L. Z.: Hydrochlorothiazide pharmacokinetics and pharmacologic effect: The influence of indomethacin. J. Clin. Pharmacol. 22:32, 1982.

88. Guidi, G., Guintoli, F., Saba, G., Diamanti, G., Checchi, M., Gabbani, S. A., Birindelli, A., and Saba, P.: Clinical investigation on efficacy of indapamide as an antihypertensive agent. Curr. Ther. Res. 31:601, 1982.

89. Berglund, G., and Andersson, O.: Beta-blockers or diuretics in hypertension? A six year follow-up on blood pressure and metabolic side effects. Lancet 1: 744, 1981.

90. Buhler, F. R., Burkart, F., Lutold, B. E., Kung, M., Marbet, G., and Pfisterer, M.: Antihypertensive beta blocking action as related to renin and age: A pharmacologic tool to identify pathogenetic mechanisms in essential hypertension. Am. J. Cardiol. 36:653, 1975.

91. Veterans Administration Cooperative Study Group on Antihypertensive Agents: Comparison of propranolol and hydrochlorothiazide for the initial treatment of hypertension. I. Results of short-term titration with emphasis on racial differences in response. J.A.M.A. 248:1996–2003, 1982.

92. Beilin, L. J., Bulpitt, C. J., Coles, E. C., Dollery, C. T., Gear, J. S. S., Harper, G., Johnson, B. F., Munro-Faure, A. D., and Turner, S. C.: Long-term antihypertensive drug treatment and blood pressure control in three hospital hypertension clinics. Br. Heart J. 43:74, 1980.

93. Kaplan, N. M.: The prognostic implications of plasma renin in essential hypertension. J.A.M.A. 231:167, 1975.

94. Langer, S. Z., and Shepperson, N. B.: Prejunctional modulation of noradrenaline release by α_2-adrenoceptors: Physiological and pharmacological implications in the cardiovascular system. J. Cardiovasc. Pharmacol. 4 (Suppl. 1):S35, 1982.

95. Veterans Administration Cooperative Study Group on Antihypertensive Agents. Propranolol in the treatment of essential hypertension. J.A.M.A. 237: 2303, 1977.

96. Finnerty, F. A., Gyftopoulos, A., Berry, C., and McKenney, A.: Step 2 regimens in hypertension. J.A.M.A. 241:579, 1979.

97. Participating Veterans Administration Medical Centers: Low dose v standard dose of reserpine. J.A.M.A. 248:2471–2477, 1982.

98. Curb, J. D., Hardy, R. J., Labarthe, D. R., Borhani, N. O., and Taylor, J. O.: Reserpine and breast cancer in the hypertension detection and follow-up program. Hypertension 4:307, 1982.

99. Corder, C. N.: Bethanidine dose, plasma levels, and antihypertensive effects. J. Clin. Pharmacol. 18:249, 1978.

100. Häusler, G.: Central α-adrenoceptors involved in cardiovascular regulation. J. Cardiovasc. Pharmacol. 4:S72, 1982.

101. Fouad, F. M., Nakashima, Y., Tarazi, R. C., and Salcedo, E. E.: Reversal of left ventricular hypertrophy in hypertensive patients treated with methyldopa. Am. J. Cardiol. 49:795, 1982.

102. Seeverens, H., deBruin, C. D., and Jordans, J. G. M.: Myocarditis and methyldopa. Acta Med. Scand. 211:233, 1982.

103. Rodman, J. A., Deutsch, D. J., and Gutman, S. I.: Methyldopa hepatitis. Am. J. Med. 60:941, 1976.

104. Dybing, E., Nelson, S. D., Mitchell, J. R., Sasame, H. A., and Gillette, J. R.: Oxidation of α-methyldopa and other catechols by cytochrome P-450–generated superoxide anion: Possible mechanisms of methyldopa hepatitis. Molec. Pharmacol. 12:911, 1976.

105. Weber, M. A., Case, D. B., Baer, L., Sealey, J. E., Drayer, J. I. M., Lopez-Ovejero, J. A., and Laragh, J. H.: Renin and aldosterone suppression in the antihypertensive action of clonidine. Am. J. Cardiol. 38:825, 1976.

106. Metz, S. A., Halter, J. B., Porte, D., Jr., and Robertson, R. P.: Suppression of plasma catecholamines and flushing by clonidine in man. J. Clin. Endocrinol. Metab. 46:83, 1978.

107. Houston, M. C.: Abrupt cessation of treatment in hypertension: Consideration of clinical features, mechanisms, prevention and management of the discontinuation syndrome. Am. Heart J. 102:415, 1981.

108. Bosanac, P., Dubb, J., Walker, B., Goldberg, M., and Agus, Z. S.: Renal effects of guanabenz: A new antihypertensive. J. Clin. Pharmacol. 16:631, 1976.

109. Fagan, T. C., Bloomfield, S. S., Cowart, T. D., Corns-Hurwitz, R. H., Lipicky, R. J., Conradi, E. C., Hsu, C., Grossman, W. J., Harmon, G. E., Degenhart, W. J., Sinkfield, A. W., and Gafney, T.: Antihypertensive effects of lofexidine in patients with essential hypertension. Br. J. Clin. Pharmacol. 13:405, 1982.

109a. Safar, M. E., Loria, Y., Weiss, Y. A., and Boutier, J. R.: Antihypertensive effects and plasma levels of guanfacine in man. J. Clin. Pharmacol. 22:385–390, 1982.

110. Davey, M. J.: The pharmacology of prazosin, an alpha 1-adrenoceptor antagonist and the basis for its use in the treatment of essential hypertension. Clin. Exper. Hyper. A4:47, 1982.

111. Jauernig, R. A., Moulds, R. F. W., and Shaw, J.: The action of prazosin in human vascular preparation. Arch. Intern. Pharmacodyn. 231:81, 1978.

112. Heagerty, A. M., Russell, G. I., Bing, R. F., Thurston, H., and Swales, J. D.: The addition of prazosin to standard triple therapy in the treatment of severe hypertension. Br. J. Clin. Pharmacol. 13:539, 1982.

113. Miller, R. R., Awan, N. A., Maxwell, K. S., and Mason, D. T.: Sustained reduction of cardiac impedance and preload in congestive heart failure with the antihypertensive vasodilator prazosin. N. Engl. J. Med. 297:303, 1977.

114. Zacharias, F. J., Cuthbertson, P. J. R., Prestt, J., Cowen, K. J., Johnson, T. B. W., Thompson, J., Vickers, J., Simpson, W. T., and Tuson, R.: Atenolol in hypertension: A study of long-term therapy. Postgrad. Med. J. 53(Suppl. 3):102, 1977.

115. Campbell, W. B., Johnson, A. R., Callahan, K. S., and Graham, R. M.: Antiplatelet activity of beta-adrenergic antagonists: Inhibition of thromboxane synthesis and platelet aggregation in patients receiving long-term propranolol treatment. Lancet 2:1382, 1981.

116. Amos, H. E., Lake, B. G., and Artis, J.: Possible role of antibody specific for a practolol metabolite in the pathogenesis of oculomucocutaneous syndrome. Br. Med. J. 1:402, 1978.

117. Wilcox, R. G.: Randomised study of six beta-blockers and a thiazide diuretic in essential hypertension. Br. Med. J. 2:383, 1978.

118. Day, J. L., Metcalfe, J., and Simpson, C. N.: Adrenergic mechanisms in control of plasma lipid concentrations. Br. Med. J. 284:1145, 1982.

119. Groop, L., Tötterman, K. J., Harno, K., and Gordin, A.: Influence of beta-blocking drugs on glucose metabolism in patients with non-insulin dependent diabetes mellitus. Acta Med. Scand. 211:7, 1982.

120. Fitzgerald, J. D.: The effect of different classes of beta-antagonists on clinical and experimental hypertension. Clin. Exper. Hyper. A4:101, 1982.

121. Henningsen, N. C., and Mattiasson, I.: Long-term clinical experience with atenolol—a new selective β-1-blocker with few side-effects from the central nervous system. Acta Med. Scand. 205:61, 1979.

122. Esler, M., Jackman, G., Leonard, P., Skews, H., Bobik, A., and Jennings, G.: Effects of propranolol on noradrenaline kinetics in patients with essential hypertension. Br. J. Clin. Pharmacol. 12:375, 1981.

123. O'Connor, D. T., and Preston, R. A.: Propranolol effects on autonomic function in hypertensive men. Clin. Cardiol. 5:340, 1982.

124. Jackson, E. K., and Campbell, W. B.: A possible antihypertensive mechanism of propranolol: Antagonism of angiotensin II enhancement of sympathetic nerve transmission through prostaglandins. Hypertension 3:23, 1981.

125. Hallberg, H., Almgren, O. L., and Svensson, T. H.: Reduced brain serotonergic activity after repeated treatment with β-adrenoceptor antagonists. Psychopharmacology 76:114, 1982.

126. Lund-Johansen, P.: Hemodynamic consequences of long-term beta-blocker therapy: A 5-year follow-up study of atenolol. J. Cardiovasc. Pharmacol. 1: 487, 1979.

127. Bolli, P., Amann, F. W., Burkart, F., and Bühler, F. R.: Role of α-adrenoceptor–mediated vasoconstriction for antihypertensive β-blockade. J. Cardiovasc. Pharmacol. 4:S162, 1982.

128. Kristensen, B. O., Brons, M., Christensen, C. K., Geday, E., Jacobsen, F. K., Jensen, S. N., and Linde, N. C.: Antihypertensive effect of atenolol (100 mg once a day) and methyldopa (250 mg thrice a day). Acta Med. Scand. 209: 267, 1981.

129. Serlin, M. M., Orme, M. L'E., Baber, N. A., Sibeon, R. G., Laws, E., and Breckenridge, A.: Propranolol in the control of blood pressure: A dose-response study. Clin. Pharmacol. Ther. 27:586, 1980.

130. Lundborg, P., Aström, H., Bengtsson, C., Fellenius, E., Von Schenck, H., Svensson, L., and Smith, U.: Effect of β-adrenoceptor blockade on exercise performance and metabolism. Clin. Sci. 61:299, 1981.

131. Laragh, J. H.: Modern system for treating high blood pressure based on renin profiling and vasoconstriction-volume analysis: A primary role for beta blocking drugs such as propranolol. Am. J. Med. 61:797, 1976.

132. Drayer, J. I. M., Keim, H. J., Weber, M. A. A., Case, D. B., and Laragh, J. H.: Unexpected pressor responses to propranolol in essential hypertension. Am. J. Med. 60:897, 1976.

133. James, I. M., Griffith, D. N. W., Pearson, R. M., and Newbury, P.: Effect of oxprenolol on stage-fright in musicians. Lancet 2:952, 1977.

134. Frishman, W. H., Christodoulou, J., Weksler, B., Smithen, C., Killip, T., and Scheidt, S.: Abrupt propranolol withdrawal in angina pectoris: Effects on platelet aggregation and exercise tolerance. Am. Heart J. 95:169, 1978.

135. Rangno, R. E., Nattel, S., and Lutterodt, A.: Prevention of propranolol withdrawal mechanism by prolonged small dose propranolol schedule. Am. J. Cardiol. 49:828, 1982.

136. Smulyan, H., Weinberg, S. E., and Howanitz, P. J.: Continuous propranolol infusion following abdominal surgery. J.A.M.A. 247:2539, 1982.

137. Wilkinson, R.: β-blockers and renal function. Drugs 23:195, 1982.

138. Gallery, E. D. M., Saunders, S. M., Hunyor, S. N., and Györy, A. Z.: Randomised comparison of methyldopa and oxprenolol for treatment of hypertension in pregnancy. Br. Med. J. 1:1591, 1979.

139. Sandstrom, B.: Adrenergic beta-receptor blockers in hypertension of pregnancy. Clin. Exper. Hyper. B1:127, 1982.

140. Leren, P., Foss, P. O., Helgeland, A., Hjermann, I., Holme, I., and Lund-Larsen, P. G.: Effect of propranolol and prazosin on blood lipids. Lancet 2:4, 1980.

141. Feely, J., Wilkinson, G. R., and Wood, A. J. J.: Reduction of liver blood flow and propranolol metabolism by cimetidine. N. Engl. J. Med. 304:692, 1981.

142. Sotaniemi, E. A., Anttila, M., Rautio, A., Stengard, J., Saukko, P., and Järvensivu, P.: Propranolol and sotalol metabolism after a drinking party. Clin. Pharmacol. Ther. 29:705, 1981.

143. Alvan, G., vonBahr, C., Seideman, P., Sjöqvist, F.: High plasma concentration of β-receptor blocking drugs and deficient debrisoquine hydroxylation. Lancet *1*:333, 1982.

144. Lund-Johansen, P., and Bakke, O. M.: Haemodynamic effects and plasma concentrations of labetolol during long-term treatment of essential hypertension. Br. J. Clin. Pharmacol. *7*:169, 1979.

145. Cumming, A. M. M., Brown, J. J., Lever, A. F., and Robertson, J. I. S.: Intravenous labetalol in the treatment of severe hypertension. Br. J. Clin. Pharmacol. *13*(Suppl. 1):93s–96s, 1982.

146. Perry, H. M., Jr., Camel, G. H., Carmody, S. E., Ahmed, K. A., and Perry, E. F.: Survival in hydralazine-treated hypertensive patients with and without late toxicity. J. Chron. Dis. *30*:519, 1977.

147. Hagstam, K., Lundgren, R., Wieslander, J.: Clinical experience of long-term treatment with minoxidil in severe arterial hypertension. Scand. J. Urol. Nephrol. *16*:57, 1982.

148. Houston, M. C., McChesney, J. A., and Chatterjee, K.: Pericardial effusion associated with minoxidil therapy. Arch. Intern. Med. *141*:69, 1981.

149. Husted, S. E., Nielsen, H. K., Christensen, C. K., and Pedersen, O. L.: Long-term therapy of arterial hypertension with nifedipine given alone or in combination with a beta-adrenoceptor blocking agent. Eur. J. Clin. Pharmacol. *22*:101, 1982.

149a. Bonaduce, D., Ferrara, N. Petretta, M., Romano, E., Postiglione, M., Rengo, F., and Condorelli, M.: Hemodynamic study of nifedipine administration in hypertensive patients. Am. Heart J. *105*:865, 1983.

149b. Hornung, R. S., Gould, B. A., Jones, R. I., Sonecha, T. N., and Raftery, E. B.: Nifedipine tablets for systemic hypertension: A study using continuous ambulatory intraarterial recording. Am. J. Cardiol. *51*:1323, 1983.

150. Anavekar, S. N., Christophidis, N., Louis, W. J., and Doyle, A. E.: Verapamil in the treatment of hypertension. J. Cardiovasc. Pharmacol. *2*:287, 1981.

151. Krebs, R., Graefe, K.-H., and Ziegler, R.: Effects of calcium-entry antagonists in hypertension. Clin. Exper. Hyper. *A4*:271, 1982.

152. Yagil, Y., Kobrin, I., Leibel, B., and Ben-Ishay, D.: Ischemic ECG changes with initial nifedipine therapy of severe hypertension. Am. Heart J. *103*:310, 1982.

153. Rubin, R. P.: Actions of calcium antagonists on secretory cells. *In* Weiss, G. B. (ed.): New Perspectives on Calcium Antagonists. Bethesda, American Physiological Society, 1981, p. 147.

154. Barbarino, A., and De Marinis, L.: Calcium antagonists and hormone release. II. Effects of verapamil on basal, gonadotropin-releasing hormone– and thyrotropin–releasing hormone–induced pituitary hormone release in normal subjects. J. Clin. Endocrinol. Metab. *51*:749, 1980.

155. Lindemann, J. P., Bailey, J. C., and Watanabe, A. M.: Potential biochemical mechanisms for regulation of the slow inward current: Theoretical basis for drug action. Am. Heart J. *103*:746, 1982.

156. Atlas, D., and Adler, M.: α-Adrenergic antagonists as possible calcium channel inhibitors. Proc. Natl. Acad. Sci. *78*:1237, 1981.

157. Weiss, G. B.: Sites of action of calcium antagonists in vascular smooth muscle. *In* Weiss, G. B. (ed.): New Perspectives on Calcium Antagonists. Bethesda, American Physiological Society, 1981, p. 83.

158. Vidt, D. G., Bravo, E. L., and Fouad, F. M.: Captopril. N. Engl. J. Med. *306*:214, 1982.

159. Gavras, H., Biollaz, J., Waeber, B., Brunner, H. R., Gavras, I., and Davies, R. O.: Effects of the new oral angiotensin converting enzyme inhibitor MK-421 in human hypertension. Clin. Exper. Hyper. *A4*:303, 1982.

160. Vlasses, P. H., Rotmensch, H. H., Swanson, B. N., Mojaverian, P., and Ferguson, R. K.: Low-dose captopril. Its use in mild to moderate hypertension unresponsive to diuretic treatment. Arch. Intern. Med. *142*:1098, 1982.

161. Atlas, S. A., Case, D. B., Sealey, J. E., Laragh, J. H., and McKinstry, D. N.: Interruption of the renin-angiotensin system in hypertensive patients by captopril induces sustained reduction in aldosterone secretion, potassium retention and natriuresis. Hypertension *1*:274, 1979.

162. Swartz, S. L., Williams, G. H., Hollenberg, N. K., Moore, T. J., and Dluhy, R. G.: Converting enzyme inhibition in essential hypertension: The hypotensive response does not reflect only reduced angiotensin II formation. Hypertension *1*:106, 1979,

163. Jenkins, A. C., and McKinstry, D. N.: Review of clinical studies of hypertensive patients treated with captopril. Med. J. Aust. (Suppl.)*2*:32, 1979.

164. Karlberg, B. E., Asplund, J., Nilsson, O. R., Wettre, S., and Öhman, P. K.: Captopril, an orally active converting enzyme inhibitor, in the treatment of primary hypertension. Acta Med. Scand. *209*:245, 1981.

165. Tarazi, R. C., Bravo, E. L., and Fouad, F. M.: Late resistance to captopril. *In* Laragh, J. H., Buhler, F. R., and Seldin, D. W. (eds.): Frontiers in Hypertension Research. New York, Springer-Verlag, 1981.

166. Waeber, B., Gavras, I., Brunner, H. R., and Gavras, H.: Safety and efficacy of chronic therapy with captopril in hypertensive patients: An update. J. Clin. Pharmacol. *21*:508, 1981.

167. Captopril Collaborative Study Group: Does captopril cause renal damage in hypertensive patients? Lancet *1*:988, 1982.

168. Case, D. B., Atlas, S. A., Mouradian, J. A., Fishman, R. A., Sherman, R. L., and Laragh, J. H.: Proteinuria during long-term captopril therapy. J.A.M.A. *244*:346, 1980.

169. Erslev, A. J., Alexander, J. C., Caro, J., and Boyd, R. L.: Hematologic side effects of captopril and associated risk factors. Cardiovasc. Rev. Rep. *3*:660, 1982.

170. Ibrahim, M. M., Tarazi, R. C., Dustan, H. P., and Gifford, R. W., Jr.: Electrocardiogram in evaluation of resistance to antihypertensive therapy. Arch. Intern. Med. *137*:1125, 1977.

171. Gavras, H., Waeber, B., Kershaw, G. R., Liang, C., Textor, S. C., Brunner, H. R., Tifft, C. P., and Gavras, I.: Role of reactive hyperreninemia in blood pressure changes induced by sodium depletion in patients with refractory hypertension. Hypertension *3*:441, 1981.

172. Cohn, J. N.: Paroxysmal hypertension and hypovolemia. N. Engl. J. Med. *275*:643, 1966.

173. Prys-Roberts, C., Meloche, R., and Föex, P.: Studies of anaesthesia in relation to hypertension. I. Cardiovascular responses of treated and untreated patients. Br. J. Anaesth. *43*:122, 1971.

174. Prys-Roberts, C., Föex, P., Biro, G. P., and Roberts, J. G.: Studies of anaesthesia in relation to hypertension. V. Andrenergic beta-receptor blockade. Br. J. Anaesth. *45*:671, 1973.

175. Lieberman, E.: Hypertension in childhood and adolescence. *In* Kaplan, N. M. (ed.): Clinical Hypertension. 3rd ed. Baltimore, Williams and Wilkins Co., 1982, pp. 411–435.

176. Management Committee: Treatment of mild hypertension in the elderly. Med. J. Aust. *2*:398, 1981.

177. Wollner, L., McCarthy, S. T., Soper, N. D. W., and Macy, D. J.: Failure of cerebral autoregulation as a cause of brain dysfunction in the elderly. Br. Med. J. *1*:1117, 1979.

178. Gifford, R. W., Jr.: Isolated systolic hypertension in the elderly. J.A.M.A. *247*:781, 1982.

179. Spence, J. D., Sibbald, W. J., and Cape, R. D.: Pseudohypertension in the elderly. Clin. Sci. Molec. Med. *55*:399s, 1978.

180. Bank, N., Lief, P. D., and Piczon, O.: Use of diuretics in treatment of hypertension secondary to renal disease. Arch. Intern. Med. *138*:1524, 1978.

181. Friedlaender, M. M., Rubinger, D., and Popovtzer, M. M.: Improved renal function in patients with primary renal disease after control of severe hypertension. Am. J. Nephrol. *2*:12, 1982.

182. Cottrell, J. E., Casthely, P., Brodie, J. D., Patel, K., Klein, A., and Turndorf, H.: Prevention of nitroprusside-induced cyanide toxicity with hydroxycobalamin. N. Engl. J. Med. *298*:809, 1978.

183. Niarchos, A. P., and Kritikou, P. E.: Cardiovascular effects of sodium nitroprusside in hypertensive patients before and during acute beta-adrenergic blockade. J. Clin. Pharmacol. *19*:31, 1979.

184. Garrett, B. N., and Kaplan, N. M.: Efficacy of slow infusion of diazoxide in the treatment of severe hypertension without organ hypoperfusion. Am. Heart J. *103*:390, 1982.

185. Alpert, M. A., and Bauer, J. H.: Rapid control of severe hypertension with minosidil. Arch. Intern. Med. *142*:2099–2104, 1982.

28 HYPOTENSION AND SYNCOPE

by Burton E. Sobel, M.D., and Robert Roberts, M.D.

The *sudden* development of hypotension, particularly when it occurs in a recumbent patient, is usually associated with impaired systemic perfusion and may be an important feature of shock, as discussed in detail in Chapter 18. In contrast, *chronic hypotension*, with systolic pressure in the range of 85 to 110 mm Hg is not pathological and may actually be associated with a longer life expectancy than a "normal" arterial pressure. This chapter deals with a variety of syndromes responsible for *episodic hypotension* and its cardinal clinical manifestation, syncope.

REGULATION OF ARTERIAL PRESSURE

Systemic arterial pressure is closely related to the product of cardiac output and systemic vascular resistance. *Cardiac output* is the product of heart rate and stroke volume, the latter being determined by interactions between preload, afterload, and contractility, as described in Chapter 14. Thus, the cardiac causes of sudden hypotension relate to abrupt reductions in ventricular rate, as occurs with atrioventricular block, or in stroke volume, as may occur in hypovolemia (reduced preload); to critical aortic stenosis (augmented afterload); or to massive myocardial infarction (impaired ventricular function). *Vascular resistance* varies inversely with the fourth power of the radius of the resistance vessels, the arterioles, and therefore is determined by the intrinsic physical characteristics of these vessels, i.e., the ratio of lumen to wall thickness; the degree of extravascular support and compression; and the extent of contraction of the smooth muscle in the vascular wall. The last-named is in turn influenced by (1) metabolic and mechanical autoregulatory mechanisms that act to maintain *nearly* constant perfusion of each vascular bed—there is substantial evidence that adenosine is a principal metabolic mediator of vascular resistance (p. 1244); (2) neurogenic vasoconstrictor influences, operating through the action of

adrenergic neurotransmitter norepinephrine on alpha-adrenergic receptors in vascular smooth muscle; (3) neurogenic vasodilator influences, operating through the action of acetylcholine on muscarinic receptors, or norepinephrine on $beta_2$ receptors, and perhaps of histamine, serotonin, and other transmitters; and (4) circulating and locally released vasoactive substances, including catecholamines, angiotensin II, bradykinin, and prostaglandins. The vascular causes of hypotension may involve any of these four mechanisms (Table 28–1).

The autonomic nervous system plays a major role in the maintenance of arterial pressure because it influences both cardiac output and the degree of constriction of the vessels of resistance (arterioles) and capacitance (venules and veins). The afferent limbs of the autonomic reflex arcs that acutely regulate arterial pressure arise in stretch receptors in the aortic arch, the carotid sinuses, ventricles, and atria. Impulses are transmitted along afferent fibers in the glossopharyngeal and vagus nerves to extensive central connections in the medulla. Synapses connect not only the sympathetic and parasympathetic nuclei and efferent arcs but also the cerebral cortex and hypothalamic nuclei, which control hormonal secretion via the pituitary gland (Fig. 28–1).

A sudden reduction of arterial and intraventricular pressure diminishes the stimulation of pressoreceptors, which in turn reflexly activates sympathetic outflow and inhibits parasympathetic activity. As a result, vascular smooth muscle in arterioles and veins constricts, whereas heart rate and myocardial contractility are augmented. In addition, as arterial pressure falls, adrenal medullary secretion increases, along with the output of antidiuretic hormone (ADH), adrenocorticotropic hormone (ACTH), renin, and aldosterone; all these effects restore the arterial pressure toward control levels. Opposite changes occur if arterial pressure rises suddenly. Thus, the operation of these baro-

TABLE 28–1 IMPORTANT CAUSES OF PROLONGED OR INTERMITTENT HYPOTENSION

1. Cardiac dysfunction
   a. Disturbances of rate and rhythm
      (1) Conduction abnormalities
      (2) Diverse dysrhythmias, including severe bradycardia and paroxysmal tachycardias
   b. Obstruction to flow
      (1) Aortic or pulmonary valvular stenosis
      (2) Hypertrophic obstructive cardiomyopathy
      (3) Atrial myxoma
      (4) Primary pulmonary hypertension
      (5) Pulmonary peripheral branch stenosis
      (6) Pulmonary emboli
      (7) Cardiac tamponade
      (8) Mitral or tricuspid stenosis
      (9) Cor triatriatum
      (10) Tetralogy of Fallot
      (11) Eisenmenger's syndrome
   c. Impaired ventricular function
      (1) Myocardial infarction
      (2) Cardiomyopathy

2. Vascular or neurological dysfunction
   a. Vasovagal
   b. Postural hypotension
      (1) Idiopathic
      (2) Acquired
      (3) Familial
   c. Hyperventilation
   d. Carotid sinus hypersensitivity
   e. Glossopharyngeal neuralgia, micturition, deglutition, or posttussive syncope

3. Metabolic and endocrine disturbances
   a. Pheochromocytoma
   b. Serotonin-secreting tumors
   c. Hyperbradykininemia

4. Drug toxicity
   a. Vasodilators
   b. Adrenergic antagonists
   c. Diuretics
   d. Phenothiazines
   e. Barbiturates and other CNS depressants
   f. Vincristine and other neuropathic drugs
   g. Quinidine and other drugs with negative chronotropic effects
   h. Digitalis

receptors and a number of hormonal systems normally serve to buffer the body from a variety of influences that would otherwise produce marked alterations in arterial pressure.

In a resting supine adult, the level of sympathetic discharge to the vasculature is low.[1] Assumption of the upright posture is accompanied by venous pooling of approximately 700 ml of blood in the legs.[1,2] Systemic arterial pressure is maintained by venous and arterial constriction mediated by sympathetic stimulation. Even modest reflex changes of this type markedly facilitate maintenance of venous return and stroke volume.[1] The initial gravitational effects associated with upright posture are compensated not only by reflex arteriolar and venous constriction but also by acceleration of heart rate and by mechanical factors that limit venous pooling in the lower extremities, including venous valves, "milking" of veins in the lower extremities by contractions of the leg musculature (Fig. 28–2), and reduced intrathoracic pressure that facilitates venous return. The increased sympathetic activity is reflected in a rise in concentration of plasma catecholamines.[3] As a consequence of these compensatory mechanisms, when a normal person assumes the upright posture, there is only a transient decline in systolic arterial blood pressure, generally of 5 to 15 mm Hg. Diastolic pressure tends to rise, and mean arterial pressure remains essentially unchanged; cardiac output and stroke volume decline; and there is reflex tachycardia and vasoconstriction, the latter reflected in a rise in systemic vascular resistance. In patients with orthostatic hypotension, by definition the decline in arterial pressure with assumption of the upright posture is more profound and persistent. Depending on the severity and duration of the hypotension, it may be accompanied by symptoms of impaired cerebral perfusion such as dizziness, presyncope, or syncope.

Hypotension may be a manifestation of impairment of any element in (1) the afferent limb, including the carotid, aortic, ventricular, and atrial baroreceptors; (2) the central

NEURAL MECHANISMS FOR PERIPHERAL VASCULAR CONTROL

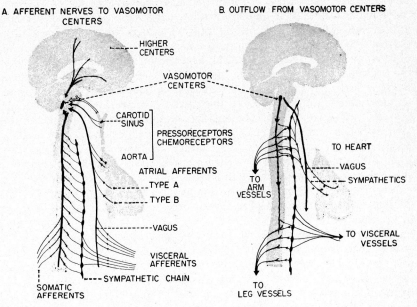

A. AFFERENT NERVES TO VASOMOTOR CENTERS

B. OUTFLOW FROM VASOMOTOR CENTERS

FIGURE 28–1 The vasomotor centers in the medulla receive afferent impulses from many different areas of the body, including the higher centers of the nervous system, heart, blood vessels, viscera, and somatic pain receptors. Efferent impulses descend via the spinal cord in the intermediolateral column and initiate sympathetic impulses to the blood vessels throughout the organism. (From Rushmer, R. F.: Cardiovascular Dynamics. Philadelphia, W. B. Saunders Co., 1961, p. 153.)

PUMPING ACTION OF MUSCLES DURING WALKING

A. COMMUNICATIONS BETWEEN
SUPERFICIAL AND DEEP VEINS

B. THE REDUCTION OF VENOUS PRESSURE
DURING WALKING

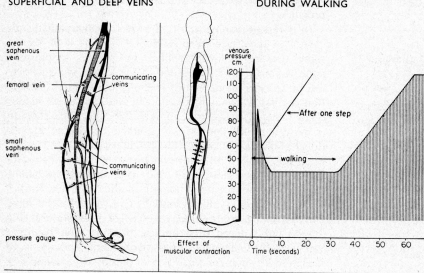

FIGURE 28-2 The venous blood from the leg may return to the heart via superficial or deep channels. Even a single step is associated with a marked reduction in venous pressure that is maintained with walking. With resumption of standing, pressure returns only gradually to control values. (From Rushmer, R. F.: Cardiovascular Dynamics, Philadelphia, W. B. Saunders Co., 1961, p. 176.)

vasomotor centers; (3) the cortical or spinal outflow efferent tracts; (4) the peripheral sympathetic or parasympathetic nerves; (5) mechanical factors that normally limit pooling in the peripheral veins; (6) intravascular blood volume; and (7) the heart's ability to maintain cardiac output.

CAUSES OF ORTHOSTATIC HYPOTENSION

Clinically, the causes of orthostatic hypotension may be classified as follows:[4]

1. *Chronic idiopathic hypotension,* a primary degenerative disorder impairing the function of the autonomic nervous system (discussed below).

2. *Vasoactive drugs,* including essentially all antihypertensive but particularly ganglionic blocking agents; depletors of catecholamines such as reserpine; and drugs that block the neuronal release of catecholamines, such as guanethidine (Chap. 27). In patients with hypertension who are treated too vigorously with antihypertensive drugs, particularly when the treatment is accompanied by dehydration and hypovolemia, postural hypotension is common. Other drugs not used in the treatment of hypertension, such as tranquilizers, sedatives, hypnotics, or antidepressants, may also induce hypotension by depressing the vasomotor center. Hypotension, although rarely seen with judicious use of calcium antagonists, may be encountered more frequently as these drugs are employed more widely in the treatment of angina, particularly when they are used in combination with nitrates and other vasodilators (p. 1351). Postural hypotension may occur in association with administration of numerous other agents, such as bromocriptine.[5]

3. *Disorders of the peripheral, autonomic, or central nervous system,* including diabetes mellitus, alcoholism, uremia, pyridoxine deficiency, multiple sclerosis, tabes dorsalis, pernicious anemia, Parkinson's disease, vascular lesions in the brain stem, neoplasms, and cysts (particularly in the parasellar region and in the posterior fossa), Wer-

nicke's encephalopathy, syringomyelia, and a number of demyelinating disorders.

4. *Cardiovascular deconditioning* after any prolonged illness with prolonged recumbency, especially in elderly patients.

5. *Diseased or varicose veins* causing pooling of blood in the lower extremities.

6. *The supine hypotensive syndrome of pregnancy* (p. 1764), resulting from obstruction of the inferior vena cava with reduction in venous return and decline in cardiac output.

7. *Infiltration of vessel walls,* which may preclude a physiological response to sympathetic stimulation, e.g., amyloidosis.

8. *Surgically induced sympathectomy* with abolition of vasopressor reflex responses.

CHRONIC IDIOPATHIC ORTHOSTATIC HYPOTENSION. This syndrome, the *Bradbury-Eggleston syndrome,* which most often occurs in older men, has also been termed *primary autonomic insufficiency* and is characterized by postural hypotension without a compensatory tachycardia, hypohidrosis, impotence, and disturbed sphincter control.[6] Hypertension in the supine position and postprandial hypotension are relatively common. Dizziness, visual disturbances, presyncope, and syncope accompanying standing or walking are typical signs and occur with distressing regularity, especially when the upright posture is assumed suddenly and during the early morning hours; the course is usually progressive. The *Shy-Drager syndrome* (also known as multiple system atrophy) is a somewhat similar disorder but exhibits prominent degeneration of the central nervous system, with involvement of the extrapyramidal tracts and basal ganglia.[7,8] The degeneration involves the dorsal nucleus of the vagus and pigmented brain stem nuclei, intermediate and lateral columns of the spinal cord, and sympathetic ganglia;[9,10] in a variant form the pathological findings resemble those of Parkinson's disease, with dementia, extrapyramidal signs, loss of facial expressions, and tremor. *Secondary orthostatic hypotension* occurs in a number of neurological disorders that involve the autonomic nervous system, including alcoholic and diabetic neuropathy, subacute combined sclerosis, spinal cord transection, syringomyelia, and tabes dorsalis.

The postural hypotension in chronic idiopathic orthostatic hypotension and in many of the forms of secondary orthostatic hypotension[11] is due primarily to impairment of peripheral vasoconstriction, acceleration of heart rate, and maintenance of cardiac output in response to the assumption of the upright posture.[3,12-14] There is a greater than normal decline in arterial pressure during the Valsalva maneuver, with a reduced or absent arterial pressure overshoot following release, as well as a paradoxical decline in arterial pressure during exercise.

Kontos et al. found that patients with idiopathic orthostatic hypotension do not exhibit vasoconstriction in the forearm and hands in response to intraarterial administration of tyramine, whereas the vasoconstrictor responses to intraarterial administration of norepinephrine are augmented. These findings strongly suggest that sympathetic nerve endings are depleted of and unable to take up norepinephrine. Depletion of norepinephrine from sympathetic nerve endings was confirmed by histochemical demonstration of the absence of catecholamine-specific fluorescence in sympathetic vasomotor nerves.[15,16]

Excretion of norepinephrine and its synthesis from precursors are reduced in this condition.[17-20] Plasma renin release and aldosterone secretion in response to assumption of the erect posture or to salt restriction are also blunted,[15,17-19] possibly contributing to the difficulty in augmenting plasma volume to compensate adequately for the impaired reflex control of vasomotor tone. Thus, blood volume in patients with these disorders is normal or only slightly increased.

While recumbent, patients with idiopathic orthostatic hypotension and multiple central nervous system defects have *normal* plasma levels of norepinephrine that fail to increase normally after standing or exertion. In contrast, patients with peripheral autonomic insufficiency *without* signs of central nervous system defects have *low* levels of plasma norepinephrine while recumbent that also fail to increase normally after standing or exercise. Both groups have low levels of plasma dopamine beta-hydroxylase.

These findings are consistent with other pathological and pharmacological observations, suggesting that patients with idiopathic orthostatic hypotension and central nervous system disease are unable to activate appropriately an otherwise intact sympathetic nervous system, whereas in patients without signs of central nervous system disease, the defect affects peripheral sympathetic nerves.[10]

Since the fundamental disorder is not amenable to therapy, the *treatment* of patients with chronic idiopathic hypotension and the Shy-Drager syndrome must be symptomatic.[20a] This involves (1) a high-salt diet and judicious and monitored administration of mineralocorticoids such as fludrocortisone to expand plasma volume; (2) hydroxyamphetamine, dihydroergotamine,[21,21a] L-dopa,[8] or other directly or indirectly acting sympathomimetic agents; combined with (3) a monoamine oxidase inhibitor, such as tranylcypromine, to augment norepinephrine concentration at nerve endings;[18,22-24] (4) propranolol, a nonselective beta blocker that may prevent adrenergically mediated vasodilation and result in unopposed vasoconstriction;[8,25] (5) indomethacin, which acts presumably by inhibiting synthesis of vasodilatory prostaglandins;[8] and (6) mechanical support by elastic stockings or, in severe cases, an antigravity suit (Fig. 28-3). The *prognosis* for survival is approximately 10 years following the development of symptoms in patients without other evident neurological disease, but it is only about 5 years in patients with associated abnormalities of the central nervous system.

Familial Dysautonomia. Familial dysautonomia (Riley-Day syndrome) is a progressive disorder inherited in a pattern consistent with an autosomal recessive trait limited primarily to Ashkenazi Jews.[26] It is characterized by the appearance at or soon after birth of autonomic instability with both postural hypotension and hypertensive episodes due to defective reflex control of vascular tone. Other features include fever; impaired perception of pain, temperature, and taste; lack of fungiform papillae on the tongue; impaired lacrimation; diminished or absent deep tendon reflexes; ataxia; loss of the histamine-flare response; feeding difficulties; and susceptibility to viral pneumonia in infancy.[26,27]

Tissue norepinephrine stores are normal or elevated;[28] the concentrations of plasma catecholamines are normal in patients who are recumbent and at rest but fail to increase normally with exercise or assumption of the upright posture. Plasma dopamine beta-hydroxylase activity and the excretion of vanillylmandelic acid (VMA) are often reduced, consistent with impaired release of catecholamines from sympathetic nerve endings.[28] The cardiovascular response to infused

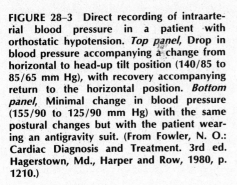

FIGURE 28-3 Direct recording of intraarterial blood pressure in a patient with orthostatic hypotension. *Top panel,* Drop in blood pressure accompanying a change from horizontal to head-up tilt position (140/85 to 85/65 mm Hg), with recovery accompanying return to the horizontal position. *Bottom panel,* Minimal change in blood pressure (155/90 to 125/90 mm Hg) with the same postural changes but with the patient wearing an antigravity suit. (From Fowler, N. O.: Cardiac Diagnosis and Treatment. 3rd ed. Hagerstown, Md., Harper and Row, 1980, p. 1210.)

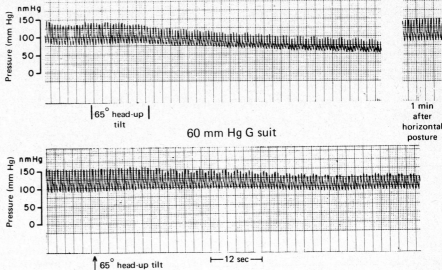

norepinephrine is exaggerated, suggesting receptor hypersensitivity or reduced uptake of the neurotransmitter by nerve endings or both.

Patients with familial dysautonomia synthesize and store norepinephrine in sympathetic nerve endings and release catecholamines from the adrenal medulla in response to stress induced by hypoglycemia.[29] Thus, the hypertensive episodes that frequently accompany even mild anxiety and are associated with increases in plasma norepinephrine may, like the response to infused catecholamines, reflect increased reactivity of vascular receptors to released adrenal catecholamines.

Although the specific abnormality responsible for familial dysautonomia remains unidentified,[26,27] defective release of norepinephrine from the nerve endings is a prominent pathophysiological component. Although it may reflect abnormalities in the afferent or efferent sympathetic system, demonstrable degeneration in the reticular formation of the brain stem suggests a primary abnormality in the central nervous system. However, in some patients the defect may be confined to the peripheral autonomic nervous system. In these patients at rest and in the recumbent position, circulating concentrations of catecholamines are low and do not rise in response to stress.[10]

Unfortunately, no specific treatment is available, and the disease progresses to death in early adult life. Symptomatic treatment involves the general measures described previously for management of postural hypotension as well as the administration of parasympathomimetic agents, such as bethanechol chloride (Urecholine), to facilitate lacrimation, reduce gastric distention and vomiting, improve esophageal motility, and improve bladder control.

Metabolic Abnormalities. Metabolic or endocrine disturbances leading to reduction of plasma volume, altered adrenergic function, or vasodilatation may underlie persistent or episodic hypotension. These include diabetes mellitus, primary systemic amyloidosis, and acute porphyria. The hypovolemia seen with adrenocortical insufficiency, hypoaldosteronism, and salt-wasting nephritis is the primary cause of hypotension in these conditions, although altered vascular responses to catecholamines may contribute in Addison's disease, and diminished levels of angiotensin may play a role in conditions in which plasma renin activity is low.[30]

Depletion of plasma volume is characteristically associated with pheochromocytoma and is a primary cause of postural hypotension in this disorder (p. 1734). However, epinephrine-induced vasodilatation contributes in some patients with epinephrine-secreting tumors. Rarely, circulatory instability results from high concentrations of circulating bradykinins. Hyperbradykininemia, a disorder that is sometimes familial, is characterized by severe tachycardia and a narrowed pulse pressure. The cause is an enzyme deficiency resulting in impaired destruction of the circulating peptides.[31] Kinins may also play a role in the hypotension and syncope sometimes seen with the carcinoid syndrome.

SYNCOPE

Syncope refers to loss of consciousness due to the impairment (usually temporary) of cerebral perfusion.[32] The metabolism of the brain, in contrast to that of many other organs, is exquisitely dependent on perfusion. In contrast to skeletal muscle, for example, storage of high-energy phosphate in the brain is limited, and energy supply depends largely on the oxidation of glucose extracted from the blood. Consequently, cessation of cerebral flow leads to loss of consciousness within approximately 10 seconds (Table 28–2).[33]

TABLE 28–2 FACTORS POTENTIALLY AFFECTING CEREBRAL PERFUSION SELECTIVELY

1. Metabolic causes
   Hypercapnia
   Hypotension
2. Decreased effective perfusion pressure
   Cerebral vascular disease (usually atherosclerotic)
   Arterial spasm
   Increased intracranial pressure
   Cerebral venospasm

A typical syncopal episode is characterized by hypotension, pallor, diaphoresis, and loss of consciousness in a motionless patient with depressed, shallow respirations and intact sphincter tone. If postural hypotension is the cause, cerebral blood flow is usually restored promptly, and consciousness is regained when the patient falls or is placed in a horizontal position. Although syncope is most often associated with the upright posture because it is frequently a manifestation of postural hypotension, it may result from conduction disturbances or other arrhythmias causing profound, sudden reductions in cardiac output in which case postural associations may be lacking.

Faintness or presyncope, a less severe but etiologically similar phenomenon, is characterized by sudden weakness, the inability to stand, visual difficulty, and the sensation of impending loss of consciousness. At this stage, frank loss of consciousness can often be averted if cerebral perfusion is restored, as by the assumption of the supine posture.

REFLEX-MEDIATED VASOMOTOR INSTABILITY. Inappropriate or excessive activation of vasomotor reflexes may initiate syncope in syndromes such as *carotid sinus hypersensitivity*. Pressure on the carotid artery was observed to slow the heart by Czermak in 1866, a reflex phenomenon shown by Hering to be initiated by pressure on the carotid sinus rather than on the vagus nerve. Under physiological conditions, afferent impulses from the carotid sinuses are transmitted via the glossopharyngeal nerve to vasomotor and cardioinhibitory centers in the medulla. The efferent limb of the carotid sinus reflex comprises vagal and cervical sympathetic fibers (Fig. 28–4).[34,35] Afferent impulses from the carotid sinus impinge on the medulla with a frequency dependent on the pressure and rate of change of pressure in the walls of the vessel. Increased pressure leads to an increased frequency of afferent stimulation of the central vasomotor (pressor) center. Consequently, parasympathetic outflow increases, sympathetic outflow is reduced, and systemic vasodilatation and bradycardia ensue.

A clinical syndrome, the hypersensitive carotid sinus syndrome, has been recognized as a cause of hypotension, bradycardia, dizziness, presyncope, and syncope.[35,35a] Two major forms of hypersensitive carotid sinus syndromes have been well delineated.[36] The most common, the *vagal* or *cardioinhibitory* type, occurring in approximately 70 per cent of patients with this syndrome, is manifested by sinus bradycardia, sinus arrest, atrioventricular block, a combination of these disturbances, or even asystole (Fig. 28–5). The second, or *vasodepressor type*, is manifested by marked hypotension without significant bradycardia or atrioventricular (AV) block. Many patients exhibit a combination of both the cardioinhibitory and the vasodepressor syndromes.[37] Carotid sinus hypersensitivity usually occurs in the elderly and is more frequent in men than in women. Arteriosclerosis, hypertension, diabetes mellitus, and local pathological changes such as scars, lymph nodes, and tumors involving the carotid body[36] predispose to a hyperactive carotid sinus. Episodes are often precipitated by turning the head or pressure on the carotid sinus area, such as during shaving. Attacks can be initiated and the diagnosis thereby confirmed by manual pressure on the carotid sinus. Occasionally, cervical lymphadenopathy, scar tissue, or a carotid body tumor may be responsible.[36] Usually, however, the underlying increased sensitivity of the

CAROTID SINUS REFLEXES

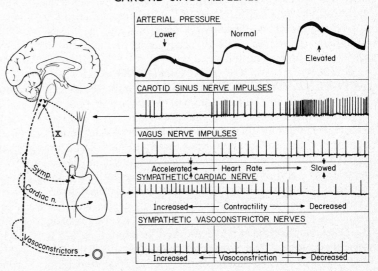

FIGURE 28–4 Relationship between carotid sinus discharge and arterial blood pressure. With a drop in blood pressure (first panel), the frequency of baroreceptor impulses decreases, afferent vagal impulses decrease, and efferent sympathetic nerve impulses increase. The sympathetic vasoconstrictor fiber impulse traffic is active, and an increase in peripheral resistance occurs, resulting in a rise in blood pressure. With an increase in blood pressure, the opposite occurs, resulting in vasodilatation and a drop in blood pressure. (From Rushmer, R. F.: Cardiovascular Dynamics. Philadelphia, W. B. Saunders Co., 1961, p. 150.)

carotid sinus to pressure accompanying specific movements of the neck or a tight collar is not associated with an overt anatomic lesion. Electrophysiological study usually reveals normal intrinsic function of the sinoatrial node and atrioventricular conduction system.[38]

Diagnosis is confirmed by applying manual pressure to the carotid artery in the region of the carotid sinus with the patient supine and the head in a neutral position.[39] Pressure should be applied only lightly at first on only one side and for a maximum of 20 seconds at a time while the electrocardiogram and blood pressure are monitored. Normal subjects exhibit mild sinus bradycardia, sometimes with first-degree atrioventricular block. Ventricular asystole with a duration of 3 seconds or more or a decrease in systolic arterial blood pressure exceeding 50 mm Hg is a definitively abnormal response. Complications of carotid sinus stimulation are rare but potentially catastrophic and include cardiac standstill and hemiplegia.[40] The risk is greatest in elderly, hypertensive patients with cerebral or extracranial vascular occlusive disease. Emergency treat-

ment with closed chest cardiac compression, intravenous atropine, epinephrine, and norepinephrine is indicated.

Other coexisting causes of syncope or episodes mimicking syncope must be excluded, since documentation of a hypersensitive carotid sinus does not prove that it is responsible for the syncopal episode in an individual case.[40] Impaired cerebral perfusion due to cerebral vascular disease may also be responsible for syncope associated with extrinsic pressure on the vessels of the neck,[37] and this condition must be differentiated from the hypersensitive carotid sinus syndrome.

If the syndrome is caused by an anatomically identifiable lesion, such as a carotid sinus tumor, excision is required. In the usual case in which no anatomical cause is recognizable and when symptoms are infrequent, reassurance, precautions to avoid rapid movements, and avoidance of tight collars usually constitute effective therapy.[37] Frequent symptoms should be evaluated by ambulatory electrocardiographic monitoring. If associated with severe bradycardia, they may be prevented by ventricular[37] or

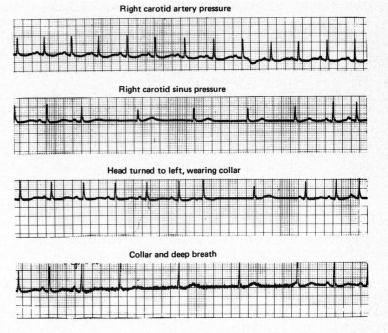

FIGURE 28–5 Electrocardiographic tracings obtained from a patient with the hypersensitive carotid sinus syndrome who presented with attacks of dizziness associated with wearing a tight collar (cardioinhibitory type). Right carotid pressure or sudden turning of the head while wearing a tight collar produced suppression of the sinoatrial node with a junctional escape rhythm. (From Fowler, N. O.: Cardiac Diagnosis and Treatment. 3rd ed. Hagerstown, Md., Harper and Row, 1980, p. 1208.)

atrioventricular pacing.[37a] Surgical resection[37] or denervation[41] of the hypersensitive carotid sinus may be required for refractory cases, particularly when syncope is due to vasodilatation rather than to bradycardia. Irradiation of the carotid sinus is not effective.[36]

OTHER CAUSES OF SYNCOPE SECONDARY TO AFFERENT STIMULATION. Afferent impulses associated with pain in the ear, soft palate, larynx, or pharynx are transmitted centrally via the glossopharyngeal and vagal nerves and may also give rise to reflex hypotension and syncope[42,43] associated with sinus bradycardia,[43] sinus arrest, or heart block.[44] *Glossopharyngeal neuralgia* is characterized by paroxysmal pain usually localized to the posterior pharynx or external auditory canal. It may be accompanied by syncope, secondary to bradycardia and systemic vasodilatation. It may be caused by tumor invasion of the glossopharyngeal nerve and may be treated by intracranial section of the glossopharyngeal nerve.[45] Syncope, often with associated severe vertigo, which follows pleural or peritoneal taps and prostatic massage, may be responsible for similar cardiovascular changes.

Syncope[46-49] or occasionally severe bradycardia without syncope[48] may be provoked by swallowing, usually in association with esophageal tumor,[46] diverticulum,[47] or spasm,[48] but sometimes occurs in patients without overt esophageal disease (*deglutition syncope*).[49] Attacks can be reproduced by inflation of a balloon at the level of an esophageal diverticulum in some patients and in others can be prevented by administration of atropine or by local anesthesia of the vagus nerve in the neck with procaine.[50,51] In some cases afferent impulses may be transmitted via the glossopharyngeal nerve, which also supplies the posterior pharynx and a portion of the esophagus. Treatment requires correction of overt esophageal disease. Palliation and reduction of recurrent syncope may be achieved with the use of an artificial pacemaker in selected patients.

Another reflex-mediated syndrome, *postmicturition syncope*, occurs typically in healthy young to middle-aged men, usually when the patient arises from bed to void. Syncope occurs during or immediately after micturition, and recovery is rapid and complete. Recurrent episodes are rare. Predisposing factors include ingestion of alcohol, diminished food intake, fatigue, and upper respiratory tract infection.[52] Increased vagal stimulation at night, vagal sensory input from the bladder during micturition and the standing position during voiding represent the most common triggering factors of this syndrome.[53]

Paroxysms of coughing may be accompanied by giddiness, vertigo, or syncope, particularly in short, stocky, middle-aged men with chronic lung disease (*post-tussive syncope*). Syncope may occur even with patients in the recumbent position. Sequelae are rare.[54] Syncope in this syndrome may result not only from reflex-mediated mechanisms but also from hydraulic factors, particularly when it follows a paroxysm of coughs, in which case it may result from increased intracranial pressure, which can sometimes be relieved by surgery of the spine.[54,55] In syncope associated with paroxysms of coughing, the intrathoracic, intraarterial, and cerebrospinal fluid pressures increase to levels as high as 300 mm Hg. During the paroxysm, pressure within the cerebral vessels declines because of the diminished cardiac output resulting from inhibition of venous return due to the elevated intrathoracic pressure

and secondary to the increased intracranial pressure reflecting the rise in cerebrospinal fluid pressure. Accordingly, cerebral perfusion declines precipitously (Table 28–2).

VASOVAGAL HYPOTENSION AND SYNCOPE (VASODEPRESSOR SYNCOPE, THE COMMON FAINT). This type of syncope is the most frequently encountered form, accounting for more than 55 per cent of cases in some series.[56] It is often precipitated by the sight of blood; the sudden loss of blood, such as that occurring with phlebotomy; a sudden stressful or painful experience, such as arterial puncture or venipuncture; surgical manipulation; or severe trauma. Vasodepressor syncope is most likely to occur in association with hunger, fatigue, or crowding, particularly in a hot room. Premonitory signs and symptoms are common, including pallor, yawning, sighing, hyperventilation, epigastric discomfort, nausea, diaphoresis, blurred vision, impaired hearing, a vague feeling of unawareness, mydriasis, and sometimes a rapid heart rate. It generally occurs with the patient in an upright position, and if the patient sits or lies down promptly, frank syncope may be aborted.[56a]

Pathophysiology. Despite intensive study of the phenomenon, its etiology has not been elucidated definitively.[57-60] Early in the process, peripheral vasodilatation appears to predominate. Blood pressure declines modestly while blood flow to the limbs, cardiac output, and heart rate remain essentially constant.[58-60] Later, resistance in the skeletal muscular beds is reduced, and skeletal blood flow rises markedly while flow through other vascular beds such as the cutaneous, mesenteric, renal, and cerebral declines as arterial pressure falls rapidly. Although cardiac output does not usually decline markedly in vasodepressor syncope, the pathophysiological mechanism must involve more than arteriolar dilation (or failure of normal arteriolar constriction in the upright position), since in normal individuals the fall in peripheral vascular resistance induced by vasodilatation would be compensated for by a compensatory increase in heart rate and cardiac output, which would limit the reduction of arterial pressure. In patients with vasodepressor syncope, however, cardiac output and heart rate fail to rise, presumably owing to some impairment of venous return, perhaps because of venous dilatation or failure of normal venous constriction. In addition, there appears to be a diminished rise in plasma renin, and presumably this reduces angiotensin-mediated vasoconstriction.

The marked vasodilatation in skeletal muscle beds may be mediated, in part, by reflexes triggered by stimulation of intracardiac receptors[61,62] in a cycle that may involve hypotension due to peripheral vasodilatation, reflex-increased sympathetic stimulation of the heart, increased intramyocardial wall tension and stimulation of intracardiac receptors, and reflex-potentiated vasodilatation.[63] The vasodilatation may also be exacerbated by efferent cholinergic sympathetic stimulation of the arterioles in skeletal muscle.[59] With syncope the electroencephalogram shows slow wave activity of large amplitude.

The hyperventilation that generally precedes and accompanies vasodepressor syncope results in a decline in arterial pCO_2, which in turn produces cerebral vasoconstriction, thereby further impairing cerebral perfusion. Later, heart rate, arterial pressure, central venous pressure, and cardiac output decline precipitously.

During the recovery period, oliguria is common, mediated by increased secretion of antidiuretic hormone (ADH).[64] This finding suggests that some of the other clinical features of the syndrome, including pallor and nausea, may be mediated in part by posterior pituitary hormones.[65]

Management. Vasovagal syncope appearing for the first time demands a thorough diagnostic evaluation, since the syncope may be caused by conditions such as valvular or subvalvular aortic stenosis, hypertrophic obstructive cardiomyopathy, carotid sinus hypersensitivity, or another unrecognized cardiac or neurological abnormality. Therapy consists of placing the patient in the recumbent position with the lower extremities elevated (reverse Trendelenburg). Removal of the offending stimuli, inhalation of spirits of ammonia, and stimulation of the face with cold water usually suffice in treatment of the acute episode. Treatment with vasopressors is not usually required. Consciousness is usually regained rapidly, with a somewhat slower regression of bradycardia. Rarely, if recovery is delayed, atropine may be helpful.

CARDIAC CAUSES OF SYNCOPE. The common denominator in syncope of cardiac cause is a transient, marked diminution of cardiac output due to an arrhythmia or reduced stroke volume.[66,67] The association of syncope and bradycardia, first described by Gerbezius in 1719 and later by Morgagni in 1769[68] and by Adams in 1827,[69] was clarified by Stokes in 1846, who recognized the etiological connections between a change in heart rate and cerebral manifestations.[70] The mechanism underlying syncope even among patients with complete heart block is often a superimposed arrhythmia (such as transient asystole or ventricular fibrillation)[71] at the time of loss of consciousness[71] rather than the heart block per se. Thus, the generic term "arrhythmia-induced syncope" may be more useful.[72]

More than 50,000 new cases of complete heart block occur annually in the United States,[72] and approximately 50 per cent of patients with acquired, complete heart block experience syncope. The causes of complete heart block are listed in Table 28–3 and discussed in detail in Chapter 22.

Arrhythmias Causing Syncope (see also Chapter 22). Arrhythmia-induced syncope may result from asystole, severe bradycardia, or tachyarrhythmia and generally conforms to one of the following categories:

1. Transitory, complete interruption of atrioventricular conduction with asystole during the "preautomatic pause" or "pacemaker warm-up" interval.

2. Asystole developing in the presence of persistent complete heart block, owing to failure of the intra- or infranodal pacemaker, accompanied by a preautomatic pause in other potential pacemakers.

3. Paroxysmal ventricular tachycardia or fibrillation precipitated by ischemia due to the slow heart rate in patients with complete heart block.

4. Paroxysmal ventricular tachycardia or fibrillation in patients with normal atrioventricular conduction, recognized increasingly more often with the use of ambulatory electrocardiographic monitoring.

5. Supraventricular tachy- or bradyarrhythmias leading to decreased cardiac output secondary to the rate itself or to the deleterious effects of the arrhythmia on myocardial perfusion already compromised by coronary artery disease.

6. Asystole due to atrial standstill with failure of automaticity in subsidiary pacemakers, commonly seen in patients with the sick sinus syndrome.[73]

7. Combinations of conduction disturbances and supraventricular arrhythmia, commonly associated with the sick sinus syndrome (p. 693).

Hemodynamic Abnormalities Predisposing to Syncope. Systemic vascular resistance ordinarily declines as a consequence of arteriolar dilatation secondary to the accumulation of vasodilator metabolites during exercise. Normally, this vasodilatation is more than compensated for by the augmentation of cardiac output and arterial pressure during heavy exertion (Chap. 8). However, in those severe forms of heart disease in which cardiac output rises proportionately less than vascular resistance falls, arterial pressure declines, sometimes to hazardous levels. Thus, exertional hypotension and syncope are characteristic features of virtually all forms of heart disease in which cardiac output is relatively fixed and fails to rise normally or even declines during exertion. It is most characteristic of severe valvular aortic stenosis and other forms of obstruction to left ventricular outflow and of coronary artery disease in which global ischemia occurs during exertion.

The mechanism responsible for exertional hypotension and syncope in patients with lesions producing right or left outflow tract obstruction probably involves peripheral vasodilatation as well as decreased cardiac output, the former reflexes resulting from high intraventricular pressure acting on ventricular baroreceptors with blunting of the compensatory carotid and aortic baroreceptor-mediated reflexes.[74,75] Patients with aortic valvular stenosis have been shown to exhibit an excessive reduction of forearm vascular resistance with exertion, with a return of the physiological vasoconstrictor response after correction of the aortic valve lesion.[74] In patients in whom syncope can be ascribed to obstruction to left ventricular outflow, surgical intervention is ordinarily necessary (p. 1103). Syncope in patients with prosthetic cardiac valves is an ominous phenomenon, often indicative of the need for urgent reoperation to relieve a mechanical obstruction caused by serious dysfunction of the prosthetic valve or formation of a thrombus.

When left ventricular outflow tract obstruction is dynamic, as in hypertrophic obstructive cardiomyopathy (Chap. 41) it is exacerbated by increased contractility, decreased chamber dimensions, or decreased afterload and

---

TABLE 28–3   CAUSES OF COMPLETE HEART BLOCK

1. Structural abnormalities of the conduction system
   a. Congenital heart block
   b. Infectious diseases such as diphtheria, syphilis, toxoplasmosis, mumps, rheumatic fever
   c. Collagen diseases
   d. Valvular heart disease
   e. Degenerative disease (Lev's disease, Lenegre's disease, Friedreich's ataxia, progressive muscular dystrophy, myotonic dystrophy, Duchenne's dystrophy)
   f. Coronary artery disease with or without infarction
   g. Tumors
   h. Endocrine and metabolic disorders (gout with urate deposition in the conduction system, hypo- and hyperthyroidism, hemochromatosis, Addison's disease)
   i. Trauma
   j. Diseases of unknown etiology (Reiter's syndrome, sarcoidosis, amyloidosis, Paget's disease)
2. Electrolyte disturbances such as hyperkalemia, acidosis, hypomagnesemia
3. Drug toxicity: Examples include digitalis, quinidine, lidocaine, aprindine, phenytoin (Dilantin), and amitriptyline (Elavil)

distending pressure. Thus, drugs with positive inotropic effects such as digitalis or arterial or venous vasodilators such as nitroglycerin may precipitate hypotension.[76]

Sustained hypotension associated with ischemic heart disease is usually due to severely impaired ventricular function, but episodic hypotension or syncope often results from conduction disturbances or arrhythmia. Sometimes, marked hypotension accompanies angina pectoris or acute myocardial infarction, owing to increased parasympathetic activity, particularly with ischemia of the inferior wall (Chap. 37). Afferent reflexes from atrial and ventricular myocardium or from the coronary vessels themselves elicit increased parasympathetic outflow, bradycardia, and hypotension, which, coupled with the decreased contractility resulting from ischemia, may precipitate syncope.[13,77,78]

Pedunculated left atrial myxoma (p. 1459) or a large thrombus may obstruct the left ventricular inflow tract and suddenly reduce cardiac output. An important clinical clue to the diagnosis is the association of syncope with specific postures (such as sitting or leaning forward) because of movement of a pedunculated or migratory tumor or clot into the left ventricular inflow tract.

Systemic hypotension may be a critical complication in patients with *congenital heart disease* characterized by right-to-left shunting (Chaps. 29 and 30). When pulmonary blood flow is reduced with right-to-left shunting through an intracardiac communication associated with obstruction to right ventricular outflow or severe pulmonary hypertension, marked arterial hypoxemia occurs; this serves as a potent vasodilatory stimulus.

Hypotension may also result from obstruction to outflow due to lesions *extrinsic* to the heart, such as massive pulmonary embolus (Chap. 46), Takayasu's disease (Chap. 45), and supravalvular aortic stenosis (Chaps. 29 and 30), all of which interfere with ventricular emptying. Syncope is a manifestation of primary pulmonary hypertension (Chap. 25) and rarely of pulmonary valvular stenosis (Chaps. 29 and 30); it may accompany cardiac tamponade (Chap. 43).

DIFFERENTIAL DIAGNOSIS OF SYNCOPE. Syncope and presyncope must be differentiated from a variety of other acute episodes. It is critical, for example, to distinguish syncopal episodes from epileptic seizures, particularly the akinetic type. In general, syncope due to vasomotor failure or impaired cardiac output occurs when the patient is in the upright position, although syncopal episodes secondary to cardiac arrhythmia may occur in any position. Syncope occurs most commonly in young women or elderly males and, in contrast to epilepsy, in most instances (1) is of gradual onset *without* aura; (2) is *not* associated with injury from falling; (3) is *not* associated with convulsive movements, biting of the lips, or urinary incontinence; (4) is *brief,* with a rapid return to consciousness; and (5) is *not* followed by a state of confusion.

Epileptic seizures, in contrast, can occur with the patient in any position and are sudden in onset; the warning aura, if it occurs at all, lasts only a few seconds. Injury from falling is frequent, as are convulsive movements with the eyes upturned. The period of unconsciousness usually lasts for minutes, and there is often urinary incontinence, biting of the lips, and a prolonged postictal state of mental confusion and drowsiness.

Attacks of *cerebral ischemia* due to cerebral arteriosclerosis may produce transient ischemic attacks characterized by neurological deficits that tend to resemble each other from attack to attack. These are often visual disturbances, hemiparesis, hemianesthesia, slurred speech, and impaired consciousness.

Anxiety attacks may produce dizziness but not frank syncope. They are usually characterized by, and can be reproduced by, hyperventilation, which results in reduction of cerebral blood flow; are not accompanied by cardiac arrhythmia; and are not relieved by recumbency. *Hysterical fainting* occurs most frequently in persons with hysterical personalities and is not accompanied by any changes in blood pressure, heart rate, or skin color. *Hypoglycemia* is manifested by confusion, sinus tachycardia, jitteriness, and other symptoms of sympathetic stimulation, ultimately leading to loss of consciousness. Loss of consciousness with this entity proceeds gradually but is often prolonged, constituting frank coma. When caused by a tumor of the islets of Langerhans, it occurs with and can be reproduced by prolonged fasting, but when hypoglycemia is reactive, it tends to occur 3 to 5 hours after meals. The diagnosis is confirmed by the finding of reduced blood glucose.

APPROACH TO DIAGNOSIS OF POSTURAL HYPOTENSION AND SYNCOPE

The cause of postural hypotension or syncope is often obvious, after a thorough history and physical examination and laboratory tests selected on the basis of positive findings have been done. In taking the patient's history, the examiner must determine the onset, frequency, and duration of premonitory symptoms; circumstances surrounding the attacks (such as relationship to meals, alcohol ingestion, cough, micturition, defecation, or movements of the head and neck); associated symptoms such as nausea, vomiting, chest pain, or dyspnea; medications utilized; the presence of potentially predisposing disorders such as diabetes mellitus, chronic illness with weight loss, prolonged bed rest, blood loss, or plasma volume depletion. Exclusion of the simple faint is important, since this condition usually requires no treatment and only minor investigation.

Physical examination should focus on the following:

1. Evaluation of blood pressure with the patient recumbent and standing after the patient has been recumbent for at least 3 minutes;
2. Evaluation of blood pressure in both arms and legs;
3. Recognition of bruits in the carotid, subclavian, supraorbital, and temporal vessels;
4. Detection of cyanosis, clubbing, and other signs of congenital heart disease; and
5. Assessment of the heart rate and blood pressure response to carotid sinus pressure and simulated movements precipitating syncope.

Accurate measure of blood pressure with the patient recumbent and sitting is all that is required to detect postural hypotension. The patient should be recumbent for at least 3 minutes before assuming an upright posture. If acceleration of heart rate accompanies postural hypotension, the syncope is more likely to be drug-induced, secondary to prolonged deconditioning, or due to old age rather than

TABLE 28-4   **EVALUATION OF AUTONOMIC FUNCTION**

PROCEDURE	MECHANISM AND NORMAL PATHWAY TESTED	NORMAL RESPONSE	USUAL CLINICAL IMPLICATIONS OF ABNORMAL RESPONSE
Standing (sometimes simulated in the laboratory with the use of a tilt table)	Systemic venous pooling of blood leads to a reduction of cardiac output, decreased baroreceptor discharge, and consequent vasomotor center stimulation in the central nervous system, sympathetic discharge, and end-organ response and vasoconstriction	$\leq$ 20 mm Hg decrease of systolic arterial blood pressure associated with modest tachycardia and an increase of $\geq$ 140 pg/ml of plasma norepinephrine	Exaggerated hypotension suggests the presence of a lesion affecting the afferent, central, or efferent adrenal system or end-organ unresponsiveness
Deep breathing	Afferent, central, and efferent vagal system	$\geq$ 10 beat/min variation in heart rate or R-R interval measured electrocardiographically	Impaired vagal function due to afferent, central, or efferent component lesions or end-organ unresponsiveness
Valsalva maneuver	Increased intrathoracic pressure diminishes systemic venous return to the heart after transitory augmentation of pulmonary venous return. Cardiac output declines, eliciting systemic hypotension, decreased baroreceptor discharge, and afferent, central, and efferent sympathoadrenal discharge with tachycardia. Sustained sympathoadrenal discharge results in a post-Valsalva overshoot of blood pressure and consequent modest bradycardia	A 4-phase response, including transitory initial blood pressure elevation, $\geq$ 50% decrease of systemic arterial blood pressure with tachycardia during the maneuver, and a blood pressure overshoot with modest tachycardia after release of Valsalva	Sympathetic lesion (afferent, central, efferent) or end-organ unresponsiveness
Hyperventilation	Vasomotor center responsivity and efferent sympathoadrenal system	A decrease of arterial pressure of 10 to 20 mm Hg	A central lesion
Cold pressor test (immersion of an extremity in ice water for 1 to 3 minutes)	Centrally mediated sympathoadrenal discharge as well as afferent pain fiber stimulation, spinal cord reflex arcs, efferent sympathetic discharge, and end-organ response	$\geq$ 15 mm Hg increase in both systolic and diastolic blood pressure	A central or efferent sympathetic lesion
Inhalation of amyl nitrite	Systemic arterial vasodilatation leads to reduction of systemic arterial blood pressure, decreased baroreceptor discharge, afferent and central nervous system stimulation, and efferent sympathetic discharge	Tachycardia in response to systemic arterial hypotension	Central or efferent sympathetic lesion
Induction of hyperthermia	Augmentation of core temperature by 1°C leads to centrally mediated sympathetic stimulation involving cholinergic postganglionic neurons	Sweating	Central or efferent sympathetic lesions. End-organ unresponsiveness can be excluded with a direct sweat test with 5 to 15 mg of pilocarpine HCl or electrical stimulation
Administration of atropine (0.02 mg/kg)	Efferent parasympathetic fibers, including vagal fibers	An increase of heart rate by $\geq$ 20% or resting rate	Central or efferent parasympathetic impairment
Administration of tyramine (200 to 6000 μg doses incrementally)	Release of catecholamine stores from adrenergic nerves	Increased systemic blood pressure by $\leq$ 20 mm Hg/1000 μg bolus	Postganglionic sympathetic lesion
Norepinephrine bitartrate (0.05 to 0.07 μg/kg/min)	End-organ response (peripheral vasculature)	An increase of systolic and diastolic blood pressures of approximately 20 mm Hg	Exaggerated hypertension implies the presence of a postganglionic sympathetic lesion or denervation hypersensitivity
Responses of the pupil to conjunctival sac instillations of 1 to 2 drops of epinephrine HCl (1:1000) or 4% phenylephrine or indirect-acting agents such as hydroxamphetamine (1%) or cocaine (4%)	End-organ response	No effect with dilute solutions of direct-acting agents; mydriasis with indirect-acting agents	Exaggerated response to epinephrine implies the presence of a postganglionic sympathetic lesion (denervation hypersensitivity). Absence of mydriasis to indirect-acting agents but not to cocaine implies a preganglionic or central lesion. A sympathetic lesion can be confirmed by absence of mydriasis induced by homatropine (5%), a cholinergic antagonist

Modified from Henrich, W. L.: Autonomic insufficiency. Arch. Intern. Med. *142*:339, 1982.

because of degenerative or familial orthostatic hypotension. Detection of bruits in the vessels of the neck may suggest vascular obstruction. Since hypotensive episodes due to congenital heart disease in adults are usually caused by intracardiac shunts, cyanosis and clubbing may be important clues. Carotid hypersensitivity is established by maneuvers that reproduce the patient's symptoms and by simulation of movements potentially precipitating syncope in a given case, such as turning movements of the head. Assessment of the blood pressure in both arms and legs is particularly helpful in detecting differences due to obstructive vascular disease such as Takayasu's disease.

Test of autonomic function may be particularly helpful (Table 28–4). In addition, assessment of the following may be useful:

1. Twenty-four–hour (ambulatory) electrocardiographic recordings (p. 632): Many patients with underlying cardiac causes of syncope have normal electrocardiograms between attacks, although some exhibit abnormalities such as premature ventricular contractions, atrial arrhythmias, or minor conduction defects. These abnormalities in themselves do not confirm the cause of syncope. Often it is necessary to monitor the patient for 24 hours, preferably during his or her usual activities. Short runs of ventricular tachycardia, transient complete heart block, or asystole may be demonstrable. If the patient develops syncope or presyncope during the recording, and the electrocardiogram reveals an arrhythmia that can account for the symptoms, appropriate treatment is instituted; this usually consists of drugs for tachyarrhythmias and permanent pacing for bradyarrhythmias. If, on the other hand, the recording is normal even though the patient concurrently develops syncope, arrhythmias can be excluded as a cause of symptoms. If the patient remains asymptomatic during a recording that shows arrhythmias, it may be desirable to repeat the 24-hour electrocardiogram, commence a trial of antiarrhythmic therapy, or carry out the electrophysiological studies described below. The last-named, in any case, are indicated when patients are asymptomatic during the recording, when the recording is normal or nearly so, and when no other medical or neurological cause of syncope or presyncope is evident.

2. Electrophysiological evaluation with programmed atrial and ventricular stimulation: This technique may be very helpful in establishing the diagnosis and selecting treatment for tachy- and bradyarrhythmias and intermittent conduction disturbances leading to syncope[79–81] (p. 634). Induction of the responsible arrhythmia by programmed ventricular stimulation and suppression of inducibility by specific pharmacological agents provide an objective means of selecting appropriate therapy. When the cause of syncope is obscure, inducibility of recurrent atrial or ventricular tachycardia accompanied by syncope or presyncope strongly suggests that the arrhythmia occurs spontaneously and is responsible for the syncope.[79,80] The presence of uni- or bifascicular block with stress-induced complete heart block by atrial pacing, a prolonged His-ventricular (HV) interval on His bundle recordings, or the demonstration of prolonged sinoatrial node recovery in patients with symptoms of hypotension or syncope may implicate conduction system disease, requiring a permanent artificial pacemaker.[82]

3. Determination of levels of plasma electrolytes, catecholamines (with the patient supine and upright), dopamine beta-hydroxylase, and urinary vanillylmandelic acid (VMA): Under physiological conditions, plasma catecholamine concentrations increase several-fold with assumption of the upright position. In contrast, among patients with idiopathic orthostatic hypotension or diabetic neuropathy, the response is markedly blunted or absent. In these patients, basal plasma dopamine beta-hydroxylase levels are low, and values do not increase with assumption of an upright posture. Urinary VMA and plasma catecholamines are elevated markedly in patients with pheochromocytoma; rarely, the tumor may secrete predominantly epinephrine, eliciting paradoxical hypotension.

4. Determination of plasma aldosterone and mineralocorticoids: Among patients with primary or secondary adrenal cortical insufficiency or hypoaldosteronism, concentrations of plasma and urinary mineralocorticoids are low.

5. Glucose tolerance test: A normal glucose tolerance test with normal plasma insulin responses will exclude functional hypoglycemia or an insulin-secreting tumor.

6. Electroencephalography: This test frequently detects abnormalities in patients with epilepsy, even when these studies are performed between attacks.

7. Ophthalmotonometry and cerebral angiography: These tests are sometimes necessary to identify a cerebral or extracranial vascular lesion.

8. Physiological stress tests, such as carotid sinus stimulation and tilt-table tests, with evaluation of the plasma catecholamine response: In patients with orthostatic hypotension or recurring vasovagal fainting episodes without obvious cause, it may be necessary to assess the hemodynamic and catecholamine responses to tilting, since hypotension without a physiological compensatory elaboration of catecholamines is common in this entity.

A combined approach that employs meticulous acquisition of historical data, thorough physical examination, and judicious utilization of selected laboratory procedures will generally delineate even the most obscure causes of recurrent hypotension and syncope.

References

1. Folkow, B.: Nervous control of the blood vessels. Physiol. Rev. 35:629, 1955.
2. Hickam, J. B., and Pryor, W. W.: Cardiac output in postural hypotension. J. Clin. Invest. 30:410, 1951.
3. Cryer, P. E., and Weiss, S.: Reduced plasma norepinephrine response to standing in autonomic dysfunction. Arch. Neurol. 33:275, 1976.
4. Hines, S., and Houston, M.: The clinical spectrum of autonomic dysfunction. Am. J. Med. 70:1091, 1981.
5. Linch, D. C., Shaw, K. M., Mohleman, M. F., and Ross, E. J.: Bromocriptine induced postural hypotension in acromegaly. Lancet 2:320, 1978.
6. Bradbury, S., and Eggleston, C.: Postural hypotension: A report of three cases. Am. Heart J. 1:73, 1925.
7. Shy, G. M., and Drager, G. A.: A neurological syndrome associated with orthostatic hypotension. A clinical pathological study. Arch. Neurol. 2:511, 1960.
8. Cohen, J. I. (ed.): Postural hypotension. Johns Hopkins Med. J. 148:127, 1981.
9. Bannister, R.: Degeneration of the autonomic nervous system. Lancet 2:175, 1971.
10. Ziegler, M. G., Lake, C. R., and Kopin, I. J.: The sympathetic nervous system defect in primary orthostatic hypotension. N. Engl. J. Med. 296:293, 1977.
11. Hilsted, J., Parving, H.-H., Christensen, N. J., Benn, J., and Galbo, H.: Hemodynamics in diabetic orthostatic hypotension. J. Clin. Invest. 68:1427, 1981.
12. Bannister, R., Ardill, L., and Fentem, P.: Defective autonomic control of blood vessels in idiopathic orthostatic hypotension. Brain 90:725, 1967.
13. Abboud, F. M., Heistad, D. D., Mark, A. L., and Schmid, P. G.: Reflex control of the peripheral circulation. Prog. Cardiovasc. Dis. 18:371, 1976.

14. Bannister, R.: Chronic autonomic failure with postural hypotension. Lancet. 2: 404, 1979.

15. Kontos, H. A., Richardson, D. W., and Norvell, J. E.: Norepinephrine depletion in idiopathic orthostatic hypotension. Ann. Intern. Med. 82:336, 1975.

16. Bannister, R., Crowe, R., Eames, R., and Brunstock, G.: Adrenergic innervation in autonomic failure. Neurology 31:1501, 1981.

17. Luft, R., and von Euler, U. S.: Two cases of postural hypotension showing a deficiency in release of norepinephrine and epinephrine. J. Clin. Invest. 32: 1065, 1953.

18. Hickler, R. B., Thompson, G. R., Fox, L. M., et al.: Successful treatment of orthostatic hypotension with 9-alpha-fluorohydrocortisone. N. Engl. J. Med. 261:788, 1959.

19. Goodall, M., Harlan, W. R., Jr., and Alton, H.: Noradrenaline release and metabolism in orthostatic (postural) hypotension. Circulation 36:489, 1967.

20. Goodall, M. C. C., Harlan, W. R., Jr., and Alton, H.: Decreased noradrenaline (norepinephrine) synthesis in neurogenic orthostatic hypotension. Circulation 38:592, 1968.

20a. Wilcox, C. S.: Current therapy for orthostatic hypotension. J. Cardiovasc. Med. 8:292, 1983.

21. Fouad, F. M., Tarazi, R. C., and Bravo, E. L.: Dihydroergotamine in idiopathic orthostatic hypotension: Short-term intramuscular and long-term oral therapy. Clin. Pharmacol. Ther. 30:782, 1981.

21a. Chobanian, A. V., Tifft, C. P., Faxon, D. P., Creager, M. A., and Sackel, H.: Treatment of chronic orthostatic hypotension with ergotamine. Circulation 67: 602, 1983.

22. Diamond, M. A., Murray, R. H., and Schmid, P. G.: Idiopathic postural hypotension: Physiological observations and report of a new mode of therapy. J. Clin. Invest. 49:1341, 1970.

23. Lubke, K. O.: A controlled study with Dihydergot on patients with orthostatic dysregulation. Cardiology 61(Suppl. 1):333, 1976.

24. Nanda, R. N., Johnson, R. H., and Keogh, H. J.: Treatment of neurogenic orthostatic hypotension with a monoamine oxidase inhibitor and tyramine. Lancet 2:1164, 1976.

25. Brevetti, G., Chiariello, M., Giudice, P., De Michele, G., Mansi, D., and Campanella, G.: Effective treatment of orthostatic hypotension by propranolol in the Shy-Drager syndrome. Am. Heart J. 102:938, 1981.

26. Riley, C. M., Day, R. L., Greeley, D. M., and Langford, W. E.: Central autonomic dysfunction with defective lacrimation. I. Report of 5 cases. Pediatrics 3: 468, 1949.

27. Dancis, J., and Smith, A. A.: Familial dysautonomia. N. Engl. J. Med. 274: 207, 1966.

28. Ziegler, M. G., Lake, C. R., and Kopin, I. J.: Deficient sympathetic nervous response in familial dysautonomia. N. Engl. J. Med. 294:630, 1976.

29. Smith, A. A., and Dancis, J.: Catecholamine release in familial dysautonomia. N. Engl. J. Med. 277:61, 1967.

30. Williams, G. H., Cain, J. P., Dluhy, R. G., and Underwood, R. H.: Studies of the control of plasma aldosterone concentration in normal man. I. Response to posture, acute and chronic volume depletion, and sodium loading. J. Clin. Invest. 51:1731, 1972.

31. Streeten, D. H. P., Kerr, L. P., Prior, J. C., Kerr, C., and Dalakos, T. G.: Hyperbradykininism: A new orthostatic syndrome. Lancet 2:1048, 1972.

32. McHenry, L. C., Jr., Fazekas, J. F., and Sullivan, J. F.: Cerebral hemodynamics of syncope. Am. J. Med. Sci. 241:173, 1961.

33. Rossen, R., Kabat, H., and Anderson, J. P.: Acute arrest of cerebral circulation in man. A.M.A. Arch. Neurol. Psychiatry 50:510, 1943.

34. Hering, H. E.: Die Sinus Reflexe vom Sinus Caroticus werden durch einen Nerven (Sinusvert) vermittelt, der ein Ast des Nervus glossopharyngeus ist. Munch. Med. Wschr. 71:1265, 1924.

35. Weiss, S., and Baker, J. P.: The carotid sinus reflex in health and disease: Its role in the causation of fainting and convulsions. Medicine 12:297, 1933.

35a. Leatham, A.: Carotid sinus syncope. Br. Heart J. 47:409, 1982.

36. Gardner, R. S., Magovern, G. J., Park, S. B., Cushing, W. J., Liebler, G. A., and Hughes, R.: Carotid sinus syndrome: New surgical considerations. Vasc. Surg. 9:204, 1975.

37. Peretz, D. I., Gerein, A. N., and Miyahishima, R. T.: Permanent demand pacing for hypersensitive carotid sinus syndrome. Can. Med. Assoc. J. 108:1131, 1973.

37a. Morley, C. A., Perrins, E. J., Grant, P., Chan, S. L., McBrien, D. J., and Sutton, R.: Carotid sinus syncope treated by pacing. Analysis of persistent symptoms and role of atrioventricular sequential pacing. Br. Heart J. 47:411, 1982.

38. Walter, P. F., Crawley, I. S., and Dorney, E. R.: Carotid sinus hypersensitivity and syncope. Am. J. Cardiol. 42:396, 1978.

39. Lown, B., and Levine, S. A.: The carotid sinus: Clinical value of its stimulation. Circulation 23:766, 1961.

40. Lesser, L. M., and Wenger, N. K.: Carotid sinus syncope. Heart Lung 5:453, 1976.

41. Trout, H. H., III, Brown, L. I., and Thompson, J. E.: Carotid sinus syndrome: Treatment by carotid sinus denervation. Ann. Surg. 189:575, 1979.

42. Lee, Y. T., Lee, T. K., and Tsai, H. C.: Glossopharyngeal neuralgia as the cause of cardiac syncope: A case report with a review of literature. J. Formosan Med. Assoc. 4:103, 1975.

43. Khero, B. A., and Mullins, C. B.: Cardiac syncope due to glossopharyngeal neuralgia. Arch. Intern. Med. 128:806, 1971.

44. Kong, Y., Heyman, A., Entman, M. L., and McIntosh, H. D.: Glossopharyngeal neuralgia associated with bradycardia, syncope, and seizures. Circulation 30:109, 1964.

45. Dykman, T. R., Montgomery, E. B., Gerstenberger, P. D., Zeiger, H. E., Clutter, W. E., and Cryer, P. E.: Glossopharyngeal neuralgia with syncope secondary to tumor: Treatment and pathophysiology. Am. J. Med. 71:165, 1981.

46. Waddington, J. K. B., Matthews, H. R., Evans, C. C., and Ward, D. W.: Carcinoma of the esophagus with swallow syncope. Br. Med. J. 3:232, 1975.

47. Wik, B., and Hillestead, L.: Deglutition syncope. Br. Med. J. 3:747, 1975.

48. Tolman, K. G., and Ashworth, W.: Syncope induced by dysphagia correction by esophageal dilatation. Am. J. Dig. Dis. 16:1026, 1971.

49. Levin, B., and Posner, J. B.: Swallow syncope. Neurology 22:1086, 1972.

50. Weiss, S., and Ferris, E. B.: Adams-Stokes syndrome with transient complete heart block of vasovagal reflex origin. Arch. Intern. Med. 54:931, 1934.

51. James, A. H.: Cardiac syncope after swallowing. Lancet 1:771, 1958.

52. Haldane, J. H.: Micturition syncope. Can. Med. Assoc. J. 101:712, 1969.

53. Godec, C. J., and Cass, A. S.: Micturition syncope. J. Urol. 126:551, 1981.

54. Larson, S. J., Sances, A., Baker, J. B., and Reigel, D.: Herniated cerebellar tonsils and cough syncope. J. Neurosurg. 40:524, 1974.

55. Corbett, J. J., Butler, A. B., and Kaufman, B.: Sneeze syncope, basilar invagination and Arnold-Chiari type I malformation. J. Neurol. Neurosurg. Psychiatry 39:381, 1976.

56. Wayne, H. H.: Syncope, physiological considerations and an analysis of the clinical characteristics in 510 patients. Am. J. Med. 30:418, 1961.

56a. Day, S. C., Cook, F., Funkenstein,, H., and Goldman, L.: Evaluation and outcome of emergency room patients with transient loss of consciousness. Am. J. Med. 73:15, 1983.

57. Barcroft, H., Edholm, O. G., McMichael, J., and Sharpey-Schafer, E. P.: Posthemorrhagic fainting: Study by cardiac output and forearm flow. Lancet 1:489, 1944.

58. Weissler, A. M., Warren, J. V., Estes, E. H., Jr., McIntosh, H. D., and Leonard, J. J.: Vasodepressor syncope: Factors influencing cardiac output. Circulation 15:875, 1957.

59. Glick, G., and Yu, P. N.: Hemodynamic changes during spontaneous vasovagal reactions. Am. J. Med. 34:42, 1963.

60. Epstein, S. E., Stampfer, M., and Beiser, G. D.: Role of the capacitance and resistance vessels in vasovagal syncope. Circulation 37:524, 1968.

61. Aviado, D. M., Jr., and Schmidt, C. F.: Cardiovascular and respiratory reflexes from the left side of the heart. Am. J. Physiol. 196:726, 1959.

62. Friedberg, C. K.: Syncope: Pathological physiology: Differential diagnosis and treatment (II). Mod. Concepts Cardiovasc. Dis. 40:61, 1971.

63. Martin, A. K., Hackel, D. B., and Sieber, H. O.: Intraventricular pressure changes in dogs during hemorrhagic shock. Fed. Proc. 22:252, 1963.

64. Brun, C., Knudsen, E. O. E., and Raaschou, F.: Kidney function and circulatory collapse, postsyncopal oliguria. J. Clin. Invest. 25:568, 1946.

65. Stead, E. A., Jr., Kunkel, P., and Weiss, S.: Effect of pitressin in circulatory collapse induced by sodium nitrate. J. Clin. Invest. 18:673, 1939.

66. Wright, K. E., Jr., and McIntosh, H. D.: Syncope: A review of pathophysiological mechanisms. Progr. Cardiovasc. Dis. 13:580, 1971.

67. MacMurray, F. G.: Stokes-Adams disease: A historical review. N. Engl. J. Med. 256:643, 1957.

68. Morgagni, J. B.: The seats and causes of disease. In Major, H. H. (ed.): Classic Descriptions of Disease. Oxford, Blackwell Scientific Publications, 1948, p. 346.

69. Adams, R.: Cases of diseases of the heart, accompanied with pathological observations. Dublin Hosp. Rep. 4:353, 1827.

70. Stokes, W.: Observations on some cases of permanently slow pulse. Dublin Q. J. Med. Sci. 2:73, 1846.

71. Parkinson, J., Papp, C., and Evans, W.: The electrocardiogram of the Stokes-Adams attack. Br. Heart J. 3:171, 1941.

72. Pomerantz, B., and O'Rourke, R. A.: The Stokes-Adams syndrome. Am. J. Med. 46:941, 1969.

73. Moss, A. J., and Davis, R. J.: Brady-tachy syndrome. Prog. Cardiovasc. Dis. 16:439, 1974.

74. Mark, A. L., Kioschos, J. M., Abboud, F. M., Heistadt, D., and Schmid, P. G.: Abnormal vascular responses to exercise in patients with aortic stenosis. J. Clin. Invest. 52:1138, 1973.

75. Flamm, M. D., Braniff, B. A., Kimball, R., and Hancock, E. W.: Mechanism of effort syncope in aortic stenosis. Circulation 35:II–109, 1967.

76. Braunwald, E., Brockenbrough, E. D., and Frye, R. L.: Studies on digitalis. V. Comparison of the effects of ouabain on left ventricular dynamics in valvular aortic stenosis and hypertrophic subaortic stenosis. Circulation 26:166, 1962.

77. Jarisch, A., and Zotterman, Y.: Depressor reflexes from the heart. Acta Physiol. Scand. 16:31, 1948.

78. Eckberg, D. L., Drabinsky, M., and Braunwald, E.: Defective cardiac parasympathetic control in patients with heart disease. N. Engl. J. Med. 285:877, 1971.

79. DiMarco, J. P., Garan, H., Harthorne, W., and Ruskin, J. N.: Intracardiac electrophysiologic techniques in recurrent syncope of unknown cause. Ann. Intern. Med. 95:542, 1981.

80. Josephson, M. D., and Seides, S. F.: Clinical Cardiac Electrophysiology: Techniques and Interpretations. Philadelphia, Lea and Febiger, 1979, p. 44.

81. Kapoor, W. N., Karpf, M., Maher, Y., Miller, R. A., and Levey, G. S.: Syncope of unknown origin: The need for a more cost-effective approach to its diagnostic evaluation. J.A.M.A. 247:2687, 1982.

82. Hauer, R. N. W., Lie, K. I., Liem, K. L., and Durrer, D.: Long term prognosis in patients with bundle branch block complicating acute anteroseptal infarction. Am. J. Cardiol. 49:1581, 1982.

INDEX

Pages in *italics* indicate illustrations. Page numbers followed by t indicate tables.